Casarett and Doull's
TOXICOLOGY

The Basic Science of Poisons

All substances are poisons; there is none which is not a poison. The right dose differentiates a poison and a remedy.

PARACELSUS
(1493–1541)

EDITED BY

Curtis D. Klaassen, Ph.D.

Professor of Pharmacology and Toxicology,
University of Kansas Medical Center,
Kansas City, Kansas

Mary O. Amdur, Ph.D.

Senior Research Scientist, Energy Laboratory and
Department of Applied Biological Sciences,
Massachusetts Institute of Technology,
Cambridge, Massachusetts; Associate
Professor of Toxicology, Harvard
School of Public Health, Boston, Massachusetts

John Doull, M.D., Ph.D.

Professor of Pharmacology and Toxicology,
University of Kansas Medical Center,
Kansas City, Kansas

Casarett and Doull's

TOXICOLOGY

The Basic Science of Poisons

THIRD EDITION

Macmillan Publishing Company
New York

Collier Macmillan Canada, Inc.
Toronto

Collier Macmillan Publishers
London

Earlier editions: *Toxicology: The Basic Science of Poisons,* edited
by Louis J. Casarett and John Doull, copyright © 1975 by Macmillan
Publishing Company. *Casarett and Doull's Toxicology: The Basic
Science of Poisons,* edited by John Doull, Curtis D. Klaassen,
and Mary O. Amdur, copyright © 1980 by Macmillan Publishing
Company.

MACMILLAN PUBLISHING COMPANY
866 Third Avenue, New York, New York 10022

Collier Macmillan Canada, Inc.
Collier Macmillan Publishers • London

Library of Congress Cataloging-in-Publication Data
Toxicology (Macmillan Publishing Company)
  Casarett and Doull's toxicology.
  Includes bibliographies and index.
  1. Toxicology. I. Casarett, Louis J. II. Doull,
John, 1923– . III. Klaassen, Curtis D. IV. Amdur,
Mary O. V. Title. [DNLM: 1. Poisoning. 2. Poisons.
QV 600 T757]
RA1211.T6338 1986 615.9 86-8683
ISBN 0-02-364650-0

Printing: 1 2 3 4 5 6 7 8   Year: 6 7 8 9 0 1 2 3 4

Preface to the Third Edition

THE GOALS of the editors for the third edition of this textbook have remained those of the earlier editions. This volume is designed to serve primarily as a textbook for, or adjunct to, courses in toxicology. Because the two previous editions have also been widely used in courses in environmental health and related areas, we have attempted to maintain those characteristics that make it useful to scientists from other disciplines. This third edition will again provide those in other professions, as well as toxicologists, with information on the many facets of toxicology and on the principles, concepts, and modes of thought that are the foundation of the discipline. Research toxicologists who have used the previous editions of this book as a reference source will find updated material in areas of their special or peripheral interests.

The overall framework of the third edition is similar to that of the second edition, with major sections covering "General Principles of Toxicology" (Unit I), "Systemic Toxicology" (Unit II), "Toxic Agents" (Unit III), "Environmental Toxicology" (Unit IV), and "Applications of Toxicology" (Unit V). In accord with a policy adopted for the second edition, we have changed the authorship of one-third of the chapters in this edition to broaden input and provide new coverage of the many aspects of toxicology. New chapters have been added on toxic responses of the immune system, the cardiovascular system, and the skin, and many other chapters have been extensively updated.

The editors are grateful to our colleagues in academia, industry, and government who have made useful suggestions for improving this third edition both as a textbook and as a reference source. We are especially grateful to the contributors, whose combined expertise has made possible a volume of this breadth. We appreciate the efforts of those who revised chapters and those who prepared new ones to limit their chapters to lengths that would keep the third edition from becoming unwieldy in size and prohibitive in cost.

C.D.K.

M.O.A.

J.D.

Preface to the First Edition

THIS VOLUME has been designed primarily as a textbook for, or adjunct to, courses in toxicology. However, it should also be of interest to those not directly involved in toxicologic education. For example, the research scientist in toxicology will find sections containing current reports on the status of circumscribed areas of special interest. Those concerned with community health, agriculture, food technology, pharmacy, veterinary medicine, and related disciplines will discover the contents to be most useful as a source of concepts and modes of thought that are applicable to other types of investigative and applied sciences. For those further removed from the field of toxicology or for those who have not entered a specific field of endeavor, this book attempts to present a selectively representative view of the many facets of the subject.

Toxicology: The Basic Science of Poisons has been organized to facilitate its use by these different types of users. The first section (Unit I) describes the elements of method and approach that identify toxicology. It includes those principles most frequently invoked in a full understanding of toxicologic events, such as dose-response, and is primarily mechanistically oriented. Mechanisms are also stressed in the subsequent sections of the book, particularly when these are well identified and extend across classic forms of chemicals and systems. However, the major focus in the second section (Unit II) is on the systemic site of action of toxins. The intent therein is to provide answers to two questions: What kinds of injury are produced in specific organs or systems by toxic agents? What are the agents that produce these effects?

A more conventional approach to toxicology has been utilized in the third section (Unit III), in which the toxic agents are grouped by chemical or use characteristics. In the final section (Unit IV) an attempt has been made to illustrate the ramifications of toxicology into all areas of the health sciences and even beyond. This unit is intended to provide perspective for the nontoxicologist in the application of the results of toxicologic studies and a better understanding of the activities of those engaged in the various aspects of the discipline of toxicology.

It will be obvious to the reader that the contents of this book represent a compromise between the basic, fundamental, mechanistic approach to toxicology and the desire to give a view of the broad horizons presented by the subject. While it is certain that the editors' selectivity might have been more severe, it is equally certain that it could have been less so, and we hope that the balance struck will prove to be appropriate for both toxicologic training and the scientific interest of our colleagues.

L.J.C.
J.D.

Although the philosophy and design of this book evolved over a long period of friendship and mutual respect between the editors, the effort needed to convert ideas into reality was undertaken primarily by Louis J. Casarett. Thus, his death at a time when completion of the manuscript was in sight was particularly tragic. With the help and encouragement of his wife, Margaret G. Casarett, and the other contributors, we have finished Lou's task. This volume is a fitting embodiment of Louis J. Casarett's dedication to toxicology and to toxicologic education.

J.D.

Contributors

Amdur, Mary O., Ph.D. Senior Research Scientist, Energy Laboratory and Department of Applied Biological Sciences, Massachusetts Institute of Technology, Cambridge, Massachusetts; Associate Professor of Toxicology, Harvard School of Public Health, Boston, Massachusetts

Andrews, Larry S., Ph.D. Senior Toxicologist, Celanese Corporation, New York, New York; formerly Toxicology Advisor, ARCO Chemical Company, Newton Square, Pennsylvania

Balazs, Tibor, D.V.M. Chief, Drug Toxicology Branch, Division of Drug Biology, Center for Drugs and Biologics, Food and Drug Administration, Washington, D.C.; Visiting Professor of Pharmacology and Toxicology, Howard University College of Medicine, Washington, D.C.

Bruce, Margaret C., Sc.D. Assistant Professor, Department of Pediatrics, Rainbow Babies and Childrens Hospital, Case Western Reserve University, Cleveland, Ohio

Call, Katherine M., Ph.D. Postdoctoral Associate, Department of Applied Biological Sciences, Massachusetts Institute of Technology, Cambridge, Massachusetts

Campbell, T. Colin, Ph.D. Professor of Nutritional Biochemistry, Division of Nutritional Sciences, Cornell University, Ithaca, New York

Dean, Jack H., Ph.D. Head, Department of Cell Biology, Chemical Industry Institute of Toxicology, Research Triangle Park, North Carolina

Dixon, Robert L., Ph.D. Director of Toxicology, Sterling-Winthrop Research Institute, Rensselaer, New York

Doull, John, M.D., Ph.D. Professor of Pharmacology and Toxicology, University of Kansas Medical Center, Kansas City, Kansas

Emmett, Edward A., M.D. Professor and Director, Division of Occupational Medicine, Schools of Hygiene and Public Health and of Medicine, Johns Hopkins University, Baltimore, Maryland

Gandolfi, A. Jay, Ph.D. Associate Professor of Anesthesiology and Pharmacology, Department of Anesthesiology, University of Arizona, Tucson, Arizona

Goyer, Robert A., M.D. Deputy Director, National Institute of Environmental Health Sciences, Research Triangle Park, North Carolina; Adjunct Professor of Pathology, University of North Carolina School of Medicine, Chapel Hill, North Carolina

Hanig, Joseph P., Ph.D. Pharmacologist–Group Leader, Food and Drug Administration, Washington, D.C.; Adjunct Associate Professor of Pharmacology and Toxicology, Howard University College of Medicine, Washington, D.C., and New York Medical College, Valhalla, New York

Hayes, Johnnie R., Ph.D. Master Toxicologist, Bowman-Gray Technical Center, R. J. Reynolds Industries, Winston-Salem, North Carolina

Herman, Eugene H., Ph.D. Research Toxicologist, Division of Drug Biology, Center for Drugs and Biologics, Food and Drug Administration, Washington, D.C.

Hewitt, William R., Ph.D. Assistant Director, Department of Investigative Toxicology, Smith Kline and French Laboratories, Philadelphia, Pennsylvania

Hobbs, Charles H., D.V.M. Assistant Director, Inhalation Toxicology Research Institute, Lovelace Biomedical and Environmental Research Institute, Albuquerque, New Mexico

Hook, Jerry B., Ph.D. Vice President, Preclinical Research and Development, Smith Kline and French Laboratories, Philadelphia, Pennsylvania

Klaassen, Curtis D., Ph.D. Professor of Pharmacology and Toxicology, University of Kansas Medical Center, Kansas City, Kansas

Lampe, Kenneth F., Ph.D. Chairman, Department of Drugs, American Medical Association, Chicago, Illinois

Lauwerys, Robert R., M.D., D.Sc. Professor and Chairman, Department of Occupational Medicine and Hygiene, Catholic University of Louvain, Brussels, Belgium

Lovejoy, Frederick H., Jr., M.D. Associate Professor of Pediatrics, Harvard Medical School, and Associate Physician-in-Chief, The Children's Hospital, Boston, Massachusetts; Director, Massachusetts Poison Control System, Boston, Massachusetts

McClellan, Roger O., D.V.M. Director, Inhalation Toxicology Research Institute, Lovelace Biomedical and Environmental Research Institute, Albuquerque, New Mexico

Manson, Jeanne M., Ph.D. Associate Director, Developmental Toxicology, Smith Kline and French Laboratories, Philadelphia, Pennsylvania

Menzel, Daniel B., Ph.D. Professor and Director, Chemical Carcinogenesis Program and Laboratory of Environmental Toxicology, Departments of Pharmacology and Medicine, Duke University Medical Center, Durham, North Carolina

Menzer, Robert E., Ph.D. Professor of Entomology, University of Maryland, College Park, Maryland

Merrill, Richard A., LL.B., M.A. Dean and Daniel Caplin Professor of Law, University of Virginia School of Law, Charlottesville, Virginia

Murphy, Sheldon D., Ph.D. Professor and Chairman, Department of Environmental Health, School of Public Health and Community Medicine, University of Washington, Seattle, Washington

Murray, Michael J., Ph.D. Research Toxicologist, Human and Environmental Safety Division, Research and Development Department, The Procter and Gamble Company, Miami Valley Laboratories, Cincinnati, Ohio

Nelson, Judd O., Ph.D. Associate Professor of Entomology, University of Maryland, College Park, Maryland

Norton, Stata, Ph.D. Professor of Pharmacology, University of Kansas Medical Center, Kansas City, Kansas

Plaa, Gabriel L., Ph.D. Professor of Pharmacology, Faculty of Medicine, University of Montreal, Montreal, Quebec, Canada

Potts, Albert M., Ph.D., M.D. Clinical Professor of Ophthalmology, University of Arizona College of Medicine, Tucson, Arizona

Rumack, Barry H., M.D. Professor of Pediatrics, University of Colorado Health Sciences Center; Director, Rocky Mountain Poison Center, Denver General Hospital, Denver, Colorado

Russell, Findlay E., M.D., Ph.D. Research Professor, University of Arizona College of Pharmacy, Tucson, Arizona; Adjunct Professor of Neurology, University of Southern California, Los Angeles, California; Adjunct Professor of Neuropharmacology, Loma Linda University, Loma Linda, California

Sipes, I. Glenn, Ph.D. Professor and Head, Department of Pharmacology and Toxicology, University of Arizona College of Pharmacy, Tucson, Arizona; Professor of Pharmacology and Anesthesiology, University of Arizona College of Medicine, Tucson, Arizona

Smith, Roger P., Ph.D. Professor and Chairman, Department of Pharmacology and Toxicology, Dartmouth Medical School, Hanover, New Hampshire

Snyder, Robert, Ph.D. Professor and Director, Joint Graduate Program in Toxicology; Professor and Chairman, Department of Pharmacology and Toxicology, College of Pharmacy—Busch Campus, Rutgers The State University of New Jersey, University of Medicine and Dentistry of New Jersey, Piscataway, New Jersey.

Sunshine, Irving, Ph.D. Chief Toxicologist, Cuyahoga County Coroner's Office, Cleveland, Ohio; Professor of Toxicology and of Clinical Pharmacology, Case Western Reserve University, Cleveland, Ohio

Thilly, William G., Sc.D. Professor of Genetic Toxicology, Department of Applied Biological Sciences, Massachusetts Institute of Technology, Cambridge, Massachusetts

Ward, Edward C., Ph.D. Late Senior Research Microbiologist, Department of

Molecular Biology, A. H. Robins Company, Richmond, Virginia

Weisburger, John H., Ph.D., M.D.(h.c.) Vice President for Research, American Health Foundation, and Director, Naylor Dana Institute for Disease Prevention, Valhalla, New York; Research Professor of Pathology, New York Medical College, Valhalla, New York

Williams, Gary M., M.D. Chief, Division of Pathology and Toxicology, Naylor Dana Institute for Disease Prevention, American Health Foundation, Valhalla, New York; Research Professor of Pathology, New York Medical College, Valhalla, New York

Contents

UNIT I
General Principles of Toxicology

UNIT II
Systemic Toxicology

UNIT III
Toxic Agents

UNIT IV
Environmental Toxicology

UNIT V
Applications of Toxicology

UNIT I
GENERAL PRINCIPLES
OF TOXICOLOGY

Chapter 1

ORIGIN AND SCOPE OF TOXICOLOGY

John Doull and *Margaret C. Bruce*

INTRODUCTION

In selecting a subtitle for this textbook of toxicology, the authors have utilized the traditional definition that defines toxicology as the basic science of poisons. To use this definition, we need to define a poison. If we define a poison as any agent that is capable of producing injury or death when ingested or absorbed, then, as pointed out by Paracelsus over 400 years ago (see first page of this text), "All substances are poisons; there is none which is not a poison. The right dose differentiates a poison and a remedy." Since all chemicals can produce injury or death under some exposure conditions, it is evident that there is no such thing as a "safe" chemical in the sense that it will be free of injurious effects under all conditions of exposure. However, it is also true that there is no chemical that cannot be used safely by limiting the dose or exposure. By defining toxicology as the study of the adverse effects of chemical agents on biologic systems, we avoid the use of the term "poison" and all of the legal and historic problems associated with attempts to provide a precise and quantifiable definition of a poison.

Toxicologists, then, are individuals who study the adverse effects of chemical agents on living organisms. With this broad definition, most biomedical scientists and many others can be considered to be toxicologists. Pharmacologists, for example, usually study the adverse effects as well as the beneficial effects of drugs, and emergency room physicians treating acute poisoning or epidemiologists investigating the effects of chronic exposure to chemicals are engaged in toxicology. What distinguishes the toxicologist is a primary focus on the adverse effects of chemical agents in his research and activity as well as in his training and experience. The important role of experience in becoming a toxicologist is illustrated by Dr. A. J. Lehman's often-quoted remark that, "Anyone can become a toxicologist in two easy lessons, each of which takes ten years."

The contributions and activity of toxicologists are diverse and widespread. In the biomedical area, toxicologists are concerned with exposure to chemical agents as a cause of both acute and chronic illness. They are involved in the recognition, identification, and quantitation of hazards resulting from occupational exposure to chemicals and the public health aspects of chemicals in air, water, food, drugs, and other parts of the environment. Toxicologists also participate in the development of standards and regulations designed to protect human health and the environment from the adverse effects of chemicals. Conversely, they also contribute to the development of new agents that are selectively toxic for microorganisms (antibiotics) and insects, weeds, fungi, and other unwanted organisms (pesticides). They explore the mechanisms by which chemicals produce adverse effects in biologic systems and develop antidotes and treatment regimes for treating such injury. Toxicologists carry out some or all of these activities as members of academic, industrial, and governmental organizations. In doing so, they share common methodologies for obtaining data on the toxicity of materials and the responsibility for using this information to make reasonable predictions regarding the hazards of the material to man and to his environment. These two different but complementary activities characterize the discipline of toxicology.

Toxicology, like medicine, is both a science and an art. Having defined toxicology as the study of the adverse effects of chemicals on biologic systems, the science of toxicology can be defined as the observational or data-gathering phase and the art of toxicology as the predictive phase of the discipline. In most cases, these two phases are linked since the "facts" generated by the science of toxicology are used to develop the prediction or "hypothesis" for the adverse effects of chemical agents in situations where there is little or no information. For example, the observation that exposure to chloroform can produce hepatomas in B6C3F1 mice is a docu-

3

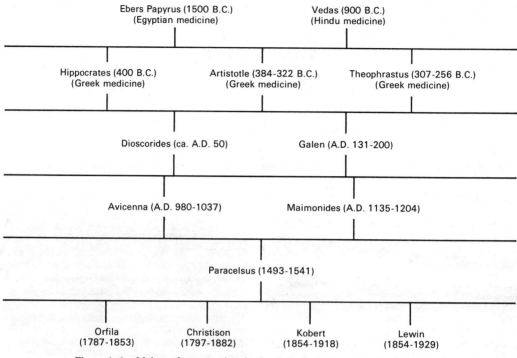

Figure 1–1. Major reference points in the evolution of toxicology as a science.

mented fact, whereas the conclusion that it will also do so in man is a prediction or hypothesis.

It is useful to distinguish the facts generated by the science of toxicology from the predictions generated by the art of toxicology as a means of testing the validity of each. When we fail to distinguish between the science and the art of toxicology, we tend to confuse our facts with our predictions and to argue that they have equal validity, which they clearly do not. In toxicology, as in other biologic sciences, theories have a higher level of certainty than hypotheses, which in turn are more certain than speculations, opinions, conjectures, and guesses.

Some insight into the development of the scope of toxicology and the roles, points of view, and activities of the toxicologist can be obtained by an examination of the historic evolution of the discipline.

HISTORY OF TOXICOLOGY

Antiquity

Toxicology, in a variety of specialized and primitive forms, has been a relevant part of the history of man (Figure 1–1). Earliest man was well aware of the toxic effects of animal venoms and poisonous plants. His knowledge was used for hunting, for waging more effective warfare, and, probably, to remove undesirables from the small groups of primitive society. The Ebers papyrus, perhaps our earliest medical record (circa 1500 B.C.), contains information extending back many centuries. Of the more than 800 recipes given, many contain recognized poisons. For example, one finds hemlock, which later became the state poison of the Greeks; aconite, an arrow poison of the ancient Chinese; opium, used as both poison and antidote; and such metals as lead, copper, and antimony. There is also an indication that plants containing substances akin to digitalis and belladonna alkaloids were known. Hippocrates, while introducing rational medicine about 400 B.C., added a number of poisons. He further wrote instructions that might be considered primitive principles of toxicology, in the form of attempts to control absorption of the toxic materials in therapy and overdosage.

In the mythology and literature of classic Greece, one finds many references to poisons and their use, and it was during this period that the first professional treatment of the subject began to appear. For example, Theophrastus (370–286 B.C.), a student of Aristotle, included numerous references to poisonous plants in *De Historia Plantarum*. Dioscorides, a Greek physician in the court of Emperor Nero, made the first attempt at a classification of poisons, which was accompanied by descriptions and drawings. The separation into plant, animal, and mineral poisons he used not only remained a standard for 16 centuries, but is still a convenient classification today (see Gunther, 1934). Dioscorides also dabbled in therapy, recognizing the use of emetics in poisoning and the use of caustic agents or cupping glasses in snakebite.

Poisoning with plant and animal toxins was quite common. Perhaps the best-known recipient of a poison used as a state method of execution was Socrates (470–399 B.C.), although he was in distinguished company. Expeditious suicide on a voluntary basis also made use of toxicologic knowledge. Demosthenes (385–322 B.C.), who took poison hidden in his pen, was only one of many examples. The mode of suicide calling for one to fall on his sword, although manly and noble, carried little appeal and less significance for ladies of the day. Cleopatra's (69–30 B.C.) knowledge of natural, primitive toxicology permitted her the more genteel method of falling on her asp instead.

The Romans too made considerable use, often political, of poisons. Much legend and myth have grown out of the skill of poisoners and the occupational hazards of political life. One such legend tells of the King Mithridates VI of Pontus whose numerous experiments on unfortunate criminals led to his eventual claim that he had discovered "an antidote for every venomous reptile and every poisonous substance" (Guthrie, 1946). He himself was so fearful of poisons that he regularly ingested a mixture of 36 ingredients (Galen reports 54) as protection against assassination. On the occasion of his imminent capture by enemies, his attempts to kill himself with poison failed because of his successful concoction and he was forced to use his own sword held by a servant. From this tale comes the term "mithridatic" referring to an antidotal or protective mixture. Another term from the Greek, "theriac," also has become a synonym for "antidote" although the word derives from a poetic treatise by Nicander of Colophon (204–135 B.C.) entitled "Theriaca," which dealt with poisonous animals. Another poem, "Alexipharmaca," was about antidotes.

This search for antidotal measures or chemicals remained a preoccupation for centuries. In addition to the terms given above, others were applied such as Alexiteria and Bezoardica, the latter referring to concretions found in the goat bladder. The practice of medicine was based largely on an "antidoting" of disease, and descriptions of therapeutic agents also were so classified. For example, an early respectable forerunner of the modern pharmacopoeia was the *Antidotarium of Nicholaus.* It was not until the seventeenth century that a commission appointed by the Pope to Matthiolus opened the horizons to a search for *Antidota specifica.*

In Rome, poisoning seemed to take on epidemic characteristics, which are described by Livy as being especially distressing to the public in the fourth century B.C. It was during this period that a conspiracy of women to remove those from whose death they might profit was uncovered, and similar large-scale poisoning continued from time to time until 82 B.C., when Sulla issued the *Lex Cornelia.* This appears to be the first law against poisoning, and it later became a regulatory statute directed at careless dispensers of drugs.

The history of poisons and their use is the basis of entertaining retrospective diagnosis, as described by Meek in his essay *The Gentle Art of Poisoning* (1928) and in a book by Thompson entitled *Poisons and Poisoners* (1931). Although most poisons used during the period were of vegetable origin, the sulfide of arsenic and arsenous acid were known to be used. It has been postulated that arsenic was the poison with which Agrippina killed Claudius to make Nero the emperor of Rome. This postulate is supported by the later use of the same material by Nero in poisoning Britannicus, Claudius's natural son. The deed was performed under the direction of Locusta, a professional poisoner attached to the family.

The mixture of fact and legend surrounding that murder illustrates the practices of the times. A first attempt to poison Britannicus failed, but the illness reported contained evidence of all the symptoms of arsenic poisoning. The failure led to suspicion and the hiring of a taster. The second, and successful, attempt involved a more devious scheme. The arsenic was placed in cold water and Britannicus was served excessively hot soup. The taster had demonstrated the safety of the soup, but it was not retested after the water had been added to cool the soup.

Here superstition and legend embellish the story. Nero claimed that Britannicus had died of epilepsy and ordered immediate burial to prevent others from seeing the blackening of the body believed to occur after poisoning. As the legend continues, the corpse was painted with cosmetics to hide the deed, but, in a raging storm, the cosmetics washed off, revealing Nero's perfidy.

Middle Ages

Prior to the Renaissance and extending well into that period, the Italians, with characteristic pragmatism, brought the art of poisoning to its zenith. The poisoner became an integral part of the scene, if not as a social being, at least as a political tool and as custodian of a common social expedient. The records of the city councils of Florence, and particularly the infamous Council of Ten of Venice, contain ample testimony of the political use of poisons. Victims were named, prices set, contracts recorded, and when the deed was accomplished, payment made. The notation *"factum"* often appeared after the entry in the archives, indicating successful accomplishment of its transaction.

In less organized but more colorful ways, the citizens of Italy in the Middle Ages also practiced the art of poisoning. A famous figure of the time was a lady named Toffana, who peddled specially prepared arsenic-containing cosmetics *(Agua Toffana)*. Accompanying the product were appropriate instructions for use. Toffana was succeeded by an imitator with organizational genius, a certain Hieronyma Spara, who provided a new fillip by directing her activity toward specific marital and monetary objectives. A local club was formed of young, wealthy, married women, which soon became a club of eligible young, wealthy widows, reminiscent of the matronly conspiracy many centuries earlier.

Among the prominent families engaged in poisoning, the Borgias are the most notorious. Although there is no doubt that they were among the leading entrepreneurs in the field, they probably received more credit than their due. Many deaths that were attributed to poisoning are now recognized as having occurred from infectious diseases such as malaria, which was sufficiently bad as to make Rome virtually uninhabitable during the summer months. It appears true, however, that Alexander VI, his son Cesare, and Lucretia were quite active. Aside from personal reasons, the deft applications of poisons to men of stature in the Church swelled the holdings of the Papacy, which was the prime heir.

A paragon of the distaff set of the period was Catherine de Medici. Catherine, although not so thoroughly fabled as her Borgia relatives and ancestors, was, in tune with her time, a practitioner of the art of applied toxicology. She also represented a formidable export from Italy to France. As appeared to be all too common in this period, the prime targets of the ladies were their husbands. However, unlike others of an earlier period, the circle represented by Catherine (and epitomized by the notorious Marchioness de Brinvillers) depended on direct evidence to arrive at the most effective compounds for their purposes. Under guise of delivering provender to the sick and the poor, Catherine tested toxic concoctions, carefully noting the rapidity of the toxic response (onset of action), the effectiveness of the compound (potency), the degree of response of the parts of the body (specificity, site of action), and the complaints of the victim (clinical signs and symptoms). Clearly, Catherine must be given credit as perhaps the earliest untrained experimental toxicologist.

Culmination of the practice in France is represented by the commercialization of the service by a Catherine Deshayes, who earned the title *La Voisine.* Her business was dissolved by her execution. Her trial was one of the most famous of those held by the Chambre Ardente, a special judicial commission established by Louis XIV to try such cases without regard to age, sex, or national origin. La Voisine was convicted of many poisonings, including over 2000 infants among the victims.

During the Middle Ages and on into the Renaissance, poisoning seems to have been accepted as one of the normal hazards of living. It had some elements of sport, with a code, unwritten rules of honor, and a fatalistic attitude on the part of the selected victim. Devices and methods of poisoning proliferated at an alarming rate. The Chambre Ardente created in France was but a mild deterrent, and it remained for the rise of scientific methods in modern times to make the practice more risky for poisoners.

Another individual whose contributions to toxicology have survived through the years was Moses ben Maimon, or Maimonides (A.D. 1135–1204). In addition to being a competent and well-respected physician, Maimonides was also a prolific writer. Of particular significance was his volume entitled *Poisons and Their Antidotes* (1198), a first-aid guide to the treatment of accidental or intentional poisonings and insect, snake, or mad dog bites. Maimonides recommended that suction be applied to insect stings or animal bites as a means of extracting the poison and advised application of a tight bandage above a wound located on a limb. He also noted that the absorption of toxins from the stomach could be delayed by ingestion of oily substances such as milk, butter, or cream. A cautious and critical observer, Maimonides rejected numerous popular remedies of the day after finding them to be ineffective (e.g., the use of unleavened bread in the treatment of scorpion stings) and mentioned his doubts concerning the efficacy of others.

Age of Enlightenment

A significant figure in the history of science and medicine in the late Middle Ages was the renaissance man, Philippus Aureolus Theophrastus Bombastus von Hohenheim-Paracelsus (1493–1541). Between the time of Aristotle and the age of Paracelsus there was little substantial change in the biomedical sciences. In the sixteenth century the revolt against the authority of the Church was accompanied by a parallel attack on the godlike authority exercised by the followers of Hippocrates and Galen. Paracelsus, personally and professionally, embodied the qualities that forced numerous changes in this period. He and his age were pivotal, standing between the philosophy and magic of classic antiquity and the philosophy and science willed to us by figures of the seventeenth and eighteenth centuries. Clearly one can identify in Paracelsus's approach, his point of view, and his breadth of interest numerous similarities to the discipline we now call toxicology.

Paracelsus formulated many then-revolutionary views that remain an integral part of the present structure of toxicology. He promoted a focus on the "toxicon," the toxic agent, as a chemical entity. A view initiated by Paracelsus that became a lasting contribution held, as corollaries, that (1) experimentation is essential in examination of responses to chemicals; (2) one should make a distinction between therapeutic and toxic properties of chemicals; (3) these properties are sometimes, but not always, indistinguishable except by dose; and (4) one can ascertain a degree of specificity of chemicals and their therapeutic or toxic effects. The latter view presaged the "magic bullet" of Paul Ehrlich and the introduction of the therapeutic index. Further, in a very real sense, this was the first sound articulation of the dose-response relation, which is a bulwark of toxicology (Pachter, 1961).

Another noteworthy contribution was his volume entitled *Bergsucht* (1533–1534), the first treatise in the medical literature to provide a comprehensive description of the occupational diseases of miners. The book contains numerous clinical observations of chronic arsenic and mercury poisoning and describes in detail the asthmatic attacks and gastrointestinal symptoms of Miners' disease (Pagel, 1958).

Modern Toxicology

Often cited as the founder of toxicology is Mattieu Joseph Bonaventura Orfila (1787–1853), a Spanish physician who held a position of respect as attending physician to Louis XVIII of France and occupied a chair at the University of Paris. Orfila was the first to attempt a systematic correlation between the chemical and biologic information of the then-known poisons. Much of his contribution was based on personal observation of the effect of poisons in several thousand dogs. Among other contributions, he singled out toxicology as a discipline distinct from others and defined toxicology as the study of poisons.

Orfila also turned attention to problems combining chemistry and jurisprudence. He pointed to the necessity of chemical analysis for legal proof of lethal intoxication and he devised methods for detecting poisons, some of which are still used. A major outcome of his activity was the emergence of autopsy material for the purpose

of detection of accidental and intentional poisonings. The introduction of this approach survives in modern toxicology as one specialty area, that of forensic toxicology.

The era of modern toxicology ushered in by Orfila marked the beginning of a number of analytic developments that made poisoning detectable. The close relationship between poisons and the occult that had evolved earlier began to dissipate with the advent of tests to determine whether a murder has been committed. For example, the test for arsenic by Marsh, in 1836, removed from the unknown and undetected one of the most widely used substances for murder.

The fascination with toxic substances was common among many leading physiologists of the eighteenth and nineteenth centuries. Francois Magendie (1783–1855) spent a significant part of his time in the study of the mechanism of action of emetine and strychnine. He was interested in "arrow poisons" used by primitive tribes and began a study of their actions (see Olmsted, 1944). Magendie transmitted this interest to his equally famous student Claude Bernard (1813–1878).

Bernard continued the study of arrow poisons and reported a classic experiment identifying the site of action of curare, confirming an earlier report of Kolliker at Würtzburg (Bernard, 1850). Bernard held and propagated the view that "the physiological analysis of organic systems . . . can be done with the aid of toxic agents." Bernard assiduously applied this principle using a number of agents besides curare, including strychnine and carbon monoxide, which he noted formed a complex with hemoglobin (Bernard, translated by Greene, 1949).

Louis Lewin (1854–1929) was a prodigious figure in toxicology. His interests were broad, leading to many publications dealing with the toxicology of methyl, ethyl, and higher alcohols, chloroform, chronic opiate use, and hallucinogenic materials contained in plants. Among his publications was a toxicologist's view of world history, and, in the year of his death, a textbook of toxicology (1920, 1929). Robert Christison (1797–1882), who studied toxicology under Orfila, produced a major work on poisons (1845), Rudolf Kobert (1854–1918), a student of Oswald Schmiedeberg and a contemporary of Lewin, also produced a textbook on toxicology (1893).

Developments in toxicology occurred rapidly in the twentieth century. On the one hand, there were many toxic and therapeutic agents that served as the starting points for fundamental studies of mechanisms, for example, the development by Rudolf Peters and colleagues (1945) of dimercaprol (BAL) as an antidote to arsenic-containing war gases and studies of the mechanism of BAL action on organic arsenicals by Carl Voegtlin and associates (1923). On the other hand, there were developments leading to discovery and understanding of toxic substances for use by man, such as the discovery and study of DDT by Paul Müller and the discovery and development of organophosphorus insecticides by Willy Lange and Gerhard Schrader. Following this refinement of analytic techniques, toxicology developed rapidly. Although the contributions are too numerous to catalog, a selective sampling of contributions to toxicology may be informative. Such a list is presented in Table 1–1.

Although it is evident from the history described above that the origins of toxicology predate those of most other biologic sciences and perhaps even those of medicine, the emergence of toxicology as a discipline and particularly as an academic scientific discipline is a much more recent phenomenon. Most of the usual characteristics of an academic discipline, such as professional societies, journals, textbooks, graduate degree programs, accreditation boards, national meetings, awards, and so forth, have come about in the last two decades and some within the past few years. Similarly, the methodology of toxicology has changed dramatically in recent years with the introduction of teratology, the Ames test and other mutation assays, and the use of mathematical models for risk extrapolation. In comparison with the other biologic science disciplines, toxicology is clearly an infant, and thus it is perhaps not surprising that the discipline is having some ''growing pains.'' During the coming decade, it is likely that toxicology will continue to experience additional evolutionary shock as new methodology for neuro- and behavioral toxicology, immunotoxicology, short-term assays for fetotoxicity, and the like are developed, validated, and incorporated into the battery of toxicity-testing protocols.

Table 1–1.   SELECTION OF DEVELOPMENTS IN TOXICOLOGY

Development of early advances in analytic methods

Marsh, 1836: development of method for arsenic analysis
Reinsch, 1841: combined method for separation and analysis of As and Hg
Fresenius, 1845; von Babo, 1847: development of screening method for general poisons
Stas-Otto, 1851: extraction and separation of alkaloids
Mitscherlich, 1855: detection and identification of phosphorus

Early mechanistic studies

F. Magendie, 1809: study of ''arrow poisons,'' mechanism of action of emetine and strychnine
C. Bernard, 1850: carbon monoxide combination with hemoglobin, study of mechanism of action of strychnine, site of action of curare
R. Bohm, ca. 1890: active anthelmintics from fern, action of croton oil catharsis, poisonous mushrooms

Introduction of new toxins, antidotes

R. A. Peters, L. A. Stocken, and R. H. S. Thompson, 1945: development of British antilewisite (BAL) as a relatively specific antidote for arsenic, toxicity of monofluorocarbon compounds
K. K. Chen, 1934: introduction of modern antidotes (nitrite and thiosulfate) for cyanide toxicity
C. Voegtlin, 1923: mechanism of action of As and other metals on the SH groups
P. Müller, 1944–1946: introduction and study of DDT (dichlordiphenyltrichloroethane) and related insecticide compounds
G. Schrader, 1952: introduction and study of organophosphorus compounds
R. N. Chopra, 1933: indigenous drugs of India

Miscellaneous toxicologic studies

R. T. Williams: study of detoxication mechanisms and species variation
A. Rothstein: effects of uranium ion on cell membrane transport
R. A. Kehoe: investigation of acute and chronic effects of lead
A. Vorwald: studies of chronic respiratory disease (beryllium)
H. Hardy: community and industrial poisoning (beryllium)
A. Hamilton: introduction of modern industrial toxicology
H. C. Hodge: toxicology of uranium, fluorides; standards of toxicity
A. Hoffman: introduction of lysergic acid and derivatives; psychotomimetics
R. A. Peters: biochemical lesions, lethal synthesis
A. E. Garrod: inborn errors of metabolism
T. T. Litchfield and F. Wilcoxon: simplified dose-response evaluation
C. J. Bliss: method of probits, calculation of dosage-mortality curves

Modern toxicology includes much more than a simple extension of the work of Orfila and other pioneers in the discipline. There is greater emphasis today on safety assessment and the use of the data from toxicologic studies as a basis for regulatory control of the hazards of chemicals. The passage of laws that require decisions as to whether the use of specific chemicals pose "an unreasonable risk to health or to the environment" challenges the ability of the toxicologist to provide accurate and relevant estimates for the risk side of the risk/benefit equation on which such decisions are based.

There are four interrelated components in the risk estimate about which the toxicologist needs information in order to make accurate and relevant predictions. The first is the chemical (or physical) agent, the second is the biologic system, the third is the effect or response, and the fourth is the exposure situation. The chemical must be capable of producing an adverse response in the test species under defined exposure conditions in order for the toxicologist to identify and characterize the hazard associated with the chemical. However, to identify and characterize the toxicity of any chemical the toxicologist must be able to identify and describe all the acute and chronic adverse effects that the agent is capable of causing and dose-response relationships for each of these adverse effects. Thus, more information may be needed to characterize the toxicity of a chemical than is needed to characterize the hazard associated with the use of the chemical in a specific situation.

The primary source for this information (the toxicology database) is animal testing, and over the years toxicologists have developed a set of testing protocol guidelines to facilitate the collection of toxicology data. The results from such tests have been and continue to be a key factor in assessing the safety of drugs, food additives, pesticides, and other chemicals in the environment and workplace. There are, however, some problems with this approach. It is quite possible, for example, to carry out tests that meet all protocol requirements yet fail to identify all possible adverse effects of an agent and the corresponding dose-response relationships. Such studies do not characterize the toxicity of the test agent even though they may establish a "safe" dosage level for the agent.

Another problem with the protocol approach is that protocols are designed to provide yes-no answers to toxicologic questions (is the agent carcinogenic? fetotoxic? hepatotoxic? etc.). In toxicology, as in most biologic sciences, answers come mostly in shades of gray rather than in black or white, and thus the most scientific answer may be a qualified no/yes or even maybe. Rigid protocols provide little opportunity to introduce the elements of judgment and experience into the selection, conduct, and evaluation of the tests, and they fail to deal with questions of "why" and "how" the effects occur (mechanism of action, kinetics, etc.). There is some concern in the toxicologic community that because of this focus on protocol-driven testing, toxicology may become a checklist of cookbook protocols. A related concern is that most risk-extrapolation models that use the results of animal tests to predict adverse effects in man ignore the relevant biology in both the test and target species. It is encouraging to note, however, that in most of the recent attempts to improve the current bioassay protocols, greater emphasis is being given to investigative toxicology and to providing increased flexibility as a means to improve both the scientific quality and the predictive value of these studies (OSTP, 1984; NTP, 1984; IARC/IPCS/CEC, 1983; US EPA, 1982; OECD, 1981; US FDA, 1982; NCI, 1976).

During the last two decades, there has been heightened public concern about the effects of chemicals, radiation, and technology in general on our health and environment. Episodes such as the methyl isocyanate (MIC) exposure in Bhopal, India, reinforce these concerns and raise questions about the possibility of similar disasters, not only in or near chemical plants but also from the transportation of hazardous chemicals. Issues such as "acid rain," ground water pollution, toxic waste dumps, "right to know," and EDB receive extensive media coverage that impacts on public confidence in both the science and the policy decisions relating to these and other environmental issues. Attempts to separate the scientific from the policy issues have led to new definitions for risk assessment and risk management (NAS/NRC, 1983) and renewed interest in the concept of a National Science Council (U.S. Congress, 1981). All of us recognize that a "zero-risk" environment is neither attainable nor desirable, but our perception of risks correlates poorly with the scientific information. We are less concerned about the risk of driving an automobile than breathing the tailpipe exhaust, and we are less concerned about the natural carcinogens in food (Ames, 1983) than about food additives and chemical contaminants. We focus on industry and technology as the cause of cancer rather than on the major factors of smoking and diet. Arguments against the linking of environmental cancer with industrialization (Handler, 1979; Totter, 1980; Effron, 1984), the influence of risk perception (Weinberg, 1972; Lowrance, 1976), and the causes of cancer (Doll and Peto, 1981) may be useful to the reader desiring a broader perspective on these environmental issues.

REFERENCES

Ames, B. N.: Dietary carcinogens and anticarcinogens. *Science*, **221**:1249–64, 1983.

Bernard, C.: Action du curare et de la nicotine sur le système nerveux et sur le système musculaire. *C.R. Séances Soc. Biol.*, **2**:195, 1850.

———: *An Introduction to the Study of Experimental Medicine*, translated by H. C. Greene. H. Schuman, New York, 1949.

Christison, R.: *A Treatise on Poisons*, 4th ed. Barrington & Howell, Philadelphia, 1845.

Doll, R., and Peto, R.: *The Causes of Cancer*. Oxford University Press, New York, 1981.

Effron, E.: *The Apocalyptics, Cancer and the Big Lie*. Simon & Schuster, New York, 1984.

Gunther, R. T.: *The Greek Herbal of Dioscorides*. Oxford University Press, New York, 1934.

Guthrie, D. A.: *A History of Medicine*. J. B. Lippincott Co., Philadelphia, 1946.

Handler, P.: Some comments on risk assessment. In *The National Research Council in 1979: Current Issues and Studies*. NAS, Washington, D.C., 1979.

IARC/IPCS/CEC: *Working Group Report: Approaches to Classifying Carcinogens According to Mechanism of Action*. IARC Internal Technical Report, 83/1. International Agency for Research on Cancer, Lyon, 1983.

IARC: *Long-term and Short-term Screening Assays for Carcinogens: A Critical Appraisal*. IARC Monographs on the Evaluation of the Carcinogenic Risk of Chemicals to Humans, Suppl. 2, International Agency for Research on Cancer, Lyon, 1980.

Robert, R.: *Lehrbuch der Intoxikationen*. Enke, Stuttgart, 1893.

Levey, M: Medieval arabic toxicology. The book on poisons of Ibn Wahshiya and its relation to early Indian and Greek texts. *Trans. Am. Philos. Soc.*, **56**:Part 7, 1966.

Lewin, L.: *Gifte und Vergiftungen*. Stilke, Berlin, 1929.

———: *Die Gifte in der Weltgeschichte. Toxikologische, allgemeinverständliche Untersuchungen der historischen Quellen*. Springer, Berlin, 1920.

Loomis, T. A.: *Essentials of Toxicology*, 3rd ed. Lea & Febiger, Philadelphia, 1978.

Lowrance, W. W.: *Of Acceptable Risk, Science and the Determination of Safety*. William Kaufmann, Inc., Los Altos, Calif., 1976.

Macht, D. J.: Louis Lewin: pharmacologist, toxicologist medical historian. *Ann. Med. Hist.*, **3**:179–94, 1931.

Meek, W. J.: *The Gentle Art of Poisoning*. Medico-Historical Papers. University of Wisconsin, Madison, 1954; reprinted from Phi Beta Pi Quarterly, May 1928.

Muller, P.: Über zusammenhange zwischen Konstitution und insektizider Wirkung. I. *Helv. Chim. Acta*. **29**:1560–80, 1946.

Munter, S. (ed.): *Treatise on Poisons and Their Antidotes*. Vol. II of the *Medical Writings of Moses Maimondides*. J. B. Lippincott Co., Philadelphia, 1966.

NAS/NRC: *Risk Assessment in the Federal Government: Managing the Process*. National Academy Press, Washington, D.C., 1983.

NAS/NRC: *Toxicity Testing, Strategies to Determine Needs and Priorities*. National Academy Press, Washington, D.C., 1984.

NCI: *Guidelines for Carcinogen Bioassay in Small Rodents*. NCI-CG-TR-1, 1976.

NTP: *Report of the Ad Hoc Panel on Chemical Carcinogenesis Testing and Evaluation*. Board of Scientific Counselors, National Toxicology Program, Research Triangle Park, N.C., 1984.

OECD: Guidelines for Testing Chemicals. Publ. #ISBN92-64-12221-4, Organization for Economic Co-operation and Development, Paris, 1981.

Olmsted, J. M. D.: *Francois Magendie. Pioneer in Experimental Physiology and Scientific Medicine in XIX Century France*. Schuman, New York, 1944.

Orfila, M. J. B.: *Traité des Poisons Tirés des Règnes Minéral, Végétal et Animal, ou, Toxicologie Générale Considérée sous les Rapports de la Physiologie, de la Pathologie et de la Médecine Légale*. Crochard, Paris, 1814–1815.

———: *Secours à Donner aux Personnes Empoisonées et Asphyxiées*. Feugeroy, Paris, 1818.

OSTP: *Chemical Carcinogens*. Federal Register May 22, Office of Science and Technology Policy, Washington, D.C., 1984.

Pachter, H. M.: *Paracelsus: Magic into Science*. Collier Books, New York, 1961.

Pagel, W.: *Paracelsus: An Introduction to Philosophical Medicine in the Era of the Renaissance*. S. Karger, New York, 1958.

Paracelsus (Theophrastus ex Hohenheim Eremita): *Von der Besucht*. Dillingen, 1567.

Peters, R. A.; Stocken, L. A.; and Thompson, R. H. S.: British anti-lewisite (*BAL*). *Nature*, **156**:616–19, 1945.

Ramazzini, B.: *De Morbis Artificum Diatriba*. Modena, 1700.

Schmiedeberg, O., and Koppe, R.: *Das Muscarin das giftige Alkaloid des Fliegenpilzes*. Vogel, Leipzig, 1869.

Siegrist, H. E.: *The Great Doctors*. Doubleday & Co. Garden City, N.Y., 1958.

Thompson, C. J. S.: *Poisons and Poisoners. With Historical Accounts of Some Famous Mysteries in Ancient and Modern Times*. H. Shaylor, London, 1931.

Totter, J. R.: Spontaneous cancer and its possible relationship to oxygen metabolism. *Proc. Natl. Acad. Sci.*, **77**:1763–67, 1980.

U.S. Congress: *House of Representatives H.R. 638*. National Science Council Act, 97th Congress, 1st Session, 1981.

US EPA: *Health Effects Test Guidelines*. EPA 560/6-82-001, U.S. Environmental Protection Agency, Washington, D.C., 1982.

US FDA: *Toxicologic Principles for the Safety Assessment of Direct Food Additives and Color Additives Used in Food*. U.S. Food and Drug Administration, Bureau of Foods, Washington, D.C., 1982.

Voegtlin, C.; Dyer, H. A.; and Leonard, C. S.: On the mechanism of the action of arsenic upon protoplasm. *Public Health Rep.*, **38**:1882–1912, 1923.

Weinberg, A. M.: Science and trans-science. *Minerva*, **10**:202–22, 1972.

SUPPLEMENTAL READING

Adams, F. (trans.): *The Genuine Works of Hippocrates*. Williams & Wilkins Co., Baltimore, 1939.

Beeson, B. B.: Orifila—pioneer toxicologist. *Ann. Med. Hist.*, **2**:68–70, 1930.

Bernard, C.: Analyse physiologique des propriétés des systèmes musculaire et nerveux au moyen du curare. *C.R. Acad. Sci. (Paris)*, **43**:325–29, 1856.

Bryan, C. P.: *The Papyrus Ebers*. Geoffrey Bales, London, 1930.

Clendening, L.: *Source Book of Medical History*. Dover, New York, 1942.

DuBois, K. P., and Geiling, E. M. K.: *Textbook of Toxicology*. Oxford University Press, New York, 1959.

Gaddum, J. H.: *Pharmacology*, 5th ed. Oxford University Press, New York, 1959.

Garrison, F. H.: *An Introduction to the History of Medicine*, 4th ed. W. B. Saunders Co., Philadelphia, 1929.

Hamilton, A.: *Exploring the Dangerous Trades*. Little, Brown & Co., Boston, 1943. (Reprinted by Northeastern University Press, Boston, 1985.)

Chapter 2

PRINCIPLES OF TOXICOLOGY

Curtis D. Klaassen

INTRODUCTION TO TOXICOLOGY

Toxicology is the study of the adverse effects of chemicals on living organisms. The *toxicologist* is specially trained to examine the nature of these adverse effects and to assess the probability of their occurrence. The variety of potential adverse effects and the diversity of chemicals present in our environment combine to make toxicology a very broad science. Therefore, toxicologists are usually specialized to work in one area of toxicology.

Different Areas of Toxicology

The professional activities of toxicologists fall into three main categories: descriptive, mechanistic, and regulatory. The *descriptive toxicologist* is concerned directly with toxicity testing. The appropriate toxicity tests (as described later in this chapter) in experimental animals are designed to yield information that can be used to evaluate the risk posed to humans and the environment by exposure to specific chemicals. The concern may be limited to effects on humans, as in the case of drugs or food additives. Toxicologists in the chemical industry, however, must be concerned not only with risk posed by the company's chemicals (insecticides, herbicides, solvents, etc.) to humans but also with potential effects on fish, birds, plants, and other factors that might disturb the balance of the ecosystem. The *mechanistic toxicologist* is concerned with elucidating the mechanisms by which chemicals exert their toxic effects on living organisms. Results of these studies often lead to the development of sensitive predictive tests useful in obtaining information for risk assessment, chemicals that are safer, or rational therapy for toxic symptoms. In addition, an understanding of the mechanisms of toxic action also contributes to the knowledge of basic physiology, pharmacology, cell biology, and biochemistry. For example, studies on the toxicity of fluoroorganic alcohols and acids contributed to the knowledge of basic carbohydrate and lipid metabolism;

knowledge of regulation of ion gradients in nerve axonal membranes has been greatly aided by studies of natural and synthetic toxins such as tetrodotoxin and DDT. Mechanistic toxicologists are active in universities, in research institutes supported by the government or by private sources, and in the pharmaceutical and chemical industries.

A *regulatory toxicologist* has the responsibility of deciding on the basis of data provided by the descriptive toxicologist if a drug or other chemical poses a sufficiently low risk to be marketed for a stated purpose. The Food and Drug Administration (FDA) is responsible for admitting drugs, cosmetics, and food additives onto the market according to the Federal Food, Drug and Cosmetic Act (FDCA). The Environmental Protection Agency (EPA) is responsible for regulating most other chemicals according to the Federal Insecticide, Fungicide and Rodenticide Act (FIFRA), the Toxic Substances Control Act (TSCA), the Resource Conservation and Recovery Act (RCRA), the Safe Drinking Water Act, and the Clean Air Act. The Occupational Safety and Health Administration (OSHA) of the Department of Labor was established to assure that safe and healthful conditions exist in the workplace. The Consumer Product Safety Commission has the responsibility of protecting the consumer from hazardous household substances, while the Department of Transportation (DOT) assures that materials shipped in interstate commerce are labeled and packaged in a manner consistent with the degree of hazard they present. Regulatory toxicologists are also involved in the establishment of standards for the amount of chemicals permitted in ambient air, in industrial atmospheres, or in drinking water. Some of the philosophic and legal aspects of regulatory toxicology are discussed in Chapter 30.

Three specialized areas of toxicology are forensic, clinical, and environmental toxicology. *Forensic toxicology* is a hybrid of analytic chemistry and fundamental toxicologic principles. It is concerned primarily with the medicolegal aspects of the harmful effects of chemicals on humans and animals. The expertise of the forensic toxicologist is primarily invoked to aid in establishing the cause of death and elucidating its circumstances in a postmortem investigation (see Chapter 27). *Clinical toxicology* designates an area of professional emphasis within the realm of medical science concerned with disease caused by, or uniquely associated with, toxic substances (see Chapter 28). Efforts are directed at treating patients poisoned with drugs or other chemicals and at development of new techniques to treat these intoxications. *Environmental toxicology* usually designates the study of the effects of pollutants on wildlife and how this might affect the ecosystem; however, it is sometimes used to designate toxicologic evaluations made in the interest of humans but dealing with environmental pollutants.

Spectrum of Toxic Dose

One could define a poison as any agent capable of producing a deleterious response in a biologic system, seriously injuring function or producing death. This is not, however, a useful working definition for the very simple reason that virtually every known chemical has the potential to produce injury or death if present in a sufficient amount. Paracelsus (1493–1541) phrased this well when he noted, "All substances are poisons; there is none which is not a poison. The right dose differentiates a poison and a remedy."

Among chemicals there is a wide spectrum of doses needed to produce deleterious effects, serious injury, or death. This is demonstrated in Table 2–1, which shows the dosage of chemical needed to produce death in 50 percent of the treated animals (LD50). Some chemicals will

Table 2–1. APPROXIMATE ACUTE LD50'S OF SOME REPRESENTATIVE CHEMICAL AGENTS

AGENT	LD50 (mg/kg)*
Ethyl alcohol	10,000
Sodium chloride	4,000
Ferrous sulfate	1,500
Morphine sulfate	900
Phenobarbital sodium	150
Picrotoxin	5
Strychnine sulfate	2
Nicotine	1
d-Tubocurarine	0.5
Hemicholinium-3	0.2
Tetrodotoxin	0.10
Dioxin (TCDD)	0.001
Botulinum toxin	0.00001

* LD50 is the dosage (mg/kg body weight) causing death in 50 percent of the exposed animals.

produce death in microgram doses and are commonly thought of as being extremely poisonous. Other chemicals may be relatively harmless following doses in excess of several grams. Categories of toxicity have been devised on the basis of the wide variation in the dosage of chemical needed to produce death. Table 2–2 illustrates an example of such a classification, which provides a toxicity rating or class based on the probable lethal oral dose for humans. Such classifications are only qualitative, but they serve a practical and useful purpose, especially to a toxicologist who is asked by someone in another discipline, "How toxic is this chemical?"

Risk and Safety

In practical situations the critical factor is not the intrinsic toxicity of a substance, but the risk or hazard associated with its use. Risk is the probability that a substance will produce harm under specified conditions. Safety, the reciprocal of risk, is the probability that harm will not occur under specified conditions. Potentially supertoxic substances can be used safely provided one controls the environment to prevent absorption of sufficient quantities of the material to produce toxicity. In such a situation, although the chemical is supertoxic, it is not hazardous in the manner in which it is being used. Therefore, depending on the conditions under which it is used, a very toxic chemical may be less hazardous than a relatively nontoxic one. Risk assessment takes into account possible harmful effects on individuals or on society from the use of a material in the quantity and in the manner proposed. It is important to consider harmful effects on the environment as well as more direct effects on human health.

The question of what constitutes an acceptable risk is a matter of judgment. Such decisions are multifaceted and complex and involve a balance of risk and benefit. High risks may be acceptable in the use of lifesaving drugs but would be unacceptable for food additives. Some of the factors considered in determining an acceptable risk are (1) benefits gained from use of the substance, (2) the adequacy and availability of alternative substances to meet the identified use, (3) the anticipated extent of public use, (4) employment considerations, (5) economic considerations, (6) effects on environmental quality, and (7) conservation of natural resources.

CLASSIFICATION OF TOXIC AGENTS

Toxic agents are classified in a variety of ways, depending on the interests and needs of the classifier. In this textbook, for example, toxic agents are discussed in terms of their target

Table 2–2. TOXICITY RATING CHART

| | PROBABLE LETHAL ORAL DOSE FOR HUMANS | |
TOXICITY RATING OR CLASS	*Dosage*	*For Average Adult*
1. Practically nontoxic	> 15 g/kg	More than 1 quart
2. Slightly toxic	5–15 g/kg	Between pint and quart
3. Moderately toxic	0.5–5 g/kg	Between ounce and pint
4. Very toxic	50–500 mg/kg	Between teaspoonful and ounce
5. Extremely toxic	5–50 mg/kg	Between 7 drops and teaspoonful
6. Supertoxic	< 5 mg/kg	A taste (less than 7 drops)

organ (liver, kidney, hematopoietic system, etc.), their use (pesticide, solvent, food additive, etc.), their source (animal and plant toxins), and their effects (cancer, mutation, liver injury, etc.). Toxic agents may also be classified in terms of their physical state (gas, dust, liquid), their labeling requirements (explosive, flammable, oxidizer), their chemistry (aromatic amine, halogenated hydrocarbon, etc.), or, as shown in Table 2–2, their poisoning potential (extremely toxic, very toxic, slightly toxic, etc.). Classification of toxic agents on the basis of their biochemical mechanism of action (sulfhydryl inhibitor, methemoglobin producer) is usually more informative than classification by general terms such as irritants and corrosives, but the more general classifications such as air pollutants, occupation-related agents, and acute and chronic poisons can provide a useful focus on a specific problem. It is evident from the above that no single classification will be applicable for the entire spectrum of toxic agents and that combinations of classification systems or classification based on other factors may be needed to provide the best rating system for a special purpose. Nevertheless, classification systems that take into consideration both the chemical and biologic properties of the agent and the exposure characteristics are most likely to be useful for legislative or control purposes and for toxicology in general.

CHARACTERISTICS OF EXPOSURE

Adverse or toxic effects in a biologic system are not produced by a chemical agent unless that agent or its biotransformation products reach appropriate sites in the body at a concentration and for a length of time sufficient to produce the toxic manifestation. Whether or not a toxic response occurs is dependent, therefore, on the chemical and physical properties of the agent, the exposure situation, and the susceptibility of the biologic system or subject. Thus, to characterize fully the potential hazard or toxicity of a specific chemical agent we need to know not only what type of effect it produces and the dose required to produce the effect, but also information about the agent, the exposure, and the subject. The major factors that influence toxicity as it relates to the exposure situation for a specific chemical are the route of administration and the duration and frequency of exposure.

Route and Site of Exposure

The major routes by which toxic agents gain access to the body are through the gastrointestinal tract (ingestion), lungs (inhalation), skin (topical), and other parenteral (other than intestinal canal) routes. Toxic agents generally elicit the greatest effect and produce the most rapid response when given by the intravenous route. An approximate descending order of effectiveness for the other routes would be: inhalation, intraperitoneal, subcutaneous, intramuscular, intradermal, oral, and topical. The vehicle and other formulation factors can markedly alter the absorption following ingestion, inhalation, or topical exposure. In addition, the route of administration can influence the toxicity of agents. For example, an agent that is detoxified in the liver would be expected to be less toxic when given via the portal circulation (oral) than when given via the systemic circulation (inhalation). Industrial exposure to toxic agents most frequently is the result of inhalation and topical exposure, whereas accidental and suicidal poisoning occurs most frequently by oral ingestion. Comparison of the lethal dose of an agent by different routes of exposure often provides useful information concerning the absorption of the agent. In instances when the lethal dose after oral or topical administration is similar to the lethal dose for intravenous administration, the assumption is that the toxic agent is absorbed readily and rapidly. Conversely, in those cases where the lethal dose by the dermal route is several orders of magnitude higher than the oral lethal dose, it is likely that the skin provides an effective barrier to poisoning by the agent. Toxic effects by any route of exposure can also be influenced by the concentration of the agent in its vehicle, the total volume of the vehicle and the properties of the vehicle to which the biologic system is exposed, and the rate at which exposure occurs. Studies in which the concentration of the chemical in the blood is determined at various times after exposure are often needed to clarify the role of these and other factors on the toxicity of a compound. For more details on the absorption of toxicants see Chapter 3.

Duration and Frequency of Exposure

Toxicologists usually divide the exposure of animals to chemicals into four categories: acute, subacute, subchronic, and chronic. Acute exposure is defined as exposure to a chemical for less than 24 hours, and examples of exposure routes are intraperitoneal, intravenous, and subcutaneous injection, oral intubation, and dermal application. While acute exposure usually refers to a single administration, repeated exposures may be given within a 24-hour period for some slightly toxic or practically nontoxic chemicals. An extreme example is acute exposure by inhalation, which refers to continuous exposure for less than 24 hours, most frequently for four hours. Repeated exposure is divided into three categories: subacute, subchronic, and chronic. Subacute exposure refers to repeated exposure to a chemical for one month or less, subchronic for one to three months, and chronic for more than three months. These three categories of repeated exposure can be by any route, but most often it is by the oral route, with the chemical added directly to the diet.

For many agents, the toxic effects following a single exposure are quite different from those produced by repeated exposure. For example, the primary acute toxic manifestation of benzene is central nervous system depression, but repeated exposures can result in leukemia. Acute exposure to agents that are rapidly absorbed is likely to produce immediate toxic effects, but acute exposure can also produce delayed toxicity that may or may not be similar to the toxic effects of chronic exposure. Conversely, chronic exposure to a toxic agent may produce some immediate (acute) effects after each administration, in addition to the long-term, low-level, or chronic effects of the agent. In characterizing the toxicity of a specific chemical agent, it is evident that information is needed not only for the single-dose (acute) and long-term (chronic) effects, but also for exposures of intermediate duration.

The other time-related factor that is important in the temporal characterization of exposure is the frequency of administration. In general, fractionation of the dose reduces the effect. A single dose of a test substance that produces an immediate severe effect might produce less than half the effect when given in two divided doses and no effect when given in ten doses over a period of several hours or days. Such fractionation effects occur when biotransformation or excretion occurs between successive doses or when the injury produced by each administration is partially or fully reversed prior to the next administration. A diagrammatic representation of these concepts is presented in Figure 2–1. It is evident that with any type of multiple dose the production of a toxic effect is not only influ-

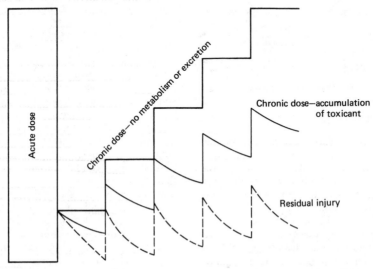

Figure 2–1. Diagrammatic view of dose and corresponding measure of effect. Acute dose is compared to the cumulative dose after multiple administration of a chemical that has limited elimination and thus accumulates, and one that produces injury, which accumulates with multiple dosing.

enced by the frequency of administration but may, in fact, be totally dependent on frequency rather than duration of exposure. Chronic toxic effects occur, therefore, if the chemical accumulates in the biologic system (absorption exceeds biotransformation and/or excretion), if it produces irreversible toxic effects, or if there is insufficient time for the system to recover from the toxic damage within the exposure frequency interval. When the rate of elimination is less than the rate of absorption, the toxic agent usually does not accumulate indefinitely, but reaches a steady state where the rate of elimination equals the rate of administration. For additional discussion of these relationships, the reader should consult Chapter 3.

SPECTRUM OF UNDESIRED EFFECTS

The spectrum of undesired effects of chemicals is broad. Some are deleterious and others are not. In therapeutics, for example, each drug produces a number of effects, but usually only one of these is associated with the primary objective of the therapy; all other effects are referred to as undesirable or side effects of that drug for that therapeutic indication. However, some of these side effects might be desired for another therapeutic indication. For example, dryness of the mouth is a side effect of atropine when used to decrease gastric secretion in the treatment of peptic ulcer but is the desired effect when used for preanesthetic medication. Some side effects of drugs are never desirable but are deleterious to the well-being of humans. These are referred to as the *adverse, deleterious,* or *toxic* effects of the drug.

Allergic Reactions

Chemical allergy is an adverse reaction to a chemical resulting from previous sensitization to that chemical or to a structurally similar one. The term *hypersensitivity* is most often used to describe this allergic state, but *allergic reaction* and *sensitization reaction* are also used to describe this situation where preexposure of the chemical is required to produce the toxic effect (Goldstein *et al.*, 1974; Loomis, 1974). Allergic reactions usually occur at low doses of chemicals, and therefore dose-response curves for allergic reactions have seldom been obtained. Because of this omission, some people have assume that allergic reactions are not dose related. Thus, they have not considered the allergic reaction to be a true toxic response. However, allergic reactions are dose related. For example, it is well known that the allergic response to pollen in sensitized individuals is related to the concen-

tration of pollen in the air. In addition, since the allergic response is an undesirable, adverse, deleterious effect, it obviously is also a toxic response. Sensitization reactions are often very severe and many are fatal.

To produce an allergic reaction most chemicals or their metabolic products function immunologically as haptens and must combine with an endogenous protein to form an antigen (or immunogen). The antigen is then capable of eliciting the formation of antibodies, and usually at least one or two weeks are required for synthesis of significant amounts of antibodies. Subsequent exposure to the chemical will result in an antigen-antibody interaction, which provokes the typical manifestations of allergy. The manifestations of allergy are numerous. They involve various organ systems and range in severity from minor skin disturbance to fatal anaphylactic shock. The pattern of allergic response differs in various species. In humans, involvement of the skin (e.g., dermatitis, urticaria, and itching) and involvement of the eyes (e.g., conjunctivitis) are most common, whereas in guinea pigs bronchiolar constriction leading to asphyxia is common. Hypersensitivity reactions are discussed in more detail in Chapter 9.

Idiosyncratic Reactions

Chemical idiosyncrasy is a genetically determined abnormal reactivity to a chemical (Goldstein *et al.*, 1974; Levine, 1978). The response observed is usually qualitatively similar to that observed in all individuals but may take the form of extreme sensitivity to low doses or extreme insensitivity to high doses of the chemical. However, while some people use the term idiosyncratic as a catchall to refer to all reactions that occur with low frequency, it should not be used in this manner (Goldstein *et al.*, 1974).

An example of an idiosyncratic reaction is provided by patients who exhibit prolonged muscular relaxation and apnea, lasting several hours, after a standard dose of succinylcholine. Succinylcholine usually produces skeletal muscle relaxation of only a short duration because of its very rapid metabolic degradation by plasma pseudocholinesterase. Patients exhibiting this idiosyncratic reaction have an atypical pseudocholinesterase. Family pedigree studies have demonstrated that the presence of atypical cholinesterase is a genetically determined characteristic. Similarly, there is a group of people who are abnormally sensitive to nitrites and other chemicals that produce methemoglobinemia. These individuals have a deficiency in NADH-methemoglobin reductase, which is inherited as an autosomal recessive trait.

Immediate Versus Delayed Toxicity

Immediate toxicologic effects can be defined as those that occur or develop rapidly after a single administration of a substance, while delayed effects are those that occur after the lapse of some time. Carcinogenic effects of chemicals usually have a long latency period, often 20 to 30 years, before tumors are observed in humans. For example, the vaginal and uterine cancer produced by diethylstilbestrol in young women was due to their exposure *in utero* to diethylstilbestrol taken by their mothers to prevent miscarriages. Also, delayed neurotoxicity is observed after exposure to some organophosphorus anticholinesterase agents. The most notorious of the compounds that produce this type of neurotoxic effect is triorthocresylphosphate (TOCP). The effect is not observed until at least several days after exposure to the toxic compound. In contrast, most substances produce immediate toxic effects but fail to produce delayed effects.

Reversible Versus Irreversible Toxic Effects

Some toxic effects of chemicals are reversible and others are irreversible. If a chemical produces pathologic injury to a tissue, the ability of the tissue to regenerate will largely determine whether the effect is reversible or irreversible. Thus, for a tissue such as liver, which has a high ability to regenerate, most injuries are reversible, whereas injury to the central nervous system is largely irreversible since differentiated cells of the central nervous system cannot divide and be replaced. Carcinogenic effects of chemicals are also irreversible toxic effects.

Local Versus Systemic Toxicity

Another distinction between types of effects is made on the general locus of action. Local effects refer to those that occur at the site of first contact between the biologic system and the toxicant. Examples of local effects are the ingestion of caustic substances or inhalation of irritant materials. The obverse of local effects is systemic effects that require absorption and distribution of the toxicant from its entry point to a distant site at which deleterious effects are produced. Most substances, except highly reactive materials, produce systemic effects. For some materials, both effects can be demonstrated. For example, tetraethyl lead produces effects on skin at the site of absorption and then is transported systemically to produce its typical effects on the central nervous system and other organs. If the local effect is marked, there may also be indirect systemic effects. For example, kidney damage following a severe acid burn is an indirect systemic effect because the toxicant does not reach the kidney.

Most chemicals that produce systemic toxicity do not cause a similar degree of toxicity in all organs but usually elicit the major toxicity in only one or two organs. These sites are referred to as the *target organs* of toxicity of a particular chemical. The target organ of toxicity is often not the site of highest concentration of the chemical. For example, lead is concentrated in bone, but its toxicity is due to the effects of lead in soft tissues. Likewise, DDT is concentrated in adipose tissue but produces no known toxic effects in this tissue.

The target organ of toxicity most frequently involved in systemic toxicity is the central nervous system. Even with many compounds having a prominent effect elsewhere, damage to the central nervous system, particularly the brain, can be demonstrated by the use of appropriate and sensitive methods. Next in order of frequency of involvement in systemic toxicity are the circulatory system, the blood and hematopoietic system, visceral organs, such as liver, kidney, and lung, and the skin. Muscle and bone are least often the target tissues for systemic effects. With substances having a predominantly local effect, the frequency with which tissues react depends largely on the portal of entry (skin, gastrointestinal tract, or respiratory tract).

INTERACTION OF CHEMICALS

In assessing the spectrum of responses, the accessibility of large numbers of toxicants creates an increasing necessity for consideration of interacting effects of toxicants. Interactions can occur in a variety of ways. Chemical interactions are known to occur by a number of mechanisms such as alterations in absorption, protein binding, and biotransformation or excretion of one or both of the interacting toxicants. In addition to these modes of interaction, the response of the organism to combinations of toxicants may be increased or decreased because of the toxicological responses at the site of action.

The effects of two chemicals given simultaneously will produce a response that may be simply additive of their individual responses or may be greater or less than that expected by addition of their individual responses. Study of these interactions often leads to a better understanding of the mechanism of toxicity of the chemicals involved. A number of terms have been used to describe pharmacologic and toxicologic interactions. An *additive* effect is the situation in which the combined effect of two chemicals is equal to the sum of the effect of each agent given alone (example: $2 + 3 = 5$). The effect most commonly observed when two chemicals are given together is an additive effect. For example, when two organic phosphate insecticides are given together, the cholinesterase inhibition is usually additive. A *synergistic* effect is the situation in which the combined effect of two chemicals is much greater than the sum of the effect of each agent given alone (example: 2 + 2 = 20). For example, both carbon tetrachloride and ethanol are hepatotoxic compounds, but together they produce much more liver injury than the mathematical sum of their individual effects on liver would suggest. *Potentiation* is the situation when one substance does not have a toxic effect on a certain organ or system, but when added to another chemical it makes the latter much more toxic (example: 0 + 2 = 10). Isopropanol, for example, is not hepatotoxic, but when isopropanol is administered in addition to carbon tetrachloride, the hepatotoxicity of carbon tetrachloride is much greater than when given alone. *Antagonism* is the situation in which two chemicals, administered together, interfere with each other's actions or one interferes with the action of the other chemical (example: 4 + 6 = 8, 4 + (−4) = 0, 4 + 0 = 1). Antagonistic effects of chemicals are often very desirable effects in toxicology and are the basis of many antidotes. There are four major types of antagonism: functional, chemical, dispositional, and receptor antagonism. *Functional antagonism* is the situation when two chemicals counterbalance each other by producing opposite effects on the same physiologic function. Advantage is taken of this principle in that the blood pressure can markedly fall during severe barbiturate intoxication, and it can be effectively antagonized by intravenous administration of a vasopressor agent, such as norepinephrine or metaraminol. Similarly, many chemicals, when given at toxic dose levels, produce convulsions and the convulsions can often be controlled by giving anticonvulsants, such as the benzodiazepines (e.g., diazepam). *Chemical antagonism* or *inactivation* is simply a chemical reaction between two compounds to produce a less toxic product. For example, dimercaprol (BAL) chelates with various metal ions such as arsenic, mercury, and lead, which decreases their toxicity. The use of antitoxins to treat various animal toxins is also an example of chemical antagonism. The use of the strongly basic low-molecular-weight protein protamine sulfate to form a stable complex with heparin, which abolishes its anticoagulant activity, is another example of chemical antagonism. *Dispositional antagonism* is the situation in which the disposition, that is, the absorption, biotransformation, distribution, or excretion of the chemical, is altered so that less toxic compound reaches the target organ or its duration at the target organ is diminished. Thus, prevention of absorption of a toxicant by ipecac or charcoal

and the increased excretion of a chemical by administration of an osmotic diuretic or by alteration of the pH of the urine are examples of dispositional antagonism. If the parent compound is responsible for the toxicity of the chemical (such as the organophosphate insecticide paraoxon) and its metabolites are less toxic than the parent compound, then increasing the compound's biotransformation by a microsomal enzyme inducer (like phenobarbital) will decrease its toxicity. However, if the chemical's toxicity is largely due to a metabolic product (such as the organophosphate insecticide parathion), then inhibiting its biotransformation by an inhibitor of microsomal enzyme activity (SKF-525A or piperonyl butoxide) will decrease its toxicity. *Receptor antagonism* is when two chemicals that bind to the same receptor produce less of an effect when given together than the addition of their separate effects (example: 4 + 6 = 8) or when one chemical antagonizes the effect of the second chemical (example: 0 + 4 = 1). Receptor antagonists are often termed blockers. This concept is used to advantage in the clinical treatment of poisoning. For example, the receptor antagonist naloxone is used for treating the respiratory depressive effects of morphine and other morphinelike narcotics by competitive binding to the same receptor. The effect of oxygen in carbon monoxide poisoning is also an example of receptor antagonism. Treatment of organophosphate insecticide poisoning with atropine is an example not of the antidote competing with the poison for the receptor (cholinesterase), but rather blocking the receptor (cholinergic receptor) for the acetylcholine that accumulates by poisoning of the cholinesterase by the organophosphate.

TOLERANCE

Tolerance is a state of decreased responsiveness to a toxic effect of a chemical resulting from prior exposure to that chemical or to a structurally related chemical. Two major mechanisms are responsible for tolerance; one is due to a decreased amount of toxicant reaching the site where the toxic effect is produced (*dispositional tolerance*) and the other is due to a reduced responsiveness of a tissue to the chemical. Comparatively less is known about cellular mechanisms responsible for altering the responsiveness of a tissue to a toxic chemical than is known about dispositional tolerance. Two chemicals known to produce dispositional tolerance are carbon tetrachloride and cadmium. Carbon tetrachloride produces tolerance to itself by decreasing formation of the reactive metabolite (trichloromethyl radical) that produces liver injury (see Chapter 10). The mechanism of cadmium tolerance is explained by induction of a metal binding protein, metallothionein. Subsequent binding of cadmium to metallothionein rather than to critical macromolecules thereby decreases its toxicity (Goering and Klaassen, 1983).

DOSE-RESPONSE

The characteristics of exposure and the spectrum of effects come together in a correlative relationship customarily referred to as the dose-response relationship. This relationship is the most fundamental and pervasive concept in toxicology. Indeed, an understanding of this relationship is essential for the study of toxic materials.

Assumptions

A number of assumptions must be considered before the dose-response relationships can be appropriately used. The first is that the response is due to the chemical administered. For example, for data such as that presented in Figure 2–2 it is usually assumed that the responses were a result of the various doses of chemical administered. However, to describe the relationship between a toxic material and an observed effect or response, one must know with reasonable certainty that the relationship is indeed a causal one. For some data, it is not always apparent that the response is the result of chemical exposure. For example, an epidemiologic study might result in discovery of an "association" between a response (e.g., disease) and one or more variables. Frequently the data are presented similarly to the "dose-response" in pharmacology and toxicology. Use of dose-response in this context is suspect. One is usually in some doubt about the identity of the specific toxic agent, the true dose to which the organism has been exposed, the site and relative specificity of the response, or all of these. In its most strict usage, then, the dose-response relationship is based on the knowledge that the effect is a result of a known toxic agent(s).

A second assumption seems simple and obvious, namely, that the response is, in fact, related to the dose. Perhaps because of its apparent simplicity, this assumption is often a source of misunderstanding. The assumption is really a composite of three others that will recur frequently.

1. There is a molecular or receptor site (or sites) with which the chemical interacts to produce the response.

2. The production of a response and the degree of response are related to the concentration of the agent at the reactive site.

3. The concentration at the site is, in turn, related to the dose administered.

Thus, the numerical and graphic dimensions of the dose-response relationship include the assumptions that (1) the response is a function of the concentration at a site, (2) the concentration at the site is a function of the dose, and (3) response and dose are causally related.

The third assumption in using the dose-response relationship is that one has both a quantifiable method of measuring and a precise means of expressing the toxicity. A great variety of criteria or end-points of toxicity could be used. The ideal criterion would be one closely associated with the molecular events resulting from exposure to the toxin. Early in the assessment of toxicity such an ideal is usually unapproachable; indeed, it might not be approachable at all even for well-known toxicants.

Failing in a mechanistic, molecular ideal criterion of toxicity, one looks to a measure of toxicity that is unequivocal and clearly relevant to the toxic effect. For example, with a new compound chemically related to the class of organophosphate insecticides, one might approach the measurement of toxicity by measuring inhibition of cholinesterase in blood. In this way one would be measuring, in a readily accessible system by a technique that is convenient and reasonably precise, a prominent effect of the chemical and one that is usually pertinent to the mechanism by which toxicity is produced.

The selection of a toxic end point for measurement is not always so straightforward. Even the example cited above may be misleading as an organophosphate may produce a decrease in blood cholinesterase, but this change may not be

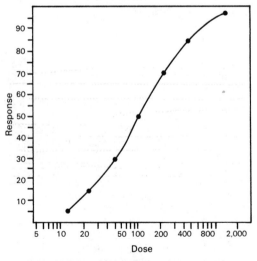

Figure 2–2. Diagram of dose-response relationship. Dosage is most often expressed as mg/kg and plotted on a log scale.

directly related to its toxicity (DuBois, 1961). As additional data are gathered to suggest a mechanism of toxicity for any substance, other measures of toxicity might be selected. Although many end-points are quantitative and precise, they are often indirect measures of toxicity. Changes in enzyme levels in blood can be indicative of tissue damage. For example, SGOT and SGPT are used to detect liver damage. Patterns of isozymes and their alteration may provide insight as to the organ or system that is the site of toxic effects. These measures may not be directly related to the mechanism of the toxic action.

Many direct measures of effects are also not necessarily related to the mechanism by which a substance produces its harm to the organism but have the advantage of permitting a causal relation to be drawn between the agent and its action. For example, measurement of the alteration of the tone of smooth or skeletal muscle for substances acting on muscles represents a rather fundamental approach to toxicologic assessment. Similarly, measures of heart rate, blood pressure, and electrical activity of heart muscle, nerve, or brain are examples of the use of physiologic functions as indices of toxicity. Measurement can also take the form of a still higher level of integration, such as the degree of motor activity or behavioral change.

The measurements used as examples all assume prior information about the toxicant, such as its target organ or site of action or a fundamental effect. Such information is usually available only after toxicologic screening and testing based on other measures of toxicity. With a new substance, the customary starting point in toxicologic evaluation utilizes lethality as an index. Measurement of lethality is precise, quantal, and unequivocal and is, therefore, useful in its own right if only to suggest the level and magnitude of the potency of the substance. Lethality provides a measure of comparison among many substances whose mechanism and sites of action may be markedly different. Furthermore, from these studies clues to the direction to be taken in further studies are obtained. This comes about in two important ways. First, simply recording a death is not an adequate means of conducting a lethality study with a new substance. A key element must be a careful, disciplined, detailed observation of the intact animal extending from the time of administration of the toxicant to death of the animal. From properly conducted observations, immensely informative data can be gathered by the trained toxicologist. Second, a lethality study ordinarily is supported by histologic examination of major tissues and organs for abnormalities. From the latter observations,

one can usually obtain more specific information about the events leading to the lethal effect, target organ(s) involved, and often a suggestion as to the possible mechanism of toxicity at a relatively fundamental level.

Calculations

Whatever response is selected for measurement, the relation between the degree of response of the biologic system and the amount of toxicant administered assumes a form that occurs so consistently as to be considered classic and fundamental and is referred to as the dose-response relationship. This is the relationship that Trevan (1927) envisioned in his introduction of lethal dose as an index (LD50). The LD50 is the statistically derived single dosage of a substance that can be expected to cause death in 50 percent of the animals. Figure 2–2 illustrates the typical sigmoid form that is found when this relationship is measured. The ordinate is simply labeled "response"; response may be the degree of response in an individual or system or the fraction of a population responding. A distinction is sometimes made between a quantal or "all-or-none" response and a "graded" response. Although the distinction may be useful for some purposes, for practical and sound conceptual reasons they can be considered to be identical. Consider the hypothetical curve in Figure 2–2 as representative of cholinesterase inhibition in the presence of an organophosphate, smooth muscle contraction with Ba^{2+}, bone marrow depression with benzene, or similar graded responses to increasing doses. Many other examples are applicable.

In toxicology the quantal dose-response is used extensively. Determination of the median lethal dose (LD50) is usually the first experiment performed with a new chemical. In practice, this is experimentally determined usually using mice or rats and using either the oral or intraperitoneal route of administration. At least ten animals are used per dose, and a range of doses is administered so that at least three and preferably more of the doses result in producing some deaths and some survivals, i.e., kill less than 100 percent and more than 0 percent. If a large number of doses is used with a large number of animals per dose, a sigmoid dose-response curve is observed, as depicted in the top panel of Figure 2–3. With the lowest dosage (6 mg/kg), 1 percent of the animals died. A normally distributed sigmoid curve, such as this one, approaches a response of 0 percent as the dose is decreased and approaches 100 percent as the dose is increased but theoretically never passes through 0 and 100 percent. However, the minimally effective dose of any chemical that evokes a stated all-or-none

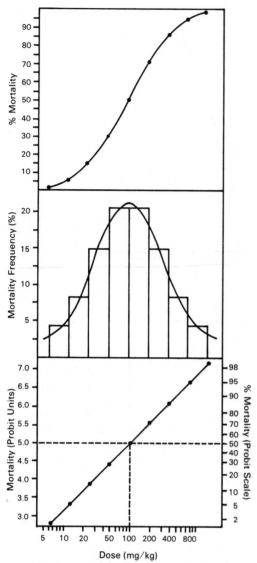

Figure 2–3. Diagram of quantal dose-response relationship. The abscissa is a log dosage of the chemical. In the top panel the ordinate is percent mortality; in the middle panel the ordinate is mortality frequency; and in the bottom panel the mortality is in probit units (see text).

sample sizes to define adequately the sigmoid curve.

The middle panel of Figure 2–3 shows that quantal dose-responses, such as lethality, exhibit a normal or gaussian distribution. The frequency histogram in this panel also shows the relationship between dose and effect. The data used to construct this histogram are the same as those used in the top panel. The bars represent the percent of animals that died at each dose minus the percent that died at the immediately lower dose. One can clearly see that only a few animals responded to the lowest dose and also only a small number at the highest dose. Larger numbers of animals responded to doses intermediate between these two extremes, and the maximum frequency of response occurred in the middle portion of the dose range. Thus, we have a bell-shaped curve known as a *normal frequency distribution*. The reason for this normal distribution is that there are differences in susceptibility among individuals to chemicals, which is known as biologic variation. Those animals responding at the left end of the curve are referred to as *hypersusceptible* and those at the right end of the curve as *resistant*.

In a normally distributed population, the mean ± 1 SD represented 68.3 percent of the population, the mean ± 2 SD represents 95.5 percent of the population, and the mean ± 3 SD equals 99.7 percent of the population. Since quantal dose-response phenomena are usually normally distributed, one can convert the percent response to units of deviation from the mean or normal equivalent deviations (NED). Thus, the NED for a 50 percent response is 0; an NED of +1 is equated with 84.1 percent response. Later it was suggested (Bliss, 1935, 1952, 1957) that units of NED be converted by the addition of 5 to the value to avoid negative numbers and that these converted units be called probit units. The probit (from the contraction of probability unit), then, is an NED plus 5. In this transformation a 50 percent response becomes a probit of 5, +1 deviation becomes a probit of 6, and −1 deviation is a probit of 4.

PERCENT RESPONSE	NED	PROBIT
0.1	−3	2
2.3	−2	3
15.9	−1	4
50.0	0	5
84.1	+1	6
97.7	+2	7
99.9	+3	8

The data given in the top two panels of Figure 2–3 are replotted in the bottom panel with the mortality plotted in probit units. The data in the

response is called the *threshold dose*, even though it cannot be determined experimentally.

The sigmoid curve has a relatively linear portion between 16 and 84 percent. These values represent the limits of 1 standard deviation (SD) of the mean (and the median) in a population with truly normal or gaussian distribution. However, it is usually not practical to describe the dose-response curve from this type of plot because one does not usually have large enough top panel (which was in the form of a sigmoid curve) and in the middle panel (a bell-shaped curve) form a straight line when transformed into probit units. In essence, what is accomplished in a probit transformation is an adjustment of mortality or other quantal data to an assumed normal population distribution, which results in a straight line. The LD50 is obtained by drawing a horizontal line from the probit unit 5, which is the 50 percent mortality point, to the dose-effect line. At the point of intersection a vertical line is drawn, and this line intersects the abscissa at the LD50 point. It is evident from the line that information with respect to the lethal dose for 90 percent or for 10 percent of the population may also be derived by a similar procedure. Mathematically, it can be demonstrated that the range of values encompassed by the confidence limits is narrowest at the midpoint of the line (LD50) and is widest at both extremes (LD10 and LD90) of the dose-response curve. In addition to the LD50, the slope of the dose-response curve can also be obtained. Figure 2–4 demonstrates the dose-response curves for mortality of two compounds. Compound A exhibits a "flat" dose-response curve showing that a large change in dosage is required before a significant change in response will be observed. However, compound B exhibits a "steep" dose-response curve where a relatively small change in dosage will cause a large change in response. It is evident that the LD50 for both compounds is the same (8 mg/kg). However, the slopes of the dose-response curves are quite different. At one-half of the LD50 of the compounds (4 mg/kg) less than 1 percent of the animals exposed to compound B would die, but 20

percent of the animals given compound A would die. For more information on the mechanics of determining the LD50 and its 95 percent confidence limits as well as the slope of probit line, the reader is referred to Litchfield and Wilcoxon (1949), Bliss (1957), and Finney (1971).

Determination of the LD50 has become a public issue because of increasing concern for the welfare and protection of laboratory animals. However, the LD50 is essential for characterizing the toxic effects of chemicals and thus determining their hazard to humans. In determination of the LD50 more than a number is obtained. Information is obtained on the types of toxic effects the chemical produces, on the onset of toxicity, on the duration of toxicity, etc. This information is essential for the rational treatment of humans exposed to the chemical, for the design of experiments to assess the toxicity of repeated exposure to the chemical, and for protection of people in the manufacture and distribution of the chemical. What is debatable is the precision to which the LD50 should be determined. The methods described above require a large number of animals (approximately 50) to obtain an LD50. Other statistical techniques are available to estimate the LD50 that can use a smaller number of animals, such as the "up-and-down method" of Brownlee and associates (1953) and the "moving-average method" of Thompson and Weil (1952; Weil, 1952). However, while these techniques require fewer numbers of animals, they do not provide confidence limits for the LD50 nor the slope of the probit line. Thus, the abbreviated techniques only provide the LD50 and not the LD10, LD90, etc.

When animals are exposed to chemicals by the air they are breathing or the water they (fish) are living in, the dose the animals received is usually not known. For these situations the lethal concentration 50 (LC50) is usually determined, that is, the concentration of chemical in the air or water that causes death to 50 percent of the animals. When reporting an LC50, it is imperative that the time of exposure be indicated.

The LD50 and LC50 are not constants. There are many factors that influence these values. For example, the LD50 can depend on the species, strain, sex, age, etc., as well as environmental factors such as temperature, exposure to other chemicals such as insecticides, the number of animals in a cage, and diet. These and other factors that influence toxicity have been discussed in earlier editions of this textbook (Doull, 1980).

The quantal or "all-or-none" response is not limited to lethality. Similar dose-effect curves can be constructed for cancer, liver injury, and other types of toxic responses, as well as for

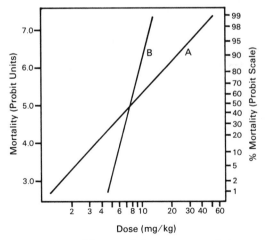

Figure 2–4. Diagram of dose-response relationships. Dose-response relationship is steeper for chemical B than chemical A.

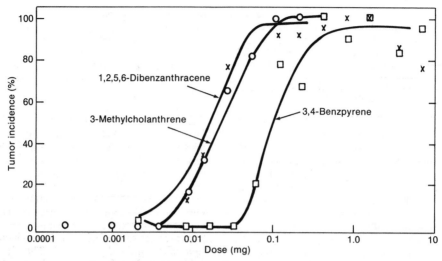

Figure 2–5. Dose-response relationship for carcinogens. Three carcinogenic polycylic aromatic hydrocarbons were administered subcutaneously in a single dose, each to a group of 20 mice. The incidence of sarcomas at the site of injection was noted. (Modified from Bryan and Shimkin, 1943.)

beneficial therapeutic responses, such as anesthesia. Figure 2–5 indicates the dose-response for three different chemical carcinogens. When higher doses were administered, higher percentages of the animals developed sarcomas. While some toxic and therapeutic responses, such as anesthesia, are all-or-none, other graded responses, such as blood pressure, can be transformed into quantal responses. This is usually performed by quantitating a particular parameter (e.g., blood pressure) in a large number of control animals and determining its standard deviation, which is a measure of its variability. Because the mean ± 3 SD represents 99.7 percent of the population, one can assign all animals that lie outside this range after treatment with a chemical as affected and those lying within this range as not being affected by the chemical. Using a series of doses of the chemical, one can thus construct a quantal dose-response curve similar to that described above for lethality.

In Figures 2–2, 2–3, and 2–4, the dosage has been given on a log basis. Although the use of the log of the dosage is empiric, log-dosage plots usually provide a more nearly linear representation of the data. It must be remembered, however, that this is not universally the situation. Some radiation effects, for example, give a better probit fit when the dose is expressed arithmetically rather than logarithmically. There are other situations in which other functions (e.g., exponentials) of dosage provide a better fit to the data than the log function. It is also conventional to express the dosage in milligrams per kilogram. It might be argued that expression of dosage on a mole-per-kilogram basis would be better, particularly for making comparisons of a series of compounds. Although such an argument has considerable merit, dosage is usually expressed as milligrams per kilogram.

One might also view dosage on the basis of body weight as being less appropriate than other bases, such as surface area, which is approximately proportional to (body weight)$^{2/3}$. In Table 2–3 selected values are given to compare the differences in dosage by the two alternatives.

Table 2–3. COMPARISON OF DOSAGE BY WEIGHT AND SURFACE AREA

	WEIGHT (g)	DOSAGE (mg/kg)	DOSE (mg/animal)	SURFACE AREA (cm^2)	DOSAGE (mg/cm^2)
Mouse	20	100	2	46	0.043
Rat	200	100	20	325	0.061
Guinea pig	400	100	40	565	0.071
Rabbit	1500	100	150	1270	0.118
Cat	2000	100	200	1380	0.145
Monkey	4000	100	400	2980	0.134
Dog	12000	100	1200	5770	0.207
Human	70000	100	7000	18000	0.388

Given a dosage of 100 mg/kg, it can be seen that the dose (mg/animal), of course, is proportional to the dosage administered per body weight. Surface area is not proportional to weight: while the weight of a human is 3500 times greater than that of a mouse, the surface area of humans is only about 390 times greater than that of mice. Chemicals are usually administered in toxicologic studies as mg/kg. The same dosage given to humans and mice on a weight basis (mg/kg) would be approximately ten times greater in humans than mice if that dosage were expressed per surface area (mg/cm²). Cancer chemotherapeutic agents are usually administered on a surface area basis.

Comparison of Dose-Responses

Figure 2–6 illustrates the quantal dose-response curve for a desirable effect of a chemical (ED), such as anesthesia, a toxic effect (TD), such as liver injury, and the lethal dose (LD). As depicted in Figure 2–6, a parallelism is apparent between the effective dose curve (ED) and the curve depicting mortality (LD). It is tempting to view the parallel dose-response curves as indicative of identity of mechanism, i.e., to conclude that the lethality is a simple extension of the therapeutic effect. While this conclusion may ultimately prove to be correct in any particular case, it is not warranted solely on the basis of the two parallel lines. The same admonition applies to any pair of parallel ''effect'' curves or any other pair of toxicity or lethality curves.

Therapeutic Index. The hypothetical curves in Figure 2–6 illustrate two other interrelated points, namely, the importance of the selection of the toxic criterion and the interpretation of comparative effect. The concept of the ''therapeutic index,'' introduced by Paul Ehrlich in 1913, can be used to illustrate this relationship. Although therapeutic index is directed toward a comparison of the therapeutically effective dose to the toxic dose of a chemical, it is equally applicable to considerations of comparative toxicity. The *therapeutic index* (TI) in its broadest sense is defined as the ratio of the dose required to produce a toxic effect and the dose needed to elicit desired therapeutic response. Similarly, an index of comparative toxicity is obtained by either the ratio of doses of two different materials to produce identical response or the ratio of doses of the same material necessary to yield different toxic effects.

The most commonly used index of effect, whether beneficial or toxic, is the median dose, i.e., the dose required to result in a response in 50 percent of a population (or to produce 50 percent of a maximal response). The therapeutic index of a drug is an approximate statement about the relative safety of a drug expressed as the ratio of the lethal or toxic dose to the therapeutic dose.

$$TI = \frac{LD50}{ED50}$$

From Figure 2–6 one can approximate a ''therapeutic index'' using these median doses. The larger the ratio, the greater the relative safety. The ED50 is approximately 20 and the LD50 about 200; thus, the therapeutic index is 10, a number indicative of a relatively safe drug. But the use of the median effective and median lethal doses is not without disadvantage, since median doses tell nothing about the slopes of the dose-response curves for therapeutic and toxic effects.

Margin of Safety. One way to overcome this deficiency is to use the ED99 for the desired effect and the LD1 for the undesired effect. These parameters are used in the calculation of the margin of safety.

$$\text{Margin of safety} = \frac{LD1}{ED99}$$

The quantitative comparisons described above have been used mainly after a single administration of chemicals. However, they can be applied to responses observed after repeated exposure. In fact, the *chronicity index* (Hayes, 1975) of a chemical is obtained by dividing its 1-dose LD50 (expressed as milligrams per kilogram per day) by its 90-dose (90 day) LD50 (expressed as milligrams per kilogram per day). The chronicity index constitutes a measure of the cumulative effect of a chemical. Theoretically, if no cumulative effect occurs over the doses, the chronicity index would be 1. If a compound were absolutely cumulative, the chronicity index would be 90.

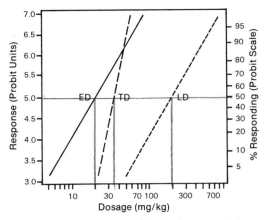

Figure 2–6. Comparison of effective dose (*ED*), toxic dose (*TD*), and lethal dose (*LD*). The plot is of log dosage versus percent of population responding in probit units.

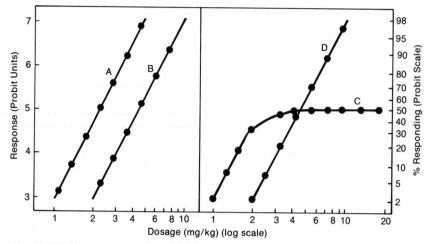

Figure 2–7. Schematic representation of the difference in the dose-response curves for four chemicals (*A–D*), to illustrate the difference between potency and efficacy (see text).

Similar statistical procedures that are used to calculate the LD50 can also be used to determine the lethal time 50 (LT50) or the time required for half the animals to die (Litchfield, 1949). The LT50 value for a chemical indicates the time course of the toxic effects but does not indicate whether one chemical is more toxic than another.

Potency Versus Efficacy. To compare the toxic effects of two or more chemicals, first the dose-response to the toxic effects of each chemical needs to be established. One can then compare the potency and maximal efficacy of the two chemicals to produce a toxic effect. These two important terms can be explained by reference to Figure 2–7, which depicts dose-response curves to four different chemicals for the frequency of a particular toxic effect, such as production of tumors. Chemical A is said to be more potent than chemical B because of their relative positions along the dosage axis. Potency thus refers to the range of doses over which a chemical produces increasing responses. Thus, A is more potent than B and C is more potent than D. Maximal efficacy reflects the limit of the dose-response relationship on the response axis to a certain chemical. Chemicals A and B have equal maximal efficacy, while the maximal efficacy of C is less than that of D. No matter how high the dosage of C administered, specific response is observed in only 50 percent of the animals.

SELECTIVE TOXICITY

Selective toxicity means that a chemical produces injury to one kind of living matter without harming some other form of life, even though the two may exist in intimate contact (Albert, 1965, 1973). The living matter that is injured is termed the *uneconomic form,* and the matter protected is called the *economic form.* They may be related to one another as parasite and host, or they may be two tissues in one organism. This biologic diversity interferes with the ability of the toxicologist to predict the toxic effects of a chemical in one species (humans) from experiments performed in another species (laboratory animals). However, by taking advantage of the biologic diversity, it is possible to develop agents that are lethal for an undesired species and harmless for other species. In agriculture, for example, there are fungi, insects, and even competitive plant life that injure the crop and thus selective pesticides are needed. Similarly, animal husbandry and human medicine require agents such as antibiotics that are selectively toxic to the uneconomic form but do not produce damage to the economic form of living matter.

Drugs and other chemical agents used for selective toxic purposes are selective for one of two reasons. Either (1) the chemical is equitoxic to both economic and uneconomic cells but is accumulated mainly by the uneconomic cells, or (2) it reacts fairly specifically with (a) a cytologic or (b) a biochemical feature that is absent from or does not play an important part in the economic form (Albert, 1965, 1973). Selectivity due to differences in distribution is usually the result of differences in absorption, biotransformation, or excretion of the toxicant. The selective toxicity of an insecticide spray may be partly due to a larger surface area per unit weight causing the insect to absorb a proportionally larger dose than the mammal being sprayed. The effectiveness of radioactive iodine in the treatment of hyperthyroidism is due to the selective ability of the thyroid gland to accumulate iodine. A major reason why chemicals are toxic to one but not to another type of tissue is that there are differences in accumulation of the ultimate toxic compound in various tissues. This, in turn, might be due to differences in the ability of various tissues to biotransform the chemical into the ultimate toxic product.

Selective toxicity due to differences in comparative cytology is exemplified by comparison of plant and animal cells. Plants differ from animals in many ways: e.g., absence of a nervous system, an efficient circulatory system, and muscles and the presence of a photosynthetic mechanism and cell walls. The fact that bacteria contain cell walls and humans do not has been utilized in developing selective toxic chemotherapeutic agents, like penicillin and cephalosporins, that kill the bacteria but are relatively nontoxic to mammalian cells.

Selective toxicity can also be a result of a difference in biochemistry of the two types of cells. For example, bacteria do not absorb folic acid but synthesize it from p-aminobenzoic acid, glutamic acid, and pteridine, while mammals cannot synthesize folic acid but have to absorb it from their diet. Thus, sulfonamide drugs are selectively toxic to bacteria because the sulfonamides, which resemble p-aminobenzoic acid in both charge and dimensions, antagonize the incorporation of p-aminobenzoic acid into the folic acid molecule, a reaction that humans do not carry out.

DESCRIPTIVE ANIMAL TOXICITY TESTS

Two main principles underlie all descriptive animal toxicity testing. The first is that the effects produced by the compound in laboratory animals, when properly qualified, are applicable to humans. This premise applies to all of experimental biology and medicine. On the basis of dose per unit of body surface, toxic effects in humans are usually in the same range as those in experimental animals. On a body weight basis, humans are generally more vulnerable than experimental animals, probably by a factor of about ten. With an awareness of these quantitative differences, appropriate safety factors can be applied to calculate relatively safe dosages for humans. All known chemical carcinogens in humans, with the possible exception of arsenic, are carcinogenic in some species but not in all laboratory animals. This species variation appears to be due in part to differences in biotrans-

formation of the procarcinogen to the ultimate carcinogen.

The second main principle is that exposure of experimental animals to toxic agents in high doses is a necessary and valid method of discovering possible hazards in humans. This principle is based on the quantal dose-response concept that the incidence of an effect in a population is greater as the dose or exposure increases. Practical considerations in the design of experimental model systems require that the number of animals used in toxicology experiments will always be small compared to the size of human populations similarly at risk. To obtain statistically valid results from such small groups of animals requires the use of relatively large doses so that the effect will occur frequently enough to be detected. For example, an incidence of a serious toxic effect, such as cancer, as low as 0.01 percent would represent 20,000 people in a population of 200 million and would be considered unacceptably high. To detect such a low incidence in experimental animals directly would require a minimum of about 30,000 animals. For this reason, there is no choice but to give large doses to relatively small groups and then to use toxicologic principles in extrapolating the results to estimate risk at low doses.

Toxicity tests are not designed to demonstrate that a chemical is safe, but rather to characterize what toxic effects a chemical can produce. There are no set toxicology tests that have to be performed on every chemical intended for commerce. Depending on the eventual use of the chemical, the toxic effects produced by structural analogs of the chemical, as well as the toxic effects produced by the chemical itself, all contribute to determine what toxicology tests should be performed. However, the FDA, EPA, and Organization for Economic Cooperation and Development (OECD) have written good laboratory practice (GLP) standards. These guidelines are expected to be followed when toxicity tests are conducted in support of the introduction of a chemical to the market.

Acute Lethality

The first toxicity test performed on a new chemical is acute toxicity. The LD50 and other acute toxic effects are determined after one or more routes of administration (one route being oral or the intended route of exposure), in one or more species. The species most often used are the mouse and rat, but sometimes the rabbit and dog are employed. In mice and rats, the LD50 is usually determined as described earlier in this chapter, but in the larger species only an approximation of the LD50 is obtained by increasing the dose in the same animal until serious toxic effects of the chemical are demonstrated. Studies are performed in both adult male and female animals. Food is often withheld the night prior to dosing. The number of animals that die in a 14-day period after a single dosage is tabulated. In addition to mortality and weight, periodic examination of test animals should be conducted for signs of intoxication, lethargy, behavioral modifications, morbidity, etc. The acute toxicity tests give (1) a quantitative measure of acute toxicity (LD50) for comparison to other substances, (2) identify the clinical manifestations of acute toxicity, and (3) give dose-ranging guidance for other studies.

If there is a reasonable likelihood of substantial exposure to the material by dermal or inhalation exposure, then acute dermal and acute inhalation studies are performed. The acute dermal toxicity test is usually performed in rabbits. The site of application is shaven. The test substance is kept in contact with the skin for 24 hours by wrapping with an impervious plastic material. At the end of the exposure period, the wrapping is removed and the skin wiped to remove any test substance still remaining. Animals are observed at various intervals for 14 days and the LD50 calculated. If no toxicity is evident at 2 g/kg, further acute dermal toxicity testing is usually not performed. Acute inhalation studies are performed similar to the other acute toxicity studies except the route of exposure is inhalation. Most often, the length of exposure is four hours.

Skin and Eye Irritations

The ability of the chemical to irritate the skin and eye after an acute exposure is usually determined in rabbits. For the dermal irritation test (Draize test), rabbits are prepared by removal of fur on a section of their backs by electric clippers. The chemical is applied to the skin (0.5 ml of liquid or 0.5 g of solid) under four covered gauze patches (1-in. square; one intact and two abraded skin sites on each animal) and usually kept in contact for a period of four hours. The degree of skin irritation is scored for erythema, eschar and edema formation, and corrosive action. These dermal irritation observations are repeated at various intervals after the covered patch is removed. To determine the degree of ocular irritation, the chemical is instilled into one eye (0.1 ml of liquid or 100 mg of solid) of each of the test rabbits. The eyes of the rabbits are then examined at various times after application.

Sensitization

Information about the potential of a chemical to sensitize skin is needed in addition to irritation testing for all materials that may repeatedly come into contact with the skin. The albino guinea pig is the preferred species. The chemical is often injected intradermally three times weekly on alternate days for three weeks, so that a total of ten treatments are administered. Following the tenth sensitizing treatment, the animals are set aside for two weeks, after which they are challenged by a final injection.

Subacute

The subacute toxicity tests are performed to obtain information on the toxicity of the chemical after repeated administration and as an aid to establish the doses for the subchronic studies. A typical protocol is to give four different dosages of the chemicals to the animals by mixing it in the feed. For rats, ten animals per sex per dose are often used, whereas for dogs three dosages and three animals per sex are used. Clinical chemistry and histopathology are performed after 14 days' exposure, as described below in the subchronic toxicity testing section.

Subchronic

The toxicity of the chemical after subchronic exposure is then determined. Subchronic exposure can last for different periods of time, but 90 days is the most common test duration. The subchronic study is usually conducted in two species (rat and dog) by the route of intended exposure (usually oral). At least three doses are employed (a high dose that produces toxicity but does not cause more than 10 percent fatalities, a low dose that produces no apparent toxic effects, and an intermediate dose) with 20 rats and six dogs of each sex per dose. Observations on the test animals include mortality, body-weight changes, diet consumption, pharmacologic and toxicologic signs, hematology, and blood chemistry measurements. Hematology and blood chemistry measurements are usually done prior to, in the middle of, and at the termination of exposure. Hematology measurements usually include hemoglobin concentration, hematocrit, erythrocyte counts, total and differential leukocyte counts, platelet count, clotting time, and prothrombin time. Clinical chemistry determinations commonly made include glucose, calcium, potassium, urea nitrogen, glutamic pyruvic transaminase, glutamic oxaloacetic transaminase, lactic dehydrogenase, alkaline phosphatase, creatinine, bilirubin, triglycerides, cholesterol, albumin, globulin, and total protein. Urinalysis is usually performed in the middle and at the termination of the testing period and often includes determination of specific gravity or osmolarity, pH, glucose, ketones, bilirubin, and urobilinogen as well as microscopic examination of formed elements. At the end of the experiments the gross and microscopic condition of the organs and tissues (about 15 to 20) and the weight of various organs (about 12) are recorded and evaluated. If humans are likely to have significant exposure to the chemical by dermal contact or by inhalation, subchronic dermal and/or inhalation experiments might also be required. The subchronic toxicity studies not only characterize the dose-response relationship of a test substance following repeated administration but also provide data for a more reasonable prediction of appropriate doses for the chronic exposure studies.

After the acute and subchronic studies are completed on an agent and after some special studies that might be required owing to known toxicity of that class of agents (and the agent is a drug), the company can file an IND (Investigational New Drug) with the FDA and, if approved, clinical trials can commence. At the same time that phase I, phase II, and phase III clinical trials are being performed, chronic exposure of the animals to the test compound can be carried out in laboratory animals as well as additional specialized tests.

Chronic

Long-term or chronic exposure studies are performed similarly to the subchronic studies except the period of exposure is longer. The length of exposure is somewhat dependent on the intended period of exposure in humans. If the agent is a drug planned to be used for short periods of time, such as an antimicrobial agent, a chronic exposure of six months might be sufficient, whereas if the agent is a food additive with the potential of lifetime exposure in humans, then a chronic study up to two years in duration is likely to be required.

Chronic exposure studies are often used to determine the carcinogenic potential of chemicals. These studies are usually performed in rats and mice and extend over the average lifetime of the species. Thus, for a rat, exposure is two years. To assure that 30 rats per dose survive the two-year study, 60 rats per group per sex are often started in the study. Both gross and microscopic pathologic examinations are made, not only on those animals that survive the chronic exposure but also on those that die early (see Chapter 5 for a more detailed discussion of the use of the chronic test for detecting carcinogens).

Teratology and Reproduction

The teratogenic effect and the effect of chemicals on reproduction and development also need to be determined. *Teratology* is the study of defects induced during development between conception and birth. General fertility and reproductive performance (phase or segment I) tests are usually performed in rats with two or three doses (20 rats per sex per dose) of the test chemical (neither produces maternal toxicity). Males are given the chemical 60 days and females 14 days prior to mating. The animals are given the chemical throughout gestation and lactation. Typical observations made are the percent of the females that become pregnant, the number of stillborn and live offspring, and the weight, growth, survival, and general condition of the offspring during the first three weeks of life.

Teratogenic potential of chemicals is also determined in laboratory animals (phase II). Teratogens are most effective when administered during the first trimester, the period of organogenesis. Thus, the animals (12 rabbits and 20 rats or mice per group) are usually exposed to one of three dosages during organogenesis (day 6 to 15 in rats and 6 to 18 in rabbits) and the fetuses removed by cesarean section a day prior to the estimated time of delivery (rabbit—day 31, rat—day 21). The uterus is excised and weighed, then examined for the number of live, dead, and resorbed fetuses. Live fetuses are weighed, and one-half of each litter is examined for skeletal abnormalities and the remaining one-half for soft tissue anomalies.

The perinatal and postnatal toxicities of chemicals are also often examined (phase III). This test is performed by administering the test compound to rats from the fifteenth day of gestation throughout delivery and lactation and determining its effect on birth weight, survival, and growth of the offspring during the first three weeks of life.

A multigeneration study is often carried out to determine the effects of chemicals on the reproductive system. At least three dosage levels are given to groups of 25 female and 25 male rats shortly after weaning (30 to 40 days of age). These rats are referred to as the F0 generation. Dosing continues throughout breeding (about 140 days of age), gestation, and lactation. The offspring (F1 generation) thus have been exposed to the chemical *in utero,* via lactation, and in the feed thereafter. When the F1 generation is about 140 days old, about 25 females and 25 males are bred to produce the F2 generation, and administration of the chemical is continued. The F2 generation is thus also exposed to the chemical *in utero* and via lactation. The F1 and F2 litters are examined as soon as possible after delivery. The percentage of F0 and F1 females that get pregnant, the number of pregnancies that go to full term, the litter size, number of stillborn, and number of livebirths are recorded. Viability counts and pup weights are recorded at birth, 4, 7, 14, and 21 days of age. The fertility index (percentage of mating resulting in pregnancy), gestation index (percentage of pregnancies resulting in live litters), viability index (percentage of animals that survive four days or longer), and lactation index (percentage of animals alive at four days that survived the 21-day lactation period) are then calculated. Gross necropsy and histopathology is performed on some of the parents (F0 and F1), with greatest attention being paid to the reproductive organs, and gross necropsy on all weanlings.

Mutagenicity

Investigation of the mutagenic potential of chemicals is being increasingly important. Mutagenesis is the ability of chemicals to cause changes in the genetic material in the nucleus of cells in ways that can be transmitted during cell division. If mutations are present at the time of fertilization in either the egg or sperm, the resulting combination of genetic material may not be viable, and death may occur in the early stages of embryonic cell division. Alternatively, the mutation in the genetic material may not affect early embryogenesis but may result in death of the fetus at a later developmental period, resulting in abortion. Congenital abnormalities may also result from mutations. Since the initiation event of chemical carcinogenesis is thought to be a mutagenic event, mutagenic tests are often used to screen for potential carcinogens.

Several *in vivo* and *in vitro* procedures have been devised for testing chemicals for their ability to cause mutations. Some genetic alterations are visible with the light microscope. In this case, cytogenetic analysis of bone marrow smears is used after the animals have been exposed to the test agent. Because some mutations are incompatible with normal development, the mutagenic potential of a chemical can also be measured by the dominant lethal test. This test is usually performed in rodents. The male is exposed to a single dose of the test compound and then mated with two untreated females weekly for eight weeks. The females are killed before term and the number of live embryos and the number of corpora lutea determined. The test for mutagens receiving the widest attention is the *Salmonella*/microsome test developed by Ames and colleagues (Ames *et al.*, 1975). This test uses a mutant strain of *Salmonella typhimurium* that lacks the enzyme phosphoribosyl ATP synthetase, which is required for histidine synthesis. This strain is unable to grow in a histidine-deficient medium unless a reverse or back mutation has occurred. Since many chemicals are not mutagenic or carcinogenic unless they are biotransformed to a toxic product by the

endoplasmic reticulum (microsomes), rat liver microsomes are usually added to the medium containing the mutant strain and the test chemical. The number of reverse mutations is then quantitated by number of bacterial colonies that grow in a histidine-deficient medium. Mutagenicity is discussed in detail in Chapter 6.

Other Tests

Most of the tests described above will be included in a "standard" toxicity testing protocol because they are required by the various regulatory agencies. Additional tests may also be required or included in the protocol to provide information relating to a special route of exposure (inhalation) or to a special effect (behavior). Inhalation toxicity tests in animals are usually carried out in a dynamic (flowing) chamber rather than in static chambers, to avoid particulate settling and exhaled gas complications. Such studies usually require special dispersing and analytic methodologies depending on whether the agent to be tested is a gas, vapor, or aerosol; additional information on methods, concepts, and problems associated with inhalation toxicology is provided in Chapters 12 and 25 of this text. A discussion of behavioral toxicology can be found in Chapter 13 of this text. The duration of exposure for both inhalation and behavioral toxicity tests can be acute, subchronic, or chronic, but acute studies are more common with inhalation toxicology and chronic studies are more common with behavioral toxicology studies. Other special types of animal toxicity tests include immunotoxicology, toxicokinetics (absorption, distribution, biotransformation, and excretion), the development of appropriate antidotes and treatment regimes for poisoning, and the development of analytic techniques to detect residues of chemicals in tissues and other biologic materials. Approximate costs of some of the descriptive toxicity tests are given in Table 2–4.

PREDICTIVE TOXICOLOGY—RISK ASSESSMENT

The main purpose of the toxicity tests described in the preceding section of this chapter is to provide a database that can be used to assess the risk (or evaluate the hazard) to humans associated with a situation in which the chemical agent, the subject, and the exposure conditions are defined. It is evident that the ideal situation is one in which the agent, the biologic system, and the exposure conditions used for the toxicity tests are identical to those for which risk assessment is desired. From the chronic toxicity studies in laboratory animals one obtains a lowest-

Table 2–4. TYPICAL COSTS OF DESCRIPTIVE
TOXICITY TESTS

Acute toxicity (rat; 2 routes)	$6,500
Acute dermal toxicity (rabbit)	3,000
Acute inhalation toxicity (rat)	6,500
Acute dermal irritation (rabbit)	700
Acute eye irritation (rabbit)	500
Skin sensitization (guinea pig)	7,000
Repeated dose toxicity	
14-day exposure (rat)	40,000
90-day exposure (rat)	100,000
1-yr (diet; rat)	200,000
1-yr (oral gavage; rat)	260,000
2-yr (diet; rat)	470,000
2-yr (oral gavage; rat)	600,000
Genetic toxicology tests	
Reverse mutation assay (*S. typhimurium*)	1,500
Mammalian bone marrow cytogenetics (*in vivo;* rat)	16,000
Micronucleus test (rat)	4,500
Dominant lethal (mouse)	15,000
Host mediated assay (mouse)	6,000
Drosophilia	20,000
Reproduction	
Phase I (rat)	30,000
Phase II (rat)	20,000
Phase II (rabbit)	30,000
Phase III (rat)	22,000
Acute toxicity in fish (LC50)	1,500
Daphnia reproduction study	1,500
Algae growth inhibition	1,500

observed-effect level (LOEL), also referred to as the lowest-observed-adverse-effect level (LOAEL), as well as the no-observed-effect level (NOEL) for the species tested, also referred to as no-effect level (NEL) and no-observed-adverse-effect level (NOAEL). The NOEL is the highest dosage administered that does not produce toxic effects. Thus, it is relatively easy to determine an approximate "safe" level of a compound for laboratory animals. However, the number obtained (NOEL) will depend on how closely the dosages are spaced (LOEL and NOEL) and the number of animals examined. The ultimate objective is usually to determine not the "safe" dosage in laboratory animals but the "safe" dosage for humans. Therefore, the extrapolation most often required of toxicologists is from high-dosage studies in laboratory animals to low doses in humans.

Safety Factor

The traditional approach for establishing safe levels or tolerances for chemical agents to which humans may be exposed is to reduce the NOEL by a safety or uncertainty factor that takes into consideration both the intraspecies and interspecies variation. A safety factor of ten is often used when valid, chronic exposure data in humans are available. The factor of ten takes into consideration the variability between humans, and its purpose is to protect the most susceptible (hypersusceptible) people. Most often, chronic exposure data in humans are not available for the chemical in question and one must extrapolate from chronic exposure studies in laboratory animals. A safety factor of 100 is often employed, ten for extrapolation from laboratory animals to humans, and ten for the variability between humans. When chemicals for which there are no good chronic exposure data available have to be regulated, an uncertainty factor of 1000 is often used.

Risk Extrapolation

Since the NOEL is considered a subthreshold dosage level, it is evident that the safety factor approach might not be applicable for agents that produce nonthreshold effects. Scientific information suggests that a single molecule of a chemical carcinogen can bind to DNA, produce a mutagenic effect, and result in tumor formation. Therefore, development of alternate approaches to the hazard evaluation process and particularly to the procedures used to extrapolate the results of animal toxicity data to provide an estimate of risks in humans has occurred. Other toxic effects, such as injury to liver cells, kidney cells, etc., theoretically also can be pro-

Table 2–5. ESTIMATED RISK OF DEATH TO AN INDIVIDUAL FROM VARIOUS HUMAN-CAUSED AND NATURAL ACCIDENTS

Automobile accident	1 in 4000
Drowning	1 in 30,000
Air travel	1 in 100,000
Lightning	1 in 2,000,000
Nuclear reactor accident	1 in 5,000,000,000

duced by a single molecule. But such an insult would result in injury and possibly death to a single cell, which would be biologically insignificant. In contrast, alterations of the DNA in a single cell can result in cloning of that cell, which in turn can lead to tumor formation and death. The major approach recently used for regulating carcinogen in the environment has been extrapolation of the dose-response curve and is often referred to as risk extrapolation.

Almost every aspect of modern living exposes people to health risks. Table 2–5 lists the estimated risk of death to an individual from various human-caused and natural accidents. In toxicology, *risk extrapolation* is a term used to describe the process of evaluating risks associated with exposure to a certain chemical substance. For the toxicologist to calculate the maximum dosage to which humans could be exposed without exceeding a certain risk, that risk first needs to be determined. An acceptable risk depends on a number of factors, including the benefits of the chemical to society. Some factors considered in establishing acceptable risk levels are given in Table 2–6. Establishment of acceptable risk levels for chemicals is a task for the entire society and not only for the scientific community. Presently, one fatality in 100,000 or one in 1,000,000 (10^{-5} or 10^{-6}) is most often considered an acceptable risk for exposure to a chemical. The dosage that is predicted to produce this low fre-

Table 2–6. SOME FACTORS CONSIDERED IN ESTABLISHING ACCEPTABLE RISK LEVELS

Beneficial aspects of the chemical

    Economic growth
    Employment
    Increased standard of living
    Increased quality of life
    Taxes generated

Detrimental aspects of the chemical

    Decreased quality of life
    Emotional difficulties
    Health effects
    Lawsuits
    Loss of environmental resources
    Loss of work
    Medical payments

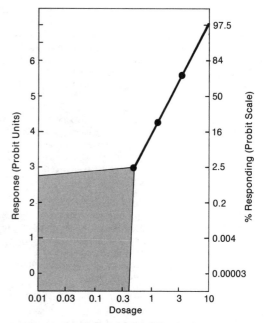

Figure 2–8. Illustration of difficulty in extrapolating from high-dose, high-frequency response to low-dose, low-frequency responses.

quency of response is often referred to as the virtual safe dose (VSD).

A major problem in risk extrapolation is determination of an appropriate mathematical model to extrapolate the dose-response curve that would produce a response in 1/10,000 percent of the exposed animals (one in 1,000,000 or 10^{-6}, see Figure 2–8). Several mathematical models have been developed for estimating the effects of exposure levels well below levels for which test data are available, with the goal that the risk will not be underestimated. The models commonly used in risk extrapolation are categorized in Table 2–7. The distribution models are based on the assumption that every member of a population has a critical dosage below which the individual will not respond to the exposure in question. It is also presumed that the critical dosage varies among individuals and that this variability can be described in terms of a probability distribution. The log-probit model, as was discussed earlier in determination of the LD50, assumes that the distribution of log dose-responses is gaussian (normal). It is therefore an extrapolation of the line obtained by plotting the experimental data on a probit versus $\log_{10}$ dosage scale to an "acceptable" level of risk such as 10^{-6} (1/10,000 percent). The log-probit model serves as the basis for the Mantel-Bryan extrapolation procedure (Mantel *et al.*, 1975). Rather than extend the slope of the observed log dose-probit

Table 2–7. MODELS USED IN RISK EXTRAPOLATION

Distribution models

Log-probit
Mantel-Bryan
Logit
Weibull

Mechanistic models

One-hit (linear)
Gamma multihit
Multistage (Armitage-Doll)
Linearized multistage

Pharmacokinetic

Time-to-tumor

response, this method uses a fixed slope of one (based on empirical knowledge of experimental carcinogenesis data that the slope is usually much greater than one) starting from the upper confidence limit of the observed proportion of animals with tumors at the experimental exposure level. The premise of this method is that the true dose-response curve lies somewhere below the extrapolation line passing through the upper confidence limit with a slope of one, thereby predicting a higher proportion of tumors than that which actually occurs at lower doses. Other distributions on which carcinogenicity dose-response models have been based include the logit and Weibull models.

Mechanistic models are based on the presumed mechanism of carcinogenesis. Each model reflects the assumption that a tumor originates from a single cell. An example of a mechanistic model is the one-hit model. The concept underlying this model is that a tumor can be induced by the exposure of DNA to a single molecule of a carcinogen. Thus, unlike the distribution models, this model is based on a specific biologic mechanism of action for carcinogens. This model is essentially equivalent to assuming that the dose-response curve is linear in the low-dose region. Consequently, extrapolation is made after the response and dosage are both plotted on an arithmetic scale. The gamma multihit model (Cornfield *et al.*, 1978) is an extension of the one-hit model, which assumes that more than one hit is required at the cellular level to initiate the process of carcinogenesis.

The biological justification for the multistage model is that cancer is believed to be a multistage process that can be approximated by a series of multiplicative linear functions (Armitage and Doll, 1961). The assumption of the multistage model and the fitting of a generalized poly-

nomial to the experimental data does not assume a particular shape of the dose-response curve. The linearized multistage model utilized by many regulatory agencies replaces the linear term of the polynomial function by its upper 95 percent confidence limit to reflect biologic variability in the observed tumor frequencies. The dose-response predicted by this model is approximately linear at low doses resulting in estimates of potential risk that are similar to those of the one-hit model.

It is known that many chemicals are only carcinogenic after they have been biotransformed. The amount of reactive metabolite formed might not be directly related to dosage because the enzyme that forms the reactive metabolite might become saturated at higher doses or there may be depletion of cosubstrate. This is referred to as nonlinear pharmacokinetics (see Chapter 3). After the reactive metabolite is formed, it is often destroyed by a second enzyme, such as epoxide hydrolase or glutathione transferase (see Chapter 4). These enzymes can also be saturated. The reactive metabolites that are not destroyed by these detoxication pathways often bind to DNA. But the metabolites bound to DNA can be removed by various DNA repair systems. These systems also can be saturated. The pharmacokinetic model therefore estimates the amount of reactive metabolites formed and bound to DNA ("effective dose") and uses this value as the dosage rather than the administered dose. Figure 2–9 shows different dose-response curves that theoretically would result if there were no saturation (simple first-order kinetics), saturation of only the activation system, satura-

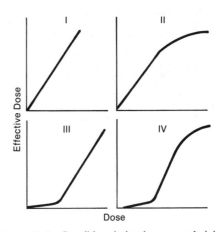

Figure 2–9. Possible relation between administered dose and effective dose for different kinetic models: *I*, simple first-order kinetics; *II*, saturation of the activation system; *III* and *IV*, combination of II and III. (See text for explanation; modified from Hoel *et al.*, 1983.)

tion of both the detoxication and repair systems, and saturation of activation, detoxication, and repair systems.

Time-to-tumor is the time at which a tumor is detected or observed by palpation or by gross or microscopic examination of an animal at the time of death. In assessing risk, the time-to-tumor method uses both the time-to-observance in addition to the proportion of animals possessing tumors.

The various models usually fit the observed data equally well, but they can predict different potential risks at low doses. The models tend to have the following rank order (from highest to lowest estimates) of potential risk at low doses.

One-hit
Linearized multistage
Multistage
Weibull
Multi-hit
Logit
Probit

Clearly the models disagree most in the low-dose region, for which little or no information is available.

Presently, these quantitative assessments provide a rough estimate of magnitude of cancer risks. They are used in the regulation of carcinogens and in obtaining a rough idea of the magnitude of the public health problem posed by a given carcinogen.

REFERENCES

Albert, A.: Fundamental aspects of selective toxicity. *Ann. N.Y. Acad. Sci.*, **123**:5–18, 1965.

——— : *Selective Toxicity*. Chapman and Hall, London, 1973.

Ames, B.; McCann, J.; and Yamasaki, E.: Methods for detecting carcinogens and mutagens with the *Salmonella*/mammalian microsome mutagenicity test. *Mutation Res.*, **31**:347–64, 1975.

Armitage, P.; and Doll, R.: Stochastic models for carcinogenesis. In Lecam, W., and Heyman, J. (eds.): *Proceedings of the Fourth Berkeley Symposium on Mathematical Statistics and Probability*, Vol. 4. University of California Press, Berkeley, Calif, 1961, pp. 19–38.

Bliss, C. L.: The calculation of the dose-mortality curve. *Ann. Appl. Biol.*, **22**:134–67, 1935.

——— : *The Statistics of Bioassay*. Academic Press, Inc., New York, 1952.

——— : Some principles of bioassay. *Am. Sci.*, **45**:449–66, 1957.

Brownlee, K. A., Hodges, J. L.; and Rosenblatt, M.: The up-and-down method with small samples. *Am. Statist. Assoc. J.*, **48**:262–77, 1953.

Bryan, W. R.; and Shimkin, M. B.: Quantitative analysis of dose-response data obtained with three carcinogenic hydrocarbons in strain C3H male mice. *J. Natl Cancer Inst.*, **3**:503–31, 1943.

Cornfield, J.; Carlborg, F. W.; and VanRyzin, J.: Setting tolerances on the basis of mathematical treatment of dose-response data extrapolated to low doses. In Plaa, G. L., and Duncan, W. A. M. (eds.): *Proceedings of the First International Congress on Toxicology*. Academic Press, New York, 1978, pp. 143–64.

Doull, J.: Factors influencing toxicity. In Doull, J.; Klaassen, C. D.; and Amdur, M. O. (eds.): *Casarett and Doull's Toxicology: The Basic Science of Poisons*, 2nd ed. Macmillan Publishing Co., New York, 1980.

DuBois, K. P.: Potentiation of the toxicity of organophosphorus compounds. *Adv. Pest Control Res.*, **4**:117–51, 1961.

Finney, D. J.: *Probit Analysis*. Cambridge University Press, Cambridge, 1971.

Goering, P. L., and Klaassen, C. D.: Altered subcellular distribution of cadmium following cadmium pretreatment: possible mechanism of tolerance to cadmium-induced lethality. *Toxicol. Appl. Pharmacol.*, **70**:195–203, 1983.

Goldstein, A.; Aronow, L; and Kalman, S. M.: *Principles of Drug Action*. John Wiley & Sons, Inc., New York, 1974.

Hayes, W. J., Jr.: *Toxicology of Pesticides*. Williams & Wilkins Co., Baltimore, 1975.

Hoel, D. G.; Kaplan, N. L.; and Anderson, M. W.: Implications of nonlinear kinetics on risk estimation in carcinogenesis. *Science*, **219**:1032–37, 1983.

Levine, R. R.: *Pharmacology: Drug Actions and Reactions*, 2nd ed. Little, Brown & Co., Boston, 1978.

Litchfield, J. T., Jr.: A method for rapid graphic solution of time-percent effective curve. *J. Pharmacol. Exp. Ther.*, **97**:399–408, 1949.

Litchfield, J. T., and Wilcoxon, F.: Simplified method of evaluating dose-effect experiments. *J. Pharmacol. Exp. Ther.*, **96**:99–113, 1949.

Loomis, T. A.: *Essentials of Toxicology*, 2nd ed. Lea & Febiger, Philadelphia, 1974.

Mantel, N.; Bohidar, N. R.; Brown, C. C.: Ciminera, J. L.; and Tukey, J. W.: An improved "Mantel Bryan" procedure for "safety testing" of carcinogens. *Cancer Res.*, **35**:865–72, 1975.

Thompson, W. R., and Weil, C. S. On the construction of tables for moving average interpolation. *Biometrics* **8**:51–54, 1952.

Trevan, J. W.: The error of determination of toxicity. *Proc. R. Soc. Lond. (Biol.)*, **101**:483–514, 1927.

Weil, C. S.: Tables for convenient calculation of median-effective dose (LD_{50} or ED_{50}) and instruction in their use. *Biometrics*, **8**:249–63, 1952.

Chapter 3

DISTRIBUTION, EXCRETION, AND ABSORPTION OF TOXICANTS

Curtis D. Klaassen

INTRODUCTION

The toxicity of a chemical, as noted in the last chapter, is dependent on the dose administered: that is, more toxicity is observed after a high dose of a chemical than after a low dose. In this chapter we will refine the concept of the dose-response, illustrating that the ultimate concept in regard to dose is not the dose of chemical administered, but rather the concentration of the toxic chemical in the target organ. The concentration attained in the target organ of toxicity depends on the disposition of the chemical, that

is, its absorption, distribution, biotransformation, and excretion. These factors are depicted in Figure 3–1 and will be discussed in detail in this chapter and Chapter 4. If the concentration of the toxic chemical remains low in the target organ of toxicity, little or no toxicity will result, whereas if high concentrations are attained, toxicity will result. For example, (1) if the fraction of the chemical absorbed is low or the rate of absorption is low, then only a low concentration of the chemical in the target organ may be obtained and thus no toxicity. (2) Similarly, the

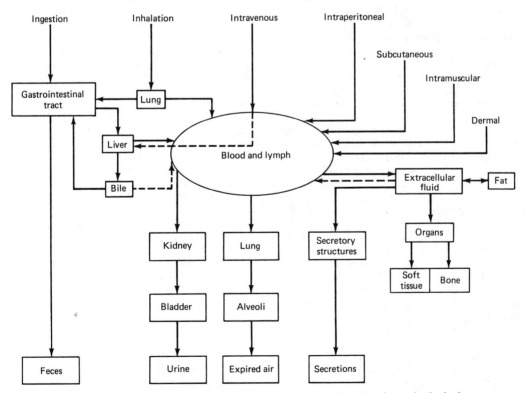

Figure 3–1. Routes of absorption, distribution, and excretion of toxicants in the body.

distribution of the chemical in the body will influence its toxicity; if most of the chemical is concentrated in an organ other than its target organ of toxicity, this will tend to decrease the toxicity of the chemical. (3) Biotransformation also markedly affects the toxicity of many chemicals. Biotransformation may result in the formation of a less toxic chemical or in a more toxic chemical. Thus, how the chemical is biotransformed by the body and the rate it is biotransformed are important factors in determining the concentration of the toxic chemical found in the target organ. (4) Of course, the more rapidly a chemical is eliminated from the body, the lower the concentration of the chemical will be in the target organ, and thus less toxicity. However, the rate at which a chemical is excreted depends on its distribution and biotransformation. If the chemical is distributed to and stored in fat, it is likely to be eliminated slowly because it is not readily available for excretion. Also, many chemicals are very lipid soluble and cannot be excreted until they are biotransformed into a water-soluble product. Thus the processes of absorption, distribution, biotransformation, and excretion are closely interrelated and very important factors in determining whether a chemical will be toxic.

Quantitation of the time course of chemical absorption, distribution, biotransformation, and excretion is referred to as the kinetics of the chemical and frequently termed *pharmacokinetics* and/or *toxicokinetics*. The use of mathematical models to describe these processes allows predictions about body burdens, duration of the toxicant in the body after termination of exposure, and other information that may aid in assessing the hazards of chemicals to humans.

The skin, lung, and alimentary canal are the main barriers that separate humans from toxic substances. However, these are not complete barriers, and toxicants do enter the body to produce damage. Before a toxicant produces its undesirable effects, it is absorbed and enters the blood. Exceptions to this rule are caustic agents, such as acids, which act topically. The major sites at which toxicants enter the body are the lungs, gastrointestinal tract, and skin. Once the chemical has entered the bloodstream, it is available to distribute to the site in the body where it produces damage. This site is often termed the target organ. The target organ depends on the toxicant. For example, mercury and lead produce damage to the central nervous system, kidney, and hematopoietic system, benzene to the hematopoietic system, carbon tetrachloride to the liver, and so forth. To produce a toxic effect in a certain organ, the toxicant must reach that organ. However, several factors in-

fluence the susceptibility of organs to toxicants; for this reason the organ in which the toxicant is most highly concentrated is not necessarily the organ where most of the tissue damage occurs. For example, the chlorinated hydrocarbon insecticides attain the highest concentration in fat depots of the body, but produce no known toxic effect in this organ. A toxicant may also exert its adverse effect directly on the bloodstream, as in the case with arsine gas, which produces hemolysis. In this case, the bloodstream itself is a target organ of toxicity.

Toxicants are eliminated from the blood by biotransformation, excretion, and accumulation at various storage sites. The relative importance of these processes depends on the physical and chemical properties of the toxicant. The kidney plays the major role in elimination of most toxicants from the body; other organs, however, are of greater importance in elimination of certain toxicants. Examples include excretion by lungs of a volatile agent such as carbon monoxide or biliary excretion of a substance such as lead. Although liver is the organ most active in the biotransformation of toxicants, enzymes in other tissues, such as the esterases in plasma and enzymes in kidney, lung, and gastrointestinal tract, may also biotransform the toxicant. Biotransformation is often a prerequisite for renal excretion of a toxicant because many toxicants are lipid soluble, and these are subsequently reabsorbed by renal tubules after filtration. After the toxicant is biotransformed, its metabolites may be excreted preferentially into bile, as are the metabolites of DDT, or they may be excreted into urine, as are the metabolites of organophosphate insecticides.

In this chapter we will discuss the distribution, excretion, and absorption of chemicals and how to quantitate these processes. However, first we will describe how chemicals pass body membranes. Then we will present information on how chemicals distribute in the body, emphasizing that chemicals do not distribute evenly throughout the body. Elimination of chemicals will follow, building on the information that the rate at which chemicals are cleared from the body depends in part on how they are distributed. Absorption of chemicals will be presented last because to quantitate absorption, one needs to understand how to quantitate distribution and excretion.

CELL MEMBRANES

A toxic agent may pass through a number of barriers before achieving a sufficient concentration in the organ where it produces its characteristic lesion. These include membranes of a num-

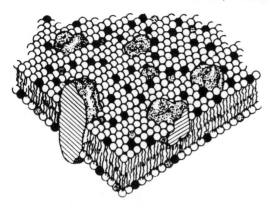

Figure 3–2. Schematic model of a biologic membrane. Spheres represent the ionic and polar head groups of the phospholipid molecules, different types being represented as black, white, or stippled. Zigzag lines represent the fatty acid chains. Proteins associated with the membrane are represented by the large bodies with cross-hatching.

ber of cells such as the stratified epithelium of the skin, the thin layer in the lung and gastrointestinal tract, the capillary endothelium, and the cells of the organ where the toxicant produces its deleterious effect. The plasma membranes that surround all of these cells are remarkably similar. The thickness of the cell membrane is on the order of 7 nm. Electron micrographic, chemical, and physiologic studies provide compelling evidence that the cell membrane as a bimolecular layer of lipid molecules coated on each side with a protein layer (Figure 3–2). Certain branches of the protein layer appear to penetrate the lipid bilayer, and others extend through the membrane. The lipid portion of the membrane consists primarily of phosphatidyl choline, phosphatidyl ethanolamine, and cholesterol. The fatty acids of the membranes do not have a rigid crystalline structure but at the physiologic temperatures are quasifluid in character. The fluid character of membranes is largely determined by the structure and relative proportion of unsaturated fatty acids. When the membranes contain more unsaturated fatty acids, they are more fluidlike, and active transport is more rapid.

A toxicant may pass through a membrane by one of two general processes: (1) diffusion or passive transfer of the chemical, in which the cell expands no energy in its transfer; and (2) specialized transport, in which the cell takes an active part in the transfer of the toxicant through the membranes.

Passive Transport

Simple Diffusion. Most toxicants cross membranes by simple diffusion. Small hydrophilic compounds diffuse across lipid membranes through aqueous channels, whereas larger organic molecules diffuse across hydropholic, lipid domains. Therefore, a lipid-soluble compound such as ethanol readily traverses cell membranes by simple diffusion. Consequently, ethanol is rapidly absorbed from the stomach and intestine by diffusion and enters the central nervous system and other organs also by the same process. The rate of transfer of toxic agents across cell membranes is dependent on their lipid solubility, as measured by the ethanol/water partition coefficient, and their concentration gradient across the membrane.

Many toxic chemicals exist in solution in both the ionized and nonionized form. The ionized form is often unable to penetrate the cell membrane because of its low lipid solubility, whereas the nonionized form may be sufficiently lipid soluble to diffuse across cell membranes. Diffusion is primarily dependent on the lipid solubility of the nonionized form of the compound.

The amount of a weak organic acid or base in the nonionized form is dependent on its dissociation constant. The pH at which an acid is 50 percent dissociated (nonionized = ionized) is called its pK_a. Like pH, pK_a is an arithmetic expression, defined as the negative logarithm of the acid dissociation constant. The degree of dissociation and ionization of a weak acid or base is dependent on the pH of the medium. When the pH of a solution is equal to the pK_a of a compound, half the chemical exists in the ionized and half in the nonionized state. Conventionally, the dissociation constant for both acids and bases can be expressed as a pK_a. An acid with a low pK_a is a relatively strong acid and one with a high pK_a is a weak acid. Conversely, a base with a low pK_a is a weak base and one with a high pK_a a relatively strong base. The pK_a value alone does not indicate whether the compound is acidic or basic because a basic compound can have a pK_a less than 7 and an acidic compound can have a pK_a greater than 7.

The degree of ionization of a compound depends both on its pK_a and on the pH of the solution in which it is dissolved, a relation described by the Henderson-Hasselbalch equations:

For acids $\qquad pK_a - pH = \log \dfrac{[\text{nonionized}]}{[\text{ionized}]}$

For bases $\qquad pK_a - pH = \log \dfrac{[\text{ionized}]}{[\text{nonionized}]}$

The effect of pH alteration on the ionization of an acid, benzoic acid, and a base, aniline, is shown in Figure 3–3. At pH 4, 50 percent of benzoic acid is ionized and 50 percent is nonionized,

pH	Benzoic Acid	% Nonionized	Aniline	% Nonionized
1	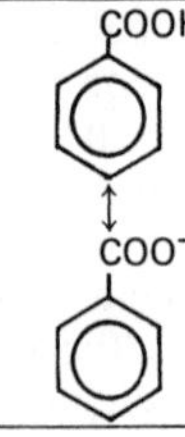 $COOH$	99.9	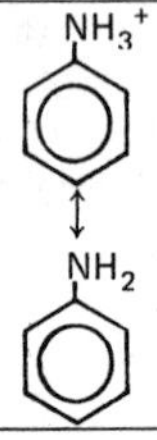 NH_3^+	—
2		99		0.1
3		90		1
4		50		10
5		10		50
6	COO^-	1	NH_2	90
7		0.1		99

Figure 3–3. Effect of pH on the ionization of benzoic acid ($pK_a = 4$) and aniline ($pK_a = 5$).

since this is the pK_a of the compound. As the pH decreases, more of the acid becomes nonionized because it has gained a proton. Conversely, as the pH increases, less of it is nonionized because it has lost a proton (an acid is a proton donor) and has become negatively charged. For an organic base like aniline, the opposite occurs. That is, as the pH decreases, less of the base becomes nonionized since it has gained a proton and thus a positive charge. When the pH increases, less of the base becomes ionized. Since the lipid-soluble form (nonionized) of a weak electrolyte is the species that crosses cell membranes, organic acids are more likely to diffuse across membranes when they are in an acidic environment whereas a basic environment favors diffusion of bases across membranes.

Filtration. When water flows in bulk across a porous membrane, any solute that is small enough to pass through the pores flows with it. Passage through these channels is called filtration, since it involves bulk flow of water due to a hydrostatic or osmotic force. One of the main differences between various body membranes is the size of these channels. In the kidney glomeruli and the capillaries of the body these pores are relatively large (70 nm) and allow molecules smaller than albumin (molecular weight 60,000) to pass through, whereas the channels in most cells are relatively small (4 nm) and allow chemicals only up to a molecular weight of 100 to 200 to pass through (Schanker, 1961, 1962).

Special Transport

There are a number of instances in which the movement of a compound across a membrane cannot be explained by a simple diffusion or filtration because the compound is too water soluble to dissolve in the cell membranes and too large to flow through the channels. To explain this phenomenon (movement), the existence of specialized systems has been postulated. Specialized transport systems are responsible for the transport of many nutrients, such as sugars, amino acids, and nucleic acids, across cell membranes as well as for the transport of some foreign molecules.

Active Transport. The following properties characterize an active transport system: (1) chemicals are moved against electrochemical gradients; (2) at high substrate concentrations the transport system is saturated and a transport maximum (Tm) exhibited; (3) the transport system is selective—therefore, certain basic structural requirements exist for chemicals to be transported by the same mechanism with the potential for competitive inhibition; and (4) the system requires the expenditure of energy so that metabolic inhibitors block the transport process.

Substances that are actively transported across a cell membrane are presumed to pass into the cell interior by forming a complex with a macromolecular carrier on one side of the membrane. The complex subsequently traverses to the other side of the membrane where the substance is released, and thereafter the carrier returns again to the original surface to repeat the transport cycle. Active transport is especially important in toxicology for the elimination of foreign compounds from the organism. To transport substances out of the cerebrospinal fluid, the central nervous system has two transport systems at the choroid plexus, one for organic acids and one for organic bases. Likewise, the kidney has two active transport systems that eliminate foreign compounds from the body, and the liver has at least four active transport systems, two for organic acids, one for organic bases, and one for neutral organic compounds.

Facilitated Diffusion. This term is applied to carrier-mediated transport exhibiting the properties of active transport except that the substrate is not moved against a concentration gradient, and the transport process is not energy dependent. The transport of glucose from the gastrointestinal tract into blood, from plasma into red blood cells, and from blood into the central nervous system is thought to occur by facilitated diffusion.

Additional Transport Processes. Additional forms of specialized transport have been proposed; however, the importance of these processes in all parts of the body is not yet known. Phagocytosis and pinocytosis are processes in which the cell membrane flows around and engulfs particles. This type of transfer across cell membranes is important for removal of particulate matter from the alveoli by alveolar phagocytes and for removal of some toxic substances from blood by the reticuloendothelial system of liver and spleen.

DISTRIBUTION

After it enters plasma, either by absorption or by direct intravenous administration, a toxicant is available for distribution (translocation) throughout the body. Distribution usually occurs rapidly, and the rate of distribution to the tissues of each organ is determined by the blood flow through the organ and the ease with which the chemical crosses the capillary bed and penetrates the cells of the particular tissue. Its eventual distribution is largely dependent on the ability of the chemical to pass through the cell membrane of the various tissues and its affinity for the various tissues. The penetration of toxicants into cells depends on diffusion and special transport processes discussed previously. Small water-soluble molecules and ions apparently diffuse through aqueous channels or pores in the cell membrane. Lipid-soluble molecules readily permeate the membrane itself. Water-soluble molecules and ions of moderate size (molecular weights of 50 or more) cannot enter cells easily except by special transport mechanisms.

Some toxicants do not readily cross cell membranes and therefore have a restricted distribution, whereas other toxicants readily pass through cell membranes and distribute throughout the body. Some toxicants actually accumulate in various parts of the body as a result of protein binding, active transport, or high solubility in fat. While the site of accumulation of a toxicant may be its site of major toxic action, more often it is not. If the toxicant accumulates at a site other than the site at which it produces toxic effects, the accumulation may serve as a protective mechanism by distributing part of the toxicant into a storage depot (which could keep the concentration of the toxicant in the target organ at a lower level). In this case the chemical in the storage depot is toxicologically inactive. However, since the chemical in the storage depot is in equilibrium with the free toxicant, it is released into the circulation as the free toxicant is eliminated.

Volume of Distribution

The total body water may be divided into three distinct compartments: (1) plasma water,

(2) interstitial water, and (3) intracellular water. Extracellular water is made up of plasma water plus interstitial water. The concentration that a toxicant will achieve in blood will depend largely on its apparent volume of distribution (V_d). For example, if 1 g of various chemicals were injected directly into the bloodstream of 70-kg humans, marked differences in their plasma concentrations would be observed depending on their distribution: a high concentration would be observed in the plasma if it distributed only in plasma water, and a much lower concentration would be reached if it distributed in a large pool like total body water. The distribution of a toxicant is usually quite complex and cannot be equated with distribution into one of the water compartments of the body, but distribution is complicated by binding to or dissolution in various storage sites in the body such as fat, liver, or bone.

If a chemical distributes rapidly into tissues, its concentration in plasma would decrease exponentially with time. When plotted as a logarithm of plasma concentration versus time, a single straight line is obtained, as shown in the top panel of Figure 3–4. The body can be considered a one-compartment system for that chemical. The concentration of the chemical in tissues reaches equilibrium with that in plasma very rapidly. However, some chemicals require longer time for their concentration in tissues to reach equilibrium with that in plasma, as depicted in the bottom panel of Figure 3–4. This results in a biexponential elimination of the toxicant from the plasma. The disposition of the chemical is said to obey a two-compartment model. A schematic representation of various compartment open model systems is given in Figure 3–5. During the distributive phase (α, Figure 3–4), concentrations of the chemical in the plasma will decrease more rapidly than in the postdistributive (also referred to as equilibrium or elimination) phase (β). The distributive phase may last for only a few minutes or for hours or days. Whether or not the distributive phase is apparent will depend on the time the first plasma samples are obtained.

The elimination of some chemicals may be too complex to be described by a one- or two-

COMPARTMENT	PERCENT OF TOTAL	LITERS IN 70-KG HUMAN	PLASMA CONCENTRATION AFTER 1 G OF CHEMICAL
Plasma water	4.5	3	333 mg/L
Total extracellular water	20	14	71 mg/L
Total body water	55	38	26 mg/L
Tissue binding	—	—	0–25 mg/L

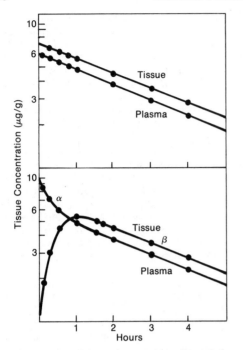

Figure 3–4. Schematic representation of the concentration of a toxicant in plasma and tissue with time in a one-compartment open model (top panel) and in a two-compartment open model (bottom panel).

compartment model, and a multicompartment model might be necessary. Multicompartmental models may be required to describe the disposition of toxicants that are slowly distributed to and released from "deep" compartments, such as that in fat and bones. For further information on multicompartmental analyses and more de-

tails on pharmacokinetics, see Gibaldi and Perrier (1982).

The apparent volume of distribution (V_d) of a chemical is mathematically defined as the quotient between the amount of chemical in the body and its plasma concentration. Determination of the V_d of a chemical is analogous to adding a known amount of a dye to a container with unknown volume of liquid. After the liquid has been well stirred, the volume of the liquid (i.e., the volume of distribution) can be determined by dividing the amount of dye added by the concentration. In the plasma, the concentration of the chemical declines because of elimination as well as distribution to tissues. Therefore, to estimate V_d, it is necessary to extrapolate the plasma disappearance curve to the zero time point. For a chemical whose distribution is rapid (one-compartment model), the apparent volume of distribution (V_d) can be determined first by plotting the logarithm of the concentration of the chemical in the plasma as a function of time after intravenous (iv) administration (Figure 3–6). C_o is the extrapolated concentration of the chemical in plasma immediately after injection, which is obtained, as shown in Figure 3–6, by extrapolation of the plasma disappearance curve to zero time. The apparent volume of distribution (V_d) can be calculated by the following equation:

$$V_d = D_{iv}/C_o$$

where D_{iv} is the intravenous dose. This equation

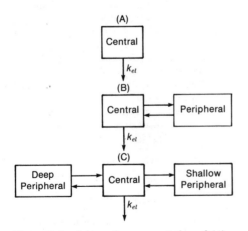

Figure 3–5. Schematic representation of (*A*) a one-compartment, (*B*) a two-compartment, and (*C*) a three-compartment open model system.

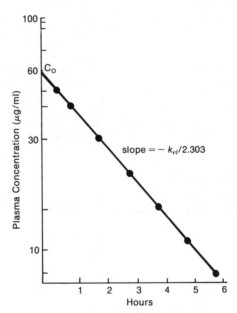

Figure 3–6. Schematic representation of the concentration of a chemical in the plasma as a function of time after intravenous injection.

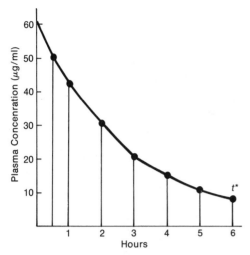

Figure 3–7. Schematic representation of the plasma concentration of a toxicant in plasma plotted on an arithmetic-arithmetic scale.

is appropriate for chemicals that are rapidly distributed (one-compartment) but is not valid for those that distribute slowly into tissues (two-compartment).

A better method for determining V_d is to use the relationship:

$$V_d = D_{iv}/(AUC_{o \to \infty} \cdot k_{el})$$

in which $AUC_{o \to \infty}$ is the total area under the plasma concentration versus time curve plotted on rectilinear graph paper, as depicted in Figure 3–7. This is usually determined by calculating the area under the curve from time zero to the last time point at which plasma was collected by adding the area of the trapezoids formed by each two successive plasma samples $[A = \frac{1}{2}(c_1 + c_2) \cdot (t_2 - t_1)$, where c_1 and c_2 are the plasma concentrations of the chemical at two consecutive time intervals and $t_2 - t_1$ is the time interval between the two plasma samples] plus the area of the curve from the last plasma sample (t^*) to infinity, which is calculated by the following relationship:

$$\text{Area from } t^* \text{ to } \infty = C_t^*/k_{el}$$

where C_t^* is the last plasma concentration data point. The elimination rate constant (k_{el}) can be obtained graphically (Figure 3–6) from the slope of the plasma disappearance (slope equal to $-k_{el}/2.303$).

The volume of distribution, a constant, has no direct physiologic meaning and usually does not refer to a real volume. Some chemicals, such as ethanol, do distribute themselves evenly in total body water. If the chemical has a high affinity

for plasma proteins or is very polar, it would be restricted to the plasma and not enter other tissues and thus would have a small volume of distribution. A chemical that has high affinity for tissues will have a large volume of distribution, indicating most of the chemical is in tissues and not in plasma. In fact, binding to tissues may be so great that the pharmacokinetic volume for a chemical may be much larger than actual body volume. The various organs in the body concentrate most toxicants to different extents, and if some organs have a high capacity to remove a toxicant from the plasma, the chemical will exhibit a large volume of distribution. If a chemical has a large volume of distribution, it is likely to be excreted slowly because little is in the plasma available for excretion.

The apparent volume of distribution (V_d) of a chemical is important in determining the body burden of a chemical. Body burden is the total amount of chemical in the body. Since the V_d is mathematically defined as the quotient of the amount of chemical in the body and its plasma concentration, it is evident that the body burden of a chemical can be determined from the product of the plasma concentration of the chemical and V_d.

Storage of Toxicants in Tissues

Toxicants are often concentrated in a specific tissue. Some toxicants achieve their highest concentration at their site of toxic action, such as carbon monoxide, which has a very high affinity for hemoglobin, and paraquat, which accumulates in the lung. Other agents concentrate at sites other than the site of toxic action. For example, lead is stored in bone, whereas the symptoms of lead poisoning are due to lead in the soft tissues. The compartment where the toxicant is concentrated can be thought of as a storage depot. While stored, the toxicant seldom harms the organism. Storage depots, therefore, could be considered as protective mechanisms, preventing the accumulation of high concentrations of the toxicants at the site of toxic action. The toxicants in these depots are always in equilibrium with free toxicant in plasma, and as the chemical is biotransformed or excreted from the body, more is released from the storage site. As a result, the biologic half-life of stored compounds can be very long. The following are the major storage sites for toxicants.

Plasma Proteins as a Storage Depot. Several plasma proteins can bind foreign compounds as well as some normal physiologic constituents. As depicted in Figure 3–8, albumin has the capacity to bind many compounds. Transferrin, a β_1-globulin, is important for transport of iron in

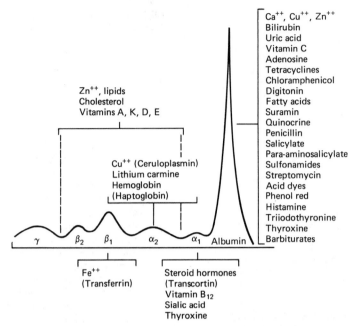

Figure 3–8. Ligand interactions with plasma proteins. Plasma proteins are depicted according to their relative amounts (y axis) and electrophoretic mobilities (x axis). Some representative interactions are listed. (From Goldstein, A.; Aronow, L.; and Kalman, S. M.: *Principles of Drug Action* [copyright © 1968, by Harper and Row; reprinted by permission of John Wiley & Sons, Inc., copyright proprietor]. Modified from Putman, F. W.: Structure and function of the plasma proteins. In Neurath, H. [ed.]: *The Proteins,* 2nd ed., Vol. III [Academic Press, Inc., New York, 1965].)

the body. The other main metal-binding protein in plasma is ceruloplasmin, which carries most of the copper in the serum. The α- and β-lipoproteins are very important for the transport of lipid-soluble compounds, such as vitamins, cholesterol, and steroid hormones. The γ-globulins are antibodies that interact specifically with antigens. Compounds possessing basic characteristics often bind to α_1-acid glycoprotein (Wilkinson, 1983).

Many therapeutic agents have been examined with respect to plasma protein binding. The extent to which toxicants are bound to plasma proteins can vary considerably. Some, such as antipyrine, are not bound; others, such as secobarbital, are bound about 50 percent; and some, like thyroxine, are 99.9 percent bound. The plasma proteins can bind acidic compounds, like phenylbutazone, basic compounds, such as imipramine, and neutral compounds, like digitoxin.

Binding of toxicants to plasma proteins is usually determined by equilibrium dialysis or by ultrafiltration. The fraction that passes through the dialysis membrane or appears in the ultrafiltrate is the unbound or free fraction, and that which is retained is the total concentration, which is the sum of the bound and free fraction. The bound

fraction thus can be determined from the difference of the total and free fraction.

The binding of toxicants to plasma proteins can be analyzed by the Scatchard plot (Scatchard, 1949). In this analysis, the ratio of bound to free ligand (toxicant) concentration is plotted on the ordinate and the concentration of bound ligand on the abscissa, as depicted in Figure 3–9. From this analysis, the number of ligand binding sites (N) per molecule of protein and the affinity constant of the protein:ligand complex can be determined. The Scatchard plot frequently exhibits nonlinearity, indicating the presence of two or more classes of binding sites with different affinity and capacity characteristics.

The majority of foreign chemicals that are bound to plasma proteins are bound to albumin. Serum albumin is the most abundant protein in plasma and serves as a depot protein and transport protein for numerous endogenous and exogenous compounds. Long-chain fatty acids and bilirubin are examples of endogenous ligands with affinity to albumin. There appear to be six binding regions on the protein (Kragh-Hansen, 1981), and protein-ligand interactions occur primarily as a result of hydrophobic forces reinforced by hydrogen bonds and Van der Waals

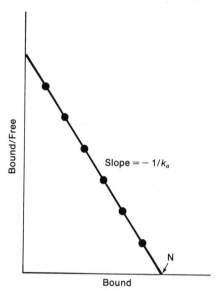

Figure 3–9. Schematic representation of the Scatchard plot for the analysis of the binding of small molecules to proteins.

(Figure axes: vertical axis labeled "Bound/Free", horizontal axis labeled "Bound". Line annotated with Slope = $-1/k_a$, and point N on the horizontal axis.)

forces. Because of their high molecular weight, plasma proteins, and any toxicants they bind, cannot cross capillary walls. Consequently, toxicants bound to plasma proteins are confined to the vascular space. The fraction of toxicant bound to plasma proteins is not immediately available for distribution into the extravascular space or for filtration by kidneys. However, the interaction of a chemical with plasma proteins is a rapidly reversible process. As unbound chemical diffuses from capillaries, bound chemical dissociates from the protein until chemical in the extravascular water equilibrates with unbound chemical in plasma. Active processes, such as those in kidney and liver, are not limited by a high degree of binding of the chemical to plasma proteins.

The binding of chemicals to plasma proteins is of special importance to toxicologists because severe toxic reactions can result if the agent is displaced from plasma proteins. The bound form of the chemical is not available to enter the target organ to produce injury. However, it has been demonstrated that another chemical agent may displace the first from plasma proteins, making it available in the free form. In this way a second chemical can induce toxicity from the first chemical. For example, if a strongly bound sulfonamide drug is given to a patient who is taking an antidiabetic drug, the sulfonamide may displace the antidiabetic drug and induce hypoglycemic coma. Foreign compounds can also compete and displace normal physiologic compounds that are bound to plasma proteins. The

importance of this fact was demonstrated in a clinical trial comparing the efficacy of tetracycline and of a penicillin-sulfonamide mixture in the management of bacterial infections in premature infants (Silverman *et al.*, 1956). It was found that the sulfonamide mixture resulted in a much higher mortality than tetracycline. The sulfonamide displaced a considerable amount of bilirubin from albumin, and the bilirubin was then able to diffuse into brain because of the less well developed blood-brain barrier of the newborn and produce a severe type of brain damage termed kernicterus.

Most of the research performed on the binding of xenobiotics to plasma proteins has been with drugs. However, other chemicals, such as the insecticide dieldrin, also avidly bind to plasma proteins (99 percent). It is likely that chemicals other than drugs also compete for these same binding sites and chemical-chemical interactions are likely to occur by this mechanism.

Liver and Kidney as a Storage Depot. Liver and kidney have a high capacity to bind chemicals, and these two organs probably concentrate more toxicants than other organs. This might be related to the fact that liver and kidney are very important in the elimination of toxicants from the body. Kidney and liver have a capacity to excrete many chemicals, and the liver has a high capacity to biotransform them. Although the precise mechanism by which the liver and kidney remove toxicants from the blood has not yet been established, active transport or binding to tissue components is likely to be involved.

Intracellular binding proteins may be important in concentrating toxicants within the liver and kidney. A protein in the cytoplasm of the liver (Y protein or ligandin) has a high affinity for many organic acids, and it has been suggested that this protein may be important in the transfer of organic anions from plasma into liver (Levi *et al.*, 1969). This protein also binds azodye carcinogens and corticosteroids (Litwack *et al.*, 1971). Another binding protein (metallothionein) has been found in the kidney and liver to bind cadmium. Hepatic uptake of lead illustrates the rapidity with which liver binds foreign compounds: 30 minutes after a single administration, the concentration of lead in liver is 50 times higher than in plasma (Klaassen and Shoeman, 1974).

Fat as a Storage Depot. Because many organic compounds entering the environment are highly lipophilic, a characteristic that permits rapid penetration of cell membranes and uptake by tissues, it is not surprising that these highly lipophilic toxicants distribute and concentrate in body fat. This has been demonstrated for a number of chemicals such as chlordane, DDT, polychlorinated biphenyls, and polybrominated biphenyls.

Toxicants appear to accumulate in fat by simple physical dissolution in the neutral fats. Neutral fats constitute about 50 percent of the body weight of an obese individual and about 20 percent of the body weight of a lean, athletic individual. Thus, a toxicant with a high lipid/water partition coefficient may be stored in the body fat to a large extent, and this storage will lower the concentration of the toxicant in the target organ and, thus, serve as a protective mechanism. One might suspect that the toxicity of compounds that concentrate in fat would be less severe in an obese person compared to a lean individual. However, of more practical concern is the possibility of a sudden increase in the concentration of the chemical in the blood and in the target organ should there occur a rapid mobilization of stored fat for energy. A number of studies have shown that signs of intoxication can be produced by short-term starvation of experimental animals previously exposed to persistent organochlorine insecticides.

Bone as a Storage Depot. Bone can also serve as a reservoir for compounds like fluoride, lead, and strontium. Bone is a major storage site for some toxicants. For example, 90 percent of lead in the body is found in the skeleton.

The phenomenon of skeletal uptake of foreign materials can be considered to be essentially a surface chemistry phenomenon, in which the exchange takes place between the bone surface and the fluid in contact with it. The fluid is the extracellular fluid, and the surface on which the exchange phenomenon takes place is that of the hydroxyapatite crystals of bone mineral. Many of these crystals are small and of such dimensions that the surface is large in proportion to the mass. Upon being brought to a crystal of bone by extracellular fluid, the toxicant enters the hydration shell of the crystal and penetrates the crystal surface. By virtue of similarities in size and charge, F^- may readily replace OH^-, whereas lead or strontium may replace calcium in the hydroxyapatite lattice structure by an exchange adsorption reaction.

The deposition and storage of toxicants in bone may or may not be detrimental. Lead is not toxic to bone, but the chronic effects of fluoride deposition (skeletal fluorosis) and radioactive strontium (osteosarcoma and other neoplasms) are well known.

Foreign compounds deposited in bone are not irreversibly sequestered by this tissue. The toxicants can be released by ionic exchange at the crystal surface and by dissolution of bone crystals through osteoclastic activity. An increase in osteolytic activity, such as that seen after para-thormone administration, can lead to an enhanced toxicant mobilization, which will be reflected by an increased plasma concentration of the toxicant.

Blood-Brain Barrier

The blood-brain barrier is not an absolute barrier to the passage of toxic materials into the central nervous system (CNS), but rather represents a site that is less permeable than most other areas of the body. Many poisons do not enter the brain in appreciable quantities.

There are three major anatomic and physiologic reasons why some toxicants have reduced capacity for entering the CNS. First, the capillary endothelial cells of the CNS are tightly joined, leaving few or no pores between the cells. Second, the capillaries of the CNS are largely surrounded by glial cell processes (astrocytes), and third, the protein concentration in the interstitial fluid of the CNS is much less than elsewhere in the body. Thus, in contrast to other tissue, the toxicant has difficulty going between capillaries and has to traverse not only the capillary endothelium itself but also the membranes of glial cells in order to gain access to the interstitial fluid. Because the interstitial fluid of the CNS is low in protein, this also decreases the distribution of chemicals to the CNS. These features together act as a protective mechanism to decrease the distribution of toxicants to the CNS and thus the toxicity.

The effectiveness of the blood-brain barrier varies from one area of the brain to another. For example, the cortex, lateral nuclei of hypothalamus, area postrema, pineal body, and posterior lobe of the hypophysis are more permeable than are other areas of the brain. It is not clear whether this is due to the increased blood supply to these areas or to a more permeable barrier or both.

In general, the entrance of toxicants into brain follows the same principle as does transfer across other cells in the body. Only the free toxicant (i.e., one not bound to plasma proteins) is free to enter the brain. Lipid solubility plays a major role in determining the rate at which a compound enters the CNS. If an agent is ionized, it will not enter the CNS readily because it is not lipid soluble. If it is not ionized, it will enter the brain at a rate proportional to its lipid/water partition coefficient. Therefore, a very lipid-soluble compound readily enters the central nervous system and a less lipid-soluble compound enters the brain with difficulty. Thus, methylmercury is taken up by the brain much more readily than is inorganic mercury. Also, since pralidoxime (2-PAM) is a quaternary nitrogen derivative, it will not readily penetrate the brain and is quite ineffective in reversing inhibition of brain cholinesterase produced by organophosphate insecticides.

The blood-brain barrier is not completely developed at birth, and this is one reason why some chemicals are more toxic to newborns than in adults. Morphine, for example, is three to ten times more toxic to the newborn rat than in the adult because of the higher permeability of the brain of the newborn to morphine (Kupferberg and Way, 1963). Lead produces encephalomyelopathy in newborn rats but not in adults, also apparently because of differences in the stages of development of the blood-brain barrier (Pentschew and Garro, 1966).

Passage of Toxicants Across the Placenta

For years the term "placental barrier" typified a concept that the main function of the placenta was to protect the fetus against passage of noxious substances from mother to fetus. However, the placenta has other functions; it provides nutrition for the conceptus, exchanges maternal and fetal blood gases, disposes of fetal excretory material, and maintains pregnancy by a variety of hormonal mechanisms. Most of the vital nutrients necessary for the development of the fetus are transported by energy-coupled specific active transport systems. For example, vitamins, amino acids, essential sugars, and ions such as calcium and iron are transported from mother to fetus against a concentration gradient (Young, 1969; Ginsburg, 1971). In contrast, most toxic materials pass the placenta by simple diffusion, except for a few antimetabolites that are structurally similar to the endogenous purines and pyrimidines that are normally actively transported from maternal to fetal circulation.

Many foreign substances can cross the placenta. In addition to chemicals, viruses (e.g., rubella virus), cellular pathogens (e.g., syphilis spirochete), antibody globulins, and even erythrocytes (Goldstein *et al.*, 1974) traverse the placenta.

Anatomically, the placental barrier is a number of layers of cells interposed between fetal and maternal circulations. The number of layers varies with the species and the state of gestation, and this probably affects the permeability of the placenta. Placentae in which all six layers are present are called epitheliochorial (Table 3–1), and those in which the maternal epithelium is absent are called syndesmochorial. When only the endothelial layer of the maternal tissue remains, it is called endothelialchorial; when even the endothelium is gone, so that the chorionic villi bathe in the maternal blood, they are called hemochorial. In some species, some of the fetal tissues are absent and then are termed hemoendothelial (Dawes, 1968). Therefore, one might suspect that a relatively thin placenta, such as in the rat, would be more permeable to toxic agents than the placenta of humans, while a thicker placenta, such as that in the goat, would be less permeable. Within a single species, the placenta may also change its histologic classification during gestation (Amaroso, 1952). For example, at the beginning of gestation the rabbit has a placenta with six major layers (epitheliochorial) and at the end of gestation it has a placenta of one layer (hemoendothelial). The relationship of the number of layers of the placenta to its permeability has not been thoroughly investigated, but presently is not thought to be of primary importance in determining the distribution of chemicals to the fetus.

As is the case in the transfer of most compounds across the body membranes, diffusion appears to be the mechanism by which most toxicants pass through the placenta. The same factors, especially lipid/water partition, are important determinants in placental transfer. It is questionable whether the placenta plays an active role in preventing the passage of noxious

Table 3–1. TISSUES SEPARATING FETAL AND MATERNAL BLOOD*

	MATERNAL TISSUE			FETAL TISSUE			
	Endo-thelium	*Connective Tissue*	*Epi-thelium*	*Tropho-blast*	*Connective Tissue*	*Endo-thelium*	*Species*
Epitheliochorial	+	+	+	+	+	+	Pig, horse, donkey
Syndesmochorial	+	+	−	+	+	+	Sheep, goat, cow
Endotheliochorial	+	−	−	+	+	+	Cat, dog
Hemochorial	−	−	−	+	+	+	Man, monkey
Hemoendothelial	−	−	−	−	−	+	Rat, rabbit, guinea pig

* Modified from Amaroso, E. C.: Placentation. In Parkes, A. S. (ed.): *Marshall's Physiology of Reproduction*, Vol. 2. Longmans, Green & Co., London, 1952.

substances from mother to fetus; however, the placenta has drug biotransformation mechanisms that may prevent some toxic substances from reaching the fetus (Juchau, 1972). Of the substances that cross the placenta by passive diffusion, the more lipid-soluble substances traverse more rapidly and attain a maternal-fetal equilibrium more rapidly. During steady-state conditions, the concentrations of a toxic compound in the plasma water of the mother and fetus will be the same. For compounds with a large volume of distribution (V_d), little will be available in the plasma of the pregnant woman to distribute into the fetus. The concentration in the various tissues of the fetus will be determined by the ability of the fetal tissue to concentrate the toxicant. For example, the concentration of diphenylhydantoin in the plasma of the fetal goat was found to be about one-half that found in the mother goat. This was due to differences in plasma protein concentration and binding affinity for diphenylhydantoin to plasma proteins (Shoeman *et al.*, 1972). Also, some organs such as the liver of the newborn (Klaassen, 1972) and fetus (Mirkin and Singh, 1972), do not concentrate some exogenous chemicals and, therefore, lower levels might be found in the liver of the fetus. In contrast, higher concentrations of some chemicals such as lead and methylmercury are found in brain of the fetus because the blood-brain barrier is immature.

Redistribution of Toxicants

The distribution of a toxic material in the body can change with time. The initial site where a chemical localizes is dependent on the blood flow to the area, the permeability of the tissue to the toxicant, and the availability of binding sites. A chemical can later redistribute to less well-perfused tissues when more binding sites are available. An example of redistribution is seen with inorganic lead. Immediately after absorption, the lead is localized in the erythrocytes, liver, and kidney. Approximately 50 percent of the dose is found in liver two hours after administration (Klaassen and Shoeman, 1974). Lead is later redistributed to bone and substitutes for calcium in the crystal lattice. A month after administration, 90 percent of lead remaining is localized in bones. Similarly, redistribution of highly lipophilic chemicals from well-perfused tissues such as brain to less well-perfused tissues such as adipose tissue occurs with time.

EXCRETION

Toxicants are eliminated from the body by various routes. The kidney is a very important organ for excretion of poisons, and more chemicals are eliminated from the body by this route than any other (see Chapter 11). Many xenobiotics have to be transformed to more water-soluble products before they can be excreted into urine (see Chapter 4). Other routes can be major pathways for excretion of specific compounds; the liver and biliary system are important for excretion of compounds like DDT and lead, whereas lungs are important for excretion of gases, such as carbon monoxide. All body secretions appear to have the ability to excrete foreign compounds; toxicants have been found in sweat, tears, and milk (Stowe and Plaa, 1968).

Figure 3–10 represents a simulation of a typical time course of concentration of a chemical in plasma after instantaneous absorption of a chemical (such as occurs with intravenous injec-

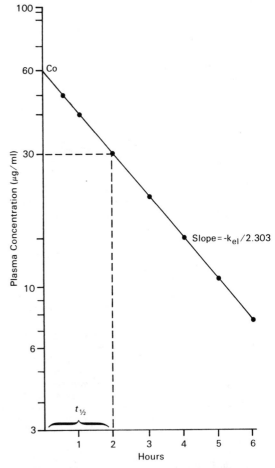

Figure 3–10. Schematic representation of the concentration of a chemical in the plasma as a function of time after intravenous injection if the body acts as a one-compartment system and elimination of the chemical obeys first-order kinetics with a rate constant (k_{el}).

tion or inhalation of a readily absorbable chemical). With this compound, points derived from a plot of the logarithm of the plasma concentration versus time can be fitted to a single straight line, suggesting a rapid distribution of the compound into a one-compartment system and elimination from the body by first-order kinetics. For compounds that are eliminated by first-order kinetics, the time required for the concentration of the chemical to decrease by one-half is known as the half-life or elimination half-life of the chemical ($t_{1/2}$) and remains constant until all the chemical is eliminated. Elimination includes all biotransformation and excretion routes. During each half-life, one-half of the chemical is eliminated. Theoretically, therefore a toxicant that is eliminated by a first-order process is never completely eliminated from the body.

The $t_{1/2}$ is frequently determined by visual inspection of a plot of the logarithm of the plasma concentrations of the chemical versus time, as shown in Figure 3–10. Small laboratory animals may not have enough blood to support closely spaced sampling required for a kinetic study and, thus, data for excretion of the chemical into the urine are often used to determine $t_{1/2}$. Urinary excretion of the parent compound can be used to determine the $t_{1/2}$ but not the volume of distribution (V_d). In practice, the concentration of a compound is measured in aliquots of timed urine samples and multiplied by the total sample volume in order to determine amount. The amount is plotted semilogarithmically against time representing the midpoint of the collection period. The accuracy of this method is highly dependent on how often urine samples are obtained. A more precise method of determining the kinetics of a chemical from urine is to plot the log of the amount yet to be excreted on the ordinate and time on the abscissa. It is necessary to collect urine for seven half-lives and not to lose any samples in order to accurately determine the total amount to be excreted into urine. From the slope of the line obtained by either of these methods, the $t_{1/2}$ can be estimated.

The half-life of a chemical obeying first-order elimination kinetics is independent of dose; a plot of chemical concentration/dose as a function of time yields a single curve independent of dose (Figure 3–11). This is known as the principle of superposition. In a one-compartment open

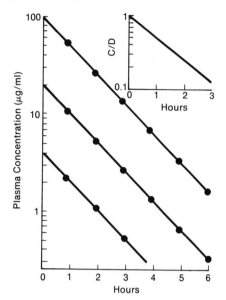

Figure 3–11. Schematic representation of the time course of elimination of different doses of a chemical after intravenous injection, assuming that the body acts as a one-compartment system and elimination obeys first-order kinetics. The inset is a semilogarithmic plot of plasma concentrations (C) divided by dose (D) as a function of time.

model (open indicating that the chemical is being eliminated from the system), the concentration of chemical in the tissues decreases with the same half-life as that in the plasma (Figure 3–12). The ratio of the concentration in the tissue to that in plasma is a constant, and once this ratio is known, the concentration of the chemical in a tissue can be calculated from the plasma concentration.

The apparent first-order rate constant for elimination (k_{el}) can be obtained graphically where the slope of the plasma disappearance curve (Figure 3–10) is equal to $-k_{el}/2.303$ or from the following relationship:

$$k_{el} = 0.693/t_{1/2}$$

The elimination rate constant has units of reciprocal time. In the example given below, k_{el} is 0.3 hr^{-1}. In this example, k_{el} equals 0.3 hr^{-1} because 30% of the chemical in the body at the beginning of each hour is eliminated each hour.

TIME (HR)	0	1	2	3	4	5	6
Chemical remaining (mg)	60	42	29.4	20.6	14.4	10.1	7.0
Chemical eliminated (mg)		18	12.6	8.8	6.1	4.3	3.1	
Chemical eliminated (% of that remaining)		30	30	30	30	30	30	

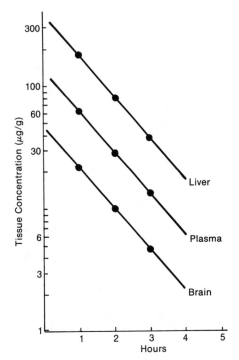

Figure 3–12. Schematic representation of the concentration of a chemical in plasma and various tissues as a function of time after intravenous injection if the body acts as a one-compartment system.

Important characteristics of first-order elimination are: (1) a semilogarithmic plot of log chemical concentration versus time yields a single straight line; (2) the rate or amount of chemical eliminated at any time is directly proportional to the concentration or amount of chemical in the body at that time; (3) the half-life ($t_{1/2}$) is independent of dose; and (4) the concentration of chemical in plasma and other tissues decrease by some constant fraction per unit time, referred to as the elimination rate constant (k_{el}) (for example, 0.3 hr^{-1} or 30 percent/hr).

If the semilogarithmic plot of the plasma concentration of a chemical versus time is best described by an exponential curve rather than a straight line, then a multicompartmental analysis of the results is required. In the simplest case, such a curve can be resolved into two exponentials (two-compartment model). The plasma concentration-time curve can be resolved into two straight lines by the method of residuals (also called "feathering"), as is depicted in Figure 3–13. By this method, the α-phase can be obtained by extrapolating the β phase to zero time, and the difference between the observed points and the extrapolated line are plotted to give the new line α. The slopes of the rapid

and slow exponential components are called $-\alpha/2.303$ and $-\beta/2.303$, respectively. The intercepts on the concentration axis are designated A and B.

A biexponential decline of a chemical from the plasma justifies, from a pharmacokinetic point of view, the representation of the body as an open, two-compartment, linear system. It is usually assumed that the chemical is removed from the central or plasma compartment as depicted in Figure 3–14. The reason for this assumption is that the liver and kidney, the major sites of biotransformation and excretion, are well perfused with blood and thus are rapidly accessible to chemical in the central compartment. The rate constants between the two compartments and excretion are given by the following equations:

$$k_{21} = \frac{\alpha B + \beta A}{A + B}$$

$$k_{el} = \frac{\alpha\beta}{k_{21}}$$

$$k_{12} = \alpha + \beta - k_{21} - k_{el}$$

It should be noted that the elimination rate constant (k_{el}) in a two-compartment model is not the

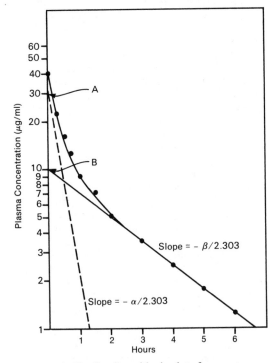

Figure 3–13. Semilogarithmic plot of concentration of chemical in plasma after intravenous injection when the body may be represented as a two-compartment, open system. The dashed line is obtained by the method of residuals (see text).

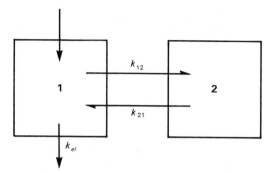

Figure 3–14. Schematic representation of the two-compartment system consisting of a central compartment (*1*) and a peripheral compartment (*2*). The numbering of the rate constants (*k*) indicates the originating compartment (first numeral) and the receiving compartment (second numeral).

same as the terminal half-life (β); as it is in a one-compartment model. Determination of these rate constants permits assessment of the relative contribution of distribution and elimination processes to the concentration versus time profile of a chemical.

The elimination of most chemicals occurs by first-order processes, but as the dosage of a chemical increases, its initial rate of elimination may decrease, as shown in Figure 3–15. This is referred to as saturation or Michaelis-Menten kinetics. Biotransformation and active transport processes, as well as protein binding, have a finite capacity and can be saturated. When the concentration of a chemical in the body is lower than the K_m for these processes, linear first-order kinetics are observed; however, when the concentration is higher than the K_m, a nonlinear elimination is observed. The transition from first-order kinetics to saturable kinetics is important in toxicology because the dose at which this occurs indicates that the body is handling the chemical differently than at lower doses. This may be the dose at which a chemical becomes hazardous.

Some criteria that indicate nonlinear pharmacokinetics are applicable for describing the elimination of a chemical from the body are: (1) decline in the levels of the chemical in the body is not exponential; (2) the $t_{1/2}$ increases with increasing dose; (3) the area under the plasma concentration versus time curve (AUC) is not pro-

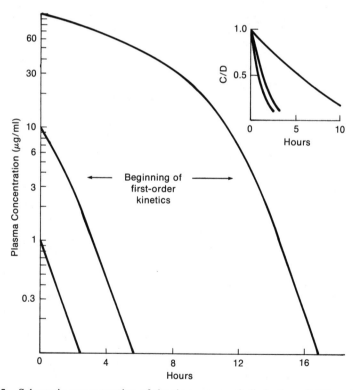

Figure 3–15. Schematic representation of the time course of elimination of different doses of a chemical after rapid intravenous administration of three different dosages, assuming the body acts as a one-compartment system and that it is easily saturated. The inset is a plot of the plasma concentrations (*C*) divided by dose (*D*).

portional to the dose; (4) the composition of the excretory products may change both quantitatively and qualitatively with dose; (5) competitive inhibition by other chemicals biotransformed or actively transported by the same enzyme system can occur; and (6) dose-response curves may show an unusually large increase in response to increasing dose, starting at the dose level where "saturation" effects become evident.

The elimination of some chemicals from the body is readily saturated. These compounds follow zero-order kinetics. Ethanol is an example where saturation of biotransformation is the rate-limiting step in its elimination. As exemplified below, a constant amount is biotransformed per unit time regardless of the amount of ethanol in the body.

TIME (HR)	0	1	2	3	4	5
Ethanol remaining (ml)	50	40	30	20	10	0
Ethanol eliminated (ml)		10	10	10	10	10
Ethanol eliminated (% of that remaining)		20	25	33	50	100

Important characteristics of zero-order processes are: (1) an arithmetic plot of chemical concentration versus time yields a straight line; (2) the rate or amount of chemical eliminated at any time is constant and is independent of concentration or amount of chemical in the body; and (3) a true $t_{1/2}$ or k_{el} does not exist.

Urinary Excretion

The kidney is a very efficient organ for the elimination of toxicants from the body. Toxic compounds are excreted into urine by the same mechanisms the kidney uses to remove end products of metabolism from the body. These processes are passive glomerular filtration, passive tubular diffusion, and active tubular secretion.

The kidney receives about 25 percent of the cardiac output, and 20 percent of this is filtered at the glomeruli. The glomerular capillaries have large pores (70 mm). Therefore, a compound will be filtered at the glomerulus unless its molecular weight exceeds about 60,000. The degree to which a toxic material binds to plasma protein affects the rate of filtration because a protein-bound toxicant is too large to pass through the pores of the glomeruli.

Once the toxicant has been filtered at the glomeruli, it may remain within the tubular lumen and be excreted with urine, or it may be passively reabsorbed across the tubular cells of the nephron into the bloodstream. The principles governing the reabsorption of a toxicant across the tubular cells are the same ones that relate to any passive diffusion across cell membrane. Therefore, toxicants with a high lipid/water partition coefficient will be passively reabsorbed, whereas polar compounds and ions will be unable to diffuse across the tubular membranes and, therefore, will be excreted into the urine. Generally, toxicants that are bases will be excreted (i.e., not reabsorbed) to a greater extent when the urine is acidic, whereas acid compounds will be excreted more readily when the urine is alkaline. A practical application of this knowledge is in the treatment of phenobarbital poisoning. Since phenobarbital is a weak acid with a pK_a of 7.2, the percentage of the drug in the ionized form in the urine can be markedly altered by changes in pH at levels obtainable in mammalian urine. Phenobarbital poisoning, therefore, can be treated by alkalinization of urine through the administration of sodium bicarbonate, resulting in a significant increase in excretion of phenobarbital (Weiner and Mudge, 1964). Similarly, acceleration of salicylate loss via the kidney can be achieved by sodium bicarbonate administration.

Toxic agents can also be excreted from the plasma into urine by passive diffusion through the tubule. This mechanism is probably of only minor significance. Since urine is normally acidic, this process may play a role in the excretion of some organic bases because an organic base is ionized in the acidic environment of urine. For organic acids, simple diffusion across the renal tubule contributes little, if any, to their excretion. In fact, after weakly acidic compounds are filtered at the glomerulus, they are reabsorbed by passive diffusion. Thus, the excretion of weakly acidic compounds by renal mechanisms would take a very long time because after they are filtered, they are passively reabsorbed. Fortunately, however, weak acids are frequently biotransformed to stronger acids, thereby increasing the percentage in the ionic form leading to reduced tubular reabsorption.

Toxic agents can also be excreted into urine by active secretion. There are two tubular secretory processes, one for organic anions (acids) and the other for organic cations (bases). p-Aminohippurate (PAH) is the prototype for an agent excreted by the organic acid transport system, and N-methylnicotinamide (NMN) is the prototypal base. Renal transport systems are located in the proximal tubules, and, in contrast to filtration, protein-bound toxicants are available for active transport. These processes have all the characteristics of an active transport system; for this reason various compounds compete with one another for secretion. This fact was put to use during World War II when penicillin was in short supply. Since penicillin is actively secreted by the organic acid system of kidneys, another acid was sought that would compete with penicillin for renal secretion and, thereby, lengthen its half-life and prolong the duration of action of the antibiotic. Probenecid was introduced for this purpose. The organic acid transport system normally excretes uric acid. Through competition, other toxicants that are transported by the organic acid transport system can produce an increase in plasma uric acid concentration and precipitate an attack of gout.

The renal excretory mechanisms (glomerular filtration, renal secretion, renal reabsorption, or any combination thereof) usually remove a constant fraction of the toxicant from the blood delivered to kidneys. It is known that the polymeric carbohydrate inulin is neither bound to plasma proteins nor secreted into tubules nor reabsorbed from tubules, but enters the urine by filtration only. In fact, all of the inulin filtered by the kidneys is excreted into urine. Thus, the kidney has "cleared" a large volume of plasma of inulin by the processes of filtration of fluid and inulin with subsequent reabsorption of fluid without inulin. This volume is termed clearance, and its units are milliliters per minute. Thus, clearance is a theoretical volume of plasma from which all of the chemical was removed per unit time. Since inulin is not reabsorbed after being filtered, its clearance (Cl_{IN}) is the same as the glomerular filtration rate (GFR).

Many substances are reabsorbed back into the circulation together with the fluid after they are filtered at the glomerulus. For these substances, the volume of plasma cleared is smaller than the filtered volume ($Cl_X < Cl_{IN}$). For substances that are secreted by the kidney, the volume of plasma cleared of the substance can be greater than the GFR because theoretically all of the chemical reaching the kidney can be cleared by active secretion ($Cl_X > Cl_{IN}$), and it must be remembered that renal plasma flow (660 ml/min) is much larger than GFR (125 ml/min). Thus, by comparing the renal clearance of a toxicant to that of inulin, one can determine how substances are excreted by kidneys. However, after the chemical is filtered or secreted into tubules, the toxicant, if in the lipid-soluble form, can be passively reabsorbed. For many toxicants, more than one process is responsible for their urinary excretion, and the use of competitive blockers of active transport systems and/or changes in acid-base balance may be necessary to elucidate fully the mechanisms of excretion. One must remember that only the portion of the toxicant that is not bound to plasma proteins is available for filtration while both bound and unbound toxicant are available for secretion.

Although clearance tells us the virtual volume of plasma cleared per minute, it tells nothing about the rate at which the plasma concentration of the toxicant is lowered by the renal excretory process. To determine this rate, it is necessary to know the apparent volume of distribution (V_d) of the toxicant. Clearly, the greater the volume of distribution, the less chemical is present in the plasma and thus available for excretion. For example, if a toxicant is excreted solely by glomerular filtration (125 ml/min), the half-life of the toxicant would be about 16 minutes if it distributed in plasma water (3 liters) but would be about 200 minutes if it distributed in total body water (38 liters).

Total body clearance (Cl_b) is a concept and a parameter that is analogous to renal clearance. This constant represents the sum of all processes by which a chemical is eliminated. Conceptually, the body as a whole is acting as a chemical elimination system. Total body clearance can be determined for a chemical whose kinetics can best be described by a one-compartment model by the following equation:

$$Cl_b = K_{el} \cdot V_d$$

However, a better equation, since it is model independent (i.e., it is valid for one-, two-, and multicompartment models), is:

$$Cl_b = \frac{D_{iv}}{AUC_{O \rightarrow \infty}}$$

Because many functions of the kidney are incompletely developed at birth, some foreign chemicals are eliminated slowly and, thus, are more toxic in newborns than adults. For example, the clearance of penicillin by premature infants is only about 20 percent of that observed in older children (Barnett et al., 1949). It has been demonstrated that development of this organic acid transport system in newborns can be stimulated by administration of substrates that are normally excreted by this system (Hirsch and Hook, 1970). Some compounds such as cephaloridine are known to be nephrotoxic in adult animals but not in newborns. The reason for this is that cephaloridine is nephrotoxic only when a high concentration is achieved in the kidney. Since the active uptake of cephaloridine by the kidneys is not well developed in newborns, the kidneys of newborns cannot concentrate cephaloridine and, thus, it is not nephrotoxic. If development of the uptake mechanism in newborn animals is stimulated by substrates, newborns will then take up cephaloridine more readily and nephrotoxicity is observed (Wold et al., 1977). Similarly, the nephrotoxicity of cephaloridine can be blocked by probenecid, which competitively inhibits the uptake of cephaloridine into kidneys (Tune *et al.*, 1977).

Biliary Excretion

The liver is in a very advantageous position for removing toxic materials from blood after their absorption from the gastrointestinal tract, because blood from the gastrointestinal tract passes through the liver before reaching the general systemic circulation. Thus, liver can remove compounds from blood and prevent their distribution to other parts of the body. Furthermore, because the liver is the main site of biotransformation of toxic agents, the metabolites may be excreted directly into bile. Biliary excretion obviates the need for metabolites to enter the bloodstream for excretion by the kidneys. A toxicant may be excreted by liver cells into bile and thus pass into the small intestine and remain there. However, when the properties of such a toxicant favor its reabsorption, an enterohepatic cycle will result.

Foreign compounds excreted into bile are often divided into three classes based on the ratio of their concentration in bile versus plasma. Class A substances have a ratio of nearly 1.0 and include sodium, potassium, glucose, thallium, cesium, and cobalt. Class B substances have a bile-to-plasma ratio greater than 1.0 and usually between 10 and 1000. Class B substances include bile acids, bilirubin, sulfobromophthalein, lead, arsenic, manganese, and many other foreign compounds. Class C substances, which have a bile-to-plasma ratio less than 1.0, include inulin, albumin, zinc, iron, gold, and chromium. Compounds rapidly excreted into bile are most likely to be class B substances. However, a compound does not have to be highly concentrated in bile for biliary excretion to be of quantitative importance. For example, mercury is not concentrated in bile, yet bile is the main route of excretion for this slowly eliminated substance.

The mechanism by which foreign substances are transported from plasma into liver and from liver into bile is not known with certainty. Little is known about the mechanism of transfer of class A and C compounds. However, it is thought that most class B compounds are actively transported across both sides of the hepatocyte. Liver has at least four transport systems for excretion of organic compounds into bile, of which two specifically transport organic acids. One organic acid whose excretion into bile has been examined thoroughly is a blue dye called sulfobromophthalein (BSP). The rate of removal of BSP has long been used as a liver function test. This test is performed by injecting the blue dye intravenously. At a certain time thereafter (usually 30 minutes), a blood sample is taken and the concentration of BSP in plasma is determined. If the liver is functioning properly, it should remove the dye from plasma and excrete it into bile. A lack of proper plasma clearance of BSP indicates reduced biliary excretion, suggesting liver injury. Bilirubin is also actively transported from plasma into bile, for which reason jaundice is often observed after liver injury.

Like the kidney, the liver also has an active transport system for the excretion of bases; procainamide ethyl bromide (PAEB) is the prototype for this transport system. The liver has a third transport system for the excretion of neutral compounds such as ouabain. In addition to these four transport systems for organic compounds, it appears that the liver has at least one transport system for the excretion of metals (Klaassen, 1976). For example, lead is excreted into the bile against a large bile/plasma concentration ratio (100), and an apparent biliary transport maximum exists. Whether other metals are excreted into bile by the same or similar mechanisms, or whether metals compete for biliary excretion, remains to be determined.

As with renal tubular secretion, toxic agents that are bound to plasma proteins are fully available for biliary excretion; in fact, many compounds of this type are excreted into bile. The relative importance of the biliary excretory route depends on the substance and species concerned. It is not known what determines whether a chemical will be excreted into bile or urine. However, low-molecular-weight compounds are poorly excreted into bile, but compounds (or their conjugates) with molecular weights exceeding about 325 are excreted in appreciable quantities into bile. The percentage of various compounds excreted into bile has been tabulated (Klaassen *et al.*, 1981). Marked species variation in the biliary excretion of foreign compounds exists and results in species variation in the biologic half-life of a compound and its toxicity. This species variation in biliary excretion is compound specific. It is difficult, therefore, to generalize as to whether a species will be a "good" or "poor" biliary excretor of a certain compound. However, in general, rats and mice are good biliary excretors (Klaassen and Watkins, 1984). This species variation makes it very difficult to extrapolate information from laboratory animals to humans.

Once a compound is excreted into bile and enters the intestine, it can either be reabsorbed or eliminated with feces. Many organic compounds are biotransformed into polar metabolites or conjugates before excretion into bile. Such polar metabolites are not sufficiently lipid soluble enough to be reabsorbed. However, intestinal microflora can hydrolyze various glucuronide and sulfate conjugates, enabling reabsorption of the toxicant. Reabsorption of a xenobiotic results in an enterohepatic cycle. A toxicant that undergoes an enterohepatic cycle might have a very long duration in the body and, thus, it might be advantageous to interrupt this cycle to hasten the elimination of the toxicant from the body. This principle has been utilized in the treatment of methylmercury poisoning; ingestion of a polythiol resin binds the mercurial and thus prevents its reabsorption (Magos and Clarkson, 1976).

When the liver is injured by disease or chemical insult, biliary excretion is often impaired. In fact, the clearance of sulfobromophthalein (BSP) and indocyanine green (ICG) is often used to assess hepatic function. The decrease in hepatic function results in an increased biologic half-life of the compound that can increase the toxicity of some compounds.

An increase in hepatic excretory function has been observed after pretreatment with some drugs (Klaassen and Watkins, 1984). For example, phenobarbital has been demonstrated to increase the plasma disappearance and biliary excretion of sulfobromophthalein, bilirubin, phenol-3,6-dibromophthalein disulfonate, amaranth, indocyanine green, ouabain, procainamide ethyl bromide, and mercury. This increase in biliary excretion is not due only to an increased biotransformation, for this effect is observed with phenol-3,6-dibromophthalein disulfonate, amaranth, and ouabain, agents that are not conjugated before excretion. The increase in bile flow produced by phenobarbital appears to be an important factor in increasing the biliary excretion of sulfobromophthalein. However, other factors, such as the increase in ligandin (an intracellular binding protein), increase in conjugating capacity of the liver, and increase in blood flow, may also be important for the enhanced plasma disappearance and biliary excretion of some drugs after phenobarbital treatment. Not all microsomal enzyme inducers increase bile flow and excretion; 3-methylcholanthrene and benzo[a]pyrene are relatively ineffective.

An increase in biliary excretion can decrease the toxicity of foreign compounds. Phenobarbital treatment of laboratory animals has been shown to enhance the biliary excretion and elimination of methylmercury from the body (Klaassen, 1975a; Clarkson and Magos, 1976). Two steroids that are known to induce microsomal enzymes, spironolactone and pregnenolone-16α-carbonitrile, have also been shown to increase bile production and biliary excretion of sulfobromophthalein (Zsigmond and Solymoss, 1972). These two steroids have been demonstrated to decrease the toxicity of a number of chemicals (Selye, 1971), including cardiac glycosides (Selye, 1969), and mercury (Selye, 1972). These steroids protect against the toxic effects of cardiac glycosides by increasing their biliary excretion, which decreases their concentration in the heart, the target organ for toxicity (Castle and Lage, 1972, 1973; Klaassen, 1974a). The protection afforded by spironolactone against mercury does not appear to be due to an increase in biliary excretion but rather an alteration in the distribution of mercury. Spironolactone is biotransformed in the body to canrenone and thioacetate. The thioacetate is a ligand of mercury in the body and reduces its concentration in the kidney, the target organ for mercury toxicity. Thus, the animal is protected against mercury toxicity (Klaassen, 1975b).

The toxicity of some compounds can be directly related to their biliary excretion. For example, indomethacin has been demonstrated to produce intestinal lesions. The sensitivity of various species to this toxic response is directly related to the amount of indomethacin excreted into bile, and the formation of intestinal lesions can be abolished by bile duct ligation (Duggan et al., 1975).

The hepatic excretory system is not fully developed in the newborn, which is another reason why some compounds are more toxic in newborns than in adults (Klaassen, 1972, 1973a). For example, ouabain is about 40 times more toxic in the newborn than in adult rats. This is due to the almost complete inability of the newborn rat liver to remove ouabain from plasma. A similar relative inability of newborn liver to excrete other foreign compounds has been demonstrated (Klaassen, 1973c). The development of the hepatic excretory mechanism can be promoted by administering microsomal enzyme inducers (Klaassen, 1974b).

Other Routes of Excretion

Lung. Substances that exist predominantly in the gas phase at body temperature are excreted principally by the lungs. Volatile liquids in equilibrium with their gas phase may also be excreted via the lungs. Thus, the amount of liquid excreted by the lungs is related to its vapor pressure. A practical application of this principle is the breathalyzer test for determining the amount of ethanol in the body. Highly volatile liquids, such as diethyl ether, are almost exclusively excreted by the lungs.

No specialized transport systems have been described for excretion of toxic substances by the lung. They are eliminated by simple diffusion. Elimination of foreign gases is nearly inversely proportional to the rate of gas uptake.

Gases with low solubility in blood, such as ethylene, are rapidly excreted, whereas chloroform, which has a much higher blood/gas solubility, is excreted very slowly by the lungs. Trace concentrations of highly soluble anesthetic gases, such as halothane and methoxyflurane, may be present in expired air for as long as two to three weeks after a few hours of anesthesia. Undoubtedly this prolonged retention results from deposition of the highly lipid-soluble agents in adipose tissue. The rate of transfer of a gas that has a very low solubility in blood will be perfusion limited, whereas for gases with a high solubility, it will be ventilation limited.

Gastrointestinal Tract. Many toxic compounds appear in feces. Appearance in feces can be due to a number of factors: (1) the chemical was not completely absorbed after oral ingestion, (2) it was excreted into bile, (3) it was secreted in saliva, in gastric or intestinal secretory fluid, or in pancreatic secretion, and/or (4) it was secreted by the respiratory tract and then swallowed.

The stomach and the intestine each normally secretes about 3 liters of fluid per day in humans, and foreign compounds can be excreted along with the fluid. While active transport has been suggested for the gastrointestinal excretion of compounds, it is generally thought that most toxicants enter the gastrointestinal contents by passive diffusion. In the past, this route of elimination has been considered to be of little significance, but recent data suggest that intestinal excretion may be a major route of elimination of highly lipophilic compounds, such as organochlorine insecticides, dioxin (TCDD), and the polychlorinated biphenyls (Rozman *et al.*, 1982). The gastrointestinal elimination of these compounds, each of which has a long biologic half-life, can be enhanced by increasing the lipid composition of the diet.

Compounds in the gastrointestinal tract are usually not toxic to the individual before absorption. This fact is of significant clinical importance because if they can be removed from the GI tract before absorption, toxicity may be prevented. Emetic agents that act either locally in the stomach or centrally at the vomiting center can be given to remove the toxicant from the gastrointestinal tract. Because rodents do not respond to emetic agents, red squill is a relatively safe rodenticide because in other species it produces vomiting, and the toxicant is removed from the body before any serious toxic effects are produced.

Cerebrospinal Fluid. A specialized route of removal of toxic materials from a specific organ is via the cerebrospinal fluid. All compounds can leave the CNS with the bulk flow of cerebrospinal fluid through the arachnoid villi. A lipid-soluble toxicant can exit across the blood-cerebrospinal fluid barrier. In addition, toxicants can also be removed from the cerebrospinal fluid by active transport similar to the transport systems of the kidneys for the excretion of organic ions.

Milk. Secretion of toxic compounds into milk is extremely important because (1) a toxic material may be passed in milk from mothers to the nursing child, and (2) compounds can be passed from cows to humans by this route. Toxic agents are excreted into milk by simple diffusion. Because milk is more acidic (pH $\approx$ 6.5) than plasma, basic compounds may be concentrated in milk while acidic compounds attain a lower concentration in milk than in plasma water (Wilson, 1983; Findlay, 1983). More important, a considerable portion of milk consists of lipid (3 to 5 percent). The concentration of lipid in colostrum following parturition is even higher. Due to the high lipid content of milk, many highly lipid-soluble xenobiotics concentrate in milk. Compounds like DDT and polychlorinated and polybrominated biphenyls are concentrated in milk, and milk can be a major route of their excretion. Metals that are chemically similar to calcium, such as lead, and chelating agents that form ligands with calcium can also be excreted into milk to a considerable extent.

Sweat and Saliva. The excretion of toxic agents by these two routes is quantitatively of minor importance. Again, excretion is dependent on diffusion of the nonionized, lipid-soluble form of an agent. Toxic compounds excreted into sweat may produce dermatitis. Substances excreted in saliva enter the mouth, where they are usually swallowed and are then available for gastrointestinal absorption.

ABSORPTION

The process by which toxicants cross body membranes and enter the bloodstream is referred to as absorption. As one might suspect, no specialized system exists in mammals for the sole purpose of absorption of toxicants. Toxicants appear to penetrate the body membranes by the same processes that effect physiologic absorption of oxygen, foodstuffs, and other nutrients. The main sites of absorption are the gastrointestinal tract, lungs and skin. However, specialized routes of administration, such as intraperitoneal and subcutaneous, are often used in toxicologic studies.

The apparent first-order rate constant for the absorption of toxicants can be determined by the method of residuals, as depicted in Figure 3–16. The method consists of back-extrapolating the terminal linear portion of the log-plasma concentration versus time curve to time zero and deter-

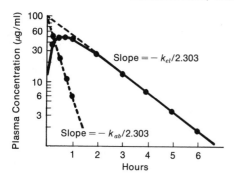

Figure 3–16. Semilogarithmic plot of concentration of chemical in plasma after oral administration of a chemical whose disposition can be described by a one-compartment, open system. The rate constant for absorption (k_{ab}) is determined by the method of residuals as discussed in the text.

mining the difference between the experimentally determined plasma concentrations and the corresponding concentrations on the extrapolated line. These differences are called residuals. A semilogarithmic plot of the residuals versus time has a slope of $-k_{ab}/2.303$ and thereby permits determination of the absorption rate constant.

Absorption of Toxicants by the Gastrointestinal Tract

The gastrointestinal tract is one of the most important routes by which toxicants are absorbed. Many environmental toxicants enter the food chain and are absorbed from the gastrointestinal tract. This site of absorption is also of interest to the toxicologist since suicide attempts frequently involve an overdose of an orally ingested drug. Oral intake tract is also the most common route by which children are poisoned.

The gastrointestinal tract may be viewed as a tube going through the body. Although it is within the body, its contents can be considered exterior to it. Therefore, poisons within the gastrointestinal tract do not produce injury to the individual until they are absorbed, unless the agent is caustic or very irritating to the gastrointestinal tract. Most toxicants that are ingested by the oral route do not produce a systemic effect unless they are absorbed.

Absorption of toxicants can take place along the entire gastrointestinal tract, even in the mouth and rectum. Therefore, some drugs such as nitroglycerin are administered sublingually and others rectally, while the majority of drugs are administered orally. If a toxicant is a weak organic acid or base, it will tend to be absorbed by diffusion in that part of the gastrointestinal tract in which it exists in the most lipid-soluble (nonionized) form. Since gastric juice is acidic,

and the intestinal contents are nearly neutral, the lipid solubility of a toxicant can differ markedly in these two areas of the gastrointestinal tract. From the Henderson-Hasselbalch equation, one can determine the percent or fraction of the toxicant that is in the nonionized lipid-soluble form (i.e., the percent available for absorption). The percent of a weak acid (benzoic) and a weak base (aniline) in the ionized form in the stomach and intestine is indicated on below. A weak organic acid is in the nonionized lipid-soluble form in the stomach and, therefore, tends to be absorbed by the stomach. In contrast, a weak organic base is not in the lipid-soluble form in the stomach, but is so in the intestine. Therefore, organic bases tend to be absorbed in the intestine rather than the stomach. The equations are misleading with respect to the ability of the small intestine to absorb weak organic acids. Since only 1 percent of benzoic acid, for example, is in the lipid-soluble form in the intestine, one might conclude that the intestine has little capacity to absorb organic acids. However, as the intestine absorbs the nonionized benzoic acid, the equilibrium will always be maintained at 1 percent in the lipid-soluble form available for absorption. Moreover, because of the very large surface area of the intestine (the villi and microvilli increase the surface area approximately 600-fold), the overall capacity of the intestine for chemical absorption is magnified.

FOR WEAK ACIDS

$$pK_a - pH = \log \frac{[\text{nonionized}]}{[\text{ionized}]}$$

Benzoic acid $pK_a \approx 4$

Stomach $pH \approx 2$

$$4 - 2 = \log \frac{[\text{nonionized}]}{[\text{ionized}]}$$

$$2 = \log \frac{[\text{nonionized}]}{[\text{ionized}]}$$

$$10^2 = \frac{[\text{nonionized}]}{[\text{ionized}]}$$

$$100 = \frac{[\text{nonionized}]}{[\text{ionized}]}$$

Ratio favors absorption

Intestine $pH \approx 6$

$$4 - 6 = \log \frac{[\text{nonionized}]}{[\text{ionized}]}$$

$$-2 = \log \frac{[\text{nonionized}]}{[\text{ionized}]}$$

$$10^{-2} = \frac{[\text{nonionized}]}{[\text{ionized}]}$$

$$\frac{1}{100} = \frac{[\text{nonionized}]}{[\text{ionized}]}$$

FOR WEAK BASES

$$pK_a - pH = \log \frac{[ionized]}{[nonionized]}$$

Aniline $pK_a \approx 5$

Stomach $pH \approx 2$

$$5 - 2 = \log \frac{[ionized]}{[nonionized]}$$

$$3 = \log \frac{[ionized]}{[nonionized]}$$

$$10^3 = \frac{[ionized]}{[nonionized]}$$

$$1000 = \frac{[ionized]}{[nonionized]}$$

Intestine $pH \approx 6$

$$5 - 6 = \log \frac{[ionized]}{[nonionized]}$$

$$-1 = \log \frac{[ionized]}{[nonionized]}$$

$$10^{-1} = \frac{[ionized]}{[nonionized]}$$

$$\frac{1}{10} = \frac{[ionized]}{[nonionized]}$$

Ratio favors absorption

The mammalian gastrointestinal tract has specialized transport systems for the absorption of nutrients and electrolytes. There is a carrier system for the absorption of glucose and galactose, three separate transport systems for the absorption of amino acids, an active transport system for the absorption of pyrimidines, and separate transport systems for the absorption of iron, calcium, and sodium.

The absorption of some of these substances is complex and depends on a number of factors. The absorption of iron, for example, is dependent on the need for iron, and its absorption takes place in two steps. Iron first enters the mucosal cells, and then moves into blood. The first step is a relatively rapid one, and the second is slow. Consequently, iron accumulates within the mucosal cells as a protein-iron complex termed ferritin. When iron in blood is decreased below normal values, some of it is liberated from the mucosal stores of ferritin-iron, triggering absorption of more iron from the gut to replenish these stores. Calcium is also absorbed by a two-step process: calcium is first absorbed from the lumen and then extruded into the interstitial fluid. The first step is faster than the second, and therefore intracellular calcium rises in mucosal cells during absorption. Vitamin D is required for both steps of calcium transport.

Some toxicants can be absorbed by these same specialized transport systems; for example, 5-fluorouracil is absorbed by the pyrimidine transport system (Schanker and Jeffrey, 1961), thallium is transported by the system that normally absorbs iron (Leopold et al., 1969), and lead may be absorbed by the system that normally transports calcium (Sobel et al., 1938). Cobalt and manganese compete for the iron transport system (Schade et al., 1970; Thomson et al., 1971a, 1971b).

Few toxicants are actively absorbed by the gastrointestinal tract; most enter the body by simple diffusion. Although lipid-soluble substances are more rapidly and extensively absorbed by this process than nonlipid-soluble substances, the latter may be absorbed to some degree. Upon oral ingestion, about 10 percent of lead is absorbed, 4 percent of manganese, 1.5 percent of cadmium, and 1 percent of chromium. If the compound is very toxic, even small amounts of absorbed material will produce serious effects. An organic compound that one would not expect to be absorbed on the basis of the pH-partition hypothesis is the fully ionized quaternary ammonium compound, pralidoxime (2-PAM), which is almost entirely absorbed from the gastrointestinal tract (Levine and Steinberg, 1966). The mechanism or mechanisms by which some lipid-insoluble compounds are absorbed are not clear.

It is interesting that even particles can be absorbed by the gastrointestinal epithelium. Particles of azo dye, variable in size but averaging several thousand nm in diameter, have been shown to be taken up by the duodenum (Barnett, 1959). Emulsions of polystyrene latex particles of 22 μm in diameter have been demonstrated to be picked up by the intestinal epithelium, carried through the cytoplasm within intact vesicles, and discharged into the interstices of the lamina propria where entrance is gained into the lymphatics of the mucosa (Sanders and Ashworth, 1961). The particles appear to enter the intestinal cell by pinocytosis, a process that is much more prominent in the newborn than the adult (Williams and Beck, 1969). These examples demonstrate that many types of toxicants can be absorbed at least to some extent by the gastrointestinal tract.

The resistance of chemicals to the acid pH in the stomach, to the enzymes in the stomach and intestine, and to the intestinal flora is of extreme importance. The toxicant may be altered by the acid, enzymes, or intestinal flora to form a new compound that may differ in toxicity from the parent compound. Relative to intravenous exposure, snake venom is nontoxic when administered orally because it is broken down by the digestive enzymes of the gastrointestinal tract.

Ingestion of well water with a high nitrate content has produced methemoglobinemia much more frequently in infants than in adults. This is due to the higher pH of the gastrointestinal tract in the newborn and the associated presence of higher flora of certain bacteria, especially *Escherichia coli,* which convert nitrate into nitrite. The nitrite formed by the bacterial action then produces methemoglobinemia (Rosenfield and Huston, 1950). The formation of carcinogenic nitrosamines can also occur in the stomach when secondary amines, such as those present in fish, vegetables, and fruit juices, come in contact with nitrite, which is often used as a food additive in meats and smoked fish (see Chapter 5). Also, the intestinal flora can reduce aromatic nitro groups to aromatic amines that may be goitrogenic or carcinogenic (Thompson *et al.,* 1954). The intestinal flora, more specifically *Aerobacter aerogenes,* have been shown to degrade DDT to DDE (Mendel and Walton, 1966).

There are many factors that alter the gastrointestinal absorption of toxicants. Ethylenediaminetetraacetic acid (EDTA) increases the absorption of a number of agents (Levine and Pelikan, 1964). This effect is nonspecific because EDTA increases the absorption of bases, acids, and neutral compounds. It appears that by chelating calcium, EDTA causes a general increase in membrane permeability.

Alteration of gastrointestinal motility can also affect the absorption of toxicants. A decreased motility tends to increase the overall absorption, whereas an increased intestinal motility tends to decrease absorption (Levine, 1970). This is due to the high absorption capacity of the proximal segment of the small intestine; almost one-half of the total mucosal area is found in the proximal one-fourth of the small intestine. Therefore, if the toxicant remains in the proximal part of the small intestine for a longer period of time, more will be absorbed.

Experiments have shown that oral toxicity of some chemicals is increased by diluting the dose (Ferguson, 1962; Borowitz *et al.,* 1971). This phenomenon, which has been shown for many xenobiotics, may be explained by the increased rapidity of stomach emptying, which is induced by the increased dosage volume, and thus more rapid absorption in the duodenum because of the larger surface area available.

The absorption of a toxicant from the gastrointestinal tract can also be dependent on the physical properties of the compound, such as lipid solubility, and dissolution rate. While it is often generalized that an increase in lipid solubility will increase the absorption of chemicals, an extremely lipid-soluble chemical will not dissolve in the gastrointestinal fluids and absorp-

tion will be low (Houston *et al.,* 1974). If the toxicant is a solid and relatively insoluble in the gastrointestinal fluids, the compound will have limited contact with the gastrointestinal mucosa and therefore will not be absorbed extensively. If the particle size is large, even less will be absorbed by diffusion since dissolution rate is proportional to particle size (Gorringe and Sproston, 1964; Bates and Gibaldi, 1970). This is the reason why metallic mercury is relatively nontoxic when ingested orally and why finely powdered arsenic trioxide is significantly more toxic than the coarse granular material (Schwartze, 1923).

The amount of chemical that enters the general systemic circulation after oral administration depends on a number of factors. First, it depends on the amount absorbed into the gastrointestinal cells. Before the chemical enters the general systemic circulation, it can be biotransformed by the gastrointestinal cells, extracted by the liver and excreted into bile, biotransformed by the liver or biotransformed by the lung. This phenomenon of removing chemicals after oral absorption before entering the general systemic circulation is referred to as presystemic elimination, or first-pass effect. The following equation, which compares the area under the curve (*AUC*) after oral and intravenous administration, can be used to determine the amount of chemical that enters the general systemic circulation after oral administration, which is termed the bioavailability of the chemical:

$$\text{Bioavailability} = \frac{AUC_{O\rightarrow\infty,\ \text{oral}}}{AUC_{O\rightarrow\infty,iv}} \times 100$$

A number of other factors have been shown to alter absorption. One metal can alter the absorption of another: cadmium decreases the absorption of zinc and copper, calcium decreases the absorption of cadmium, zinc decreases the absorption of copper, and magnesium decreases the absorption of fluoride (Pfeiffer, 1977). Milk has been found to increase lead absorption (Kello and Kostial, 1973), and starvation enhances the absorption of dieldrin (Heath and Vandekar, 1964). The age of the animal also appears to affect absorption. For example, two-hour-old rats absorb 12 percent of a dose of cadmium while adult rats absorb only 0.5 percent (Sasser and Jarboe, 1977). While lead and many other heavy metals are not readily absorbed from the gastrointestinal tract, EDTA and other chelators will increase the solubility and absorption of metals. Thus it is important not to give a chelator orally while metal is still present in the gastrointestinal tract.

Absorption of Toxicants by Lungs

It is well known that toxic responses to chemicals can result from their absorption from lungs. The most frequent cause of death from poisoning, carbon monoxide, and probably the most important occupational disease, silicosis, are results of the absorption or deposition of airborne poisons by lungs. This site of absorption has even been used in chemical warfare (chlorine gas, phosgene gas, lewisite, mustard gas) and for executing criminals in gas chambers (hydrogen cyanide).

Toxicants that are absorbed by the lungs are usually gases, such as carbon monoxide, nitrogen dioxide, and sulfur dioxide, vapors of volatile or volatilizable liquids such as benzene and carbon tetrachloride, and aerosols. The site of deposition of aerosols is highly dependent on the size of the particles. This relationship is discussed in detail in Chapter 12. Particles of 5 μm or larger are usually deposited in the nasopharyngeal region (Figure 3–17). Those deposited on the unciliated anterior portion of the nose tend to remain at the site of deposition until they are removed by nose wiping, blowing, or sneezing. The mucous blanket of the ciliated nasal

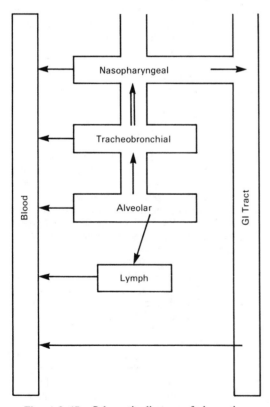

Figure 3–17. Schematic diagram of absorption and translocation of chemicals by lungs.

surface carries with it insoluble particles as it is propelled by beating of the cilia. These particles as well as particles inhaled through the mouth are swallowed within minutes and passed to the gastrointestinal tract. Soluble particles may dissolve in the mucus and be carried to the pharynx or be absorbed through the epithelium into blood.

Particles of 2 to 5 μm are deposited in the tracheobronchiolar regions of the lungs, where they are cleared by the upward movement of the mucus layer in the ciliated portions of the respiratory tract. The rate of ciliary movement of the mucus varies in different parts of the respiratory tract but is a rapid and efficient removal mechanism. Measurements have shown transport rates between 0.1 and 1 mm/min resulting in removal half-lives between 30 and 300 min. Coughing and sneezing result in a rapid movement of the mucus and particular matter toward the mouth. Particles may eventually be swallowed and absorbed from the gastrointestinal tract.

Particles 1 μm and smaller penetrate to the alveolar sacs of the lung. They may be absorbed into blood or may be cleared by scavenging action of alveolar macrophages.

The alveolar zone is an area of the lung where toxicants are readily absorbed. The surface area is large (50 to 100 m^2), and blood flow to the lung is high and in close proximity to the alveolar air (10 μm). Gas in the alveoli equilibrates almost instantaneously with blood passing through the pulmonary capillary bed. The concentration of the gas in blood as it leaves the lung is dependent on the solubility of the gas in blood, where solubility is defined according to Henry's law as the ratio of the concentration of dissolved gas in fluid (blood) to the concentration in the gas phase at equilibrium. By this definition, it can be shown that chloroform has a high solubility (15) and ethylene a low solubility (0.14) in blood. For a substance with low solubility, such as ethylene, only a small percentage of the total gas in the lung is removed by blood during each breath. Because blood is saturated with gas, an increase in the respiratory rate or minute volume does not change the transfer of the gas to blood. However, an increase in the rate of cardiac output would markedly increase the rate of uptake of gas. Blood as a potential reservoir for an insoluble gas such as ethylene would be small and filled quickly. It has been calculated that the time for blood and gas to equilibrate for a relatively insoluble gas would be 8 to 21 minutes.

For a very highly soluble gas such as chloroform, so much is transferred to blood during each breath that little, if any, remains in the alveoli just before the next inspiration. The more soluble a toxic agent is in blood, the more of it must be dissolved in blood to reach equilibrium. Naturally, the time required to equilibrate with body water will be very much longer with high-than with low-solubility gases and has been calculated to take a minimum of one hour. This can be prolonged considerably if the gas has a high tissue solubility (i.e., high solubility in fat), as do many toxic agents. With these highly soluble gases, the principal factor that limits the rate of absorption is respiration. Because the blood is already removing virtually all the gas from the lungs, increasing the cardiac output does not substantially increase the rate of absorption, but the rate can be substantially accelerated by increasing the rate or depth of respiration.

Thus the rate of absorption of gases is variable and dependent on the toxicant's blood:gas solubility. If a gas has a very low solubility, the rate of transfer is mainly dependent on blood flow through the lung (perfusion limited), whereas for gases with a high solubility, it is primarily dependent on the rate and depth of respiration (ventilation limited). Of course, there is a transition zone between the two types of extreme behavior, which centers at a blood-gas solubility of about 1.2.

In addition to gases, liquid aerosols and particles are often absorbed in the alveoli. Liquid aerosols, if lipid soluble, will readily cross the alveolar cell membranes by passive diffusion. Mechanisms responsible for the removal or absorption of particulate matter that reaches the alveolus (usually less than 1 μm in diameter) are less clearly defined than those responsible for removal of particles deposited in the tracheobronchial tree discussed above. Alveolar removal is a slow process and is in no way comparable to the effective and rapid action of the bronchial mucociliary system. Removal of toxic agents from the alveoli appears to occur by three major routes. The first is physical removal of particles from the alveoli. It is thought that particles deposited on the fluid layer of the alveoli are aspirated onto the mucociliary escalator of the tracheobronchial region to the gastrointestinal tract. The origin of the thin fluid layer in the alveoli is probably the transudation of lymph and the secretion of lipid and other components by alveolar epithelium. The alveolar fluid flows to the terminal bronchioles by some unknown mechanism, but seems to be dependent on lymphatic flow, capillary action, respiratory motion of the alveolar walls, the cohesive nature of the respiratory tract fluid blanket, and the propelling power of the ciliated bronchioles. The second route of removal of particles from the alveoli is by phagocytosis. The principal cell responsible for engulfing alveolar debris is the mononuclear phagocyte or macrophage. These cells are found in large quantities in normal lungs and contain many phagocytized particles of both exogenous and endogenous origin. They then apparently migrate to the distal end of the mucociliary escalator. The third route of removal is via the lymphatics. Normally water, together with electrolytes and soluble proteins up to the size of albumin, passes freely back and forth from capillary to interstitial and alveolar space and back via the lymphatic system. Both free and phagocytized particles can migrate via the lymphatic system. Particulate material can remain in the lymphatic tissue for long periods of time, and for this reason, has been termed the dust stores for the lungs.

The overall removal of particulates from the alveolus is relatively inefficient. Within the first day only about 20 percent is removed from the alveoli, and that which remains longer than 24 hours is very slowly removed. The rate of this clearance can be predicted by the compounds' solubility in lung fluids. The least soluble compounds are removed at a slower rate than the soluble compounds. Thus, it appears that removal is largely due to dissolution and vascular removal. Some particles may remain in the alveolus indefinitely. This can occur when alveolar cells ingest dust particles that do not desquamate but instead proliferate and, in association with a developing network of reticulin fibers, form an alveolar dust plaque or nodule.

Absorption of Toxicants Through the Skin

Human skin comes into contact with many toxic agents. Fortunately, the skin is not very permeable and, therefore, is a relatively good lipoid barrier separating humans from their environment. However, some chemicals can be absorbed by the skin in sufficient quantities to produce systemic effects. For example, nerve gases, such as sarin, are readily absorbed by the intact skin. Also, carbon tetrachloride can be absorbed by the skin in sufficient quantities to produce liver injury, and various insecticides have produced death in agricultural workers after absorption through the intact skin.

In order to be absorbed through the skin, a toxicant must either pass through the epidermal cells, the cells of the sweat or sebaceous glands, or enter through the hair follicles. The sweat glands and hair follicles are scattered throughout the skin in varying numbers but are comparatively sparse; their total cross-sectional area is probably between 0.1 and 1.0 percent of the area of the skin. Although follicular pathways may enable immediate entry of small amounts of toxicants, most chemicals pass through the epidermal cells, which constitute the major surface area of skin.

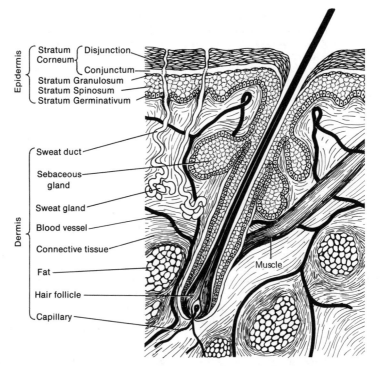

Figure 3–18.   Diagram of a cross-section of human skin.

Absorption of a chemical to be absorbed by the percutaneous route requires passage through the densely packed outer layer of horny, keratinized epidermal cells, through the germinal layer of the epidermis, through the dermis, and on into the systemic circulation (Figure 3–18). In contrast, when toxicants are absorbed by the lung and gastrointestinal tract, the chemical may pass through only two cells.

The first phase of percutaneous absorption is diffusion of the toxicant through the epidermis, which is the rate-limiting barrier for the cutaneous absorption of toxicants. More specifically, the barrier is the stratum corneum—the thin, cohesive, multicellular membrane that comprises the dead surface layer of skin. Studies have shown that the stratum corneum is replenished about every two weeks in adults. This complex process includes a gross dehydration and polymerization of the intracellular material, resulting finally in a keratin-filled, biologically inactive, dried cell layer. In the course of keratinization the cell walls apparently double in thickness owing to the inclusion, or deposition, of chemically resistant material. Thus a change in the physical state of the tissue and a commensurate change in its diffusion occur, that is, a transformation from an aqueous fluid medium characterized by liquid state to a dry, semisolid, keratin membrane characterized by a much lower rate of diffusion.

It appears that all toxicants move across the stratum corneum of mammals by passive diffusion and not by active transport. Kinetic measurements support the postulate that polar and nonpolar toxicants diffuse through the stratum corneum by different molecular mechanisms. Polar substances appear to diffuse through the outer surface of protein filaments of the hydrated stratum corneum, while nonpolar molecules dissolve in and diffuse through the nonaqueous lipid matrix between the protein filaments (Blank and Scheuplein, 1969). The rate of diffusion of nonpolar toxicants is related to the lipid solubility and inversely related to the molecular weight (Marzulli *et al.*, 1965).

In human stratum corneum there are significant differences in structure and chemistry from one region of the body to another, which affects the permeability of the skin to chemicals. Skin from the plantar and palmar regions of the body is much different from that in other areas; the horny layer of the palms and soles is adapted for weight bearing and friction. The membranous horny layer of the rest of the body surface is adapted for flexibility, impermeability, and fine sensory discrimination. While the stratum corneum is much thicker on the palms and soles (being 400 to 600 μm in callous areas) than on the arms, back, legs, and abdomen (8 to 15 μm), it has much more diffusivity per unit thickness. Permeability of the skin is dependent on both the diffusivity of the stratum corneum and its thickness. Thus toxicants readily cross the scrotum since it is extremely thin and has high diffusivity; toxicants cross the abdominal skin less rapidly since it is both thicker and exhibits less diffusivity; and toxicants cross the sole with the greatest difficulty because it has such a great distance to traverse even though it exhibits the greatest diffusivity.

The second phase of percutaneous absorption is diffusion of the toxicant through the dermis, which is far inferior to the stratum corneum as a diffusion barrier. In contrast to the stratum corneum, the dermis contains a porous, nonselective, watery diffusion medium. Toxicants pass through this area by diffusion into the systemic circulation, and the diffusion is dependent on sufficient blood flow, interstitial fluid movement, lymphatics, and perhaps other factors including interactions with dermal constituents.

The absorption of toxicants through the skin varies under a number of conditions. Since the stratum corneum plays a critical role in determining cutaneous permeability, abrasion or removal of this layer causes an abrupt increase in the permeability of the epidermis for all kinds of molecules, large or small, lipid soluble and water soluble (Malkinson, 1964). Injurious agents such as acids, alkalis, and mustard gases likewise will injure the barrier cells and increase permeability (Malkinson, 1964). Water plays an extremely important role in skin permeability. Under normal conditions the stratum corneum is always partially hydrated. Skin normally contains about 90 g of water per gram of dry tissue. This amount of water increases the permeability of the stratum corneum approximately tenfold over that when it is perfectly dry. Upon additional contact with water the stratum corneum can maximally increase its weight of tightly bound water three to five times, which results in an additional two- to threefold increase in permeability. Studies on dermal absorption of toxicants often utilize the method of Draize and associates (1944) in which plastic is wrapped around the animal and the chemical placed between the plastic and the skin. This hydrates the stratum corneum and enhances the absorption of toxicants.

Solvents such as dimethyl sulfoxide (DMSO) can also facilitate the penetration of toxicants through the skin. DMSO increases the permeability of the skin barrier layer, the stratum corneum. Little information is available concerning the mechanism by which DMSO enhances the permeability. However, it has been suggested that DMSO (1) removes much of the lipid fraction of the stratum corneum, which makes holes or artificial shunts in the membrane, (2) produces reversible configurational changes in protein structure brought about by substitution of integral water molecules by DMSO, and (3) functions as a swelling agent (Allenby et al., 1969; Dugard and Embery, 1969).

Various species have been employed in studying the absorption of toxicants, and species variation in the cutaneous permeability have been observed. The skin of the rat and rabbit is more permeable, the skin of the cat is less permeable, while the cutaneous permeability characteristics of the guinea pig, pig, and monkey are similar to those observed in humans (Scala et al., 1968; Coulston and Serrone, 1969; Wester and Maibach, 1977). Species differences in percutaneous absorption account for the fact that many insecticides are more toxic to insects than to humans. For example, the LD50 of DDT is approximately equal in an insect and mammal when the insecticide is injected but is much less toxic to the mammal than to the insect when applied to the skin. This appears to be due to the fact that DDT is poorly absorbed through the skin of a mammal but passes readily through the chitinous exoskeleton of the insect and the fact that insects have a much greater body surface area relative to weight than do mammals (Winteringham, 1957; Albert, 1965; Hayes, 1965).

Absorption of Toxicants After Special Routes of Administration

Toxic agents usually enter the bloodstream of humans after absorption from the skin, lungs, or gastrointestinal tract. However, in studying chemical agents, toxicologists frequently administer these chemicals to laboratory animals by special routes, the most common of which are (1) intraperitoneal, (2) subcutaneous, (3) intramuscular, and (4) intravenous. The intravenous route of administration introduces the toxicant directly into the bloodstream, and thus the process of absorption is eliminated. The intraperitoneal route of administration of toxicants to laboratory animals is also a common procedure. This method results in rapid absorption of toxicants owing to the rich blood supply to the peritoneal cavity and to the large surface area. Compounds administered intraperitoneally are absorbed primarily through the portal circulation and, therefore, must pass through the liver before reaching other organs (Lukas et al., 1971). Toxicants administered subcutaneously and intramuscularly are usually absorbed at a slower rate. The rate of absorption by these two routes can be altered by changing the blood flow to the area and by altering the solution in which the toxicant is administered. For example, epinephrine will cause vasoconstriction and decrease the rate of absorption of a toxicant. The formulation of the toxicant may also affect the rate of absorption;

toxicants are absorbed more slowly from suspensions than from solutions.

The toxicity of a chemical may or may not be dependent on the route of parenteral administration. If a toxicant is injected intraperitoneally, most of the chemical will enter the liver via the portal circulation before it reaches the general circulation of the animal. Therefore, an intraperitoneally administered compound might be completely biotransformed or extracted by the liver and excreted into the bile and never gain access to the remainder of the animal. Propranolol (Shand and Rangno, 1972) and lidocaine (Boyes et al., 1970) are two such drugs that are efficiently extracted during the first pass through the liver. Any toxicant that has a selective toxicity for an organ other than the liver and gastrointestinal tract would be expected to be much less toxic when administered intraperitoneally than when injected subcutaneously or intramuscularly. Compounds that are not biotransformed by the liver or excreted into bile should have a toxicity independent of route of administration, provided rates of absorption are equal. Therefore, it is possible to obtain some preliminary information on the biotransformation and excretion of a toxicant by comparing its toxicity when given by various routes.

KINETICS OF REPEATED EXPOSURE

The concentration of a chemical in plasma as well as in other tissues and the amount of chemical in the body (body burden) after repeated exposure or administration are obviously important factors to be considered in the toxicologic evaluation of a substance. If the half-life is short in relation to the exposure interval, the substance may be almost completely eliminated during this interval, and the amount after consecutive doses would be practically equal to that after the initial dose. When the half-life is about the same as or larger than the exposure interval, an appreciable amount of toxicant will remain in the body prior to the second and subsequent exposures, and the toxicant will accumulate (Figure 3–19). Assuming that the first-order elimination processes following a single dosage do not change (that is, biotransformation and excretion pathways are not induced or saturated), the cumulative concentration or amount in the body, as shown in Figure 3–19, fluctuates between the exposures. The time required to attain 90 percent of the plateau value is about 3.5 times the biologic half-life; for 99 percent of the plateau values it requires about seven times the biologic half-life.

The "average" plateau concentration C_∞^{av} can be determined by the following equation:

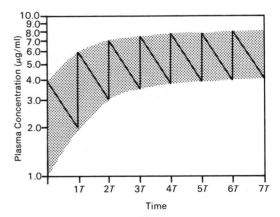

Figure 3–19. Concentration of toxicant in plasma as a function of time during repeated exposure to the toxicant at constant time intervals (τ).

$$C_\infty^{av} = \frac{f \cdot D_{oral}}{V_d k_{el} \tau}$$

where f is the fraction absorbed, D_{oral} is the oral dose, and τ is the constant time interval between administration or exposure. Since $k_{el} = 0.693/t_{1/2}$, another useful equation to determine the average plasma concentration at infinity (C_∞^{av}) is:

$$C_\infty^{av} = \frac{1.44 \cdot t_{1/2} \cdot f \cdot D_{oral}}{V_d \cdot \tau}$$

Although the preceding equations describe the average concentration of chemical in plasma or tissue, the equations can be multiplied by V_d to obtain the amount of chemical in the body. Thus, the "average" body burden at steady state (X_∞^{av}) is described by the following relationship:

$$X_\infty^{av} = C_\infty^{av} \cdot V_d$$

CONCLUSIONS

Humans are in continuous contact with toxic agents. Toxicants are in the food we eat, the water we drink, and the air we breathe. Depending on their physical and chemical properties, toxic agents may be absorbed by the gastrointestinal tract, lungs, and/or skin. Fortunately, the body has the ability to biotransform and to excrete these compounds into urine, feces, and air. However, when the rate of absorption exceeds the rate of elimination, the toxic compound may accumulate to a critical concentration in the body, and toxic effects are then observed (Figure 3–20). A toxicant may produce toxicity through a pharmacologic or pathologic effect or

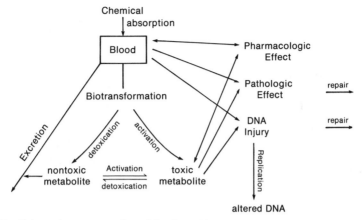

Figure 3–20. Schematic representation of the disposition and toxic effects produced by chemicals.

genotoxic (alter DNA) effect. An example of a pharmacologic effect leading to toxicity is depression of the central nervous system by barbiturates, an example of a pathologic effect is kidney injury produced by mercury, and an example of a genotoxic effect is cancer produced by mustard gas. Generally, if the concentration of chemical in the tissues does not exceed a critical level, the effects may be reversible. The pharmacologic effects are usually reversed when the concentration of chemical in the tissues is decreased by excretion from the body. Pathologic and genotoxic effects can be repaired. If the pharmacologic and pathologic effects are severe, death may ensue within a short time, whereas if DNA is not repaired, cancer may result in a few months in laboratory animals or in a decade or more in humans.

Many chemicals are not toxic themselves but have to be activated by biotransformation into toxic metabolites; the toxic response then is dependent on the balance of the rate at which the toxic metabolite is produced and detoxified. Toxic effects are related to the concentration of the "toxic chemical" in the body, either the chemical administered or that generated by biotransformation in the body. Thus, the toxic response produced by a chemical is largely determined by its rate of absorption, distribution, biotransformation, and excretion.

REFERENCES

Albert, A.: *Selective Toxicity,* 3rd ed. Meuthuen & Co., London, 1965.
Allenby, A. C.; Creasey, N. H.; Edginton, J. A. G.; Fletcher, J. A.; and Schock, C.: Mechanism of action of accelerants on skin penetration. *Br. J. Dermatol.,* **81** (Suppl. 4):47–55, 1969.
Amoroso, E. C.: Placentation. In Parks, A. S. (ed.): *Marshall's Physiology of Reproduction,* Vol. 2, 3rd ed. Longmans, Green & Co., London, 1952, pp. 127–311.

Barnett, H. L.: McNamara, H.; Schultz, S.; and Tompsett, R.: Renal clearances of sodium penicillin G, procaine penicillin G, and inulin in infants and children. *Pediatrics,* 3:418–22, 1949.
Barnett, R. J.: The demonstration with the electron microscope of the end-products of histochemical reactions in relation to the fine structure of cells. *Exp. Cell Res.* (Suppl. 7):65–89, 1959.
Bates, T. R., and Gibaldi, M.: Gastrointestinal absorption of drugs. In Swarbrick, J. (ed.): *Current Concepts in the Pharmaceutical Sciences: Biopharmaceutics.* Lea & Febiger, Philadelphia, 1970.
Blank, I. H., and Scheuplein, R. J.: Transport into and within the skin. *Br. J. Dermatol.,* 81 (Suppl. 4):4–10, 1969.
Borowitz, J. L.: Moore, P. F.; Him, G. K. W.; and Miya, T. S.: Mechanism of enhanced drug effects produced by dilution of the oral dose. *Toxicol. Appl. Pharmacol.,* 19:164–68, 1971.
Boyes, R. N.; Adams, H. J.; and Duce, B. R.: Oral absorption and disposition kinetics of lidocaine hydrochloride in dogs. *J. Pharmacol. Exp. Ther.,* 174:1–8, 1970.
Castle, M. C., and Lage, G. L.: Effect of pretreatment with spironolactone, phenobarbital or β-diethylaminoethyl diphenylpropylacetate (SKF 525-A) on tritium levels in blood, heart and liver of rats at various times after administration of [³H] digitoxin. *Biochem. Pharmacol.,* 21:1449–55, 1972.
——: Enhanced biliary excretion of digitoxin following spironolactone as it relates to the prevention of digitoxin toxicity. *Res. Commun. Chem. Pathol. Pharmacol.,* 5:99–108, 1973.
Coulston, F., and Serrone, D. M.: The comparative approach to the role of nonhuman primates in evaluation of drug toxicity in man: a review. *Ann. N.Y. Acad. Sci.,* 162:681–704, 1969.
Dawes, G. S.: *Foetal and Neonatal Physiology: A Comparative Study of the Changes at Birth.* Year Book Medical Publishers, Inc., Chicago, 1968.
Dowling, R. H.: Compensatory changes in intestinal absorption. *Br. Med. Bull.,* 23:275–78, 1967.
Draize, J. H.: Woodard, G.; and Calvery, H. O.: Methods for the study of irritation and toxicity of substances applied topically to the skin and mucous membranes. *J. Pharmacol. Exp. Ther.,* 82:377–90, 1944.
Dugard, P. H., and Embery, G.: The influence of dimethyl sulphoxide on the percutaneous migration of potassium butyl [³⁵S] sulphate, potassium methyl [³⁵S] sulphate and sodium [³⁵S] sulphate. *Br. J. Dermatol.,* 81 (Suppl. 4):69–74, 1969.

Duggan, D. E.; Hooke, K. F.; Noll, R. M.; and Kwan, K. C.: Enterohepatic circulation of indomethacin and its role in intestinal irritation. *Biochem. Pharmacol.,* **24:**1749–54, 1975.

Ferguson, H. C.: Dilution of dose and acute oral toxicity. *Toxicol. Appl. Pharmacol.,* **4:**759–62, 1962.

Findlay, J. W. A.: The distribution of some commonly used drugs in human breast milk. *Drug. Metab. Rev.,* **14:**653–686, 1983.

Gibaldi, M., and Perrier, D.: Pharmacokinetics, Marcel Dekker, Inc., New York, 1982.

Ginsburg, J.: Placental drug transfer. *Annu. Rev. Pharmacol.,* **11:**387–408, 1971.

Goldstein, A.; Aronow, L.; and Kalman, S. M. (eds.): *Principles of Drug Action: The Basis of Pharmacology,* 2nd ed. John Wiley & Sons, Inc., New York, 1974.

Gorringe, J. A. L., and Sproston, E. M.: The influence of particle size upon the absorption of drugs from the gastrointestinal tract. In Binns, T. B. (ed.): *Absorption and Distribution of Drugs.* Williams & Wilkins Co., Baltimore, 1964, pp. 128–39.

Hayes, W. J., Jr.: Review of the metabolism of chlorinated hydrocarbon insecticides especially in mammals. *Annu. Rev. Pharmacol.,* **5:**27–52, 1965.

Heath, D. F., and Vandekar, M.: Toxicity and metabolism of dieldrin in rats. *Br. J. Ind. Med.,* **21:**269–79, 1964.

Hirsch, G. H., and Hook, J. B.: Maturation of renal organic acid transport: substrate stimulation by penicillin and *p*-aminohippurate (PAH). *J. Pharmacol. Exp. Ther.,* **171:**103–108, 1970.

Houston, J. B.; Upshall, D. G.; and Bridges, J. W.: A re-evaluation of the importance of partition coefficients in the gastrointestinal absorption of nutrients. *J. Pharmacol. Exp. Ther.,* **189:**244–54, 1974.

Juchau, M. R.: Mechanisms of drug biotransformation reactions in the placenta. *Fed. Proc.,* **31:**48–51, 1972.

Kello, D., and Kostial, K.: The effect of milk diet on lead metabolism in rats. *Environ. Res.,* **6:**355–60, 1973.

Klaassen, C. D.: Immaturity of the newborn rat's hepatic excretory function for ouabain. *J. Pharmacol. Exp. Ther.,* **183:**520–26, 1972.

———: Comparison of the toxicity of chemicals in newborn rats to bile duct-ligated and sham-operated rats and mice. *Toxicol. Appl. Pharmacol.,* **24:**37–44, 1973a.

———: Hepatic excretory function in the newborn rat. *J. Pharmacol. Exp. Ther.,* **184:**721–28, 1973b.

———: Effect of microsomal enzyme inducers on the biliary excretion of cardiac glycosides. *J. Pharmacol. Exp. Ther.,* **191:**201–11, 1974a.

———: Stimulation of the development of the hepatic excretory mechanism for ouabain in newborn rats with microsomal enzyme inducers. *J. Pharmacol. Exp. Ther.,* **191:**212–18, 1974b.

———: Biliary excretion of mercury compounds. *Toxicol. Appl. Pharmacol.,* **33:**356–65, 1975a.

———: Effect of spironolactone on the distribution of mercury. *Toxicol. Appl. Pharmacol.,* **33:**366–75, 1975b.

———: Biliary excretion of metals. *Drug. Metab. Rev.,* **5:**165–96, 1976.

Klaassen, C. D.; Eaton, D. L.; and Cagen, S. Z.: Hepatobiliary disposition of xenobiotics. In Bridges, J. W., and Chasseaud, L. F. (ed.): *Progress in Drug Metabolism.* John Wiley & Sons, Inc., New York, 1981, pp. 1–75.

Klaassen, C. D., and Shoeman, D. W.: Biliary excretion of lead in rats, rabbits and dogs. *Toxicol. Appl. Pharmacol.,* **29:**434–46, 1974.

Klaassen, C. D., and Watkins, J. B.: Mechanisms of bile formation, hepatic uptake, and biliary excretion. *Pharmacol. Rev.,* **36:**1–67, 1984.

Kragh-Hansen, U.: Molecular aspects of ligand binding to serum albumin. *Pharmacol. Rev.,* **33:**17–53, 1981.

Kupferberg, H. J., and Way, E. L.: Pharmacologic basis for the increased sensitivity of the newborn rat to morphine. *J. Pharmacol. Exp. Ther.,* **141:**105–12, 1963.

Leopold, G.; Furukawa, E.; Forth, W.; and Rummel, W.: Comparative studies of absorption of heavy metals *in vivo* and *in vitro.* *Arch. Pharmacol. Exp. Pathol.,* **263:**275–76, 1969.

Levi, A. J.; Gatmaitan, Z.; and Arias, I. M.: Two hepatic cytoplasmic protein fractions, Y and Z, and their possible role in the hepatic uptake of bilirubin, sulfobromophthalein, and other anions. *J. Clin. Invest.,* **48:**2156–67, 1969.

Levine, R. R.: Factors affecting gastrointestinal absorption of drugs. *Am. J. Dig. Dis.,* **15:**171–88, 1970.

Levine, R. R., and Pelikan, E. W.: Mechanisms of drug absorption and excretion. Passage of drugs out of and into the gastrointestinal tract. *Annu. Rev. Pharmacol.,* **4:**69–84, 1964.

Levine, R. R., and Steinberg, G. M.: Intestinal absorption of pralidoxime and other aldoximes. *Nature (Lond.),* **209:**269–71, 1966.

Litwack, G.; Ketterer, B.; and Arias, I. M.: Ligandin: A hepatic protein which binds steroids, bilirubin, carcinogens and a number of exogenous organic anions. *Nature (Lond.),* **234:**466–67, 1971.

Lukas, G.; Brindle, S. D.; and Greengard, P.: The route of absorption of intraperitoneally administered compounds. *J. Pharmacol. Exp. Ther.,* **178:**562–66, 1971.

Magos, L., and Clarkson, T. W.: The effect of oral doses of a polythiol resin on the excretion of methylmercury in mice treated with cysteine, D-penicillamine or phenobarbitone. *Chem.-Biol. Interactions,* **14:**325–35, 1976.

Malkinson, F. D.: Permeability of the stratum corneum. In Montagna, W., and Lobitz, W. C., Jr. (eds.): *The Epidermis.* Academic Press, Inc., New York, 1964.

Marzulli, F. N.: Callahan, J. F.; and Brown, D. W. C.: Chemical structure and skin penetrating capacity of a short series of organic phosphates and phosphoric acid. *J. Invest. Dermatol.,* **44:**339–44, 1965.

Mendel, J. L., and Walton, M. S.: Conversion of *p,p*-DDT to *p,p*-DDD by intestinal flora of the rat. *Science,* **151:**1527–28, 1966.

Mirkin, B. L., and Singh, S.: Placental transfer and pharmacokinetics of digoxin in the pregnant rat. *Proceedings of the Fifth International Congress of Pharmacology* (abstract), 949, 1972.

Pentschew, A., and Garro, F.: Lead encephalo-myelopathy of the suckling rat and its implication on the porphyrinopathic nervous diseases. *Acta Neuropathol. (Berl.),* **6:**266–78, 1966.

Pfeiffer, C. J.: Gastroenterologic response to environmental agents—absorption and interactions. In Lee, D. H. K. (ed.): *Handbook of Physiology. Section 9: Reactions to Environmental Agents.* American Physiological Society, Bethesda, Md., 1977, pp. 349–74.

Rosenfield, A. B., and Huston, R.: Infant methemoglobinemia in Minnesota due to nitrates in well water. *Minn. Med.,* **33:**787–96, 1950.

Rozman, T.; Ballhorn, L.; Rozman, K.; Klaassen, C.; and Greim, H.: Effect of cholestyramine on the disposition of pentachlorophenol in rhesus monkeys, *J. Toxicol. Env. Hlth,* **10:**277–83, 1982.

Sanders, E., and Ashworth, C. T.: A study of particulate intestinal absorption of hepatocellular uptake. Use of polystyrene latex particles. *Exp. Cell Res.,* **22:**137–45, 1961.

Sasser, L. B., and Jarboe, G. E.: Intestinal absorption and retention of cadmium in neonatal rat. *Toxicol. Appl. Pharmacol.,* **41:**423–31, 1977.

Scala, J.; McOsker, D. E.; and Reller, H. H.: The percutaneous absorption of ionic surfactants. *J. Invest. Dermatol.,* **50:**371–79, 1968.

Scatchard, G.: The attraction of proteins for small molecules and ions. *Ann. N.Y. Acad. Sci.*, **51**:660–72, 1949.

Schade, S. G.; Felsher, B. F.; Glader, B. E.; and Conrad, M. E.: Effect of cobalt upon iron absorption. *Proc. Soc. Exp. Biol. Med.*, **134**:741–43, 1970.

Schanker, L. S.: Mechanisms of drug absorption and distribution. *Annu. Rev. Pharmacol.*, **1**:29–44, 1961.

———: Passage of drugs across body membranes. *Pharmacol. Rev.*, **14**:501–30, 1962.

Schanker, L. S., and Jeffrey, J.: Active transport of foreign pyrimidines across the intestinal epithelium. *Nature (Lond.)*, **190**:727–28, 1961.

Schwartze, E. W.: The so-called habituation to "arsenic:" variation in the toxicity of arsenious oxide. *J. Pharmacol. Exp. Ther.*, **20**:181–203, 1923.

Selye, H.; Krajny, M.; and Savoie, L.: Digitoxin poisoning: Prevention by spironolactone. *Science*, **164**:842–43, 1969.

———: Hormones and resistance. *J. Pharm. Sci.*, **60**:1–28, 1971.

———: Mercury poisoning: prevention by spironolactone. *Science*, **169**:775–76, 1970.

Shand, D. G., and Rangno, R. E.: The deposition of propranolol. I. Elimination during oral absorption in man. *Pharmacology*, **7**:159–68, 1972.

Shoeman, D. W.; Kauffman, R. E.; Azarnoff, D. L.; and Boulos, B. M.: Placental transfer of diphenylhydantoin in the goat. *Biochem. Pharmacol.*, **21**:1237–43, 1972.

Silverman, W. A.; Andersen, D. H.; Blanc, W. A.; and Crozier, D. N.: A difference in mortality rate and incidence of kernicterus among premature infants allotted to two prophylactic antibacterial regimens. *Pediatrics*, **18**:614–25, 1956.

Sobel, A. E.: Gawron, O.; and Kramer, B.: Influence of vitamin D in experimental lead poisoning. *Proc. Soc. Exp. Biol. Med.*, **38**:433–35, 1938.

Stowe, C. M., and Plaa, G. L.: Extrarenal excretion of drugs and chemicals. *Annu. Rev. Pharmacol.*, **8**:337–56, 1968.

Thompson, R. Q.; Sturtevant, M.; Bird, O. D.; and Glazko, A. J.: The effect of metabolites of chloramphenicol (Chloromycetin) on the thyroid of the rat. *Endocrinology*, **55**:665–81, 1954.

Thomson, A. B. R.; Olatunbosun, D.; and Valberg, L. S.: Interrelation of intestinal transport system for manganese and iron. *J. Lab. Clin. Med.*, **78**:642–55, 1971a.

Thomson, A. B. R.; Valberg, L. S.; and Sinclair, D. G.: Competitive nature of the intestinal transport mechanism for cobalt and iron in the rat. *J. Clin. Invest.*, **50**:2384–94, 1971b.

Tune, B. M.; Wu, K. Y.; and Kempson, R. L.: Inhibition of transport and prevention of toxicity of cephaloridine in the kidney. Dose-responsiveness of the rabbit and the guinea pig to probenecid. *J. Pharmacol. Exp. Ther.*, **202**:466–71, 1977.

Weiner, I. M., and Mudge, G. H.: Renal tubular mechanisms for excretion of organic acids and bases. *Am. J. Med.*, **36**:743–62, 1964.

Wester, R. C., and Maibach, H. I.: Percutaneous absorption in man and animal: a perspective. In Drill, V. A., and Lazar, P. (eds.): *Cutaneous Toxicity*. Academic Press, Inc., New York, 1977.

Wilkinson, G. R.: Plasma and tissue binding considerations in drug disposition. *Drug. Metab. Rev.*, **14**:427–65, 1983.

Williams, R. M., and Beck, F.: A histochemical study of gut maturation. *J. Anat.*, **105**:487–501, 1969.

Wilson, J. T.: Determinants and consequences of drug excretion in breast milk. *Drug Metab. Rev.*, **14**:619–52, 1983.

Winteringham, F. P. W.: Comparative biochemical aspects of insecticidal action. *Chem. Ind. (Lond.)*, 1195–1202, 1957.

Wold, J. S.; Joost, R. R.; and Owen, N. V.: Nephrotoxicity of cephaloridine in newborn rabbits: role of the renal anionic transport system. *J. Pharmacol. Exp. Ther.*, **201**:778–85, 1977.

Young, M.: Three topics in placental transport: amino transport; oxygen transfer; placental function during labour. In Klopper, A., and Diczfalusy, E. (eds.): *Foetus and Placenta*. Blackwell Scientific Publications, Oxford, 1969.

Zsigmond, G., and Solymoss, B.: Effect of spironolactone, pregnenolone-16α-carbonitrile and cortisol on the metabolism and biliary excretion of sulfobromophthalein and phenol-3,6-dibromophthalein disulfonate in rats. *J. Pharmacol. Exp. Ther.*, **183**:499–507, 1972.

Chapter 4

BIOTRANSFORMATION OF TOXICANTS

I. Glenn Sipes and A. Jay Gandolfi

INTRODUCTION

Humans and other animals are constantly exposed in their environment to a vast array of chemicals that are foreign to their bodies. These foreign chemicals, or xenobiotics, can be of natural origin or they can be man-made. In general, the more lipophilic compounds are readily absorbed through the skin, across the lungs, or through the gastrointestinal tract. Constant or even intermittent exposure to these lipophilic chemicals could result in their accumulation within the organism, unless effective means of elimination are present. Indeed, chemicals can be excreted unchanged into urine, bile, feces, expired air, and perspiration. Except for exhalation, the ease with which compounds are eliminated from the body largely depends on their water solubility. This is particularly true for nonvolatile chemicals that are eliminated in urine and feces, the predominant routes of elimination. Lipophilic compounds that are present in these excretory fluids tend to diffuse into cellular membranes and are reabsorbed, whereas water-soluble compounds are excreted. Therefore, it is apparent why lipophilic xenobiotics could accumulate within the body: they are readily absorbed, but poorly excreted.

Fortunately, animal organisms have developed a number of biochemical processes that convert lipophilic compounds to more hydrophilic metabolites. These biochemical processes are termed *biotransformation* and are usually enzymatic in nature. It should be stressed that biotransformation is the sum of the processes by which a foreign chemical is subjected to chemical change by living organisms (Figure 4–1). This definition implies that a particular chemical may undergo a number of chemical changes. It may mean that the parent molecule is chemically modified at a number of positions or that a particular metabolite of the parent compound may undergo additional modification. The end result of the biotransformation reaction(s) is that the metabolites are chemically distinct from the parent compound. Metabolites are usually more hydrophilic than the parent compound. This enhanced water solubility reduces the ability of the metabolite to partition into biologic membranes and thus restricts the distribution of the metabolites to the various tissues, decreases the renal tubular and intestinal reabsorption of the metabolite(s), and ultimately promotes the excretion of the chemical by the urinary and biliary fecal routes.

Phase I and Phase II Biotransformation

A number of enzymes in animal organisms are capable of biotransforming lipid-soluble

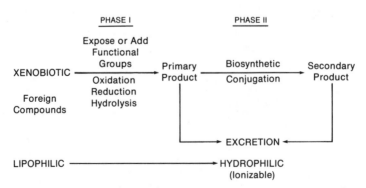

Figure 4–1. Integration of phase I and phase II biotransformation reactions.

xenobiotics in such a way as to render them more water soluble. These enzymic reactions are of two types: phase I reactions, which involve oxidation, reduction, and hydrolysis; and phase II reactions, which consist of conjugation or synthetic reactions. Although phase I reactions generally convert foreign compounds to derivatives that are more water soluble than the parent molecule, a prime function of these reactions is to add or expose functional groups (e.g., —OH, —SH, —NH$_2$, —COOH). These functional groups then permit the compound to undergo phase II reactions. Phase II reactions are biosynthetic reactions where the foreign compound or a phase I-derived metabolite is covalently linked to an endogenous molecule, producing a conjugate. In these cases, the endogenous moieties (e.g., glucuronic acid, sulfate) usually confer upon the lipophilic xenobiotic or its metabolite increased water solubility and the ability to undergo significant ionization at physiologic pH. These conjugating moieties are normally added to endogenous products to promote their secretion or transfer across hepatic, renal, and intestinal membranes. The transport mechanisms that have developed recognize the conjugating moiety. Thus, the excretion of conjugated xenobiotics is enhanced by their ability to participate in transport systems that have evolved for the conjugated products of endogenous molecules. The relationship between phase I and phase II reactions is summarized in Figure 4–1.

Organ and Cellular Location of Biotransformation

The enzymes or enzyme systems that catalyze the biotransformation of foreign compounds are localized mainly in the liver. This is not surprising, since a primary function of the liver is to receive and process chemicals absorbed from the gastrointestinal tract before they are distributed to other tissues. Liver receives all the blood that has perfused the splanchnic area, which contains nutrients and other foreign substances. Because of this the liver has developed the capacity to extract these substances readily from the blood and to modify chemically many of these substances before they are stored, secreted into bile, or released into the general circulation. Other tissues can also biotransform foreign compounds. Nearly every tissue tested has shown activity toward some foreign chemicals. However, they are limited with respect to the diversity of chemicals they can handle and, thus, their contribution to the overall biotransformation of xenobiotics is limited. However, biotransformation of a chemical within an extra-

LUNG   Skin

LIVER

KIDNEY   Gonads

INTESTINE
Gut Flora

Figure 4–2. Organs involved in biotransformation.

hepatic tissue may have an important toxicologic implication for that particular tissue (Figure 4–2).

Subcellular Localization of Biotransformation Enzymes

Biotransformation of foreign compounds within the liver is accomplished by several remarkable enzyme systems. These can chemically modify a wide variety of structurally diverse drugs and toxicants that enter the body through ingestion, inhalation, the skin, or by injection. The phase I enzymes, those that add or expose functional groups, are located primarily in the endoplasmic reticulum, a network of interconnected channels present in the cytoplasm of most cells. These enzymes are membrane bound, since the endoplasmic reticulum is basically a contiguous membrane composed of lipids and proteins. The presence of enzymes within a lipoprotein matrix is critical, since the lipophilic substrates will preferentially partition into the lipid membranes, the site of biotransformation.

When liver is removed and homogenized, the tubular endoplasmic reticulum breaks up and fragments of the membrane are sealed off (vesicle) to form microvesicles. These are referred to as microsomes, which can be isolated by differential centrifugation of the liver homogenate. If the supernatant fraction that results from centrifugation of the homogenate at 9000 × g (to remove nuclei, mitochondria, and lysosomes as well as unbroken cells and large membrane fragments) is subjected to centrifugation at 105,000 × g, a pellet highly enriched in microsomes is obtained The resulting supernatant, which contains a number of soluble enzymes, is referred to as the cytosol. This cytosol contains many of the enzymes of phase II biotransformation. Many of the important biotransformation enzymes are referred to as cytosolic or microsomal to indicate the subcellular location of the enzymes.

The microsomal enzymes that catalyze the phase I reactions were characterized primarily by their ability to metabolize drugs. Thus, much of the literature refers to these enzymes as the microsomal drug metabolizing enzymes. Indeed, the microsomal enzymes will convert drugs to more polar products, but they also act on innumerable chemicals. Therefore, the word biotransformation is preferred to drug metabolism, since it conveys the more universal nature of the reactions. In addition, it delineates the normal process of metabolism of endogenous nutrients from that of biotransformation of foreign chemicals.

Detoxication–Toxication

Inasmuch as both phase I and phase II enzymes convert foreign chemicals to forms that can be more readily excreted, they are often referred to as detoxication enzymes. However, it should be emphasized that biotransformation is not strictly related to detoxication. In a number of cases the metabolic products are more toxic than the parent compounds. This is particularly true for some chemical carcinogens, organophosphates, and a number of compounds that cause cell necrosis in the lung, liver, and kidney. In many instances a toxic metabolite can be isolated and identified. In other cases, highly reactive intermediates are formed during the biotransformation of a chemical. The term toxication or bioactivation is often used to indicate the enzymatic formation of reactive intermediates. These reactive intermediates are thought to initiate the events that ultimately result in cell death, chemically induced cancer, teratogenesis, and a number of other toxicities.

Characterization of Biotransformation

The biphasic nature of biotransformation is best presented by considering phase I and phase II reactions separately. These will be discussed with emphasis on the nature of the reaction, the cofactors required, a general example of the type of reactions catalyzed, the mechanism of the reaction, the predominant tissue and subcellular localization of the enzymes, and the importance of each enzyme in detoxication/toxication. However, it must be remembered that each xenobiotic is presented to a variety of the enzymes at any given time; for this reason the biotransformation of a foreign compound is one of an integrated approach.

The second consideration will focus on factors affecting biotransformation of xenobiotics. These include such factors as nutritional and disease status, age, route, dose, time of day/year, enzyme induction or inhibition, sex, and species differences as they relate to rates of biotransformation of foreign compounds and to toxicity.

Finally, the process of bioactivation will be discussed to explain its role in the toxicity of xenobiotics. Particular emphasis will be placed on the balance that exists between formation and detoxication of reactive intermediates.

PHASE I ENZYME REACTIONS

Characteristics of Microsomal Phase I Enzymes

Phase I is the predominant biotransformation pathway. These reactions may add functional groups by two oxidative enzymes systems: the cytochrome P-450 system (which is also referred to as the polysubstrate monooxygenase system, or the mixed function oxygenase [MFO] system) and the mixed-function amine oxidase (which is a flavin-monooxygenase). Basically, both enzyme systems add a hydroxyl moiety to the foreign substrate by mechanisms that will be outlined later.

Preexisting functional groups are exposed by a family of hydrolytic enzymes, esterases and amidases. The cleavage of the ester or amide bond, regardless of the remaining chemical structure, will produce two functional groups for further biotransformation, a carboxylic acid plus either an amine (from an amide) or an alcohol (from an ester).

Finally, a variety of oxidation-reduction systems can be considered part of the phase I enzymes since these are redox enzymes and often alter the oxidation state of a carbon to allow it to be more readily excreted or biotransformed by the phase II enzymes.

Cytochrome P-450

The most important enzyme systems involved in phase I reactions are the cytochrome P-450-containing monooxygenases. The cytochrome P-450 system is actually a coupled enzyme system composed of two enzymes: NADPH-cytochrome P-450 reductase, and a heme-containing enzyme, cytochrome P-450. As illustrated in Figure 4–3, these enzymes are embedded in the phospholipid matrix of the endoplasmic reticulum. The phospholipids play a crucial role in cytochrome P-450 reactions since they facilitate the interaction between the two enzymes. Accompanying this complex is another cytochrome called cytochrome b_5 and its associated reductase. The function of the cytochrome b_5 and cytochrome b_5 reductase in cytochrome P-450-mediated reactions is not clearly established.

The NADPH-cytochrome P-450 reductase has a preference for NADPH as its cofactor (Figure 4–4). It is a flavoprotein capable of transferring one or two electrons to cytochrome P-450. Cytochrome P-450 is actually a b-type cytochrome with a unique redox potential and spectral properties. It receives its name from the fact that when reduced cytochrome P-450 (Fe^{2+}) forms a ligand with carbon monoxide, the maximal absorbance of light occurs at 450 nm. This spectral

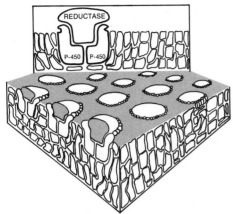

Figure 4–3. Schematic demonstration of the interaction of cytochrome P-450, reductase, and lipid. Note the low ratio of reductase to cytochrome P-450. (From Nebert, D. W.; Eisen, H. J.; Negishi, M.; Lang, M. A.; and Hjelmeland, L. M.: Genetic mechanisms controlling the induction of polysubstrate monooxygenase (P-450) activities. *Ann. Rev. Pharmacol. Toxicol.*, **21**:431–62, 1981.)

property is present only when the cytochrome P-450 is intact and catalytically functional. When denatured, cytochrome P-450 loses its unique spectral peak at 450 nm and produces only a 420-nm absorbance maximum, similar to other hemoproteins.

Components of the Cytochrome P-450 System
In early studies it was noted that treatment of rats and mice with certain chemicals produced a shift in the spectral maximum of cytochrome P-450. This shift was to 448 nm, and thus the cytochrome became known as cytochrome P-448. Other evidence for different forms came

from the fact that cytochrome P-450 and cytochrome P-448 displayed different substrate specificity or they biotransformed similar substrates at different rates.

These differences prompted attempts to isolate and characterize the cytochrome P-450 components. Isolation was accomplished by solubilizing the microsomes with ionic and nonionic detergents and stabilizing the hemoproteins with sulfhydryl agents, glycerol, and metal chelators. The solubilized microsomes can then be resolved into their components by column chromatography. The resolved components are then characterized by electrophoresis, immunochemical analysis, peptide mapping, and amino acid analysis. When the cytochrome P-450 enzymes are recombined with NADPH-cytochrome P-450 reductase in the presence of the natural microsomal phospholipids or dilauroyl phosphatidyl choline, they reconstitute to form a complex capable of the biotransformation reactions observed with microsomes.

These studies provided evidence for more then two forms of cytochrome P-450. To date at least ten forms of cytochrome P-450 have been isolated from rat liver microsomes. These differ in both the structure of the polypeptide chain and the specificity of the reactions they catalyze. The cytochrome P-450 composition of liver microsomes is altered by treatment of animals with different chemicals. In addition, the types and amounts of cytochrome P-450 vary with species, organ, age, health, sex, stress, and chemical exposure.

In contrast to cytochrome P-450, only one NADPH cytochrome P-450 reductase has been isolated from a single source. Its concentration is usually one-tenth to one-thirtieth that of cyto-

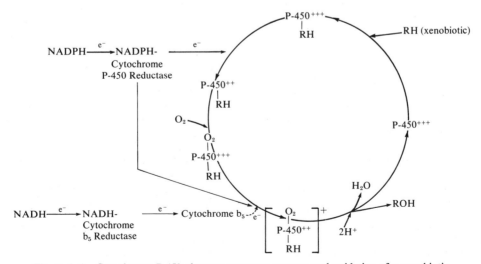

Figure 4–4. Cytochrome P-450 electron transport systems and oxidation of a xenobiotic.

chrome P-450. Therefore, this enzyme must mediate the reduction of the many different forms of cytochrome P-450 (Figure 4–3). The composition of the phospholipids has received considerable attention. Dilauroylphosphatidylcholine can be substituted for the natural phospholipids.

Substrate Interaction. In some instances, substrates for cytochrome P-450 can be tentatively identified by their ability to interact with the cytochrome P-450 and produce characteristic difference spectra. Difference spectra are measured by recording the absorbance differences between the cytochrome alone and the cytochrome with the substrate. Most substrates interact with cytochrome P-450 to produce a type I spectrum, with a peak at 385 to 390 nm and a trough at 420. The opposite spectrum (trough at 390 nm with a peak at 420 nm) is produced by reverse type I substrates. Both type I and reverse type I substrates are believed to bind at or near the catalytic site of cytochrome P-450. Type I substrates (e.g., cyclohexane) cause a conversion of low-spin ferricytochrome P-450 to the high-spin form, whereas reverse type I substrates (e.g., aliphatic alcohols) cause the opposite conversion (i.e., high spin to low spin). Other compounds, especially those containing a nitrogen atom such as octylamine, produce a type II spectrum, characterized by a peak at 425 to 435 nm and a trough at 390 to 405 nm. These compounds are thought to bind directly to the heme iron.

Microsomal Electron Transfer. In reactions catalyzed by this enzyme system the substrate (RH) combines with the oxidized form of cytochrome P-450 (Fe^{3+}) to form a substrate-cytochrome P-450 complex (Figure 4–4). This complex then accepts an electron from NADPH (via NADPH-cytochrome P-450 reductase) which reduces the iron in the cytochrome P-450 heme moiety to the Fe^{2+} state. The reduced (Fe^{2+}) substrate-cytochrome P-450 complex combines with molecular oxygen, which then accepts another electron from NADPH. In a series of steps that are not completely understood, both electrons are thought to be transferred to molecular oxygen. The resulting oxygen species is highly reactive and unstable. One atom of this reactive oxygen is introduced into the substrate, while the other is reduced to water. The oxygenated substrate then dissociates, regenerating the oxidized form of cytochrome P-450. Carbon monoxide is a strong inhibitor of cytochrome P-450-catalyzed reactions because it competes with oxygen for binding to the reduced cytochrome P-450.

Oxidative Reactions Catalyzed by the Cytochrome P-450 System. Examples of the reactions catalyzed by the microsomal cytochrome P-450 system are shown in Table 4–1. The participation of cytochrome P-450 in a reaction can be established by several criteria, some of which are outlined in Table 4–2. First, the *in vivo* and *in vitro* reaction rates can be altered by the use of inducing or inhibiting agents, which will be discussed later. Second, the demonstration that the substrates interact with the microsomal cytochrome P-450 to produce difference spectra indicates a probable substrate. Finally, the use of isolated and reconstituted cytochrome P-450 systems to show that the reaction is specific for these components is essential.

Aliphatic hydroxylation of the ω-carbon (CH_3 group) or ω-1 (next to last carbon) occurs with compounds such as *n*-hexane, *n*-pentane, and compounds that contain aliphatic side chains (i.e., pentobarbital). The reaction occurs as a result of the insertion of an oxygen atom into a carbon-hydrogen bond, either directly or following hydrogen abstraction. *Aromatic hydroxylation* is also a common reaction. The hydroxyl is thought to be incorporated by one of two mechanisms: One mechanism involves direct insertion of an oxygen atom into the carbon-hydrogen bond. A more prevalent mechanism involves addition of the oxygen to the carbon-carbon double bond to produce an arene oxide intermediate, which then rearranges to form an aromatic hydroxyl compound. Depending on the ring substituents, the latter reaction leads to intramolecular migration and retention of groups attached to the two carbons being hydroxylated. These arene oxide intermediates are important in determining the possible toxicity of aromatic compounds. *Alkene epoxidation* proceeds via cytochrome P-450-mediated reaction analogous to arene oxide formation. The oxygen is added to the carbon-carbon double bond to produce an epoxide intermediate. Both the arene oxides and aliphalic epoxides are capable of being hydrolyzed by another microsomal enzyme, epoxide hydrolase to dihydrodiol products.

Oxidative dealkylation proceeds via a cytochrome P-450-mediated aliphatic hydroxylation. The alpha carbon of the alkyl group attached to an N, O, or S atom is hydroxylated by the insertion of an oxygen atom into its carbon-hydrogen bond. The resulting hydroxylalkyl moiety adjacent to the electronegative N, O, or S is unstable and decomposes into an aldehyde or ketone (the alkyl moiety) and a metabolite containing a free amino, hydroxyl, or sulfhydryl group.

Oxidative deamination can occur for xenobiotics that contain an aliphatic moiety with a primary amino group. The reaction is similar to that of *N*-dealkylation. In this case, the alpha carbon adjacent to the primary amine is hydrox-

Table 4–1. EXAMPLE OF THE GENERAL TYPE OF OXIDATION REACTIONS CATALYZED BY THE CYTOCHROME P-450-CONTAINING MONOOXYGENASES*

REACTION	EXAMPLE
Aliphatic hydroxylation	$R—CH_2—CH_2—CH_2 \longrightarrow R—CH_2—CHOH—CH_3$
Aromatic hydroxylation	$R—\langle\bigcirc\rangle \longrightarrow R—\langle\bigcirc\rangle—OH$
Epoxidation	$R—CH{=}CH—R' \longrightarrow R—\overset{\displaystyle O}{CH{-}CH}—R'$
N-, O-, or S-dealkylation	$R—(N, O, S)—CH_3 \longrightarrow R—(NH_2, OH, SH) + CH_2O$
Deamination	$R—CH_2—NH_2 \longrightarrow R—\overset{O}{\overset{\|}{C}}—H + NH_3$
N-hydroxylation	$R—NH—\overset{O}{\overset{\|}{C}}—CH_3 \longrightarrow R—NOH—\overset{O}{\overset{\|}{C}}—CH_3$
Sulfoxidation	$R—S—R \longrightarrow R—\underset{O}{\overset{\|}{S}}—R'$
Desulfuration	$R_1R_2\overset{S}{\overset{\|}{P}}—X \longrightarrow R_1R_2\overset{O}{\overset{\|}{P}}—X + S$
Oxidative Dehalogenation	$R—\overset{X}{\underset{H}{\overset{\|}{\underset{\|}{C}}}}—H \longrightarrow R—\overset{X}{\underset{H}{\overset{\|}{\underset{\|}{C}}}}—OH \longrightarrow R—\overset{O}{\overset{\|}{C}}—H + HX$

* X = halogen.

ylated and the resulting unstable intermediate abstracts a hydride ion to form ammonia and the oxidized alpha carbon rearranges to an aldehyde or ketone.

Oxidation of sulfur and *nitrogen* or *desulfuration* also occur by the addition of oxygen via cytochrome P-450 to the unshared electron pair on the sulfur or nitrogen atom. In the case of nitrogen, the product often is a hydroxylamine that may be further oxidized. The addition of the oxygen to sulfur in a carbon-sulfur-carbon bond forms a stable sulfoxide metabolite. If the sulfur is in the form of a carbon-sulfur or phosphorus-

Table 4–2. CRITERIA FOR CYTOCHROME P-450-MEDIATED BIOTRANSFORMATION

1. Enzymatic activity increased by induction
2. Enzymatic activity decreased by inhibitors
3. Substrates produce characteristic difference spectra
4. Enzymatic activity reconstituted with individual purified components

sulfur double bond, the oxygen attaches to the double-bonded sulfur, which then converts to a resonance form in which the oxygen has a full negative charge. This oxygen atom then forms a three-component cyclic intermediate by attacking the carbon/phosphorus attached to the sulfur. The cyclic structure collapses to yield inorganic sulfur and a carbonyl or phosphoryl metabolite. In total, the reaction is considered a substitution reaction.

In *oxidative dehalogenation,* the activated oxygen does not attack the carbon-halogen bond, but inserts at the carbon-hydrogen bond. The resultant product is an unstable aliphatic halohydrin, which undergoes dehalogenation. Thus, the carbon-halogen bond is broken during the rearrangement phase of the reaction and is not the site of attack of the activated oxygen. If the carbon contained a single halogen, the resulting product would be an aldehyde. If it contained two halogens, the dihalohydrin moiety would rearrange to an acid halide. Both the aldehyde and acid halide are unstable and can react

Table 4–3. REDUCTIVE BIOTRANSFORMATION BY THE CYTOCHROME P-450 SYSTEM

REACTION	EXAMPLE
Azo reduction	$R—N=N—R' \longrightarrow R—NH_2 + R'NH_2$
Aromatic nitro reduction	$R—\langle\bigcirc\rangle—NO_2 \longrightarrow R—\langle\bigcirc\rangle—NH_2$
Reductive dehalogenation	$R—\overset{\overset{\textstyle X}{\mid}}{\underset{\underset{\textstyle X}{\mid}}{C}}—X \longrightarrow R—\overset{\overset{\textstyle X}{\mid}}{\underset{\underset{\textstyle X}{\mid}}{C}}—H + HX$

nonenzymatically with functional groups on biologic macromolecules.

Microsomal-Mediated Reductive Metabolism. Even though the microsomal cytochrome P-450 is classed as an oxygenase, it also catalyzes the *reductive biotransformation* of certain xenobiotics (Table 4–3). These reactions proceed most readily under conditions of low oxygen tension. Owing to the transfer to reducing equivalents in cytochrome P-450-catalyzed reactions, certain xenobiotic substrates may accept one or two of these electrons. In effect, the substrate rather than molecular oxygen accepts the electrons and is reduced. In fact, oxygen acts as an inhibitor of these reactions since it competes for the reducing equivalents. The classic inhibitors of the cytochrome P-450 system are also inhibitors of these reductive reactions since they either compete for the substrate binding sites or complex with the iron in the heme and thus stop electron flow.

The nitro or azo groups are reduced enzymatically in much the same manner as they would be reduced chemically. By accepting reducing equivalents (hydride ions), the oxidation state of the nitrogen is decreased. The nitro group progresses in sequential steps to a nitrone, a hydroxylamine, and finally an amine. The nitrogen-nitrogen double bond of azo compounds is progressively reduced until it is cleaved into two amine metabolites. Besides the reduction of azo and nitro compounds, other chemical groups are now known to be reduced by this system, such as arene oxides, *N*-oxides, and alkyl halides. Both the flavoprotein enzyme, NADPH-cytochrome P-450 reductase, and the terminal oxidase, cytochrome P-450, are involved in these reductions. The very low redox potential, broad substrate specificity, and strong ligand binding of these systems allow the donation of electrons to electron-accepting xenobiotics, which results in a reduction rather than the predominant oxidative biotransformation.

This route of biotransformation may detoxify a xenobiotic, but it often results in more toxic products or reactive intermediates. For example, numerous nitro compounds undergo reduction to amino derivatives, which can then be oxidized to toxic *N*-hydroxyl metabolites. Polyhalogenated alkanes accept electrons to become radical anions that fragment into carbon-centered free radicals upon cleavage of the carbon-halogen bond. Carbon tetrachloride and halothane ($CF_3CHBrCl$) are two classic examples of cytochrome P-450-catalyzed reductive bioactivation to free radical intermediates.

Intestinal microflora are also known to mediate the reduction of a number of chemicals, particularly those with azo and nitro groups. These microbes have virtually all the enzymatic machinery to mimic the cytochrome P-450-mediated reactions observed in mammalian systems. Owing to the anaerobic environment and the high concentration of chemical seen upon ingestion or biliary excretion, these microbes can have a substantial effect on the *in vivo* biotransformation of xenobiotics. These microbes may also further modify metabolites of xenobiotics that were produced by hepatic cytochrome P-450. In some instances, a new reductive metabolite may be reabsorbed and further processed by hepatic enzymes.

Importance of the Cytochrome P-450 System. The cytochrome P-450-containing monooxygenases have been found in the hepatic endoplasmic reticulum of every animal species so far examined. The wide distribution of this enzyme system in various organs of a single species and among the various animal species, coupled with its versatility in catalyzing the introduction of oxygen atoms into foreign compounds of widely different structure, makes it, without question, the most important group of enzymes involved in the biotransformation of foreign compounds.

Amine Oxidase

Another oxidative enzyme that is rapidly gaining recognition as an important contributor to

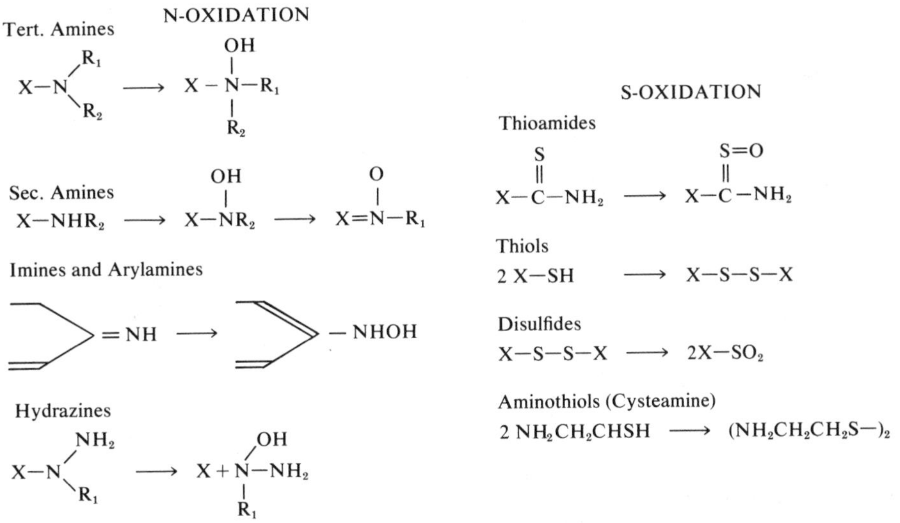

N-OXIDATION

Tert. Amines

$$X-N\begin{smallmatrix}R_1\\[2pt]\\R_2\end{smallmatrix} \longrightarrow X-\underset{\underset{R_2}{|}}{\overset{\overset{OH}{|}}{N}}-R_1$$

Sec. Amines

$$X-NHR_2 \longrightarrow X-\underset{}{\overset{\overset{OH}{|}}{N}}R_2 \longrightarrow X=\overset{\overset{O}{|}}{N}-R_1$$

Imines and Arylamines

$=NH \longrightarrow$ $-NHOH$

Hydrazines

$$X-N\begin{smallmatrix}NH_2\\[2pt]\\R_1\end{smallmatrix} \longrightarrow X+\underset{\underset{R_1}{|}}{\overset{\overset{OH}{|}}{N}}-NH_2$$

S-OXIDATION

Thioamides

$$X-\overset{\overset{S}{\|}}{C}-NH_2 \longrightarrow X-\overset{\overset{S=O}{\|}}{C}-NH_2$$

Thiols

$$2\,X-SH \longrightarrow X-S-S-X$$

Disulfides

$$X-S-S-X \longrightarrow 2X-SO_2$$

Aminothiols (Cysteamine)

$$2\,NH_2CH_2CHSH \longrightarrow (NH_2CH_2CH_2S-)_2$$

Figure 4–5. Oxidations catalyzed by the flavin-containing monooxygenase.

phase I biotransformation is an enzyme historically referred to as mixed-function amine oxidase. This FAD-flavoprotein is present in the endoplasmic reticulum and is capable of oxidizing nucleophilic nitrogen and sulfur atoms. Thus, it is not solely an amine oxidase and should be termed a microsomal flavin-containing monooxygenase. This enzyme activity is exceptionally high in humans and pigs while low in rats. Flavin-containing monooxygenase competes with the cytochrome P-450 system in the oxidation of amines. It converts tertiary amines to amine oxides, secondary amines to hydroxyl amines and nitrones, and primary amines to hydroxylamines and oximes (Figure 4–5). The oxidation of nucleophilic divalent sulfur atoms by the flavin-containing monooxygenase is an interesting feature. Further studies are necessary to determine its role in the biotransformation of other sulfur-containing chemicals, but thiocarbamides and thioureas are already known substrates.

It is believed that the endogenous substrate for the flavin-containing monooxygenase is cysteamine, which is oxidized to cystamine. The endogenous cystamine-cysteamine balance may then be controlled by this enzyme, and it thus may be involved in disulfide generation during peptide synthesis.

The flavin-containing monoxygenase is not under the same regulatory control as cytochrome P-450. In fact, it is repressed rather than induced by phenobarbital or 3-methylcholanthrene treatment. It appears the concentration of the enzyme is regulated by steroid sex hormones, with testosterone decreasing and progesterone increasing its concentration. The role

the flavin-containing monooxygenase has in other biotransformation processes and the toxicity of xenobiotics is still being elucidated.

Epoxide Hydrolase

An important hydrolytic enzyme thought to be located in close proximity to the microsomal cytochrome P-450 monooxygenases is epoxide hydrolase, formerly known as epoxide hydrase or epoxide hydratase. The enzyme catalyzes the hydration of arene oxides and aliphatic epoxides to their corresponding *trans*-1,2-dihydrodiols (Figure 4–6). An important toxicologic aspect of the reaction is that the corresponding diols are less electrophilic and, therefore, less chemically reactive than the epoxides. Arene oxides (epoxides of aromatic compounds) are generally unstable and rearrange to the corresponding phenol. The phenol is then available to participate in various phase II conjugation reactions.

Epoxide hydrolase has been found in a wide variety of tissues, including liver, testis, ovary, lung, kidney, skin, intestine, colon, spleen, thymus, brain, and heart. Its distribution among tissues with multiple cell types is heterogenous. For example, the pulmonary clara cells possess

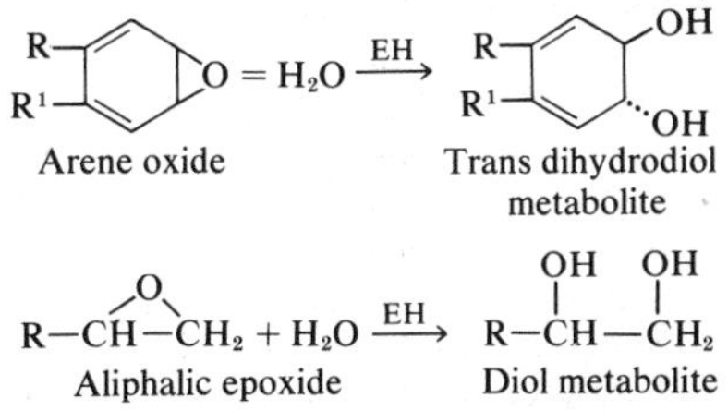

Arene oxide   Trans dihydrodiol metabolite

Aliphatic epoxide   Diol metabolite

Figure 4–6. Dihydrodiol formation catalyzed by epoxide hydrolase (EH).

three to four times more epoxide hydrolase activity than the alveolar type I cells. These are also the two cell types of the lung that contain the majority of the cytochrome P-450-dependent monooxygenase activity. From the nature of the reaction catalyzed by epoxide hydrolase, it is not surprising that the bulk of the activity is located in the endoplasmic reticulum of the various cell types that possess the enzyme. This close proximity to the site of formation of its substrates suggests that epoxide hydrolase may have evolved as an important means of detoxifying arene oxides and aliphatic epoxides.

A distinct cytosolic epoxide hydrolase exists in a number of animal tissues. This activity appears to be high in tissues from mice and rabbits, but low in rats. The cytosolic and microsomal hydrolase enzymes are immunologically distinct and have different substrate specificities. Their role in detoxication of various epoxides is under investigation.

Available evidence indicates that epoxide hydrolase-catalyzed hydration of oxides occurs by activation of water to a nucleophilic species. The resulting nucleophilic species attacks the least hindered carbon atom from the side opposite to the oxide ring. Consequently, ring opening is directed away from the hydroxylation and the resulting diols have a *trans* configuration.

In general, epoxide hydrolase is considered a detoxication enzyme, since it inactivates a number of highly reactive oxides that have been implicated in tissue injury (bromobenzene 3,4-oxide) and mutagenicity (benzo[a]pyrene 4,5-oxide). However, the hydration of benzo(a)pyrene 7,8-oxide by epoxide hydrolase can be considered an activation reaction. The diol derivative (*trans*-7,8-dihydroxy-7,8-dihydrobenzo[a]pyrene) can be epoxidated by the cytochrome P-450 system to yield the highly reactive and carcinogenic species benzo(a)pyrene 7,8-dihydrodiol-9,10-oxide. This, and other reactive diol epoxides of polycyclic aromatic hydrocarbons, are poor substrates for epoxide hydrolase. Therefore, they cannot be readily deactivated and, thus, interact with critical tissue macromolecules.

Microsomal epoxide hydrolase activity is regulated by a number of factors. In rats, epoxide hydrolase activity in the liver becomes detectable at about four days before birth and then steadily increases to adult levels. Its activity in liver of male rats is about twice that in female rats. Inducers of the microsomal mixed-function oxygenases also induce epoxide hydrolase activity. No specific inducer has been identified. Several alcohols, ketones, and imidazoles stimulate microsomal epoxide hydrolase activity *in vitro*. Similarly, certain epoxides are known to inhibit

$$R-\overset{\overset{\displaystyle O}{\|}}{C}-O-R' + H_2O \rightarrow R-\overset{\overset{\displaystyle O}{\|}}{C}-OH + HOR'$$
Ester hydrolysis

$$R-\overset{\overset{\displaystyle O}{\|}}{C}-\underset{\underset{\displaystyle R}{|}}{N}-R' + H_2O \rightarrow R-\overset{\overset{\displaystyle O}{\|}}{C}-OH + HNR'R''$$
Amide hydrolysis

$$R-\overset{\overset{\displaystyle O}{\|}}{C}-S-R' + H_2O \rightarrow R-\overset{\overset{\displaystyle O}{\|}}{C}-OH + HSR'$$
Thioester hydrolysis

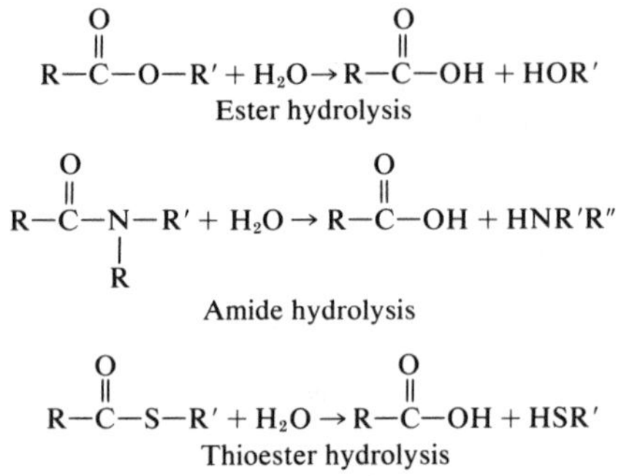

Figure 4–7. Hydrolytic biotransformation reactions.

the enzyme. The most widely used are 1,1,1-trichloropropane oxide and cyclohexene oxide.

Esterases and Amidases

Mammalian tissues contain a large number of nonspecific esterases and amidases that can hydrolyze ester and amide linkages in foreign compounds. This hydrolytic cleavage of ester and amide linkages liberates carboxyl groups and an alcohol function in the case of esters and an amine or NH_3 in the case of amides (Figure 4–7). These carboxyl, alcohol, and amine groups may undergo a variety of conjugations (phase II reactions). In certain cases even thioesters can be hydrolyzed by this group of enzymes.

As summarized in Table 4–4 esterases may be broadly categorized into four main classes: (1) arylesterases, which preferentially hydrolyze aromatic esters (ArCOOR'; Ar = aromatic), (2) carboxylesterases, which hydrolyze aliphatic esters (RCH_2COOR'), (3) acetylesterases, in which the acid moiety of the ester is acetic acid (CH_3COOR'), and (4) cholinesterases, which hydrolyze esters in which the alcohol moiety is choline $(CH_3)_3N^+$—CH_2—CH_2—OOCR). It should be noted that there is considerable overlap in substrate specificity among these classes of esterases. For example, a carboxyl esterase may hydrolyze an aromatic ester at a detectable rate. Therefore, these classifications should not be considered to be absolute.

Table 4–4.   SIMPLIFIED CLASSIFICATION OF ESTERASES

ESTERASE	PREFERRED SUBSTRATES
A-esterases (arylesterases)	Aromatic ester
B-esterases (carboxylesterases)	Aliphatic ester
C-esterases (acetylesterases)	Acetyl ester
Cholinesterases	Choline esters

In general, enzymatic hydrolysis of amides occurs more slowly than with esters. Enzyme specificity for the various amides may be partially responsible for this slower rate of biotransformation. However, electronic factors are also important. Thus, substituent groups in primary, secondary, and tertiary amides that have electron-withdrawing properties will cause a weakening of the amide bond, making it more susceptible to enzymatic hydrolysis.

The esterases/amidases are both cytosolic and microsomal enzymes. The cytosolic esterases are usually associated with a specific reaction, such as acetyl cholinesterase and pseudocholinesterase, whereas the microsomal-associated esterases handle a diverse array of xenobiotic esters.

The esterases/amidases can be inhibited when substrates bind tightly to the active sites or when the resulting products are very reactive. This is the case with organophosphates, where metabolites bind to the active site following hydrolysis.

There is evidence for considerable genetic influence in certain of the esterase enzymes. For example, pseudocholinesterase detoxifies many of the aliphatic ester/amide muscle relaxants. However, the subunit makeup, enzymatic activity, and sensitivity to inhibition are under genetic control. Thus extremes of high/low enzyme activity and resistance/susceptibility to inhibition are known.

Alcohol, Aldehyde, Ketone Oxidation-Reduction Systems

Aldehydes, ketones, and alcohols are functional groups that occur from the oxidation of carbon or the hydrolysis of ester linkages. In addition, they are frequent functional groups that appear in drugs and other xenobiotics. These functional groups are often further biotransformed in the body by oxidation or reduction. The principal enzymatic systems involved in this redox reaction, which are listed in Figure 4–8, are: alcohol dehydrogenase, aldehyde reductase, ketone reductase, and a variety of aldehyde oxidizing systems (such as aldehyde dehydrogenase and aldehyde oxidase). These soluble enzymes are present in a number of mammalian tissues. NAD^+ is frequently the cofactor for oxidation and NADH or NADPH is the cofactor for reduction. Since alcohol, aldehyde, or ketone moieties often impart pharmacologic properties, the oxidation or reduction of these groups is a means of detoxication. However, in some cases more reactive functional groups may be produced that can lead to toxicity (i.e., oxidation of alcohols to reactive aldehydes).

One of the most important enzymes of this group is alcohol dehydrogenase, which oxidizes

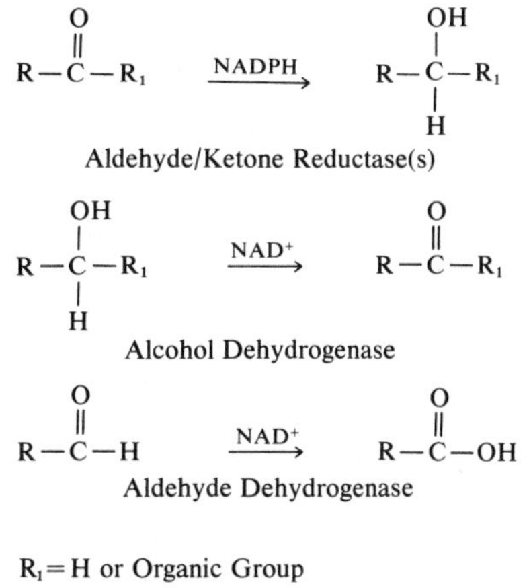

Figure 4–8. Alcohol, aldehyde, ketone oxidation-reduction systems.

ethanol ($CH_3CH_2OH + NAD^+ \rightarrow CH_3CHO + NADH + H^+$). This cytosolic enzyme, located primarily in liver, is responsible for the biotransformation of ethanol. The resulting acetaldehyde is then oxidized to acetic acid by aldehyde dehydrogenase. Some alcohol dehydrogenase activity is associated with the endoplasmic reticulum. Other alcohols may also act as substrates for alcohol dehydrogenase, as may polyalcohols (methanol, ethylene glycol, and allyl alcohol).

While most of the alcohol dehydrogenase reactions detoxify the alcoholic substance, there are cases where the product is more toxic. Such is the case with the oxidation of methanol and ethylene glycol to their ultimate metabolic products formate and oxalate, respectively. In addition, the aldehyde products have also been found to react under physiologic conditions with primary amine groups to form Schiff's bases. Such interactions often alter the functional ability of that macromolecule. Pyrazole and certain of its derivatives inhibit alcohol dehydrogenase.

Aldehyde dehydrogenase oxidizes aldehydes to carboxylic acids with NAD^+ as the cofactor. There are two major types of aldehyde dehydrogenases in mammals. One specifically oxidizes formaldehyde that is complexed with glutathione and is called formaldehyde dehydrogenase. The other oxidizes free aldehydes and has broad substrate specificity. This latter enzyme is the aldehyde dehydrogenase involved in most xenobiotic aldehyde oxidation. Isozymes of this enzyme are found in hepatic cytosol, mitochondria, and microsomes with characteristic specificities. For example, acetaldehyde is mainly oxidized by the mitochondrial enzyme, whereas xenobiotic aldehydes are oxidized mainly by the cytosolic and microsomal dehydrogenases.

It is the inhibition of the aldehyde dehydrogenase that usually results in toxicity of xenobiotics requiring this route of biotransformation. When *in vivo* inhibitors of aldehyde dehydrogenase activity (such as disulfiram and cyanamide) are present, the concentration of the aldehyde increases and, hence, is more likely to react with nucleophiles such as endogenous amines.

Aldehyde and ketones can be reduced to alcohols by aldehyde/ketone reductases. These are soluble enzymes that typically use NADPH as the source of reducing equivalents. Since cells typically have an overall potential for oxidation, with a high ratio of NAD^+ to NADH, the selective use of NADPH, which is present in excess of $NADP^+$, allows for the conversion of lipid-soluble carbonyls to less reactive and soluble alcohols in an oxidizing environment.

PHASE II ENZYME REACTIONS

The phase II biotransformation reactions are biosynthetic and thus require energy to drive the reaction. This is accomplished by activating the cofactors, or in one case the substrate, to high-energy intermediates. Since the cofactors are activated either directly or indirectly with ATP, the energy status of the organ is important in determining cofactor availability.

Glucuronosyltransferases

Glucuronidation represents one of the major conjugation phase II reactions in the conversion of both exogenous and endogenous compounds to polar, water-soluble compounds. The resulting glucuronides are eliminated from the body in the urine or bile. The widespread species occurrence, the broad range of substrates that are accepted, and the diversity in the nature of acceptor groups make conjugation with glucuronic acid qualitatively and quantitatively the most important conjugation reaction.

The enzyme that carries out the reaction is uridine diphosphate glucuronosyltransferase or UDP-glucuronosyltransferase. It catalyzes the interaction between the high-energy nucleotide, UDP-glucuronic acid (UDP-GA, Figure 4–9), and the functional group on the acceptor molecule (the substrate or aglycone). Glucuronosyltransferase activity is localized in the endoplasmic reticulum of numerous tissues, whereas most phase II enzymes are cytosolic enzymes. Quantitatively, the liver is the most important tissue, but activity is also present in the kidney, intestine, skin, brain, and spleen. The location of glucuronosyltransferase in the microsomal membrane is important physiologically, since it may have direct access to the

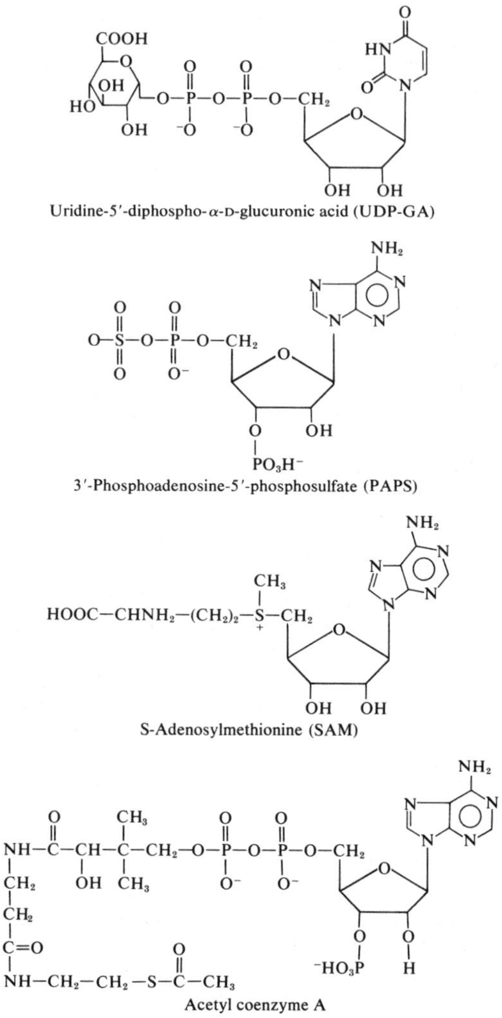

Figure 4–9. High-energy cofactors of phase II enzymes.

products formed by the action of microsomal cytochrome P-450. Thus, one can envision a highly integrated system within the microsomal membrane that results in the sequestration of highly lipophilic compounds, the addition or unmasking of a functional group, and the conjugation of this functional group with the highly polar glucuronic acid moiety.

There are several distinct forms of UDP-glucuronosyltransferase. Enzyme heterogeneity explains in part the differential increases in enzyme activities toward different aglycones following treatment with known microsomal enzyme inducing agents, differential decreases in activities with respect to inhibition, and species differences that lead to defects in glucuronidation of only certain classes of glucuronic acid acceptors.

Table 4–5. EXAMPLES OF THE DIFFERENT CLASSES OF GLUCURONIDE CONJUGATES*†

| TYPES OF GLUCURONIDES* | ACCEPTOR | |
	Functional Group	*Example*
O-Glucuronide		
—C—O—G	Alcohol	
	Aliphatic	Trichloroethanol
	Alicyclic	Hexobarbital
	Benzylic	Methylphenylcarbinol
	Phenolic	Estrone
—C—O—G (with =O)	Carboxylic acid	
	Aliphatic	α-Ethylhexanoic acid
	Aromatic	*o*-Aminobenzoic acid
—CH=C—O—G	α,β-Unsaturated ketone	Progesterone
—N—O—G	*N*-Hydroxy	*N*-Acetyl-*N*-phenyl-hydroxylamine
N-Glucuronide		
—O—C—N—G (with ‖O, H)	Carbamate	Meprobamate
Ar—N—G (with H)	Arylamine	2-Naphthylamine
$(R)_3$—N^+—G	Aliphatic tertiary amine	Tripelennamine
R—SO_2—N—G (with H)	Sulfonamide	Sulfadimethoxine
S-Glucuronide		
Ar—S—G	Aryl thiol	Thiophenol
—C—S—G (with ‖S)	Dithiocarbamic acid	*N,N*-Diethyldithio-carbamic acid
C-Glucuronide		
—C—G	1,3-Dicarbonyl system	Phenylbutazone

* G = glucuronic acid.
† Modified from Jakoby, W. E. (ed.): *Enzymatic Basis of Detoxication,* Vol. 2. Academic Press, Inc., New York, 1980.

The number of distinct forms of the enzyme is unknown at this time. Purification studies have revealed the presence of at least three forms in rat liver. One form shows preferential catalytic activity toward such hydroxylated substrates as 4-nitrophenol, 2-aminophenol, and 1-naphthol. However, it is only partially active toward the glucuronidation of morphine and chloramphenicol and is inactive toward testosterone and bilirubin. Clearly, additional studies on the protein chemistry of purified glucuronosyltransferases are needed to establish structural heterogeneity.

Numerous functional groups present in both foreign and endogenous compounds that undergo conjugation with glucuronic acid are listed in Table 4–5. These include aliphatic and aro-

matic alcohols, carboxyl acids, primary and secondary aromatic and aliphatic amines, and free sulfhydryl groups. These form *O*-, *N*-, and *S*-glucuronides, respectively. Certain nucleophilic carbon atoms have also been shown to form *C*-glucuronides.

During the conjugation reaction, the UDP-glucuronic acid cofactor, which is in the α configuration, undergoes inversion leading to glucuronides that have a β configuration. It is important to note that glucuronidation contributes a carboxyl group, which exists primarily in the ionized form at physiologic pH (Figure 4–10). This group promotes excretion not only because of the water solubility it confers, but also because it can participate in biliary and renal or-

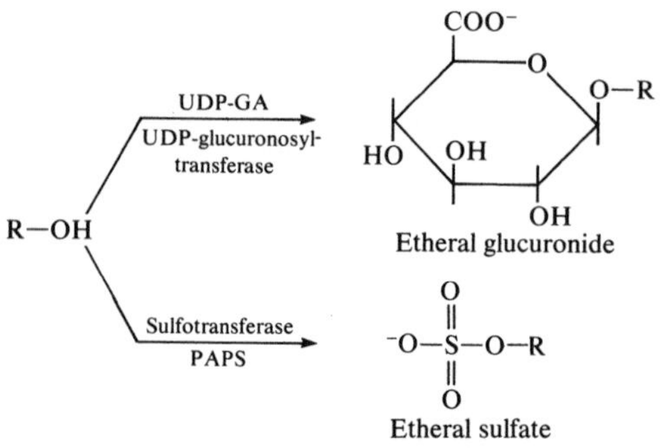

Figure 4–10. Glucuronidation and sulfation of a hydroxyl functional group.

ganic anion transport systems that recognize this group.

Glucuronides are excreted from the body in either the bile or urine depending on the size of the aglycone (Table 4–6). If this moiety has a molecular weight below about 250, the glucuronide will be cleared by renal tubular organic acid secretion into urine. If the structure has a molecular weight greater than 350, the conjugate is often secreted into bile. From 250 to 350 molecular weight, the conjugate may be excreted by either pathway.

Glucuronide conjugates of xenobiotics are substrates for β-glucuronidase. Although present in the lysozomes of some mammalian tissues, considerable β-glucuronidase activity is present in the intestinal microflora. Thus, this enzyme can release the aglycone, which can be reabsorbed and enter a cycle called the enterohepatic recirculation. Compounds involved in this cycle tend to have a longer lifetime in the body and may undergo more extensive biotransformation before being eliminated. N-glucuronides are more slowly hydrolyzed by β-glucuronidase than O- or S-glucuronides. Glucuronides can also be hydrolyzed in the presence of acid or bases (e.g., 0.2 N HCl or NaOH), an important point that must be considered when attempting to extract glucuronides from a biologic matrix.

Table 4–6. PREFERRED ROUTE OF EXCRETION OF CONJUGATES OF XENOBIOTICS

Glucuronides	<250 M.W.—kidney
	>350 M.W.—bile
Sulfates	Kidney
Glutathione conjugates	Bile
Acetylated conjugates	None
Amino acid conjugates	Kidney
Mercapturic acids	Kidney

Because of the susceptibility of certain glucuronides to enzymatic and chemical degradation, glucuronides may serve to transport potentially reactive compounds from the liver to the target tissue. The most widely cited examples are N-glucuronides of N-hydroxy-arylamines. These derivatives have been implicated in bladder cancer produced by 2-naphthylamine, 4-aminobiphenyl, and related compounds. It is proposed that these arylamines undergo N-hydroxylation in the liver, with the subsequent formation of the N-glucuronide of the N-hydroxyarylamine. The N-glucuronides, which accumulate in the urine of the bladder, are unstable in acidic pH, and thus are hydrolyzed to the corresponding unstable carcinogenic N-hydroxylamine.

Sulfotransferase

In mammals, an important conjugation reaction for hydroxyl groups is sulfation. This reaction is catalyzed by the sulfotransferases, a group of soluble enzymes found primarily in liver, kidney, intestinal tract, and lungs. Their primary function is to transfer inorganic sulfate to the hydroxyl group present on phenols and aliphatic alcohols. The resulting products are referred to as sulfate esters or ethereal sulfates (Figure 4–10). In addition, sulfation of aromatic amines and hydroxylamines to form the corresponding sulfamate and N-O-sulfates is occasionally seen.

As a detoxication process, sulfation is considered an effective means of decreasing the pharmacologic and toxicologic activity of compounds. The products of this reaction are ionized organic sulfates and, therefore, are more readily excreted than the parent compound or hydroxylated metabolite. In addition, if the hydroxyl or amine function is important in expression of the toxicologic activity, sulfation would mask this functional group and prevent its interaction with some critical cellular component. Numerous low-molecular-weight endogenous compounds, such as catecholamines, hydroxy steroids, and bile acids, are known to undergo sulfation.

There are four classes of sulfotransferases involved in detoxication processes (Table 4–7). Aryl sulfotransferase conjugates phenols, catecholamines, and organic hydroxylamines. Hydroxysteroid sulfotransferase conjugates hydroxysteroids and certain primary and secondary alcohols. Estrone sulfotransferase is active with phenolic groups on the aromatic ring of steroids, and finally, bile salt sulfotransferases catalyze the sulfation of both conjugated and unconjugated bile acids. The activity of these enzymes is known to vary considerably with the sex and age of animals.

Table 4–7. CLASSIFICATION OF SULFOTRANSFERASES

Aryl sulfotransferase	Phenols
	Catechols
	Hydroxylamines
Hydroxysteroid sulfotransferase	Hydroxysteroids
	Some primary/secondary alcohols
Estrone sulfotransferase	Phenolic steroids
Bile salt sulfotransferase	Bile acids

The sulfate donor for these reactions is 3'-phosphoadenosine-5'-phosphosulfate (PAPS, Figure 4–9). This cofactor is synthesized from inorganic sulfate and ATP. The major source of sulfate required for the synthesis of PAPS appears to be derived from cysteine through a complex oxidation sequence. Since the concentration of free cysteine is limited, an important determinant in the extent of sulfation of foreign chemicals is the availability of the cofactor, PAPS. In reactions catalyzed by the sulfotransferases, the SO_3^- group of PAPS is readily transferred in a reaction involving nucleophilic attack of the phenolic oxygen or the amine nitrogen on the sulfur atom with the subsequent displacement of adenosine-3',5'-diphosphate.

Sulfation seems to have a high affinity but low capacity for conjugation of phenols. The major alternative reaction for phenols, glucuronidation, has low affinity but a much higher capacity (Table 4–8, Figure 4–10). Therefore, following administration of low doses of phenols, the major phenolic conjugate may be the sulfate ester. However, as the dose of the phenol is increased, the percent of dose and, occasionally, the absolute amount excreted as the sulfate may actually decrease, with a disproportionate increase in the amount excreted as the glucuronide. Although depletion of inorganic sulfate can explain a reduction in the percent of dose excreted as the sulfate with increasing doses of phenol, it does not explain the reduction in absolute amount. The most likely explanation for the reduced rate of sulfate conjugation is substrate

Table 4–8. RELATIVE CAPACITIES OF THE CONJUGATION REACTIONS*

CAPACITY	REACTION
High	Glucuronidation
Medium	Amino acid conjugation
Low	Sulfation, glutathione conjugation
Variable	Acetylation

* From Caldwell. In Jenner, P., and Testa, B. (eds.): *Concepts in Drug Metabolism.* Marcel Dekker, Inc., New York, 1981. Reprinted by courtesy of the publisher.

inhibition of the transferase, as has been observed *in vitro* with preparations of purified acyl sulfotransferase. Because of the generally greater activity of the glucuronosyltransferase reactions in most animal species, sulfate conjugation is considered to be of lesser importance in facilitating the excretion of hydrophobic alcohols and phenols.

Although sulfate conjugation usually results in detoxication, examples exist where conjugation results in toxication. Certain sulfate conjugates are chemically unstable and degrade to form potent electrophilic species. The most notable example is the N-O sulfate esters of N-hydroxy-2-acetylaminofluorene, which will be discussed later.

Sulfate conjugates of xenobiotics are excreted mainly in urine (Table 4–6). Some of these conjugates can also be degraded enzymatically. Aryl sulfatases are present in gut microflora, but some activity is associated with the endoplasmic reticulum and lysozomes. Although these primarily degrade sulfates of endogenous compounds, they also possess activity toward sulfate conjugates of xenobiotics. Their role on the subsequent disposition of sulfate conjugates is poorly understood.

Methylation

Methylation is a common biochemical reaction for the biotransformation of endogenous compounds, but is not usually a quantitatively important pathway for xenobiotic metabolism. Methylation differs from most other conjugation reactions in that it actually masks functional groups. This may reduce the water solubility of the chemical and/or impair its ability to participate in other conjugation reactions.

The functional groups involved in methylation reactions are aliphatic and aromatic amines, N-heterocyclics, mono- and polyhydric phenols, and sulfhydryl-containing compounds. In particular, methylthio metabolites of aromatic and aliphatic substances are being detected more routinely.

The nature of the methylation reaction is similar to that for the other conjugation processes in that the methyl group is transferred to the xenobiotic from a high-energy cofactor, S-adenosyl methionine (SAM, Figure 4–9). The methyl group bound to the sulfonium ion in SAM has the characteristics of a carbonium ion and is transferred by nucleophilic attack of the alcohol oxygen, the amine nitrogen, or the thiol sulfur on the methyl group giving S-adenosylhomocysteine and the methylated substrate as products.

The O-methylation reaction of primary importance is catalyzed by catechol-O-methyl transferase (Table 4–9). This soluble enzyme is ubiquitous but concentrated in liver and kidney. It

Table 4–9. EXAMPLES OF PRODUCTS OF METHYLATION REACTIONS

SUBSTRATE	PRODUCT
1. Pyridine	(pyridine N-methylated, CH_3)
2. Catechol (OH, OH)	(OCH_3, OH)
3. $(C_2H_5)_2N-\overset{\displaystyle S}{\overset{\|}{C}}-SH$ Diethyldithiocarbamate	$(C_2H_5)_2N-\overset{\displaystyle S}{\overset{\|}{C}}-S-CH_3$

will catalyze this reaction only with catechols and will not methylate monohydric phenols.

Various specific (histamine and indole) and nonspecific N-methyl transferases have been described. The nonspecific N-methyl transferases are of most concern since these enzymes are capable of methylating a variety of primary, secondary, and tertiary exogenous and endogenous amines such as serotonin, benzylamine, amphetamine, and pyridine.

S-methyl transferases are believed to have evolved in the liver to handle the evolution and uptake of hydrogen sulfide produced by anaerobic bacteria in the intestinal tract. The hydrogen sulfide is methylated to methane thiol, which is further methylated to dimethylsulfide. Other free sulfhydryl compounds also appear to be handled by this system.

The largest source of substrates for this S-methyl transferase appears now to be the thio ethers of glutathione conjugates. Certain glutathione thio ethers are hydrolyzed to cysteine conjugates in the kidney prior to acetylation and excretion. Those conjugates escaping acetylation are substrates for cysteine conjugate β-lyase, an enzyme that cleaves cysteine thioethers. Owing to the large variety of xenobiotics proceeding through the glutathione conjugation pathway, a variety of organic sulfhydryl compounds can be produced that will ultimately be available for S-methylation.

N-Acetyl Transferases

A major route of biotransformation for arylamines found in most species is acetylation of the amine function. Examples of substrates for the N-acetyl transferases include aromatic primary amines, hydrazines, hydrazides, sulfon-amides, and certain primary aliphatic amines (Table 4–10).

The enzymes that catalyze the acetylation of amines are designated as acetyl CoA: amine N-acetyl transferases. The cofactor for these reactions is acetyl coenzyme A (Figure 4–9). N-acetyl transferases are cytosolic enzymes found in many tissues of a number of species. It appears that multiple forms of the transferase occur in most tissues, but the number of different enzymes that contribute to acetylation of foreign compounds is yet to be determined. The dog and related species are deficient in the major N-acetyl transferase and thus are unable to acetylate a wide number of substrates. Polymorphism of acetylation for selected substrates has been reported in humans, mice, rabbits, and

Table 4–10. EXAMPLES OF PRODUCTS OF N-ACETYL TRANSFERASE REACTIONS

SUBSTRATE	PRODUCT
1. (NH_2 on benzene ring)	$NH-\overset{\displaystyle O}{\overset{\|}{C}}-CH_3$ (on benzene ring)
2. $R-NH-NH_2$ substituted hydrazine	$R-NH-NH-\overset{\displaystyle O}{\overset{\|}{C}}-CH_3$
3. $R-SO-NH_2$ aryl-substituted sulfonamide	$R-SO-NH-\overset{\displaystyle O}{\overset{\|}{C}}-CH_3$

squirrel monkeys. This polymorphism is of genetic origin. Subjects are classified as "rapid" or "slow" acetylators based on their ability to acetylate isoniazid. Data from a number of biochemical studies suggest that the transferases from rapid and slow acetylator rabbits are structurally different and that they possess different substrate specificity. Sulfanilamide and *p*-aminobenzoic acid are monomorphic substrates, since the capacity for *N*-acetylation of these amines displays a unimodal distribution, at least in the human population.

Acetylation of arylamines occurs in two sequential steps. Initially the acetyl group from acetyl CoA is transfered to the *N*-acetyl transferase to form acetyl-*N*-acetyl transferase as an intermediate. The second step is acetylation of the amino group of the arylamine substrate with regeneration of the enzyme. The interaction between the amine and the acetyl group results in formation of an amide bond.

Although the amide bond is relatively stable, a number of deacetylases/amidases are present in the mitochondrial, microsomal, and soluble fractions. Thus, the overall production of *N*-acetyl conjugates in a particular species will depend on the relative rates of acetylation and deacetylation.

For *N*-acetylated amines that undergo *N*-hydroxylation, an arylhydroxamic acid: acyl transferase has been identified. This enzyme can remove the acetyl group from the aryl hydroxamic acid and transfer it to oxygen of the hydroxylamine. The resulting product is the highly unstable *N*-acyloxyarylamine, which degrades to the highly reactive arylnitrenium ion. The role of this enzyme in tumor induction of aromatic amines is currently being delineated. It is widely distributed throughout species and has been located in a number of tissues.

Acetylation is another example of a conjugation reaction that masks a functional group. Many *N*-acetyl derivatives are less water soluble than the parent compound. *N*-acetyl derivatives of certain sulfonamides have been reported to precipitate in the kidney tubules, an event that can result in kidney damage.

Amino Acid Conjugation

An important reaction for xenobiotics containing a carboxylic acid group is conjugation with one of a variety of amino acids. These reactions result in the formation of an amide (peptide) bond between the carboxylic acid group of the xenobiotic and the amino group of the amino acid. Substrates for conjugation include aromatic carboxylic acids, arylacetic acids, and aryl-substituted acrylic acids (Table 4–11). Al-

Table 4–11. EXAMPLES OF AMINO ACID CONGUGATES OF ORGANIC ACIDS*

ORGANIC ACID SUBSTRATE	AMINO ACID	PEPTIDE PRODUCT
(Aryl acid) Benzoate	Glycine	Hippurate
(Arylacetic acid) Phenylacetate	Glutamine	Phenylacetylglutamine
(Bile acid) Cholate	Taurine	Taurocholate

* Modified from Jakoby, W. E. (ed.): *Enzymatic Basis of Detoxication*, Vol. 2. Academic Press, Inc., New York, 1980.

though the most common reaction involves gly-cine, conjugation with glutamine is more preva-lent in humans and certain monkeys, and conjugation with ornithine is seen in birds and reptiles. Taurine serves as an acyl acceptor for bile acid conjugation.

The formation of the peptide bond is a two-step coupled reaction catalyzed by different en-zymes. The first reaction involves activation of the acid to a thioester derivative of coenzyme A. The energy for this reaction is supplied by ATP. The enzymes that catalyze this activation are called ATP-dependent acid:CoA ligases. The coenzyme A thioester then transfers its acyl moiety to the amino group of the acceptor amino acid. The ligase and the N-acyltransferase are soluble enzymes, but there is also activity within the matrix of hepatic and renal mitochondria. The number and specificity of the activating and acylating enzymes in all species is not known. In mammals evidence exists for two acid:CoA li-gases that can activate benzoic acid. Two differ-ent types of N-acyl transferases have been puri-fied from mammalian hepatic mitochondria. One prefers benzoyl CoA as substrate, while the other prefers arylacetyl CoA.

The formation of amino acid conjugates of aromatic acids is quantitatively an important reaction in a number of animal species. Since carboxylic acids are also subjected to glucuroni-dation, competition between the glucuronosyl-transferases and the amino acid transferases is expected. The degree to which glucuronide formation or amino acid conjugation predomi-nates depends on both the animal species and the structure of the acid. For example, the major conjugate of phenylacetic acid in the rat, ferret, and monkey is the amino acid conjugate. How-ever, diphenylacetic acid undergoes only glucu-ronidation in these three species. Other struc-ture-activity comparisons also indicate the importance of structure in determining the de-gree of amino acid conjugation.

Amino acid conjugation can be classified as a system with high affinity and medium-to-low capacity (Table 4–8). As the dose increases, the pathway becomes readily saturated and other means of elimination predominate (i.e., glucu-ronidation, or phase I reactions). Amino acid conjugates are eliminated primarily in urine. The addition of an endogenous amino acid to xenobiotics may facilitate this elimination by increasing their ability to interact with the tubu-lar organic anion transport system (Table 4–6).

Glutathione S-Transferases

The glutathione S-transferases are a family of enzymes that catalyze the initial step in the for-mation of N-acetylcysteine (mercapturic acid) derivatives of a diverse group of foreign com-pounds. At least seven different glutathione S-transferases have been isolated from the cytosol of rat livers with a broad display of overlapping substrate specificity (Table 4–12).

Glutathione S-transferases are localized in both the cytoplasm and the endoplasmic reticu-lum. However, the cytosolic glutathione trans-ferase activities are usually 5 to 40 times greater than the microsomal activity. The enzymes are ubiquitous, with the greatest activity found in the testis, liver, intestine, kidney, and adrenal gland.

The cofactor for reactions catalyzed by these enzymes is the tripeptide glutathione (GSH), which is composed of glycine, glutamic acid, and cysteine (Figure 4–11). The glutathione S-transferases catalyze the reaction of the nucleo-philic sulfhydryl of glutathione with compounds containing electrophilic carbon atoms. The reac-tion of the glutathione thiolate anion (GS$^-$) re-sults in formation of a thioether bond between the carbon atom and the sulfhydryl group of glu-tathione (Figure 4–11).

Compounds that are substrates for the gluta-thione S-transferases share three common fea-tures: they must be hydrophobic to some de-gree, they must contain an electrophilic carbon atom, and they must react nonenzymatically with glutathione at some measurable rate. It is important to note that these transferases also serve as ligands for a number of compounds that are not substrates for the enzymic reactions. Lipophilic domains of the transferases serve as binding sites for a number of endogenous and exogenous chemicals. Thus, the glutathione S-transferases may serve as storage or transport proteins as well as enzymes.

The glutathione (GSH) conjugates are subse-quently cleaved to cysteine derivatives, primar-ily by enzymes located in the kidney. These de-rivatives are then acetylated to give the N-acetylcysteine (mercapturic acid) conjugates (Figure 4–11). Mercapturic conjugates are read-ily excreted into urine. The loss of glutamic acid from the glutathione conjugate is catalyzed by the enzyme γ-glutamyltranspeptidase, a mem-brane-associated enzyme found in high concen-trations in cells that exhibit absorptive or excre-tory functions. Cysteinyl glycinase catalyzes the loss of glycine from the conjugate to yield the cysteine conjugate. Finally, N-acetyl transferase enzymes acetylate the amino group of cysteine to form the mercapturic acid derivative. The cofactor for the acetylation reaction is acetyl-CoA. In the rat, a microsomal acetyl transferase present in the kidney exhibited the highest activ-ity toward S-substituted cysteines.

The importance of the nucleophilic reactions

Table 4–12. GLUTATHIONE-S-TRANSFERASE REACTIONS

Substitution Reaction

Glutathione *S*-alkyltransferase:

$$CH_3I + GSH \longrightarrow CH_3\text{-}SG + HI$$

Methyl iodide

Glutathione *S*-aryltransferase:

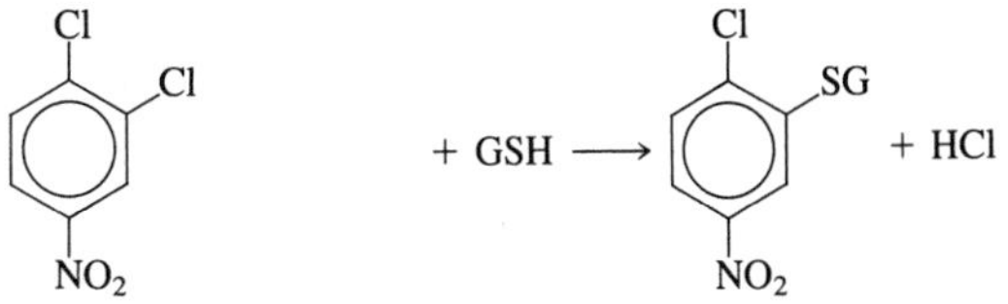

3,4-Dichloronitrobenzene

Glutathione *S*-aralkyltransferase:

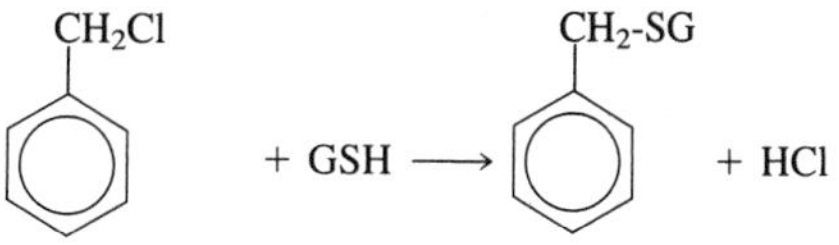

Benzyl chloride

Addition Reaction

Glutathione *S*-alkenetransferase:

$$\begin{matrix} CHCOOC_2H_5 \\ \| \\ CHCOOC_2H_5 \end{matrix} + GSH \longrightarrow \begin{matrix} CH_2COOC_2H_5 \\ | \\ GS\text{-}CHCOOC_2H_5 \end{matrix}$$

Diethyl maleate

Glutathione *S*-epoxidetransferase:

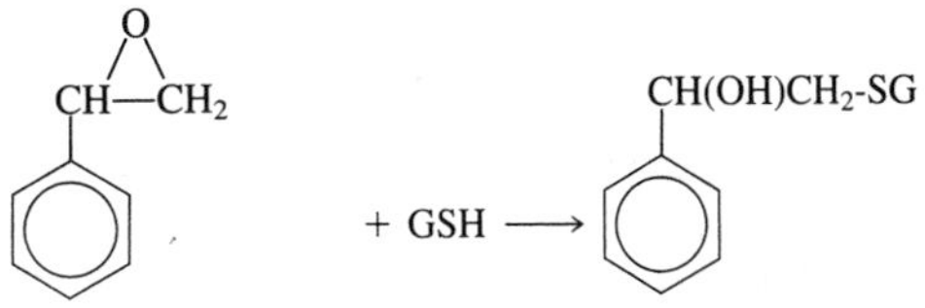

1,2-Epoxyethylbenzene

catalyzed by glutathione *S*-transferases has become increasingly apparent over the last few years. The glutathione *S*-transferase enzymes provide a means of reacting the diverse array of electrophilic xenobiotics with the endogenous nucleophile glutathione, thus preventing, to a degree, the reaction of these compounds with essential constituents of the cell. Considerable evidence indicates that glutathione *S*-transferases act to detoxify reactive intermediates produced by the cytochrome P-450 system. For example, bromobenzene, chloroform, and acetaminophen are biotransformed by the cytochrome P-450-containing monooxygenase enzyme system of the liver to highly reactive intermediates. These reactive intermediates may bind covalently to various macromolecule constituents in hepatocytes or react with GSH. The latter reaction prevents covalent binding of reactive intermediates to vital cellular constituents.

There is a delicate balance within cells between the rate of formation of the reactive metabolites and their inactivation by GSH. Thus, factors that affect this balance can dramatically alter the toxic potential of chemicals that produce toxicity via reactive intermediates. Reactive intermediates may also deplete cellular stores of GSH. Since GSH is a cofactor for glutathione peroxidase, its depletion can promote

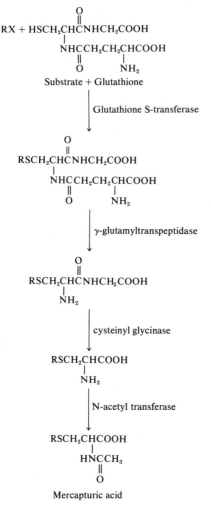

Figure 4–11. Glutathione conjugation and mercapturic acid biosynthesis.

lipid peroxidation, a process that leads to deleterious results.

Rhodanese

An important reaction in the detoxication of cyanide is catalyzed by the mitochondrial enzyme rhodanese (Figure 4–12). Thiosulfate can act as the donor of sulfur; however, it is unclear at this time which of the components of the sulfite pool is the true cofactor. Since the product of the reaction, thiocyanate, is far less toxic than cyanide, rhodanese catalyzes an unmistakable detoxication reaction.

$$CN^- \; + \; S_2O_3{}^{2-} \; \longrightarrow \; SCN^- \; + \; SO_3{}^{2-}$$
Cyanide   Thiosulfate   Thiocyanate   Sulfite

Figure 4–12. Detoxication reaction of cyanide catalyzed by rhodanese.

EXTRAHEPATIC BIOTRANSFORMATION

Other Organs

Although biotransformation of xenobiotics occurs predominantly in the liver, biotransformation in extrahepatic tissues is important in regulating the fate of foreign compounds such as environmental pollutants in air and water, food additives and contaminants, industrial chemicals, or cigarette smoke. The major tissues of extrahepatic biotransformation are those involved in absorption or excretion of chemicals, such as lung, kidney, skin, and gastrointestinal mucosa. The rate of extrahepatic biotransformation may not be as high as in liver, and the total capacity is usually lower. However, humans are primarily exposed to low levels of environmental and occupational chemicals over long periods of time. Thus, biotransformation by these tissues may have a marked effect on the ultimate disposition of selected chemicals. Clearly, extrahepatic biotransformation has been implicated as a factor in toxicant-induced tissue injury.

Compared to extrahepatic tissues, the liver is a relatively homogenous mixture of cells, with all parenchymal cells having some biotransformation capacity. In most extrahepatic tissues the biotransformation enzymes are usually concentrated within one or two cell types that comprise only a small percentage of the total cell population in an organ (Table 4–13). For example, the Clara and type II cells of the lung and the cells of the S_3 segment of the renal proximal tubules contain essentially all of the cytochrome P-450 in these tissues. Phase II conjugation enzymes are more widely distributed among the tissues than is cytochrome P-450. In fact, certain phase II reactions are equivalent to or higher than cytochrome P-450 reactions in extrahepatic tissues.

Intestinal Microbial Biotransformation

An aspect of *in vivo* extrahepatic biotransformation of xenobiotics frequently overlooked is

Table 4–13. BIOTRANSFORMATION ENZYME-CONTAINING CELLS IN VARIOUS ORGANS

ORGAN	CELL(S)
Liver	Parenchymal cells (hepatocytes)
Kidney	Proximal tubular cells (S₃ segment)
Lung	Clara cells, type II cells
Intestine	Mucosa lining cells
Skin	Epithelial cells
Testes	Seminiferous tubules, Sertoli's cells

modification by intestinal microbes. It has been estimated that the gut microbes have the potential for biotransformation of xenobiotics equivalent to or greater than the liver. With over 400 bacterial species known to exist in the intestinal tract, differences in gut flora content as a result of species variation, age, diet, and disease states would be expected to influence xenobiotic modification.

Intestinal microbial biotransformation is of interest because bacterial reactions often produce less water-soluble metabolites and because the anaerobic state of the intestinal tract promotes reductive reactions. In addition, the presence of deconjugating enzymes (i.e., β-glucuronidases and arylsulfatases) leads to major modifications of metabolites produced in the liver and excreted in the bile. Such deconjugation usually promotes enterohepatic recycling.

FACTORS AFFECTING RATES OF BIOTRANSFORMATION OF FOREIGN COMPOUNDS

Intrinsic Factors Related to the Chemical

One of the important factors controlling the rate and/or route of enzymatic modification of foreign compounds is the concentration of the compound at the active center of enzymes involved in its biotransformation. The concentration at the active centers of these enzymes depends on the physicochemical properties of the compound as well as dose (Table 4–14).

Lipophilicity is an important property since it can govern the rate of absorption of a xenobiotic from its portal of entry (skin, intestine, lung). Lipophilic chemicals are more readily absorbed into the blood, while water-soluble substances are less rapidly absorbed. Similarly, the ease with which a compound crosses the cell membrane to reach the active sites of intracellular enzymes is governed by its lipid solubility. An important factor controlling the water solubility of foreign compounds is whether they contain ionizable groups in the molecule. Thus, compounds containing amine, carboxyl, phosphate, sulfate, phenolic hydroxyl, and other groups that are ionized at physiologic pH values are generally more water soluble and are less readily

transferred across cell membranes than compounds not containing these groups.

Another factor controlling the absorption and penetration of xenobiotics to the intracellular biotransformation enzymes is protein binding. Intra- and extracellular proteins have the capacity to bind foreign compounds and to reduce the concentrations of these compounds at the active sites of enzymes involved in their biotransformation. This capacity to bind foreign compounds results from the presence in proteins of hydrophobic regions that will bind lipid-soluble compounds and hydrophilic regions that contain polar side chains of amino acids capable of forming hydrogen and electrostatic bonds with polar groups in water-soluble foreign compounds. Thus, proteins and particularly serum proteins (albumin) have a capacity for nonspecific binding of foreign compounds. This binding reduces the availability of these compounds for biotransformation and has a definite effect on the intrinsic clearance of a xenobiotic by the biotransformation enzymes.

Another important factor is the dose or exposure concentration. Dose often has an effect on the pathway of biotransformation. Certain enzymes have a high affinity, but low capacity for xenobiotic biotransformation. These pathways will quickly become saturated as the dose increases. Thus, the percentage of dose undergoing biotransformation by this pathway will decrease. However, low-affinity, high-capacity enzymatic pathways will now biotransform a larger percentage of the administered dose. Acetaminophen is an excellent example. At low doses (15 mg/kg in rats) over 90% of the dose is excreted as the sulfate conjugate. At high doses (300 mg/kg) only 43% is excreted as the sulfate, but larger amounts of parent compound, glucuronide, and mercapturic acids are now excreted in the urine.

Host Variables That Affect Xenobiotic Biotransformation

A number of physiologic, pharmacologic, and environmental factors affect rates of xenobiotic biotransformation (Table 4–15). Some of these factors are unique to laboratory animals, but for the most part can be considered as broad factors that affect biotransformation in all species. Key

Table 4–14. FACTORS AFFECTING INTRACELLULAR CONCENTRATION OF XENOBIOTICS

Lipophilicity
Protein binding
Dose
Route administration

Table 4–15. VARIABLES AFFECTING XENOBIOTIC METABOLISM

Species	Enzyme induction
Strain	Enzyme inhibition
Age	Nutrition
Sex	Disease states
Time of day	

factors to be addressed are induction and inhibition of the biotransformation enzymes, species-strain variations in xenobiotic metabolism, gender differences in biotransfermation, alteration in metabolism with respect to age, role of genetics in biotransformation ability, nutritional status relative to biotransformation ability, and the effects of environment and disease states on xenobiotic disposition.

Induction of the Biotransformation Enzymes

A striking feature of the biotransformation enzymes is the fact that their activities can be enhanced following treatment of animals or humans with chemicals. These chemicals can be drugs, pesticides, industrial chemicals, natural products, and even ethanol. In general, this enhanced activity results from an increase in the rate of synthesis of the biotransformation enzymes. Therefore, this process has been termed "enzyme induction," an event requiring *de novo* protein synthesis. Previously, induction was considered to be limited to cytochrome P-450-dependent monooxygenases, but certain conjugating enzymes can also be induced following exposure to selected chemicals. Literally hundreds of chemicals have been shown to induce monooxygenase activity and have been termed microsomal-inducing agents. Most of these chemicals have not been widely tested, and thus the extent of their inducing effects has not been well characterized.

The onset, magnitude, and duration of increases in monooxygenase activities are known to vary with the inducing agent and its dose, the substrates used to assay the activity of the enzymes, the species, strain, or sex of the animal, the duration of exposure, and the tissue in which enzyme activity is measured. When induction occurs in the liver, the net effect may be an increase in the rate of excretion of chemicals from the body. Although induction of monooxygenases can occur in extrahepatic tissues, the impact on the biologic half-lives of chemicals is generally much less pronounced.

Morphologic and Biochemical Results of Induction The most widely studied inducing agents are phenobarbital and the polycyclic aromatic hydrocarbons [benzo(a)pyrene and 3-methylcholanthrene]. Although both classes of compounds induce certain monooxygenase activities, they produce different morphologic and biochemical effects in the liver. These are summarized in Table 4–16. Phenobarbital pretreatment results in marked hepatic hypertrophy, an increase in the concentration of microsomal protein (mg/g of liver), and a proliferation of the smooth endoplasmic reticulum. Accompanying these morphologic changes are increases in protein and phospholipid synthesis as well as induction of the synthesis of NADPH-cytochrome P-450 reductase (threefold) and selected cytochrome P-450 isozymes (up to 70-fold). The major cytochromal P-450 isozymes induced by

Table 4–16. CHARACTERISTICS OF THE HEPATIC EFFECTS OF PHENOBARBITAL AND POLYCYCLIC AROMATIC HYDROCARBONS

CHARACTERISTICS	PHENOBARBITAL	POLYCYCLIC HYDROCARBONS
Onset of effects	8–12 hours	3–6 hours
Time of maximum effect	3–5 days	24–48 hours
Persistence of induction	5–7 days	5–12 days
Liver enlargement	Marked	Slight
Protein synthesis	Large increase	Small increase
Phospholipid synthesis	Marked increase	No effect
Liver blood flow	Increase	No effect
Biliary flow	Increase	No effect
Enzyme components		
Cytochrome P-450	Increase	No effect
Cytochrome P-448	No effect	Increase
NADPH-cytochrome-c reductase	Increase	No effect
Substrate specificity		
N-Demethylation	Increase	No effect
Aliphatic hydroxylation	Increase	No effect
Polycyclic hydrocarbon hydroxylation	Small increase	Increase
Reductive dehalogenation	Increase	No effect
Glucuronidation	Increase	Small increase
Glutathione conjugation	Small increase	Small increase
Epoxide hydrolase	Increase	Small increase
Cytosolic receptor	None identified	Identified

phenobarbital are virtually absent from liver microsomes of untreated laboratory animals. Interestingly, these changes occur predominantly in hepatocytes located in the centrilobular region of the liver. The net effect of these morphologic and biochemical changes is enhanced biotransformation of a large number of chemicals. Those substrates with high affinity for the induced cytochrome P-450 isozymes show the greatest increase in rates of biotransformation. However, the increased liver size and proliferation of components of the smooth endoplasmic reticulum explain the smaller increases in the rates of biotransformation of substrates with less affinity for the induced P-450 isozymes.

The pattern of induction in the liver following pretreatment with 3-methylcholanthrene or benzo(a)pyrene is dramatically different. The marked increase in liver weight, protein and phospholipid synthesis, and NADPH-cytochrome P-450 reductase does not occur (Table 4–16). Instead there is a selective induction (up to 70-fold) of cytochrome P-450 isozymes with spectral and catalytic properties different than those from the phenobarbital-inducible cytochrome P-450 isozymes. As with phenobarbital, the 3-methylcholanthrene-inducible cytochrome P-450 isozymes are virtually absent from liver microsomes of untreated laboratory animals. One of the 3-methylcholanthrene-inducible forms of cytochrome P-450 has a high catalytic turnover for benzo(a)pyrene. This form of cytochrome P-450 has long been called cytochrome P-448, cytochrome P_1-450 or aryl hydrocarbon hydroxylase (AHH). Unlike phenobarbital, specificity of induction to a particular region of the liver lobule is not observed following administration of 3-methylcholanthrene or similar types of inducing agents.

Other major classes of inducing agents include halogenated pesticides (DDT, aldrin, hexachlorobenzene, lindane, chlordane); polychlorinated and polybrominated byphenyls; steroids and related compounds (testosterone, spironolactone, pregnenolone-16α-carbonitrile); and chlorinated dioxins (2,3,7,8-tetrachlorodibenzo-p-dioxin, or TCDD). Certain of these produce a spectrum of induction similar to phenobarbital or the polycyclic aromatic hydrocarbons whereas some induce the synthesis of other forms of cytochrome P-450. Selective induction of cytochrome P-450 may occur at low doses, while high doses may also result in liver hypertrophy.

Mechanism of Induction. In recent years the actual mechanism of microsomal enzyme induction by the polycyclic aromatic hydrocarbons has become much clearer. Using TCDD, an extremely potent 3-methylcholanthrene-type inducer of AHH activity, Poland and his colleagues (1976) identified a high-affinity binding site for TCDD in the cytosol of liver and other tissues. This binding protein has the properties of a receptor in that it provides stereospecific recognition of the inducing compound. When the inducing agent (i.e., TCDD) interacts with this receptor, the resulting receptor-ligand complex translocates to the nucleus. Following interaction of this complex with specific genomic recognition sites, transcription and translation of the specific genes that code for cytochrome P-448 activity are initiated. Benzo(a)pyrene, 3-methylcholanthrene, other polycyclic aromatic hydrocarbons, and 3,3′,4,4′-tetrachlorobiphenyl were found to displace TCDD from this receptor. Therefore, these agents appear to interact with this common receptor and induce the synthesis of cytochrome P-448 by an identical mechanism. Critical requirements for interaction with the receptor include lipophilicity and a planar configuration. Other classes of inducers including phenobarbital and 2,2′,4,4′,5,5′-hexachlorobiphenyl will not displace TCDD from this receptor. To date, no analogous receptor for phenobarbital-type inducers has been identified, although the induction of specific cytochrome P-450 isozymes by phenobarbital is regulated at the transcriptional level and involves a dramatic increase in the mRNA's encoding these enzymes.

Time Course for Induction. Maximal induction following parenteral administration of hypnotic doses of phenobarbital occurs within three to five days. Induction following administration of 3-methylcholanthrene is more rapid, with maximal induction being achieved by 48 hours (Table 4–16). Induction is a reversible event. Withdrawal of the inducing agent results in a return to basal enzymic activity. Again, the duration of the induced state is a function of the dose and the inducing agent. Following withdrawal of phenobarbital, these induced activities return to basal level by seven to ten days. However, inducing agents that are highly lipophilic and poorly biotransformed (highly chlorinated PCBs) will be retained by the body and lead to prolonged induction because of their continued presence.

Induction of Other Microsomal Biotransformation Enzymes. Microsomal UDP-glucuronosyltransferases and epoxide hydrolase are induced by phenobarbital, 3-methylcholanthrene, and related compounds. *Trans*-stilbene oxide, acetylaminofluorene, and certain polychlorinated biphenyls are good inducers of epoxide hydrolase. Antioxidants, such as butylated hydroxyanisole (BHA) and butylated hydroxytoluene (BHT), are potent inducers of epoxide hydrolase in mice, but not in rats. Glucuronosyltransferase activities toward naphthol and *p*-nitrophenol are induced preferentially by 3-methylcholanthrene, whereas activities toward morphine and chloramphenicol are preferentially induced by phenobarbital. The major form(s) of cytochrome P-450 and UDP-glucuronosyltransferase inducible by pregnenolone-16α-carbonitrile are distinct from those induced by phenobarbital and 3-methylcholanthrene.

Induction of Extrahepatic Biotransformation Enzymes. Cytochrome P-450 enzymes in extrahepatic tissues are not readily induced by phenobarbital and compounds that produce a similar pattern of induction. However, the polycyclic aromatic hydrocarbons are known to be effective in such extrahepatic tissues as lung, kidney, intestinal tract, and skin. The cytosolic binding protein that complexes with polycyclic aromatic compounds is present in these tissues. It has been postulated that this rapidly inducible enzyme system at these portals of entry serves as a defense against noxious chemicals. In fact, this enzyme system, as measured by benzo(a)pyrene hydroxylation, can be decreased to undetectable levels in extrahepatic tissues if rats are maintained on highly purified diets and kept in isolated rooms that receive highly filtered air.

Induction of Cytosolic Enzymes. Except for the GSH-*S*-transferases, the major cytosolic conjugating enzymes are not readily induced. Specific inducers of the sulfotransferases, *N*-acetyltransferases, or amino acid conjugating enzymes are not known. In addition, these enzymes do not respond to the previously described inducers of the microsomal phase I and phase II enzymes. In rats, cytosolic glutathione-*S*-transferases are induced by 3-methylcholanthrene, phenobarbital, and *trans*-stilbene oxide. Depending on the isozyme, GSH-*S*-transferase induction may be as high as two- or three-fold. Butylated hydroxyanisole (BHA) is the most effective inducer of cytosolic transferase activity in the mouse but is less effective in the rat.

Inhibition of the Biotransformation Enzymes

According to Testa and Jenner (1981), "inhibition of xenobiotic metabolism is said to occur when under *in vivo*, *ex vivo* or in *in vitro* conditions, a given factor (endogenous or exogenous) decreases the ability of an enzyme or enzyme system to metabolize an exogenous substrate relative to control activity. Such a broad and operational definition has the advantage of including all possible inhibitory mechanisms, such as competition for active sites or cofactors of the enzymes, inhibition of transport components in multienzymic systems, decreased biosynthesis or increased breakdown of enzymes or their co-

factors'' as well as allosteric changes in enzyme conformation and even loss of functional tissue (i.e., hepatic necrosis). Some of these mechanisms of inhibition are briefly discussed in order to familiarize the reader with the chemicals used to inhibit various biotransformation reactions.

Obviously, agents that affect *protein synthesis* will ultimately inhibit biotransformation reactions. This occurs because of reduced synthesis of the actual biotransformation enzymes as well as the enzymes necessary for the production of cofactors. However, certain chemicals are more specific in that they are not general inhibitors of protein synthesis. For example, 3-amino-1,2,3-triazole decreases cytochrome P-450 synthesis, probably via its inhibitory affect on porphyrin synthesis. Acute administration of cobalt also decreases the hepatic concentration of cytochrome P-450 by its inhibitory effect on heme synthesis as well as its inductive effect on heme oxygenase, the enzyme that converts hemoproteins to biliverdin. Both chemicals have been shown to inhibit cytochrome P-450-catalyzed reactions.

Chemicals may also affect the tissue levels of necessary cofactors or conjugating species. For example L-methionine-*S*-sulfoximine and buthionine sulfoximine inhibit the synthesis of glutathione, while diethylmaleate, glycidol, and selected other chemicals conjugate with and rapidly reduce tissue stores of glutathione. Similarly, galactosamine inhibits the synthesis of UDP-glucuronic acid by depleting hepatic stores of uridine, while borneol and salicylamide conjugate with and deplete UDP-glucuronic acid. The ultimate effect of treatment with these chemicals would be a reduction in the capacity to form glutathione or glucuronide conjugates of subsequently administered xenobiotics or their metabolites.

A number of chemicals have been shown to have inhibitory effects in the cytochrome P-450 system. These are illustrated in Figure 4–13. Carbon monoxide (CO) and ethylisocyanide act as ligands for the reduced heme moiety and thus compete with the endogenous ligand, molecular oxygen. These are potent inhibitors of oxidative reactions. CO also inhibits P-450-mediated reductive reactions. By far the most common type of inhibition is competition of two different substrates (xenobiotics) for the substrate binding site of cytochrome P-450. This competition will result in mutual metabolic inhibition. The degree of inhibition will depend on the relative affinities of the xenobiotics for the binding site. Individual forms of cytochrome P-450 show different sensitivities to the inhibitory action of selected chemicals. For example, 7,8-benzoflavone is a direct-acting, competitive inhibitor that is highly spe-

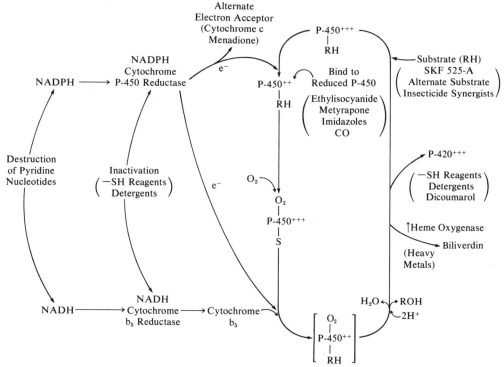

Figure 4–13. Inhibitors of the microsomal cytochrome P-450 system. (Modified and reprinted by permission of the publisher from Figure 8, page 117, Chapter 1 in *Extrahepatic Metabolism of Drugs and Other Foreign Compounds* by Theodore E. Gram (ed.). Copyright 1980, Spectrum Publications Inc., Jamaica, N.Y.)

cific for cytochrome P-448, while SKF 525-A and metyrapone are more specific for the phenobarbital inducible form of cytochrome P-450. SKF 525-A, piperonyl butoxide, and many other inhibitors produce a mixed type of inhibition. The parent molecule produces a competitive inhibition, while a metabolite forms a stable complex with cytochrome P-450 and results in noncompetitive inhibition.

Recently, several chemicals have been identified that act as suicide inhibitors of cytochrome P-450. Following activation of the chemical by the cytochrome P-450 system, reactive metabolites bind covalently to the pyrrole nitrogens present in the heme moiety. This interaction results in the destruction of heme and a loss of cytochrome P-450 activity. Various halogenated alkanes (CCl_4), alkenes (vinyl chloride, trichloroethylene), and compounds containing allylic (allylisopropylacetamide, secobarbital) and acetylenic (norethindrone acetate, acetylene) derivatives inhibit P-450-catalyzed reactions by suicide inactivation.

Inhibition of xenobiotic biotransformation *in vivo* is a complex situation. Many chemicals produce multiple effects, such as inhibition of both phase I and phase II reactions. Inhibitors

may show pronounced effects on only certain cytochrome P-450 isozymes, and therefore, the degree of inhibition will vary in untreated animals versus those treated with inducing agents. The degree of inhibition is also time dependent. For example, many agents that initially inhibit cytochrome P-450 also result in its induction at later time points (e.g., SKF 525-A, piperonyl butoxide). Chronic treatment with metal ions may result in adaptive biochemical responses in heme synthesis and metal-binding proteins, such as metallothionein. Clearly, these factors must be considered when evaluating the effect of inhibitors on xenobiotic biotransformation.

Species, Strain, Genetic Variations

Variations in biotransformation between species may be readily divided into qualitative and quantitative differences. *Qualitative* differences involve metabolic routes and are due either to a species defect or to a reaction peculiar to a species. *Quantitative* variations may result from differences in enzymic levels or natural inhibitors, in the balance of reverse enzyme reactions, or in the extent of competing reactions. It appears that qualitative differences occur mainly in conjugative phase II systems and that differ-

Table 4–17. CHARACTERIZATION OF
QUANTITATIVE AND QUALITATIVE
DIFFERENCES OBSERVED IN
BIOTRANSFORMATION AMONG SPECIES AND
STRAINS

QUALITATIVE
Predominantly associated with phase II reactions
Defective enzymes in certain species
Unique species reactions
Evolutionary
Some genetic aspects

QUANTITATIVE
Predominantly associated with phase I reactions
Differences in enzyme concentration
Different cytochrome P-450 isozymes
Differences in regiospecific reactions
Genetic

ences in phase I processes are restricted to quantitative alterations (Table 4–17).

Species differences in phase I reaction are most readily explained by differences in the profile of cytochrome P-450 isozymes. Although these isozymes may have overlapping substrate specificity, they usually have a marked regiospecificity. An excellent example of this is the observed species variation in the biotransformation of N-acetylaminofluorene. This carcinogenic amine undergoes several biotransformations. Two routes are N-hydroxylation and aromatic hydroxylation, which lead, respectively, to the hepatocarcinogenic N-hydroxy derivative and to the noncarcinogenic 7-hydroxy derivative. Marked species variations exist in the extent of these pathways. The guinea pig does not produce the N-hydroxy derivative *in vivo* or *in vitro,* and in this species the compound is not carcinogenic. On the other hand, the carcinogenic activity of 2-acetylaminofluorene is apparent in such species as mouse, rabbit, and

dog, which generate the N-hydroxy metabolite. Since these two reactions are catalyzed by two different forms of cytochrome P-450 isozymes, the species differences can be explained by differences in the activity or amount of the particular enzyme.

Species variation in phase I biotransformation is also apparent with amphetamine and 2,2',4,4',5,5'-hexachlorobiphenyl. In rats, amphetamine is primarily biotransformed by aromatic hydroxylation, while in rabbits it is primarily deaminated. Of all species studied to date only the dog can readily hydroxylate 2,2',4,4',5,5'-hexachlorobiphenyl, which explains why dogs can reduce their body burden of what in most species is an extremely persistent xenobiotic.

Species variation in phase II reactions are more apparent and appear to be associated with evolutionary development. These variations can result from differences in the ability of an animal to synthesize and/or activate the necessary cofactor, the nature and amount of the transferase, the occurrence of the conjugating agent, and the nature of the xenobiotic involved. Certain species lack a widespread conjugative process or perform a peculiar reaction (Table 4–18). For example, conjugation with glucuronic acid is one of the most important conjugation reactions in mammals. However, the cat and a few closely related species have a defective glucuronide-forming system. Although they can conjugate bilirubin with glucuronic acid, they cannot form glucuronides of phenol, naphthol, and other phenolic derivatives.

The dog cannot acetylate aromatic amino compounds because it lacks the appropriate isozyme of N-acetyl transferase. Similarly, the pig is deficient in sulfate conjugation. Finally, conjugation with amino acids is phylogenetically determined. Primates utilize glycine and glutamine, while some birds utilize ornithine.

Strain differences in biotransformation are also under genetic control. These differences often account for variations in the observed bio-

Table 4–18. SPECIES DEFECTS IN FOREIGN
COMPOUND METABOLISM*

REACTION	DEFECTIVE SPECIES
Aliphatic amine N-hydroxylation	Rat, marmoset
Arylacetamide N-hydroxylation	Guinea pig,
Arylamine N-acetylation	Dog
Glucuronidation	Cat, lion, lynx, Gunn rat
Sulfation	Pig, opossum, brachymorphic mice
Hippuric acid formation	African fruit bat
Mercapturic acid formation	Guinea pig

* Modified from Jakoby, W. E. (ed.): *Enzymatic Basis of Detoxication,* Vol. 1. Academic Press, Inc., New York, 1980.

logic responses to xenobiotics. Unusual pharmacologic responses can result from genetic defects and may be associated with altered enzyme activity. These hereditary variations in biotransformation are apparent in humans as well as in animals and are referred to as pharmacogenetics.

Homozygous strains are routinely used in toxicological studies to avoid the added complications involved in the use of heterozygous animal groups. To ensure that an observed difference results from a genetic variation, care must be taken to eliminate environmental influences, which may produce greater or lesser degrees of enzyme induction or inhibition in one strain versus another.

Examples of strain variation in phase I biotransformation include the differences in the rates of oxidation of hexobarbital among Holtzman, Sprague-Dawley, and Wistar rats. The duration of sleep after hexobarbital is inversely related to these rates of biotransformation. Each strain can be further divided into short and long sleepers, and the activity of cytochrome P-450-mediated enzyme activities correlates with sleep time. Similar differences were found among inbred strains of mice. Marked strain differences in hepatic cytochrome P-450-related enzyme activities have been noted among various strains of rabbits. Genetically controlled polymorphism in the regiospecific hydroxylation of drugs is well established in humans. For example 7 to 9 percent of British subjects are deficient in the 4-hydroxylation of debrisoquine. This same genetic polymorphism is apparently responsible for the interindividual variability observed in the biotransformation of propranolol, phenytoin, phenacetin, and other drugs. Studies that compared the plasma half-lives of drugs in identical versus fraternal twins found little or no differences between identical twins, but large differences (two to three-fold) between fraternal twins. Even larger variations are observed among unrelated individuals. Much of these variations can be attributed to genetic differences.

Genetic differences in the ability of animals to respond to enzyme-inducing agents are well known. The most notable example is the difference in response to 3-methylcholanthrene between C57BL6J and DBA2 mice. The C57 mice respond with a marked induction of hepatic microsomal benzo(a)pyrene hydroxylase activity and are termed "responsive." The DBA2 mice are classified as "nonresponsive," since the induction in this species is minimal. The difference between the two strains is linked to the *Ah* locus, which codes for the cytosolic receptor that regulates certain cytochrome P-450 isozymes. This binding protein is defective in the nonresponsive DBA2 mice. These strain differences in enzyme induction can lead to strain differences in rates and routes of biotransformation following exposure to the inducing agent.

Individual or strain variations in phase II reactions are also known. The defect in glucuronide formation observed in the Gunn rat is similar to the inherited human metabolic disorder congenital familial nonhemolytic jaundice. This disorder is associated with reduced glucuronosyltransferase activity. Differences in glucuronide formation are considered to originate mainly from genetic deficiencies and affect only a few strains. On the other hand, differences in acetylation ability show a much wider distribution and are not associated with the concept of genetic deficiency or disorder, but rather with genetic heterogeneity. In humans large individual variations exist in the acetylation of the antituberculosis drug isoniazid. The population is generally considered to be bimodally distributed into rapid and slow acetylators. The inheritance of the rapid inactivator phenotype has been shown to be autosomal dominant. The incidence of slow and rapid activators is not the same in all racial groups.

Sex Differences in Biotransformation

A marked difference between male and female rats in the pharmacologic and toxicologic response to a number of xenobiotics has been noted. For example, female rats sleep considerably longer than male rats when treated with equivalent doses of hexobarbital. Similarly, the widely used organophosphate insecticide parathion is approximately twice as toxic to female rats as to males. These potentiated responses in female rats result from a reduced capacity of their livers to biotransform these as well as other chemicals. In these cases the parent compound has a prolonged biologic half-life in females that leads to a prolonged response. If a metabolite or reactive intermediate produces the biologic response, then male rats will usually show the greater response. This is the reason male rats are more susceptible to hepatic injury produced by carbon tetrachloride and halothane. Male rats convert these chemicals to reactive intermediates at faster rates than female rats.

Sex differences in biotransformation also occur in extrahepatic tissues. Chloroform is converted to a reactive intermediate (phosgene) ten times faster by microsomes obtained from the kidneys of male mice than those from female mice. Male mice are susceptible to chloroform-induced nephrotoxicity, whereas female mice are resistant.

The balance between male and female sex

Table 4–19. EFFECT OF SEX ON BIOTRANSFORMATION IN THE RAT

ANALYSIS	RATIO OF MALE/FEMALE
Cytochrome P-450	1.4
NADPH–cytochrome P-450 reductase	1.3
Benzphetamine N-demethylation	5.6
Aniline hydroxylation	5.5

hormones is important in determining the activity of cytochrome P-450 enzymes. Administration of testosterone to female rats increases their ability to biotransform a number of drugs and other xenobiotics. Following treatment, rates of biotransformation in female rats approach the activity observed in their male counterparts. Similarly, castration of male rats reduces their capacity to biotransform xenobiotics.

Measurements of cytochrome P-450 concentration and NADPH-cytochrome P-450 reductase activity in hepatic microsomes have shown preparations from male rats to contain 20 to 30 percent more of these components (Table 4–19). It is now established that the differences between the sexes reflect differences in the profile of cytochrome P-450 isozymes in liver microsomes from male and female rats. Both male-specific and female-specific forms of cytochrome P-450 have been identified.

Despite the large sex variations observed in the biotransformation of xenobiotics by rats and certain strains of mice, such variations are not common in other species. There are, however, random examples of such differences in other species. In humans, for example, sex-dependent differences in the biotransformation of nicotine, acetylsalicyclic acid, and heparin have been reported. If sex differences in a biologic response to a xenobiotic are observed, differences in rates of biotransformation should always be considered as a possible cause.

Effect of Age on Biotransformation

Fetal and newborn animals have been shown to be severely limited in their ability to biotransform xenobiotics, which provides a basis for the increased toxicity of xenobiotics in young animals. However, not all pathways of biotransformation are absent or limited in newborn animals.

In rats the low or negligible activity of cytochrome P-450-catalyzed reactions observed at birth develops rapidly and reaches maximal activity by 30 days of age. Enzyme activities then begin to decrease gradually with age. By 600 days of age, these activities are only 50 to 60 percent of maximum. In humans, cytochrome P-450 activities are 20 to 50 percent of adult activities by the second trimester of gestation. However, the isozyme pattern is qualitatively different from that observed in adults. This pattern of ontogenetic development appears to be common to diverse species and has been characterized with several substrates.

The age-related changes observed in the activity of the biotransformation enzymes is correlated with biochemical differentiation of hepatocytes. Comparison of rat hepatic microsomal preparations from one- and three-day-old animals shows a marked increased in the quantity of both rough and smooth endoplasmic reticulum. The increase in smooth elements is far more pronounced and appears to arise from transformation of rough endoplasmic reticulum by loss of ribosomes. It is only at birth, however, that many of the constitutive membrane-bound enzymes appear, and it is unknown whether these enzymes are integrated into existing membranes or whether de novo synthesis occurs. The smooth endoplasmic reticulum appears in human hepatocytes around the third month of gestation, the time at which cytochrome P-450 activities appear.

Since a low level of biotransformation activity in neonates is due to an actual enzyme deficiency, activity can be increased by inducing agents. Polycylic aromatic hydrocarbons and certain polychlorinated biphenyls are effective transplacental inducing agents. In humans, prolonged administration of phenytoin, phenobarbital, and perhaps alcohol leads to pharmacokinetic alterations in the newborn. These alterations have been related to the enzyme-inducing effects of these agents. Newborn animals also respond to enzyme inducers. Indeed, the increase in activity produced by inducing agents administered to immature animals is greater than that seen in adults.

A similar pattern of development in rats exists for some of the phase II conjugation enzymes. Both glutathione and glycine conjugation develop slowly after birth to adult levels by 30 days, while sulfation is almost at adult levels at birth. In the case of UDP-glucuronosyltransferase, activity toward bilirubin reaches adult levels by five to seven days, whereas 30 days are required for activity toward ortho-aminophenol to reach adult values.

Increased toxicity of xenobiotics often occurs in older animals and is often explained in terms of increased tissue sensitivity to the toxicant. Serum levels of some toxicants are known to reach higher values and to persist for longer periods in old rats (27 months) than in younger ones (six months). In addition, hepatic microsomes from older rats show decreased biotransformation capacity. Increased toxicologic activity of these xenobiotics with age parallels a decrease in *in vitro* biotransformation. Thus, compounds generating toxic metabolites will be associated with decreased toxicity in both the young and old. For example, inhibitors of cholinesterase are less effective in the elderly, while carbon tetrachloride is not hepatotoxic in newborn rats. Both these agents require biotransformation to exert these toxic effects.

Decreased capacity for biotransformation correlates with a reduction in the concentration of cytochrome P-450 and the activity of its associated reductase. It should be emphasized that, in the elderly, the observed increases in the biological half-lives of drugs may be related not only to decreased enzyme activities but also to decreased renal and hepatic blood flows, decreased liver size, decreased efficiency of urinary/biliary excretory systems, increased mass of adipose tissue, etc. Clearly many biochemical and physiologic functions decrease in the elderly, and these changes can affect their response to xenobiotics.

Effect of Diet on Biotransformation

The nutritional status of experimental animals is an important factor influencing biotransformation. A number of examples are outlined in Table 4–20. Mineral deficiencies (calcium, copper, iron, magnesium, and zinc) decrease both cytochrome P-450-catalyzed oxidation and reduction reactions. Decreases in basal cytochrome P-450 concentrations can partly account for the lower biotransformation activity. A return to normal dietary mineral intake returns the enzyme activities to normal levels.

Table 4–20. DIETARY CONDITIONS AFFECTING BIOTRANSFORMATION

DIETARY ALTERATION	USUAL EFFECT
Mineral deficiencies	
Calcium	↓
Copper	↓
Iron	↓
Magnesium	↓
Zinc	↓
Vitamin deficiencies	
Ascorbic acid	↓
Tocopherol	↓
B complex	↓
Protein deficiencies	↓
Lipid composition	↑↓
Fasting (12 hours)	↑↓ *
Starvation (>48 hours)	↓
Natural substances	↑↓

* Certain phase II reactions.

Vitamin deficiencies (C, E, and B complex) reduce the rates of xenobiotic biotransformation. These vitamins are directly or indirectly involved in the regulation of the cytochrome P-450 system. In addition, their deficiencies can alter the energy and redox state of the cells, thus hindering the production of the high-energy cofactors required for phase II biotransformation. Reintroduction of the vitamins to the diet will result in a return to basal enzyme activities.

Low-protein diets have been found to increase markedly the toxicity of a number of xenobiotics that are active as the parent compound, but to reduce the toxicity of those that require biotransformation to express their toxicities. For example, the lethality and severity of hepatotoxicity produced by dimethylnitrosamine are markedly reduced in rats maintained on a low-protein diet. Correlated with these decreases in toxicity is a reduction in the *N*-demethylation of dimethylnitrosamine, the initial step in its conversion to an alkylating agent. Dietary lipids are important in determining the activity of biotransformation enzymes, particularly those enzymes that are membrane bound. In rats, diets high in polyunsaturated fats decrease the concentration of hepatic cytochrome P-450. This reduction results from the increased susceptibility of unsaturated fatty acids to undergo peroxidation. Thus, the microsomal membranes degrade with a concomitant loss of cytochrome P-450. The nature of the fatty acids present in the membrane may also affect its fluidity.

Overnight food deprivation is a common technique used in toxicologic studies. It decreases the volume of material present in the gut and, thus, promotes the absorption of orally administered chemicals. Since rodents are nocturnal feeders, they will have been deprived of food longer than the anticipated 12 to 16 hours. This procedure stimulates a number of biotransformation enzymes and can have a marked affect on toxicity. Food deprivation has been shown to increase the dealkylation of dimethylnitrosamine and to potentiate the liver injury it produces. Food deprivation can also reduce the concentration of cofactors and conjugating agents. The concentration of hepatic glutathione is reduced by 50% during an overnight fast, an event known to potentiate the hepatotoxicity of acetaminophen, bromobenzene, and other compounds that are detoxified by glutathione. If the animals are starved (i.e., without food for 48 hours), xenobiotic biotransformation is suppressed *in vivo*. However, until the starvation is severe, the biotransformation enzymes are present, but not functioning appropriately owing to the reduced energy state of the animals.

Natural substances present in the diets can

also affect biotransformation enzymes. For example, the indoles in certain vegetables enhance the phase I biotransformation activity in the intestinal lining cells and the liver. Charcoal-broiled meat, because of the presence of polycyclic aromatic hydrocarbons, also induces enzymic activities in these tissues. Dietary chemicals that inhibit certain biotransformation reactions are also known. We are just beginning to understand how diet can affect xenobiotic biotransformation. Clearly, this is an important area that may explain the pronounced interindividual variation observed in the biologic response to xenobiotics.

Effect of Hepatic Injury on Biotransformation

Since the liver is the principal site of xenobiotic biotransformation, any disease state that severely interferes with the normal function of this organ can influence the processes of biotransformation. Similarly, chemically induced hepatic injury will decrease biotransformation.

Schistosomiasis, viral infections, carcinomas, obstructive jaundice, hepatitis, and cirrhosis compromise the liver and reduce hepatic biotransformation (Figure 4–14). In toxicologic studies, a toxicant can injure the liver or irreversibly inhibit the biotransformation enzymes. The impairment observed is related to the degree of damage. After such injuries, there will be a rapid regeneration phase, which often results in enzyme activities that are temporarily higher than the preinjury activities.

Conditions that decrease hepatic blood flow (i.e., delivery of the xenobiotic to the liver) suppress the biotransformation and clearance of a xenobiotic. These include cardiac complications, shock, and hypotension. Renal injury also reduces the clearance of xenobiotics. Such injury often leads to a decrease in hepatic function and a reduced biotransformation capacity.

Circadian Rhythms

An influence of the time of day on the rate of biotransformation of foreign compounds is often seen within a given animal species. This variation in the rate of biotransformation is often correlated with variations in endocrine functions as influenced by the light-dark cycle to which the animal is exposed. Thus, the *in vitro* biotransformation of aminopyrine and hexobarbital by the hepatic cytochrome P-450 monooxygenase system of rats is variable, depending on when during the day the animals are terminated. This variation in enzyme activity is thought to be largely the result of a variation in the activities of the cytochrome P-450 isozymes.

Concentrations of hepatic glutathione also

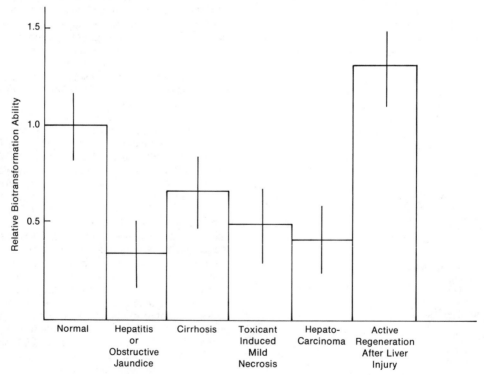

Figure 4–14. Effects of liver disease on biotransformation.

exhibit circadian rhythmicity, with concentrations being highest at the end of the dark cycle. Thus, during the feeding period glutathione accumulates, but during the light period it declines. This circadian rhythmicity in glutathione can affect the toxicity of xenobiotics that are detoxified by glutathione conjugation. The number of animals dying from acetaminophen and 1,1-dichloroethylene is greater when these toxicants are administered to animals at periods of low hepatic glutathione levels.

BIOACTIVATION

In the previous sections it was emphasized that the biotransformation enzymes can produce reactive intermediates. These are defined as chemical species that are more reactive than the parent compound or its metabolites that are subsequently eliminated from the body. For convenience the enzymatic formation of reactive intermediates is termed bioactivation. It is important to emphasize that the nature of the reactive intermediate is dependent on the chemical and the biotransformation process. The insertion of an oxygen, addition of oxygen, acceptance of a reducing equivalent, or a conjugation process can produce a chemical structure that is a reactive intermediate or that rearranges to the unstable reactive intermediate. Thus, formation of reactive intermediates can be considered part of the overall biotransformation process. Reactive intermediates can interact with nucleophilic sites on tissue constituents, such as the sulfhydryl group of glutathione and cysteine, or the amino or hydroxyl groups present in DNA, RNA, or protein. This covalent interaction with tissue macromolecules is thought to be a key factor in the toxic effects produced by the xenobiotics. For many chemicals these reactive intermediates can be detoxified. Provided there is a balance between rates of formation and rates of detoxication, the formation of reactive intermediates may not lead to adverse cellular events. When this balance is disturbed, either by enhanced production of reactive intermediates or diminished capacity for their detoxication, formation of reactive intermediates can be associated with cellular injury.

There are many conditions that can disturb the balance between the rates of formation and detoxication of reactive intermediates. Enzyme induction can increase the overall rate of biotransformation of a chemical, which can in turn lead to an excess production of reactive intermediates. Large doses of a xenobiotic can rapidly deplete cellular defense mechanisms. Large doses can also lead to saturation of the major nontoxic biotransformation pathways. Minor pathways, which form reactive intermediates, may now become operative. Finally, conditions may exist in which detoxication pathways are compromised and nontoxic doses of a xenobiotic can now result in cellular injury.

The factors and variables that are known to affect normal biotransformation also affect the bioactivation of xenobiotics. These have been covered in detail earlier. It is important to emphasize that bioactivation is not limited to the liver. Extrahepatic bioactivation of xenobiotic explains why numerous toxic foreign compounds produce organ-specific toxicities.

Table 4–21 lists a few examples of chemicals that undergo bioactivation. Reactive intermediates have been implicated in the toxicities that they produce. From this table it is apparent that epoxides, free radicals, and N-hydroxy derivatives are often encountered as reactive intermediates. Certain of these examples will be discussed in greater detail to illustrate the nature of reactive intermediate formation and its role in xenobiotic-induced toxicities.

The cytochrome P-450 system produces reactive intermediates by either oxidative or reductive reactions. With polycyclic aromatic compounds, aromatic compounds, heterocyclic aromatic compounds, or olefinic compounds, the addition of an oxygen molecule to the carbon-carbon double bond can produce an epoxide. The epoxide may nonenzymatically react with macromolecular nucleophiles resulting in an opening of the oxide and the formation of a covalent bond to the macromolecule. Numerous compounds with carbon-carbon double bonds proceed through arene oxide or epoxide intermediates during biotransformation. Not all, though, result in covalent binding. This, again, relates to the intrinsic reactivity of the specific epoxide and its steady-state concentration, since there are natural mechanisms that can defend against a certain quantity of these reactive intermediates.

The cytochrome P-450-mediated oxidative biotransformation of other xenobiotics can also produce reactive intermediates, primarily following a change in the resonance in the structure or a rearrangement of the initial metabolite. For example, the N-demethylation of dimethylnitrosamine is a common phase I biotransformation for secondary amines (Figure 4–15). Following loss of the alkyl group, the remaining unstable nitroso structure proceeds through resonance changes that result in an unstable intermediate. This decomposes and releases a reactive alkylating, carbonium ion. Similar examples exist for compounds undergoing O-dealkylation, N-hydroxylation, sulfur oxidation, etc. Cytochrome P-450-mediated reactions produce an

Table 4–21.   EXAMPLES OF XENOBIOTICS KNOWN TO UNDERGO BIOACTIVATION

COMPOUND	REACTIVE PATHWAY OR INTERMEDIATE	ADDITIONAL FACTORS THAT ENHANCE TOXICITY
Acetaminophen	N-hydroxylation	Sulfate and gluta-thione depletion
2-Acetylaminofluorene	N-hydroxylation	Conjugation
Acetylhydrazine	N-hydroxylation and subsequent rearrangement	
Aflatoxin B$_1$	Epoxidation	
Allyl alcohol	Oxidation to a reactive aldehyde	Glutathione depletion
Benzene	Epoxidation and further metabolism	
Benzo(a)pyrene and related compounds	Epoxidation, and other pathways	Secondary biotransformation of of diol to diol epoxide
Bromobenzene	Epoxidation	Glutathione depletion
Bromotrichloro-methane	Free radical formation	
Carbon disulfide	Oxidation with release of sulfur	
Carbon tetrachloride	Free radical formation	Reductive metabolism
Chloramphenicol	Formation of oxamyl chloride intermediate	
Chloroform	Carbonylchloride (phosgene) formation	Glutathione depletion
Cyclophosphamide	4-Hydroxylation and subsequent rearrangement	
Dimethylnitrosamine	α-Hydroxylation; rearrangement to yield a carbonium ion—CH$^+_3$	
Furosemide	Epoxidation of furan ring	
Halothane	Free-radical formation	Reductive metabolism
4-Ipomeanol	Oxidation of furan ring	
Isoniazide	Acetylation, N-hydroxylation	Fast/slow acetyletor
Parathion	Oxidation with release of sulfur	
Polychlorinated and polybrominated biphenyls	Epoxidation and ring hydroxylation with subsequent oxidation of catechol nucleus	Glutathione depletion
Thioacetamide	S-oxidation and subsequent further metabolism	
Trichloroethylene	Epoxidation	
Vinyl chloride	Epoxidation and other pathways	

entity that subsequently rearranges or degrades to an intermediate that covalently binds to tissue macromolecules.

Oxidative dehalogenation often leads to reactive chemical species. For example, when the carbon undergoing oxidation contains two halogens (usually chlorines or bromines), the product of oxygen insertion is a dihalohydrin, which undergoes dehydrohalogenation to a carbonyl halide entity (Figure 4–16). These acid halides are reactive and acylate macromolecules. A similar reaction is known to occur for chloroform. The initial reactive intermediate is phosgene, which can act as a bifunctional alkylating agent.

Thus, in almost all cases where a xenobiotic has a terminal carbon with two halides attached, side-chain oxidation mediated by cytochrome P-450 will produce a toxic, reactive intermediate.

Biotransformation of xenobiotics by the flavin-containing monooxygenase also produces reactive intermediates. Oxidation of amines to N-hydroxides produces, in some cases, metabolites that rearrange to reactive nitrogen centers or aryl imines. These reactive intermediates behave similarly to those produced by cytochrome P-450-mediated oxidative metabolism and result in covalent binding to cellular macromolecules.

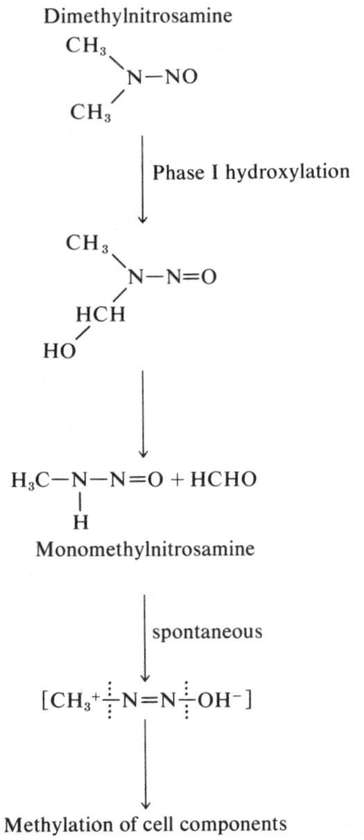

Dimethylnitrosamine

$$\begin{array}{c} CH_3 \\ \diagdown \\ N-NO \\ \diagup \\ CH_3 \end{array}$$

Phase I hydroxylation ↓

$$\begin{array}{c} CH_3 \\ \diagdown \\ N-N=O \\ HCH \diagup \\ HO \end{array}$$

↓

$$\begin{array}{c} H_3C-N-N=O + HCHO \\ | \\ H \end{array}$$
Monomethylnitrosamine

↓ spontaneous

$$[CH_3 \overset{.}{\underset{.}{+}} N=N \overset{.}{\underset{.}{-}} OH^-]$$

↓

Methylation of cell components

Figure 4–15. Bioactivation of dimethylnitrosamine.

$$\begin{array}{c} O \\ \parallel \\ CH_2=CH-CH_2-O-C-R \end{array}$$
Allyl esters

Esterases ↓

$$CH_2=CH-CH_2-OH$$
Allyl alcohol

Alcohol dehydrogenase ↓

$$CH_2=CH-CHO$$
Acrolein

Non-enzymatic ↓

Covalent binding to tissue macromolecules

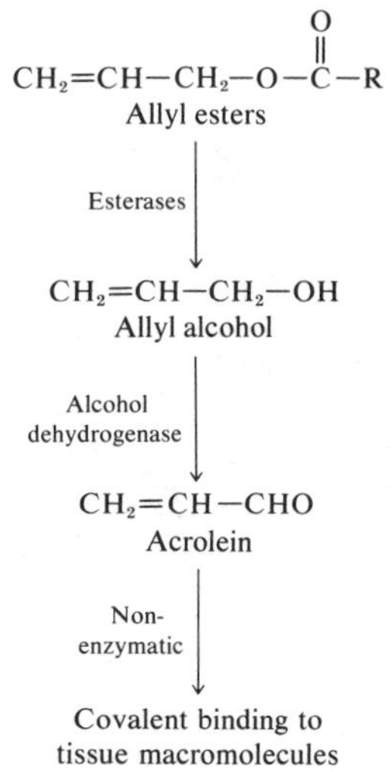

Figure 4–17. Bioactivation of allyl esters. (Modified from Jenner, P., and Testa, B. [eds.]: *Concepts in Drug Metabolism,* Part B. Marcel Dekker, Inc., New York, 1981.)

Reductive metabolism of xenobiotics by the cytochrome P-450 enzymes also produces reactive intermediates. The reductive dehalogenation of specific halogenated aliphatics results in production of free-radical intermediates owing to the uptake of the reducing equivalent (electron). Carbon tetrachloride ($CCl_4 \xrightarrow{e^-}$ $\cdot CCl_3 + Cl^-$), bromotrichloromethane, and halothane are examples of chemicals that undergo reductive cleavage to toxic intermediates.

Often the product of one reaction can lead to a substrate for another enzyme that produces a toxic product. Biotransformation of allyl esters is a good example (Figure 4–17). These esters are cleaved by nonspecific esterases to allyl al-

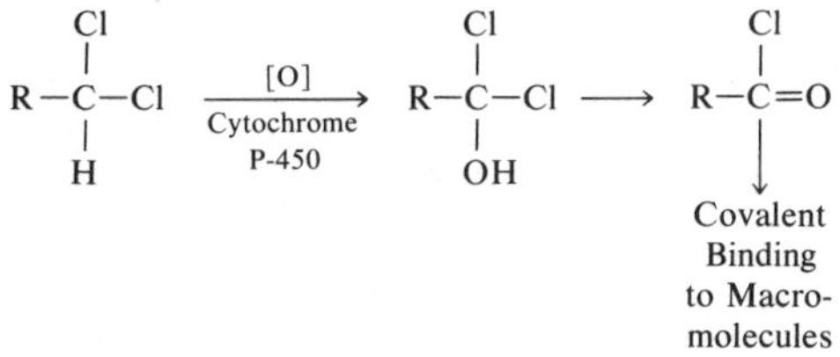

$$\begin{array}{c} Cl \\ | \\ R-C-Cl \\ | \\ H \end{array} \xrightarrow[\text{Cytochrome}]{[O]} \begin{array}{c} Cl \\ | \\ R-C-Cl \\ | \\ OH \end{array} \longrightarrow \begin{array}{c} Cl \\ | \\ R-C=O \end{array}$$

Covalent Binding to Macromolecules

Figure 4–16. Bioactivation of a dihalocarbon moiety.

cohol, which is then oxidized by alcohol dehydrogenases to the reactive allyl aldehyde. This aldehyde reacts with macromolecules or may be detoxified by glutathione conjugation. The rapid reactions catalyzed by the esterase and alcohol dehydrogenase produce a concentration of the aldehyde that overwhelms the detoxication pathways and results in the observed toxicities with these compounds.

The phase II biotransformation enzymes can also produce reactive intermediates. These usually result from rearrangement of unstable conjugates. When the unstable conjugate rearranges, the fragments are often reactive moieties that covalently bind to macromolecules. For example, conjugates of the phase I metabolite of 2-acetylaminofluorene are mutagenic and carcinogenic (Figure 4–18). The phase I-derived metabolite, *N*-hydroxy-2-acetylaminofluorene, can be converted via sulfate conjugation to a highly reactive electrophilic *N-O*-sulfate ester. This sulfate ester rearranges and fragments into a reactive intermediate that covalently binds to nucleic acids and proteins. The *N*-hydroxyl metabolite can form a glucuronide, which is also unstable and reactive. Acetyl transferases form an unstable *O*-acetyl conjugate (i.e., an *N*-acetoxy-2-aminofluorene), which results in a toxic reactive intermediate. Thus, conjugation of the *N*-hydroxy metabolite of 2-acetylaminofluorene with three separate conjugating species can lead to a reactive, potentially carcinogenic product.

Acetylation of drugs and xenobiotics can lead to toxic reactive products. A classic example is

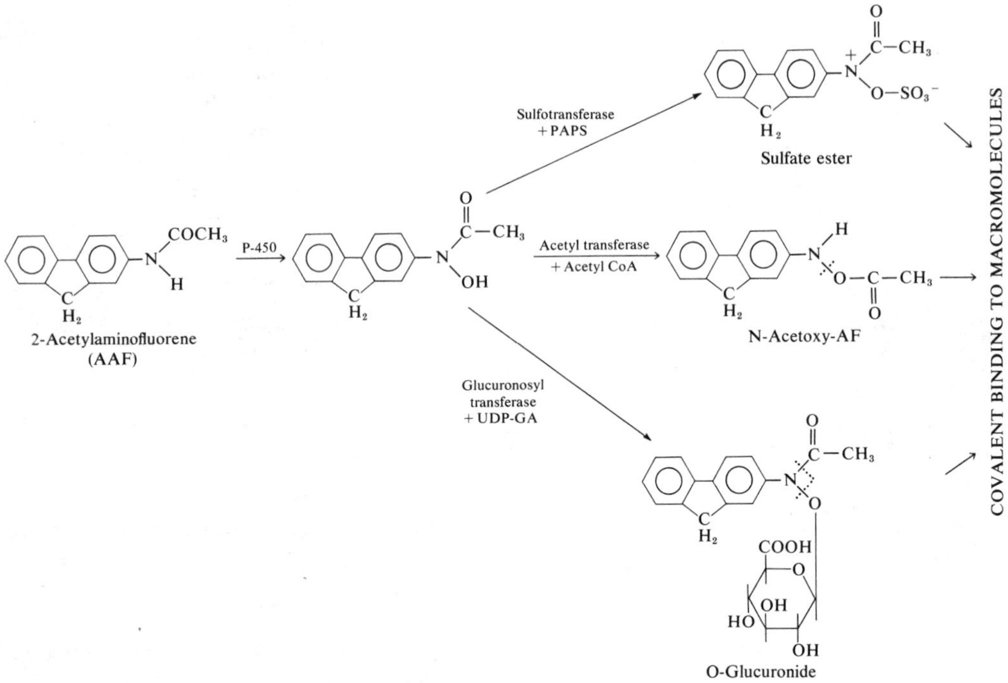

Figure 4–18. Bioactivation of 2-acetylaminofluorene.

the acetylation of isoniazid (Figure 4–19) to form acetylisoniazid. This unstable metabolite rearranges to produce acetylhydrazine, which is oxidized by cytochrome P-450 to *N*-hydroxylacetyl hydrazine. This unstable derivative fragments to an acetyl radical or carbonium ion, which can acylate tissue macromolecules. Thus, the acetylation reaction produces a product that subsequently degrades and, in conjunction with cytochrome P-450-mediated *N*-hydroxylation, produces a toxic covalent-binding species.

Even the glutathione *S*-transferases can produce conjugates that can rearrange to reactive intermediates. For example, glutathione *S*-transferases can mediate the conjugation of 1,2-dihaloethanes with glutathione (Figure 4–20). In this reaction a halogen (usually chloride or bromide) is displaced and *S*-(2-haloethyl)-glutathione is formed. Since the sulfur is still nucleophilic, it can displace the halogen on the adjacent carbon to form a highly strained, three-membered-ring intermediate called an episulfonium or thiiranium ion. This electrophilic species has been shown to alkylate nucleic acids, an event associated with mutagenicity and carcinogenicity.

Some glutathione conjugates that are hydrolyzed to cysteine conjugates by the kidney are

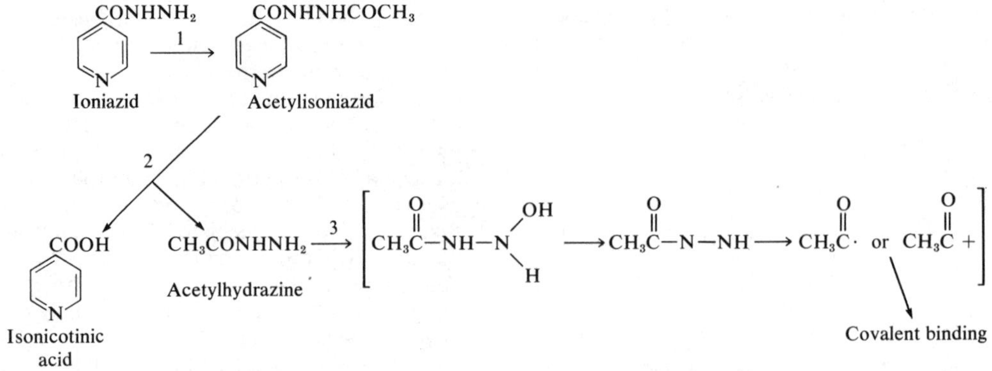

Figure 4–19. Bioactivation of isoniazid. *1*, *N*-acetyltransferase; *2*, hydrolysis; *3*, cytochrome P-450.

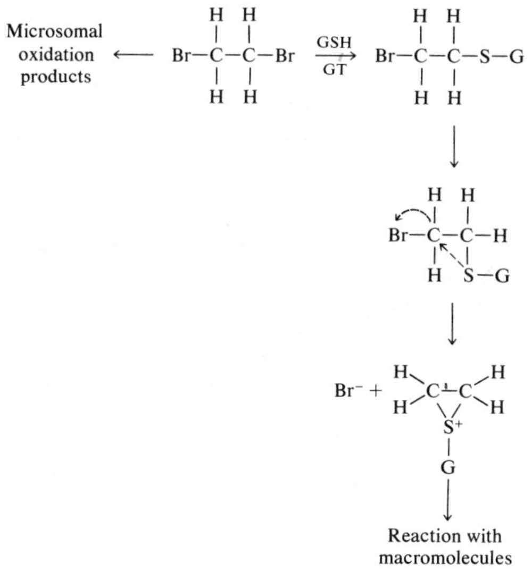

Microsomal oxidation products ←

Reaction with macromolecules

Figure 4–20. Bioactivation of 1,2-dibromoethane via glutathione transferase *(GT)*.

then bioactivated by a cysteine β-lyase. The cleavage of the β-carbon-sulfur bond by this enzyme produces a sulfhydryl-containing moiety that can react with kidney macromolecules or be conjugated by methylation. Hexachlorobutadiene and various fluorinated ethylenes are toxic by this pathway.

The biotransformation of acetaminophen is a good example of how a minor metabolic pathway can result in tissue injury. This analgesic is quite safe, and only under abnormal conditions does acetaminophen administration result in hepatotoxicity. Acetaminophen (*N*-acetyl-4-aminophenol) is readily conjugated with sulfate and glucuronic acid (Figure 4–21). Following large doses, the sulfate pool becomes exhausted before much of the compound is biotransformed. Since the glucuronidation pathway is rate limited, more of the parent compound is available for biotransformation by the cytochrome P-450 system. This minor pathway produces *N*-hydroxy-acetaminophen, which converts to a quinoneimine resonance form. The carbon atom ortho to the phenolic group is electrophilic and reacts with the nucleophilic sulfhydryl of glutathione. As long as sufficient gluta-

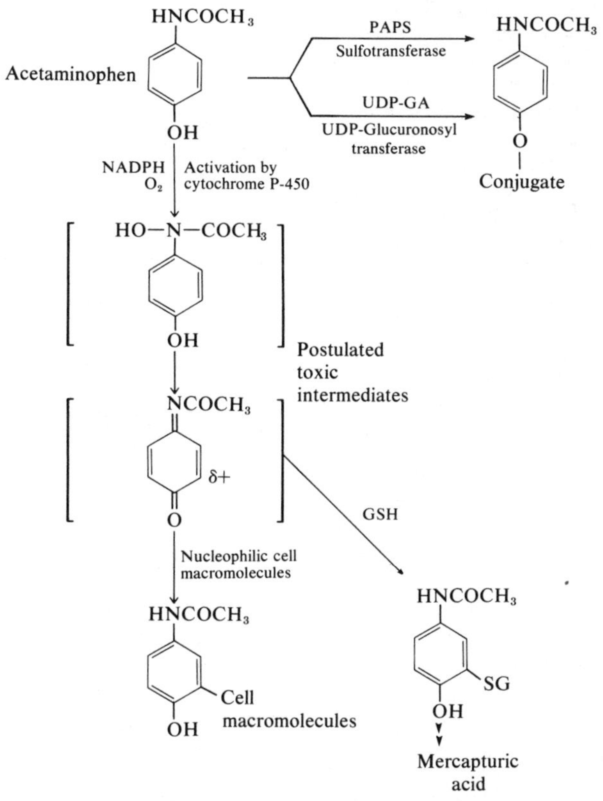

Figure 4–21. Bioactivation of acetaminophen.

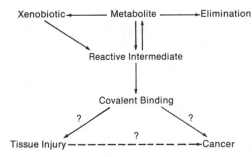

Figure 4–22. Proposed relationship between biotransformation, bioactivation, and toxicity of a xenobiotic. (From Plaa, G. L., and Hewitt, W. R. [eds.]: *Toxicology of the Liver.* Raven Press, New York, 1982.)

thione is available, this reactive intermediate can be detoxified. However, the pool of glutathione is limited and is depleted. When this occurs, the electrophilic intermediate reacts covalently with nucleophilic substituents present on macromolecules, an event associated with hepatotoxicity. If the cytochrome P-450 pathway is enhanced by previous induction or if the sulfate and/or glutathione pools are depleted by a previous stress (fasting, another xenobiotic, etc.), the toxicity of a given dose of acetaminophen will be enhanced. Early administration of compounds containing a sulfhydryl group, such as cysteamine, cysteine, *N*-acetycysteine, and methionine, can decrease the severity of liver injury.

In summary, the toxicity of acetaminophen requires a dose or doses such that there is a depletion of the sulfate pool, overwhelming of glucuronidation, increased biotransformation by the cytochrome P-450 system and ultimately depletion of glutathione. Only this combination of events results in an overwhelming of defense mechanisms and increased covalent binding of toxic intermediates to cellular macromolecules. Acetaminophen is not a unique example. Most chemicals follow a similar sequence of events in that some critical pathway becomes over-

whelmed by continued production of reactive intermediates.

Figure 4–22 summarizes the proposed relationship between biotransformation, bioactivation, and toxicity of a xenobiotic. It is seen that the parent compound or its metabolite may be converted to a reactive intermediate. Reactive intermediates can be detoxified and thus become metabolites that are eliminated. Indeed, only a small portion of these reactive intermediates may become covalently bound to tissue macromolecules. The relationship between covalent binding of xenobiotics to cellular components and tissue injuries remains to be established.

REFERENCES

Caldwell, J., and Jakoby, W. B.: *Biological Basis of Detoxification.* Academic Press, Inc., New York, 1983.

Gillette, J. R.: Significance of mixed function oxygenases and nitroreductase in drug metabolism. *Ann. N.Y. Acad. Sci.,* **160:**558–70, 1969.

Gram, T. E., and Gillette, J. R.: Biotransformation of drugs. In Bacq. Z.M. (ed.): *Fundamentals of Biochemical Pharmacology.* Pergamon Press, Ltd., New York, 1971, pp. 571–609.

Jakoby, W. B. (ed.): *Enzymatic Basis of Detoxication,* Vols. 1–2 Academic Press, Inc., New York, 1980.

Jakoby, W. B.; Bend, J. R.; and Caldwell, J.: *Metabolic Basis of Detoxification: Metabolism of Functional Groups.* Academic Press, Inc., New York, 1982.

Jenner, P., and Testa, B. (eds.): *Concepts in Drug Metabolism,* Parts A–B. Marcel Dekker, Inc., New York, 1981.

La Du, B. N.; Mandel, H. G.; and Way, E. L.: *Fundamentals of Drug Metabolism and Drug Disposition.* Williams & Wilkins Co., Baltimore, 1971.

Poland, A.; Glover, E.; and Kende, A. S.: Stereospecific, high affinity binding of 2,3,7,8-tetrachlorodibenzo-*p*-dioxin by hepatic cytosol. Evidence that the binding species is the receptor for the induction of aryl hydrocarbon hydroxylase. *J. Biol. Chem.,* **251:**4936–46, 1976.

Schenkman, J. B., and Kupfer, D. (eds.): *Hepatic Cytochrome P-450 Monooxygenase System.* Pergamon Press, Ltd., New York, 1982.

Testa, B., and Jenner, P.: *Drug Metabolism: Chemical and Biochemical Aspects.* Marcel Dekker, Inc., New York, 1976.

Testa, B., and Jenner, P.: Inhibitors of cytochrome P-450s and their mechanism of action. *Drug Metab. Rev.,* **12:**1–117, 1981.

Chapter 5

CHEMICAL CARCINOGENS

Gary M. Williams and John H. Weisburger

INTRODUCTION

Chemical carcinogens are a type of toxic agent that exhibits a specific, defining adverse effect—the production of cancer in animals or humans. In many respects, chemical carcinogens are similar to drugs and other toxic agents: for example, carcinogens in a given experimental setting show dose-response relationships. Carcinogens undergo biotransformation, as would any similarly structured xenobiotic. In addition, the effects of chemical carcinogens vary with the species, strain, and sex of the experimental animal, as is the case with other chemicals. Carcinogens interact with other environmental agents; their effects are sometimes enhanced and sometimes decreased, as occurs with drugs. Yet, some very important differences render chemical carcinogenesis a specialized field of toxicology. Chemical carcinogens of the type that have the ability to react with DNA differ from most other kinds of toxins in that (1) their biologic effect is persistent, cumulative, and delayed; (2) divided doses are in some cases more effective than an individual large dose; and (3) the underlying mechanisms, particularly with respect to interaction and alteration of genetic elements and other macromolecules, are distinct.

Early Discoveries in Chemical Carcinogenesis

Several types of chemicals were discovered to be carcinogenic in experimental animals after having first been suspected of causing cancer in man (Shimkin, 1980; Becker, 1982; Schottenfeld and Fraumeni, 1982). The association between exposure to soot and coal tars and cancer was identified in the late eighteenth century by the English physician Percival Pott who observed that many of his patients who had cancer of the scrotum were chimney sweeps. That coal tar could cause cancer at the point of application in rabbits was reported by Yamagiwa and Ichikawa in 1916. In the 1920s, English investigators, directed by Kennaway, fractionated coal tar and discovered the carcinogenic potency of pure

polynuclear aromatic hydrocarbons, including dibenz[a,h]anthracene and benzo[a]pyrene.

The aromatic amines are another type of chemical carcinogen whose study also stems from the discovery of cancer in humans exposed to them. In the late 1800s, the German physician Rehn noted a cluster of cases of cancer of the urinary bladder among workers in the dye industry. The experimental evidence for the carcinogenicity of amines to which these workers were exposed did not appear until 1937, when Hueper and associates found that 2-naphthylamine could cause bladder cancer in dogs, reproducing the lesions seen in humans.

A third important type of carcinogen, azo dyes, has not been implicated in human cancer. In this case, the illustrious pharmacologist Ehrlich discovered that exposure to a related chemical, scarlet red, led to a reversible proliferation of liver cells. It was not until 25 years later, 1932–1934, that in pioneering studies Kinosita and Yoshida independently discovered the carcinogenic effect of some azo dyes in rodents.

In the years since, many other classes and types of chemicals were found to be carcinogenic (Searle, 1984; Arcos et al., 1968–1983; IARC Monogr. series, 1971–1983). Some, such as vinyl chloride, were discovered after they were suspected of being involved in the development of cancer in humans. Others, such as dimethylhydrazine, were identified as a result of their structural similarity to known carcinogens. Some chemicals were found to be carcinogenic in the course of routine bioassays for the detection of adverse effects in chronic toxicity studies; this was the case with N-2-fluorenylacetamide and dimethylnitrosamine. Some chemicals were also discovered to be carcinogenic during investigations that attempted to reproduce in laboratory animals adverse effects that had been observed in humans or domestic animals. A study dealing with the possible causative factors of amyotrophic lateral sclerosis prevalent on Pacific islands led to the finding that the plant product cycasin was a potent carcinogen. Other tests delving into the factor responsible for turkey x disease, which accounted for extensive losses of livestock, pinpointed aflatoxin B_1 and, later, other mycotoxins as hepatotoxins and potent carcinogens. The powerful carcinogenicity of *bis*(chloromethyl)ether was observed first in the laboratory, and a few years later lung cancer was noted in individuals exposed occupationally.

DEFINITION OF CHEMICAL CARCINOGENS

Chemical carcinogens are defined operationally by their ability to induce neoplasms. Four types of response have generally been accepted as evidence of induction of neoplasms: most importantly (1) the presence of types of tumors not seen in controls; (2) an increase in the incidence of the tumor types occurring in controls; (3) the development of tumors earlier than in controls; and (4) an increased multiplicity of tumors. For agents producing any of these effects, the term "carcinogen" is generally used, although it literally means giving rise to carcinomas, i.e., epithelial malignancies. For agents producing sarcomas of mesenchymal origin, the term "oncogen" is more correct. As evidence of carcinogenicity, production of even benign neoplasms is accepted, a practice justified by the fact that no chemical has yet been identified that produces exclusively benign neoplasms.

The application of these criteria must, of course, be made by experienced investigators as part of a full evaluation of the properties of the chemical (see section on Bioassay, p. 164). Otherwise artifacts and inadequate results can lead to misclassification, an error appropriately described by Roe (1983) as "pseudocarcinogenesis."

Chemicals capable of eliciting one of the four responses described, and which are thereby classified as carcinogens, comprise a highly diverse collection of agents, including organic and inorganic chemicals, solid-state materials, cytotoxins, hormones, and immunosuppressants. For some of these chemicals, such as neoplasm enhancers or promoters, the designation "carcinogen" is perhaps unfortunate, but necessary, since these chemicals in specific situations do increase the yield of cancers, albeit usually those that occur spontaneously. Nonetheless, the diverse agents that can be considered carcinogens have different properties and appear to produce neoplasms through different modes of action. In turn, these distinct mechanisms of action necessitate appropriate health risk analyses.

MODE OF ACTION OF CHEMICAL CARCINOGENS

The elucidation of the mechanism of action of a carcinogen entails establishing how the effects of the chemical on a cell or tissue lead to the evolution of cells with abnormalities essential to the neoplastic phenotype. Carcinogens interact with numerous tissue constituents and produce a number of effects, which are covered in the section on Reactions of Carcinogens (p. 138). To identify actions that are necessary or contributory to the production of neoplasms, an understanding of the neoplastic process is required. Although this has not yet been completely achieved, current knowledge provides considerable insight, which points to certain effects of chemicals as being crucial to carcinogenicity.

The induction of cancer in humans and in animals by chemicals proceeds through a complex series of individual reactions, which usually involve a protracted expression time from onset of exposure to manifestation of a neoplasm. These events are subject to and controlled by a number of modifying factors. The events can be divided into two sequences, one in which the normal cell is converted to a neoplastic cell and a second in which the neoplastic cell develops into an overt neoplasm (Figure 5–1). Chemicals are involved in diverse ways in both sequences.

1. Neoplastic Conversion

i. Biotransformation by host enzyme systems. Numerous distinct enzyme systems carry out the detoxication and elimination of xenobiotics. As part of this biotransformation, many carcinogens undergo enzymatic activation to a reactive ultimate carcinogen. A small number of carcinogens, mostly industrial intermediates and chemotherapeutic drugs, are reactive in their parent form and, therefore, do not require activation. In addition, there seem to be carcinogens that, while not reactive themselves, generate reactive moieties intracellularly.

ii. Interaction of the ultimate carcinogen with cellular constituents. Carcinogens that form reactive species undergo covalent reactions with most cellular macromolecules, including DNA. The damaged DNA is subject to removal and restoration by repair enzyme systems. Other altered macromolecules are disposed of and replaced. Thus, under these conditions, the cell can recover from most of the immediate effects of carcinogen interaction.

iii. Fixation of carcinogen damage. If the cell replicates while DNA damage is persistent, permanent alterations in the genome can be pro-

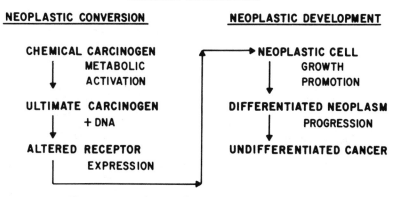

Figure 5–1. Main steps in the carcinogenic process.

duced in several possible ways, including the mispairing of bases leading to point mutations, errors in replication yielding frame-shift mutations, transpositions resulting in codon rearrangement (Cairns, 1981), combinations of these alterations in sequential steps, and their amplification. Codon rearrangement may involve sequences known as oncogenes, which are emerging as critical gene sequences for transformation (Land *et al.*, 1983; Bishop, 1985; Reynolds *et al.*, 1986). At least five distinct mechanisms have been identified as being responsible for conversion of proto-oncogenes to active oncogenes, including point mutation. The gene products of many oncogenes have been identified and most function in biochemical processes that could be involved in transformation.

Interactions with proteins that regulate gene expression (Rubin, 1980) or alteration of enzymatic methylation of DNA (Boehm and Drahovsky, 1983; Nyce *et al.*, 1983) have also been suspected to be able to permanently alter cell function. In the case of interactions with the mitotic apparatus, chromosomal mutations and aneuploidy could result. All these alterations can generate a permanently abnormal cell with altered genotype and phenotype. The abnormal cell may possess only some properties of neoplastic cells or, if the alterations are sufficient, may be fully neoplastic.

iv. Multiplication of the altered cells. Abnormal cells that are not fully neoplastic may be held in check by tissue homeostatic factors or, if the conditions of carcinogen exposure or abnormalities generated in the cells permit, they may undergo limited proliferation to form "preneoplastic" lesions (Farber, in Becker, 1982). During these processes, further alterations of DNA as a result of transpositions and other error-prone processes are possible and would lead to the formation of a neoplastic cell.

2. Neoplastic Development and Progression

i. Progressive growth to neoplasm formation (promotion). Cells that have undergone neoplastic conversion may remain dormant, presumably being controlled by tissue homeostatic factors. The regulatory factors are probably transmitted by one of several types of intercellular communication. Some neoplastic cells with the requisite abnormalities may be capable of progressive growth to form neoplasms. For suppressed neoplastic cells, their proliferation is facilitated by promoters, possibly by the interruption of tissue growth control, leading to neoplastic development.

ii. Progression. Some neoplasms undergo qualitative changes in their phenotypic properties, possibly including transition from benign to malignant behavior (Foulds, 1969). This probably reflects the selection during growth of a population with a genotype coding for advantageous phenotypic properties. New genotypes could arise in neoplasms through errors in DNA replication, alterations in chromosome constitution, or hybridization of different cell types. The neoplasm that ultimately emerges is in most cases the progeny of a single cell; that is, it is a clonal population. Nevertheless, neoplasms display abnormalities in expression of numerous gene products.

3. Overall Mechanisms

Many of the specific steps in carcinogenesis are controlled and modified by numerous endogenous and exogenous factors. Thus, species, strain, sex, and age affect the processes in certain of these steps, particularly biotransformation and DNA repair. In addition, hormonal, immunologic, and other endogenous factors may enhance or diminish the extent and rate of the carcinogenic process. For example, cocarcinogens enhance neoplastic conversion, while promoters enhance neoplastic development (see section on Modifiers of Carcinogenesis, p. 141). Among the exogenous elements, nutritional factors are heavily involved. Furthermore, many interactions occur between all of these elements as well as between synthetic and also naturally occurring chemicals that can augment or decrease the overall effectiveness of the administered agent in leading to cancer.

The neoplastic state is heritable at the cellular level (i.e., the progeny of the division of a neoplastic cell inherit the neoplastic potential), and thus theories on the mechanisms by which chemicals convert normal cells to malignant ones must ultimately explain how the effect becomes permanent. In the 1920s, Boveri suggested that cancer arose from an imbalance of chromosomes. The important discovery that carcinogens interact with DNA provided a basis on which the permanent neoplastic state could be explained by alterations in the genotype. A number of considerations support the view that DNA is a critical target of carcinogens (Table 5–1). Nevertheless, studies on the interactions of carcinogens with proteins and RNA have led to the alternate postulate that effects on these macromolecules could eventually be rendered permanent through epigenetic mechanisms on gene expression creating a new stable state of differentiation (Rubin, 1980; Nyce et al., 1983).

Although these two distinct mechanisms for neoplastic conversion, i.e., genetic and epigenetic, have often been thought of as alternatives for the action of carcinogens generally, the fact that carcinogens are an extremely diverse group of agents, both structurally and in terms of biologic effects, makes it likely that chemical carcinogens operate in a variety of different ways.

Table 5–1. CONSIDERATIONS INDICATING THAT DNA IS A CRITICAL TARGET FOR CARCINOGENS

1. Many carcinogens are or can be biotransformed to electrophiles that react covalently with DNA. Consequently, such carcinogens are mutagens.
2. Defects in DNA repair such as in xeroderma pigmentosum predispose to cancer development.
3. Several heritable or chromosomal abnormalities predispose to cancer development.
4. Initiated dormant tumor cells are persistent, which is consistent with a change in DNA.
5. Cancer is heritable at the cellular level and, therefore, may result from an alteration of DNA.
6. Most, if not all, cancers display chromosomal abnormalities.
7. Many cancers display aberrant gene expression.
8. Cells from many cancers contain activated oncogenes.

The pioneering studies of Elizabeth and James Miller (1981, 1983) revealed that many structurally different types of carcinogens could give rise to electrophilic reactants that interacted with cellular macromolecules. Such carcinogens that interact with DNA are mutagenic, as revealed in the early studies of Auerbach, Tatum, and Demerec and firmly established by many investigators in the last decade (see Ames, in Ramel et al., 1986; Rosenkranz and Mermelstein, in Williams et al., 1980; Sugimura et al., 1982). However, a number of carcinogenic substances such as plastics, asbestos, and hormones have structures that do not suggest an obvious reactive form (i.e., an electrophile), and have not been documented to alter DNA, nor to be gene mutagens. Thus, it has been recognized that various modes of action seem to be involved in the overall carcinogenic effects of chemicals (IARC, 1983; ICPEMC, 1983). Accordingly, several distinctions between different types of carcinogens have been proposed (Kolbye, in Williams et al., 1980; Kroes, in Williams et al., 1983; Stott and Watanabe, 1982; Weisburger and Williams, 1981). In one of these, first proposed by Williams in 1977 as a working hypothesis to call attention to possible differences in the properties of carcinogens, two major types, genotoxic and epigenetic, were described.

Carcinogens that interact with and alter DNA were categorized as genotoxic or DNA-reactive. These carcinogens are, of course, mutagenic. DNA alteration leading to neoplastic conversion of cells in the first sequence in carcinogenesis is the likely basis for their carcinogenicity. Considering the variety of abnormalities in cancer cells, it seems that such carcinogens would have to produce multiple alterations of the gene mutation type, alterations in major regulatory genes, or changes in expression of large regions of the genome. The latter could come about through chromosomal mutations or activation of oncogenes (Bishop, 1985; Land et al., 1983; Harris and Autrup, 1983).

Carcinogens designated as epigenetic were those for which no evidence of DNA reactivity had been found and for which there was evidence of another biologic effect that could be the basis for carcinogenicity. Possible mechanisms may involve cytotoxicity and chronic tissue injury, intracellular generation of reactive species, hormonal imbalance, immunologic effects, or promotional activity. In some cases, these agents could indirectly cause genetic alterations and neoplastic conversion by means of the production of inaccurate DNA synthesis, reactive oxygen free radicals, aberrant methylation, and chromosomal abnormalities (Williams, in Williams et al., 1983). Alternatively, they could produce neoplastic conversion by epigenetic effects on gene expression (Rubin, 1980; Nyce *et al.,* 1983). For many of these, however, they probably do not produce neoplastic conversion at all, but rather act in the sequence of neoplastic development to facilitate tumor development by cells that are either genetically altered or have been independently altered by genotoxic carcinogens.

As will be detailed in this chapter, it now seems likely that there is no single mode of action by which all carcinogens produce cancer. Nevertheless, the ultimate effect, the establishment of a neoplastic population with a permanently altered phenotype, is the same. Whether that comes about by totally diverse actions or actions that are initially diverse, but which culminate in a final common step (e.g., oncogene activation) is not yet known. To completely elucidate the essential effects of any particular agent, it will be necessary to determine at what steps in the overall process of carcinogenesis the agent functions.

CLASSES OF CHEMICAL CARCINOGENS

The classification of carcinogens described in the previous edition of this text separates them into classes based on their chemical or biologic properties. These, in turn, can be placed in the two general categories: DNA-reactive (genotoxic) and epigenetic (Table 5–2), where available information is sufficient. Otherwise, specific carcinogens or classes are left unassigned.

The proposal of different types of carcinogens has been regarded as premature by some, even to the present, although the idea has now received a measure of acceptance from international groups (IARC, 1983; ICPEMC, 1983). The scientific facts in support of mechanistically distinct types of carcinogens have increased greatly since 1977 when the proposal was first advanced, and we now consider it to be established. Also, the organization of carcinogens according to their properties provides a useful structure for the presentation of this complex subject and, therefore, will be used in this chapter.

The DNA-reactive (genotoxic) category comprises carcinogens that chemically interact with DNA. The defining characteristic is a biochemical property and, therefore, biochemical assays are most definitive for identifying such agents. In the absence of such data, DNA reactivity can be indirectly assessed in short-term tests, but clearly the reliability of such evidence depends on the characteristics and performance of the tests. This category consists mainly of carcinogens that function as electrophilic reactants, as originally postulated by the Millers (1981). Also,

Table 5–2. CLASSIFICATION OF CARCINO-GENIC CHEMICALS

CATEGORY AND CLASS	EXAMPLE
A. *DNA-Reactive (Genotoxic) Carcinogens*	
1. Activation-independent	Alkylating agent
2. Activation dependent	Polycyclic aromatic hydrocarbon, nitrosamine
3. Inorganic*	Metal
B. *Epigenetic Carcinogens*	
1. Promoter	Organochlorine pesticide
	Saccharin
2. Cytotoxic	Nitrilotriacetic acid
3. Hormone-modifying	Estrogen
	Amitrole
4. Immunosuppressor	Purine analog
5. Solid state	Plastics
C. *Unclassified*	
1. Peroxisome proliferators	Clofibrate
	Phthalate esters
2. Miscellaneous	Dioxane

* Some are tentatively categorized as genotoxic because of evidence for damage of DNA; others may operate through epigenetic mechanisms such as alterations in fidelity of DNA polymerases.

because some metals have displayed genotoxic effects suggestive of DNA interaction, these have been tentatively placed in this category. However, the studies of Loeb and colleagues (Loeb and Mildvan, in Eichhorn and Marzilli, 1981; Hansen and Stern, 1984) on effects of metals on the fidelity of DNA polymerases suggest that these might yield abnormal DNA by a mechanism distinct from the electrophilic DNA-damaging compounds. For an agent that has both DNA-reactive and epigenetic properties, assignment is made to the DNA-reactive category.

The second broad category, designated as epigenetic carcinogens, comprises those carcinogens for which there is evidence of a lack of direct interaction with genetic material and for which another biologic effect has been delineated that could be the basis for carcinogenicity. This category contains chemicals with diverse modes of action (Table 5–2). Agents producing effects that might be indirectly genotoxic are presently left unclassified or grouped with epigenetic agents because of the fact that genotoxicity (if ultimately established) still is secondary to another biologic effect.

It is important to note that this scheme does not preclude genotoxic carcinogens as such or as metabolites from also having epigenetic effects. Indeed, the potency of some carcinogens may reside in their genotoxic as well as promoting actions.

The recognition of different types of carcinogens has major implications for human risk extrapolation from data on experimental carcinogenesis (Weisburger and Williams, in Pereira, 1983). Genotoxic carcinogens, because of their effects on genetic material, pose a clear qualitative hazard to humans. These carcinogens are occasionally effective after a single exposure, act in a cumulative manner, and act together with other genotoxic carcinogens having the same organotropism. Thus, the level of human exposure acceptable for "no risk" to ensue needs to be evaluated most stringently in the light of existing data and relevant mechanisms. Often, with powerful carcinogens, zero exposure is the goal, even though with some agents there is evidence for practical no-effect levels. Further discussion will deal with these quantitative aspects.

On the other hand, some classes of epigenetic carcinogens have carcinogenic effects occurring only with high and sustained levels of exposure that lead to prolonged physiologic abnormalities, hormonal imbalances, or tissue injury. Consequently, the risk from exposure may be of a quantitative nature. This is almost certainly the case with estrogens, which are carcinogenic at high, unphysiologic chronic exposure levels in animal studies and in humans. Lower levels are obviously innocuous, for otherwise every individual would develop cancer. Thus, for epigenetic carcinogens, it may be possible to establish a "safe" threshold of exposure once their mechanism of action is elucidated. For example, for promoters, a threshold can be determined in several experimental systems involving a series of dose levels of promotion following an initiating treatment with a genotoxic carcinogen. Such a threshold level permits assignment of a maximum safe dose using a safety factor (see section on Quantitative Aspects, p. 150).

The types of chemicals found in each of the ten major classes (Table 5–2) are reviewed in the following discussion. It will be noted that not all carcinogens can be precisely categorized, pointing to the need for additional data (unclassified group). Also, in some instances, structurally related chemicals fall into different classes as a consequence of their differing biologic or toxicologic properties.

A. DNA-Reactive (Genotoxic) Carcinogens

This category contains most of the "classic" organic carcinogens. These can be subdivided according to whether they are active in their parent form or require metabolic activation.

1. DIRECT-ACTING OR ACTIVATION-INDEPENDENT CARCINOGENS

The types of activation-independent genotoxic agents are listed in Table 5–3 together with typical examples of each type. Inherent in the chemical structure of these agents is the property of chemical reactivity; they are electrophilic reactants that can interact with nucleophilic molecules, including DNA. The adducts formed in DNA have been identified for many of these (Rajalakshmi et al., in Becker, 1982).

These agents are not found in nature, but rather, are synthetic products used in chemical production and as cytostatic agents. The direct-acting carcinogens include strained lactones, such as β-propriolactone, propane sulfone, and α,β-unsaturated larger-ring lactones, epoxides, imines, alkyl and other sulfate esters, and some active halogen derivatives, such as bis(chloromethyl)ether (Fox and Scott, 1980; Goldschmidt, in Sontag, 1981; Arcos et al., 1983; Van Duuren et al., 1983). Although such reactive chemicals might be thought to be carcinogenic under a variety of conditions, some agents, such as methyl methanesulfonate, are not highly carcinogenic in animals, mainly because they undergo secondary hydrolytic decomposition, or their reactive groupings provide ready targets for specific detoxication reactions. Nevertheless, these reagents can be potent carcinogens. Several, including ethylnitrosourea, produce cancer in the offspring of treated female animals (Rice, 1979). Dimethyl sulfate was reported to induce cancer in humans after laboratory handling without adequate precautions (Hoffmann, 1980).

Halo Ethers and Other Active Haolgen Compounds. Chemicals such as certain halo ethers in which the halogen-carbon bond is chemically activated through electron transfer are extremely powerful alkylating agents and carcinogens. The most important example is bis(chloromethyl)ether, discovered first to be carcinogenic by Van Duuren, Laskin, and their associates in laboratory experiments (see Arcos et al.,1982). It was subsequently found that this highly reactive alkylating agent, an important chemical intermediate in industry, led to cancer of the upper respiratory tract in humans exposed to apparently low levels of this chemical. In animal models inhalation of 0.1 ppm was carcinogenic.

The higher homologs appear to be less active. Bis(chloroethyl)ether induces tumors of liver and other organs in mice by mechanisms perhaps not related to direct-acting genotoxicity, especially since it appears to be inactive in rats. The related bis(2-chloro-1-methylethyl)ether also was not carcinogenic in rats.

Table 5–3. EXAMPLES OF DIRECT-ACTING OR PRIMARY CARCINOGENS

Alkyl Imines
Ethylene imine

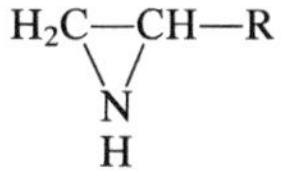

$$H_2C—CH—R$$
(N, H ring — aziridine structure)

Alkylene Epoxides
1,2,3,4-Butadiene epoxide

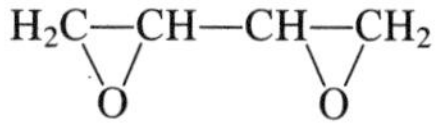

$$H_2C—CH—CH—CH_2$$ (each with O epoxide)

Small-Ring Lactones
β-Propiolactone

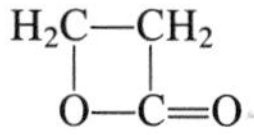

$$H_2C—CH_2$$
$$O—C=O$$

Propane sultone

$$CH_2—CH_2$$
$$CH_2—SO_2$$ O

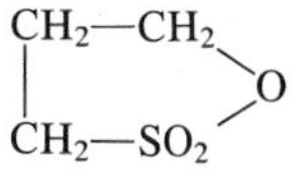

Sulfate Esters
Dimethyl sulfate
Methyl methanesulfonate
1,4-Butanediol dimethanesulfonate (Myleran)

$CH_3OSO_2OCH_3$
$CH_3SO_2OCH_3$
$CH_3SO_2O(CH_2)_4OSO_2CH_3$

Mustards
Bis(2-Chloroethyl)sulfide (mustard gas, Yperite)

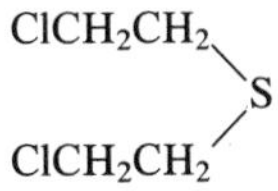

$ClCH_2CH_2$
$ClCH_2CH_2$ S

Bis(2-Chloroethyl)amine (nor-nitrogen mustard; R=H
nitrogen mustard; R=CH$_3$)

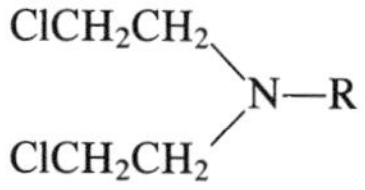

$ClCH_2CH_2$
$ClCH_2CH_2$ N—R

Cyclophosphamide (Cytoxan)

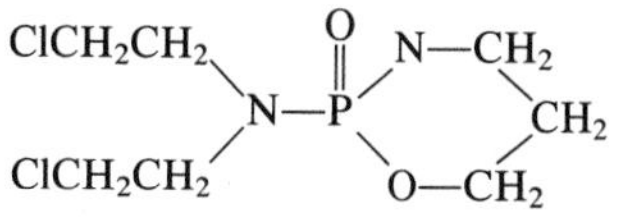

$ClCH_2CH_2$ N—P (with O, N—CH$_2$, CH$_2$, O—CH$_2$ ring)
$ClCH_2CH_2$

2-Naphthylamine mustard (Chlornaphazine)

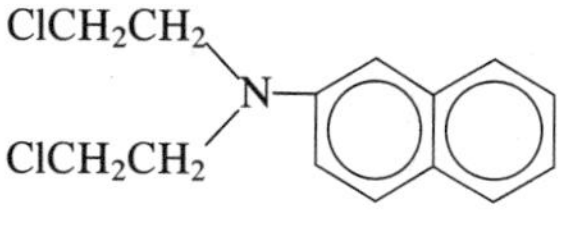

$ClCH_2CH_2$
$ClCH_2CH_2$ N (naphthalene ring)

Triethylenemelamine

$H_2C—CH_2$ (N ring; with H$_2$C—N, H$_2$C and CH$_2$—N, CH$_2$ on benzene ring)

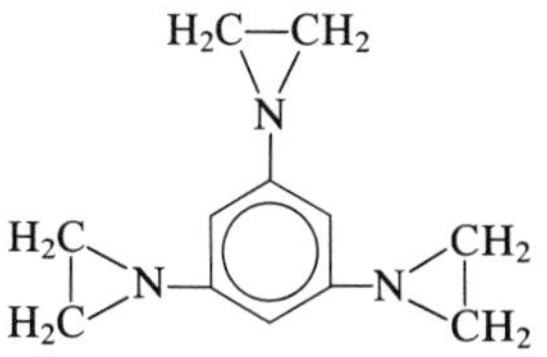

Active Halogen Compounds
Bis(chloromethyl)ether
Benzyl chloride
Methyl iodide
Dimethylcarbamyl chloride

$ClCH_2OCH_2Cl$
$C_6H_5CH_2Cl$
CH_3I
$(CH_3)_2NCOCl$

Nitrosamides and Nitrosoureas. Agents such as *N*-methylnitrosourea, *N*-methylnitroso-urethan, and *N*-methyl-*N'*-nitro-*N*-nitroso-guanidine (Table 5–11), unlike sulfate esters or imines, for example, are chemically stable in the anhydrous state. However, under aqueous conditions they undergo hydrolytic decomposition, possibly modified by specific enzymes, to liberate an alkylating moiety. The carcinogenicity of these compounds is further discussed in

Table 5–4. PLATINUM (II) AMINE CHELATES

These compounds were developed as antineoplastic drugs. They are direct-acting mutagens and carcinogens. The *cis* isomers are usually more active than the *trans* compounds.

cis-Dichlorodiamine-platinum(II) or DDP

trans-DDP

cis-Dichlorobis (pyrrolidine)-platinum (II)

cis- or *trans*(−)-or *trans*(+)-Dichloro-1,2-diaminocyclohexane-platinum(II) complexes

the section on Nitrosamines and Nitrosamides (p. 117) together with other carcinogens to which they are structurally related.

Cis-Platinum(II) Coordination Complexes. This group of chemicals structurally represents a complex chelate of divalent platinum and an appropriate anion that most of the time is chloride with two molecules possessing amino groups (Table 5–4). These structures can assume *cis* or *trans* configurations. The simplest compound in the series is the one in which R is ammonia to form *cis*-dichlorodiamineplatinum (II). This and related compounds have found use as drugs in cancer therapy. Other compounds of this series involve structures where the amine is pyrrolidine, cyclopentylamine, and 1,2-diaminocyclohexane. Several of these chemicals exist as *cis* and *trans* isomers and the cyclohexane compound as *cis, trans*(−), and *trans*(+). These chemicals are direct-acting mutagens in the *Salmonella typhimurium* system of Ames, and they also exhibit activity in various other genetic tests such as inactivation of transforming DNA, which is typical of direct-acting genotoxic chemicals. In addition, they are powerfully carcinogenic as measured by a number of tests such as induction of lung tumors in mice, initiation of skin tumors when applied to skin of mice followed by phorbol ester promotion, and induction of sarcomas upon subcutaneous injection. The *cis* stereoisomer is more active than the *trans* compound. With the diaminocyclohexane derivative, the *cis* compound also was more ac-

tive than the *trans* compound, although the latter did exhibit activity, depending on the chemical, that was much less mutagenic than the *trans*(+) or *cis* derivative (Leopold *et al.,* 1981). The reactive intermediate derived from the chloride derivatives appears to be an aquo species. The geometry of the stereoisomers of the *cis* isomer is such that they chelate the O^6 and the N^7 positions of guanine, which may account for their mutagenic and carcinogenic effects.

2. PROCARCINOGENS OR ACTIVATION-DEPENDENT CARCINOGENS

Most of the known chemical carcinogens are in the form of precursor compounds, often called parent, pre-, or procarcinogens. These activation-dependent carcinogens usually do not produce cancer at the site of application (except for certain skin carcinogens such as the polycyclic aromatic hydrocarbons), but rather are carcinogenic to distant tissues where metabolic activation occurs. The capacity for biotransformation varies greatly between species and organs, accounting largely for the species differences and organotropism of these agents (Weisburger and Williams, in Becker, 1982.)

The large class of procarcinogens includes both naturally occurring substances and synthetic chemicals.

Polycyclic or Heterocyclic Aromatic Hydrocarbons. These chemicals consist of annelated aromatic (benzene) rings (Table 5–5). They occur in

Table 5–5. SEVERAL TYPICAL CARCINOGENIC
POLYCYCLIC AROMATIC HYDROCARBONS

These chemicals are all derived from the anthracene molecule. Anthracene itself is not carcinogenic, but in some tests benz[a]anthracene is carcinogenic. 7,12-Dimethylbenz[a]anthracene is a widely used synthetic hydrocarbon. Chemicals such as benzo[a]pyrene and dibenz[a,h]anthracene and similar structures occur in products of incomplete combustion, including coal and petroleum tars, and exhausts of combustion engines. They are also important components of tobacco smoke.

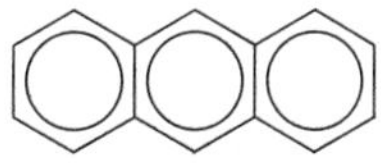

Anthracene

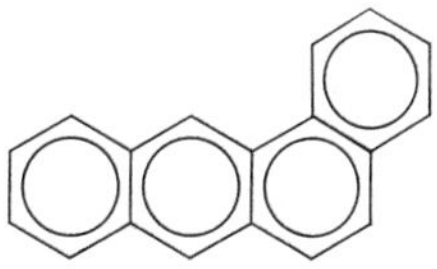

benz[a]anthracene

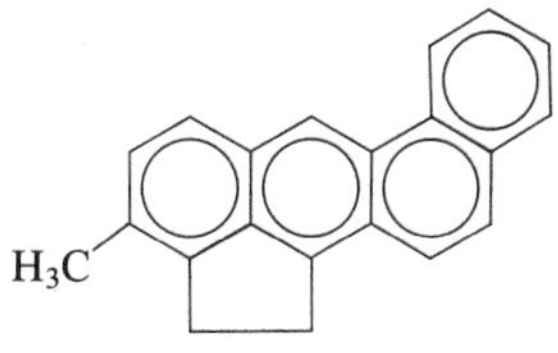

3-Methylcholanthrene

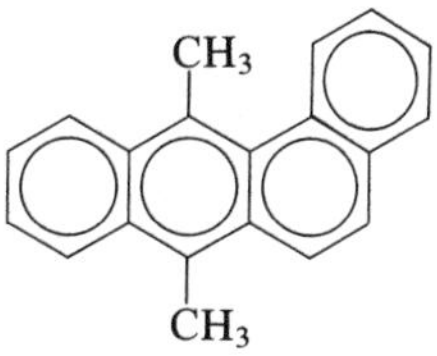

7,12-Dimethylbenz[a]anthracene

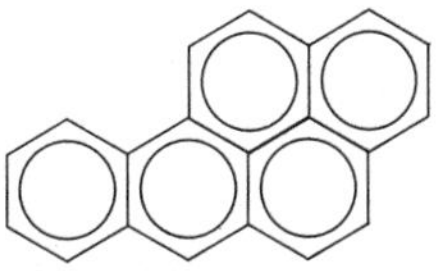

Benzo[a]pyrene

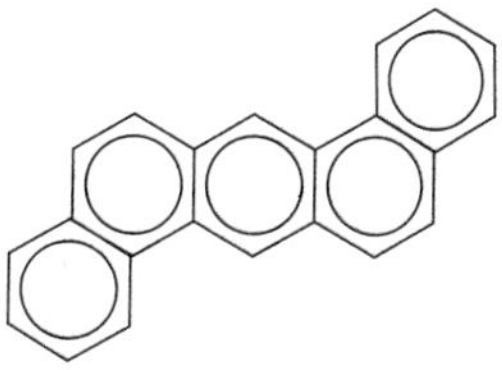

Dibenz[a,h]anthracene

a variety of environmental products such as soot, coal, tar, tobacco smoke, petroleum, and cutting oils. The isolation of pure aromatic hydrocarbons from coal tar and the demonstration of their carcinogenicity by English investigators led by Kennaway in the 1930s was one of the milestones in chemical carcinogenesis (*see* Shimkin, 1980; Phillips, 1983). There is good reason to suspect that these carcinogens are involved, for example, in lung cancer seen in cigarette smokers or tar-roofing workers (Surgeon General Rept., 1982). Nevertheless, it is also clear that in complex mixtures such as tar and smoke, other agents including promoters contribute to overall carcinogenicity (Hoffmann *et al.,* in Pereira, 1983).

Many rodent species are exquisitely sensitive to chemical carcinogens of this type. In mice, skin application of the more powerful agents such as 3-methylcholanthrene, 7,12-dimethyl-

benz[a]anthracene, and benzo[a]pyrene (Table 5–5) leads rather quickly to carcinoma formation. Subcutaneous injection produces sarcomas in rats or mice. Oral administration in sesame oil to 50-day-old female Sprague-Dawley rats results in the rapid induction of breast cancer, a model influenced by endocrine control, as is the disease in human females. However, administration of polycyclic aromatic hydrocarbons to rhesus monkeys and other primates has so far not been highly successful in yielding tumors (Adamson and Sieber, 1983). On the other hand, application of a crude petroleum oil to monkeys has induced cancer.

Within the large class of polycyclic hydrocarbons, many structure-activity studies have been done. Data so generated have led to theoretic developments relating chemical electronic structure to carcinogenic activity. For detailed discussions of these aspects, the reader is referred to reviews by Arcos (1978; 1985) and specialized monographs (T'so and Di Paolo, 1974; Cooke and Dennis, 1985; IARC Monogr. series). Suffice it to say that many of the results obtained can be interpreted, in the light of contemporary concepts, in terms of chemical structure and susceptibility to biochemical activation and detoxification.

Briefly, the situation can be summarized as follows. Many of the carcinogenic polycyclic aromatic hydrocarbons are derived from an angular benz[a]anthracene skeleton (Table 5–5). Anthracene itself is not carcinogenic, but benz[a]anthracene appears to have weak carcinogenicity. Addition of another benzene ring in select positions results in agents with powerful carcinogenicity such as dibenz[a,h]anthracene or benzo[a]pyrene, which are "natural" products resulting from incomplete combustion processes of carbonaceous materials. In addition, substitution of methyl groups on specific carbons of the ring also enhances carcinogenicity. Thus, 7,12-dimethylbenz[a]anthracene (DMBA) is one of the most powerful synthetic, polycyclic aromatic hydrocarbon carcinogens known.

As a result of the efforts of Lacassagne, Buu-Hoi, and others who synthesized and tested a number of polynuclear heterocyclic compounds, a wide variety has been found to be carcinogenic, usually at the point of injection. (Arcos, in Ts'o and DiPaolo, 1974; Woo and Arcos, in Sontag, 1981; Cooke and Dennis, 1983).

Biotransformation of Polycyclic Aromatic Hydrocarbons. Historically, on the basis of theoretic developments related to the electronic structure of these hydrocarbons, a certain area of the molecule, called the K region, was postulated to be related to the carcinogenic potential of a given compound (Pullman, in T'so and DiPaolo, 1974). On the other hand, substitution at another portion of the molecule, the L region, such as the 7 and 12 carbons in benz[a]anthracene, increased carcinogenic potency. If these positions were free, there was a decrease in carcinogenicity. This simple scheme was a strong stimulus to research in structure-activity relationships for over 20 years. However, exceptions appeared for polycyclic aromatic hydrocarbons composed of other than five rings, and the scheme failed when chemicals with alkyl and, in particular, methyl substitution were involved. As noted above, because the polycyclic hydrocarbons are powerful local carcinogens, it was thought that they were direct acting. This was so, even though Boyland in England proposed as early as 1950 that an epoxide might be an active metabolite (*see* Brookes, 1980; Phillips, 1983). In 1968, based on the fact noted by Gelboin in the United States, and independently

by Sims in England, that binding to DNA of isotope from a labeled polycyclic hydrocarbon is higher in the presence of a microsome fraction of liver, the view of investigators changed, and extensive research on the reactive metabolites from polycyclic hydrocarbons began. It was already known that with several other classes of carcinogens, especially the carcinogenic arylamines and nitrosamines, biotransformation led to reactive intermediates. Sims proposed the now well-established concept that activation of polycyclic hydrocarbons was not likely to be on the K region, but rather stems from a two-step oxidation with the eventual formation of a dihydrodiol epoxide. Several groups in Europe and North America have rounded out this picture. Collaboration between the organic chemist Jerina and the pharmacologist Conney (1982) in the United States elucidated the actual sequence of steps for several polycyclic hydrocarbons leading to formation of the reactive sites in the part of the molecule they called the Bay region (Table 5–6). The adducts produced in DNA by covalent binding of these sites have been identified.

Thus far, this activation process appears to be broadly applicable to many polycyclic hydrocarbons, including benzofluoranthrenes and methyl-substituted chemicals such as 12-methylcyclopentenophenanthrene, 5-methylchrysene, and 7,12-dimethylbenz[a]anthracene. Even a three-ring analog, 9,10-dimethylanthracene, and, more so, the 1,2-epoxide have shown mutagenic activity, thus reflecting a likely genotoxic intermediate. However, these simple epoxides are probably readily detoxified in mammalian cells, and therefore of low carcinogenic activity (LaVoie *et al.*, 1980a, 1982b; Oesch, 1980; Conney, 1982). It is possible that the metabolic conversion to other epoxides might also play a role and that there may be multiple active forms, especially with respect to distinct target organs. Nonetheless, the main active ultimate carcinogen is a diol epoxide, probably in the specific form of one of the several possible stereoisomers since cancer induction is the result of a highly stereospecific chemical interaction. For any polycyclic aromatic hydrocarbon, however, the bulk of biotransformation leads to detoxified metabolites that are conjugated and rapidly excreted. Inhibition of the carcinogenicity of this class of compounds by xenobiotics depends on increasing the level of detoxication reactions (Conney, 1982).

Aromatic and Heterocyclic Amines. Aromatic amines or arylamines are chemicals composed of single or multiple ring systems with an exocyclic amino group. These do not occur in nature, except for complex heterocyclics that

**Table 5–6.   CARCINOGENIC POLYCYLIC
AROMATIC HYDROCARBONS**

These hydrocarbons require a multistep metabolic activation by the
complex cytochrome P-450 enzyme system. The first reaction is an
epoxidation. With benzo[a]pyrene, the product is the corresponding
7,8-epoxide that, in turn, is subject to epoxide hydrolases to form
stereoisomeric diols. These are converted further to the 9,10-epoxide.
The diol epoxide can exist in four stereoisomeric forms of which
the key carcinogenic product is (+)-benzo[a]pyrene-7,8-diol-9,10-
epoxide 2.

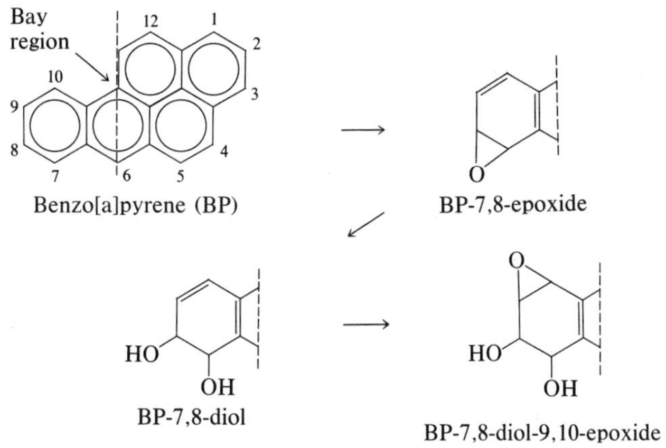

Benzo[a]pyrene (BP)

BP-7,8-epoxide

BP-7,8-diol

BP-7,8-diol-9,10-epoxide

are generated during pyrolysis. They are synthetics used in dye and drug manufacturing and
as antioxidants (Lotlikar, in Sontag, 1981).

The prototype aniline, a single aromatic ring
with amino substituent (Table 5–7), was long
considered to be noncarcinogenic, but in a recent study, feeding at high doses for a long term
resulted in a low yield of splenic sarcomas. The
relevant mechanism has not yet been clarified
but may not involve DNA reaction. At high dose
levels, aniline, through its metabolite phenylhydroxylamine, is a powerful hematopoietic poison producing methemoglobinemia. This has
been postulated by Goodman et al. (1984) to lead
to chronic splenic congestion and sarcoma formation. Careful tests of the N-acetylated derivative, acetanilide, have not given any evidence of
carcinogenicity, probably because little of the
N-hydroxy metabolite is formed. p-Hydroxy-
acetanilide (paracetamol or acetaminophen) at
high chronic doses can be hepatotoxic in rats
and in humans (suicidal doses). One study in
mice involving severely toxic chronic intake
reported limited induction of hepatomas, in addition to evidence of hepatotoxicity. Moderate
and intermittent intake as a drug has not yielded
any reports of liver toxicity despite widespread
use. Chronic bioassays in mice and rats at nontoxic doses have not yielded evidence of carci-

**Table 5–7.   TYPICAL MONOARYLAMINES WITH
CARCINOGENIC POTENTIAL**

The prototype, aniline, has induced splenic sarcomas
in rats, perhaps because it is a powerful hematopoietic
poison. The other arylamines are genotoxic upon metabolic activation and induce specific types of neoplasms.

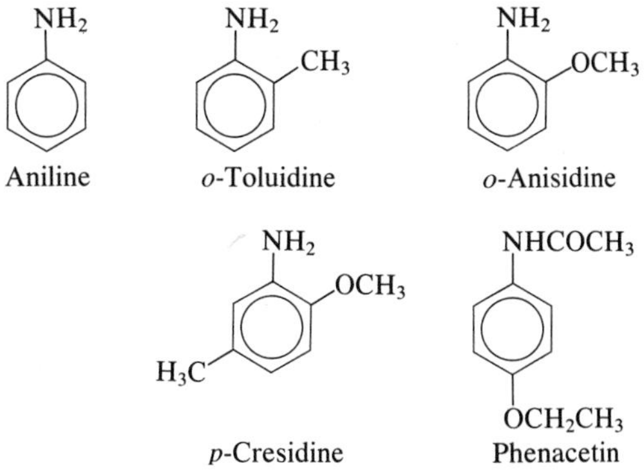

Aniline

o-Toluidine

o-Anisidine

p-Cresidine

Phenacetin

nogenicity (Amo and Matsuyama, 1985; Hiraga and Fujii, 1985).

A number of substituted anilines, particularly where the substitution is by an ortho-methyl group, are weakly carcinogenic. Like aniline they induce splenic sarcomas and, in addition, *ortho*-toluidine (2-methylaniline) and, more so, *ortho*-anisidine and *para*-cresidine (Table 5–7) also induced cancer in the urinary bladder, though at high dose levels. It should be noted that *o*-toluidine and 2,6-dimethylaniline can be released from the local anesthetics prilocaine and lidocaine, respectively (Nelson *et al.*, 1978).

The significance of the carcinogenic effects of single-ring aromatic amines in relation to human exposures to these relatively weak carcinogens requires evaluation. Even in situations of occupational exposure they have not been associated with human cancer. High-level chronic abuse, but not ordinary intermittent drug use, of phenacetin (4-ethoxyacetanilide) has led to human bladder cancer (Piper *et al.*, 1985). This finding has been reproduced in rats, where chronic dietary intake of 2.5 percent phenacetin induced bladder cancer, but the lower dose of 1.25 percent was virtually inactive in the bladder (Isaka *et al.*, 1979). In the mouse kidney and bladder, neoplasms were found (Nakanishi *et al.*, 1982). Thus, in man and in rats moderate levels of phenacetin yield detoxified metabolites, whereas continuing high intake produces a carcinogenic intermediate. Administration of the probably proximate carcinogen, *N*-hydroxyphenacetin, causes liver cancer in rats (Calder *et al.*, 1976). Two aniline moieties linked by a sulfonyl group, 4,4'-sulfonyldianiline or dapsone, a drug used to treat leprosy, upon bioassay in rats and mice did not induce epithelial neoplasms but instead led to splenic sarcomas, as did aniline, probably secondary to methemoglobinemia (see above).

The prototype two-annelated-ring aromatic amine 2-naphthylamine (Table 5–8) has demonstrated carcinogenicity in several species, including humans, rhesus monkey, dog, mouse, rat, and hamster (Arcos *et al.*, 1982; Hicks *et al.*, 1982; Adamson and Sieber, 1983). 1-Naphthylamine, an important industrial intermediate, has been thought to cause human cancer, but animal experimentation has not revealed carcinogenicity. Processes for the production of 1-naphthylamine can also generate 2-naphthylamine as well as other possibly carcinogenic aromatic amines. Thus, it would seem that the suspected carcino-

Table 5–8.　TYPICAL DICYCLIC OR POLYCYCLIC ARYLAMINES

These arylamines exhibit organ- and species-specific carcinogenic action, in part, because of a series of metabolic activation steps, including *N*-oxidation. 1-Naphthylamine undergoes this key step only to a limited extent and is not carcinogenic. 6-Aminochrysene is not active when fed, but can act as an initiator on mouse skin, probably because of biochemical activation in the chrysene ring, modified by the amino group at the α carbon.

2-Naphthylamine　　　　1-Naphthylamine　　　　4-Aminobiphenyl

Benzidine
(4,4'-diaminobiphenyl)　　　　2-Fluorenamine　　　　2-Anthramine

2-Phenanthrylamine　　　　6-Aminochrysene　　　　4-Aminostilbene

genicity of 1-naphthylamine in humans may not in fact be due to this particular pure chemical entity but may relate to carcinogenic impurities.

Polycyclic arylamines in which the amino group is in an α position to the adjoining ring are not usually carcinogenic because such compounds easily yield detoxified ring-hydroxy metabolites and undergo the activation reaction of N-hydroxylation only with difficulty, in contrast to arylamines with an amino group in other parts of the ring. However, it appears that such inactive arylamines become weakly, but definitely, active if a methyl group is inserted in the *ortho* position as, for example, 1-amino-2-methylanthraquinone. The reason is not yet understood, but might hinge on an effect of this substitution in directing metabolic activation in a manner similar to that for larger polycyclic aromatic hydrocarbons. Thus, the active forms of such chemicals might be an epoxide or dihydrodiol epoxide. It is noteworthy, however, that arylamines bearing a substitution by an electron-donating methyl group or by certain halogens in a position ortho to the amino group appear to be more powerful carcinogens than the unsubstituted compounds.

The biphenyl series, which consists of two phenyl rings joined by a carbon to carbon bond and an exocyclic amino group, consists entirely of synthetic products used mainly as chemical intermediates in dyestuff and antioxidant production. The prototype amino derivative 4-aminobiphenyl (4-biphenylamine or xenylamine) is carcinogenic in humans and in a number of laboratory animal species (Table 5–8). It is no longer manufactured in most countries because of this hazard. On the other hand, 2-aminobiphenyl is not genotoxic, and most tests indicate that it is not carcinogenic. However, at high dose levels for long duration, it did produce angiosarcomas, as did aniline, possibly through indirect effects. Among the higher *para*-substituted homologs, 4-aminoterphenyl is also carcinogenic, as would be expected.

The biphenyl derivative benzidine that has a *para* amino group on each ring (Table 5–8) is an important industrial chemical intermediate. It is carcinogenic in several animal species under a variety of conditions, as are substituted benzidines such as *o*-tolidine, the *ortho*-dimethyl derivative, and also the 3,3'-dichloro compound. In the same class are methylenedianiline (or 4,4'-diaminodiphenylmethane) and its derivatives. Benzidine, but not the other diamino compounds, has induced cancer in production workers under unhygienic conditions formerly prevailing. In most countries, benzidine is no longer made.

Among the tricyclic arylamine derivatives, a number of interesting structure-activity relationships have been found. 2-Aminofluorene (or 2-fluorenamine), a good but never-used experimental insecticide, and its acetyl derivative were discovered to be carcinogenic in most species except the guinea pig and the steppe lemming (E. K. Weisburger, in Sontag, 1981). Tests in rhesus monkeys are negative so far, even though exposures have been underway for more than ten years (Adamson and Sieber, 1983). The 1- and 3-isomers of fluorenamine compounds are weakly carcinogenic, if at all, and the 4-isomer does not seem to be carcinogenic in rodents.

In the anthracene and phenanthrene series, similar observations are recorded. Thus, 1-anthramine and 1-phenanthrylamine are not carcinogenic, whereas the 2-isomers are highly active. 2-Anthramine, in addition to causing a variety of tumor types distant from the point of application, also induces skin cancer in rats upon cutaneous application. 2-Phenanthreneamine is a good leukemogen and leads to a variety of other tumors in rats.

Not many tests of the higher homologs have been conducted. However, 6-aminochrysene, an α-substituted arylamine, appears to be carcinogenic to liver when administered to newborn mice and induces skin tumors in mice after cutaneous application. This compound has been used in the chemotherapy of splenomegaly secondary to malaria and also of human cancer, particularly breast cancer. Chronic feeding to rats gave no evidence of carcinogenicity (Lambelin *et al.*, 1975). The reason for the activity of 6-aminochrysene in mice may be due to the fact that it reacts similarly to a substituted polycyclic hydrocarbon rather than an aromatic amine.

Many, but not all, carcinogenic aromatic amines administered to rodents cause cancer of the liver or the urinary bladder, especially in male animals. In females, breast cancer is often the result. Depending on the specific structure of the aryl moiety, lesions at a number of other target sites are seen. For example, 4-aminostilbene usually leads to cancer of the external ear duct, and 3-methyl-2-naphthylamine and 3-methyl-4-aminobiphenyl derivatives frequently cause intestinal, particularly colon, cancer as well as breast and prostate cancer (Weisburger and Fiala, in Autrup and Williams, 1983). In the dog, and even in the hamster, these agents produce cancer in the urinary bladder (Brookes 1980; Kadlubar and Beland, 1983). The evidence thus far is that the urinary bladder is also the site affected in humans exposed occupationally to certain of the carcinogenic aromatic amines.

Biotransformation of Aromatic and Heterocyclic Amines. The metabolism of aromatic or heterocyclic amines can lead to ring epoxy derivatives, which, in turn, can be reduced to dihydrodiols or rearranged to phenols. For certain specific arylamines, ring epoxidation may play a role in carcinogenesis at certain target organs as, for example, mouse skin or mammary gland. This reaction seems to be involved even in liver carcinogenesis with certain chemicals such as quinoline, where epoxidation has been linked to activation (LaVoie *et al.*, 1983a). While not fully demonstrated, this kind of activation mechanism may also bear on the effect of certain polycyclic nitroaryl compounds such as 1-nitropyrene.

Nevertheless, it seems clear that the major activation reaction of arylamines depends on *N*-hydroxylation with the production of the corresponding hydroxylamine, or in the case of the *N*-acetyl derivative, of the *N*-hydroxy acetyl compounds (Miller and Miller, 1981; Weisburger, in Sontag, 1981; Kadlubar and Beland, 1983). Usually the exocyclic amino group needs to be in a β position in an annellated ring system or in a para position in linked benzene ring systems such as biphenyl. When the amino group is in either the α or in the ortho position, relatively little *N*-hydroxylation occurs, and such compounds are usually not carcinogenic. The *N*-hydroxy compounds or the corresponding facile oxidation product, the nitroso derivative, also exerts a strong action on the hematopoietic system, and for these reasons virtually all such compounds, beginning with aniline or phenylhydrazine, are strong hematopoietic poisons.

Most laboratory animals have the necessary enzymes belonging to the cytochrome P-450 system that can perform the *N*-oxidation reaction. However, in the steppe lemming and especially in the guinea pig, the cytochrome P-450 system isozymes tend to *C*-hydroxylate such compounds preferentially, and for that reason relatively small amounts of the reactive *N*-hydroxylation compound are formed. In turn, most studies have demonstrated that arylamine derivatives, including azo dyes, are not carcinogenic in the guinea pig or the steppe lemming. Humans have the ability to *N*-hydroxylate arylamines, but there are quantitative differences between individuals.

Once formed, arylhydroxylamines, under some conditions such as the acidic pH of urine or through enzymic oxidation, yield the reactive nitrenium ions that can combine with cellular macromolecules, especially with DNA, thus leading to toxicity and carcinogenicity. With the often used *N*-acyl and especially *N*-acetyl derivatives, the corresponding *N*-hydroxy-*N*-acetyl compounds require additional activation reactions. In rodent liver, one such activation reaction is performed by the PAPS-linked sulfotrans-

ferase to yield the ultimate carcinogen, the *N*-hydroxy sulfate ester. Another reaction involves an arylhydroxamic acid acyl transferase that shifts the acetyl group from the nitrogen to the oxygen of the hydroxylamine group.

Another important enzyme system in the disposition of aromatic amines is *N*-acetyltransferase (Weber and Glowinski, 1980). This activity has a polymorphic distribution in humans such that individuals are either rapid or slow acetylators. The rabbit also displays polymorphic expression while other species can be classified as rapid (e.g., hamster) or slow (e.g., dog, rat) acetylators. For many *N*-containing xenobiotics, acetylation is a detoxication reaction, but certain aromatic amines appear to be directed toward activation in the liver by acetylation (McQueen and Williams, in Bartsch *et al.*, 1982). Conversely, slow acetylation disposes some animals and humans to bladder cancer. This could stem from activation in other tissues, in which case aromatic amine target organs such as liver and breast might be at higher risk. Also, acetylation may block other activation reactions.

In tissues other than liver, other biotransformation processes seem to be involved in aromatic amine carcinogenicity. For example, a prostaglandin H synthetase that uses arachidonic acid as a cofactor (Eling *et al.*, 1983; Lambeir *et al.*, 1985) appears to play a role in bladder activation. This system does not utilize acetylated aromatic amines very well, which may in part explain the higher risk of slow acetylator individuals to bladder cancer. In addition, there are deacetylases yielding the corresponding hydroxylamines. While many tissues have an *N*-oxidation capability, most such biotransformation occurs in liver. These metabolites are converted by type II conjugation reactions to metabolites such as glucuronic acid derivatives that serve as transport forms, and the occurrence of urinary bladder cancer has been traced to the enzymatic or acid-catalyzed splitting of conjugates in the bladder followed by additional specific activation reactions in this target tissue. Similar considerations may apply to processes of cancer induction in other target organs susceptible to carcinogenesis by certain of these aromatic amines.

Quinolines and Azarenes. Whereas the field of cancer research has led to many studies of structure-activity relationships among aromatic homocyclic compounds, relatively few such investigations have been done with the heterocyclic analogs even though the latter represent fundamental structures on which many important drugs are based. Quinoline (Table 5–9) itself does have carcinogenic properties, leading to hepatocellular cancer and hemangioendothelio-

Table 5–9. QUINOLINES AND AZARENES

Quinoline and benzo[g]quinoline can act as initiators in mouse skin carcinogenesis. Quinoline induces liver cancer upon oral feeding to rats. 2-Amino-3-methylimidazo[4,5-f]quinoline is one of the important components found in fried foods. 4-Nitroquinoline-N-oxide is carcinogenic in several tissues upon biochemical reduction to the 4-hydroxylamino metabolite. 2,4- and 2,6-dinitrotoluene are carcinogenic in animal models. The intestinal bacterial flora mediates, in part, their reductive metabolism. 1-Nitropyrene found in exhausts of diesel engines is carcinogenic. The effect depends in part on microbiologic nitroreduction and can also involve appropriate ring epoxidation. The nitrofuran FANFT is a typical carcinogen of this class. FANFT induces bladder cancer, but other nitrofurans have other specific target organs. AF-2, formerly used as a food preservative in Japan, was first found to be mutagenic, then carcinogenic, to the forestomach in rodents.

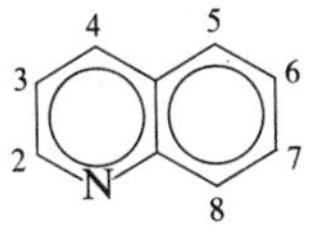

Quinoline

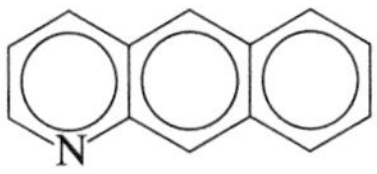

Benzo[g]quinoline

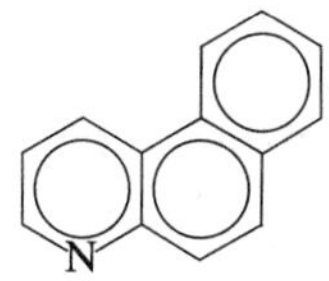

Benzo[f]quinoline

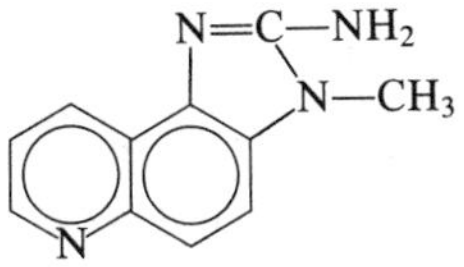

2-Amino-3-methyl-imidazo[4,5-f]quinoline

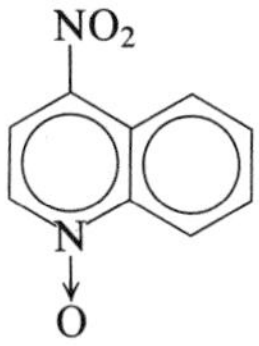

4-Nitroquinoline-N-oxide

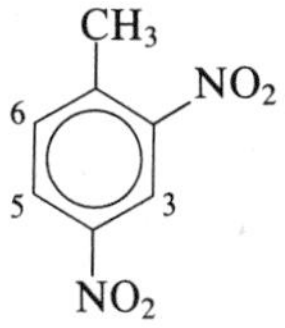

2,4-Dinitrotoluene

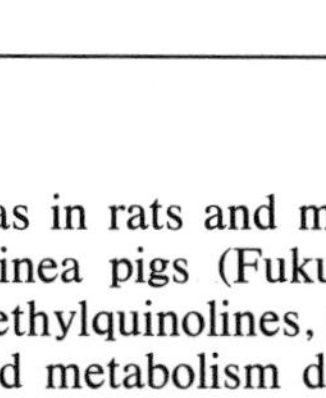

1-Nitropyrene

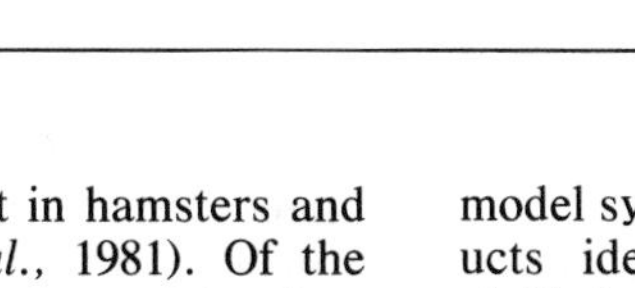

2-Formamido-4-(5-nitro-2-furyl)thiazole (FANFT)

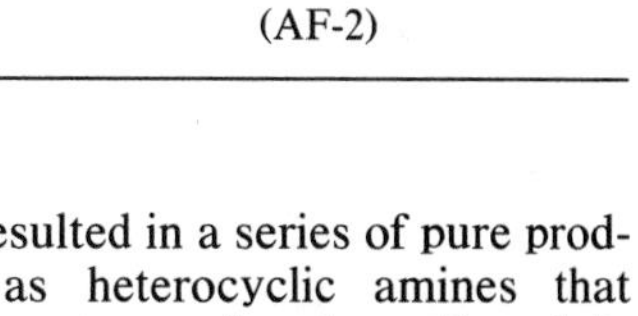

2-(2-Furyl)-3-(5-nitro-2-furyl)acrylamide (AF-2)

mas in rats and mice, but not in hamsters and guinea pigs (Fukushima et al., 1981). Of the methylquinolines, the 4-isomer was most active, and metabolism data indicate that quinoline is converted to an epoxide, a reactive product. Isoquinoline is nongenotoxic and not carcinogenic (LaVoie et al., 1983a). Quinoline is not only an industrial product but is found in tobacco smoke. Benzoquinolines or azarenes exhibit mutagenicity through metabolic formation of reactive epoxides, as would be true for homocyclic hydrocarbons (LaVoie et al., 1983b).

Recently, new mutagenic heterocyclic chemicals have been found in "nature," as a result of the pyrolysis or cooking of protein-containing materials (Sugimura and Sato, 1983; Knudsen, 1985). The pyrolysis of individual amino acids in

model systems resulted in a series of pure products identified as heterocyclic amines that yielded mainly liver tumors in mice, although in rats several compounds exhibited carcinogenic action at select organs such as ear duct, intestine, breast, and bladder, similar to the action of the corresponding homocyclic compound 3,2'-dimethyl-4-aminobiphenyl. Among chemicals obtained from the action of frying or broiling meat under realistic home cooking conditions were several compounds based on an imidazoquinoline or quinoxaline ring system. These chemicals were among the most mutagenic chemicals found so far in the Salmonella typhimurium TA98 system and required metabolic activation by a liver S9 fraction. The carcinogenicity of several of these chemicals has been established, and it is postulated that they might represent the agents associated with major human cancers such as cancer of the colon (Weisburger *et al.,* 1982; Knudsen, 1985). Most of these chemicals have an exocyclic amino function, and it is likely that their mutagenicity and possible carcinogenicity stem from the biochemical conversion of the amino group to the corresponding hydroxylamino group followed by appropriate target organ specific conversion to the alkylating intermediate (Kato *et al.,* 1983; Barnes *et al.,* 1983).

An interesting carcinogen is 4-nitroquinoline-*N*-oxide, a nitroazarene (Sugimura *et al.,* 1979) (Table 5–9). Investigation of the mechanism of action of this compound showed that the required activation reaction is reduction to the corresponding 4-hydroxylaminoquinoline-*N*-oxide, accomplished *in vivo* and *in vitro* by the soluble enzyme xanthine oxidase. The hydroxylamine derivative can induce pancreatic cancer, especially together with azaserine. The corresponding amino derivative, or a compound lacking the *N*-oxide function, is not carcinogenic. 4-Nitroquinoline-*N*-oxide is carcinogenic under many different conditions. It yields papillomas and carcinomas when painted on the skin of mice, especially if followed by a promoting agent such as croton oil. When the compound is injected subcutaneously in rodents, sarcomas result. When it is given parenterally by intraperitoneal or intravenous injection, tumors are seen at a variety of sites, testifying to the potency of this agent and to the capability of many tissues to convert it to the active intermediate. The corresponding 4-nitropyridine-*N*-oxides require 3-alkyl substitution to be carcinogenic, implying a stabilized quinoid structure of an intermediate hydroxylamino compound as key reactant for neoplastic potential.

Nitroaryl Compounds. Nitro analogs of carcinogenic aromatic amines have also been found to lead to tumor formation (Table 5–9). More information in this area is essential because certain of these nitro derivatives are still used extensively as industrial chemical intermediates, some have been found in diesel engine exhausts, and some exist in certain commercial products in low concentrations (Claxton, 1983; Wei and Shu, 1983; Holmberg and Ahlborg, 1983). Nitro compounds can be reduced fairly readily to hydroxylamino derivatives and thence to the amines. The enzymatic systems performing such reductions are less stereospecific than those for the biochemical hydroxylation of amines. Hence, it may be that nitro derivatives would exhibit less stringent structural requirements for carcinogenicity than the corresponding amines. In the few instances where this hypothesis was tested, arylhydroxylamines, except phenyl-

hydroxylamine, have been found uniformly carcinogenic. For example, whereas 1-naphthylamine is inactive, 1-naphthylhydroxylamine is carcinogenic, in fact more so than the 2-isomer. Interestingly 1-nitronaphthalene has not been found active, which suggests that the rate of the *in vivo* reduction of the hydroxylamine is much faster than its formation from the nitro compound. Likewise, in the fluorene series, *N*-acetyl-1-hydroxylamino- and 3-hydroxylamino-fluorene are carcinogenic, whereas the corresponding amines are not (Kadlubar and Beland, 1983).

Technical dinitrotoluene fed to rats induced liver cancer, but the *para*-2,4-dinitrotoluene was much less active. Attention was drawn to the 2,4-isomer, because of the known liver carcinogenicity of 2,4-diaminotoluene. However, examination of the potential to initiate hepatocellular-altered foci showed that the 2,6-dinitrotoluene, present in the technical product to about 20 percent, was much more active than the 2,4-isomer (Leonard *et al.,* 1983). Biotransformation by the intestinal microflora seems to bear on the effect of these compounds (DeBethizy *et al.,* 1983).

A number of analytic studies on the exhaust of functioning diesel engines have revealed that components of this mixture have mutagenic activity for *Salmonella typhimurium* (McCoy *et al.,* 1983; Rosenkranz and Mermelstein, 1983). Among other chemicals, the compounds associated with the mutagenic activity were nitro derivatives of polycyclic aromatic hydrocarbons such as 1-nitropyrene. By analogy with tests of other nitro compounds, a hydrocarbon in which the nitro group is substituted in a position for which the corresponding amino compound would be carcinogenic (for example, 2-nitropyrene) can reasonably be assumed to be a carcinogenic nitro compound. For compounds such as 1-nitropyrene where the corresponding amine might not be carcinogenic, the effect would depend on the polycyclic aromatic hydrocarbon moiety, as discussed for 6-aminochrysene, and yield carcinogenicity at target organs in species under conditions appropriate for the substituted hydrocarbon (McCoy *et al.,* 1983). And indeed, Hirose *et al.* (1984) found that 1-nitropyrene could induce mammary cancer in female rats. It is not yet known whether the intestinal microflora contributes to this effect, as appears true for dinitrotoluene. 2,4,7-Trinitrofluorenone, used in some dry-copying processes, was found mutagenic (Rosenkranz and Mermelstein, 1983). This chemical is related to the carcinogenic arylamine 2-fluorenamine, and hence, these biologic properties are not unexpected since the bacterial flora can reduce the nitro function to amino. The contribution of these chemicals in, for example, diesel exhaust or industrial products to human health risk remains to be defined because of the great dilution of diesel exhaust and low-level use of other nitro compounds, except at the place of manufacture.

Nitrofurans and Nitroheterocyclics. Many nitrofuran derivatives have been synthesized because this particular structure has demonstrated practical use for drugs, particularly compounds with antibacterial activities, which are used in agricultural practices as well as in medical applications such as against urinary tract infections. A number of such compounds are very potent carcinogens for several distinct target organs, depending on the structure of the chemical and the test system (for general review, see Bryan, 1978). For example, nitrofuran derivatives are known to quickly induce mammary cancer in rats or cancer of the urinary bladder in several species (Table 5–9). AF-2 or furylfuramide was used as a food additive mainly in Japan, until it was found to be mutagenic and carcinogenic (Sugimura *et al.*, 1982). As a rule, many 2-nitrofuran compounds are carcinogenic (Arcos *et al.*, 1968–1985). It seems probable that these chemicals are converted biochemically to the corresponding reactive hydroxylamino derivatives as carcinogenic intermediates. Thus, any such chemical requires detailed testing prior to widespread public use.

Azo Compounds. Simple azo compounds consist of two aromatic rings joined by an azo (—N=N—) bond. More complex compounds can have two such azo bonds (tetraazo compounds) with a central benezene ring, or more often a biphenyl system. The azo acts as a chromophore, and hence azo compounds are colored and, depending on substituents, are widely used dyes (Table 5–10).

Azo compounds are synthetic chemicals not found in nature. In the early 1930s, Yoshida and Kinosita, working in separate laboratories in Japan, discovered the carcinogenicity of some azo dye derivatives, including 4-dimethylaminoazobenzene (formerly commonly called butter yellow because it was used in the 1930s in some countries to color butter) and *o*-aminoazotoluene, which induced liver and bladder cancer after feeding (Table 5–10). Many azo dyes were synthesized and examined for carcinogenic activity for the purpose of establishing structure-activity relationships. One of the salient conclusions drawn from these pioneering studies was that not all agents belonging to a given class of chemicals are carcinogenic. In fact, very minor alterations in structure modified the carcinogenic potential considerably. For instance, 4′-methyl-4-dimethylaminoazobenzene is carcinogenic, but the 4′-ethyl analog is not. 4-Dimethylaminoazobenzene is the highly active standard carcinogen, but the 4-diethyl derivative is not carcinogenic. (For a detailed discussion of these structure-activity relationships *see* Arcos *et al.*, 1968–1983; Lotlikar, in Sontag, 1981; IARC Sci. Publ. No. 40). Briefly, some of the variations in activity as a function of structure stem from the susceptibility of the specific molecule to detoxication enzyme systems or, in reverse, to biochemical activation systems. The carcinogenic azo compounds typically have a 4-substituted exocyclic amino group, and sometimes a required *N*-methyl-4-amino substitution. As for the carcinogenic arylamines, biochemical activation is required, and involved *N*-oxidation and further conversion to reactive electrophils, capable of forming covalent bonds, often at the 8-position of guanine in DNA.

An important detoxication process is splitting of the azo bond. This is readily performed by a bacterial azo reductase. In fact, the activity of this system under adequate nutritional conditions initially resulted in a failure by Western researchers to confirm the earlier studies of Japanese investigators. This, in turn, led to the discovery by Kensler and co-workers in 1941 that riboflavin was involved in protecting against azo dye liver carcinogens and by Mueller and Miller in 1950 that the underlying mechanisms depended on control of the detoxifying azo dye reductase by riboflavin, one of the first clear demonstrations of the role of nutrition in carcinogenesis (see National Research Council, 1982). Mutagenicity tests provide reasonable agreement with carcinogenicity, reflecting the potential of a given dye to yield a reactive metabolite (Ashby *et al.*, 1983; Brown and Dietrich, 1983). Most of the azo dyes studied are compounds with one azo link. All other things being equal, they are usually not carcinogenic if they contain polar substituents such as sulfonic acid residues. Thus, pure amaranth (FD&C Red No. 2), with such a structure, is neither mutagenic nor carcinogenic, in spite of suggestions to the contrary.

Bioassays in rodents of some monoazo dyes have yielded no evidence of carcinogenicity, in contrast to the fairly potent series of aminoazobenzene compounds discussed above, except for the induction of splenic sarcomas. For example, azobenzene caused splenic sarcomas, like aniline, the metabolite stemming from reductive splitting of the azo bond. More complex, unsymmetric azo dyes like D and C Red No. 9 upon high dose chronic intake also led to splenic sarcomas (Goodman *et al.*, 1984). The biochemical split products, most likely generated by the intestinal bacterial enzymes, are (*a*) a polar sulfonated substituted aniline, which

Table 5–10. AZO COMPOUNDS

4-Dimethylaminoazobenzene (or butter yellow) has been used as a laboratory hepato-carcinogen to study the mode of action of this class of compounds, including structure-activity relationships. Because of its characteristic color change as a function of pH, it was the first carcinogen that demonstrated binding to cellular macromolecules. Because of the flavin-dependent azo dye reductase, it was also one of the first carcinogens with a clear-cut nutritional modulation of its activity. Substitution with polar groups such as sulfonic acid in simple azo dyes usually abolishes carcinogenicity and mutagenicity. Thus, molecules such as FD and C Red No. 2 (amaranth) are not mutagenic or carcinogenic. On the other hand, tetrazo dyes such as direct black 38 or direct blue 6, which are not mutagenic and are quite polar, can release the mutagenic and carcinogenic benzidine upon reduction of the azo link by bacteria. Such dyes are highly carcinogenic.

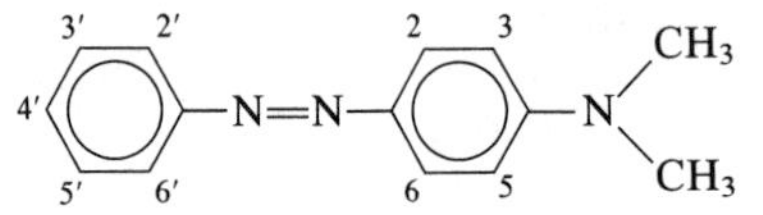

4-Dimethylaminoazobenzene

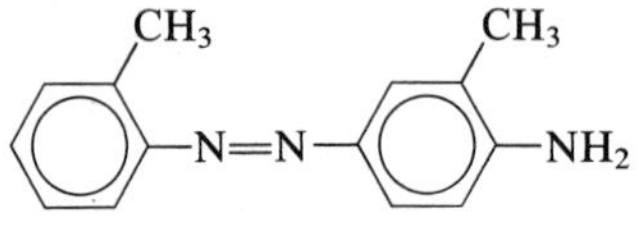

o-Aminoazotoluene

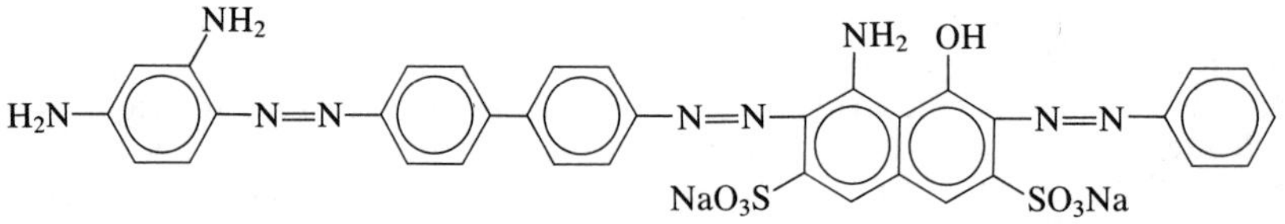

Direct black 38
(Disodium 2,7-Naphthalenedisulfonate-4-amino-3-{[4'-((2,4-diamino phenyl)azo)(1,1'-biphenyl)-4-yl]azo}-5-hydroxy-6-(phenylazo)-

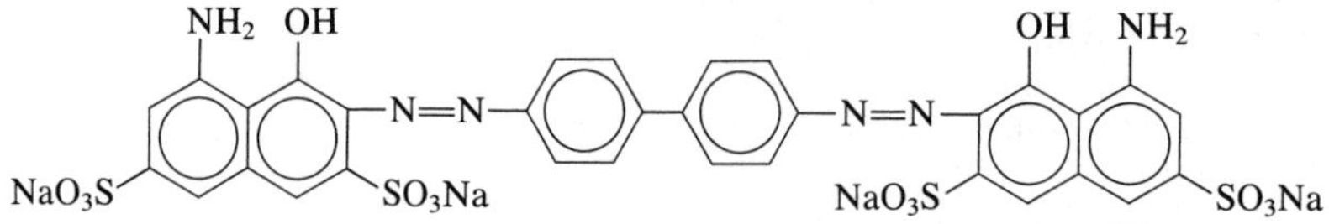

Direct blue 6
(Tetrasodium 2,7-naphthalenedisulfonate-3,3'[(1,1'-biphenyl)-4,4'-diylbis(azo)*bis*(5-amino-4-hydroxy)-

because of its structure would be expected to be readily eliminated in urine, and (*b*) 1-amino-2-napthol, an easily oxidized product. These oxidizable amines are the likely intermediate affecting the hematopoietic system as such, or, through H_2O_2 produced during co-oxidation, leading to methemoglobinemia. The prolonged methemoglobinemia affects splenic function, possibly leading to sarcoma development. These events typically arise during high-level administration when normal detoxication and excretion capabilities are overwhelmed.

Complex tetraazo dyes consist of polycyclic structures linked by azo groups. Metabolic splitting of such compounds by reduction of the azo bonds has the opposite effect from splitting of simple azo dyes; namely, the complexed carcinogenic aromatic amine, such as benzidine, is released (Nony *et al.*, 1983). Because such dye-stuffs can be biotransformed not only by mammalian enzymes but also to a greater extent by bacterial enzymes in the gut, exposure to them is potentially harmful (Cerniglia *et al.*, 1982; Chung, 1983). Thus, dyes such as direct blue 6, black 38, and brown 95 have been active as rat liver carcinogens (Table 5-10). With few exceptions, the carcinogenic complex azo dyes do not cause tumors at the point of injection. In rats, the usual end-point is liver cancer and in mice or hamsters, liver or urinary bladder tumors. Thus far, no known case of human cancer can be traced to exposure to such dyes, albeit heavy occupational contact with arylamines such as 2-naphthylamine or benzidine used as intermediates in dyestuff manufacture has led to bladder cancer.

Table 5–11. TYPICAL ALIPHATIC AND CYCLIC NITROSAMINES, REQUIRING METABOLIC ACTIVATION, AND NITROSAMIDES, DIRECT-ACTING CARCINOGENS

N-Nitrosodiphenylamine is not genotoxic, but induces bladder cancer through unknown mechanisms. Proline yields noncarcinogenic *N*-nitrosoproline that can be found in urine, as is *N*-nitroso-L-thioproline, as indicator of *in vivo* nitrosation.

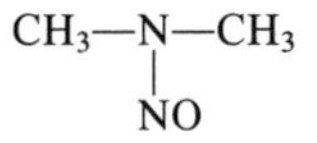

CH₃—N—CH₃ | NO Dimethylnitrosamine (or *N*-nitrosodimethyl- amine)	R—N—R' | N=O Dialkyl nitrosamine	*N*-Nitroso- pyrrole	*N*-Nitroso- piperidine

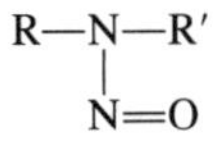

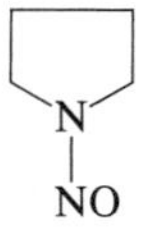

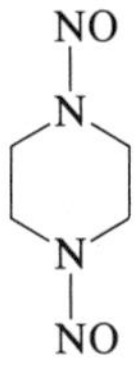

CH₃—N—CH₃ | NO — Dimethylnitrosamine (or *N*-nitrosodimethylamine)

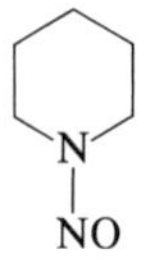

R—N—R' | N=O — Dialkyl nitrosamine

N-Nitrosopyrrole (NO)

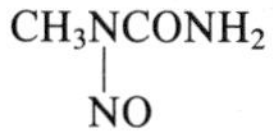

N-Nitrosopiperidine (NO)

N-dinitroso piperazine (NO···N···NO)

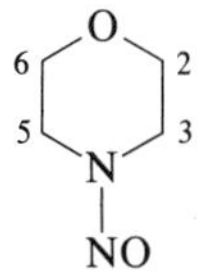

N-Nitroso morpholine (O, positions 6,2,5,3; N; NO)

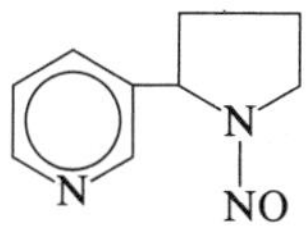

N-Nitrosonornicotine (NO)

CH₃NCONH₂ | NO — *N*-Methyl-*N*-nitroso-urea

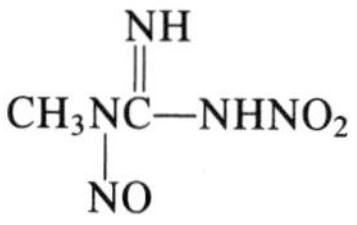

CH₃NC—NHNO₂ | NH | NO — *N*-Methyl-*N'*-nitro-*N*-nitrosoguanidine

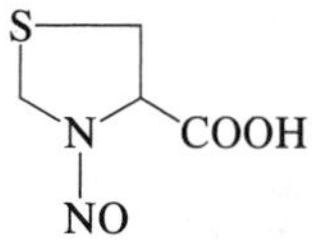

N-nitroso-α-thioproline (S, N, COOH, NO)

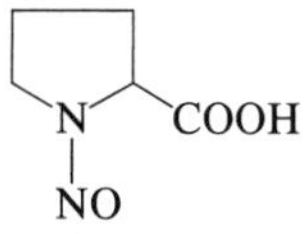

N-Nitrosoproline 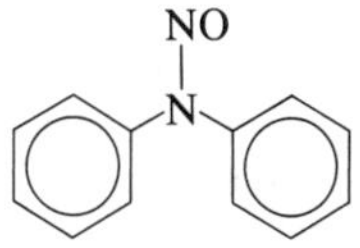 (N, COOH, NO)

N-Nitrosodiphenylamine (diphenylnitrosamine) (NO)

N-Nitroso Compounds. This major class of important chemical carcinogens is characterized by chemicals derived from secondary amines or amides by nitrosation (Table 5–11). The corresponding nitrosamines and nitrosamides are synthetic as well as naturally occurring substances. The prototype nitrosamine, dimethylnitrosamine, was discovered to be carcinogenic only in the last 30 years beginning with the finding by Barnes and Magee in England (see Shimkin, 1980) that this chemical, an industrial solvent that caused jaundice and liver damage in workmen exposed to it, was highly hepatotoxic in rodents, where it reproduced the lesions seen in man. Subsequently, these investigators demonstrated that this agent was among the most carcinogenic materials then known. Some of the first studies on alteration of DNA by carcinogens were performed with nitrosamines, and their patterns of alkylation of DNA have now been extensively documented.

The discovery of the carcinogenicity of dimethylnitrosamine led to an intensive effort to establish structure-activity relationships in this class of chemicals with the typical structure

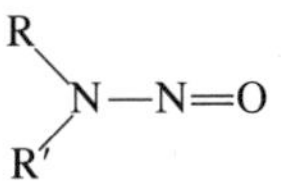

$$\begin{matrix} R \\ R' \end{matrix}\!\!>\!\!N—N=O \quad \text{(Table 5–11)}.$$ Virtually all nitrosamines are carcinogenic (Preussmann and Stewart, in Searle, 1984; O'Neill *et al.*, 1984).

In rodents, the symmetric dialkyl nitrosamines under some conditions exhibit highly specific organotropism; i.e., they preferentially cause cancer in a given organ. For example, dimethyl- and diethylnitrosamine usually cause liver cancer in rats, while the dibutyl derivative causes cancer of the urinary bladder, and the diamyl compound cancer of the lung. The dose rate also plays a role. Dimethylnitrosamine administered to rats in relatively low doses for a long time leads to cancer of the liver, whereas fewer doses or, indeed, a single large dose results in renal carcinomas. Asymmetric nitrosamines, especially those with at least one methyl group, often result in cancer of the esophagus, as do some nitrosamines based on cyclic secondary amines. In hamsters, on the other hand, diethylnitrosamine also causes cancer in the respiratory tract, and diketopropylnitrosamine or 2,6-dimethylnitrosomorpholine in the ductal pancreas, a model for this important type of human cancer. The hamster, because it is characterized by a deficiency in liver activity of the alkyl acceptor protein involved in repair of O^6-alkylation of guanine, is extremely sensitive to liver carcinogenesis by dimethylnitrosamine.

The antibiotic streptozotocin, a drug used mainly in cancer chemotherapy, has the structure of an N-methylnitrosamine. As expected, this drug is carcinogenic, interestingly to the pancreas islet cells. It is also diabetogenic, unless nicotinamide is administered at the same time. In rats, on the other hand, diketopropylnitrosamine leads to colon cancer, the only nitrosamine to do so reliably.

Similar in structure and probable mechanism of action are the alkyl and dialkylaryltriazeno derivatives containing the —N=N—N=O group. These materials, some of which are industrial products, have potent carcinogenic properties including induction of brain, kidney, and mammary cancer in rats.

Hoffmann and colleagues (Hoffmann et al. and Hecht et al., in Magee, 1982) discovered that several nitrosamines derived from nicotine, in particular nitrosonornicotine, are found in tobacco and are formed by bacterially mediated nitrosation of nicotine during the curing process. These and related nitrosamines are found also in tobacco smoke. In rats they cause mainly cancer of the esophagus, in hamsters cancer of the upper respiratory tract. The contribution of these chemicals to carcinogenesis in humans who smoke cigarettes or chew tobacco products is not yet known but is likely to be an important factor (Surgeon General Rept., 1982). Individuals who smoke and excessively drink alcoholic beverages have a high risk of cancer of the oral cavity and esophagus (Wynder, in Pereira, 1983). The relevant mechanism may be an induction by alcohol of enzymes capable of biotransforming nitrosamines such as nitrosonornicotine, or polycyclic aromatic hydrocarbons found in smoke, in the target tissues.

The role of nitrosamines in human cancer has been under extensive study (Magee, 1982). As noted above, the most likely carcinogens of this class that might have an effect in humans are those found in tobacco and tobacco smoke. The properties of the smaller dialkylnitrosamines, such as dimethyl- or diethylnitrosamine, categorize them as very powerful, versatile carcinogens in animals. In the last 20 years, highly sensitive and specific techniques, such as those utilizing the thermal electron analyzer, have permitted the reliable determination of nitrosamines in the environment at the parts-per-billion and even parts-per-trillion level (IARC Sci. Publ. No. 45, 1983). In order to induce cancer in rats and mice, continuing exposure to alkylnitrosamines at the parts-per-million level or infrequent exposure to an amount of parts per thousand are required. There exists a specific DNA repair activity, the alkyl acceptor protein system, for removing the alkyl group inserted in DNA by nitrosamines. Humans display a greater activity of this system than do rats (Pegg et al., 1985). Thus, the biologic significance of concentrations of parts per billion or lower is obscure, yet these are the amounts found, for example, in certain foodstuffs, such as bacon. In fact, it is quite likely that larger amounts of such carcinogens were present in the food chain in previous years or decades, before the potential hazards due to such chemicals were known. Therefore, the cancer risks of such nitrosamines present in trace amounts seem to be quite minimal compared to those inherent in other kinds of exposures, for example, nitrosonornicotine and analogs in tobacco products.

The nitrosamines, which are nitroso derivatives of alkylureas, alkylamides, and esters are some of the most remarkable carcinogens known (Table 5–11). Many of these agents are chemically quite stable in the anhydrous state and do not require specific enzymic activation but spontaneously release an active intermediate in the presence of aqueous, preferably alkaline, systems. Such materials are carcinogenic in virtually all living systems, even under in vitro conditions (Preussmann and Stewart, in Searle 1984). Odashima et al. (1975) discovered that in several species N-butylnitrosourea causes leukemia, mainly the granulocytic type also seen in humans. Certain of these materials were actually used commercially in industry and in chemical laboratories because of their property to undergo alkali hydrolysis and yield reactive intermediates. For example, methylnitrosourea was the classic reagent for the laboratory preparation of diazomethane, itself utilized to esterify carboxylic acids, phenols, and the like. Since its carcinogenicity was demonstrated, methylnitrosourea has not been used for this purpose, but has been replaced by methylnitrosotoluenesulfonamide, which is not carcinogenic. Diazomethane itself is a highly carcinogenic chemical, yielding tumors in the respiratory tract, especially the lung, in rats and mice.

Given by oral administration, alkylnitrosoureas, such as methylnitrosourethan, and the closely related *N*-methyl-*N'*-nitro-*N*-nitrosoguanidine, nitrosobiuret, and *N*-methyl-*N*-nitroso-*N'*-acetylurea produced tumors in the gastrointestinal tract (Sugimura *et al.* 1982). In fact, these compounds are the chemicals of choice to induce experimental cancer of the glandular stomach, mimicking one of the most frequent human cancers in Japan, parts of Latin America, Iceland, Scandinavia, and certain other countries of Europe (Magee, 1982). Treatment of certain foods with nitrite, especially fish or beans frequently eaten in areas where stomach cancer is high, yields an extract with mutagenic activity that, in turn, induces cancer of the glandular stomach in rats. Other foods eaten in areas such as China, where the risk for cancer in the upper respiratory and the upper gastrointestinal tract is high, also contain specific nitrosamines. Thus, there may be a relationship between nitrite, nitrosamines, nitrosamides, and similar compounds, and certain human cancers prevalent in diverse parts of the world.

Nitrosamines and related materials are synthesized by reaction of nitrous acid with a secondary amine. Sound evidence shows that in biologic systems, including humans, nitrosamines, nitrosoureas, and similar hazardous materials can be formed following oral administration of nitrite and the appropriate amine or amide (see Magee, 1982; Searle, 1984).

In many places, nitrite is utilized as a deliberate food additive but also occurs adventitiously in food supplies through reduction of nitrate. Nitrate is ubiquitous in the environment and is also used as a component of food preservatives. Under some conditions, nitrate is reduced to nitrite, particularly by microbiologic systems. This reduction is likely to occur in food stored at room temperature, a relatively common occurrence in less-advanced countries where household refrigeration is uncommon (Weisburger *et al.*, 1982). The reduction also occurs readily mediated by oral bacterial flora, in individuals having eaten foods, especially plants, high in nitrate. Secondary amines and similar nitrosatable substrates likewise are widespread in the environment (food) and they also arise by digestive processes. Potential exposure to exogenous nitrite or endogenous formation of nitrite can be assessed by the sensitive and specific procedure of Bartsch and co-workers (see Magee, 1982) that measures the presence of the noncarcinogenic nitrosoproline in individuals given a dose of proline. Gumbar *et al.* (1983) proposed measurement of urinary 7-methylguanine for the same purpose.

These nitrosation reactions can be inhibited by preferential, competitive neutralization of nitrite with naturally occurring and synthetic materials such as vitamin C, vitamin E, sulfamate, and certain antioxidants such as butylated hydroxytoluene, butylated hydroxyanisole, gallic acid, and even amino acids or proteins (Mirvish, in Scanlan and Tannenbaum, 1981; Mirvish, 1983). Practical use has been made of these inhibitory reactions; for example, certain meats preserved with nitrite are at the same time treated with ascorbate or erythrobate, thereby appreciably lowering the amount of detectable dimethylnitrosamine, nitrosopyrrolidine, and other nitrosamines in the treated meats (NRC/NAS 1982). In addition, this interaction may bear on the considerable decrease in the incidence of stomach cancer in the United States during the last 40 years (Weisburger *et al.,* 1982). This property of neutralization of nitrite by vitamin C is also being used in certain pharmaceutical preparations with a potential nitrosatable substituent by formulating such drugs with vitamin C or vitamin E (Mirvish, in Scanlan and Tannenbaum, 1981; Mergens and Newmark, in Zedeck and Lipkin, 1981).

Some of the alkylnitrosoureas, particularly the ethyl derivative, yield brain tumors upon parenteral, especially intravenous, injection. These alkylnitrosoureas provide unique means of specifically inducing neurogenic tumors and related lesions. Chemicals of this type are also active transplacentally, yielding a high incidence of cancer in the offspring after a single dose to a pregnant female given in the last trimester (Rice, 1979; Müller and Rajewsky, 1983). The question can be asked whether the relatively rare cancers of the human brain and nervous system stem from a similar transplacental effect with as-yet-unknown compounds.

Tertiary and quarternary amines, and, in particular, dimethylamino derivatives, can react with nitrite under similar conditions releasing dimethylnitrosamine (Lijinsky, in Magee, 1982). Many drugs have a structure permitting nitrosation, and this remains to be explored in regard to the possible human risk. Cimetidine, a widely used drug in the management of gastric or duodenal ulcers, can form a nitroso compound with a structure mimicking that of the alkyl nitrosoureas. Although the compound is mutagenic, two tests for carcinogenicity have been totally negative suggesting that under *in vivo* conditions this nitroso compound can be detoxified (Jensen, 1983).

Biotransformation of Nitrosamines. Nitrosamines as a class are converted to active electrophilic reactants through oxidation (Arcos *et al.,* 1982; Scanlan and Tannenbaum, 1982; Preussmann and Stewart, in Searle, 1984). The active species alkylate DNA at various sites, which have been determined for several nitrosamines.

With the prototype dimethylnitrosamine, an active intermediate has been thought to be the unstable hydroxymethyl compound, which is converted to a reactive methyl carbonium ion. Longer-chain or cyclic nitrosamines can conceptually be metabolized by hydroxylation α or β to the N-nitroso function. Recent developments demonstrate that the key activation reaction appears to be α-hydroxylation (see Magee, in IARC Sci. Publ. 41, 45, 1982). Thus, such steps with a typical cyclic nitrosamine, N-nitrosopyrrolidine, eventually yield 4-hydroxybutanal via a reactive diazohydroxide and/or a carbonium ion (see Hecht et al., in above monographs). With an asymmetric nitrosamine such as the important tobacco-specific nitrosonornicotine (see Hoffmann et al., in above monographs), both α positions are attacked, depending on the organ-specific enzymes, and thus distinct reactive intermediates are obtained that may account for the species, strain, and organ selectivity. Aliphatic longer-chain nitrosamines such as dibutylnitrosamine can undergo α, β, or ω hydroxylation, and these yield specific products, including some derived from such chain-shortening β-oxidation (Suzuki et al., 1983; IARC Publ. Co., 1984; O'Neill et al., 1984). As is true for the polycyclic aromatic hydrocarbons, there is a stereospecificity for nitrosamines as noted in the distinct carcinogenicity of 2-isomers of N-nitroso-2,6-dimethylmorpholine (Lijinsky, in Magee, 1982).

Biochemical activation of these nitrosamines appears to take place in all species so far studied. Whereas even the highly potent polycyclic hydrocarbons, such as 3-methylcholanthrene, have so far failed to reliably cause cancer in monkeys, a number of nitrosamines led to cancer relatively rapidly in rhesus monkeys. For example, diethylnitrosamine induced liver cancer in less than two years and in more recent experiments in less than one year (Adamson and Sieber, 1983). Species differences appear in relation to the tissue primarily affected. Diethylnitrosamine leads chiefly to liver cancer in rats and mice, but in the hamster, lung cancer is the main lesion, although liver and esophageal tumors also result. There is also a dramatic species difference in the capacity to repair the DNA damage produced by alkylating nitrosamines; in particular, the hamster is deficient in the removal of O^6 alkylation.

Diphenylnitrosamine has been thought to be not carcinogenic because of the substitution of two bulky phenyl groups in this nitrosamine, and it is difficult to visualize the metabolic production of a reactive alkylating agent through the normally expected mechanism, as is also true for the di-t-butyl derivative. Yet high-level, long-term administration of diphenylnitrosamine has induced urinary bladder cancer (Lijinski, in Magee, 1982). It is possible that (1) there is metabolic transfer of the nitroso function to a substrate that would yield bladder cancer, or (2) there is metabolic epoxidation or hydroxylation of the phenyl ring yielding the corresponding phenol, which in turn might have promoting activity in the urinary bladder, as has been found with other phenolic compounds.

Dialkylhydrazines. Laqueur in the United States discovered that flour made from the cycad nut led to a variety of cancers in the liver, kidney, and digestive tract of rats. Cycasin, the active ingredient, is the β-glucoside of methylazoxymethanol (Table 5–12). It is a powerful carcinogen for liver, kidney, and digestive tract upon oral intake in conventional rats but is inactive both in germ-free rats and after intraperitoneal injection, because of the requirement for the bacterial enzyme β-glucosidase to hydrolyze the cycasin and release the active principle, methylazoxymethanol.

Methylazoxymethanol itself leads to cancer in various species of conventional and germ-free animals, irrespective of the mode of administration. Interestingly, in rodents, mainly colon cancer is induced, although duodenal, liver, kidney, and ear duct cancers also occur. Methylazoxymethanol is not entirely stable at physiologic pH, but its organospecificity suggested the need to search for enzymatically mediated activation mechanisms such as are present in microsomal fractions of appropriate cell homogenates (Fiala et al., 1984). These reactions yield reactive metabolites. The natural product cycasin yields the same ultimate carcinogen, as does synthetic dimethylnitrosamine after biochemical oxidation by host systems. Yet, dimethylnitrosamine does not yield colon cancer because the organospecificity of each carcinogen depends on specific activation and repair enzyme systems in each tissue and cell type.

Based on the effects of cycasin, Druckrey in Germany examined the carcinogenic properties of 1,2-dimethylhydrazine (Table 5–12), which was postulated to be oxidized to methylazoxymethanol via azomethane and azoxymethane. 1,2-Dimethylhydrazine and azoxymethane, in fact, were found to be highly carcinogenic in many species, yielding the same types of neoplasms as methylazoxymethanol. Of considerable interest is the fact that in rodents these compounds cause a high incidence of cancer of the lower intestinal tract, colon, and rectum, thereby providing models to study the types of

Table 5–12. ALKYL HYDRAZINES, NITRO ALKYL COMPOUNDS, URETHANE, ETHIONINE

In mice, rats, and hamsters, 1,2-dimethylhydrazine (*1*) causes large bowel cancer, and to a lesser extent, cancer in the kidney and liver. *1* is metabolized to azomethane *2*, then azoxymethane *3*, then methylazoxymethanol *4*, and *3* or *4* also induce the same types of cancers as *1*. 1-Methyl-1-formylhydrazine (*6*), found in certain mushrooms, is more carcinogenic than the synthetic prototype, 1-methylhydrazine (*5*), which causes mostly blood vessel neoplasms, especially in liver. Inhalation of 2-nitropropane (*7*) induced liver cancer, but 1-nitropropane (*8*) seems not carcinogenic. Urethane or ethyl carbamate (*9*) is carcinogenic in many species including the nonhuman primate; metabolic activation involves dehydrogenation to the vinyl derivative (*10*), followed by epoxidation. Ethionine (*11*) may undergo a similar sequence via vinylhomocysteine (*12*), and methionine (*13*) is an antagonist to the effect of *11*.

human cancers prevalent in the United States and the Western world (*see* Autrup and Williams, 1983). Curiously, the closely related 1,2-diethylhydrazine has an entirely different organotropism, yielding primarily cancer of lung and liver (Preussman and Stewart, in Searle, 1984). More information is required to understand the specific localization of the effect of this series of compounds.

Hydrazine (NH_2NH_2) itself, when administered at high dose levels, has been shown to reliably induce pulmonary tumors in mice, although the effect in rats is much less pronounced, resulting in a low incidence of liver tumors (Lotlikar, in Sontag, 1981). It is interesting to note that in the C3H strain of mouse, a strain prone to develop spontaneous mammary tumors, hydrazine inhibits the occurrence of mammary tumors while simultaneously inducing lung tumors. The mechanism of this dual effect is not understood. The structurally related but noncarcinogenic hydroxylamine also inhibits mammary tumor formation in C3H mice. Under the influence of hydrazine, incorporation of one-carbon compounds to yield O^6-methylguanine and a 7-*N*-methyl analog in DNA was observed. Barrows (1986) has examined the conditions surrounding the biotransformation of *S*-adenosylmethionine,

the likely source of the methyl group incorporated into DNA.

Some substituted hydrazines, including the important drug isoniazid, also lead to pulmonary tumors in specific strains of mice (Swiss or strain A), because of metabolic release of hydrazine. Tests of isoniazid in other strains of mice or in other rodent species have afforded dubious evidence of carcinogenicity. A number of other drugs and chemicals that possess this type of structure, potentially giving rise to hydrazine during biotransformation, have induced pulmonary tumors in susceptible strains of mice (Shimkin and Stoner, 1975). 1,1-Dimethylhydrazine and similar unsymmetric hydrazines often induce vascular tumors in rodents (Toth, 1980).

Among substituted methylhydrazine derivatives, the antitumor agent Natulan (procarbazine) has been found to be highly carcinogenic in several test systems. Although the exact mechanism is not known, it is presumed to depend on the metabolic liberation of methyl carbonium ions, as is true for symmetric 1,2-dimethylhydrazine. The parent compound, 1-methyl-2-benzylhydrazine, has a similar pattern of carcinogenicity.

1,2-Dimethylhydrazine is biotransformed to

the gas azomethane, which is exhaled in part in the breath of animals given the carcinogen. A subsequent step yields azoxymethane, and thence methylazoxymethanol (Weisburger and Fiala, In Autrup and Williams, 1983). Under some conditions, such as administration of low levels of 1,2-dimethylhydrazine in the drinking water, the tumor distribution seen, namely, vascular tumors, particularly in liver, is different than when high doses are given orally or subcutaneously, which produces intestinal cancer. In hamsters, oral administration of 1,2-dimethylhydrazine leads also to blood vessel tumors, mainly in liver (Toth, 1980). It is presumed that the metabolic activation is different and proceeds via monomethylhydrazine, a chemical that induces mostly such vascular neoplasms, although under some circumstances tumors in the cecum but not in other parts of the intestinal tract are noted. The metabolic activation of methylhydrazine is unknown. A highly carcinogenic natural product found in some types of mushrooms is N-methyl-N-formylhydrazine (Toth, 1980).

Nitro Alkyl Compounds. Nitro alkyl compounds have important industrial uses as solvents or intermediates. A number of tests show that nitromethane, nitroethane, and 1-nitropropane appear to be noncarcinogenic. However, inhalation of 2-nitropropane (Table 5–2) caused liver cancer in rats through mechanisms that remain to be defined (Lewis et al., 1979). One possible mode of action proposes the displacement of the nitro groups through release of nitrite postulated as carcinogen, an unlikely event. Another possibility involves direct alkylation via the reactivity of the nitro compound with cellular macromolecules, again of low probability. A third possibility is the intermediary metabolic formation of an azoxy compound that structurally would be similar to the highly carcinogenic azoxymethane (Fiala, unpublished data). 2-Nitropropane is mutagenic (Speck et al., 1982).

Aldehydes. In inhalation tests, formaldehyde, a widely used chemical in medicine as well as in industrial applications, induced tumors in the nasopharynx at two of three dose levels, 15 and 8 ppm, but not at 2 ppm in rats (Clary et al., 1983; Starr and Gibson, 1985). Thus far tests in mice have been negative. Formaldehyde is genotoxic in a number of in vitro test systems. Even though formaldehyde has been used extensively for decades as a tissue fixative in pathology and in embalming practices, so far there appears to be no documented record of a higher incidence of respiratory tract neoplasia in the many humans exposed to it occupationally or generally (Walrath and Fraumeni, 1983). None-theless, there is a report of a single case (Halperin et al., 1983), and this area needs extensive epidemiologic studies.

Similarly to formaldehyde, inhalation of acetaldehyde also induced tumors in the nasal cavity in rats (Feron et al., 1982). Other tests of acetaldehyde appear negative. Acetaldehyde is not clearly genotoxic by the standards of in vitro tests. Both acetaldehyde and formaldehyde occur as ephemeral intermediates in the physiologic metabolism of one- and two-carbon compounds, including widely used alcoholic beverages (Lieber, 1983). In some countries where consumption of alcoholic beverages is high, there is a finding of liver cancer together with more widespread cirrhosis. It is not known whether neoplasia stems from the alcohol or from other components in the dietary environment, such as mycotoxins, the action of which would be potentiated by the alcoholic cirrhosis. It appears that the amounts of aldehydes prevailing under physiologic conditions as part of the biochemistry of metabolism of two-carbon compounds do not exert a carcinogenic effect. There are well-developed means of detoxifying aldehydes by oxidation to acids or reduction to alcohols. Perhaps it is only in specialized organs such as the nasal cavity that inhalation of appreciable amounts may overcome the local defense mechanisms.

Aldehydes further occur during the biotransformation of a number of aliphatic nitrosamines. It is not known whether these play a role in the expression of the carcinogenicity of these compounds.

Hexamethylphosphoramide (HMPA) This chemical is a good solvent in various applications in the laboratory and in industry. It has a low acute toxicity but has a number of chronic effects including kidney damage and testicular atrophy. Inhalation of 50 to 4000 ppb led to a dose-related incidence of nasal cancer of varied histologic types that began to appear after approximately eight months. At the highest dose level of 4000 ppb, 83 percent of rats had nasal cancers, but at a dose of 50 ppb only 26 percent of the rats had cancer. Interestingly, the animals exposed to 400 ppb exhibited the same time trend in the occurrence of cancer, which suggests a saturation phenomenon (Lee and Trochimowicz, 1982).

As with other N-methyl compounds, HMPA is oxidized by a cytochrome P-450 system, and it appears that the key intermediate, formaldehyde, may be produced in the nasal cavity, an observation further supporting the view that inhalation of formaldehyde, or of substances yielding formaldehyde by metabolism in the nasal cavity, would constitute a carcinogenic risk at that site (Dahl and Hadley, 1983). As is true for formaldehyde itself, the critical factor is the production of the carcinogenic intermediate versus its detoxication by reduction or oxidation. Thus, the presence of a rather low level of HMPA that yields cancer upon continuing inhalation may be due to the production of the carcinogenic intermediate within the cell, and this may be more effective than the exogenous induction of formaldehyde, which is more likely to be detoxified further by cytoplasmic or microsomal enzymes (Dahl and Hadley, 1983). Similarly, other N-methyl or O-methyl compounds of sufficient volatility that could be inhaled might likewise constitute carcinogenic risks in the nasal cavity.

Carbamates. These are synthetic chemicals comprised of esters or derivatives of carbamic acid (Table 5–12). This class includes many important industrial chemicals, among which are pesticides and agricultural chemicals. Ethyl carbamate (urethan) was used as a veterinary anesthetic until its carcinogenicity was discovered in 1943. In mice, this agent readily induces pulmonary tumors, even with a single large dose (Arcos et al., 1982; Miller and Miller, 1983). Different strains of mice exhibit variable responsiveness. Most sensitive are strain A mice, whereas C57BL mice are among the strains responding less readily. Depending on conditions and strain, other organs such as liver and other parts of the hematopoietic system are also affected. Cutaneous application or oral administration followed by a promoting skin treatment (see below) with croton oil or pure phorbol esters leads to skin tumors. In rats, urethan is also active as a multi-potent carcinogen for several target organs. In hamsters, this agent has produced melanotic lesions on the skin and also neoplasms in liver, forestomach, and lung. In monkeys, urethan caused neoplasms in several organs (Adamson and Sieber, 1983). In mice, urethan is active by the transplacental route and is passed to offspring in the milk. Thus administered, it leads to a variety of neoplasms in different organs.

In a series of related carbamates, the methyl ester, an industrial intermediate, is not carcinogenic and fails to inhibit the effect of the active ethyl ester. The propyl, isopropyl, and butyl esters are weakly active, while the higher homologs are inactive. N-Hydroxyurethane exhibits the same degree of carcinogenicity as does urethan. The structure-activity relationships and the inactivity of the methyl derivative may relate to the fact that the biotransformation pathway involves a dehydrogenation of the ethyl group, with formation of vinyl carbamate, a key proximate carcinogen, which can then further un-

dergo epoxidation (Table 5–12). Of course, this would not be possible for the methyl ester and hence accounts for its inactivity. Vinyl carbamate is more active than ethyl carbamate in several test systems, and hence is a good candidate for the metabolic intermediate, even though it has not yet been possible to demonstrate the direct formation of the vinyl compound from ethyl carbamate (Miller and Miller, 1983).

A series of diaryl acetylenic carbamates were synthesized as possible drugs, and a number were found highly carcinogenic. Thus, chemicals such as 1,1-bis-(4-fluorophenyl)-2-propynyl-N-cycloactyl carbamate and the cycloheptyl or cyclohexyl esters induced leukemias rapidly and also neoplasms in the intestines, ear duct, mammary gland, liver, and even in the heart (see Arcos et al., 1982).

Arcos et al. (1982) provide a detailed review of carbamate pesticides and reach the conclusion that although a few may be carcinogenic, most are not. In Japan, the group directed by Shirasu has performed extensive work on the mutagenicity of such compounds in S. typhimurium and note that some of the chemicals with $(CH_3)N-R$ structures are positive (Moriya et al., 1983).

Ethionine. This agent (Table 5–12) was synthesized as an antimetabolite to L-methionine and used in the study of transmethylation reactions in relation to the biochemistry of this essential amino acid. The hepatotoxic and carcinogenic effect of ethionine was discovered many years later by Farber in the United States. The mechanism underlying the chronic action of ethionine leading to liver tumors in rats has not yet been explained. Whereas ethionine is not mutagenic, the vinyl analog is highly mutagenic and binds to cellular macromolecules, including DNA (Leopold et al., 1982). Thus, the activation pathway of ethionine may proceed via S-vinyl-homocysteine, further converted to an epoxide, in a manner similar to the documented example of urethan converted to vinyl carbamate and of aflatoxin B_2 biotransformed to aflatoxin B_1 (Table 5–12; Miller and Miller, 1983). Interestingly, methionine inhibits the development of mutagenicity of vinylhomocysteine and in later stages delays the occurrence of liver cancer (Brada et al., 1982). No doubt, the mechanisms involved are different.

Halogenated Hydrocarbons. Among this group of chemicals are many industrially important agents used as solvents, chemical intermediates, and consumer products. Many of them are nonflammable and, therefore, safe under conditions where other solvents would be risky to use. They are often chemically quite stable, and their toxicologic properties have been extensively studied (Chapter 20). Many of the chlorinated hydrocarbons are powerful liver (Chapter 10) and kidney (Chapter 11) toxins in many species, including humans (Hayes *et al.,* 1982). In this chapter, chlorinated hydrocarbons are discussed in several sections based on the currently known properties of these chemicals relating to their carcinogenicity.

The chlorinated hydrocarbons with one carbon, specifically chloroform and carbon tetrachloride, have induced mainly liver neoplasms in mice. However, these chemicals are not genotoxic by virtue of their failure to exhibit binding to DNA and their inactivity in tests for genotoxicity. Likewise, in the series of two- or three-carbon alkanes or alkenes, those with three or more chlorine atoms also do not appear to be DNA reactive by these same criteria. These agents are discussed under the section on Unclassified Carcinogens (p. 134) because of unresolved questions on their mode of action. Certain polyhalogenated cyclic compounds, including the important pesticides aldrin, dieldrin, heptachlor, chlordane, DDT, and the class of polychlorinated biphenyls and tetrachlordibenzodioxin, are similarly nongenotoxic, but for these, evidence of promoting activity exists, and consequently, they are classified as epigenetic carcinogens of the promoter type (see p. 132).

Tests for genotoxicity, however, provide evidence that vinyl chloride, 1,2-dichloroethane, 1,2-dibromoethane, and 1,2-dibromo-3-chloropropane (Table 5–13) are DNA reactive (Laib, 1982; Van Duuren *et al.,* 1983). In addition, a formerly widely used flame retardant, *tris*(2,3-dibromopropyl)phosphate or tris, was discovered to be active in the Ames test, and subsequently its carcinogenic activity was discovered. This might have been expected based on the already known carcinogenicity of dibromochloropropane. Tris is no longer used as a flame retardant for clothing. With equal chemical structure, bromo derivatives are generally more toxic than the corresponding chloro compounds.

Vinyl chloride or monochloroethylene (Table 5–13) is a very important intermediate in the production of products made of polyvinylchloride. Several papers appeared early in 1970 demonstrating that vinyl chloride was carcinogenic in animal models. The younger the animal at first exposure, the more sensitive it was, especially for hamsters (Drew *et al.,* 1983). The reactive intermediate is the epoxide, or oxirane, which is mutagenic and yields several metabolites eventually excreted in the urine of exposed animals (Lijinsky and Andrews, 1980; Waxweiler *et al.,* 1981; Eder *et al.,* 1982). Vinyl chloride was also identified as a human carcinogen when it was discovered that individuals charged with clean-

Table 5–13. HALOGENATED HYDROCARBONS

Typical halogenated saturated and unsaturated genotoxic alkanes and alkenes. *1*, vinyl chloride; *2*, acrylonitrile (not halogenated but structurally analogous to *1*); *3*, 1,2-dichloroethane; *4*, *trans*-1,2-dichloroethylene; *5*, *cis*-1,2-dichloroethylene (not genotoxic or carcinogenic); *6*, 1,1,1-trichloroethane or methylchloroform (not genotoxic or carcinogenic); *7*, 1,2-dibromoethane (or ethylene dibromide); *8*, 1,2-dibromo-3-chloropropane.

1 H—C=C—Cl (with H on each carbon)

2 H—C=C—C≡N (with H on each carbon)

3 Cl—C—C—Cl (with H, H above and H, H below)

4 C=C, *trans*-1,2-dichloroethylene (Cl, H / H, Cl)

5 C=C, *cis*-1,2-dichloroethylene (Cl, Cl / H, H)

6 Cl—C—C—H (with Cl, H and Cl, H)

7 Br—C—C—Br (with H, H above and H, H below)

8 Br—C—C—C—Cl (with H, H, H above and H, Br, H below)

ing the reactor vessels in the polymerization plants, who presumably were exposed at that time to relatively large concentrations of vinyl chloride, developed angiosarcomas of the liver as a main kind of neoplasm. There are some suggestions that such individuals might also be at higher risk for other cancers, including lung cancer, but the data for that target organ are not striking and are difficult to interpret because of the possible influence of cigarette smoking. It is interesting that thus far it has been only the reactor cleaners who have exhibited disease but not other individuals involved in the production or use of vinyl chloride.

1,2-Dichloroethane is an important solvent, used also in the petroleum industry as a gasoline additive, as well as in agricultural applications as a fumigant. 1,2-Dichloroethane is a powerful liver and kidney toxin. It is also carcinogenic, leading to lung and liver tumors in mice, angiosarcomas in male rats, and, interestingly, mammary adenocarcinomas in female rats when the compound was administered in corn oil chronically by mouth. On the other hand, inhalation studies with rats or mice so far are negative. This suggests that there might be concentration effects and that lower levels such as might be absorbed from inhaled air might not be adequate to induce neoplasia (Laib, 1982). This chemical is genotoxic. Whereas with most chemicals and drugs, conjugation with glutathione catalyzed by glutathione transferase is a detoxication reaction, with dichloroethane, this conjugation leading to the production of a vinyl chloride analog appears to be an effective activation pathway to reactive metabolites having a sulfur mustard structure (*see* Hathaway, 1981; White *et al.*, 1983).

1,2-Dichloroethylene occurs in *cis* and *trans* forms. The commercially used material is usually a mixture of the two. In contrast to the saturated alkane, the alkenes are less toxic, and they do not appear to be mutagenic or carcinogenic. Their metabolism yields dichloroacetylaldehyde, presumably via an epoxide, although the exact intermediary metabolism has not been worked out. The aldehyde is further converted by reduction to the corresponding alcohol or by oxidation to the dichloroacetic acid.

The asymmetric 1,1-dichloroethane or vinylidene chloride is toxic to liver and kidney in rodents as well as in dogs and monkeys. Vinylidene chloride was carcinogenic in mice, leading to kidney and liver tumors, particularly in males, as well as lung and liver angiosarcomas. However, tests in rats appeared to be negative. Also, the closely related 1,1,1-trichloroethane or methylchloroform is not carcinogenic. Vinylidene chloride is mutagenic in the presence of S9 fractions from mouse and rat liver, more so from males, and male mouse kidney. Vinylidene chloride is biotransformed to the epoxide that, like the other compounds in this series, rearranges and eventually leads to chloroacetic acid that reacts further with glutathione yielding thioacetic acid. Radioactivity from labeled vinylidene chloride is bound to protein as well as to DNA. 1,1-Dichloroethane has a specific effect on a number of key enzymes in liver and kidney, particularly cytochrome P-450 monooxygenases, epoxide hydrolase, and glutathione transferase. Chronic intake of the chemical has little effect on the basal level of these enzymes in the sensitive strain of mice, but in the less sensitive rats, there is a progressive increase in the level of epoxide hydrolase and glutathione transferase that may account for the increasing resistance of rats to this chemical. In addition, in the sensitive strains of mice chronic administration of the chemical is cytotoxic. Thus, the carcinogenic effect noted in kidney and liver may be the result of production of reactive intermediate epoxide and tissue regeneration consequent to cytotoxicity that would tend to fix the effect of the carcinogen (Oesch *et al.*, 1983; Maltoni *et al.*, 1985).

Acrylonitrile or vinyl nitrile is a commercially important monomer in the plastics industry. It has a structure similar to that of vinyl chloride. Its metabolism involves an epoxide intermediate that would constitute the genotoxic and mutagenic product (Geiger *et al.*, 1983). Inhalation tests have indicated carcinogenicity in rodents, and there are suggestions that some conditions of human exposure have led to cancer.

In general, 1,2-dibromoethane or ethylene dibromide has similar properties to dichloroethane but is more mutagenic and carcinogenic than the chloro analog. Oral administration induces squamous cell carcinoma of the stomach in addition to a similar tumor pattern exhibited by the chloro compound. The expression time is shorter, testifying to its greater potency. Inhalation induces cancer in the nasal cavity.

1,2-Dibromo-3-chloropropane exhibits an identical behavior to 1,2-dibromoethane and appears more powerful. These dibromo compounds are also important industrially, although less so than the dichloro compounds, and find applications in the agricultural industry. The dibromo compounds appear to undergo the same type of activation mechanisms as the dichloro compound (Van Bladeren *et al.*, 1981). In addition, they appear to be able to react directly with important cellular receptors since they are mutagenic in assays without a liver S-9 fraction. These dibromo derivatives lead to sterility in rodents and also in men exposed during manufacture (Wong *et al.*, 1982; Huff, 1983). The use of these two compounds must be carefully controlled.

Microbiologic Carcinogens. A number of carcinogens are formed in nature by microorganisms or plants (Tables 5–14, 5–15). The mechanism of action of many of these, particularly the antibiotics, is unknown. However, most of these naturally occurring carcinogens clearly undergo

Table 5–14. CARCINOGENS PRODUCED IN NATURE

MICROORGANISMS	PLANTS
Aflatoxins	Tobacco, snuff
Sterigmatocystin	Betel nut
Luteoskyrin	Cycasin
Islanditoxin	Pyrrolizidine (*Senecio*)
Griseofulvin	alkaloids
Actinomycins	Coltsfoot
Mitomycin C	Bracken fern
Adriamycin	Mushroom toxins
Daunomycin	Safrole
Elaiomycin	β-Asarone (calamus oil)
Ethionine	Thiourea, goitrogens
Azaserine	Phorbol esters
Nitrosonornicotine	
Streptozotocin	

Table 5–15.　MYCOTOXINS

Aflatoxin B_1　　　　　　　　Aflatoxin G_1

metabolic activation to a DNA-reactive ultimate carcinogen. The structures of these agents are diverse, but they are described together because of their similar origins.

Mycotoxins. Investigations of the cause of an enormous loss of turkey poults with fulminating liver necrosis in Great Britain early in 1960 led to the discovery of a mold toxin produced on feeds contaminated with a strain of *Aspergillus flavus* and related molds. The toxin accounted for the pronounced hepatotoxicity of such contaminated meals (Busby and Wogan, in Searle, 1984; Linsell, 1982). These active components exhibit characteristic fluorescence patterns; they were isolated and their structure established in record time, a significant achievement in the area of toxicologic studies. The key compound, named aflatoxin B_1 (Table 5–15), not only is highly hepatotoxic but is one of the most powerful carcinogens known, inducing liver tumors in several species after dietary intake of very low levels, of the order of ppb. The mold usually produces four types of aflatoxin: B_1, B_2, G_1, and G_2, so labeled because of a blue (B) or green (G) fluorescence. The B_2 and G_2 compounds are the dihydro derivatives of the B_1 and G_1 analogs, respectively. Among the four isomers found, aflatoxin B_1 is much more toxic and carcinogenic than the G_1 analog. The G_2 derivative is virtually not carcinogenic. Aflatoxin B_2, on the other hand, is definitely but slightly carcinogenic, probably because there is an enzyme that converts aflatoxin B_2 to B_1 to a small extent (Roebuck *et al.*, 1978). The carcinogenicity depends on the double bond in the furan portion of the molecule. The ultimate carcinogenic metabolite of the various aflatoxins is an epoxide that reacts with DNA at N-7 in guanine (Essigman *et al.*, 1982). Inasmuch as there are many other competing biotransformation steps, including the production of ring-hydroxylated metabolites and of the demethylated phenol, it seems that the epoxide is indeed a highly active carcinogen. The other parts of the molecule, including the potentially reactive lactone ring, do not contribute directly to carcinogenic activity but apparently provide bulk, since molecules such as the difuran rings alone, for example, are not active.

Aflatoxin B_1 is highly hepatocarcinogenic in rats and in trout and is also appreciably carcinogenic in a number of other experimental species, including nonhuman primates (Adamson and Sieber, 1983). In highly sensitive species such as rats, or trout, aflatoxin B_1 exhibits carcinogenicity when fed in the diet at levels as low as 1 ppb. The major target organ is liver, but under some conditions, kidney and colon tumors have been seen in rodents. Interestingly, the strains of mice treated thus far do not seem to manifest an effect in liver, except in newborn mice. Adult mice develop lung tumors. The relatively low sensitivity of mice may relate to a high level of GSH-transferase, providing an effective detoxication pathway for the epoxide. Also, it has been reported that subcellular fractions from mouse liver activate AFB_1 to mutagenic metabolites less readily than fractions from rat liver.

In certain African and Asian countries, where staple foods have been contaminated by high levels of aflatoxins on the order of ppm, primary liver cancer is one of the principal neoplastic diseases. In this region, hepatitis B antigen is also endemic, and it is thought that there might be a potentiating effect between this antigen and mycotoxicosis, accounting not only for the high incidence, but also for the fact that the disease is seen at a young age, 20 to 30 years, especially in males (see Blumberg and London, 1982; Omata *et al.*, 1983).

Sterigmatocystin is a related mycotoxin, which is likewise found in mold-contaminated food crops. It is also carcinogenic and may also play a role in human liver cancer.

Antibiotics. These mold products enter the human environment for a variety of uses, mainly as drugs. Several agents, such as doxorubicin, daunomycin, and dactinomycin, are carcinogenic (Schmähl *et al.*, 1977; Uraguchi and Yamazaki, 1978; Bucciarelli, 1981; Clayson, in Sontag, 1981; Westendorf *et al.*, 1983). Streptozotocin is a drug developed for antineoplastic therapy. It is a glucopyranose derivative of methylnitrosourea. It also is diabetogenic unless administered together with nicotinamide. Such molecular structures have been shown in part to bind strongly, but often reversibly, to DNA, perhaps by intercalation. Adriamycin and daunomycin, which cause cancer at several target organs including the mammary gland in rats, give evidence of covalent binding.

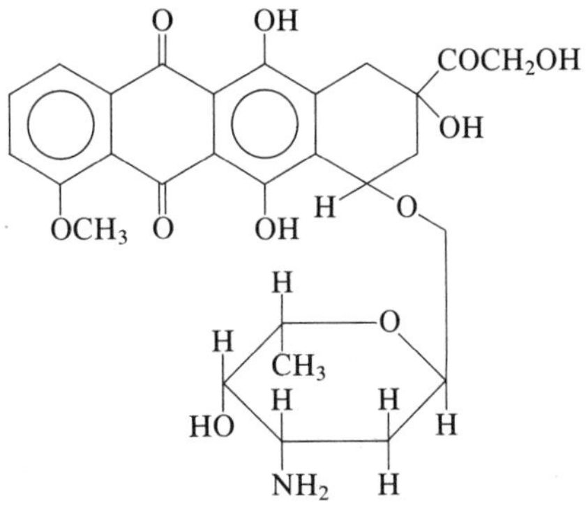

Doxorubicin (Adriamycin)

Adriamycin has caused cardiopathy in clinical application, a condition mimicked in rodents and remedied by vitamin E.

Azaserine or serine diazoacetate, which is produced by *Streptomyces,* has been of interest as an antitumor agent.

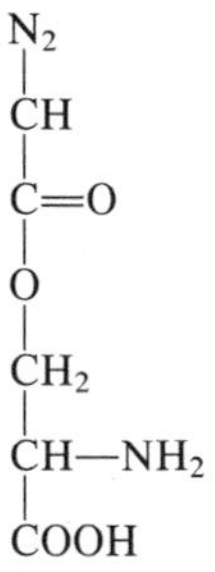

Azaserine

It inhibits purine biosynthesis through inhibition of the enzyme 2-formamido-N-ribosylacetamide 5'-phosphate: L-glutamine amido-ligase. Azaserine was shown to produce primarily pancreas and kidney cancer in rats. This organotropism correlates with localization of the agent (Longnecker, 1983). The mechanism of action is not clear, but the enzyme inhibition has been shown to be due to alkylation of the sulfhydryl group of a cysteine residue in the enzyme, and azaserine is mutagenic without metabolic activation. Thus, a genotoxic action seems probable.

Carcinogens from Plants. A variety of structurally different types of carcinogens are produced by plants (Table 5–14). The best known of these with a major impact as a cause of human cancer, accounting for at least 23% of all cancers in the United States, are the chemicals that come from the tobacco plant (Surgeon General Rept., 1982). Tobacco contains certain carcinogens such as nitrosonornicotine and related agents even before burning and pyrolysis. Tobacco smoke is an exceedingly complex chemical mixture that contains diverse types of carcinogens, cocarcinogens, accelerators, and promoters. The carcinogens include polycyclic aromatic hydrocarbons, heterocyclic compounds, phenolic derivatives, etc. (Hoffmann *et al.,* 1983). The increase in human cancer in men, especially cancer of the respiratory tract, since 1930, and in women since 1960, can be accounted for by the increase in smoking of manufactured cigarettes—by men since about 1915, and by women since about 1940. Newer low-tar products now on the market have a lower, but not zero, risk. Chewing tobacco and snuff are also hazardous and cause cancer in the oral cavity and upper gastrointestinal tract. The reader is referred to specialized reviews for this important area of toxicology (Surgeon General Rept., 1982; Hoffmann *et al.,* 1983).

In India and Asia generally, betel chewing likewise leads to human cancer in the mouth and upper gastrointestinal tract. Current evidence on the carcinogenic constituents implicates both tobacco and certain constituents from the betel nut. Arecoline, the major alkaloid of the betel nut, for example, can be nitrosated to form a carcinogenic nitrosamine.

Safrole. This chemical is typical of a number of related propenyl or allylbenzenes, which are natural and synthetic flavoring agents.

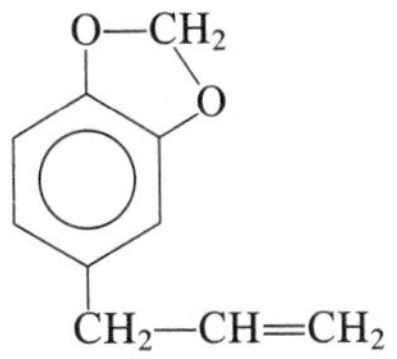

Safrole

These also include β-asarone, methyleugenol, estragole, and isosafrole (Rogers, in Sontag, 1981; Eder *et al.,* 1982; Miller and Miller, 1983). Safrole is carcinogenic to the liver of rats only when rather appreciable amounts, 0.5 percent, are given in the diet. Also, it is difficult to demonstrate genotoxicity for this class of compounds (Sekiwaza and Shibamoto, 1982). This may be because the biochemical activation reactions, involving 1'-hydroxylation, oxidation, or sulfation of this 1'-hydroxy metabolite, or epoxidation on the exocyclic double bond, occur to a relatively small extent. Of those, the 1'-hydroxy sulfate ester appears the likely ultimate carcinogen since its reaction products with gua-nine and adenine have been identified in the liv-ers of rats given labeled safrole. In a study in-volving the elegant use of brachymorphic mice, deficient in sulfate ester synthesis, mice given 1'-hydroxysafrole had a lower liver cancer inci-dence and less DNA-bound carcinogen than normal mice (Fennel *et al.*, 1985).

Senecio Alkaloids. These interesting natural products, consisting mainly of monocrotaline, lasiocarpine, heliotrine, and the basic skeleton retronecine, are complex, aliphatic, hydroxyl-ated fatty acid esters used extensively as teas or as drugs in some civilizations.

Pyrrolizidine alkaloids
(*Senecio, Crotolaria, Heliotropium*)

They have a distinct effect on liver (Rogers, in Sontag, 1981). There is no question that pro-longed administration of these agents leads to hepatomegalocytosis, mainly because they exert a pronounced antimitotic effect. Certain of these alkaloids have a carcinogenic effect in rat liver. It is thought that the intake of such alkaloids in some areas of the world, perhaps together with mycotoxins and in the presence of viral agents such as hepatitis B, may contribute to the liver cancer prevalent in these areas. These chemicals require metabolic activation to pyrrole deriva-tives in which, upon biochemical oxidation of the ring, the exocyclic ester as a leaving group splits to yield an electrophilic compound.

Bracken Fern. In investigations of the cause of hematuria and bladder cancers in cattle in Turkey and other regions, it was found that the consumption of bracken fern was etiologically related to the development of these lesions (Rogers, in Sontag, 1981). In rats, administration of bracken fern has an effect not only on the uri-nary bladder but also on the upper intestinal tract. Human exposure to the carcinogen in bracken fern may occur through drinking the milk of cows who have consumed the plant, or, in some areas of the world, eating the fern itself as part of traditional dietary patterns. The active principle is a complex glucoside (van der Hoeven *et al.*, 1983; Hirono, in Knudsen, 1986).

3. INORGANIC CARCINOGENS

Compounds of uranium, polonium, radium, and radon gas have demonstrated carcinogenic-ity, attributable chiefly to their radioactive prop-erties. Uranium, radium, and the derived radon gas have been implicated in the occurrence of lung cancer in individuals engaged in mining ores. Miners who smoke cigarettes are at higher risk, indicating a possible synergistic effect be-tween ore dust, radiation, and cigarette smoking (Schottenfeld and Fraumeni, 1982).

Connections have been established with delib-erate or inadvertent intake of radioactive ele-ments or their compounds that concentrate in certain organs or tissues. Thus, intake of labeled iodine and derivatives, concentrating in thyroid gland, has been known to give rise to cancer in that organ. Chemicals that concentrate in bone, such as strontium derivatives, in their labeled forms can induce osteosarcomas. These ele-ments are the main contributors to the cancer hazard associated with radioactive fallout, con-sequent to the above-ground use of nuclear weapons. Medical use of thorotrast is known to induce liver cancer (Schmähl *et al.*, 1977).

Among the inorganic chemicals, titanium, nickel, chromium, cobalt, lead, manganese, be-ryllium, and certain of their derivatives have been found carcinogenic under specific experi-mental conditions (Friberg and Nelson, 1981; Heck and Costa, 1982; Sunderman, 1984). Among these, salts of nickel and titanium appear to be most powerful. Manganese antagonizes the effect of the nickel salts. In most instances, these chemicals lead to cancer formation at the point of application, for example, the rapid for-mation of sarcoma after subcutaneous injection of nickel sulfide in rats; on the other hand, oral intake of large amounts of lead acetate induces kidney cancer in rats, and inhalation of beryl-lium salts or ores has induced pulmonary carci-noma in rats and rhesus monkeys.

In humans, small-molecule inorganic com-pounds have been shown definitely carcinogenic only in the case of certain nickel derivatives ob-tained by a process that was abandoned in the mid-1930s (Doll *et al.*, 1977). Workmen on the job since that time appear not to have apprecia-ble risk, an impressive demonstration of preven-tion of occupational cancer by altering exposure conditions without detracting from commercial production.

In addition, human exposure to certain com-plex ores such as chromates, hematite, or nickel apparently has a high risk, particularly of cancer in the respiratory tract. The question of interac-tion with tobacco smoke needs consideration in interpreting these data. It is not certain whether the disease process is due to a direct carcino-genic reaction by the ore (likely for nickel ore, but perhaps not for hematite) or whether the neoplastic effect is due more to a type of solid-state carcinogenesis, akin to that of asbestos discussed below.

Selenium derivatives have had a controversial history as regards carcinogenicity. Years ago suggestions were made that such compounds may be hepatocarcinogenic, but it is clear now that inorganic selenium derivatives are extremely hepatotoxic but do not appear to be carcinogenic. In fact, it seems that selenium is an essential element that controls the function of glutathione peroxidase, among other key enzymes. Also, selenium derivatives inhibited carcinogenicity in several experimental systems and interfered with the mutagenicity of other carcinogens (Griffin and Jacobs, in Zedeck and Lipkin, 1981). There have been suggestions that soil geochemistry, especially in relation to a deficiency of selenium, coincides with a higher incidence of several important cancers, an obvious subject for more research.

Arsenic likewise has been called carcinogenic (Leonard and Lauwerys, 1980). There seems to be an association between trivalent inorganic arsenic exposure of humans through drinking water or certain occupations and the development of lung and skin cancer and lymphomas. However, the exposure situation may not be to arsenic alone but simply to a complex environment containing excess arsenic together with other materials. Some regions where water contains arsenic apparently have no excess of cancer. Also, so far animal tests of arsenic derivatives have not yielded firm evidence that inorganic arsenic compounds can cause cancer, a truly exceptional situation. Rossman et al. (1977) have noted that arsenic compounds can affect fidelity of DNA biosynthesis.

Little is known about the mechanisms of the oncogenic action of inorganic chemicals. They do not seem to operate directly as electrophiles, as do the corresponding ultimate, organic molecule carcinogens. There are certain indications that they are active in rapid bioassay systems and thus may be genotoxic (Hansen and Stern, 1984; Sunderman, 1984). However, a potentially important conceptual advance stems from the research of Loeb (Loeb and Mildvan, in Eichhorn and Marzilli, 1981; Zakour et al., 1981; Sunderman, 1984) indicating that certain metal ions affect the fidelity of the polymerases involved in the biosynthesis of DNA, thus yielding abnormal DNA through this indirect mechanism.

B. Epigenetic Carcinogens

This category is by definition comprised of agents that have been reliably demonstrated not to react with DNA and that exert another kind of biologic effect that appears to be the basis for their carcinogenicity.

1. CYTOTOXINS

One of the oldest theories of cancer causation implicated chronic irritation. It now seems likely that agents that produce cell death leading to compensatory proliferation can indeed give rise to cancer by this means (Stott and Watanabe, 1982). The exact mechanisms are not yet clear, but could involve enhanced susceptibility to environmental carcinogens, mutations during DNA replication, aberrant methylation (Barrows 1986), or chromosome effects. A number of chlorinated hydrocarbons classified as promoters may also involve cytotoxic mechanisms.

Nitrilotriacetic Acid (NTA). This chelating agent is used for a number of industrial purposes and as a replacement for phosphates in household detergents. It was shown to produce kidney and urinary bladder neoplasms in rats and mice when given at high levels in the diet or in drinking water (see Anderson et al., 1985). NTA is not biotransformed and is excreted almost entirely in urine. It is not DNA reactive, and thus, studies of its mode of action have focused on its toxic effects in kidney and bladder as a consequence of its chelating activity. In a series of studies, Anderson and co-workers (Anderson et al, 1985) have shown that NTA carries zinc into the renal tubular ultrafiltrate, where it is reabsorbed by the tubular epithelium. Zinc is toxic to these cells, producing cell injury and death leading to a hyperplastic, and, eventually, neoplastic response. The NTA in urine chelates calcium, extracting it from the urothelium of the renal pelvis and bladder, thereby stimulating cellular proliferation, apparently leading to neoplastic development.

2. SOLID-STATE MATERIALS

Plastics implanted subcutaneously in rodents can lead to sarcoma formation after a long latent period (see Brand, in Becker, 1982). The chemical composition of the implanted material is relatively unimportant. Indeed, thin disks or sheets of metal (such as gold) were as effective as a variety of polymers. The important factors were the size and shape of the insert. Smooth materials were more effective than rough, perforated disks, and sheets were less effective than more solid types. Although the detailed mechanism is not yet known, it seems clear that the solid materials provide a substrate for proliferation of dermal fibroblasts. There are a few reports of sarcomas occurring at the site of vascular grafts in humans, but the cases have in common the fact that the individuals involved were young at the time of implant, which may provide a clue to further epidemiologic investigations as well as laboratory studies (Schmähl et al., 1977).

Asbestos. Asbestos alone, in the pleural cavity in animal models and in humans, leads to mesotheliomas, usually with a long expression period. The latent period is usually long. Importantly, other fibers, such as fine fibrous glass, have a similar effect (Stanton *et al.*, 1981). Thus, the effect has features of solid-state carcinogenesis, especially since the lesion obtained is not epithelial, but mesenchymal. Apart from weak clastogenic effects at high concentrations, no firm evidence for DNA reactivity of asbestos has been developed from *in vitro* tests.

The mechanism of action of asbestos is unknown. However, asbestos is similar to other solid-state materials insofar as it is not biotransformed and excreted but remains permanently in the body. It produces a fibroblastic pleural reaction in advance of pleural mesothelioma. As a consequence of its persistence, even limited exposure to high levels of asbestos, as used to be the case in occupational situations, leads to its continued presence in the body. Men exposed to asbestos during mining operations or in the large-scale shipbuilding effort in the United States in the early 1940s are currently at high risk for this disease. This is apparent from the geographic "hot spots" of lung cancer in counties or areas in the United States where shipbuilding was a major industry (Schottenfeld and Fraumeni, 1982).

In addition, a major health problem stems from the·fact that asbestos particles, and other mineral ores, such as in uranium or hematite mining, potentiate the action of other carcinogens, such as cigarette smoke, reaching the same organ. This cocarcinogenic or promoting effect is discussed in the section on Modification of Carcinogenesis (p. 141). Cases of disease have been seen even in relatives of workmen, who, through frequent indirect exposures such as laundering work clothing, inhaled this material, especially at young ages. Thus, asbestos is in some respects more dangerous than organic carcinogens, although the latter are genotoxic.

There have been suggestions that asbestos fibers ingested during high-level occupational exposure could contribute to cancer in the gastrointestinal tract. Although more information in this area is required, animal studies so far have not demonstrated any effects in these target organs, not even when asbestos was fed at high levels together with the appropriate carcinogen for the gastrointestinal tract.

Iron-Carbohydrate Complexes. Subcutaneous injection in rodents of iron dextran or iron dextrin yielded local sarcomas. Schmähl *et al.*, (1977) have recorded a few reports of subcutaneous tumors, which may have been associated with iron dextran injection in humans, but noted that no direct association has been established between drug injection and oncogenesis in millions of patients treated.

3. HORMONE MODIFERS

Over 40 years ago, hormones, especially of the estrogen type, were shown to cause cancer in laboratory animals. Subsequently, it was found that agents that perturb the physiology of endocrine organs also lead to an increase in neoplasia in those organs.

Estrogens. The naturally occurring hormone estradiol has caused cancer in animals and is suspected to do so in humans when administered chronically at high levels or when present in unphysiologic amounts for long periods of time because of disturbances in normal endocrine balances and receptor systems (see Armstrong, in Bartsch *et al.*, 1982; Rose, 1982). Postmenopausal women, maintained on pharmacologic levels of estrogen preparations, had a high risk of endometrial cancer that disappeared once this phenomenon was recognized and drug use was discontinued (Austin and Roe, 1982). Among users of oral contraceptives, rare cases (considering the widespread use of these agents) of hemorrhagic liver neoplasms have occurred. The mechanism of action of estrogen in these situations is not known. It seems likely that the hormones and endocrine balances have promoting effects. This complex situation may involve systemic effects, including changes in pituitary hormones, e.g., prolactin, or growth hormone, and also adrenal and thyroid hormones. As a rule, hormones need to be present in abnormal amounts for a long time in order to induce neoplasia in endocrine-sensitive tissue.

The synthetic estrogen diethylstilbestrol (DES), when used as a drug at substantial dose rates in pregnant women, has led to clear cell cancer in the vagina of their female offspring, usually about the time of puberty (Robboy, 1983). This finding has been reproduced in rodent models (Forsberg, in Rice, 1979). The underlying mechanism in this instance is also complex and may depend on the production of abnormal tissue elements in the genital tract and faulty differentiation of the complex endocrine apparatus in the fetus, which become apparent at the time of sexual maturation (Iguchi *et al.*, 1986). In addition to these endocrine-related effects, it has also been proposed that DES can act via a genetic mechanism through its metabolites (Metzler, 1984: Ross *et al.*, 1985). This matter has not yet been resolved.

Androgens. In contrast to estrogens, these hormones have rarely caused cancer. A few cases of liver cancer were reported in males taking large amounts of androgens as anabolic agents or muscle builders for athletes.

3-Aminotriazole. This herbicide is still used under some conditions.

3-Aminotriazole

It induces thyroid tumors in rodents and in some studies was associated with liver tumors (IARC Monogr. 7, 1974). The mechanism for induction of thyroid neoplasms appears to be due to interference with the synthesis of thyroxine and thus alteration in the pituitary-thyroid feedback system. 3-Aminotriazole is not established to be DNA reactive, and in a comprehensive study it produced thyroid tumors in rats but not in mice or hamsters, and did not induce liver tumors (Steinhoff *et al.*, 1983).

Ethylenethiourea. This synthetic chemical has been used in the rubber industry.

Ethylenethiourea

It induces thyroid neoplasms in a dose-related fashion. Interestingly, and as might be expected for early lesions due to endocrine imbalances in the thyroid-pituitary axis (Furth, in Becker, 1982; Rose, 1982), there was evidence of reversibility (Arnold *et al.*, 1983).

4. IMMUNOSUPPRESSIVE DRUGS

Immune processes can influence carcinogenesis in a variety of ways (Melief and Schwartz, in Becker, 1982). Animals given immunosuppressive sera or drugs such as azathioprine or 6-mercaptopurine have developed leukemias and lymphomas (IARC Monographs; Clayson, in Sontag, 1981). Likewise, patients so treated developed cancers, usually leukemias or sarcomas but rarely solid tumors (Adamson and Sieber, 1981; Hoover and Fraumeni, 1981). Some of these drugs may alter DNA synthesis or even be incorporated into DNA, but none react with DNA.

In animal models, the underlying causative agent is often an oncogenic virus, and the same may be true in humans. Thus, it is thought that the carcinogenicity of immunosuppressants may stem from an epigenetic phenomenon, by which immunosuppression allows development of tu-

mors initiated by a distinct genetic event (Tarr and Olsen, 1985). Interestingly, a newly developed immunosuppressive drug, cyclosporin A, that operates via a selective inhibition of the activation of lymphocytes did not seem to induce hematopoietic malignancies in chronic toxicity and carcinogenicity tests (Ryffel *et al.*, 1983).

5. PROMOTERS

Promoters, as originally defined by Berenblum (1974), are agents that facilitate the growth of dormant neoplastic cells into tumors. As such, promoters were not considered to be carcinogens. This assertion was initially questioned by Nakahara and others (*see* Nakahara, 1970) who viewed "promotion" as merely representing the effect of a weak carcinogen in producing the synergistic effect of two carcinogens given in sequence (*see* Modifying Factors, p. 141). The argument of those supporting promotion as delineated in the skin model was that the carcinogenic effects of promoters were due to their promotion of spontaneously transformed cells. Consequently, the idea grew that promoters were noncarcinogenic, in spite of their production of neoplasms by themselves. As described earlier, carcinogens are defined operationally by the production of tumors. Accordingly, many agents that have promoting activity are also "carcinogenic." In the section on Modifying Factors (p. 141), the phenomenon of promotion and noncarcinogenic promoters are discussed. This section describes non-DNA reactive "carcinogens" whose mode of action appears to be promotion.

Tetradecanoyl Phorbol Acetate (TPA). This component of croton oil, also known as phorbol myristate acetate, has been the classic "promoter" used in two-stage skin carcinogenesis experiments. However, TPA by itself produces a low incidence of skin cancer even under conventional promoting conditions (Van Duuren, 1982). Moreover, when applied to hairless mice, it elicits a 100% incidence of skin cancer (Iversen and Iversen, 1979). These carcinogenic effects may be due to the promotional activity of the agent binding to specific receptors, and certainly that seems to be involved (Ashendel *et al.*, 1983). However, it has also been shown that TPA produces chromosomal effects (Kinsella and Radman, 1978) possibly through generation of reactive oxygen (Cerutti, 1985). Thus, TPA may be in fact an indirect genotoxin. The phorbol esters are distinct from other carcinogens of the promoting classes by virtue of binding to a membrane receptor (Blumberg, in Williams *et al.*, 1983).

Phenobarbital. The antiseizure drug phenobarbital and other chemicals to be discussed next increase the incidence of mouse liver tumors but cause cancer in the rat liver infrequently, if at all. By most measures, phenobarbital is nongenotoxic, although some positive results have been recorded in the Ames test. It enhances the effects of hepatocarcinogens when administered after them (Peraino *et al.*, in Hecker *et al.*, 1982). Moreover, phenobarbital has been shown to enhance the development of preneoplastic lesions in rat liver (*see* Williams in Pereira, 1983), from which it can be postulated that the carcinogenicity of phenobarbital occurs by a mechanism of promotion exerted on preexisting abnormal liver cells, such as in foci, that eventually give rise to the "spontaneously" occurring liver lesions and neoplasms in old mice and rats (Williams, 1981; Schulte-Hermann *et al.*, 1983). The basis for this effect may be an inhibition of intercellular communication (see section on Promotion, p. 143), which liberates abnormal cells from growth control by surrounding normal cells. The nature of the "inducing" agent yielding the abnormal cells is obscure; it could be genetic in the inbred strains of mice, such as proximity of a proto-oncogene to a fragile site in a chromosome. A high frequency of activated oncogene has been found in mouse liver neoplasms (Fox and Watanabe, 1985; Reynolds *et al.*, 1986). Also, variations in incidence between different colonies raise the possibility of an exogenous factor, such as nitrosamines. Detailed epidemiologic studies on humans using phenobarbital have not revealed evidence of carcinogenicity (Clemmensen and Hjalgrim-Jensen, 1978).

Chlorinated Hydrocarbons. As was discussed earlier, this important class of widely used chlorinated hydrocarbons has been subdivided for the purpose of discussing their apparently distinct actions. One group comprises those chemicals that appropriate tests and the underlying chemistry show to be endowed with genotoxic properties that may lead to cancer at select and specific target organs (see p. 104). The class of chlorinated hydrocarbons includes, however, a substantial number of commercially important chemicals that appropriate tests for genotoxicity indicate are not genotoxic within the limitations of such tests. Thus, assays such as bacterial mutagenesis, DNA repair in various cell systems including liver cells, and detailed biochemical studies on the possible binding of metabolic products to DNA were basically negative (Williams, in Pereira, 1983).

DDT and a variety of organochlorine pesticides, polychlorinated and polybrominated biphenyls, and tetrachlorodibenzodioxin (Table 5–16) have all produced predominantly or exclusively liver cancer in rodents (Guzelian, 1982;

IARC, 1982; Poland and Kimbrough, 1986). Interestingly, DDT tested many times under widely different conditions has not been found carcinogenic in the hamster or in nonhuman primates, and indeed, despite the fact that the pesticide has been used extensively for almost 40 years, has given no evidence of cancer risk in humans (Hayes, 1982). This includes not only the general public, where trace amounts of DDT have been found in body fat, but also individuals exposed to higher levels during its production or spraying. While DDT is innocuous in hamsters, a lifetime test of the metabolite DDE induced a small number of neoplastic nodules (not cancer) (Rossi *et al.*, 1983).

Highly chlorinated aromatic compounds such as polychlorinated biphenyls contain a number of isomers after the technical production process (Kimbrough, 1983; Poland and Kimbrough, 1986). This includes molecules containing from three to six chlorines, polybrominated biphenyls with an identical distribution of bromine in the technical material, or tetrachlorodibenzo-*p*-dioxin (TCDD), which has been found in small but definite amounts in formulations of 2,4,5-T, a valuable herbicide. All of these chemicals are highly toxic to liver and kidney. In fact, TCDD is one of the most toxic chemicals known, giving adverse effects with as little as parts per trillion and certainly at the parts-per-billion level. There appears to be a specific cytosolic receptor protein with a high affinity for TCDD that translocates to the nucleus of liver and other cells (Poellinger *et al.*, 1982; Poland and Knutson, 1982). These chemicals also induce liver tumors in mice and to a definite but small amount in rats. Thus, ingestion by rats of 2000 ppt or 0.1 μg/kg/day induced squamous cancer in the respiratory tract and in the oral cavity, and liver cancer, the latter in females only (Kociba, in Poland and Kimbrough, 1986). Halogenated benzopyranes and benzofurans are also suspected to be carcinogenic. The carcinogenicity of polychlorinated biphenyls (PCB) may stem in part from such contaminants, together with promoting effects by PCB (Kimbrough, 1983).

Tests for genotoxicity in diverse prokaryotic and eukaryotic systems reliably positive for known genotoxic hepatocarcinogens are uniformly negative for these compounds (Pereira *et al.*, 1982; Pereira, 1983; Poland and Knutson, 1982). Liver tumor-enhancing activity has been identified for DDT (see IARC, 1982), PCB (see IARC, 1982), polybrominated biphenyl (Jensen *et al.*, 1982), chlordane and heptachlor (Williams and Numoto, 1984), and TCDD (Pitot and Sirica, 1980). Although highly suggestive, none of these studies rigorously excluded syncarcinogenesis as the basis for enhancement. Nevertheless, it

Table 5–16. CHLORINATED POLYCYCLIC HYDROCARBONS

These hydrocarbons were formerly of great commercial importance, such as the pesticides DDT, aldrin, endrin, and chlordane, or the industrial nonflammable solvents and transformer fluids, PCB. TCDD is a highly toxic contaminant, found in some batches of PCB and 2,4,5-T. These chemicals are fat soluble and for that reason have a long residence time in the body. They are toxic to the liver and kidney and are promoters in liver cancer induction. They also are good inducers of the cytochrome P-450 enzyme system.

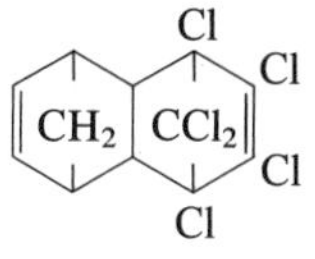

Aldrin

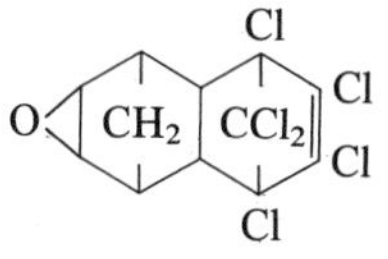

Endrin

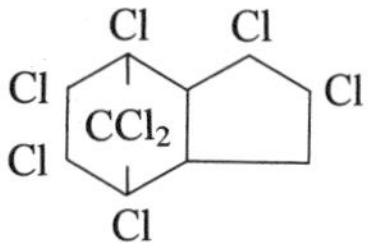

Chlordane

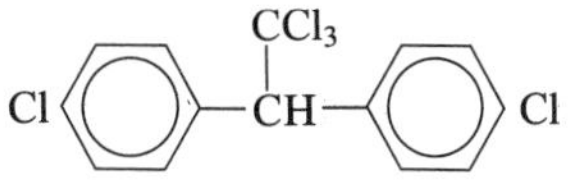

1,1'-(2,2,2-Trichloroethylidene)bis(4-chloro benzene), or 2,2'-bis(p-chlorophenyl)-1,1,1-trichloroethane or DDT

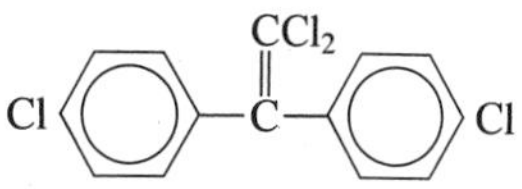

1,1-Dichloro-2,2'-bis(p-chlorophenyl)ethylene or DDE

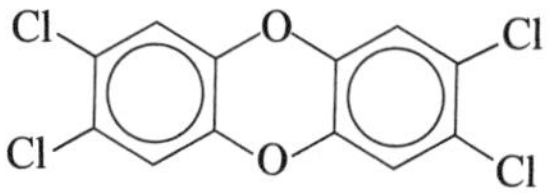

Tetrachlorodibenzo-p-dioxin (TCDD)

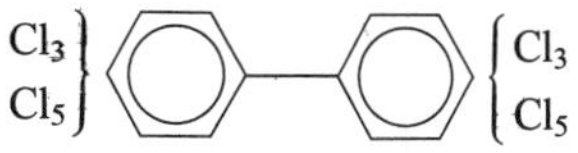

Polychlorobiphenyls (PCB, Arochlor)

seems likely that, as in the case of phenobarbital, the chemicals are carcinogenic though promoting mechanisms on preexisting abnormal cells. This is further supported by the observations that these agents act on cell membranes producing inhibition of intercellular communication (Trosko et al., in Milman and Weisburger, 1985; Williams, 1981).

Saccharin. The artificial sweetener saccharin has been extensively studied as a carcinogen. In 1974, two studies reported an increased incidence of bladder tumors in the first-generation male offspring of rats fed 5 percent or 7.5 percent saccharin throughout pregnancy and for lifetime in the first generation. These early studies were complicated by the presence of ortho-toluene sulfonamide in the saccharin and bladder parasites *Trichosomoides crassicaudum* and bladder stones in the test animals. A subsequent multigeneration experiment with Swiss mice in which saccharin was given at 0.5 percent in the diet for six generations did not reveal a carcinogenic effect. However, in a two-generation study in which rats were fed 5 percent saccharin, a small increase in bladder tumors in male rats in the F_1 generation was found. A series of papers

has reviewed this field (various authors, 1985). Saccharin is not biotransformed and has not been shown to be genotoxic, although some impurities have been noted to be mutagenic. Several studies have shown that saccharin enhances the development of bladder cancer when administered after a bladder carcinogen. Sims and Renwick (1983) have shown that dietary saccharin produces a dose-related increase in the urinary excretion of indole metabolites, as a result of altered metabolism of protein in the cecum. Tryptophan is a promoter in bladder carcinogenesis (p. 143), and thus the action of saccharin may be quite indirect. Also, the sodium ion of the saccharin salt tested may be involved. Hence, saccharin itself may not be the active agent.

Butylated Hydroxyanisole (BHA) and Butylated Hydroxytoluene (BHT). These antioxidants have been utilized safely as food additives in many countries. Indeed, several tests of chronic toxicity have not revealed any adverse effects. Recently, however, Ito et al. (1983) have reported that dietary administration of 20,000 ppm of BHA led to hyperplasia and neoplasia in the forestomach of Fischer strain rats in a lifetime study. They noted that 5000 ppm BHA had a much lower effect. Olsen *et al.* (1983) observed that the first generation offspring in a two-generation study involving dietary intake of 250 mg/kg body weight BHT produced a small, but significant, yield of hepatocellular adenoma and carcinoma, more so in males than in females. The structure of these agents does not suggest a likely electrophile, and tests for genotoxicity have been uniformly negative.

Peraino (in Slaga *et al.*, 1978) found that dietary intake of 500 ppm BHT following an initiating treatment with the carcinogen 2-acetylaminofluorene appeared to exert a promoting effect, which was, however, not as strong as that of phenobarbital. This was subsequently confirmed (Maeura and Williams, 1984). Witschi and Lock (in Slaga *et al.*, 1978) observed that BHT enhanced pulmonary carcinogenesis in mice. In a study on BHT inhibition of liver carcinogenesis, Williams *et al.* (1983) noted that with rats fed 2-acetylaminofluorene, liver carcinogenesis was inhibited, as previously reported by Wattenberg (*see* 1983), but that, at high levels of BHT, induction of bladder cancer was seen. Probably, metabolic shifts are involved that protect the liver and yield a higher level of excretion of metabolites that could affect the bladder, but a promoting effect may also be involved. The findings of Ito and of Olsen are consistent with a promoting effect of these antioxidants, but more work needs to be done before assignment can be confidently made.

If the carcinogenic effects of BHA and BHT are due to a promoting action, dose-response studies will be important in assessing human risk since Maeura and Williams (1984) have reported a threshold for the liver neoplasm-promoting effect of BHT. In many instances, those antioxidants have exhibited cancer-protective effects (Prochaska *et al.*, 1985).

C. Unclassified Carcinogens

There are a number of carcinogens that have not been demonstrated to react covalently with DNA, but whose mode of action is not sufficiently well understood to permit assignment to a specific class of epigenetic agents.

Dioxane. This important commercial solvent induced liver cancer in rats when administered at sizable dosages, 1 percent in drinking water.

Dioxane

In some tests it was also noted that animals had nasopharyngeal cancers, possibly caused by the introduction of the solution or the vapors from the solution into the air passages. The mechanism of action has not been completely clarified, but would depend on an α-hydroxylation with formation of an active electrophile (Woo *et al.*, 1978; Young *et al.*, 1978). However, genotoxicity has not been demonstrated.

Benzene. Occupational exposure to benzene under quantitatively ill-defined conditions has led to a number of cases of leukemia (Adamson and Sieber, 1981; IARC Monogr. 29, 1982; Arp *et al.*, 1983). The prevailing hygienic conditions led to the suspicion that the air concentrations were high. Recently, the threshold limit value was set at 1 ppm.

Benzene is not genotoxic (Dean, 1985). Chronic inhalation of high levels of benzene in rats induced thymic and nonthymic lymphoma and several solid neoplasms, including neoplasms in the ear duct (Cronkite *et al.*, 1985; Maltoni *et al.*, 1985). Specific antecedent effects on the bone marrow were noted as a result of exposure to benzene or an oxidative metabolite (Gaido and Wierda, 1985; Wallin *et al.*, 1985). Inasmuch as leukemias in animals can be readily induced by viruses, or by immunosuppressive drugs in animals and in humans (see comment in this chapter), the question as to the mode of action of benzene in inducing leukemia in specific occupational groups remains open, but may also involve an indirect immunosuppressive action by a benzene metabolite such as catechol (Bolcsak and Nerland, 1983).

Thioamides. In connection with the determination of the safety of certain food additives, it was discovered that thiourea, thioacetamide, thiouracil, and similar thioamides were carcinogenic.

Thiourea   Thioacetamide

Thiouracil

The main target organs are the thyroid and in some instances the liver (Neal and Halpert, 1982). The action on the thyroid is thought to be due to an interference with the synthesis of thyroxine leading to an imbalance of the pituitary–thyroid gland relationships. Thus, an increased flow of thyrotropic hormone is generated by the pituitary, stimulating thyroid growth and contributing to tumor formation. In addition, a direct, local effect of the carcinogen or a metabolite in the thyroid appears necessary. The action on the liver by agents such as thiouracil and thioacetamide has not yet received a sound fundamental explanation. Biotransformation studies suggest oxidation on the sulfur atom to thiono and sulfone derivatives might yield reactive compounds, involving a charge separation between the sulfur-oxygen and the carbon, the latter thus being electrophilic.

Acetamide, a related chemical, when given to rats in doses as large as 1 to 5 percent in the diet, elicits hepatocellular carcinomas in approximately one year. The mechanism of action of this chemical on the liver is quite different from that of the corresponding thioacetamide, the latter being effective in much lower dosages in a shorter span of time.

Halogenated Hydrocarbons. Among this class of widely used industrial chemicals there are a number of agents whose mode of action remains unclear. Among these, carbon tetrachloride, chloroform, and several polychlorinated alkanes or alkenes yield negative or equivocal results in current test systems for genotoxicity (Table 5–17). Furthermore, biotransformation in mammalian systems *in vivo* or *in vitro* does not provide any evidence that they give rise to reactive electrophilic metabolites. These experiments include utilizing highly isotopically labeled chemicals in attempts to verify reaction with DNA.

On the other hand, one element that is quite clear is that these chlorinated hydrocarbons are cytotoxic after a single dose or upon chronic intake. For the most part, the toxicity is expressed mainly in liver and kidney of rodents. With some

agents, where accidental or suicidal ingestion occurred, there was evidence of liver or kidney damage in humans.

There is no question but that halogenated hydrocarbons can be toxic and in some instances carcinogenic in mouse liver. The important finding was made that administration in an edible oil appeared to be more toxic than when equivalent amounts were administered in drinking water. Thus, the role of the vehicle will have to be defined. In addition, of course, this distinction is important in evaluating the possible effect of halogenated hydrocarbons present in small amounts in drinking water.

Methylene chloride, or dichloromethane, is a useful solvent and chemical with broad chemical application, especially since it is nonflammable, as are most of the halogenerated hydrocarbons. Methylene chloride is active in bacterial mutagenesis tests without requiring metabolic activation. However, it is inactive in most systems involving mammalian cells and has not been found to alkylate DNA. Therefore, methylene chloride may not justify classification as a genotoxin. Yet, chronic inhalation by mice led to the development of neoplasms in lung and liver, but a similar test in rats led to equivocal results. On the other hand, administration in drinking water of rats and mice gave no evidence of carcinogenicity (see a series of papers, Kirschman et al., 1986; National Toxicology Program, 1986).

Carbon tetrachloride is a high volume, nonflammable solvent. In virtually all species, it is severely hepatotoxic, and in mice of certain strains, it induces liver tumors. During liver intoxication, it has been proposed that lipid

Table 5–17. HALOGENATED HYDROCARBONS

Simple polychlorinated aliphatic compounds typified by carbon tetrachloride are highly hepatotoxic and nephrotoxic. In addition, they induce liver cancer in mice but, with the exception of carbon tetrachloride, not in rats or hamsters. Their mode of action remains to be clarified. Carbon tetrachloride may be somewhat different from the other chemicals in this series since it also leads to peroxidation processes that may be involved in its capacity to damage the liver.

Cl—C—Cl with Cl above and H below	H above; Cl—C—Cl; Cl—C—Cl with H below	Cl—C—Cl (double bond) Cl—C—H	Cl—C—Cl (double bond) Cl—C—Cl
Chloroform	Tetrachloroethane	Trichloroethylene	Tetrachloroethylene (or perchloroethylene)

peroxidative processes might play a role. Plaa's group (Hewitt *et al.*, 1982) has noted potentiation of toxicity of carbon tetrachloride in rats by 1,3-butanediol.

Chloroform (Table 5–17) was formerly used in human anesthesia and is an important industrial solvent. Specific sensitive chemical analytic procedures have revealed that chloroform is the main chlorinated hydrocarbon produced during chlorination of drinking water and, thus, is present in small but definite amounts in water supplies. Similarly to carbon tetrachloride, chloroform causes liver and kidney damage, somewhat more in kidney and somewhat less in liver as compared to carbon tetrachloride. Chronic oral intake in mice leads to liver tumors, and lifetime administration to rats has induced a smaller yield of renal neoplasms, in addition to being severely nephrotoxic. It has been proposed that there was an association between liver and kidney toxicity and the occurrence of neoplasms (Moore *et al.*, 1982).

Administration of trichlorethylene, trichlorethane, and tetrachloroethane (perchloroethane) (Table 5–17) to mice induces neoplasms in the liver, as is typical of virtually all chlorinated hydrocarbons. These chemicals are highly toxic to kidneys in mice and even more so in rats.

Even though an epoxide seems to be the critical genotoxic metabolite derived from vinyl chloride, it has been much more difficult to demonstrate the formation of a reactive epoxide from a polychloroethylene such as trichloroethylene (Eder *et al.*, 1982; van Duuren *et al.*, 1983; Miller and Guengerich, 1983). This chemical can form an epoxide or oxirane, as seen by the properties of the synthetic epoxide. However, formation of the epoxide in biologic systems would appear to be difficult because of the steric highly hindered position of the ethylene bond owing to the three neighboring chlorine atoms. It may be that the kinetics of the formation of the epoxide are considerably slower than that of its reaction with a nucleophilic component in the cell other than DNA. Thus far, it has not been possible to demonstrate a covalent binding of the reactive metabolite to DNA (Magee, 1982). Importantly, the saturated trichloro or tetrachloroethanes exhibit the same kind of toxicity and tumor spectrum as do the ethylene derivatives, so that the hindered double bond apparently is biochemically equivalent to the single bond in the polychlorinated ethanes.

Peroxisome Proliferators. A variety of agents having in common the ability to increase the numbers of peroxisomes in rodent liver have produced liver tumors, leading to the hypothesis that peroxisome proliferators as a class are carcinogenic (Reddy and Lalwani, 1983). Per-oxisome proliferators that have been found to be hepatocarcinogenic in rodents include the hypolipidemic drugs, clofibrate, fenofibrate, gemfibrozil, tibric acid, the plasticizer di(2-ethylhexyl)phthalate, and the organic solvent 1,1,2-trichloroethylene (Cohen and Grasso, 1981; Elcombe *et al.*, 1984; Reddy and Lalwani, 1983; Kluwe *et al.*, 1985). These agents have been proven to be generally negative in short-term tests for genotoxicity, and di(2-ethylhexyl)phthalate does not bind to liver DNA *in vivo*. Some evidence for a liver tumor-promoting effect with certain of these agents has also been reported (Mochizuki *et al.*, 1982; Ward *et al.*, 1983), but this has not been found for all agents of this type (Numoto *et al.*, 1984) and does not seem likely to be the mechanism of their carcinogenicity. Alternatively, it has been proposed by Reddy (Reddy and Lalwani, 1983) that, as a consequence of the increase in the numbers of peroxisomes, increased H_2O_2 could lead to the formation of reactive oxygen species that have the capability to damage DNA and initiate carcinogenesis. Substantiation of this indirect mechanism of neoplastic conversion would place these agents in the category of epigenetic carcinogens.

Methapyrilene. This antihistaminic was widely used in sleep aids in the United States, until it was reported in 1980 that it produced liver tumors in rats (Lijinsky *et al.*, 1980). Methapyrilene has also been shown to enhance liver tumor development when administered either before or after a genotoxic liver carcinogen (Furuya and Williams, 1984). Methapyrilene is negative in most short-term tests for genotoxicity, but some positive results have been noted. An unusual finding, as yet unexplained, is the considerable increase in the number of mitochondria in liver cells of rats given this drug (Reznik-Schuller and Lijinsky, 1982). This indicates the possibility of excess production of reactive oxygen species, as has been proposed for the peroxisome proliferators.

BIOTRANSFORMATION OF CHEMICAL CARCINOGENS

Enzyme systems that have evolved for the biotransformation of endogenous substrates are capable of metabolizing most chemical carcinogens (Weisburger and Williams, in Becker, 1982; Searle 1984; Miller and Miller, 1981; 1983; Snyder *et al.*, 1982; Jakoby, 1984; Anders, 1985; Flamm and Lorentzen, 1985). Within the broad category of genotoxic carcinogens, the biotransformation of direct-acting or activation-independent carcinogens often leads to less active, or inactive, products and hence represents detoxication. With procarcinogens, the biotransformation of most is likewise in the direction of detoxified products, but in this process certain biotransformation steps result in the generation of reactive species in the form of electrophilic or radical cation compounds, which constitute the proximate carcinogen, sometimes via an intermediary step. The study of these steps is greatly facilitated by examining the mutagenicity of products. For example, a direct-acting, electrophilic or radical cation compound would appear positive in the Ames test without additional biochemical activation with a liver enzyme fraction (assuming that the bacteria cannot activate it, for example, a nitroaryl compound), whereas a procarcinogen or a proximate carcinogen would require such a biochemical activation.

Direct-Acting Carcinogens

Biotransformation leads to loss of activity in the case of the primary direct-acting electrophilic carcinogens. In view of their reactive nature, such reactions can be straightforward chemical processes, involving an SN_1 or an SN_2 type of chemical interaction with cellular nucleophiles. Other reactions, which differ as a function of the structure of the carcinogen, can be enzyme mediated. The relative effectiveness of agents depends in part on the relative rates of interaction between the chemical and genetic material, DNA, versus competing reactions with other cellular nucleophiles. Thus, the relative activity in a given series of chemicals hinges principally on such competing interactions and also on enzymic detoxication reactions. Stability during transport, permeability across membranes, and similar factors also play a role.

The detoxication of compounds, as is true for drugs and other chemicals, depends on the chemical structure, species, and strain in which tested, and environmental conditions. Alkylating agents such as methyl methanesulfonate are detoxified via an SN_2-type reaction by nucleophiles such as proteins, by water itself, by sulfhydryl compounds, and by esterases. Oxidative reactions on the alkyl group are also possible. Aromatic rings are likely to undergo a hydroxylation reaction yielding phenolic compounds that are conjugated with glucuronic or sulfuric acid, and then excreted. In addition, the metabolic introduction of hydroxy groups on the phenyl ring may modify hydrolysis of the alkyl or arylalkyl esters and decrease carcinogenic potency.

Similar considerations with respect to the detoxication reactions and mechanisms apply to the nitrogen mustard type of compound, even though they also undergo biochemical activation reactions. In general, a mustard derived from an aromatic or heterocyclic ring system has some-

what longer half-time *in vivo* as compared to an aliphatic mustard. For this reason, the former has greater systemic effects.

Reactivity toward nucleophilic reactants also controls hydrolytic destruction of lactone and similar structures built on strained ring systems. Thus, β-propiolactone is more carcinogenic than higher homologs because of its reactivity. Ethylene oxide likewise hydrolyzes readily in mammalian cells and is detoxified. Inhalation of substantial quantities can overcome local hydrolytic capability and hence induce neoplasia in the nasal septum.

In general, the rate of hydrolytic attack on these direct-acting chemicals either by water in the host or mediated, in the case of esters, by enzymes affects carcinogenic potency. Such agents are also detoxified readily by chemical or enzyme-mediated reactions with sulfur amino acids and peptides such as glutathione, yielding eventually the corresponding mercapturic acids. Reactions such as these produce compounds that appear more toxic because of their reaction with specific life-supporting enzymes, and of lower carcinogenicity than might be expected from the reactive nature of these type of carcinogens.

Carcinogens Requiring Biochemical Activation: Procarcinogens

Most of the chemical carcinogens in the environment belong to this class. In contrast to direct-acting carcinogens, which are chemically reactive and therefore do not persist in the environment, procarcinogens are often chemically stable entities. They are subject to a great variety of biotransformation reactions by mammalian as well as bacterial systems. Most of these biochemical reactions yield detoxified metabolites, but in the process toxication or activation reactions take place (Brookes, 1980; Conney, 1982; Miller and Miller, 1981, 1983; Weisburger and Williams, in Becker, 1982; Anders, 1985, Lambeir *et al.*, 1985). The activated metabolites usually account for only a small portion of a dose of a procarcinogen. Therefore, in order to detect such active metabolites, all the metabolites of a given agent must be accounted for quantitatively as accurately as possible. A determination of only the main metabolites, as is often performed in studies of drug, food additive, or pesticide metabolism, would probably fail to identify the key active metabolites.

A combination of the techniques of biochemical pharmacology through *in vivo* and *in vitro* studies of genetic toxicology testing constitutes a most useful approach to assess whether a given chemical is converted even in small yield to a potentially harmful DNA reactive metabolite. If such a reactive product is detected, separation techniques can be directed toward isolating it for the purpose of structural identification. These procedures are useful not only for academic purposes, but in general to assess whéther or not under certain circumstances a potentially harmful product is present or has been generated through biotransformation. As noted above, because the major metabolites of chemicals are often of little consequence with regard to toxic effects, this approach would permit a decision to be made as to possible adverse effects stemming from a given material. As will be discussed, not all such indications of electrophile characteristics necessarily imply hazard. Nevertheless, the presence of this property is a warning signal that must be investigated in detail.

It is outside the scope of this chapter to elaborate on all the known enzymic activation reactions for chemical carcinogens. Specific details have been provided for certain major and historically important classes, polycyclic aromatic hydrocarbons, aromatic amines, and nitrosamines. Here, only the general principles of these activation reactions will be discussed. Most of these reactions consist of biochemical oxidation or hydroxylation (Table 5–18), performed by enzyme systems associated with the endoplastic reticulum. The main enzymes, including the complex cytochromes, protaglandin synthetases, and specific cofactors, exist in virtually all tissues in all species, but in differing amounts and often with a specificity for certain substrates. It is this feature that accounts often in a major way for the organ-specific localization of the action of individual chemical carcinogens. Carcinogens are active at certain sites under specific conditions because of the presence of the necessary activation enzyme system (Conney, 1982; Bartsch et al., 1982; Snyder et al., 1982; Langenbach et al., 1983; Morton et al., 1983; Marnett and Eling, 1983; Anders, 1985; Nebert et al., 1985).

Liver is the organ with the greatest capacity for biotransforming chemical carcinogens. Nevertheless, other organs, particularly kidney, lung, and the gastrointestinal tract, have a definite capability. In addition, the metabolic fate of several carcinogens is dependent on, or influenced by, the action of the bacterial flora in the gut. Cycasin, the β-glucoside of methylazoxymethanol, is split only by the mediation of bacterial enzymes. With other agents, such as simple azo dyes, the bacterial flora may assume mainly a detoxifying role, by virtue of its reducing capability. Inasmuch as diet and other conditions modify the gut microflora, the biotransformation of carcinogens, drugs, and chemicals affected by the flora could thus be indirectly modulated (see Brookes, 1980; Reddy et al., 1980; Ashby et al., 1983; Autrup and Williams, 1983).

In some cases reductive enzymes yield activated intermediates, for example, the conversion of nitroaryl or nitroheterocyclic compounds to the corresponding hydroxylamino derivatives. Thus, the active intermediate of 4-nitroquinoline N-oxide is the corresponding 4-hydroxylamino derivative, stemming from the action of soluble xanthine oxidase. In other cases, the active intermediate is released from a transport form such as glucuronide conjugate by enzymic systems or a suitable pH in certain target organs, for example, the urinary bladder.

Some carcinogens require a series of activation steps that involves not only the cytochrome systems, but also other oxidative, reductive, or conjugative type I or type II enzymes (Jakoby, 1984). Examples discussed in detail above are the aromatic amines and polycyclic aromatic hydrocarbons.

When organic chemicals can be transformed to electrophilic reagents within cells, they are almost certain to act as genotoxic carcinogens. However, administration of the same chemicals in their reactive form may be innocuous, for they can react with competing nucleophilic substrates such as water or select protein or peptide end groups such as glutathione. Thus, the sulfate ester of N-hydroxy-N-2-fluorenylacetamide is not carcinogenic when administered to animals, simply because it undergoes rapid side reactions prior to reaching targets where it could be carcinogenic. Certain alkylating agents undergo similar reactions and are less carcinogenic than might be surmised on the basis of their structure. On the other hand, agents such as alkylnitrosoureas or alkylnitrosourethan that, because of their chemical configuration, can readily penetrate organ and cellular membranes and release the active alkyl carbonium ions inside cells by spontaneous or enzyme-mediated hydrolytic processes are among the most dangerous carcinogenic chemicals. Thus, intracellular activation is a major factor in the carcinogenicity of many chemicals.

REACTIONS OF CHEMICAL CARCINOGENS

A. Cellular Macromolecules

The study of the interaction of carcinogens with cellular constituents began with the observation by the Millers in the United States in 1947 of the detectable color produced in rat liver when carcinogens of the azo dye type reacted with liver proteins. The hues of the dyes bound to tissue proteins were pH dependent. Subse-

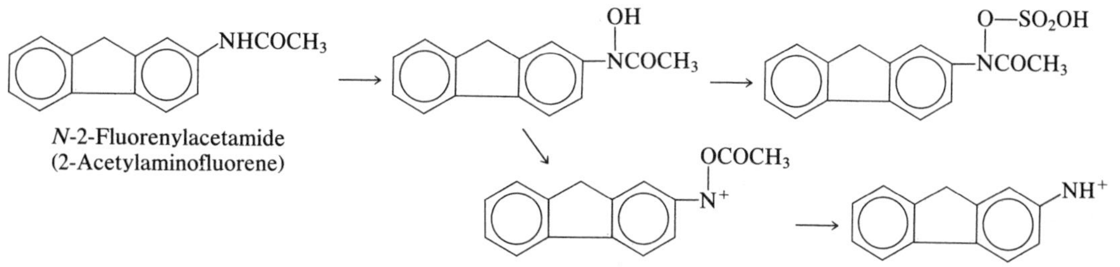

N-2-Fluorenylacetamide
(2-Acetylaminofluorene)

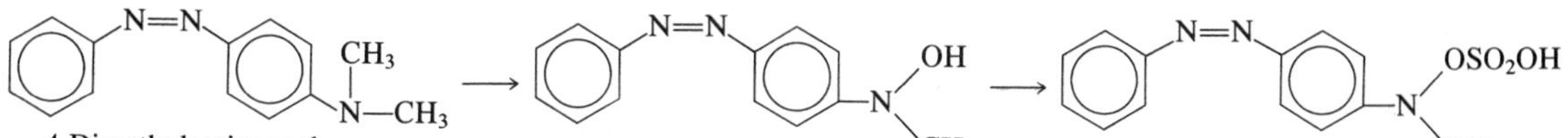

4-Dimethylaminoazobenzene

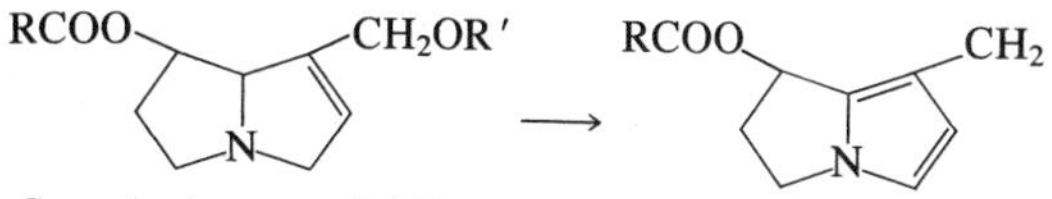

Senecio (or pyrrolizidine)
alkaloids

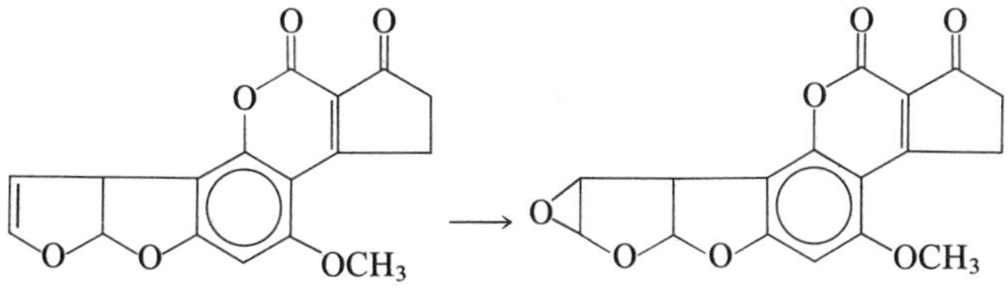

Aflatoxin B_1

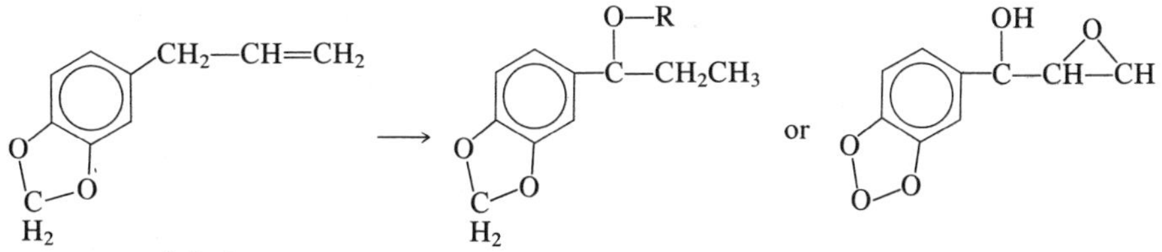

Safrole

$$CH_3NCH_3 \longrightarrow \left[CH_3NCH_2OH \right] \longrightarrow CH_3^+$$
$$\quad | \qquad\qquad\quad |$$
$$\quad NO \qquad\qquad\quad NO$$

Dimethyl-
nitrosamine

$$CH_3NHNHCH_3 \longrightarrow CH_3N{=}NCH_3 \longrightarrow CH_3\overset{O}{\overset{\uparrow}{N}}{=}NCH_3$$

1,2-Dimethylhydrazine   Azomethane   Azoxymethane

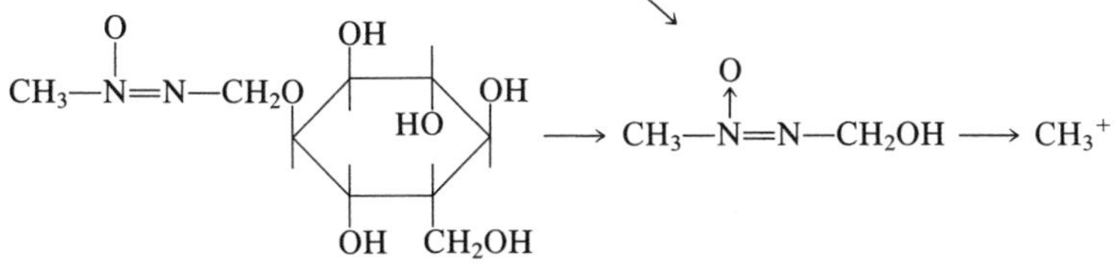

$$CH_3{-}N{=}N{-}CH_2O\text{–(sugar)} \longrightarrow CH_3{-}\overset{O}{\overset{\uparrow}{N}}{=}N{-}CH_2OH \longrightarrow CH_3^+$$

Cycasin   Methylazoxymethanol

$$C_2H_5SCH_2CH_2\underset{\underset{NH_2}{|}}{C}HCOOH \longrightarrow CH_2{=}CHSCH_2CH_2\underset{\underset{NH_2}{|}}{C}HCOOH \longrightarrow CH_2{-}CHSCH_2CH_2\underset{\underset{NH_2}{|}}{C}HCOOH$$

Ethionine   Vinylhomocysteine   Epoxyvinylhomocysteine

$$CH_3CSNH_2 \longrightarrow CH_3{-}\underset{\underset{O{\leftarrow}\overset{\text{S}}{}{\rightarrow}O}{\overset{\|}{C}}}{}{-}NH_2$$

Thioacetamide

quently, with the development of sensitive and specific techniques, mainly the use of carcinogens tagged with isotope, and as new knowledge on the function, isolation, and purification of other key cellular macromolecules such as various types of RNA and DNA became available, it was discovered that many chemical carcinogens associate with a variety of cellular entities (*see* Ts'o and DiPaolo, 1974).

Early work focused on the binding to proteins, leading to the recognition that there are two types of binding: reversible binding to acceptor proteins such as albumin or a specific globulin serving as transport carriers and nonspecific irreversible covalent binding. Intracellular transport from cytoplasm or endoplasmic reticulum to nucleus may also involve a transport protein. The binding to acceptor proteins may be very important for certain of the effects of carcinogens.

Carcinogens that form reactive electrophilic species bind covalently to macromolecules and, indeed, to any nucleophilic center in the cell. In proteins, the main reactive sites appear to be tryptophan, tyrosine, methionine, and perhaps histidine, all of which are nucleophilic reactants. In one instance, reaction with glycogen has been documented. These chemical interactions relate not only to the carcinogenic process but also to other toxic reactions.

As with protein, RNA is also a target for electrophilic reactants. Interactions have been demonstrated with transfer RNA, messenger RNA, and ribosomal RNA. Such interactions are probably involved in the inhibition of protein synthesis that occurs with toxic doses of carcinogens.

The ability of carcinogens to interact with DNA was disputed in the early years when protein interactions were of principal interest. However, the demonstration of the interaction of polycyclic aromatic hydrocarbons with DNA by Brookes, Lawley, Heidelberger, Sims, and Gelboin (*see* Ts'o and DiPaolo, 1974) opened this area of investigation. Subsequently, numerous carcinogens of the electrophilic reactant type have been found to bind to DNA. This, in turn, led to the development of tests for genetic effects to detect such carcinogens. Current interest has turned to examination of the bases to which carcinogens bind and the nature of the adducts. The overall chemistry of many of these interactions has been established (see Rajalakshmi *et al.*, in Becker, 1982; Hemminki, 1983). For example, methyl carbonium ions from several sources, such as the direct-acting alkylating agent methyl methanesulfonate, from the nitrosourea methylnitrosourea, from the procarcinogen nitrosamine dimethylnitrosamine, or from the hydrazine 1,2-dimethylhydrazine, all alkylate guanine bases in DNA at

several positions. Current information suggests that the interaction at the O-6 position is associated with mutagenicity and carcinogenicity. Alkylation at N-7 often occurs to a greater extent with the methyl carbonium ions but does not seem to relate to carcinogenesis. With aflatoxin B_1 through the metabolically produced epoxide, reaction at N-7 in guanine seems relevant (Essigmann *et al.*, 1982). The active product derived from *N*-2-fluorenylacetamide forms adducts on guanine at N-2 and C-8, as is true for a number of other arylamines (Kadlubar and Beland, 1983). With the polycylic aromatic hydrocarbon benzo(a)pyrene, through its activated form, the 7,8-dihydrodiol-9,10-epoxide, the main reaction is through the 10 carbon of the benzo(a)pyrene metabolite to the 2-amino position in guanine (Weinstein, 1981; Conney, 1982). In addition, there are also minor interactions with other purines and pyrimidines in DNA, as a function of the type of carcinogen and the tissue and cells affected (Waring, 1982; Monnat and Loeb, 1983).

As a result of interaction with DNA, DNA-reactive carcinogens generally exhibit genotoxicity in cellular systems (Ames 1983; Hollaender, 1971–1983; Sugimura *et al.*, 1982), where appropriate activation is provided. However, because of their high reactivity and electrophilic character, direct-acting genotoxic carcinogens are often more active in the *in vitro* systems but less carcinogenic in animal bioassays because of rapid detoxication *in vivo*.

Certain chemicals that can intercalate into the DNA strands in the absence of covalent binding are mutagenic to phage and bacteria. However, there is no documentation that carcinogenicity in mammalian systems arises from pure intercalation without covalent binding. On the other hand, it is clear that the molecular size and shape of covalently bound carcinogens can play a role in determining quantitative responses such as DNA repair or the events involved in mutagenesis and carcinogenesis. Thus, stereochemical molecular attractions are involved that facilitate the attachment of carcinogen to DNA mainly prior to and also after covalent bonds are formed. This is especially true with aromatic or heterocyclic compounds where potency increases with the number of rings up to an optimum of five to six benzene rings, or equivalent. Even here, specific stereoisomers of reactive molecules are the key active metabolites (Conney, 1982).

Thus, considerable knowledge has accrued on the interaction with DNA of genotoxic carcinogens. However, the altered steric and chemical properties of DNA with covalently bound carcinogen adducts in relation to transcription of the genetic code into phenotypic characteristics are not known as yet. The molecular consequences of the presence of specific carcinogen-DNA adducts are currently under active study (*see* Schaaper *et al.*, 1983, as an example). In a nonreplicating cell, the damaged DNA can be repaired by several distinct systems (Roberts, in Brookes, 1980; Morgan and Cleaver, 1983; Park *et al.*, 1983). The efficacy of repair bears on the organ specificity of the carcinogen. For example, methylnitrosourea reacts readily with DNA of kidney, liver, and brain, but the damage is repaired readily in liver and somewhat less readily in kidney, and very slowly in brain. This accounts for the fact that under certain experimental conditions methylnitrosourea or ethylnitrosourea induces brain cancer in rodents (Müller and Rajewsky, 1983). Pegg *et al.* (1985) have described some properties of an enzyme concerned with transfer of a methyl group of guanine methylated at $O = 6$ to cysteine in protein, thus effecting DNA repair. In a replicating cell, the damaged DNA can lead to a number of serious consequences during the duplicative process, including cell death, point mutations, or translocation and amplification of codons that may include oncogene sequences (see p. 101). Creation of permanently abnormal DNA represents a mutation that may be the basis for the evolution neoplastic cells.

New means of detecting DNA adducts of carcinogens are being developed, such as the use of monoclonal antibodies (Poirier *et al.*, 1983; Berlin *et al.*, 1984), the ^{32}P–postlabeling technique (Everson *et al.*, 1986), and mass spectrometric determinations (Wiebers *et al.*, 1981). These may eventually permit detection of DNA damage in humans exposed to environmental carcinogens (see Bartsch *et al.*, 1982; Teo *et al.*, 1983).

B. Chemical-Viral Interactions

Although sufficient human data have not yet been accumulated, excellent experimental evidence shows that some types of cancer in animals have a viral etiology, e.g., certain leukemias, lymphomas, and mammary tumors in mice (Gross, 1981). An antecedent viral hepatitis has been postulated to account for the occurrence of human liver cancer in certain tropical countries (Blumberg and London, 1982), where this disease has a high incidence at a young age, especially in males. There is a replicate of this phenomenon in animals (Omata *et al.*, 1983). In these areas of the world, consumption of foodstuffs contaminated with mycotoxins or *Senecio* alkaloids, which are liver carcinogens, also occurs, suggesting that both a virus and a chemical may be involved.

Some experiments have permitted the conclusion that an antecedent or existing viral infection with specific nononcogenic viruses may potentiate the effect of chemical carcinogens (see Fischer and Weinstein, in Sontag, 1981). There are a number of possible explanations for such interactions. One concept is that cells or tissues containing viruses may have greater sensitivity, perhaps because their rate of cell multiplication is altered or their cellular receptors are more exposed. Another possible explanation is that cells containing viruses have an altered metabolic capability and hence different metabolic activation potential for carcinogens. From the pragmatic point of view of evaluating the possible carcinogenic risk attached to environmental chemicals, the possible augmenting action of viral elements in animals and even in humans (case of benzene?) needs to be considered.

Indeed, drugs with immunosuppressive properties induce in animals and in humans mainly leukemias, lymphomas, or sarcomas (Adamson and Sieber, 1981; Hoover and Fraumeni, 1981; Milief and Schwartz, in Becker, 1982; Tarr and Olsen, 1985), which can also be induced by oncogenic viruses. In an animal model, spontaneous and chemically induced leukemias have been inhibited through a form of vaccination, an interesting and possibly fruitful lead (Pottathil *et al.*, 1978).

MODIFYING FACTORS IN CHEMICAL CARCINOGENESIS

A. Enhancement of Carcinogenesis

Syncarcinogenesis. A number of studies involving mixtures of chemical carcinogens of the type designated here as genotoxic have indicated that, when these agents act on the same target organ, the effects are additive and sometimes synergistic (Nakahara, 1970; Schmähl, 1980). For example, administration of a carcinogenic azo dye and diethylnitrosamine, both of which affect the liver, results in an increased incidence of liver tumors. On the other hand, agents that have distinct organ specificity often exert their carcinogenic effect independently. The tumor incidence in the various target organs is the same as when the two agents are administered separately. The latent period, too, is the same, provided it is similar for both agents. For example, a carcinogenic azo dye that affects the liver and 4-dimethylaminostilbene, which affects the ear duct, do not interact, since, when they are given jointly, both types of neoplasms are seen in similar yields to what occurs when the carcinogens are administered individually.

The additive or synergistic effect of two carcinogens is designated as syncarcinogenesis. Two types may be distinguished: combination syncarcinogenesis in which the two agents are given together and sequential syncarcinogenesis in which they are given one after another (Williams, 1984). It is important that initiation/promotion be distinguished from the latter, the sequential action of carcinogens. Two principal features distinguish these phenomena: (1) in syncarcinogenesis, both carcinogens are usually DNA reactive, whereas promoters are not; and (2) in syncarcinogenesis the sequence of compound administration can be reversed, whereas promotion must follow initiation.

More detailed and realistic studies of the interactions between carcinogens are needed in order to shed light on possible interactions between agents in the complex environment in which humans exist.

Distinction between Cocarcinogenesis and Promotion. There are also noncarcinogenic chemicals that augment, sometimes very appreciably, the effect of a primary carcinogen. Originally, Berenblum (1974) defined all such agents as cocarcinogens. Thus, promoters were one type of cocarcinogen. However, more commonly a distinction has been made whereby cocarcinogens modify the effectiveness of a carcinogen present at the same time (Van Duuren et al., 1982), whereas promotion occurs subsequent to the exposure to a carcinogen. According to this differentiation, cocarcinogens would enhance the first sequence of the carcinogenic process (Figure 5–1), neoplastic conversion, while promoters would produce their effects in the second sequence, neoplastic development. To maintain this mechanistic distinction, it must be recognized that cocarcinogens can also act after exposure to a DNA-reactive carcinogen at a time when DNA damage is still persistent. Also, promotion can take place during carcinogen administration if neoplastic conversion has occurred. Thus, to distinguish between these forms of enhancement requires detailed mechanistic studies.

Cocarcinogenesis. Cocarcinogens are agents that enhance the overall carcinogenic process initiated by a genotoxic carcinogen when administered before or together with the carcinogen or at a time when carcinogen damage to DNA is still persistent. Accordingly, cocarcinogenesis applies to events occurring during neoplastic conversion (Figure 5–1). The relevant mechanisms can be one or more of several possibilities: (1) increased uptake or availability of a carcinogen; (2) enhanced metabolic activation of a genotoxic carcinogen or decreased detoxication; (3) inhibition of DNA repair processes; and (4) increased proliferation of cells with DNA damage, thereby facilitating mutation, codon translocation, or amplification (Williams, 1984).

The demonstration of cocarcinogenesis was made over 40 years ago in the laboratories of Berenblum and Shubik and of Shear (see Berenblum, 1974). Berenblum and Shubik noted that application of a carcinogenic polycyclic aromatic hydrocarbon to mouse skin together with croton oil, an oil extracted from the seed of euphorbiacea *Croton tiglium L.*, induced a much higher incidence of skin cancer than in controls given the carcinogen alone. The cocarcinogic action of croton oil was found to be species specific, not being demonstrable in rabbits, rats, or guinea pigs. The active constituents in croton oil eventually isolated and identified by Hecker and by Van Duuren (see Hecker et al., 1982; Pereira, 1983) were shown to be phorbol esters. The mechanism of action of phorbol esters as enhancers when given together with polycyclic aromatic hydrocarbons is unknown. Subsequent studies showed that they produced enhancement long after cessation of carcinogen exposure, which was interpreted to show that they promoted growth of dormant neoplastic cells into tumors. It could be that they act as promoters even during concurrent administration of a carcinogen, if neoplastic conversion has occurred. However, they may also act as carcinogens in the terms used here by stimulating cell proliferation at the time of DNA damage

In the mouse skin system not all cocarcinogens are promoters, catechol being an example (Van Duuren, 1982; Yoshida and Fukuhara, 1983). However, not many thorough studies have been done in other systems to distinguish mechanistically between cocarcinogenesis and promotion. Various forms of chemical or physical injury occurring before carcinogen exposure are cocarcinogenic by virtue of stimulating cell proliferation such that more cells are in DNA synthesis at the time of carcinogen damage to DNA and are, therefore, more susceptible to genetic alteration.

Cocarcinogens are important agents in human cancer. Asbestos, which by itself produces pleural and peritoneal mesotheliomas, but infrequently yields lung cancer, contributes not additively but synergistically to the development of bronchogenic lung cancer in cigarette smokers who have occupational exposure. The asbestos and similar products thus have the properties of a cocarcinogen or promoter. In support of this point, asbestos has potentiated the effects of carcinogens in cell cultures (Mossman et al., 1983; Reiss et al., 1983). It is important, therefore, to control extensive exposure to asbestos and other mineral dusts. For those individuals who were unfortunately exposed to asbestos years or decades ago, efforts to reduce their risk for disease, particularly lung cancer, should involve smoking withdrawal programs.

Tobacco smoke, as described, contains relatively small amounts of genotoxic carcinogens such as polycyclic aromatic hydrocarbons, certain nitrosamines, and possibly certain pyrolysis products of proteins in the form of α- or β-carbolines and related materials (DeMarini, 1983; Hoffmann *et al.*, 1983). However, the cocarcinogenic factors such as catechols in tobacco smoke are thought to play an important role in the overall effect of the smoke in leading to human cancer (van Duuren, 1982; Hoffmann *et al.*, in Pereira, 1983; Wynder, in Pereira, 1983).

In addition, it has been shown that individuals who smoke and also drink alcoholic beverages regularly in appreciable amounts have a higher risk of head and neck cancers. It is likely that under these conditions, ethanol functions as a cocarcinogen in augmenting the metabolic conversion of tobacco procarcinogens such as polycyclic aromatic hydrocarbons or nitrosamines to the reactive electrophilic products in the target organs. Such a mechanism is demonstrated by the finding that the conversion of the model compound nitrosopyrrolidine to a mutagen is increased in rodents given alcohol and nitrosopyrrolidine, and in hamsters a higher yield of nasal cavity and tracheal cancers was obtained (McCoy *et al.*, 1981). Curiously, so far this same finding has not been made for the tobacco-specific nitrosamine (Hoffmann and Hecht, 1985). A greater conversion of benzo[a]pyrene to its proximate carcinogenic metabolites occurred in rats on alcohol. Thus, cocarcinogenicity represents a major factor in determining human disease risk.

Promotion. This phenomenon was first demonstrated in the laboratories of Rous and of Berenblum and Shubik in studies of skin carcinogenesis. In these experiments, croton oil was shown to have a highly specific and exquisite enhancing effect on cancer development in mouse skin when applied after a known carcinogen. In an impressive series of experiments it was shown that the genotoxic event, application of a polycyclic aromatic hydrocarbon, can be followed months later and, in fact, one year later by a promoting stimulus, such as the application of phorbol esters from croton oil, and still result in the production of skin tumors (van Duuren, 1982; Loerke *et al.*, 1983). From these observations developed the "two-stage" concept of carcinogenesis: initiation and promotion. In these studies, promotion designated the facilitation of growth of a latent neoplastic cell into a tumor. Conceptually then, promotion applies to events occurring after the completion of neoplastic conversion of the cell (Figure 5-1). However, in many other studies, particularly current ones,

promotion has been used broadly to describe any situation yielding an increased development of neoplasms. The active constituents of croton oil, certain phorbol esters, are true promoters as well as carcinogens. Sulfur, sulfur compounds, aldehydes, phenols, and dodecane represent other examples of enhancers of the effect of polycyclic aromatic hydrocarbons and other carcinogens for mouse skin. In some of these instances, it is not certain whether the dramatic increase in carcinogenicity results from a true promoting effect or from a more effective action of the primary carcinogen as a result of effects on carcinogen-damaged cells with persistent DNA adducts, an effect that is described here as cocarcinogenesis. Such sizable enhancing effects may account for the carcinogenicity of petroleum products, cutting oils, and the like, which may be much greater than might be suspected from their content of carcinogenic polycyclic aromatic hydrocarbons. The same applies to roofing-tar workers exposed to fumes of asphalt. To distinguish promotion from cocarcinogenesis, the agent must be tested at a sufficient duration after carcinogen application to allow for complete DNA repair.

Although, phorbol esters remain a popular experimental model, a number of other promoters for different organ systems have been discovered (Hecker *et al.*, 1982; Pereira, 1983). Hormones increase carcinogenicity through a mechanism of promotion when present in abnormal amounts (Rose, 1982). Bile acids have been shown to be promoters in colon carcinogenesis (Reddy *et al.*, 1980). In bladder carcinogenesis, saccharin and tryptophan are promoters (Hicks, in Hecker *et al.*, 1982; Cohen, in Pereira, 1983). Peraino and co-workers (in Slaga *et al.*, 1978) observed that certain inducers of liver metabolic enzyme systems, such as phenobarbital, DDT, and BHT, exerted enhancing effects when administered after small doses of 2-acetylaminofluorene. In most instances, these same chemicals when administered together with hepatocarcinogens decrease carcinogenicity, most likely by increasing detoxication reactions, especially those concerned with conjugation (Weisburger and Williams, in Becker, 1982).

The mechanism of the promoting effect of chemicals when administered after a primary carcinogen is complex and there are a number of possibilities. Numerous studies have shown that phorbol esters exert various types of effects on cellular membranes (Hecker *et al.*, 1982). Recent studies using phorbol esters also indicate an ability to produce gene derepression and repression (Slaga, in Pereira, 1983; Huberman *et al.*, in Hecker *et al.*, 1982).

Studies in other systems have led to a concept

of promotion, which is consistent with the original definition of Berenblum, and the mechanistic distinction developed above. Following neoplastic conversion of cells by a genotoxic carcinogen, these latent tumor cells can be visualized to be held in check by regulatory processes that maintain normal tissue homeostasis. Cells are able to interact with one another through specialized membrane structures, known as gap junctions, that permit the transfer of small-molecular-weight substances that may have a growth regulatory function. Possibly these gap junctions serve to transfer the factors that inhibit the growth of latent tumor cells. The groups of Trosko in the United States (Trosko *et al.,* in Milman and Weisburger, 1985) and Murray and Fitzgerald in Australia (Murray *et al.,* in Hecker *et al.,* 1982) have shown in cell culture studies that tumor promoters are capable of inhibiting intercellular molecular exchange through gap junctions. Such inhibition *in vivo,* if it impeded transfer of regulatory factors, would serve to release dormant neoplastic cells for growth into tumors. It has been shown in the laboratories of Kitagawa, Pitot, and Williams that liver tumor promoters enhance the development of preneoplastic liver lesions (see Pitot and Sirica, 1980). This action could reflect the release of abnormal cells from regulatory control.

Sound data now indicate that in humans, cancer of the large bowel, breast, prostate, ovary, and endometrium may depend to a very considerable extent not only on a carcinogen but also on promoting phenomena (Reddy *et al.,* 1980; Miller, in Bartsch *et al.,* 1982; Pereira, 1983). The evidence stems from a consideration of the diverse incidence of these diseases in various parts of the world as well as studies of the relevant mechanisms in animal models. A high-risk region for the types of neoplasms enumerated above, such as the United States, typically has a dietary intake high in fat. On the other hand, the population of a country where the incidence is low usually consume diets low in fat. Simulation of such conditions in animal models shows that animals on a high-fat diet develop, for example, colon or breast cancer in higher yield after similar doses of the appropriate carcinogens. In the case of colon cancer, a high-fat diet has been shown to lead to a high flow of bile acids through the gut, and further that bile acids are good promoters in colon carcinogenesis. Humans on a high-fat diet also have higher intestinal levels of bile acids. Further evidence supporting this phenomenon comes from an explanation for the lower risk of Finnish people for colon cancer because of their simultaneous intake of a high-fiber bran diet while consuming high levels of fat, in which the fiber acts as a nonspecific diluent and possibly specific absorbent of bile acids.

In regard to the endocrine-related cancers such as breast, endometrium, and prostrate, current data show that dietary fat modulates hormonal balances, which in turn may act as promoters (*see* Rose, 1982). However, thus far, no synthetic chemical promoter, apart from hormones, has been implicated in human cancer.

A better understanding of the phenomenon of promotion may provide additional means to reduce cancer risk, complementing procedures to lower exposure to carcinogens. This may be a fruitful approach insofar as animal experiments have indicated that with the same level of carcinogens, the incidence of cancer induced can be influenced very powerfully by changing the promotional stimulus.

B. Inhibition of Carcinogenesis

In a variety of experimental situations, the effect of chemical carcinogens has been decreased by antagonistic influences (*see* Zedeck and Lipkin, 1981; Wattenberg, 1983; Williams, 1984). The joint administration of a chemical carcinogen and a structurally analogous noncarcinogenic chemical has sometimes resulted in inhibitory effects, especially if the noncarcinogenic analog was present in large excess. For example, non- or weakly carcinogenic, partially hydrogenated polycyclic hydrocarbons have reduced the carcinogenicity of the fully aromatic structure. A 20 molar excess of acetanilide reduced the carcinogenicity of N-2-fluorenylacetamide on the liver and several other target organs in several species. The underlying mechanisms may be different in each case (E. K. Weisburger, in Sontag, 1981).

The mechanism accounting for such antagonistic effects could involve (1) competitive displacement at the level of the target, (2) variation in the effectiveness of an activating enzyme system, or (3) a more general systemic effect leading to altered detoxication mechanisms or changed receptor ratios. The carcinogenic effect of a given chemical is dependent on the rate of bioactivation of the chemical. This metabolic rate can be influenced by environmental or host-controlled factors, other carcinogens, or noncarcinogenic agents (see Zedeck and Lipkin, 1981; Conney, 1982). A variation in these factors will alter the ratio of activated product over detoxified metabolites. Obviously, an increase in this ratio is likely to yield a picture of increased or synergistic effect, a decrease, one of reduced or antagonistic action. Most such studies have dealt with an evaluation of effects at the level of liver microsomal enzymes, others with effects on organs such as skin, lung, breast, and intestinal tract, and others yet with carcinogens in tissue culture.

In the last few years, the understanding of the

operation of microsomal enzymes has increased considerably, in connection with the study not only of the biotransformation of chemical carcinogens, but of drugs and exogenous chemicals generally. A number of recent reviews deal with these complex reaction systems (see Chapter 3). In general, agents that augment the effectiveness of phase II microsomal enzymes lead to increased detoxication reactions and thus often, but not always, decrease carcinogenicity (Wattenberg, 1983; Prochaska et al., 1985). An exception could be the case of certain halogenated hydrocarbons that seem to undergo activation by conjugation with glutathione, as discussed herein.

The pioneering experiment of Conney, Miller, and Miller (see Conney, 1982) demonstrated that dietary 3-methylcholanthrene increased the level of an enzyme system concerned with reduction of the azo link in the carcinogenic dyestuff 4-dimethylaminoazobenzene yielding noncarcinogenic split products and, thus, explained the inhibition of the dye's carcinogenicity by the hydrocarbon. Indeed, it is this experiment, which gave insight into the relationship between chemicals capable of increasing the levels of such enzyme systems and the subsequent physiologic effects, that laid the foundation for the entire field of enzyme induction in relation to drug metabolism and, in part, drug addiction.

Since that time numerous other chemicals, such as DDT, BHT, phenobarbital, and benzoflavones, were found to induce enzymes and thus reduce the carcinogenicity not only of these azo dyes but of many types of carcinogens (Conney, 1982; Williams, 1984). Also, a number of natural components of foods produce similar effects (Wattenberg, 1983). These studies on interactions have been performed mainly in rats; experimentation with other species is needed because of species differences. For example, administration of 3-methylcholanthrene decreases the ratio of N-hydroxy-N-2-fluorenylacetamide, an activated carcinogenic intermediate derived from N-2-fluorenylacetamide, to detoxication metabolites in rats, but increases the ratio in hamsters. Parallel to these findings are the biologic and toxicologic findings that in rats 3-methylcholanthrene reduced the carcinogenicity of N-2-fluorenylacetamide, but increased it in hamsters (E. K. Weisburger, in Sontag, 1981).

C. Immunologic Factors

Immunologic factors have been found in some instances to alter the rate and extent of tumor development. There are tumor-related antigens produced during transformation of normal to neoplastic cells that provide possible tools to detect and diagnose, and also specifically treat, neoplasms (Fish et al., 1981; Haugen et al., 1981; Baldwin and Price; Melief and Schwartz, in Becker, 1982). Immunologic mechanisms have been thought to play a role in the greater sensitivity of newborn animals to chemical carcinogens, for in some species and strains the immunologic competence in newborns is either totally lacking or considerably less than that present in adult animals. Immunologic status appears to play a role in the development of metastases, more so than in the early effects in the carcinogenic process. Several carcinogens (apart from immunosuppressant agents) have been shown to suppress the immune system, but this has not been established to be critical to their carcinogenicity (Tarr and Olsen, 1985).

D. Environmental Factors

Diet. Developments in the area of azo dye carcinogenesis many years ago drew attention to the fact that diet can modify the effectiveness of chemical carcinogens. Rats fed a rice diet, low in protein and riboflavin, were highly sensitive to liver tumor formation when treated with 4-dimethylaminoazobenzene, but a diet containing adequate amounts of protein and vitamin B_2 reduced, and in some cases prevented, the carcinogenic effect. Mueller and Miller (see Conney, 1982) found that this diet-mediated change in carcinogenicity stemmed from an alteration in the level of a flavin adenine dinucleotide-dependent azo dye reductase, which, in turn, altered the effective dosage of the carcinogen.

Other, more recent examples can be given in which diet exerted an effect on the outcome of the carcinogenic process by controlling the effectiveness of enzymes concerned with activation versus detoxication of chemical carcinogens (Parke and Ioannides, 1981; Wattenberg, 1983). For example, administration of the potent liver carcinogen dimethylnitrosamine to rats on a protein-free diet has virtually no toxic effect on the liver, mainly because of a severe decrease of microsomal enzymes in this organ. However, rats so treated exhibit tumors in the kidneys after a fairly long latent period. The acute toxicity of the mycotoxin aflatoxin B_1 is considerably reduced when rats are on a low-lipotrope diet, but the carcinogenicity to the liver is enhanced (Rogers, 1983).

Tumor induction in the mammary gland of rats is decreased when the animals are fed fat-restricted diets, but is augmented on high-fat diets (see Reddy et al., 1980). Skin tumor formation in mice is decreased when the food intake is low. In this instance the degree of tumor formation was dependent on the amount of food intake during the promoting phase. When the animals were placed on a restricted food intake during the application of the primary carcinogen, but were fed *ad libitum* during the promotion phase, the tumor incidence was identical to that seen in well-fed control animals. On the other hand, normal food intake during initiation by carcinogen, followed by dietary restriction during the promotion phase, reduced tumor incidence, pointing clearly to the fact that in this instance, the developmental phases of cancer cells are inhibited by lower food intake (Boutwell, 1983a).

Restricted food intake, especially during the developmental phases, reduces the incidence of all neoplasms, but especially that in the endocrine-sensitive organs, and increases overall longevity (Tucker, 1979; Beauchene *et al.*, 1986).

There is now an extensive literature on this subject (NAS, 1982) indicating that diet exerts a major modifying role in many types of experimental and human cancer.

Protein. Most rodent diets contain 18 to 25 percent protein. As the protein content increases above 50 percent, a voluntary reduction in the number of total calories consumed takes place. Thus, in situations where caloric intake influences tumor induction, animals fed diets with elevated protein levels have been found to have fewer tumors. A diet restricted in protein, on the other hand, has a lesser effect. In fact, in the case of the carcinogenic azo dyes mentioned earlier, a protein-restricted (12 percent) diet appears to increase the relative efficiency of the carcinogen. Diets completely devoid of protein, which can be administered only for limited periods of time, may decrease the effectiveness of certain carcinogens in specific target organs because of a significant decrease in the amount of enzymes bound to the endoplasmic reticulum, especially the cytochrome systems, and a consequent decrease in the biochemical activation of carcinogens.

Fats. For several types of chemical carcinogens, especially those affecting the endocrine-sensitive organs or affecting the colon, the effectiveness of the carcinogen can be increased appreciably by a high-fat diet. As discussed previously, these considerations also appear to hold for humans (Reddy *et al.*, 1980). The relevant mechanisms appear identical; they depend on increased promotion (see Promoters, p. 143). This factor appears most important in providing rational approaches to the prevention of important types of human cancer (Weisburger *et al.*, 1982).

Carbohydrates and Starches. The starches contained in most commercial experimental diets exert relatively little influence on tumor induction. Semipurified diets, on the other hand, containing highly soluble carbohydrates, such as glucose and sucrose, may enhance absorption of a carcinogen fed in the diet, thus enhancing toxicity. In humans, the risk of colon cancer has been related to low-residue, highly digestible foods, in contrast to diets high in roughage and residues (Reddy *et al.*, 1980).

Animal experiments have confirmed that certain fibers such as bran or pectin reduce the carcinogenicity of certain colon carcinogens. For many other types of carcinogens, a difference is seen when animals are placed on a low-residue semipurified diet, compared to a diet composed of natural foodstuffs. In most instances, the carcinogen is somewhat less effective on the latter diet although there are exceptions for reasons that are not clear but may involve the presence of enzyme inducers leading to better detoxication (Wattenberg, 1983).

Micronutrients. A number of specific vitamins and minerals are essential cofactors for the effective operation of many key enzymes. Thus, a deficiency in these specific micronutrients would obviously have an effect on the physiology of the host and on the pharmacologic and toxicologic responses to exogenous agents, including carcinogens. The effect of riboflavin on the carcinogenicity of azo dyes in rat liver has already been discussed. In addition, riboflavin appears to be involved in tumor induction processes at other sites, such as the oral cavity, by a mechanism that has not yet been determined (Correa, 1982).

Vitamin A has been implicated in the differentiation of epithelial tissues. Saffiotti and coworkers, Sporn, DeLuca and associates, Bjelke, Cone, and Nettesheim have reported that vitamin A levels may affect the induction of pulmonary tumors in rodent systems and in humans. Additional data indicate that some types of human cancer, such as cancer of the cervix, bladder, or lung, arise somewhat more frequently in people with limited vitamin A levels. Vitamin A analogs or retinoic acid derivatives have been shown to inhibit carcinogenesis in several target organs, especially the mammary gland and the urinary bladder (see Moon *et al.*, 1983).

Vitamin E and other synthetic antioxidants, such as butylated hydroxytoluene (BHT), propyl gallate, and ethoxyquin, have modified tumor induction by certain carcinogens in a number of target organs (Mergens and Newmark, in Zedeck and Lipkin, 1981; Wattenberg, 1983). However, inhibition was achieved at high doses at which induction of biotransformation enzymes also occurs, and, therefore, it is not certain that inhibition can be attributed to antioxidant effects.

Selenium derivatives also appear to decrease

tumor incidence (Combs and Clark, 1985). In some cases when high levels of the antioxidants were administered, the effect was traced directly to modification of enzyme levels, mainly in liver, which led to changes in activation and detoxication of the metabolites of carcinogens. Dietary elements, particularly micronutrients such as vitamins A, E, and B_2, may provide some degree of protection against carcinogens. As was discussed above, vitamins C and E prevent the formation of nitrosamines and nitrosamides and thus reduce or eliminate cancer risk at various target organs such as the liver and upper gastrointestinal and respiratory tract (*see* Magee, 1982). Further study of the mechanisms of action of dietary factors may suggest means of reducing the prevalence of certain types of human cancers (NRC/NAS, 1982).

E. Host Factors

Species, Strain, and Organ Sensitivity. Human cancers were first found to relate to exposure to specific chemical carcinogens at the workplace. Even though, in time, a large fraction of those exposed developed a specific cancer, not all of those at risk were affected. Also, the expression period (the time to overt cancer presentation) differed widely from individual to individual. For cancers related to life-style, such as those due to cigarette smoking or nutrition, whether it is the high gastric cancer risk of the Japanese or Latin Americans, or the high colon or breast cancer risk seen in the Western world, it is fortunately true that not everyone in a given environment is affected to the same extent. To be sure, there are competitive risks; someone on a high-fat diet might die of a heart attack and be withdrawn from the pool of those susceptible to colon or prostatic cancer. Likewise, in animal models utilizing random-bred animals or highly inbred animals, variations in sensitivity or in target organs occur to a given carcinogenic challenge. Even a spontaneous cancer seen in an aging, untreated population of animals occurs to different extents in different species and strains (Bartosek *et al.*, 1982; Nunziata and Storino, 1982).

There are many inbred strains of mice, some of which, such as the strain A mouse, eventually develop a high incidence of pulmonary neoplasms; this strain is also very sensitive to the chemical induction of these tumors. The C3H strain readily develops spontaneous or induced neoplasms of the liver. On the other hand, the C57 black strain mouse is resistant to induced or spontaneous visceral neoplasms, but cutaneous cancer can be induced fairly readily. Identical considerations apply to rat strains. The young female Sprague-Dawley is exquisitely sensitive to

the development of mammary gland cancer by the use of specific carcinogens, whereas the Long-Evans strain is not; the latter develops leukemia. Within the class of broadly acting alkyl nitrosamines, quantitative differences in response appear as regards tumor yield and latent period with a given amount of a specific nitrosamine. Distinct target organs are also affected. Whereas in rats diethylnitrosamine readily induces primary liver cancer, in hamsters a good yield of cancer in the esophagus is obtained. That does not mean that esophageal cancer is not induced in rats with diethylnitrosamine, but simply reflects the fact that liver is a much more sensitive target organ so that the animals die of primary liver cancer before they have a chance to develop cancer in the esophagus. If liver carcinogenesis can be inhibited in rats, then more cancer of the esophagus is seen. The same kind of differential sensitivity applies for *N*-2-fluorenylacetamide, which usually causes primary liver cancer with Wistar or Fischer strain rats, but in the presence of tryptophan, which delays liver carcinogenesis and promotes urinary bladder carcinogenesis, cancer in the urinary bladder is seen more frequently. For 1,2-dimethylhydrazine given as large doses orally or subcutaneously to rats or mice, the primary target organ is the large bowel. However, oral administration of lower dosages usually does not affect the large bowel but leads to hemangioendotheliomas.

In animal models and in some human cases, it has been possible to delineate the complex mechanisms accounting in part for such species differences (Gelboin *et al.*, 1980; Nebert *et al.*, 1981; Nettesheim *et al.*, 1981; Bartsch *et al.*, 1982; Conney, 1982; Miwa *et al.*, 1982, Langenbach *et al.*, 1983). Sensitivity or resistance finds one explanation in the metabolic capability to convert procarcinogen to the reactive electrophilic, ultimate carcinogen. A well-known example is the relative resistance of the guinea pig to the induction of any kind of cancer by a typical aromatic amine, *N*-2-fluorenylacetamide, because in guinea pigs the required metabolic activation to the proximate carcinogen, the *N*-hydroxy derivative, occurs to a minor extent, and the major *in vivo* metabolite is a detoxified 7-hydroxy derivative. Parenthetically, it is interesting that a microsome fraction from guinea pig liver can convert the related deacetylated 2-fluorenamine to a mutagenic compound to a greater extent than the microsomes from rat liver, testifying to the need to be cautious in translating the results of *in vitro* tests to *in vivo* behavior by utilizing mutagenicity. However, as a first approximation to species- and strain-related differences in metabolic activation, the large differences found in rodents appear to be linked to the Ah locus, which, in turn, reflect the presence and/or inducibility of distinct forms of cytochrome P-450 (Nebert *et al.*, 1981).

Similar considerations apply in regard to the organotropism of carcinogens in specific hosts, with the additional consideration that some agents have transport forms such as glucuronic acid conjugates often generated in liver that release a reactive proximate carcinogen in a specific target organ such as urinary bladder or large bowel.

Both species differences and organotropism are also dependent on the operation of the multistep DNA repair systems. For example, hamsters are more susceptible than rats to liver cancer by dimethylnitrosamine because of its deficiency in repair of O^6-alkylation of guanine in DNA. In rats a single large dose of dimethylnitrosamine induces kidney, but not liver, cancer because of the capability of liver repair enzymes to remove alkylated forms of DNA from liver (Pegg *et al.*, 1985). Likewise, ethylnitrosourea initially forms DNA adducts in liver, kidney, and brain, but because of the limited repair capacity in brain tissue, the animals eventually develop cancer there, but do not develop liver, and rarely kidney, cancer (Müller and Rajewsky, 1983).

In nonhuman primates, as in rhesus monkeys, some chemicals such as dimethyl- or diethylnitrosamine lead to primary liver cancer amazingly rapidly (in some instances in about one year), considering the greater longevity of this animal (Adamson and Sieber, 1983). On the other hand, administering the very powerful mycotoxin aflatoxin B_1, the first liver cancer was seen after only five years and usually required an average of ten years. Powerful rodent carcinogens such as aromatic amines have not yet led to any cancer, even though a number of these studies have been underway for over 15 years. In humans, aromatic amines usually lead to cancer in an occupational setting after 15, and more likely 25, years of exposure. In some instances, however, a larger dosage, such as might occur with exposure to certain drugs (e.g., chlornaphazine), occasionally can lead to cancer after five years. But in most instances, more than 10 to 15 years are needed (Williams *et al.*, in Flamm and Lorentzen, 1985). As we noted elsewhere, most known human carcinogens can be detected by the appropriate high dosing in rodent models that have the required biotransformation capability (Weisburger and Williams, in Searle, 1984). Thus, rodents are suitable tools to delineate potential cancer risks with unknown carcinogens especially, as will be discussed, if collateral data as to mechanisms are generated.

Animals models have also been found suitable to mimic the operation of other factors in the nongenotoxic human environment such as the role of dietary fat in augmenting the development of breast or colon cancer, thereby paralleling the situation seen in humans (Reddy *et al.*, 1980, NRC/NAS, 1982). Nevertheless, rodent models do have genetically determined critical differences between each other and, indeed, humans.

Age. Age is an important variable in studies on carcinogenesis. Newborn animals exhibit higher sensitivity to certain carcinogens than older animals. Thus, injection of newborn mice with any one of a number of chemical carcinogens results in tumors, primarily of the liver and lung, approximately a year after administration of the carcinogen (Rice, 1979). Carcinogens may be effective when administered to young animals but ineffective when administered to older animals. For example, the polycyclic aromatic hydrocarbons do not usually induce liver cancer when administered to young adult mice or rats, but do so when given to newborn animals because of the then rapid growth of the liver. Likewise, aflatoxin B_1 fails to induce liver tumors in mice when administered after weaning, but does induce tumors when given at birth. Hamsters, too, appear to be more sensitive to aflatoxin B_1 at birth than after weaning, but the difference in sensitivity is not as great as that in rats (Homburger, 1983).

Many investigators utilize weanling animals in experiments with chemical carcinogens. Such animals are quite sensitive, and with agents of low carcinogenicity requiring a long latent period for tumor development, it is useful to begin with animals as young as possible. However, in some instances weanling animals are considerably more sensitive to the toxic effect of an agent. Hence, failure to adjust dosages upward as the animal develops the capability of tolerating higher levels may result in fewer neoplasms and a longer experimental period.

The greater susceptibility of young animals to carcinogenesis may also be seen in humans. Existing data on lung cancer incidence as a function of number of cigarettes smoked per day currently indicate that the average incidence is lower in Japan than in the United States, perhaps because the habit of chronic smoking begins at an older age in Japan than in the United States.

Transplacental Exposure. Some carcinogens cross the placental barrier and are carcinogenic following *in utero* exposure (Rice, 1979). In certain cases, the enzyme system necessary to produce activated products is sufficiently developed in the fetus to give an adequate level of the required reactive intermediates. In other cases, the mother may generate the active intermediate in a transportable form, which is released in the fetus by select enzyme systems. Certain types of carcinogens that do not require enzymes to develop the reactive ultimate carcinogen, such as alkylnitrosoureas, are sometimes extremely effective transplacentally. However, for reasons that are not yet clear, methylnitrosourea is less effective than the ethyl homolog as a transplacental carcinogen. The method of experimental transplacental carcinogenesis has been developed by several investigators, including Druckrey, Napalkov, Tomatis, and Rice (*see* Rice, 1979), as a means of detecting possible environmental carcinogens. In addition, *in vivo–in vitro* systems, in which the agent is given to a pregnant female and the fetuses are explanted into tissue culture, can yield abnormal transformed tumor cells that are visualized after a short period of time.

It is quite probable that cancers occurring in childhood are the result of transplacental exposure. An important series of cases were discovered by Herbst *et al.* (*see* Williams *et al.*, in Flamm and Lorentzen, 1985) in young prepubertal girls with a rare form of vaginal cancer that was traced to the fact that their mothers had been treated with sizable doses of the hormone diethylstilbestrol in order to maintain a successful pregnancy.

Sex and Endocrine Balance. Epidemiologic data show that some types of cancer occur more frequently in one sex than the other (American Cancer Society, 1986; Schottenfeld and Fraumeni, 1982). In experimental animals, likewise, some chemical carcinogens affecting specific target organs appear to induce cancer more frequently in one than the other sex, even when a nonendocrine organ is involved (IARC Monogrs.; Arcos *et al.*, 1968–1985). For example, N-2-fluorenylacetamide induces liver cancer primarily in male rats although females of certain strains are not entirely resistant (E. K. Weisburger, in Sontag, 1981). On the other hand, o-aminoazotoluene is somewhat more active in female mice than in males in leading to liver cancer. Dimethyl- or diethylnitrosamine produces liver cancer often, but not always, with similar efficiency in males and females. On the other hand, a variety of carcinogens cause pulmonary tumors in male and female mice with equal frequency (Shimkin and Stoner, 1975). In nonendocrine target organs, the sex-linked effectiveness of a given carcinogen stems mostly from a sex-dependent activity of enzyme systems necessary for the conversion of a procarcinogen to the active ultimate carcinogen. For example, in the case of N-2-fluorenylacetamide-induced liver cancer in males, the key difference

resides in the levels of the enzyme sulfotransferase giving rise to the active sulfate ester of N-hydroxide-N-2-fluorenylacetamide (Miller and Miller, 1981). Levels of enzyme are six to eight times higher in male than in female rats. Alternatively, a sex difference in carcinogenic susceptibility may stem from varying ratios of detoxication enzymes. For example, for some substrates glucuronide formation is higher in females than in males.

The endocrine system is important in relation to tumor growth in endocrine-sensitive tissues such as the gonads, adrenals, prostate, and breast (Rose, 1982). Also, alteration in the hormonal balance, e.g., by gonadectomy or hypophysectomy, may affect the carcinogenic process even in nonendocrine organs if endocrine-sensitive enzyme systems are required for activation or detoxication of the carcinogen or for the growth and development of the tumor, as noted above. In any case, the situation is quite complex, for endocrine glands and their target organs are interconnected by delicately balanced feedback pathways. Alteration in one hormone level usually leads to repercussions in the entire system, yielding a new equilibrium. In females of most species, regular and periodic oscillations occur, corresponding to the normal estrus cycle. Age, in turn, plays a role in endocrine responsiveness. Thus, superimposition of an exogenous toxicant with an affinity for any of the endocrine-susceptible organs may also indirectly affect other organs in the body. Addition of a hormone may have an even more complex action. The long-term effect of chemicals on the endocrine balance and the periodicity of the system must also be considered. Hormones such as those contained in oral contraceptives may have an entirely different action in animals such as rodents or dogs with an estrus cycle quite unlike that of the human female. Continuous administration of hormonally active preparations to rodents often results in the development of tumors, especially in the mammary gland. This may not necessarily constitute a carcinogenic risk for sexually mature human females receiving the same preparation in low dosages on a rhythmic basis tailored to the normal menstrual cycle. In fact, such treatment may serve to maintain the individual in hormonal balance and reduce the risk of cancer development in endocrine-responsive organs. On the other hand, exposure of fetuses, newborn or immature animals, or humans to an exogenous agent may permanently affect the differentiation of endocrine organs by leading to imprinting, and thus lead to cancer later in life due to either hormonal imbalance or aberrant tissue receptor response to prevailing hormone levels. Such processes may have been involved in the etiology of vaginal cancer in young, pubertal girls, whose mothers were given large doses of the estrogenic drug diethylstilbestrol during pregnancy.

QUANTITATIVE ASPECTS OF CARCINOGENESIS

DNA-Reactive Carcinogens

Extensive experimentation with a variety of chemical carcinogens has established the fact that, as is the case with other pharmacologic agents, the response to chemical carcinogens is dose related (see Eckhardt, 1959; Druckrey, 1967; Conning *et al.*, 1980). Chemical carcinogens of the electrophilic, reactive type, however, are quite distinct from ordinary pharmacologic agents in one way. Drugs and toxic chemicals generally exert their action rapidly, depending, of course, on mode of exposure. As the drug is biotransformed and excreted, the effect diminishes to the vanishing point, and in most instances, no residual effect persists. In general, subsequent exposures act anew in the same manner without any long-lasting effects. In contrast, while the onset of the interaction between a reactive carcinogen and cells is fundamentally similar in that the chemical may undergo biotransformation, the key, often biochemically activated, ultimate carcinogen reacts with tissue macromolecules, of which DNA appears to be critical. During DNA synthesis and cell duplication, altered DNA can lead to gene or chromosomal mutations and thereby imprint a permanent effect in the cell.

Thus, with DNA-reactive (genotoxic) carcinogens, a given dose can result in permanent abnormalities of cells. Subsequent dosages can add to such a change. After a sufficient number of such alterations have been produced, the multiplication of abnormal cells results in a detectable lesion and eventually a neoplasm. Because the effects vary with the carcinogen and the tissue in which it exerts its action, the time required for a neoplasm to appear varies. Thus, time as well as dose is a factor in assessing the properties of chemical carcinogens. It is primarily in this way that DNA-reactive carcinogens differ from ordinary toxic agents; a number of small doses may give no immediate evidence of their action, but in time they can yield neoplasms within the lifespan of the host. Indeed, there are carcinogens of the DNA-reactive type that can induce cancer in animal models with a single dose. With noncarcinogenic toxins, comparably subthreshold dosages for acute effects would probably be completely innocuous.

DNA-reactive carcinogens are further distinct from other types of toxins, insofar as the same total dose, when administered as smaller doses over a longer period of time, can actually be more effective than when given as larger, yet fewer, individual doses in a shorter period of time. In the extreme, several chemicals that are potent carcinogens when administered chronically are not carcinogenic at all when given as a single large dose. Also, administration of small single doses can be disproportionately effective compared to large doses, especially when accompanied by promotion (Stenbäck *et al.*, 1981).

In quantifying carcinogenic effects, the most superficial information is the overall incidence of neoplasms in exposed groups compared to the control group. More sensitivity is obtained if the parameters for evaluation include the expression period (time to tumor), often expressed as the time when the experimental group has reached a 50 percent incidence of neoplasms or the total time required for all animals to manifest neoplasms. Other relevant parameters of effect include the type of neoplasm and the multiplicity of neoplasms, which, when considered in relationship to dosage, yields a more refined estimation of dose-response effects.

Also, the expression of the dose is important. Often, it is given only as the concentration in diet or drinking water. Better quantitation is obtained if it is expressed as the amount administered per unit body weight. Suggestions have been made to express dose per unit surface area of the animal, as is often done with cancer chemotherapeutic drugs, but this has not been demonstrated to provide better quantification. All of these measures, however, describe only the administered dose. A more refined expression would be the effective dose actually taken in by the animal or, even better, that reaching the target site.

In numerous experiments using appropriate quantitative parameters, detailed dose-response relationships have been demonstrated. Two effects are usually observed: with increasing dose (1) the percent yield and multiplicity of neoplasms increases and (2) time required for neoplasm appearance decreases. In most cases the overall neoplasm yield in any specific organ is proportional to the total dose, but the speed or rate of neoplasm appearance is related to the amount in an individual dose or dose rate (Druckrey, 1967).

A controversial issue in dose-response relationships is whether no-effect or threshold levels exist for chemical carcinogens. In a classic study by Bryan and Shimkin (1943), 12 doses of each of three polycyclic aromatic hydrocarbons were injected subcutaneously in mice. There were 40 to 80 animals in the lower dose groups and 20 in the higher. The actual data show that two or three of the lower exposure levels yielded no evidence of tumor. Such observations, although clearly demonstrating no-observed-effect levels (NOEL) within the context of the experiment, have not been accepted as evidence of thresholds for large numbers of subjects at risk because of statistical limitations. To develop some information on the actual shape of the dose-response curve at low levels of exposure, several relatively large-scale studies have been conducted. In one study conducted at the National Center for Toxicological Research mice were fed 2-acetylaminofluorene at seven doses ranging between 30 and 150 ppm (see Staffa and Mehlman, 1979). The data were interpreted to show a linear dose-response for liver neoplasms, but yielded evidence of no-effect levels at 45, 35, and 30 ppm for bladder cancer. Another large-scale study performed at the British Industrial Biological Research Association (Peto, in O'Neill *et al.*, 1984) involved administration of 15 dose levels of several nitrosamines to rats using doses as low as 0.033 ppm in the diet. This study also has been interpreted to show a linear response for liver neoplasms, but with no-effect level for esophageal cancer. These studies, thus, suggest carcinogenic effects at low-level exposures in liver, but not other tissues.

DNA-reactive carcinogens vary greatly in their potency. For example, among liver carcinogens, a greater than 50 percent incidence is produced by lifetime administration to rats of aflatoxin B_1 at 1 ppb, by diethylnitrosamine at 5 ppm, by safrole at 1000 to 5000 ppm, and by acetamide at 12,500 ppm. Relatively few studies have been done on the effect of dose rate or even dose-response with the weaker DNA-reactive carcinogens. Shimkin *et al.* (1966; *see* Shimkin and Stoner, 1975) examined the potential of alkylating drugs of diverse structures to induce pulmonary tumors in mice. They found that the strong carcinogens were active over a broad dose range, whereas weaker ones gave evidence of some carcinogenicity only at the highest, but not at lower dose levels. Long *et al.* (1963) fed safrole in the diet to groups of 50 rats at levels of 100, 500, 1000, and 5000 ppm. Malignant liver cancers were obtained only at the highest dose level, and benign adenomas at the two highest, but not the lower doses. Thus, available data show that a threshold or no-observed-effect level can be observed with DNA-reactive carcinogens under standard bioassay conditions. However, the question can always be raised whether such thresholds would be seen if larger numbers of animals were used, as in the two large-scale studies. Based on considerations of

metabolism, the barriers to electrophiles in reaching critical targets in DNA, DNA repair processes, etc., it seems almost certain that for every carcinogen there must be a threshold. It may be very low for powerful carcinogens, as suggested by the two studies on 2-acetylaminofluorene and the nitrosamines, but seems to be correspondingly higher for weak carcinogens.

These dose-response studies on DNA-reactive carcinogens have provided the data for mathematical modeling. A number of models have been proposed (Office of Technology Assessment, 1982), and there is active debate on which of these is most appropriate. One that is widely used by regulatory agencies because it is "conservative" is a linear-no threshold extrapolation. As noted, proof has not been provided for any carcinogen that no threshold exists and, in fact, no-observed-effect levels have been documented in many studies, particularly with weak carcinogens. The assumption of linearity at low doses is also not well founded. Indeed, even for the less complicated process of chemical mutagenesis *in vivo*, a drop below linearity at low doses has been demonstrated (Russel *et al.*, 1982). Therefore, a "hockey stick"-shaped curve (Hoel *et al.*, 1985) would appear to best fit current data and concepts on carcinogenic effects at low levels of exposure to DNA-reactive carcinogens.

Dose-dependent carcinogenic effects have also been observed with human exposures to carcinogens. The most reliable quantitative data on human cancer resulting from exposure to specific carcinogens come from studies of occupational or therapeutic exposures (Williams *et al.*, in Flamm and Lorentzen, 1985). In these situations, adequate data exist on several carcinogens to show that human cancer incidence is proportional to dose, often measured by length of employment, since there are virtually no actual data on prevailing levels of any chemical in the industrial environment, especially in the past. The cancer incidence in workmen exposed to benzidine, vinyl chloride, or *bis*(chlormethyl)ether had a general relationship between exposure and disease occurrence. Workmen engaged in uranium or asbestos mining exhibited a risk of cancer broadly related to the length of time an individual was engaged in these particular occupations. Likewise, with the drug chlornaphazine, where intake was reasonably well established, the percentage of treated patients who subsequently developed bladder cancer was proportional to the amount of drug consumed (Williams *et al.*, in Flamm and Lorentzen, 1985). Many of the available dose-response relationships were observed in limited populations of people exposed iatrogenically (Schmähl et al., 1977).

As in experimental studies, the question of thresholds for human exposures to carcinogens is controversial. The issue has great contemporary importance in light of the capability of analytic chemists to measure accurately, at the parts-per-billion and even the parts-per-trillion level, the presence of several types of carcinogens in the food chain and in the environment generally. Several chemicals such as nitrosopyrrolidine, found in bacon, can induce liver cancer in several species with appropriate higher dosages, of the order of parts per million to parts per thousand (IARC Sci. Publ. 45, 1982; Preussmann and Stewart, in Searle, 1984). Primary liver cancer is rarely seen in populations that consume fried bacon. Is this evidence for a no-effect level? Similar questions can be raised for the trace amounts of mycotoxins currently permitted in food. Such considerations are controversial; opinions abound and facts are few. It must be accepted that the issue is currently beyond the reach of exact science.

Nevertheless, several lines of evidence suggest that in the human context there are thresholds for DNA-reactive carcinogens. For example, hepatocellular carcinoma is relatively rare in much of the Western world even though unavoidable contamination of foods with the liver carcinogens aflatoxin and dimethylnitrosamine has occurred for decades and continues to be found. Thus, there may be practical no-effect levels even for strong carcinogens, especially in the absence of promoting factors. A recent, additional documentation on this point is an evaluation of the effect of the powerful pulmonary carcinogen chloromethylmethylether. In one factory, evidence for a carcinogenic effect to workers was observed, but in another it was not (McCallum et al., 1983). Nonetheless, prudent policy dictates avoidance, wherever possible, of exposure to genotoxic carcinogens.

Epigenetic Carcinogens

In the case of carcinogens that are not DNA reactive and operate by the production of other biologic effects, it would be expected that their carcinogenic effects would parallel dose-response relationships for their relevant biologic effects. Unfortunately, relatively few dose-response studies have been done with carcinogens of the epigenetic type and almost none with regard to underlying toxicologic or pharmacologic effects. Reasonable data exist for the chelating agent nitrilotriacetic acid showing that kidney and bladder tumors are produced by exposures to about 75 mmoles/kg diet and that this diminishes dramatically, in a nonlinear fashion, when the exposure is reduced below 50 mmoles/kg diet (Anderson et al., 1985). A recent dose-response study in which saccharin was fed to large numbers of rats over two generations (various authors, 1985) shows that a 37 percent yield of bladder carcinoma plus papilloma was induced with 7.5 percent, 20 percent with 6.25 percent, 15 percent with 5 percent, 12 percent with 4 percent, 8 percent with 3 percent, 5 percent with 1 percent and 8 percent with 0 percent, the controls. Thus, the data show a two-thirds drop in neoplasm incidence with less than a one-half reduction of dose; 3 percent and 1 percent saccharin appear to be no-effect levels.

For several types of epigenetic carcinogens, especially promoters, theoretical considerations as well as available data from experimental studies strongly support the existence of no-effect levels or thresholds. When such agents as DDT, phenobarbital, or butylated hydroxyanisole were tested by themselves for carcinogenicity, an effect was evident only at the highest dose levels given in lifetime studies. These observations are supported by promoting studies with these agents where results can be obtained in shorter time with smaller numbers of animals. No-effect levels have been observed in promotion assays after exposures to the appropriate tissue-specific genotoxic carcinogens for saccharin in bladder cancer promotion (Nakanishi et al., 1980), and BHT and phenobarbital in liver cancer promotion (Maeura and Williams, 1984; Goldsworthy et al., 1984).

These observations on dose-response for nongenotoxic agents apply also to the human setting. Relatively few epigenetic agents have been carcinogenic to humans; examples are asbestos and diethylstilbestrol. There are no real dose-response data on the carcinogenic effects of these, although it is apparent that risk diminishes rapidly with reduction of exposures from the high levels associated with cancer causation.

Better data exist for dose-response of promoting agents. Bile acids are demonstrated promoters for colon cancer. In Western populations at high risk for colon cancer, the prevailing concentration of bile acids is 12 mg/g of feces. In Japan, with a low fat intake or in Finland, with a high cereal fiber intake, the risk for colon cancer is low, and the concentration of fecal bile acids is about 4 mg/g, only one-third of the concentration associated with high risk (Reddy et al., 1980). Complex tobacco smoke contains relatively small amounts of genotoxic polycyclic aromatic hydrocarbons, nicotine-derived nitrosamines, and certain heterocyclic amines. The major effect of tobacco stems from the promoting effect of the acidic fraction of the smoke

(Hoffmann *et al.,* in Surgeon General Report, 1982). It is established that an individual chronically smoking 40 cigarettes per day is at high risk, but with ten cigarettes per day the risk is much lower, and with four cigarettes per day the risk is most difficult to evaluate accurately. This represents evidence that enhancing factors have steep dose-response curves in humans, as in experimental animals.

Humans have been exposed to significant levels of a variety of epigenetic carcinogens such as organochlorine pesticides, BHA, BHT, phenobarbital, and natural estrogens without evidence of cancer causation (Clemmesen *et al.,* 1980; International Agency for Research on Cancer, 1982; Hayes, 1982). Nevertheless, carcinogens that are not DNA-reactive have produced cancer in humans, such as with asbestos through occupational exposure and diethylstibestrol at high pharmacologic levels. The negative findings with other epigenetic agents, therefore, suggest that their exposure levels have been below the thresholds for cancer production.

In summary, carcinogens, both DNA-reactive and epigenetic, act in a dose-dependent fashion, although the dose-response relations appear to be different. There are observed thresholds for both types of carcinogens in experimental animals and humans. The thresholds for DNA-reactive carcinogens vary greatly and may be low. Those for epigenetic carcinogens, particularly of the promoter class, have been fairly high. These observations have implications regarding the type of carcinogen testing that should be done to delineate human risk. This is discussed in the next section.

BIOASSAY OF CHEMICAL CARCINOGENS

The testing of chemicals for possible carcinogenic effects has as its aim the detection of those that may be harmful to humans. Although the induction of cancer in animals defines a chemical as a carcinogen, evaluation of the basis for carcinogenicity cannot be based exclusively on chronic testing because chemical carcinogens exhibit varied modes of action (see p. 103 and Table 5-2), which are not necessarily revealed by chronic bioassay. Of prime importance, evidence of genotoxic versus epigenetic effects is not obtained in such chronic tests although inferences can sometimes be made from the nature of the carcinogenic effect, including the type of dose-response pattern.

Carcinogen testing involves many approaches. Some are based on traditional practices, others on regulatory requirements. Several of these have been previously discussed (Williams and Weisburger, 1981; Weisburger and Williams, in Searle, 1984) and will not be repeated here. The essential information for a comprehensive risk extrapolation to humans can be obtained through a "decision point approach" to carcinogenicity evaluation (Weisburger and Williams, in Searle, 1984), which is based entirely on established toxicologic methods applied in a systematic manner. In addition to providing a framework within which the information required for risk extrapolation can be obtained, this approach also offers a guide to the elimination of unnecessary procedures. It utilizes systems that yield definitive data with reduced animal usage, and thus is more economical and humane than routine large-scale bioassays (Kushner *et al.,* 1982). Specific applications to testing of pharmaceuticals have recently been discussed (Williams and Weisburger, 1985). A recent monograph reviews aspects of carcinogen assays along these lines (Milman and Weisburger, 1985).

Based on established mechanisms of carcinogenesis, the Decision Point Approach takes the two main classes of DNA-reactive carcinogens and nongenotoxic, epigenetic agents into account in two ways:

1. A battery of short-term tests is structured with the aim of identifying genotoxic carcinogens at an early stage. The battery also includes systems that may respond to epigenetic agents.

2. Test methods are offered with the realization that all types of subchronic testing may not detect some chemicals that can produce neoplasms in animals under specific conditions upon chronic administration.

For the decision point approach, a series of sequential steps is followed in a stepwise progression (Table 5-19), and a critical evaluation of the information obtained and its significance in relation to the testing objective is performed at the end of each phase. A decision is made as to whether the data generated are sufficient to reach a definitive conclusion or whether a higher level of testing is required. There are four such decision points. Attention is paid to qualitative—yes or no—answers, and to quantitative—high, medium, or low—effects, in relation to known positive control compounds.

A. Structure of Chemical

As detailed above, structure-activity studies have provided considerable information upon which predictions as to whether or not a given chemical might be carcinogenic can be made with fair success within certain classes of chemicals, particularly those that include known carcinogens (Arcos *et al.,* 1968–1985). Structure must always be evaluated in the light of known species differences in biotransformation, which can render a weak or a noncarcinogenic agent in one species a powerful carcinogen in another (see p. 136) (Weisburger and Williams, in Becker, 1982; Langenbach *et al.*, 1983).

The induction of neoplasms by chemicals is quite specific and structure-related. Literally hundreds of polycyclic aromatic hydrocarbons have been studied after skin application or subcutaneous injection resulting in many structure-activity correlations. These demonstrate very clearly that structures that are closely related chemically, and even stereoisomers, may show quite divergent carcinogenic properties under identical exposure conditions (Brookes, 1980; Conney 1982; Arcos *et al.*, 1968–1985; Cooke and Dennis, 1985). Similar observations have been made for other types of chemical carcinogens.

Information on structure and biotransformation also provides a guide to the selection among limited bioassays at stage D and, as more infor-

mation accrues, may eventually contribute to selection of specific short-term tests at stage B.

B. In Vitro *Short-Term Tests*

The objective at this stage is to obtain information on the chemical reactivity of the test material. A crucial set of data needed is whether the chemical undergoes covalent reaction with DNA (see section on Reactions, p. 138). If radiolabeled material is available, definitive determination of adduct formation can be made. Other biochemical and biophysical techniques are also available, but vary in specificity and sensitivity. Highly sensitive techniques for identifying adducts include pyrolysis-electron impact mass-analyzed ion kinetic energy spectrometry (Wiebers *et al.*, 1981) and ^{32}P postlabeling (Everson *et al.*, 1986). In place of definitive biochemical techniques, a select battery of short-term tests for genotoxicity can be used.

Short-term tests are discussed in detail in Chapter 6 on Genetic Toxicology, but their application in that context is somewhat different than for mutagen testing. Among *in vitro* assays, no individual test, which has been studied adequately, has detected all carcinogens tested. In many cases, as described, this is because the "carcinogens" are not DNA-reactive. Another important factor is the complexity of biotransformation of chemical carcinogens. Known species differences in response to carcinogens can be related to a large extent (but not exclusively) to biotransformation, and thus, tests with different metabolic capabilities are extremely useful. Moreover, in addition to tests that identify genetic effects, newer procedures, still in the research stage, to detect epigenetic carcinogens are becoming available.

A number of reviews of aspects of short-term tests have appeared (IARC Monogr. Suppl. 2, 1980; Garattini *et al.*, 1982; Williams *et al.*, 1983; Ramel *et al.*, 1986). The two critical elements of a test are the end-point and the metabolic parameters. The end-point should be reliable and of definite biologic significance. The metabolic parameters of a test should be complementary to others in the battery, and the battery should include some tests that mimic as closely as possible *in vivo* characteristics of biotransformation.

A screening battery must include microbial mutagenesis tests because these have been the most sensitive, effective, and readily performed screening tests thus far. However, the bacterial mutagenesis tests require a mammalian enzyme preparation to provide for activation of most procarcinogens, and hence, other tests to be included should expand the biotransformation capability of the battery since this factor is often the most limiting aspect of a test series. Among available short-term tests, several employing intact hepatocytes (McQueen and Williams, in Flamm and Lorentzen, 1985) and other cell types (Langenbach *et al.,* 1983) have been developed. Since whole cell biotransformation is closer to the *in vivo* condition, such systems are included. In particular, the hepatocyte primary culture/DNA repair test (McQueen and Williams, in Flamm and Lorentzen, 1985) is useful because DNA repair is a specific response to DNA damage and, unlike other effects on DNA, cannot be attributed to toxicity. Mutagenesis of mammalian cells is a definitive end-point, as is bacterial mutagenesis, and is included to complement the latter end-point in a eukaryotic system. Sister chromatid exchange is included to provide a measurement of effects at the highest level of genetic organization. Its sensitivity, ease, and objectivity of measurement exceeds that of clastogenicity, although in some instances its significance is not yet fully understood. Clastogenicity does not correlate well with carcinogenicity. Cell transformation is included because this alteration is potentially the most relevant to carcinogenesis. This test is considered optional because much more needs to be done to standardize systems and clarify the significance of the end-point. Both sister chromatid exchange and transformation may have the potential to detect also epigenetic agents.

1. Bacterial Mutagenesis. Widely used bacterial screening tests have been developed in the laboratories of Ames (Maron and Ames, 1983) and Rosenkranz (in Williams *et al.,* 1980; Ramel *et al.,* 1986). The Ames test measures backmutation to histidine independence of histidine mutants of *Salmonella typhimiurium* and can be conducted with strains that are also repair-deficient, possess abnormalities in the cell wall to make them permeable to carcinogens, and carry an R factor enhancing mutagenesis. Recently, strains responsive to oxidative mutagens have been introduced. Hence, these organisms are highly susceptible to mutagenesis, making them sensitive indicators. Other bacterial and microbial mutagenicity systems are available (*see* Hollaender, 1971–1983). In a different type of test developed by Rosenkranz and associates, DNA repair-deficient *Escherichia coli* are used to measuring their enhanced susceptibility to cell killing by carcinogens. In this system a chemical that interacts with DNA is more toxic to the repair-deficient strain than to wild-type *E. coli* because the mutant strain cannot repair the damage. Thus, by measurement of relative toxicity, an indication of DNA interaction is obtained. These tests are dependent on mammalian enzyme preparations for biotransformation of carcinogens. The capability of the Ames test to

detect certain carcinogens has been enhanced by application of preincubation of the compound and the activation system with the test organism, or by a sensitive variant involving turbidity measurement, the flocculation test. A limitation of the Ames test is that several chemicals not known to be carcinogenic, such as quercetin, or those not likely to be carcinogenic, such as glutathione and cystine, have been positive in this system.

2. Mammalian Mutagenesis. A variety of end-points for mutational assays in mammalian cells are available, including resistance to purine analogs, bromodeoxyuridine, ouabain, or diphtheria toxin. Of these, purine analog and bromodeoxyuridine resistance are the most widely used. In purine analog resistance assays, mutants lacking the purine salvage pathway enzyme hypoxanthine-guanine phosphoribosyl transferase are identified by their resistance to toxic purine analogs such as 8-azaguanine or 6-thioguanine, which kill cells that utilize the analogs. This assay has the advantage over the measurement of thymidine kinase-deficient mutants by resistance to bromodeoxyuridine in that the gene for the affected enzyme is on the X chromosome rather than a somatic chromosome, as with thymidine kinase, and consequently the gene is highly mutable without having to construct and maintain heterozygous mutants (Clive in Williams *et al.,* 1980). The target cells used in purine analog resistance assays have almost all been fibroblastlike, such as the V79 line, and have displayed little ability to activate carcinogens. This deficiency has been overcome by providing exogenous biotransformation mediated by either cocultivated cells or enzyme preparations (Hsie, in Williams *et al.,* 1980). The latter again offer no extension in metabolic capability over that used for bacterial systems. However, the use of freshly isolated hepatocytes as a feeder system offers additional possibilities since the metabolic capability of hepatocytes has been shown to be superior to that of liver enzyme preparations as regards replicating *in vivo* biotransformation. Another interesting development is the finding that liver epithelial cultures can be mutated by activation-dependent carcinogens and may therefore provide another system with additional self-contained metabolic potential.

3. Hepatocyte Primary Culture DNA Repair Test. DNA repair synthesis is a specific response to various types of DNA damage and can be measured in a variety of ways (Williams, in Williams *et al.,* 1980). Several of the definitive procedures are technically sufficiently demanding that they have not been widely used for screening purposes. Of the two procedures that have, autoradiographic measurement of repair synthesis has an advantage over liquid scintillation counting in that it excludes cells in replicative synthesis, whereas these are part of the background with liquid scintillation counting. In addition, with liquid scintillation counting, increases in incorporation can result from changes in uptake or the pool size of thymidine without any repair occurring. Furthermore, autoradiography affords a determination of the percentage of cells in the affected population that responds. Two features that complicated early repair assays were that they required suppression of replicative DNA synthesis because continuously dividing lines were used, and the cell systems were dependent on enzyme preparations for biotransformation. Both of these complications were overcome with the introduction of the hepatocyte primary culture/DNA repair assay of Williams (in McQueen and Williams, in Flamm and Lorentzen, 1985; in Milman and Weisburger, 1985), which uses freshly isolated, nondividing liver cells that can biotransform carcinogens and respond with DNA repair synthesis measured autoradiographically. This assay has demonstrated substantial sensitivity and reliability with activation-dependent procarcinogens. It also offers the advantages of expanded biotransformation capability in the battery and clear biologic significance of its end-point. An *in vivo/in vitro* version of the test has been developed by Butterworth and colleagues (1982) that permits detection of agents that require biotransformation by enteric organisms. An alternative to this approach is simply to supplement the *in vitro* system with bacterial enzymes.

4. Sister Chromatid Exchange. Sister chromatid exchange is an exchange at one locus between the sister chromatids of a chromosome, which does not result in an alteration of overall chromosome morphology (Evans, in Williams *et al.*, 1983). The most widely used method for differentiating sister chromatids combines staining with a fluorescent dye plus Giemsa, the FPG, or harlequin methods. Using this technique, the observation of sister chromatid exchanges induced by chemicals is one of the quickest, easiest, and most sensitive tests for genetic damage (Wolff, in Williams *et al.*, 1983). Sister chromatid exchanges are suspected to be due to a recombination event that may occur at the DNA replication fork, but at present, the lesions responsible for exchanges are unknown. Thus far, this response has not been validated with a very extensive array of chemicals. Also, certain noncarcinogens or promoters have been positive (Kinsella and Radman, 1978). Nevertheless, this is still a useful complement to the other end-points in the battery.

5. Cell Transformation. The first reliable system for transformation of cultured mammalian cells was introduced by Sachs and associates. This system utilizing hamster fibroblasts was subsequently developed into a colony assay for quantitative studies by DiPaolo and has been adapted as a screening test by Pienta and co-workers (in Williams *et al.*, 1980). In addition, a quantitative focus assay for transformation using mouse cells has been devised (Heidelberger *et al.*, 1983). The correlation between transformation and malignancy appears to be good in these systems. Also, they provide an indication of the activity of chemicals, which could be due to either genotoxic or epigenetic mechanisms. Other approaches under development include the use of epithelial systems (Borek, in Williams *et al.*, 1983) and cell systems carrying oncogenic viruses as a more sensitive means of detecting transforming chemicals (Fischer and Weinstein, in Sontag, 1981).

DECISION POINT 1

The six steps (A, and B, 1–5) recommended thus far provide a basis for decision making at this stage. If clear-cut evidence of genotoxicity in more than one test has been obtained, the chemical is highly suspect. Positive results in both the bacterial mutagenicity test of Ames and the hepatocyte-DNA repair test of Williams reflect probable carcinogenicity. Confirmation of carcinogenicity may be sought in the limited *in vivo* bioassays without the necessity of resorting to the more costly and time-consuming chronic bioassay.

Evidence of genotoxicity in only one test must be evaluated with caution. In particular, several types of chemicals such as intercalating agents are mutagenic to bacteria, but are not reliably carcinogenic. Positive results in bacterial tests also have been obtained with synthetic phenolic compounds or natural products with phenolic structures such as flavones. *In vivo,* such compounds are likely to be conjugated and readily excreted. Their carcinogenicity thus would depend on *in vivo* splitting of such conjugates, which may occur more readily in laboratory rodents than in humans. Therefore, positive evidence of bacterial mutagenesis must be evaluated further with regard to chemical structure and biotransformation.

If all the preceding test systems yield no indication of genotoxicity, the chemical should be evaluated according to two principal criteria: (a) the structure and known physiologic properties (e.g., hormone) of the material, and (b) the potential human exposure. If the chemical structure suggests a need for sequential bacterial-mammalian cell biotransformation, then an *in vitro* system supplemented with bacterial enzymes could be used, or an *in vivo* assay. Where substantial human exposure is likely, careful consideration should be given to the necessity for additional testing with the likelihood of a standard chronic bioassay. The chemical structure and the properties of the material provide guidance on the appropriate course of action. Thus, organic chemicals with structures suggesting possible sites of activation may reveal their carcinogenicity in limited *in vivo* bioassays. On the other hand, substances such as solid-state materials, hormones, possibly some metal ions, and promoters that are negative in tests for genotoxicity operate by complex and as yet poorly understood mechanisms. For these, it is unlikely that the limited *in vivo* bioassays would yield any results when such materials are tested alone. The next step that is recommended for such chemicals is specific mechanistic studies or assay for promoting activity, depending on structure.

Taking advantage of the concept proposed by Loeb (*see* Eichhorn and Marzilli, 1981; Loeb and Mildvan, 1983) that certain metal ions affect the fidelity of enzymes concerned with DNA synthesis, such ions may be tested in rapid bioassay. In addition, certain metal ions can be detected in tests for mutagenicity (Heck and Costa, 1982). It seems reasonable that the nature of the metal ion, of which there are only a limited number, would provide the necessary insight for further testing in the type of assay most likely to reveal any adverse effects (Sunderman, 1984).

Compounds other than the strictly androgen and estrogen type can nevertheless exert effects on endocrine glands, e.g., amitrole. Such chemicals are potential cancer risks mainly because they interfere with the normal, physiologic endocrine balances. More research is required on methods to test quickly for such properties. It is known, for example, that certain drugs lead to release of prolactin or other hormones from the pituitary gland. Chronic intake of such drugs causing a permanently higher serum and tissue peptide hormone level might, in turn, alter the relative ratio of other hormones. At this time, any substance with such properties needs to undergo a chronic bioassay with carefully and appropriately selected doses or an initiation-promotion test with a suitable initiator so as to evaluate whether endocrine-sensitive tissues would be at higher risk. The interpretation of data needs to take into account the normal diurnal, monthly, and even seasonal cycles of the endocrine system and whether the test might have led to interference in this balanced, rhythmic system.

The implications of a positive response in specific chronic bioassays coupled with convincing data of the absence of genotoxicity are discussed under the final evaluation.

C. Tests for Promoting Agents

A major group of epigenetic agents are those that facilitate the development of neoplastic cells into tumors and are thus carcinogenic in animals with "spontaneously" or cryptogenically transformed cells. A variety of synthetic chemicals, certain drugs, immunosuppressants, and hormones belong to this group. Thus, tests for promoting activity are essential in the safety evaluation of chemicals. In assessing promotion the tumor-enhancing activity of an agent is indicative of promotion only for nongenotoxic chemicals since those with DNA-damaging capability can augment carcinogenicity (syncarcinogenesis) in a sequential protocol as a result of summation of DNA damage.

1. *In Vitro* Tests for Tumor-Promoting Agents. A great deal of information has accumulated dealing with the effects of the classic tumor promoters, the phorbol esters, in *in vitro* systems (Hecker *et al.,* 1982; Pereira, 1983). A variety of responses related to interactions with specific membrane receptors has been noted. Some suggested approaches to the identification of promoters include the induction of plasminogen activator, ornithine decarboxylase, gene amplification, production of sister chromatid exchange, and aneuploidy. For most of these, effects have not been found with nonphorbol types of promoters.

The transformation systems can be modified to test for promoting substances if a limited amount of a genotoxic carcinogen is used as initiator followed by, or even together with, another agent (cocarcinogenesis).

Based on the concept that important informational molecules are exchanged between cells in contact through gap junctions, several systems have been developed to detect promoting agents by their ability to block intercellular molecular exchange through gap junctions (Murray *et al.,* in Hecker *et al.,* 1982; Trosko, in Williams *et al.,* 1983). A similar approach using liver cells has been devised by Williams (in Pereira, 1983). This effect *in vitro* would cause cells with an abnormal genome to be isolated from the growth-controlling elements provided by neighboring normal cells and thus released for progressive growth. These relatively new techniques for detecting promotion *in vitro* shows considerable promise, but need extension and validation.

2. *In Vivo* Promoting Assays. Promoters of neoplastic development often display a high degree of organ specificity. Consequently, *in vivo* assays involve the administration of a genotoxic-initiating agent that affects the organ in which the promoting activity of the test substance is to be examined.

The most widely used system involves testing for promoting activity on mouse skin initiated with small doses of benzo(a)pyrene or 7,12-dimethylbenz(a)anthracene. Also, induction of ornithine decarboxylase in the absence of initiation has been proposed as an assay (Boutwell, 1983b). New promoters have been discovered by this means (Sugimura et al., 1982).

A material exhibiting endocrine properties or one affecting endocrine balances in general likewise may show an effect in modifying breast or endometrial cancer induction in animals given limited amounts of methylnitrosourea as an initiating dose, or utilizing mice with or without the mammary tumor virus. Similarly, promoters for urinary bladder or colon cancer may be identified by specific enhancing effects subsequent to pretreatment with limited amounts of a bladder or colon carcinogen.

To test for promoting activity by a chemical in liver carcinogenesis, rapid in vivo bioassay tests have been designed by giving a few doses of a limited amount of an appropriate genotoxic hepatocarcinogen such as diethylnitrosamine or N-2-fluorenylacetamide followed by the test chemical. An increase in number or size of carcinogen-induced altered foci can be identified as evidence of promotion with histochemical markers such as γ-glutamyl transpeptidase or iron exclusion (Williams, 1982; Pereira, in Milman and Weisburger, 1985).

Drugs or other chemicals that appear to be enzyme inducers that in a chronic bioassay in rats and mice have given some evidence of liver tumor induction in mice but not in rats and that have been negative for genotoxicity in appropriate in vitro test batteries have shown promoting activity in such systems. The response of liver of certain mouse strains appears to be such as would reflect an abnormal genome. With rats this is somewhat different, although chronic tests with nongenotoxic promoters have often yielded a low incidence of liver tumors, perhaps related to the presence in the diet of mycotoxins or nitrosamines. Many of the more complex polychlorinated aliphatic and cyclic hydrocarbons also fall into the class of enhancing substances.

These initiation-promotion schemes, when designed with a number of dose levels, including the possible prevailing environmental level, help provide the necessary background information for the establishment of a threshold level and for health risk analysis.

DECISION POINT 2

A positive response in the in vitro test for inhibition of intercellular molecular exchange is highly suggestive of a promoting potential. However, this test has not yet been sufficiently validated, largely because of the paucity of proven neoplasm promoters outside of the class of phorbol compounds. Therefore, a positive response in this system indicates the advisability of an in vivo test for neoplasm promotion.

A nongenotoxic chemical that is active in an in vivo test for neoplasm promotion must be regarded as a potential hazard, depending on dose or exposure rates. Therefore, the finding of a positive effect indicates the need for further safety testing. This should include a multidose administration following a short course of the appropriate genotoxic carcinogen, which may permit the determination of a relative no-effect level.

Neoplasm promoters are almost certain to be negative in the limited in vivo bioassays (see below) for carcinogenicity. Therefore, no point is served by submitting the chemical to testing of this type; instead it should undergo chronic bioassay if the potential human exposure warrants it. Since a finding of promoting activity indicates a possible contribution to cancer risk, the chronic bioassay should be undertaken with a view to establishing a possible no-effect level by means of testing over a broad dose range. The finding of a no-effect level in chronic bioassay coupled with lack of genotoxicity and evidence for a promoting action would lead to a health risk assessment distinctly different from that of genotoxic carcinogens.

D. Limited In Vivo Bioassays

This stage of evaluation employs tests that will provide further evidence of any potential hazard of chemicals giving limited evidence of genotoxicity without the necessity of undertaking a full-scale chronic bioassay (Weisburger and Williams, 1981). Also, certain of the tests will provide relative potency ratings when the design includes known carcinogens.

The in vivo tests at this stage provide evidence of carcinogenicity, in a relatively short period (i.e., 40 weeks or less). The sensitivity of some of the systems can be enhanced by using a known promoter for a specific organ to detect an unknown initiator. However, the latter kind of agent should have been positive in tests for genotoxicity, and this set of tests and approach would rapidly provide semiquantitative data on relative potency in these in vivo tests. Unlike the in vitro tests, these are not applied as a battery, but rather selected according to the information available on the chemical. Negative results in any of these systems cannot be taken as strong evidence of noncarcinogenicity, since all are limited in their end point.

1. Skin Neoplasm Induction in Mice. The carcinogenicity of a limited number of chemicals and crude products can be revealed readily upon continuous application to the skin of mice, producing papillomas or carcinomas, or upon subcutaneous injection, yielding sarcomas. Also, initiating activity can be rapidly determined by the concurrent or sequential application of a specific promoter, such as one of the phorbol esters (*see* Hecker *et al.*, 1982; Slaga, 1983). Tars from coal, petroleum, or tobaccos are active in such systems, as are the pure polycyclic aromatic hydrocarbons and congeners contained in such products. Mouse skin responds positively because it appears to have the necessary enzymes to yield the active intermediates leading to initiation, especially in the presence of cocarcinogens or promoters in the crude products. On the other hand, such mixtures rarely yield visceral neoplasms, mainly because the liver can detoxify these chemicals quickly. However, lung and lymphoid neoplasms in sensitive mouse strains can be a secondary tumor site.

Mouse skin is useful primarily, therefore, for chemicals such as polycyclic hydrocarbons, also direct-acting chemical carcinogens such as sulfur or nitrogen mustard, *bis*(chloromethyl) ether, propiolactone, as well as alkylnitrosoureas. Arylamines and related carcinogens by themselves usually do not provide a positive response on mouse skin, although some exceptions are 2-anthramine and 3-methyl-2-naphthylamine, which are active in this system perhaps because these chemicals are converted to active epoxy intermediates, in the same manner as the polycyclic aromatic hydrocarbons. On the other hand, mouse skin does not appear to yield a positive result with a basic fraction of tobacco tar, even though this fraction is mutagenic and leads to cell transformation. Some arylamines and urethane, however, provide a positive indication but only upon promotion with phorbol ester.

2. Pulmonary Neoplasm Induction in Mice. Andervont and Shimkin pioneered with the model involving the development of lung tumors in specific sensitive strains of mice, especially the A/Heston and related strains such as A/J. As Shimkin and Stoner (1975) point out, a singular advantage of the assay system is that, in addition to an end-point measuring the percentage of animals with neoplasms compared to controls, the multiplicity of tumors is an additional parameter

expressing the "strength" of any carcinogenic action. Most chemicals that are active in this system are also carcinogenic in other longer, chronic animal tests. Another useful aspect of this assay is that significant results are obtained in as short a time as 30 to 35 weeks, and sometimes faster. Extension of the test for a longer period is not desirable since the incidence of pulmonary tumors in control animals increases rapidly after 35 weeks, and thus the test loses sensitivity. Positive results are obtained with polycyclic aromatic hydrocarbons, certain nitrosamines and nitrosamides, aflatoxin B_1, ethyl carbamate, hydrazines, alkylating agents, and, much less sensitive, arylamines.

3. Breast Cancer Induction in Female Sprague-Dawley Rats. This model is based on the finding that polycyclic hydrocarbons rapidly induce cancer in the mammary gland of young, female, random-bred Wistar rats and still better in Sprague-Dawley rats. With powerful carcinogens, especially select polycyclic hydrocarbons, arylamines, certain chloroalkanes such as 1,2-dichloroethane, or nitrosoureas, a positive result is obtained rapidly, in less than nine months. As in the case of lung tumor induction in mice, the multiplicity of mammary tumors provides an additional quantitative criterion to denote relative strength of the carcinogenic stimulus. A positive response in this system often correlates with results in other animal bioassay models.

4. Altered Foci Induction in Rodent Liver. During liver carcinogenesis several distinct liver cell lesions precede the development of carcinomas. The earliest of these, the altered focus, when sufficiently developed, can be demonstrated in routine histologic tissue sections. Also, foci are abnormal in a number of properties that permit their reliable and objective identification at early stages by more sensitive techniques. Altered foci in rat liver display abnormalities in the enzymes gamma-glutamyl transpeptidase, glucose-6-phosphatase, and adenosine triphosphatase, which have been used for their histochemical detection (Pitot and Sirica, 1980; Williams, 1982). Another important marker for foci that permits histochemical identification is their resistance to iron accumulation (Williams, 1982). This latter property is sometimes more sensitive than the enzyme abnormalities and also, unlike the enzyme abnormalities, characterizes rat and mouse liver lesions. Therefore, induction of iron-excluding altered foci in mouse or rat liver can be used as a limited bioassay.

With known carcinogens, foci have been detected within three weeks of carcinogen exposure and in high numbers by 12 to 16 weeks of exposure (Williams, 1982). Therefore, the recommended approach is that of exposure for 12 weeks to the test chemical with injection of subcutaneous iron during the last two weeks to produce the iron load that delineates the foci resistant to iron accumulation. A number of carcinogens have been detected using this regimen (Pereira, in Milman and Weisburger, 1985).

Another approach to detecting altered foci employs their resistance to the cytotoxic effect of carcinogens (Tatematsu *et al.*, 1983). In this approach, administration of the test chemical is followed by exposure to *N*-2-fluorenylacetamide and partial hepatectomy or, instead of the latter, a necrogenic dose of CCl_4. The selective agent is biotransformed by normal liver cells and affects them so that they cannot proliferate in response to the partial hepatectomy. In contrast, the cells in altered foci proliferate and become extremely conspicuous. The current complexity of this approach, involving administration of a known carcinogen and surgical manipulation, appears to be a disadvantage compared to the demonstration of foci resulting from repeat application. However, future developments in this active field may lead to significant improvements in all these approaches.

DECISION POINT 3

Proven activity in more than one of the limited *in vivo* bioassays may be considered unequivocal qualitative evidence of carcinogenicity. A definite positive result in one of the limited *in vivo* bioassays, together with two positive results in a battery of rapid *in vitro* bioassay tests reliable for genotoxicity, also indicates potential carcinogenicity. This is true especially if the *in vivo* results were obtained with moderate dosages, and more so if there was evidence of a good dose response, particularly as regards the multiplicity of the skin, lung, or mammary gland neoplasms, or of the liver foci.

Positive results in one *in vivo* bioassay and in only one *in vitro* test makes the agent highly suspect, but further testing is indicated. A negative result in any of these assays does not constitute proof of noncarcinogenicity since they all have some limitations.

E. Chronic Bioassay

In the systematic approach described, chronic bioassay is used as a last resort (1) for confirming questionable results in the more limited testing, or (2) for chemicals that are negative in the preceding stages of testing but where extensive human exposure is likely, or (3) for the acquisition of data on possible carcinogenicity through indirect epigenetic mechanisms. Multispecies

and dose-response data are most important if the data are to be applied to risk assessment. For chemicals found nongenotoxic in the *in vitro* tests (decision point 1), but with some indication of promoting potential (decision point 2), it may be worthwhile and efficient to include an initiation-promotion test using an initiating agent with broad tissue responses such as some of the nitrosamines or nitrosamides to secure solid data on promoting properties.

It is important to keep in mind that chronic tests for carcinogenicity are highly time and money consuming and are not exercises in theoretic estimations of response of animals to chemicals. Rather the deliberate aim of carcinogen test systems should be the acquisition of data that permit evaluation of the carcinogenic risk for humans. Therefore, a key issue regarding chronic bioassays is the degree to which data obtained in such systems actually reflect a human carcinogenic risk (Richmond *et al.*, 1980; Conning *et al.*, 1981; Pitot, 1982; Hoel *et al.*, 1985). About 29 chemicals or mixtures have been demonstrated unambiguously to have induced cancer in humans (IARC Monogr. Suppl. 4, 1982). Almost everyone of these chemicals that has led to cancer in humans is also highly carcinogenic in several animal models. Therefore, the reverse may very likely be true; that is, a chemical that is carcinogenic in animal models would also affect humans. This certainly seems to be true for chemicals that are active over several dose ranges in a number of species and that induce a high yield of neoplasms at a given site and possibly several select sites within a reasonably short latent period (15 months or shorter). Such chemicals are unquestionably human risks, especially if collateral data show them to be also genotoxic. The known human carcinogens are typically endowed with such properties. A key exception is arsenic in the form of inorganic arsenite, where animal models have failed to provide convincing evidence of carcinogenicity and where the underlying mechanisms are unknown.

Bioassay systems primarily use rats, mice, and for some specific purposes hamsters (Sontag, 1981; Robens *et al.*, 1982; Weisburger and Williams, in Searle, 1984; Milman and Weisburger, 1985). Because younger animals are often more sensitive, exposure begins at weaning or shortly thereafter. Newborn mice, and in some cases newborn rats and hamsters, have been recommended because they appear to show even higher sensitivity to some carcinogens.

Certain bioassays have involved exposure of males and females of a parent generation that are mated during treatment, thus providing for possible transplacental exposure. The exposure is then continued during infancy. Advantages and limitations of two-generation tests require definition. At this time, and in the framework of a systematic Decision Point Approach as described here, these two-generation tests are probably no more useful for delineating human cancer risk than is a standard bioassay. In fact, they could yield misleading data and interpretations, if the fetus and newborn during rapid growth and differentiation are exposed to high levels of an xenobiotic.

Many types of chemical carcinogens show dose-response effects, but the time factor needs to be considered because cancer induction under a variety of conditions, even with powerful carcinogens, requires a certain minimum period of time. This is because the entire process is very complicated, from the biochemical activation of the agent leading to neoplastic conversion of cells in specific tissues, to the growth and development of abnormal cells to a visible neoplasm. This entire process has been thought to take at least one-eighth the life-span of a species. Thus, mice, rats, and hamsters, with an average life of two to three years, usually develop detectable cancer in no less than three months after treatment with most carcinogens. With longer-lived species, including primates, the process may be expected to take much longer. For example, diethylnitrosamine induces malignant liver cancer in rats in as little as three to five months, whereas in the rhesus monkey the same point is reached in one to three years. High levels of 2-naphthylamine induce cancer in the urinary bladder of hamsters in about a year, but two or more years are required in the dog or the monkey. Hence, the trend has been to use even shorter-lived species as a means to decrease the time required for bioassays (Weisburger and Williams, in Searle, 1984).

A high dose usually induces a certain yield of cancers in a given target organ more rapidly than a low dose, even though the latter, given sufficient time, may eventually induce the same yield of neoplasms. In addition, varying the dosage may lead to shifts in target organs, mainly because of alterations in biotransformation pathways, and possibly also to tissue-related factors such as cell turnover times and repair mechanisms. For example, a few large doses of dimethylnitrosamine induce cancer of the kidneys after a fairly long expression period, whereas continuous low dosing with the same agent consistently results in a high incidence of liver cancer with a shorter expression period. The relevant mechanism involves DNA repair capability, which is expressed more in rat liver than in kidney tissue.

Potent carcinogens, such as those with demonstrated activity in humans, can be detected in mice or rats rather quickly, often in less than one year (Squire, 1981). Weaker agents take longer, even at high dose levels, and it may be necessary to observe the animals for their entire lifetime. Similar relationships can be demonstrated to hold for humans. For example, it has been shown that the development of human pulmonary carcinoma as a result of cigarette smoking is proportional to the number of cigarettes smoked per day, and the age of appearance is inversely related to cigarette consumption (Hoffmann et al., 1983).

During studies of the pathogenesis of certain cancers, antecedent precancerous lesions could be detected in some organs, sometimes long before a definitive neoplasm could be diagnosed. If this were true for all chemical carcinogens, their early detection by rapid examination of tissues for such specific cellular lesions would be greatly facilitated, and, indeed, the reliable detection of such lesions in the liver is the basis for a proposed limited in vivo bioassay (see above). However, in some tests, autopsies performed one year after the beginning of treatment have given no diagnostic signs although neoplasms were present after 18 months. Thus, in a study lasting less than two years or a lifetime, a negative finding would not necessarily mean that an agent was not carcinogenic, and collateral data from other tests are important. On the other hand, the interpretation of the two-year or lifetime tests can be difficult. As animals age, they (1) die from causes unrelated to carcinogen treatment and are thus lost to the experiment without necessarily exhibiting cancer and (2) exhibit spontaneous tumors, most often in the endocrine-sensitive organs, again not related to the treatment. The incidence of these spontaneous neoplasms is not constant and varies sometimes with fairly large limit values, for example, with neoplasms in the pituitary or adrenal glands. Thus, it is necessary to compare the incidence in an experimental group not only to simultaneous controls, but also historic controls.

Some investigators recommend lifetime studies, which, when animal colonies are carefully maintained, permit some strains of rats to live as long as three years and mice to live as long as two and one-half years. Most current procedures, however, involve exposure of groups of male and female rats, mice, or hamsters in experiments that terminate after two years for rats and 21 to 24 months for mice and hamsters, depending on strain, thus allowing optimum survival time for nonexposed controls. An advantage of this scheme is that 70 to 90 percent of the experimental animals live to the end of the test. Thus, tissues from scheduled necropsies are secured for subsequent microscopic study. In lifetime studies, it is sometimes difficult to avoid losses of valuable material due to autolysis when the animals die spontaneously, and of course, evaluation may find a high incidence of neoplasms in controls.

Furthermore, the question of the length of administration of the test compound requires consideration. With food additives and related materials, where humans are conceivably exposed during their life-span, it is useful to administer the compound throughout the test series, or even through a partial two-generation study, discussed above. For industrial chemicals and other materials where the potential exposure may be intermittent, a period of 18 months might be more useful. This seems sufficiently long, since even with a weak carcinogen, it is logical to assume that the processes leading to tumor induction have been initiated, although no accurate comparative study to ascertain this point experimentally has been performed. Thus, discontinuing administration of the compound after 18 months and maintaining the animals for three to six additional months may be useful to support the development of any tumor produced and lead to regression of many abnormal, yet noncancerous lesions. At the same time, the toxic stress of compound administration is removed, and thus a beneficial, more prolonged survival of the animals might actually be facilitated.

An important aspect of bioassays involves the dosage and mode of compound administration. The maximally tolerated dose (MTD) is established in preliminary assays, under the same conditions selected for the test series. The need for high-level testing at the MTD has been discussed in detail (Weisburger and Williams, in Searle, 1984). Acute LD50 determinations do not necessarily contribute information that will be useful in determining doses tolerated under chronic conditions. If a chemical leads to changes in the processing enzymes, the chronically tolerated dose could be higher or lower than an acute toxic dosage, depending on how the balance of activation or toxication over detoxication metabolites is altered.

With DNA-reactive carcinogens, the induction of tumors may be seen at several dose levels. Such studies have shown that even with powerful carcinogens there are doses at which no effect is obtained within the normal life-span of the animals. The entire problem of testing in bioassays very small doses, approximately those prevailing in the environment, is still unresolved. Analytic chemistry has advanced impressively, permitting accurate determinations of chemicals at parts-per-billion and even parts-

per-trillion levels. Even with powerful carcinogens and with consideration of possibly synergistic interactions, the question remains whether levels in this range have any biologic significance, especially in defining human risk. This subject is discussed in the section on Quantitative Aspects (p. 150).

Even in simplified test series it is advisable to utilize at least one dose level below the MTD. The main reason is to ensure adequate survival of at least one of the groups of animals for the planned experimental period. If the preliminary toxicology leads to the selection of a high-dose level that is tolerated for six to nine months but then results in death of the experimental group without cancer or adverse effects, the entire study will have to be repeated. Thus, to save time, a similar group of animals is started simultaneously at a lower dose level; one-half or one-third of the MTD generally is adequate and usually permits survival of the animals for the necessary length of time. An active carcinogen would show a response, proportional to dose, at both dosages. If the MTD shortens life-span, that group of test animals, by dying sooner, might exhibit a lower cancer incidence than those on the reduced dosage who live longer. However, in any case, the results of the battery of the short-term tests and the limited *in vivo* bioassays will have yielded information essential for the design of the chronic tests. Often, the latter will not be necessary since adequate information for decision making will have been obtained in the preceding set of short-term and limited bioassays. When the importance of the chemical in view of the possible extensive human contact mandates a chronic bioassay, this should be designed with three to five dose levels from the MTD to one approximating the highest probable human exposure.

With weaker carcinogens, active when given at the MTD, it has been found that the second dose level fails to induce statistically significant rates of cancer in a chronic test with the usual number of animals at risk. Hence, careful selection of dosages is necessary in order to detect relatively low degrees of carcinogenicity, unless, of course, larger numbers of animals are used. Such a pattern of activity is indicative not only of weaker genotoxic carcinogens but even more so of nongenotoxic promoters that under some conditions at high dose levels can induce a low, but significant, yield of neoplasms in two-year or lifetime tests.

Modes of Administration and Selection of Animal Type. The primary direct-acting carcinogens will almost always cause cancer in any tissue to which they are directly applied. On the other hand, procarcinogens, which require metabolic or chemical conversion, are rarely active at the site of application and, in contrast, sometimes exhibit quite specific organotropic affinity, depending on the biochemical potential of a given tissue. Even so, the mode of administration can influence the tumor yield at a given site, since it dictates pathways of internal distribution and biotransformation and hence the concentration in a tissue. For example, dibutylnitrosamine given subcutaneously to rats leads almost exclusively to tumors in the urinary bladder. After subcutaneous injection, absorption leads to direct passage via the blood into renal pathways. On the other hand, oral administration produces tumors in liver, lung, and urinary bladder because these additional organs receive a sufficient concentration of the agent.

In general, the mode of administration should logically mimic the potential human exposure. Thus, food additives would normally be fed or given by gavage. Cosmetics would be applied to the skin. Drugs given by parenteral injection would be thus tested. However, if the only question asked is whether a given chemical structure has carcinogenic potential that, as discussed previously, is a highly specific, nonrandom property, then the mode of administration may depend more on such mechanistic aspects. The mode used is the one that would most likely reveal a carcinogenic effect based on the chemical structure of the agent. In any case, with many chemical carcinogens, particularly the more powerful agents, an effect is observed, irrespective of the mode of intake. This statement does not imply, however, that there is not an optimal procedure for each chemical.

Certain modes of administration are clearly in need of further study. For example, the daily administration of corn oil as a vehicle for garage adds sizable fat calories that have specific metabolic effects and may, in turn, alter the action of a test compound. It apparently influences the background of pancreatic neoplasms (Eustis and Boorman, 1985).

The induction of tumors in rodents at the site of single or repeated subcutaneous injection requires careful interpretation. With this proviso, this technique offers advantages. With direct-acting carcinogens, tumors are formed at the site of injection, often quickly and with small amounts of chemical. Any systemic effects can also be observed. However, some chemicals induce local sarcomas, but this finding is not evidence of oncogenic potential. In fact, such materials may not be a hazard to humans who should be exposed to such chemicals by some way other than the parenteral route. An example is the induction of sarcoma upon subcutaneous injection or implantation of polymers or certain chemicals as in detergents, soaps, emulsifiers, or organic salts into rats or mice. This would normally not reflect a human oncogenic risk (see Schmähl et al., 1977). Again, it is important to consider collateral data from tests for genotoxicity in judging risk from extrapolation of bioassays in rodents.

Within the numerous strains of mice, rats, and hamsters, strains should be selected that are readily available, have good breeding performance, are disease-free, with extended survival, and have good sensitivity to carcinogens. Some investigators prefer to use random-bred animals, others inbred animals. Because the variability is less and the reproducibility of tests is somewhat better in inbred animals, and also because certain transplantation experiments and related immunologic considerations are performed more readily or possibly exclusively in inbred animals, or F_1 hybrid descendants of two inbred strains, the trend has been toward the use of such inbred animals. However, even with random-bred animals, properly conducted tests can be executed reproducibly. The induction of mammary gland cancer is reliably performed in the random-bred Sprague-Dawley rat.

The number of animals to be used depends on several factors, including the need to generate sufficient data for a dependable statistical evaluation. For a known carcinogen giving a high incidence of tumors in less than one year, the loss of animals due to treatment-unrelated causes may be minimal, and groups of 20 to 30 suffice. For an unknown agent or where the effect is weak, and therefore requires a lengthy experimental period, a larger number of animals is used to compensate for deaths unrelated to treatment. If the experiment calls for killing some of the animals prior to termination of the main tests, for example, to delineate any early effects, the initial number would have to be increased, so as to take into account this reduction in the group size of the animals at risk in any set. Current practice is to use 50 or even more animals per group, for specific tests such as dose-response studies. Such tests are best planned with the advice and continuing consultation of professional statisticians.

Once an animal has been in any test series longer than a year, it becomes a valuable specimen. Every effort must be made not to lose it because of poor husbandry practices or inadequate professional supervision. Animals must be inspected every day and toward the end of an experiment, twice a day. Animals in poor health should be examined to establish whether survival is possible. If this is unlikely, proper necropsy procedures should be instituted immediately. After a substantial time on test, little is gained by maintaining an animal already in poor health for a few more days or weeks.

Autopsies should be performed by highly trained personnel, capable of detecting even minor grossly visible lesions. A complete autopsy includes opening of the skull and examination of the tissues of the nervous system, the brain, and the pituitary gland, as well as the other viscera. Proper fixation of tissues in suitable fluids, trimming of select tissues for histologic processing, and finally microscopic study of stained sections should be supervised or performed by trained professionals. The entire assay hinges on accurate execution of the total test series, but in particular it depends on correct diagnosis and interpretation of the significance of any lesions noted. Again, individuals trained in experimental pathology should be part of the team designing and monitoring a test series. An experienced pathologist using correct diagnostic procedures will be in the best position to successfully conclude the study.

Control groups are as important as experimental groups. In smaller studies evaluating the carcinogenicity of only one or two compounds, the control group must be of the same size as each experimental group. Some effort can be saved if a number of chemicals or drugs are studied simultaneously, for then one control group can serve as reference point for a number of contemporary experimental groups. The control group should involve a number of animals, $A\sqrt{n}$, where A is the size of each group and n is the number of simultaneous experimental groups. If a vehicle is used, control groups treated with the vehicle alone, in addition to untreated control groups, are required in order to assess the possible influence of the treatment with the vehicle. In addition, it is desirable to give a positive control carcinogen at two dose levels, one known to be effective quickly, as a means of assessing the responsiveness of the specific type of animals used. The other dose level could be lower to mimic any possible weaker effect of the unknown compounds.

F. Final Evaluation

Chronic bioassays stemming from systematic application of the decision point approach would be expected to yield definitive data on carcinogenicity. In any case, the results from biochemical studies and short-term tests *must* be considered for evaluation of possible mechanisms of action and risk extrapolation to humans (Squire, 1981; Weisburger and Williams, 1981). Convincing evidence of DNA-reactivity or genotoxicity tests coupled with documented *in vivo* carcinogenicity permit classification of the chemical as a DNA-reactive carcinogen. It would, therefore,

be anticipated that the chemical could display the properties characteristic of such carcinogens, which include the ability under some circumstances to be effective at a single dose, cumulative effects, and synergism or at least additive effects with other DNA-reactive carcinogens that affect the same tissues although they may demonstrate thresholds (see Quantitative Effects, p. 150). DNA-reactive carcinogens, nevertheless, in the absence of information to the contrary, must be regarded as qualitative hazards to humans. Accordingly, the level of exposure permitted must be rigorously evaluated and controlled.

If appropriate studies yield no convincing evidence for DNA reactivity, but nonetheless the chemical is carcinogenic in animal bioassays, it is possible that the agent is an epigenetic carcinogen. The strength of this conclusion depends on the relevance of the negative evidence for DNA reactivity and the degree to which an alternative mode of action has been established. For instance, the sensitive techniques of ^{32}P postlabeling (Everson *et al.*, 1986) and pyrolysis-electron impact mass-analysis ion kinetic energy spectrometry (Wiebers *et al.*, 1981) can provide compelling evidence for the absence of DNA adduct formation in the target organ of the carcinogen. A biologic approach is to assess for syncarcinogenesis between the agent in question and a DNA-reactive carcinogen with the same target organ (Williams and Furuya, 1984).

The nature of epigenetic mechanisms is not completely understood at present, but they appear to be different for the different classes. They may involve chronic tissue injury and cell proliferation, generation of reactive species, immunosuppressive effects, hormonal imbalances, blocks in differentiation, promotion of preexisting genetically altered cells, or processes as yet unknown. In any event, many epigenetic carcinogens have displayed carcinogenicity only at the MTD in bioassays. Detailed dose-response studies would be informative with such agents since it seems likely that they may represent only quantitative hazards to humans, and safe levels of exposure may be established by carrying out proper toxicologic and pharmacologic dose-response studies.

The question has often been asked as to how animal carcinogenicity data can be extrapolated to humans. *Homo sapiens*, unlike many experimental species, is genetically heterogenous. In addition, humans have wide variations in environment, diet, and life-style. Thus, one would not expect a uniform response to exogenous agents such as carcinogens. In pharmacology and medicine, it is a well-accepted fact that patients need to be considered as individuals when prescribing dosages of drugs. Animal systems, on the other hand, can be controlled much more effectively. Indeed, highly inbred strains of genetically uniform rodents, mice, rats, and hamsters, are available. Animals can be housed under standard conditions, fed uniform purified diets, and, in essence, treated identically. Thus, it can be expected that the carcinogenic response would be more uniform in experimental animals than in humans. Nonetheless, cancer induction processes are very complex. Many chemical carcinogens undergo biochemical detoxication and need biochemical activation. The active forms of some carcinogens attack specific molecular and cellular receptors, especially DNA. Repair processes operate to limit key alterations. Cell duplication leads to a newly structured heritable genome, which is expressed as neoplastic behavior of the cell. Latent neoplastic cells must increase in number to form a tumor, a process that can be modulated considerably by host factors. All of these steps are, of course, strain and species dependent, and thus, the response to a given chemical carcinogen is a function of the experimental system. Humans are not uniform, and it is probably true that some people will respond some of the time to a given carcinogenic challenge. One of the key elements in the response of any species, including *Homo sapiens,* would appear to be the biochemical potential in activating or deactivating exogenous carcinogens. Promoting stimuli, stemming from elements such as the biosynthesis of cholesterol and bile acids, hormonal balances, immune competence, and endogenous viral profiles and intestinal flora, also are distinct as a function of species and strain. Nonetheless, with the curious exceptions of benzene and arsenic, all DNA-reactive carcinogens and promoting agents now known to play a role in human cancer causation have been reproduced reasonably well in animal models, provided the dose rate and time elements were taken into account. Thus, animal models do provide a basis for assessing human risk. The process, however, is complicated since collateral mechanistic information is essential to determining which animal model is predictive (Williams *et al.,* in Flamm and Lorentzen, 1985).

EPILOGUE

During the last decade, much progress had been made in the basic sciences underlying toxicology with specific reference to chronic effects, including carcinogenesis. Thus, we have come to realize that the great diversity of chemical structures capable of causing cancer depends for some on the specific property of such structures to be either electrophilic reactants or to become such after metabolic activation. At the same time, further insight into the molecular target of such carcinogens as electrophilic reactants implicates the genetic material in the cell—DNA. It has also been discovered that DNA with covalently bound carcinogens can be repaired and that some of the observed biologic effects, including organotropism, depend as much on such repair processes, or the lack thereof, as on the metabolic activation and interaction of intermediates with DNA.

The recognized interaction of some carcinogens with DNA has provided the necessary scientific background for relating mutagenicity to carcinogenicity. In turn, this connection has provided a sound basis for utilizing short-term tests measuring genotoxicity in the assessment of the carcinogenic potential of a chemical. In this chapter, we have organized chemical carcinogens as DNA-reactive agents, and as agents capable of inducing cancer through other mechanisms referred to as epigenetic. Inasmuch as current evidence shows that the carcinogenic properties of chemicals of these two categories differ, especially that most classes of epigenetic agents act in a reversible, highly dose-dependent fashion, attention needs to be directed toward developing distinct risk management procedures for different types of carcinogens. It is expected that further research on methods of detection in the light of the systematic classification described will provide a rational and scientific approach to the elimination of risk of potentially harmful substances. This is important inasmuch as there are sound data, with respect to the causes of the main human cancers, that they are due as much to the presence of agents operating via epigenetic mechanisms as to genotoxic carcinogens. For example, epigenetic agents play a major role in the development of cancer of the lung due to cigarette smoking, or of cancers of the colon, breast, prostate, and perhaps pancreas that are contributed to by certain dietary habits. Thus, some leads such as the lower risk of lung cancer after smoking cessation, or of endometrial cancer upon reduction in body weight or less use of estrogen, indicate that these major types of cancer can be controlled by modifying the environment not only with respect to DNA-reactive carcinogens but also with respect to epigenetic carcinogens. In fact, public health programs to decrease the habit of smoking, or to lower total dietary fat intake, actually depend on the property of reversibility of promotion.

Nowadays the public is much more aware of environmental cancer risks, and their concern has led to legislation and regulation at many levels. Public involvement has also provided increased resources in toxicology from both private and public funds, which have contributed to the base of knowledge. At the same time, however, the public, while concerned with cancer, is not well informed as to the actual risk factors. The facts and principles described in this chapter will hopefully not only assist professionals involved in toxicology and oncology, but can be translated into activities that will provide the public with better information and protection against avoidable cancer hazards.

REFERENCES

The references have been confined in the main to reviews or monographs so as to comply with editorial policy to limit the number of citations. Detailed references to the research literature can be found in the reports quoted. The reader is referred also to the continuing series below as source material.

Advances in Cancer Research
Methods in Cancer Research
Progress in Experimental Tumor Research
International Agency for Research on Cancer (IARC):
  Monograph and scientific publications series
National Cancer Institute Monographs
Proceedings, Symposium of the Princess Takamatsu Cancer Research Fund, Tokyo
Recent Results in Cancer Research (Springer-Verlag, Berlin)
Annual Review of Pharmacology and Toxicology

Adamson, R. H., and Sieber, S. M.: Chemically induced leukemia in humans. *Environ. Health Perspect.*, 39:93–103, 1981.
Adamson, R. H., and Sieber, S. M.: Chemical carcinogenesis studies in nonhuman primates. In Langenbach, R.; Nesnow, S.; and Rice, J. M. (eds.): *Organ and Species Specificity in Chemical Carcinogenesis.* Plenum Publishing Corp., New York, 1983, pp. 129–56.
American Cancer Society: *1986 Facts and Figures.* American Cancer Society, Inc., New York, 1986.
Ames, B. N.: Dietary carcinogens and anticarcinogens. *Science,* 221:1256–63, 1983.
Amo, H., and Matsuyama, M.: Subchronic and chronic effects of feeding of large amounts of acetaminophen in B6C3F1 mice. *Jpn. J. Hyg.* 40:567–74, 1985.
Anders, M. W. (ed.): *Bioactivation of Foreign Compounds.* Academic Press, New York, 1985.
Anderson, R. L.; Bishop, W. E.; and Campbell, R. L. A review of the environmental and mammalian toxicology of nitrilotriacetic acid. *CRC Crit. Rev. Toxicol.,* 15:1–102, 1985.
Arcos, J. C.: Criteria for selecting chemical compounds for carcinogenicity testing: an essay. *J. Env. Pathol. Toxicol.,* 1:433–58, 1978.
Arcos, J. C.; Woo, Y-T.; Argus, M. F.; and Lai, D. Y.: *Chemical Induction of Cancer,* Vols. I, IIA, IIB, IIIA, IIIB. Academic Press, Inc., New York, 1968–1985.
Arnold, D. L.; Krewski, D. R.; Junkins, D. B.; McGuire, P. F.; Moodie, C. A.; and Munro, I. C.: Reversibility of ethylenethiourea-induced thyroid lesions. *Toxicol. Appl. Pharmacol.,* 67:264–73, 1983.
Arp, E. W., Jr.; Wolf, P. H.; and Checkoway, H.: Lymphocytic leukemia and exposures to benzene and other solvents in the rubber industry. *J. Occup. Med.,* 25:598–602, 1983.
Ashby, J.; Lefevre, P. A.; and Callander, R. D.: The possible role of azoreduction in the bacterial mutagenicity of 4-dimethylaminoazobenzene (DAB) and 2 of its analogues (6BT and 5I). *Mutat. Res.,* 116:271–79, 1983.
Ashendel, C. L.; Staller, M. N.; and Boutwell, R. K.: Solubilization, purification, and reconstitution of a phorbol ester receptor from the particulate protein fraction of mouse brain. *Cancer Res.,* 43:4327–32, 1983.
Austin, D. F., and Roe, K. M.: The decreasing incidence of endometrial cancer: public health implications. *Am. J. Public Health,* 72:65–68, 1982.
Autrup, H., and Williams, G. M.: *Experimental Colon Carcinogenesis.* CRC Press, Boca Raton, Fl., 1983.
Barnes, W. A., Spingarn, N. E.; Garvie-Gould, C.; Vuolo, L. L.; Wang, Y. Y.; and Weisburger, J. H.: Mutagens in cooked foods: possible consequences of the Maillard reaction. In Waller G. R., and Feather, M. S. (eds.): *The Maillard Reaction in Foods and Nutrition.* ACS Symposium Series 215, American Chemical Society, Washington, D.C., 1983, pp. 485–506.
Barrows, L. R.: Methylation of DNA guanine via the 1-carbon pool in dimethylnitrosamine-treated rats. *Mutat. Res.,* 173:73–79, 1986.
Bartosek, I.; Guaitaini, A.; and Pacei, E. (eds.): *Animals in Toxicological Research.* Raven Press, New York, 1982.
Bartsch, H.; Armstrong, B.; and Davis, W. (eds.): *Host Factors in Human Carcinogenesis.* IARC Sci. Publ. 39. Internatl. Agency for Res. on Cancer, Lyon, 1982.
Becker, F. F. (ed.): *Cancer: A Comprehensive Treatise,* Vol. 1, 2nd ed. Plenum Publishing Corp., New York, 1982.
Berenblum, I.: *Carcinogenesis as a Biological Problem.* Frontiers of Biology, Vol. 34. North-Holland Publishing Co., Amsterdam, 1974.
Berlin, A.; Draper, M.; Hemminki, K.; et al. (eds.) *Monitoring Human Exposure to Carcinogenic and Mutagenic Agents,* IARC Sci. Publ. 59. Internatl. Agency for Res. on Cancer, Lyon, 1984.
Beauchene, R. E.; Bales, C. W.; Bragg, C. S.; Hawkins, S. T.; and Mason, R. L.: Effect of age of initiation of feed restriction on growth, body composition, and longevity of rats. *J. Gerontol.,* 41:13–19, 1986.
Bishop, J. M.: Viral oncogenes. *Cell,* 42:23–38, 1985.
Blumberg, B. S., and London, W. T.: Hepatitis B virus: pathogenesis and prevention of primary cancer of the liver. *Cancer,* 50:2657–65, 1982.
Boehm, T. L. J., and Drahovsky, D.: Alteration of enzymatic methylation of DNA cytosines by chemical carcinogens: a mechanism involved in the initiation of carcinogenesis. *J. Natl Cancer Inst.,* 71:429–33, 1983.
Bolcsak, L. E., and Nerland, D. E.: Inhibition of erythropoiesis by benzene and benzene metabolites. *Toxicol. Appl. Pharmacol.,* 69:363–68, 1983.
Boutwell, R. K.: Diet and anticarcinogenesis in the mouse skin two-stage model. *Cancer Res.,* 43:2465s–68s, 1983a.
————: Evidence that an elevated level of ornithine decarboxylase activity is an essential component of tumor promotion. *Adv. Polyamine Res.,* 4:127–34, 1983b.
Brada, Z.; Altman, N. H.; Hill, M.; and Bulba, S.: The effect of methionine on the progression of hepatocellulars carcinoma induced by ethionine. *Res. Commun. Chem. Pathol. Pharmacol.,* 38:157–60, 1982.
Brookes, P. (ed.): Chemical carcinogenesis. *Br. Med. Bull.,* 36:1–100, 1980.
Brown, J. P., and Dietrich, P. S.: Mutagenicity of selected sulfonated azo dyes in the *Salmonella*/microsome assay: use of aerobic and anaerobic activation procedures. *Mutat. Res.,* 116:305–15, 1983.
Bryan, G. T. (ed.): *Nitrofurans.* Raven Press, New York, 1978.
Bryan, W. R., and Shimkin, M. B.: Quantitative analysis of dose-response data obtained with three carcinogenic

hydrocarbons in strain C3H male mice. *J. Natl Cancer Inst.*, 3:503–31, 1943.

Bucciarelli, E.: Mammary tumor induction in male and female Sprague-Dawley rats by adriamycin and daunomycin. *J. Natl Cancer Inst.*, 66:81–84, 1981.

Butterworth, B. E.; Doolittle, D. J.; Working, P. K.; Strom, S. C.; Jirtle, R. L.; and Michalopoulos, G.: Chemically-induced DNA repair in rodent and human cells. *Banbury Rep.*, 13:101–14, 1982.

Cairns, J.: The origins of human cancer. *Nature*, 289:353–57, 1981.

Calder, I. C.; Goss, D. E.; Williams, P. J.; Funder, C. C.; Green, C. R.; Ham, K. N.; and Tange, J. D.: Neoplasia in the rat induced by *N*-hydroxy-phenacetin, a metabolite of phenacetin. *Pathology*, 8:1–6, 1976.

———: A decision tree approach to the regulation of food chemicals associated with irreversible toxicities. *Regul. Toxicol. Pharmacol.*, 1:193–201, 1981.

Cerniglia, C. E.; Freeman, J. P.; Franklin, W.; and Pack, L. D.: Metabolism of azo dyes derived from benzidine, 3,3'-dimethylbenzidene and 3,3'-dimethoxybenzidine to potentially carcinogenic aromatic amines by intestinal bacteria. *Carcinogenesis*, 3:1255–60, 1982.

Cerutti, P. A.: Prooxidant states and tumor promotion. *Science*, 227:375–81, 1985.

Chung, K-T.: The significance of azo-reduction in the mutagenesis and carcinogenesis of azo dyes. *Mutat. Res.*, 114:269–81, 1983.

Clary, J. J.; Gibson, J. E.; and Waritz, R. S. (eds.): *Formaldehyde: Toxicology, Epidemiology, Mechanisms*. Marcel Dekker, Inc., New York, 1983.

Claxton, L. D.: Characterization of automotive emissions by bacterial mutagenesis bioassay: a review. *Environ. Mutagenesis*, 5:609–31, 1983.

Clemmesen, J., and Hjalgrim-Jensen, S.: Is phenobarbital carcinogenic? A follow-up of 8078 epileptics. *Ecoltoxicol. Environ. Safety*, 1:457–70, 1978.

Cohen, A. J., and Grasso, P.: Review of the hepatic response to hypolipidaemic drugs in rodents and assessment of its toxicological significance to man. *Food. Cosmet. Toxicol.*, 19:585–605, 1981.

Combs, G. F., Jr., and Clark, L. C.: Can dietary selenium modify cancer risk? *Nutr. Rev.*, 43:325–31, 1985.

Conney, A. H.: Induction of microsomal enzymes by foreign chemicals and carcinogens by polycyclic aromatic hydrocarbons. *Cancer Res.*, 42:4875–4917, 1982.

Conning, D. M.; Magee, P.; Oesch, F.; and Clemmesen, J. (eds.): Quantitative aspects of risk assessment in chemical carcinogenesis. *Arch. Toxicol.*, Suppl. 3:1–330, 1980.

Cooke, M., and Dennis, J. J. (eds.): *Seventh International Symposium on Polynuclear Aromatic Hydrocarbons: Mechanisms, Methods and Metabolism*. Battelle Press, Columbus, Ohio, 1985.

Cornfield, J.: Carcinogenic risk assessment. *Science*, 198:693–99, 1977.

Correa, P.: Precursors of gastric and esophageal cancer. *Cancer*, 50:2554–65, 1982.

Cronkite, E. P.; Drew, R. T.; Inoue, T.; and Bullis, J. E.: Benzene hematotoxicity and leukemogenesis. *Am. J. Industr. Med.*, 7:447–56, 1985.

Dahl, A. R., and Hadley, W. M.: Formaldehyde production promoted by rat nasal cytochrome P-450-dependent monooxygenases with nasal decongestants, essences, solvents, air pollutants, nicotine, and cocaine as substrates. *Toxicol. Appl. Pharmacol.*, 67:200–205, 1983.

Dean, B. J.: Recent findings on the genetic toxicology of benzene, toluene, xylenes and phenols. *Mutat. Res.*, 154:153–81, 1985.

deBethizy, J. D.; Sherrill, J. M.; Rickert, D. E.; and Hamm, T. E., Jr.: Effects of pectin-containing diets on the hepatic macromolecular covalent binding of 2,6-dinitro-[³H]toluene in Fischer-344 rats. *Toxicol. Appl. Pharmacol.*, 69:369–76, 1983.

Degen, G. H.; Metzler, M.; and Sivarajah, K. S.: Co-oxidation of diethylstilbestrol and structural analogs by prostaglandin synthase. *Carcinogenesis*, 7:137–42, 1986.

Deichmann, W. B.: The chronic toxicity of organochlorine pesticides in man. In McKee, W. D. (ed.): *Environmental Problems in Medicine*. Charles C Thomas, Pub., Springfield, Ill., 1974, pp. 568–642.

DeMarini, D. M.: Genotoxicity of tobacco smoke and tobacco smoke condensate. *Mutat. Res.*, 114:59–89, 1983.

Doll, R.; Mathews, J. D.; and Morgan, L. G.: Cancers of the lung and nasal sinuses in nickel workers: a reassessment of the period of risk. *Br. J. Ind. Med.*, 34:102–105, 1977.

Drew, R. T.; Boorman, G. A.; Haseman, J. K.; McConnell, E. E.; Busey, W. M.; and Moore, J. A.: The effect of age and exposure duration on cancer induction by a known carcinogen in rats, mice, and hamsters. *Toxicol. Appl. Pharmacol.*, 68:120–30, 1983.

Druckrey, H: Quantitative aspects in chemical carcinogenesis. *UICC Monogr.*, 7:60–77, 1967.

Eckardt, R. K.: *Industrial Carcinogens*. Grune & Stratton, New York, 1959.

ED₀₁ Workshop Program: A report on the workshop on biological and statistical implications of the ED₀₁ study and related data bases. *Fund. Appl. Toxicol.*, 3:127–60, 1983.

Eder, E.; Henschler, D.; and Neudecker, T.: Mutagenic properties of allylic and α-β-unsaturated compounds: consideration of alkylating mechanisms. *Xenobiotica*, 12:831–48, 1982.

Eichhorn, G. L., and Marzilli, L. G. (eds.): *Metal Ions in Genetic Information Transfer*. Elsevier/North-Holland, New York, Amsterdam, 1981.

Elcombe, C. R.; Rose, M. S.; and Pratt, I. S.: Biochemical and histological changes in rat and mouse liver following the administration of trichloroethylene: possible relevance to species differences in hepatocarcinogenicity. *Toxicol. Appl. Pharmacol*, 79:365–76, 1985.

Eling, T.; Boyd, J.; Reed, G.; Mason, R.; and Sivarajah, K.: Xenobiotic metabolism by prostaglandin endoperoxide synthetase. *Drug Metab. Rev.*, 14:1023–53, 1983.

Essigmann, J. M.; Croy, R. G.; Bennett, R. A.; and Wogan, G. N.: Metabolic activation of aflatoxin B₁: patterns of DNA adduct formation, removal, and excretion in relation to carcinogenesis. *Drug Metab. Rev.*, 13:581–602, 1982.

Eustis, S. L., and Boorman, G. A.: Proliferative lesions of the exocrine pancreas: relationship to corn oil gavage in the National Toxicology Program. *J. Natl Cancer Inst.*, 75:1067–73, 1985.

Everson, R. B.; Randerath, E.; Santella, R. M.; Cefalo, R. C.; Avitts, T. H.; and Randerath, K.: Detection of smoking-related covalent DNA adducts in human placenta. *Science*, 231:54–57, 1986.

Fennell, T. R.; Wiseman, R. W.; Miller, J. A.; and Miller, E. C.: Major role of hepatic sulfotransferase activity in the metabolic activation, DNA adduct formation, and carcinogenicity of 1'-hydroxy 2',3'-dehydroestragole in infant male C57BL/6J × C3H/HeJF₁ mice. *Cancer Res.*, 45:5310–20, 1985.

Feron, V. J.; Kruysse, A.; and Woutersen, R. A.: Respiratory tract tumours in hamsters exposed to acetaldehyde vapour alone or simultaneously to benzo(a)pyrene or diethylnitrosamine. *Eur. J. Cancer Clin. Oncol.*, 18:13–31, 1982.

Fiala, E. S.; Caswell, N.; Sohn, O. S.; Felder, M. R.; McCoy, G. D.; and Weisburger, J. H.: Nonalcohol dehydrogenase-mediated metabolism of methylazoxymethanol in the deer mouse, *Peromyscus maniculatus*. *Cancer Res.*, 44:2885–91, 1984.

Fish, D. C.; Demarais, J. T.; Djurickovic, D. B.; and Huebner, R. J.: Prevention of 3-methylcholanthrene-induced fibrosarcomas in rats pre-inoculated with endogenous rat retrovirus. *Proc. Natl Acad. Sci. USA,* **78:**2526–27, 1981.

Flamm, W. G., and Lorentzen, R. J. (eds.): *Mechanisms and Toxicity of Chemical Carcinogens and Mutagens.* Princeton Sci Publ., Princeton, N.J., 1985.

Foulds, L.: *Neoplastic Development.* Academic Press, Inc., New York, 1969.

Fox, M., and Scott, D.: The genetic toxicology of nitrogen and sulphur mustard. *Mutat. Res.,* **75:**131–68, 1980.

Fox, P. G., and Watanabe, P. G.: Detection of a cellular oncogene in spontaneous liver tumors of B6C3F1 mice. *Science,* **228:**596–97, 1985.

Friberg, L., and Nelson, N. (eds.): Conference on the role of metals in carcinogenesis. *Environ. Health Perspect.,* **40:**1–252, 1981.

Fukushima, S.; Ishihara, Y.; Nishio, O.; Ogiso, T.; Shirai, T.; and Ito, N.: Carcinogenicities of quinoline derivatives in F344 rats. *Cancer Lett.,* **14:**115–23, 1981.

Furuya, K.; and Williams, G. M.: Neoplastic conversion in rat liver by the antihistamine methapyrilene demonstrated by a sequential syncarcinogenic effect with N-2-fluorenylacetamide. *Toxicol. Appl. Pharmacol.,* **74:**63–69, 1984.

Gaido, K. W., and Wierda, D.: Modulation of stromal cell function in DBA/2J and B6C3F1 mice exposed to benzene or phenol. *Toxicol. Appl. Pharmacol.,* **81:**469–75, 1985.

Garattini, S.; Mazue, G.; Roncucci, R.; and Williams, G. M. (eds.): *Quo Vadis? Short-Term Tests for Carcinogenesis.* Excerpta Medica, Amsterdam, 1983.

Geiger, L.; Hogy, L. L.; and Guengerich, F. P.: Metabolism of acrylonitrile by isolated rat hepatocytes. *Cancer Res.,* **43:**3080–87, 1983.

Gelboin, H.; MacMahon, B.; Matsushima, T.; Sugimura, T.; Takayama, S.; and Takebe, H.: *Genetic and Environmental Factors in Experimental and Human Cancer.* Jap. Sci. Soc. Press, Tokyo, 1980.

Goldworthy, T.; Campbell, H. A.; and Pitot, H. C.: The natural history and dose-response characteristics of enzyme-altered foci in rat liver following phenobarbital and diethylnitrosamine administration. *Carcinogenesis,* **5:**67–71, 1984.

Gombar, C. T.; Zubroff, J.; Strahan, G. D.; and Magee, P. N.: Measurement of 7-methylguanine as an estimate of the amount of dimethylnitrosamine formed following administration of aminopyrine and nitrite to rats. *Cancer Res.,* **43:**5077–80, 1983.

Goodman, D. G.; Ward, J. M.; and Reichardt, W. D.: Splenic fibrosis and sarcomas in F344 rats fed diets containing aniline hydrochloride, *p*-chloroaniline, azobenzene, *o*-toluidine hydrochloride, 4,4′-sulfonyldianiline, or D and C red No. 9. *J. Natl. Cancer Inst.,* **73:**265–70, 1984.

Griffin, A. C., and Shaw, C. R.: *Carcinogens: Identification and Mechanisms of Action.* Raven Press, New York, 1979.

Gross, L.: *Oncogenic Viruses,* 3rd ed. Pergamon Press, New York, 1981.

Gupta, R. C.; Reddy, M. V.; and Randerath, K.: ^{32}P-postlabeling analysis of non-radioactive aromatic carcinogen—DNA adducts. *Carcinogenesis,* **3:**1081–92, 1982.

Guzelian, P. S. Comparative toxicology of chlordecone (Kepone) in humans and experimental animals. *Ann. Rev. Pharmacol.,* **22:**89–113, 1982.

Hagan, E. C.; Jenner, P. M.; Jones, W. I.; Fitzhugh, O. G.; Long, E. L.; Brouwer, J. G.; and Webb, W. K.: Toxic properties of compounds related to safrole. *Toxicol. Appl. Pharmacol.,* **7:**18–24, 1965.

Halperin, W. E.; Goodman, M.; Stayner, L.; Elliott, L. J.; Keenlyside, R. A.; and Landrigan, P. J.: Nasal cancer in a worker exposed to formaldehyde. *JAMA,* **249:**510–12, 1983.

Hansen, K., and Stern, R. M. A survey of metal-induced mutagenicity *in vitro* and *in vivo. J. Am. Coll. Toxicol.* **3:**381–430, 1984.

Harris, C. C., and Autrup, H. (eds.): *Human Carcinogenesis.* Academic Press, Inc., New York, 1983.

Hathway, D. E.: *Foreign Compound Metabolism in Mammals,* Vol. 6, *A Specialist Periodical Report.* The Royal Society of Chemistry, London, 1981. (See also previous volumes in this series.)

Haugen, A.; Groopman, J. D.; Hsu, I-C.; Goodrich, G. R.; Wogan, G. N.; and Harris, C. C.: Monoclonal antibody to aflatoxin B_1-modified DNA detected by enzyme immunoassay. *Proc. Natl Acad. Sci. USA,* **78:**4124–27, 1981.

Hayes, W. J., Jr.: *Pesticides Studied in Man.* Williams & Wilkins, Baltimore, 1982.

Hayes, A. W., and the SOT Technical Committee: Correlation of human hepatotoxicants with hepatic damage in animals. *Fund. Appl. Toxicol.,* **2:**55–66, 1982.

Heck, J. D., and Costa, M: *In vitro* assessment of the toxicity of metal compounds. II. Mutagenesis. *Biol. Trace Element Res.,* **4:**319–30, 1982.

Hecker, E.; Fusenig, N. E.; Kunz, W.; Marks, F.; and Thielmann, H. W. (eds.): *Cocarcinogenesis and Biological Effects of Tumor Promoters,* Vol. 7, *Carcinogenesis—A Comprehensive Survey.* Raven Press, New York, 1982.

Heidelberger, C.; Freeman, A. E.; Pienta, R. J.; Sivak, A.; Bertram, J. S.; Casto, B. C.; Dunkel, V. C.; Francis, M. W.; Kakunaga, T.; Little, J. B.; and Schechtman, L. M.: Cell transformation by chemical agents—a review and analysis of the literature. *Mutat. Res.,* **114:**283–385, 1983.

Hemminki, K.: Nucleic acid adducts of chemical carcinogens and mutagens. *Arch. Toxicol.,* **52:**249–85, 1983.

Hewitt, W. R.; Miyajima, H.; Cote, M. G.; Hewitt, L. A.; Cianflone, D. J.; and Plaa, G. L.: Dose-response relationships in 1,3-butanediol-induced potentiation of carbon tetrachloride toxicity. *Toxicol. Appl. Pharmacol.,* **64:**529–40, 1982.

Hicks, R. M.; Wright, R.; and Wakefield, J. St. J.: The induction of rat bladder cancer by 2-naphthylamine. *Br. J. Cancer,* **46:**646–50, 1982.

Hiraga, K., and Fujii, T.: Carcinogenicity testing of acetaminophen in F344 rats. *Jpn. J. Cancer Res. (Gann),* **76:**79–85, 1985.

Hirose, M.; Lee M.-S.; Wang, C. Y.; and King, C. M.: Induction of rat mammary gland tumors by 1-nitropyrene, a recently recognized environmental mutagen. *Cancer Res.,* **44:**1158–62, 1984.

Hoel, D. G.; Merrill, R. A.; and Perera, F. P. (eds.): *Risk Quantitation and Regulatory Policy, Banbury Rept. 19.* Cold Spring Harbor Lab., Cold Spring Harbor, N.Y., 1985.

Hoffmann, D., and Hecht, S. S.: Nicotine-derived *N*-nitrosamines and tobacco-related cancer: current status and future directions. *Cancer Res.,* **45:**935–44, 1985.

Hoffmann, D.; Hecht, S. S.; and Wynder, E. L.: Tumor promoters and cocarcinogens in tobacco carcinogenesis. *Environ. Health Perspect.,* **50:**247–57, 1983b.

Hoffmann, D.; Wynder, E. L.; Rivenson, A.; LaVoie, E. J.; and Hecht, S. S.: Skin bioassays in tobacco carcinogenesis. *Prog. Exp. Tumor Res.,* **26:**43–67, 1983a.

Hoffmann, G. R.: Genetic effects of dimethyl sulfate, diethyl sulfate, and related compounds. *Mutat. Res.,* **75:**63–129, 1980.

Hollaender, A. (eds.): *Chemical Mutagens, Principles, and Methods for their Detection.* Plenum Press, New York, 1971–1983.

Holmberg, B., and Ahlborg, U. (eds.): Consensus report: mutagenicity and carcinogenicity of car exhausts and coal combustion emissions. *Environ. Health Perspect.,* **47:**1–30, 1983.

Homburger, F. (ed.): *Skin Painting Techniques and In*

Vivo *Carcinogenesis Bioassays.* Progr. in Exper. Tumor Res. Vol. 26. Karger, Basel, 1983.

Hoover, R., and Fraumeni, J. F., Jr.: Drug-induced cancer. *Cancer,* **47**:1071–80, 1981.

Huff, J. E.: 1,2-Dibromo-3-chloropropane. *Environ. Health Perspect.,* **47**:365–69, 1983.

IARC Monographs, Supplement 4: *Evaluation of the Carcinogenic Risk of Chemicals to Humans.* Internatl. Agency for Res. on Cancer (WHO), Lyon, France, October, 1982.

IARC Monograph series, Vol. 1–38: *Evaluation of the Carcinogenic Risk of Chemicals to Humans.* Internatl. Agency for Res. on Cancer (WHO), Lyon, France, 1972–1985.

IARC Scientific Publications, Vol. 1–68: Internatl. Agency for Res. on Cancer (WHO), Lyon, France, 1971–1985.

Iguchi, T.; Takase, M.; and Takasugi, N.: Development of vaginal adenosis-like lesions and uterine epithelial stratification in mice exposed perinatally to diethylstilbestrol (422224). *Proc. Soc. Exp. Biol. Med.,* **181**:59–64, 1986.

International Commission for Protection Against Environmental Mutagens and Carcinogens (ICPEMC): Report of ICPEMC Task Group on the differentiation between genotoxic and non-genotoxic carcinogens. *Mutat. Res.,* **133**:1–49, 1984.

International Symposium: Threshold doses in chemical carcinogenesis. *Oncology,* **33**:49–100, 1976.

Isaka, H.; Yoshii, H.; Otsuji, A.; Koike, M.; Nagai, Y.; Koura, M.; Sugiyasu, K.; and Kanabayashi, T.: Tumors of Sprague-Dawley rats induced by long-term feeding of phenacetin. *Gann,* **70**:29–36, 1979.

Ito, N.; Fukushima, S.; Hagiwara, A.; Shibata, M.; and Ogiso, T.: Carcinogenicity of butylated hydroxyanisole in F344 rats. *J. Natl Cancer Inst.,* **70**:343–52, 1983.

Iversen, U. M., and Iversen, O. H.: The carcinogenic effect of TPA (12-0-tetradecanoylphorbol-13-acetate) when applied to the skin of hairless mice. *Virchows Arch.,* **30**:33–42, 1979.

Jakoby, W. B. (ed.): *Metabolic Basic of Detoxication: Metabolism of Functional Groups.* Academic Press, New York, 1984.

Jensen, D. E.: Denitrosation as a determinant of nitrosocimetidine *in vivo* activity. *Cancer Res.,* **43**:5258–67, 1983.

Jensen, R. K.; Sleight, S. D.; Goodman, J. I.; Aust, S. D.; and Trosko, J. E.: Polybrominated biphenyls as promoters in experimental hepatocarcinogenesis in rats. *Carcinogenesis,* **3**:1183–86, 1982.

Kadlubar, F. F., and Beland, F. A. (eds.): Second internatl. conference on carcinogenic and mutagenic N-substituted aryl compounds. *Environ. Health Perspect.,* **49**:1–232, 1983.

Kato, R.; Kamataki, T.; and Yamazoe, Y.: N-hydroxylation of carcinogenic and mutagenic aromatic amines. *Environ. Health Perspect.,* **49**:21–25, 1983.

Kimbrough, R. D. (ed.): *Halogenated Biphenyls, Terphenyls, Naphthalenes, Dibenzodioxins and Related Products,* Vol. 4. Elsevier/North Holland, Amsterdam, New York, 1983.

Kinsella, A. R., and Radman, M.: Tumor promoter induces sister chromatid exchanges: Relevance to mechanisms of carcinogenesis. *Proc. Natl Acad. Sci. USA,* **75**:6149–53, 1978.

Kirschman, J. C.; Brown, N. M.; Coots, R. H.; and Morgareidge, K.: Review of investigations of dichloromethane metabolism and subchronic oral toxicity as the basis for design of chronic oral studies in rats and mice. *Food Chem. Toxicol.,* in press, 1986.

Kluwe, W. M.; Huff, J. E.; Matthews, H. B.; Irwin, R.; and Haseman, J. K.: Comparative chronic toxicities and carcinogenic potentials of 2-ethylhexyl-containing compounds in rats and mice. *Carcinogenesis,* **6**:1577–83, 1985.

Knudsen, I. (ed.): *Genetic Toxicology of the Diet. Progress in Clinical and Biological Research,* Vol. 206. Alan R. Liss, Inc., New York, 1986.

Kraybill, H. F., and Mehlman, M. A. (eds.): *Environmental Cancer,* Vol. 3. Halsted Press, New York, 1977.

Kushner, L. M.; Butcher, A. M.; Pienta, R.; and Russell, S.: *The Application of Decision Theory to Toxicological Testing Requirements Under FIFRA.* The Mitre Corp., McLean, Va., 1982.

Laib, R. J.: Specific covalent binding and toxicity of aliphatic halogenated xenobiotics. *Rev. Drug Metab. Drug Interact.,* **4**:2–48, 1982.

Lambeir, A.-M.; Markey, C. M.; Dunford, H. B.; and Marnett, L. J.: Spectral properties of the higher oxidation states of prostaglandin H synthase. *J. Biol. Chem.,* **260**:14894–96, 1985.

Lambelin, G.; Roba, J.; Roncucci, R.; and Parmentier, R.: Carcinogenicity of 6-aminochrysene in mice. *Eur. J. Cancer,* **11**:327–34, 1975.

Land, H.; Parada, L. F.; and Weinberg, R. A.: Cellular oncogenes and multistep carcinogenesis. *Science,* **222**:771–78, 1983.

Langenbach, R.; Nesnow, S.; and Rice, J. M.: *Organ and Species Specificity in Chemical Carcinogenesis.* Plenum Press, New York, 1983.

LaVoie, E. J.; Adams, E. A.; Shigematsu, A.; and Hoffmann, D.: On the metabolism of quinoline and isoquinoline: possible molecular basis for differences in biological activities. *Carcinogenesis,* **4**:1169–73, 1983a.

LaVoie, E. J.; Adams, E. A.; and Hoffmann, D.: Identification of the metabolites of benzo(f)quinoline and benzo(h)quinoline formed by rat liver homogenate. *Carcinogenesis,* **4**:1133–38, 1983b.

LaVoie, E. J.; Bedenko, V.; Tulley-Freiler, L.; and Hoffman, D.: Tumor-initiating activity and metabolism of polymethylated phenanthrenes. *Cancer Res.,* **42**:4045–49, 1982a.

LaVoie, E. J.; Hecht, S. S.; Bedenko, V.; and Hoffmann, D.: Identification of the mutagenic metabolites of fluoranthene, 2-methylfluoranthene, and 3-methylfluoranthene. *Carcinogenesis,* **3**:841–46, 1982b.

Lee, K. P., and Trochimowicz, H. J.: Induction of nasal tumors in rats exposed to hexamethylphosphoramide by inhalation. *J. Natl Cancer Inst.,* **68**:157–64, 1982.

Leonard, A., and Lauwerys, R. R.: Carcinogenicity, teratogenicity and mutagenicity of arsenic. *Mutat. Res.,* **75**:49–62, 1980.

Leonard, B. J. (ed.): Toxicologic aspects of food safety. *Arch. Toxicol.,* Suppl. 1:1–200, 1978.

Leonard, T. B.; Lyght, O.; and Popp, J. A.: Dinitrotoluene structure-dependent initiation of hepatocytes *in vivo. Carcinogenesis,* **4**:1059–61, 1983.

Leopold, W. R.; Miller, J. A.; and Miller, E. C.: Comparison of some carcinogenic, mutagenic, and biochemical properties of S-vinylhomocysteine and ethionine. *Cancer Res.,* **42**:4364–74, 1982.

Leopold, W. R.; Batzinger, R. P.; Miller, E. C.; Miller, J. A.; and Earhart, R. H.: Mutagenicity, tumorigenicity, and electrophilic reactivity of the stereoisomeric platinum(II) complexes of 1,2-diaminocyclohexane. *Cancer Res.,* **41**:4368–77, 1981.

Lewis, T. R.; Ulrich, C. E.; and Busey, W. M.: Subchronic inhalation toxicity of nitromethane and 2-nitropropane. *J. Environ. Pathol. Toxicol.,* **2**:233–49, 1979.

Lieber, C. S.: Ethanol metabolism and toxicity. In Hodgson, E.; Bend, J. R.; and Philpot, R. M. (eds.): *Reviews in Biochemical Toxicology,* Vol. 5, Elsevier, New York, 1983, pp. 267–312.

Lijinsky, W.; Reuber, M. D.; and Riggs, C. W.: Dose response studies of carcinogenesis in rats by nitrosodiethylamine. *Cancer Res.,* **41**:4997–5003, 1981.

Littlefield, L. A.; Farmer, J. H.; Sheldon, W. G.; and Gaylor, D. W.: Effects of dose and time in a long-term, low-dose carcinogenic study. *J. Environ. Pathol. Toxicol.*, 33:17, 1979.

Loehrke, H.; Schweizer, J.; Dederer, E.; Hesse, B.; Rosenkranz, G.; and Goerttler, K.: On the persistence of tumor initiation in two-stage carcinogenesis on mouse skin. *Carcinogenesis*, 4:771–75, 1983.

Long, E. L.; Nelson, A. A.; Fitzhugh, O. G.; and Hansen, W. H.: Liver tumors produced in rats by feeding safrole. *Arch. Pathol.*, 75:595–604, 1963.

Longnecker, D. S.: Carcinogenesis in the pancreas. *Arch. Pathol. Lab. Med.*, 107:54–58, 1983.

Maeura, Y., and Williams, G. M.: Enhancing effect of butylated hydroxytoluene on the development of liver altered foci and neoplasms induced by N-2-fluorenylacetamide in rats. *Food Chem. Toxicol.*, 22:211–15, 1984.

Magee, P. (ed.): *Nitrosamines and Human Cancer*. Banbury Rept. 12. Cold Spring Harbor Lab., Cold Spring Harbor, N.Y., 1982.

Maltoni, C.; Conti, B.; Cotti, G.; and Belpoggi, F.: Experimental studies on benzene carcinogenicity at the Bologna Institute of Oncology: current results and on-going research. *Am. J. Industr. Med.*, 7:415–46, 1985.

Maltoni, C.; Lefemine, G.; Cotti, G.; Chieco, P.; and Patella, V.: *Experimental Research on Vinylidene Chloride Carcinogenesis. Archives of Research on Industrial Carcinogenesis*, Vol. III. Princeton, Sci, Publ., Princeton, N.J., 1985.

Marnett, L. J., and Eling, T. E.: Cooxidation during prostaglandin biosynthesis: a pathway for the metabolic activation of xenobiotics. In Hodgson, E.; Bend, J. R.; and Philpot, R. M. (eds.): *Reviews in Biochemical Toxicology*, Vol. 5. Elsevier, New York, 1983, pp. 135–72.

Maron, D. M., and Ames, B. N. Revised methods for the *Salmonella* mutagenicity test. *Mutat. Res.*, 113:173–215, 1983.

McCallum, R. I.; Woolley, V.; and Petrie, A.: Lung cancer associated with chloromethyl methyl ether manufacture: an investigation at two factories in the United Kingdom. *Br. J. Ind. Med.*, 40:384–89, 1983.

McCoy, E.; De Marco, G.; Rosenkranz, E. J.; Anders, M.; Rosenkranz, H. S.; and Mermelstein, R.: 5-Nitroacenaphthene: a newly recognized role for the nitro function in mutagenicity. *Environ. Mutagen.*, 5:17–22, 1983.

McCoy, G. D.; Hecht, S. S.; Katayama, S.; and Wynder, E. L.: Differential effect of chronic ethanol consumption on the carcinogenicity of N-nitrosopyrrolidine and N'-nitrosonornicotine in male Syrian golden hamsters. *Cancer Res.*, 41:2849–54, 1981.

Metzler, M.: Diethylstilbestrol: reactive metabolites derived from a hormonally active compound. In Greim, H.; Jung, R.; Kramer, M.; Marquardt, H.; and Oesch, F. (eds.): *Biochemical Basis of Chemical Carcinogenesis*. Raven Press, New York, 1984, pp. 69–75.

Meyer, A. L.: *In vitro* transformation assays for chemical carcinogens. *Mutat. Res.*, 115:323–38, 1983.

Miller, E. C.; Miller, J. A.; Hirono, I.; Sugimura, T.; and Takayama, S. (eds.): *Naturally Occurring Carcinogens-Mutagens and Modulators of Carcinogenesis*. Japan Sci. Soc. Press, Tokyo; University Park Press, Baltimore, 1979.

Miller, E. C., and Miller, J. A.: Mechanisms of chemical carcinogenesis. *Cancer*, 47:1055–64, 1981.

Miller, J. A., and Miller, E. C.: The metabolic activation and nucleic acid adducts of naturally-occurring carcinogens: recent results with ethyl carbamate and the spice flavors safrole and estragole. *Br. J. Cancer*, 48:1–15, 1983.

Miller, R. E., and Guengerich, F. P.: Metabolism of trichloroethylene in isolated hepatocytes, microsomes, and reconstituted enzyme systems containing cytochrome P-450. *Cancer Res.*, 43:1145–52, 1983.

Milman, H. A., and Weisburger, E. K. (eds.): *Handbook of Carcinogen Testing*. Noyes Publ., Park Ridge, N.J., 1985.

Mirvish, S. S.: The etiology of gastric cancer. *J. Natl Cancer Inst.*, 71:631–47, 1983.

Mishra, N.; Dunkel, V.; and Mehlman, M. (eds.): *Advances in Modern Environmental Toxicology*. Vol. 1, *Mamammalian Cell Transformation by Chemical Carcinogens*. Senate Press, Inc., N.J., 1980.

Miwa, M.; Nishimura, S.; Rich, A.; Söll; and Sugimura, T. (eds.): *Primary and Tertiary Structure of Nucleic Acids and Cancer Research*. Japan Sci. Soc. Press, Tokyo, 1982.

Mochizuki, Y.; Furukawa, K.; and Sawada, N.: Effects of various concentrations of ethyl-α-p-chlorophenoxyisobutyrate (clofibrate) on diethylnitrosamine-induced hepatic tumorigenesis in the rat. *Carcinogenesis*, 3:1027–29, 1982.

Monnat, R. J., Jr., and Loeb, L. A.: Mechanisms of neoplastic transformation. *Cancer Invest.*, 1:175–83, 1983.

Moon, R. C.; McCormick, D. L.; and Mehta, R. G.: Inhibition of carcinogenesis by retinoids. *Cancer Res.*, 43:2469s–75s, 1983.

Moore, D. H.; Chasseaud, L. F.; Majeed, S. K.; Prentice, D. E.; and Roe, F. J. C.: The effect of dose and vehicle on early tissue damage and regenerative activity after chloroform administration to mice. *Food Chem. Toxicol.*, 20:951–54, 1982.

Morgan, W. F., and Cleaver, J. E.: Effect of 3-aminobenzamide on the rate of ligation during repair of alkylated DNA in human fibroblasts. *Cancer Res.*, 43:3104–3107, 1983.

Moriya, M.; Ohta, T.; Watanabe, K.; Miyazawa, T.; Kato, K.; and Shirasu, Y.: Further mutagenicity studies on pesticides in bacterial reversion assay systems. *Mutat. Res.*, 116:185–216, 1983.

Morton, K. C.; King, C. M.; Vaught, J. B.; Wang, C. Y.; Lee, M. S.; and Marnett, L. J.: Prostaglandin H synthase-mediated reaction of carcinogenic arylamines with tRNA and homopolyribonucleotides. *Biochem. Biophys. Res. Commun.*, 3:96–103, 1983.

Mossman, R.; Light, W.; and Wei, E.: Asbestos: mechanisms of toxicity and carcinogenicity in the respiratory tract. *Ann. Rev. Pharmacol. Toxicol.*, 23:595–615, 1983.

Müller, R., and Rajewsky, M. F.: Elimination of O^6-ethylguanine from the DNA of brain, liver, and other rat tissues exposed to ethylnitrosourea at different stages of prenatal development. *Cancer Res.*, 43:2897–2904, 1983.

Nakahara, W.: *Chemical Tumor Problems*. Japanese Society for Promotion of Science, Tokyo, 1970.

Nakanishi, K.; Hagiwara, A.; Shibata, M.; Imaida, K.; Tatematsu, M.; and Ito, N.: Dose response of saccharin in induction of urinary bladder hyperplasias in Fischer 344 rats pretreated with N-butyl-n-(4-hydroxybutyl)nitrosamine. *J. Natl Cancer Inst.*, 65:1005–10, 1980.

Nakanishi, K.; Kurata, Y.; Oshima, M.; Fukushima, S.; and Ito, N. Carcinogenicity of phenacetin: long-term feeding study in B6C3F₁ mice. *Int. J. Cancer*, 29:439–44, 1982.

National Research Council, National Academy of Science (NRC/NAS): *Diet, Nutrition, and Cancer*. National Academy Press, Washington, D.C., 1982.

National Toxicology Program: *Technical Report on the Toxicology and Carcinogenesis Studies of Dichloromethane (Methylene Chloride) in F344/N rats and B6C3F1 Mice*. NIH Publ. (Bethesda,) 1986.

Neal, R. A., and Halpert, J.: Toxicology of thiono-sulfur compounds. *Ann. Rev. Pharmacol. Toxicol.*, 22:321–39, 1982.

Nebert, D. W.; Kimura, S.; and Gonzalez, F. J.: In Boobis, A.; Caldwell, J.; and Davies, D., (eds.): *Microsomes and Drug Oxidations*. Taylor and Francis Ltd, London, 1985.

Nelson, S. D.; Nelson, W. L.; and Trager, W. F.: *N*-hydroxyamide metabolites of lidocaine, synthesis, characterization, quantitation and mutagenic potential. *J. Med. Chem.*, 21:721–25, 1978.

Nettesheim, P.; Topping, D. C.; and Jamasbi, R.: Host and environmental factors enhancing carcinogenesis in the respiratory tract. *Ann. Rev. Pharmacol. Toxicol.*, 21:133–63, 1981.

Nohmi, T.; Yoshikawa, K.; Nakadate, M.; Miyata, R.; and Ishidate, M., Jr.: Mutations in *Salmonella typhimurium* and inactivation of bacillus subtilis transforming DNA induced by phenylhydroxylamine derivatives. *Mutat. Res.*, 136:159–68, 1984.

Nony, C. R.; Althaus, J. R.; and Bowman, M. C.: Chromatographic assays for traces of potentially carcinogenic metabolites of two azo dyes, direct red 2 and direct blue 15, in rat, hamster and human urine. *J. Analyt. Toxicol.*, 7:40–48, 1983.

Numoto, S.; Mori, H.; Furuya, K.; Levine, W. G.; and Williams, G. M.: Absence of a promoting or sequential syncarcinogenic effect in the rat liver by the hypolipidemic drug nafenopin given after *N*-2-fluorenylacetamide. *Toxicol. Appl. Pharmacol.*, 77:76–85, 1985.

Nunziata, A., and Storino, A. A.: Spontaneous neoplastic pathology in control rats—a review. *Vet. Hum. Toxicol.*, 24:243–47, 1982.

Nyce, J.; Weinhouse, S.; and Magee, P. N.: 5-Methylcytosine depletion during tumour development: an extension of the miscoding concept. *Br. J. Cancer*, 48:463–75, 1983.

Odashima, S.; Takayama, S.; and Sato, H. (eds.): *Recent Topics in Chemical Carcinogenesis*. GANN Monogr. 17, University Park Press, Baltimore, 1975.

Oesch, F.: Influence of foreign compounds on formation and disposition of reactive metabolites. In Ciba Fnd. Symp. 73: *Environmental Chemicals, Enzyme Function and Human Disease*. Excerpta Medica, Amsterdam/New York, 1980, pp. 169–189.

Oesch, F.; Protic-Sabljic, M.; Friedberg, T.; Kimisch, H. J.; and Glatt, H. R.: Vinylidene chloride: changes in drug-metabolizing enzymes, mutagenicity and relation to its targets for carcinogenesis. *Carcinogenesis*, 4:1031–38, 1983.

Office of Technology Assessment: *Cancer Risk: Assessing and Reducing the Dangers in our Society*. Westview Press, USA, 1982.

Olsen, P.; Bille, N.; and Meyer, O.: Hepatocellular neoplasms in rats induced by butylated hydroxytoluene (BHT). *Acta Pharmacol. Toxicol.*, 53:433–34, 1983.

Omata, M.; Uchiumi, K.; Ito, Y.; Yokosuka, O.; Mori, J.; Terao, K.; Wei-Fa, Y.; O'Connell, A. P.; London, W. T.; and Okuda, K.: Duck hepatitis B virus and liver diseases. *Gastroenterology*, 85:260–67, 1983.

O'Neill, I. K.; Von Borstel, R. C.; Miller, C. T.; Long, J.; and Bartsch, H.: *N-Nitroso Compounds: Occurrence, Biological Effects and Relevance to Human Cancer*. IARC Sci. Publ. 57. Internatl. Agency for Research on Cancer, Lyon, 1984.

Park, S. D.; Kim, C. G.; and Kim, M. G.: Inhibitors of poly(ADP-ribose) polymerase enhance DNA strand breaks, excision repair, and sister chromatid exchanges induced by alkylating agents. *Environ. Mutagen.*, 5:515–25, 1983.

Parke, D. V., and Ioannides, C.: The role of nutrition in toxicology. *Ann. Rev. Nutr.*, 1:207–34, 1981.

Pegg, A. E.; Dolan, M. E.; Scicchitano, D.; and Morimoto, K.: Studies of the repair of O^6-alkylguanine and O^4-alkylthymine in DNA by alkyltransferases from mammalian cells and bacteria. *Environ. Health Perspect.*, 62:109–14, 1985.

Pereira, M. A. (ed.): International symposium on tumor promotion. *Environ. Health Perspect.*, 50:3–370, 1983.

Pereira, M. A.; Lin, L-H. C.; Lippitt, J. M.; and Herren, S. L.: Trihalomethanes as initiators and promoters of carcinogenesis. *Environ. Health Perspect.*, 46:151–56, 1982.

Phillips, D. H.: Fifty years of benzo(a)pyrene. *Nature*, 303:468–72, 1983.

Piper, J. M.; Tonascia, J.; and Matanoski, G. M.: Heavy phenacetin use and bladder cancer in women aged 20 to 49 years. *N. Engl. J. Med.*, 313:292–95, 1985.

Pitot, H. C.: The natural history of noeplastic development: the relation of experimental models to human cancer. *Cancer*, 49:1206–11, 1982.

Pitot, H. C., and Sirica, A. E.: The stages of initiation and promotion in hepatocarcinogenesis. *Biochim. Biophys. Acta*, 605:191–215, 1980.

Poellinger, L.; Kurl, R. N.; Lund, J.; Gillner, M.; Carlstedt-Duke, J.; Högberg, B.; and Gustafsson, J.-A.: High-affinity binding of 2,3,7,8-tetrachlorodibenzo-*p*-dioxin in cell nuclei from rat liver. *Biochim. Biophys. Acta*, 714:516–23, 1982.

Poirier, M. C.; Nakayama, J.; Perera, F. P.; Weinstein, I. B.; and Yuspa, S. H.: Identification of carcinogen-DNA adducts by immunoassays. In Milman, H. A., and Sell, S. (eds.): *Application of Biological Markers to Carcinogen Testing*. Plenum Press, New York, 1983; pp. 427–40.

Poland, A., and Kimbrough, D. (eds.): *Biological Mechanisms of Bioxin Action. Banbury Rep. 18*. Cold Spring Harbor Lab., Cold Spring Harbor, N.Y., 1986.

Poland, A., and Knutson, J. C.: 2,3,7,8-Tetrachlorodibenzo-*p*-dioxin and related halogenated aromatic hydrocarbons: examination of the mechanism of toxicity. *Ann Rev. Pharmacol.*, 22:517–54, 1982.

Pottathil, R.; Huebner, R. J.; and Meier, H.: Suppression of chemical (DEN) carcinogenesis in SWR/J mice by goat antibodies against endogenous murine leukemia viruses. *Proc. Soc. Exp. Biol. Med.*, 159:65–68, 1978.

Prochaska, H. J.; De Long, M. J.; and Talalay, P.: On the mechanisms of induction of cancer-protective enzymes: a unifying proposal. *Proc. Natl. Acad. Sci.*, 82:8232–36, 1985.

Ramel, C.; Lambert, B.; and Magnusson, J. (eds.): *Genetic Toxicology of Environmental Chemicals*. Alan R. Liss, New York, 1986.

Reddy, B. S.; Cohen, L. A.; McCoy, G. D.; Hill, P.; Weisburger, J. H.; and Wynder, E. L.: Nutrition and its relationship to cancer. *Adv. Cancer Res.*, 32:237–345, 1980.

Reddy, J. K., and Lalwani, N. D.: Carcinogenesis by hepatic peroxisome proliferators: evaluation of the risk of hypolipidemic drugs and industrial plasticizers to humans. *CRC Crit. Rev. Toxicol.*, 12:1–58, 1983.

Reddy, M. V.; Gupta, R. C.; Randerath, E.; and Randerath, K.: Postlabeling test for covalent DNA binding of chemicals in vivo: application to a variety of aromatic carcinogens and methylating agents. *Carcinogenesis*, 5:231–43, 1984.

Reiss, B.; Tong, C.; Telang, S.; and Williams, G. M.: Enhancement of benzo(a)pyrene mutagenicity by chrysotile asbestos in rat liver epithelial cells. *Environ. Res.*, 31:100–104, 1983.

Reynolds, S. H.; Stowers, S. J.; Maronpot, R. R.; Anderson, M. W.; and Aaronson, S. A.: Detection and identification of activated oncogenes in spontaneously occurring benign and malignant hepatocellular tumors of the B6C3F1 mouse. *Proc. Natl Acad. Sci. USA*, 83:33–37, 1986.

Reznik-Schüller, H. M., and Lijinsky, W.: Ultrastructural changes in the liver of animals treated with methapyrilene and some analogs. *Ecotoxicol. Environ. Safety*, 6:328–35, 1982.

Rice, J. M. (ed.): *Perinatal Carcinogenesis*, NCI Monogr. 51. DHEW Publ. No. (NIH) 79-1622. U.S. Government Printing Office, Washington, D.C., 1979.

Richmond, C. R.; Walsh, P. J.; and Copenhaver, E. D. (eds.): *Health Risk Analysis*. Franklin Institute Press, Philadelphia, 1980.

Robboy, S. J.: A hypothetic mechanism of diethylstilbestrol[DES]-induced anomalies in exposed progeny. *Hum. Pathol.*, **14**:831–33, 1983.

Robens, J. F.; Joiner, J. J.; and Schueler, R. L.: Methods in testing for carcinogenicity. In Hayes, A. W. (ed.): *Principles and Methods of Toxicology.* Raven Press, New York, 1982, pp. 79–105.

Roe, F. J. C.: Testing for carcinogenicity and the problem of pseudocarcinogenicity. *Nature,* **303**:657–58, 1983.

Roebuck, B. D.; Siegel, W. G.; and Wogan, G. N.: *In vitro* metabolism of aflatoxin B_2 by animal and human liver. *Cancer Res.,* **38**:999–1002, 1978.

Rogers, A. E.: Influence of dietary content of lipids and lipotropic nutrients on chemical carcinogenesis in rats. *Cancer Res.,* **43**:2477s–84s, 1983.

Rose, D. P. (ed.): *Endocrinology of Cancer,* Vols. I–III. CRC Press, Boca Raton, Fl., 1979–1982.

Rosenkranz, H. S., and Mermelstein, R.: Mutagenicity and genotoxicity of nitroarenes: All nitro-containing chemicals were not created equal. *Mutat. Res.,* **114**:217–67, 1983.

Ross, D.; Mehlhorn, R. J.; Moldeus, P.; and Smith, M. T.: Metabolism of diethylstilbestrol by horseradish peroxidase and prostaglandin-H synthase. *J. Biol. Chem.,* **260**:16210–14, 1985.

Rossi, L.; Barbieri, O.; Sanguineti, M.; Cabral, J. R. P.; Bruzzi, P.; and Santi, L.: Carcinogenicity study with technical-grade dichlorodiphenyltrichloroethane and 1,1-dichloro-2,2-*bis*(*p*-chlorophenyl)ethylene in hamsters. *Cancer Res.,* **43**:776–81, 1983.

Rossman, T. G.; Meyn, M. S.; and Troll, W.: Effects of arsenite on DNA repair in *Escherichia coli. Environ. Health Perspect.,* **19**:229–33, 1977.

Rubin, H.: Is somatic mutation the major mechanism of malignant transformation? *J. Natl Cancer Inst.,* **64**:995–1000, 1980.

Ryffel, B.; Donatsch, P.; Madörin, M.; Matter, B. E.; Rüttimann, G.; Schön, H.; Stoll, R.; and Wilson, J.: Toxicological evaluation of cyclosporin A. *Arch. Toxicol.,* **53**:107–41, 1983.

San, R. H. C., and Stich, H. F. (eds.): *Short Term Tests for Chemical Carcinogens.* Springer-Verlag, New York, 1980, pp. 581–609.

Scanlan, R. A., and Tannenbaum, S. R. (eds.): N-*Nitroso Compounds,* ACS Symposium Series 174, American Chemical Society, Washington, D.C., 1981.

Schaaper, R. M.; Kunkel, T. A.; and Loeb, L. A.: Infidelity of DNA synthesis associated with bypass of apurinic sites. *Proc. Natl Acad. Sci. USA,* **80**:487–91, 1983.

Schmähl, D.: Combination effects in chemical carcinogenesis. *Arch. Toxicol.,* Suppl. **4**:29–40, 1980.

Schmähl, D.; Thomas, C.; and Auer, R.: *Iatrogenic Carcinogenesis.* Springer-Verlag, Berlin, Heidelberg, 1977.

Schottenfeld, D., and Fraumeni, J. F., Jr.: *Cancer Epidemiology and Prevention.* W. B. Saunders Co., Philadelphia, 1982.

Schulte-Hermann, R.; Timmermann-Trosiener, I.; and Schuppler, J.: Promotion of spontaneous preneoplastic cells in rat liver as a possible explanation of tumor production by nonmutagenic compounds. *Cancer Res.,* **43**:839–44, 1983.

Searle, C. E. (ed.): *Chemical Carcinogens,* 2nd ed. ACS Monogr. 173, American Chemical Society, Washington, D.C., 1984.

Selikoff, I. J., and Hammond, E. C.: Health hazards of asbestos exposure. *Ann. N.Y. Acad. Sci.,* **330**:1–814, 1979.

Shimkin, M. B.: *Some Classics of Experimental Oncology.* NIH Publ. No. 80-2150, U.S. Government Printing Office, Washington, D.C., 1980.

Shimkin, M. B., and Stoner, G. D.: Lung tumors in mice: application to carcinogenesis bioassay. *Adv. Cancer Res.,* **21**:2–58, 1975.

Sims, J., and Renwick, A. G.: The effects of saccharin on the metabolism of dietary tryptophan to indole, a known carcinogen for the urinary bladder of the rat. *Toxicol. Appl. Pharmacol.,* **67**:132–51, 1983.

Slaga, T. J.: Overview of tumor promotion in animals. *Environ. Health Perspect.,* **50**:3–13, 1983.

Slaga, T. J.; Sivak, A.; and Boutwell, R. K. (eds.): *Mechanisms of Tumor Promotion and Cocarcinogens.* Raven Press, New York, 1978.

Snyder, R.; Jollow, D. J.; Parke, D. V.; Gibson, C. G.; Kocsis, J. J.; and Witmer, C. M. (eds.): *Biological Reactive Intermediates—I. Chemical Mechanisms and Biological Effects,* Part B. Plenum Press, New York, 1982.

Sontag, J. M. (ed.): *Carcinogens in Industry and the Environment.* Marcel Dekker, Inc., New York, 1981.

Speck, W. T.; Meyer, L. W.; Zeiger, E.; and Rosenkranz, H. S.: Mutagenicity and DNA-modifying activity of 2-nitropropane. *Mutat. Res.,* **104**:49–54, 1982.

Squire, R.: Ranking animal carcinogens: a proposed regulatory approach. *Science,* **214**:877–80, 1981.

Staffa, J. A., and Mehlman, M. A. (eds.): *Innovations in Cancer Risk Assessment (ED$_{01}$ Study).* Pathotox Publishers, Inc., Ill., 1979.

Stanton, M. F.; Layard, M.; Tegeris, A.; Miller, E.; May, M.; Morgan, E.; and Smith, A.: Relation of particle dimension to carcinogenicity in amphibole asbestoses and other fibrous minerals. *J. Natl Cancer Inst.,* **67**:965–75, 1981.

Starr, T. B., and Gibson, J. E.: The mechanistic toxicology of formaldehyde and its implications for quantitative risk estimation. *Annu. Rev. Pharmacol. Toxicol.,* **25**:745–67, 1985.

Steinhoff, D.; Weber, H.; Mohr, U.; and Boehme, K.: Evaluation of amitrole (aminotriazole) for potential carcinogenicity in orally dosed rats, mice, and golden hamsters. *Toxicol. Appl. Pharmacol.,* **69**:161–69, 1983.

Stenbäck, F.; Peto, R.; and Shubik, P.: Initiation and promotion at different ages and doses in 2200 mice II. Decrease in promotion by TPA with ageing. *Br. J. Cancer,* **44**:15–23, 1981.

Stott, W. T., and Watanabe, P. G.: Differentiation of genetic versus epigenetic mechanisms of toxicity and its application to risk assessment. *Drug Metab. Rev.,* **13**:853–73, 1982.

Sugimura, T.; Endo, H.; Ono, T.; and Sugano, H. (eds.): *Progress in Cancer Biochemistry.* GANN Monogr. on Cancer Res. 24, Japan Sci. Soc. Press, Tokyo; University Park Press, Baltimore, 1979.

Sugimura, T.; Kondo, S.; and Takebe, H. (eds.): *Environmental Mutagens and Carcinogens.* Univ. Tokyo Press, Tokyo; Alan R. Liss, Inc., New York, 1982.

Sugimura, T., and Sato, S.: Mutagens-carcinogens in foods. *Cancer Res.,* **43**:2415s–21s, 1983.

Sunderman, F. W., Jr.: Recent advances in metal carcinogenesis. *Ann. Clin. Lab. Sci.,* 1984 (in press).

Surgeon General Report: *The Health Consequences of Smoking. Cancer.* U.S. Govt. Pub. No. DHHS (PHS)82-50179, U.S. Government Printing Office, Washington, D.C., 1982.

Suzuki, E.; Mochizuki, M.; Wakabayashi, Y.; and Okada, M.: *In vitro* metabolic activation of *N,N*-dibutylnitrosamine in mutagenesis. *Gann,* **74**:51–59, 1983.

Swenberg, J. A.; Barrow, C. S.; Boreiko, C. J.; Heck, H.; Levine, R. J.; Morgan, K. T.; and Starr, T. B.: Nonlinear biological responses to formaldehyde and their implications for carcinogenic risk assessment. *Carcinogenesis,* **4**:945–52, 1983.

Takigawa, M.; Verma, A. K.; Simsiman, R. C.; and Boutwell, R. K.: Inhibition of mouse skin tumor promotion and of promoter-stimulated epidermal polyamine biosynthesis by α-difluoromethylornithine. *Cancer Res.,* **43**:3732–38, 1983.

Tarr, M. J., and Olsen, R. G.: Species variation in susceptibility to methylnitrosourea-induced immunosuppression. *J. Environ. Pathol. Toxicol. Oncol.* **6**:261–70, 1985.

Tatematsu, M.; Hasegawa, R.; Imaida, K.; Tsuda, H.; and Ito, N.: Survey of various chemicals for initiating and promoting activities in a short-term *in vivo* system based on generation of hyperplastic liver nodules in rats. *Carcinogenesis,* **4**:381–86, 1983.

Teo, I. A.; Lehmann, A. R.; Müller, R.; and Rajewsky, M. F.: Similar rate of O^6-ethylguanine elimination from DNA in normal human fibroblast and xeroderma pigmentosum cell strains transformed by SV 40. *Carcinogenesis,* **4**:1075–77, 1983.

Toth, B.: Actual new cancer-causing hydrazines, hydrazides, and hydrazones. *J. Cancer Res. Clin. Oncol.,* **97**:97–108, 1980.

Ts'o, P. O. P., and DiPaolo, J. A. (eds.): *Chemical Carcinogenesis.* Marcel Dekker, Inc., New York, 1974.

Tucker, M. J.: The effect of long-term food restriction on tumours in rodents. *Int. J. Cancer,* **23**:803–807, 1979.

Uraguchi, K., and Yamazaki, M. (eds.): *Toxicology, Biochemistry and Pathology of Mycotoxins.* Halsted Press, New York, 1978.

van Bladeren, P. J.; Hoogeterp, J. J.; Breimer, D. D.; and van der Gen, A.: The influence of disulfiram and other inhibitors of oxidative metabolism on the formation of 2-hydroxyethyl-mercapturic acid from 1,2-dibromoethane by the rat. *Biochem. Pharmacol.,* **30**:2983–87, 1981.

van der Hoeven, J. C. M.; Lagerweij, W. J.; Posthumus, M. A.; van Veldhuizen, A.; and Holterman, H. A. J.: Aguilide A, a new mutagenic compound isolated from bracken fern *(Pteridium aquilinum (L.) Kuhn). Carcinogenesis,* **4**:1587–90, 1983.

van Duuren, B. L.: Cocarcinogens and tumor promoters and their environmental importance. *J. Am. Coll. Toxicol.,* **1**(1):17–27, 1982.

van Duuren, B. L.; Kline, S. A.; Melchionne, S.; and Seidman, I.: Chemical structure and carcinogenicity relationships of some chloroalkene oxides and their parent olefins. *Cancer Res.,* **43**:159–62, 1983.

Various authors: Saccharin: current Status: *Food Chem. Toxicol.,* **23**:417–546, 1985.

Wallin, H.; Melin, P.; Schelin, C.; and Jergil, B.: Evidence that covalent binding of metabolically activated phenol to microsomal proteins is caused by oxidised products of hydroquinone and catechol. *Chem.-Biol. Interact.,* **55**:335–46, 1985.

Walrath, J., and Fraumeni, J. F., Jr.: Mortality patterns among embalmers. *Int. J. Cancer,* **31**:407–11, 1983.

Ward, J. M.; Rice, J. M.; Creasia, D.; Lynch, P.; and Riggs, C.: Dissimilar patterns of promotion by di(2-ethylhexyl)phthalate and phenobarbital of hepatocellular neoplasia initiated by diethylnitrosamine in B6C3F1 mice. *Carcinogenesis,* **4**:1021–29, 1983.

Waring, M. J.: DNA modification and cancer. *Ann. Rev. Biochem.,* **50**:159–92, 1981.

Wattenberg, L. W.: Inhibition of neoplasia by minor dietary constituents. *Cancer Res.,* **43**:2448s–53s, 1983.

Waxweiler, R. J.; Landrigan, P. J.; Infante, P.; and Shapiro, R.: Conference on vinyl chloride. *Environ. Health Perspect.,* **41**:1–231, 1981.

Weber, W. W., and Glowinski, I. B.: Acetylation. In *Enzymatic Basis of Detoxication,* Vol. II. Academic Press, Inc., New York, 1980.

Wei, E. T., and Shu, H. P.: Nitroaromatic carcinogens in diesel soot: a review of laboratory findings. *Am. J. Public Health,* **73**:1085–88, 1983.

Weinstein, I. B.: Scientific basis for carcinogen detection and primary cancer prevention. *Cancer,* **47**:1133–41, 1981.

Weisburger, J. H., and Williams, G. M.: Carcinogen testing. Current problems and new approaches. *Science,* **214**:401–407, 1981.

Weisburger, J. H.; Wynder, E. L.; and Horn, C. L.: Nutritional factors and etiologic mechanisms in the causation of gastrointestinal cancers. *Cancer,* **50**:11–19, 1982.

Westendorf, J.; Marquardt, M.; Ketkar, M. B.; Mohr, U.; and Marquardt, H.: Tumorigenicity *in vivo* and induction of mutagenesis and DNA repair *in vitro* by aclacinomycin A and marcellomycin: Structure-activity relationship and predictive value of short-term tests. *Cancer Res.,* **43**:5248–51, 1983.

White, R. D.; Gandolfi, A. J.; Bowden, G. T.; and Sipes, I. G.: Deuterium isotope effect on the metabolism and toxicity of 1,2-dibromoethane. *Toxicol. Appl. Pharmacol.,* **69**:170–78, 1983.

Wiebers, J. L.; Abbott, P. J.; Coombs, M. M.; and Livingston, D. C.: Mass spectral characterisation of the major DNA-carcinogen adduct formed from the metabolically activated carcinogen 15,16-dihydro-11-methyl-cyclopenta[a]phenanthren-17-one. *Carcinogenesis,* **2**:637–43, 1981.

Williams, G. M.: Liver carcinogenesis: the role for some chemicals of an epigenetic mechanism of liver tumor promotion involving modification of the cell membrane. *Food Cosmet. Toxicol.,* **19**:577–83, 1981.

Williams, G. M.: Phenotypic properties of preneoplastic rat liver lesions and applications to detection of carcinogens and tumor promoters. *Toxicol. Pathol.,* **10**:3–10, 1982.

Williams, G. M.: Modulation of chemical carcinogenesis by xenobiotics. *Fund. Appl. Toxicol.,* **4**:325–44, 1984.

Williams, G. M.; Dunkel, V. C.; and Ray, V. A. (eds.): Cellular systems for toxicity testing. *Ann. NY Acad. Sci.,* **407**:1–484, 1983.

Williams, G. M., and Furuya, K.: Distinction between liver neoplasm promoting and syncarcinogenic effects demonstrated by reversing the order of administering phenobarbital and diethylnitrosamine either before or after *N*-2-fluorenylacetamide. *Carcinogenesis,* **5**:171–74, 1984.

Williams, G. M.; Kroes, R.; Waaijers, H. W.; and van de Poll, K. W. (eds.): *The Predictive Value of Short-Term Screening Tests in Carcinogenicity Evaluation.* Elsevier/North Holland, Amsterdam, 1980.

Williams, G. M.; Maeura, Y.; and Weisburger, J. H.: Simultaneous inhibition of liver carcinogenicity and enhancement of bladder carcinogenicity of *N*-2-fluorenylacetamide by butylated hydroxytoleune. *Cancer Lett.,* **19**:55–60, 1983.

Williams, G. M., and Numoto, S.: Promotion of mouse liver neoplasms by the organochlorine pesticides, chlordane and heptachlor in comparison to dichlorodiphenyltrichloroethane. *Carcinogenesis,* **5**:1689–96, 1984.

Williams, G. M., and Weisburger, J. H.: Systematic carcinogen testing through the decision point approach. *Annu. Rev. Pharmacol. Toxicol.,* **21**:393–416, 1981.

Williams, G. M., and Weisburger, J. H.: Carcinogenicity testing of drugs. *Prog. Drug Res.,* **29**:155–213, 1985.

Wogan, G. N.; Paglialunga, S.; and Newberne, P. M.: Carcinogenic effects of low dietary levels of aflatoxin B_1 in rats. *Food Cosmet. Toxicol.,* **12**:681–85, 1974.

Wong, L. C. K.; Winston, J. M.; Hong, C. B.; and Plotnick, H.: Carcinogenicity and toxicity of 1,2-dibromoethane in the rat. *Toxicol. Appl. Pharmacol.,* **63**:155–65, 1982.

Woo, Y.-T.; Argus, M. F.; and Arcos, J. C.: Effect of mixed-function oxidase modifers on metabolism and toxicity of the oncogen dioxane. *Cancer Res.,* **38**:1621–25, 1978.

Yoshida, D., and Fukuhara, Y.: Mutagenicity and co-mutagenicity of catechol on *Salmonella. Mutat. Res.,* **120**:7–11, 1983.

Young, J. D.; Braun, W. H.; and Gehring, P. J.: Dose-dependent fate of 1,4-dioxane in rats. *J. Toxicol. Environ. Health,* **4**:709–26, 1978.

Zedeck, M. S., and Lipkin, M. (eds.): *Inhibition of Tumor Induction and Development.* Plenum Publishing Corp., New York, 1981.

Chapter 6

GENETIC TOXICOLOGY

William G. Thilly and *Katherine M. Call*

INTRODUCTION

Genetic toxicology is the study of the interaction of chemical and physical agents with the processes of heredity. Three levels of study are well established in this field: (1) epidemiologic classification of the kinds and frequencies of human hereditary disorders, (2) mechanistic studies of the means by which chemicals and physical agents cause genetic change in experimental systems, and (3) testing of compounds and mixtures to which people are exposed to assess potential genetic hazards.

There is a growing awareness of the great diversity of genetically active agents that exist in the human environment as determined by assays in small animals or single-cell systems. In considering the kinds of genetic damage that may occur in humans, we have incorporated material in this chapter illustrating some experimental approaches and examples of assays developed to detect each particular kind of genetic aberration. This chapter also discusses the role of genetic damage in heritable diseases, particularly birth defects. A summary of estimated frequencies of different chromosome abnormalities and some of their resulting diseases in newborns and spontaneous abortuses, presented in Figure 6–1, shows the impact of various types of genetic damage in the human population. Equally important, although not shown in this figure, is the contribution of point mutations to heritable diseases. If somatic diseases, such as cancer or atherosclerosis, are demonstrated to arise via genetic errors, then the discussions presented here might apply to their etiology as well.

GENETIC DISEASE: A CASCADE OF PROCESSES

Chemical induction of genetic change is not simply the reaction of a chemical with DNA. A series or cascade of processes separates an environmental chemical from the appearance of a genetic disease in humans. The probability that a particular chemical will cause genetic damage is affected by its concentration in the environment; its entry into and distribution within the body; the metabolic systems in the tissues to which the compound is distributed; the reactivity of the compound or its metabolites with cellular target molecules, especially DNA; the capacity of the cell to rectify or amplify the damage; the opportunity for expression of whatever potential genetic change has been caused; and the ability of the tissue to recognize and suppress the multiplication of cells with aberrant properties (see Figure 6–2).

To design test systems that faithfully assess the effects of environmental chemicals on people, all of the relevant pharmacokinetic, metabolic, biochemical, and genetic characteristics of humans should ideally be taken into account. This is difficult because many important facts about these processes in humans are not well understood. Many differences between organisms are already known in the processes of foreign compound biotransformation and DNA repair; thus, in the development of an experimental test system involving, for instance, *Salmonella typhimurium* or *Mus musculus*, biochemical differences between these species and humans must be taken into account. Another problem in designing suitable test systems is presented by the biochemical differences in processes involved in fixation of error among the many cell types in humans. For example, repair differences among types of human cells or tissues *in vivo* may be anticipated, comparable to the variation in repair of DNA reaction products recently found in different cell types in rats and other rodents (Kleihues *et al.*, 1982).

In addition, there are important differences in the duration and concentration of chemical exposure between humans and test systems. Human exposures to a wide variety of chemicals generally occur in amounts that rarely raise concentrations in body fluids above the nanomolar range for any given chemical, while nearly all

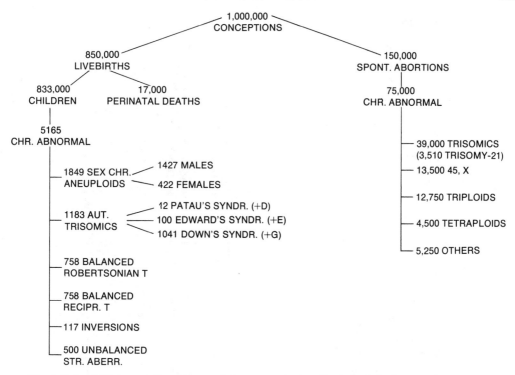

Figure 6–1. A diagrammatic summary of chromosomal anomalies in both liveborns and spontaneous abortuses. (From Sankaranarayanan, K.: The role of nondisjunction in aneuploidy in man. An overview. *Mutat. Res.*, **61**:1–28, 1979.)

experiments expose test animals or cells to effective concentrations in the micromolar-to-millimolar range for periods rarely exceeding one day. Thus, conclusions drawn from studies at high concentrations may not reflect responses at a more biologically relevant dose. An example of this problem may be drawn from our studies showing that a single 24-hour treatment with ethyl methanesulfonate at a concentration of greater than 100 μM induced mutation more efficiently in human lymphoblasts than 20 daily treatments at concentrations below 16 μM (Penman *et al.*, 1983).

CLASSIFICATION OF GENETIC LESIONS

Human genetic diseases arise from *at least* three separate modes of failure to transmit genetic information accurately and quantitatively: aneuploidization, clastogenesis, and mutagenesis. The gain or loss of whole chromosomes is termed *aneuploidization*. The term *clastogenesis* is used to designate the process of genetic change that appears as microscopically observable addition, deletion, or rearrangement

of parts of the chromosomes in eukaryotic species. However, some authors include the processes resulting in the gain or loss of whole chromosomes in their use of the term clastogenesis. Chromosome breakage and aneuploidization should be distinguished from one another, since the molecular mechanisms and induction by chemical and physical agents are probably quite different.

Gene-locus mutation or ''point mutations'' are small changes in a DNA sequence. Addition or deletion of a small number of base pairs or substitution of an incorrect base pair constitutes a mutation. The process of forming gene-locus mutations is called *mutagenesis,* although this term is also used less stringently to refer to all genetic changes. In this chapter, *mutagenesis* is used *solely* to designate the production of gene-locus mutations.

The terms aneuploidization, clastogenesis, and mutagenesis each define specific kinds of structural changes in the eukaryotic genome (see Table 6–1). Each definition should be used in its most general sense, keeping in mind that each of these types of genetic alteration may be caused by more than one mechanism.

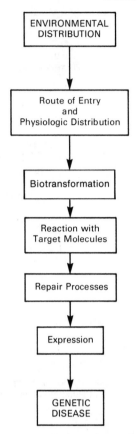

Figure 6–2. Toxicologic paradigm.

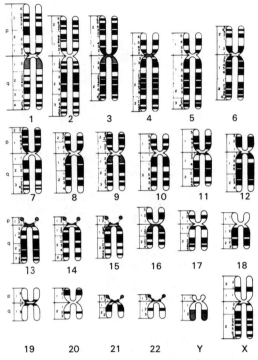

Figure 6–3. Diagrammatic representation of metaphase chromosome bands as observed with the Q- and G-staining methods; centromere representative of Q-banding method only. (From Paris Conference [1971]: Standardization in human cytogenetics. In Bergsma, D. (ed.): *Birth Defects. Original Article Series,* Vol. 8, No. 7. The National Foundation, New York, 1972.)

The Normal Human Karyotype

The normal human chromosomal complement or "karyotype" contains 46 chromosomes: 22 pairs of autosomes designated 1, 2, 3 . . . 22; and two sex chromosomes, XX in females and XY in males (Figure 6–3). Morphologically, the chromosomes are best characterized at mitosis, when they assume an extremely condensed conformation and thus become visible in the light microscope. At mitosis they can be described as

Table 6–1. DEFINITIONS

Mutagenesis:	Occurrence of "point" or "gene-locus" mutation (base-pair substitutions and small additions or deletions)
Clastogenesis:	Occurrence of chromosomal breaks resulting in gain, loss, or rearrangement of pieces of chromosomes
Aneuploidization:	Gain or loss of one or more intact chromosomes

X-shaped objects consisting of two biarmed chromatids in which the two pairs of arms join at the region called the centromere (Figure 6–4). The short arm of a chromosome is called p (for petite), while the long arm is designated q. The length (both relative and absolute) of each chromatid arm is constant for each chromosome but varies among chromosomes. This variation in size is the basis for the first level of discrimination among chromosomes, in which seven groups (A to G) are described. Chromosomes can be readily identified by staining techniques that reveal each chromosome to have a characteristic series of light and dark bands (Figure 6–3). For example, Q bands refer to the banding patterns seen with quinacrine and G bands with Giemsa stains, under specified protocols.

As techniques for describing normal chromosomal morphology have become more refined, it has become possible to recognize chromosomal damage at a finer level. An example is the use of chromosome banding to detect exchange of chromosomal material between two nonhomolo-

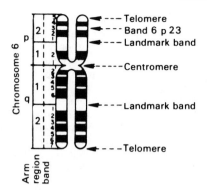

Figure 6–4. Diagrammatic representation of chromosome 6 in metaphase. (From Sanchez, O., and Yunis, J. J.: New chromosomal techniques and their medical applications. In Yunis, J. J. [ed.]: *New Chromosomal Syndromes*. Academic Press, Inc., New York, 1977.)

gous chromosomes (translocation), which does not visually affect the size of the chromosomes involved.

Abnormal Karyotypes

An abnormal karyotype can be defined as having a cytogenetically (light microscopy) detectable alteration in chromosome number or structure compared to the normal complement of chromosomes. Abnormal karyotypes are designated by giving the total number of chromosomes observed, followed by the number of the aberrant chromosome, if known. For instance, Down's syndrome is associated with an additional chromosome 21, and the karyotype is designated (47, 21+), while Turner's syndrome, in which only one X chromosome is found, is designated (45, XO). If an addition or deletion is noted in part of a chromosome, the convention is to indicate the chromosomes involved and, if possible, the arm affected. A syndrome with a deletion in part of the long arm of chromosome 18 is designated (46, 18q-) according to this convention. Structural abnormalities are classified by an ordered six-character designation citing the chromosome, the arm, the region, band, and subbands involved, according to the Paris Conference (1972). 05p140 would indicate an aberration in the *short* arm (p) of chromosome 5 in region *1* (there is only one) in the *4*th band, but without any designation of subband position *0*. (Subbands indicate relative positions within bands and are not seen as distinguishable microscopic entities.)

Aneuploidization

Aneuploidy is a condition in which the karyotype is increased or decreased by one or more chromosomes compared to the normal human diploid (2n) karyotype. Monosomy is the loss (2n − 1) and trisomy is the gain (2n + 1) of a chromosome. Other aberrant conditions, such as a double trisomy (2n + 1 + 1) or tetrasomy (2n + 2) involving the gain of two chromosomes, are also possible, as is the loss of two chromosomes (nullisomy, 2n − 2). Polyploidy is a special aneuploid condition in which the entire complement of chromosomes in a cell is increased. Polyploid karyotypes can be triploid (3n), tetraploid (4n), or in some cases can exist with even greater ploidy. A haploid condition (n) is one in which only one copy of each chromosome is present.

Role of Aneuploidy in Genetic Disease. Aneuploidy is responsible for several of the most common heritable genetic diseases. Klinefelter's (47, XXY) and Down's (47, 21+) syndromes are generally due to trisomies, while Turner's (45, XO) is due to a monosomy. These syndromes result from aneuploidy in either a germ cell or early embryonic somatic cell. Aneuploidy in somatic cells is observed in some forms of tumors; the most common abnormality is that of an extra chromosome 8, 17, or 17q (reviewed by Yunis, 1983). In these cases, however, it is not clear whether aneuploidy is the primary cause of tumor formation or whether it occurs as the tumor progresses, possibly conferring a growth advantage.

Extensive epidemiologic investigations have been made to determine the prevalence, effects, and possible causes of aneuploidy in abortuses and newborns. Hook and Hamerton (1977) have summarized the results of seven studies of chromosomal abnormalities and found 0.62 percent of newborns (353/56,952) to have a microscopically detectable lesion. As shown in Table 6–2, 189 of these abnormalities were due to aneuploidization, of which 107 involved sex chromosomes and 82 involved autosomes. This total frequency of 0.4 percent for abnormalities of chromosome number in newborns can be contrasted with a frequency of 60 percent in spontaneous abortuses less than 12 weeks of age (Boué et al., 1975) and 30 percent for spontaneous abortuses up to 27 weeks of age (Creasy and Alberman, as reported by Carr and Gedeon, 1977).

There is apparently a strong intrauterine selection process in determining the frequency of particular chromosomal number abnormalities in liveborn infants. Of the chromosome anomalies found in spontaneous abortuses, about half are trisomies. When trisomies in spontaneous abortuses were examined for each of the 22 autosomes, an extra chromosome 16 accounted for 116/368, while no examples of extra chromo-

Table 6–2. FREQUENCY OF ANEUPLOIDY IN HUMAN NEWBORN*

	TOTAL OBSERVED	PERCENT
Sex Chromosomes		
47,XYY	35	0.061
47,XXY	35	0.061
47,XXX	28	0.049
45,XO	2	0.004
Other	7	0.012
Autosomes		
+D	3	0.005
+E	7	0.012
+G	71	0.125
Other	1	0.002
Total examined = 56,952		

* Summarized from Hook and Hamerton (1977).

somes 1 or 5 were found (Carr and Gedeon, 1977). This contrasts with the predominance of an extra chromosome 21 (Down's syndrome) among trisomies in newborns.

There generally appears to be less selective pressure *in utero* against sex-chromosomal than autosomal aneuploidies. Table 6–3 shows that the frequency of sex-chromosomal aneuploidies in newborns is 0.22 percent compared to 0.14 percent for autosomal aneuploidies (Hook and Hamerton, 1977). Given 3.2 million live births per year, these percentages extrapolate to approximately 7100 sex chromosomal and 4600 autosomal aneuploidies in newborns each year in the United States. Generally, phenotypic abnormalities are less severe and life expectancy longer in liveborns with sex chromosome aneuploidies than autosomal aneuploidies. The degree of expression of aneuploid chromosomal material may affect the severity of the defect and

hence the probability that the fetus survives to term. Thus, chromosome aberrations involving heterochromatin, which is thought to be inactive, may have less effect on gene dosage and be more tolerable. Trisomies in liveborns involve chromosomes 8, 13, 18, and 21, all containing large regions of heterochromatin, and the sex chromosomes X and Y. An extra copy of the X chromosome becomes heterochromatic, while the extra gene dosage of the relatively small Y chromosome does not appear to have severe enough effects to prevent the fetus surviving to term.

Of the many etiologic factors examined in attempts to determine causes of aneuploidization, only maternal age has yielded a statistically positive correlation. Vogel's (1970) summary of the maternal age dependence of trisomies 13 (Patau's syndrome) and 18 (Edward's syndrome) is redrawn in Figure 6–5. A correlation with maternal age has also been reported for Down's syndrome resulting from an extra chromosome 21. The continuous interaction of the parent with the chemical and physical environment might be expected to yield a monotonic increase in total genetic insults, and thus these data on the age-dependent incidence of aneuploidization are particularly important in considering possible causes of genetic change.

The correlations with maternal age, however, do not mean that the events of aneuploidization occur only in female gametogenesis. Ayme and Lippman-Hand (1982) report data indicating that the age of mothers of Down's syndrome offspring is elevated regardless of whether the extra chromosome is of maternal or paternal origin. They suggest that the elevated incidence of Down's syndrome offspring with increasing maternal age may be due to a decreased *in utero* selection against abnormal fetuses.

Table 6–3. FREQUENCIES OF CHROMOSOME STRUCTURE ABNORMALITIES IN LIVEBORNS

TYPE OF ABNORMALITIES	FREQUENCY/100,000 LIVE BIRTHS*	U.S. LIVE BIRTHS/ YEAR[†]
Sex chromosome aneuploidies	223	7136
Autosomal trisomies	144	4608
Structural rearrangements		
Balanced	195	6240
Unbalanced	60	1920
(Translocations)	(19)	(608)
(Inversions)	(2)	(64)
(Deletions)	(9)	(288)
(Supernumerary)	(18)	(576)
(Other)	(12)	(384)
Total	622	19,904

* Summarized from Hook and Hammerton (1977).
[†] Summarized from Milunsky (1979).

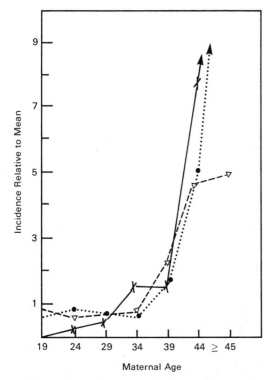

Figure 6–5. Chromosomal abnormalities and maternal age: (∇) D_1 trisomy (Patau's syndrome, 172 cases); ($\bullet$) trisomy 18 (Edward's syndrome, 153 cases); (X) $E_{18}q$ (35 cases). (Redrawn from Vogel, F.: Spontaneous mutation in man. In Vogel, F., and Rörhborn, G. [eds.]: *Chemical Mutagenesis in Mammals and Man.* Springer-Verlag, New York, 1970, pp. 16–68.)

Assays for Aneuploidy. Several assay systems have been developed in fungi to detect both meiotic and mitotic aneuploidy. For example, in yeast, nondisjunction can be detected by the emergence of a recessive characteristic after loss of a sister chromosome containing the dominant variant (Parry and Zimmerman, 1976). Using this type of system, Parry *et al.* (1979) reported that 14 chemical and physical agents, including caffeine, heat, ethyl methanesulfonate, saccharin, ultraviolet light, and x-rays, significantly increased mitotic aneuploidy in the yeast *Saccharomyces cerevisiae*. Griffiths (1979) tested 57 agents in *Neurospora crassa* and found that eight, including caffeine, γ-rays, and amethopterin, induced meiotic aneuploidy. Surveys of the status of systems for detecting chemically induced aneuploidy in *Neurospora* (Griffiths *et al.*, 1986) and *Saccharomyces cerevisiae* (Resnick *et al.*, 1986) have been published.

Although these fungal assays yield valuable information and are relatively simple to perform,

the importance of examining mammalian cells should be emphasized because the mechanisms of nondisjunction, and therefore the response to a given chemical, may differ between fungi and humans. This is illustrated by the finding that the plant alkaloid colchicine, which disrupts microtubules, does not induce meiotic aneuploidy in *Neurospora*, yet drastically alters chromosome segregation in cultured mammalian cells.

Nondisjunction has also been examined cytogenetically (light microscopy) in mammalian cells, although to date relatively little information regarding the effect of chemicals has been amassed. One reason for this is the difficulty in eliminating artificial loss of chromosomes that may occur in some cells during cytogenetic preparation. Tates (1979) has examined meiotic nondisjunction and diploid gamete induction in male germ cells of the vole *Microtus oeconomus* and found increases caused by several chemicals tested. However, a more recent study did not confirm that x-ray treatment caused an increase in aneuploidy, illustrating the difficulty of assaying this genetic end point in mammalian cells (Tates and de Vogel, 1981). Studies have shown that x-rays can induce nondisjunction in male mice (Szemere and Chandley, 1975). In this study, 23/1000 meiotic cells from irradiated animals were trisomic, as compared to 0/200 in controls. Galloway and Ivett (1986) have assessed *in vitro* mammalian cell systems for detecting chemically induced aneuploidy.

Mammalian assays are more time consuming than are microbial systems, since visual chromosome scoring is performed as opposed to selection of a phenotype indicative of aneuploidy, as in the fungal systems. However, improved methods for measuring aneuploidy, such as fluorescent detection for the presence of two Y chromosomes in human sperm (Kapp, 1979), are presently being developed that may eliminate the need for visual scoring. This assay, however, is practiced in relatively few laboratories (Allen *et al.*, 1986).

Clastogenesis

Cytogenetic analyses of chromosome structural aberrations have been performed on cells from many eukaryotic species. The method is straightforward: the desired cells are collected and their growth halted in metaphase by colcemid or colchicine; they are then fixed, stained, and examined under the microscope (see Cohen and Hirschhorn, 1971). The types of abnormalities scored include (1) single chromatid gap, an unstained region on a single chromatid without a definite boundary whose dimensions are no more than the width of the chromatid; (2) single chromatid break, a clean, unstained region with a definite boundary with space between boundaries greater than the width of the chromatid; (3) isochromatid gap, an unstained region on *both* chromatids without a definite boundary whose dimensions are no more than the width of the chromatids; (4) isochromatid break, a clean, unstained region on *both* chromatids with a definite boundary and space between the boundaries greater than the width of the chromatids; (5) dicentric and exchange chromosomes, the rejoining of two chromosomes by either short or long arms, resulting in various exchange figures with *two centromeres;* and (6) translocations, the exchange of material between two chromosomes (e.g., Cohen and Hirschhorn, 1971; Kihlman, 1971; Bender *et al.*, 1973).

Role of Clastogenesis in Genetic Disease. Hook and Hamerton (1977) have summarized data (Table 6–3) regarding microscopically detectable chromosomal breaks in newborns and reported that the total number of balanced (total chromosomal material appears unchanged) and unbalanced (loss or gain of some chromosomal material is evident) rearrangements is 144 in the six studies of 56,952 infants, for a frequency of 0.25 percent. Thus, approximately 8200 newborns per year in the United States suffer from chromosome structure rearrangements.

As with trisomy, an intrauterine selective pressure seems to be operative. Carr and Gedeon (1977) have summarized a number of studies involving spontaneous abortuses and reported a range of 1.3 to 3.8 percent for detectable translocations. A conservative estimate indicates that the intrauterine selective pressure permits only 0.54 percent (0.0033/0.605) of the errors in chromosomal number arising during or shortly after gametogenesis to survive to term. This estimate should be compared to the apparently smaller intrauterine selective pressure allowing 6.6 percent (0.0025/0.038) of fetuses carrying a recognizable chromosomal *break* to survive to term. Hook (1982) suggests that although there appears to be more *in utero* selection against numerical abnormalities, there may be a higher ratio of structural to numerical abnormalities associated with stillbirths and infant and later mortality. As a generalization, it appears that the greater the amount of DNA involved in a lesion, the smaller the possibility that the affected fetus will survive to term. However, it should be remembered that the activity or gene dosage of the genetic material affected by chromosome aberrations may also be significant factors.

Similar to aneuploidy, a higher probability of occurrence for some categories of chromosome breaks is found in infants of older mothers. Cenani and Pfeiffer (reported by Vogel, 1970) found that a syndrome associated with deletion of the long arm of chromosome 18 increased markedly with maternal age (Figure 6–5). No association of chromosomal breaks with paternal age has been found.

Clastogenesis Assays. Numerous studies have examined the frequency of chromosomal aberrations in cells exposed to a chemical or physical agent. Several different types of systems, all using dividing cells, are summarized below.

1. *In vivo* studies: Cells (e.g., bone marrow cells, spermatogonia, spermatocytes, oocytes, or early developing embryos) from chemically treated animals, usually rodents, are isolated, prepared for cytogenetic (light microscopy) observation, and then scored for frequency and types of chromosomal aberrations.

2. *In vivo* host-mediated assays: This type of assay, although not commonly used, involves implanting a sterilized chamber containing the cells (e.g., lymphocytes, fibroblasts, or lymphoid lines) into the peritoneal cavity of the host animal, generally a rodent. The animal is chemically treated, later the implanted chamber is removed, and the cells are recovered and prepared for cytogenetic analysis.

3. *In vivo* F_1 studies (heritable translocation test): To determine whether a chemical induces translocations, male and/or female animals are chemically treated, mated, and the fertility of the F_1 offspring is subsequently examined (Generoso *et al.*, 1978). Reciprocal translocations have been shown to cause partial or full sterility in mice. In this assay, reciprocal translocations are presumed to have occurred if the fertility of the F_1 mice is decreased. Major drawbacks of this assay are the time and cost involved and the indirect nature of the measurement. The validity of this assay can be strengthened by cytogenetic analysis of F_1 mice with decreased fertility.

4. Micronucleus test: This *in vivo* assay measures a type of chromosome aberration termed micronuclei. These are small nuclei containing those chromosome fragments or chromosomes not incorporated into the main nucleus at mitosis owing to a spindle defect or lack of centromere for spindle attachment. To simplify scoring, micronuclei are usually measured in a population of bone marrow erythrocytes in which the main nucleus has been expelled (Schmid, 1976). Studies have shown a strong correlation between chemical ability to induce micronuclei and chromosomal breakage by karyotype analyses (Heddle *et al.*, 1983).

5. Human studies: Human peripheral lymphocytes can easily be obtained and examined for chromosomal damage. Groups examined

usually include industrial workers exposed to chemicals (e.g., Bauchinger *et al.*, 1976; Meretoja *et al.*, 1977) and patients undergoing treatment with various drugs (Watson *et al.*, 1976).

6. *In vitro* studies: Many different cell types have been used for *in vitro* clastogenesis work. Cells suitable for these studies should have a fairly rapid doubling time, a relatively stable karyotype, and be easy to score. An advantage of *in vitro* use of human cells is the possibility of controlled chemical treatment, which cannot be performed in humans.

7. Sister chromatid exchange: Sister chromatid exchanges (SCE), although not necessarily chromosomal aberrations, are believed to be caused by strand breakage resulting in apparently homologous strand interchange and reunion during DNA replication. The actual mechanisms by which SCE's are caused is not known, but models have been postulated (e.g., Painter, 1980). Procedures for measuring SCE involve labeling dividing cells *in vivo* or *in vitro* with bromodeoxyuridine (BrdUrd) for either one or two cell cycles and then analyzing chromosomes at the second metaphase following BrdUrd incorporation. Various fluorescent or nonfluorescent dyes or fluorescent antibodies, all of which differentially label strands of DNA based on BrdUrd incorporation, are used to visualize SCE's. If no strand exchange occurs, the two chromosomes will stain differently along their entire length at the second metaphase, since BrdUrd is incorporated only in the newly synthesized chromatid. However, if an SCE occurs, a "harlequin" staining pattern is observed, in which regions of the differentially staining sister chromatids have exchanged. SCE production has been employed as both an *in vitro* and *in vivo* test for clastogenic agents. A wide variety of mutagens and carcinogens have been reported to induce SCE formation, as evaluated and summarized by Latt *et al.* (1981).

Fragile Sites. A discussion of clastogenesis would be incomplete without inclusion of a unique type of heritable defect, a fragile site, in which a specific position(s) on the chromosome is found to have an abnormally high frequency of breakage. Sutherland (1979) ascribed the following characteristics to a chromosomal fragile site: (1) a nonstaining gap of variable width, usually involving both chromatids, (2) fixed occurrence at the same point on a given chromosome in individuals or their relatives, (3) (co)dominant Mendelian inheritance, and (4) acentric fragments, deleted chromosomes, triradial figures, and other clastogenic aberrations. Fragile sites are postulated to be chromosomal areas that do not condense properly during mitosis, but the

reasons for this defect and its site specificity are unknown.

The presence of a fragile site(s) in a given individual can be determined by culturing lymphocytes *in vitro* under defined media conditions and analyzing chromosome breakage by light microscopy. Fifteen fragile sites have been identified and grouped into three categories, according to what conditions induce breakage (Figure 6–6). Group 1 fragile sites are sensitive to the removal of folic acid and thymidine from the medium; Group 2 sites are not sensitive to any known media conditions, but can be induced by distamycin A; and Group 3 contains only one fragile site (10q25), which is expressed after bromodeoxyuridine treatment.

Nonrandomly distributed breaks and "hotspots" have been observed in chemically treated lymphocytes (e.g., Honeycombe, 1978; Reeves and Margoles, 1974), but these sites are not classified as fragile sites for two reasons. First, breaks at fragile sites can be induced at a frequency as high as 100 percent in metaphase cells, whereas breaks at "hotspots" can be in-

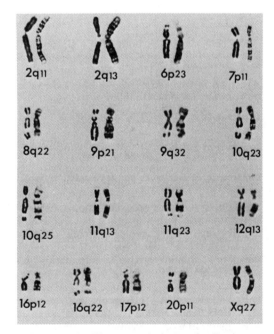

Figure 6–6. The presently known fragile sites. Group 1 sites are located at 2q11, 2q13, 6p23, 7p11, 8q22, 9p21, 9q32, 10q23, 11q13, 11q23, 12q13, 16p12, 20p11, and Xq27. Group 2 sites are located at 16q22 and 17p12. Group 3 is located at 10q25. (From Opitz, J. R., and Sutherland, G. R.: Conference report: International workshop on the fragile X and X-linked mental retardation. *Am. J. Med. Gen.*, **17**:5–94, 1984. Reprinted with permission.)

duced at a frequency of at most 3 to 5 percent. Second, fragile sites result in the production of unique triradial fragments.

The chromosome fragile site Xq27, also known as the fragile X, is associated with a type of X-linked mental retardation with symptoms varying from mild to severe (reviewed by Sutherland, 1983). Sutherland has estimated the incidence of the fragile X in males to be approximately 0.40 per 1000. The heterozygous effect of a fragile X in females is generally less severe and is expressed in varying degrees, possibly owing to selective pressure against or inactivation of an active fragile X chromosome during development.

Fragile sites may also be involved in other human diseases. Sutherland has found a tenfold greater frequency of autosomal fragile sites in institutionalized mentally retarded persons compared to random newborns. In addition, several types of tumors frequently exhibit rearrangements at three autosomal fragile sites (Yunis et al., 1981, 1982). Further studies of fragile sites are needed to understand their cause(s) and assess their role in genetic disease.

MUTAGENESIS

Mutagenesis involves one of the six possible base-pair substitutions (i.e., two transitions AT → GC, GC → AT; and four transversions AT → TA or CG, GC → CG or TA) or the addition or deletion of any number of base pairs in a sequence (e.g., $\frac{-AAAAAA-}{-TTTTT-}$ → $\frac{-AAAXXAAA-}{-TTTYYTTT-}$, an addition of two base pairs). Base-pair mutation at the DNA or genotypic level would be expected to be phenotypically observed only under several specific conditions: (1) if formation of a new triplet codon causes an amino acid substitution that changes some important property of the protein, for example its catalytic activity or resistance to protease attack; (2) if instead of a triplet codon for an amino acid, a premature protein synthesis termination sequence is generated in the mRNA (DNA coding sequences ATC, ACT, and ACC) severely modifying biologic activity of the observed protein; (3) if DNA transcription is prevented; or (4) if RNA maturation is prevented.

Although nascent RNA is transcribed from a continuous sequence of DNA, often specific RNA sequences are spliced out to produce the final version of the message. Mutations at specific sequences may prevent mRNA maturation and hence protein translation by befouling the splicing reactions. Although relatively little is known about how different mutations may affect RNA processing, it has been reported that the human genetic disease, α-thalessemia, can be due to a pentanucleotide deletion (Felber et al., 1982) and β-thalessemia to a GC → AT transition (Treisman et al., 1982), causing a splicing defect in the α- and β-globin mRNA, respectively.

Addition or deletion of base pairs, when the number of base-pair changes is not a multiple of three, will alter the reading frame and change the amino acid sequence, often causing a dramatic effect on protein function. These base-pair changes are called *frameshift mutations*. Addition or deletion of three base pairs (or multiples of three) would *add or delete* one (or more) amino acid(s) from a coded protein. Addition or deletion of three base pairs would probably mimic base-pair substitution, and thus only changes in protein structure affecting catalysis, protease resistance, or RNA processing, etc., would be observed as a phenotypic change.

There is some imprecision in our definition of addition or deletion mutations, in that it is usually applied to a small number of base pairs. Events involving, for example, ten or more bases are usually termed "large additions" or "large deletions" and, if sufficiently large (greater than 10^4 base pairs, for instance), enter the undefined realm between point mutation and chromosomal abnormality in eukaryotic cells.

Role of Mutations in Genetic Disease

Several problems confound accurate estimates of the frequency of genetic disease caused by gene locus mutation. It is assumed that many heritable diseases with no detectable chromosomal abnormalities result from mutation(s), since they behave similarly to well-studied microbiologic examples of point or gene-locus mutants. This subclass of diseases includes, but is not limited to, disorders in which a change in protein structure or function has been detected or for which heritability has been demonstrated. However, we must emphasize that molecular evidence indicating a gene-locus mutational origin is available for only a small portion of the diseases known to behave in a Mendelian manner without any microscopically evident chromosomal malformation.

Point mutations may also be involved in diseases inherited in a non-Mendelian fashion for which cytogenetic abnormalities have been eliminated as a cause. These diseases, which include congenital malformations, idiopathic mental retardation, and syndromes with variable age of clinical onset, appear to be caused by more than one factor. They may result from a genetic predisposition, possibly caused by a mutation, in conjunction with other genetic or environmental influences. However, it is presently difficult to estimate the contribution of point mutations to such genetic diseases that display multifactorial causality.

Yet another consideration in calculating incidence rates is that many genetic defects may not become evident until a considerable time after birth. Despite these uncertainties, we will cite estimates of total genetic damage incurred by mutagenesis based on the data available for disease in newborns inherited in a Mendelian manner with no apparent chromosomal abnormalities.

Carter (1977) estimated that some 7/1000 newborns in European populations suffered from diseases behaving as autosomal dominants, 2.5/1000 from autosomal recessive diseases, and 0.4/1000 from X-linked diseases, yielding a total incidence of about 1 percent for disorders with putative mutagenic origin. McKusick (1981, as cited in Matsunaga, 1982) has catalogued human disease syndromes that behave as Mendelian traits and lists a total of 3303; new syndromes continue to be reported. Frequencies of occurrence for autosomal dominant and X-linked recessive syndromes range from a high of about 10^{-4} for the X-linked Duchenne-type muscular dystrophy, about 10^{-5} for acondroplasia (autosomal dominant), to less than 10^{-6} for rare syndromes of which only one or two cases have ever been identified. Vogel and Rathenberg (1975) summarized data showing that many of the diseases associated with mutagenesis do not display any increasing frequency with advanced maternal age, but, in contrast to the syndromes associated with chromosomal number and structure abnormalities, display a strong positive correlation with paternal age. Several of Vogel's (1970) examples are redrawn for summary in Figure 6–7.

Assays to Measure Chemically Induced Mutation

Basic Principles. In contrast to chromosomal aberrations, which are observed microscopically, the results of gene mutation are usually detected indirectly. In general, some phenotypic property of the cell or colony of cells, altered as a result of mutation, is observed under defined conditions. Commonly used phenotypic changes include the loss of the function of a particular enzyme (forward mutation, i.e., away from the wild phenotype) and the regaining of the function of an enzyme (reversion, i.e., toward the wild phenotype). The existence of mutations in the DNA coding for the structure of the protein phenotypically scored is inferred by demonstrating that (1) the frequency is affected by mutagenic stimuli, (2) the occurrence is a spontaneous event independent of selective conditions,

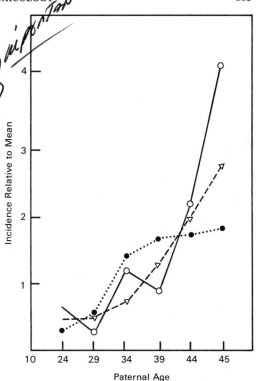

Figure 6–7. Gene-locus mutation and paternal age: (▽) achondroplasia ($n = 175$); (●) hemophilia A, maternal grandfathers ($n = 77$); (○) myositis ossificans ($n = 40$). (Redrawn from Vogel, F.: Spontaneous mutation in man. In Vogel, F., and Röhrborn, G. [eds.]: *Chemical Mutagenesis in Mammals and Man.* Springer-Verlag, New York, 1970, pp. 16–68.)

and (3) the phenotype is heritable. In a growing number of experimental systems, the genetic basis of the observed phenotypic changes has been demonstrated by sequencing the affected protein or the DNA from various mutants.

Still other assays are based on observations of morphologic changes in phenotype, such as colony size, shape, or color in microbiologic systems; wing veination or absence of bristles in *Drosophila;* or coat color or marking in mice. In most cases, the enzyme or functional protein associated with these phenotypic changes is unknown. The genetic basis of these phenotypes is demonstrated by classic genetic techniques such as mating and back crossing. Hollaender (1971a, 1971b, 1973, 1976) and de Serres and Hollaender (1978, 1980, 1982) have edited a series of volumes, each containing detailed descriptions of a wide variety of genetic assays involving species from bacteria to human cells.

While most of the mutagenesis literature involves the measurement of change in one or a small number of genetic loci by detecting an associated phenotypic change, it is also possible to examine the products of hundreds of soluble proteins and note the appearance or disappearance of electrophoretic bands, indicative of mutation. This approach has been discussed by Harris (1980) and applied broadly to the study of genetic diversity in human populations. At the biochemical level, Harris summarized the amino acid sequences associated with the hemoglobin variants in humans and pointed out that all of the possible transition and transversion base-pair substitution mutations are represented.

Target Theory. Underlying the use and understanding of mutation assays is the primary assumption that mutation at the locus scored and death are independently occurring events. When a sufficient concentration of a noxious agent is introduced into a large population of organisms or cells, some individuals are mutated at a given genetic locus and some individuals die. Death and mutation caused by a test agent can be modeled as independent events, since mutations in the loci generally chosen do not confer a selective disadvantage.

There are four kinds of individuals in a population following treatment with a test agent:

Fraction A, dead and mutated;
Fraction B, not dead and mutated;
Fraction C, dead and not mutated;
Fraction D, not dead and not mutated.

The fraction of dead cells is simply A + C, and the fraction that are mutant for the selected phenotype is A + B. The independence of death and mutation is a fundamental assumption, since the determination of mutant fraction would not be an accurate reflection of the whole population unless the fraction of mutant cells among surviving cells (B/[B + D]) is equal to the fraction of all cells mutated ([A + B]/[A + B + C + D]).

Both mutation and death can be modeled as occurring from one or more chemical reactions with a fixed number of cellular target molecules. For this discussion, we will use the simplest example, that of a single fixed target requiring one reaction (hit) to cause mutation. This kind of modeling, known as "target theory," has been used in radiation biology (e.g., Elkind and Whitmore, 1967) for decades.

The fraction of all cells that are mutated by the treatment can be designated M and the fraction killed designated T. It is possible that any cell might be hit in the death target 0, 1, 2, 3 . . . times, and this is equally true for hits in the mutation target. The situation can be described in terms of the Poisson distribution, since the requirements of a discrete variable, having an infinite number of possible integral values, independ-

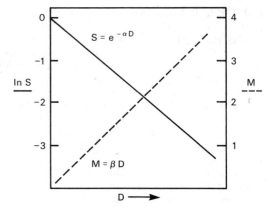

Figure 6–8. Survival and mutation as a function of dose when killing and mutation are modeled as simple first-order reactions between a cellular target and the agent tested.

dence of events, and statistical equilibrium, are fulfilled (Wadsworth and Bryan, 1960). The probability of surviving, $S = 1 - T$, can be derived from the Poisson distribution as the probability of not having any lethal hits:

$$S = e^{-\alpha D}$$

which is applicable even as T approaches 1. Mutation can be modeled in the same way as killing. The only adjustment is that an independent target parameter β must be chosen so that $M = \beta D$. D, dose, is a parameter depending on the concentration and duration of exposure of the target to the test agent. These arithmetic models would give results as in Figure 6–8, in which the surviving fraction S decreases as an exponential function of D, and the mutant fraction increases linearly with D. However, as will be discussed later in the section on Fixation of Genetic Error (p. 186), experimental results do not always yield such linear dose responses.

Examples of Mutagenesis Assay Systems

Salmonella **Tests.** Bruce Ames and his colleagues at the University of California at Berkeley have developed a number of mutant strains in the *his* operon of *S. typhimurium* that can be reverted by base-pair substitution or addition or deletion mutations (Ames *et al.*, 1975). To date over 5000 compounds have been tested in the Ames/*Salmonella* assay, and Ames and McCann (1981) estimate the correlation between mutagenicity and carcinogenicity to be approximately 83 percent. McCann and associates (1984) have outlined statistical procedures for evaluating mutagenicity data reported in the literature for this assay. The standard tester strains presently recommended by Ames are

TA97, TA98, TA100, and TA102 (Maron and Ames, 1983). All these strains carry the pK$_m$101 plasmid; in addition, TA97, TA98, and TA100 carry the *uvrB* and *rfa* mutations to enhance sensitivity. The TA100 strain and its predecessor TA1535 can be reverted to wild type by certain base-pair substitution mutations. The TA98 strain possesses a single base-pair deletion and detects frameshift mutagens that restore the reading frame. A $\frac{-GCGCGCGC-}{-CGCGCGCG-}$ sequence, which is postulated to be a "hotspot" for frameshift mutation, is near the site of the one-base-pair deletion. The TA97 strain, which has been reported to have an added cytosine residue in a run of six cytosines in the *hisD* gene, also detects frameshift mutagens. An additional strain, TA102, containing an ochre mutation, is employed to test a wide variety of mutagens (e.g., formaldehyde, glyoxal, cross-linking agents, UV) which are detected only poorly by the other strains.

An assay for forward mutation to 8-azaguanine drug resistance, presumed to be due to mutation inactivating one of the several enzymes necessary for metabolizing the base analog to a form that can be incorporated into RNA, has been developed in a *S. typhimurium* strain (Skopek *et al.*, 1978a). Our own experience suggests that this single forward assay can effectively replace the set of reversion assays in detecting the activity of a broad spectrum of chemical mutagens without compromising the sensitivity of the Ames/*Salmonella* assay (Skopek *et al.*, 1978b; Skopek and Thilly, 1983). In general, bacterial mutation assays have gained widespread use because they are relatively simple to perform, are inexpensive, and results can be obtained quickly.

Rodent and Human Cell Mutation Assays. The advent of techniques for growing mammalian cells in culture worked out by Puck and his colleagues (Puck and Marcus, 1955) has made possible the development of mammalian cell mutation assays. These assays are similar in principle to those performed in bacteria. Generally, forward mutation has been scored as resistance to a particular drug or, in some cases, as temperature sensitivity. Reverse mutation from amino acid auxotrophy (amino acid required) to prototrophy (amino acid not required) has also been used in some systems.

The two primary loci employed to measure forward mutation in mammalian cells are the X-linked gene hypoxanthine guanine phosphoribosyltransferase (*hgprt*) and the autosomal marker thymidine kinase (*tk*). Selection conditions for the presence or absence of HGPRT activity were initially developed by Szybalski

(1964). The toxic purine analogs 8-azaguanine and 6-thioguanine have been employed in a variety of rodent and human cell lines to select for HGPRT deficient mutants.

Several considerations, depending on the cell line used, have to be taken into account when a mutation assay is performed at the *hgprt* locus. Some mammalian cells, when plated in contact with one another, have the ability to form intercellular junctions that allow the transfer of small molecules between cells. The junction of an HGPRT$^+$ cell and an HGPRT$^-$ cell would create a two-cell unit with an HGPRT$^+$ phenotype. Thus, an underestimation of the HGPRT$^-$ mutant fraction would be made at densities permitting intercellular junction formation (Fujimoto *et al.*, 1971). Also, accurate determination of mutant fraction at the *hgprt* or any other locus cannot be properly performed without knowledge of the time interval necessary for expression of the selected phenotype in the cell line employed. For instance, the development of phenotypic resistance to 6-thioguanine can be delayed for as many as 14 generations after chemical treatment, presumably owing to the requirement for loss of essentially all HGPRT enzyme by degradation and dilution by cell division (Thilly *et al.*, 1978).

The autosomal *tk* locus is useful for mutation assays because the period of phenotypic lag is considerably shorter than for the *hgprt* locus (two versus about seven days). Since the *tk* gene is located on autosome 17 in humans, the assay requires isolation of a cell line heterozygous for thymidine kinase activity. Clive *et al.* (1973) achieved this by selecting for a rare presumptive homozygous-deficient (TK$^{-/-}$) cell line, then counterselecting for a thymidine kinase-proficient cell line, which behaved as a heterozygote. Construction of various heterozygous TK$^{+/-}$ cell lines has more readily permitted the detection of TK-deficient mutants (at frequencies generally $\geq 10^{-6}$) in cultured mammalian cells.

Dominant resistance to the drug ouabain is used in a number of mutation assays. Ouabain resistance is hypothesized to be due to base-pair substitution mutations in the gene for Na$^+$K$^+$-ATPase that alter the ouabain binding site without interfering with enzyme activity. Additional loci, such as adenosine phosphoribosyltransferase, adenosine kinase, and uridine kinase, as well as drug resistance conferred by mutation in many other unknown loci are candidates for incorporation into various preexisting mammalian cell mutation assays.

Mutation assays have been developed at the *hgprt* locus in Chinese hamster ovary (CHO) cells (Baker *et al.*, 1974; Hsie *et al.*, 1975;

O'Neill *et al.*, 1977) and for both the *hgprt* locus (Parodi and Brambilla, 1977) and ouabain resistance (Huberman and Sachs, 1976; Parodi and Brambilla, 1977) in V79 cells. Clive and colleagues have developed mutation assays at the *hgprt* and *tk* loci and for ouabain resistance in L5178Y lymphoma cells (reviewed by Clive *et al.*, 1973). These lymphoma cells have a rapid doubling time, are suspension grown, and can be cloned in agar.

Mutation assays have also been developed in diploid human lymphoblast and fibroblast cell lines. Our laboratory has developed mutation assays at the *tk* and *hgprt* loci and for ouabain resistance (reviewed by Thilly *et al.*, 1980). Human lymphoblast lines have a rapid doubling time (15 to 18 hours), are grown in suspension, and can be plated easily on microwell plates. Anchorage-dependent human fibroblasts, obtained from both normal and xeroderma pigmentosum (a skin condition resulting from an inherited hypersensitivity to the carcinogenic effect of ultraviolet light) patients, have been used in mutation assays at the *hgprt* locus.

Improvements in mammalian cell mutation assays that better approximate *in vivo* conditions, increase limits of detection, decrease time needed to test a compound, or lower costs can be anticipated in the future. It is also probable that full understanding of human cell genetics will eventually depend on studies of a wide variety of primary human tissues.

FIXATION OF GENETIC ERROR

The production of genetic damage, whether errors in chromosome number, structure, or at the gene level, appears to occur by complex mechanisms and to involve cellular processes that may differ depending on the agent, species, or cell type. The following discussion explores how spontaneous or chemically induced damage may cause different types of genetic errors and how cellular processes may ultimately act as determinants in the fixation of these genetic errors. While there is presently only a rudimentary understanding of aneuploidization, more extensive progress has been made in unraveling the mechanisms and cellular processes involved in clastogenesis and, in particular, mutagenesis. Although the following discussion on the fixation of genetic error is focused on mutagenesis, it should be kept in mind that some of the discussion may apply to clastogenesis and possibly aneuploidization as well.

Aneuploidization

At least one of the mechanisms by which either aneuploid germ-line or somatic cells arise is thought to be nondisjunction, in which chromosomes do not separate and thus are unequally distributed to daughter cells. In the case of mitotic cells, one daughter would become monosomic and the other trisomic for the chromosome not distributed properly. It is also theoretically possible for a single chromosome to be replicated twice in a mitotic cycle and give rise to two trisomic daughter cells via normal segregation of chromosomes. Polyploidy, which is almost always lethal in mammals, may result from improper reduction division during gametogenesis, blockage of cell division, or even fertilization by more than one sperm.

The actual physical and molecular mechanisms by which aneuploidies result and how chemicals may cause these aberrations are obscure. Functions involved in cell division are in all probability major determinants in many cases of aneuploidization. For example, colchicine is believed to cause aneuploidization in mammalian cells by disrupting microtubule formation necessary for cell division. Improper chromosome condensation, spindle formation and attachment, or chromosome alignment, as well as lagging of chromosomes during segregation, are a few of the errors that might be envisioned to contribute to aneuploidy.

Clastogenesis

DNA damage and the action of replication and repair systems upon these lesions are regarded as causal factors in the induction of many clastogenic events. Bender *et al.* (1973) have proposed models by which ultraviolet (UV)-induced photoproducts, pyrimidine dimers in particular, may result in the formation of chromosomal aberrations. These models have also been extended to the induction of chromosomal aberrations by chemicals. According to these models, achromatic gaps or lesions would be formed on the newly synthesized strand owing to the inability of DNA replication to bypass an unrepaired lesion. Incision, whether repair mediated, spontaneous, or otherwise, of the DNA damage opposite a gap may account for chromatid breaks involving both strands of DNA. Other types of chromosomal aberrations may be explained by additional models, involving DNA replication, repair, and recombination.

Evidence that repair functions can influence production of various chromosomal aberrations is evident in studies of UV-sensitive cell lines with a putative defect in excision repair. Xeroderma pigmentosum (XP) is a hereditary disorder marked by an increased sensitivity to UV light, a greatly elevated incidence of skin cancer, and a deficiency in excision repair. XP cells exhibit elevated chromosomal aberrations in response to UV light (Parrington *el al.*, 1971; Marshall and Scott, 1976). A UV-sensitive mouse cell line with a putative excision repair defect has also been reported to show an elevated incidence of chromatid breaks in response to UV light (Takahashi *et al.*, 1983). The studies of chromosomal aberrations in these repair deficient cell lines indicate that repair processes play an important role in clastogenesis.

Mutagenesis

Insight into processes and mechanisms involved in the fixation of genetic error has been gained from the study of mutagenesis. James and Elizabeth Miller (1969) postulated that many chemical mutagens are either electrophilic species, or are converted to such, which react with nucleophilic macromolecules within the cell. Prodigious research in this field has led to a better understanding of the biotransformation of mutagens to reactive metabolites and the interaction of these species with cellular macromolecules (reviewed by Miller and Miller, 1981). These reactive compounds have been shown to bind covalently to DNA, RNA, and protein, forming what has been termed adducts. DNA adducts are generally regarded as an important determinant in mutagenesis and, as previously discussed, in clastogenesis. Compounds such as aflatoxin and benzo[a]pyrene are believed to be activated to reactive epoxides that can bind covalently to DNA, forming bulky adducts. Other mutagens such as alkylating agents can act as donors of methyl and ethyl groups to DNA. Attempts have been made to ascertain relationships between chemical structure of adducts and the types of genetic damage induced (reviewed by Brendel and Ruhland, 1984). Identifying and quantifying potentially mutagenic adducts and correlating these data with the type and amount of mutation induced have been an active area of research for determining which DNA adducts cause mutation and by what mechanisms they do so.

Role of DNA Replication and Repair in Mutagenesis. At least two major cellular processes, DNA replication and DNA repair, have been identified as important determinants in the fixation of spontaneous and chemically induced mutation. One mechanism hypothesized to result in fixation of mutation is misreplication. This may be caused by spontaneous or chemically induced template alterations, such as modification of base structure, formation of rare base tautomeric forms, depurination, deamination, or looping out of bases from the helix. For example, the fidelity of *in vitro* DNA synthesis on synthetic templates has been shown to decrease in a manner directly proportional to the degree of depurination (Shearman and Loeb, 1979).

DNA replication *in vivo* is catalyzed by enzymes, each assigned different tasks. Mutations in genes coding for these proteins may alter the rate of spontaneous or induced mutation. The effect of replication machinery on mutation has been studied both *in vivo*, with mutants defective in various replication enzymes, and *in vitro* in systems using synthetic templates. Mutants with known or putative repair defects have proven valuable in the study of DNA repair and mutagenesis. While these rare mutants are relatively easy to select in prokaryotes and lower eukaryotes, limitations on the number of mammalian cells that can be cultured and screened make isolation more difficult. In many cases, the identification of repair mechanisms and pathways has been made possible by comparing the repair ability, measured by a number of biochemical methods, and mutation response of a normal organism with repair-deficient mutants. The effect of DNA repair in response to damage may generally be viewed as increasing survival and decreasing mutation, except in the case of a misrepair system, which enhances survival coincident with an increased frequency of mutation.

Several modes of DNA repair have been identified and studied in both prokaryotic and eukaryotic organisms. Some damaged bases, such as thymidine dimers, have been shown to be fixed by a group of excision repair enzymes, which produce a nick near the lesion, excise an area of DNA containing the lesion, resynthesize the DNA, and then ligate (seal) the gap between the newly repaired region and the preexisting DNA on the same strand. Another form of excision repair is performed by glycosylases that catalyze the excision of a single base from the sugar backbone (reviewed by Lindahl, 1979). These two types of excision repair are illustrated in Figure 6–9. Yet another gene product, a methyltransferase, restores the putative premutagenic alkylated base O^6 methylguanine to a guanine (reviewed by Yarosh, 1985).

Other modes of repair, which may be either inducible or constitutive, have been postulated to excise mismatched bases, correct errors following replication, or involve genetic recombination. Uncharacterized repair systems also exist to correct single-strand breaks, double-strand breaks, cross-linked DNA strands, and other damage. The examples cited by no means enumerate all possible modes of repair, but rather illustrate the complexity and variety of DNA repair systems.

Analysis of Dose Responses. How does DNA replication and repair affect the fate of premutagenic DNA adducts? How would the

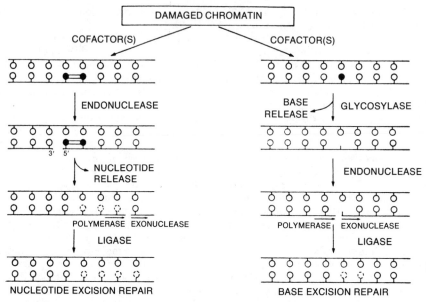

Figure 6–9. Two types of excision repair. (From Cleaver, J. E.: DNA repair and its coupling to DNA replication in eukaryotic cells. *Biochim. Biophys. Acta*, **516**:489–516, 1978.)

behavior of such processes influence the shape of mutation dose-responses for a given agent? Three assumptions underlie our analysis of the process of mutagenesis: (1) some DNA adducts are premutagenic lesions; (2) these premutagenic lesions will be repaired, misrepaired, or remain unrepaired by the time DNA synthesis occurs; and (3) during DNA synthesis, unrepaired DNA may be replicated, misreplicated, or unreplicated. By definition, if DNA is correctly repaired, the base sequence is restored to its original composition and no mutation occurs. Mutation results if the DNA is misrepaired either at the site of the lesion or at a site encompassed within the repaired region.

A lesion may also remain unrepaired if repair enzymes do not have the capacity to act on it prior to DNA synthesis or if it is not recognized. The genetic consequence of an unrepaired lesion would not be determined until replication occurs; the affected DNA would then be replicated, correctly or incorrectly, or remain unreplicated. Correct replication would result in the proper base sequence, whereas misreplication would result in the fixation of a genetic change in the newly synthesized daughter strand. If the lesion prevented replication, then cell death might eventually ensue.

We outline here how replication and repair processes may be responsible for nonlinear dose responses. Since a finite number of enzymes is involved in repair, it is theoretically a saturable

process. Thus, the repair capacity, defined as amount of DNA damage that a cell can repair, may be limited by such factors as the rate or ability of the repair enzymes to ameliorate premutagenic damage and the amount of time to do so before replication occurs. The repair system(s) may also possess a capacity to misrepair a DNA lesion prior to replication, which may result in a detectable mutation.

Mutation resulting solely from the misreplication of nonrepaired lesions would be predicted to increase as the repair system saturates with increasing dose. Mutation resulting from a nonrepaired lesion can be described as the probability of three independent events: (1) the probability that a premutagenic lesion is formed, (2) the probability of nonrepair, and (3) the probability that a nonrepaired, premutagenic lesion is misreplicated.

In contrast, since the capacity of repair systems should be finite, mutation–dose-response curves that plateau can be modeled to result from the saturable misrepair of premutagenic lesions. The probability that a lesion is acted on by a repair or misrepair system is simply 1 − (probability of not being repaired). Therefore, the probability of a mutation resulting from misrepair may be described as the joint probability of two events: the probability of a premutagenic lesion and the probability that such a lesion is misrepaired. A more complete discussion of how nonlinear mutation dose responses may be explained by nonrepair and misrepair mechanisms can be found in Thilly (1983).

Additional explanations potentially exist to explain nonlinear mutation–dose-responses. For example, Haynes and colleagues (1985) propose models in which nonlinear mutation-dose responses may be attributed to (1) two-hit events in molecular mechanisms of mutagenesis, or (2) a dependence between mutation and survival as a result of differential survival of mutants and nonmutants. Alternatively, concave upward mutation–dose-responses might be due to an inducible misrepair system. In this case, a misrepair system might be induced after a critical level of DNA damage had occurred, and this induced misrepair system might then cause mutation in the process of repairing the damage. According to this scenario, mutation would not be caused until a dose level sufficient for misrepair induction was attained.

Another consideration is that mutation–dose-responses are typically plotted as a function of exogenously administered mutagen, in most cases without knowledge of either the extent or profile of DNA adducts incurred as a function of dose. Any saturable function limiting the formation of premutagenic lesions might yield a concave upward dose-response with an apparent threshold. Saturation of an enzyme system necessary to activate a compound to a reactive intermediate might result in a plateauing dose-response. However, in these illustrative cases, had the mutation response been plotted with respect to the dose (defined as the number of chemical DNA adducts formed) rather than exogenous concentration, a linear dose-response might have been obtained. Examining the dose-response behavior of a mutagen together with other important parameters, such as DNA binding, adduct formation, and removal

profiles, is a valuable approach for probing mechanisms involved in the fixation of mutation and understanding dose-response behavior.

SPECIFICITY OF GENETIC DAMAGE CAUSED BY PHYSICAL AND CHEMICAL AGENTS

Review of the vast literature on genetic damage shows that, while an agent may effectively cause one kind of genetic damage, it will not necessarily cause all kinds. Barthelmess (1970) reviewed the available data regarding the ability of environmental chemicals to cause gene mutations in viruses and bacteria and their ability to cause chromosomal defects of structure and/or number in plants, insects, and mammals at the cellular or organismal level. Examples of chemical specificity with regard to the type of genetic damage caused can readily be cited. For instance, 2-aminopurine is an active mutagen in bacteria but causes no chromosomal defects in insects. Colchicine, which affects mitotic spindle formation, has been examined in a number of cell types and found to cause errors of chromosome number but relatively few errors of chromosome structure. Table 6–4 reduces the data of Kao and Puck (1969) to a comparison of the relative ability of several agents to cause chromatid exchanges and gene-locus mutation in cultured Chinese hamster ovary cells. Methylnitronitrosoguanidine was found to be about four times *less* mutagenic but seven times *more* clastogenic than ethyl methanesulfonate. Caffeine, a potent clastogen in *in vitro* assays, was found to be nonmutagenic. On the other hand, ICR-191, a half-mustard substituted acridine, had substantial mutagenic activity but little clastogenic potency. The differences cited point out the diversity of action spectra of different chemicals.

Table 6–4. RELATIVE CLASTOGENIC VERSUS MUTAGENIC ACTIVITY AMONG CHEMICAL AND PHYSICAL AGENTS*[†]

AGENT	RELATIVE MUTAGENIC ACTIVITY (GLY LOCUS)	RELATIVE CLASTOGENIC ACTIVITY (CHROMATID EXCHANGES)
Ethyl methanesulfonate	100	100
Methylnitronitrosoguanidine	27	710
Ultraviolet light	12	350
ICR-191	3	<13
Caffeine	0	340
Hydroxylamine	0	88

* Summarized from Kao and Puck (1969).
[†] All compared at a survival of approximately 14 percent.

SOCIAL CONSIDERATIONS AND THE PRACTICE OF GENETIC TOXICOLOGY

The major goal of genetic toxicology is to identify causes of human genetic disease initiated in both somatic and germ cells and to suggest means to decrease their incidence. To reach this goal, the identity and relative impact of environmental agents that induce genetic change in people must be determined. This approach is based on the fundamental assumption that, in fact, environmental chemicals cause a significant proportion of genetic disease afflicting humans.

The historical development of this important assumption can be traced to observations that humans suffer a significant amount of disease stemming from genetic errors and that the environment contains many chemicals that induce all known kinds of genetic damage in experimental systems, including human cells and rodent germ cells. The premise that environmental agents contribute substantially to genetic disorders, while suggested by present knowledge, remains untested in humans. Today this assumption has attained an important status, reflected in the regulatory laws and policies of many nations.

We discuss below four combined strategies to assess the contribution of environmental agents to genetic disease in the human population: (1) further testing of environmental chemicals and complex mixtures in short-term genetic assays, (2) measurements of in vivo human exposure to chemicals capable of causing genetic errors, (3) measurements of in vivo genetic damage occuring in humans, and (4) continued epidemiologic studies of genetic disease.

The use of short-term genetic assays to test chemicals and complex mixtures is a common first step toward identifying agents that may cause genetic disease in humans. Improvements in these short-term assays that better approximate conditions of in vivo human exposure and genetic damage can be anticipated. Ideally, environmental exposure to any agent deemed a potential hazard in a battery of short-term tests should be eliminated or minimized until further risk analysis can be performed.

The second strategy, to determine to what chemicals and at what levels humans are exposed, is often concentrated on those environmentally encountered agents shown to induce genetic errors in short-term tests. The development of highly sensitive techniques, based on high-performance liquid chromatography, fluorimetry, monoclonal antibodies, and DNA labeling, for the detection and quantitation of the binding of chemicals to DNA, RNA, or proteins in human cells or body fluids, holds great potential for ascertaining in vivo exposure. This type of study may also facilitate identification of groups or individuals who may be at increased risk of genetic damage owing to high exposures.

Development of methods for measuring chromosomal errors and gene-locus mutations in human cells with sufficient ease and accuracy for widespread application will permit determination of in vivo genetic damage in humans. The B and T lymphocytes circulating in the blood are prime candidates for such studies because they are available in sufficient quantity and can be obtained with little risk to the donor. Methods for cloning and measuring genetic damage in human T lymphocytes have been developed (Morley et al., 1983a, 1983b; Albertini and Sylvester, 1984; Vijayalaxmi and Evans, 1984a, 1984b; Albertini, 1982, 1985). One approach to reaching this goal is to examine cells of individuals having known or suspect exposure to high levels of specific chemicals to determine whether genetic errors are significantly elevated.

Another approach being developed in our laboratory (Thilly et al., 1982) to determine whether chemically induced genetic change is prevalent in the human population is based on the recognition by Benzer (1961) that chemically induced gene mutations are specific with regard to type and position in bacteriophage. The observation that the distributions, or "mutational spectra," of detectable spontaneous and induced mutations at the DNA sequence level differ for a wide variety of chemicals was extended to bacteria by Miller and co-workers (Miller et al., 1977; Coulondre and Miller, 1977a, 1977b; Schmeissner et al., 1977; Miller et al., 1978; Calos and Miller, 1981) and seems to be applicable to gene mutations induced in cultured rodent and human cells. The goal is to determine whether the mutational spectra in human blood cells display a pattern indicative of spontaneous or chemically induced mutation. This approach would provide a means to test the central premise of the field and, if it is substantiated, to suggest identities of the most active mutagens causing human genetic alterations.

Although studies of in vivo genetic damage and exposure should yield valuable information regarding the role of environmental exposure in human genetic error, epidemiologic studies are necessary to determine whether environmental exposure and genetic errors can be linked causally to genetic disease. Furthermore, continual accurate monitoring of the frequency of spontaneous abortion and genetic defects in abortuses and liveborns should aid in identifying groups of individuals at increased risk as well as in detecting any changes in incidences of birth defects. The cascade of complicated and as yet not fully understood processes involved in the eventual appearance of genetic disease should not be forgotten. Although genetic error may eventually lead to genetic disease, the contribution of other intervening steps remains to be elucidated. Epidemiologic studies are fundamental in that they may serve to identify factors, other than or in addition to environmental agents, that exert a causal role in genetic disease.

Reducing Genetic Disease

The present legal and regulatory attitude is that environmental agents contribute to genetic disease, cancer, and other health problems. It follows that, in the case of industrially and medically utilized substances believed to pose a health problem, safer substitutes should be found or exposure should be greatly minimized. Efforts should also be concentrated on reducing exposure to or detoxifying sources of potentially hazardous chemicals present in the environment. These measures may be of great benefit in reducing genetic diseases, should the central premise concerning the role of chemical and physical agents in the development of genetic maladies prove true.

The goal of reducing genetic disease in humans may also be reached by a number of technologic paths, such as gene or enzyme replacement therapy for afflicted individuals. It is not beyond present technical ability to develop transport vectors that might carry specific genetic information to a sufficient fraction of tissues or cells to eliminate or ameliorate disease symptoms. Another approach of demonstrated use in reducing genetic disease is to augment intrauterine surveillance through cytogenetic and biochemical analysis of fetal cells collected by amniocentesis or chorionic cell sampling. Recent progress has already been made in surgically correcting some structural abnormalities *in utero*. Intrauterine detection of genetic error places upon the parents the decision whether to bring to term a fetus with an uncorrectable defect. A variation on this approach is genetic counseling for parents identified to be at increased risk to voluntarily forego parenthood. These approaches have in common the advantage that they deal with genetic disease independent of the cause of error.

In summary, reaching the goal of reducing genetic diseases depends on identifying and reducing important causal factors in conjunction with developing means of screening for and correcting genetic defects.

REFERENCES

Albertini, R. J.: Studies with T-lymphocytes: An approach to human mutagenicity monitoring. In Bridges, B. A.; Butterworth, B. E.; and Weinstein, I. B. (eds.): *Banbury Conference Report 13, Indicators of Genotoxic Exposure in Man and Animals.* Cold Spring Harbor Laboratory, Cold Spring Harbor, N.Y., 1982, pp. 453–65.

Albertini, R. J.: Somatic gene mutations *in vivo* as indicated by the 6-thioguanine-resistant T-lymphocytes in human blood. *Mutat. Res.,* **150**:411–22, 1985.

Albertini, R. J., and Sylvester, D. L.: 6-Thioguanine-resistant lymphocytes in human blood. In Kilbey, B. J.; Legator, M.; Nichols, W.; and Ramel, C. (eds.): *Handbook of Mutagenicity Test Procedures.* Elsevier, Amsterdam, 1984, pp. 357–72.

Allen, J. W.; Liang, J. C.; Carrano, A. V.; and Preston, R. J.: Review of literature on chemically-induced aneuploidy in mammalian male germ cells. *Mutat. Res.,* **167**:123–37, 1986.

Ames, B. N., and McCann, J.: Validation of the *Salmonella* test: a reply to Rinkus and Legator. *Cancer Res.,* **41**:4192–4203, 1981.

Ames, B. N.; McCann, J.; and Yamasaki, E.: Methods for detecting carcinogens and mutagens with the *Salmonella*/mammalian-microsome mutagenicity test. *Mutat. Res.,* **31**:347–64, 1975.

Ayme, S., and Lippman-Hand, A.: Maternal-age effect in aneuploidy: does altered embryonic selection play a role? *Am. J. Hum. Genet.,* **34**:558–65, 1982.

Baker, R.; Brunette, D.; Mankovitz, R.; Thompson, L.; Whitmore, G.; Siminovitch, L.; and Till, J.: Ouabain-resistant mutants of mouse and hamster cells in culture. *Cell,* **1**:9–21, 1974.

Barthelmess, A.: Mutagenic substances in the human environment. In Vogel, F., and Röhrborn, G. (eds.): *Chemical Mutagenesis in Mammals and Man.* Springer-Verlag, New York, 1970, pp. 69–147.

Bauchinger, M.; Schmid, E.; Einbrodt, H. J.; and Dresp, J.: Chromosome aberrations in lymphocytes after occupational exposure to lead and cadmium. *Mutat. Res.,* **40**:57–62, 1976.

Bender, M. A.; Griggs, H. G.; and Walker, P. L.: Mechanisms of chromosomal aberration production. I. Aberration induction by ultraviolet light. *Mutat. Res.,* **20**:387–402, 1973.

Benzer, S.: On the topography of the genetic find structure. *Proc. Natl Acad. Sci. (USA),* **47**:403–15, 1961.

Boué, J.; Boué, A.; and Lazar, P.: Retrospective and prospective epidemiological studies of 1500 karyotyped spontaneous human abortions. *Teratology,* **12**:11–26, 1975.

Brendel, M., and Ruhland, A.: Relationships between functionality and genetic toxicology of selected DNA-damaging agents. *Mutat. Res.* **133**:51–85, 1984.

Calos, M. P., and Miller, J. H.: Genetic sequence analysis of frameshift mutations induced by ICR-191. *J. Mol. Biol.,* **153**:39–64, 1981.

Carr, D. H., and Gedeon, M.: Population cytogenetics of human abortuses. In Hook, E. B., and Porter, I. H. (eds.): *Population Cytogenetics. Studies in Humans.* Academic Press, Inc., New York, 1977, pp. 1–9.

Carter, C. O.: Monogenic disorders. *J. Med. Genet.,* **14**:316–20, 1977.

Clive, D.; Flamm, W. G.; and Patterson, J. B.: Specific-locus mutational assay systems for mouse lymphoma cells. In Hollaender, A. (ed.): *Chemical Mutagens: Principles and Methods for their Detection,* Vol. 3. Plenum Press, New York, 1973, pp. 79–104.

Cleaver, J. E.: DNA repair and its coupling to DNA replication in eukaryotic cells. *Biochim. Biophys. Acta,* **516**:489–516, 1978.

Cohen, M. M., and Hirschhorn, K.: Cytogenetic studies in animals. In Hollaender, A. (ed.): *Chemical Mutagens: Principles and Methods for their Detection,* Vol. 2. Plenum Press, New York, 1971, pp. 515–34.

Coulondre, C., and Miller, J. H.: Genetic studies of the lac repressor: III. Additional correlation of mutational sites with specific amino acid residues. *J. Mol. Biol.,* **117**:525–75, 1977a.

——: Genetic studies of the lac repressor: IV. Mutagenic specificity in the lacI of *Escherichia coli. J. Mol. Biol.,* **117**:577–606, 1977b.

de Serres, F. J., and Hollaender, A.: *Chemical Mutagens: Principles and Methods for Their Detection,* Vol. 5. Plenum Press, New York, 1978.

——: *Chemical Mutagens: Principles and Methods for Their Detection,* Vol. 6. Plenum Press, New York, 1980.

——: *Chemical Mutagens: Principles and Methods for Their Detection,* Vol. 7. Plenum Press, New York, 1982.

Elkind, M. M., and Whitmore, G. F.: *The Radiobiology of Cultured Mammalian Cells.* Gordon & Breach, New York, 1967.

Felber, B. K.; Orkin, S. H.; and Hamer, D. H.: Abnormal RNA splicing causes one form of α-thalassemia. *Cell,* **29**:895–902, 1982.

Fujimoto, W. Y.; Subak-Sharpe, J. H.; and Seegmiller, J. E.: Hypoxanthene-guanine phosphoribosyltransferase deficiency: chemical agents selective for mutants or normal cultured fibroblasts in mixed and heterozygote cultures. *Proc. Natl Acad. Sci. (USA),* **68**:1516–19, 1971.

Galloway, S. M., and Ivett, J. L.: Chemically induced aneuploidy in mammalian cells in culture. *Mutat. Res.,* **167**:89–105, 1986.

Generoso, W. M.; Cain, K. T.; Huff, S. W.; and Gosslee, D. G.: Heritable translocation test in mice. In de Serres, F. J., and Hollaender, A. (eds.): *Chemical Mutagens, Principles and Methods for their Detection,* Vol. 5. Plenum Press, New York, 1978, pp. 55–77.

Griffiths, A. J. F.: *Neurospora* prototroph selection system for studying aneuploid production. *Environ. Health Perspect.,* **31**:75–80, 1979.

Griffiths, A. J. F.; Brockman, H. E.; DeMarini, D. M.; and de Serres, F. J.: The efficacy of *Neurospora* in detecting agents that cause aneuploidy. *Mutat. Res.,* **167**:35–45, 1986.

Harris, H.: *The Principles of Human Biochemical Genetics,* 3rd ed. North Holland/American Elsevier, New York, 1980.

Haynes, R. H.; Eckardt, F.; and Kunz, B. A.: Analysis of non-linearities in mutation frequency curves. *Mutat. Res.,* **150**:51–59, 1985.

Heddle, J. A.; Hite, M.; Kirkhart, B.; Mavournin, K.; MacGregor, J. T.; Newell, G. W.; and Salamone, M. F.: The induction of micronuclei as a measure of genotoxicity. A report of the U.S. Environmental Protection Agency Gene-Tox Program (MTR 07162). *Mutat. Res.,* **123**:61–118, 1983.

Hollaender, A. (ed.): *Chemical Mutagens: Principles and Methods for Their Detection,* Vol. 1. Plenum Press, New York, 1971a.

——: *Chemical Mutagens: Principles and Methods for Their Detection,* Vol. 2. Plenum Press, New York, 1971b.

——: *Chemical Mutagens: Principles and Methods for Their Detection,* Vol. 3. Plenum Press, New York, 1973.

——: *Chemical Mutagens: Principles and Methods for Their Detection,* Vol. 4. Plenum Press, New York, 1976.

Honeycombe, J. R.: The effects of busulphan on the chromosomes of normal human lymphocytes. *Mutat. Res.,* **57**:35–49, 1978.

Hook, E. B.: Contribution of chromosome abnormalities to human morbidity and mortality and some comments upon surveillance of chromosome mutation rates. In Bora, K. C.; Douglas, G. R.; and Nestmann, E. R. (eds.): *Progress in Mutation Research.* Vol. 3, *Chemical Mutagenesis, Human Population Monitoring and Genetic Risk Assessment.* Elsevier Biomedical Press, Amsterdam, 1982, pp. 9–38.

Hook, E. B., and Hamerton, J. L.: The frequency of chromosome abnormalities detected in consecutive newborn studies—differences between studies—results by sex and severity of phenotype involvement. In Hook, E. B., and Porter, I. H. (eds.): *Population Cytogenetics: Studies in Humans.* Academic Press, Inc., New York, 1977, pp. 63–80.

Hsie, A. W.; Brimer, P. A.; Mitchell, T. J.; and Gosslee, D. G.: The dose-response relationship for ethyl methanesulfonate-induced mutations at the hypoxanthine-guanine phosphoribosyl transferase locus in Chinese hamster ovary cells. *Somatic Cell Genet.,* **1**:247–61, 1974.

Huberman, E., and Sachs, L.: Mutability of different genetic loci in mammalian cells by metabolically activated carcinogenic polycyclic hydrocarbons. *Proc. Natl Acad. Sci. (USA),* **73**:188–92, 1976.

Kao, F. T., and Puck, T. T.: Genetics of somatic mammalian cells. IX. Quantitation of mutagenesis by physical and chemical agents. *J. Cell. Physiol.,* **74**:245–58, 1969.

Kapp, R. W., Jr.: Detection of aneuploidy in human sperm. *Environ. Health Perspect.,* **31**:27–32, 1979.

Kihlman, B. A.: Root tips for studying the effects of chemicals on chromosomes. In Hollaender, A. (ed.): *Chemical Mutagens, Principles and Methods for their Detection,* Vol. 2. Plenum Press, New York, 1971, pp. 489–514.

Kleihues, P.; Patzchke, K.; and Doerjer, G.: DNA modification and repair in the experimental induction of nervous system tumors by chemical carcinogens. *Ann. NY Acad. Sci.,* **381**:290–303, 1982.

Latt, S. A.; Allen, J.; Bloom, S. E.; Carrano, A.; Falke, E.; Kram, D.; Schneider, E.; Schreck, R.; Tice, R.; Whitfield, B.; and Wolff, S.: Sister-chromatid exchanges: a report of the gene-tox program. *Mutat. Res.,* **87**:17–62, 1981.

Lindahl, T.: DNA glycosylases, endonucleases for apurinic/apyrimidinic sites, and base-excision repair. In Cohn, W. E. (ed.): *Progress in Nucleic Acid Research and Molecular Biology,* Vol. 22. Academic Press, Inc., New York, 1979, pp. 135–92.

Maher, V. M.; Ouellette, L. M.; Curren, R. D.; and McCormick, J. J.: Frequency of ultraviolet light–induced mutations is higher in xeroderma pigmentosum variant cells than in normal human cells. *Nature (London),* **261**:593–94, 1976.

Maron, D. M., and Ames, B. N.: Revised methods for the *Salmonella* mutagenicity test. *Mutat. Res.,* **113**:173–215, 1983.

Marshall, R. R., and Scott, D.: The relationship between chromosomal damage and cell killing in UV-irradiated normal and xeroderma pigmentosum cells. *Mutat. Res.,* **36**:397–400, 1976.

Matsunaga, E.: Perspectives in mutation epidemiology. I. Incidence and prevalence of genetic disease (excluding chromosomal aberrations) in human populations. *Mutat. Res.,* **99**:95–128, 1982.

McCann, J.; Horn, L.; and Kaldor, J.: An evaluation of *Salmonella* (Ames) test data in the published literature: application of statistical procedures and analysis of mutagenic potency. *Mutat. Res.,* **134**:1–47, 1984.

Meretoja, T.; Vainio, H.; Sorsa, M.; and Härkönen, H.: Occupational styrene exposure and chromosomal aberrations. *Mutat. Res.,* **56**:193–97, 1977.

Miller, E. C., and Miller, J. A.: Searches for ultimate

chemical carcinogens and their reactions with cellular macromolecules. *Cancer*, **47**:2327–45, 1981.

Miller, J. A., and Miller, E. C.: Metabolic activation of carcinogenic aromatic amines and amides via *N*-hydroxylation and *N*-hydroxy esterification and its relationship to ultimate carcinogens as electrophilic reactants. In *The Jerusalem Symposia on Quantum Chemistry.* Vol. I. *Physiochemical Mechanisms of Carcinogenesis.* The Israel Academy of Sciences and Humanities, Jerusalem, 1969, pp. 237–62.

Miller, J. H.; Ganem, D.; Lu, P.; and Schmitz, A.: Genetic studies of the Lac repressor. I. Correlation of mutational sites with specific amino acid residues: Construction of colinear gene-protein map. *J. Mol. Biol.*, **109**:275–98, 1977.

Miller, J. H.; Coulondre, C.; and Farabaugh, P. J.: Correlation of nonsense sites in the lacI gene with specific codons in the nucleotide sequence. *Nature (London)*, **274**:770–75, 1978.

Milunsky, A.: The prenatal diagnosis of chromosomal disorders. In Milunsky, A. (ed.): *Genetic Disorders and the Fetus: Diagnosis, Prevention, and Treatment.* Plenum Press, New York, 1979, pp. 93–156.

Morley, A. A.; Cox, S.; Wismore, D.; Seshadri, R.; and Dempsey, J. L.: Enumeration of thioguanine-resistant lymphocytes using autoradiography. *Mutat. Res.*, **95**:363–75, 1983a.

Morley, A. A.; Trainor, K. J.; Seshadri, R.; and Ryall, R. B.: Measurement of *in vivo* mutation in human lymphocytes. *Nature (London)*, **302**:155–56, 1983b.

O'Neill, J. P.; Couch, D. B.; Machanoff, R.; Hirsch, G. P.; and Hsie, A. W.: A quantitative assay of mutation induction at the hypoxanthine-guanine phosphoribosyltransferase locus in Chinese hamster ovary cells (CHO/HGPRT system): Development and definition of the system. *Mutat. Res.*, **45**:91–101, 1977.

Opitz, J. R., and Sutherland, G. R.: Conference report: International workshop on the fragile X and X-linked mental retardation. *Am. J. Med. Gen.*, **17**:5–94, 1984.

Painter, R. B.: A replication model for sister-chromatid exchange. *Mutat. Res.*, **70**:337–41, 1980.

Paris Conference (1971): Standardization in human cytogenetics. In Bergsma, D. (ed.): *Birth Defects. Original Article Series*, Vol. 8, No. 7. The National Foundation, New York, 1972.

Parodi, S., and Brambilla, G.: Relationships between mutation and transformation frequencies in mammalian cells treated *in vitro* with chemical carcinogens. *Mutat. Res.*, **47**:53–74, 1977.

Parrington, J. M.; Delhanty, J. D. A.; and Baden, H. P.: Unscheduled DNA synthesis, UV-induced chromosome aberrations and SV40 transformation in cultured cells from xeroderma pigmentosum. *Ann. Hum. Genet.*, **35**:149–60, 1971.

Parry, J. M., and Zimmerman, F. K.: The detection of monosomic colonies produced by mitotic chromosome non-disjunction in the yeast *Saccharomyces cerevisiae.* *Mutat. Res.*, **36**:49–66, 1976.

Parry, J. M.; Sharp, D.; and Parry, E. M.: Detection of mitotic and meiotic aneuploidy in the yeast *Saccharomyces cerevisiae. Environ. Health Perspect.*, **31**:97–111, 1979.

Penman, B. W.; Crespi, C. L.; Komives, E. A.; Liber, H. L.; and Thilly, W. G.: Mutation of human lymphoblasts exposed to low concentrations of chemical mutagens for long periods of time. *Mutat. Res.*, **108**:417–36, 1983.

Puck, T. T., and Marcus, P. I.: A rapid method for viable cell titration and clone production with HeLa cells in tissue culture: The use of x-irradiated cells to supply conditioning factors. *Proc. Natl Acad. Sci. (USA)*, **41**:432–37, 1955.

Reeves, B. R., and Margoles, C.: Preferential location of chlorambucil-induced breakage in the chromosomes of normal human lymphocytes. *Mutat. Res.*, **26**:205–208, 1974.

Resnick, M. A.; Mayer, V. W.; and Zimmermann, F. K.: The detection of chemically induced aneuploidy in *Saccharomyces cerevisiae:* an assessment of mitotic and meiotic systems. *Mutat. Res.*, **167**:47–60, 1986.

Sanchez, O., and Yunis, J. J.: New chromosomal techniques and their medical applications. In Yunis, J. J. (ed.): *New Chromosomal Syndromes.* Academic Press, Inc., New York, 1977.

Sankaranarayanan, K.: The role of non-disjunction in aneuploidy in man: An overview. *Mutat. Res.*, **61**:1–28, 1979.

Schmid, W.: The micronucleus test for cytogenetic analysis. In Hollaender, A. (ed.): *Chemical Mutagens: Principles and Methods for their Detection*, Vol. 4. Plenum Press, New York, 1976, pp. 31–53.

Schmeissner, U.; Ganem, D.; and Miller, J. H.: Genetic studies of the lac repressor. II. Fine structure deletion map of the lacI gene, and its correlation with the physical map. *J. Mol. Biol.*, **109**:303–26, 1977.

Shearman, C. W., and Loeb, L. A.: Effects of depurination on the fidelity of DNA synthesis. *J. Mol. Biol.*, **128**:197–218, 1979.

Skopek, T. R.; Liber, H. L.; Krolewski, J. J.; and Thilly, W. G.: Quantitative forward mutation assay in *Salmonella typhimurium* using 8-azaguanine resistance as a genetic marker. *Proc. Natl Acad. Sci. (USA)*, **75**:410–14, 1978a.

Skopek, T. R.; Liber, H. L.; Kaden, D. A.; and Thilly, W. G.: Relative sensitivities of forward and reverse mutation assays in *Salmonella typhimurium. Proc. Natl Acad. Sci. (USA)*, **75**:4465–69, 1978b.

Skopek, T. R., and Thilly, W. G.: Rate of induced forward mutation at 3 genetic loci in *Salmonella typhimurium. Mutat. Res.*, **108**:45–56, 1983.

Sutherland, G. R.: Heritable fragile sites on human chromosomes. I. Factors affecting expression in lymphocyte culture. *Am. J. Hum. Genet.*, **31**:125–35, 1979.

————: The fragile X chromosome. In Bourne, G. H., and Danielli, J. F. (eds.): *International Review of Cytology*, Vol. 81. Academic Press, Inc., New York, 1983, pp. 107–43.

Szemere, G., and Chandley, A. C.: Trisomy and triploidy induced by x-irradiation of mouse spermatocytes. *Mutat. Res.*, **33**:229–38, 1975.

Szybalski, W.: Chemical reactivity of chromosomal DNA as related to mutagenicity: Studies with human cell lines. *Cold Spring Harbor Symp. Quant. Biol.*, **29**:151–60, 1964.

Takahashi, E.-I.; Tobari, I.; Shiomi, T.; and Sato, K.: Chromosomal hypersensitivity in mutant M10 and Q31 mouse cells exposed to ultraviolet radiation (UV) and 4-nitroquinoline-1-oxide (4NQO). *Mutat. Res.*, **109**:207–17, 1983.

Tates, A. D.: *Microtus oeconomus* (Rodentia), a useful mammal for studying the induction of sex-chromosome nondisjunction and diploid gametes in male germ cells. *Environ. Health Perspect.*, **31**:151–59, 1979.

Tates, A. D., and de Vogel, N.: Further studies on effects of X-irradiation on prespermatid stages of the Northern vole *Microtus oeconomus.* Low induction of sex-chromosome nondisjunction and diploid gametes in vole germ cells. *Environ. Health Perspect.*, **31**:151–59, 1981.

Thilly, W. G.: Analysis of chemically induced mutation in single cell populations. In Lawrence, W. (ed.): *Induced Mutagenesis: Molecular Mechanisms and their Implications for Environmental Protection.* Plenum Press, New York, 1983, pp. 337–73.

Thilly, W. G.; DeLuca, J. G.; Furth, E. E.; Hoppe IV, H.; Kaden, D. A.; Krolewski, J. J.; Liber, H. L.; Skopek, T. R.; Slapikoff, S.; Tizard, R. J.; and Penman, B. W.: Gene locus mutation assays in diploid human lymphoblast lines. In de Serres, F. J., and Hollaender, A. (eds.): *Chemical Mutagens,* Vol. 6. Plenum Press, New York, 1980, pp. 331–64.

Thilly, W. G.; DeLuca, J. G.; Hoppe IV, H.; and Penman, B. W.: Phenotypic lag and mutation to 6-thioguanine resistance in diploid human lymphoblasts. *Mutat. Res.,* **50:**137–44, 1978.

Thilly, W. G.; Leong, P.-M.; and Skopek, T. R.: Potential of mutational spectra for diagnosing the cause of genetic change in human cell populations. In Bridges, B. A.; Butterworth, B. E.; and Weinstein, I. B. (eds.): *Banbury Report 13. Indicators of Genotoxic Exposure in Man and Animals,* Cold Spring Harbor Laboratory, Cold Spring Harbor, N.Y., 1982, pp. 453–65.

Treisman, R.; Proudfoot, N. J.; Shandler, M.; and Maniatis, T.: A single-base change at a splice site in a β-thalassemic gene causes abnormal RNA splicing. *Cell,* **29:**903–11, 1982.

Vijayalaxmi, and Evans, H. J.: Measurement of spontaneous and X-irradiation induced 6-thioguanine resistant human blood lymphocytes using a T-cell cloning technique. *Mutat. Res.,* **125:**87–94, 1984a.

Vijayalaxmi, and Evans, H. J.: Induction of 6-thioguanine-resistant mutants and SCEs by 3 chemical mutagens (EMS, ENU and MNC) in cultured human blood lymphocytes. *Mutat. Res.,* **129:**283–89, 1984b.

Vogel, F.: Spontaneous mutation in man. In Vogel, F., and Rörhborn, G. (eds.): *Chemical Mutagenesis in Mammals and Man.* Springer-Verlag, New York, 1970, pp. 16–68.

Vogel, F., and Rathenberg, R.: Spontaneous mutation in man. *Adv. Hum. Genet.,* **5:**223–318, 1975.

Wadsworth, G. P., and Bryan, J. G.: *Introduction to Probability and Random Variables.* McGraw-Hill Book Co., Inc., New York, 1960.

Watson, W. A. F.; Petrie, J. C.; Galloway, D. B.; Bullock, I.; and Gilbert, J. C.: *In vivo* cytogenic activity of sulphonylurea drugs in man. *Mutat. Res.,* **38:**71–80, 1976.

Yarosh, D. B.: The role of O^6-methylguanine-DNA methyltransferase in cell survival, mutagenesis and carcinogenesis. *Mutat. Res.,* **145:**1–16, 1985.

Yunis, J. J.: The chromosomal basis of human neoplasia. *Science,* **221:**227–36, 1983.

Yunis, J. J.; Bloomfield, C. D.; and Ensrud, K.: All patients with acute nonlymphocytic leukemia may have a chromosomal defect. *N. Engl. J. Med.,* **305:**135–39, 1981.

Yunis, J. J.; Oken, M. M.; Kaplan, M. E.; Ensrud, K. M.; Howe, R. R.; and Theologides, A.: Distinctive chromosomal abnormalities in histologic subtypes of non-Hodgkin's lymphoma. *N. Engl. J. Med.,* **307:**1231–36, 1982.

Chapter 7

TERATOGENS

Jeanne M. Manson

HISTORY

Teratology is concerned with the investigation of birth defects and is a field of study with roots going back to early primitive times. Abnormal births are events that have stimulated responses of awe, horror, and curiosity, and records of their occurrence have been transmitted in many forms. Legends, artistic renderings, and written descriptions of malformed infants can be found in cultural artifacts of many civilizations and provide a history of human perception of this event. It is believed that many mythologic figures originated with the birth of severely malformed infants (Thompson, 1930; Warkany, 1977). The similarities between some descriptions of mythologic beings and gods of antiquity to what we now recognize as patterns of human congenital malformations are remarkable. Births of abnormal infants have also been considered to be portents for events to come, and the word "monster" comes from a Latin root meaning "to warn" (Thompson, 1930). The most extensive early records of congenital malformations appear to have been kept for purposes of divination or foretelling the future, a practice that became so firmly established that a systematic record of congenital malformations was kept by many early civilizations (Warkany, 1977). Cross-breeding between humans and animals has been used as an explanation for abnormal births in offspring with hybrid features. An alternative belief, which still survives today in some parts of the world, is that the visual impressions and emotions of a woman during pregnancy can have a formative influence on fetal development. Unlike the situation in animals, which often cannibalize malformed offspring, the reaction of human populations to malformations has varied according to the belief of the culture. Responses have varied from practices of infanticide to natural death and from protective rearing to deification (Warkany, 1977). Today, scientific explanations are sought for the causes of birth defects, but there is no doubt that these strange, awesome, and terrifying variations of human form are still a great mystery to us. Our reactions to them are not so different from those of our ancestors, and profound ethical and legal questions concerning the causation and survival of defective children remain.

Experimental teratology first began in the late nineteenth century in studies of nonmammalian species. A variety of environmental conditions (temperature, microbial toxins, drugs) were found to perturb development in avian, reptile, fish, and amphibian classes. Mammalian embryos were thought to be immune to induction of malformations, and to be either killed outright or protected by the maternal system from adverse environmental conditions. The primary causal explanation for malformations in humans was genetic inheritance, and the terms "congenital" and "hereditary" were used interchangeably (Warkany, 1965). The first reports of induced birth defects in mammalian species came out in the 1930s to 1940s and involved maternal nutritional deficiencies (i.e., vitamin A and riboflavin). These were followed by many other studies in which a number of chemical and physical agents that caused malformations in mammalian species were identified—e.g., nitrogen mustard, trypan blue, hormones, antimetabolites, alkylating agents, hypoxia, and x-rays, to name a few (Warkany, 1965).

The field of modern teratology has taken shape in the last 40 years with the development of animal models for producing birth defects, and with the occurrence of human epidemics of malformations induced by exogenous agents. The first such reported epidemic was that identified by Gregg in 1941 on rubella virus infection in pregnant women (Gregg, 1941). The eye, heart, and ear defects, as well as mental retardation, produced by rubella remained unrecognized until an epidemic of rubella infections in Austria elevated their incidence to the level where a clinical syndrome became apparent, and the etiology was identified. When rubella infection occurred during the first or second month of pregnancy, heart and eye defects predominated, while hearing defects were most commonly associated with infection in the third month. The risk of congenital anomalies with rubella infection in the first four weeks of pregnancy was estimated to be 61 percent; in weeks 5 to 8, 26 percent; and in weeks 9 to 12, 8 percent (Sever, 1967; Warkany, 1971b). Approximately 16 to 18 percent of pregnancies complicated by early rubella infections ended in miscarriage or stillbirth. Infections after the 14th week did not result in malformations but did carry risk for hearing and speech deficits, as well as mental retardation in the offspring (Warkany, 1971b). Rubella infections have not influenced the overall incidence of malformations to a great extent, but their impact on pregnancy outcome has been severe at times of rubella epidemics. It has been estimated that in the United States approximately 20,000 children have become malformed owing to rubella infections alone (Cooper and Krugman, 1966).

In a relatively short time the embryos of mammals, including humans, were found to be susceptible to common environmental influences such as nutritional deficiencies and intrauterine infections. The full impact of these findings, however, was not brought to bear upon the public consciousness until 1961, when the association between thalidomide ingestion by pregnant women and the birth of severely malformed infants was established. In contrast to the situation with rubella, the teratogenicity of thalidomide in humans was recognized relatively quickly because a syndrome of severe and rare limb defects was involved. If more common malformations of the skeleton and viscera had been induced by thalidomide, it might have taken much longer to recognize the syndrome and to identify the cause.

Thalidomide was introduced in 1956 by the drug manufacturer Chemie Grünenthal as a sedative/hypnotic, and was used throughout the world to ameliorate nausea and vomiting in pregnancy. It had no apparent toxicity or addictive properties in humans and adult animals at therapeutic exposure levels. The drug was widely prescribed under a variety of trade names (e.g., Contergan, Distaval, Kevadon), at an oral dose of 50 to 200 mg/day. There were a few reports of peripheral neuritis attributable to thalidomide, but only in patients with long-term use of up to 18 months (Fullerton and Kremer, 1961). In 1960, a large increase in newborns with rare limb malformations was recorded in West Germany. The affected children had amelia (absence of the limbs) or various degrees of phocomelia (preaxial reduction of the long bones of the limbs), usually affecting the arms more than the legs, and usually involving left and right sides, although to different degrees. At the University Pediatric Clinic in Hamburg, for example, no cases of phocomelia were seen in the decade 1949–1959. In 1959, there was a single case; in 1960, 30 cases; and in 1961, 154 cases (Taussig, 1962). Comparable increases in the frequency of these rare limb anomalies occurred in other parts of the world where thalidomide was in use. Congenital heart disease, ocular, intestinal, and renal anomalies, and malformations of the external ears were also involved, but the limb defects were the most characteristic element of the malformation pattern (Warkany, 1971a). In 1961, Lenz in Germany (Lenz, 1963) and McBride in Australia (McBride, 1961) independently identified thalidomide as the causative agent. The drug was withdrawn from the market at the end of 1961, and by August of 1962 the epidemic subsided. Subsequent studies indicated that 70 percent of mothers with characteristically affected children had taken thalidomide during the first three months of pregnancy, 14 percent had taken it without being able to accurately identify the time of ingestion, 8 percent had possibly taken it, and 8 percent had a definite negative history of thalidomide ingestion (Weicker, 1963). The critical period for developmental toxicity was found to be during the sixth and seventh weeks of pregnancy (35 to 50 days from the first day of the last menstrual period or 23 to 38 days after conception) (Nowack, 1965). Exposure beyond this period could result in minor defects such as hypoplastic thumbs and anorectal stenosis. The malformation rate was extremely high in infants exposed during the sensitive period, and some studies have indicated that every woman ingesting the drug during this period had an offspring with some type of malformation, ranging from major to minor defects (Knapp, 1963). No relationship has been established between the severity of the malformations and the amount of drug taken during the sensitive period (Schardein, 1976b). Projections of the number of children deformed by thalidomide range upward to 10,000, while more conservative estimates place the number between 7000 and 8000 (Lenz, 1966). West Germany, England, Wales, and Japan were the countries most affected, while only a few cases were reported from the United States where sale of thalidomide was delayed by Dr. Frances Kelsey of the Food and Drug Administration. While malformations of the limbs were the most conspicuous element of thalidomide embryopathy, defects of the cardiovascular, intestinal, and urinary systems have most often been the cause of death in affected children (Warkany, 1971a).

After the discovery of the teratogenic effects

of thalidomide in humans, experimental studies in animals were undertaken to reproduce the syndrome of malformations. An unexpected finding was that the mouse and rat were resistant, the rabbit and hamster variably responsive, and certain strains of primates were sensitive to thalidomide developmental toxicity. Different strains of the same species of animals were also found to have highly variable sensitivity to thalidomide. Factors such as differences in absorption, distribution, biotransformation, and placental transfer have been ruled out as causes of the variability in species and strain sensitivity. The New Zealand white rabbit had been the most widely used animal owing to its relatively consistent response, and thalidomide exposure during the sensitive period (days 8 to 10 of pregnancy) results in a wide spectrum of malformations, particularly of the limbs (reviewed in Fabro, 1981).

The chemical structure of thalidomide [(±)-3′phthalimidoglutarimide] is shown in Figure 7–1. The compound is relatively insoluble and unstable in aqueous solutions. Primary hydrolysis products are formed by cleavage of the four amidic bonds, and these products then undergo additional nonenzymatic breakdown to form secondary, tertiary, and quarternary hydrolysis products (Schumacher et al., 1965). The relatively lipophilic parent compound is found at

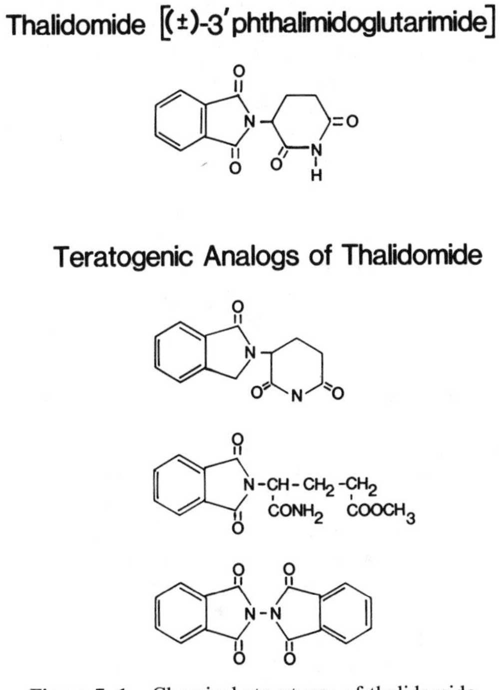

similar concentration is maternal plasma and embryonic tissue and is believed to cross the placenta by simple diffusion (Fabro et al., 1967). Several of the hydrolysis products are found at higher concentrations in the embryo than in the maternal plasma, a finding that has given rise to the "trapping" hypothesis. According to this theory, the lipophilic parent compound crosses the placenta and enters the embryonic compartment where it undergoes spontaneous cleavage to the highly charged hydrolysis products. These products are then trapped in the embryonic compartment because they are too polar to pass back into the maternal circulation (Keberle et al., 1965). Even though bioaccumulation of the hydrolysis products in the embryo has been well established, the hydrolysis products themselves do not appear to possess significant teratogenic activity. Extensive structure-activity studies have been carried out with over 60 compounds stereochemically related to thalidomide (Schumacher, 1975). The structural requirements for teratogenicity appear to be quite strict insofar as only thalidomide itself and three other analogs (Figure 7–1) are clearly teratogenic in the rabbit. An intact phthalimide or phthalimidine group appears to be essential for teratogenic activity, and the glutarimide moiety can be replaced by a glutarimide ester group or a structure that can be converted into a glutarimide ring.

A number of theories have been proposed to explain the biochemical and cellular mechanisms of thalidomide teratogenicity (reviewed in Schumacher, 1975, and Fabro, 1981). These have included interference with folic acid or glutamic acid metabolism, depurination of DNA through intercalation between base pairs, and acylation of polyamines. Potential sites of cellular toxicity that have been examined include direct toxic effects on limb mesenchyme tissue, inhibition of mesonephric-limb tissue interaction, and damage to the developing neural crest tissue leading to segmental sensory peripheral neuropathy. Despite intense efforts made over the past 20 years, none of these hypotheses have been adequately substantiated, or definitively disproved, and the mode of action remains unknown. A more fundamental understanding of the mechanisms of normal morphogenesis will need to be achieved before there is an explanation for the teratogenic effects of thalidomide.

After the thalidomide episode and the recognition of species differences in response and sensitivity, the emphasis shifted from genetic inheritance as a primary causal explanation for birth defects to chemical exposures during pregnancy. There has been a tremendous increase in research on chemical teratogens since the thalidomide episode, much of which has been influ-

Thalidomide [(±)-3′phthalimidoglutarimide]

Teratogenic Analogs of Thalidomide

Figure 7–1. Chemical structures of thalidomide and analogs with teratogenic activity.

enced by the characteristic and perhaps unique events associated with the human response to this drug.

Chronic ingestion of alcohol during pregnancy has also been implicated in causing substantial risk to human pregnancy. It was not until 1973 that the embryotoxic effects of alcohol were placed into a category and termed fetal alcohol syndrome, or FAS. Chronic ingestion of alcohol produces variable and nonspecific embryotoxicity, most frequently manifested as intrauterine growth retardation, psychomotor dysfunction, and craniofacial anomalies (Jones and Smith, 1973). These features are not unique, and accurate diagnosis of FAS is often not possible without a priori knowledge of maternal alcohol consumption. It is estimated that full expression of FAS occurs in 1 to 2 live births/1000, and that partial expression is present in an additional 3 to 5 live births/1000 (Abel, 1980).

Intrauterine growth retardation is the most sensitive measure of prenatal alcohol exposure and is characterized by deficiencies in height and weight and a lack of postnatal catchup. Risk of intrauterine growth retardation increases with maternal consumption of at least 1 oz absolute alcohol per day (Kaminski et al., 1981). For comparison, 1 g/kg absolute alcohol is equal to 80 ml (2.7 oz) absolute alcohol or five drinks. Heavy alcohol consumption, defined as consumption of five or more drinks per occasion and a consistent daily intake of more than 45 ml absolute alcohol, is clearly associated with a threefold increase in small-for-gestation-age infants (Sokol et al., 1980). The risk is significantly decreased if alcohol consumption is reduced during the third trimester (Rosett et al., 1980).

Psychomotor dysfunction characterized by IQs more than 2 standard deviations below the mean has been found in 85 percent of FAS children. Learning disabilities are manifested as impulsiveness, restlessness, shortened attention span, distractability, and speech and language disorders (Streissguth et al., 1978). Craniofacial anomalies include shortened palpebral fissures, epicanthal folds, broadened nasal bridge, upturned nose, and thinned upper lips. Additional and more severe neuropathologic effects are microcephaly, hydrocephaly, and cerebral and cerebellar disorganization. The risk of congenital anomalies is not as well defined as for intrauterine growth retardation. Consumption in excess of 2 oz absolute alcohol/day is necessary to significantly increase the incidence of malformations (Sokol et al., 1980). Consumption levels associated with these adverse outcomes have been obtained by self-reporting, and under-reporting of consumption by heavy drinkers is a likely source of bias. The potential synergistic

effects of caffeine and cigarette smoking must also be taken into consideration.

Many species of laboratory animals have been treated with ethanol during pregnancy with varying degrees of success in reproducing human FAS. Attempts to develop a model of FAS in nonhuman primates have yielded equivocal results, and at present primates are not suitable for replicating the human syndrome (Scott and Fradkin, 1981). The most consistent findings in rats are intrauterine growth retardation, embryolethality, and behavioral deficits (Henderson et al., 1979). The mouse appears to be the best species for producing birth defects with alcohol (Chernoff, 1980). The high exposure levels (4 to 8 g/kg) required to produce these developmental toxicities can cause prolonged maternal sedation. Consequently, the confounding role of food and water deprivation should be considered in animal models of FAS. Whether the human fetus is at risk from moderate social drinking or only from severe chronic alcoholism cannot be accurately determined at this time, leading to the recommendation that alcohol consumption be reduced to the greatest extent possible during pregnancy.

Another agent implicated in a spectrum of developmental toxicities in humans is diethylstilbestrol (DES). Between 1966 and 1969, seven young women between the ages of 15 and 22 were seen at the Massachusetts General Hospital with clear-cell adenocarcinoma of the vagina. This tumor had previously never been seen in patients below the age of 30, with a primary occurrence in women over 50. An epidemiologic case-control study was carried out to identify etiologic factors, and an association was found with maternal ingestion of DES in the first trimester of pregnancy (reviewed in Poskanzer and Herbst, 1977). DES was widely used from the mid-1940s to 1970 in the United States to prevent threatened miscarriage and was believed to stimulate the placenta to synthesize higher levels of estrogen and progesterone. A study of the therapeutic value of DES was carried out in 1953, and administration of DES in graduated amounts prior to the 20th week up to the 35th week of pregnancy was found to have no effect on the incidence of abortion, prematurity, postmaturity, perinatal mortality, or toxemia of pregnancy (Dieckmann et al., 1953). Despite these findings, DES treatment continued to be regarded as appropriate, and in the 1960s a committee of the National Academy of Science rated the drug as "possibly effective" for the treatment of high-risk pregnancies.

After the association was made between maternal ingestion of DES during the first trimester and vaginal adenocarcinoma in female offspring, a Registry of Clear Cell Adenocarcinoma of the Genital Tract in Young Females was established in 1971. Reports from this registry have indicated that treatment prior to the 18th week of pregnancy is necessary for genital tract abnormalities. The incidence of genital cancer peaked in DES-exposed female offspring at age 19 and declined through age 22. The absolute risk for developing clear-cell adenocarcinoma of the vagina and cervix with prenatal exposure was low, in the range of 0.14 to 1.4/1000 through age 24 (Herbst *et al.,* 1977). A high proportion of DES-exposed female offspring had other disorders of the vagina and cervix, including vaginal adenosis, cervical erosion, transverse fibrous ridges of the vagina and cervix, and cervical pseudopolyps. In one study of approximately 100 female offspring per group, vaginal adenosis was found in 35 percent of exposed versus 1 percent of control subjects. Fibrous ridges of the vagina and cervix were found in 22 percent of exposed and none in the controls. Overall, abnormalities of a benign nature were found in about 75 percent of female offspring exposed to DES *in utero* (Poskanzer and Herbst, 1977).

Abnormal physical findings have also been identified in male offspring exposed *in utero* to DES (reviewed in Bibbo *et al.,* 1977). In one study with approximately 165 male offspring per group, epididymal cysts, hypotrophic testes, and capsular induration were found in 25 percent of exposed versus 6 percent of control males. Low ejaculate volume was found in 26 percent, and poor semen quality in 28 percent of exposed men and none in controls. Malignant lesions have not been observed in male offspring. The primary lesion induced in both sexes is believed to be persistence of Mullerian duct derivatives in the genital tract with DES exposure between 6 and 16 weeks of gestation in humans. The persistence of embryonic, columnar Mullerian epithelium is believed to occur in areas of the vagina that are normally transformed to squamous cells in female fetuses. In male fetuses, the Mullerian ducts normally regress, but derivatives participate in formation of the prostate and other accessory organs. Incomplete regression of Mullerian derivatives or abnormal participation of the derivatives in formation of the male genital tract may give rise to the genital lesions observed (McLachlan and Dixon, 1977).

PROTOCOL TESTING

Following the thalidomide episode, a reexamination and expansion of testing procedures for developmental toxicity of drugs was carried out by the Food and Drug Administration. In 1966,

the document *Guidelines for Reproduction Studies for Safety Evaluation of Drugs for Human Use* (FDA, 1966) was issued. Similar documents have been issued for evaluation of food additives, pesticides, and household products (FDA, 1970; CPSC, 1977). A brief description of these protocols will be given here, and additional information can be obtained from more comprehensive reviews (Collins, 1978; Adams and Buelke-Sam, 1981; Palmer, 1981; Manson *et al., 1982*).

In the multigeneration study, animals are continuously exposed to the test agent in the food or water throughout three generations. This test protocol was developed to assess chemical agents that are likely to accumulate in the body with long-term exposures, such as food additives and pesticides, and provides an overview of reproductive function. Parental animals are first exposed shortly after weaning (30 to 40 days) and, when reproductively mature, are mated to produce the F_1 generation. F_1 offspring are selected to produce F_2 offspring, and the same procedure is followed for production of the F_3 generation, all of which are killed at weaning. Three treatment groups and one control group are employed, and a minimum of 20 pregnant females per group and per generation are included. Rodent species are most frequently used, allowing completion of the three generation study within 20 months. The influence of the test agent on fertility, litter size, sex ratio, neonatal viability, and growth is monitored throughout each generation.

Testing procedures for evaluation of short-term exposures are the three-segment single-generation studies. These consist of three phases: I, evaluation of fertility and general reproductive performance; II, assessment of developmental toxicity; and III, peri- and postnatal evaluation. Phase I tests include treatment of male rodents for 70 days and female rodents for 14 days, and treatment of females is continued during mating, pregnancy, and lactation. At mid-pregnancy half of the females are killed and uterine contents examined for preimplantation and postimplantation death. The other half are allowed to deliver and wean their offspring. Weanlings are killed and autopsied for gross and visceral abnormalities. This study phase provides an overview of effects on fertility, conception rates, pre- and postimplantation survival, parturition, and lactation.

Phase II studies include the treatment of inseminated females during the organogenesis period alone. One day prior to birth, females are killed and fetuses are delivered by cesarean section. Developmental toxicity is assessed in terms of the occurrence of early or late embryo (fetal) deaths, reduced fetal body weight, and the presence of gross, visceral, and skeletal malformations. In phase III studies, effects on perinatal and postnatal development are measured. Pregnant females are exposed during the last third of gestation and through weaning. The purpose of this study is to determine effects on late fetal development, labor and delivery, lactation, neonatal viability, and growth of the offspring. Common variants of this test are to allow weanlings to survive to adulthood for assessment of neurobehavioral deficits, fertility, and the occurrence of perinatally induced cancer.

Much controversy exists today about the adequacy of these test protocols. They were based on the understanding of reproductive toxicology 20 years ago, which was strongly influenced by the thalidomide episode. As basic knowledge has improved, recommendations have been made for alterations of these protocols and for inclusion of *in vitro* tests. At best, these protocols have served as a "norm" for safety evaluation of chemicals for reproductive effects. They have provided a uniform format for compilation of extensive historical data. At worst, the protocols have inhibited development of new approaches for understanding reproductive toxicity. This is perhaps best exemplified in preclinical testing of drugs, where emphasis is placed on the "safety" of the drug, or whether it will produce developmental toxicity when given to normal animals at multiples of the human therapeutic dose. The potential therapeutic effect of drugs in ameliorating diseases of pregnancy and adverse outcomes (i.e., hypertension, premature labor, fetal growth retardation) is seldomly explored, resulting in a critical shortage of information about drugs that could be used to improve the course of pregnancy. This is a topic of active consideration in academic, regulatory, and industrial sectors and one that should result in a reexamination of how to determine both safety and therapeutic efficacy of drugs intended for use by pregnant women.

DIMENSION OF THE PROBLEM

In the remainder of this chapter, the importance of xenobiotics as factors contributing to adverse pregnancy outcome is explored. Those outcomes associated with prenatal insult alone will be emphasized even though damage to the adolescent and adult reproductive and neuroendocrine systems can also result in reproductive dysfunction. These aspects are covered in Chapter 16 ("Toxic Responses of the Reproductive System"). Extensive data are available on reproductive performance in the human population that provide useful information on the fre-

quency but not the cause of reproductive failure. Although early spontaneous abortions often go unreported, particularly among pregnancies of less than 20 weeks' duration, their frequency has been estimated to be 15 percent of all recognized pregnancies (Warburton and Fraser, 1964). This figure is generally considered to be an underestimate insofar as most spontaneous abortions occur early in gestation, often before the pregnancy is recognized. Of approximately three million infants born alive each year, 13.1 per 1000 die within the first year (NCHS, 1980). Approximately 2 to 3 percent of infants born alive have major congenital malformations recognized within the first year of life (National Foundation, 1981a). When defects that only become apparent later in life are included, the frequency of major and minor malformations increases to about 16 percent (Chung and Myrianthopoulos, 1975). Approximately 7 percent of newborns are born prematurely (before the 37th week) and 7 percent of infants born at full term have low birth weights (2.5 kg or less) (USDHEW, 1972).

In very few cases has it been possible to separate the impact of a specific chemical exposure on human reproduction from the background rate of spontaneous defects or from other causes such as radiation, infection, nutritional deficiencies, or maternal diseases. Wilson (1973) has estimated that 23 to 35 percent of birth defects have an identifiable genetic component, and 7 to 11 percent have an identifiable external factor, such as radiation, drugs, environmental chemicals, infections, and maternal metabolic imbalances. For 55 to 70 percent of birth defects, no causal associations can presently be made. Correlation between exposure to a specific chemical agent and adverse pregnancy outcome is also complicated by the magnitude of chemical agents in the environment. The Chemical Abstract Service of the American Chemical Society listed 4,039,906 individual chemical entities as of November 1977, with an average growth rate of 6000 new entries per week (Maugh, 1978). In the NIOSH Registry of Toxic Substances (NIOSH, 1977), there were 37,860 entries of agents in common industrial use, of which 585 had notations of teratogenic activity. Schardein (1976a) estimated that a total of 1930 compounds had been tested for teratogenicity as of 1976, with 580 compounds showing positive effects. In the *Catalog of Teratogenic Agents* compiled by Thomas Shepard (1980), over 600 agents causing congenital anomalies in laboratory animals are listed, with only 20 known to cause defects in humans. Many gaps exist in our understanding of how to predict which chemicals among the millions in the environment possess teratogenic activity, of the correlation between responses of laboratory animals and humans, and of the mechanisms of action of teratogens in any species. The following discussion of some well-established principles of teratology should indicate, however, that much progress has been made in these areas since the thalidomide episode.

PRINCIPLES OF TERATOLOGY

Definition of Terms

The term "developmental toxicity" covers any detrimental effect produced by exposures to developing organisms during embryonic stages of development. Such lesions can be either irreversible or reversible. Embryolethal lesions are incompatible with survival of the conceptus and result in resorption, spontaneous abortion, or stillbirth. Irreversible lesions that are compatible with survival may result in structural or functional anomalies in live offspring, and these are called teratogenic. Persistent lesions that cause overall growth retardation or delayed growth of specific organ systems are generally referred to as embryotoxic. For a chemical to be labeled a teratogen, it must significantly increase the occurrence of structural or functional abnormalities in offspring after it is administered to either parent before conception, to the female during pregnancy, or directly to the developing organism.

Many teratologists believe that any chemical administered under appropriate conditions of dose and time of development can cause some disturbances in embryonic development in some laboratory species (Karnofsky, 1965; Staples, 1975). For an agent to be classified as a developmental toxicant, it must produce adverse effects on the conceptus at exposure levels that do not induce severe toxicity in the mother (e.g., substantial reduction in weight gain, persistent emesis, hypo- or hyperactivity, or convulsions). Adverse effects on development under these conditions may be secondary to stress in the maternal system. The main reason for conducting developmental toxicity studies is to ascertain whether an agent causes specific or unique toxicity to pregnant animals or to the conceptus. If these studies are conducted under extreme conditions of maternal toxicity, then identification of exposures uniquely toxic to the conceptus or pregnant animal is not possible. Chemical agents can be deliberately administered at maternally toxic doses to determine the threshold level for adverse effects on the offspring. In such cases conclusions can be qualified to indicate that adverse effects on the conceptus were obtained at maternally toxic exposure levels, and may not be indicative of selective or unique developmental toxicity.

Influence of Time of Exposure

Compared to adults, developing organisms undergo rapid and complex changes within a relatively short period. Consequently, the susceptibility of the conceptus to chemical insult varies dramatically within the narrow time span of the major developmental stages, i.e., the preimplantation, embryonic, fetal, and neonatal periods. The embryologic characteristics of each of these stages and the types of spontaneous and chemically induced adverse outcomes associated with each stage will be described.

The major morphogenic events occurring during preimplantation development are formation of a compact mass of cells (the morula) and of the blastocyst. Development of the blastocyst involves differentiation of the trophectoderm, which is necessary for implantation, and the inner cell mass (ICM), which differentiates into primary endoderm and ectoderm before implantation. The ICM gives rise to the embryo and the extraembryonic membranes but cannot implant or survive in the uterus in the absence of trophectoderm.

As shown in Table 7–1, considerable similarity exists in the timing of preimplantation development across several mammalian species, regardless of the total length of gestation (Brinster, 1975). Shortly after fertilization, the mammalian embryo has a low oxygen consumption and metabolic capacity. At the time of blastocyst formation, there is a dramatic increase in cell division and metabolic capacity. Both the total synthetic rate as well as the types of RNAs and proteins synthesized are markedly increased. During the preimplantation period, biochemical changes in the uterine endometrium controlled by progesterone and estrogen result in the development of endometrial sensitivity to the blastocyst. It is now well established that the same basic hormonal sequence, i.e., low levels of estrogen in a progesterone-primed uterus, initiates uterine receptivity. The blastocyst must implant within 24 hours after the progesterone-estrogen regimen when the uterus is in the peak receptive phase. One of the earliest signs of blastocyst implantation in all species investigated is a localized increase in endometrial vascular permeability, which is believed to be mediated by prostaglandins (Kennedy and Armstrong, 1981). Alterations in the hormonal milieu, as well as direct excretion of drugs into uterine secretions during this period, can interfere with implantation and result in embryolethality. The preimplantation embryo appears to be susceptible

Table 7–1. TIMING OF EARLY DEVELOPMENT IN SOME MAMMALIAN SPECIES*

	BLASTOCYST FORMATION	IMPLANTATION	ORGANOGENESIS PERIOD	LENGTH OF GESTATION
Mouse	3–4	4–5	6–15	19
Rat	3–4	5–6	6–15	22
Rabbit	3–4	7–8	6–18	33
Sheep	6–7	17–18	14–36	150
Monkey (rhesus)	5–7	9–11	20–45	164
Human	5–8	8–13	21–56	267

* Developmental ages are days from the time of ovulation.

to lethality but rarely to teratogenicity with chemical insult. In studies utilizing preimplantation embryo cultures, severe toxicity is manifested by rapid death of the embryo, while less severe effects are measured by decreases in cleavage rates and arrested development (Brinster, 1975). There have been few studies of the effects of sublethal exposures on preimplantation embryos, and the possibilities of persistent biochemical or morphologic alterations have not been adequately explored.

Following implantation, organogenesis takes place. The organogenesis period is characterized by the division, migration, and association of cells into primitive organ rudiments. The basic structural templates for organization of tissues and organs are established on the molecular, cellular, and morphologic level. The most characteristic susceptibility of the embryo to chemical insult during the organogenesis period is the induction of structural birth defects, although these are often accompanied by embryo-

lethality. Within the organogenesis period, individual organ systems possess highly specific periods of vulnerability to teratogenic insult. Figure 7–2 depicts the sensitive periods of the major embryonic organ systems to teratogenic insult. Administration of a teratogen on day 10 of rat gestation would result in a high level of brain and eye defects, with intermediate levels of heart and skeletal defects, and a low level of urogenital defects. If the same agent was administered on day 11, a different spectrum of malformations would be anticipated, with brain and palate malformations predominating. Consequently, the exact time of exposure has a strong influence on the final pattern of malformation. Figure 7–2 also illustrates that exposure to teratogens usually results in a spectrum of malformations involving a number of organ systems, reflecting the overlap of critical periods for individual organ systems. This situation is more evident in species with short gestation periods, such as rodents. Most human teratogens, how-

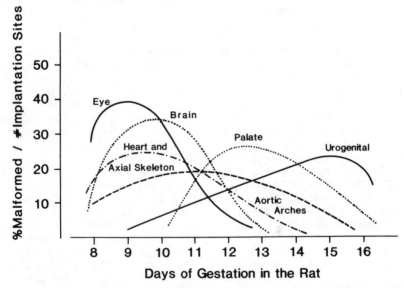

Figure 7–2. Pattern of susceptibility of embryonic organ rudiments to teratogenic insult. (Modified from Wilson, J. G.: *Environment and Birth Defects*. Academic Press, Inc., New York, 1973.)

ever, have been found to influence the development of several organ systems and induce syndromes of malformations rather than just single anomalies, as described for rubella and thalidomide.

The critical phase for inducing anomalies in individual organ systems may be as short as one day or may extend throughout organogenesis. Urogenital defects, for example, can result from drug treatment from the 9th to 18th days of gestation in the rat. This implies that development of the urogenital system is multiphasic, and that individual stages may have different sensitivities to chemical insult. Renal anomalies can be induced by irradiation on day 9 of rat gestation, for example, while the earliest primordium of the pronephric kidney is not present until day 10 (Wilson, 1973). Presumably, this is due to interference with molecular or cellular events preceding structural differentiation of the kidney. Chemical insult on day 11.5 could interfere with formation of the mesonephric kidney, or on day 12 to entrance of the mesonephric duct into the urogenital sinus. On day 12.5, the metanephric kidney is first formed, and this is followed by formation of the definitive genital ducts and indifferent gonads from days 12 to 20 of gestation (Hoar and Monie, 1981). Depending on the mechanism of action of the agent and the time of administration, it is likely that only one or a few of these steps will be affected, but succeeding steps will be disrupted as a result of the original alteration. Processes governing embryonic differentiation are not well understood, yet most likely determine the intrinsic susceptibility of individual organs to teratogenic insult. The mechanism of action and the persistence of the toxic effect also influence the malformation pattern, as discussed in the next section.

Histogenesis, functional maturation, and growth are the major processes occurring during the fetal and neonatal (i.e., perinatal) periods. Insult at these late developmental stages leads to a broad spectrum of effects that can be generally manifested as growth retardation or more specifically manifested as functional disorders and transplacental carcinogenesis. The fetus is more resistant to lethal effects than is the embryo, but the incidence of stillbirths is measurable. The perinatal period of life is a time of high susceptibility to carcinogenesis. At least three factors contribute to this enhanced susceptibility: high cellular replication rates, ontogeny of xenobiotic biotransforming enzymes, and low immunocompetence. Several childhood tumors occur so early after birth that prenatal origin is considered likely. Among these are acute lymphocytic (but not myelogenous) leukemia, Wilms' tumor, neuroblastoma, primary carcinoma of the liver,

and presacral teratoma (Miller, 1973). Cancer was the chief cause of death by disease in children under the age of 15 in the United States in 1976, accounting for 11.3 percent of all deaths. Leukemia and lymphoma account for approximately half of these deaths followed by cancers of the brain and central nervous system, soft tissues, kidney, and bone (ACS, 1980).

Studies with direct-acting transplacental carcinogens such as ENU (ethylnitrosourea) indicate that susceptibility to carcinogens begins after completion of the organogenesis period in rodents. Tumors in offspring occurred primarily when ENU was given during the fetal period, whereas birth defects and embryolethality predominated with exposures earlier in organogenesis. (Ivankovic, 1979). This is not to imply that teratogenesis and carcinogenesis are mutually exclusive processes, however. Birth defects and neoplasias occur together in the same offspring with unusually high frequency, but not necessarily at the same site. Teratogenesis and carcinogenesis are viewed as graded responses of the embryo to injury, with teratogenesis representing the grosser response involving major tissue necrosis. Bolande (1977) has postulated that certain agents cause teratogenic damage in early, relatively undifferentiated embryos, combined carcinogenic-teratogenic damage in older embryos, and finally, carcinogenic damage alone in the perinatal period. Alternatively, it has been suggested that embryotoxic insult may predispose the offspring to secondary tumor induction in later life.

Patterns of Dose-Response

Functional deficits and perinatally induced cancers are not manifested until adolescence or later. They are usually examined as end-points in themselves without correlation to the outcomes observable at the time of birth. The major effects from prenatal exposure measured at the time of birth in developmental toxicity studies are embryolethality, malformations, and growth retardation. Embryolethality is reported as the ratio of resorptions or dead fetuses in the litter at term to the number of implantation sites. Growth retardation is measured by weighing and taking crown-rump measurements of live fetuses at term. The frequency and type of malformations are determined by gross inspection of fetuses and detailed skeletal and soft tissue analysis. The occurrence of embryolethality precludes measurements of growth retardation or malformation because the latter two endpoints are made on live fetuses only. The relationship between embryolethality, malformations, and growth retardation is quite complex and varies with the type of agent, the time of exposure, and the dose. In order to simplify the situation, for the time being conditions will be restricted to administration of agents at a single time point during organogenesis, and at exposure levels not severely toxic to the mother. Even under these strict conditions, diverse patterns of response for the three major end-points occur, three of which will be described.

Some developmental toxicants can cause malformations of the entire litter at exposure levels that do not cause embryolethality. A depiction of the dose-response pattern for such agents is given in Figure 7–3,A. If the dose is increased beyond that malforming the entire litter, embryolethality can occur, but often in conjunction with severe maternal toxicity. Malformed fetuses are often growth retarded, and the curve for growth retardation is often parallel to and slightly displaced from the curve for teratogenicity. Such a pattern of response is rare and is indicative of agents with high teratogenic potency.

A more common dose-response pattern involves embryolethality, malformations, and growth retardation of surviving fetuses (Figure 7–3,B). For agents producing this response pattern, exposure within the embryotoxic range of doses results in a combination of resorbed, malformed, growth-retarded, and "normal" fetuses within the litter. Depending on the teratogenic potency of the agent, lower doses may cause predominantly resorptions or malformations. As the dosage increases, however, embryolethality predominates until the entire litter is resorbed. Agents with high teratogenic potency would produce a pattern where the teratogenicity curve was to the left but still overlapping the embryolethality curve, while agents that were predominantly embryolethal would produce the pattern shown in Figure 7–3,B, where embryolethality was the most prominent outcome throughout the range of doses. Growth retardation can precede both these outcomes or parallel the teratogenicity curve.

A third dose-response pattern consists of growth retardation and embryolethality without malformations (Figure 7–3,C). The dose-response curve for embryolethality in this case is usually steep, implying the existence of a sharp threshold for survival of the embryo. Growth retardation of surviving fetuses usually precedes significant embryolethality. Agents producing this pattern of response would be considered embryotoxic or embryolethal, but not teratogenic. When such a pattern is observed, it is necessary to conduct additional studies with doses within the range causing growth retardation and embryolethality. Results obtained at these intermediary doses can indicate whether teratogenicity has been masked by embryolethality (Neubert et al., 1980).

The existence of these three general patterns of response indicate that for some agents embryolethality and teratogenicity are different degrees of manifestations of the same primary insult (Figure 7–3,B). For other agents, there is a qualitative difference in response, and the primary insult leads to embryolethality alone (Figure 7–3,C) or teratogenicity alone (Figure 7–3,A). Separate evaluation of growth retardation, teratogenicity, and embryolethality, with increasing dose must be carried out to arrive at conclusions about the primary mode of action of the agent.

With agents of unknown developmental toxicity, the sequence of testing begins with a dose range-finding study containing relatively small numbers of pregnant rodents. They are exposed on days 6 through 15 of gestation to the test agent at doses up to and including those causing limiting maternal toxicity and/or developmental toxicity (death, severe growth retardation). The purpose of the dose-range study is to obtain a qualitative yes/no signal about the potential developmental toxicity of the agent, and information on doses causing extreme maternal toxicity. At the next level of testing, larger numbers of animals are exposed on days 6–15 of gestation to obtain quantitative information on dose-

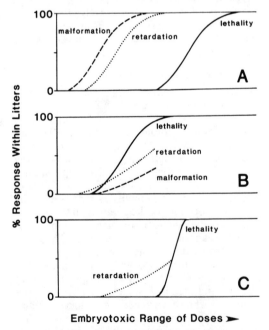

Figure 7–3. Dose-response patterns for different types of developmental toxicants. (Modified from Neubert, D.; Barrach, H. J.; and Merker, H. J.: Drug-induced damage to the embryo or fetus. *Curr. Top. Pathol.,* **69:**242–324, 1980.)

response relationships. The highest dose should cause measurable but slight maternal toxicity (i.e., significant depression of weight gain) or developmental toxicity (i.e., significant depression of fetal body weight or increased embryolethality), and the low dose should cause no observable effects. If evidence of selective developmental toxicity is obtained from this study, it is necessary to conduct a third study exposing dams on single days during organogenesis at doses that are not maternally toxic to obtain a clear definition of the dose-response pattern of developmental toxicity.

If an agent with selective developmental toxicity is administered throughout the organogenesis period (days 6 to 15 in the rat), it becomes difficult to identify the most sensitive target organs and to produce a consistent pattern of malformation. In addition, teratogenic effects induced by agents acting according to pattern B can be masked by embryolethality with repeated dosing during the organogenesis period. If the agent is administered at levels sufficiently toxic to the mother, then all responses can revert to pattern C, embryolethality or growth retardation, but rarely malformations.

It is generally accepted that developmental toxicity in the form of increased resorption and decreased fetal body weight can occur at maternally toxic dose levels. The role of maternal toxicity in causing congenital malformations, however, is not clear. Khera (1984) reviewed over 85 published studies in mice to examine the relationship between maternal toxicity, embryotoxicity, and birth defects. He noted that doses of test agents that caused maternal toxicity, as indicated by reduced maternal body weight, clinical signs of toxicity, or deaths, commonly caused reduction in fetal body weight, increased resorption, and, rarely, fetal deaths. He identified three patterns of association between maternal toxicity and malformations: (1) for some compounds, maternal toxicity was not associated with malformations; (2) for others, maternal toxicity was associated with a diverse pattern of malformations, which often include cleft palate; and (3) the maternal toxicity of still others was associated with a characteristic and unique pattern of malformation.

Compounds in the second category are the most difficult to classify in terms of teratogenic potential. Cleft palate has been reported as the principal malformation resulting from food and water deprivation during pregnancy in mice (Szabo and Brent, 1975); however, cleft palate is also a malformation specifically induced in mice by a number of teratogens, most notably the glucocorticoids, without any apparent maternal toxicity. Complete ascertainment of food and

water consumption, maternal body weights, and, occasionally, alterations in maternal homeostasis (i.e., organ histopathology, kidney or liver dysfunction, hematologic alterations, pharmacologic reactions, and other possible toxic effects) are necessary to distinguish between cleft palate caused by a teratogenic effect of a chemical on the embryo and a nonspecific toxic effect on the dam that secondarily influences embryonic development.

Compounds in the third category were structurally unrelated to test agents administered at maternally toxic doses that caused increased resorptions and decreased fetal body weight. The characteristic pattern of defects caused by these agents was exencephaly; open eyes; fused, missing, or supernumerary ribs; and fused or scrambled sternebrae. The severity and incidence of these defects could be directly related to the degree of maternal toxicity. They were absent or rare at doses that were nontoxic to the dam. Khera (1984) concluded that these defects resulted from maternal toxicity and did not reflect the teratogenic potential of the compounds. While most investigators accept that maternal toxicity can be the cause of minor variants in the ribs and sternebrae, not all accept it as the cause of major malformations such as exencephaly and open eyes.

The timing of exposure and patterns of dose-response obtained in animal studies have important implications for extrapolating the resultant data to humans. The major implication is that a spectrum of end points can be produced, even under the controlled conditions of timing and exposure that can be achieved in animal studies. In some cases, the spectrum comprises a continum of response, with depressed birth weight or functional impairment occurring at low doses, birth defects at intermediate doses, and lethality at high doses. Less commonly, birth defects alone or lethality alone are produced. Consequently, in estimating human risk, all exposure-specific adverse outcomes must be taken into consideration, and not just birth defects.

A similar spectrum of response has been observed in humans after prenatal exposure to developmental toxicants. The spectrum of response is determined by the time and duration of exposure, magnitude of exposure, interindividual differences in sensitivity, interactions with other types of exposure, and interactions among all these factors (Fraser, 1977). Consequently, manifestations of developmental toxicity cannot be presumed to be constant or specific across species; i.e., an animal model cannot be expected to forecast exactly the human response to a given exposure. For instance, an agent that induces cleft palate in the mouse may elevate the

**Table 7-2. FREQUENCY OF SELECTED ADVERSE PREGNANCY
OUTCOMES IN HUMANS***

EVENT	FREQUENCY PER 100	UNIT
Spontaneous abortion, 8–28 weeks	10–20	Pregnancies or women
Chromosomal anomalies in spontaneous abortions, 8–28 weeks	30–40	Spontaneous abortions
Chromosomal anomalies from amniocentesis	2	Amniocentesis specimens
Stillbirths	2–4	Stillbirths and livebirths
Low birthweight <2500 g	7	Livebirths
Major malformations	2–3	Livebirths
Chromosomal anomalies	0.2	Livebirths
Severe mental retardation	0.4	Children to 15 years of age

* Modified from National Foundation/March of Dimes: Report of Panel II. Guidelines for reproductive studies in exposed human populations. In Bloom, A. D. (ed.): *Guidelines for Studies of Human Populations Exposed to Mutagenic and Reproductive Hazards.* The Foundation, New York, 1981, pp. 37–110.

frequency of spontaneous abortion or intrauterine growth retardation in humans. *Any* manifestation of exposure-related developmental toxicity in animal studies can be indicative of a spectrum of response in humans (Kimmel *et al.*, 1984).

Table 7–2 illustrates an important factor to be considered in extrapolation of animal data to humans. The most prevalent adverse pregnancy outcome in humans is spontaneous abortion or early fetal loss prior to 28 weeks of pregnancy, occurring in at least 10 to 20 percent of all recognized pregnancies. Estimates from prospective studies range even higher, on the order of 20 to 25 percent of conceptions (National Foundation, 1981b). The frequency of spontaneous abortion is highest in early pregnancy, especially during the first 12 weeks, and gradually decreases to 20 weeks, after which fetal loss is uncommon. Approximately one-third of specimens obtained from spontaneous abortions occurring between 8 and 28 weeks of gestation contain chromosomal aberrations. The frequency of aberrations is at least 60-fold higher in spontaneous abortions than term births. Of the remaining two-thirds of spontaneous abortions that do not have chromosomal aberrations, approximately half have structural malformations (National Foundation, 1981b). The occurrence of malformations in abortuses is not as well documented as that for chromosomal aberrations because of the difficulty in observing malformations in specimens that are often macerated or incomplete. The remaining one-third of specimens lack chromosomal and morphologic abnormalities, but the incidence of placental inflammations suggestive of uterine infections can be high in these "normal" abortuses (Ornoy *et al.*, 1981).

These figures suggest that the majority of human embryos bearing chromosomal and/or morphologic abnormalities are lost through early miscarriage, and that relatively few survive to term. Consequently, examination of adverse outcomes at the time of birth alone (malformations, stillbirths, low birthweight) is likely to result in a substantial underestimate of the true risk, insofar as the occurrence of embryolethality would be missed. It is possible that developmental toxicants operating according to pattern A in Figure 7–3 could be picked up by monitoring malformations at the time of birth in humans, especially if the malformations were rare (thalidomide) or if the exposed population was large (rubella). Those agents operating according to patterns B and C would most likely be missed and would require detailed examination of the frequency of early fetal loss and the presence of chromosomal and structural malformations in abortuses for their detection.

Mechanism of Action

Despite the influence of time of exposure and the complex interaction between maternal toxicity and embryolethality on pregnancy outcome, there are examples of agent specificity. This encompasses the mechanism whereby classes of agents interact with differentiating tissues to produce birth defects. Agent specificity is discussed in the framework of the three patterns of dose-response described in the previous section.

Cytotoxic Teratogens. The majority of well-known developmental toxicants produce the second pattern of response, i.e., both malformations and embryolethality. Such a pattern or response is typical of agents that are cytotoxic to replicating cells via alterations in replication, transcription, translation, or cell division. Examples of these chemicals include alkylating agents, antineoplastic agents, and many mutagens. The rationale for susceptibility of the embryo to these agents is that the rate of cell division is extremely high during the organogenesis period. Within days 8 to 11 of gestation in rats, the DNA content of the embryo increases 1000-fold (Neubert et al., 1980). Therefore, it is not surprising that many agents known to interfere with cellular proliferation are embryotoxic. A characteristic, early response of embryonic tissues to these agents is the occurrence of excessive cell death in target organs destined to become malformed (Scott, 1977). Although cell death cannot be invoked as the initial event in the cause of teratogenicity, at some point it becomes an important intermediate or final manifestation of the primary insult. The increased necrosis must occur selectively and within a critical period of time for malformations to be found. Low doses of cytotoxic agents administered relatively early in the critical period may produce levels of cell death that can be replaced through compensatory hyperplasia of surviving cells, resulting in the formation of growth-retarded but morphologically normal fetuses at term. Higher doses administered later during the critical period may cause substantial depletion of cell number, leaving insufficient time for replacement prior to the occurrence of critical morphogenetic events. The resulting hypoplasia of the organ rudiments, as well as reduced proliferative rate of surviving cells, are important events related to the induction of malformations. High levels of exposure may damage too many cells and organ systems to be compatible with survival, and result in embryolethality (Ritter, 1977). A single exposure to a cytotoxic agent during organogenesis can result in all three outcomes both within and between litters. Some litters may be totally resorbed, others may contain only growth-retarded fetuses at term, while others may have a mixture of malformed and/or growth retarded fetuses and resorption sites at term. The variation in response has been ascribed to differences in pharmacokinetics of the agent in the maternal system, differential delivery of chemicals to individual embryos according to uterine position, as well as variations in developmental age of embryos within the litter (Neubert et al., 1980).

An example of an agent that produces this response is MNNG (N-methyl-N'-nitro-N-nitroso-guanidine), an alkylating agent that induces replication-dependent mutations and inhibition of DNA synthesis (Mandel, 1960). When administered on days 7 to 12 of gestation, a spectrum of malformations involving the brain, palate, vertebral column, ribs, and limbs is produced (Inouye and Murakami, 1978). Limb defects are prominent, but not unique, with exposure on day 10 or 11. Table 7–3 contains data on the dose-response pattern for induction of limb malformations, growth retardation, and embryolethality with maternal exposure on day 11. Teratogenicity predominates under these exposure conditions, but embryolethality is elevated at all dose levels (Manson and Miller, 1983). When the types of limb malformations were examined, an unusual pattern was observed. Hindlimbs were more frequently malformed than forelimbs, and limbs on the left side were malformed more frequently than limbs on the right side (Table 7–4). The forelimb-hindlimb response is not unusual insofar as the hindlimbs (HL) develop a day behind the forelimbs (FL) with peak susceptibility for forelimb malformation on day 10, and for hindlimbs on day 11. The left-right (L-R) asymmetry is somewhat more unusual, although there are a few other chemical teratogens known to cause asymmetric limb malformations in rodents (reviewed in Manson and Miller, 1983).

The differential susceptibility of each of the four limb types to MNNG-induced malformations has been utilized to determine whether there was a correlation between the level and persistence of cell death in limb buds shortly

Table 7–3. PATTERN OF DOSE-RESPONSE WITH THE CYTOTOXIC TERATOGEN MNNG*[†]

DOSE	% IMPLANTS DEAD/RESORBED	FETAL BODY WT. (g)	% LIVE FETUSES WITH LIMB MALFORMATION
Control	4.7	1.18	2.5
25 mg/kg	10.4[‡]	1.05	24[§]
50 mg/kg	8.9[‡]	0.87[‡]	58[§]
75 mg/kg	19.4[‡]	0.59[‡]	87[§]
100 mg/kg	46.1[‡]	0.47[‡]	100[§]

* Pregnant mice were injected ip with MNNG or with the vehicle 10 percent ETOH (control) on day 11, and uterine contents were examined on day 18.
[†] Modified from Manson, F. M., and Miller, M. L.: Contribution of mesenchymal cell death and mitotic alteration to assymetric limb malformations induced by MNNG. Teratogenesis Carcinog. Mutagen., 3:335–53, 1983.
[‡] Significantly depressed relative to controls, $p < 0.01$.
[§] Significantly elevated relative to controls, $p < 0.001$.

Table 7–4. FREQUENCY OF MALFORMATION (POSTAXIAL ECTRODACTYLY) BY LIMB POSITION WITH MNNG EXPOSURE*[†]

	RFL	LFL	RHL	LHL
Control	0.0	0.0	0.0	0.0
Treated	8.6 ± 3.1	40.1 ± 4.2	23.5 ± 4.6	51.6 ± 4.5

* Results are presented as the mean litter frequency of fetuses with absence of digits 3 to 5 for each limb type.

[†] Modified from Manson, J. M., and Miller, M. L.: Contribution of mesenchymal cell death and mitotic alteration to asymmetric limb malformations induced by MNNG. *Teratogenesis Carcinog. Mutagen.*, 3:335–53, 1983.

after exposure and the frequency of malformations at term. Figure 7–4 contains results of this analysis, where the percentage of necrotic cells in the subridge mesenchyme of limb buds from 1 to 72 hours after maternal exposure to MNNG on day 11 was measured. An increase in the number of necrotic cells in limb buds was first detected at four hours, was elevated at 18 hours, peaked at 24 hours, and began declining at 48

hours to reach the control baseline at 72 hours. The necrotic index values at 24 hours, when the level of cell death was the highest for all limb types, correlated with the pattern of limb malformations. The level of necrosis was highest in hindlimbs, and limbs on the left side had higher levels of necrosis than limbs on the right side. At all time points examined, left-sided limbs had higher levels of cell death than right-sided limbs. Thus, with MNNG, the level and persistence of cell death are quantitatively related to the frequency of limb malformations. Additional studies have indicated that the asymmetry in limb malformations and necrosis observed with MNNG are not related to the uptake of the chemical into each of the four limb types. Rather, it appears that the limb buds have different intrinsic susceptibility to MNNG, possibly based on the percentage of cells undergoing proliferation in each limb type.

Studies performed by Kochhar (1978) with a different cytotoxic agent, cytosine arabinoside, have indicated that there is also a qualitative re-

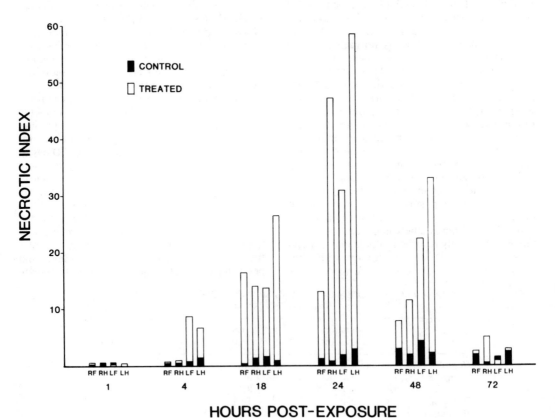

Figure 7–4. Necrotic index of control and MNNG-treated limbs. *RF*, right forelimb; *RH*, right hindlimb; *LF*, left forelimb; *LH*, left hindlimb. (From Manson, J. M., and Miller, M. L.: Contribution of mesenchymal cell death and mitotic alteration to asymmetric limb malformations induced by MNNG. *Teratogenesis Carcinog., Mutagen.*, **3**:335–53, 1983.)

lationship between the location of necrotic areas in limb buds and the final morphologic pattern of malformation. The selective, regional susceptibility of limb mesenchyme cells to death after cytosine arabinoside exposure correlated with the proliferation rate; as proliferation zones moved from proximal to distal regions of the limb bud, so did the areas where cell death was the highest after exposure. A substantial body of literature exists (reviewed in Scott, 1977) indicating that sites of high proliferative activity in the embryo are susceptible to cell death after exposure to cytotoxic teratogens, and that the frequency and morphologic pattern of the malformations are related to the localization and extent of necrosis in embryonic organ rudiments. Depression in DNA synthesis or DNA damage does not appear to be as important. The embryo can tolerate substantial depressions in DNA synthesis, which, unless accompanied by excessive necrosis, do not lead to malformations (Ritter, 1977; Kochhar et al., 1978). Likewise, chromosomal aberrations have been observed in embryonic cells after exposure to a variety of alkylating agents during the organogenesis period (Adler, 1983; Meyne and Legator, 1983; Theiss et al., 1983). Cells bearing chromosomal aberrations appear to be rapidly eliminated, usually within 24 hours after transplacental exposure, indicating that chromosomal aberrations may contribute to cell death but not to heritable mutations in surviving cells. Even stable chromosomal aberrations (i.e., small deletions, inversions, and reciprocal translocations) do not persist after several cell divisions with prenatal exposure to ENU (Theiss et al., 1983). There may be insufficient time for repair of DNA damage with the rapid rate of cell division during organogensis. Depressions in DNA synthesis and cell death are more likely outcomes of DNA damage in embryonic tissues than are heritable mutations (Manson, 1981).

With cytotoxic teratogens, the embryo is usually far more susceptible than is the mother, although rapidly proliferating maternal tissues (hematopoietic, intestinal mucosa) can be affected. A full spectrum of malformations can be induced by these agents, and site specificity is primarily determined by the time of exposure. Those organ rudiments undergoing rapid proliferation at the time of exposure are likely to be the sites of future malformation. Many of the resulting malformations involve reduction deformities, or missing elements, presumably because insufficient cells were available to form the organ rudiment. There is often a narrow dose-response curve for teratogenicity with these agents because there is little difference in doses that will malform the embryo and those

that kill the embryo. Malformations are often induced at doses that cause death in a significant portion of the litter.

Teratogens Affecting Specific Events in Differentiation. While necrosis is a common event in the developmental toxicity of cytotoxic agents, it is not a universal mechanism. There are agents that disrupt development by highly specific mechanisms of action not involving excessive necrosis or embryolethality. These are characterized by the dose-response pattern exhibited in Figure 7–3,A, where malformations occur without embryolethality. These specific teratogens usually induce a subset of all possible malformations at a given time of exposure, and usually at narrow time points within the organogenesis period. A well-defined structural anomaly or a distinct malformation syndrome occurs from prenatal exposure to these agents. It is not possible to make generalities about the mechanism of action of agents falling within this class. Rather, each agent appears to operate according to its own unique mechanism of action.

Thalidomide is the classic example of such a teratogen, but insofar as relatively little is understood about its mechanism of action, it will not be described further. Glucocorticoids, both natural and synthetic, are another example. Physiologic levels of glucocorticoids are required for normal growth and differentiation of embryonic tissue, while pharmacologic doses administered at midgestation in laboratory animals induce malformations primarily of the palate, and less frequently of the limbs. Different strains of inbred mice exhibit different degrees of susceptibility to glucocorticoid-induced cleft palate. The level of cytoplasmic glucocorticoid receptors in the maxillary mesenchyme cells of embryo correlates with the strain susceptibility; i.e., higher receptor levels are found in responsive strains, and lower levels in nonresponsive strains (Pratt and Salomon, 1981). High levels of glucocorticoids cause significant growth inhibition in maxillary mesenchyme cells and subsequent alteration in production of extracellular matrix. The target organ specificity of glucocorticoids is also related to the concentration of the receptor protein, which is higher in the craniofacial region than in other parts of the embryo (Pratt and Salomon, 1981). Glucocorticoid induction of cleft palate alone in the absence of embryolethality, extensive necrosis, and overall growth retardation is a good example of a teratogen operating through a specific mechanism of action involving receptor-mediated events.

Another example of a teratogen that produces a distinct malformation syndrome through what appears to be a specific mechanism of action is the herbicidal agent nitrofen (2,4-dichloro-4′-

Table 7–5. PATTERN OF DOSE-RESPONSE WITH THE SPECIFIC TERATOGEN NITROFEN*†

DOSE	% IMPLANTS DEAD/RESORBED	FETAL BODY wt. (g)	% LIVE FETUSES MALFORMED
Control	3.7	5.63	0
75 mg/kg	3.1	5.46	45[§]
150 mg/kg	3.5	5.49	83[§]
250 mg/kg	4.1	5.37	96[§]
400 mg/kg	5.8	4.70[‡]	100[§]

* Nitrofen was dissolved in corn oil, administered by gavage on day 11 to pregnant rats, and uterine contents examined on day 22. Results are the mean litter frequency of 10 to 12 litters per group.

† Modified from Costlow, R. D., and Manson, J. M.: The heart and diaphragm: Target organs in the neonatal death induced by nitrofen (2,4-dichlorophenyl-*p*-nitrophenyl ether). *Toxicology*, 20:209–27, 1981.

‡ Significantly depressed relative to controls, $p < 0.05$.

§ Significantly elevated relative to controls, $p < 0.001$.

nitro diphenyl ether). Exposure of pregnant rats by the oral route results in neonatal lethality due to cardiac, diaphragm, and kidney malformations as well as lung immaturity (Stone and Manson, 1981; Costlow and Manson, 1981). The dose-response pattern for malformations, embryolethality, and growth retardation with maternal exposure on day 11 is given in Table 7–5. The major difference in these data and those for MNNG in Table 7–3 is that doses of nitrofen at and above those causing malformation of the entire litter did not significantly increase the incidence of embryolethality and had a relatively minor effect on fetal body weight. Histologic observations of the embryonic heart, the major target organ, failed to reveal indications of excess vacuolization, pyknosis, or cytoplasmic inclusions up to four days after exposure, but did reveal an overall reversible delay in growth and septation within 24 hours after exposure.

Several lines of evidence have indicated that nitrofen may exert a teratogenic effect via alterations in thyroid hormone status (Manson *et al.*, 1983). One is that nitrofen, as a diphenyl ether compound, has a stereochemical structure similar to thyroxine. When administered on day 11 of pregnancy, maternal TSH and T_4 levels are lowered, and fetal T_4 levels are depressed at term. Coadministration of T_4 with nitrofen results in a significant protection against nitrofen-induced malformations, especially of the heart (Table 7–6). A metabolite of nitrofen (4-hydroxy-2,5-dichloro-4'-amino diphenyl ether) found in maternal and embryonic tissues after teratogenic exposure has been found to cross-react with antibodies for T_3. A potential mechanism of action is that nitrofen exerts a teratogenic effect through production of a T_3-active metabolite which, unlike maternal thyroid hormones, is able to enter the embryonic compartment. The resulting premature and pharmacologic exposure of the embryo to a T_3-active substance may stimulate putative T_3 responses, such as enhanced amplification of the β-adrenergic signal of the heart. Heart anomalies, especially of the arterial outflow tract, have been induced in other systems with known β agonists, presumably due to altered cardiovascular hemodynamics (Hodach *et al.*, 1975). Consequently, the target organ specificity of nitrofen, at least in regard to the heart, may also be due to receptor-mediated tissue interactions as it was for glucocorticoid-induced cleft palate.

Nonspecific Developmental Toxins. The third pattern of response is one in which growth retardation and embryolethality occur without tera-

Table 7–6. PROTECTION AGAINST NITROFEN TERATOGENICITY BY THYROXINE*†

	NITROFEN	NITROFEN+T_4
$\overline{X}$% Fetuses with		
Heart anomalies (total)	26.7 ± 2.8	2.4 ± 1.6[‡]
Aortic arch anomalies	12.4 ± 2.7	2.4 ± 1.6
Ventricular septal defect	10.3 ± 3.7	0
Tetralogy of Fallot	4.8 ± 2.9	1.3 ± 1.3
Truncus arteriosus communis	1.6 ± 1.6	0
Kidney anomalies	17.0 ± 4.0	8.6 ± 3.3
Diaphragmatic hernias	4.6 ± 2.4	3.1 ± 2.1
$\overline{X}$% Malformed fetuses	39.9 ± 5.3	12.3 ± 3.9[‡]

* Dams were thyroidectomized on day 1 of pregnancy and treated with nitrofen (25 mg/kg, days 9 to 11) or nitrofen plus T_4 (4 μg/100 g body wt, days 2 to 21). Results are presented as the mean litter frequency of fetuses with the indicated anomalies.

† Modified from Manson, F. M.; Brown, T.; and Baldwin, D. M.: Teratogenicity of nitrofen (2,4-dichloro-4'-nitro diphenyl ether) and its effects on thyroid function in the rat. *Toxicol. Appl. Pharmacol.*, 73:323–35, 1983.

‡ Significantly depressed relative to nitrofen alone, $p < 0.002$.

togenicity (Figure 7–3,*C*). Examples of agents that fall within this class are the mitochondrial protein synthesis inhibitors chloramphenicol and thiamphenicol (Neubert *et al.*, 1980). After treatment on days 10 and 11, the dose response for embryolethality is steep, increasing from control levels to 100 percent mortality at doses between 100 and 125 mg/kg/day for thiamphenicol (Bass *et al.*, 1978). Dose-dependent inhibition of mitochondrial respiration, ATP content, and cytochrome oxidase activity in embryonic tissue correlated with growth retardation and death of embryos. Inhibition of cellular processes as fundamental as mitochondrial function is believed to result in nonspecific effects such as overall growth retardation and lethality. There is no basis for target organ susceptibility in the early embryo for perturbation of such a fundamental cellular process, and consequently all tissues appear to be affected to an equal extent. The early signs of perturbation are overall growth retardation progressing to complete lethality of the litter once a critical threshold for cellular energy depletion was crossed. These conditions are incompatible with teratogenicity in which some tissues are permanently damaged and others are spared, permitting survival of abnormal embryos to term.

Developmental Toxicity Mediated by Perturbations in Maternal and Placental Homeostasis. The agents discussed so far are believed to exert developmental toxicity through a direct effect on the conceptus, either by killing proliferating cells or by altering differentiative processes. There are examples of agents and conditions that are embryotoxic through indirect effects on the conceptus resulting from alterations in the maternal system. The best example of these are perturbations that lead to maternal nutritional deficiencies. Generalized malnutrition, caloric restriction, and protein deficiency during pregnancy lead to severe growth retardation, thyroid deficiencies, and delays in CNS maturation that are not reversible with augmentation of the food supply to the neonate (Shrader *et al.*, 1977). Deprivation of specific nutrients in the maternal diet, i.e., vitamin A (Warkany and Roth, 1948), zinc (Hurley *et al.*, 1971), and folic acid (Johnson and Chepenik, 1981), can lead to malformations, growth retardation, and embryolethality. Treatment of the mother with agents that reduce availability of essential nutrients to the embryo, i.e., EDTA for trace metals, aminopterin for folic acid, results in syndromes similar to those obtained with restriction in the maternal diet.

Agents that reduce the transport of nutrients from the maternal to embryonic compartment through specific interference with placental function can have an indirect embryotoxic effect. Trypan blue is believed to be teratogenic through interference with histiotrophic nutrition of the embryo by the yolk sac placenta (Beck, 1981). This type of nutrition involves pinocytosis/phagocytosis of maternal macromolecules and hydrolytic breakdown by lysosomal enzymes in cells of the yolk sac placenta, followed by passage of soluble nutrients to the embryo. Trypan blue inhibits the process of pinocytosis and the lysosomal enzymes involved in the hydrolysis of macromolecules. Teratogenic activity of the dye ceases between days 10 to 11 of gestation in rats, which coincides with the transition from a yolk sac placenta to a chorioallantoic placenta. Hemotrophic nutrition, or the simple diffusion of nutrients between closely apposed maternal and embryonic circulations, is characteristic of the chorioallantoic placenta and is not influenced by trypan blue. Demonstration that developmental toxicants do not penetrate into embryonic tissues is the usual approach taken to defining the "indirect" mode of action. This can prove to be difficult insofar as few analytic techniques are sufficiently sensitive to detect low levels of chemical agents in the early embryo. A more accurate approach may be to utilize cultures of postimplantation rat embryos where test agents are either added directly to the culture medium, or control embryos are cultured in serum derived from treated mothers. This approach has recently been taken by Steele *et al.* (1983) to determine whether hypolipidemic agents that were embryotoxic *in vivo* were so due to maternal hypolipidemia or to direct effects on the embryo. Results indicated that the culture of embryos in hypolipidemic serum had no adverse effects, while direct exposure of embryos to the agents themselves in normal serum was embryotoxic.

Alteration of uteroplacental blood flow is an important factor in indirect effects of developmental toxicants. Uteroplacental blood flow is reduced in women with hypertension, a condition that is associated with the birth of growth-retarded infants. In rats, the effects of short-term but total arrest of circulation have been studied by uterine vascular clamping (Barr and Brent, 1978). When conducted prior to the 6th day of gestation, embryolethality in the clamped horn is high, but survivors are not growth retarded. Clamping during the organogenesis period for up to an hour can produce a spectrum of malformations specific for the developmental age at the time of obstruction, but negligible lethality or growth retardation. Partial but permanent reduction in uteroplacental blood flow by uterine artery ligation is generally associated with growth retardation, especially when performed at later stages of gestation (Barr and Brent, 1978). Vasoactive drugs such as serotonin, epinephrine, and ergotamine have been shown to cause malformations, embryolethality, and growth retardation (Neubert *et al.*, 1980). Intravenous infusion of epinephrine into pregnant rabbits elevated maternal blood pressure and caused extensive uterine vasoconstriction, placental cyanosis, and functional cardiovascular alterations in the fetus. The placental cyanosis coincided with, or slightly preceded, the fetal hemodynamic changes (Dornhorst and Young, 1952).

Hydroxyurea, an agent whose teratogenicity has been attributed to inhibition of DNA synthesis and cytotoxicity, was found to have a dramatic effect on uteroplacental blood flow in pregnant rabbits. Within two to five minutes after maternal exposure, uteroplacental blood flow decreased 77 percent and uterine vascular resistance increased 400 percent compared to controls. (Millicovsky *et al.*, 1981). Immediately thereafter, craniofacial and cardiac hemorrhages were observed in rabbit embryos. The same effects were produced in rabbit embryos after clamping the uterine vessels for ten minutes. These findings indicate that the developmental toxicity of hydroxyurea may be partly attributed to alteration of maternal and uterine hemodynamics, which cause an immediate pathologic effect on the embryo. Inhibition of DNA synthesis and cell death may constitute secondary effects that compromise the recovery of the embryo from the initial vascular insult. This example indicates that developmental toxicity is a far more complex process than mutagenicity or cytotoxicity. Assumptions cannot be made that the mode of embryotoxic action is identical to the mode of cellular action, even for agents with well-defined cellular mechanisms of action such as hydroxyurea, given the complex interchange that occurs between maternal, placental, and embryonic systems.

CHEMICAL DISTRIBUTION AND BIOTRANSFORMATION IN PREGNANCY

The manner in which chemicals are absorbed during pregnancy, whether or not they reach the conceptus, and in what form, is an area of unique and highly specialized research in pharmacokinetics. It is now accepted that every aspect of xenobiotic disposition and biotransformation is modified by the physiologic changes associated with pregnancy. The maternal, placental, and fetal compartments comprise independent, yet interacting, systems that undergo profound changes throughout the course of pregnancy. Each of these components will first be considered separately, and then attempts will be made to describe their interactions at different stages of pregnancy, i.e., the organogenesis

and fetal periods, to determine whether the balance is in favor of or against protection of the conceptus. More detailed information on xenobiotic disposition and biotransformation during pregnancy can be found in a number of reviews (Neims *et al.*, 1976; Nau and Neubert, 1978; Green *et al.*, 1979; Juchau, 1980, 1981; Krauer *et al.*, 1980; Pelkonen, 1980).

Physiologic Changes in Pregnancy That Alter the Pharmacokinetics of Chemical Agents

Several pregnancy-related physiologic alterations favor increased absorption of drugs. Gastric emptying and transport through the small intestine are delayed, leading to more complete absorption. Likewise, increased tidal volume and reduced residual lung volume favor increased absorption of volatile and soluble substances through the lung. The uptake of particles and aerosols is also increased with the elevation in airstream velocity. Early in pregnancy the cardiac output increases by about 30 percent owing to an elevation in both heart rate and stroke volume. This results in increased tissue concentrations of absorbed toxicants, especially in organs that are highly perfused, such as the placenta and uterus (reviewed in Krauer *et al.*, 1980).

Pregnancy alters several factors that influence the distribution of xenobiotics. These include an increase in total body water and body fat, and a decrease in plasma binding proteins (reviewed in Krauer *et al.*, 1980). Plasma volume is elevated by 50 percent, while the increase in red cell volume is only approximately 18 percent, leading to borderline anemia. The generalized edema characteristic of normal pregnancy is due to a 70 percent elevation of the extracellular fluid space, which represents an increased area for distribution of drugs and other chemicals. The average pregnant woman stores 3 to 4 kg of body fat in subcutaneous depots. This fat is gained in the first six months of pregnancy and tends to be mobilized in the last trimester. The increase in body fat can act as a reservoir for fat-soluble compounds, which, when released during late pregnancy, can result in increased xenobiotic exposure to both mother and fetus.

Many xenobiotics are bound to plasma proteins, predominantly albumin. This binding is usually reversible, saturable, and relatively nonspecific. The concentration of plasma albumin declines in the first half of pregnancy by approximately 20 percent owing to an increase in maternal plasma volume and actual decrease in total plasma albumin content (reviewed in Krauer *et al.*, 1980). For highly bound xenobiotics, the hypoalbuminaemia of pregnancy results in a decrease in the bound and a corresponding increase in the free plasma fraction. The mobilization of fat stores in the last trimester and subsequent competition for albumin binding sites by free fatty acids enhances the fraction of unbound xenobiotic. As the maternal plasma albumin concentration falls during pregnancy, levels of albumin in fetal plasma gradually increase. Since the toxicologic activity of a compound is usually related to the concentration of the unbound molecule, i.e., the free fraction in the plasma, changes in the degree of maternal and fetal binding of xenobiotics can influence toxicity of absorbed compounds. Thus, for a compound absorbed in early pregnancy, if lower fetal plasma albumin concentration is combined with a high free xenobiotic fraction in maternal plasma, a net accumulation of unbound compound in the fetal compartment will occur, ever at lower-than-normal maternal plasma drug concentrations.

Pregnancy alters many aspects of hepatic xenobiotic biotransformation. During phase I reactions, the compound is oxidized, reduced, or hydrolyzed and is generally rendered less lipid soluble. The decrease in lipid solubility is rather slight, and the addition of one hydroxyl group into a molecule decreases the octanol:water partition coefficient by a factor of only 0.5 to 0.8 (Pelkonen, 1977). The toxicologic properties of the parent compound may be increased, decreased, or unchanged as a result of phase I reaction. During phase II reactions, the compound itself or a phase I metabolite is conjugated with endogenous agents (glucuronic acid, sulfate, glutathione), which results in a large increase in water solubility and usually a decrease in toxicologic activity due to rapid excretion. Conjugation of a lipid-soluble compound with glucuronic acid decreases the octanol:water partition coefficient by a factor of at least 10. The result is that phase I metabolites are still somewhat lipid soluble, and if they possess sufficient stability and do not bind at the site of generation in maternal tissues, they could theoretically cross the placenta. Phase II metabolites are so polar that it is unlikely they would be able to cross the placenta and would probably be rapidly excreted from the maternal system.

Although several studies have been published, little is known about the effect of pregnancy on the relative rates of activating and detoxifying reactions for any given substrate (Juchau, 1981). The human liver is not enlarged in pregnancy as it is in rats, which have a 40 percent increase in absolute liver weight (Neims et al., 1976). When expressed in units of hepatic microsomal protein or wet weight of hepatic tissue, rates of most phase I and phase II reactions are decreased during pregnancy in rats. The lowered specific

activity of these reactions is counteracted by the increase in maternal liver weight, however, so that the total activity in the whole liver can be comparable to that in the nonpregnant female. The decreased level of monooxygenase activity in maternal liver has been attributed to decreased enzyme levels as well as to competitive inhibition by circulating steroids (Neims et al., 1976). Another factor that could contribute to the lower monooxygenase activities is that pregnant rats appear to be less responsive to induction of hepatic P-450 systems by phenobarbital (but not 3-methylcholanthrene) than are nonpregnant females (Guenther and Mannering, 1977). Despite the absence of a comprehensive literature on this subject, there appears to be an overall decrease in hepatic xenobiotic biotransformation during pregnancy. There is not sufficient information on extrahepatic biotransformation during pregnancy to generalize about their contribution to maternal biotransformations.

Excretion by the kidneys accounts for a major portion of xenobiotic elimination, and during pregnancy renal function undergoes a greater change than any other maternal system. In humans, the renal plasma flow and the glomerular filtration rate double in early pregnancy and continue to increase until term. The effect of the increased glomerular filtration rate on drug elimination will depend on the concentration of free drug in plasma. It is likely that the increase in filtration will have a major effect on elimination of those drugs excreted unchanged in urine and of conjugates. In summary, the physiologic changes that occur in the maternal system during pregnancy are increased absorption and distribution of xenobiotics, accompanied by decreased hepatic biotransformation. These alterations will tend to favor retention of xenobiotics, but may be offset by the increase in renal function.

Transport and Biotransformation of Xenobiotics by the Placenta

The placenta should be viewed as a lipid membrane that permits bidirectional transfer of substances between maternal and fetal compartments rather than as a ''barrier.'' The transfer depends on three major elements: the type of placentation, the physiochemical properties of the compound, and placental biotransformation. There are two distinctly different placentas in most mammalian species during organogenesis. In most laboratory animals, the yolk sac placenta predominates during organogenesis, while in primate species including humans, the chorioallantoic placenta is dominant. Except for cases where chemical agents are selectively toxic to one type of placenta over another (i.e., trypan blue), few correlations have been made between anatomic classification of the placenta and transfer of chemicals between mother and fetus (Waddell and Marlowe, 1981). Although earlier work suggested that placental membrane thickness or the number of placental layers limited diffusion, it is now clear that the situation is more complex. For example, the observed decrease in tissue layers and thickness of the trophoblast does not predict the decrease in placental permeability between the 7th and 14th days of rodent pregnancy (Green *et al.*, 1979). The fetal endothelium, which is not markedly altered during pregnancy, is believed to be the layer responsible for diffusional resistance to larger-molecular-weight substances in rabbits (Thornburg and Faber, 1976). For smaller polar molecules, diffusion through sheep and rabbit placentas has been associated with the presence of interstitial water-filled pores of fixed diameter. Species differences in this parameter are great, however, and the calculated pore radii are 0.4 nm for sheep and approximately 30 nm for rabbits (Thornburg and Faber, 1976). Blood flow constitutes the major rate-limiting factor in placental transfer of the more lipid-soluble compounds. Placental blood flow progressively increases throughout pregnancy at a rate that is proportional to fetal size even though placental mass, relative to fetal mass, is reduced (Green *et al.*, 1979).

The movement of xeonbiotics from maternal to fetal circulation primarily occurs by diffusion. Active transport, facilitated diffusion, and carrier-mediated transfer are important for endogenous molecules and seem to play a much more limited role for xenobiotics. Lipid solubility, ionic charge, molecular weight, and structural configuration influence transport. Xenobiotics with molecular weights less than 500 can readily cross the placenta, while those with molecular weights higher than 1000 cannot. The most rapid transplacental passage occurs with compounds that are lipophilic and nonionized at physiologic pH. The net result of protein binding on placental transfer is also dependent on lipid solubility and degree of ionization; i.e., the transfer of lipophilic nonpolar compounds is not influenced by protein binding while the diffusion rate of non-lipophilic, polar compounds can be greatly affected. The different possibilities of xenobiotic transfer based on lipid solubility are illustrated in Figure 7–5. In panel A, the parent compound is lipid soluble and crosses the placenta without difficulty. Polar metabolites (i.e., conjugates) are formed in the mother, but do not cross the placenta and are excreted from the maternal compartment. Another possibility is illustrated

in panel B, where nonpolar metabolites (i.e., products of phase I reactions) are formed in the mother and the parent compound, and stable, nonpolar metabolites cross the placenta. Additional biotransformation to polar metabolites and subsequent excretion occur primarily in the maternal compartment. A third possibility is that the lipid-soluble parent compound and nonpolar metabolites equilibrate across the placenta, and polar metabolites formed in either maternal or fetal compartments do not cross the placenta. Excretion occurs to a greater extent on the maternal side, and polar metabolites may accumulate on the fetal side (Figure 7–5,*C*). A fourth possibility is that the parent compound is so polar that it does not cross the placenta and is excreted unchanged from the maternal compartment (Figure 7–5,*D*).

The human placenta appears to contain the enzyme systems for classical xenobiotic biotransformation, i.e., oxidation, reduction, hydrolysis, and conjugations. Cytochrome P-450-dependent reactions have been most extensively studied in human term placentas, and at least five human placental cytochromes P-450 have been identified to date, which are listed in Table 7–7. Virtually all of the spectrally visible cytochrome P-450 in the human placenta is involved in the conversion of steroidal precursors to estrogen. Compared to hepatic tissues, the xenobiotic biotransforming capacity of the placenta is negligible unless the mother has been exposed to 3-methylcholanthrene-type inducing agents during pregnancy. Cigarette smoking, for example, is positively correlated with increased AHH (aryl hydrocarbon hydroxylase) activity in the placenta. A high, dose-related correlation ($r = 0.9$) between placental AHH activity and smoking of 1 to 40 cigarettes a day during pregnancy has been found (Gurtoo *et al.*, 1983). Saturation of AHH induction occurred with smoking more than 20 to 25 cigarettes per day. Xenobiotics not biotransformed through 3-methylcholanthrene-type inducible pathways are, in general, poorly biotransformed by the placenta. Phenobarbital or "phenobarbital-type" inducing agents do not appear to affect placental enzyme systems. Epoxide hydrolase activity is relatively low in placentas of humans and laboratory animals, as are conjugation reactions involving glucuronidation and sulfation, while glutathione conjugation occurs at levels comparable to those in liver. Overall, placental biotransformation of xenobiotics appears to make little difference in the transplacental passage of xenobiotics. As a result, the placenta is not a metabolic barrier, and xenobiotics possessing sufficient lipid solubility can pass unchanged to the fetus. Generation of reactive metabolites by the placenta that could

MATERNAL COMPARTMENT   FETAL COMPARTMENT

PLACENTA

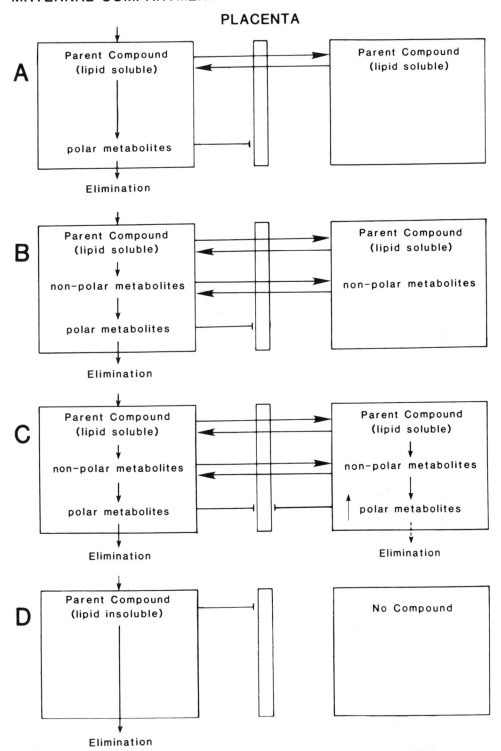

Figure 7–5. Influence of lipid solubility on the distribution and accumulation of xenobiotics in maternal and fetal compartments. See text for explanation. (Modified from Krauer, B.; Krauer, F.; and Hytten, F. E.: Drug disposition and pharmacokinetics in the maternal-placental-fetal unit. *Pharmacol. Ther.*, **10**:301–28, 1980.)

Table 7–7. SUBSTRATES BIOTRANSFORMED BY SEPARATE FORMS OF HUMAN PLACENTAL CYTOCHROME P-450*

SUBSTRATE	CELLULAR SUBFRACTION	SITE OF MONO OXYGENASE REACTION	INDUCER
Benzo(a)pyrene	Microsomal	3- and 9-hydroxylation	MC-type[†‡]
N-2-fluorenylacetamide	Microsomal	N-hydroxylation	MC-type[†]
Androstenedione	Microsomal	Aromatization	—
β-Estradiol	Microsomal	2-hydroxylation	PB-type[‡]
Cholesterol	Mitochondrial	Side-chain cleavage	—

* Modified from Juchau, M. R.: Drug biotransformation in the placenta. *Pharmacol. Ther.*, 8:501–24, 1980.
[†] Induced by cigarette smoking during pregnancy.
[‡] MC,3-methylcholanthrene; PB, phenobarbital.

subsequently result in developmental toxicity does not seem to be a major concern except in the case of exposure to 3-methylcholanthrene-type inducing agents (Juchau, 1980, 1981).

Fetal Disposition and Biotransformation of Xenobiotics

Xenobiotics that have crossed the placenta enter the fetal circulation via the umbilical vein. The fetal liver is located between the umbilical vein and the inferior vena cava so that xenobiotics passing the placenta must traverse the fetal liver before entering the heart and the systemic circulation. The umbilical venous flow is diverted in the fetal liver so that substantial amounts of blood may enter the ductus venosus and bypass the liver, while the remainder flows into the portal vein and perfuses the hepatic parenchymal cells. In the human fetus, approximately 60 percent of the fetal blood flow is shunted through the ductus venosus, although wide intrasubject variation has been observed (Green *et al.*, 1979). The development of the ductus venosus and hepatic vasculature occurs by approximately 10 to 11 weeks of age, just beyond the organogenesis period in human embryos.

Amniotic fluid has the potential for being a slowly equilibrating reservoir for xenobiotics with the characteristics of a deep compartment (Kraven *et al.*, 1980). Up to 20 weeks of human development, the fetal epidermis is highly permeable and amniotic fluid has the same composition as fetal extracellular fluid. After 20 weeks the fetal skin becomes keratinized, limiting the exchange between amniotic fluid and extracellular fluid. The composition and volume of amniotic fluid then represent a balance between fetal urine production and fetal swallowing, and entry of xenobiotics into amniotic fluid is dependent on excretion via fetal urine. The major route of removal for xenobiotics in amniotic fluid is for the fluid to be swallowed by the fetus, filtered

out by the fetal kidney, and returned to the maternal system via the umbilical artery.

The biotransformation of xenobiotics by embryonic and fetal tissue is a subject that has received considerable experimental attention, (Pelkonen, 1980; Neims *et al.*, 1976; Nau and Neubert, 1978; Juchau, 1981). The appearance of cytochrome P-450-mediated xenobiotic biotransformation in fetal liver has been correlated with development of the smooth endoplasmic reticulum (SER). As indicated in Table 7–8, the SER does not appear in fetal liver of most laboratory animal species until the end of gestation. In humans the SER is first observed at 40 to 60 days of gestation. These ultrastructural findings correlate with measurements of enzyme activity, which is low in most laboratory animals just prior to birth and increases to adult levels within several days (guinea pigs) or several weeks (rat) after birth. In humans, enzyme activity is first detectable at six to seven weeks of gestation, at the end of the organogenesis period. At 12 to 14 weeks, enzyme activity reaches a relatively constant level (20 to 40 percent of adult levels for some substrates), and adult levels may not be reached until a year after birth.

Most conjugation pathways appear to be poorly developed in fetuses of laboratory animals, and low to nonexistent levels of glucuronidation, sulfation, and glutathione formation have been observed. There are important differences between species and substrates, however, with some inbred strains of mice exhibiting high levels of glucuronidation at midgestation (Pelkonen, 1980). Steroid glucuronidation occurs with different isomeric forms of the enzyme UDP-GT (uridine diphospho-glucuronosyltransferase) than xenobiotic glucuronidation (Lucier *et al.*, 1979). Most studies of glucuronidation in human fetal tissues have indicated low to nonexistent activity, while conjugations with glutathione, glycine, and sulfate are fairly well developed in fetal liver. Whether these systems

Table 7–8. APPEARANCE OF XENOBIOTIC BIOTRANSFORMING ENZYMES IN FETAL LIVER*

SPECIES	ORGANOGENESIS PERIOD (DAYS)	APPEARANCE OF SER (DAYS)	CYTOCHROME P-450 (% OF ADULT CONCENTRATION)[†]	BIRTH (DAYS)
Rat	6–15	18–22	0–5	22
Mouse	6–15	19–20	0–4	19
Rabbit	6–18	25–30	0–5	33
Guinea pig	10–18	50–60	6–30	66
Hamster	8–12	14–15	0–5	15
Macaque	20–45	80–100	10–20	170
Human	21–56	40–60	20–40	267

* Data from Nau and Neubert (1978) and Pelkonen (1980).

[†] Presented as the percent of adult values at birth in nonprimate species, at 120 to 160 days in macaques and at 84 to 98 days in humans.

function exclusively in steroid conjugation or also participate in xenobiotic conjugation is not known. Conjugates formed in the fetus may accumulate in the fetal compartment, either in fetal tissues themselves or in amniotic fluid.

Cytochrome P-450 in the human fetal liver has relatively broad substrate specificity and will biotransform substrates such as aniline and ethylmorphine, but not benzo[a]pyrene. Even with heavy maternal smoking, benzo[a] pyrene hydroxylase activity is not induced in the human fetal liver as it is in the placenta. The fetal adrenal gland has high cytochrome P-450 content, exceeding that of the liver at all developmental stages examined (Pelkomen, 1977). Other fetal organs such as the lung, kidney, and intestine have low to undectectable levels of cytochrome P-450 activity.

Table 7–9 contains a summary of xenobiotic biotransformation during pregnancy in maternal, placental, and fetal tissues. Induction of cytochrome P-450 activity in embryonic tissues can occur under some conditions. In humans, it is probable that drug-biotransforming enzymes are inducible during late pregnancy, but available information is fragmentary. Lack of induction in the fetal liver with chronic maternal exposure to cigarette smoke, alcohol, and certain drugs may indicate that the fetal enzymes are intrinsically noninducible or that insufficient substrate concentrations reach the fetal tissues for induction to occur. Xenobiotic biotransformation in laboratory animals is not easily induced during pregnancy in laboratory animals. Exposure during the perinatal period to agents such as 3-methylcholanthrene, TCDD, or certain polychlorinated

Table 7–9. BIOTRANSFORMATION OF XENOBIOTICS IN LABORATORY ANIMALS AND HUMANS DURING PREGNANCY

TISSUE	LABORATORY ANIMALS	HUMANS
Maternal Liver		
Phase I reactions	Reduced in pregnancy	Reduced in pregnancy
Phase II reactions	Reduced in pregnancy	Reduced in pregnancy
Placenta		
Phase I reactions	Low to nonexistent unless exposed to 3-MC-type inducing agents	Low to nonexistent except with heavy maternal smoking
Phase II reactions	Low to nonexistent	Glutathione conjugation predominates
Fetal Liver		
Phase I reactions	Enzymes appear at the end of gestation, can be prematurely induced with 3-methylcholanthrene-type inducers	20 to 40 percent of adult values by midgestation; phenobarbital-type substrate specificity; not apparently inducible
Phase II reactions	Low to nonexistent, but large species and substrate variations	Glucuronidation low; enzyme systems for sulfate, glycine, and glutathione conjugation

* See text for explanation 3-MC,3-methylcholanthrene; PB, phenobarbital.

[†] Data from Pelkonen (1977) and Manson *et al.* (1982).

biphenyls can elevate cytochrome P-450 levels, while agents like phenobarbital, pregnenolone, 16 α-carbonitrile and alcohol are not effective (Pelkonen, 1980).

SUMMARY AND CONCLUSIONS

The field of teratology has evolved from an experimental science concerned with anatomic description of malformations. As advances were made in the basic understanding of embryology, xenobiotics were used as tools for disrupting normal development to achieve a greater understanding of differentiation. This still constitutes the major underpinning of experimental research in teratology and is the critical factor in any advances made in the field. Today, additional demands are placed on teratologists to predict the risk of xenobiotic exposure on human pregnancy outcome. The necessity of evaluating risks to the conceptus from xenobiotic exposure has been forcefully demonstrated in epidemics of human birth defects induced by nutritional deficiencies, infectious agents, and xenobiotic exposure of the population. Consequently, the objectives of teratology research are increasingly oriented to an understanding of developmental toxicology, or how xenobiotics are taken up, distributed, accumulated, and biotransformed by pregnant mammals. The methodologies for carrying out this type of research are relatively well established and principles of general systemic toxicology in adult animals can be applied. Disciplined application of these principles will no doubt reveal that xenobiotics can interfere with the state of pregnancy and the process of development by unique and highly complex mechanisms. The key to understanding how some xenobiotics specifically interfere with the successful completion of pregnancy, however, ultimately depends on a more complete comprehension of the basic processes of development.

REFERENCES

Abel, E.: Fetal alcohol syndrome: Behavioral teratology. *Psychol. Bull.*, 87:29–50, 1980.

Adams, J., and Buelke-Sam, J.: Behavioral assessment for the postnatal animal: Testing and methods development. In Kimmel, C. A., and Buelke-Sam, J. (eds.): *Developmental Toxicology*. Raven Press, New York, 1981, pp. 233–58.

Adler, I-D.: New approaches to mutagenicity studies in animals for carcinogenic and mutagenic agents. II. Clastogenic effects determined in transplacentally treated mouse embryos. *Teratogenesis Carcinog. Mutagen.*, 3:321–34, 1983.

American Cancer Society (ACS): *Cancer Facts and Figures*. The Society, New York, 1980.

Barr, M., and Brent, R.: Uterine vascular interruption and combined radiation and surgical procedures. In Wilson, J. G., and Fraser, F. C. (eds.): *Handbook of Teratology*, Vol. 4. Plenum Press, New York, 1978, pp. 275–304.

Bass, R.; Oerter, D.; Krowke, R.; and Speilmann, H.: Embryonic development and mitochondrial function. III. Inhibition of respiration and ATP generation in rat embryos by thiamphenicol. *Teratology*, 18:93–102, 1978.

Beck, F.: Comparative placental morphology and function. In Kimmel, C. A. and Buelke-Sam, J. (eds.): *Developmental Toxicology*. Raven Press, New York, 1981, pp. 35–54.

Bibbo, M.; Gill, W.; Azizi, F.; Blough, R.; Fang, V.; Rosenfield, R.; Schumacher, G.; Sleeper, K.; Sonek, M.; and Wied, G.: Follow-up study of male and female offspring of DES-exposed mothers. *Obstet. Gynecol.*, 49:1–8, 1977.

Bolande, R. P.: Teratogenesis and oncogenesis. In Wilson, J. G., and Fraser, F. C. (eds.): *Handbook of Teratology*, Vol. 2. Plenum Press, New York, 1977, pp. 293–328.

Brinster, R. L.: Teratogen testing using preimplantation mammalian embryos. In Shepard, T. H.; Miller, J. R.; and Marois, M. (eds.) *Methods for Detection of Environmental Agents that Produce Congenital Defects*. American Elsevier Publishing Co., Inc., New York, 1975, pp. 113–24.

Chernoff, G.: The fetal alcohol syndrome in mice: Maternal variables. *Teratology*, 22:71–75, 1980.

Chung, C. S., and Myrianthopoulos, N. C.: Factors affecting risks of congenital malformations. *The National Foundation March of Dimes Original Articles Series*, Vol. XI, No. 10, 1975.

Collins, T. F.: Multigeneration studies of reproduction. In Wilson, J. G., and Fraser, F. C. (eds.): *Handbook of Teratology*, Vol. 4. Plenum Press, New York, 1978, pp. 191–214.

Consumer Product Safety Commission (CPSC): *Toxicity Testing of Household Products*. Document 1138. Washington, D.C., 1977.

Cooper, L. Z., and Krugman, S.: Diagnosis and management: congenital rubella. *Pediatrics*, 37:335–42, 1966.

Costlow, R. D., and Manson, J. M.: The heart and diaphragm: Target organs in the neonatal death induced by nitrofen (2,4-dichlorophenyl-*p*-nitrophenyl ether). *Toxicology*, 20:209–27, 1981.

Dieckmann, W. J.; Davis, M. E.; and Rynkiewicz, L. M.: Does administration of diethylstilbestrol during pregnancy have therapeutic value? *Am. J. Obstet. Gynecol.*, 66:1062–81, 1953.

Dornhorst, A. C., and Young, M. I.: The action of adrenalin and noradrenaline on the placental and foetal circulations in the rabbit and guinea pig. *J. Physiol. (Lond.)*, 118:282–91, 1952.

Fabro, S.: Biochemical basis of thalidomide teratogenicity. In Juchau, M. R. (ed.): *The Biochemical Basis of Chemical Teratogenesis*. Elsevier/North-Holland, New York, 1981, pp. 159–78.

Fabro, S.; Smith, R. L.; and Williams, R. T.: Fate of ^{14}C-thalidomide in the pregnant rabbit. *Biochem. J.*, 104:565–69, 1967.

Food and Drug Administration (FDA): *Guidelines for Reproduction Studies for Safety Evaluation of Drugs for Human Use*. Washington, DC, 1966.

———: Advisory Committee on Protocols for Safety Evaluation, Panel on Reproduction: Report on reproduction studies in the safety evaluation of food additives and pesticide residues. *Toxicol. Appl. Pharmacol.*, 16:264–96, 1970.

Fraser, F. C.: Relation of animal studies to the problem in man. In Wilson, J. G., and Fraser, F. C. (eds.): *Handbook of Teratology*, Vol. 1. Plenum Press, New York, 1977, pp. 75–96.

Fullerton, P. M., and Kremer, M.: Neuropathy after intake of thalidomide (Distaval). *Br. Med. J.*, 2:855–58, 1961.

Green, T. P.; O'Dea, R. F.; and Mirkin, B. L.: Determinants of drug disposition and effect in the fetus. *Annu. Rev. Pharmacol. Toxicol.*, **19**:285–322, 1979.

Gregg, N. M.: Congenital cataract following German measles in the mother. *Trans. Opthalmol. Soc. Aust.*, **3**:35–46, 1941.

Guenther, T. M., and Mannering, G. T.: Induction of hepatic monooxygenase systems of pregnant rats with phenobarbital and 3-methylcholanthrene. *Biochem. Pharmacol.*, **26**:577–84, 1977.

Gurtoo, H. L.; Williams, C. J; Gottlieb, K.; Mulhern, A.; Caballes, L.; Vaught, J.; Marinello, A.; and Bansal S.: Population distribution of placental benzo(a)pyrene metabolism in smokers. *Int. J. Cancer*, **31**:29–37, 1983.

Henderson, G.; Hoyumpa, A.; McClain, C.; and Shenker, S.: The effects of chronic and acute alcohol administration on fetal development in the rat. *Alcoholism: Clin. Exp. Res.*, **3**:99–106, 1979.

Herbst, A. L.; Cole, P.; Colton, T.; Robboy, S.; and Scully, R.: Age-incidence and risk of diethylstilbestrol-related clear cell adenocarcinoma of the vagina and cervix. *Am. J. Obstet. Gynecol.*, **128**:43–50, 1977.

Hoar, R. M., and Monie, I. W.: Comparative development of specific organ systems. In Kimmel, C. A., and Buelke-Sam, J. (eds.): *Developmental Toxicology*. Raven press, New York, 1981, pp. 13–33.

Hodach, R. J.; Hodach, A. E.; Fallon, J. D.; Bruyere, H. J.; and Gilbert, E. F.: The role of β-adrenergic activity in the production of cardiac and aortic arch anomalies in chick embryos. *Teratology*, **12**:33–46, 1975.

Hurley, L. S.; Gowan, J.; and Swenerton, H.: Teratogenic effects of short-term and transitory zinc deficiency in rats. *Teratology*, **4**:199–204, 1971.

Inouye, M., and Murakami, U.: Teratogenic effect of *N*-methyl-*N'*-nitronitrosoguanidine. *Teratology*, **18**:263–68, 1978.

Ivankovic, S.: Teratogenic and carcinogenic effects of some chemicals during prenatal life in rats, Syrian Golden hamsters and minipigs. In *Perinatal Carcinogenesis*. National Cancer Institute Monograph 51, DHEW Publication No. (NIH) 7a-1063, 1979, pp. 103–16.

Johnson, E. M. and Chepenik, K. P.: Teratogenicity of folate antagonists. In Juchau, M. R. (ed.), *The Biochemical Basis of Chemical Teratogenesis*. Elsevier/North Holland, New York, 1981, pp. 137–78.

Jones, K., and Smith, D.: Recognition of the fetal alcohol syndrome in early infancy. *Lancet*, **2**:999–1001, 1973.

Juchau, M. R.: Drug biotransformation in the placenta. *Pharmacol. Ther.*, **8**:501–24, 1980.

———: Enzymatic bioactivation and inactivation of chemical teratogens and transplacental carcinogens/mutagens. In Juchau, M. R. (ed.): *The Biochemical Basis of Chemical Teratogenesis*. Elsevier/North Holland, New York, 1981, pp. 63–94.

Kaminski, M.; Le Bouvier, F.; du Mazanbrun, C.; and Runzeau-Rouquette, C.: Moderate alcohol use and pregnancy outcome. *Neurobehav. Toxicol. Teratol.*, **3**:173–81, 1981.

Karnofskey, D. A.: Mechanism of action of certain growth-inhibiting drugs. In Wilson, J. G., and Warkany, J. (eds.) *Teratology: Principles and Techniques*. University of Chicago Press, Chicago, 1965, pp. 185–93.

Keberle, H.; Faigle, J. W.; Fritz, H.; Knuesel, F.; Loustalot, P.; and Schmid, K.: Theories on the mechanism of action of thalidomide. In Robson, J. M.; Sullivan, F. M.; and Smith, R. L. (eds.): *Embryopathic Activity of Drugs*. Churchill Ltd., London, 1965, pp. 210–33.

Kennedy, T. Q., and Armstrong, D. T.: The role of prostaglandins in endometrial vascular changes at implantation. In Glasser, S. R., and Bullock, D. W. (eds.): *Cellular and Molecular Aspects of Implantation*. Plenum Press, New York, 1981, pp. 349–61.

Khera, K. S.: Maternal toxicity—a possible factor in fetal malformations in mice. *Teratology*, **29**:411–16, 1984.

Kimmel, C. A.; Holson, J. F.; Hogue, C. J.; and Carlo, G. L.: Reliability of experimental studies for predicting hazards to human development. Final report. *NCTR Technical Report for Experiment No. 6015*. National Center for Toxicological Research, Jefferson, Ark., 1984, p. 56.

Knapp, K.: Das thalidomid-syndrom. *Bull. Soc. Roy. Belge. Gynec. Obst.*, **33**:37–42, 1963.

Kochhar, D. M.; Penner, J. D.; and McDay, J. A.: Limb development in mouse embryos. II. Reduction defects, cytotoxicity and inhibition of DNA synthesis produced by cytosine arabinoside. *Teratology*, **18**:71–92, 1978.

Krauer, B.; Krauer, F.; and Hytten, F. E.: Drug disposition and pharmacokinetics in the maternal-placental-fetal unit. *Pharmacol. Ther.*, **10**:301–28, 1980.

Lenz, W.: Das Thalidomid-syndrom. *Fortschr. Med.*, **81**:148–53, 1963.

———: Malformations caused by drugs in pregnancy. *Am. J. Dis. Child.*, **112**:99–106, 1966.

Lucier, G. W.; Lui, E.; and Lamartiniere, C.: Metabolic activation/deactivation reactions during perinatal development. *Environm. Health Perspect.*, **29**:7–16, 1979.

Mandel, J. D.: A new chemical mutagen for bacteria, 1-methyl-3-nitro-1-nitrosoguanidine. *Biochem. Biophys. Res. Commun.*, **3**:575–77, 1960.

Manson, J. M.: Developmental toxicity of alkylating agents: Mechanism of action. In Juchau, M. R. (ed.): *The Biochemical Basis of Chemical Teratogenesis*. Elsevier/North-Holland, New York, 1981, pp. 95–136.

Manson, J. M.; Brown, T.; and Baldwin, D. M.: Teratogenicity of nitrofen (2,4-dichloro-4'-nitro diphenyl ether) and its effects on thyroid function in the rat. *Toxicol. Appl. Pharmacol.*, **73**:323–35, 1984.

Manson, J. M., and Miller, M. L.: Contribution of mesenchymal cell death and mitotic alteration to asymmetric limb malformations induced by MNNG. *Teratogenesis Carcinog. Mutagen.*, **3**:335–53, 1983.

Manson, J. M.; Zenick, H.; and Costlow, R.: Teratology test methods for laboratory animals. In Hayes, A. W. (ed.): *Principles and Methods of Toxicology*. Raven Press, New York, 1982, pp. 141–84.

Maugh, T. H.: Chemicals: How many are there? *Science*, **199**:162, 1978.

McBride, W. G.: Thalidomide and congenital anomalies. *Lancet*, **2**:1358, 1961.

McLachlan, J., and Dixon, R.: Toxicologic comparisons of experimental and clinical exposure to diethylstilbestrol during gestation. *Adv. Sex Horm. Res.*, **3**:309–36, 1977.

Meyne, J., and Legator, M.: Clastogenic effects of transplacental exposure of mouse embryos to nitrogen mustard or cyclophosphamide. *Teratogenesis, Carcinog., Mutagen.*, **3**:281–87, 1983.

Miller, R. W.: Prenatal origins of cancer in man: Epidemiological evidence. In Tomatis, L., and Mohr, E. (eds.): *Transplacental Carcinogenesis*. IARC Pub. #4, 1973, p. 175.

Millicovsky, G.; DeSesso, J.; Kleinman, L.; and Clark, K.: Effects of hydroxyurea on hemodynamics of pregnant rabbits: A maternally mediated mechanism of embryotoxicity. *Am. J. Obstet. Gynecol.*, **140**:747–52, 1981.

National Center for Health Statistics (NCHS): *Births, marriages, divorces, and deaths for 1979*. Monthly Vital Statistics Report. U.S. Department of Health, Education and Welfare, 1980.

National Foundation/March of Dimes: *Facts 1980*. The Foundation, New York, 1981a.

———: Report of Panel II. Guidelines for reproductive studies in exposed human populations. In Bloom, A. D. (ed.): *Guidelines for Studies of Human Populations*

Exposed to Mutagenic and Reproductive Hazards. The Foundation, New York, 1981b, pp. 37–110.

National Institute for Occupational Safety and Health (NIOSH): *Registry of Toxic Substances,* 1977.

Nau, H., and Neubert, D.: Development of drug-metabolizing monooxygenase systems in various mammalian species including man. Its significance for transplacental toxicity. In Neubert, D.; Merker, H. J.; Mau, H.; and Langman, J. (eds.): *Role of Pharmacokinetics in Prenatal and Perinatal Toxicology.* Georg Theime Publishers, Stuttgart, 1978, pp. 13–44.

Neims, A. H.; Warner, M.; Loughnan, P. M.; and Aranda, J. V.: Developmental aspects of the hepatic cytochrome P_{450} monooxygenase system. *Annu. Rev. Pharmacol. Toxicol.,* 16:427–44, 1976.

Neubert, D.; Barrach, H. J.; and Merker, H. J.: Drug-induced damage to the embryo or fetus. *Curr. Top. Pathol.,* 69:242–324, 1980.

Nowack, E.: Die sensible phase bei der thalidomid-embryopathie. *Humangenetik,* 1:516–22, 1965.

Ornoy, A.; Salamon-Aron, J.; Ben-Zur, A.; and Kohn, G.: Placental findings in spontaneous abortions and stillbirths. *Teratology,* 24:243–51, 1981.

Palmer, A. K.: Regulatory requirements for reproductive toxicology: Theory and practice. In Kimmel, C. A., and Buelke-Sam, J. (eds.): *Developmental Toxicology.* Raven Press, New York, 1981, pp. 259–87.

Pelkonen, O.: Transplacental transfer of foreign compounds and their metabolism by the foetus. In Bridges, J. W., and Chasseaud, L. F. (eds.): *Progress in Drug Metabolism,* Vol. 2. John Wiley & Sons, Inc., New York, 1977, pp. 119–61.

——— : Biotransformation of xenobiotics in the fetus. *Pharmacol. Ther.,* 10:261–81, 1980.

Poskanzer, D., and Herbst, A.: Epidemiology of vaginal adenosis and adenocarcinoma associated with exposure to stilbestrol *in utero. Cancer,* 39(4):1892–95, 1977.

Pratt, R. M., and Salomon, D. S.: Biochemical basis for the teratogenic effects of glucocorticoids. In Juchau, M. R. (ed.): *The Biochemical Basis of Chemical Teratogenesis.* Elsevier/North-Holland, New York, 1981, pp. 179–99.

Ritter, E. J.: Altered biosynthesis. In Wilson, J. G., and Fraser, F. C. (eds.): *Handbook of Teratology,* Vol. 2. Plenum Press, New York, 1977, pp. 99–116.

Rosett, H.; Weiner, L.; Zuckerman, B.; McKinlay, S.; and Edelin, K.: Reduction of alcohol consumption during pregnancy with benefits to the newborn. *Alcoholism: Clin. Exp. Res.,* 4:178–84, 1980.

Schardein, J.: Introduction. In *Drugs as Teratogens.* CRC Press, Cleveland, 1976a, p. 6.

——— : Sedatives-hypnotics. In *Drugs as Teratogens.* CRC Press, Cleveland, 1976b, pp. 145–153.

Schumacher, H. J.: Chemical structure and teratogenic properties. In Shepard, T.; Miller, R.; and Marois, M. (eds.): *Methods for Detection of Environmental Agents that Produce Congenital Defects.* American Elsevier Publishing Co., New York, 1975, pp. 65–77.

Schumacher, H.; Smith, R. L.; and Williams, T. T.: The metabolism of thalidomide: The spontaneous hydrolyses of thalidomide solutions. *Br. J. Pharmacol. Chemother.,* 25:324–37, 1965.

Scott, W. J.: Cell death and reduced proliferative rate. In Wilson, J. G., and Fraser, F. C. (eds.): *Handbook of Teratology,* Vol. 2. Plenum Press, New York, 1977, pp. 81–98.

Scott, W. J., and Fradkin, R.: Effects of alcohol on non-human primate pregnancy. *Teratology,* 24:31A, 1981.

Sever, J. L.: Rubella as a teratogen. *Adv. Teratol.,* 2:127–38, 1967.

Shepard, T. H.: *Catalog of Teratogenic Agents,* 3rd ed., Johns Hopkins University Press, Baltimore, 1980.

Shrader, R. E.; Ferlatte, M. I.; Hastings-Roberts, M. H.;

Schoenborne, B. M.; Hoernicke, C. A.; and Zeman, F. J.: Thyroid function in prenatally protein-deprived rats. *J. Nutr.,* 107:221–29, 1977.

Sokol, R.; Miller, S.; and Reed, G.: Alcohol abuse during pregnancy: an epidemiologic study. *Alcoholism: Clin. Exp. Res.,* 4:178–84, 1980.

Staples, R. E.: Definition of teratogenesis and teratogens. In Shepard, T. H.; Miller, J. R.; and Marois, M. (eds.) *Methods for Detection of Environmental Agents That Produce Congenital Defects.* American Elsevier Publishing Company, Inc., New York, 1975, pp. 25–26.

Steele, C. E.; New, D. A. T.; Ashford, A.; and Copping, G. P.: Teratogenic action of hypolipidemic agents: An *in vitro* study with postimplantation embryos. *Teratology,* 28:229–36, 1983.

Stone, L. C., and Manson, J. M.: Effects of the herbicide 2,4-dichlorophenyl-*p*-nitrophenyl ether (nitrofen) on fetal lung development in rats. *Toxicology,* 20:195–207, 1981.

Streissguth, A.; Herman, C.; and Smith, D.: Intelligence, behavior, and dysmorphogenesis in the fetal alcohol syndrome: a report on 20 patients. *J. Pediatr.,* 92:363–67, 1978.

Szabo, K., and Brent, R. L.: Reduction of drug-induced cleft palate in mice. *Lancet,* 1:1296–97, 1975.

Taussig, H. B.: A study of the German outbreak of phocomelia. The thalidomide syndrome. *JAMA,* 180:1106, 1962.

Theiss, I.; Basler, A.; and Röhrborn, G.: Transplacental and direct exposure of mouse and marmoset to ethylnitrosourea: analysis of chromosomal aberrations. *Teratogenesis, Carcinog. Mutagen.,* 3:219–30, 1983.

Thompson, C. J. S.: *The Mystery and Lore of Monsters.* Bell Publishing Co., New York, 1930.

Thornburg, K. C., and Faber, J.: The steady-state concentration gradients of an electron dense marker (ferritin) in the three-layered hemochorial placenta of the rabbit. *J. Clin. Invest.,* 58:912–25, 1976.

U.S. Department of Health, Education and Welfare (USDHEW): The women and their pregnancies. *The Collaborative Perinatal Study of the National Institute of Neurological Diseases and Strokes.* DHEW Publication No. (NIH) 73-379, 1972.

Waddell, W. J., and Marlowe, C.: Biochemical regulation of the accessibility of teratogens to the developing embryo. In Juchau, M. R. (ed.): *The Biochemical Basis of Chemical Teratogenesis.* Elsevier/North Holland, New York, 1981, pp. 1–62.

Warburton, D., and Fraser, F. C.: Spontaneous abortion risks in man: Data from reproductive histories collected in a medical genetics unit. *Hum. Genet.,* 16:1–12, 1964.

Warkany, J.: Development of experimental mammalian teratology. In Wilson, J. G., and Warkany, J. (eds.): *Teratology: Principles and Techniques.* University of Chicago Press, Chicago, 1965, pp. 1–11.

——— : Drugs. In *Congenital Malformations: Notes and Comments.* Year Book Medical Publishers, Chicago, 1971a, pp. 84–96.

——— : Environmental factors, infection. In *Congenital Malformations: Notes and Comments.* Your Book Medical Publishers, Chicago, 1971b, pp. 62–70.

——— : History of teratology. In Wilson, J. G., and Fraser, F. C., (eds.): *Handbook of Teratology,* Vol. I. Pelnum Press, New York, 1977, pp. 3–46.

Warkany, J., and Roth, C. B.: Congenital malformations induced in rats by maternal vitamin A deficiency. II. Effect of varying the preparatory diet upon the yield of abnormal young. *J. Nutr.,* 35:1–12, 1948.

Weicker, H.: Klinik und epidemiologie der thalidomid-embryopathie. *Bull. Soc., Roy. Belge. Gynec. Obst.,* 33:21–32, 1963.

Wilson, J. G.: *Environment and Birth Defects.* Academic Press, Inc., New York, 1973, pp. 11–35.

UNIT II
SYSTEMIC TOXICOLOGY

Chapter 8

TOXIC RESPONSES OF THE BLOOD

Roger P. Smith

INTRODUCTION

For many years hematology concerned itself exclusively with the study of the formed elements of the blood, namely red cells, white cells, and platelets. An immense body of knowledge has accrued from the microscopic study of smears of peripheral blood (Bessis, 1977). The formed elements alone constitute a complex organ with a total mass equivalent to that of the liver. Gradually the field expanded to include other essential parts of the system such as the bone marrow, spleen, lymph nodes, and the reticuloendothelial tissue consisting of phagocytic macrophages in the reticulum of various organs and lining many sinuses. Obviously, the formed elements have a functional interrelationship with the blood plasma and with the heart and the lungs. Most of the biochemical and hematologic parameters used in this chapter apply to man; Mitruka and Rawnsley (1977) have compiled an extensive anthology of biochemical and hematologic reference values for normal experimental animals. Less elaborate but readily accessible compendia are also available (Burns and de Lannoy, 1966; Calsey and King, 1980) and include data on proteins, enzymes, electrolytes, and other constituents of plasma.

HEMATOPOIESIS

In the human fetus several organs are involved in the production of the formed elements of the blood. For a very brief period the yolk sac produces nucleated red cells containing a special embryonic hemoglobin designated as $\alpha_2\epsilon_2$. Subsequent crops of red cells are furnished by the liver, the spleen, and eventually the bone marrow. The liver is also the first organ to produce white cells and platelets. These primitive red cells are not nucleated, but they contain fetal hemoglobin, $\alpha_2\gamma_2$. The oxygen affinity of human fetal blood is higher than that of human adult blood although that difference does not extend to the purified hemoglobins. As noted below, other constituents in red cells influence the affinity of hemoglobin for oxygen.

At birth only the marrow is still producing red cells. A slow "switchover" from the synthesis of fetal to adult hemoglobin ($\alpha_2\beta_2$) begins at that time and it is usually completed by the fourth to sixth month of age. Up to the age of about four years hepatic and splenic red cell production can be reactivated in response to the demands of normal growth, but beyond that age these extramedullary sites are activated only in pathophysiologic states. It is also abnormal beyond that age to find nucleated red cells in the systemic circulation of mammals. However, birds, fish, reptiles, and amphibians always have nucleated red cells in peripheral blood (Prankerd, 1961).

The Bone Marrow

Bone marrow contains stem cells, which are the immature precursors of the formed elements of the blood (Figure 8–1). This multipotential stem cell pool is stimulated to differentiate into unipotential (or committed) cells, which eventually mature into red cells (erythrocytes), platelets (thrombocytes), or one of several series of white cells (leukocytes). Decreased numbers of these elements in peripheral blood (as determined by actual counts usually with an electronic cell counter) are referred to respectively as anemia, thrombocytopenia, and leukopenia. Stimulation of the stem cell pool is carried out by blood-borne factors called "poietins." It is highly likely that each circulating cell type has its own or more than one poietin.

Erythropoiesis refers to the process by which red cells are produced. Control over the rate of erythropoiesis is exerted primarily through changes in tissue oxygen tension, which in turn regulate the activity of a plasma hormone, erythropoietin. The kidney is critical in the production of erythropoietin, but it is not clear whether the kidney secretes erythropoietin *per se* or whether it secretes an enzyme that activates a plasma proerythropoietin produced by the liver.

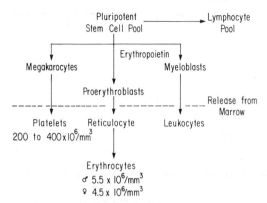

Figure 8–1. Bone marrow differentiation into the formed elements of peripheral blood. See also Figure 8–2 for further differentiation and classification of lymphocytes and leukocytes.

In the marrow erythropoietin apparently acts on the differentiation process at the stage in which a stem cell is converted to a proerythroblast (Figure 8–1). Therefore, erythropoietin may be thought of as regulating the size of the committed red cell pool. After several additional stages, the immature red cell is released from the marrow as a reticulocyte. By then the cell has extruded its nucleus and lost its ability to divide. It still possesses an endoplasmic reticulum (hence its name), and it can synthesize small amounts of hemoglobin. Cytochrome systems and the tricarboxylic acid cycle are still functional in the reticulocyte, but all of these are absent in the mature mammalian red cell. Maturation of reticulocytes occurs over the first 24 to 36 hours in the systemic circulation.

The presence of an abnormally large number of reticulocytes in the peripheral blood (more than 1 percent of the erythrocytes) is called reticulocytosis, and it indicates an accelerated replacement function of the bone marrow such as might occur in chronic hemolytic disease, exposure to hypoxia, or following an acute episode of intravascular hemolysis. Reticulocytes are easily distinguished after supravital staining of peripheral blood smears. It is common to correct the crude percentage count of reticulocytes for any abnormality in the hematocrit or to present the absolute count where the normal is about $60,000/mm^3$.

The presence of nucleated "blast" forms in peripheral blood may indicate an even greater demand for replacement. Megaloblastic anemia may also be a sign of either vitamin B_{12} or folic acid deficiency. Folic acid antagonist drugs used in cancer chemotherapy (methotrexate) or as antimalarials (pyrimethamine, chlorguanide) may induce megaloblastic anemia as a side effect because they interfere with DNA synthesis

(Stebbins and Bertino, 1976). Traditionally megaloblastic anemia is thought of as being associated with red cells, but all formed elements can be shown to be affected.

Bone marrow failure is characterized by inadequate production of red cells and/or other formed elements. Chemicals toxic to bone marrow can result in a decrease in the circulating numbers of all three major groups of formed elements, a condition known as pancytopenia. A diagnosis of pancytopenia is based on actual cell counts in peripheral blood. Agents regularly associated with pancytopenia provided that the exposure is sufficiently intense include ionizing radiation, benzene, antimetabolites, lindane or chlordane, mustards, arsenic, chloramphenicol, trinitrotoluene, gold, hydantoin derivatives, and phenylbutazone (Harris and Kellermeyer, 1970).

Damage to bone marrow may be so severe that it fails to proliferate, a condition described in morphologic terms as aplastic anemia. This diagnosis is made after microscopic examination of bone marrow biopsy specimens. On the other hand, the marrow can have a normal cellularity or even hypercellularity but still fail to deliver normal formed elements or normal numbers of formed elements. Ineffective erythropoiesis is a functional description of a normal-appearing but unresponsive marrow.

Most authorities agree that biotransformation is essential for benzene-induced bone marrow damage. The toxic metabolite(s), however, are still unknown, and there is disagreement about whether benzene is activated in the marrow or in other tissues such as the liver for transport to the marrow (e.g., Gosselin et al., 1984). In addition to direct cytotoxic effects of chemicals on the marrow, which are usually mediated through disturbances in DNA structure or function, bone marrow damage may have an allergic basis involving antibodies to precursor cells and a sensitizing chemical. Chloramphenicol-induced bone marrow damage may sometimes involve immune mechanisms. Although the spleen can be activated to serve as a reserve source of erythropoietic effort in rats and mice exposed to extreme altitude (Ou et al., 1980), in man and most animals it cannot support life in the event of bone marrow failure; thus, chemical or physical damage to this vital organ is always a grave threat to survival.

Thrombocytes. Differentiation into thrombocytes, the smallest of the formed elements of the blood, is a unique process because it involves the largest cell type in the marrow, the megakaryocyte. One megakaryocyte results in the release of large numbers of thrombocytes. The spent form of this giant cell is then phagocytized in the marrow.

Platelets are the first line of defense against accidental blood loss. They accumulate almost instantaneously where vascular injury has exposed collagen fibers. Within seconds the normally nonsticky circulating platelets will adhere to these fibers, undergo degranulation, and release ADP, which in turn causes adhesion and aggregation of new platelets. In addition, another platelet factor is unmasked on the thrombocyte surface that augments thrombin formation. The platelet plug is then coated with fibrin resulting in a white thrombus. This process of intravascular coagulation also involves many other plasma factors as well. Platelet aggregation *in vitro* can be studied by turbidimetric techniques where an aggregating agent such as ADP, epinephrine, or collagen is added to platelet-rich plasma. As the platelets aggregate, the optical density decreases (Born, 1962).

Increasing knowledge about the mechanism of clot formation has suggested that the control of platelet aggregation by drugs may be useful in preventing the thromboembolic complications of such diseases as atherosclerosis and hypertension. Considerable interest has been focused on aspirin since epidemiologic evidence has suggested that its use may prevent a second myocardial infarction in patients who have already experienced one. Aspirin inhibition of platelet aggregation depends on its ability to suppress prostaglandin synthesis since thromboxane A_2 is known to promote platelet aggregation. Nitroprusside, hydroxylamine, azide, and nitroglycerin are also known to block platelet aggregation at least *in vitro*.

Normal platelet counts in man are shown in Figure 8–1. Thrombocytopenia is manifested by hemorrhagic disorders the most common of which is leakage from capillaries following minor injury (purpura). Petechiae, prolonged bleeding time, and impaired clot retraction are also consequences. Thrombocytopenia accompanies a bewildering array of congenital and acquired disorders, but drugs are the most common cause. The myelosuppressive anticancer drugs may cause thrombocytopenia as part of a generalized depression of bone marrow function, but cytosine arabinoside is said to affect platelet production somewhat specifically. Quinidine and phenacetin are widely recognized as causes of autoimmune thrombocytopenia, which results in increased peripheral platelet destruction. Thrombocytosis (an increased number of circulating platelets) has not as yet been associated with chemical injury.

Leukocytes. Leukocytes have the most complex organization of the formed elements. They differ from other formed elements in that they perform important functions outside of the vascular compartment. Although each subtype seems to have some unique duties, the primary purpose for their existence appears to be to defend the body against "foreignness." Defense against foreign organisms or extraneous materials involves two mechanisms: (1) phagocytosis as carried out by the phagocytic series, and (2) antibody production as carried out by the immunocytic series Figure 8–2).

Phagocytes. The phagocytic series can be divided into the granulocytes (neutrophils, eosinophils, and basophils) and the monocyte-macrophages. Subdivision of the granulocytes

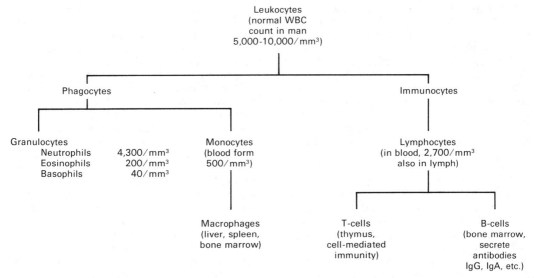

Figure 8–2. A classification of leukocytes and their normal values in man.

can be accomplished on the basis of their reaction with Wright's stain (Figure 8–2), but these distinctions would be more valuable if their various functions were more clearly understood. Eosinophilia occurs in some allergic diseases and in infestations with large parasites whereas basophilia occurs in polycythemia vera, but the significance of these associations is unknown.

Granulocytes spend less then a day in the circulation before they become marginated (attached to blood vessel walls); they then pass between vascular epithelial cells by diapedesis and are disposed of in various tissues. Specific leukotaxines that increase capillary permeability are released from inflammatory lesions, and these induce local migration of granulocytes. The actual bactericidal activity appears to involve a destruction of bacterial membranes and the release of lysosomal enzymes. Pyrogens and other degradation products may temporarily exacerbate the local inflammation. It is interesting that one effect of pharmacologic doses of glucocorticoids is to decrease the number of granulocytes that will diapedese and enter an exudate. Presumably this phenomenon accounts for increased susceptibility to infections of patients on steroids without a decrease in their rate of granulocyte production.

Monocytes exist in the blood for three to four days. After they migrate into reticuloendothelial tissues like liver, spleen, and bone marrow, they are called macrophages, and they survive in these sites for several months. Macrophages play a role in the phagocytic response to inflammation and infection, but they are also responsible for the ongoing destruction of senile blood cells. Denatured plasma proteins and plasma lipids are disposed of by pinocytosis. Macrophages are also involved in iron metabolism and possess inducible heme oxidase activity for the catabolism of hemoglobin.

The term "granulocytopenia" is used when the absolute granulocyte count is less than $3,000/mm^3$. When the count reaches $1,000/mm^3$, the patient becomes vulnerable to infection and at $500/mm^3$ the risk is very serious. The confusing term "agranulocytosis" is reserved for the serious granulocytopenias in which both the marginated pool and the bone marrow are devoid of neutrophils (also called neutropenia).

Granulocytopenia to varying degrees is the most common manifestation of chemically induced bone marrow damage, and many drugs as well as ionizing radiation can induce the reaction. Alkylating agents and antimetabolites regularly cause granulocytopenia, and phenothiazines, nonsteroidal anti-inflammatory drugs, antithyroid drugs, and some anticonvulsants sometimes elicit the reaction (Pisciotta, 1973). Peripheral destruction of granulocytes although an uncommon reaction has occurred via drug haptens after exposure to aminopyrine, phenylbutazone, and methyluracil. Granulocytes coated with the antigen-antibody complex are destroyed by the reticuloendothelial system.

An excess of granulocytes (granulocytosis is the term for counts greater than $10,000/mm^3$) occurs transiently after the administration of epinephrine, cortisone, and some endotoxins, but it is not believed to be of any physiologic significance. Chronic granulocytosis has not been associated with exposure to specific chemicals. When the count is greater than $30,000/mm^3$, the term "leukemia" is employed. In patients far advanced with the disease the white cell "crit" may actually exceed the red cell "crit" and the blood will appear pale. Chronic granulocytic leukemia has a better prognosis than the acute form of the disease. The former more commonly occurs in middle age, and although chemicals are suspected as etiologic agents, clear-cut associations have been difficult to make. The acute leukemias are often rapidly fatal in the absence of chemotherapy. They are usually classified into two groups: (1) acute lymphocytic leukemia (below) and (2) the acute myelogenous leukemias, which include all other bone marrow–derived leukocytes. Benzene, chloramphenicol, and phenylbutazone have been associated with acute myelogenous leukemia.

Neither monocytosis nor monocytopenia appears to be specifically induced by chemical injury, but either can be part of a generalized syndrome of bone marrow damage.

Immunocytes. The immunocytic series of leukocytes work in concert with the phagocytic series to defend the body against foreign invaders. Both the bone marrow and the thymus are primary lymphocyte-producing organs, and from these sites the cells are dispatched to populate secondary lymphatic tissue in the gastrointestinal tract (Peyer's patches) and the bursa of Fabricius in birds. Circulating pools of lymphocytes exist in both blood and lymph.

Immunocytic defense mechanisms are of two types. One is associated with the cell itself as in the case of the thymus lymphocytes (T cells). The other is humoral in the form of antibodies as in the case of the bone marrow-derived lymphocytes (B cells). Other characteristics distinguish between these cells such as the bizarre "hairy" appearance of B lymphocytes when viewed by scanning electron microscopy. Perhaps these structures are associated with the greater complement of surface immunoglobulins and receptors for antigen-antibody complexes of B cells. T cells can be distinguished by their ability to stick to sheep red cells and form rosettes.

T cell–mediated immunity is responsible for

delayed hypersensitivity, homograft rejection, graft vs. host reactions, and defense against viral, fungal, bacterial, and, perhaps, neoplastic invasion. After receiving a specific antigenic stimulus, T cells are activated to perform several functions: (1) they appear to inhibit the migration of macrophages from the area, (2) they secrete cytotoxic factors, (3) they recruit other T cells, and (4) they form subpopulations of small nondividing lymphocytes that may remain dormant over the lifetime of the host but retain a "memory" of the event and can respond on reexposure to the initial antigen.

B cells must also be programmed with a specific antigen, and T cells appear to cooperate in the activation of B cells to plasma cells. Plasma cells cannot divide, but they can initiate antibody synthesis. A family of five immunoglobulins is produced of which IgG is by far the major type (Figure 8–2), yet these five molecules exhibit both remarkable diversity and specificity in terms of antigenic reactions. See Chapter 9 for a more thorough discussion of T cell–mediated immunity.

Lymphocytopenia is induced transiently by corticosteroids, but the significance of that response is unknown. Lymphocytosis and acute lymphocytic leukemia have not been associated with specific chemical insults.

Erythrocytes. No cell type in the human body has been studied as extensively as the red blood cell (Surgenor, 1974, 1975). This unique disk-shaped element has a diameter of about 8 μm, and its biconcave sides make it more than twice as thick at the periphery (about 2.4 μm) as it is in the center. Although devoid of intracellular organelles, special techniques in combination with scanning electron microscopy suggest that an internal structure may exist. As much as 30 percent of the wet weight of red cells consists of hemoglobin, which, in turn, is the most extensively studied protein in the world.

Erythrocytes (Figure 8–1) perform the essential function of transporting oxygen from the alveoli of lungs to peripheral tissue, where it is used to support aerobic metabolism. Nor is the return trip wasted, since it serves as the means for the transport of waste carbon dioxide for excretion via the lungs. A small amount of carbon dioxide is transported in simple solution within the cell, but the bulk (75 percent) is transported as bicarbonate anion by virtue of the activity of carbonic anhydrase in the red cell. It is of interest that the remainder combines directly with free amino groups on hemoglobin to form carbaminohemoglobin (Hb-NH-COOH). An analogous reaction occurs with cyanate, which can carbamylate the N-terminal valine residues resulting in a hemoglobin with an increased oxygen affinity (Cerami and Manning, 1971; see also

below). Hemoglobin can also accept hydrogen ions, and it accounts for about 85 percent of the buffer capacity of the blood.

Acute damage to the red cell or its hemoglobin content can result in an impairment of oxygen transport with consequent peripheral hypoxia. The signs and symptoms in such cases are due secondarily to damage to the central nervous system and/or the heart, the organs most sensitive to oxygen lack. Normally the human erythrocyte remains in the blood for an average of 120 days before it ends its life in the spleen. Common laboratory animals (rabbits, rats, and especially guinea pigs and mice) have much shorter red cell survival times than man (Prankerd, 1961).

Anemia can arise if for any reason the rate of red cell destruction in peripheral blood exceeds the normal rate of production in bone marrow. Some chemicals are recognized as having acute and direct hemolytic effects *in vivo*, e.g., saponin, phenylhydrazine, arsine, and naphthalene. Other chemicals, such as primaquine among many others, produce hemolysis only in red cells congenitally deficient in glucose-6-phosphate dehydrogenase (cf. Figure 8–5). Finally, peripheral destruction of red cells may involve an allergic mechanism (autoimmune hemolytic anemia) after sensitization by a chemical such as acetanilid.

Laboratory evidence for an accelerated rate of hemolysis includes decreases in red cell lifespan and plasma haptoglobin concentration, increases in plasma bilirubin and hemoglobin (hemoglobinemia), and decreases in hematocrit and red cell counts (Rifkind et al., 1980). An unusual hematologic condition is a hemoglobinemia in the face of a greatly elevated hematocrit. This reaction is elicited in several laboratory species, and perhaps in man, at extreme altitude. Under these conditions it appears that the demand for additional red cells exceeds the ability to produce normal ones. Some imperfectly formed cells seem to hemolyze even before reaching the systemic circulation (Ou and Smith, 1978). When the red cell contents are released into plasma, hemoglobin (or its heme groups) are rapidly trapped by albumin, haptoglobin, or hemopexin (Muller-Eberhard, 1970) and then transported to reticuloendothelial tissues. If the rate of hemolysis is such as to saturate these systems, free hemoglobin may be found in urine, and hemoglobinuria is a further sign of a hemolytic crisis.

An abnormally increased number of red cells in blood is called polycythemia. Polycythemia vera is a disease in which there is an overproduction of red cells, perhaps because of an unusual sensitivity of the stem cell pool to erythropoietin. Polycythemia is an adaptive response to hypoxia whether it is due to altitude, cardiopulmonary disease, or anemic hypoxia (see below). In most mammals, polycythemia is one of the manifestations of cobalt toxicity. It was regularly observed together with other signs in the epidemics of beer drinker's cardiomyopathy in the 1960s. The onset of these epidemics coincided with the introduction of minute amounts of cobalt into some brands of beer to stabilize the "head" (Gosselin et al., 1984). This effect of cobalt is said to be secondary to an action in the central nervous system that results in respiratory alkalosis. In turn, alkalosis increases the affinity of hemoglobin for oxygen (below), which is interpreted by tissue "sensors" as hypoxia. These then act to increase the activity of erythropoietin (Miller et al., 1974).

ANEMIC HYPOXIA

Hypoxia refers to any condition in which there is an inadequate supply of oxygen to the tissues, but it is often useful to classify hypoxias on the basis of three quite different causes. Arterial or anoxic hypoxia is characterized by a lower-than-normal P_{O_2} in arterial blood when the oxygen capacity and rate of blood flow are normal or elevated. In toxic insults this type of hypoxia results from exposure to pulmonary irritants or drugs that depress the respiration. Anemic hypoxia is characterized by a lowered oxygen capacity when the arterial P_{O_2} and rate of blood flow are normal or elevated. Stagnant (hypokinetic) hypoxia is characterized by a decreased rate of blood flow. Sometimes a fourth condition, histotoxic hypoxia, is included in the classification (see below).

Oxygen Binding to Hemoglobin

Hemoglobin is an oligomeric protein with four separate peptide chains: two alpha chains and two beta chains $(\alpha_2\beta_2)$; its molecular weight is about 67,000 daltons. Each peptide chain has a porphyrinic heme group bound in a noncovalent linkage (Figure 8–3). The protein chains (globin) have irregularly folded conformations that enclose the heme group in a hydrophobic pocket. Hemoglobin is one of a handful of proteins for which the complete tertiary structure is known (Perutz et al., 1968).

The structure of a single heme group may be represented diagrammatically as a square planar complex with the four nitrogens of the porphyrin ring at the angles. The central iron atom has a hexavalent coordination shell analogous to the inorganic iron complex, ferrocyanide. The two remaining coordination bonds are closely associated with imidazole (histidyl) residues from the particular globin chain to which the heme group

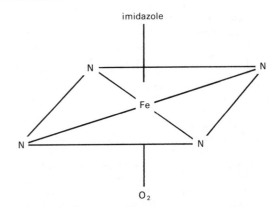

Figure 8–3. A stylized representation of a single heme group.

is attached. One of these bonds is available for reversible combination with molecular oxygen, which apparently binds between the iron and the histidyl residue. No ligand is known to occupy this latter site in the case of deoxyhemoglobin. The reversible binding of oxygen by hemoglobin is called oxygenation, and the tertiary structures of the oxygenated and deoxygenated forms of hemoglobin are known to differ. Since conformational changes do not occur on oxygenation of a single globin chain-heme unit such as myoglobin, it follows that there are interactions between the four subunits comprising a hemoglobin molecule. These interactions are referred to as cooperativity.

There are two physiologic regulators of the affinity of hemoglobin for oxygen, which is usually defined in terms of the P_{50}, or that partial pressure of oxygen necessary to half-saturate the hemoglobin present. These two regulators are hydrogen ion (responsible for the Bohr effect) and 2,3-diphosphoglycerate (2,3-DPG). Increasing concentrations of either of these tend to decrease the affinity of hemoglobin for oxygen, and decreasing concentrations of either have the converse effect. Thus, as noted above, cobalt-induced alkalosis decreases the concentration of hydrogen ion and increases the affinity of hemoglobin for oxygen. The red cell has the capability for both the synthesis and degradation of 2,3-DPG (Figure 8–5), and 2,3-DPG is normally present in red cells in about the same molar concentration as hemoglobin. One molecule of 2,3-DPG can bind reversibly with one hemoglobin tetramer. The bound form tends to stabilize hemoglobin in the deoxy form so that 2,3-DPG and oxygen could be regarded as competitive ligands for hemoglobin although they bind to different sites. A decreased affinity of hemoglobin for oxygen shifts the oxygen dissociation curve (Figure 8–4) in a parallel fashion to

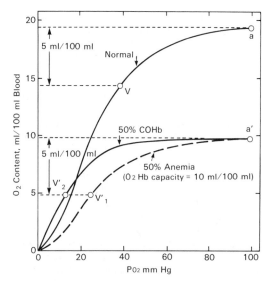

Figure 8–4. Normal oxyhemoglobin dissociation curve and curves for the case of a 50 percent anemia and the case of a 50 percent carboxyhemoglobinemia. The delivery of 25 percent of the total oxygen content of fully oxygenated arterial blood (5 ml/100 ml blood) requires a drop in the P_{O_2} of about 60 mm Hg (from point *a* to point *V* on the normal curve). Delivery of a comparable volume of oxygen in the case of a 50 percent anemia requires a drop in the P_{O_2} of more than 75 mm Hg (from point *a'* to point V_1'), but an even greater fall in the P_{O_2} is required to deliver the same volume of oxygen in the case of the curve distorted by the presence of carboxyhemoglobin (from point *a'* to point V_2'). See text for an explanation for this phenomenon. (From Bartlett, D., Jr.: Effects of carbon monoxide in human physiological processes. *Proceedings of the Conference on Health Effects of Air Pollutants,* Washington, D.C. U.S. Government Printing Office, Serial 93–15, pp. 103–26, Nov., 1973).

the right (increases the P_{50}) whereas an increased affinity produces a left-shifted dissociation curve. A number of drugs, chemicals, and manipulations are now known to result in such shifts (Norton and Smith, 1981).

Normal adult human hemoglobin binds 2,3-DPG more tightly than does fetal hemoglobin, accounting for the higher oxygen affinity of fetal blood, which presumably favors extraction of oxygen from the maternal circulation by the fetus. In sickle cell anemia hemolytic crises are triggered by hypoxia because only the deoxy form of hemoglobins can form the polymeric structures that distort the shape of the red cell. Carbamylation of the end-terminal valines on globin chains also increases the oxygen affinity of hemoglobin and prevents hemolytic crises. Unfortunately, cyanate (above), which has been

tested for that purpose, proved to be too toxic for chronic use in humans. Fetal hemoglobin with its higher oxygen affinity in the presence of 2,3-DPG might be advantagous to the sickle cell patient if some safe means could be devised to switch back on its synthesis in adult life. In one patient with thalassemia where there is a deficiency in the synthesis of one of the two types of globin chains, the immunosuppresent drug 5-azacytidine was able to turn on selectively the gene for γ-globin synthesis (Ley *et al.*, 1982).

A large body of experimental evidence now supports the concept that the deoxygenation process occurs in four separate steps, each with a different dissociation constant because of cooperativity changes that accompany the release of each successive oxygen molecule:

$$Hb_4O_8 \longrightarrow Hb_4O_6 + O_2 \quad K_1$$
$$Hb_4O_6 \longrightarrow Hb_4O_4 + O_2 \quad K_2$$
$$Hb_4O_4 \longrightarrow Hb_4O_2 + O_2 \quad K_3$$
$$Hb_4O_2 \longrightarrow Hb_4 + O_2 \quad K_4$$

It has not yet been possible to determine the exact values for each individual dissociation constant, K_1 through K_4. Both dissociation and association constants are defined here as equilibrium constants, the distinction between the two being merely the way in which the chemical equation is written. For the first equation shown above the dissociation constant has the value:

$$K_1 = \frac{[Hb_4O_6][O_2]}{[Hb_4O_8]}$$

with units of moles. The association constant would be the reciprocal expression with units of $moles^{-1}$. Obviously, the smaller the dissociation constant (or the larger the association constant), the more tightly the oxygen is bound and the more stable is the complex.

When the hemoglobin molecule is fully saturated, all of the oxygens may be thought of as equivalent since it is not known whether the two types of globin chains play a role in sequencing deoxygenation. A fall in the ambient P_{O_2} results in the release of the first oxygen molecule. Its release in turn triggers a cooperativity change that greatly facilitates the release of the second oxygen molecule. Thus, K_1 is considerably smaller than K_2. In the same manner the release of the second oxygen facilitates the release of the third oxygen. Release of the fourth oxygen does not occur under normal physiologic conditions.

The above sequence of events is responsible for the sigmoid shape of the normal oxygen dissociation curve (Figure 8–4). Since the total oxygen content of normal blood is about 20 ml/

100 ml, the release of 5 ml/100 ml (or ¼ of the total) is analogous to the release of one oxygen molecule from a single hemoglobin tetramer. That release requires a change in the P_{O_2} of about 60 mm Hg (from point *a* to point *V*). The release of an additional 5 ml/100 ml, which is analogous to the dissociation of the second oxygen molecule, requires a further decrease in the P_{O_2} of only about 15 mm Hg (from about 40 down to 25 mm Hg) because of cooperativity. The release of the third increment of 5 ml/100 ml blood can then be effected by a decrease in the P_{O_2} of only 10 mm Hg. Thus, the properties of the hemoglobin molecule facilitate the loading and unloading of large amounts of oxygen over a physiologically critical range of P_{O_2}.

Carbon Monoxide Binding to Hemoglobin

Carbon monoxide is the best-known example of an agent that can decrease the oxygen transport capability of blood and produce an anemic hypoxia. The elucidation of its mechanism of action by Claude Bernard in 1865 is a classic example of the successful application of the experimental method.

Claude Bernard's deductions about the mechanism of action of carbon monoxide were formalized by Douglas and the Haldanes in 1912. The so-called Haldane equation quantitatively defines the competition between oxygen and carbon monoxide for the same ferrous heme-binding sites on hemoglobin:

$$\frac{[COHb]}{[HbO_2]} = M \frac{[P_{CO}]}{[P_{O_2}]}$$

The constant, M, has the value of 245 at pH 7.4 for human blood. Therefore, if the $P_{CO} = 1/245 \times P_{O_2}$, the blood at equilibrium will be half-saturated with oxygen and half-saturated with carbon monoxide. Since air contains 21 percent oxygen by volume, it is obvious that exposure to a gas mixture of 0.1 percent carbon monoxide in air would result in a 50 percent carboxyhemoglobinemia in man at equilibrium and at sea level. For this reason carbon monoxide is potentially dangerous at very low concentrations. However, the rate at which the arterial blood approaches equilibrium with the inspired concentration depends on such factors as the diffusion capacity of the lungs and the alveolar ventilation both of which in turn depend on the level of exercise of the subject.

Some species variation is recognized with respect to the value of M, but this is not necessarily a major determinant of the species sensitivity to carbon monoxide. For example, the alleged sensitivity of the canary to carbon monoxide cannot be due to a higher affinity of canary blood for the gas; the M value for canary blood is less than half the value for human blood. Instead, more rapid breathing in support of a higher rate of aerobic metabolism allows canaries to reach equilibrium between blood and inspired CO more rapidly than humans. On the other hand, the canary brain appears to be less sensitive than the human brain to hypoxia. Because of these two opposing factors, canaries are more sensitive than humans to short exposures at high concentrations, but with long exposures to low concentrations the roles can be reversed (Spencer, 1962).

If, instead of oxygen, hemoglobin is exposed to pure carbon monoxide, a gradual decrease in the P_{CO} would allow one to describe a series of dissociation constants for carboxyhemoglobin analogous to those for oxyhemoglobin. If the absolute value for each of the latter were known, the former could be derived, e.g., $K_{10_2}/245 = K_{1CO}$, by correcting for the more tenacious binding of carbon monoxide. In actual experience this principle holds as a first approximation. Thus, the hemoglobin molecule has no intrinsic mechanism for distinguishing between oxygen and carbon monoxide, and carboxyhemoglobin exhibits the phenomenon of cooperativity as does oxyhemoglobin.

When carbon monoxide and oxygen are present together, another phenomenon is observed that has profound physiologic significance (Figure 8–4). If deoxyhemoglobin is exposed to a gas mixture in which the $P_{CO} = 1/245 \, P_{O_2}$, at equilibrium and 1 atmosphere total pressure, half the heme groups will be occupied by carbon monoxide and half by oxygen. The distribution of the two ligands among the four heme groups on any one hemoglobin molecule, however, is random. Thus, the blood will contain a distribution of hybrid species in which most molecules will contain both oxygen and carbon monoxide. Chance would dictate that the most common species would be a molecule with two oxygens and two carbon monoxides, e.g., $Hb_4(O_2)_2(CO)_2$.

In Figure 8–4 the experimental conditions have been contrived in such a way that the P_{CO} is held constant while the P_{O_2} is reduced. Therefore, half the total number of heme-binding sites are always occupied by carbon monoxide irrespective of the degree of oxygen saturation. For the most common hybrid species, $Hb_4(O_2)_2(CO)_2$, only two oxygen molecules are available for dissociation, and there can be only one opportunity for cooperativity to facilitate the dissociation of oxygen. In effect, only the top half of the dissociation curve can be called into play, and it is displaced downward because of the loss of half the total oxygen capacity. Since cooperativity cannot be utilized to facilitate the dissociation of a third oxygen molecule, the result is an apparent increase in the mean binding strength for oxygen (a shift to the left of the curve) and a distortion in the shape of the curve from its normal sigmoid appearance.

The physiologic significance of this phenomenon may be grasped from Figure 8–4, where a change in the P_{O_2} of about 75 mm Hg is required to deliver 5 ml O_2/100 ml of blood to peripheral tissue in the case of a 50-percent anemia. Here the residual hemoglobin functions normally with respect to the influence of cooperativity even though the total oxygen content is only half that of normal. In the case of a 50-percent carboxyhemoglobinemia, however, a change of 85 mm Hg or more in the P_{O_2} is required to deliver the same 5 ml O_2/100 ml of blood. Obviously, the latter individual would be more severely compromised in terms of peripheral hypoxia.

Carbon Monoxide Poisoning. Although the above model is felt to be useful for understanding the molecular events at work in carbon monoxide poisoning, other factors influence the course of events in intact animals and man. Changes in regional blood flow will shunt the perfusion toward the more critical organs. Changes in ventilation will result in changes in the rate of hemoglobin saturation with carbon monoxide. Exposure to very high ambient concentrations can result in sufficient hemoglobin saturation to produce death in minutes with almost no premonitory signs, but the attainment of equilibrium between hemoglobin saturation and ambient P_{CO} occurs slowly on exposure to low concentrations of the gas. For these reasons a poor correlation exists between the blood content of carboxyhemoglobin and signs and symptoms in poisoned humans.

The presence of carboxyhemoglobin can result in a significant decrease in the oxygen content of blood, but the ambient concentration is rarely high enough to result in a detectable decrease in the arterial P_{O_2}. Thus, chemoreceptor mechanisms may not be triggered, and the usual respiratory parameters may remain within normal limits. Peripheral vasodilatation in response to a slowly developing hypoxia may exceed the compensatory ability to increase the cardiac output. For this reason fainting is more common than dyspnea in victims of carbon monoxide poisoning, and consciousness may be lost for long periods before death. Tachycardia and ECG changes suggestive of hypoxia have been observed at carboxyhemoglobin saturations of 30 percent or more. Other symptoms include headache, weakness, nausea, dizziness, and dimness of vision. Lactic acidemia may result from impaired aerobic metabolism. Unconsciousness, coma, convulsions, and death are associated with 50-to-80-percent saturation.

Carbon monoxide is not a cumulative poison in the usual sense. Carboxyhemoglobin is fully dissociable, and, once an acute exposure has been terminated, the pigment will eventually revert to oxyhemoglobin and the carbon monoxide will be excreted via the lungs. Certain individuals occupationally exposed to carbon monoxide, such as garage workers or traffic policemen, may suffer acute recurring toxic episodes during each working day. Without an adequate medical history, the unwary physician may be presented with a baffling symptom complex. Sometimes in cases of single massive exposure, permanent sequelae may result from hypoxic damage to neural structures.

Carboxyhemoglobin is a cherry red color, and its presence in high concentrations in capillary blood may impart an abnormal red color to skin, mucous membranes, and nail beds. Carbon monoxide combines with other heme proteins such as myoglobin and cytochromes, including P-450 but these reactions have no significance in acute poisoning. This point was made by Haldane in 1895 by placing mice in a high concentration of carbon monoxide together with 2 atmospheres of oxygen. Even though the circulating blood pigment in these animals was totally in the form of carboxyhemoglobin enough oxygen was carried in physical solution in their blood to prevent signs of poisoning.

Management of Carbon Monoxide Poisoning. The obvious and specific antagonist to carbon monoxide is oxygen. After termination of the exposure, respirations must be supported artificially if necessary. By increasing the ambient P_{O_2}, advantage can be taken of the mass law to increase significantly the rate of conversion of carboxyhemoglobin to oxyhemoglobin *in vivo*. For example, the half-recovery time in terms of blood carboxyhemoglobin levels for resting adults breathing air at 1 atmosphere is 320 minutes. When oxygen is given at 1 atmosphere, the time is decreased to 80 minutes. By the use of hyperbaric chambers developing 3 atmospheres of oxygen, this time can be further reduced to 23 minutes, although such measures carry some risk of oxygen poisoning. Exchange transfusion has also been used for moribund victims.

The addition of 5 to 7 percent carbon dioxide to oxygen to serve as a respiratory stimulant (with precautions against rebreathing) does hasten the pulmonary excretion of carbon monoxide. At the same time it entails some risk of compounding the metabolic acidosis arising from tissue hypoxia. (Gosselin *et al.,* 1984).

Endogenous and Environmental Carbon Monoxide. Nonsmoking human adults normally do not have more than 1 percent of their total circulating blood pigment in the form of carboxyhemoglobin, but heavy smokers may show values as high as 5 to 10 percent saturation. Combustion of fossil fuels and automobile exhaust (4 to 7 percent carbon monoxide) are other key environmental sources. For many years it was presumed that environmental exposure was responsible for the low levels of carboxyhemoglobin found in the general population, but in 1967 Coburn and coworkers established that carbon monoxide is generated endogenously in normal humans. A major source of this endogenous carbon monoxide arises from the catabolism of heme proteins, principally hemoglobin, although catalase and cytochromes contribute small amounts.

The alpha-methane bridge of the heme porphyrin is the group metabolized, and carbon monoxide is generated in amounts that are equimolar to the bile pigment produced or to the heme catabolized. The average rate of production (0.4 ml/hr) is increased in hemolytic disease because of increased heme catabolism. The physiologic significance of this source in combination with environmental exposure is not well defined at present (National Academy of Sciences, 1977a).

Methemoglobinemia

The heme iron of hemoglobin is susceptible to a true chemical oxidation involving a valence change from the ferrous to the ferric state. The resulting pigment is called methemoglobin. It is greenish brown to black in color, and it cannot combine reversibly with oxygen or with carbon monoxide. Therefore, methemoglobinemia is another potential cause of anemic hypoxia. As in the oxidation of simple inorganic coordination complexes like ferrocyanide, the oxidation of the heme iron does not change the total number (six) of the bonds in the coordination shell (Fig. 8–3). The additional positive charge on the heme iron itself is satisfied in physiologic solutions by hydroxyl or chloride anions. The ferric heme iron can also combine with a variety of nonphysiologic anions, a property that has been exploited for therapeutic purposes (see below).

Unlike the case of carboxyhemoglobinemia, it is known with certainty that methemoglobin as generated in vivo or in vitro by partial oxidation consists of a mixture of the hybrid species $(\alpha^{3+}\beta^{2+})_2$ and $(\alpha^{2+}\beta^{3+})_2$. Complete oxidation to $(\alpha^{3+}\beta^{3+})_2$ can be forced by an excess of oxidant in vitro, but that would be fatal in vivo.

Methemoglobin has at least one additional property that is of toxicologic interest, namely, its ability to dissociate complete heme groups as units. When methemoglobin is free in plasma instead of in intact red cells, the transfer of heme groups to albumin results in methemalbumin, an abnormal pigment found during acute hemolytic

crises such as transfusion reactions, severe malaria, paroxysmal nocturnal hemoglobinuria, and poisonings by some chemicals such as chlorate salts. Methemalbumin in a blood sample that is abnormally dark in color can be easily distinguished from methemoglobin after centrifugation. The plasma will be dark and the cells their normal red color if methemalbumin is present. With a true methemoglobinemia the plasma will be a normal color, and the cells will be dark. In neither case will the blood samples change in color if oxygenated, whereas the blood would turn rapidly to a bright red if deoxyhemoglobin were responsible for the dark color.

Spontaneous Hemoglobin Oxidation. Although the rate of hemoglobin oxidation is greatly increased by exposure to a variety of chemicals, heme group oxidation occurs spontaneously in air. Presumably spontaneous or autoxidation accounts for the very low concentrations (less than 2 percent) found in normal circulating blood. As studied in vitro autoxidation appears to be a first-order process with respect to the concentrations of the ferrous forms of either hemoglobin or myoglobin. The first order rate constants, however, depend in a complex manner on the partial pressure of oxygen. The rate constants are maximal at partial pressures of oxygen that correspond to half-saturation of the heme groups. Since a reaction mechanism in which a deoxygenated molecule (or heme group) interacts with an oxygenated one would not exhibit first-order kinetics, a multistep mechanism is inferred. The quasi-first-order kinetics can then be explained as arising from an algebraic artifact rather than any single intramolecular, rate-determining step. The complexity of these reactions is illustrated by studies on their stoichiometry. Both myoglobin and hemoglobin oxidation consume many times more oxygen than can be accounted for on the basis of the reduction of an appropriate amount of oxygen to water (Smith and Olson, 1973). It has been suggested that such autoxidation reactions involve the participation of the superoxide anion, O_2^- (Fridovich, 1983).

Methemoglobin-Generating Chemicals. Some chemicals capable of mediating the oxidation of hemoglobin are active both in vivo and in vitro. Others are active only in vivo, and a third group are active only in lysates or solutions of hemoglobin. Among chemicals active both in vivo and in vitro, sodium nitrite is the best known. Inorganic hydroxylamine has some similarities to nitrite, but these two agents appear to oxidize hemoglobin by different mechanisms (Cranston and Smith, 1971).

The mechanism of the reaction between hemoglobin and nitrite is still not understood.

Under strictly anaerobic conditions 1 mole of nitrite yields 1 mole of ferric heme and 1 mole of the ferroheme-NO complex. Under physiologic conditions and in the presence of an excess of nitrite complete conversion to methemoglobin occurs, but the heme oxygen is largely consumed. Whether or not O_2^- is involved in the reaction has been disputed. After a lag phase, the reaction proceeds with a pronounced autocatalytic phase that is not observed when nitrite reacts with deoxyhemoglobin (e.g., Smith and Olson, 1973). Nitrite is also included among those anions that can complex with ferric heme groups. Thus, excess nitrite first generates methemoglobin then forms a nitrite-methemoglobin complex. The latter has significance for the spectrophotometric determination of methemoglobin (van Assendelft and Ziljstra, 1965), and it may account partially for the uniquely protracted nitrite methemoglobinemia observed in some species as compared with other chemicals active *in vivo* (Smith, 1967; but see also below).

Organic compounds active both *in vivo* and *in vitro* include some simple aminophenols, certain *N*-hydroxyarylamines, amyl nitrite, and other aliphatic nitrites and nitrates (Kiese, 1974). As tested in mice, phenylhydroxylamine, *N*-hydroxy-*p*-aminotoluene, and *N*-hydroxy-*p*-acetophenone were all about equipotent, i.e., generated equivalent peak concentrations of methemoglobin at equal doses. At the same time all these were ten or more times more potent than nitrite, hydroxylamine, or simple aminophenols (Smith *et al.*, 1967).

It is now clear that intraerythrocytic recycling accounts for the high potency of phenylhydroxylamine to produce methemoglobinemia relative to other compounds. According to Kiese (1974), phenylhydroxylamine and hemoglobin react to form methemoglobin and nitrosobenzene. In the intact normal red cell provided with substrate, mechanisms exist for the reduction of nitrosobenzene to regenerate phenylhydroxylamine. The requirement of this reaction for glucose (as opposed to lactate) suggests that some component of the pentose phosphate shunt such as NADPH is involved in the cycle (*cf.* Figure 8–5). Although phenylhydroxylamine is active in lysates, under those conditions it is no more potent than nitrite. Similarly aminophenols and inorganic hydroxylamine are not recycled in red cells so they are equipotent in intact red cells and in lysates.

Among agents active only *in vivo* the aromatic amines and arylnitro compounds are best known. Obviously these substances must be metabolized *in vivo* to active forms presumably by mixed-function oxidase activity in liver. It has long been suspected that the active metabo-

lites are either aminophenols or *N*-hydroxy derivatives. For some compounds such as aniline and nitrobenzene the relative importance of these two possible metabolites still has not been clarified. In contrast, conclusive evidence has established that the active metabolite of *p*-aminopropiophenone (PAPP) in several species is the *N*-hydroxy metabolite. In the case of nitrobenzene some evidence suggests that the active metabolite in rats is generated by nitroreductases in the intestinal microflora rather than in the liver (Reddy *et al.*, 1976). For this group of chemicals prominent species differences may be anticipated that depend on differences in the rates of activation and detoxication of the parent compounds and their metabolites.

Two compounds with widely different chemical properties are active only in lysates. The first of these is potassium ferricyanide, which cannot penetrate the intact red cell membrane. Even so, it is widely used in the laboratory as a reagent for generating methemoglobin standards in solution. One mole of ferricyanide mediates the oxidation of one mole of heme whether or not oxygen is present. Ferricyanide is unique in that it is the only agent that quantitatively releases the heme oxygen during its reaction with oxyhemoglobin. The oxygen evolved can be measured manometrically or polarographically as an estimate of the amount of oxyhemoglobin in the sample. Ferrocyanide is also generated, which can bind tenaciously to the globin moiety of the methemoglobin.

An interesting contrast with phenylhydroxylamine is the paradoxic methemoglobin-generating activity of methylene blue, which is prominent only in lysates (Smith and Thron, 1972). The products of this reaction are methemoglobin and leucomethylene blue. The latter is spontaneously reoxidized by molecular oxygen so that a cyclic mechanism is established in this case also. The potency of methylene blue as a methemoglobin-generating agent in lysates is roughly equivalent to that of phenylhydroxylamine in intact cells provided with substrate. Although methemoglobin does not accumulate in mammalian red cells exposed to methylene blue, the increased rate of hemoglobin-methemoglobin turnover accounts for the weak antagonistic effects of methylene blue against cyanide (see below). Molecular oxygen is analogous to methylene blue in that it generates methemoglobin in a sustained fashion only in lysates. Hemolysis results in a loss of the activity of both methemoglobin reducing systems in the red cell (see below.)

Susceptibility of Mammalian Hemoglobins to oxidation. Inherent differences are recognized among hemoglobins in their susceptibility

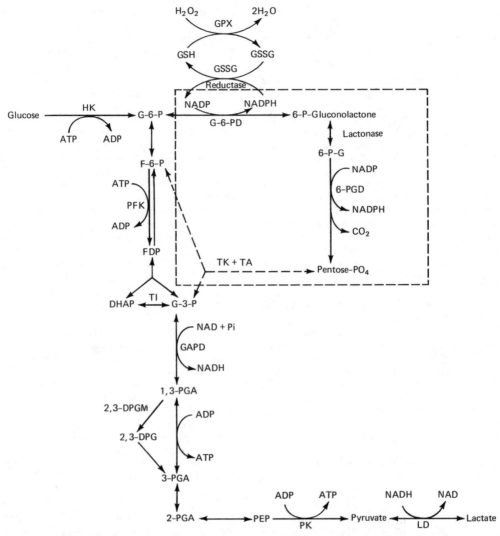

Figure 8–5. The metabolic resources of the mature mammalian red cell. *GSH*, reduced glutathione; *GSSG*, oxidized glutathione; *G-6-P*, glucose-6-phosphate; *F-6-P*, fructose-6-phosphate; *FDP*, fructose-1,6-diphosphate; *DHAP*, dihydroxyacetone phosphate; *G-3-P*, glyceraldehyde-3-phosphate; *LD*, lactic dehydrogenase; *NADP*, oxidized triphosphopyridine nucleotide; *NADPH*, reduced triphosphopyridine nucleotide; *NAD*, oxidized diphosphopyridine nucleotide; *NADH*, reduced diphosphopyridine nucleotide; *6-P-G*, 6-phosphogluconate; *G-6-PD*, glucose-6-phosphate dehydrogenase; *TK*, transketolase, *TA*, transaldolase; *Pi*, inorganic phosphate; *ADP*, adenosine diphosphate; *ATP*, adenosine triphosphate; *PEP*, phosphoenolpyruvate; *PK*, pyruvic kinase; *1,3-PGA*, 1,3-phosphoglyceric acid; *3-PGA*, 3-phosphoglyceric acid; *2-PGA*, 2-phosphoglyceric acid; *2,3-DPG*, 2,3-diphosphoglyceric acid; *6-PGD*, 6-phosphogluconate dehydrogenase; *PFK*, phosphofructokinase; *HK*, hexokinase; *TI*, trioseisomerase; *GPX*, glutathione peroxidase; *GAPD*, glyceraldehyde-3-phosphate dehydrogenase; *2,3-DPGM*, 2,3-diphosphoglycerate mutase. (Modified from Harris, J. W., and Kellermeyer, R. W.: *The Red Cell—Production, Metabolism, Destruction: Normal and Abnormal,* rev. ed. Harvard University Press, Cambridge, Mass., 1970.)

to oxidation by various agents (Bartels *et al.*, 1963). Such differences undoubtedly reflect structural or conformational variations, but their contribution to the overall methemoglobinemic response seems necessarily small. For example, Smith and Beutler (1966a) found the conversion half-times in minutes for hemoglobin solutions exposed to identical concentrations of nitrite to be about two for sheep, goat, and bovine hemoglobin, three for human hemoglobin, four for equine hemoglobin, and up to seven for porcine hemoglobin. Such differences cannot play a major role since even in species resistant to nitrite an acute methemoglobinemia can be expected to last for several hours.

Pathophysiology of Methemoglobinemias. Impairment of the oxygen transport capability of blood is not the only analogy between carboxyhemoglobin and methemoglobin. The presence of a certain fraction of methemoglobin distorts the oxygen dissociation curve of residual hemoglobin in a manner analogous to the presence of a certain fraction of carboxyhemoglobin. Presumably this analogy extends also to the mechanism for the distortion, as discussed above for carbon monoxide. Indeed, hybrid species, $(\alpha^{2+}\beta^{3+})_2$ and $(\alpha^{3+}\beta^{2+})_2$, have been isolated by electrofocusing techniques (Banergee and Cessoly, 1969). The distortion with a given fraction of methemoglobin, however, is said to be less drastic than with an identical fraction of carboxyhemoglobin.

As an experimental tool for the study of the effects of peripheral hypoxia, methemoglobinemia is less satisfactory than simulated altitude, oxygen replacement, or exposure to carbon monoxide. Unless the methemoglobin-generating chemical is continuously infused, it is impossible to maintain stable circulating levels of the pigment for prolonged periods of time. If death does not intervene, a variety of intraerythrocytic reductive mechanisms are activated to reduce methemoglobin back to hemoglobin. With a single dose of the agent, methemoglobin levels tend to rise abruptly and then decline toward normal at rates that vary widely with the species (Table 8–1). These fluctuating levels of circulating methemoglobin undoubtedly lead to wide variations in peripheral oxygen tensions.

Moreover, all chemical agents used to generate methemoglobin have additional toxic effects, and, unlike carbon monoxide, these side effects may make important contributions to the toxic syndrome. Some aromatic amino and nitro compounds, such as aniline and nitrobenzene, have central and cardiac effects that in some species, including man, appear to be the proximal cause of death. Chlorate salts produce intravascular hemolysis, and the "methemoglobin" formed appears to be largely extracellular. Hydroxylamine, inorganic salts of nitrite, and organic nitrates and nitrites also act directly as peripheral vasodilators. A stagnant (hypokinetic) hypoxia due to orthostatic hypotension, reflex tachycardia, circulatory inadequacy, and cardiovascular collapse certainly compound the effects of the methemoglobinemia. Unsubstituted hydroxylamine and even p-aminopropiophenone (PAPP) in large doses produce Heinz bodies, sulfhemoglobin, and hemolysis as well as methemoglobin (Cranston and Smith 1971). The herbicide paraquat, which has adverse effects on

many organs, also generates methemoglobin (Ng *et al.*, 1982.)

It is doubtful that any chemical agent produces an otherwise uncomplicated methemoglobinemia, although PAPP in moderate doses has very few other effects. Large differences among various agents can be shown to exist for the methemoglobin levels measured at the time of death, even when tested in a single species (Smith and Olson, 1973). Therefore, it is inappropriate and misleading to suggest that there is a "lethal level of methemoglobin" without account to the particular agent and species involved.

Metabolic Resources of the Mature Mammalian Red Cell. Unlike carboxyhemoglobin, which spontaneously dissociates in accord with the ambient partial pressures of oxygen and carbon monoxide, metabolic energy must be expended by the red cell to reduce methemoglobin to hemoglobin. Indeed, a major share of the total metabolic energy of the red cell is directed toward that end and toward the maintenance of the integrity of the cell membrane. As shown in Figure 8–5, however, the metabolic resources of the mature mammalian red cell are rather limited. Only two anaerobic alternatives are available for glucose metabolism: (1) the Embden-Meyerhof (glycolytic) pathway and (2) the pentose phosphate (phosphogluconic acid, hexosemonophosphate) shunt (enclosed by dashed lines in Figure 8–5).

The enzyme glucose-6-phosphate dehydrogenase occupies a key position in red cell metabolism. It introduces the shunt and participates in the reduction of NADP. An additional mole of NADP is reduced in the next reaction by 6-phosphogluconate dehydrogenase. Since the shunt is the only source of NADPH in the mature human red cell, the appropriate selection of substrates can thwart NADP reduction while permitting NAD reduction. If lactate is substituted for glucose, NADH is generated via the activity of lactic dehydrogenase. In some mammalian erythrocytes stereospecificity of glucose-6-phosphate dehydrogenase prevents the utilization of galactose as a substrate in the shunt although it is available for glycolysis (Smith and Beutler, 1966b).

Methemoglobin Reducing Systems. *Spontaneous Methemoglobin Reduction.* The major system responsible for methemoglobin reduction in mammalian red cells (to the extent of at least 60 percent) is methemoglobin reductase or diaphorase, which has been identified as cytochrome b_5. As indicated in Figure 8–6, this intracellular enzyme requires NADH as a cofactor.

Chronic methemoglobinemia in rare individuals without exposure to suspect chemicals has been recognized for more than a century. In

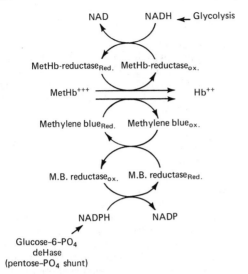

Figure 8–6. The spontaneous (*NADH*) and the dormant (*NADPH*) methemoglobin reductase systems. Methemoglobin (*MetHb*) reductase is active in intact red cells in the presence of substrates that can provide for NAD reduction. The NADPH system requires intact red cells, glucose or its metabolic equivalent, a functioning pentose phosphate shunt, and methylene blue (*M.B.*). M.B.-reductase reduces M.B., which in turn nonenzymatically reduces MetHb.

1959 Scott and Griffith demonstrated that the erythrocytes of some chronically methemoglobinemic individuals were deficient in NADH-methemoglobin reductase. From 10 to 50 percent of their total circulating blood pigment existed as methemoglobin. Since their methemoglobin levels remain at a steady state throughout life, alternative mechanisms for methemoglobin reduction must be available but deficient individuals are extremely sensitive to methemoglobin-generating chemicals. So are newborns, although high concentrations of fetal hemoglobin may contribute as much to their sensitivity as the recognized transient deficiency in NADH-reductase.

The congenital methemoglobinopathies due to abnormal amino acid substitutions in the globin chain constitute a separate disease entity. These abnormalities as in the hemoglobins M or H apparently enhance heme dissociation, rendering the iron more susceptible to molecular oxygen. Such individuals are also sensitive to oxidant chemicals despite a normal NADH-reductase activity.

The duration of methemoglobinemia after an acute challenge with sodium nitrite is largely determined by the methemoglobin reductase activity in the erythrocytes of that species. An exception may be sodium nitrite in red cells of species with high rates of methemoglobin reductase activity, e.g., mice. The uniquely prolonged response in such cells as compared with all other agents suggests that nitrite or some product of the nitrite-hemoglobin reaction may transiently inhibit the NADH reductase system (Kruszyna et al., 1982). In human red cells the reductase system is so sluggish under normal circumstances that all agents produce about the same duration of methemoglobinemia.

As shown in Table 8–1, a greater than tenfold difference exists among the listed species with respect to methemoglobin reductase activity. It is presumed that these data represent primarily NADH-reductase activity, although the contributions from alternative pathways for the most part have not been evaluated. In each case glucose was the substrate, and the data have been expressed as a ratio of the species activity to that in human cells. In order to place these ratios in some perspective, estimates of the reduction half-time for high (80 to 100 percent) levels of methemoglobin in normal human red cells under similar conditions range from 6 to about 24 (Bolyai et al., 1972) hours. In general, rates of reduction tend to decrease with decreasing methemoglobin levels.

Table 8–1 shows that pig and horse red cells have considerably lower rates of methemoglobin reduction than human red cells. Both these species are said to utilize plasma lactate in preference to glucose to drive reduction (Rivkin and Simon, 1965; Robin and Harley, 1967). Rat, guinea pig, mouse, and rabbit red cells have relatively high rates of methemoglobin reductase activity. The significance of these differences remains unknown.

The Dormant NADPH-Reductase System. Normal human and most mammalian erythrocytes possess a second reductive system that requires NADPH as a cofactor. The physiologic role of this system is not understood. In most species the system appears to be dormant, and it is activated only in the presence of exogenously added electron carriers such as methylene blue. According to Sass and co-workers (1969), the enzyme involved reduces methylene blue to the leuco form, which in turn nonenzymatically reduces methemoglobin (Figure 8–6).

The evidence that this system plays no important physiologic role in methemoglobin reduction is compelling. What may be an extremely rare congenital deficiency of this enzyme has been found (Sass et al., 1967), and the propositus had normal levels of methemoglobin. Moreover, in cases of a far more common congenital deficiency, namely that of glucose-6-phosphate dehydrogenase, individuals are not methemoglobinemic despite decreased shunt activity and

Table 8–1. SPONTANEOUS METHEMOGLOBIN REDUCTASE ACTIVITY OF MAMMALIAN ERYTHROCYTES*

| SPECIES | INVESTIGATORS | | | | |
	(1)	(2)	(3)	(4)	(5)
	Activity in Species/Activity in Man				
Pig	0.37	0.37		0.09	
Horse	0.75	0.50		0.64	
Cat		0.50	0.85	1.2	1.0
Cow	0.80	0.75		1.1	
Goat	1.1	0.75			
Dog		0.88	1.4	1.3	1.0
Sheep	1.4	1.0		2.1	
Rat		1.4	1.3	1.9	5.0
Guinea pig		1.2	2.4	1.9	4.5
Rabbit		3.5	3.3	3.8	7.5
Mouse					9.5

* Data from various investigators using nitrited red cells with glucose as a substrate have been normalized by making a ratio of the activity of the species to the activity in human red cells. The indicated investigators are: (1) Smith and Beutler, 1966a; (2) Malz, 1962; (3) Kiese and Weis, 1943; (4) Robin and Harley, 1966; (5) Stolk and Smith, 1966; Smith et al., 1967; Bolyai et al., 1972.

impaired NADP-reductive capacity. The therapeutic activation of this system is an important procedure for the management of acute acquired methemoglobinemia. It cannot be activated, however, in either of the deficiency states noted above.

Species differences are also recognized in terms of the magnitude of the response to added methylene blue (Table 8–2), but all species tested responded to the dye (1 to 2 × 10⁻⁵ M) by an increase in reductase activity over that observed with glucose alone. The data are expressed as a ratio of the species increase to the increase observed in human cells under the same conditions. To place these ratios in some perspective, estimates of the reduction half time of high (70 to 90 percent) levels of methemoglobin in normal human red cells with methylene blue range from 45 to 90 minutes (Layne and Smith, 1969). A certain parallelism is noted between Tables 8–1 and 8–2 in that species with high spontaneous rates of reductase activity respond more vigorously to methylene blue, with the possible exception of the rabbit. The nucleated red cells of reptiles and birds have both NADH and NADPH reductase activity, but in this case the tricarboxylic acid cycle appears to be the source of the NADH (Board et al., 1977).

Minor Pathways for Methemoglobin Reduction. Several minor pathways exist in red cells for methemoglobin reduction, which are at least in part nonenzymatic. Reduced glutathione slowly reduces methemoglobin, but it can ac-

count only for 12 percent of the total erythrocyte reductive capacity (Scott et al., 1965). Ascorbic acid (vitamin C) has been used to reduce methemoglobin levels in individuals with NADH-reductase deficiency, but this reaction is too sluggish to be of value in an acute methemoglobinemic crisis. It accounts for no more that 16 percent of the reductive effort of red cells. Methemoglobinemia is not found in subjects with frank ascorbate deficiency (scurvy) or in subjects with abnormally low levels of reduced glutathione in their red cells (glucose-6-phosphate dehydrogenase deficiency). The guinea pig is one of the few nonprimate mammals unable to synthesize ascorbate. Oddly, methemoglobinemic guinea pig red cells do not respond to ascorbate as do human red cells (Bolyai et al., 1972). NADH, NADPH, cysteine, and ergothioneine also have limited capacities for direct methemoglobin reduction.

Management of Acquired Methemoglobinemias. Although all methemoglobin-generating chemicals have additional toxic effects, it is generally agreed that a reduction in the circulating titer of the abnormal pigment is a desirable therapeutic goal. For agents that produce hemolysis as well as methemoglobin and methemalbumin (e.g., chlorate salts) exchange transfusion is the only present approach to that goal. If the methemoglobin is contained within intact, normal, and functional erythrocytes, the intravenous administration of methylene blue (1 to 2 mg/kg) usually

Table 8–2. STIMULATION OF METHEMOGLOBIN REDUCTASE ACTIVITY OF MAMMALIAN ERYTHROCYTES BY METHYLENE BLUE*†

| SPECIES | INVESTIGATORS | | | | |
	(1)	(2)	(3)	(4)	(5)
	Increased Activity, Species/Increased Activity, Man				
Pig	0.05	0.03		0.15	
Horse	0.10	0.06		0.25	
Goat	0.50	0.03			
Sheep	0.38	0.28		0.45	
Cow	0.42	0.34		1.0	
Cat		0.69	0.16	0.65	1.0
Dog		0.41	0.24	0.85	1.0
Rabbit		0.50	1.4	0.70	0.50
Mouse					1.1
Guinea pig		1.3	0.94	2.4	
Rat		2.1	1.0	2.2	1.9

* Data from various sources using nitrited red cells with glucose as a substrate have been normalized by the ratio:

$$\frac{(\text{activity M.B. and glucose} - \text{activity glucose})_{\text{species}}}{(\text{activity M.B. and glucose} - \text{activity glucose})_{\text{human}}}$$

† See footnote to Table 8–1 for literature citation.

evokes a dramatic response (Gosselin *et al.*, 1984). Although a spectrum of efficacy can be shown experimentally in human red cells exposed to various agents, methylene blue provides unequivocal protection against death in animals, with all methemoglobin generating agents tested (Smith and Layne, 1969).

A suggested alternative that would bypass the lesion in the oxygen-transport function of the blood is hyperbaric oxygen. Goldstein and Doull (1971) found that oxygen at 4 atmospheres decreased mortality and methemoglobin levels after nitrite in rats. After *p*-aminopropiophenone (PAPP) administration to rats, however, methemoglobin levels were actually increased (Goldstein and Doull, 1973). Since PAPP is a model for compounds metabolized to N-hydroxylarylamines, hyperbaric oxygen would appear to be contraindicated for related structures. The mechanism of the effect on nitrite is not understood, but hyperbaric oxygen seems to block acetylation of PAPP, which is a major route for its detoxication. In reversing nitrite poisoning in mice, methylene blue and hyperbaric oxygen appear to have at least additive effects (Way and Sheehy, 1971).

Oxidative Hemolysis

Sulfhemoglobin. The term "sulfhemoglobin" was coined more than a century ago to describe a pigment generated *in vitro* by exposing oxyhemoglobin to high concentrations of hydrogen sulfide. This phenomenon plays no role in acute hydrogen sulfide poisoning, which is described below. When generated in that way, sulfhemoglobin is unstable and solutions are so turbid that visible absorption spectra must be derived indirectly (Drabkin and Austin, 1935–1936). It appears to have a weak absorption maximum at about 620 nm, which overlaps to some extent the absorption maximum of methemoglobin at about 630 nm. This similarity was responsible for much confusion in the early literature. In contrast to methemoglobin, however, the absorption band for sulfhemoglobin is not abolished by the addition of cyanide, and this difference serves as the basis for methods for determining both pigments in the same solution (Evelyn and Malloy, 1938; Van Kampen and Zijlstra, 1965). In recent years so-called sulfhemoglobins of high purity have been generated with hydrogen sulfide under special conditions (e.g., Nichol *et al.*, 1968), but their relationship to the originally described pigment has not been clarified.

When the criteria of an absorption band at 620 nm, which is stable toward cyanide, were applied to large numbers of human blood samples in clinical laboratories, positive results were encountered in some patients (Evelyn and Malloy, 1938). By definition these patients were said to have "sulfhemoglobinemia" even though no source of exposure to hydrogen sulfide could be documented and even though all previous attempts to generate sulfhemoglobin *in vivo* by exposure to hydrogen sulfide had failed. In retrospect it appears likely that two unrelated phenomena have been identified for years by the same name because of a coincidence in the position of an absorption maxima and its failure to shift with cyanide (National Academy of Sciences, 1977b).

Over the years the term "sulfhemoglobin" has come to be used almost exclusively in the literature for the abnormal pigment(s) generated *in vivo* in the apparent absence of hydrogen sulfide. This phenomenon, which might better be called pseudosulfhemoglobinemia, is associated with at least three clinical situations: (1) the ingestion of "oxidant" drugs, which may also generate methemoglobin in normal subjects, (2) the presence of an abnormal hemoglobin (Tönz, 1968) such as one of the hemoglobins M, and (3) the exposure of individuals congenitally deficient in glucose-6-phosphate dehydrogenase to certain drugs or chemicals. It seems likely that the phenomenon represents nonspecific oxidative damage, including partial hemoglobin denaturation (Beutler, 1969).

No mechanism exists in red cells for the reversal of a sulfhemoglobinemia. Because it is irreversible, sulfhemoglobinemia would appear to constitute a more serious toxicologic threat than methemoglobinemia. Sulfhemoglobin, however, has never been generated in sufficient concentrations *in vivo* to constitute a serious threat to life. The disorder is either self-limiting as damaged cells are replaced by erythropoiesis, or it forms one part of a more serious condition as indicated below.

Heinz Body Hemolytic Anemia. Heinz bodies (Figure 8–7) are dark-staining, refractile granules found in red cells. They are thought to consist of denatured hemoglobin, possibly sulfhemoglobin. Heinz bodies lie on or near the interior surface of red cell membranes and appear to be firmly attached to membrane thiol groups. Sulfhydryl groups on the denatured hemoglobin may form disulfide bonds with the membrane surface (Jacob *et al.*, 1968). This process leads to an impairment of membrane functions involving active and passive ion transport. Hyperpermeability and hemolysis may result due to osmotic pressure. Actual distortion in the shape of the cell may occur, resulting in premature splenic capture (see below). Sulfhemoglobin, Heinz bodies, and hemolysis may,

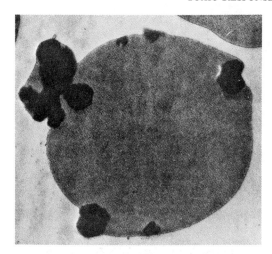

Figure 8–7. End-stage Heinz bodies lying under and distorting the plasma membrane of a mature erythrocyte. ×26,000. (From Rifkind, R. A., and Danon, D.: Heinz body anemia–An ultrastructural study. I. Heinz body formation. *Blood,* **25**:885–96, 1965.)

therefore, be regarded as a continuum of oxidative stress to the red cell.

According to Jandl and co-workers (1960), however, this process is preceded by a transient methemoglobinemia. Not all authorities agree that methemoglobin is an obligatory or even an important precursor. There is a rather poor correlation (almost in inverse one) between the ability of a given chemical to generate methemoglobin and its ability to produce Heinz bodies (Rentsch, 1968), although some overlap is recognized. Methemoglobinemia per se does not lead to hemolysis (Beutler, 1969) but in some cases this may simply be a matter of dose or concentration. The presence of molecular oxygen is required. The hydroxylamine-deoxyhemoglobin reaction results only in methemoglobin formation, whereas the hydroxylamine-oxyhemoglobin reaction results in both methemoglobin and sulfhemoglobin (Cranston and Smith, 1971).

Mechanisms of Heinz Body Formation. Congenital Heinz body hemolytic anemia occurs in individuals who have hemoglobins with certain abnormal amino acid substitutions. A rather convincing body of evidence (Jacob *et al.,* 1968; Rieder, 1970) now indicates that in such cases dissociation of the heme group is enhanced in these abnormal pigments. Dissociation of heme presumably results in decreased solubility and precipitation of the pigment as a Heinz body. Stabilization of the heme group by the addition of cyanide or carbon monoxide inhibits Heinz body formation *in vitro.*

Heme dissociation, however, has not been convincingly demonstrated in acquired Heinz body anemias, such as the reaction of normal erythrocytes to phenylhydrazine or the reaction of glucose-6-phosphate dehydrogenase-deficient cells to primaquine. Heme loss did not occur during hemoglobin denaturation by hydroxylamine (Cranston and Smith 1971).

According to Cohen and Hochstein (1964) oxidant drugs like phenylhydrazine generate peroxide in the red cell either by reaction with molecular oxygen or by a coupled reaction with oxyhemoglobin. Hydrogen peroxide is detoxified by glutathione peroxidase (Figure 8–5), resulting in the oxidation of reduced glutathione. Oxidized glutathione is reduced by the activity of glutathione reductase, which requires the NADPH generated by glucose-6-phosphate dehydrogenase. These three enzymes work in concert, and a deficiency in any one of them carries with it an increased sensitivity to oxidant chemicals. A necessary part of this hypothesis is that glutathione peroxidase plays the major role in red cell disposal of peroxide instead of catalase, which is also present in abundance.

The peroxide hypothesis is attractive because, whether the reaction is induced in normal or in glucose-6-phosphate dehydrogenase-deficient cells, an early event is a precipitous fall in red cell levels of reduced glutathione. Allen and Jandl (1961) suggest that oxidized glutathione forms mixed disulfides with free thiol groups on hemoglobin, contributing to its instability and denaturation. The possible involvement of other forms of "active oxygen" such as O_2^- in these reactions has not been explored.

Agents Producing Heinz Bodies. As in the case of methemoglobin-generating agents, prominent species differences are recognized or are to be expected because of different patterns of biotransformation of suspect Heinz body-producing chemicals. The nature of the active metabolites of agents producing Heinz bodies only *in vivo* is unknown. Aromatic amino (aniline) and nitro (nitrobenzene) compounds produce Heinz bodies in many species, but nonnitrogenous structures have also been implicated: phenols, propylene glycol, ascorbic acid, sulfite, dichromate, arsine, stibine, and others. Hydroxylamine and chlorate salts were among the earliest agents to be recognized as eliciting the response. Ingestion of crude oil has resulted in Heinz body hemolytic anemia in marine birds (Leighton *et al.,* 1983), and dimethyl disulfide produces the reaction in chickens (Maxwell, 1981). At present no single unifying hypothesis links these diverse structures to red cell damage.

Species Differences. Cat, mouse, dog, and human erythrocytes are said to be particularly susceptible to Heinz body formation, whereas rabbit, monkey, chick, and guinea pig are among the least responsive. These impressions, however, are based on a variety of compounds, some of which were not tested in all species. Moreover, they are based at least in part on *in vivo* observations, which have the limitations mentioned above.

The morphology and ultrastructure of Heinz bodies also show some variations with species and with agents. Under certain conditions a large number of small bodies are seen. It has been suggested that these eventually coalesce into larger and perhaps multibodied inclusions. In the nucleated turkey erythrocyte, phenylhydrazine Heinz bodies were smaller than those produced under identical conditions in dog or horse red cells, and they were present in both the nucleoplasm and the cytoplasm. Extraerythrocytic Heinz bodies were observed with suspensions of horse erythrocytes but not dog or turkey red cells (Simpson, 1971).

The Spleen. Although many lines of evidence indicate that the red cell normally ends its life in the spleen, splenectomy in man does not result in a significant increase in red cell survival time. Thus, other segments of the reticuloendothelial system such as the bone marrow and liver, in addition to the spleen, must play important roles in senescent red cell destruction.

With respect to the spleen, however, its anatomic ultrastructure appears particularly well suited to the above task. Numerous fine arterial vessels arise from the central splenic artery and form a rich plexus in the white pulp. These appear to run to the periphery of the white pulp and terminate in the marginal zone or the contiguous red pulp, although some communicate with cordal vessels. The latter are vascular spaces in the red pulp and lie between the splenic sinuses, which collect blood for the venous return. The splenic cords communicate with the sinuses through mural apertures or fenestrations smaller than the diameter of a red cell. The apertures are lined with reticular cells that have a phagocytic function. Red cells are believed to move through these apertures by diapedesis.

At this point senescent or damaged erythrocytes may be trapped and phagocytized. This concept is supported by the demonstration that red cell deformability has a metabolic dependence (Weed *et al.*, 1969). Thus, cells with impaired metabolic resources or physical impediments may be subject to hemolysis. After hemolysis, hemoglobin is catabolized and the heme groups degraded to bilirubin. Splenic engorgement is, therefore, another sign of hemolytic disease where there is an increased demand for these functions.

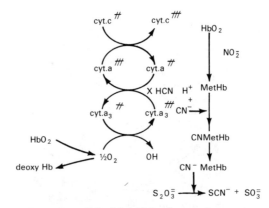

Figure 8-8. Principles of the therapeutic management of cyanide poisoning. Although the exact chemical details are still unknown, the undissociated form (HCN) appears to block electron transfer in the cytochrome a-a₃ complex, which is isolated *in vitro* as a single unit. As a consequence oxygen utilization is decreased and oxidative metabolism may slow to the point that it cannot meet metabolic demands. At the level of the brainstem nuclei this effect may result in central respiratory arrest and death. On injection of sodium nitrate methemoglobin is generated, which can complete effectively with cytochrome aa₃ for free cyanide. Note that it is the ionic form that complexes with methemoglobin. The injection of thiosulfate provides substrate for the enzyme rhodanese, which catalyzes the biotransformation of cyanide to thiosulfate.

HISTOTOXIC HYPOXIA

Semantic purists object to the term histotoxic "hypoxia" since the critical lesion does not involve an inadequate supply of oxygen to peripheral tissues. Instead the peripheral tissue P_{O_2} is often normal or even greater than normal, but the cells are unable to utilize oxygen. Two chemicals are thought to act by this mechanism: hydrogen sulfide and hydrogen cyanide. The biochemical lesion is illustrated for the case of cyanide in Figure 8-8, but sulfide probably has the same mechanism of action. Some evidence suggests that it is the undissociated acid, hydrogen cyanide, which interrupts electron transport down the cytochrome chain by inhibiting at the cytochrome a-cytochrome a₃ step (Smith *et al.*, 1977). Since these cytochromes are isolated as a single unit, they are referred to as cytochrome aa₃ or cytochrome oxidase. As a result of cyanide inhibition, oxidative metabolism and phosphorylation are compromised. Electron transfer from cytochrome aa₃ to molecular oxygen is blocked, peripheral tissue oxygen tensions begin to rise, and the unloading gradient for oxyhemoglobin (Figure 8-8) is decreased. Sometimes high concentrations of oxyhemoglobin are found in the venous return, imparting a flush to skin and mucous membranes.

Cyanide directly stimulates the chemoreceptors of the carotid and aortic bodies with a resultant hyperpnea. Cardiac irregularities are often noted, but the heart invariably outlasts the respirations. Death is due to respiratory arrest of central origin. It can occur within seconds or minutes of the inhalation of high concentrations of hydrogen cyanide gas. Because of slower absorption, death may be delayed after the ingestion of cyanide salts, but the critical events still occur within the first hour.

Other sources of cyanide have been responsible for human poisoning. One of these is amygdalin, a cyanogenic glycoside found in apricot, peach, and similar fruit pits and in sweet almonds. Amygdalin is a chemical combination of glucose, benzaldehyde, and cyanide from which the latter can be released by the action of β-glucosidase or emulsin. Although these enzymes are not found in mammalian tissues, the human intestinal microflora appears to possess these or similar enzymes capable of effecting cyanide release resulting in human poisoning. For this reason amygdalin may be as much as 40 times more toxic by the oral route than by intravenous injection. Amygdalin is the major ingredient of Laetrile, and this alleged anticancer drug has also been responsible for human cyanide poisoning.

An ethical drug that may also cause cyanide poisoning in overdose is the potent vascular smooth muscle relaxant sodium nitroprusside. Fortunately, the therapeutic margin for nitroprusside appears to be quite large. The acute toxic and teratogenic effects of a series of low-molecular-weight aliphatic nitriles appears to be due to biotransformation reactions leading to the release of free cyanide (Willhite and Smith, 1981; Doherty *et al.*, 1982).

Treatment of Cyanide Poisoning

The treatment regimen consists first of the intravenous injection of sodium nitrite (300 mg for an adult). A modest and tolerable fraction of the circulating blood pigment is converted to methemoglobin (Figure 8–8). The newly generated ferric heme groups act as competitors with cytochrome aa_3 for cyanide by complexing with the ionic form. The affinity of methemoglobin for cyanide exceeds that of cytochrome aa_3, leading to a dissociation of the cyanide-cytochrome complex and a resumption of oxidative metabolism. Obviously, in the intact animal or man this competition for free cyanide occurs across a number of biologic barriers, yet it is rapidly efficacious.

At this point a certain fraction of the total circulating hemoglobin exists as cyanmethemoglobin, which is inert in terms of oxygen transport. Although the cyanide is bound very tenaciously, cyanmethemoglobin is a somewhat dissociable complex, and there is some risk of the release of free cyanide. Therefore, the second prong of the therapeutic approach involves the intravenous administration of sodium thiosulfate. Thiosulfate serves as a substrate for the enzyme rhodanese, which mediates the conversion of cyanide to the much less toxic thiocyanate, which is excreted in the urine. Although ubiquitously distributed in the body, liver rhodanese is said to play the major role in cyanide detoxification. The enzyme serves as an endogenous mechanism for cyanide metabolism, but the provision of exogenous sulfur greatly accelerates the rate of detoxication. Methemoglobin is restored to functional blood pigment by the intracellular reductase systems (Figure 8–6). In the red cells of species with brisk rates of methemoglobin reductase activity (e.g., mice, rabbits), it appears that cyanmethemoglobin is also a substrate for the enzyme. Thus, agents that produce the typical short-lasting methemoglobinemia, such as hydroxylamine or PAPP, are not as effective as nitrite in preventing death by cyanide. Although the cyanide is at first trapped and inactivated, the activity of the reductase releases cyanide to cause delayed deaths. This phenomenon would not be observed in man or species with slower rates of reductase activity (Kruszyna *et al.*, 1982).

From the principles summarized in Figure 8–8, it appears that the administration of oxygen in cyanide poisoning would serve no useful purpose. Since the lesion is one of oxygen utilization instead of oxygen transport, peripheral tissue oxygen tensions are normal or even supranormal. It has been demonstrated that even hyperbaric oxygen has no effect on cyanide poisoning in mice (Way *et al.*, 1972). However when oxygen at 1 atmosphere is given in combination with nitrite and thiosulfate, a significantly greater protective effect is obtained than when the two chemicals are given in combination with air at the same pressure (Way *et al.*, 1966). Rhodanese itself is not known to be sensitive to oxygen so the mechanism for this phenomenon is unknown.

Hydrogen Sulfide Poisoning

Hydrogen sulfide is also an established inhibitor of cytochrome oxidase *in vitro* (Smith *et al.*, 1977). Signs and symptoms of poisoning on exposure to hydrogen sulfide gas or after the administration of soluble sulfide salts to animals are similar in almost all respects to those produced by cyanide. The only notable exceptions are due to the irritancy of hydrogen sulfide, which on chronic exposure to low concentrations may produce conjunctivitis (gas eye) or occasionally pulmonary edema.

The hydrosulfide anion (HS^-) also forms a complex with methemoglobin known as sulfmethemoglobin, which is analogous to cyanmethemoglobin. Sulfmethemoglobin is a well-characterized entity as distinct from the confusion noted above surrounding the nature of sulfhemoglobin. The dissociation constant for sulfmethemoglobin has been estimated as 6×10^{-6} moles/liter whereas the dissociation constant for cyanmethemoglobin is about 2×10^{-8} moles/liter. Despite the lower binding affinity for sulfide, an induced methemoglobinemia provides unequivocal protection against death from acute sulfide poisoning in animals (Smith and Gosselin, 1964). The induction of methemoglobinemia was successful in the resuscitation of two humans severely poisoned by hydrogen sulfide (Peters, 1981; Stine et al., 1976). No rationale is seen for the use of thiosulfate in sulfide poisoning. As in the case of cyanide, oxygen does not affect the course of acute sulfide poisoning (Smith et al., 1976), but oxygen would be specifically indicated if pulmonary edema occurs. Unfortunately, hydrogen sulfide poisoning rarely occurs under circumstances in which a rapid intravenous injection of nitrite is possible.

Because of its ability to react with disulfide bonds under physiologic conditions, the hydrosulfide anion can be inactivated by oxidized glutathione and other simple disulfides (Smith and Abbanat, 1966). Sulfide in vivo is biotransformed rapidly to sulfate and other sulfur oxides. Human hydrogen sulfide poisoning is invariably the result of occupational exposure to the gas. It is encountered in some natural gas deposits and in volcanic gases in high concentrations. Hydrothermal vents in some locations on the ocean floor continually release huge amounts of hydrogen sulfide. Vent tube worms thriving in the vicinity may have lethal concentrations in their blood. A unique blood factor that binds sulfide and transports it to symbiotic bacteria for metabolic detoxication prevents poisoning of their respiration (Powell and Somero, 1983). A synonym, sewer gas, refers to the presence of hydrogen sulfide wherever organic matter undergoes putrefication. It is a pollutant in the atmosphere in the proximity of industrial paper plants using the kraft process. The leather industry uses sodium sulfide to remove the hair from hides prior to tanning, and ton quantities are employed in the production of

heavy water for nuclear reactors (National Academy of Sciences, 1977b). Interestingly, carbonyl sulfide, a by-product of coal hydrogenation and gasification, is metabolized in vivo by carbonic anhydrase to yield hydrogen sulfide (Chengelis and Neal, 1980).

REFERENCES

Allen, D. W., and Jandl, J. H.: Oxidative hemolysis and precipitation of hemoglobin. II. Role of thiols in oxidant drug action. J. Clin. Invest., 40:454–75, 1961.

Banerjee, R., and Cassoly, R.: Oxygen equilibria of human hemoglobin valency hybrids. J. Mol. Biol. 42:351–61, 1969.

Bartels, H.; Hilpert, P.; Barbey, K.; Betke, K.; Riegel, K.; Lang, E. M.; and Metcalfe, J.: Respiratory functions of blood of the yak, llama, camel, Dybowski deer, and African elephant. Am. J. Physiol., 205:331–36, 1963.

Bernard, C.: An Introduction to the Study of Experimental Medicine (first published in 1865). Reprinted by Dover, New York, 1957.

Bessis, M.: Blood Smears Reinterpreted, translated by G. Brecher. Springer-Verlag, Berlin, 1977.

Beutler, E.: Drug-induced hemolytic anemia. Pharmacol. Rev., 21:73–103, 1969.

Board, P. G.; Agar, N. S.; Gruca, M.; and Shine, R.: Methaemoglobin and its reduction in nucleated erythrocytes from reptiles and birds. Comp. Biochem. Physiol., 57B:265–67, 1977.

Bolyai, J. Z.; Smith, R. P.; and Gray, C. T.: Ascorbic acid and chemically induced methemoglobinemias. Toxicol. Appl. Pharmacol., 21:176–85, 1972.

Born, G. V. R.: Aggregation of blood platelets by adenosine diphosphate and its reversal. Nature, 194:927–29, 1962.

Burns, K. F., and de Lannoy, C.W., Jr.: Compendia of normal blood values of laboratory animals, with indications of variations. I. Random-sexed populations of small animals. Toxicol. Appl. Pharmacol., 8:429–37, 1966.

Calsey, J. D., and King, D. J.: Clinical chemical values for some common laboratory animals. Clin. Chem., 26:1877–79, 1980.

Cerami, A., and Manning, J. M.: Potassium cyanate as an inhibitor of the sickling of erythrocytes in vitro. Proc. Natl Acad. Sci. USA, 68:1180–83, 1971.

Chengelis, C. P., and Neal, R. A.: Studies of carbonyl sulfide toxicity: Metabolism by carbonic anhydrase. Toxicol. Appl. Pharmacol., 55:198–202, 1980.

Coburn, R. F.; Williams, W. J.; White, P.; and Kahn, S. B.: The production of carbon monoxide from hemoglobin in vivo. J. Clin. Invest., 46:346–56, 1967.

Cohen, G., and Hochstein, P.: Generation of hydrogen peroxide in erythrocytes by hemolytic agents. Biochemistry, 3:895–900, 1964.

Cranston, R. D., and Smith, R. P.: Some aspects of the reactions between hydroxylamine and hemoglobin derivatives. J. Pharmacol. Exp. Ther., 177:440–46, 1971.

Doherty, P. A.; Smith, R. P.; and Ferm, V. H.: Tetramethyl substitution on succinonitrile confers pentylenetetrazole-like activity and blocks cyanide release in mice. J. Pharmacol. Exp. Ther., 223:635–41, 1982.

Douglas, C. G.; Haldane, J. S.; and Haldane, J. B. S.: The laws of combination of haemoglobin with carbon monoxide and oxygen. J. Physiol. (Lond.), 44:275–304, 1912.

Drabkin, D. L., and Austin, J. H.: Spectrophotometric studies. II. Preparations from washed blood cells; nitric oxide hemoglobin and sulfhemoglobin. J. Biol. Chem., 112:51–65, 1935–1936.

Evelyn, K. A., and Malloy, H. T.: Microdetermination of oxyhemoglobin, methemoglobin and sulfhemoglobin in a single sample of blood. *J. Biol. Chem.*, **126**:655–62, 1938.

Fridovich, I.: Superoxide radical, an endogenous toxicant. *Ann. Rev. Pharmacol. Toxicol.*, **23**:239–57, 1983.

Goldstein, G. M., and Doull, J.: Treatment of nitrite-induced methemoglobinemia with hyperbaric oxygen. *Proc. Soc. Exp. Biol. Med.*, **138**:137–39, 1971.

———: The use of hyperbaric oxygen in the treatment of p-aminopropiophenone-induced methemoglobinemia. *Toxicol. Appl. Pharmacol.*, **26**:247–52, 1973.

Gosselin, R. E.; Smith, R. P.; and Hodge, H. C.: *Clinical Toxicology of Commercial Products*, 5th ed. Williams & Wilkins Co., Baltimore, 1984.

Haldane, J.: The relation of the action of carbonic oxide to oxygen tension. *J. Physiol.*, **18**:201–17, 1895.

Harris, J. W., and Kellermeyer, R. W.: *The Red Cell Production, Metabolism, Destruction: Normal and Abnormal*, rev. ed. Harvard University Press, Cambridge, Mass., 1970.

Jacob, H. S.; Brain, M. C.; and Dacie, J. V.: Altered sulfhydryl reactivity of hemoglobins and red blood cell membranes in congenital Heinz body hemolytic anemia. *J. Clin. Invest.*, **47**:2644–77, 1968.

Jandl, J. H.; Engle, L. K.; and Allen, D. W.: Oxidative hemolysis and precipitation of hemoglobin. I. Heinz body anemias as an acceleration of red cell aging. *J. Clin. Invest.*, **39**:1818–36, 1960.

Kiese, M.: *Methemoglobinemia: A Comprehensive Treatise.* CRC Press, Cleveland, 1974.

Kiese, M., and Weis, B.: Die Ruduktion des Hämiglobins in den Erythrocyten verschiedener Tiere. *Naunyn Schmiedebergs Arch. Pharmacol.*, **202**:493–501, 1943.

Kruszyna, R.; Kruszyna, H.; and Smith, R. P.: Comparison of hydroxylamine, 4-dimethylaminophenol and nitrite protection against cyanide poisoning in mice. *Arch. Toxicol.*, **49**:191–202, 1982.

Layne, W. R., and Smith, R. P.: Methylene blue uptake and the reversal of chemically induced methemoglobinemias in human erythrocytes. *J. Pharmacol. Exp. Ther.*, **165**:36–44, 1969.

Leighton, F. A.; Peakall, D. B.; and Butler, R. G.: Heinz body hemolytic anemia from the ingestion of crude oil, a primary toxic effect in marine birds. *Science*, **220**:871–73, 1983.

Ley, T. J.; DeSimone, J.; and Anagou, N. P.: 5-Azacytidine selectively increases γ-globin synthesis in a patient with β^+-thalassemia. *N. Engl. J. Med.*, **307**:1469–75, 1982.

Malz, E.: Vergleichende Untersuchungen über die Methämoglobinreduktion in kernhaltigen und kernlosen Erythrozyten. *Folia. Haematol. (Leipz.)*, **78**:510–15, 1962.

Maxwell, M. H.: Production of a Heinz body anemia in the domestic fowl after ingestion of dimethyl disulphide: A haematological and ultrastructural study. *Res. Vet. Sci.*, **30**:233–38, 1981.

Miller, M. E.; Howard, D.; Stohlman, F., Jr.; and Flanagan, P.: Mechanism of erythropoietin production by cobaltous chloride. *Blood*, **44**:339–46, 1974.

Mitruka, B. M., and Rawnsley, H. M.: *Clinical Biochemical and Hematological Reference Values in Normal Experimental Animals.* Masson Publishing USA, Inc., New York, 1977.

Müller-Eberhard, U.: Hemopexin. *N. Engl. J. Med.*, **283**:1090–94, 1970.

National Academy of Sciences: *Carbon Monoxide.* Committee on Medical and Biological Effects of Environmental Pollutants, National Research Council, Washington, D.C., 1977a.

———: *Hydrogen Sulfide.* Committee on Medical and Biological Effects of Environmental Pollutants, National Research Council, Washington, D.C., 1977b.

Ng, L. L.; Naik, R. B.; and Polak, A.: Paraquat ingestion with methaemoglobinaemia treated with methylene blue. *Br. Med. J.*, **284**:1445, 1982.

Nichol, A. W.; Hendry, I.; and Morell, D. B.: Mechanism of formation of sulphhaemoglobin. *Biochim. Biophys. Acta*, **156**:97–108, 1968.

Norton, J. M., and Smith, R. P.: Drugs affecting the oxygen transport function of hemoglobin. In *Respiratory Pharmacology, Section 104, International Encyclopedia of Pharmacology and Therapeutics* (Section Editor J. Widdicombe), Pergamon Press, Oxford, 1981.

Ou, L. C., and Smith, R. P.: Hemoglobinuria in rats exposed to high altitude. *Exp. Hematol.*, **6**:473–78, 1978.

Ou. L. C.; Kim, D.; Layton, W. M., Jr.; and Smith, R. P.: Splenic erythropoiesis in polycythemic response of the rat to high altitude exposure. *J. Appl. Physiol.: Respirat. Environ. Exercise Physiol.*, **48**:857–61, 1980.

Perutz, M. F.; Muirhead, H.; Cox, J. M.; and Goaman, L. C. G.: Three-dimensional Fourier synthesis of horse oxyhaemoglobin at 2.8Å resolution: The atomic model. *Nature (London)*, **219**:131–39, 1968.

Peters, J. W.: Hydrogen sulfide poisoning in a hospital setting. *JAMA*, **246**:1588–89, 1981.

Pisciotta, A. V.: Immune and toxic mechanisms in drug-induced agranulocytosis. *Semin. Hematol.*, **10**:279–310, 1973.

Powell, M. A., and Somero, G. N.: Blood components prevent sulfide poisoning of respiration of the hydrothermal vent tube worm *Rifitia pachytila. Science*, **219**:297–99, 1983.

Prankerd, T. A. J.: *The Red Cell. An Account of Its Chemical Physiology and Pathology.* Blackwell Scientific Publications, Oxford, England, 1961.

Reddy, B. G.; Pohl, L. R.; and Krishna, G.: The requirement of the gut flora in nitrobenzene-induced methemoglobinemia in rats. *Biochem. Pharmacol.*, **25**:1119–22, 1976.

Rentsch, G.: Genesis of Heinz bodies and methemoglobin formation. *Biochem. Pharmacol.*, **17**:423–27, 1968.

Rieder, R. F.: Hemoglobin stability: Observations on the denaturation of normal and abnormal hemoglobins by oxidant dyes, heat and alkali. *J. Clin. Invest.*, **49**:2369–76, 1970.

Rifkind, R. A.; Bank, A.; Marks, P. A.; Nossell, H. L.; Ellison, R. R.; and Lindenbaum, J.: *Fundamentals of Hematology*, 2nd ed. Year Book Medical Publishers, Inc., Chicago, 1980.

Rivkin, S. E., and Simon, E. R.: Comparative carbohydrate catabolism and methemoglobin reduction in pig and human erythrocytes. *J. Cell. Comp. Physiol.*, **66**:49–56, 1965.

Robin, H., and Harley, J. D.: Factors influencing response of mammalian species to the methaemoglobin reduction test. *Aust. J. Exp. Biol. Med. Sci.*, **44**:519–26, 1966.

———: Regulation of methaemoglobinaemia in horse and human erythrocytes. *Aust. J. Exp. Biol. Med. Sci.*, **45**:77–88, 1967.

Sass, M. D.; Caruso, C. J.; and Axelrod, D. R.: Mechanism of the TPNH-linked reduction of methemoglobin by methylene blue. *Clin. Chim. Acta*, **24**:77–85, 1969.

Sass, M. D.; Caruso, C. J.; and Farhangi, M.: TPNH-methemoglobin reductase deficiency: A new red-cell enzyme defect. *J. Lab. Clin. Med.*, **70**:760–67, 1967.

Schwerin, F. T.; Rosenstein, R.; and Smith, R. P.: Cyanide prevents the inhibition of platelet aggregation by nitroprusside, hydroxylamine and azide. *Thromb. Haemostas.*, **50**:780–83, 1983.

Scott, E. M.; Duncan, I. W.; and Ekstrand, V.: The reduced pyridine nucleotide dehydrogenases of human erythrocytes. *J. Biol. Chem.*, **240**:481–85, 1965.

Scott, E. M., and Griffith, I. V.: Enzymatic defect of hereditary methemoglobinemia: The diaphorase. *Biochim. Biophys. Acta*, **34**:584–86, 1959.

Simpson, C. F.: The ultrastructure of Heinz bodies in

horse, dog, and turkey erythrocytes. *Cornell Vet.*, **61**:228–38, 1971.

Smith, J. E., and Beutler, E.: Methemoglobin formation and reduction in man and various animal species. *Am. J. Physiol.*, **210**:347–50, 1966a.

——— : Anomeric specificity of human erythrocyte glucose-6-phosphate dehydrogenase. *Proc. Soc. Exp. Biol. Med.*, **122**:671–73, 1966b.

Smith, L.; Kruszyna, H.; and Smith, R. P.: The effect of methemoglobin on the inhibition of cytochrom *c* oxidase by cyanide, sulfide and azide. *Biochem. Pharmacol.*, **26**:2247–50, 1977.

Smith, R. P.: The nitrite methemoglobin complex—Its significance in methemoglobin analyses and its possible role in methemoglobinemia. *Biochem. Pharmacol.*, **16**:1655–64, 1967.

Smith, R. P., and Abbanat, R. A.: Protective effect of oxidized glutathione in acute sulfide poisoning. *Toxicol. Appl. Pharmacol.*, **9**:209–17, 1966.

Smith, R. P., and Gosselin, R. E.: The influence of methemoglobinemia on the lethality of some toxic anions. II. Sulfide. *Toxicol. Appl. Pharmacol.*, **6**:584–92, 1964.

Smith, R. P.; Alkaitis, A. A.; and Shafer, P. R.: Chemically induced methemoglobinemias in the mouse. *Biochem. Pharmacol.*, **16**:317–28, 1967.

Smith, R. P., and Layne, W. R.: A comparison of the lethal effects of nitrite and hydroxylamine in the mouse. *J. Pharmacol. Exp. Ther.*, **165**:30–35, 1969.

Smith, R. P., and Olson, M. V.: Drug-induced methemoglobinemia. *Semin. Hematol.*, **10**:253–68, 1973.

Smith, R. P., and Thron, C. D.: Hemoglobin, methylene blue and oxygen interactions in human red cells. *J. Pharmacol. Exp. Ther.*, **183**:549–58, 1972.

Smith, R. P., and Kruszyna, H.: Nitroprusside produces cyanide poisoning *via* a reaction with hemoglobin. *J. Pharmacol. Exp. Ther.*, **191**:557–63, 1974.

Smith, R. P.; Kruszyna, R.; and Kruszyna, H.: Management of acute sulfide poisoning. Effects of oxygen, thiosulfate, and nitrite. *Arch. Environ. Health*, **31**:166–69, 1976.

Spencer, T. D.: Effects of carbon monoxide on man and canaries. *Ann. Occup. Hyg.*, **5**:231–40, 1962.

Stebbins, R., and Bertino, J. R.: Megaloblastic anemias produced by drugs. *Clin. Haematol.*, **5**:619–30, 1976.

Stine, R. J.; Slosberg, B.; and Beacham, B. E.: Hydrogen sulfide intoxication. A case report and discussion of treatment. *Ann. Intern. Med.*, **85**:756–58, 1976.

Stolk, J. M., and Smith, R. P.: Species differences in methemoglobin reductase activity. *Biochem. Pharmacol.*, **15**:343–51, 1966.

Surgenor, D. M.: *The Red Blood Cell*, 2nd ed. Academic Press, Inc., New York, Vol. I, 1974; Vol. II, 1975.

Tönz, O.: *The Congenital Methemoglobinemias. Physiology and Pathophysiology of the Hemiglobin Metabolism*. S. Karger, Basel, 1968. Published simultaneously as Bibliotheca Haematologica No. 28.

van Assendelft, O. W., and Zijlstra, W. G.: The formation of haemoglobin using nitrites. *Clin. Chim. Acta*, **11**:571–77, 1965.

van Kampen, E. J., and Zijlstra, W. G.: Determination of hemoglobin and its derivatives. In Sobotka, H., and Steward, C. P. (eds.): *Advances in Clinical Chemistry*, Vol. 8. Academic Press, Inc., New York, 1965.

Way, J. L.; Gibbon, S. L.; and Sheehy, M.: Effect of oxygen on cyanide intoxication. I. Prophylactic protection. *J. Pharmacol. Exp. Ther.*, **153**:381–85, 1966.

Way, J. L., and Sheehy, M. H.: Antagonism of sodium nitrite intoxication. *Toxicol. Appl. Pharmacol.*, **19**:400–401, 1971.

Way, J. L.; End, E.; Sheehy, M. H.; de Miranda, P.; Feitknecht, U. F.; Bachand, R.; Gibbon, S. L.; and Burrows, G. E.: Effect of oxygen on cyanide intoxication. IV. Hyperbaric oxygen, *Toxicol. Appl. Pharmacol.*, **22**:415–21, 1972.

Weed, R. I.; LaCelle, P. L.; and Merrill, E. W.: Metabolic dependence of red cell deformability. *J. Clin. Invest.*, **48**:795–809, 1969.

Willhite, C. C., and Smith, R. P.: The role of cyanide liberation in the acute toxicity of aliphatic nitriles. *Toxicol. Appl. Pharmacol.*, **59**:589–602, 1981.

Chapter 9

TOXIC RESPONSES OF THE IMMUNE SYSTEM*

Jack H. Dean, Michael J. Murray, and *Edward C. Ward*

INTRODUCTION

The immune system functions in resistance to infectious agents, homeostasis of leukocyte maturation, immunoglobulin production and immune surveillance against arising neoplastic cells. Cells of the immune system providing these functions are termed leukocytes, and they arise from pluripotent stem cells within the bone marrow, where they undergo highly controlled proliferation and differentiation before giving rise to functionally mature cells. The functionally mature cells are divided into granulocytes, lymphocytes, and macrophages. Lymphocytes can be subdivided into thymus-derived (T lymphocytes) and bursa-equivalent (B lymphocytes) depending on the primary lymphoid tissue where maturation occurs. The interaction of environmental chemicals or drugs with lymphoid tissue may alter the delicate balance of the immune system and result in four types of undesirable effects: (1) immunosuppression, (2) uncontrolled proliferation (i.e., leukemia and lymphoma), (3) alterations of host defense mechanisms against pathogens and neoplasia, and (4) allergy or autoimmunity.

* Abbreviations used in this chapter include the following: AIDS = Acquired Immunodeficiency Syndrome; Ab = Antibody; ADCC = Antibody-Dependent Cellular Cytotoxicity; CMI = Cell-Mediated Immunity; CF = Chemotactic Factor; C' = Complement; Con A = Concanavalin A; Fc = Constant Portion of Ab Molecule; Cy = Cyclophosphamide; CYA = Cyclosporin A; CTL = Cytotoxic T Lymphocyte; DTH = Delayed-Type Hypersensitivity; ELISA = Enzyme-Linked Immunosorbent Assay; GALT = Gut-Associated Lymphoid Tissue; HI = Humoral Immunity; Ig = Immunoglobulin; IFN = Interferon; K Cell = Killer Cell; LPS = Lipopolysaccharide; MØ = Macrophage; MAF = Macrophage-Activating Factor; MIF = Migration Inhibition Factor; MLC = Mixed Leukocyte Culture; NK Cell = Natural Killer Cell; PHA = Phytohemagglutinin; PFC = Plaque-Forming Cell; PWM = Pokeweed Mitogen; PMN = Polymorphonuclear Leukocyte; PGs = Prostaglandins; RAST = Radioallergsorbent Test; RBC = Red Blood Cell; SRBC = Sheep Red Blood Cell; SRS-A = Slow-Reacting Substance of Anaphylaxis.

Traditional methods for toxicologic assessment have implicated the immune system as a target organ of toxic insult following chronic or subchronic exposure to some chemicals and drugs. Alterations in lymphoid organ weight or histology; quantitative changes in peripheral leukocyte counts and differentials; depressed cellularity of lymphoid tissues; and increased susceptibility to infections by opportunistic organisms may reflect potential immune alterations and have been observed in animals exposed to chemicals at doses where overt toxicity was not apparent. Increased incidence of allergy and autoimmunity has also been associated with exposure to chemicals and drugs in both animals and humans. It is becoming increasingly apparent that the immune system represents an important target organ for studying the toxicology of chemical exposure for the following reasons: immunocompetent cells are required for host resistance, and thus exposure to immunotoxicants can result in increased susceptibility to disease; immunocompetent cells require continued proliferation and differentiation for self-renewal and are thus sensitive to agents that affect cell proliferation; the cellular and molecular biology of the immune system is better understood than in many other target organ systems, and thus the mechanism(s) by which toxicants are immunoalterative can be determined; functional assessment or enumeration of leukocytes can be easily achieved using a small volume of blood or lymphoid tissue; and finally, observations obtained in experimental animals can be confirmed in humans using leukocytes obtained by minimally invasive methods (i.e., venipuncture). Now that sensitive and reproducible assays of immune function and host resistance are available, attention has focused on the usefulness of immunotoxicity as an adjunct in the routine safety evaluation of chemicals and drugs under development.

This chapter will provide an overview of the current concepts regarding the organization and function of the immune system and its cellular elements; dysfunctions of the immune system; approaches and methods for assessing immunotoxicity induced by chemicals and drugs; and a partial listing of chemicals, metals, and drugs that have been found to produce immunosuppression, allergy, or autoimmunity.

CELLS OF THE IMMUNE SYSTEM AND THEIR FUNCTION

The immune system is a highly evolved organ system involved in rejection of foreign tissue grafts and host defense against infectious agents and neoplastic cells. These functions are provided by two major mechanisms: a *nonspecific* or *constitutive* mechanism not requiring prior contact with the inducing agent and lacking specificity; and a *specific* or *adaptive* mechanism directed against and specific for the eliciting agent (Table 9–1). Mononuclear phagocytes (i.e., blood monocytes and tissue macrophages) and granulocytes are phagocytic cells involved with nonspecific resistance. Lymphoid cells, as well as macrophages, are responsible for specific host resistance.

Pluripotent stem cells comprise a unique group of cells that are unspecialized and have renewal capacity. During fetal development, pluripotent stem cells are found in the blood islands of the yolk sac in the embryo, in the liver of the fetus, and later in the bone marrow. The pluripotent stem cell differentiates along several different pathways giving rise to erythrocytes, myeloid series cells (i.e., macrophages, and granulocytes or polymorphonuclear leukocytes [PMNs]), megakaryocytes (which produce platelets), or lymphocytes. Maturation generally occurs within the bone marrow. Lymphoid progenitor cells are, however, disseminated by the vasculature to the primary lymphoid organs where they differentiate under the influence of the microenvironment of these organs (Figure 9–1).

Nonspecific and Specific Mechanisms of Immunity

Two categories of phagocytic leukocytes, the polymorphonuclear phagocyte or granulocyte and the mononuclear phagocyte or macrophage (MØ), are involved with nonspecific mechanisms of host resistance. Both cell types originate from the same myeloid progenitor in bone marrow, pass through several developmental stages, and enter the bloodstream where they circulate for one to three days. PMNs can traverse blood vessels and represent the primary line of defense against infectious agents. Both PMNs and MØs exhibit phagocytic activity toward foreign material, especially in the presence of specific opsonic antibodies and complement (see below for description), and can destroy most microorganisms. In the event that PMNs either cannot contain or are destroyed by the infectious agent, as is the case with certain bacteria such as *Listeria monocytogenes,* macrophages are recruited to the site. Macrophages can be activated to a state of enhanced bactericidal activity by soluble mediators (lymphokines) produced by T lymphocytes sensitized to a specific microbial antigen. Macrophages are unique since they can adhere to glass or plastic, can be recruited by sensitized T lymphocytes to a specific tissue location, and can be activated to become more efficient killers of intracellular microorganisms and tumor cells.

The immune response involved with adaptive host resistance represents a series of complex events that occur after the introduction of a foreign material (i.e., antigen) into an immunocompetent host. There are two major types of immune responses: (1) *cell-mediated immunity* (CMI), which is a response by specifically sensitized, thymus-dependent lymphocytes and is generally associated with delayed-type hypersensitivity, graft rejection, and resistance to persistent infectious agents (e.g., certain viruses, bacteria, protozoa, and fungi); and (2) *humoral*

Table 9–1. **DIFFERENCES BETWEEN NONSPECIFIC AND SPECIFIC MECHANISMS OF HOST RESISTANCE**

PARAMETER	NONSPECIFIC	SPECIFIC
Exogenous stimulation	Not required	Required
Specificity of reaction	None	High degree
Cell types involved	Polymorphonuclear leukocytes	T lymphocytes
		B lymphocytes
	Monocytes/macrophages (effector cells)	Monocytes/macrophages (accessory cells)

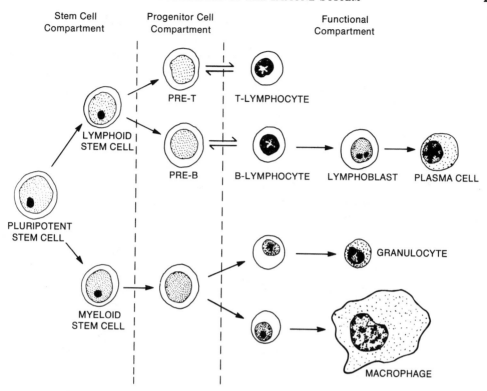

Figure 9–1. Differentiation pathways of lymphomyeloid pluripotent stem cells.

immunity (HI), which involves the production of specific antibodies (immunoglobulins) by bursa-equivalent lymphocytes or plasma cells following sensitization to a specific antigen.

Lymphocyte Differentiation

The primary lymphoid organs include the thymus in all vertebrates and the bursa of Fabricius in birds, or bursa-equivalent tissue in mammals. Primary lymphoid organs are lymphoepithelial in origin, derived from ectoendodermal junctional tissue in association with gut epithelium. During the second half of embryogenesis (days 12 to 13 in the mouse), stem cells migrate into the epithelia of the thymus and bursa-equivalent areas and begin their differentiation into T cells and B cells, respectively (Figure 9–2). The development of lymphocytes in the primary lymphoid organs is independent of antigenic stimulation.

Lymphocytes that differentiate from lymphoid stem cells in the thymus are termed thymus-dependent lymphocytes (T cells). The thymus, which is derived embryologically from the third and fourth pharyngeal pouches, is an organization of lymphoid tissue located in the chest (above the heart). Thymus development occurs during the sixth week of embryologic development in humans and day 9 of gestation in the mouse. The thymus reaches its maximum size (approximately 0.27 percent of body weight) at birth or shortly thereafter in most mammals and then begins a gradual involution until at 5 to 15 years in humans it represents only 0.02 percent of body weight.

Histologically, the thymus consists of many lobules, each containing a cortex and medulla. Lymphocyte precursors from bone marrow proliferate in the cortex of the lobules and then migrate to the medulla, where they further differentiate under the influence of thymic epithelium into mature T lymphocytes before emigrating to secondary lymphoid tissues. The neonatal/postnatal thymus has an endocrine function associated with the nonlymphoid thymic epithelium cells. These cells are believed to produce hormones essential for T-lymphocyte maturation and differentiation. A role for the adult thymus as an endocrine organ responsible for maintaining immune system homeostasis is also speculated.

In birds, B-cell differentiation occurs in the

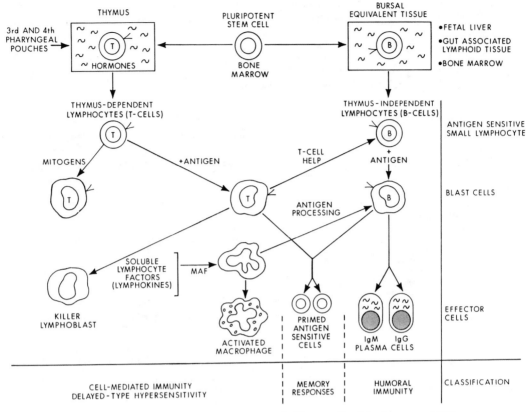

Figure 9–2. Development, interactions, and effector cells of the immune system.

bursa of Fabricius, a lymphoepithelial organ that develops from a diverticulum of the posterior wall of the cloaca. It is divided into a medullary region, containing lymphoid follicles, and a cortical region. Bursectomy in young birds results in impairment of germinal center formation (see below), plasma cell formation, and immunoglobulin production. The mammalian bursa-equivalent is believed to be the fetal liver, the neonatal spleen, gut-associated lymphoid tissue, and adult bone marrow. Mature B lymphocytes migrate from the bursa-equivalent tissue to populate the B-dependent areas of the secondary lymphoid tissues.

Neonatal removal or chemical destruction of primary lymphoid organs prior to the maturation of lymphocytes into T or B cells or prior to their population of secondary lymphoid tissue dramatically depresses the immunologic capacity of the host. However, removal of these same organs in adults has little influence on immunologic capacity. In addition, neonatal thymectomy in mammals dramatically impairs the development of CMI, but does not generally influence the generation of immunoglobulin-producing cells involved in humoral antibody responses unless they require T lymphocyte help for induction of antibody production. In contrast to the removal of primary lymphoid organs, removal of secondary lymphoid organs does not inhibit the development of immunocompetence although it may suppress the magnitude or alter the tissue location of the responsive cells (Table 9–2).

Markers of Differentiation

T lymphocytes, B lymphocytes, and MØs can be identified by a distinct pattern of cell surface-associated markers and receptors found on each of these cell types (Table 9–3). B cells, for example, have a high density of immunoglobulin on their surface, whereas T cells lack immunoglobulin. Conversely, B cells lack specific alloantigens that are found on T cells at different stages of differentiation. In humans, but not in mice, T lymphocytes can also be distinguished by their ability to form rosettes with sheep erythrocytes, while B cells lack this characteristic. Macrophages, granulocytes, killer cells, and plasma cells possess a receptor for the Fc region of antibody molecules.

Table 9–2. ORIGIN AND CHARACTERISTICS OF LYMPHOID ORGANS

PARAMETER	PRIMARY LYMPHOID ORGANS	SECONDARY LYMPHOID ORGANS
Lymphoid organs	Thymus Bursa of Fabricius (birds) Fetal liver (mammals) Adult bone marrow	Spleen Lymph nodes Gut-associated lymphid tissue (GALT)
Embryonic origin and development	Ectoendodermal junction Thymus—day 9 to 10 mouse, week 6 man Bursa-equivalent—day 10 to 13 mouse, week 10 man	Mesoderm
Lymphoid cell proliferation	Independent of antigenic stimulation	Dependent on antigenic stimulation
Germinal center formation	Nonexistent	Occurs after antigenic stimulation
Cells repopulating after depletion	Stem cells only	Differentiated lymphocytes
Early surgical or drug removal	Depressed numbers of T and B cells, depressed immune responses	No significant effect on immune function

Table 9–3. DIFFERENTIAL CHARACTERISTICS OF LYMPHOID CELLS

PARAMETER	T CELLS	B CELLS	MACROPHAGES
Phagocytosis	No	No	Yes
Adherence	No (blasts only)	No (plasma cells)	Yes
Surface receptors:			
Antigens	Yes	Yes	No
Fc region of Ig	Some	Yes	Yes
Complement	No	Yes	Yes
Differentiation antigen:			
Mouse	Thy-1 (pan-T cell) Lyt-1 (helper) Lyt-2,3 (suppressor, cytotoxic)		MAC-1
Man	OKT-3 (pan-T cell) OKT-4 (helper) OKT-5,8 (suppressor, cytotoxic)	Ig	—
Proliferation to:			
Phytohemagglutinin	Yes	No	No
Concanavalin A	Yes	No	No
Lipopolysaccharide of gram-negative bacteria	No	Yes (mouse only)	No
Allogeneic leukocyte antigens in mixed leukocyte culture	Yes	No	No
Effector functions:			
Immunologic memory	Yes	Yes	No
Tumor cell cytotoxicity	Yes	No	Yes
Bactericidal activity	No	No	Yes
Immunoglobulin production	No	Yes	No
Cytokine production	Yes (lymphokines)	No	Yes (monokines)

In contrast to T and B lymphocytes, macrophages and blood monocytes have the ability to phagocytose bacteria and other foreign particles. A group of mononuclear cells has been described that lack well-defined cell surface markers and are nonphagocytic. These cells possess a receptor for the Fc region of the immunoglobulin molecule and, when mixed with antibody and tumor target cells, are able to lyse the tumor target cells. They have been termed killer cells (K cells) and are believed to mediate cytolytic reactions against tumors and foreign tissue grafts in the presence of antibody, a process termed antibody-dependent cellular cytotoxicity (ADCC) (Perlmann *et al.*, 1975). Other subpopulations of lymphocytes have been described that possess spontaneous cytolytic activity toward neoplastic cells, but not normal cells. These are termed natural killer (NK) cells (see review by Herberman and Holden, 1978) and natural cytotoxic (NC) lymphocytes (Stutman and Cuttito, 1981).

Organization of Secondary Lymphoid Organs

The organized areas of secondary lymphoid tissues consist of the lymph nodes, spleen, and gut-associated lymphoid tissue (Table 9–2). The anatomic organization of these tissues provides a microenvironment for functional development of lymphocytes.

Lymph Nodes. Lymph nodes are discrete, organized secondary lymphoid organs and serve as filtering devices for lymphatic fluid. Lymph nodes are divided structurally into three areas: the cortex, paracortex, and medulla (Figure 9–3). Each lymph node is served by several afferent lymphatic vessels collecting lymphatic fluid from distal sites, and this fluid or lymph may contain foreign antigens. The efferent lymphatic vessel, which drains lymph from the node, contains antibodies, lymphokines, and lymphocytes produced in response to foreign antigenic stimulation. The cortex is located beneath the subcapsular sinus and receives the afferent lymph. It is the major site of B-lymphocyte localization. In the absence of antigenic stimulation, the cortex consists of a narrow rim of small lymphocytes. Also located in the cortex are aggregations of small lymphocytes, termed lymphoid follicles, which contain dendritic reticulum cells capable of retaining antigens on their plasma membranes. When the lymphocytes comprising the lymphoid follicles are stimulated by antigen, they undergo proliferation giving rise to dense aggregations of lymphocytes, termed germinal centers, which serve as sites for differentiation of B lymphocytes to plasma cells capable of antibody production. Following antigenic stimulation, germinal centers are easily detectable as spherical or ovoid structures containing many large and medium-sized lymphocytes. Histologically the germinal center is predominantly a B lymphocyte area and contains three principal regions termed the densely populated, thinly populated, and lymphocyte cuff regions. In the densely populated region, the lymphocytes are actively mitotic, while in the thinly populated area one finds an accumulation of large to medium-sized lymphocytes. The cuff

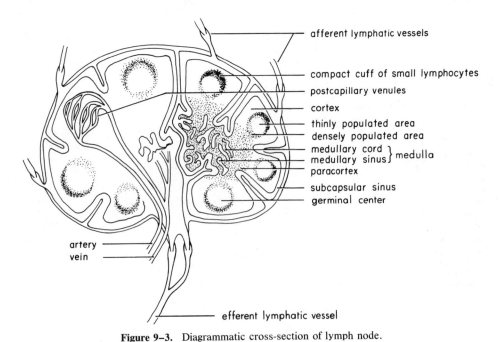

Figure 9–3. Diagrammatic cross-section of lymph node.

contains many small to medium-sized lymphocytes that are part of the recirculating B lymphocyte memory cell pool.

The paracortex, lying between the cortex and the medulla, is predominantly a T-lymphocyte area (Figure 9–3) and is a major area of macrophage/T-cell interactions. Neonatal thymectomy or short-term lymphocyte depletion by thoracic duct cannulation reduces paracortical lymphocytes, leading to depressed immune capacity. In addition, the paracortex contains specialized blood vasculature, termed postcapillary venules, which serve as points of entry for recirculating lymphocytes from the bloodstream.

The medulla of the lymph node is primarily composed of networks of cords and sinuses. The sinuses are continuations of the subcapsular space passing through the cortex and medulla and are interspersed between the medullary cords. They ultimately merge in the hilus of the lymph node to form an efferent lymphatic vessel (Figure 9–3). The medullary cords consist of a structural network of dendritic cells surrounded by dense aggregations of lymphocytes. Together, this system of cords and sinuses serves as an effective filter for removing particulate material from lymphatic fluid. Following antigenic stimulation a major portion of the antibody is produced by plasma cells found within these medullary cords.

Spleen. Lymph nodes serve as a major filter for lymph, while the spleen serves a similar function for blood. Since the spleen is the major filter of bloodborne antigens, it is also the major site of immunologic responses to these antigens.

In addition, the spleen is a site of extramedullary erythropoiesis and removal of damaged blood cells. There are two major histologic regions within the spleen: the red and the white pulp (Figure 9–4). These areas have been named for their color in a freshly cut spleen. The white pulp consists of numerous white blood cell aggregates and lymphoid follicles. The red pulp contains cords and venous sinuses analogous to the medullary region of lymph nodes. The spleen has no afferent lymphatic vessels; thus, all antigenic material or cells enter the spleen through the blood vasculature. The marginal sinus in the spleen is structurally and functionally similar to the subcapsular sinus of the lymph node.

Gut-Associated Lymphoid Tissue (GALT). The lamina propria of the intestinal tract represents another secondary lymphoid tissue and, on a volume basis, is a major source of lymphoid tissue. Lymphocytes within the GALT are scattered in loose connective tissue or organized into lymphoid follicles (i.e., Peyer's patches) which contain germinal centers and diffuse concentrations of T lymphocytes analogous to the cortex and paracortex of the lymph node. As in all other lymphoid tissue, the lymphocyte cuff of the germinal center in the GALT is located nearest the source of antigenic stimulation (i.e., lumen of the intestine).

Antigen Recognition and Induction of Immunity

In 1959, Burnet proposed the clonal selection theory to describe the recognition of foreign antigens by lymphocytes, the induction of the

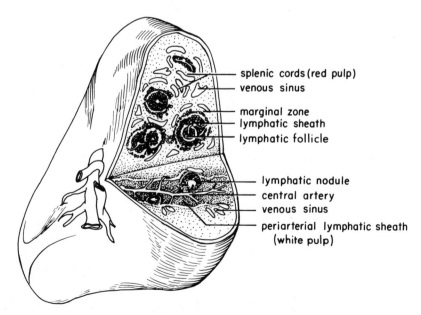

splenic cords (red pulp)
venous sinus

marginal zone
lymphatic sheath
lymphatic follicle

lymphatic nodule
central artery
venous sinus
periarterial lymphatic sheath
(white pulp)

Figure 9–4. Diagrammatic cross-section of spleen.

immune response that followed, and the discrimination by the immune system of between self and nonself. In this theory, a specific antigen was believed to be nonstimulatory to all but a few lymphocytes possessing receptors with a surface structure complementary to the configuration of the antigen. Following interaction with specific antigen, the receptor-bearing cell was stimulated to undergo proliferation and differentiation, producing a clone of progeny cells that were derived from a single ancestral cell. There is convincing evidence in support of Burnet's hypothesis. Immunoglobulin (Ig) molecules are thought to represent the primary cell membrane receptor on B lymphocytes. However, it is unclear what type of receptors are involved with T-lymphocyte antigen recognition and subsequent differentiation.

Whether or not an antigen induces CMI, antibody production, or both presumably depends on a multitude of factors, including the physical and chemical nature of the antigen, the mode of presentation of the antigen to lymphocytes, the localization pattern of the antigen within lymphoid tissue, and the molecular configuration of the antigen. Those antigens generally found to elicit CMI include tissue antigens present on cells; chemical agents and drugs that conjugate with autologous proteins; and antigenic determinants on persistent intracellular microorganisms. In contrast, some antigens, for example the pneumococcal polysaccharides, predominantly elicit antibodies. The route of exposure also plays a role in the type of response generated. Sheep erythrocytes, for example, will elicit antibodies when injected intravenously or will elicit both antibodies and CMI if injected intracutaneously. It is now established that intradermal presentation of antigen favors the development of CMI.

The induction of CMI proceeds by small lymphocytes differentiating into large pyroninophilic cells, that do not contain rough endoplasmic reticulum and are thus distinct from plasma cells. These large lymphocytes ultimately divide, giving rise to cells responsible for immunologic memory and effector function. T cells can further differentiate into effector cells endowed with cytotoxic potential (i.e., cytotoxic T-cells); helper cells (T_H), which facilitate antibody responses by B lymphocytes and aid in some T-lymphocyte responses; or T-suppressor cells (T_S) capable of inhibiting both T- and B-cell responses. The steps involved in T-cell activation and the several humoral factors elaborated by T-cells are shown in Figure 9–5. These factors, termed lymphokines, include interferon (IFN), chemotactic factor (CF), and macrophage activation factor (MAF), which represent nonspecific effectors of cell-mediated immunity and are responsible for amplification and regulation of the CMI response.

The main function of B lymphocytes is production of antibody molecules in response to

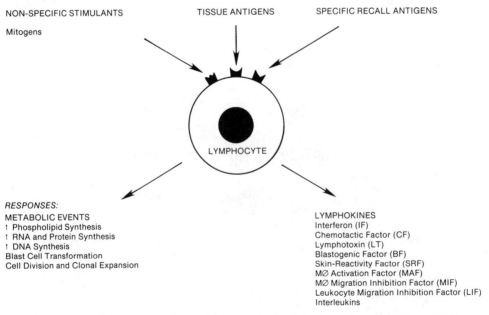

Figure 9–5.   Cellular events and lymphokine production following antigen induction of CMI.

Table 9–4. BIOLOGIC PROPERTIES OF IMMUNOGLOBULIN CLASSES

CLASS	MOLECULAR WEIGHT	HALF-LIFE (DAYS)	BIOLOGIC FUNCTION
IgG	150,000	23	Fix complement Cross placenta Heterocytotropic antibody
IgA	170,000	6	Secretory antibody Properdin pathway
IgM	890,000	5	Fix complement Efficient agglutination
IgD	150,000	2.8	Lymphocyte receptor?
IgE	196,000	1.5	Reaginic antibody Homocytotropic antibody

antigenic stimulation. Antibody molecules are serum proteins synthesized in response to an antigen, which react specifically with that antigen. Based on chemical structure and biologic function, there are five classes of antibody molecules: IgM, IgG, IgA, IgD, and IgE. Table 9–4 lists the principal physical and biologic characteristics of each of the classes.

Over a period of three to five days following the introduction of antigens into an immunocompetent host, B lymphocytes differentiate into lymphoblasts, immature plasma cells, and finally antibody-secreting plasma cells. There is an early rise in IgM antibody titer in the serum, followed several days later by the appearance of IgG antibodies. The production of IgM antibodies precedes that of IgG antibodies. Figure 9–6 depicts the time course of detectable serum antibody following immunization. During this differentiation process, lymphocytes are committed to immunologic memory so that when the same antigen is encountered a second time, an enhanced response is observed, characterized by a shorter latency to the appearance of serum IgG, increased production of Ig, and sustained production of IgG antibodies.

Figure 9–7 is a diagrammatic representation of an immunoglobulin molecule. It consists of four peptide chains, two light chains, and two heavy chains, held together by disulfide bonds. Furthermore, each heavy and light chain is subdivided into a variable and constant region. It is the variable region that determines the molecular specificity for antigen while the constant region of the heavy chains is responsible for the biologic activities of the molecule. For example, the constant region contains the sites that allow IgE to bind to mast cells or allow IgG to bind complement. All antibody molecules are variations of this basic structure and may occur as monomers, or in some instances as dimers (some IgA molecules) or pentamers (IgM).

Antibody molecules have four basic functions in protecting the host from infectious agents. The first is virus neutralization. If antibodies are made to viral antigens, they may bind to the virus particles and prevent them from infecting target cells. Antibodies also aid in the elimination of foreign agents by opsonization. Antibody molecules can coat an infectious agent (i.e., bacteria or virus), and the antibody-antigen complex can bind to PMNs or macrophages via their Fc receptors, resulting in enhanced phagocytosis of the antibody-coated agent. The third way in which antibody molecules may function is via antibody-dependent cellular cytotoxicity (ADCC). Some leukocytes have receptors for the constant portion (Fc) of the molecule. Following interaction of the antibody with antigens

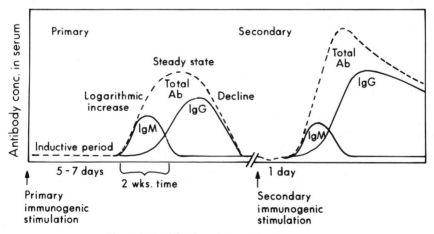

Figure 9–6. Kinetics of the antibody response.

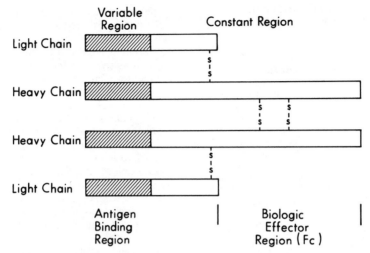

Figure 9–7.   Structure of an immunoglobulin molecule.

on target cells, the Fc portion binds to the leukocyte, which can then lyse the target cell. In this way, the antibody molecule provides the specificity for the action of the effector cell. The last way in which antibody molecules can protect the host from infectious agents is through cell lysis mediated by the complement (C') system. This cascading system consists of 20 chemically and immunologically distinct serum proteins (see review by Muller-Eberhard, 1975). The initial protein in this cascade can combine with antibody following its interaction with antigen. Subsequently C' components interact with other proteins in a sequential fashion to generate biologic activities, that result in lysis of red blood cells, foreign or transplanted cells, lymphocytes, platelets, bacteria, and certain enveloped viruses (Figure 9–8). Many of the products of complement activation mediate inflammatory reactions (e.g., the C5 cleavage products). Evidence for the biologic importance of this system of proteins comes from the markedly increased susceptibility to infections in individuals with congenital or acquired deficiencies in complement components.

Cellular Regulation of Immune Responses

Macrophages are required for activation of some antigen-specific T cells, in particular T helper cells and T cells involved in delayed cutaneous type hypersensitivity (DTH), but not for activation of T suppressor cells. The physical interaction between lymphocytes and macrophages has been well documented. In addition, T-helper cells are required for the induction of B cells to synthesize antibodies (Ab) to certain T-dependent antigens such as foreign red blood cells or serum proteins. In contrast, a variety of

antigens do not require T-helper cells for induction of antibody synthesis and are termed T-independent antigens. It has been postulated that T-independent antigens can trigger B cells in the absence of T cells because their structure allows them to bind multivalently to the immunoglobulin receptor on the B-cell surface. T-dependent antigens are believed to lack this characteristic and can only bind to individual antigen recognition sites on B cells. Macrophages are required for triggering some T and B cells because the surface of the macrophage may act as a matrix to concentrate the relevant antigenic determinants (epitopes) in a manner similar to the multivalent antigens. T cells are also responsible for switching from IgM to IgG antibody expression in B cells. There is now ample data suggesting that certain T cells may exert a suppressive influence on immune responses and that these cells belong to a distinct subset of T cells with the Lyt-2,3 phenotype in mice and OKT-5,8 phenotype in humans (i.e., suppressor T cell). In contrast, T-helper cells have the Lyt-2,3 phenotype in mice and the OKT-4 phenotype in humans. Helper and suppressor T cells exist in the circulation of humans and mice in a ratio of approximately 2:1 helper to suppressor cells. An imbalance in the ratio of helper to suppressor cells is observed in the newly recognized acquired immune deficiency syndrome (AIDS).

IMMUNE DYSFUNCTION

Hypersensitivity, and Allergy

The function of the immune system is to recognize and eliminate agents that are harmful to the host. When the immune system is functioning properly, the foreign agents are eliminated

ANTIGEN–ANTIBODY

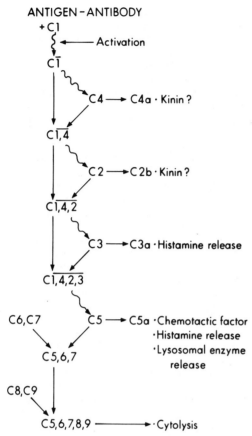

Figure 9–8. Schematic diagram of the classic complement activation cascade. (Modified from Cooper, N. R.: The complement system. In Stites, D. P.; Stobo, J. D.; Fudenberg, H. H.; and Wells, J. V. (eds.): *Basic and Clinical Immunology,* 4th ed. Lange Medical Publications, Los Altos, Calif., 1980, pp. 124–35.)

quickly and efficiently. Occasionally the immune system responds adversely to environmental agents, resulting in an allergic reaction. Coombs and Gell (1975) have divided allergic responses into four general categories based on the mechanism of immunologic involvement. These are summarized in Table 9–5 (for review, see Wells, 1982).

The type I or anaphylactic reactions are mediated by homocytotropic antibodies (IgE in man). The Fc portion of IgE antibodies can bind to receptors on mast cells and basophils. If the antibody molecule then binds antigen, pharmacologically active amines such as slow-reacting substance of anaphylaxis and histamine are released from the mediator cell (e.g., mast cell, basophil). These agents result in vasodilation, edema, and generation of an inflammatory response. The main targets of this type of reaction are the gastrointestinal tract (food allergies), the skin (urticaria and atopic dermatitis), the respiratory system (rhinitis and asthma), and the vasculature (anaphylactic shock). These responses tend to occur quickly after rechallenge with an antigen to which the individual has been sensitized and are termed immediate hypersensitivity.

The type II or cytolytic reactions are mediated by both IgG and IgM antibodies. These reactions are usually attributed to the antibody's ability to fix complement, opsonize particles, or function in an antibody-dependent cellular cytotoxicity reaction. The major target is often tissues of the circulatory system including red and white blood cells and platelets. The interaction of cytolytic antibody with these cells or their progenitors results in depletion and the production of hemolytic anemia, leukopenia, or thrombocytopenia. Additional target organs include the lungs and kidneys, as observed in Goodpasture's disease. In these type II reactions, an in-

Table 9–5. GELL AND COOMBS CLASSIFICATION SCHEME OF ALLERGY

CLASSIFICATION	EXAMPLES	MECHANISM
Type 1 Anaphylaxis (immediate hypersensitivity)	Asthma, urticaria rhinitis, atopic dermatitis	IgE bound to mast cell/basophil triggers release of soluble mediators (e.g., histamine).
Type II Cytolytic	Hemolytic anemia, Goodpasture's disease	IgG and/or IgM binds to cells and results in destruction via complement, opsonization, or ADCC
Type III Arthus	Systemic lupus erythematosus, glomerular nephritis, rheumatoid arthritis, serum sickness	Antigen-antibody complexes deposit in various tissues and may then fix complement
Type IV Delayed-type hypersensitivity	Contact dermatitis, tuberculosis	Sensitized T lymphocytes induce a DTH response

dividual may develop antibodies to respiratory and glomerular basement membranes, resulting in glomerulonephritis and pulmonary hemorrhaging.

The type III or Arthus reactions are mainly mediated by IgG through a mechanism involving the generation of antigen-antibody complexes that subsequently fix complement. The complexes become deposited in the vascular endothelium, where a destructive inflammatory response occurs. This is contrasted to the type II reaction, where the inflammatory response is induced by antibodies directed against the tissue antigens. The main target tissues are the skin (lupus), the joints (rheumatoid arthritis), the kidneys (glomerulonephritis), the lungs (hypersensitivity pneumonitis), and the circulatory system (serum sickness). The antigens responsible for these types of reactions may be self-antigens, as is thought to occur in lupus and rheumatoid arthritis, or foreign antigens, as in serum sickness.

The type IV or delayed-hypersensitivity response is not mediated by antibodies, but rather by macrophages and sensitized T lymphocytes. When sensitized T lymphocytes come in contact with the sensitizing antigen, an inflammatory reaction is generated: lymphokines are produced followed by an influx of granulocytes and macrophages. The target for this type of reaction can be almost any organ, the classic example being skin.

Autoimmunity

For the immune system to function properly, it must be able to distinguish self-antigens from nonself-antigens. Occasionally, the delicate balance that prevents an individual from elaborating an immune response to self-antigens becomes perturbed, resulting in an inappropriate response to self. This phenomenon is known as autoimmunity and can be manifested by the production of antibodies to self- or modified self-antigens, or by tissue destruction from T lymphocytes or macrophages. (For a review of autoimmunity, see Theofilopoulos, 1982.)

Autoimmune diseases can belong to any of the four Gell and Coombs classifications (see Table 9–5). There are several hypotheses to explain the pathogenesis of autoimmune responses. During embryonic development, it is thought that the immune system becomes tolerized to the tissues and antigens to which it is exposed either by eliminating those lymphocytes that react with self-antigens or by generating suppressor T cells that inhibit the production of an immune response to self-antigens. If effector cells arise that are specific for self-antigens, or specific suppressor T cells are lost or become nonfunctional, an immune response directed against self may occur, resulting in tissue destruction. Alternatively, during development of the immune system there are many sequestered self-antigens to which the immune system is not exposed and thus are not perceived as self-antigens. Some examples of these types of antigens are found in the tissue of the central nervous system, the lens of the eye, the thyroid gland, and the testes, as well as antigens such as DNA or RNA sequestered within cells. If these antigens become exposed, an autoimmune response may develop. Some examples of autoimmune diseases include systemic lupus erythematosus (SLE) (type III, IV), rheumatoid arthritis (type III), Goodpasture's disease (type II), serum sickness (type III), and hemolytic anemia and thrombocytopenia (type IV).

Autoimmune diseases are not necessarily the result of an immune response to self-components. Environmental agents may bind to tissue or serum proteins, and an immune response may be generated against these modified self-antigens, resulting in cell injury or death. Many drugs, chemicals, and metals have been implicated as causative agents in autoimmune diseases. For example, hydralazine and procainamide can induce an SLE-like syndrome, α-methyldopa and the pesticide Dieldrin have been shown to cause an autoimmunelike hemolytic anemia, and metals (gold, mercury) have induced a glomerular nephritis similar to that seen in Goodpasture's disease.

Immunodeficiency

Pathogenic states of decreased immunoresponsiveness can be illustrated using examples of well-characterized, naturally occurring immunodeficiency disorders. These disorders may be subdivided according to etiology into primary and secondary deficiencies. Primary immunodeficiencies are genetic or congenitally acquired and can affect either specific or nonspecific components of the immune response. Patients with these disorders are subject to characteristic alterations in resistance to various types of infections depending on the cell types or other lesions involved. In some instances the study of immunodeficient patients has helped clarify many of the mechanisms involved in resistance to infectious agents. The majority of primary immunodeficiencies involve defects in either cellular or humoral immune responses, or both, subsequent to a loss of immune cell function or absence of a particular immune cell population (Table 9–6).

Secondary or acquired immunodeficiency disorders are more common than primary immunodeficiencies and have varied etiologies (see Table 9–7). Viral infection, malnutrition, can-

Table 9–6.   EXAMPLES OF CONGENITAL IMMUNODEFICIENCY

TYPE	DEFECT	TREATMENT
Thymic hypoplasia (DiGeorge's syndrome)	T lymphocytes	Fetal thymus transplant thymosin?
Infantile X-linked agammaglobulinemia	B lymphocytes	γ-Globulin
Severe combined immunodeficiency	T and B lymphocytes	Bone marrow transplant Fetal liver transplant Fetal thymus transplant
Chronic granulomatous disease	Enzyme deficiency in granulocytes	Early and prolonged antibiotic therapy
C3 deficiency	Deficiency of C3 activator	Infusion of normal plasma

cer, renal diseases, and aging are a few examples of potential causes of secondary immunodeficiency; however, in many instances the underlying cause of the condition remains obscure. Acquired as well as primary immunodeficiencies can be life-threatening. Immunosuppressive drugs may also lead to immunodeficiency and are often clinically exploited for this characteristic.

Immunosuppression is of particular clinical importance in the prolongation of allograft survival and in the treatment of autoimmune disorders. In general, primary immune responses are amenable to suppression, and secondary responses are not. Drug-induced immunosuppression depends on the characteristics of the drug and the time of its administration relative to the generation of an immune response. In this regard, the immune response can be subdivided into two phases: the inductive phase, which follows antigen exposure and is characterized by lymphoproliferation; and the productive or effector phase, characterized by antibody production and cell-mediated effector function. Most immunosuppressive agents are maximally active when administered during or just prior to the

inductive phase of the immune response. An alternative classification of immunosuppressive drugs is based on their mode of action. In general, these drugs are effective because of their antiproliferative or lympholytic and lymphomodulatory actions. They usually function as general rather than specific immunosuppressants.

Many immunosuppressive drugs were originally developed as cytoreductive cancer chemotherapeutic agents because of their ability to interfere with cell growth and proliferation. Because of the high rate of proliferation in antigen-stimulated lymphocytes, these cells are sensitive to many of the same drugs as rapidly dividing tumor cells, and the use of antiproliferative drugs in transplant patients or patients with certain autoimmune diseases has become almost routine. Azathioprine is a commonly utilized antiproliferant whose active metabolite interferes with the synthesis of compounds required for cell metabolism, growth, and division. Therefore, this drug and other antiproliferatives are most effective when administered following antigen stimulation, during the inductive portion of the immune response.

Lympholytic or lymphomodulatory agents generally act by directly destroying the lymphocyte or lethally damaging their ability to undergo mitosis; thus, as immunosuppressants these agents are most successfully used when administered just prior to the introduction of antigen. Common examples include the corticosteroids, which cause massive lympholysis in some species and act primarily through modulation of lymphocyte trafficking and effector functions in other species, including man. In contrast, alkylating agents such as cyclophosphamide crosslink DNA, causing immediate cell death or cytolysis during mitosis. Since these effects are similar to radiation-induced cell injury, alkylating agents are often referred to as radiomimetic drugs. Cyclosporin A is a relatively new immu-

Table 9–7.   CAUSATIVE AGENTS THAT MAY RESULT IN SECONDARY IMMUNODEFICIENCY

Drugs	Immunosuppressants, anticonvulsants, corticosteroids, chemotherapeutic agents
Infections	Acute viral, coccidioidomycosis, measles, tuberculosis, leprosy
Neoplasia	Acute leukemia, Hodgkin's disease, chronic leukemia, lymphosarcoma, thymoma, multiple myeloma, reticulum cell sarcoma
Autoimmune disease	Systemic lupus erythematosus, rheumatoid arthritis
Others	Aging, genetic disorders, malnutrition, radiation, nephrotic syndrome

nosuppressant that appears to act by mechanisms dissimilar to those previously discussed (for review see White, 1982). Although its mode of action is not completely understood, immunosuppression by Cyclosporin A may involve altered lymphokine release or blocking of lymphocyte membrane receptors for an interleukin (IL2) required to stimulate lymphocyte proliferation. Its major benefit is its apparent specificity for T-helper cells and its minimal effects on other immunoresponsive cells.

Immunosuppression may also be achieved through methods other than drug administration. Common approaches involve the use of radiation, antilymphocyte serum, and antigen (e.g., allergic desensitization). Immunosuppression, as evidenced by depressed antibody-mediated immunity and/or cell-mediated immunity, has also been observed in rodents exposed to sublethal levels of several chemicals of environmental concern. Chemicals that have produced immune alterations in rodents include: 2,3,7,8-tetrachlorodibenzo-p-dioxin (TCDD);

diethylstilbestrol (DES); polychlorinated biphenyls (PCB); polybrominated biphenyls (PBB); dimethyl vinyl chloride (DMVC); gallic acid; hexachlorobenzene (HCB); orthophenylphenol; organometals; and heavy metals. The observation that residents of Michigan, Japan, and China accidentally exposed to polybrominated biphenyl or polychlorinated biphenyl exhibited immune alterations similar to those observed in rodent studies has increased concern over the effects of xenobiotic agents on suppression of the immune system.

IMMUNOLOGIC MECHANISMS OF HOST RESISTANCE

The eradication and control of most bacterial agents that produce acute infections (e.g., *Staphylococcus*, *Streptococcus*) is facilitated by the production of specific antibodies. These antibodies enhance phagocytosis and killing of pathogenic microorganisms by granulocytes and macrophages through opsonization (Figure 9–9).

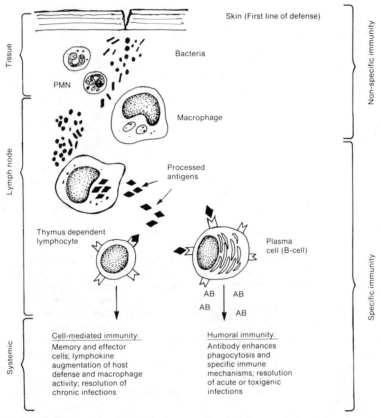

Figure 9–9. Diagrammatic representation of host resistance to bacteria indicating the roles of cell-mediated and humoral immunity. (Modified from Dean, J. H.; Luster, M. I.; Boorman, G. A.; and Laver, L. D.: Procedures available to examine the immunotoxicity of chemicals and drugs. *Pharmacol. Rev.*, **34**:137–48, 1982.)

In contrast, chronic bacterial infections are usually caused by organisms such as *Listeria monocytogenes* or *Mycobacterium tuberculosis,* which are facultative intracellular pathogens that can multiply within the phagocytic cell and thus escape antibody-mediated reactions. CMI enhances granulocyte phagocytosis or macrophage-mediated killing of such intracellular pathogens through the production of lymphokine (see Figure 9–9). Toxigenic infections, which result from the production of toxins by certain bacteria, require the production of specific antibody for toxin neutralization (e.g., tetanus toxin). CMI plays little, if any, role in managing toxigenic infections. Antibodies responsible for neutralization of bacterial toxins often prevent binding of the toxin to specific receptors, thus preventing their harmful effects.

Viral antigens expressed on the surface of infected cells may also serve as targets for cytotoxic T lymphocyte-mediated cytolysis. CMI is also instrumental in eliminating viral infections through the production and release of the lymphokine interferon by lymphocytes. Interferon signals adjacent cells to produce an antiviral protein that blocks virus replication. Interferon does not have direct antiviral activity, but causes adjacent cells to manufacture antiviral proteins.

An increased incidence of infectious disease and neoplasia has been frequently associated with primary immunodeficiency diseases and immunosuppressive therapy. Gatti and Good (1971) observed a significant frequency of lymphoreticular neoplasia in patients with primary immunodeficiency diseases (Table 9–8) and suggested that the incidence would have been higher had not most of the patients died of bacterial or fungal infections before they developed neoplasia. Immunosuppressive therapy has been widely used to prevent rejection of transplanted organs and to treat certain autoimmune diseases, collagen-vascular diseases, and chronic inflammatory disorders. Nonspecific therapeutic depression of immunity has frequently caused serious complications with bacterial, viral, fungal, and parasitic infections, and less frequently has been associated with an increased incidence of certain malignancies. One important complication in transplant patients on immunosuppressive therapy is the inadvertent transplantation of malignant cells in an organ obtained from a cadaver or living donor suffering from cancer. Of 89 patients who received organs from donors who had been diagnosed for neoplasia within five years of donation, 42 percent of the recipients developed the transplanted neoplasia (Penn, 1978). Currently, transplantation of cancer is a rare event as surgeons avoid using organs from donors with cancer.

A second and more important complication in immunosuppressed transplant patients has been the high frequency of *de novo* cancer. In a sampling of renal transplant patients (Table 9–8) who survived one year, 26 percent had developed cancer, while at ten years 47 percent were so affected (*see* Penn, 1985). The types of tumors observed included skin and lip cancer (21-fold increase over general population), non-Hodgkin's lymphomas (28- to 49-fold increase), Kaposi's sarcoma (400 to 500-fold increase), and carcinomas of the cervix (14-fold increase) (Penn, 1985).

Cell-mediated immune responses are believed to be important in controlling spontaneously arising tumors and limiting the growth of estab-

Table 9–8. EVIDENCE OF INCREASED CANCER INCIDENCE IN CONGENITALLY IMMUNODEFICIENT AND RENAL TRANSPLANT PATIENTS*

DISEASE	IMMUNE ALTERATION	% CANCER INCIDENCE	TUMOR TYPE
Congenital (Bruton's) agammaglobulinemia	B cells†	6 (10,000 × normal)	Acute lymphatic leukemia
Severe combined immunodeficiency	T and B cells	2	Lymphoreticular
Common variable immunodeficiency	B cells†	10	Lymphoreticular and carcinomas
Ataxia-telangiectasia	T cells	10	Lymphoreticular, sarcoma, and carcinomas
Renal transplant patients	T and B cells	26 (by 1 year) 47 (by 10 years)	Skin and lip cancer, non-Hodgkin's lymphoma, Kaposi's sarcoma, carcinoma of cervix

* Data from Gatti and Good (1971) and Penn (1985).
† Recent evidence of excessive suppressor cell activity.

lished neoplasms. In this regard, an imbalance or transient dysfunction of the immune surveillance mechanism is thought to facilitate development of neoplastic disease. Most tumor cells have unique cell-surface antigens that clearly distinguish them from normal cells, although immune responses to these antigens may vary considerably. In rodents, for example, chemically and virally induced tumors evoke strong antitumor immune responses, which may result in regression or elimination of the developing tumor, while spontaneously arising tumors are generally less immunogenic. The weight of the evidence, however, suggests that cell-mediated immune responses are important in recognition and destruction of arising neoplasms. Indeed, this hypothesis is the basis for the concept of immune surveillance, which views CMI as the effector mechanism for eliminating spontaneously arising neoplastic clones.

The principal methods of tumor cytolysis have been elucidated through in vitro studies and involve direct T cell–mediated cytotoxicity, antibody-dependent cell-mediated cytotoxicity (ADCC), and natural killer cell cytolysis of tumor cells. Cytotoxic T lymphocytes (CTL) can be generated in response to specific membrane-associated antigens on tumor cells or foreign grafts. CTLs are capable of lysing the sensitizing tumor cells through direct cellular contact. In vitro studies with rodents have clearly shown the effector cell to be the T lymphocyte and have also demonstrated the tumor specificity of cytolysis.

In contrast, the macrophage can be considered as both an antigen-specific and nonspecific cellular mediator of tumor cytolysis. Macrophages may specifically lyse tumor targets following interactions with lymphokines, or by serving as the effector cell in antibody-dependent cellular cytotoxicity (ADCC). In ADCC, specific antibodies to tumor membrane antigens serve to focus the effector cell on the tumor cell. Several cell types may participate as effectors of ADCC including killer (K) cells, which are lymphoid in origin but are devoid of the usual B- and T-cell surface markers, macrophages, and granulocytes. In addition, fully activated macrophages are capable of nonspecific tumoricidal activity without the requirement of an interposed antibody, through a nonphagocytic mechanism of cytolysis.

An additional subpopulation of lymphocytes with tumoricidal activity, called natural killer or NK cells, has been functionally characterized in humans and rodents (see reviews by Herberman and Holden, 1978; Herberman and Ortaldo, 1981). These blood cells have unique cell surface markers distinguishing them from other cytolytic effectors and are constitutively present in nonimmune animals. They are capable of spontaneously lysing tumor cells in vitro and respond to different immunomodulators than either T cells, B cells or macrophages. NK cells are circulating lymphocytes whose activity may be potentiated by a variety of chemical and biologic agents including interferon and interferon inducers.

THE TIER APPROACH TO ASSESSMENT OF IMMUNOLOGIC FUNCTION

Since a single immune function assay cannot be used to comprehensively evaluate deleterious effects on the immune system following exposure to chemicals or drugs, a flexible tier of sensitive in vivo and in vitro assays has been proposed to assess immunotoxicity in rodents (Dean et al., 1982a) and is currently being further refined and evaluated. The tier approach to immunotoxicity assessment consists of a screening panel assessing three parameters (TIER I), which enables the identification of compounds that may produce immune alterations. Agents testing positive in TIER I assays can be further evaluated with assays selected from a more comprehensive panel (TIER II). TIER II assays allow an in-depth evaluation of the underlying mechanism(s) of immunotoxicity. Since most immune function assays require a working knowledge of the complex interactions and functions of the immune system, it is recommended that a competent immunologist assist with any evaluation of immunotoxicity.

Immunocompetency assessment should include the evaluation of immunopathology, CMI function, humoral immunity, MØ function, and host resistance. These parameters form the basis for the assays used in the TIER I screening panel (Table 9–9). If warranted by data obtained in the preliminary TIER I screen, additional immunologic tests can be selected from TIER II (Table 9–10) to examine the underlying mechanism(s) of a particular chemical or drug-induced immune alteration. If the pathophysiologic mechanism responsible for the deleterious effect on the target cell can be defined, it may be possible to synthesize new analogs of the compound that produce the desirable effects, but lack the immunoalterative effects.

The number of immunologic tests available or under development to study altered immune function is extensive. The procedures in general use to evaluate immune function following exposure to chemicals and drugs have been described in detail (Dean et al., 1979b; Luster et al.,

Table 9–9. SCREENING PANEL (TIER I) FOR DETECTING IMMUNE ALTERATION FOLLOWING CHEMICAL AND DRUG EXPOSURE IN RODENTS

PARAMETER	PROCEDURES PERFORMED
Immunopathology	Hematology—complete blood count and white blood cell differential Weights—body, spleen, thymus, kidney, adrenal Histology—spleen, thymus, bone marrow, lymph node, adrenal Spleen and bone marrow cellularity
Cell-mediated immunity	Lymphocyte blastogenesis in response to mitogens (PHA or Con A and LPS) and allogeneic leukocytes (mixed leukocyte response) Natural killer cell activity
Humoral immunity	Antibody plaque forming cell response to sheep erythrocytes (IgM) or specific antibody level

1982b). Assays in TIER I represent a general immunologic screen and offer a means of assessing compounds for their immunotoxic potential. These methods in TIER I are well defined for both mice and rats, and are frequently used in the clinical immunologic evaluation of humans. If the immune function data obtained from the TIER I panel are negative, there can be reasonable confidence regarding the safety of the drug or chemical for the immune system under the conditions and dosages defined in the screen. If conservative extrapolations are made using data from appropriate and clinically relevant immune function and host challenge assays, the most accurate estimate possible of chemical safety relative to the immune system will be obtained.

The following is a brief description of the tests currently utilized to assess the immunomodulatory potential of a suspect agent.

Immunopathology

Lymphoid organ weight, cellularity, and histopathology are useful in initially screening the immunomodulatory potential of an environmental agent or drug in rodents. Thymic and splenic weights, which are best expressed as organ-to-body-weight ratios, may be indicators of immune dysfunction. Thymic atrophy occurs following exposure to many chemicals and appears to be a useful indicator of chemical insult to the immune system; however, thymic atrophy alone is not necessarily a specific indicator of immu-

Table 9–10. COMPREHENSIVE PANEL (TIER II) FOR FURTHER CHARACTERIZING IMMUNE ALTERATIONS FOLLOWING CHEMICAL OR DRUG EXPOSURE

PARAMETER	PROCEDURES PERFORMED
Immunopathology	Cell surface marker profile (% T, B, MØ; T-cell subsets)
Host resistance	*Listeria monocytogenes* challenge Susceptibility to transplantable syngeneic tumor (TD 10–20 of PYB6 sarcoma or B16F10 melanoma) *Streptococcus* challenge Influenza challenge
Cell-mediated immunity	Lymphokine quantitation Cytotoxic T lymphocyte function Antibody-dependent cellular cytotoxicity
Humoral immunity	B-cell progenitor-cell quantitation Primary antibody response (IgM) to T-independent (LPS) antigen and secondary antibody response (IgG) to T-dependent antigen (SRBC) Mishell-Dutton assay
Macrophage function*	Quantitation of peritoneal macrophase cell number and phagocytosis ability Macrophage ectoenzyme levels Cytolysis of tumor target cells Bactericidal activity
Granulocyte function	NBT reduction
Bone marrow	Pluripotent stem cell quantitation Granulocyte/macrophage progenitor quantitation

* Utilizes both resident and activated peritoneal macrophages.

nosuppression since stress, severe weight loss, or general toxicity can also induce similar thymic lesions. Cellularity and histologic studies of bone marrow, spleen, and lymph nodes are also recommended. Splenic weights and cellularity may be decreased as a result of lymphoid depletion or markedly increased by extramedullary hematopoiesis since the spleen retains its hematopoietic potential during adult life. Histologic evaluation of the spleen is often helpful in determining the nature of a weight change. For example, following the introduction of an antibody-inducing antigen, there is a rapid increase in both the size and number of germinal centers. Lack of a germinal center reaction is a common finding following the administration of certain immunosuppressive drugs, chemicals and radiation, and is accompanied by a decreased ability of the animal to produce IgG antibodies. In contrast, the induction of cell-mediated immunity by antigen results in a massive proliferation (i.e., 50- to 100-fold increase) in the cells within the paracortex of lymph nodes. Both proliferation and recruitment of new cells to the paracortex occur. The use of drugs that suppress CMI depresses this massive cellular expansion within the paracortical region.

Another potentially useful procedure in immunopathology is quantitation of lymphocyte subpopulations. Specific surface markers and receptors on macrophages and lymphocytes are well characterized in rodents and humans (see Table 9–3). One method for quantitating splenic leukocyte subpopulations in mice uses fluorochrome-conjugated antisera against specific cell surface antigens identifying B cells (Ig), T cells (Thy-1 and Lyt-1,2,3), and MØs (MAC-1).

Cell-Mediated Immunity

While the previously mentioned procedures allow quantitation of leukocyte populations, they do not allow an assessment of the functional capacity of these cells. Several assays are available to examine cell-mediated immunologic functions (for detailed methods see Luster et al., 1982b). These include both in vivo (e.g., delayed hypersensitivity, graft-versus-host reactions, or skin graft rejection) and in vitro techniques (e.g., lymphoproliferation and lymphokine production). Historically, CMI has been examined using delayed-type cutaneous hypersensitivity (DTH) responses. Current approaches include measuring the in vitro lymphoproliferative responses to mitogens and allogeneic leukocytes in mixed leukocyte cultures (MLC). Values obtained from animals exposed to several doses of chemical are analyzed and compared with values from vehicle-treated controls.

Lymphoproliferative responses are widely used in assessing CMI. The lymphocyte proliferation assay utilizes mitogens (e.g., stimulants such as plant lectins and bacterial products) or antigens (e.g., tissue or soluble antigens) to stimulate proliferation in selective lymphocyte populations. Proliferation is quantitated by incorporation of tritiated thymidine into lymphoblast DNA. In some instances animals treated with immunosuppressants will exhibit depressed proliferative responses can be seen when normal numbers of lymphocytes are present, thus indicating a failure of cell function. Recent studies have demonstrated that altered responsiveness may also occur through suppression by regulatory subpopulations of macrophages and T lymphocytes (Katz, 1977). Other factors may also cause depressed proliferative responses. These include chemically induced cytotoxicity of lymphocytes or accessory cells; redistribution of lymphocyte subpopulations (i.e., T, B, or null cells), and maturational defects in lymphocyte development. The lymphoproliferative assays are reliable predictors of immune alteration and are widely used in clinical medicine.

Assessment of Humoral Immunity

There are a variety of methods to quantitate immunoglobulins (Igs) and specific antibodies. A disadvantage of merely quantitating Ig levels is that the half-life of some immunoglobulins may exceed the subchronic (14-day) exposure period, thus rendering the method insensitive to change in short-term studies. However, quantitating immunoglobulin levels is an acceptable procedure for chronic dosing studies, although it may lack the predictive ability of methods that measure specific antibody responses following antigenic challenge.

Assessment of a specific immune response following challenge with a novel antigen such as sheep erythrocytes (SRBC) or bovine gamma globulin has more commonly been used in immunotoxicity assessment. Antigenic challenge is usually performed following exposure to the chemical or drug. The immune response to the antigen can be quantitated either by measuring serum antibody titers or by determining the number of splenic lymphocytes producing antibody to the specific eliciting antigen. Both methods are acceptable, and the former methodology can be quantitated by hemagglutination, complement lysis, or antibody precipitin procedures. Enzyme-linked immunosorbent assays (ELISA) and radioimmunoassay methodology provide even more sensitive methods for quantitating specific serum antibodies and, in addition, lend themselves to automation.

We prefer the method of quantitating numbers of splenic lymphocytes producing antibody to a specific eliciting antigen. In this procedure, single cell suspensions of splenocytes from animals previously exposed to sheep erythrocytes (SRBC) are mixed with complement and SRBC in a specialized hemocytometer. After incubation, plaques (clear areas) indicative of sheep erythrocyte lysis occur circumscribing the cells producing the specific antibody. If one adds an anti-IgG antisera to the mixtures described above, the number of cells producing IgG type antibodies can be quantitated as well. These assays are sensitive, simple, and useful in characterizing a variety of chemical- and drug-induced lesions in the humoral immune response.

Macrophage Function Assays

Macrophages not only provide nonspecific phagocytic functions but are also specifically directed and regulated by lymphocytes through lymphokines. In addition, they are involved in cellular interactions and the elaboration of products (i.e., prostaglandins and monokines) that have feedback and regulatory roles in immune responses. Macrophage functions include phagocytosis, intracellular killing of infectious agents, antigen processing and presentation, interferon production, ecotoenzyme production, and cytostasis and cytolysis of virally infected or neoplastically transformed cells. Obviously, an evaluation of MØ function is essential in immune assessment. Chemical exposure may alter basal activity or the ability of MØ to respond to activation stimulants. Thus, macrophage function in chemical- or drug-exposed mice should be assessed in resident and activated macrophages. Assays quantitating phagocytosis and inhibition of tumor cell growth are preferred for TIER I analysis of MØ function. Assays defining MØ activation can be utilized to further characterize impairment of MØ function. Most of these functional tests can be readily quantitated and are described in a recent review (Adams and Dean, 1982).

Granulocyte Function

Granulocyte function can be assessed by measuring physiologic activities such as phagocytosis, chemotactic activity, bactericidal activity, or nitro blue tetrazolium (NBT) dye reduction. Perhaps the best single assay is the NBT dye reduction procedure, which has been extensively employed in the diagnosis of persons with chronic granulomatous disease. Failure of granulocytes to reduce NBT was found to correlate with an impaired enzymatic ability to kill phagocytosed bacteria. The number of granulocytes reducing dye can be easily quantitated histo-

chemically. This procedure is included in the TIER II panel and can be utilized if altered bacterial resistance is observed in the presence of normal CMI, HI, and macrophage function.

Bone Marrow Progenitors

Bone marrow hypoplasia is a significant complication of cancer chemotherapy and has also been implicated as a result of exposure to numerous drugs and environmental agents. The bone marrow contains pluripotent stem cells capable of differentiating along hematopoietic lines giving rise to lymphocytes, macrophages, or granulocytes. Chemical toxicity to progenitor cells, which ordinarily possess impressive proliferative capacity, can result in a magnification of chemically induced lesions, which may ultimately be expressed as altered host resistance. During the past decade, a variety of in vitro culture techniques have been developed for quantitating precursors for all the hematopoietic cell lines. Examination of colony formation by hematopoietic progenitor cells following exposure to various agents has proven to be a sensitive indicator of toxicity; therefore, bone marrow cellularity (TIER I) and progenitor cell assays (TIER II) are included as an integral part of the panels.

One method for quantitating murine pluripotent stem cells is by injecting bone marrow cells into irradiated recipients and subsequently counting the number of colonies forming in the spleen. In vitro assays quantitating progenitor cells are also available. Committed progenitor cells can be stimulated to form colonies in semisolid media by adding appropriate growth factors to the culture medium. Currently, clonal progenitor assays exist for quantitating B lymphocyte, T lymphocyte, macrophage-granulocyte, megakaryocyte, eosinophil, and erythroid precursors.

Challenge Models

A simple method for detecting immunomodulatory chemicals or drugs is to challenge the chemically exposed animal with an infectious agent. This procedure provides a general approach to determine whether the chemical interferes with host resistance to pathogens. Analysis of host susceptibility to carefully selected pathogens constitutes a holistic approach that can aid in characterizing immune dysfunctions.

Challenge with Salmonella typhimurium, Klebsiella pneumoniae, Escherichia coli, Streptococcus pneumoniae or pyogenes, and Staphylococcus aureus; with facultative intracellular organisms such as Listeria monocytogenes and Candida albicans; or with influenza or herpes virus, allows assessment of humoral or cell-mediated immune resistance. Immune defense to extracellular organisms requires the interaction of T lymphocytes, B lymphocytes, and macrophages for the production of specific antibodies that may activate the complement system to aid in phagocytosis and/or lysis. Antibodies also can directly neutralize some bacteria and viruses. Resistance to intracellular organisms requires induction of CMI through T-lymphocyte and macrophage interactions, which results in the production of lymphokines and further facilitates the bactericidal activities of macrophages. A chemical- or drug-induced lesion in any of these cells or a disruption of their activation or ability to interact with each other could result in an enhanced susceptibility.

Resistance to transplantable syngeneic or semisyngeneic tumor cells is also a sensitive parameter for detecting altered host resistance following chemical exposure (Dean *et al.*, 1982a). The tumor models used include PYB6 fibrosarcoma and B16F10 melanoma. Almost any tumor model in which resistance is dependent on T-cell immunity or natural cytotoxicity can be employed.

APPROACHES TO HYPERSENSITIVITY ASSESSMENT

Another consideration in immunotoxicity assessment involves evaluating the potential of drugs and chemicals to induce allergic responses. There are three principal experimental models for evaluating the allergenic potential of an agent. The first is the Draize test (described in Klecak, 1983). In this assay, guinea pigs are exposed to the agent in question intradermally, rested, and then rechallenged by intradermal injection of the agent at a virgin site. Allergic responses, indicated by erythema and edema, are subsequently quantitated. The Buehler occluded-patch test (Ritz and Buehler, 1980) is similar, except the test agent is applied by an occluded patch rather than by an intradermal injection.

A more rigorous method for experimentally determining the allergenic potential of a compound is the Magnusson and Kligman guinea pig maximization test (Magnusson and Kligman, 1969). Animals are sensitized by subcutaneous injection with and without complete Freund's adjuvant followed by further sensitization by occluded patch. Rechallenge is by topical application with an occluded patch two weeks following the last challenge. The site is evaluated for a response 24 hours after removal of the patch. For a more complete discussion of the various testing procedures see Klecak (1983).

Two principal clinical tests are utilized for detecting immediate hypersensitivity in humans. The most common is skin testing (reviewed by Norman, 1976) in which a patch of skin is scratched or pricked followed by topical application of the suspect agent. Alternatively, the agent can be administered intradermally or by an occluded patch and the individual monitored for the development of an allergic reaction. By monitoring of both the time course and appearance of the elicited reactions, these assays can be used to distinguish between type I, II, or IV allergic reactions.

In humans, immediate hypersensitivity responses are mediated by IgE; thus, as an alternative to actual challenge with a suspected allergen, the individual can be evaluated for the presence of specific IgE antibodies in a radioallergosorbent test (RAST). Briefly, suspected allergens are immobilized on filter paper disks and the disks incubated with serum from the individual. This is followed by addition of radiolabeled anti-IgE antiserum. If an individual has IgE antibodies directed against the test agent, they will bind to the allergin-impregnated disk, and these bound antibodies will subsequently bind the radiolabeled anti-IgE antibodies. By determination of the amount of radioactivity bound to the disk, the level of specific IgE antibody to the test allergen in the patients serum can be determined.

AGENTS THAT ALTER THE IMMUNE RESPONSE

Allergy Induced by Chemicals and Metals

The problem of occupational and environmental hypersensitivity is now widely recognized. Industrial workers and consumers are exposed to many materials capable of inducing asthma, hypersensitivity, and contact dermatitis. This section will deal with the problems of sensitization to environmental contaminants followed by a detailed discussion of some of the classes of compounds of most concern.

Immunologic Lung Disease. One of the major types of hypersensitivity observed in an industrial setting is asthma. In the United States, the exact proportion of asthma cases with an occupational or environmental link is unknown. However, estimates from other industrialized nations suggest that 2 percent of asthma cases are of industrial origin. The Japanese have determined that 15 percent of asthma in men may be directly attributable to industrial exposure. Since 3 to 5 percent of the U.S. population suffers from asthma, the question of occupational-induced asthma is of concern.

Table 9–11.   **EXAMPLES OF AGENTS THAT INDUCE ALLERGIC REACTIONS**

COMPOUND	EXPOSURE	TYPE OF REACTION	REFERENCE
Formaldehyde	Disinfectants, cosmetics, deodorants, paper, dyes, photography, textiles, inks, wood products, resins	Type IV	Maibach, 1983
Phthalic anhydrides	Saccharin production	Type I	Bernstein et al., 1982
B. subtilis	Detergents	Type I	Luster and Dean, 1982
Pesticides	Food, exterminators	Type I, IV	Ercegovich, 1973
Ethylenediamine	Plastic industry	Type I	Popa et al., 1969
Food additives (azodyes, BHT, BHA)	Ingestion of processed foods	Type I	Juhlin, 1980
Antimicrobials (e.g., Parabene, EDTA, mercurials)	Cosmetics, shampoos, creams, lotions	Type IV	Schorr, 1971; Baer et al., 1973
Resins and plasticizers (toluene diisocyanate, trimellitic anhydride)	Plastics, glues, nail lacquers, wood products, resins	Type I, IV	Patterson et al., 1982 Bernstein, 1982
Platinum compounds	Metal refining	Type I	Luster and Dean, 1982
Nickel	Jewelry, garment fastners	Type I, IV	Baer et al., 1973 Wahlberg, 1976
Chromium	Leather products, printing	Type IV	Peltonen and Fräki, 1983
Gold, mercury	Medicinal treatments, photography	Type II, III, IV	Druet et al., 1982 Baer et al., 1973
Beryllium	Manufacture of alloys	Type I, IV	Reeves and Preuss, 1984
Drugs (penicillin, quinidine, tetracycline)	Medicinal treatments	Type I, II, III, or IV	DeWeck, 1978 Parker, 1982 Van Arsdel, 1981

While there are no overall figures for the United States, some data are available concerning asthma induction by industrial exposure to specific compounds (for review, *see* Luster and Dean, 1982). For example, 5 percent of workers exposed to the chemical toluene diisocyanate (TDI) develop asthma. Studies in the detergent industry indicate that 2 percent of workers exposed to enzymes from *Bacillus subtilis,* which is used in the manufacture of enzyme-containing detergents, develop asthma. In addition, it has been found that direct industrial exposure in the workplace is not necessary for development of this condition. Living near a plant utilizing these agents may result in sufficient exposure to develop allergy (e.g., TDI). Table 9–11 lists several agents that have been shown to induce allergic reactions along with the most common sources of exposure.

Allergic Contact Dermatitis. Another major type of allergic reaction to environmental agents is allergic contact dermatitis, a type IV reaction (see discussion of Gell and Coombs classification) mediated by sensitized T lymphocytes. Symptoms include a red rash, swelling, itching, and possibly blisters. A variety of substances may evoke this type of reaction, including poison ivy, drugs, cosmetics, certain metals (i.e.,

nickel, chromates), and other chemicals (see Table 9–11). In allergic contact dermatitis, symptoms may appear seven to ten days following the initial exposure to the allergen, but more often the reaction develops after several years of continued low-level exposure. Once sensitized, contact with the offending agent will produce symptoms within 24 to 48 hours. Patch tests (see above) are the preferred assay for diagnosing the specific causative agent(s).

A common criterion of most agents inducing contact hypersensitivity is a low molecular weight, usually less than 500 to 1000 MW. In most cases, the offending agent is not sufficient to induce the allergic reaction itself, but must be conjugated to a protein to induce sensitization. This process is known as haptenization, and the small-molecular-weight compound is known as a *hapten,* while the protein to which it is conjugated is known as a *carrier.* The plasticizer, TDI, sensitizes in this manner. Presumably, the sensitizing agent acts *in vivo* to haptenate self-proteins, and this haptenated self-protein serves as the stimulus for generation of the allergic immune response. Some chemicals may induce contact hypersensitivity only after interacting with sunlight (i.e., photoallergy). This topic has been recently reviewed by Morison and

Kochevar (1983). In photo-induced allergies, the immune response is thought to be directed against antigens that arise after the chemical, one of its metabolites, or an altered host molecule absorbs light energy. The prototype photoallergic chemical is tetrachlorosalicylanilide, an antibacterial agent in soaps.

Chemicals That Are Allergenic. *Plastics and Resins.* Toluene diisocyanate (TDI) is representative of a class of compounds used in the manufacture of plastics and resins. TDI is highly reactive with amino groups and can readily haptenate self-proteins and produce allergic reactions. Indeed, both asthma and contact dermatitis have been demonstrated in workers exposed to TDI. Recently, an animal model for TDI sensitization using both dermal and inhalation exposure was developed in guinea pigs (Karol *et al.*, 1980). In this model, sensitization was dependent on exposure to a threshold concentration of TDI vapor for the induction of pulmonary sensitivity and reaginic antibody production. When animals were exposed to the same total amount of TDI as those developing hypersensitivity, but at a lower level for a longer period of time, no allergic responses were noted (Karol, personal communication). This correlated well with human findings where workers exposed to high levels of TDI (i.e., spills or splashes) developed a pulmonary response, while workers exposed to continuous low levels of TDI remained free from TDI-induced allergic reactions. Inhalation exposure did not appear to be mandatory for the development of pulmonary hypersensitivity, since dermal exposure sensitized guinea pigs such that subsequent inhalation of TDI resulted in a pulmonary response (Karol *et al.*, 1981).

With most allergens, removal of the offending agent abrogates the allergic response. Interestingly, patients with TDI-induced asthma continue to be symptomatic for months and even years after cessation of TDI exposure. The reason for this is unknown, but it is thought that TDI may cause the airways to become hyperreactive to many agents such as smoke and other air pollutants. In addition, some individuals susceptible to TDI-induced asthma develop crossreactivity to other diisocyanates (e.g., diphenylmethane diisocyanate) to which they have never been exposed.

Textile Finishes. Another class of chemicals that has been demonstrated to induce allergy is the resin finishes used in the textile industry to improve the wrinkle resistance and durability of fabrics. Probably the most prevalent and best studied compound in this field has been formaldehyde. This highly reactive, low-molecular-weight compound is extremely soluble in water and haptenates human proteins quite easily (Maibach, 1983). When formaldehyde resins

were first used in the garment industry to provide wrinkle-resistant finishes, many workers developed allergic reactions due to the free formaldehyde. Fabrics are now allowed time to gas-off the formaldehyde or are washed prior to being used.

Sensitization with formaldehyde can induce type IV (contact dermatitis) reactions. Sensitive individuals may have difficulty avoiding formaldehyde exposure. There have been reports of individuals so sensitive that they will react to formaldehyde found in the newsprint dyes (free formaldehyde of 0.02 percent) and photographic films and papers. When one considers the ubiquitous nature of formaldehyde and its increasing usage in everyday products (furniture, auto upholstery, cosmetics, resins), the magnitude of the problem becomes apparent (for review, *see* Cronin, 1980).

Cosmetics. Another group of chemicals that induces hypersensitivity is the antimicrobials used in cosmetics. These include paraben esters, sorbic acid, phenolics (e.g., hexachlorophene), organic mercurials, quaternary ammonia compounds, ethylenediamine tetraacetate (EDTA), and formaldehyde (for review, *see* Schorr, 1971). Cosmetics are applied topically; thus, the major type of reaction is a contact dermatitis (type IV) reaction.

Metals. Metals have also been implicated in many hypersensitivity responses. Some individuals exposed to nickel in costume jewelry and metal garment fasteners have developed contact hypersensitivity. It has been estimated that 5 percent of all eczema can be linked to contact with nickel-containing compounds. Occupational hypersensitivity to beryllium has also been noted. Beryllium was previously used to coat fluorescent lamps, which led to skin sensitization when shards of broken lamps became embedded under the skin. This use of beryllium has since been discontinued. Another reaction associated with beryllium exposure thought to involve immune hypersensitivity is the chronic pulmonary syndrome berylliosis. This disease is frequently fatal and involves cough, chest pain, and a chronic progressive pneumonitis. Upon biopsy, interstitial granulomas are found. Other metals known to cause hypersensitivity responses include platinum, chromium (from the tanning of the leather products and the printing industry), and mercury and gold (usually from the medicinal use of gold salts). This subject has been extensively reviewed by IARC (1981).

Autoimmunity Induced by Chemicals and Metals

Haptenization of proteins is the most probable mechanism by which chemicals and metals cause allergic sensitization. It is interesting to note that many drugs may also haptenate self-proteins and result in autoimmune reactions rather than hypersensitivity. This difference is probably attributed to the different routes of exposure, since individuals are exposed to metals and chemicals mainly through contact or inhalation. This type of exposure results in haptenization of cells in the skin and mucous membranes and leads to the development of hypersensitivity or dermatitis. The main exposure to drugs, however, is systemically, which may predispose to development of an autoimmune response. This is not to imply that chemicals and metals are devoid of autoimmune-inducing potential. For example, an individual who had been exposed to the pesticide Dieldrin developed immune hemolytic anemia. When blood from this person was analyzed, it was found to contain anti-Dieldrin antibodies bound to the red blood cells (RBCs). Presumably, the Dieldrin was binding to the RBCs, and this subsequently led to the autoimmune destruction of the RBCs (Hamilton *et al.*, 1978).

Heavy metals have also been implicated in autoimmune processes that may be classified as type II or type IV reactions. For example, gold salts and mercury-containing compounds can induce an immune complex glomerulonephritis (Druet *et al.*, 1982), or they may induce antiglomerular basement membrane antibodies resulting in glomerulonephritis similar to that seen in Goodpasture's disease. The mechanism by which heavy metals produce autoimmunity is unknown. One hypothesis views metals as haptens, while the second hypothesis suggests that metals alter the antigenicity of cellular proteins, rendering them "foreign" to the host. However, in mercury-induced glomerulonephritis in rabbits and gold salt-induced glomerulonephritis in humans, metals have not been observed localized at the site of the lesion (Druet *et al.*, 1982). These observations have led to a third hypothesis, which perceives metals as interfering with immune regulatory cells, resulting in the generation of an anti-self response. There is experimental evidence in support of the latter hypothesis. Weening *et al.* (1981) found that mercury was able to significantly inhibit the generation of suppressor T lymphocytes in PVG/c rats. It is plausible that metals may decrease the suppressor T lymphocyte balance necessary for preventing the formation of anti-self antibodies, thus leading to autoimmunity.

Many people are being exposed to chemicals, metals, and drugs, some of which are capable of inducing allergic reactions and autoimmunity. Therefore, an increasing amount of research emphasis should be placed on developing predictive rodent models, on a better understanding of types of agents that haptenate self-proteins,

and on mechanistic studies of how these compounds exhibit their effects.

Allergy and Autoimmunity Induced by Drugs

Clinically it is difficult to distinguish between immunologic and nonimmunologic reactions to drugs. In clinical diagnosis of drug or chemical allergy, certain guidelines strongly suggest an immunologic basis for an adverse drug reaction. These have been summarized by de Weck (1978) as follows: The reaction should (1) not resemble the pharmacologic reaction of the drug; (2) be elicited by minute amounts of the drug; (3) occur only after an induction period of at least five to seven days following primary exposure to the drug; (4) include symptoms classic for allergic reactions to natural macromolecular antigens (e.g., anaphylaxis, urticaria, serum sickness syndrome, asthma); (5) reappear promptly on readministration of the drug in small amounts; and (6) be reproduced by drugs possessing similar and cross-reacting chemical structure. Immunologic testing can in some instances verify the existence of drug hypersensitivity through the detection of antibodies or sensitized lymphocytes specific for the suspected allergen. More commonly, however, the immunologic basis for the reactivity is difficult to establish since an appropriate test antigen or reactive metabolite may be difficult to identify.

Penicillin. The β-lactam antibiotics (penicillin, semisynthetic penicillin, and cephalosporins) share a common molecular structure and are responsible for the majority of allergic reactions to drugs (for reviews, *see* de Weck, 1978; Ahlstedt *et al.*, 1980). Penicillin allergy has been studied in detail and much of our current knowledge on the induction and elicitation of drug hypersensitivity has been based on results obtained from studies of penicillin hypersensitivity.

There is a high frequency of anaphylactic reactions in patients demonstrating adverse reactions to penicillin, although these individuals do not usually have detectable serum antibody titers to penicillin itself. Instead, it appears that the biotransformation product of penicillin (e.g., the penicilloyl group) is capable of combining with self-proteins, which then act as effective inducers of an antibody response (Parker, 1982). Penicillin, itself, does not appear to be sufficiently immunogenic to elicit a response. Alternatively, commercially prepared penicillin solutions may contain high-molecular-weight contaminants that could serve as carriers for penicillin antigens, thereby increasing the immunogenicity of penicillin (Ahlstedt *et al.*, 1980). Additional sources of carrier molecules might include the gastrointestinal contents, bacteria or bacterial products, and autologous proteins.

Route of administration also appears to be an important consideration in development of penicillin allergy. There is, for example, a higher frequency of allergic reactions following intramuscular compared to oral administration (Ahlstedt et al., 1980; Van Arsdel, 1981).

Penicillin allergy can be of either the immediate or delayed type. Of these, the immediate type, particularly those involving anaphylaxis, can be life-threatening. Penicillin hypersensitivity is the most frequent cause of anaphylaxis in man. Therefore, it is of clinical importance to be able to identify those patients at risk for possible adverse reactions to penicillin. Usually a patient's history concerning drug allergy provides the major basis for this assessment; however, skin testing and, more recently, radioallergosorbent tests (RAST) and enzyme-linked immunosorbent assays (ELISA) measuring serum IgE to penicilloyl-polylysine, penicillin, and penicilloic acid have been used to identify individuals at risk (Ahlstedt et al., 1980; Parker, 1982). In addition to anaphylaxis, penicillin and other β-lactams have been implicated in the clinical incidence of several types of hypersensitivity reactions including serum sickness, urticaria, allergic fever, hemolytic anemia, rashes, allergic contact dermatitis, and possible renal disease following the administration of antibiotics containing β-lactam rings. Penicillin may, in fact, produce nephropathy in renal tubules suggestive of a drug-induced autoimmune reaction in which autoantibodies to tubular epithelial basement membranes can be demonstrated (Border et al., 1974; Parker, 1982).

Methyldopa. Methyldopa is extensively used in the treatment of essential hypertension. Allergic reactions may occur in patients receiving methyldopa over extended periods. Perhaps the most serious of these are a number of reported cases of hemolytic anemia. This drug-induced autoimmune reaction usually regresses upon discontinuation of the drug (Parker, 1982; Van Arsdel, 1981). In contrast to penicillin-induced hemolytic anemia, where penicillin acts as a hapten, methyldopa is not haptenic (Parker, 1982), but appears instead to modify erythrocyte surface antigens. IgG against modified erythrocyte surface antigens can be demonstrated in the blood of these patients. Although this autoantibody response is present in only about 1 percent of patients receiving chronic high dosages of methyldopa, other indications of immune reactivity have been more prevalent, in particular, the development of positive direct antiglobulin Coombs reactivity. There have also been reports of positive tests for lupus and rheumatoid factor (Parker, 1982) in patients receiving methyldopa.

Salicylates. Aspirin (acetylsalicylic acid) is one of the most widely used drugs in the world. It is utilized extensively for its analgesic, antipyretic, and antiinflammatory properties. Aspirin may occasionally produce symptoms such as urticaria, rhinitis, and bronchospasm, which mimic drug allergy (e.g., pseudoallergy), although the immunologic bases for these symptoms remain doubtful. Even though commercial aspirin contains potentially immunogenic compounds to which patients could become sensitized, and despite the eosinophilia usually observed in aspirin-intolerant patients, no distinct immunologic mechanisms for this reactivity have been demonstrated (de Weck, 1978). The weight of the evidence indicates a nonimmunologic basis for aspirin intolerance. This includes the observation that molecularly unrelated drugs produce responses similar to aspirin in aspirin-sensitive individuals while molecularly similar drugs (e.g., sodium salicylate) do not (Settipane, 1981). Many of the symptoms of aspirin intolerance appear to be related to an inhibition of the cyclooxygenase oxidative pathway for prostaglandin synthesis, which results in alterations in the relative amounts of prostaglandins and leukotrienes formed (Flower et al., 1980).

Immunosuppression

Benzene. Benzene exposure has frequently been associated with myelotoxicity expressed as leukopenia, pancytopenia, anemia, aplastic or hypoplastic bone marrow, lymphocytopenia, granulocytopenia, and thrombocytopenia (see review, IARC Monograph, 1982). In workers occupationally exposed to benzene, a strong correlation was noted between the most frequently cited symptom, lymphocytopenia, and abnormal immunologic parameters. Benzene exposure in rabbits, rats, and mice resulted in anemia, hypoplastic bone marrow, and dose-related lymphocytopenia. Myelotoxicity was also correlated with the appearance of benzene metabolites in the bone marrow, and it is now evident that bone marrow can metabolize benzene (see review, IARC Monograph, 1982).

Studies in benzene-exposed rabbits have described increased susceptibility to tuberculosis and pneumonia as well as a reduced antibody response to bacterial antigens (IARC Monograph, 1982). Wierda et al. (1981) observed that exposure of C57B16 mice to benzene inhibited both antibody production and the mitogenic response of lymphocytes. Thus, the altered immune parameters reported in experimental animals may explain why the terminal event in severe benzene toxicity is often an acute, overwhelming infection.

Evaluation of a large number of workers exposed to benzene revealed depressed levels of

Table 9–12. EFFECT OF POLYHALOGENATED AROMATIC HYDROCARBONS ON HOST RESISTANCE AND IMMUNE FUNCTIONS IN RODENTS*

PARAMETER	CHEMICAL			
	PCB	PBB	TCDD	TCDF
Host resistance to challenge with				
Bacteria	D	NE	D	—
Endotoxin	D	NE	D	—
Virus	D	—	D	—
Parasite	D	NE	—	—
Tumor cells	D	—	D	—
Cell-mediated immunity				
DTH	D	—	D	D
Lymphocyte proliferation	I	D	D	D
Humoral immunity				
PFCs (T-dependent antigen)	D	D	D	—
Antibody titer or Ig levels	D	D	D	—
Macrophage function	—	NE	NE	—

* Modified from Dean, J. H.; Luster, M. I.; Boorman, G. A.; Leubke, R. W.; and Laver, L. D.: Application of tumor, bacterial, and parasite susceptibility assays to study immune alterations induced by environmental chemicals. *Environ. Health Perspect.*, **43**:81–88, 1982.
I = increased; D = decreased; NE = no effect; — = not done; PBB = polybrominated biphenyls; PCB = polychlorinated biphenyls; TCDD = 2,3,7,8-tetrachlorodibenzo-*p*-dioxin; TCDF = tetrachlorodibenzofuran.

serum complement, IgG, and IgA, but not IgM. Thus, benzene appears to be an immunotoxicant for humans, although the magnitude of this effect and the exposure threshold for immunotoxicity remain to be established.

Halogenated Aromatic Hydrocarbons. There is substantial evidence that a number of isomers of polyhalogenated aromatics are carcinogenic, teratogenic, neurotoxic, and immunotoxic (*see* review, Kimbrough, 1980). Both mixtures and individual isomers of halogenated aromatic hydrocarbons have been studied, and their immunologic effects are summarized in Table 9–12 and described in the following sections.

Polychlorinated Biphenyls. Polychlorinated biphenyls (PCBs) have been used for over a half-century in plasticizers and other industrial applications and as a heat transfer medium in transformers. PCB mixtures have been reported to suppress immune responses and alter host defense mechanisms. The most common findings in laboratory animals exposed orally or cutaneously to sublethal levels of various PCB mixtures (e.g., Aroclors) have been severe atrophy of primary and secondary lymphoid organs, lower circulating immunoglobulin levels, and decreased specific antibody responses following immunization with antigens (Loose *et al.*, 1978; Thomas and Hinsdill, 1978; Vos *et al.*, 1980).

Effects of PCBs on CMI are inconclusive; both augmentation and suppression have been reported. Prenatal and adult exposure to PCBs

have been found to depress delayed-type cutaneous hypersensitivity (DTH) (Thomas and Hinsdill, 1980). However, graft-versus-host reactivity, T lymphocyte responses to mitogens, and proliferation of leukocytes in mixed leukocyte cultures (Silkworth and Loose, 1978, 1979) have been enhanced after PCB exposure. The augmentation of selected CMI assays may reflect a relative increase in T-cell numbers due to selective depletion of B cells or, alternatively, alterations in immunoregulation through alteration of the helper/suppressor cell balance.

Studies in which PCB-exposed animals were challenged with infectious agents have indicated decreased resistance in ducks to hepatitis virus and in mice to challenge with herpes simplex virus, ectromelia virus, *Plasmodium berghei*, *Listeria monocytogenes*, or *Salmonella typhimurium* (*see* review, Dean *et al.*, 1982c). The effect of PCB on tumor resistance in rodents is unclear since both augmentation and suppression have been reported (Koller, 1975; Kerkvliet and Kimeldorf, 1977).

Human exposure to PCB has been reported in Japan and China where PCB-contaminated rice oil was consumed. In Japan (Yusho accident), PCB-exposed individuals exhibited chloracne and were more susceptible to respiratory infections (Shigematsu *et al.*, 1978). Decreased serum Ig levels were also observed. In a clinical study of individuals exposed to PCB-contaminated rice oil in China (Chang *et al.*, 1980), a decreased

DTH response to *Streptococcus* antigens was observed as well as altered T-cell numbers and function.

Polybrominated Biphenyls. Firemaster BP-6 and FF-1 are commonly used flame retardants that consist of mixtures of polybrominated biphenyls (PBBs) containing primarily 2,4,5,2′,4′,5′-hexabromobiphenyl and 2,3,4,5,2′,4′,5′-heptabromobiphenyl. In Michigan, in 1973, Firemaster BP-6 was accidentally substituted for a magnesium oxide food supplement for livestock (Dunckel, 1975) and widespread pollution of the food chain occurred over a period of several months. There was prolonged PBB contamination of meat and dairy products in the area. These contaminated products were widely consumed, and high levels of PBB were subsequently found in the serum and adipose tissues of many Michigan dairy farmers, chemical workers, and local residents (Bekesi et al., 1978). A high percentage of Michigan dairy farm residents had abnormalities in a number of immune parameters that were not evident in Wisconsin control farm families. These included decreased peripheral T-cell numbers, increased numbers of lymphocytes without detectable membrane markers (i.e., so-called "null cells"), increased Ig levels, and hyperreactivity to recall antigens upon skin testing. Lymphoproliferative responses were depressed in some Michigan dairy farm residents. PBB plasma concentrations did not correlate with depressed immune responses in these individuals, although all had significantly elevated plasma PBB levels. Bekesi and associates (1986) have now confirmed their original observations in the 1976 study groups and have extended analysis to include 333 Michigan farm residents. A similar frequency of immunologic abnormalities was observed in the expanded population.

Animals experimentally exposed to PBB demonstrated depressed CMI and antibody responses to a wide variety of antigens. However, the CMI effects, which included suppression of lymphoproliferative responses and DTH, were not as severe as the suppression of antibody responses, since CMI effects occured only at near toxic dosages (Luster et al., 1978; Luster et al., 1980b) while antibody suppression occurred at lower concentrations. Host resistance to parasitic and bacterial challenge in PBB-exposed mice was not affected (*see* review, Dean et al., 1982c).

Dibenzodioxins. Rodents exposed to 2,3,7,8-tetrachlorodibenzo-p-dioxin (TCDD) (reviewed by McConnell, 1980, Vos et al., 1980) demonstrate severe thymus atrophy. Histologic evaluation of the thymus reveals cortical lymphoid depletion similar to cortisone-induced thymus atrophy. Depressed antibody responses, DTH, graft-versus-host, and lymphoproliferative responses were observed at slightly higher dosages of TCDD (see review, Thomas and Faith, 1985). In addition, increased susceptibility to challenge with the bacteria *Salmonella bern*, but not *Listeria monocytogenes* or *Pseudorabies* virus, was noted at low dosages (Thigpen et al., 1975). Depressed antibody responses and DTH were also observed in guinea pigs receiving cumulative dosages as low as 0.32 μg/kg over an eight-week period (Vos et al., 1973). Clark et al. (1983) observed depressed T-cell function following exposure of adult mice to TCDD, which was associated with an increase in suppressor T-lymphocyte expression and loss of T-lymphocyte cytotoxicity for tumor target cells. In recent studies of adult B6C3F1 mice exposed to TCDD, we observed depressed antibody (PFC) responses and depressed lymphoproliferative responses to mitogens without alterations in cytotoxicity for tumor cells or susceptibility to bacterial or tumor cell challenge (Dean and Lauer, 1984).

Exposure to TCDD during thymic organogenesis in rodents has resulted in more severe CMI suppression than that occurring following adult exposure. In some species, *in utero* exposure (via maternal dosing) appears to be necessary to induce maximum immunosuppression (Luster et al., 1981). At higher dosages, antibody responses and bone marrow stem cell numbers are depressed in most species. Administration of TCDD *in utero* also results in decreased resistance of offspring to bacterial and tumor cell challenge, which correlates with altered CMI (Luster et al., 1980b) in these mice.

In a recent study of 44 schoolchildren residing in the TCDD-contaminated area of Seveso, Italy (Reggiani, 1980) it was revealed that 20 children exhibited chloracne (a classic sign of TCDD toxicity), although their serum immunoglobulin levels and circulating complement levels were normal. Lymphoproliferative responses to T- and B-cell mitogens were significantly elevated, a finding frequently reported following low-level TCDD exposure in rodents. In an earlier clinical study of British workers from a chemical manufacturing plant who were accidentally exposed to TCDD, reduced levels of serum IgD and IgA and depressed lymphocyte responses to T-lymphocyte mitogens were observed (Ward, unpublished report). A correlation was suggested between chloracne and altered immune status in this study. The Air Force has recently completed the preliminary evaluation of the health and immune status of individuals involved in the aerosol use of Agent Orange in Vietnam (Ranch/Hand II study) to establish or refute health effects of TCDD exposure in humans (Lathrop et al., 1984). Immunologic abnormalities were not apparent in these studies.

Currently it is believed that TCDD-induced immunosuppression is mediated through a cytosolic receptor for TCDD. The TCDD receptor was originally described by Poland and Glover (1976) in hepatic cytosol and subsequently in thymic cytosol (Poland and Glover, 1980). Both genetic and structure-activity data indicate that TCDD-induced thymic atrophy is mediated through the TCDD cytosolic receptor protein since thymic atrophy segregates with the *Ah* locus; and halogenated congeners of TCDD that compete with [^{3}H]-TCDD for specific binding sites in thymic cytosol fractions produce thymic atrophy *in vivo* (Poland and Glover, 1980). The target for immunotoxicity is thought to principally be the thymic epithelial cells, as suggested by Clark et al. (1983) and Greenlee et al. (1985). TCDD receptor-mediated events in the thymus may include altered T-cell maturation and differentiation and may be the molecular basis for the thymus atrophy and immunotoxicity observed. Since the endocrine influence of thymic epithelium in adult animals and humans is poorly understood, immunosuppression observed in rodents following adult exposure to TCDD may also involve toxicity to the thymic epithelium.

TCDBF (2,3,7,8-tetrachlorodibenzofuran), another dibenzodioxin, has been identified in various preparations of commercial Aroclors (Vos et al., 1970) and shares the same magnitude of toxicity as TCDD. The similarity between TCDD and TCDBF in chemical structure suggests competition of these substances for the putative TCDD cytosol receptor. One might expect, therefore, that TCDBF would also be immunotoxic. In animal studies, TCDBF produced severe thymic atrophy in most species studied (Moore et al., 1976) and suppressed lymphocyte responses to mitogens, DTH to novel antigens, and lymphokine (MIF) production in adult guinea pigs (Luster et al., 1979a).

Polycyclic Aromatic Hydrocarbons (PAH). Polycyclic aromatic hydrocarbons are a ubiquitous class of chemicals produced during the combustion of fossil fuels. As a class, PAHs consist of three or more benzene rings fused in linear, angular, or cluster arrangements containing only carbon and hydrogen atoms. Exposure of mice to 3-methylcholanthrene (MCA), 1,2-benzanthrene, or 1,2,5,6-dibenzanthracene produces a marked depression in the serum antibody response to sheep erythrocytes (SRBC) (Malmgren et al., 1952). Subsequent studies have confirmed that MCA suppresses immune responses, resulting in long-lasting reductions in antibody-producing cells. A similar long-term

reduction in the response to SRBC was observed in mice exposed to 7,12-dimethylbenz[a]anthracene (DMBA) and benzo[a]pyrene (B[a]P): this depression persisted for more than 32 days after exposure (Stjernsward, 1966).

In our laboratory, B[a]P-exposed mice have been observed to have depressed responses to T- and B-cell mitogens, but not to alloantigenic stimulation (Dean et al., 1983a). Exposure to the noncarcinogenic congener, B[e]P, did not alter mitogen responses. Host susceptibility following challenge with syngeneic PYB6 tumor cells and the bacterium *Listeria monocytogenes* was also unaltered in B[a]P-exposed mice, as were DTH and allograft rejection following B[a]P exposure. These data suggest that T-cell immunocompetence was minimally affected. In contrast, the primary antibody plaque-forming cell responses to both T-dependent and T-independent antigens were severely depressed. Zwilling (1977) similarly noted unaltered skin graft rejection in hamsters following inhalation exposure to B[a]P-Fe$_2$O$_3$, despite severely depressed humoral antibody responses. *In utero* exposure to B[a]P resulted in a depressed anti-SRBC response, which persisted for up to eight weeks. Urso and Gengozian (1980) also found that exposure of pregnant mice to a single dose (100 to 150 μg/g body weight) of B[a]P resulted in severe suppression of antibody responses in pups shortly after birth. This suppression persisted for at least 78 weeks and was accompanied by an increased frequency of tumors in these mice during adulthood.

There are recent data suggesting that 3-methylcholanthrene exposure in mice suppresses T-cell proliferative responses to mitogens and the generation of cytotoxic T lymphocytes (Wojdani and Alfred, 1983). Prolongation of skin graft survival, an additional measure of CMI, has also been reported following administration of MCA (DiMarco et al., 1971), but was only observed if the grafting occurred 11 or more weeks after exposure, a time that corresponded to the appearance of tumors. Thus, it was not possible to ascertain whether this was a tumor or chemical-related effect.

Neonatal exposure of mice to another PAH, DMBA, suppressed both the primary (IgM) and secondary (IgG) antibody response, to SRBC, while exposure of adult mice to DMBA resulted in a kinetic shift in the IgM PFC response, although no change in magnitude of the response was observed (Ball, 1970). This observation conflicts with our recent studies in which murine exposure to DMBA suppressed the number of antibody-producing cells and CMI functions including NK and CTL cytotoxicity for up to two months (Ward et al., 1986). Therefore, DMBA exposure appears to result in long-lasting immunosuppression of CMI, HMI, and tumor resistance mechanisms.

There is a rapidly increasing body of evidence supporting the conclusion that carcinogenic PAHs produce severe, long-term immunotoxicity. This may be related to the structure of the carcinogenic PAHs, since immune alterations have not been observed following exposure to noncarcinogenic congeners.

Urethane. Urethane (ethyl carbamate) is a potent multipotential carcinogen in mice, rats, and hamsters, producing leukemia, lymphomas, lung adenomas, hepatomas, and melanomas (IARC Monograph, 1974). Exposure of mice to tumorigenic dosages of ethyl carbamate caused severe myelotoxicity, led to a marked suppression of natural killer cell activity, inhibited immune elimination of B16F10 melanoma cells, and increased metastatic tumor growth in the lungs (Luster *et al.*, 1982a). Exposure to the noncarcinogenic congener methyl carbamate did not alter immune parameters. Previous studies have demonstrated that exposure to aliphatic carcinogens, especially urethane, inhibited antibody response to SRBC (Malmgren *et al.*, 1952). Gorelik and Herberman (1981) found that exposure to urethane suppressed natural killer cell activity, which was accompanied by an increased frequency of spontaneous lung adenomas in susceptible mouse strains.

Phorbol Diesters. Phorbol diesters are a family of chemicals with potent tumor-promoting potential that produce adverse effects on lymphoid cells. 12-*O*-tetradecanoylphorbol-13-acetate (TPA) is the most active of the croton oil-derived phorbol diester tumor promoters. TPA is a potent promoter of multiple skin tumors *in vivo* and enhances transformation of fibroblast and rat embryo cell cultures *in vitro* following exposure to PAH carcinogens or oncogenic viruses. TPA produces multiple effects in leukocytes following *in vivo* (Dean *et al.*, 1982b; Murray *et al.*, 1984) and *in vitro* exposure. These effects include enhanced lymphocyte mitogenesis (Touraine *et al.*, 1977), macrophage membrane alterations, enhanced pinocytosis, increased tumor cell cytostasis (Grimm, *et al.*, 1980), and suppression of NK activity (Keller, 1979).

Depression of immunosurveillance has been suggested as an important etiologic factor in neoplasia and tumor development (Burnet, 1970). A decrease in thymus weight, T-cell numbers, lymphoproliferative responses to T- and B-cell mitogens, or allogeneic leukocytes (MLC), and decreased resistance to transplantable tumors in mice following TPA exposure was observed (Dean *et al.*, 1983b). Spontaneous NK cytotoxicity was reduced by >90 percent while the number of antibody PFCs per spleen, bone marrow cellularity, and progenitor cell numbers were unaffected. Recently, evidence has been presented for a cell surface receptor for TPA on murine T lymphocytes that may account for the selective toxicity of TPA for T cells. These effects are not observed when nonpromoting phorbols are used. It is our belief that TPA may alter lymphocyte differentiation, thus accounting for these immunologic alterations.

Insecticides. Insecticides examined for immunotoxicity in rodents can be grouped into three general classes: the organophosphates, including parathion, methylparathion, dichlorophos, and malathion; the carbamates, of which carbaryl (Sevin) has been primarily studied; and the organochlorine insecticides, which include DDT, Mirex, and representatives of the chlorinated cyclodines, aldrin, and lindane. Increasing evidence suggests that certain insecticides can alter immune function (*see* review by Street, 1981).

Organophosphate insecticides, for example, have been shown to be immunosuppressive in certain species. Street and Sharma (1974) and Street (1981) observed that a 28-day oral exposure of rabbits to methylparathion (1.5 mg/kg/day) produced a marked reduction in splenic germinal centers following antigenic stimulation, as well as thymus cortical atrophy, and a reduced DTH response to tuberculin. Similarly, Fan (*see* Street, 1981) noted a dose-related increase in mortality following challenge with *Salmonella typhimurium,* and a depressed response to mitogens following methylparathion exposure. In contrast, Wiltrout (see Street, 1981) observed that another member of this class of insecticides, parathion, produced depression of humoral immunity, but only when administered at near-lethal levels. Studies by Desi *et al.* (1978) found that exposure to malathion depressed antibody responses to *Salmonella typhi.* Along quite different lines, Vijay (*see* Street, 1981) found that rats immunized with malathion developed reaginic antibodies but not antibodies of the IgG class. Desi *et al.* (1980) found that rabbits exposed to dichlorophos had depressed humoral antibody responses and tuberculin skin test reactivity. The dosage utilized in this study was near the LD50, and no general toxicity data were provided; thus, it is difficult to separate the immunosuppression observed from general toxicity in these animals.

In general, the evidence is quite good that organophosphate insecticides can suppress the immune response. As pesticides are stable, remaining for long periods in the environment, and can become concentrated in the food chain, it is prudent to be concerned about their potential for immunotoxicity.

The carbamate insecticide carbaryl (Sevin) has been frequently studied as an immunotoxicant. As early as 1971, Perelygin (*see* Street, 1981) observed that exposure of albino rats and rabbits to carbaryl at 20 mg/kg depressed antibody responses and phagocytosis by granulocytes. Subsequent studies in rats and chickens reported that orally administered Sevin resulted in an acute and sometimes prolonged depression of splenic germinal center formation and antibody production (*see* Street, 1981). Previously reported effects of carbaryl on granulocyte phagocytosis were confirmed and found to be prolonged for up to nine months following exposure to the chemical. In contrast to studies from Soviet or western European laboratories, which have demonstrated that carbaryl is immunosuppressive, most studies performed in this country have found no consistent indication of immunosuppression except at near-lethal doses (Street and Sharma, 1974; Street, 1981). In general, carbamate insecticides have little or no immunotoxicity.

Accumulating data suggest that the organochlorine insecticides may alter immune function (*see* review by Koller, 1979). Class representatives examined in rodents include DDT, Mirex, aldrin, and lindane. Depressed serum antibody titers against ovalbumin were observed in rats orally exposed to 200 ppm of DDT (*see* Street, 1981). In contrast, guinea pigs and rats fed DDT had normal levels of antitoxin antibody and γ-globulin, and a reduced propensity to develop anaphylaxis, which correlated with a decreased number of mast cells (Gabliks *et al.*, 1975). Likewise, chickens exposed to DDT or Mirex had significantly depressed levels of IgG and IgM, although specific antibody responses were normal (Street, 1981). In the studies of Street and Sharma (1974) and Street (1981), a four-week exposure to DDT resulted in a reduced number of germinal centers in lymph nodes, thymus cortical atrophy, and suppression of CMI. Most studies have focused on the effects of DDT on specific antibody responses. It appears that DDT produces slight to negligible immunotoxicity. However, the effects of DDT on macrophage function, CMI, and host resistance have not been intensively investigated and appear to be an open question.

Studies by Rao and Glick (1977) of chickens exposed to DDT or Mirex revealed a marked reduction in total antibody production and serum IgG level, although serum IgM levels were elevated. The alteration in IgG levels was thought to be related to altered T-cell function. Likewise, studies of rabbits exposed to lindane demonstrated a depressed antibody response to *Salmonella typhi* antigen (Desi *et al.*, 1978). Leukopenia and impaired leukocyte phagocytosis were also observed following the oral administration of lindane (Evdokimov, 1974).

Airborne Pollutants. The lungs are a primary target organ for insult by airborne chemicals of environmental and immunologic concern and have been shown to be vulnerable to a wide range of substances producing damage to tissue involved in respiratory exchange and/or nonrespiratory functions such as host defense (see review Gardner, 1984). Since the resident alveolar (pulmonary) macrophage population is the primary cell involved in pulmonary resistance to harmful agents, compounds disrupting host defense might be suspected of altering macrophage function.

Ozone. Numerous studies demonstrate that exposure to ozone (O_3) at levels as low as 0.1 ppm alter susceptibility of mice to challenge by pathogenic bacteria (Coffin and Gardner, 1972). Further studies have shown that mice forced to exercise during O_3 exposure suffer a greater mortality on challenge with pathogenic bacterial, presumably owing to an enhanced minute volume resulting in an increased O_3 uptake. This has implications for individuals exercising in areas of high ozone levels (e.g., joggers running along roadways). Similarly, mice exposed to nitrogen dioxide (NO_2) for less than three hours and challenged with a *Streptococcus*-containing aerosol have a significantly increased mortality at doses of NO_2 above 2 ppm (Ehrlich *et al.*, 1977). The increased mortality was potentiated and occurred at lower levels upon continuous long-term exposure to NO_2. While NO_2 and O_3 have produced adverse effects on host resistance following aerosol challenge with bacteria, exposure to other gaseous pollutants such as sulfur dioxide has not altered host resistance. In cases of decreased resistance, the impairment is believed to be related to a decreased phagocytic and bactericidal activity of pulmonary macrophages following exposure to these gases (*see* review, Gardner, 1984). These experimental observations in rodents correlate with epidemiologic studies in humans that emphasize a positive correlation between an increased concentration of gaseous pollutants and a higher incidence of acute respiratory disease. For example, an increased incidence of acute respiratory disease has been observed in humans in association with exposure to NO_2, cigarette smoke, O_3, and suspended nitrates and sulfates (*see* review, Gardner, 1982).

Airborne Metals. There is also evidence suggesting that a number of trace metals that alter the physiology or function of macrophages can cause a significant increase in susceptibility to infection. Animals exposed to airborne nickel, cadmium, zinc, magnesium, and lead have modified susceptibility to aerosol challenge with bacteria (Ehrlich, 1980). Increased susceptibility to challenge with pneumonia-producing bacteria in animals exposed to airborne metals was correlated with an alteration of phagocytic and enzymatic activity in alveolar macrophages (Aranyi et al., 1979). Inhalation of airborne nickel and cadmium not only altered alveolar macrophage function but also depressed primary humoral immunity (Graham et al., 1979). In addition, increased mortality has been observed in animals exposed to copper smelter flyash samples, but not in mice exposed to coal flyash samples. These results correlated with the adverse effects of metals on alveolar macrophages (Aranyi et al., 1981).

In summary, inhalation exposure to gaseous pollutants, airborne metals, and complex metallic mixtures has been shown to alter susceptibility to bacterial challenge in mice that correlates with impairment of phagocytic, enzymatic, and bactericidal activity in alveolar macrophages. With some agents, systemic immune depression can also be observed.

Metals. Systemic metal exposure may also adversely affect the immune response and alter host resistance to infectious agents and tumors (Koller, 1979, 1980; Dean et al., 1982a; Lawrence, 1985). Immunotoxic effects of metal pollutants will be discussed using lead as the prototype, since metals may share a common mechanism and the immunotoxicity of lead has been best characterized.

Lead. Several studies assessing the influence of lead on susceptibility to infectious agents have consistently shown that lead impairs both CMI and antibody-mediated host resistance (summarized in Table 9–13). Mice injected with lead nitrate intraperitoneally (ip) for 30 days and subsequently challenged with the bacterium *Sal-*

monella typhimurium had significantly higher mortality than controls (Hemphill et al., 1971). Similar results were observed in rats exposed intravenously to lead and challenged with *Escherichia coli* (see review, Cook et al., 1975). In these two studies, lead may have interfered with the clearance or detoxication of endotoxin, resulting in death. In another study, mice exposed orally to lead for four weeks and challenged with *Listeria* were assayed for viable *Listeria* 48 and 72 hours following challenge (Lawrence, 1981a). The highest dose of lead caused significant inhibition of early bactericidal activity, and the medium and high doses produced 100 percent mortality within ten days.

Lead exposure also increased host susceptibility to viral infections. Gainer (1977) observed that mice administered lead in drinking water for two weeks had a significantly increased mortality to encephalomyocarditis (EMC) viral challenge. It has been speculated that the enhanced susceptibility of lead-treated mice to viral challenge might be due to a decreased capacity of these animals to develop an immune response or to produce interferon (IFN). Studies by Gainer (1977) indicated that exposure of mice to lead did not inhibit the antiviral action of IFN *in vivo* or *in vitro*, although it appeared to suppress viral IFN production *in vivo*. Recently, Blakely et al. (1982) found that mice exposed to lead acetate in drinking water produced similar amounts of IFN as controls when both were given the viral IFN inducer Tilorone. Similarly, the *in vitro* induction of immune IFN by the T-cell mitogens, phytohemagglutinin, concanavalin A, and staphylococcal enterotoxin in lymphocytes from lead-exposed mice was unaltered compared to controls (Blakley et al., 1982). Thus, lead exposure does not appear to significantly alter the ability of lymphocytes to produce immune interferon.

There is evidence suggesting that host resistance in humans may be altered by lead exposure. It has been noted that children with persistently elevated blood lead levels and infected with *Shigella enteritis* had prolonged diarrhea

Table 9–13. **LEAD EXPOSURES FOUND TO IMPAIR HOST RESISTANCE TO INFECTIOUS AGENTS**

SPECIES	INFECTIOUS AGENT	LEAD DOSE AND EXPOSURE	REFERENCE
Mouse	*S. typhimurium*	200 ppm/ip/30 days	Hemphill et al. (1971)
Mouse	EMC virus	2000 ppm/orally/2 wk	Gainer (1977)
Mouse	Langat virus	50 mg/kg/orally/2 wk	Thind and Kahn (1978)
Mouse	EMC virus	13 ppm/orally/10 wk	Exon et al. (1979)
Mouse	*L. monocytogenes*	80 ppm/orally/4 wk	Lawrence (1981a)
Rat	*E. coli*	2 mg/100 g/iv/1 day	Cook et al. (1975)
Rat	*S. epidermidis*	2 mg/100 g/iv/1 day	Cook et al. (1975)

(Sachs, 1978). In addition, lead smelter workers have been reported to have more colds and influenza infections per year (Ewers *et al.,* 1982) than people not exposed to lead. Secretory IgA, a major factor in immune defense against respiratory and gastrointestinal infections, was found to be suppressed in lead workers with a median blood lead level of 52 µg/100 g or greater.

Alterations in antibody-mediated immunity have also been reported in rodents following lead exposure. Reduced antibody titers in animals exposed to lead might explain the decreased host resistance to infectious agents observed, since specific antibodies can directly neutralize viruses, activate complement, and enhance opsonic phagocytosis. Lead has little effect on the serum immunoglobulin levels in rabbits, in children with >40 µg Pb/dl of blood (Reigart and Garber, 1976), or in lead-exposed workers (Ewers *et al.,* 1982). Rats pre- and postnatally exposed to lead have significantly reduced numbers of IgM PFC (Luster *et al.,* 1978). In contrast, CBA/J mice exposed to lead for one to ten weeks had unaltered IgM PFC responses to SRBC (Lawrence, 1981a). Acute oral lead exposure produces a decreased titer of specific antibodies in rabbits immunized with typhus vaccine or with pseudorabies virus. Likewise, lead-poisoned children had reduced specific antitoxoid antibody titers following booster immunizations with tetanus toxoid (Reigart and Garber, 1976). Tetraethyl lead (organic lead) also results in reduced specific antibody titers in mice and a significant reduction in IgM and IgG PFCs against sheep red blood cells (Blakley *et al.,* 1980). Although it appears likely that lead can affect antibody production, these variable data suggest that suppression may be genetically based.

The influence of inorganic lead exposure on the development of antibody responses has been further assessed by removal of splenic lymphocytes from lead-exposed mice for *in vitro* plasma cell development (Blakley and Archer, 1981). Lead exposure consistently inhibited plasma cell development. Through *in vitro* reconstitution experiments, it was concluded that inhibition of HI by lead was caused by a macrophage defect. This finding was supported by studies where 2-mercaptoethanol (2-ME), a sulfhydryl reagent that substitutes for macrophage function, was found to reverse HI inhibition by lead. These data may explain why results of studies following *in vivo* lead exposure have been variable as some of the test systems utilized 2-ME in the *in vitro* assays of immune function.

In summary, lead exposure appears to inhibit the development of antibody-producing cells and serum antibody titers. It should be noted that the dose, route of lead exposure, and genetic constitution of the host may influence immunomodulation by lead. The adverse effects of lead on humoral immunity may be due to either interference with macrophage antigen processing or antigen presentation to lymphocytes, rather than to a direct effect on B lymphocytes.

The effect of lead exposure on CMI is less clearly characterized. In a comprehensive study in Sprague-Dawley rats (Faith *et al.,* 1979), chronic low-level pre- and postnatal exposure suppressed several CMI parameters, including DTH and lymphoproliferation in response to mitogens. Gaworski and Sharma (1978) also noted that splenic lymphocytes from mice exposed orally to lead for 30 days, but not 15 days, had significantly depressed proliferative responses to T- and B-cell mitogens. In contrast, several laboratories have reported that lead exposure does not suppress T-cell proliferation (Koller *et al.,* 1979; Lawrence, 1981b; Blakley and Archer, 1982). These differences are not easily reconciled since the lead dosages and exposure periods employed do not appear to account for the differences observed.

The mechanism of lead-induced toxicity to lymphoid cells is complex. Lead, like many metals, is a sulfhydryl alkylating agent with a high affinity for subcellular sulfhydryl groups. Thus, the immunomodulatory effects of lead on immune cells may involve its association with cellular thiols since several studies have indicated that membrane and intracellular thiols are important in lymphocyte activation, proliferation, and differentiation. The study by Blakley and Archer (1982) supports this hypothesis since the inhibitory effects of lead were overcome by the addition of an exogenous thiol reagent.

Cadmium. Cadmium, like lead, is a widespread environmental pollutant producing alterations in host resistance and immune function in rodents similar to those produced by lead. Cadmium has been found to alter host susceptibility to bacterial endotoxins, *E. coli* challenge, and EMC viral challenge in mice (*see* review, Koller, 1980). Some groups, however, have reported cadmium-exposed mice to be more resistant to tumor and EMC virus challenges. Chronic cadmium exposure can result in decreased numbers of antibody-producing cells and depressed serum antibody titers in rabbits (Koller, 1973) and mice (Koller *et al.,* 1975), which is consistent with effects of other heavy metals on humoral immunity.

Gaworski and Sharma (1978) observed depressed lymphoproliferative responses to the mitogens PHA and PWM, no effect with Con A, and an enhanced response to LPS in lymphocytes from mice exposed to cadmium. Koller *et al.* (1979) confirmed that cadmium produced no effect on Con A or MLC-induced lymphoproliferation although there was enhanced proliferative responses to LPS stimulation. T-cell-mediated tumor cell cytotoxicity was found to be enhanced in cadmium-exposed mice (Kerkvliet *et al.*, 1979). The data regarding effects on T-cell and macrophage function following cadmium exposure are ambiguous owing to conflicting findings between different laboratories; however, there is a consensus that humoral immune responses are depressed following cadmium exposure, results similar to those obtained with lead.

Organic and Inorganic Mercury. Several groups have reported altered host resistance in rodents following mercury exposure. Mice exposed for 84 days to 1 or 10 ppm of methylmercury chloride in food had increased mortality following challenge with EMC virus (Koller, 1975). This observation was confirmed using inorganic mercury (Gainer, 1977).

Koller (1973) and associates (1977) examined humoral immunity in rabbits after inorganic mercury exposure and in mice following methylmercury exposure. They found significantly depressed primary antibody (IgM) PFC responses. Likewise, Ohi *et al.* (1976) observed that methylmercury suppressed both the IgM and IgG antibody PFC responses in rodents when it was administered pre- and postnatally but not when given at weaning or after. Recent studies (Blakley *et al.*, 1980) have confirmed that subchronic, low-level mercury exposure in rodents results in thymic cortex and splenic follicular atrophy with concomitant depression of IgM as well as IgG antibody PFC responses.

The effect of mercury exposure on lymphocyte function and CMI has been less clearly defined. Gaworski and Sharma (1978) found that exposure of mice for 30 days to 10 ppm mercury in drinking water produced depressed lymphocyte responses to mitogens. Likewise, Hirokawa and Hayashi (1980) reported that acute exposure to nonlethal levels of methylmercury (70 mg/kg) resulted in severely depressed lymphocyte responses to T-cell mitogens. Thus, methylmercury exposure depresses polyclonal activation of lymphocytes by T-cell mitogens and antibody responses to specific antigenic stimulation.

Organotins. The immunotoxicity of organotin compounds that are used primarily as heat stabilizers, catalytic agents, and antifungal/antimicrobial compounds has been extensively reviewed (Seinen and Penninks, 1979). In long-term subchronic feeding studies of triphenyltin acetate in guinea pigs, lymphoid depletion and antibody suppression were observed. Studies by

Seinen and Penninks (1979) have demonstrated that di-*n*-octyltindichloride (DOTC) or di-*n*-butyltindichloride (DBTC) exposure can selectively depress thymus cellularity and weight as well as T-lymphocyte function in rats without causing myelotoxicity or nonlymphoid toxicity. Depressed CMI evidenced by increased skin graft rejection time, reduced DTH, reduced graft-versus-host responses, and decreased responses to T-cell mitogens (*see* review, Seinen and Penninks, 1979) was observed in rats exposed to DOTC and DBTC. Inhibition of HI was also observed, expressed as reduced PFC numbers and antibody titers to sheep erythrocytes. The antibody response to *E. coli* was not affected in DOTC- or DBTC-exposed mice, suggesting that the dialkyltins do not directly affect B-lymphocyte function, but that they may alter T-helper-cell function. As with most immunotoxic chemicals, immunosuppression following DOTC or DBTC exposure is more pronounced in animals exposed immediately after birth rather than as adults.

Immune function is not impaired in mice or guinea pigs fed dialkyltins, which correlates with the absence of lymphoid tissue atrophy observed in these species following exposure (Seinen and Penninks, 1979). No species specificity is apparent following *in vitro* treatment since DOTC or DBTC added to rat or human thymocytes causes decreases in cell survival, responses to mitogens, and E-rosette formation (Seinen *et al.*, 1979) in cell cultures from both species. The data suggest that immunotoxicity produced by organotin compounds may be through an interaction of dialkyltins with plasma membrane sulfhydryl groups essential for amino acid transport.

Other Metals. Toyama and Kolmer (1918) reported over 60 years ago that feeding animals low concentrations of arsenic enhances antibody production, while antibody suppression occurs following high-level exposure. Recently, similar observations have been reported in mice fed various arsenate compounds. While high levels of arsenicals increased susceptibility to viral infection and decreased interferon activity, low levels had the opposite effect, causing increased viral resistance and viral interferon production (Gainer, 1972; Gainer and Pry, 1972). General toxicity occuring at higher levels of arsenical exposure may be, in part, responsible for the increased viral susceptibility. It appears that further studies with arsenicals are warranted.

There is evidence in laboratory animals that nickel exposure results in altered resistance to virus and bacteria (Adkins *et al.*, 1979). A direct effect on macrophage function has also been attributed to nickel (Graham *et al.*, 1978). Zinc, in

Table 9–14.   CHEMICALS AND METALS REPORTED TO ALTER IMMUNE FUNCTION AND HOST RESISTANCE IN RODENTS*

CHEMICAL	RESISTANCE TO CHALLENGE WITH			
	TUMOR	BACTERIA	VIRUS	PARASITE
Arsenic	↓	—	↓	—
Cadmium	↓	↓	↓	—
Cannabinoids	—	↓	↓	—
Cyclophosphamide	↓	↓	↓	↓
Diethylstilbestrol	↓	↓	↓	↓
Dimethylvinyl chloride	↓	NE	—	↓
DDT	—	—	↓	↓
Ethyl carbamate (urethane)	↓	NE	—	↓
Lead	↓	↓	↓	—
Methylmercury	—	—	↓	—
NO$_2$	↓	↓	↓	—
Ozone	—	↓	—	—
Polyhalogenated biphenyls	↓	↓	↓	↓
2,3,7,8-Tetrachlorodibenzo-p-dioxin	↓	↓	↓	—
12-O-tetradecanoyl-phorbol-13-acetate	↓	NE	—	↓

* ↑ = Increased; ↓ = depressed; — = not determined; NE = no effect.

contrast, is a metal essential for maintaining the integrity of the immune response. Several laboratories have found that zinc deficiency depresses antibody responses, possibly owing to a loss of T-helper-cell function (Fernandes et al., 1979). The underlying requirement of zinc in maintaining immunocompetence requires further study, but may be a result of its requirement in many enzyme systems, or its ability to stabilize biologic membranes.

Some of the chemicals and metals discussed in the previous sections that have been demonstrated to alter immune function and host resistance are summarized in Table 9–14.

Drugs. The majority of drugs clinically utilized for immunosuppressive purposes were initially developed for alternative reasons. Suppression of the immune response, in many instances, was an undesirable side effect. Recently, certain abused drugs have also been shown to cause immune alterations. A partial listing of drugs that suppress the immune response along with their proposed mechanisms of action is given in Table 9–15. A limited number of these agents will be discussed below to illustrate prototype agents having quite different mechanisms of immunosuppression.

Alkylating Agents. Alkylating agents are chemicals that form covalent linkages (alkylation) with biologically important molecules, including DNA, which result in disruption of cell functions, especially mitosis. Thus, these agents are particularly toxic to rapidly proliferating cells including neoplastic, lymphoid, bone mar-

row, intestinal mucosal, and germinal cells. The alkylating agents are effective at any part of the cell cycle, although cytotoxicity is usually expressed during S phase as the cell prepares to divide. Cyclophosphamide is representative of this class of drugs and is the most widely used of the nitrogen mustards. Interestingly, the feasibility of using nitrogen mustards as chemotoxic agents for neoplastic cells was based on early observations of their cytotoxicity to lymphoid tissues; their use as immunosuppressants occurred later.

As a chemotherapeutic agent, cyclophosphamide alone or in combination with other drugs has been effective in treating Hodgkin's disease, lymphosarcoma, Burkitt's lymphoma, and acute lymphoblastic leukemia (Calabresi and Parks, 1985). As an immunosuppressant, cyclophosphamide is beneficial in reducing symptoms of certain autoimmune diseases (Calabresi and Parks, 1985), although its major use has been in pretreatment of bone marrow transplant recipients in an effort to prevent subsequent graft rejection (Shand, 1979).

Several reports indicate that there may be subpopulations of lymphocytes preferentially affected by cyclophosphamide treatment, at least in certain species (Shand, 1979; Webb and Winkelstein, 1982). B cells in guinea pigs, chickens, and mice, for example, have been demonstrated to be more sensitive than T cells to cyclophosphamide-induced toxicity (Shand, 1979). In contrast, higher dosages of cyclophosphamide can also suppress T-cell function in

Table 9–15. IMMUNOSUPPRESSIVE DRUGS

Therapeutic Drugs

Alkylating agents
  Nitrogen mustards: Cyclophosphamide, L-phenylalanine mustard, chlorambucil
  Alkyl sulfonates: Busulfan
  Nitrosoureas: Carmustine (BCNU), lomustine (CCNU)
  Triazenes: Dimethyltriazenoimidazolecarboxamide (DTIC)
Antiinflammatory agents
  Aspirin, indomethacin, penicillamine, gold salts
  Adrenocorticosteroids—prednisone
Antimetabolites
  Purine antagonists: 6-mercaptopurine, azathioprine, 6-thioguanine
  Pyrimidine antagonists: 5-fluorouracil, cytosine arabinoside, bromodeoxyuridine
  Folic acid antagonists: Methotrexate (amethopterine)
Natural products
  Vinca alkaloids: Vinblastine, vincristine, procarbazine
  Antibiotics: Actinomycin D, adriablastine, bleomycin, daunomycin, puromycin, mitomycin C, mithramycin
  Antifungal agents: Griseofulvin
  Enzymes: L-Asparaginase
  Cyclosporin A
Estrogens—diethylstilbestrol, ethinyl estradiol

Abused Drugs

Ethanol
Cannabinoids
Cocaine
Opiates

mice (Dean *et al.,* 1979b). Both T-helper and T-suppressor cells have at times been implicated as targets; however, recent evidence indicates that certain T-suppressor-cell populations are extremely sensitive to cyclophosphamide (Shand, 1979). Thus, cyclophosphamide-induced immunosuppression may involve alteration in lymphocyte function as well as cytoreduction.

As is observed with other conventional immunosuppressants, treatment with cyclophosphamide can increase the risk of cancer and infection, which may relate to the lymphopenia and neutropenia seen following cyclophosphamide therapy (Webb and Winkelstein, 1982). In addition, exposure of experimental animals to cyclophosphamide increases host susceptibility to transplantable tumors (Dean *et al.,* 1979a).

Corticosteroids. Corticosteroids and their synthetic analogs can suppress both inflammatory and immune responses. The synthetic corticosteroids prednisone and methylprednisolone are common adjuncts in immunosuppressive therapy in transplant recipients and individuals with extreme hypersensitivity. Although the precise basis for their immunologic effects is unknown, corticosteroids cause a transient lymphopenia (Webb and Winkelstein, 1982), alter phagocytosis, and depress T- and B-lymphocyte function (Santiago Delpin, 1979). In rodents, a dramatic lymphopenia due to lympholysis can

be demonstrated following corticosteroid therapy; however, lymphocytes from humans are relatively resistant to lympholysis by corticosteroids (Webb and Winkelstein, 1982). Thus, suppression in humans may be due to other diverse corticosteroid-induced effects such as alterations in leukocyte mobility, production and/or responses to lymphokines, and immune cell interactions. Part of these effects, as well as many of the antiinflammatory properties of corticosteroids, might be attributed to their stabilization of biomembranes, including plasmalemmal and lysosomal membranes (Santiago Delpin, 1979). At a molecular level, these changes may be mediated through steroid-receptor complexes capable of interacting with DNA, thereby modifying enzyme synthesis, and ultimately resulting in the immunomodulatory properties of this group of compounds (Santiago Delpin, 1979).

Antimetabolites. The antimetabolites are frequently used clinically in transplant patients as immunosuppressive drugs and can be categorized as folate, purine, pyrimidine, and amino acid analogs. The most widely used antimetabolite is the purine antagonist azathioprine. It is a derivative of 6-mercaptopurine (6-MP) and was originally synthesized with the intent of preventing the rapid methylation and oxidation common to 6-MP, thus improving its therapeutic:toxic ratio. Azathioprine is more effective in cycling cells and is maximally active as an immunosuppressant when given following antigenic stimulation (Santos, 1974). Immunosuppression may result from azathioprine-induced inhibition of purine synthesis; however, other mechanisms have been suggested, including the binding of azathioprine to T lymphocytes and the subsequent inactivation of surface antigen receptors (Webb and Winkelstein, 1982).

Azathioprine is also an antiinflammatory agent and can reduce numbers of neutrophils, monocytes, and large lymphocytes. The question of specificity of this drug remains unclear. Regarding lymphocytes, there is evidence that cell-mediated immunity and T-cell functions are the main target of azathioprine-mediated suppression, which is consistent with the clinical picture (Santiago Delpin, 1979). However, recent *in vitro* studies demonstrate substantial toxicity of azathioprine for both T and B cells, although the drug concentrations used in these experiments were higher than plasma levels commonly obtained in therapeutic situations (Kazmers *et al.*, 1983).

The major clinical complication of azathioprine therapy is bone marrow toxicity and leukopenia, which may predispose to secondary infection. In addition, long-term administration of azathioprine may increase the risk of developing certin malignancies.

Natural Products. Drugs of the natural products group have a variable range of immunosuppressive actions. Cyclosporin A (CyA), a relatively new compound in this group, is isolated from fermentation products of two fungi, *Trichoderma polysporum* and *Cylindrocarpon lucidum,* and has a very narrow range of antibiotic activity against fungi and yeast. CyA was found to inhibit lymphocyte proliferation in early tests designed to detect nonspecific cellular toxicity, which further increased the doubt of its potential value as an antibiotic. Fortunately, its lymphostatic and immunologic properties were further characterized. The result has been the development of a family of cyclosporins. Cyclosporin A is the most widely known of these drugs; however, cyclosporins C and G have also been shown to be effective immunosuppressants.

An important characteristic of CyA is its relative lack of secondary toxicity at therapeutic dosages sufficient to maintain immunosuppression in transplant recipients. For example, CyA does not appear to be myelotoxic, an important consideration, particularly in bone marrow transplant recipients, although some cases of hepato- and nephrotoxicity have been reported in patients receiving CyA. The incidence of secondary infection also appears to be less frequent in transplant patients receiving CyA compared

to those receiving more conventional immunosuppressants, although this point is still controversial. Perhaps the greatest concern regarding its therapeutic use is a possible increased frequency of malignancies, especially lymphomas, in transplant patients receiving CyA (*see* review, White, 1982).

Part of the success obtained with CyA undoubtedly involves its unique mechanism of immunosuppression. Unlike lympholytic or antiproliferative/antimetabolic immunosuppressants, CyA appears to act through modulation of mechanisms regulating immunoresponsiveness (*see* review, White, 1982). In addition, its effects seem to be somewhat specific for T-cell function, predominantly sparing B-cell function. This could, in part, account for the reported decreased incidence of infection in transplant recipients receiving CyA (Calne *et al.*, 1981). The specificity of action of CyA seems to be partly mediated through a decreased production of lymphokines requisite for the generation of cytotoxic T lymphocytes. CyA may also act by either masking or preventing the expression of receptors required in triggering lymphocyte proliferation, maturation, and differentiation. The specificity of such a mechanism might also favor the functional predominance of T-suppressor cells in immunoregulation, thus further inducing transplantation tolerance (*see* review, White, 1982).

Estrogens. Diethylstilbestrol (DES) is a synthetic nonsteroidal compound possessing estrogenic activity which has widespread commercial usage. Mice exposed to DES during prenatal (Luster *et al.*, 1979a) or adult (Boorman *et al.*, 1980) life exhibited severe thymic cortical lymphoid depletion along with depressed MLC responses, DTH, and mitogen-induced lymphocyte blastogenesis (Kalland *et al.*, 1979; Luster *et al.*, 1979b; Luster *et al.*, 1980a). The usual ratios of T-cell subpopulations in neonatally DES-exposed mice were altered, suggesting a defect in maturation of T cells. A subsequent report has related the reduced proportion of T-helper cells to suppressed antibody PFC responses to T-dependent antigens (Kalland, 1980). Suppressed antibody responses following immunization with T-independent antigens also occur in rodents treated with DES and are consistent with the depressed *in vitro* proliferative response to LPS, a polyclonal B-cell mitogen (Kalland *et al.*, 1979; Luster *et al.*, 1979b; Luster *et al.*, 1980a). Macrophage functions, assessed by phagocytosis and tumor growth inhibition by adherent peritoneal cells, are potentiated by DES exposure (Boorman *et al.*, 1980), while macrophage suppressor cell activity is enhanced (Luster *et al.*, 1980a).

The effects of DES on immune surveillance and host resistance to disease are well characterized. Exposure of adult mice to DES resulted in increased mortality following challenge with the bacterium *Listeria monocytogenes,* the parasite *Trichinella spiralis,* and a transplantable syngeneic tumor, suggesting a lesion in CMI and/or macrophage function (Dean *et al.,* 1980).

DES probably exerts its immunosuppressive effects via estrogen receptors on lymphoid cells and thymic epithelial cells. The immunosuppressive effects of DES may be mediated through selective depletion or functional impairment of T lymphocytes and/or the induction of suppressor macrophages. The exact relationship between the putative thymic epithelial receptor for DES, DES-induced thymic atrophy, macrophage activation, and T-cell immunosuppression has yet to be clarified.

Abused Drugs. Chronic alcohol abuse in humans has been associated with impaired T-lymphocyte function (Berenyi *et al.,* 1975), myelosuppression, and defective humoral immunity (Gluckman *et al.,* 1977) as well as with a higher and more severe incidence of infections (Tapper, 1980). In studies by Loose *et al.* (1975), the primary, but not secondary, humoral response was reduced in rats chronically dosed with ethanol. In another study, rats chronically fed ethanol exhibited suppressed DTH, thymic and splenic atrophy, and suppressed secondary HI (Tennenbaum *et al.,* 1969).

Naturally occurring cannabinoids, unique to the plant *Cannabis sativa* and constituting 15 percent of the cannabis by weight, are also implicated as immunomodulatory (see review, Holsapple and Munson, 1985). The natural cannabinoids may be subdivided into psychoactive, with Δ9-tetrahydrocannabinol (Δ-9-THC) as the major constituent, and nonpsychoactive, of which there are five known constituents. Both psychoactive and nonpsychoactive cannabinoids have been examined to characterize their immunosuppressive properties, and several studies have shown that they suppress both humoral and cell-mediated immunity in experimental animals (for review, *see* Munson and Fehr, 1983).

The effective dose for 50 percent suppression (ED50) of the antibody plaque response to SRBC in mice was 70, 14, 13, and 8 mg/kg for Δ-9-THC, Δ-8-THC, 1-methyl-Δ8-THC (nonpsychoactive), and abnormal Δ-8-THC (nonpsychoactive), respectively (Smith *et al.,* 1978). In the same studies, at a dose of 100 mg/kg the cannabinoids suppressed the DTH response 35 to 64 percent. Studies in humans have been less conclusive, although Δ-9-THC has been found to suppress CMI, but not humoral immunity (*see* Munson and Fehr, 1983). Nonpsychoactive cannabinoids have also been synthesized in attempts to develop novel immunosuppressants (Smith *et al.,* 1978).

FUTURE DIRECTIONS

The application of the discipline of immunology to the toxicologic assessment of drugs and chemicals is progressing rapidly, and developmental, methods selection, and validation stages are nearly complete. The preceding few years of research have provided new models; data on correlations of immune function and host resistance; a better understanding of the biologic relevance of certain immune function parameters; and a better standardized panel of methods for immunotoxicity assessment. Future research is needed to develop and refine relevant host resistance models; to evaluate *in vitro* methods using microsomal activation systems as screens for detecting chemically induced immunotoxicity; to determine the distribution and function of specific receptors for chemicals; to develop better methods for evaluating chemical hypersensitivity and autoimmunity; and to develop immunologic data on humans occupationally or environmentally exposed to chemicals shown to be immunotoxic in laboratory animals.

REFERENCES

Adams, D. O., and Dean, J. H.: Analysis of macrophage activation and biological response modifier effects by use of objective markers to characterize the stages of activation. In Herberman, R. (ed.): *Natural Cell-Mediated Immunity. II.* Academic Press, Inc., New York, 1982, pp. 511–18.

Adkins, B.; Richards, J. H.; and Gardner, D. E.: Enhancement of experimental respiratory infections following nickel-inhalation. *Environ. Res.,* 20:33–42, 1979.

Ahlstedt, S.; Ekstrom, B.; Svard, P. O.; Sjoberg, B.; Kristofferson, A.; and Ortengren, B.: New aspects on antigens in penicillin allergy. *CRC Crit. Rev. Toxicol.,* 7(3):219–77, 1980.

Aranyi, C.; Miller, F. J.; Andres, S.; Ehrlich, R.; Fenters, J.; Gardner, D.; and Waters, M.: Cytotoxicity to alveolar macrophages of trace metals absorbed on fly ash. *Environ. Res.,* 20:14–23, 1979.

Aranyi, C.; Gardner, D. E.; and Huisingh, J. L.: In Dunnam, D. D. (ed.): *Evaluation of Potential Inhalation Hazard of Particulate Silicous Compounds by In Vitro Alveolar Macrophage Test. Application to Industrial Particulates Containing Hazardous Impurities.* American Society for Testing Materials, Philadelphia, 1981.

Baer, R. L.; Ramsey, D. L.; and Bondi, E.: The most common contact allergens. *Arch. Dermatol.,* 108:74–78, 1973.

Ball, J. K.: Immunosuppression and carcinogenesis: Contrasting effects with 7,12-dimethylbenz(a)anthracene, benz[a]pyrene, and 3-methylcholanthrene. *J. Natl Cancer Inst.,* 44:1, 1970.

Bekesi, J. G.; Holland, J. F.; Anderson, H. A.; Fischbein, A. S.; Rom, W.; Wolff, M. S.; and Selikoff, I. J.: Lymphocyte function of Michigan dairy farmers exposed to polybrominated biphenyls. *Science,* 199:1207–1209, 1978.

Bekesi, J. G.; Roboz, J. P.; Fischbein, A.; and Selikoff, I. J.: Clinical immunology studies in individuals exposed to environmental chemicals. In *Proceedings of the International Seminar on the Immunological System as a Target for Toxic Damage.* Luxembourg, 1986.

Berenyi, M. R.; Straus, B.; and Avila, L.: T-rosettes in alcoholic cirrhosis of the liver. *JAMA*, 232:44–46, 1975.

Bernstein, D. I.; Patterson, R.; and Zeiss, C. R.: Clinical and immunologic evaluation of trimellitic anhydride- and phtalic anhydride-exposed workers using a questionnaire with comparative analysis enzyme-linked immunosorbent and radioimmunoassay studies. *J. Allergy Clin. Immunol.*, 69:311, 1982.

Blakley, B. R., and Archer, D. L.: The effect of lead acetate on the immune response in mice. *Toxicol. Appl. Pharmacol.*, 61:18–26, 1981.

Blakley, B. R., and Archer, D. L.: Mitogen stimulation of lymphocytes exposed to lead. *Toxicol. Appl. Pharmacol.*, 62:183–89, 1982.

Blakley, B. R.; Archer, D. L.; and Osborne, L.: The effect of lead on immune and viral interferon production. *Can. J. Comp. Med.*, 46:43–46, 1982.

Blakley, B. R.; Sisodia, C. S.; and Mukkur, T. K.: The effect of methylmercury, tetraethyl lead, and sodium arsenite on the humoral immune response in mice. *Toxicol. Appl. Pharmacol.*, 52:245–54, 1980.

Boorman, G. A.; Luster, M. I.; Dean, J. H.; and Wilson, R. E.: The effect of adult exposure to diethylstilbestrol in the mouse on macrophage function. *J. Reticuloendothel. Soc.*, 28:547–59, 1980.

Border, W. A.; Lehmann, D. H.; Egan, J. D.; Sass, H. J.; Glode, J. E.; and Wilson, C. B.: Antitubular basement-membrane antibodies in methicillin associated interstitial nephritis. *N. Engl. J. Med.*, 291:381–82, 1974.

Burnet, F. M.: *The Clonal Selection Theory of Acquired Immunity*, Cambridge University Press, London, 1959.
———: The concept of immunological surveillance. *Prog. Exp. Tumor Res.*, 13:1–27, 1970.

Calabresi, P., and Parks, R.: Antiproliferative agents and drugs used for immunosuppression. In Gilman, A. G.; Goodman, L. S.; Rall, T. W.; and Murad, F. (eds.): *Goodman and Gilman's The Pharmacological Basis of Therapeutics*, 7th ed. Macmillan Publishing Co., New York., 1985, pp. 1247–1306.

Calne, R. Y.; Rolles, K.; White, D. J.; Thiru, S.; Evans, D. B.; Henderson, R.; Hamilton, D. L.; Boone, N.; McMaster, P.; Gibby, O.; and Williams, R.: Cyclosporin A in clinical organ grafting. *Transplant. Proc.*, 13:349–58, 1981.

Chang, K. J.; Ching, J. S.; Huang, P. C.; and Tung, T. C.: Study of patients with PCB poisoning. *J. Mormosan Med. Assoc.*, 79:304–12, 1980.

Clark, D. A.; Sweeney, G.; Safe, S.; Hancock, E.; Kilburn, D. G.; and Gauldie, J.: Cellular and genetic basis for suppression of cytotoxic T-cell generation by haloaromatic hydrocarbons. *Immunophramacology*, 6:143–53, 1983.

Coffin, D. L., and Gardner, D. E.: Interaction of biological agents and chemical air pollutants. *Ann. Occup. Hyg.*, 15:219–35, 1972.

Cook, J. A.; DiLuzio, N. R.; and Hoffman, E. O.: Factors modifying susceptibility to bacterial endotoxin: The effect of lead and cadmium. *CRC Crit. Rev. Toxicol.*, 3:201–29, 1975.

Coombs, R. R. A., and Gell, P. G. H.: Classification of allergic reactions responsible for clinical hypersensitivity and disease. In Gell, P. G. H.; Coombs, R. R. A.; and Lachman, P. J. (eds.): *Clinical Aspects of Immunology*, 1975, p. 761.

Cooper, N. R.: The complement system. In Stites, D. P.; Stobo, J. D.; Fudenberg, H. H.; and Wells, J. V. (eds.): *Basic and Clinical Immunology*, 4th ed. Lange Medical Publications, Los Altos, Calif., 1980, pp. 124–35.

Cronin, E.: *Contact Dermatitis*. Churchill Livingston, London, 1980.

Dean, J. H.; Padarathsingh, M. L.; Jerrells, T. R.; Keys, L.; and Northing, J. W.: Assessment of immunobiological effects induced by chemicals, drugs, or food additives. II. Studies with cyclophosphamide. *Drug Chem. Toxicol.*, 2:133–53, 1979a.

Dean, J. H.; Padarathsingh, M. L.; and Jerrells, T. R.: Assessment of immunobiological effects induced by chemicals, drugs, and food additives. I. Tier testing and screening approach. *Drug Chem. Toxicol.*, 2:5–17, 1979b.

Dean, J. H.; Luster, M. I.; Boorman, G. A.; Luebke, R. W.; and Lauer, L. D.: The effect of adult exposure to diethylstilbestrol in the mouse: Alterations in tumor susceptibility and host resistance parameters. *J. Reticuloendothel. Soc.*, 28:571–83, 1980.

Dean, J. H.; Luster, M. I.; Boorman, G. A.; Leubke, R. W.; and Lauer, L. D.: Application of tumor, bacterial, and parasite susceptibility assays to study immune alterations induced by environmental chemicals. *Environ. Health Perspect.*, 43:81–88, 1982a.

Dean, J. H.; Luster, M. I.; Boorman, G. A.; and Lauer, L. D.: Procedures available to examine the immunotoxicity of chemicals and drugs. *Pharmacol. Rev.*, 34:137–48, 1982b.

Dean, J. H.; Luster, M. I.; and Boorman, G. A. Immunotoxicology. In Sirois, P., and Rola-Pleszgyski, M. (eds.): *Immunopharmacology*. Elsevier Biomedical Press, 1982c, pp. 349–97.

Dean, J. H.; Luster, M. I.; Boorman, G. A.; Lauer, L. D.; Luebke, R. W.; and Lawson, L. D.: Immune suppression following exposure of mice to the carcinogen benzo(a)pyrene but not the non-carcinogenic benzo(e)pyrene. *Clin. Exp. Immunol.*, 52:199–206, 1983a.

Dean, J. H.; Luster, M. I.; Boorman, G. A.; Lauer, L. D.; and Ward, E. C.: Immunotoxicity of tumor promoting environmental chemicals and phorbol diesters. In Hadden, J. W., et al. (eds.): *Advances in Immunopharmacology 2*. Pergamon Press, Oxford, 1983b, pp. 23–31.

Dean, J. H., and Lauer, L. D.: Immunological effects following exposure to 2,3,7,8-tetrachlorodibenzo-p-dioxin: a review. In Lowrance, W. W. (ed.): *Public Health Risk of the Dioxins*. William Kaufmann, Los Altos, Calif., 1984, pp. 275–94.

Desi, I.; Varga, L.; and Farkas, I.: Studies on the immunosuppressive effect of organochlorine and organophosphoric pesticides in subacute experiments. *J. Hyg. Epidemiol. Microbiol. Immunol.*, 22:115–22, 1978.

Desi, I.; Varga, L.; and Farkas, I.: The effect of DDVP, an organophosphate pesticide, on the humoral and cell-mediated immunity of rabbits. *Arch. Toxicol. Suppl.*, 4:171–74, 1980.

de Weck, A. L.: Drug reactions. In Samter, M. (ed.): *Immunological Diseases, Volume I*. Little Brown & Co., Boston, 1978, pp. 413–39.

DiMarco, A. T.; Francheschi, C.; Xerri, L.; and Prodi, G.: Depression of homograft rejection and graft-versus-host reactivity following 7,12-dimethylbenz(a)thracene exposure in the rat. *Cancer Res.*, 31:1446–50, 1971.

Druet, P.; Bernard, A.; Hirsch, F.; Weening, J. J.; Gengoux, P.; Mahieu, P.; and Brikeland, S.: Immunologically mediated glomerulonephritis by heavy metals. *Arch. Toxicol.*, 50:187–94, 1982.

Dunckel, A. E.: An updating on the polybrominated biphenyl disaster in Michigan. *J. Am. Vet. Med. Assoc.*, 167:838–43, 1975.

Ehrlich, R.: Interaction between environmental pollutants and respiratory infections. *Environ. Health Perspect.*, 35:89–100, 1980.

Ehrlich, R.; Findlay, J. C.; Fenters, J. D.; and Gardner, D. E.: Health effects of short-term inhalation of nitrogen dioxide and ozone mixtures. *Environ. Res.*, **14**:223, 1977.

Ercegovich, C. D.: Relationship of pesticides to immune responses. *Fed. Proc.*, **32**(9):2010–16, 1973.

Evaluation of the carcinogenic risk of chemicals to humans. *IARC Monogr.*, **29**:93–148, 1982.

Evdokimov, E. S.: Effect of organochlorine pesticides on animals. *Veterinariya*, **12**:94–95, 1974.

Ewers, U.; Stiller-Winkler, R.; and Idel, H.: Serum immunoglobulin, complement C3, and salivary IgA levels in lead workers. *Environ. Res.*, **29**:351–57, 1982.

Exon, J. H.; Koller, L. K.; and Kerkvliet, N. I.: Lead-cadmium interaction: Effects on viral-induced mortality and tissue residues in mice. *Arch. Environ. Health*, **34**:469–75, 1979.

Faith, R. E.; Luster, M. I.; and Kimmel, C. A.: Effect of chronic developmental lead exposure on cell mediated immune function. *Clin. Exp. Immunol.*, **35**:413–24, 1979.

Fernandes, G.; Nair, M.; Onoe, K.; Tanalsa, T.; Floyd, R.; and Good, R. A.: Impairment of cell-mediated immune function by dietary zinc deficiency in mice. *Proc. Natl Acad. Sci. USA*, **76**:457–61, 1979.

Flower, R. J.; Moncada, S.; and Vane, J. R.: Analgesic-antipyretics, anti-inflammatory agents; drugs employed in the therapy of gout. In Gilman, A. G.; Goodman, L. S.; and Gilman, A. (eds.): *Goodman and Gilman's The Pharmacological Basis of Therapeutics*, 6th ed. Macmillan Publishing Co., New York, 1980, pp. 682–728.

Gabliks, J.; Al-Zubaidy, T.; and Askari, E.: DDT and immunological responses. 3. Reduced anaphylaxis and mast cell population in rats fed DDT. *Arch. Environ. Health*, **30**:81–84, 1975.

Gainer, J. H.: Effects of arsenicals on interferon formation and action. *Am. J. Vet. Res.*, **33**:2579–86, 1972.

———: Effects of heavy metals and of deficiency of zinc on mortality rates in mice infected with encephalomyocarditis virus. *Am. J. Vet. Res.*, **38**:869–73, 1977.

Gainer, J. H., and Pry, T. W.: Effects of arsenicals on viral infection in mice. *Am. J. Vet. Med. Res.*, **33**:2299–2309, 1972.

Gardner, D. E.: Effect of gases and airborne particles on lung infections. In McGrath, J. J., and Barnes, C. D. (eds.): *Air Pollution-Physiological Effects*. Academic Press, Inc., New York, 1982, pp. 47–79.

———: Alterations in macrophage function by environmental chemicals. *Environ. Health Perspect.*, 1984 (in press).

Gatti, R. A., and Good, R. A.: Occurrence of malignancy in immunodeficiency disease: A literature review. *Cancer*, **28**:89–98, 1971.

Gaworski, C. L., and Sharma, R. R.: The effects of heavy metals on ^{3}H-thymidine uptake in lymphocytes. *Toxicol. Appl. Pharmacol.*, **46**:305–13, 1978.

Gluckman, S. J.; Dvorak, V. C.; and MacGregor, R. R.: Host defenses during prolonged alcohol consumption in a controlled environment. *Arch. Intern. Med.*, **137**:1539–43, 1977.

Gorelik, E., and Herberman, R.: Susceptibility of various strains of mice to urethane-induced lung tumors and depressed natural killer activity. *J. Natl Cancer Inst.*, **67**:1317–22, 1981.

Graham, J. A.; Miller, F. J.; Daniels, M. J.; Payne, E. A.; and Gardner, D. E.: Influence of cadmium, nickel, and chromium on primary immunity in mice. *Environ. Res.*, **16**:77–87, 1978.

Graham, J. A.; Gardner, D. E.; Waters, M. D.; and Coffin, D. L.: Effect of trace metals on phagocytosis by alveolar macrophages. *Infect. Immun.*, **11**:1278–83, 1979.

Greenlee, W. F.; Dold, K. M.; Irons, R. D.; and Osborne, R.: Evidence for direct action of 2,3,7,8-tetrachlorodibenzo-*p*-dioxin (TCDD) on thymic epithelium. *Toxicol. Appl. Pharmacol.*, **79**:112–20, 1985.

Grimm, W.; Barlin, E.; Leser, H. G.; Kramer, W.; and Gemsa, D.: Induction of tumor cytostatic macrophages by 12-o-tetradecanoyl phorbol-13-acetate (TPA). *Clin. Immunol. Immunopathol.*, **17**:617–28, 1980.

Hamilton, H. E.; Morgan, D. P.; and Simmons, A.: A pesticide (Dieldrin)-induced immunohemolytic anemia. *Environ. Res.*, **17**:155–64, 1978.

Hemphill, R. E.; Kaeberle, M. L.; and Buck, W. B.: Lead suppression of mouse resistance to *Salmonella typhimurium*. *Science*, **172**:1031–32, 1971.

Herberman, R. B., and Holden, H. T.: Natural cell-mediated immunity. *Adv. Cancer Res.*, **27**:305–72, 1978.

Herberman, R. B., and Ortaldo, J. R.: Natural killer cells: Their role in defenses against disease. *Science*, **214**:24, 1981.

Hirokawa, K., and Hayashi, Y.: Acute methyl mercury intoxication in mice. *Acta Pathol. Jpn.*, **30**:23–32, 1980.

Holsapple, M. P., and Munson, A. E.: Immunotoxicology of abused drugs. In Dean, J. H.; Luster, M. I.; Munson, A. E.; and Amos, H. E. (eds.): *Immunotoxicology and Immunopharmacology*. Raven Press, New York, 1986, pp. 381–92.

Juhlin, L.: Incidence of intolerance to food additives. *Int. J. Dermatol.*, **19**:548–51, 1980.

Kalland, T.: Decreased and disproportionate T cell population in adult mice after neonatal exposure to diethylstilbestrol. *Cell. Immunol.*, **51**:55–63, 1980.

Kalland, T.; Strand, O.; and Forsberg, J.: Long term effects of neonatal estrogen treatment on mitogen responsiveness of mouse spleen lymphocytes. *J. Natl Cancer Inst.*, **63**:413–21, 1979.

Karol, M. H.; Dixon, C.; Brady, M.; and Alarie, Y.: Immunologic sensitization and pulmonary hypersensitivity by repeated inhalation of aromatic isocyanates. *Toxicol. Appl. Pharmacol.*, **53**:260–70, 1980.

Karol, M. H.; Hauth, B. A.; Riley, E. J.; and Magrem, C. M.: Dermal contact with toluene di-isocyanate (TDI) produces respiratory tract hypersensitivity in guinea pigs. *Toxicol. Appl. Pharmacol.*, **58**:221–30, 1981.

Katz, D. H.: Lymphocyte differentiation, recognition and regulation. In Dixon, F. J., and Kunkel, H. G. (eds.): *Immunology: An International Series of Monographs and Treatises*, Academic Press, Inc., New York, 1977, pp. 40–69.

Kazmers, I. S.; Doddona, P. E.; Dalke, A. P.; and Kelley, W. H.: Effect of immunosuppressive agents on human T and B-lymphocytes. *Biochem. Pharmacol.*, **32**:805–10, 1983.

Keller, R.: Suppression of natural antitumor defense mechanisms by phorbol esters. *Nature (Lond.)*, **282**:729–31, 1979.

Kerkvliet, N. I., and Kimeldorf, D. J.: Antitumor activity of a polychlorinated biphenyl mixture, Aroclor 1254, in rats innoculated with Walker 256 carcinosarcoma cells. *J. Natl Cancer Inst.*, **59**:951–55, 1977.

Kerkvliet, N. I.; Koller, L. D.; Beacher, L. G.; and Brauner, J. A.: Effect of cadmium exposure on primary tumor growth and cell-mediated cytotoxicity in mice bearing MSB-6 sarcomas. *J. Natl Cancer Inst.*, **63**:479–86, 1979.

Kimbrough, R. D.: *Halogenated Biphenyls, Terphenyls, Naphthalenes, Dibenzodioxins and Related Products*. Elsevier/North-Holland Biomedical Press, New York, 1980.

Klecak, G.: Identification of contact allergens: Predictive tests in animals. In Murzull, F. N., and Maibach, H. I. (eds.): *Dermatotoxicology*. Hemisphere Publishing Corp., New York, 1983, pp. 143–236.

Koller, L. D.: Immunosuppression produced by lead,

cadmium, and mercury. *Am. J. Vet. Res.*, **34**:1457–58, 1973.

————: Methylmercury: Effect on oncogenic and nononcogenic viruses in mice. *Am. J. Vet. Res.*, **36**:1501–1504, 1975.

————: Effects of environmental contaminants on the immune system. *Adv. Vet. Sci. Comp. Med.*, **23**:267–95, 1979.

————: Immunotoxicology of heavy metals. *Int. J. Immunopharmacol.*, **2**:269–79, 1980.

Koller, L. D.; Exon, J. H.; and Roan, J. G.: Antibody suppression by cadmium. *Arch. Environ. Health*, **30**:598–601, 1975.

Koller, L. D.; Exon, J. H.; and Arbogast, B.: Methylmercury: Effect on serum enzymes and humoral antibody. *J. Toxicol. Environ. Health*, **2**:1115–23, 1977.

Koller, L. D.; Roan, J. G.; and Kerkvliet, N. I.: Mitogen stimulation of lymphocytes in CBA mice exposed to lead and cadmium. *Environ. Res.*, **19**:177–88, 1979.

Lathrop, G. D.; Wolfe, W. H.; Albanese, R. A.; and Moynahan, P. M.: *Airforce Health Study (Project Ranch Hand II). An Epidemiologic Investigation of Health Effects in Air Force Personnel Following Exposure to Herbicides, Baseline Morbidity Study Results.* USAF School of Aerospace Medicine, Brooks Air Force Base, Texas, 1984, pp. XVI–2–1–2–12.

Lawrence, D. A.: Heavy metal modulation of lymphocyte activities—II. Lead, an *in vitro* mediator of B-cell activation. *Int. J. Immunopharmacol.*, **3**:153–61, 1981a.

————: *In vivo* and *in vitro* effects of lead on humoral and cell mediated immunity. *Infect. Immun.*, **31**:136–43, 1981b.

————: Immunotoxicity of heavy metals. In Dean, J. H.; Luster, M. I.; Munson, A. E.; and Amos, H. E. (eds.): *Immunotoxicology and Immunopharmacology.* Raven Press, New York, 1985, pp. 341–53.

Loose, L. D.; Silkworth, J. B.; Pittman, K. A.; Benitz, K. F.; and Mueller, W.: Impaired host resistance to endotoxin and malaria in polychlorinated biphenyl- and hexachlorobenzene-treated mice. *Infect. Immun.*, **20**:30–35, 1978.

Loose, L. D.; Stege, T.; and DiLuzio, N. R.: The influence of acute and chronic ethanol or bourbon administration on phagocytic and immune responses in rats. *Exp. Mol. Pathol.*, **23**:459–72, 1975.

Luster, M. I., and Dean, J. H.: Immunological hypersensitivity resulting from environmental or occupational exposure to chemicals: A state-of-the-art workshop summary. *Fundamental Appl. Toxicol.*, **2**:327–30, 1982.

Luster, M. I.; Faith, R. E.; and Moore, J. A.: Effects of polybrominated biphenyls (PBB) on immune response in rodents. *Environ. Health Perspect.*, **23**:227–32, 1978.

Luster, M. I.; Faith, R. E.; and Lawson, L. D.: Effects of 2,3,7,8-tetrachlorodibenzofuran (TCDF) on the immune system in guinea pigs. *Drug Chem. Toxicol.*, **2**:49–60, 1979a.

Luster, M. I.; Faith, R. E.; McLachlan, J. A.; and Clark, G. C.: Effect of *in utero* exposure to diethylstilbestrol on the immune system in mice. *Toxicol. Appl. Pharmacol.*, **47**:287–93, 1979b.

Luster, M. I.; Boorman, G. A.; Dean, J. H.; Luebke, R. W.; and Lawson, L. D.: The effect of adult exposure to diethylstilbestrol in the mouse. Alterations in immunological function. *J. Reticuloendothel. Soc.*, **28**:561–69, 1980a.

Luster, M. I.; Boorman, G. A.; Harris, M. W.; and Moore, J. A.: Laboratory studies on polybrominated biphenyl-induced immune alterations following low-level chronic or pre/postnatal exposure. *Int. J. Immunopharmacol.*, **2**:69–80, 1980b.

Luster, M. I.; Dean, J. H.; Boorman, G. A.; Archer, D. L.; Lauer, L.; Lawson, L. D.; Moore, J. A.; and Wilson, R. E.: The effects of orthophenylphenol, tris(2,3-dichloropropyl)phosphate and cyclophospha-

mide on the immune system and host susceptibility of mice following subchronic exposure. *Toxicol. Appl. Pharmacol.*, **58**:252–61, 1981.

Luster, M. I.; Dean, J. H.; Boorman, G. A.; Lawson, L.; Lauer, L.; Hayes, T.; Rader, J.; and Dieter, M.: Host resistance and immune functions in methyl and ethyl carbamate treated mice. *Clin. Exp. Immunol.*, **50**:223–30, 1982a.

Luster, M. I.; Dean, J. H.; and Moore, J. A.: Evaluation of immune functions in toxicology. In Hayes, W. (ed.): *Methods in Toxicology.* Raven Press, New York, 1982b, pp. 561–86.

Magnusson, B., and Kligman, A. M.: The identification of contact allergens by animal assay. The guinea pig maximization test. *J. Invest. Dermatol.*, **52**:268, 1969.

Maibach, H.: Formaldehyde: Effects on animal and human skin. In Gibson, J. (ed.): *Formaldehyde Toxicity.* Hemisphere Publishing Corp., New York, 1983, pp. 166–74.

Malmgren, R. A.; Bennison, B. E.; and McKinley, T. W., Jr.: Reduced antibody titers in mice treated with carcinogenic and cancer chemotherapeutic agents. *Proc. Soc. Exp. Biol. Med.*, **70**:484–88, 1952.

McConnell, E. E.: *Acute and Chronic Toxicity, Carcinogenesis, Reproduction, Teratogenesis, and Mutagenesis in Animals.* Elsevier/North-Holland Biomed. Press, New York, 1980, pp. 241–66.

Moore, J. A.; Gupta, B. N.; and Vos, J. G.: Toxicity of 2,3,7,8-tetrachlorodibenzofuran—Preliminary results. In *Proc. Natl Conf. on Polychlorinated Biphenyls,* Environmental Protection Agency, Washington, D.C., 1976, pp. 77–79.

Morison, W. L., and Kochevar, I. P.: Photoallergy. In Parrish, J. A.; Kriphe, M. L.; and Morison, W. L. (eds.): *Photoimmunity.* Plenum Publishing Corp., New York, 1983, pp. 227–54.

Muller-Eberhard, H. J.: Complement. *Annu. Rev. Biochem.*, **44**:697, 1975.

Munson, A. E., and Fehr, K. O.: Immunological effects of cannabis. In Fehr, K. O., and Kalant, H. (eds.): *Adverse Health and Behavioral Consequences of Cannabis Use.* Working Papers for the ARS/WHO Scientific Meeting, Toronto, 1981; Addiction Research Foundation, Toronto, pp. 257–353, 1983.

Murray, M. J.; Lauer, L. D.; Luster, M. I.; Luebke, R. W.; Adams, D. O.; and Dean, J. H.: Correlation of murine susceptibility to tumor, parasite and bacterial challenge following systemic exposure to the tumor promoter phorbol myristate acetate. *Int. J. Immunopharmacol,* **7**:491–500, 1985.

NIEHS Contract NO1-ES90004, 1983. *Investigation of the Immunological, Toxicological Effects of PBB in Michigan Farmers and Chemical Workers, Progress Report.*

Norman, P. S.: Skin testing. In Rose, N. R., and Frailman, H. (eds.): *Manual of Clinical Immunology.* American Society for Microbiology, Washington, D.C., 1976, p. 585.

Ohi, G.; Fukunda, M.; Seta, H.; and Yagyu, H.: Methylmercury on humoral immune responses in mice under conditions stimulated to practical situations. *Bull. Environ. Contam. Toxicol.*, **15**:175–90, 1976.

Parker, C. W.: Allergic reactions in man. *Pharmacol. Rev.*, **34**(1):85–104, 1982.

Patterson, R.; Zeiss, C. R.; and Pruzansky, J. J.: Immunology and immunopathology of trimellitic anhydride pulmonary reactions. *J. Allergy Clin. Immunol.*, **70**:19–23, 1982.

Peltonen, L., and Fraki, J.: Prevalence of dichromate sensitivity. *Contact Dermatitis*, **9**:190–94, 1980.

Penn, I: Tumors occurring in organ transplant recipients. In Klein, G., and Weinhouse, S. (eds.): *Advances in Cancer Research,* Vol. 28. Academic Press, Inc., New York, 1978, pp. 31–61.

————: Neoplastic Consequences of immunosuppression. In Dean, J. H.; Luster, M. I.; Munson, A. E.; and Amos, H. E. (eds.): *Immunotoxicology and Immunopharmacology*. Raven Press, New York, 1985, pp. 79–89.

Perlmann, P.; Perlmann, H.; Larsson, A.; and Wahlin, B.: Antibody-dependent cytolytic effector lymphocytes (K cells) in human blood. *J. Reticuloendothel. Soc.*, **17**:241, 1975.

Poland, A., and Glover, E.: Stereospecific, high affinity binding of 2,3,7,8-tetrachlorodibenzo-*p*-dioxin by hepatic cytosol. *J. Biol. Chem.*, **251**:4936–45, 1976.

Poland, A., and Glover, E.: 2,3,7,8-tetrachlorodibenzo-*p*-dioxin: Segregation of toxicity with the Ah locus. *Mol. Pharmacol.*, **17**:86–94, 1980.

Popa, V.; Teculescu, D.; Stanescu, D.; and Gavrilescu, N.: Bronchial asthma and asthmatic bronchitis determined by simple chemicals. *Dis. Chest*, **56**(5):395–404, 1969.

Rao, D. S. V. S., and Glick, B.: Pesticide effects on the immune response and metabolic activity of chicken lymphocytes. *Proc. Soc. Exp. Biol. Med.*, **154**:27–29, 1977.

Reeves, A. L., and Preuss, O. P.: The immunotoxicity of beryllium. In Dean, J. H.; Luster, M. I.; Munson, A. E.; and Amos, H. E. (eds.): *Immunotoxicology and Immunopharmacology*. Raven Press, New York, 1985, pp. 441–55.

Reggiani, G.: Acute human exposure to TCDD in Seveso, Italy. *J. Toxicol. Environ. Health*, **6**:27–43, 1980.

Reigart, J. R., and Garber, C. D.: Evaluation of the humoral immune response of children with low level lead exposure. *Bull. Environ. Contam. Toxicol.*, **16**:112–17, 1976.

Ritz, H. L., and Buehler, E. V. Planning, conduct, and interpretation of guinea pig sensitization patch tests. In Drill, J. A., and Lazur, P. (eds.): *Concepts in Cutaneous Toxicity*. Academic Press, Inc., New York, 1980, pp. 25–40.

Sachs, H. K.: Intercurrent infections in lead poisoning. *Am. J. Dis. Child.*, **32**:315–16, 1978.

Santiago Delpin, E. A.: Principles of clinical immunosuppression. In Simmons, R. L. (ed.): *Surgical Clinics of North America*, Vol. 59. W. B. Saunders Co., Philadelphia, 1979, pp. 283–98.

Santos, G. W.: Immunological toxicity of cancer chemotherapy. In Mathe, G., and Oldham, R. K. (eds.): *Complications of Cancer Chemotherapy*. Springer Verlag, New York, 1974, pp. 20–23.

Schorr, W. F.: Cosmetic allergy. A comprehensive study of the many groups of chemical antimicrobial agents. *Arch. Dermatol.*, **104**:459–65, 1971.

Seinen, W., and Penninks, A.: Immune suppression as a consequence of a selective cytotoxic activity of certain organometallic compounds on thymus and thymus-dependent lymphocytes. *Ann. NY Acad. Sci.*, **320**:499–517, 1979.

Seinen, W.; Vos, J. G.; Brands, R.; and Hooykaas, H.: Lymphocytotoxicity and immunosuppression by organotin compounds. Suppression of GVH reactivity, blast transformation and E. rosette formation by di-*n*-butyldichloride and di-*n*-octyldichloride. *Immunopharmacology*, **1**:343–53, 1979.

Settipane, G. A.: Adverse reactions to aspirin and related drugs. *Arch. Intern. Med.*, **141**:328–32, 1981.

Shand, F. L.: Review/commentary: The immunopharmacology of cyclophosphamide. *Int. J. Immunopharmacol.*, **1**:165–71, 1979.

Shigematsu, N.; Ishmaru, S.; Saito, R.; Ikeda, T.; Matsuba, K.; Sugiyams, K.; and Masuda, Y.: Respiratory involvement in PCB poisoning. *Environ. Res.*, **16**:92–100, 1978.

Silkworth, J. B., and Loose, L. D.: Cell-mediated immunity in mice fed either Aroclor 1016 or hexachlorobenzene. *Toxicol. Appl. Pharmacol.*, **45**:326–27, 1978.

Silkworth, J. B., and Loose, L. D.: PCB and HCB induced alteration of lymphocyte blastogenesis. *Toxicol. Appl. Pharmacol.*, **49**:86, 1979.

Smith, S. H.; Sanders, V. M.; Barrett, B. A.; Borzelleca, J. E.; and Munson, A. E.: Immunotoxicology evaluation on mice exposed to polychlorinated biphenyls. *Toxicol. Appl. Pharmacol.*, **45**:A336, 1978.

Some metals and metallic compounds. *IARC Monogr.*, **23**:143–204, 1981.

Stjernsward, J.: Effect of noncarcinogenic and carcinogenic hydrocarbons on antibody-forming cells measured at the cellular level *in vitro*. *J. Natl Cancer Inst.*, **36**:1189–95, 1966.

Street, J. C.: Pesticides and the Immune System. In Sharma, R. P. (ed.): *Immunologic Considerations in Toxicology*. CRC Press, Inc., Boca Raton, Fl., 1981, pp. 46–66.

Street, J. C., and Sharma, R. P.: Quantitative aspects of immunosuppression by selected pesticides. *Toxicol. Appl. Pharmacol.*, **29**:135–36, 1974.

Stutman, O., and Cuttito, M. J.: Normal levels of natural cytotoxic cells against solid tumors in NK-deficient beige mice. *Nature*, **270**:254–57, 1981.

Tapper, M. L.: Infections complicating the alcoholic host. In Grieco, M. H. (ed.): *Infections in the Abnormal Host*. Yorke Medical Books, New York, 1980, pp. 474.

Tennenbaum, J. I.; Ruppert, R. D.; St. Pierre, R. L.; and Greenberger, N. J.: The effect of chronic alcohol administration on the immune responsiveness of rats. *J. Allergy*, **44**:272–78, 1969.

Theofilopoulos, A. N.: Autoimmunity. In Stites, D. P.; Stobo, J. D.; Fudenberg, H. H.; and Wells, J. V. (eds.): *Basic and Clinical Immunology*. Lange Medical Pub., Los Altos, Calif., 1982, pp. 156–88.

Thigpen, J. E.; Faith, R. E.; McConnell, E. E.; and Moore, J. A.: Increased susceptibility to bacterial infection as a sequela of exposure to 2,3,7,8-tetrachlorodibenzo-*p*-dioxin. *Infect. Immun.*, **12**:1319–24, 1975.

Thind, I. S., and Kahn, M. Y.: Potentiation of the neurovirulence of Langat virus infection by lead intoxication in mice. *Exp. Mol. Pathol.*, **29**:342–47, 1978.

Thomas, P. J., and Hinsdill, R. D.: Effect of polychlorinated biphenyls on the immune responses of Rhesus monkeys and mice. *Toxicol. Appl. Pharmacol.*, **44**:41–52, 1978.

Thomas, P. T., and Hinsdill, R. D.: Perinatal PCB exposure and its effects on the immune system of young rabbits. *Drug Chem. Toxicol.*, **3**:173–84, 1980.

Thomas, P. T., and Faith, R. E.: Adult and perinatal immunotoxicity induced by halogenated aromatic hydrocarbons. In Dean, J. H.; Luster, M. I.; Munson, A. E.; and Amos, H. E. (eds.): *Immunotoxicology and Immunopharmacology*. Raven Press, New York, 1985, pp. 305–13.

Touraine, J. L.; Hadden, J. W.; Touraine, F., Hadden, E. M.; Estensen, R.; and Good, R. A.: Phorbol myristate acetate: A mitogen selective for a T-lymphocyte subpopulation. *J. Exp. Med.*, **145**:460–65, 1977.

Toyama, I., and Kolmer, J. A.: The influence of arsphenamine and mercuric chloride upon complement and antibody production. *J. Immunol.*, **3**:301–16, 1918.

Urethane: Evaluation of carcinogenic risk of chemicals to man. *IARC Monogr.*, **7**:111, 1974.

Urso, P., and Gengozian, N.: Depressed humoral immunity and increased tumor incidence in mice following *in utero* exposure to benzo(a)pyrene. *J. Toxicol. Environ. Health*, **6**:569–76, 1980.

Van Arsdel, P. P., Jr.: Drug allergy, an update. *Med. Clin. North Am.*, **65**(5):1089–1103, 1981.

Vos, J. G.; Koeman, J. H.; Van Der Maas, H. L.; Ten Noever De Braaw, M. C.; and De Vos, R. H.: Identification and toxicological evaluation of chlorinated dibenzofuran and chlorinated naphthalene in two commercial polychlorinated biphenyls. *Toxicology*, **8**:625–73, 1970.

Vos, J. G.; Moore, J. A.; and Zinkl, J. G.: Effects of 2,3,7,8-tetrachlorodibenzo-*p*-dioxin on the immune system of laboratory animals. *Environ. Health Perspect.*, **5**:149–62, 1973.

Vos, J. G.; Faith, R. E.; and Luster, M. I.: *Immune Alterations*. Elsevier/North-Holland Biomedical Press, New York, 1980, pp. 241–66.

Wahlberg, J. E.: Sensitization and testing of guinea pigs with nickel sulfate. *Dermatologica*, **152**:321–30, 1976.

Ward, E. C.; Murray, M. J.; Lauer, L. D.; House, R. V.; and Dean, J. H.: Persistent suppression of humoral and cell-mediated immunity in mice following exposure to the polycyclic aromatic hydrocarbon, 7,12-dimethylbenz[a]anthracene. *Int. J. Immunopharmacol.*, **8**:13–22, 1986.

Webb, D. R., and Winkelstein, A.: Immunosuppression, immunopotentiation and anti-inflammatory drugs. In Stites, D. P.; Stobo, J. D.; Fudenberg, H. H.; and Wells, J. V. (eds.): *Basic and Clinical Immunology*, 4th ed. Lange Medical Pub., Los Altos, Calif., 1982, pp. 277–92.

Weening, J. J.; Hoedemuekinr, P. J.; and Bukker, W. W.: Immunoregulation and antinuclear antibodies in mercury induced glomerulopathy in the rat. *Clin. Exp. Immunol.*, **45**:64–71, 1981.

Wells, J. V.: Immune mechanisms in tissue damage. In Stites, D. P.; Stobo, J. D.; Fudenberg, H. H.; and Wells, J. V. (eds.): *Basic and Clinical Immunology*. Lange Medical Publications, Los Altos, Calif., 1982, pp. 136–50.

White, D. J.: *Cyclosporin A: Proc. Int. Conf.* Elsevier Biomedical, Amsterdam, 1982.

Wierda, D.; Irons, R. D.; and Greenlee, W. F.: Immunotoxicity in C57BL/6 mice exposed to benzene and Aroclor 1254. *Toxicol. Appl. Pharmacol.*, **60**:410–17, 1981.

Wojdani, A., and Alfred, L. J.: *In vitro* effects of certain polycyclic hydrocarbons on mitogen activation of mouse T-lymphocytes: Action of histamine. *Cell. Immunol.*, **77**:132–42, 1983.

Zwilling, B. S.: The effect of respiratory carcinogenesis on systemic humoral and cell-mediated immunity of Syrian Golden hamsters. *Cancer Res.*, **37**:250–52, 1977.

Chapter 10

TOXIC RESPONSES OF THE LIVER

Gabriel L. Plaa

INTRODUCTION

Liver injury induced by chemicals has been recognized as a toxicologic problem for close to 100 years (Zimmerman, 1978). Around 1880 scientists were concerned about the mechanisms involved in the hepatic deposition of lipids following exposure to yellow phosphorus. Hepatic lesions produced by arsphenamine, carbon tetrachloride, and chloroform were also studied in laboratory animals in the first 40 years of the twentieth century. During the same period the correlation between hepatic cirrhosis and excessive ethanol consumption became recognized.

It was recognized early that "liver injury" is not a single entity, that the lesion observed depends not only on the chemical agent involved but also on the period of exposure. After acute exposure one usually finds lipid accumulation in the hepatocytes, cellular necrosis, or hepatobiliary dysfunction, whereas cirrhotic or neoplastic changes are usually considered to be the result of chronic exposures. Different biochemical alterations may lead to the same end-point: no single mechanism seems to govern the appearance of degenerative changes in hepatocytes or alterations in its function. Some forms of liver injury have been found to be reversible while others result in a permanently deranged organ. The mortality associated with various forms of liver injury varies. The incidence of injury differs among species, and the presence of a dose-response relationship may not always be apparent. It is no wonder that today the phrase "produces liver injury" has little meaning to the toxicologist; the form of injury requires precision before its consequences can be assessed.

MORPHOLOGIC AND FUNCTIONAL CONSIDERATIONS

The classic manner of presenting the relationships between the hepatic cell, its vascular supply, and the biliary system has been the configuration of the hexagonal lobule (Figure 10–1), as introduced by Kiernan in 1833. In the center of

this lobule, one finds the terminal hepatic venule (central vein) and at the periphery the portal space, containing a branch of the portal vein, an hepatic arteriole, and a bile duct. Based on this configuration, pathologic lesions of the hepatic parenchyma have been classified as centrilobular, midzonal, or periportal.

The evidence is now quite clear that the hexagonal lobule configuration does not correspond to the functional unit of the liver. The hexagonal lobule is not conspicuous under microscopic examination. Injection of colored gelatin mixtures into the portal vein or the hepatic artery has shown that terminal afferent vessels supply blood to only sectors of adjacent hepatic lobules. These sectors are found to be situated around terminal portal branches and extend from the central vein of one hexagon to the cen-

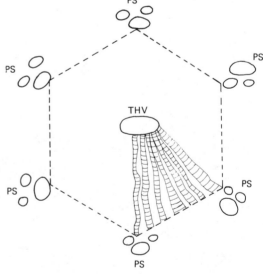

Figure 10–1. Schematic representation of the classic hexagonal lobule. *PS* is the portal space, consisting of a branch of the portal vein, an hepatic arteriole, and bile duct; *THV* is the terminal hepatic venule (central vein).

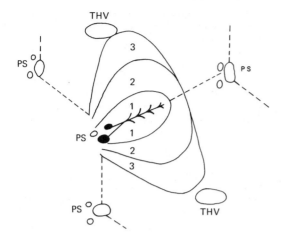

Figure 10–2. Schematic representation of a simple hepatic acinus. *PS* is the portal space, consisting of a branch of the portal vein, an hepatic arteriole, and a bile duct; *THV* is the terminal hepatic venule (central vein); *1, 2,* and *3* represent the various zones drifting off the terminal afferent vessel (in black). (Modified from Rappaport, A. M.: Anatomic considerations. In Schiff, L., (ed.): *Diseases of the Liver,* 3rd ed. J. B. Lippincott Co., Philadelphia, 1969.)

tral vein of an adjacent hexagon. This led Rappaport and co-workers to define the parenchymal mass in terms of functional units called the liver acini (Rappaport, 1979). The simple liver acinus consists of a small parenchymal mass that is irregular in size and shape and is arranged around an axis consisting of a terminal portal venule, an hepatic arteriole, a bile ductule, lymph vessels, and nerves (Figure 10–2). This acinus lies between two or more terminal hepatic venules (central veins) with which its vascular and biliary axis interdigitates. There is no physical separation between two liver acini. The hepatic cells of the simple acini are in cellular and sinusoidal contact with the cells of adjacent or overlapping acini. Even with this extensive communication, the hepatic cells of one particular acinus are preferentially supplied by their parent vessels.

The simple acinus concept also shows that there are circulatory zones within each acinus. Rappaport (1979) has divided these into three, depending on their distance from the supplying terminal vascular branch (Figure 10–2). Three or more simple acini can constitute what is called a "complex acinus." This unit consists of the three simple units and a sleeve of parenchyma around the preterminal afferent vessels, the lymph vessels, and the nerves that eventually give origin to the terminal axial channels of the simple acini.

Although it was assumed for quite some time

that the various hepatic parenchymal cells within the liver lobule have the same kind of functional specificity, it is now becoming clear that there is a lack of uniformity. Gumucio and Miller (1982) have reviewed the current knowledge on zonal differences in hepatic function within the liver acinus. The content of cytochrome P-450, epoxide hydrolase, and glutathione transferase is higher in zone 3 (Figure 10–2) hepatocytes than in other zones (Bentley and Oesch, 1982). Sweeney and co-workers (1978a, 1978b) employed sedimentation velocity analysis as a means of studying hepatocytic heterogeneity in rats. They found significant heterogeneity among populations of hepatocytes and suggested that the larger cells were richer in mixed-function oxidase activity. Furthermore, enhancement of mixed-function oxidase by two different inducers (phenobarbital and 3-methylcholanthrene) resulted in quite different sedimentation-velocity patterns. The concept of heterogeneity in various hepatic cells and in various zones is only in a state of early development. However, one can already see that the concept may permit the rationalization of differing mechanisms of action in the development of hepatic lesions associated with hepatotoxic agents.

The classic descriptions of focal, midzonal periportal, and centrilobular lesions are compatible with Rappaport's zonal acinar configuration (Rappaport, 1979). It is possible to visualize that centrilobular necrosis, for instance, is located in a region that corresponds to the distal acinar zone (zone 3 in Figure 10–2). It has also been said that regeneration occurs from cells located in the midzonal region of the classic representation; this would correspond to the acinar zone closest to the terminal afferent vessel (zone 1), a zone shown to be particularly high in cytogenic enzyme activity. Therefore, it would appear that the acinar circulatory visualization of the hepatic lobule does not come in conflict with the earlier descriptions of pathologic lesions.

Morphologically, chemical-induced injury can manifest itself in different ways. The acute effects can consist of an accumulation of lipids (fatty liver) and the appearance of degenerative processes leading to death of the cell (necrosis). The necrotic process can affect small groups of isolated parenchymal cells ("focal necrosis"), groups of cells located in zones ("centrilobular, midzonal, or periportal necrosis"), or virtually all the cells within an hepatic lobule ("massive necrosis"). The accumulation of lipids can also be zonal or more widespread. While the acute injury caused by the haloalkanes, carbon tetrachloride and chloroform, usually consists of both necrosis and fat accumulation, it is not necessary that both features be present to constitute liver injury. For example, tannic acid, when administered acutely, produces centrilobular necrosis, but extensive fat accumulation does not occur. Thioacetamide also produces centrilobular necrosis without a marked accumulation of lipids. Ethionine, on the other hand, produces fatty livers upon acute administration with little or no necrosis.

Chemical-induced liver injury resulting from chronic exposure can produce marked alterations of the entire liver structure with degenerative and proliferative changes observed in the different forms of cirrhosis. Neoplastic changes may be another end-point of chemical liver injury.

CLASSIFICATION OF CHEMICAL-INDUCED LIVER INJURY

There are a variety of ways of classifying hepatic lesions induced by various chemical substances. In addition to acute hepatic necrosis

and lipid accumulation (Table 10–1), one sees growing interest in the cholestatic type of response (Table 10–2). This latter lesion results in diminution or cessation of bile flow, with ensuing retention of bile salts and bilirubin. The retention of bilirubin leads to production of jaundice. Industrial chemicals are not usually associated with this type of response, although a large number of drugs are (Table 10–2). In addition to the cholestatic lesion, one finds another one, a type of chemical-induced hepatitis that resembles closely that produced by viral infections. The drugs associated with this lesion are less numerous (Table 10–2). A number of drugs are also associated with a mixed type of lesion, that is, one that possesses both cholestatic and hepatocellular components (Zimmerman, 1978).

In 1979 the U.S. Public Health Service promulgated a set of guidelines for the detection of hepatotoxicity due to drugs and chemicals (Davidson *et al.,* 1979). A classification scheme for drug- and chemical-induced liver injury was for-

Table 10–1. EXAMPLES OF ACUTE HEPATOTOXIC CHEMICALS

CHEMICAL	PRODUCES NECROSIS	PRODUCES FATTY LIVER	REFERENCE*
Acetaminophen	x		1
Allyl alcohol	x		2
Allyl formate		x	3
Aflatoxin	x	x	4
Amanita phalloides	x	x	1
Azaserine	x	x	1
Beryllium	x		1
Bromobenzene	x		1
Bromotrichloromethane	x	x	1
Carbon tetrachloride	x	x	1
Cerium		x	5
Chloroform	x	x	1
Cycloheximide		x	1
Dimethylaminoazobenzene	x	x	2
Dimethylnitrosamine	x	x	1
Emetine		x	1
Ethanol		x	1
Ethionine		x	1
Furosemide	x		1
Galactosamine	x	x	1
Methotrexate		x	1
Mithramycin	x		1
Mitomycin C		x	1
Penicillium islandicum	x	x	6
Phosphorus	x	x	1
Puromycin		x	1
Pyrrolizidine alkaloids	x	x	1
Tannic acid	x	x	1
Tetrachloroethane	x	x	3
Tetracycline		x	1
Thioacetamide	x		1
Trichloroethylene	x	x	2
Urethane	x		1

* (1) Zimmerman, 1978; (2) Rouiller, 1964; (3) Rees and Tarlow, 1967; (4) Raisfeld, 1974; (5) Lombardi and Recknagel, 1962; (6) Uraguchi *et al.,* 1961.

Table 10–2.   EXAMPLES OF DRUG-ASSOCIATED LIVER INJURY

DRUG	REFERENCE*	DRUG	REFERENCE*
Intrahepatic Cholestasis			
Ajmaline	1	Methyltestosterone	1
p-Aminobenzylcaffeine	1	Methylthiouracil	1
p-Aminosalicylic acid	2	Nitrofurantoin	1
Amitriptyline	3	Norethandrolone	1
Arsphenamine	1	Norethyndrol	1
Azathioprine	1	Oxacillin	1
Carbamazepine	1	Oxandrolone	1
Carbarsone	2	Oxymetholone	1
Carbimazole	1	Oxyphenisatin	1
Chlordiazepoxide	1	Penicillamine	1
Chlorpromazine	1	Perphenazine	1
Chlorpropamide	1	Phenindione	1
Chlorthiazide	2	Prochlorperazine	1
Diazepam	1	Promazine	1
Erythromycin estolate	1	Propoxyphene	1
Estradiol	1	Propylthiouracil	1
Ethacrynic acid	1	Quinethazone	1
Fluphenazine	1	Thiobendazol	1
Haloperidol	1	Thioridazine	1
Imipramine	1	Thiothixene	1
Mepazine	1	Thiouracil	1
Mestranol	1	Tolazamide	1
Methandrostenolone	1	Tolbutamide	1
Methimazole	1	Triacetyloleandomycin	1
17-Methylnortestosterone	1	Triflupromazine	1
Viral-like Hepatitis			
Acetohexamide	3	Methoxyflurane	1
p-Aminosalicyclic acid	4	α-Methyldopa	1
Carbamazepine	4	Nialamide	3
Cinchophen	1	Oxyphenisatin	1
Colchicine	4	Papaverine	1
Dantrolene	1	Phenelzine	3
Ethacrynic acid	4	Phenindione	4
Ethionamide	1	Phenylbutazone	1
Halothane	1	Phenylisopropylhydrazine	3
Ibufenac	1	Pyrazinamide	1
Indomethacin	1	Sulfamethoxazole	4
Imipramine	1	Sulfisoxazole	4
Iproniazid	1	Tranylcypromine	4
Isoniazid	1	Trimethobenzamide	4
6-Mercaptopurine	1	Zoxazolamine	1

* (1) Zimmerman, 1978; (2) Popper and Schaffner, 1959; (3) Schaffner and Raisfeld, 1969; (4) Perez et al., 1972.

mulated and the hepatic lesions were divided into two categories. *Type I* lesions are those which are "predictable, dose- and time-dependent, occurring in most, if not all, subjects exposed to appropriate doses of the causative substance; the lesions are usually readily reproducible in animals." *Type II* lesions are those which are "nonpredictable, dose- and time-independent, occurring sporadically and often becoming apparent only after monitoring a large number of exposed individuals; the lesions usually are not reproducible in animals." It is important to note that the distinction between a

type I or a type II lesion is made on the basis of predictability, dose and time dependency, frequency of appearance, and reproducibility in animals; the actual morphologic characteristics of the liver injury are not used for classification in this scheme.

For a morphologic classification, the system elaborated by Popper and Schaffner (1959) is still quite appropriate. Five groups of reactions were described. The first was called "zonal hepato-cellular alterations without inflammatory reaction." The substances included in this category all produce zonal changes, either necrosis or fat accumulation (Table 10–1). These authors point out that because of its great reproducibility in several animals species, its dose dependence, and its predictable character, this type of lesion is probably the best understood type of hepatic injury (a type I lesion).

The second group described was called "intra-hepatic cholestasis." This category contained drugs, without common chemical structural characteristics, what were capable of producing, in a very small percentage of the population, a jaundice resembling that produced by extrahepatic biliary obstruction (Table 10–2). The important histologic features associated with this response are the presence of bile stasis, dilation of the canaliculi with subsequent loss of the microvilli, and the occurrence of focal necrosis. There appeared to be no relationship between dose and response, and production of the lesion in animals was not possible with these substances (a type II lesion).

The third category was called "hepatic necrosis with inflammatory reaction." The prominent feature here is the progression to a massive necrosis characteristic of viral hepatitis (Table 10–2). Again it was found that the incidence was extremely low, that dose dependency did not seem to exist, and that reproducibility of these lesions in animals was not possible (a type II lesion).

The fourth group was called an "unclassified group." This category contained a variety of hepatic injuries that did not fit into any type of scheme. For a few of these, the lesions were associated with manifestations of pathology in several other organs.

The fifth group consisted of those producing "hepatic cancer." No drugs were contained in this last category. However, a number of chemicals are now recognized as being hepatocarcinogens in animals.

It is clear that a variety of pathologic processes are involved in what is called, in general terms, "liver injury." Furthermore, many different kinds of substances can cause injury. The question that continually arises is whether the lesion is a manifestation of the hepatotoxic property of the substance in question or whether it is a manifestation of the host's response to the agent. When one considers host response, one must consider not only hypersensitivity (allergic) reactions but also exaggerated responses to minor alterations in hepatic function. With some anabolic steroids, jaundice develops only sporadically in humans, yet diminished biliary excretory capacity is a regular occurrence. It is not known whether the jaundice seen on occasion is a result of an allergic response or whether it is an exaggerated manifestation of diminished biliary excretion. This leads one to emphasize the idea that classification schemes are extremely helpful, but they are only a means of sorting out the state of current views on liver function. As knowledge accumulates, conceptions can change and so must classifications.

CELLULAR SITES OF LIVER INJURY

For the last 50 years, many investigators have been interested in unraveling the hepatotoxic mechanisms involved in carbon tetrachloride-induced liver injury. The amount of information accumulated for this substance is much greater than that available for other substances. Also, in many studies with other agents, comparisons have been made with the effects obtained with carbon tetrachloride. In this sense, carbon tetrachloride has become a reference substance. The major interest in the early periods was devoted to the accumulation of fat associated with exposure to carbon tetrachloride. Consequently, early research efforts were oriented toward fat metabolism. The determination of biochemical mechanisms of action was limited by the analytic techniques available at the time. Consequently, the efforts that were made to determine mechanisms of action centered around the evolution of biochemical approaches to the functioning of various organelles in the hepatocyte. The early work centered on the mitochondria since this was one of the first organelles whose biochemistry became well understood. As the elements of protein synthesis became better known, and with the discovery of the role of the endoplasmic reticulum in this event, investigations were carried out with this particular organelle. The various organelles that can be affected are summarized in Table 10–3.

Carbon tetrachloride can affect cellular membranes. Christie and Judah (1954) showed that carbon tetrachloride altered the permeability of the mitochondria; the activity of the enzymes involved in the Krebs cycle was found to be diminished in these preparations. In addition, others (Dianzani, 1954; Dianzani and Bahr, 1954) demonstrated uncoupling of oxidative phosphorylation in mitochondria. Shifts of electrolytes, in particular calcium ion, were shown to occur early in the intoxication. The results of these observations led to the conclusion that the mitochondrial effects probably produced the fatty livers. This hypothesis no longer seems tenable (Recknagel, 1967; Judah, 1969) because the mitochondrial changes occur much later than does the appearance of fat accumulation. However, the eventual role of the mitochondrial changes in the development of necrosis has yet to be investigated fully.

Table 10–3. **EXAMPLES OF HEPATOTOXICANTS AFFECTING
VARIOUS ORGANELLES**

ORGANELLES AFFECTED	COMPOUND	REFERENCE*
Plasma membrane	*Amanita phalloides*	1
	Phalloidin	1
Endoplasmic reticulum	Allyl formate	2
	Carbon tetrachloride	3
	Dimethylaminoazobenzene	2
	Dimethylnitrosamine	4
	Ethionine	1
	Galactosamine	5
	Phosphorus	2
	Pyrrolizidine alkaloids	6
	Tannic acid	1
	Thioacetamide	1
Mitochondria	*Amanita phalloides*	1
	Allyl formate	2
	Carbon tetrachloride	3
	1,1-Dicholoroethylene	7
	Dimethylnitrosamine	2
	Ethionine	1
	Hydrazine	8
	Phosphorus	2
	Pyrrolizidine alkaloids	6
Lysosomes	*Amanita phalloides*	1
	Beryllium	9
	Carbon tetrachloride	1
	Ethionine	10
	Phosphorus	10
	Pyrrolizidine alkaloids	6
Nucleus	Aflatoxin	1
	Beryllium	11
	Dimethylnitrosamine	1
	Ethionine	10
	Galactosamine	5
	Hydrazine	8
	Pyrrolizidine alkaloids	6
	Tannic acid	1
	Thioacetamide	1

* (1) Zimmerman, 1978; (2) Rouiller, 1964; (3) Recknagel, 1967; (4) Magee and Swann, 1969; (5) Decker and Keppler, 1974; (6) McLean, 1970; (7) Reynolds *et al.*, 1975; (8) Ganote and Rosenthal, 1968; (9) Witschi and Aldridge, 1968; (10) Dianzani, 1976; (11) Witschi, 1970.

Later experiments show that carbon tetrachloride can also affect the membranes of the endoplasmic reticulum. Recknagel and Lombardi (1961) were the first to demonstrate that glucose-6-phosphatase, an enzyme associated with this structure, was markedly depressed very early after carbon tetrachloride administration. By electron microscopy, the cisternae of the endoplasmic reticulum were shown to be dilated. Furthermore, protein synthesis associated with this structure was inhibited (Smuckler *et al.*, 1961). Recknagel and Ghoshal (1966) demonstrated that carbon tetrachloride affects the lipid structure of microsomes, derived from the endoplasmic reticulum, and proposed that peroxidative decomposition of lipids in this organelle occurs early in the intoxication. Altered

phospholipids and toxic aldehydes were observed by Benedetti and co-workers (1982). The endoplasmic reticulum calcium pump is also markedly depressed very early after carbon tetrachloride or chloroform administration; this action appears to be independent of lipid peroxidation (Moore, 1980). Depression of the calcium pump also occurs with carbon disulfide and 1,1-dichloroethylene (Moore, 1982a, 1982b).

Another organelle that has been investigated is the lysosome. Dianzani (1963) showed that carbon tetrachloride and dimethylnitrosamine had little effect on lysosomes at a time when necrotic changes were already developing. In 1965, Baccino and co-workers demonstrated that, *in vitro*, carbon tetrachloride could cause lysosomal damage with the concomitant release of enzymes into the suspending medium. However, this effect could not be prevented by the administration of promethazine and diphenhydramine, two substances that exert protective effects against carbon tetrachloride *in vivo*. Alpers and Isselbacher (1967) also showed that release of lysosomal enzymes occurs at carbon tetrachloride concentrations that inhibit leucine incorporation into protein. They found that lipid peroxidation seemed to be independent of this effect since carbon tetrachloride did not enhance peroxide formation in lysosomal fractions at a time when its effect on enzyme activity was maximal. Witschi and Aldridge (1967, 1968) demonstrated that beryllium is taken up by rat lysosomes *in vivo* and that lysosomal enzymes are released. Since the release of enzymes is a late phenomenon, it is not known whether this effect is the cause of the liver injury. For the moment, it appears that lysosomes play a relatively minor role in the development of necrosis.

Changes in membrane permeability have been demonstrated by a number of investigators. Work by Judah (1969) showed that treatment with promethazine or EDTA could remove the inhibition of enzymes owing to a loss of semipermeable properties of the cells. Promethazine could protect against carbon tetrachloride necrosis (Rees *et al.*, 1961). An interesting finding was that, while treatment with this substance protected against the necrosis, the fatty alterations were not affected. This important observation clearly showed that the two changes could be dissociated in the case of carbon tetrachloride. There is other evidence that suggests that altered permeability exists. Calcium can accumulate in necrotic tissues (Farber, 1982). Disturbances in liver cell calcium homeostasis may be a critical secondary pathologic mechanism in liver injury (Farber, 1982; Recknagel *et al.*, 1982; Bellomo and Orrenius, 1985).

Altered membrane permeability of the hepatic cell can also lead to increased enzyme activity in plasma. The plasma activity of a number of hepatic cytoplasmic and mitochondrial enzymes is increased following carbon tetrachloride hepatotoxicity. The plasma activities of aminotransferase, lactic acid dehydrogenase, aldolase, and isocitric dehydrogenase, among others, are used as diagnostic indicators of hepatic injury. Generally speaking, the plasma activities of cytoplasmic enzymes increase more rapidly than those of mitochondrial enzymes. Because of the time sequence involved, there is some doubt that the appearance of enzymes in plasma results from necrosis; the early appearance of nonmitochondrial enzymes is thought to result from altered cell permeability. It should be pointed out that whether these increases are associated with changes in permeability or whether they reflect prenecrotic changes has little bearing on the empiric use of these enzymes for determining the presence of dysfunction.

MECHANISMS OF LIVER INJURY

Accumulation of Lipids

A number of agents that produce liver injury also cause the accumulation of abnormal amounts of fat, predominantly triglyceride, in the parenchymal cells (Table 10–1). Triglyceride accumulation is the result of an imbalance between the rate of synthesis and the rate of release of triglyceride by the parenchymal cells into the systemic circulation.

Several investigators showed that a block of the secretion of hepatic triglyceride into plasma is the major mechanism underlying the fatty liver induced in rats by carbon tetrachloride, ethionine, phosphorus, puromycin, or tetracycline, by feeding a choline-deficient diet, or by feeding orotic acid (Lombardi, 1966; Hoyumpa *et al.*, 1975; Dianzani, 1979). The accumulation of triglyceride in the hepatic cells is paralleled by a decrease in the concentration of plasma lipids and plasma lipoproteins. The plasma concentration of triglyceride in fasted rats can be diminished to almost one-half its normal value within 30 minutes after exposure to carbon tetrachloride. By two hours, triglycerides have begun to accumulate abnormally in the liver. Tetracycline induces fatty livers and interferes with triglyceride secretion (Hoyumpa *et al.*, 1975).

When hepatic triglyceride is released into the plasma, it is not released as such, but is combined with a lipoprotein. Carbon tetrachloride and ethionine can lower the level of circulating lipoprotein. The very-low-density lipoproteins are principally affected. This fraction is involved in the transport of hepatic triglycerides to extrahepatic tissues. A decrease in the proportion of triglyceride combined with lipoprotein can occur if (1) synthesis of triglyceride and the other lipid moieties increases, (2) synthesis of the protein moiety is decreased, (3) the two moieties are formed but do not associate, and (4) the formed lipoprotein is normal but cannot be secreted by the cell. Carbon tetrachloride, ethionine, phosphorus, and puromycin can interfere with the synthesis of the protein moiety (Dianzani, 1979). Although there is evidence that all these substances can affect synthesis of lipoproteins, it is by no means clear that this is the only mechanism involved. With ethionine and phosphorus, this factor is most likely the key defect; however, with carbon tetrachloride, Recknagel (1967) has pointed out that the coupling phase of triglyceride secretion is probably affected. With tetracycline, impaired release of very-low-density lipoprotein occurs, but it is not known whether synthesis, conjugation, or secretion is the phase affected (Hoyumpa *et al.*, 1975).

The function of the lipoproteins seems to be one of a vehicle, containing protein, phospholipid, and cholesterol; a defect could thus occur in the synthesis of the phospholipid or cholesterol moieties. In choline-deficient animals, a situation that results in the development of fatty liver, phospholipid synthesis is impaired. This effect of choline deficiency can result in impaired release of very-low-density lipoproteins (Lombardi and Oler, 1967). Orotic acid can produce fatty livers when fed to rats and also results in a block in the secretion of low-density lipoproteins (Windmueller and von Euler, 1971).

It was shown by electron microscopy that the accumulation of triglycerides results in the formation of droplets in the endoplasmic reticulum. Baglio and Farber (1965) coined the term "liposomes" for these droplets. They speculated that these liposomes may represent the morphologic expression of a block in the release of triglyceride; they postulate that a defective synthesis or secretion of lipoproteins may result in the accumulation of triglyceride in the cisternae of the endoplasmic reticulum. The major portion of the esterified fatty acids released by the liver appears as triglycerides in the very-low-density lipoprotein fraction. Recently microtubules have been suggested as playing a role in the secretion of very-low-density lipoprotein; a tubulin assembly-disassembly cycle exists in the liver, and interruption of the cycle by colchicine administration results in a blockade of very-low-density lipoprotein secretion (Jeanrenaud *et al.*, 1977). Hepatotoxicants have not been tried on this system, although microtubules are thought to play a major role in the secretion of lipoproteins (Dianzani, 1979).

It is possible that elevated triglyceride could result because of an increase in the rate of synthesis of this substance. Since there is evidence that the rate of synthesis is directly proportional to the concentration of the substrates present (fatty acids and glycerophosphate), it is theoretically possible that increased hepatic triglyceride synthesis could occur because of increased fatty acids or increased glycerophosphate. However, there is little evidence to support the idea that fatty acid synthesis is involved in the development of fatty liver following the administration of hepatotoxicants.

Increased mobilization of free fatty acids from adipose tissue has also been proposed as a possible mechanism for the development of fatty livers. However, after close scrutiny of the experimental evidence, it does not appear that such a mechanism could play a major role. For instance, with ethionine, where it was shown that the plasma concentration of fatty acids doubles, the net uptake by liver is still normal (Lombardi, 1966). In the case of carbon tetrachloride, Recknagel (1967) concluded that accelerated movement of fatty acids from peripheral stores is not a factor to be considered. It must be remembered that in the case of mobilization of fatty acids from adipose stores, the question is not whether this source of fat is needed for the accumulation of liver triglycerides, but whether an excessive amount of fatty acids is actually being released to the liver for uptake. Everyone agrees that fatty acids must be available from adipose tissue for the liver to synthesize triglycerides. In addition, the role of circulating free fatty acids has been amply demonstrated by interruption of the pituitary-adrenal axis with resulting diminution of plasma free fatty acids. This leads to a block in the accumulation of triglycerides. However, in this situation, the peripheral stores play a permissive role rather than a controlling role.

One can raise the question whether fat accumulation itself always represents an injurious response for the hepatocyte. As previously pointed out, a fatty liver does not necessarily lead to death of the hepatocytes; ethionine, puromycin, and cycloheximide all cause fat accumulation without producing necrosis. Promethazine protects rats against the necrogenic effects of carbon tetrachloride but does not abolish the fatty liver (Rees *et al.*, 1961). Bucher and Malt (1971) reviewed the biochemical and morphologic events associated with liver regeneration. Following partial hepatectomy in rats, there is a largely hormone-mediated mobilization of fat from adipose tissue. Neutral fat accumulates in the remainder of the liver within 18 to 24 hours, reaching a value ten times that of normal livers and bringing about distortion of the normal lobular pattern. The capacity to secrete triglycerides increases, but liposomes begin to appear along with intracellular fat globules, indicating a relative delay in triglyceride secretion when compared with triglyceride accumulation. The hepatic cells, in the presence of this fat, still function as well as normal, if not more efficiently, while preparing for cell division at the same time. As Ingelfinger (1971) points out, in the face of this, can one say that excessive fat accumulation in itself is damaging?

Protein Synthesis

With many of the hepatotoxicants that have been shown to produce necrosis, relatively similar morphologic changes have been reported to occur rapidly after the administration of the substance. Light microscopic examination reveals a loss of cytoplasmic basophilic material well before the appearance of necrosis in the hepatocyte. By electron microscopy, one sees vacuoles in the cytoplasm within one hour after the injection of carbon tetrachloride. At this time, the endoplasmic reticulum is also abnormal; the membranes are less well defined and dilated. Similar observations were reported when rats were administered dimethylnitrosamine, carcinogenic azo dyes, ethionine, and thioacetamide (Magee, 1966).

Magee (1966) doubts that these changes actually represent early changes leading to necrosis. He feels that they are merely related to the inhibitory effects of these substances on protein synthesis. Ethionine, dimethylnitrosamine, carbon tetrachloride, thioacetamide, and galactosamine inhibit incorporation of amino acids into liver proteins. While a number of investigators have thought that inhibition of protein synthesis is the cause of liver necrosis, Magee (1966) points out that this cannot be considered to be entirely correct since, for at least ethionine, protein synthesis can be inhibited without inducing liver necrosis. Cycloheximide also inhibits protein synthesis for many hours, but does not result in liver necrosis (Farber, 1971). In fact, cycloheximide treatment can protect rats against hepatocytic necrosis induced by carbon tetrachloride and against acute necrosis of the biliary epithelium following α-naphthylisothiocyanate (Farber, 1975). Furthermore, Witschi and Aldridge (1967) showed that beryllium, a substance that produces midzonal necrosis, does not cause early inhibition of protein synthesis.

Extensive work has been carried out to determine how various agents affect protein synthesis (Dianzani, 1976). Ethionine inhibits amino acid incorporation into microsomal proteins. Ethionine replaces methionine and forms S-adenosylethionine, which leads to a trapping of cellular adenine, a diminution in the rate of ATP synthesis, and inhibition of RNA synthesis. Thus, ethionine, by its adenine-trapping effect, leads to accumulation of triglycerides in liver within a few hours; this fatty liver appears to be a secondary consequence to the interference with protein metabolism (Farber, 1971).

Dimethylnitrosamine can inhibit protein synthesis, and the effects are quite striking three hours after administration of the substance (Magee, 1966). The effects also occur in the microsomes rather than in the soluble supernatant fraction of liver homogenates. Mizrahi and Emmelot (1962) claim that dimethylnitrosamine probably affects protein synthesis by causing a loss of messenger RNA from the polyribosomes. They tentatively concluded that this loss of messenger RNA from the ribosomes may be due to methylation of RNA. Mager and co-workers (1965) have reported results with dimethylnitrosamine that are consistent with the destruction of ribosome bound messenger RNA.

Inhibition of protein synthesis in rat liver by carbon tetrachloride was reported by Smuckler and co-workers (1961). A marked reduction of incorporation of amino acids into lipoproteins was observed as early as two hours after administration of carbon tetrachloride by Seakins and Robinson (1963). Smuckler and Benditt (1965) found no evidence for inhibition of RNA synthesis after carbon tetrachloride; however, they did find that there were changes in the proportions of the various subunits found in ribosomal preparations.

Farber and co-workers (1971) showed that pretreatment of rats with cycloheximide protects the liver against the ribosomal changes induced by carbon tetrachloride. This protection occurs during a time in which the changes induced by carbon tetrachloride on the endoplasmic reticulum still occur. These authors have interpreted their results to indicate that carbon tetrachloride exerts its effect on protein synthesis on single-unit ribosomes and not on the polysomes. It would thus appear that carbon tetrachloride can exert no effect when the ribosomes are aggregated in polysomes but only when they are present as monomers. In addition, these investigators showed that damage to protein synthesis induced by carbon tetrachloride appears to be irreversible in contrast to the observations made with ethionine or puromycin. These observations may explain in part why carbon tetrachloride results in cell death whereas this does not occur with the other two substances.

Galactosamine also inhibits protein synthesis; reduced synthesis of RNA and plasma proteins, particularly coagulation factors, has been observed (Decker and Keppler, 1974). Uridine prevents or reverses the inhibition, which indicates that the depression is the result of the UTP deficiency induced by galactosamine. The galactosamine-1-phosphate formed in the liver leads to the accumulation of UDP derivates of galactosamine; in turn, this results in a depletion of hepatic UTP, UDP hexoses, and a depression of uracil nucleotide-dependent biosynthesis of macromolecules. This is believed to result in injury to cellular organelles and necrosis of liver cells. Galactosamine-induced liver injury passes through several stages depending on the dosage schedule (reversible acute hepatitis, chronic progressive hepatitis, cirrhosis, production of liver tumors), but is highly specific to this amino sugar. In addition, morphologic studies indicate that all hepatocytes are affected, to a varying degree, so that the result is an experimental model of diffuse liver cell injury (Medline *et al.,* 1970).

Lipid Peroxidation

Butler (1961) demonstrated that carbon tetrachloride was biotransformed to chloroform and concluded that this transformation was caused by homolytic cleavage, yielding free radicals that could alkylate sulfhydryl groups of enzymes. In 1966, Slater published a brief review concerning the necrogenic action of carbon tetrachloride. He proposed that homolytic cleavage of the carbon-chlorine bond occurred in the endoplasmic reticulum and that this resulted in production of free radicals, which could then interact with neighboring lipid-rich material causing alterations in structure and function. Working independently, Recknagel arrived at the same conclusion (Recknagel and Ghoshal, 1966).

Recknagel and Ghoshal (1966) hypothesized that free radicals arising from the homolytic cleavage of carbon tetrachloride attacked the methylene bridges of unsaturated fatty acid side chains of microsomal lipids, resulting in morphologic alteration of the endoplasmic reticulum, loss of activity of drug-metabolizing enzymes, loss of glucose-6-phosphatase activity, loss of protein synthesis, and loss of the capacity of the liver to form and excrete low-density lipoprotein. They were able to demonstrate that *in vitro* carbon tetrachloride could act as a prooxidant and that this effect of carbon tetrachloride was limited to the liver. They demonstrated the appearance of conjugated dienes, typical of peroxidized polyenoic fatty acids. In subsequent work, the appearance *in vivo* of conjugated dienes was observed in animals and in humans subjected to intoxicating doses of carbon tetrachloride. Phenobarbital treatment resulted in increased lipid peroxidation in vivo, and SKF 525-A resulted in a diminution of the appearance of microsomal lipid peroxidation. The extensive investigative work carried out by Recknagel and his co-workers (Recknagel and Glende, 1973) has been the foundation of the lipid peroxidation theory as it concerns carbon tetrachloride liver injury.

Comporti and co-workers (1965) also provided evidence that carbon tetrachloride *in vitro* stimulates lipid peroxidation of rat liver microsomes. These authors were unable to find similar results with chloroform. DiLuzio and Hartman (1969) demonstrated that animals treated with carbon tetrachloride had lower microsomal lipid-soluble antioxidant activity and concluded that this was consistent with enhanced lipid peroxidation.

Gordis (1969) showed that five minutes after the intravenous injection of [^{14}C]- or [^{36}Cl] carbon tetrachloride, liver lipids were labeled. Most of the radioactivity was found in the phospholipid fraction. His results were compatible with the formation of free radicals and offered an alternative to the lipid peroxidation theory of Recknagel (1967). Gordis visualized the possibility that free radicals derived from carbon tetrachloride would form chlorinated lipids that may be unsuitable as membrane components. Benedetti and co-workers (1977a, 1977b) described the alterations induced by carbon tetrachloride in the lipids of the membranes of the hepatic endoplasmic reticulum one hour after treatment. Both the simple addition of carbon tetrachloride free radicals to fatty acids and a chain termination addition reaction of carbon tetrachloride free radicals to fatty acid free radicals containing conjugated dienes occurred; the latter products were quite abnormal in physical characteristics. In subsequent work, Benedetti and co-workers (1977c) produced these alterations *in vitro* using liver microsomes incubated in the presence of carbon tetrachloride; in addition, they followed the production of malonic dialdehyde and monitored glucose-6-phosphatase activity under aerobic and anaerobic environments. The binding of carbon tetrachloride free radicals to microsomal lipids occurred in both environments. However, the lipids underwent peroxidation (production of malonic dialdehyde), and depression of glucose-6-phosphatase activity occurred only in the aerobic environment. These investigators concluded that peroxidative breakdown of unsaturated lipids, rather than covalent binding, was responsible for the inactivation of glucose-6-phosphatase. The peroxidative cleavage of unsaturated fatty acids can result in the release of carbonyl compounds or the formation of carbonyl functions in the acyl residue (Benedetti *et al.,* 1982). Some of these substances are toxicologically active and have been identified as 4-hydroxyalkenals (Benedetti *et al.,* 1981; Comporti, 1985).

Alpers and co-workers (1968) studied the role of lipid peroxidation in the pathogenesis of carbon tetrachloride-induced inhibition of protein synthesis. They found that, *in vivo,* the administration of antioxidants did prevent the appearance of fatty livers and necrosis; however, protein synthesis, studied by the incorporation of leucine into hepatic proteins, was not altered by the administration of the antioxidant. These authors concluded that the demonstration of lipid peroxidation *in vitro* may not always imply functional damage to the subcellular component affected. They raised the possibility that *in vivo* inhibition of protein synthesis may not have a direct relationship to the degree of lipid peroxidation. There is still some controversy regarding the relative importance of carbon tetrachloride-induced lipid peroxidation in the subsequent pathologic changes, and there are inconsistent results reported in the literature (Plaa and Witschi, 1976). It is clear that additional events are involved in the pathologic changes that result in fat accumulation, breakup of the cell membrane, and cellular necrosis (Recknagel et al., 1982; Recknagel, 1983). Lipid peroxidation, in itself, is unable to account for all these events.

Klaassen and Plaa (1969) studied the dose-response relationships involved in carbon tetrachloride and chloroform hepatotoxicity. They confirmed the presence of conjugated dienes in vivo after the administration of carbon tetrachloride, and also the depression of glucose-6-phosphatase activity as described previously. However, these authors were unable to show the presence of conjugated dienes after the administration of chloroform in doses that resulted in fatty livers and necrosis. Furthermore, they could find no depression of glucose-6-phosphate after administration of chloroform. Brown and co-workers (1974) reported that rats pretreated with phenobarbital, but not untreated rats, will produce conjugated dienes during chloroform anesthesia; depression of glucose-6-phosphatase activity also occurs after chloroform only in phenobarbital-pretreated rats (Lavigne and Marchand, 1974). Since chloroform-induced liver injury is more severe in phenobarbital-pretreated rats, the possibility exists that the initial lesion induced by chloroform in these animals is only aggravated by the appearance of lipid peroxidation. These findings cast doubt on the general applicability of lipid peroxidation as a mechanism for necrogenic haloalkanes.

Lipid peroxidation was reported to occur after the administration of tetrachloroethane in mice (Tomokuni, 1970). This substance increases liver triglycerides under these experimental conditions. Sell and Reynolds (1969) compared the lesion produced by iodoform to that produced by carbon tetrachloride. They found that, morphologically, the lesions were quite comparable. In addition, lipid peroxidation occurred within 30 minutes, being associated with a depression in glucose-6-phosphatase activity and calcium flux. There was also an increase in cell sap RNA. These findings are essentially identical to those observed after carbon tetrachloride intoxication. Lipoperoxidation also occurs after phosphorus poisoning in rats (Ghoshal et al., 1969). Elevation of triglyceride levels was observed as well; however, the elevation of triglycerides occurred after the increases in lipid peroxidation.

Several other hepatotoxicants were shown to produce acute liver necrosis in the absence of in vivo demonstration of lipid peroxidation (Plaa and Witschi, 1976). 1,1-Dichloroethylene causes liver injury that is quite comparable to that produced by carbon tetrachloride; yet lipid peroxidation has not been observed. Dimethylnitrosamine and thioacetamide also do not seem to produce lipid peroxidation in vivo. There are also doubts about the importance of the phenomenon in ethylene dibromide-induced liver injury. With halothane the results obtained by Brown and co-workers (1974) are comparable to those observed with chloroform. DiLuzio (1973) proposed that lipid peroxidation also plays a role in acute ethanol-induced fatty liver. The subject is still controversial and the matter is yet to be resolved (Plaa and Witschi, 1976; Dianzani, 1979; Comporti, 1985). While there is no doubt that lipid peroxidation does occur with some substances, it is evident that with others this factor is either absent or of doubtful significance.

Necrosis

Despite the great advances that have been made in understanding the morphologic and biochemical alterations associated with chemical-induced liver injury, it has to be realized that the knowledge acquired is still incapable of establishing which of the changes observed lead to cell death and which are secondary disturbances (Judah, 1969; Farber, 1979); current knowledge can inform the interested person as to what can be done to a cell and yet not destroy it. As stated by Judah (1969), "this advance in knowledge by attrition will continue."

This state of affairs led Farber (1975) to suggest that perhaps our concepts of cell death are in error. Cell death has been considered to be a degenerative phenomenon, a "running down" of the metabolic activity of the cell. He suggests that under some conditions cell death may not be a passive event but may rather be the result of a more active process, like the overproduction of some enzyme or other protein ("cell suicide" instead of "cell homicide"). As support for this interesting concept Farber (1975) points out that cycloheximide, an inhibitor of protein synthesis, can protect certain cells against the necrogenic properties of carbon tetrachloride and α-naphthylisothiocyanate. Obviously, more work is needed to test the validity of this novel hypothesis.

Recently, altered calcium homeostasis and accumulation of intracellular calcium have been shown to be intimately involved in the necrogenic responses induced by phalloidin, carbon tetrachloride, and galactosamine (Farber, 1982). The processes involved represent a sequential series of cellular alterations that are poorly understood. The general applicability to other necrogenic hepatotoxicants is yet to be established.

Cholestasis

The mechanisms involved in drug-induced cholestasis are still very poorly understood. One of the major reasons for this deficiency lies in that fact that, with the possible exception of the steroids, it has been extremely difficult to reproduce in animals the drug-induced cholestatic syndrome seen in humans. However, it is possible to produce cholestatic responses in animals with certain chemicals that have no therapeutic utility. The induction of intrahepatic cholestasis in animals following the administration of certain bile salts, α-naphthylisothiocyanate (ANIT), certain steroids, and manganese has provided important contributions to the understanding of the characteristics, and perhaps the causes, of the cholestatic syndrome (Plaa and Priestly, 1976).

Lithocholic acid is a naturally occurring monohydroxy bile acid. Javitt (1966) demonstrated that the taurine conjugate of lithocholic acid (taurolithocholic acid), when administered intravenously in the rat, results in a prompt diminution of bile flow. The cessation of bile flow is dose dependent, and bile flow usually returns to normal within six hours. Prolonged infusions result in hyperbilirubinemia. Schaffner and Javitt (1966) found that the canalicular microvilli were greatly reduced in size and number after administration of taurolithocholate; the Golgi apparatus was dilated and vacuolated. Taurocholate can compete with taurolithocholate and can antagonize the cholestatic response induced by the latter substance. Taurolithocholate is poorly soluble in water and can precipitate in the biliary tract (Javitt and Emerman, 1968). However, studies (Boyer et al., 1977) indicate that this bile salt also modifies the structure and permeability of the membrane of the bile canaliculus by directly binding to components of the membrane. Lithocholate causes an increase in cholesterol in canalicular membrane, resulting in an increased inner viscosity and decreased permeability of the membrane (Kakis et al., 1980). Lithocholate can interact with cholesterol and accumulate in bile canalicular membranes in vitro; interestingly, an unidentified hepatocellular cytosolic protein appears to be involved in this process (Yousef et al., 1984). Others (Fisher et al., 1971; Miyai et al., 1971) have demonstrated cholestasis in isolated rat livers perfused with lithocholic, chenodeoxycholic, glycholithocholic, or taurolithocolic acid. The three α-sulfate esters of taurolithocholic acid and glycolithocholic acid were less cholestatic than the nonsulfated conjugates. Chenodeoxycholate causes hepatocellular necrosis in rats. Lithocholate and chenodeoxycholate differ in the mechanism by which they produce cholestasis (Plaa and Priestly, 1976). Chenodeoxycholate is cytotoxic, and cholestasis seems to result from a generalized hepatocellular dysfunction, whereas lithocholate seems to interact directly with the bile secretory function of the canalicular membrane.

A single oral dose of ANIT produces both bile stasis and hyperbilirubinemia in the rat, and the cessation of bile flow occurs within 24 hours (Plaa and Priestly, 1976). Electron microscopic studies also indicate alterations of hepatocyte membrane. ANIT can affect several hepatocyte functions. In addition to the development of hyperbilirubinemia, sulfobromophthalein (BSP) retention and inhibition of microsomal drug-metabolizing activity have also been demonstrated. The bilirubin retention induced by ANIT could be due to a number of defects in hepatic cell function. The maximal rate of biliary bilirubin excretion is diminished in ANIT-treated animals. ANIT can increase the synthesis of bilirubin from nonerythropoietic sources; this effect can be demonstrated two hours after the administration of ANIT. While all these mechanisms could participate in the response, it is predominantly the decrease in biliary excretion of bilirubin that contributes to the hyperbilirubinemia observed.

There is a considerable amount of indirect evidence that indicates that the cholestatic properties of ANIT may be due to a metabolite (Plaa and Priestly, 1976). There is marked species variation; both the cholestatic and hyperbilirubinemic responses can be potentiated if the animals are pretreated with enzyme inducers; inhibitors of microsomal enzyme activity can diminish the ANIT response; temperature can also affect the response; inhibitors of protein synthesis have been shown to markedly reduce the cholestatic and hyperbilirubinemic responses to ANIT.

The cholestatic reaction associated with the clinical use of anabolic and contraceptive steroids has prompted experimental studies designed to characterize the response in animals. Although some canalicular dilatation has been observed in rats after administration of norethandrolone (Schaffner et al., 1960), definite manifestations of intrahepatic cholestasis, such as hyperbilirubinemia and canalicular bile plugs, have not been established as norethandrolone effects in rats. Imai and Hayashi (1970) reported that large doses of norethisterone produce jaundice consistently in mice. Canalicular bile plugs were observed after treatment with norethisterone, methyltestosterone, oxymetholone, mestranol, or norethandrolone. No plugs were observed when testosterone proprionate, progesterone, or 17β-estradiol was administered. Electron microscopy revealed dilatation of the bile canaliculi and a decrease in the appearance of microvilli. Various strains of male mice were shown to respond similarly; DS and C57BL strains were the most sensitive, whereas ICR mice were the least sensitive. Sprague-Dawley rats did not exhibit cholestasis, even when treated with larger doses of norethisterone. These observations indicate a species variation and even a difference between strains. Anabolic steroids do cause BSP retention in rabbits (Lennon, 1966). With ethinyl estradiol, reduced bile flow was observed in rats (Gumucio and Valdivieso, 1971). Estrogens can affect the permeability of the biliary tree, reduce bile salt-independent bile flow, and decrease the clearance of infused bile salts (Plaa and Priestly, 1976; Schreiber and Simon, 1983); it is not clear which parameter is of major importance in producing the cholestatic reaction. With various oral contraceptive steroids, decreased bile flow and a decrease in biliary excretory maximum for bilirubin have been reported (Heikel and Lathe, 1970), but the mechanism has not been elucidated. Certain glucuronide conjugates of naturally occurring estrogens can produce a dose-dependent, reversible cholestasis in rats or monkeys (Meyers et al., 1980, 1981; Slikker et al., 1983). D-ring glucuronide conjugates are active, whereas A-ring conjugates are not. The canalicular membrane appears to be the site of action; both bile salt-dependent and bile salt-independent bile flow are depressed. Whether during pregnancy these D-ring conjugates can attain concentrations sufficient to induce intrahepatic cholestasis remains to be determined.

Intrahepatic cholestasis can also be produced in rats by the administration of an intravenous load of manganese sulfate (Witzleben, 1972). Recently, manganese ingestion has been associated with hepatotoxicity in humans (Lustig et al., 1982). In the rat, this response is associated with the development of necrotic lesions, which varies from focal necrosis to subtotal midzonal necrosis. Widespread dilatation of bile canaliculi with loss of microvilli is observed 20 hours after treatment. The maximum biliary excretion of bilirubin is markedly diminished in the manganese-loaded rats; there is no correlation between the extent of necrosis and the cholestatic response. Manganese treatment followed by bilirubin infusion can cause a more severe cholestasis; recovery of bile flow is partial at 24 hours and essentially complete at 48 hours. Small doses of manganese produce cholestasis only if followed by an injection of bilirubin; a close relationship exists between manganese and bilirubin in order to elicit the fully developed cholestatic response (de Lamirande and Plaa, 1979). The manganese-bilirubin model is particularly interesting since the degree and duration of cholestasis are dose-dependent on bilirubin, whereas the dose of manganese regulates the time period during which bilirubin can exert its effect (de Lamirande and Plaa, 1979). Recent work indicates that the site of action of the manganese-bilirubin combination is the bile canalicular membrane (de Lamirande et al., 1981; Plaa et al., 1982). Manganese enters into the bile canalicular membrane in a dose-related manner, and bilirubin facilitates this incorporation (Ayotte and Plaa, 1985). During manganese-bilirubin cholestasis, bilirubin accumulates in bile canalicular membranes (de Lamirande et al., 1981; Plaa et al., 1982). It is postulated (Ayotte and Plaa, 1985) that this incorporation of manganese and bilirubin may disrupt bile canalicular membrane fluidity and permeability.

There is still considerable controversy as to whether phenothiazines and tricyclic antidepressants cause cholestasis in humans because of a direct toxic effect or because of a hypersensitivity reaction. These compounds have been the subject of extensive investigation in animals (Plaa and Priestly, 1976; Plaa and Hewitt, 1982). An important species variation exists in chlorpromazine-induced hepatobiliary dysfunction. In the dog and rhesus monkey, a reduction in bile flow occurs after its acute intravenous administration, whereas chronic administration does not result in cholestasis in rats. Chlorpromazine rapidly inhibits bile flow in a dose-dependent manner in isolated perfused rat livers. Phenothiazines, thioxanthenes, and tricyclic antidepressants are hepatocytotoxic (Plaa and Hewitt, 1982). With chlorpromazine, demethylation, multiple ring hydroxylations, and free-radical generation appreciably increase its toxicity. Sulfoxidation results in a striking reduction of toxicity. These observations appear to be more consistent with a direct, hepatotoxic action rather than an indirect, hypersensitivity response.

With erythromycin estolate the data obtained with animals are very limited (Plaa and Preistly, 1976). Cytotoxicity, related to surfactant properties, was observed in vitro using preparations of isolated hepatocytes; reduced bile flow in the isolated perfused rat liver was also reported.

A number of mechanisms leading to cholestasis have been proposed based on various experimental results, but these are far from being definitive (Plaa and Priestly, 1976; Plaa and

Hewitt, 1982; Schreiber and Simon, 1983). These include impaired bile salt-independent canalicular bile flow (chlorpromazine, ethinylestradiol, ethacrynic acid), canalicular membrane function (ANIT, taurocholate, cytochalasin B), altered ductular cell permeability (ANIT), hypertrophic hypoactive smooth endoplasmic reticulum (bile salts, ANIT), and intracanalicular precipitation (taurolithocholate, chlorpromazine, erythromycin lactobionate).

The hepatocyte contains actin, a contractile protein, but its role in hepatocellular function has not been established (Phillips et al., 1983). However, phalloidin and cytochalasin, which affect actin filaments, can cause cholestasis and this is attributed to microfilament dysfunction. Recently, liver cells in culture were shown to exhibit regular contractions of the bile canaliculi (Phillips et al., 1982); liver cells obtained from rats pretreated with phalloidin or cytochalasin exhibited irregular contractions (Watanabe et al., 1983). These important observations uncover a whole new array of possible sites and mechanisms of action for cholestatic agents.

Cirrhosis

Cirrhosis is a chronic morphologic alteration of the liver that has received a great amount of attention. Histologically cirrhosis is characterized by the presence of septae of collagen distributed throughout the major portion of the liver (Schinella and Becker, 1975). These appear to form fibrous sheaths in a three-dimensional network, which appear as bands in a two-dimensional histologic section; the circumscribed areas of aggregated liver cells appear as nodules. Invariably the pattern of hepatic blood flow is altered. In the majority of cases, single-cell necrosis appears as the major element in its pathogenesis. This necrotic process is associated with a deficiency in the repair mechanism of the residual cells; this deficiency leads to fibroblastic activity and scar formation. The pathogenesis of cirrhosis is not at all clearly understood. Other factors, such as intrahepatic vascular alterations, may play a contributory role in the development of cirrhosis.

Cirrhosis can be induced in animals by chronic administration of carbon tetrachloride, aflatoxin, or the administration of several chemical carcinogens. In humans, however, the single most important cause of cirrhosis is chronic ingestion of alcoholic beverages (Lelbach, 1975; Rankin et al., 1975). In the usual laboratory animal the production of cirrhosis, as seen in humans, is not possible by the chronic feeding of ethanol alone (Schinella and Becker, 1975). However, precirrhotic changes (increased hydroxyproline, increased proline incorporation into collagen, and increased collagen proline hydroxylase activity) can be observed after ethanol ingestion. Lieber and DeCarli (1976) reported the production of cirrhosis in baboons after long-term feeding of ethanol.

For a number of decades a controversy has existed whether ethanol itself causes cirrhosis in humans by a direct hepatotoxic effect or whether the nutritional deficiency, which is closely associated with alcoholism, is the primary cause (Hartroft, 1975; Lieber, 1975). In part, the major reason for evoking the element of nutritional deficiency has been the lack of success experienced when attempting to produce cirrhosis by feeding ethanol to animals maintained on an otherwise nutritionally adequate diet. The proponents of the nutrition theory (Hartroft, 1975) indicate that in dogs and rats the development of cirrhosis depends on the duration of the consumption of ethanol, the percentage of total calories provided by ethanol, and the composition of the accompanying diet; diets that are inadequate in choline, proteins, methionine, vitamin B_{12}, and folic acid favor the development of cirrhosis. Supplementation of the diets with these nutrients appears to abolish the effect of long-term feeding of ethanol. The proponents of the direct hepatotoxic theory (Lieber, 1975) emphasize the requirement of long-term ingestion of large quantities of ethanol by animals on nutritionally adequate diets and the demonstrated effects of precirrhotic changes in the various animal models. Perhaps the usual laboratory species employed are more resistant to ethanol than are humans. The development of cirrhosis in the baboon (Lieber and DeCarli, 1976) maintained on an otherwise nutritionally adequate diet lends considerable weight in favor of the direct hepatotoxic theory. In any event, this animal model may permit a better understanding of the pathogenesis of ethanol-induced cirrhosis.

Carcinogenesis

The problem of chemical carcinogenesis is covered elsewhere in detail (see Chapter 5). Consequently, only a cursory view of hepatocarcinogenesis will be described in this section.

A wide variety of chemicals can elicit carcinogenic changes in laboratory animals (Wogan, 1976). Among naturally occurring substances that are liver carcinogens in animals one finds aflatoxin B_1 and other mycotoxins, some pyrrolizidine alkaloids, cycasin, and safrol. Among synthetic substances one finds some dialkylnitrosamines, some organochlorine pesticides, certain polychlorinated biphenyls, carbon tetrachloride, chloroform, vinyl chloride, dimethylaminoazobenzene, acetylaminofluorene, thioacetamide, urethane, ethionine, dimethylbenzanthracene, and galactosamine.

There is increasing evidence that chemical hepatocarcinogens do not induce cancer but rather initiate a chain of events that results in cancer (Farber, 1976, 1982). The initiating event may be a mutation, but perturbations in cell differentiation may also be involved. Many hepatocarcinogens intereact with virtually all cell organelles; yet evidence is lacking that these changes play a major role as the precursor lesion. The acute inhibition of cell proliferation is suggested to be of importance; perhaps this leads to an altered cell population that can grow in the presence of a cytotoxic environment (cell selection). Organizationally, the hepatocytes are not arranged as in the normal adult liver, but assume a "pseudofetal" configuration; this organizational difference also expresses itself in biochemical patterns (emergence of fetal isozymes, production of α-fetoprotein and fetal antigens). Each individual neoplasm is unique (pattern of enzymes, antigenic composition, morphologic appearance), and this property is consistent with the hypothesis of an origin from a single clone of cells.

After initiation, a long latent period (6 to 24 months in the rat) occurs before the liver cancer becomes evident. Farber (1976, 1982) proposes that the histogenesis of hepatocellular carcinoma involves a series of altered or new hepatocytic populations that evolve into malignant neoplasia; each population develops from its immediate precursor by a process of selection. At least four such populations appear as likely steps: enzyme-deficient foci, early hyperplastic nodules, late hyperplastic nodules, and hyperbasophilic foci. These could be pictured as proceeding in an ordered sequence from the target cell. However, an alternative scheme states that each new cell population is derived from the target cell, but is independent and unrelated to the others. The validity of either hypothesis is yet to be determined.

Little is known about the selection process that favors the development of malignant hepatocytes. Perhaps resistance to necrosis develops (selective cytotoxicity). Endogenous and exogenous modulating factors are known to affect the incidence and time of appearance of liver cancers; these include nutrients, hormones, drugs, and other chemicals. Their roles are very poorly understood, as are immunologic factors and the presence of cirrhosis. The absence of such knowledge greatly limits extrapolation of results obtained in animals under controlled conditions to humans exposed in undefined conditions.

FACTORS INVOLVED IN LIVER INJURY

Biotransformation of Toxicants

The phenomenon of biotransformation to a more active metabolite is well known in pharmacology. It is now known to occur with hepatotoxic substances. There is considerable evidence that carbon tetrachloride is biotransformed in the liver. McCollister and associates (1951) showed that a nonvolatile product could be detected in urine of monkeys treated with carbon tetrachloride. They also demonstrated the formation of CO_2 from this substance. Butler (1961) showed that carbon tetrachloride was reduced to chloroform in vivo. It is now clear that the toxicity of carbon tetrachloride depends on cleavage of the carbon-chlorine bond. In rabbits, chloroform, hexacloroethane, and two other chlorinated metabolites were found in various tissues 48 hours after administration of carbon tetrachloride (Fowler, 1969). The work of a number of investigators (Recknagel and Glende, 1973) has led to the following observations: the cleavage occurs in the endoplasmic reticulum and is mediated by the mixed function oxidase system; carbon tetrachloride forms a type I binding spectrum with cytochrome P-450; NADPH-dependent flavoproteins do not appear to be involved; the products of the homolytic cleavage can become incorporated into microsomal lipids; free-radical scavengers and lipid antioxidants protect against the liver injury; inducers of cytochrome P-450 can enhance liver injury. Recently, Noguchi and associates (1982) characterized a form of cytochrome P-450 (52,000 daltons) that exhibits high activity for the generation of the trimethyl radical from carbon tetrachloride.

Chloroform is also metabolized enzymatically by the liver, and glutathione activates this oxidation (Rubinstein and Kanics, 1964). The hepatotoxicity of chloroform is augmented by phenobarbital pretreatment, and concomitantly chloroform markedly depletes hepatic glutathione in phenobarbital-treated rats, but not in normal animals (Docks and Krishna, 1976). Covalent binding of radiolabel derived from chloroform to microsomal proteins was shown in vitro, and glutathione diminished the response. Free-radical intermediates have also been proposed to arise during chloroform activation (Brown et al., 1974). Two groups of investigators (Mansuy et al., 1977; Pohl et al., 1977) demonstrated that in vitro microsomes derived from phenobarbital-treated rats were capable of converting chloroform to phosgene, a highly reactive electrophilic compound. They proposed that this activation proceeds through the hydroxylation of chloroform to tri-chloromethanol, which spontaneously dehydro-chlorinates to produce phosgene. It was concluded that the site of activation is cytochrome P-450 rather than NADPH cytochrome c reductase (Sipes *et al.*, 1977).

A number of other haloalkanes are bioactivated *in vitro* by rat hepatic microsomes (Sipes and Gandolfi, 1982); some of these proceed to a greater degree under nitrogen than under oxygen (carbon tetrachloride, bromotrichloromethane, halothane). *In vivo*, hypoxia augments the liver injury produced by carbon tetrachloride and halothane (Shen *et al.*, 1982; de Groot and Noll, 1983). Furthermore, there are important differences among the haloalkanes regarding inducibility and covalent binding properties to microsomal protein, microsomal lipid, or calf thymus DNA (Sipes and Gandolfi, 1982).

Biotransformation is a key event in halothane-induced hepatotoxicity (Sipes and Gandolfi, 1982; de Groot and Noll, 1983). This substance undergoes reductive metabolism mediated by cytochrome P-450, which is enhanced *in vivo* by hypoxia. A reactive metabolite is formed that causes lipid peroxidation and is closely associated with the hepatotoxic process.

Biotransformation is also important in the case of hepatic lesions produced by bromobenzene. In 1953, Koch-Weser and co-workers demonstrated that bromobenzene in rats produced centrilobular necrosis. The lesion could be prevented by coadministration of cysteine and methionine, whereas the lesion was aggravated by prior fasting. When the animals were protected, urinary mercapturic acid rose. Brodie and co-workers (1971) postulated that the necrosis was produced by an active metabolite of bromobenzene, presumably an epoxide, capable of reacting covalently with macromolecules in liver cells. They showed that liver microsomes could convert bromobenzene into a compound that reacted covalently with glutathione. Furthermore, inhibitors of microsomal drug-metabolizing enzymes, SKF 525-A or piperonyl butoxide, prevented the liver necrosis and phenobarbital induction enhanced the liver injury (Reid *et al.*, 1971). With phenobarbital, increased formation of mercapturic acids was seen. It was postulated that the epoxide formation is so great that normal amounts of glutathione cannot protect the tissue proteins from the alkylating agent. In this regard, diethyl maleate, which depletes hepatic glutathione, increases the incidence of hepatic lesions produced by low doses of bromobenzene. It appears that the toxic metabolite is bromobenzene epoxide; this metabolite is further degraded through the action of glutathione

transferase and epoxide hydrolase (Mitchell *et al.*, 1976a).

Acetaminophen-induced hepatotoxicity is also caused by a chemically reactive metabolite (Mitchell *et al.*, 1976a; Hinson *et al.*, 1981). The formation of this metabolite can be followed by the irreversible binding of radiolabel, derived from the acetaminophen, to liver protein. Little covalent binding occurs after subtoxic doses, but it increases as the dose approaches the toxic range. Inducers of mixed-function oxidase enhance formation of the reactive metabolite and liver toxicity, whereas inhibitors reduce metabolite formation and toxicity. The reactive intermediate is further conjugated with glutathione and excreted as a mercapturic acid.

The experimental work carried out to unravel acetaminophen- and bromobenzene-induced liver injury has led to some very important observations. One is that hepatoxicity need not be correlated with the pharmacokinetics of the parent substance or even its major metabolites, but may be correlated with the formation of quantitatively minor, highly reactive, intermediates. A second concept is that a threshold tissue concentration must be attained before liver injury is elicted; if it is not attained, injury does not occur. Third, endogenous substances like glutathione play an essential role in protecting hepatocytes from injury by chemically reactive intermediates; this provides the cell with a means of preventing the reactive metabolite from attaining a critical, effective concentration. Finally, other enzymic pathways, like glutathione transferase and epoxide hydrolase, also play a role in protecting the hepatocyte by catalyzing the further degradation of the toxic reactive intermediates. Furthermore, these studies have provided investigators relatively simple biochemical procedures for uncovering the possible existence of potentially toxic chemically reactive metabolites or intermediates in new compounds.

The production of reactive metabolites that bind irreversibly to hepatic proteins is observed in animals with furosemide and acetylisoniazid (Mitchell *et al.*, 1976a). With furosemide a dose threshold exists for both necrosis and covalent binding, but the threshold in mice is not due to depletion of hepatic glutathione. Apparently the threshold is caused by a change in the proportion of unchanged compound that is eliminated. At subthreshold doses most of the furosemide is highly bound to plasma proteins and eventually eliminated unchanged, whereas with high doses plasma binding becomes saturated and more furosemide becomes available for hepatic biotransformation. In the case of acetylisoniazid, the major metabolite of isoniazid, increased covalent binding to liver proteins and enhanced hepatotoxicity were observed in phenobarbital-pretreated rats; enhanced covalent binding was also observed with iproniazid. In both cases the reactive metabolites are thought to be free radicals arising from monoalkyl diazenes (Mitchell et al., 1976b).

Other hepatonecrogenic responses appear to be due to the production of a toxic metabolite. The hepatotoxic effect of dimethylnitrosamine is linked to its biotransformation (Magee and Swann, 1969). The pyrrolizidine alkaloids in "bush teas" made from Crotalaria fulva result in venoocclusive haptic disease. These substances are said to be converted to toxic metabolites in the liver (Mattocks, 1968). Allyl alcohol and its precursor allyl formate produce periportal necrosis (Rouiller, 1964; Reid, 1972). Rees and Tarlow (1967) showed that allyl formate is converted to a highly reactive aldehyde, acrolein, by alcohol dehydrogenase. Hepatotoxic reactive metabolites have been proposed (Hunter et al., 1977) for thioacetamide and thioacetamide sulfite, the major metabolite of thioacetamide, to account for their acute necrogenic effects. The formation of a reactive epoxide has been proposed to account for the acute focal necrosis seen in rats given aflatoxin B_1; the biochemical characteristics of this epoxide are said to be similar to those described for bromobenzene epoxide (Mgbodile et al., 1975).

Biotransformation also appears to be involved in cholestatic reactions although the evidence is less striking (Plaa and Hewitt, 1982). With α-naphthylisothiocyanate the toxicity can be modified by inducers and inhibitors of mixed-function oxidase; the presence of reactive metabolites has been demonstrated, although no correlation with toxicity is apparent. Chlorpromazine metabolites vary in their hepatotoxic properties, as do those of the tricyclic antidepressants. Some estradiol conjugates possess cholestatic properties. Indirect evidence indicates that the cholestatic response elicited in rats by dantrolene is caused by a metabolic product.

Glutathione

When it was discovered that glutathione could markedly affect the hepatotoxicity of bromobenzene and acetaminophen, a new role for glutathione was uncovered. Its cysteinyl residue provides a nucleophilic thiol important for the detoxication of electrophilic metabolites and metabolically produced oxidizing agents (Ketterer et al., 1983). Thus, this tripeptide could protect tissue macromolecules from alkylating, arylating, acylating, or peroxidizing metabolites

generated by the bioactivation of potential hepatotoxicants. If glutathione is depleted or markedly reduced in the liver, the hepatotoxicity would be expected to be enhanced.

Although this situation prevails for bromobenzene and acetaminophen (Mitchell et al., 1976a), it is not observed with all hepatotoxicants. Mitchell and associates (1982) described the distinguishing features of different categories of chemically reactive metabolites; this scheme employs three parameters (other than protein or lipid alkylation) to differentiate the chemicals: (1) preferential glutathione depletion by the hepatotoxicant, (2) enhanced necrosis by prior glutathione depletion; and (3) diminished necrosis by prior treatment with glutathione precursors. Three categories of hepatotoxicants have been proposed (Mitchell et al., 1982): (group I) electrophilic substrates for glutathione-S-transferase (e.g., acetaminophen, bromobenzene), which exhibit preferential glutathione depletion, enhances necrosis by prior depletion of glutathione, or reduced necrosis by prior treatment with glutathione precursors; (group II) electrophilic nonsubstrates for glutathione-S-transferase (e.g., furosemide, nitrosoamines), which do not deplete glutathione preferentially and are not markedly affected by depletion of glutathione or by prior treatment with glutathione precursors; (group III) alkylating radicals (e.g., carbon tetrachloride, halothane), which do not deplete glutathione preferentially and are minimally affected by alterations in glutathione content. The role of glutathione in the hepatotoxic process is now clearer. Recent developments in the determinants of hepatic glutathione turnover (Lauterburg et al., 1982) can be expected to add to a better understanding of the overall process.

Alteration of Hepatic Blood Flow

With some hepatotoxicants alterations in hepatic blood flow are observed as a result of the injury. These alterations manifest themselves 24 hours or more after the injury. Hemorrhagic necrosis occurs in rats after the administration of beryllium (Cheng, 1956). Dimethylnitrosamine produces hemorrhagic necrosis, where the center of the lobule becomes entirely occupied by blood (Barns and Magee, 1954). This "venoocclusive" lesion can be observed ten days after administration of the substance (Magee and Swann, 1969). Similar lesions have been observed in animals and children ingesting Crotalaria, a pyrrolizidine alkaloid (McLean, 1970). This lesion seems to be a characteristic of those substances that produce hemorrhagic necrosis and are not typically found after administration of carbon tetrachloride. Butler and Hard (1971) attribute this to the fact that carbon tetrachloride induces a coagulative necrosis of the hepatocytes that does not affect the sinusoid lining cells, permitting the retention of an intact vascular pattern; however, dimethylnitrosamine affects both the parenchymal cells and the sinusoid lining cells, resulting in hemorrhage and a collapse of the trabecular reticulin framework around the central veins.

Himsworth (1954) postulated that carbon tetrachloride could act directly on hepatic cells and that this would cause swelling, resulting in a mechanical obstruction of sinusoidal blood flow. He felt that the cells distal to the swelling would become hypoxic and this would result in necrosis. However, in cats, the data indicate that diminished hepatic blood flow is not a causative factor in the initial phase of carbon tetrachloride liver injury, and at later times increased hepatic arterial blood flow is observed (Lautt and Plaa, 1974).

In 1960, Calvert and Brody proposed that hepatic vasoconstriction, due to the elaboration of catecholamines, was the primary effect of carbon tetrachloride. The hypothesis was based on indirect evidence. High spinal cord transection at the level of C6 or C7 protected rats against the necrotic effects of carbon tetrachloride. Larson and Plaa (1965) showed that cordotomy resulted in hypothermia. They also showed that if cord-transected animals were placed in an incubator to maintain their body temperature, carbon tetrachloride produced its hepatic necrotic effects. Oxygen consumption of transected rats maintained at room temperature dropped markedly. It thus appears that in hypothermic rats metabolic activity of the liver is diminished, and this would explain the apparent protective effects of cervical cordotomy. Large infusions of norepinephrine, epinephrine, or mixtures of these substances did not result in lesions similar to those produced by carbon tetrachloride. Finally, in rats sympathectomized immunologically the hepatic lesion induced by carbon tetrachloride was still present (Larson et al., 1965). Therefore, it appears that the vascular role attributed to carbon tetrachloride via release of catecholamines must be rejected as a primary cause of hepatic injury.

Potentiation of Hepatotoxicity

It is now well established that subjects exposed to several chemical agents simultaneously or sequentially can exhibit altered pharmacologic or toxicologic responses. In the field of therapeutics such drug interactions are well known. With hepatotoxicity, interactions have

been observed. Many of these have led to the discovery that biotransformation to a more active metabolite is involved in the hepatotoxic process.

In addition, other instances of potentiation of hepatotoxicity have been described. Individuals recovering from an acute ingestion of ethanol are more susceptible to the liver-damaging properties of the haloalkanes than are individuals not ingesting ethanol. Since the early investigators studying this phenomenon in animals used simultaneous administration of both agents, the explanation seemed to be that ethanol enhanced the absorption of the hydrocarbon (Stewart et al., 1960). However, Guild and co-workers (1958) reported that ingestion of ethanol several hours before exposure to the hydrocarbons caused an enhanced toxic response. The latter phenomenon occurs in mice, rats, and dogs. The haloalkanes shown to exert an enhanced hepatotoxic response after ethanol pretreatment include carbon tetrachloride, chloroform, trichloroethylene, and 1,1-2-trichloroethane (Klaassen and Plaa, 1967).

Cornish and Adefuin (1967) showed that several aliphatic alcohols, such as methanol, ethanol, isopropanol, n-butanol, sec-butanol, and tert-butanol, also exert a similar potentiating effect on the acute inhalation toxicity of carbon tetrachloride. Several examples of potentiation are depicted in Figure 10–3. The remarkable potentiating effect of isopropanol has been studied in detail (Plaa et al., 1975), and the biotransformation of isopropanol to acetone plays a crucial role. Acetone itself can potentiate carbon tetrachloride hepatotoxicity, and the response can be correlated with blood acetone concentrations (Plaa et al., 1982). The interaction between isopropanol and carbon tetrachloride was documented in an industrial accident in an isopropanol packaging plant, where workers exposed to both agents exhibited hepatotoxicity (Folland et al., 1976).

With ethanol the potentiation seems to be due to the presence of the unmetabolized alcohol; however, with isopropanol the effect seems to be caused by the presence of both unmetabolized alcohol and acetone. The results obtained with n-butanol resemble those of ethanol, whereas with 2-butanol they resemble those of isopropanol; 2-butanol is also metabolized to a ketone (2-butanone; methyl ethyl ketone) (Traiger and Bruckner, 1976). The mechanisms underlying the potentiations are not known. However, it appears that the interaction occurs within the enzyme systems associated with the endoplasmic reticulum. With isopropanol and acetone one could attempt to explain the poten-

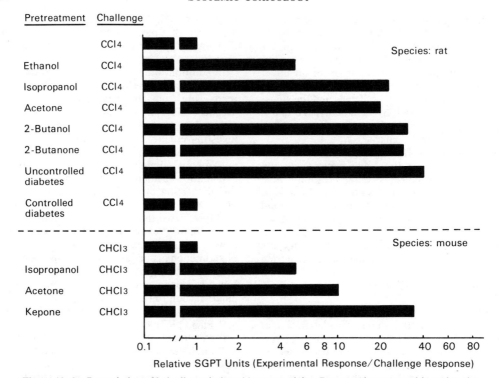

Figure 10–3. Potentiation of haloalkane-induced hepatotoxicity. Rats or mice were subjected to the specified various pretreatments before receiving a challenge dose of carbon tetrachloride or chloroform. Diabetes was produced by administering alloxan, either alone (*Uncontrolled*) or with insulin (*Controlled*). The severity of the liver injury was assessed 24 hours after the haloalkane challenge using serum glutamic pyruvic transaminase (SGPT) activity. Relative SGPT units were obtained by dividing the activity in the experimental group (*Pretreatment plus Challenge*) by the activity in the respective control group (*Challenge Alone*). The details can be found in the following references: Hewitt *et al.*, 1979; Traiger and Bruckner, 1976; Plaa *et al.*, 1975; Hanasono *et al.*, 1975a; Hewitt *et al.*, 1980.

tiation on the basis of enhanced bioactivation of carbon tetrachloride (Sipes *et al.*, 1973), but other possible mechanisms are under consideration (Hewitt *et al.*, 1980).

Isopropanol and acetone also cause enhanced hepatotoxicity with chloroform, trichloroethylene, 1,1,2-trichloroethane, or 1,1,1-trichloroethane (Plaa *et al.*, 1975). Acetone potentiates the responses to 1,1-dichloroethylene, bromodichloromethane, and dibromochloromethane (Hewitt and Plaa, 1983; Hewitt *et al.*, 1983b).

The potentiation of haloalkane hepatotoxicity occurs with a number of different ketonic solvents (methyl *n*-butyl ketone, methyl ethyl ketone, 2,5-hexanedione) (Hewitt *et al.*, 1980); experiments conducted with acetone, 2-butanone, 2-pentanone, 2-hexanone, and 2-heptanone indicate that the carbon skeleton chain length plays a role in determining the relative potentiating capacity of ketonic solvents (Hewitt *et al.*, 1983c). *n*-Hexane, which is bio-

transformed to methyl *n*-butyl ketone (2-hexanone) and 2,5-hexanedione, also potentiates chloroform toxicity (Hewitt *et al.*, 1980). Chlordecone (Kepone), a ketonic pesticide, exhibits remarkable potentiating properties with chloroform, carbon tetrachloride, bromodichloromethane, and dibromochloromethane (Hewitt *et al.*, 1979; Curtis *et al.*, 1979; Klingensmith and Mehendale, 1981); mirex, the nonketonic analog of chlordecone, does not possess this property. 1,3-Butanediol, which is metabolized to the ketone bodies β-hydroxybutyrate and acetoacetate, also potentiates carbon tetrachloride hepatotoxicity (Hewitt *et al.*, 1980, 1982) in a dose-related manner, and the effect is associated with the development of the ketotic state. Thus, it appears that the potentiation phenomenon observed with these various substances is closely related to the presence of exogenous or endogenous ketones. The mechanisms involved are not completely known, but enhanced bioactivation of a toxic haloalkane metabolite appears to play a major role (Sipes *et al.*, 1973; Hewitt *et al.*, 1980; Branchflower and Pohl, 1981; Hewitt *et al.*, 1982). With chlordecone potentiation, enhanced formation of haloalkane-derived reactive metabolites, as well as changes in their macromolecular binding in hepatic tissue, have been demonstrated (Hewitt *et al.*, 1983a).

The diabetic state induced in rats by either alloxan or streptozotocin enhances the hepatotoxic properties of carbon tetrachloride (Figure 10–3); reversal of the diabetic state by insulin treatment can prevent the potentiated response (Hanasono *et al.*, 1975a). Alloxan-induced diabetes can also enhance the response to chloroform, 1,1,2-trichloroethane, galactosamine, or thioacetamide (Hanasono *et al.*, 1975b; Elhawari and Plaa, 1983). However, Price and Jollow (1982) observed no potentiation of acetaminophen liver injury in streptozotocin-diabetic rats; instead an increased resistance to the hepatotoxicant was observed. The mechanisms involved have yet to be resolved.

Potentiation of the liver injury is not limited to necrogenic hepatotoxicants. With cholestatic agents, such interactions are less frequent, but have been observed (Plaa and Hewitt, 1982). Inducers of mixed-function oxidase can enhance the acute cholestatic or hyperbilirubinemic response to α-naphthylisothiocyanate; isopropanol and acetone potentiate its hyperbilirubinemic effect. Recently, de Lamirande and Plaa (1981) demonstrated that rats maintained on 1,3-butanediol exhibited potentiated cholestatic responses to taurolithocholate or manganese-bilirubin injections; with α-naphthylisothiocyomate the hyperbilirubinemia was enhanced, but not the depression in bile flow. Methyl *n*-butylketone and methyl *iso*-butyl ketone can aggravate taurolithocholate-induced cholestasis in rats (Plaa and Ayotte, 1985). Thus, ketones and a ketogenic chemical (1,3-butanediol) enhance some types of cholestatic reactions. The mechanisms are not known. Some unpredictable cholestatic drug reactions in humans indicate that other associated predisposing conditions (altered metabolic state, interacting chemicals) may be involved. This concept warrants further investigation in light of the results obtained experimentally.

REFERENCES

Alpers, D. H., and Isselbacher, K. J.: The effect of carbon tetrachloride on rat-liver lysosomes. *Biochim. Biophys. Acta*, **137**:33–42, 1967.

Alpers, D. H.; Solin, M.; and Isselbacher, K. J.: The role of lipid peroxidation in the pathogenesis of carbon tetrachloride-induced liver injury. *Mol. Pharmacol.*, **4**:566–73, 1968.

Ayotte, P., and Plaa, G. L.: Hepatic subcellular distribution of manganese in manganese and manganese-bilirubin induced cholestasis. *Biochem. Pharmacol.*, **21**:3857–65, 1985.

Baccino, F. M.; Rita, G. A.; and Dianzani, M. U.: Further experiments on the action of CCl₄ on lysosomes *in vitro. Enzymologia*, **29**:169–84, 1965.

Baglio, C. M., and Farber, E.: Reversal by adenine of the induced lipid accumulation in the endoplasmic reticulum of the rat liver. *J. Cell Biol.*, **27**:591–601, 1965.

Barnes, J. M., and Magee, P. N.: Some toxic properties of dimethylnitrosamine. *Br. J. Ind. Med.*, **11**:167–74, 1954.

Bellomo, G., and Orrenius, S.: Altered thiol and calcium homeostasis in oxidative hepatocellular injury. *Hepatology*, **5**:876–82, 1985.

Benedetti, A.; Barbieri, L.; Ferrali, M.; Casini, A. F.; Fulceri, R.; and Comporti, M.: Inhibition of protein synthesis by carbonyl compounds (4-hydroxyalkenals) originating from the peroxidation of liver microsomal lipids. *Chem.-Biol. Interact.*, **35**:331–40, 1981.

Benedetti, A.; Casini, A. F.; Ferrali, M.; and Comporti, M.: Early alterations induced by carbon tetrachloride in the lipids of the membranes of the endoplasmic reticulum of the liver cell. I. Separation and partial characterization of altered lipids. *Chem.-Biol. Interactions*, **17**:151–66, 1977a.

———: Early alterations induced by carbon tetrachloride in the lipids of the membranes of the endoplasmic reticulum of the liver cell. II. Distribution of the alterations in the various lipid fractions. *Chem.-Biol. Interactions*, **17**:167–83, 1977b.

———: Studies on the relationships between carbon tetrachloride-induced alterations of liver microsomal lipids and impairment of glucose-6-phosphatase activity. *Exp. Mol. Pathol.*, **27**:309–23, 1977c.

Benedetti, A.; Fulceri, R.; Ferrali, M.; Ciccoli, L.; Esterbauer, H.; and Comporti, M.: Detection of carbonyl functions in phospholipids of liver microsomes in CCl₄- and BrCCl₃-poisoned rats, *Biochim. Biophys. Acta*, **712**:628–38, 1982.

Bentley, P., and Oesch, F.: Foreign compound metabolism in the liver. In Popper, H. and Schaffner, F. (eds.): *Progress in Liver Diseases*, Vol. 7. Grune & Stratton, New York, 1982, pp. 157–78.

Boyer, J. L.; Layden, T. J.; and Hruban, Z.: Mechanisms of cholestasis-taurolithocholate alters canalicular membrane composition, structure and permeability. In Popper, H.; Bianchi, L.; and Reutter, W. (eds.): *Membrane Alterations as Basis of Liver Injury*. MTP Press Ltd., Lancaster, 1977, pp. 353–69.

Branchflower, R. V., and Pohl, L. R.: Investigation of the mechanism of the potentiation of chloroform-induced hepatoxicity and nephrotoxicity by methyl *n*-butyl ketone. *Toxicol. Appl. Pharmacol.*, **61**:407–13, 1981.

Brodie, B. B.; Reid, W. D.; Cho, A. K.; Sipes, G.; Krisha, G.; and Gillette, J. R.: Possible mechanism of liver necrosis caused by aromatic organic compounds. *Proc. Natl Acad. Sci. USA*, **68**:160–64, 1971.

Brown, B. R., Jr.; Sipes, I. G.; and Sagalyn, A. M.: Mechanisms of acute hepatic toxicity: chloroform, halothane, and glutathione. *Anesthesiology*, **41**:554–61, 1974.

Bucher, N. L. R., and Malt, R. A.: *Regeneration of Liver, and Kidney*, Little, Brown & Co., Boston, 1971, pp. 135–37.

Butler, T. C.: Reduction of carbon tetrachloride *in vivo* and chloroform *in vitro* by tissues and tissue constituents. *J. Pharmacol. Exp. Ther.*, **134**:311–19, 1961.

Butler, W. H., and Hard, G. C.: Hepatotoxicity of dimethylnitrosamine in the rat with special reference to veno-occlusive disease. *Exp. Mol. Pathol.*, **15**:209–19, 1971.

Calvert, D. N., and Brody, T. N.: Role of the sympathetic nervous system in CCl₄ hepatotoxicity. *Am. J. Physiol.*, **198**:669–76, 1960.

Cheng, K. K.: Experimental studies on the mechanism of the zonal distribution of beryllium liver necrosis. *J. Pathol. Bacteriol.*, **71**:265–76, 1956.

Christie, G. S., and Judah, J. D.: Mechanism of action of carbon tetrachloride on liver cells. *Proc. Roy. Soc. Ser. B*, **142**:241–57, 1954.

Comporti, M.: Lipid peroxidation and cellular damage in toxic liver injury. *Lab. Invest.*, **53**:599–623, 1985.

Comporti, M.; Saccocci, C.; and Dianzani, M. U.: Effect of CCl₄ *in vitro* and *in vivo* on lipid peroxidation of rat liver homogenates and subcellular fractions. *Enzymologia*, **29**:185–204, 1965.

Cornish, H. H., and Adefuin, J.: Potentiation of carbon tetrachloride toxicity by aliphatic alcohols. *Arch. Environ. Health*, **14**:447–49, 1967.

Curtis, L. R.; Williams, W. L.; and Mehendale, H. M.: Potentiation of the hepatotoxicity of carbon tetrachloride following preexposure to chlordecone (Kepone) in the male rat. *Toxicol. Appl. Pharmacol.*, **51**:283–93, 1979.

Davidson, C. S.; Leevy, C. M.; and Chamberlayne, E. C.: *Guidelines for Detection of Hepatotoxicity Due to Drugs and Chemicals*. NIH Publication No. 79-313, U.S. Department of Health, Education, and Welfare, Washington, D.C., 1979.

Decker, K., and Keppler, D.: Galactosamine hepatitis: key role of the nucleotide deficiency period in the pathogenesis of cell injury and cell death. *Pharmacol. Rev. Physiol. Biochem.*, **71**:77–106, 1974.

de Groot, H., and Noll, T.: Halothane hepatotoxicity: relation between metabolic activation, hypoxia, covalent binding, lipid peroxidation, and liver cell damage. *Hepatology*, **3**:601–606, 1983.

de Lamirande, E., and Plaa, G. L.: Dose and time relationships in manganese-bilirubin cholestasis. *Toxicol. Appl. Pharmacol.*, **49**:257–63, 1979.

de Lamirande, E., and Plaa, G. L.: 1,3-Butanediol pretreatment on the cholestasis induced in rats by manganese-bilirubin combination, taurolithocholic acid, or α-naphthylisothiocyanate. *Toxicol. Appl. Pharmacol.*, **59**:467–75, 1981.

de Lamirande, E.; Tuchweber, B.; and Plaa, G. L.: Hepatocellular membrane alteration as a possible cause of manganese-bilirubin-induced cholestasis. *Biochem. Pharmacol.*, **30**:2305–12, 1981.

Dianzani, M. U.: Toxic liver injury by protein synthesis inhibitors. In Popper, H., and Schaffner, F. (eds.): *Progress in Liver Diseases*, Vol. 5. Grune & Stratton, New York, 1976, pp. 232–45.

————: Uncoupling of oxidative phosphorylation in mitochondria from fatty livers. *Biochim. Biophys. Acta*, **14**:514–32, 1954.

————: Lysosome changes in liver injury. In de Reuck, A. V. S., and Cameron, M. P. (eds.): *Ciba Symposium on Lysosomes*. Little, Brown & Co., Boston, 1963, pp. 335–52.

————: Reactions of the liver to injury: fatty liver. In Farber, E., and Fisher, M. M. (eds.): *Toxic Injury of the Liver*, Part A. Marcel Dekker, Inc., New York, 1979, pp. 281–331.

Dianzani, M. U., and Bahr, G. F.: Electron microscope investigation of mitochondria isolated from normal and steatotic livers by differential centrifugation. *Acta Pathol. Microbiol. Scand.*, **35**:25–38, 1954.

DiLuzio, N. R.: Antioxidants, lipid peroxidation and chemical-induced liver injury. *Fed. Proc.*, **32**:1875–81, 1973.

DiLuzio, N. R., and Hartman, A. D.: The effect of ethanol and carbon tetrachloride administration on hepatic lipid-soluble antioxidant activity. *Exp. Mol. Pathol.*, **11**:38–52, 1969.

Docks, E. L., and Kirshna, G.: The role of glutathione in chloroform-induced hepatotoxicity. *Exp. Mol. Pathol.*, **24**:13–22, 1976.

El-hawari, A. M., and Plaa, G. L.: Potentiation of thioacetamide-induced hepatotoxicity in alloxan- and streptozotocin-diabetic rats. *Toxicol. Lett.*, **17**:293–300, 1983.

Farber, E.: Biochemical pathology. *Annu. Rev. Pharmacol.*, **11**:71–96, 1971.

————: Some fundamental aspects of liver injury. In Khanna, J. M., Israel, Y., and Kalant, H. (eds.): *Alcoholic Liver Pathology*. Addiction Research Foundation, Toronto, 1975, pp. 289–303.

————: The pathology of experimental liver cell cancer. In Cameron, H. M.; Linsell, D. A.; and Warwick, G. P. (eds.): *Liver Cell Cancer*. Elsevier, Amsterdam, 1976, pp. 243–77.

————: Chemical carcinogenesis: a biologic perspective. *Am. J. Pathol.*, **106**:271–96, 1982.

Farber, E.; Liang, H.; and Shinozuka, H.: Dissociation of effects on protein synthesis and ribosomes from membrane changes induced by carbon tetrachloride. *Am. J. Pathol.*, **64**:601–22, 1971.

Farber, J. L.: Calcium and the mechanisms of liver necrosis. In Popper, H. and Schaffner, F. (eds.): *Progress in Liver Diseases*, Vol. 7. Grune & Stratton, New York, 1982, pp. 347–60.

————: Reactions of the liver to injury: necrosis. In Farber, E., and Fisher, M. M. (eds.): *Toxic Injury of the Liver*, Part A. Marcel Dekker, Inc., New York, 1979, pp. 215–41.

Fisher, M. M.; Magnusson, R.; and Miyai, K.: Bile acid metabolism in mammals. I. Bile acid-induced intrahepatic cholestasis. *Lab. Invest.*, **21**:88–91, 1971.

Folland, D. S.; Schaffner, W.; Grinn, H. E.; Crofford, O. B.; and McMurray, D. R.: Carbon tetrachloride toxicity potentiated by isopropyl alcohol. *JAMA*, **236**:1853–56, 1976.

Fowler, J. S. L.: Carbon tetrachloride metabolism in the rabbit. *Br. J. Pharmacol.*, **37**:733–37, 1969.

Ganote, C. E., and Rosenthal, A. S.: Characteristic lesions of methylazoxy-methanol-induced liver damage. *Lab. Invest.*, **19**:382–98, 1968.

Ghoshal, A. K.; Porta, E. A.; and Hartroft, W. S.: The role of lipoperoxidation in the pathogenesis of fatty livers induced by phosphorus poisoning in rats. *Am. J. Pathol.*, **54**:275–91, 1969.

Gordis, E.: Lipid metabolites of carbon tetrachloride. *J. Clin. Invest.*, **48**:203–209, 1969.

Guild, W. R.; Young, J. V.; and Merrill, J. P.: Anuria due to carbon tetrachloride intoxication. *Ann. Intern. Med.*, **48**:1221–27, 1958.

Gumucio, J. J., and Miller, D. L.: Zonal hepatic function: solute-hepatocyte interactions within the liver acinus. In Popper, H. and Schaffner, F. (eds.): *Progress in Liver Diseases*, Vol. 7. Grune & Stratton, New York, 1982, pp. 17–30.

Gumucio, J. J., and Valdivieso, V. D.: Studies on the mechanism of the ethynylestradiol impairment of bile flow and bile salt excretion in the rat. *Gastroenterology*, **61**:339–44, 1971.

Hanasono, G. K.; Côté, M. G.; and Plaa, G. L.: Potentiation of carbon tetrachloride-induced hepatotoxicity in alloxan- or streptozotocin-diabetic rats. *J. Pharmacol. Exp. Ther.*, **192**:592–604, 1975a.

Hanasono, G. K.; Witschi, H. P.; and Plaa, G. L.: Potentiation of the hepatotoxic responses to chemicals in alloxan-diabetic rats. *Proc. Soc. Exp. Biol. Med.*, **149**:903–907, 1975b.

Hartroft, W. S.: On the etiology of alcoholic liver cirrhosis. In Khanna, J. M.; Israel, Y.; and Kalant, H. (eds.): *Alcoholic Liver Pathology*. Addiction Research Foundation, Toronto, 1975, pp. 189–97.

Heikel, T. A. J., and Lathe, G. H.: The effect of oral

contraceptive steroids on bile secretion and bilirubin Tm in rats. *Br. J. Pharmacol.*, **38**:593–601, 1970.

Hewitt, L. A.; Hewitt, W. R.; and Plaa, G. L.: Fractional hepatic localization of $^{14}CHCl_3$ in mice and rats treated with chlordecone or mirex. *Fund. Appl. Toxicol.*, 3:489–95, 1983a.

Hewitt, W. R.; Brown, E. M.; and Plaa, G. L.: Acetone-induced potentiation of trihalomethane toxicity in male rats. *Toxicol. Lett.*, 16:285–96, 1983b.

Hewitt, W. R.; Brown, E. M.; and Plaa, G. L.: Relationship between carbon skeleton length of ketonic solvents and potentiation of chloroform-induced hepatotoxicity in rats. *Toxicol. Lett.*, 16:297–304, 1983c.

Hewitt, W. R., and Plaa, G. L.: Dose-dependent modification of 1,1-dichloroethylene toxicity by acetone. *Toxicol. Lett.*, 16:145–52, 1983.

Hewitt, W. R.; Miyajima, H.; Côté, M. G.; and Plaa, G. L.: Modification of haloalkane-induced hepatotoxicity by exogenous ketones and metabolic ketosis. *Fed. Proc.*, 13:3118–23, 1980.

———: Acute alteration of chloroform-induced hepato- and nephrotoxicity by mirex and Kepone. *Toxicol. Appl. Pharmacol.*, 48:509–27, 1979.

Hewitt, W. R.; Miyajima, H.; Côté, M. G.; Hewitt, L. A.; Cianflone, D J.; and Plaa, G. L.: Dose-response relationships in 1,3-butanediol-induced potentiation of carbon tetrachloride toxicity. *Toxicol. Appl. Pharmacol.*, 64:529–40, 1982.

Himsworth, H. P.: *Liver and Its Diseases,* 2nd ed. Harvard University Press, Cambridge, Mass., 1954.

Hinson, J. A.; Pohl, L. R.; Monks, T. J.; and Gillette, J. R.: Acetaminophen-induced hepatotoxicity. *Life Sci.*, 29:107–16, 1981.

Hoyumba, A. M., Jr.; Greene, H. L.; Dunn, G. D.; and Schenker, S.: Fatty liver: biochemical and clinical considerations. *Dig. Dis.*, 20:1142–70, 1975.

Hunter, A. L.; Holscher, M. A.; and Neal, R. A.: Thioacetamide-induced hepatic necrosis. I. Involvement of the mixed-function oxidase enzyme system. *J. Pharmacol. Exp. Ther.*, 200:439–48, 1977.

Imai, K., and Hayashi, Y.: Steroid-induced intrahepatic cholestasis in mice. *Jpn. J. Pharmacol.*, 20:473–81, 1970.

Ingelfinger, F. J.: Foreword. In Butcher, N. L. R., and Malt, R. A.: *Regeneration of Liver and Kidney*. Little, Brown & Co., Boston, 1971.

Javitt, N. B.: Cholestasis in rats induced by taurolithocholate. *Nature (Lond.)*, 210:1262–63, 1966.

Javitt, N. B., and Emerman, S.: Effect of sodium taurolithocholate on bile flow and bile acid excretion. *J. Clin. Invest.*, 47:1002–14, 1968.

Jeanrenaud, B.; LeMarchand, Y.; and Patzelt, C.: Role of microtubules in hepatic secretory processes. In Popper, H.; Bianchi, L.; and Reutter, W. (eds.): *Membrane Alterations as Basis of Liver Injury*. MTP Press, Lancaster, 1977, pp. 247–55.

Judah, J. D.: Biochemical disturbances in liver injury. *Br. Med. Bull.*, 25:274–77, 1969.

Kakis, G.; Phillips, M. J.; and Yousef, I. M.: The respective roles of membrane cholesterol and of sodium-potassium adenosine triphosphatase in the pathogenesis of lithocholate-induced cholestasis. *Lab. Invest.*, 43:73–81, 1980.

Ketterer, B.; Coles, B.; and Meyer, D. J.: The role of glutathione in detoxication. *Environ. Health Perspect.*, 49:59–69, 1983.

Klaassen, C. D., and Plaa, G. L.: Relative effects of various chlorinated hydrocarbons on liver and kidney function in dogs. *Toxicol. Appl. Pharmacol.*, 10:119–31, 1967.

———: Comparison of the biochemical alterations elicited in livers from rats treated with carbon tetrachloride, chloroform, 1,1,2-trichloroethane and 1,1,1-trichloroethane. *Biochem. Pharmacol.*, 18:2019–27, 1969.

Klingensmith, J. S., and Mehendale, H. M.: Potentiation of brominated halomethane hepatotoxicity in the male rat. *Toxicol. Appl. Pharmacol.*, 61:378–84, 1981.

Koch-Weser, D.; de la Huerga, J.; Yesinick, C.; and Popper, H.: Hepatic necrosis due to bromobenzene as an example of conditioned amino acid deficiency. *Metabolism*, 11:248–60, 1953.

Larson, R. E., and Plaa, G. L.: A correlation of the effects of cervical cordotomy, hypothermia, and catecholamines on carbon tetrachloride-induced hepatic necrosis. *J. Pharmacol. Exp. Ther.*, 147:103–11, 1965.

Larson, R. E.; Plaa, G. L.; and Brody, M. J.: Immunological sympathectomy and CCl_4 hepatotoxicity. *Proc. Soc. Exp. Biol. Med.*, 116:557–60, 1965.

Lauterburg, B. H.; Smith, C. V.; Hughes, H.; and Mitchell, J. R.: Determinants of hepatic glutathione turnover: toxicological significance. *Trends Pharmacol. Sci.*, 3:245–48, 1982.

Lautt, W. W., and Plaa, G. L.: Hemodynamic effects of CCl_4 in the intact liver of the cat. *Can. J. Physiol. Pharmacol.*, 52:727–35, 1974.

Lavigne, J. G., and Marchand, C.: The role of metabolism in chloroform hepatotoxicity. *Toxicol. Appl. Pharmacol.*, 29:312–26, 1974.

Lelbach, W. K.: Quantitative aspects of drinking in alcoholic liver cirrhosis. In Khanna, J. M.; Israel, Y.; and Kalant, H. (eds.): *Alcoholic Liver Pathology*. Addiction Research Foundation, Toronto, 1975, pp. 1–18.

Lennon, H. D.: Relative effects of 17-alkylated anabolic steroids on sulfobromophthalein (BSP) retention in rabbits. *J. Pharmacol. Exp. Ther.*, 151:143–50, 1966.

Lieber, C. S.: Alcohol and the liver: Transition from metabolic adaptation to tissue injury and cirrhosis. In Khanna, J. M.; Israel, Y.; and Kalant, H. (eds.): *Alcoholic Liver Pathology*. Addiction Research Foundation, Toronto, 1975, pp. 171–88.

Lieber, C. S., and DiCarli, L. M.: Animal models of ethanol dependence and liver injury in rats and baboons. *Fed. Proc.*, 35:1232–36, 1976.

Lombardi, B.: Considerations on the pathogenesis of fatty liver. *Lab. Invest.*, 15:1–20, 1966.

Lombardi, B., and Oler, A.: Choline deficiency fatty liver. Protein synthesis and release. *Lab. Invest.*, 17:308–21, 1967.

Lombardi, B., and Recknagel, R. O.: Interference with secretion of triglycerides by the liver as a common factor in toxic liver injury. *Am. J. Pathol.*, 40:571–86, 1962.

Lustig, S.; Pitlik, S. D.; and Rosenfeld, J. B.: Liver damage in acute self-induced hypermanganemia. *Arch. Intern. Med.*, 142:405–406, 1982.

McCollister, D. D.; Beamer, W. H.; Atchison, G. J.; and Spencer, H. C.: Distribution and elimination of radioactive CCl_4 by monkeys upon exposure to low vapor concentration. *J. Pharmacol. Exp. Ther.*, 102:112–24, 1951.

McLean, E. K.: The toxic actions of pyrrolizidine (senecio) alkaloids. *Pharmacol. Rev.*, 22:429–83, 1970.

Magee, P. N.: Toxic liver necrosis. *Lab. Invest.*, 15:111–31, 1966.

Magee, P. N., and Swann, P. F.: Nitroso compounds. *Br. Med. Bull.*, 25:240–44, 1969.

Mager, J.; Bornstein, S.; and Halbreich, A.: Enhancement of the polyuridylic acid-directed phenylalamine polymerization in liver-microsome preparations from rats treated with carbon tetrachloride or dimethylnitrosamine. *Biochim. Biophys. Acta*, 95:682–84, 1965.

Mansuy, D.; Beaune, P.; Cresteil, T.; Lange, M.; and Leroux, J. P.: Evidence for phosgene formation during liver microsomal oxidation of chloroform. *Biochem. Biophys. Res. Commun.*, 79:513–17, 1977.

Mattocks, A. R.: Toxicity of pyrrolizidine alkaloids. *Nature (Lond.)*, 217:723–28, 1968.

Medline, A.; Schaffner, F.; and Popper, H.: Ultrastructural features in galactosamine-induced hepatitis. *Exp. Mol. Pathol.*, **12**:201–11, 1970.

Meyers, M.; Slikker, W.; Pascoe, G.; and Vore, M.: Characterization of cholestasis induced by estradiol-17βD-glucuronide in the rat. *J. Pharmacol. Exp. Ther.*, **214**:87–93, 1980.

Meyers, M.; Slikker, W.; and Vore, M.: Steroid D-ring glucoronides: characterization of a new class of cholestatic agents in the rat. *J. Pharmacol. Exp. Ther.*, **218**:63–73, 1981.

Mgbodile, M. U. K.; Holscher, M.; and Neal, R. A.: A possible protective role for reduced glutathione in aflatoxin B₁ toxicity: effect of pretreatment of rats with phenobarbital and 3-methylcholanthrene on aflatoxin toxicity. *Toxicol. Appl. Pharmacol.*, **34**:128–42, 1975.

Mitchell, J. R.; Hughes, H.; Lauterburg, B. H.; and Smith, C. V.: Chemical nature of reactive intermediates as determinant of toxicologic responses. *Drug Metab. Rev.*, **13**:539–53, 1982.

Mitchell, J. R.; Nelson, S. D.; Thorgeirsson, S. S.; McMurty, R. J.; and Dybing, E.: Metabolic activation: biochemical basis for many drug-induced liver injuries. In Popper, H., and Schaffner, F. (eds.): *Progress in Liver Diseases*, Vol. 5. Grune & Stratton, New York, 1976a, pp. 259–79.

Mitchell, J. R.; Snodgrass, W. R.; and Gillette, J. R.: The role of biotransformation in chemical-induced liver injury. *Environ. Health Perspect.*, **15**:27–38, 1976b.

Miyai, K.; Price, V. M.; and Fisher, M. M.: Bile acid metabolism in mammals: ultrastructural studies on the intrahepatic cholestasis induced by lithocholic and chenodeoxycholic acids in the rat. *Lab. Invest.*, **24**:292–302, 1971.

Mizrahi, I. J., and Emmelot, P.: The effect of cysteine on the metabolic changes produced by two carcinogenic *n*-nitrosodiakylamines in rat liver. *Cancer Res.*, **22**:339–51, 1962.

Moore, L.: Inhibition of liver-microsome calcium pump by *in vivo* administration of CCl₄, CHCl₃ and 1,1-dichloroethylene (vinylidene chloride). *Biochem. Pharmacol.*, **29**:2505–11, 1980.

——: 1,1-Dichloroethylene inhibition of liver endoplasmic reticulum calcium pump function. *Biochem. Pharmacol.*, **31**:1463–65, 1982a.

——: Carbon disulfide hepatotoxicity and inhibition of liver microsome calcium pump. *Biochem. Pharmacol.*, **31**:1465–67, 1982b.

Noguchi, T.; Fong, K. L.; Lai, E. K.; Alexander, S. S.; King, M. M.; Olson, L.; Poyer, J. L.; and McCay, P. B.: Specificity of a phenobarbital-induced cytochrome P-450 for metabolism of carbon tetrachloride to the triochloromethyl radical. *Biochem. Pharmacol.*, **31**:615–24, 1982.

Perez, V.; Schaffner, F.; and Popper, H.: Hepatic drug reactions. In Popper, H., and Schaffner, F. (eds.): *Progress in Liver Disease*, Vol. 4. Grune & Stratton, New York, 1972, pp. 597–625.

Phillips, M. J.; Oshio, C.; Miyairi, M.; Katz, H.; and Smith, C. R.: A study of bile canalicular contractions in isolated hepatocytes. *Hepatology*, **2**:763–68, 1982.

Phillips, M. J.; Oshio, C.; Miyari, M.; Watanabe, S.; and Smith, C. R.: What is actin doing in the liver cell? *Hepatology*, **3**:433–36, 1983.

Plaa, G. L., and Ayotte, P.: Taurolithocholate-induced intrahepatic cholestasis: potentiation by methyl isobutyl ketone and methyl *n*-butyl ketone in rats. *Toxicol. Appl. Pharmacol.*, **80**:228–34, 1985.

Plaa, G. L.; de Lamirande, E.; Lewittes, M.; and Yousef, I. M.: Liver cell plasma membrane lipids in manganese-bilirubin-induced intrahepatic cholestasis. *Biochem. Pharmacol.*, **31**:3698–3701, 1982.

Plaa, G. L., and Hewitt, W. R.: Biotransformation products and cholestasis. In Popper, H. and Schaffner, F. (eds.): *Progress in Liver Diseases*, Vol. 7. Grune & Stratton, New York, 1982, pp. 179–94.

Plaa, G. L.; Hewitt, W. R.; du Souich, P.; Caillé, G.; and Lock, S.: Isopropanol and acetone potentiation of carbon tetrachloride-induced hepatotoxicity: single versus repetitive pretreatment in rats. *J. Toxicol. Environ. Health*, **9**:235–50, 1982.

Plaa, G. L., and Priestly, B. G.: Intrahepatic cholestasis induced by drugs and chemicals. *Pharmacol. Rev.*, **28**:207–73, 1976.

Plaa, G. L.; Traiger, G. J.; Hanasono, G. K.; and Witschi, H. P.: Effect of alcohols on various forms of chemically induced liver injury. In Khanna, J. M.; Israel, Y.; and Kalant, H. (eds.): *Alcoholic Liver Pathology*. Addiction Research Foundation, Toronto, 1975, pp. 225–44.

Plaa, G. L., and Witschi, H. P.: Chemicals, drugs, and lipid peroxidation. *Annu. Rev. Pharmacol. Toxicol.*, **16**:125–41, 1976.

Pohl, L. R.; Bhooshan, B.; Whittaker, N. F.; and Krishna, G.: Phosgene: a metabolite of chloroform. *Biochem. Biophys. Res. Commun.*, **79**:684–91, 1977.

Popper, H., and Schaffner, F.: Drug-induced hepatic injury. *Ann. Intern. Med.*, **51**:1230–52, 1959.

Price, V. F., and Jollow, D. J.: Increased resistance of diabetic rats to acetaminophen-induced hepatotoxicity. *J. Pharmacol. Exp. Ther.*, **220**:504–13, 1982.

Raisfeld, I. H.: Models of liver injury: the effect of toxins on the liver. In Becker, F. F. (ed.): *The Liver: Normal and Abnormal Functions*, Part A. Marcel Dekker, Inc., New York, 1974, pp. 203–23.

Rankin, J. G.; Schmidt, W.; Popham, R. E.; and de Lint, J.: Epidemiology of alcoholic liver disease-insights and problems. In Khanna, J. M.; Israel, Y.; and Kalant, H. (eds.): *Alcoholic Liver Pathology*. Addiction Research Foundation, Toronto, 1975, pp. 31–41.

Rappaport, A. M.: Physioanatomical basis of toxic liver injury. In Farber, E., and Fisher, M. M. (eds.): *Toxic Injury of the Liver*, Part A. Marcel Dekker, Inc., New York, 1979, pp. 1–57.

Recknagel, R. O.: Carbon tetrachloride hepatotoxicity. *Pharmacol. Rev.*, **19**:145–208, 1967.

——: A new direction in the study of carbon tetrachloride hepatotoxicity. *Life Sci.*, **33**:401–08, 1983.

Recknagel, R. O., and Ghoshal, A. K.: Lipoperoxidation as a vector in carbon tetrachloride hepatotoxicity. *Lab. Invest.*, **15**:132–48, 1966.

Recknagel, R. O., and Glende, E. A., Jr.: Carbon tetrachloride hepatotoxicity: an example of lethal cleavage. *CRC Crit. Rev. Toxicol.*, **2**:263–97, 1973.

Recknagel, R. O.; Glende, E. A., Jr.; Waller, R. L.; and Lowrey, K.: Lipid peroxidation: biochemistry, measurement, and significance in liver cell injury. In Plaa, G. L. and Hewitt, W. R. (eds.): *Toxicology of the Liver*. Raven Press, New York, 1982, pp. 213–41.

Recknagel, R. O., and Lombardi, B.: Studies of biochemical changes in subcellular particles of rat liver and their relationship to new hypothesis regarding pathogenesis of carbon tetrachloride fat accumulation. *J. Biol. Chem.*, **236**:564–69, 1961.

Rees, K. R.; Sinha, P.; and Spector, W. G.: The pathogenesis of liver injury in carbon tetrachloride and thioacetamide poisoning. *J. Pathol. Bacteriol.*, **81**:107–18, 1961.

Rees, K. R., and Tarlow, M. J.: The hepatotoxic action of allyl formate. *Biochem. J.*, **104**:757–61, 1967.

Reid, W. D.: Mechanism of allyl alcohol-induced hepatic necrosis. *Experientia*, **28**:1058–61, 1972.

Reid, W. D.; Christie, B.; Krishna, G.; Mitchell, J. R.; Moskowitz, J.; and Brodie, B. B.: Bromobenzene metabolism and hepatic necrosis. *Pharmacology*, **6**:41–55, 1971.

Reynolds, E. S.; Moslen, M. T.; Szabo, S.; Jaeger, R. J.; and Murphy, S. D.: Hepatotoxicity of vinyl chloride and 1,1-dichloroethylene. *Am. J. Pathol.*, **81**:219–32, 1975.

Rouiller, C.: Experimental toxic injury of the liver. In

Rouiller, C. (ed.): *The Liver*, Vol. 2. Academic Press, Inc., New York, 1964, pp. 335–476.

Rubinstein, D., and Kanics, L.: The conversion of carbon tetrachloride and chloroform to carbon dioxide by rat liver homogenates. *Can. J. Biochem.*, **42**:1577–85, 1964.

Schaffner, F., and Javitt, N. B.: Morphologic changes in hamster liver during intrahepatic cholestasis induced by taurolithocholate. *Lab. Invest.*, **15**:1783–92, 1966.

Schaffner, F.; Popper, H.; and Perez, V.: Changes in bile canaliculi produced by norethandrolone: electron microscopic study of human and rat liver. *J. Lab. Clin. Med.*, **56**:623–28, 1960.

Schaffner, F., and Raisfeld, I. H.: Drugs and the liver: a review of metabolism and adverse reactions. *Adv. Intern. Med.*, **15**:221–51, 1969.

Schinella, R. A., and Becker, F. F.: Cirrhosis. In Becker, F. F. (ed.): *The Liver: Normal and Abnormal Functions*, Part B. Marcel Dekker, Inc., New York, 1975, pp. 711–23.

Schreiber, A. J., and Simon, F. R.: Estrogen-induced cholestasis: clues to pathogenesis and treatment. *Hepatology*, **3**:607–13, 1983.

Seakins, A., and Robinson, D. S.: The effect of the administration of carbon tetrachloride on the formation of plasma lipoproteins in the rat. *Biochem. J.*, **86**:401–407, 1963.

Sell, D. A., and Reynolds, E. A.: Liver parenchymal cell injury. VIII. Lesions of the membranous cellular components following iodoform. *J. Cell Biol.*, **41**:736–52, 1969.

Shen, E. S.; Garry, V. F.; and Anders, M. W.: Effect of hypoxia on carbon tetrachloride hepatotoxicity. *Biochem. Pharmacol.*, **31**:3787–93, 1982.

Sipes, I. G., and Gandolfi, A. J.: Bioactivation of aliphatic organohalogens: Formation, detection, and relevance. In Plaa, G. L., and Hewitt, W. R. (eds.): *Toxicology of the Liver*. Raven Press, New York, 1982, pp. 181–212.

Sipes, I. G.; Krishna, G.; and Gillette, J. R.: Bioactivation of carbon tetrachloride, chloroform and bromotrichloromethane: Role of cytochrome P-450. *Life Sci.*, **20**:1541–48, 1977.

Sipes, I. G.; Stripp, B.; Krishna, G.; Maling, H. M.; and Gillette, J. R.: Enhanced hepatic microsomal activity by pretreatment of rats with acetone or isopropanol. *Proc. Soc. Exp. Biol. Med.*, **142**:237–40, 1973.

Slater, T. F.: Necrogenic action of carbon tetrachloride in the rat: a speculative mechanism based on activation. *Nature (Lond.)*, **209**:36–40, 1966.

Slikker, W., Jr.; Vore, M.; Bailey, J. R.; Meyers, M.; and Montgomery, C.: Hepatotoxic effects of estradiol-17-D-glucuronide in the rat and monkey. *J. Pharmacol. Exp. Ther.*, **225**:138–43, 1983.

Smuckler, E. A., and Benditt, E. P.: Studies on carbon tetrachloride intoxication. III. A subcellular defect in protein synthesis. *Biochemistry*, **4**:671–79, 1965.

Smuckler, E. A.; Iseri, O. A.; and Benditt, E. P.: Studies on carbon tetrachloride intoxication. I. The effect of carbon tetrachloride on incorporation of labelled amino acids into plasma proteins. *Biochem. Biophys. Res. Commun.*, **5**:270–75, 1961.

Stewart, R. D.; Torkelson, T. R.; Hake, C. L.; and Erley, D. S.: Infrared analysis of carbon tetrachloride and ethanol in blood. *J. Lab. Clin. Med.*, **56**:148–56, 1960.

Sweeney, G. D.; Garfield, R. E.; Jones, K. G.; and Latham, A. N.: Studies using sedimentation velocity on heterogeneity of size and function of hepatocytes from mature male rats. *J. Lab. Clin. Med.*, **91**:432–43, 1978a.

Sweeney, G. D.; Jones, K. D.; and Krestynski, F.: Effects of phenobarbital and 3-methylcholanthrene pretreatment on size, sedimentation velocity, and mixed function oxygenase activity of rat hepatocytes. *J. Lab. Clin. Med.*, **91**:444–54, 1978b.

Tomokuni, K.: Studies on hepatotoxicity induced by chlorinated hydrocarbons. II. Lipid metabolism and absorption spectrum of microsomal lipid in mice exposed to 1,1,2,2,-tetrachloroethane. *Acta Med. Okayama*, **24**:315–22, 1970.

Traiger, G. J. and Bruckner, J. V.: The participation of 2-butanone in 2-butanol-induced potentiation of carbon tetrachloride hepatotoxicity. *J. Pharmacol. Exp. Ther.*, **196**:493–500, 1976.

Uraguchi, K.; Sakai, F.; Tsukioka, M.; Noguchi, Y.; and Tatsuno, M.: Acute and chronic toxicity in mice and rats of the fungus mat of *Penicillium islandicum* sopp added to the diet. *Jpn. J. Exp. Med.*, **31**:435–61, 1961.

Watanabe, S.; Miyairi, M.; Oshio, C.; Smith, C. R.; and Phillips, M. J.: Phalloidin alters bile canalicular contractility in primary monolayer cultures of rat liver. *Gastroenterology*, **85**:245–253, 1983.

Windmueller, H. G., and von Euler, L. H.: Prevention of orotic acid-induced fatty liver with allopurinol. *Proc. Soc. Exp. Biol. Med.*, **136**:98–101, 1971.

Witschi, H. P.: Effects of beryllium on deoxyribonucleic acid-synthesizing enzymes in regenerating rat liver. *Biochem. J.*, **120**:623–34, 1970.

Witschi, H. P., and Aldridge, W. N.: Biochemical changes in rat liver after acute beryllium poisoning. *Biochem. Pharmacol.*, **16**:263–78, 1967.

———: Uptake, distribution and binding of beryllium to organelles of the rat liver cell. *Biochem. J.*, **106**:811–20, 1968.

Witzleben, C. L.: Physiologic and morphologic natural history of a model of intrahepatic cholestasis (manganese-bilirubin overload). *Am. J. Pathol.*, **66**:577–82, 1972.

Wogan, G. N.: The induction of liver cell cancer by chemicals. In Cameron, H. M.; Linsell, D. A.; and Warwick, G. P. (eds.): *Liver Cell Cancer*. Elsevier, Amsterdam, 1976, pp. 121–52.

Yousef, I. M.; Lewittes, M.; Tuchweber, B.; Roy, C. C.; and Weber, A.: Lithocholic acid–cholesterol interactions in rat liver plasma membrane fractions. *Biochim. Biophys. Acta*, **796**:345–53, 1984.

Zimmerman, H. L.: *Hepatotoxicity*. Appleton-Century-Crofts, New York, 1978.

SUPPLEMENTAL READING

Arias, I. M.; Popper, H.; Schachter, D.; and Shafritz, D. A.: *The Liver—Biology and Pathology*. Raven Press, New York, 1982.

Cameron, H. M.; Linsell, D. A.; and Warwick, G. P.: *Liver Cell Cancer*. Elsevier, Amsterdam, 1976.

Farber, E., and Fisher, M. M.: Toxic Injury of the Liver, Part A. Marcel Dekker, Inc., New York, 1979.

Farber, E., and Fisher, M. M.: *Toxic Injury of the Liver*, Part B. Marcel Dekker, Inc., New York, 1979.

Khanna, J. M.; Israel, Y.; and Kalant, H.: *Alcoholic Liver Pathology*. Addiction Research Foundation, Toronto, 1975.

Plaa, G. L., and Hewitt, W. R.: *Toxicology of the Liver*. Raven Press, New York, 1982.

Popper, H.; Bianchi, L.; and Reutter, W.: *Membrane Alterations as Basis of Liver Injury*. MTP Press Ltd., Lancaster, 1977.

Zimmerman, H. J.: *Hepatotoxicity*. Appleton-Century-Crofts, New York, 1978.

Chapter 11

TOXIC RESPONSES OF THE KIDNEY

Jerry B. Hook and *William R. Hewitt*

INTRODUCTION

The mammalian kidney is an extremely complex organ, both anatomically and functionally. A primary renal function is excretion of wastes. In addition, the kidney plays a significant role in the regulation of total body homeostasis; it is the predominant organ involved in regulation of extracellular fluid (ECF) volume and electrolyte composition. The kidney is also the major site of formation of hormones that influence systemic metabolic functions: erythropoietin is a potent stimulus to erythrocyte formation; the relatively inactive 25-hydroxy-vitamin D_3 is metabolized to the active 1,25-dihydroxy-vitamin D_3; renin, the trigger to the formation of angiotensin and aldosterone, is formed in the kidney; and recent evidence indicates that the kidney produces several vasoactive prostaglandins and kinins. A toxicologic insult to the kidney could affect any or all of these functions. Nevertheless, the effects usually reported following toxic insult reflect decreased elimination of wastes, i.e., an increase in blood urea nitrogen (BUN) or an increase in plasma creatinine. This does not necessarily mean that excretory functions are primarily affected by nephrotoxicants; rather, these are renal functions that are measured rapidly and reliably. Thus, the use of BUN and plasma creatinine as clinical indices of nephrotoxicity reflects the state of technology, not necessarily the primary sites of nephrotoxicity.

RENAL PHYSIOLOGY AND PATHOPHYSIOLOGY

Functional Anatomy

Gross examination of a sagittal section of the kidney clearly demonstrates the demarcation between the two major anatomic areas, the cortex and the medulla (Figure 11–1). The cortex constitutes the major portion of the kidney and consequently receives most of the total nutrient blood flow to the organ. Thus, when a blood-borne toxicant is delivered to the kidney, a high percentage of the material will reach sites in the cortex. In a single pass through the kidney most chemicals will have a greater propensity to influence cortical, rather than medullary, function. A smaller percentage of the total chemical delivered to the kidney would reach the medulla. However, because of the low blood flow to the medulla and because of the anatomic arrangement of the *vasa rectae* and loops of Henle (Figure 11–1), the possibility of a chemical being trapped by the countercurrent mechanism is high. Thus, a foreign compound could remain in the medulla and achieve relatively high concentrations.

A discussion of the functional anatomy of the kidney is most appropriately based on the functional unit of the kidney, the nephron (Figure 11–1). The nephron may be considered in three portions: the vascular element including the afferent and efferent arterioles, the glomerulus, and the tubular element. All nephrons have their primary vascular elements and glomeruli in the cortex. The proximal convoluted tubule is localized in the cortex and sends the *pars recta* (straight portion) of the proximal tubule and loops of Henle deep into the substance of the kidney. Those glomeruli close to the medulla (juxtamedullary glomeruli) are associated with nephrons that send their loops of Henle deep into the medulla. Other glomeruli closer to the surface of the kidney often form nephrons whose loops of Henle are contained within the cortex (Figure 11–1). The relative proportion of nephrons with long versus short loops varies with species.

Each element of the nephron unit has specific functions, all of which may be influenced by nephrotoxicants. The vascular element serves to: (1) deliver waste and other materials to the tubule for excretion; (2) return reabsorbed and synthesized materials to the systemic circulation; and (3) deliver oxygen and metabolic substrates to the nephron. It is within the vascular element of the afferent arteriole that renin is formed. The glomerulus is a specialized capil-

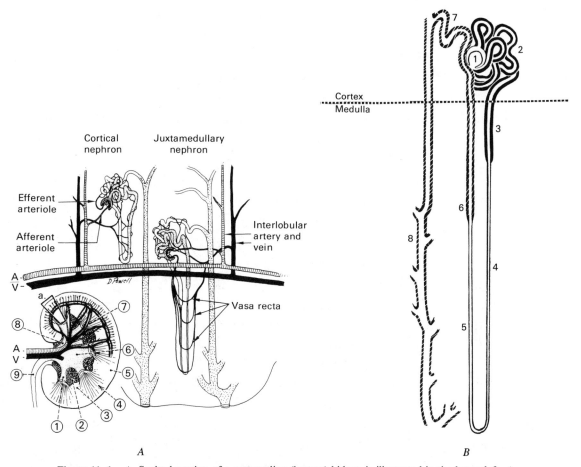

Figure 11–1. *A.* Sagittal section of a mammalian (human) kidney is illustrated in the lower left. *A* and *V* refer to renal artery and vein, respectively; (*1*) minor calix; (*2*) fat in sinus; (*3*) renal column of Bertin; (*4*) medullary ray; (*5*) cortex; (*6*) pelvis; (*7*) interlobar artery; (*8*) major calix; (*9*) ureter. Insert (a) from the upper pole of the kidney is enlarged to illustrate the relationships between the nephrons and the vasculature. (From Tisher, C. C.: Anatomy of the kidney. In Brenner, B. B., and Rector, F. C., Jr. [eds.]: *The Kidney.* W. B. Saunders Co., Philadelphia, 1976.)

B. Anatomy of a juxtamedullary nephron. Note the demarcation between cortex and medulla: (*1*) glomerulus; (*2*) proximal convoluted tubule; (*3*) proximal straight tubule (*pars recta*); (*4*) descending limb of the loop of Henle; (*5*) thin ascending limb of the loop of Henle; (*6*) thick ascending limb of the loop of Henle; (*7*) distal convoluted tubule; (*8*) collecting duct. (Modified from Gottschalk, C. W.: Osmotic concentration and dilution of the urine. *Am. J. Med., 36:670–85, 1964.*)

lary bed; it is unique in that it is the only capillary bed in the body positioned between vasoactive arterioles. The glomerulus is a relatively porous capillary and acts as a selective filter of the plasma. Based on molecular size and net charge, certain materials will be filtered into the lumen of the tubule and others will be retained in the circulation (Figure 11–2). The tubular element of the nephron selectively reabsorbs the bulk of the filtrate; approximately 98 to 99 percent of the salts and water is reabsorbed. There is virtually complete reabsorption of filtered sugars and amino acids and selective elimination

of waste materials. Furthermore, the tubular element, particularly the proximal tubule, actively secretes material into urine. Secretory activity is responsible for most excretion of certain organic compounds and for the elimination of hydrogen and potassium ions.

The tubular element is also actively involved in the synthesis of ammonia and glucose and the activation of vitamin D. (For a more detailed consideration of renal structure and function see Valtin [1973] or Brenner and Rector [1981].)

The cellular response to a toxic insult may vary from an imperceptible biochemical aberra-

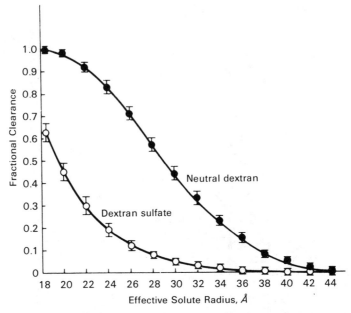

Figure 11-2. Fractional clearances (clearance compared to inulin clearance) of neutral dextran and dextran sulfate by rat kidney plotted as a function of effective molecular radius. As effective molecular radius increases, the fractional clearance, which reflects glomerular permeability, decreases. The permeability to neutral dextran is considerably greater than that of the charged dextran sulfate. (From Brenner, B. M., *et al.*: Determinants of glomerular permselectivity: Insights derived from observations *in vivo. Kidney Int.*, **12:**229–37, 1977. Reprinted with permission.)

tion to cell death with resulting necrosis. Functionally, toxicity may be reflected as a minor alteration in transport capability (e.g., transient glucosuria, aminoaciduria), as polyuria with decreased concentrating capacity, or as frank renal failure with anuria and elevated blood urea nitrogen (BUN). Depending on the magnitude of the insult, these changes may be reversible or permanent and may be lethal. Theoretically, these effects may be brought about in one of several ways: (1) Vasoconstriction could decrease renal blood flow and glomerular filtration rate, reducing urine flow, eventually resulting in an increase in BUN. If prolonged, vasoconstriction would lead to tissue ischemia with resultant loss of function and, eventually, tissue destruction. (2) The nephrotoxicant could affect the glomerular element directly, altering permeability such that filtration at the glomerulus is compromised. (3) Alternatively, or in combination with these other possibilities, the administration of a nephrotoxicant could influence tubular function directly. Either specific reabsorptive or secretory mechanisms could be influenced by the toxicant, or the general permeability of the tubule could be influenced such that the normal ability of the tubule to act as a barrier to diffusion could be altered.

Reason for Susceptibility of the Kidney

The kidney is a highly dynamic organ. Renal blood flow is quite high; the two kidneys together receive about 25 percent of the cardiac output. Approximately one-third of the plasma water reaching the kidney is filtered, and from this material approximately 98 to 99 percent of the salt and water is reabsorbed. Maintenance of normal function requires delivery of large amounts of metabolic substrates and oxygen to the kidney. Because of the high blood flow, any drug or chemical in the systemic circulation will be delivered in relatively high amounts to this organ. As salt and water are reabsorbed from the glomerular filtrate, the materials remaining (including the potential toxicant) in the urine may be concentrated in the tubule. Thus, a nontoxic concentration of a chemical in the plasma could become toxic in the kidney subsequent to concentration within the urine. Furthermore, a chemical reaching the kidney might be concentrated in the cells in one or both of the following ways: If the material is actively secreted into the tubular urine, it will first be accumulated within the cells of the proximal tubule in concentrations higher than in plasma. This process will expose these cells to very high concentrations of the agent, which could produce toxicity. Similarly, a material that is reabsorbed (even by passive means) from the urine into the blood will pass through the cells of the nephron in a relatively high concentration, potentially leading to intracellular toxicity.

As pointed out above, the renal medulla offers unique problems concerning nephrotoxicity. Because of the low blood flow to the medulla, relatively less potential toxicant might enter this region by the bloodstream than would enter the cortex. However, any materials in the tubular urine will by necessity pass through the loop of Henle and the collecting duct in the medulla. The countercurrent mechanisms within the medulla may trap the compound, leading to establishment of a high concentration within the lumen of the nephron.

The kidney is sensitive to extrarenal factors that would decrease blood pressure or blood volume, as in shock or hemorrhage. Such changes may induce signs of ischemia and functional deficit in this highly active metabolic organ. The kidney is under the influence of the sympathetic nervous system, and changes in neural activity can markedly influence renal function. Direct effects of the renal sympathetic nerves on renal vascular resistance and on renin secretion have been documented many times. More recent evidence suggests that renal nerve activity might directly influence proximal tubular function as well. Therefore, any change in systemic homeostasis that would alter sympathetic nerve activity could also influence the kidney. Similarly, dehydration may occur due to decreased water intake, elevated body temperature, or as a secondary effect of a chemical. This could lead to decreased plasma volume, which could decrease glomerular filtration. Probably of greater importance in this case is the fact that in the presence of antidiuretic hormone the urine would be maximally concentrated and the possibility of a chemical reaching excessively high concentrations in the urine would be maximized.

Assessment of Renal Function

Evaluation of the effect of a chemical on renal function can be accomplished by several methods. The methods used depend on the complexity of the question to be answered. For instance, to determine whether there had been *an* effect on kidney function, unanesthetized intact animals could be used. More information can probably be gained by quantifying renal function in anesthetized animals, where renal function can be determined in a steady state. To learn about specific biochemical or functional lesions, investigations are often conducted *in vitro*. Finally, histopathologic techniques can provide a great deal of information about renal integrity.

There are many advantages to determining the effect of a chemical agent in the intact, unanesthetized animal. These studies can be conducted serially during the course of a feeding program to monitor possible alterations in renal function. The standard battery of tests includes measurement of urine volume, urinary pH, and excretion of sodium and potassium. The appearance of sugar and/or excess protein in the urine would indicate abnormalities in renal function, as would changes in urine sediment. Abnormalities in urine osmolality might indicate a deficit in renal medullary function. Small blood samples can be drawn from the tail or from the orbital sinus of the eye and the BUN and plasma creatinine concentration estimated. A relatively simple test is the ability of the animal to eliminate a load of compound whose mechanism of renal handling is known. The compound most commonly used is phenolsulfonphthalein (PSP). These are all relatively general tests and can provide information about abnormalities of total kidney function. More recently, attempts have been made to develop noninvasive tests that might provide more specific information. Several groups have attempted to utilize the appearance of enzymes in the urine as indices of renal function. Enzymuria in general can indicate abnormality of function, and the specific enzymes involved might provide information about selective sites of damage. The appearance in the urine of enzymes of renal origin (enzymes that are specific to the kidney, such as maltase or trehalase) could indicate specific destruction of the renal proximal tubules (Berndt, 1982), whereas alkaline phosphatase in the urine could arise from renal or prerenal (e.g., hepatic) damage.

The use of anesthetized animals provides more information concerning toxic insult to the kidney. The commonly used animals are dogs, rabbits, and rats. In anesthetized preparations, systemic blood pressure and glomerular filtration rate in the steady state can be monitored. Glomerular filtration rate is usually estimated from the clearance of inulin. The clearance of urea as estimated by BUN is not particularly definitive because urea is a by-product of protein metabolism and any toxic insult that would influence protein metabolism (poor nutrition, hepatotoxicity) could influence BUN. Clearance of the polysaccharide inulin provides information about glomerular filtration rate regardless of the state of protein metabolism.

Renal blood flow can be estimated from renal plasma flow using the renal clearance and/or renal extraction of para-aminohippuric acid (PAH). Alternatively, radiolabeled microspheres or an electromagnetic flowmeter may be used to measure renal blood flow specifically. The ability of the kidney to reabsorb or secrete electrolytes is estimated as the fractional excretion of sodium, potassium, bicarbonate, chloride, etc. Fractional excretion takes into account the filtered load, thus allowing comparisons of electrolyte transport between treated and control animals even if renal hemodynamics have changed. Another estimate of nephron function in terms of the ability to remove electrolyte and water from specific sites along the nephron is to quantify the clearance of free water (which reflects the ability of the kidney to remove almost all sodium from the urine). In addition, urinary concentrating capacity in the anesthetized animal can be used to estimate medullary function (Berndt, 1982a).

Very elegant studies have been conducted in dogs and rats using micropuncture. Using this technique, individual nephron or vascular segments are punctured and fluid collected and pressures monitored. Such a technique can be used to distinguish between vascular, tubular, and glomerular changes following nephrotoxic insult (Biber *et al.*, 1968; Oken, 1976).

To quantify the effects of a nephrotoxicant more specifically, a variety of *in vitro* techniques may be employed. *In vivo* techniques might demonstrate that the renal clearance of a particular compound is diminished, but it may be difficult to distinguish between effects directly on hemodynamics, biotransformation, or transport if all are altered by a nephrotoxicant. The toxic effects of chemicals may be evaluated *in vitro* by adding the agent directly to the preparation or following administration to the animal. This allows a distinction to be made between an effect on the kidney due to direct chemical insult and secondary effects, such as those subsequent to alterations in biotransformation, for example. The renal cortical slice technique has been used extensively to evaluate the influence of nephrotoxicants on the transport of organic anions such as PAH and organic cations such as *N*-methylnicotinamide (NMN) or tetraethylammonium (TEA). Attempts have been made to evaluate transport in a reabsorptive direction using the nonmetabolized amino acid analog α-aminoisobutyric acid and the nonmetabolized sugar α-methyl-*d*-glucoside. In addition, the ability of the kidney to produce ammonia and glucose from added substrates *in vitro* can provide more specific information about metabolic alterations produced by a nephrotoxicant. Isolated tubular preparations may be employed to evaluate the influence of nephrotoxicants on selected areas of the nephron. Micropuncture and microperfusion techniques have also been uti-

lized in attempts to identify specific loci of action of nephrotoxicants (Berndt, 1982a).

Histopathologic examination of tissue can demonstrate structural changes that have occurred in response to nephrotoxicants and can often identify selected areas that have been affected. For instance, light microscopy can demonstrate the papillary necrosis produced by nonnarcotic analgesics and can isolate the proximal tubular damage induced by mercury, chromium, and other heavy metals. Histopathology will often show that an injury has occurred even in a situation in which function was not noticeably altered. The use of standard light microscopy can also provide information concerning the appearance in the tubule of protein casts, of sloughed brush border, and of crystals or stones in the kidney and urine. Very elegant experiments have been conducted using microdissection techniques. Following nephrotoxic insult, entire tubules have been carefully dissected and specific areas of damage have been identified by light microscopy (Biber *et al.*, 1968). Many histochemical techniques are also available to evaluate renal response to poisons. Electron microscopy provides information concerning subcellular localization of tubular injury. Changes in mitochondria can be identified very easily, as can alterations in other organelles. Electron microscopy has been employed extensively in efforts to understand the changes in glomerular structure that might account for changes in permeability following nephrotoxicants.

Compensation for Renal Damage

The kidney has a remarkable ability to compensate following loss of renal mass. Within a short time after surgical removal of one kidney, the remaining kidney hypertrophies to such an extent that standard clinical signs of renal function provide no indication of tissue loss (Figure 11–3). This ability to compensate becomes a problem when attempting to evaluate the effect of nephrotoxicants and points out that distinctions must be made between acute and chronic renal injury. A single dose of nephrotoxicant may produce profound, acute changes in renal function, but if the injury is not lethal and if no other insult is forthcoming, the kidney may compensate and regain normal function in a short time (Figure 11–4). Similarly, chronic administration of a low dose of a nephrotoxicant may bring about significant changes in structure of the kidney, but during the course of administration, the kidney may compensate so that marked changes are not seen in the standard renal function tests. The consequences of these effects are

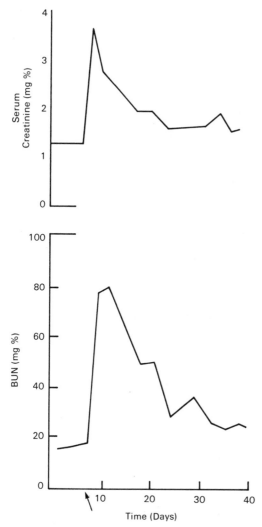

Figure 11–3. The effect of a three-fourths nephrectomy on renal function tests in a dog. BUN was measured on alternate days for eight days. At the arrow the animal was anesthetized and one kidney removed. Approximately 50 percent of the branches of the renal artery entering the renal pelvis of the remaining kidney were ligated. The surgical wound was closed and the animal allowed to recover. In the immediate postoperative period there was a significant increase in BUN, but within a short time this estimate of renal function returned to within normal limits.

profound, for if kidney function is evaluated at a time far removed from single injury, a standard function test might reveal no changes, even though there had been a great deal of tissue damage. Following chronic administration, no change in kidney function may be detected until

the ability of the kidney to compensate is exceeded. Then, within a short period of time the animal might develop life-threatening renal failure.

SITES OF ACTION OF NEPHROTOXICANTS

Few data are available that define specific cellular or subcellular sites of action of nephrotoxicants. Only rarely have specific receptors (in the classic sense of the word) for specific nephrotoxicants been identified. Rather, in many cases it appears that several tissue constituents may be influenced by toxic agents. There are two interrelated reasons for this apparent lack of specificity: (1) In contrast to a specific pharmacologic effect of a chemical that requires activation or inhibition of a specific endogenous receptor, cell damage may follow interruption of one or several of the many required cellular functions; (2) certain kidney cells may be more susceptible to damage merely because they are exposed to concentrations of chemicals many times higher than are other cells of the body, leading to nonspecific cellular damage. For instance, many nephrotoxicants appear to have their primary site of action on (in) the proximal tubule. This is reasonable, since most blood flow to the kidney is delivered to the cortex, which is predominantly proximal tubule. In addition, active secretion of compounds occurs in the proximal tubule, and changes brought about by concentrating a chemical within the tubular lumen would be expected to produce their effects first in the proximal nephron. There appear to be differences in sensitivity along various segments within the proximal nephron. The proximal convolution is the primary site of reabsorption of glucose and amino acids and seems to be more sensitive to certain metals like chromium. The *pars recta* (or straight portion) has a greater capacity to secrete organic compounds, and it is in this area where damage due to mercury, cephaloridine, and other organic compounds appears first.

This is not to say, however, that there are not specific targets for certain nephrotoxicants in the kidney. Localization of sites of action of nephrotoxicants to areas of the tubule other than the proximal nephron strongly argues for specific biochemical targets for some types of nephrotoxic agents. For instance, the loop of Henle appears to be the site of damage produced by chronic administration of analgesic mixtures (aspirin and phenacetin) and other materials that act in the medulla, such as fluoride ion. The distal convoluted tubule is a relatively small part of

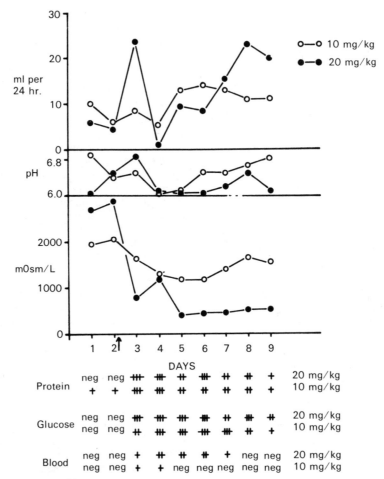

Figure 11–4. The effect of two doses of subcutaneous potassium dichromate (at the arrow) in rats. The rapidity of response and the quick return of function are illustrated. (From Berndt, W. O.: The effect of potassium dichromate on renal tubular transport processes. *Toxicol Appl Pharmacol.*, **32**:40–52, 1975.)

the total nephron and appears not to be selectively damaged by most nephrotoxicants. However, compounds such as amphotericin have been shown to influence the ability of the kidney to acidify the urine, which is probably a distal tubular event. The collecting duct appears to be relatively insensitive to most nephrotoxicants. For instance, following intoxication with analgesic mixtures, histologic evaluation of the medulla showed that most of the ascending limbs of the loop of Henle had been destroyed, whereas the collecting ducts appeared to be unaffected. Damage due to outdated tetracyclines may occur in this area.

The glomerulus is a primary site of action of several chemicals and is also susceptible to immunologic injury. The glomerulus acts as both a size-selective and charge-selective filtration barrier (Brenner *et al.*, 1981). This barrier function involves all structural aspects of the capillary wall. The sialoprotein-rich endothelium and lamina rara interna of the glomerular basement membrane (GBM) appear to be the primary impediments to filtration of large polyanionic molecules such as albumin. The GBM is the primary filtration barrier to neutral polymers whereas the filtration of large, cationic molecules is restricted by the lamina rara externa of the GBM and the slit diaphragm (Brenner *et al.*, 1981). Following toxic insult, changes in glomerular permeability may occur, leading to loss of proteins in the urine. It had previously been suggested that nephrotoxicants might change the diameter of pores in the glomerulus, allowing larger materials to pass through. However, by light microscopy the tissue does not appear to be more porous, but appears to be somewhat thicker after a toxic insult. Recent evidence suggests that several nephrotoxicants can reduce the number of fixed anionic charges on glomerular structural elements. This reduces the charge-selective properties of the glomerulus and allows circulating polyanions such as albumin to be excreted in the urine in excessive amounts. In addition, maintenance of normal glomerular ultrastructure appears to be dependent on anion-anion charge repulsion. Reduction of fixed anionic charges allows the terminal divisions of the glomerular podocytes to fuse and accounts for the characteristic thickening of the glomerulus as observed by light microscopy (Brenner *et al.*, 1981).

SPECIFIC NEPHROTOXICANTS

As indicated above, not all compounds that influence renal function affect the kidney directly. Renal function may be altered secondarily to change in blood pressure, blood volume, neural or hormonal influences and to a variety of destructive systemic effects. The focus in this section will be on compounds that produce specific effects on the kidney. Many of these compounds affect the kidney directly. In other cases, the ultimate toxicant might be a metabolic product formed within the kidney or produced in an extrarenal organ and transported to the kidney where it acts directly or requires further biotransformation to a nephrotoxic product.

Heavy Metals

Most heavy metals are potent nephrotoxicants. Relatively low doses of a variety of metals produce a similar set of signs and symptoms characterized by glucosuria, aminoaciduria, and polyuria (Figure 11–4). If the dose of the metal is increased, renal necrosis, anuria, increased BUN, and death will follow. Most metals probably produce their nephrotoxicity by a similar mechanism. Following a toxic metal insult the histologic picture is one of necrotic proximal tubules with lumens filled with proteinaceous material. It has been suggested that tissue destruction could lead to sloughing of proximal tubular cells into the lumen, resulting in tubular occlusion. Occlusion could be of sufficient magnitude to increase intratubular pressure, resulting in decreased glomerular filtration rate. However, this is probably an oversimplistic explanation. Oken (1976) has observed that when tubules are occluded after several nephrotoxicants, intraluminal pressure is reduced, not elevated. The apparently low glomerular filtration rate may be partially explained by an increased permeability of the tubule to glomerular markers such as inulin, suggesting that the filtered inulin may leak back across the tubule membrane into the peritubular blood thereby producing an artifactual decrease in glomerular filtration rate. Oken (1976), however, suggested that little leakage of inulin occurs. Rather, the fall in glomerular filtration rate is due to decreased glomerular permeability or reduced glomerular blood flow. Indeed, there appears to be a significant vascular component of the nephrotoxicity of heavy metals. The severity of the renal damage produced by several heavy metals is reduced by feeding animals a high-salt diet prior to challenge with the poison. Since the high salt would decrease renin release by the kidney, a renin-angiotensin mechanism has been proposed to explain vasoconstriction. This interpretation has not, however, been universally accepted. Several investigators have recently suggested an involvement of renal prostaglandins in this vasoconstriction. However, even in the absence of vasoconstriction, changes in renal function, particularly in the proximal tubule, occur following heavy metals. Probably the frank nephrotoxicity that occurs in response to heavy metals is due to a combination of ischemia secondary to vasoconstriction and direct cellular toxicity of these materials. The direct cellular toxicity of metals is supported by *in vitro* studies demonstrating metal-induced damage to the proximal tubule.

Several mechanisms exist that tend to protect the kidney from heavy metal damage. Following low-dose exposure, significant concentrations of metal are found in renal tissue prior to development of physiologic signs of toxicity. Renal lysosomes appear to play an active role in such a protective mechanism (Fowler *et al.*, 1975). This binding of metals by lysosomes may be stimulated by chronic low-dose exposure, and the accumulation may be due to one of several mechanisms, including lysosomal endocytosis of a metal-protein complex, autophagy of intoxicated organelles such as mitochondria, and/or binding of the metal to acidic lipoproteins within the lysosome. In addition, the smooth endoplasmic reticulum proliferates in the *pars recta* cells following exposure to mercury, and apical extrusion of endoplasmic reticulum packets may eliminate mercury from the kidney (Fowler, 1972). Exposure to very high concentrations of metals may inundate these mechanisms, resulting in detectable cellular injury.

Mercury. The toxicity of mercury has been recognized since antiquity. Mercury may be introduced into the body as elemental mercury, as inorganic mercury, or as organic mercury, such as diuretics. More recently, organic mercury as an environmental pollutant, methylmercuric chloride, has produced renal damage in man and animals. Extensive data have accumulated on the nephrotoxicity of mercury because it has been used frequently as a model compound to produce acute renal failure in animals. Functional toxicity probably results from both vasoconstriction and direct cellular effects. Both organic and inorganic mercurials are toxic *in vitro*.

Gottschalk and his collaborators (Biber *et al.*, 1968) administered mercuric chloride to rats and then evaluated individual nephron function by micropuncture and structural integrity by microdissection. Nephrotoxic doses produced relatively selective histopathologic and functional alterations in the *pars recta* of the proximal tubule. They suggested that this localization of effect was consistent with the relatively normal appearance of the surface of the poisoned kidney and the rather modest effect of $HgCl_2$ on glucose excretion (most glucose reabsorption occurs in the convoluted portion of the proximal nephron). The majority of PAH secretion occurs in the *pars recta*, and PAH transport appears to be extremely sensitive to Hg^{2+} (Phillips *et al.*, 1977). As the dose of mercury is increased, toxicity occurs throughout the proximal nephron.

The basic biochemical mechanism whereby mercury produces renal cellular damage is not completely clear. However, mercury combines with sulfhydryl groups and inhibits a great number of enzyme systems. Mitochondrial enzyme systems seem to be particularly sensitive to mercury, and the pathophysiologic effects often seen suggest inhibition of oxidative pathways. However, mitochondrial effects of mercury might not be the initiating events in mercury nephrotoxicity. Ganote *et al.* (1974) attempted to evaluate the time course of the effect of mercuric chloride on the ultrastructure of the kidney and to correlate these changes with several parameters of metabolic integrity. Within 24 hours, a low dose of mercuric chloride (1 mg/kg) to rats produced a relatively selective necrosis of proximal tubular cells in the inner cortex, consistent with an effect within the *pars recta*. However, as early as eight hours after the mercury they were able to identify a variety of other morphologic changes including loss of brush border, dispersion of ribosomes, and formation of clumps of smooth membranes in the cytoplasm of the proximal tubule. These changes were followed by the appearance of vacuoles and other changes, including rupture of the plasma membrane and mitochondrial changes characteristic of cell necrosis. As early as eight hours there were alterations in water and ion movement in renal cortical tissue, consistent with some of the morphologic changes. However, the ability of the tissue to accumulate PAH was not depressed

until after 16 hours. Oxygen consumption of tissue slices was not reduced until 24 hours after the poison, when the cells were frankly necrotic. Thus, these data suggest that mitochondrial injury does not play a primary role in the pathogenesis of mercury toxicity; rather, the data suggest that the mitochondrial damage occurred only at about the same time as general disruption of the plasma membrane.

Platinum. Nephrotoxicity is frequently a complication of therapy with cisplatin, a platinum coordination complex with antineoplastic properties (Goldstein and Mayor, 1983). Cisplatin renal dysfunction has several distinguishing characteristics. Although proximal tubular damage (primarily of the *pars recta*) has been observed in humans and animals, cisplatin also appears to attack the distal tubule and collecting duct (Daley-Yates and McBrien, 1982; Goldstein and Mayor, 1983). In addition to the functional deficits associated with acute proximal tubular necrosis (enzymuria, proteinuria, altered organic ion transport), cisplatin produces a polyuric renal failure characterized by a urinary concentrating defect, reduced glomerular filtration rate, and wastage of magnesium; the inappropriate urinary losses of magnesium may be sufficient to produce hypomagnesemia (Goldstein and Mayor, 1983; Weiner and Jacobs, 1983). Clifton *et al.* (1982) suggested that cisplatin inhibits the release of antidiuretic hormone from the posterior pituitary; this may contribute to the cisplatin-induced polyuric state. The onset and repair of the cisplatin renal lesion is delayed, and persistent tubular damage has been observed following a single administration of cisplatin (Dobyan *et al.*, 1980). Chronic cisplatin therapy may produce irreversible renal injury (Goldstein and Mayor, 1983). In contrast to other heavy metals, the platinum atom may not mediate cisplatin toxicity; the *trans* isomer of cisplatin is not nephrotoxic at dosages that produce comparable renal platinum concentrations. Similarly, cisplatin toxicity can be modified by changing the chemical nature of its ligands. Thus, a metabolite of the cisplatin complex, rather than the platinum atom itself, may mediate the nephrotoxicity of this drug.

Cadmium. Cadmium is an interesting metal in that following administration of the metal there is enhanced synthesis in the liver of the metal-binding protein, metallothionein. This compound seems to have a paradoxical effect on the systemic toxicity of cadmium. Metallothionein appears to bind cadmium and in this way protect certain organs such as the testes from cadmium toxicity. Yet, at the same time, metallothionein may enhance cadmium nephrotoxicity, possibly because the cadmium-metallothionein complex is taken up by the kidney more readily than is the free ion (Nordberg *et al.*, 1975; Nordberg, 1982). Injury produced by administration of the cadmium-metal-lothionein complex is localized to the first and second segments of the proximal tubule and is manifested by proteinuria, aminoaciduria, glucosuria, and decreased tubular reabsorption of phosphate (Goyer, 1982). The proteinuria is predominantly tubular in nature as indicated by an increased excretion of low-molecular-weight proteins (e.g., β-2 microglobulin); high-molecular-weight proteins have also been observed in the urine, suggesting a glomerular effect of cadmium as well (Goyer, 1982).

Other Metals. Another of the widely studied metal nephrotoxicants is chromium, usually administered as potassium dichromate. In sublethal doses, chromium produces a proximal tubular necrosis similar to that of mercury except for its localization. Low doses of chromium produce a relatively specific necrosis of the proximal convoluted tubule. Functionally, this leads to pronounced glucosuria (Figure 11–4). After low doses of chromium the surface of the kidney shows marked signs of ischemia and tissue damage. As with mercury, when the dose of chromium is increased, toxicity is seen throughout the proximal tubule. Renal damage has also been observed following administration of arsenic, gold, iron, antimony, and thallium (Maher, 1976). Acute or chronic administration of lead produces tissue damage and decreased transport of PAH and NMN.

Halogenated Hydrocarbons

Carbon tetrachloride (CCl_4) and chloroform ($CHCl_3$) are both hepatotoxic and nephrotoxic. The magnitude of the nephrotoxicity varies with species, strain, and sex. With both hydrocarbons the functional lesion in the kidney appears to be due primarily to proximal tubular damage, although structural alterations are seen in other portions of the nephron as well. Functionally, the nephropathy appears similar to other types of acute renal insult with polyuria, glucosuria, and proteinuria at low doses, leading to anuria and complete renal failure with higher doses. Inhibition of PAH uptake by renal cortical slices appears to be one of the most sensitive indices of toxicity (Watrous and Plaa, 1972).

There is considerable evidence to indicate that in the liver, CCl_4 and $CHCl_3$ are metabolically activated to toxic reactants. Activation of $CHCl_3$ and CCl_4 by mixed-function oxidases involves formation of reactive metabolites that covalently bind to hepatic or renal tissue. Striker *et al.* (1968) have shown in kidneys of rats that early signs of damage occur long after CCl_4 has

been eliminated, suggesting that in the kidney, as in the liver, a metabolite of CCl_4 is responsible for inducing tissue damage. Presumably, metabolic activations of $CHCl_3$ and CCl_4 are renal phenomena. Only recently have definitive data been available to rule out the formation of toxic material in the liver being transported to the kidney.

Chloroform. The mechanism of $CHCl_3$-induced hepatotoxicity has been relatively well defined within the past decade. In the liver, $CHCl_3$ is biotransformed to the highly reactive metabolite phosgene ($COCl_2$) by a cytochrome P-450-dependent reaction (Pohl, 1979). Since $CHCl_3$ is also nephrotoxic in most species including humans, it has been employed in mechanistic studies as a model compound for nephrotoxicants requiring metabolic activation. There are dramatic species differences in the degree of $CHCl_3$ nephrotoxicity; certain strains of mice seem to be especially susceptible to $CHCl_3$-induced renal damage (Kluwe, 1981). Only males exhibit a nephrotoxic response to $CHCl_3$, while the hepatotoxic response is similar in both sexes (Smith *et al.*, 1983).

The renal lesions induced by acute administration of nephrotoxic doses of $CHCl_3$ include increased kidney weight, swelling of tubular epithelium, fatty degeneration, tubular casts, and/or marked necrosis of proximal tubular epithelium. There is no glomerular damage and little involvement of the distal tubules. Functional changes include proteinuria, glucosuria, decreased secretion of organic ions, and increased BUN (Rush *et al.*, 1984a).

The agent responsible for $CHCl_3$-induced nephrotoxicity may be: (1) $CHCl_3$ itself; (2) a hepatic metabolite that travels to the kidney; (3) a hepatic metabolite that is biotransformed further in the kidney to a nephrotoxic compound; or (4) a nephrotoxic metabolite produced from $CHCl_3$ within the kidney. Most of the experimental evidence supports the third or fourth possibility. For example, following administration of $^{14}CHCl_3$ to mice, autoradiography indicated that radiolabel was localized to necrotic proximal tubular cells and centrilobular hepatocytes—the regions of highest cytochrome P-450 activity in these organs (Kluwe, 1981).

Renal necrosis in the absence of liver necrosis occurs following low concentrations of $CHCl_3$ in male mice, and functional studies have also detected renal toxicity at dosages that produced no hepatotoxicity. Phenobarbital pretreatment enhanced hepatoxicity, biotransformation of $CHCl_3$, and covalent binding by the liver, but phenobarbital did not alter renal mixed-function oxidases or nephrotoxicity in mice or rats (Rush *et al.*, 1984a). Polychlorinated biphenyls and

3-methylcholanthrene increased mixed function oxidases in both organs, but reduced $CHCl_3$ nephrotoxicity without appreciably altering hepatotoxicity. On the other hand, polybrominated biphenyls increased mouse hepatic and renal mixed-function oxidases and increased $CHCl_3$ toxicity in both organs (Kluwe, 1981). Clearly, the renal toxicity did not parallel the alterations in hepatotoxicity. All of these data suggest the *in situ* formation of a nephrotoxic $CHCl_3$ metabolite.

The observations that deuterated $CHCl_3$ ($CDCl_3$) was significantly less nephrotoxic than $CHCl_3$ in both rats (Branchflower and Pohl, 1981) and mice (Ahmadizadeh *et al.,* 1981) suggested that cleavage of the C—H bond was the rate-limiting step in biotransformation of $CHCl_3$ to a reactive metabolite. This suggests that $COCl_2$ could be involved in nephrotoxicity as well as hepatotoxicity. Possibly $COCl_2$ formed in the liver is transported to the kidney where it produces tissue damage. However, since the half-life of $COCl_2$ in water at 37°C is extremely short (Nash and Pattle, 1971), this is highly unlikely.

Alternatively, a chemically stable nephrotoxic conjugate of $COCl_2$ could be formed in the liver and transported to the kidney. However, when several of these metabolites were isolated and tested, they were not nephrotoxic *in vivo* or when added to mouse renal cortical slices *in vitro* (Branchflower *et al.,* 1983).

There is clear evidence that, at least in mice, renal biotransformation of $CHCl_3$ is a requisite step in nephrotoxicity. Incubation of renal cortical slices with $CHCl_3$ from male, but not female, mice resulted in dose-related decreases in PAH and TEA accumulation (Smith and Hook, 1983). These effects were blocked by incubation of slices with CO or in the cold, suggesting involvement of P-450 in $CHCl_3$ biotransformation. Subsequent experiments demonstrated that $^{14}CHCl_3$ was biotransformed to $^{14}CO_2$ and covalently bound radioactivity by male renal cortical microsomes. This biotransformation required O_2, an NADPH-regenerating system, and was blocked by CO (Smith and Hook, 1983, 1984). Addition of reduced glutathione (GSH) to incubations of renal microsomes and $^{14}CHCl_3$ increased the amount of aqueous soluble metabolites detected and decreased other indices of metabolism, suggesting that a $COCl_2$ conjugate similar to that described for hepatic $CHCl_3$ biotransformation had been formed (Smith and Hook, 1984). Finally, biotransformation of $CHCl_3$ via a P-450 mechanism in the kidney to $COCl_2$ was confirmed in the rabbit, a species in which phenobarbital enhances renal P-450 (Rush *et al.,* 1983a, 1983b). In rabbits, phenobarbital

pretreatment enhanced *in vitro* renal biotransformation and nephrotoxicity of $CHCl_3$. Addition of L-cysteine reduced covalent binding of $^{14}CHCl_3$ in renal microsomes and was associated with the formation of the radioactive phosgene-cysteine conjugate, 2-oxothiazolidine-4-carboxylic acid (OTZ). Renal microsomal formation of OTZ was enhanced in microsomes from phenobarbital-pretreated rabbits (Bailie, *et al.,* 1984). Thus, *in vitro* data strongly support the hypothesis that the kidney biotransforms $CHCl_3$ to the nephrotoxic metabolite phosgene.

Though the data above argue strongly for the formation of phosgene as the nephrotoxic metabolite of $CHCl_3$ in mouse and rabbit kidney, extrapolation of this mechanism to nephrotoxicity in other species should be made with caution. For other species, particularly humans and rats, the primary target of chloroform is the liver, and nephrotoxicity has been seen in human females as well as in female rats and dogs (Kluwe, 1981), suggesting possible alternate mechanisms of toxicity in these species. In addition, the chronic renal damage and tumor formation that may occur in humans and laboratory species following long-term exposure to low concentrations of chloroform and other halogenated hydrocarbons may be produced by mechanisms entirely distinct from those described above.

Other halogenated hydrocarbons have also been shown to be toxic to the kidney, producing effects similar to those of CCl_4 and $CHCl_3$ (Kluwe, 1981). Interestingly, the nephrotoxicity of several of the halogenated hydrocarbons may be related to renal activation of a conjugate formed in the liver.

Hexachlorobutadiene.   Hexachloro-1,3-butadiene (HCBD) is a widespread environmental pollutant that is a relatively potent nephrotoxicant in rats, mice, and other mammalian species. The kidneys appear to be the primary target of HCBD toxicity, with relatively few hepatic effects (Lock and Ishmael, 1982). In rats the compound produces a well-defined lesion in the pars recta of the proximal tubule, characterized by a loss of brush border accompanied by decreased urinary concentrating ability, glucosuria, proteinuria, and reduction of the renal clearances of inulin, PAH, and TEA (Rush *et al.,* 1984a).

Renal necrosis is observed in both mice and rats within 16 hours of HCBD administration. Interestingly, the site of the renal lesion varied with species. In rats, damage was confined to the corticomedullary region, specifically, the *pars recta.* In mice, the lesion was more widespread through the cortex and, while localized to the proximal tubule, was not restricted to a specific cell type.

Reports on the effects of pretreating animals with inducers and/or inhibitors of drug-metabolizing enzymes are conflicting. Early studies indicated that pretreatment of rats with such compounds had little or no effect on the toxicity of HCBD, suggesting that HCBD may not be metabolically activated by a cytochrome P-450 (Lock and Ishmael, 1981, 1982; Hook et al., 1982).

Formation of a GSH conjugate of HCBD has been demonstrated in rat liver microsomes and occurred under N_2 and CO in the absence of NADPH (Lock et al., 1982). This suggests that the reaction is a substitution of the halogen catalyzed by GSH-S-transferase, rather than cytochrome P-450. Metabolites of HCBD-GSH damage the proximal tubule (Lock et al., 1982). Thus, hepatic metabolites of HCBD-GSH may be nephrotoxic after activation to a nephrotoxic species via a renal enzyme (C-S lyase). Gandolfi and colleagues (Gandolfi et al., 1981; Hassall et al., 1983) suggested that renal C-S lyase is also involved in the nephrotoxic action of halogenated vinyl cysteine conjugates. For example, dichlorovinyl cysteine (DCVC) is thought to be formed by peptidase cleavage of a trichloroethylene-glutathione conjugate formed in the liver. Acetylation of DCVC by the kidney does not lead to formation of toxic metabolites. In contrast, DCVC biotransformation via C-S lyase forms a highly reactive toxic metabolite capable of injuring the proximal tubule (Hassall et al., 1981). A C-S lyase capable of activating such conjugates is present in liver as well as kidney; it is possible that the unique renal sensitivity to HCBD and DCVC is related to the ability of the kidney to accumulate these ionic conjugates (Rush et al., 1984a).

Bromobenzene. Bromobenzene is nephrotoxic as well as hepatotoxic. Recent evidence suggests that the nephrotoxic effects of bromobenzene in cats and mice is due to a hepatic metabolite(s) rather than intrarenal activation of bromobenzene (Lau and Zannoni, 1979; Monks et al., 1982; Rush et al., 1984b). Mice metabolize bromobenzene to ortho-, meta-, and parabromophenol and 4-bromocatechol. These metabolites are nephrotoxic in vivo and when added to renal cortical slices in vitro; bromobenzene is not nephrotoxic in vitro (Rush et al., 1984b). Rat liver microsomes convert bromobenzene and o-bromophenol to 2-bromohydroquinone. Renal microsomes do not form this metabolite. o-Bromophenol gives rise to covalently bound material in the kidney, is nephrotoxic, and the toxicity is reduced by piperonyl butoxide. Thus, these data suggest that 2-bromohydroquinone is formed in the liver and may be transported to the kidney and contribute to renal damage.

Therapeutic Agents

Analgesics. Analgesic mixtures containing aspirin and phenacetin taken by humans in large doses over prolonged periods produce a classic picture of medullary interstitial nephritis, papillary damage, and chronic renal failure with loss of concentrating ability. Histologically, the kidney demonstrates a loss of renal papillae, a medullary inflammatory response with interstitial fibrosis, and nephron atrophy (Kincaid-Smith, 1978). Proximal tubular damage may also be seen. Large quantities of analgesics must be given to experimental animals for long periods of time (i.e., weeks to months) to induce papillary necrosis similar to that produced by analgesic abuse. Molland (1978) fed rats relatively moderate doses of analgesics for extended times and observed that aspirin had a greater nephrotoxic effect than either phenacetin or acetaminophen, although aspirin toxicity was less alone than in combination with one of the nonsalicylates. Following aspirin alone, the earliest changes occurred in the medullary interstitial cells. Interestingly, the cortical lesions induced by this aspirin regimen did not depend on the presence of medullary necrosis, suggesting that the papillary and cortical damage might be separate events. This is consistent with the observation that medullary damage is a chronic event whereas cortical damage alone is seen following acute ingestion of these nephrotoxicants.

BEA (2-bromoethylamine) is proving to be a useful model of the morphologic and functional aberrations associated with papillary injury. This halogenated hydrocarbon produces complete papillary necrosis in virtually 100 percent of rats within one month (Sabatini, 1984). Histologic abnormalities are observed in the thin limbs and collecting ducts of the papilla in 24 hours, with complete necrosis of the thin limbs and more extensive collecting duct injury observable in 48 hours. The percentage of filtering juxtamedullary nephrons is markedly reduced by BEA, and the juxtamedullary glomeruli become sclerotic (Sabatini, 1984). BEA produces a marked polyuria associated with a urine-concentrating defect resistant to antidiuretic hormone. Renal wastage of Na^+ and Cl^- occurs and can result in extracellular fluid (ECF) volume contraction and metabolic alkalosis. Patients with analgesic nephropathy frequently become hyperkalemic, and potassium homeostasis is abnormal in BEA-treated rats. Phosphate, but not magnesium, wastage occurs in BEA-treated rats; however, papillary necrosis did not impair the adaptation to phosphate or magnesium deprivation. In contrast, urinary acidification remained normal in BEA-treated rats, suggesting that the hyperchloremic metabolic acidosis observed in some patients with papillary necrosis may not be related to a selective defect in acid excretion as a result of damage to the collecting duct (Sabatini, 1984). Thus, BEA-induced papillary necrosis in rats mimics several of the clinical features associated with analgesic nephropathy in humans. This feature, coupled with rapid production and reproducibility of the papillary injury, suggests that BEA will become a major tool for examination of factors capable of ameliorating papillary necrosis as well as mechanisms important to the pathogenesis of this disease.

Considerable controversy has arisen concerning the specific agent(s) in analgesic mixtures containing aspirin and phenacetin that is responsible for the nephrotoxicity and the mechanism(s) by which it might act. It was suggested that the early papillary changes produced by aspirin might be due to vasospasm in the *vasa recta* and thus represent an ischemic injury. Such an effect is consistent with the ability of aspirin to inhibit prostaglandin synthesis. Theoretically, inhibition of renal medullary prostaglandin synthesis might remove an endogenous vasodilator prostaglandin, leading to localized vasoconstriction. Significantly, other inhibitors of prostaglandin synthesis will produce renal medullary lesions in rats (Nanra, 1974). Phenacetin or one of its metabolites, primarily *N*-acetyl-para-aminophenol (APAP, acetaminophen, paracetamol), has been implicated as a major contributor to the toxicity in humans; however, removal of phenacetin from analgesic mixtures has not eliminated the problem (Kincaid-Smith, 1978). Acetaminophen, however, remains a frequently used analgesic and is capable of producing analgesic nephropathy in animals (Molland, 1978). Although neither aspirin nor phenacetin achieves increased concentrations in the medulla, acetaminophen and its conjugates appear to concentrate in the renal medulla (Duggin and Mudge, 1976). Dehydration of animals leads to maximal concentrations of these materials in the medulla, a fact consistent with the enhanced toxicity that occurs during dehydration. Thus, trapping of acetaminophen (or its metabolites) in the medulla by the countercurrent mechanism may play a role in the medullary toxicity produced by acetaminophen.

Recent studies have shown that APAP is biotransformed to an arylating metabolite *in vitro* by an arachidonic-acid-dependent pathway (Boyd and Eling, 1981; Mohandas *et al.*, 1981; Moldeus and Rahimtula, 1980). *In vitro*, arachidonic acid-dependent covalent binding of acetaminophen was greatest in the papilla and least in the cortex, whereas NADPH-dependent binding was greatest in the cortex and undetectable

in the papilla. Prostaglandin endoperoxide synthetase (PES)-dependent covalent binding of acetaminophen to rabbit renal medullary microsomes was reduced by inhibitors of prostaglandin synthetase and antioxidants (Moldeus *et al.*, 1982; Moldeus and Rahimtula, 1980; Mohandas *et al.*, 1981). GSH also reduced the PES-dependent covalent binding of acetaminophen; some of this was due to the generation of a GSH conjugate, but most could be accounted for by the oxidation of GSH to GSSG (Moldeus *et al.*, 1982). The hydroperoxidase component of PES appeared to be responsible for the metabolic activation of acetaminophen, and the inhibitory effect of antioxidants as well as the rapid oxidation of GSH supports the hypothesis that a radical intermediate of acetaminophen is formed in the renal papilla and may be responsible for initiating toxicity.

Renal cortical necrosis following acute acetaminophen overdose has been reported to occur in patients with hepatic damage and may even occur in patients without apparent hepatic insufficiency (Boyer and Rouff, 1971; Cobden *et al.*, 1982). Renal ultrastructural damage, similar to that found with other forms of toxic nephropathy in the cortex, includes loss of luminal brush borders, mitochondrial disarray, sloughing of cells, and disruption of tubular basement membranes (Kleinman *et al.*, 1980).

In the liver, most acetaminophen is detoxified by biotransformation to glucuronide or sulfate conjugates. A small amount appears to go through a cytochrome P-450-dependent reaction leading to a chemically reactive intermediate(s). Normally, this metabolite is conjugated with GSH and rendered nontoxic, presumably owing to direct combination of the nucleophilic GSH with electrophilic metabolites of acetaminophen (Hinson, 1980; Nelson, 1982). Binding would occur only after significant reduction of GSH (e.g., due to larger doses of acetaminophen or previous exposure to another GSH-depleting compound) and toxicity may then ensue (Hinson, 1980; Nelson, 1982).

Biotransformation of acetaminophen to a reactive arylating intermediate is also believed to be a requisite step in the pathogenesis of acetaminophen-induced renal cortical necrosis (McMurtry *et al.*, 1978). At least two different mechanisms for the generation of reactive intermediates from acetaminophen within the renal cortex have been proposed. McMurtry and coworkers (1978) suggested that the generation of a reactive electrophile within the proximal tubular cell is a cytochrome P-450-dependent process. Evidence for this mechanism included the demonstration of NADPH-dependent covalent binding of acetaminophen to renal microsomes *in vitro* (McMurtry *et al.*, 1978). Second, formation of certain reactive intermediates from acetaminophen within the kidney appears to be dependent on deacetylation prior to the renal biotransformation of the deacetylated product, *p*-aminophenol, to an electrophilic intermediate (Newton *et al.*, 1982a, 1983a, 1983b). Evidence for this mechanism of activation included identification of *p*-aminophenol as a urinary metabolite of acetaminophen (Newton *et al.*, 1982b) and demonstration of NADPH-independent covalent binding of ^{14}C-ring-acetaminophen to renal, but not hepatic, homogenates. ^{14}C-acetyl-acetaminophen did not bind to renal homogenates, indicating that acetaminophen was deacetylated prior to biotransformation to the reactive intermediate (Newton *et al.*, 1983c).

p-Aminophenol formation *in vivo* can account, at least in part, for acetaminophen-induced cortical necrosis. Bis-(*p*-nitro-phenyl)phosphate (BNPP), an acyl amidase inhibitor, reduced acetaminophen deacetylation and covalent binding in Fisher-344 rat renal cortical homogenates in a concentration-dependent manner and reduced acetaminophen nephrotoxicity, but not *p*-aminophenol nephrotoxicity. BNPP pretreatment reduced the fraction of acetaminophen excreted as *p*-aminophenol after nephrotoxic doses of acetaminophen but did not alter excretion of *p*-aminophenol or its metabolites after *p*-aminophenol administration.

Anesthetics. Several of the halogenated hydrocarbon anesthetics have been suggested to produce nephrotoxicity, but only one agent, methoxyflurane, has been documented to produce reproducible renal failure. In both laboratory animals and humans, methoxyflurane produced a high-output renal failure, negative fluid balance, and increases in serum sodium, osmolality, and BUN. Patients or animals were unable to concentrate urine despite fluid deprivation and vasopressin administration, pointing to a defect in the renal concentrating mechanism. This toxicity had not originally been seen in animal studies. When Mazze (1981) and his collaborators studied a series of five rat strains, however, they found that the Fischer-344 and the Buffalo strains biotransformed methoxyflurane to a greater extent than the other strains studied. The Fisher-344, which biotransformed methoxyflurane the most, was the only strain that evidenced nephrotoxicity. Methoxyflurane appears to be biotransformed primarily to inorganic fluoride and oxalate. Enhanced biotransformation and nephrotoxicity were seen following phenobarbital treatment, whereas enzyme inhibition decreased biotransformation and reduced nephrotoxicity. Subsequent studies indicated that it was the generation of the fluoride ion (acting in the ascending limb of the loop of Henle or in the collecting duct) that rendered the medulla ADH resistant.

Antibiotics. Several antibiotics have been shown to produce nephrotoxicity. For example, at least 10 percent of all cases of acute renal failure have been attributed to use of aminoglycoside antibiotics (Humes *et al.*, 1982; Bennett, 1983). The aminoglycosides consist of various sugars in glycosidic linkage with amino-containing side chains. The nephrotoxic potential of an aminoglycoside is related to the number of ionizable amino groups it contains. The clinically relevant aminoglycosides are neomycin (six amino groups), gentamicin (five), tobramycin (five), netilmicin (five), kanamycin (four), amikacin (four), and streptomycin (three). These polycationic antibiotics are primarily excreted by glomerular filtration, and aminoglycoside nephrotoxicity is often associated with changes in glomerular ultrastructure and function. Reduction in the glomerular capillary ultrafiltration coefficient and the number and size of glomerular endothelial fenestrae have been observed in aminoglycoside-treated animals (Bayliss *et al.*, 1977; Luft *et al.*, 1981; Cojocel *et al.*, 1983). These alterations may result, in part, from aminoglycoside neutralization of fixed anionic charges on the glomerular endothelium. The primary target of aminoglycoside toxicity, however, is the proximal tubular cell. After filtration, a small fraction of the cationic antibiotic binds to anionic phospholipids on the brush border of the proximal tubule. The bound aminoglycoside is engulfed by adsorptive endocytosis and stored in secondary lysosomes. This charge-mediated process results in accumulation of antibiotic in proximal tubular cells, where it may persist for days. Basolateral-membrane binding and uptake represent a minor contribution to cellular aminoglycoside concentration. Aminoglycosides produce numerous biochemical and functional aberrations in proximal tubular cells. They alter membrane phospholipid composition, permeability, Na^+-K^+-ATPase activity, adenylate cyclase activity, and cation (K^+, Ca^{2+}, Mg^{2+}) transport (Humes *et al.*, 1982; Kaloyanides, 1984). Mitochondrial oxidative phosphorylation is depressed by these antibiotics. Sequestration of aminoglycoside in lysosomes leads to myeloid body formation by impairment of phospholipid degradation (Humes *et al.*, 1982; Kaloyanides, 1984). Lysosomal membrane integrity is reduced, and release of lysosomal enzymes into the cytosol with subsequent digestion of cytoplasmic components and organelles may occur (Humes *et al.*, 1982; Kaloyanides, 1984). Significantly, the relative potency of the aminoglycosides producing these aberrations correlates with the number of ionizable amino groups and, thus, the cationic charge of the aminoglycoside molecule (Humes *et al.*, 1982). However, additional structural features must be involved since clinical comparisons suggest that the propensity of the various aminoglycosides to produce renal dysfunction is not strictly correlated with the number of ionizable amino groups.

Members of the cephalosporin class of antibiotics are also capable of producing acute proximal tubular injury. The compound most commonly associated with nephrotoxicity is cephaloridine. Like the aminoglycosides, cephaloridine has a relatively short half-life in plasma, although its renal elimination is not particularly high. Cephaloridine accumulates in the kidney to a much higher degree than in other organs, most of it within the cortex (Wold, 1981; Tune, 1982). Following administration to rabbits, guinea pigs, and rats, the cortical cephaloridine concentration was highest in rabbit and lowest in rat kidneys, which paralleled the susceptibility to nephrotoxicity. It was actively accumulated by the cells of the proximal tubule, apparently by the same organic anion transport system that transports PAH. However, minimal secretion of cephaloridine into the tubular fluid was observed, and it was subsequently determined that efflux of cephaloridine from the cell is very slow compared to other organic acids. Probenecid, which blocks organic anion transport, reduced cortical concentrations of cephaloridine and protected against nephrotoxicity. Similarly, in newborn animals, when development of anionic transport is incomplete, the renal toxicity of cephaloridine is low; enhancement of transport increases toxicity. Thus, the toxicity of cephaloridine may be due, in part, to its accumulation and retention within the cells of the proximal tubule (Wold, 1981; Tune 1982).

Cephaloridine has been suggested to act via a reactive intermediate, possibly formed by the action of cytochrome P-450 (Wold, 1981; Tune, 1982; Kuo and Hook, 1982). Inhibitors of cytochrome P-450 protected against cephaloridine-induced nephrotoxicity in rats and mice, and phenobarbital potentiated the toxicity in rabbits, but not in rats or mice. However, these agents also affected the intracellular concentration of cephaloridine; phenobarbital increased, and piperonyl butoxide decreased, renal cortical cephaloridine concentrations in rabbit (Kuo *et al.*, 1982). Cephaloridine administration depletes GSH in the renal cortex but not the medulla or the liver (Kuo *et al.*, 1983), consistent with studies localizing the nephrotoxicity to the cortex. Pretreatment with agents that deplete GSH also potentiated the nephrotoxicity of cephaloridine,

suggesting a protective role for GSH (Kuo and Hook, 1982); however, no sulfur-containing conjugates of cephaloridine could be found. It was subsequently demonstrated that while the concentration of GSH was decreased, that of total glutathione (including GSSG) was elevated; i.e., the total glutathione pool shifted from the reduced to the oxidized state (Kuo *et al.*, 1983). An increase in renal lipid peroxidation following cephaloridine treatment could account for these observations, and it has been suggested that the superoxide anion is generated during the biotransformation of cephaloridine (Kuo *et al.*, 1983). In support of this hypothesis, animals fed vitamin E- and selenium-free diets were more susceptible to the nephrotoxicity of cephaloridine.

Tetracyclines, particularly demeclocycline, have on occasion produced renal medullary toxicity. Outdated tetracyclines may produce proximal tubular damage with polyuria, glucosuria, and aminoaciduria. In humans, penicillins and sulfonamides have been implicated in an inflammatory interstitial nephritis that is not dose related, apparently due to an immunologic-type mechanism (Appel and Neu, 1977a, 1977b). Amphotericin B has been shown to be markedly nephrotoxic, producing histopathologic changes in the proximal and distal tubules. The functional alteration implicating a distal tubular lesion is decreased acidification of the urine. Decreased PAH transport is an early indication of proximal tubule damage (Appel and Neu, 1977c).

The aminonucleoside of puromycin has been used as an experimental tool to produce an animal model of the nephrotic syndrome in humans. Functionally, there appears to be an increased permeability of the glomerulus to proteins such as albumin. Although several hypotheses have been suggested considering the nature of the defect, little has been documented until recently, when Brenner *et al.* (1981) demonstrated that glomerular permeability to a series of charged dextrans was markedly increased, suggesting that there had been a pathologic alteration in net electrical charge of the glomerular basement membrane (Figure 11–5).

Environmental Contaminants

A variety of pesticides and herbicides have reached sufficient concentrations in the environment to constitute potential hazards to humans and animals. 2,4,5-Trichlorophenoxyacetic acid (2,4,5-T) was a widely used herbicide. This compound has not been shown to be directly nephrotoxic, but it may influence renal function. The compound appears to be actively transported by

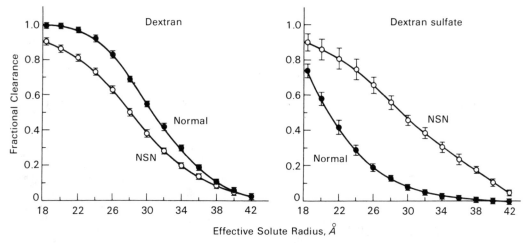

Figure 11–5. The effect of nephrotoxic serum nephritis (NSN) on glomerular permeability to neutral dextran and dextran sulfate. NSN, like puromycin aminonucleoside, appears to alter the charge on the glomerular membrane, thereby producing a net increase in permeability to dextran sulfate. (From Brenner, B. M., *et al.*: Determinants of glomerular permselectivity: Insights derived from observation *in vivo. Kidney Int.*, **12**:229–37, 1977. Reprinted with permission.)

the organic anion secretory system and is capable of inhibiting organic anion transport. Furthermore, in high concentrations the compound appears to inhibit organic cation transport as well (Berndt, 1982). The herbicide paraquat produces profound pulmonary damage following acute intoxication. In sublethal doses, paraquat appears to be actively secreted by the organic cation transport system of the kidney and is fairly rapidly removed from the body. Following high doses, however, paraquat produces direct renal damage, thereby reducing its own elimination. This leads to prolonged high plasma concentrations of this agent that enhance the lung damage (Ecker *et al.*, 1975).

A number of industrial and agricultural chemicals may influence kidney function. Several of these compounds have a profound metabolic effect on the liver, and it is these abnormalities that have received most attention. However, it is not unlikely that in the future heretofore unrecognized abnormalities in renal function could be attributed to one or more of these agents. Polychlorinated biphenyls (PCBs) are a mixture of chemicals used in a wide variety of manufacturing processes, notably in the plastics industry, and as insulators. These compounds are ubiquitous contaminants of the environment. The PCBs have been shown to have marked stimulating effects on drug metabolism in the liver and to increase liver size and liver weight. PCBs also have been shown to enhance drug-metabolizing enzyme activity in the kidney (Vainio, 1974). The polybrominated biphenyls (PBBs), although not so widespread, are also significant environ-

mental contaminants. The PBBs similarly induce drug-metabolizing enzyme activity in the liver and kidney and thereby present a potential hazard (McCormack *et al.*, 1978). Tetrachlorodibenzo-*p*-dioxin (TCDD) is an extremely toxic agent that has been known to produce a wide variety of toxic symptoms in animals and humans. Like the polyhalogenated biphenyls, TCDD has not been shown to have a profound direct toxic effect on the adult kidney but does alter drug metabolism in this organ and could pose a potential hazard (Fowler *et al.*, 1977). The presence of such potential stimulators of drug metabolism in the environment could lead to difficulty in interpreting experimental data. For instance, following accidental exposure to one of these stimulators, a relatively innocuous substance could be metabolically altered within the kidney and produce nephrotoxicity.

Mycotoxins are secondary fungal metabolites that can damage various organ systems upon injestion of contaminated foodstuffs or feeds. Several mycotoxins have been reported to be nephrotoxicants (Hayes, 1980; Berndt, 1982b). For example, rubratoxin B, aflatoxin B1, and sterigmatocystin induce renal lesions (Hayes, 1980). In rats, ochratoxin A and citrinin produced proteinuria, glucosuria, and reduction in urine osmolality. Proximal tubular transport of organic ions was also reduced by these mycotoxins. Interestingly, these mycotoxins may produce proximal tubular injury via different mechanisms. A single large dose of citrinin produced proximal tubular dysfunction and necrosis in rats. In contrast, repeated administration of small doses of ochratoxin A were required to elicit renal damage; a single large dose of this mycotoxin resulted in severe diarrhea and death without obvious effects on the kidney. Citrinin decreased rat renal cortical GSH concentration and appeared to bind covalently to renal constituents. Thus, citrinin (or a hepatic metabolite) may be activated to a toxic reactive metabolite within the kidney. Ochratoxin A and citrinin have been implicated in the production of porcine nephropathy. In addition, one or both of these mycotoxins may be involved in endemic Balkan nephropathy (EBN), a disease that is endemic to isolated rural populations of Bulgaria, Romania, and Yugoslavia (Hall, 1982). The renal pathology of EBN is characterized by extensive interstitial fibrosis and proximal tubular degeneration. This disease is comparable in many ways to porcine nephropathy, and ochratoxin A has been isolated from serum of patients with EBN (Hall, 1982).

Miscellaneous Nephrotoxicants

On occasion, chemicals may reach such high concentrations in the tubular urine that they exceed their solubilities and are precipitated as crystals. These crystals may be eliminated from the kidney or may be deposited in the collecting system, leading to the formation of larger crystals or stones. The stones may mechanically obstruct the tubules, leading to an increase in intratubular pressure. This could lead to diminution in glomerular filtration rate and renal blood flow, resulting in tissue ischemia and subsequent loss of renal tissue. Such effects have been seen with sulfonamide drugs and oxalate (metabolically derived from glycols). In some cases uric acid may form stones (Bluestone et al., 1975). The synthetic amino acid α-methyltyrosine may achieve sufficiently high concentrations to form stones in the kidney (Hook and Moore, 1969).

Dimethylnitrosamine has been reported to produce renal carcinoma in appropriately conditioned animals (Swann et al., 1976). Diphenylamine has been used as a tool to produce cystic kidneys in adult animals (Gardener et al., 1976). Maleic acid has been used as a tool to study reabsorptive pathways for amino acids and glucose because of its ability to produce reproducible nephropathy in the proximal tubule (Segal and Thier, 1973). A vasopressin-resistant concentrating defect has been produced in animals with 2-amino-4,5-diphenylthiazole (Carone et al., 1974).

Apparent nephropathy may also be caused as a secondary effect of several pharmacologic agents. For instance, long-term treatment of animals with diuretics may lead to loss of total body potassium, resulting in potassium depletion nephropathy. Similarly, drugs that reduce blood pressure or increase renal vascular resistance may produce effects reminiscent of ischemia, yet the drugs themselves are not directly nephrotoxic (Maher, 1976).

NEPHROTOXICITY IN NEWBORNS

Administration of several chemical agents during the prenatal period has been shown to produce profound alterations in kidney structure at birth. Agents like methylsalicylate and TCDD have been shown to produce teratogenic effects to the kidney, primarily hydronephrosis. Hypervitaminosis A during gestation has been suggested to produce hydronephrosis in offspring. Diphenylamine, when fed to pregnant rats, has been reported to produce polycystic kidneys in newborn animals. Similarly, large doses of steroid hormones to newborn or weanling rabbits produced polycystic kidneys. However, as pointed out by McCormack et al. (1981), these reports must be viewed with some caution in that traditional teratogenic studies are performed on animals derived by cesarean section. An apparent abnormality in structure might not constitute permanent structural damage, but only reflect delayed maturation. Considerably more investigation needs to be made into the functional sequelae in newborn animals of prenatal administration of chemicals. Preliminary data have suggested that prenatal dinoseb, paraquat, and TCDD can produce alterations in PAH transport in kidney slices from newborn animals even when no structural lesion is apparent (McCormack et al., 1981). Further studies are necessary to evaluate the significance of these changes and to determine whether they are maintained throughout the life of the animals or whether the animals may compensate for these changes during normal growth and development.

REFERENCES

Ahmadizadeh, M.; Kuo, C. H.; and Hook, J. B.: Nephrotoxicity and hepatotoxicity of chloroform in mice: effect of deuterium substitution. J. Toxicol. Environ. Health, 8:105–11, 1981.

Appel, G. B., and Neu, H. C.: The nephrotoxicity of antimicrobial agents: part 1. N. Engl. J. Med., 296:663–70, 1977a.

Appel, G. B., and Neu, H. C.: The nephrotoxicity of antimicrobial agents: part 2. N. Engl. J. Med., 296:722–28, 1977b.

Appel, G. B., and Neu, H. C.: The nephrotoxicity of antimicrobial agents: part 3. N. Engl. J. Med., 296:784–87, 1977c.

Bailie, M. B.; Smith, J. H.; Newton, J. F.; and Hook, J. B.: Mechanism of chloroform nephrotoxicity. IV. Phenobarbital potentiation of in vitro chloroform metabolism and toxicity in rabbit kidneys. Toxicol. Appl. Pharmacol., 74:285–92, 1984.

Bayliss, C.; Rennke, H. R.; and Brenner, B. M.: Mechanism of the defect in glomerular ultrafiltration associated with gentamicin administration. *Kidney Int.* 12:344–53, 1977.

Bennett, W. M.: Aminoglycoside nephrotoxicity. *Nephron,* 35:73–77, 1983.

Berndt, W. O.: Renal methods in toxicology. In Hayes, A. W. (ed.): *Principles and Methods of Toxicology.* Raven Press, New York, 1982a, pp. 447–74.

———— : Nephrotoxicity of natural products. Mycotoxin-induced nephropathy. In Porter, G. A. (ed.): *Nephrotoxic Mechanisms of Drugs and Environmental Toxins.* Plenum Publishing Corp., New York, 1982b, pp. 241–54.

Biber, T. U. L.; Mylle, M.; Baines, A. D.; Gottschalk, C. W.; Oliver, J. R.; and MacDowell, M. C.: A study in micropuncture and microdissection of acute renal damage in rats. *Am. J. Med.,* 44:664–705, 1968.

Bluestone, R.; Waisman, J.; and Klinenberg, J. R.: Chronic experimental hyperuricemic nephropathy. *Lab. Invest.,* 33:273–79, 1975.

Boyd, J. A., and Eling, T. E.: Prostaglandin endoperoxide synthetase-dependent cooxidation of acetaminophen to intermediates which covalently bind *in vitro* to rabbit renal medullary microsomes. *J. Pharmacol. Exp. Ther.,* 219:659–64, 1981.

Boyer, T. D., and Rouff, S. L.: Acetaminophen-induced hepatic necrosis and renal failure. *JAMA,* 218:440–41, 1971.

Branchflower, R. V.; Nunn, D. S.; Highet, R. J.; Smith, J. H.; Hook, J. B.; and Pohl, L. R.: Nephrotoxicity of chloroform: metabolism to phosgene by the mouse kidney. *Toxicol. Appl. Pharmacol.,* 72:159–68, 1984.

Branchflower, R. V., and Pohl, L. R.: Investigation of the mechanism of the potentiation of chloroform-induced hepatotoxicity and nephrotoxicity by methyl *n*-butyl ketone. *Toxicol. Appl. Pharmacol.,* 61:407–13, 1981.

Brenner, B. M.; Ichikawa, I., and Deen, W. M.: Glomerular filtration. In: Brenner, B. M.; and Rector, F. C., Jr. (eds.): *The Kidney,* Vol. 1. W. B. Saunders Co., Philadelphia, 1981, pp. 289–327.

Brenner, R. M., and Rector, F. C., Jr. (eds.): *The Kidney,* 3rd ed. Vols. 1 and 2. W. B. Saunders Co., Philadelphia, 1986.

Carone, F. A.; Stolarczyk, J.; Krumlovsky, F. A.; Perlman, S. G.; Roberts, T. J.; and Rowland, R. G.: The nature of a drug-induced renal concentrating defect in rats. *Lab. Invest.,* 31:658–64, 1974.

Clifton, G. G.; Pearce, C.; O'Neill, W. M., Jr.; and Wallin, J. D.: Early polyuria in the rat following single-dose *cis*-dichlorodiammineplatinum (II). Effects on plasma vasopressin and posterior pituitary function. *J. Lab. Clin. Med.,* 100:659–70, 1982.

Cobden, I.; Record, C. O.; Ward, M. K.; and Kerr, D. N. S.: Paracetamol-induced acute renal failure in the absence of fulminant liver damage. *Br. Med. J.,* 284:21–22, 1982.

Cojocel, C.; Dociu, N.; Maita, K.; Sleight, S. D.; and Hook, J. B.: Effects of aminoglycosides on glomerular permeability tubular readsorption, and intracellular catabolism of the cationic low-molecular-weight protein lysozyme. *Toxicol. Appl. Pharmacol.,* 68:96–109, 1983.

Daley-Yates, P. T., and McBrien, D. C. H.: Cisplatin (cis-dichloro diammine platinum II) Nephrotoxicity. In Bach, P. H.; Bonner, F. W.; Bridges, J. W.; and Lock, E. A. (eds.): *Nephrotoxicity Assessment and Pathogenesis.* John Wiley Sons, Inc., New York, 1982, pp. 356–70.

Dobyan, D. C.; Levi, J.; Jacobs, C.; Kosek, J.; and Weiner, M. W.: Mechanism of *cis*-platin nephrotoxicity. II. Morphologic observations. *J. Pharmacol. Exp. Ther.,* 213:551–56, 1980.

Duggin, G. D., and Mudge, G. H.: Analgesic nephropathy: Renal distribution of acetaminophen and its conjugates. *J. Pharmacol. Exp. Ther.,* 199:1–9, 1976.

Ecker, J. L.; Hook, J. B.; and Gibson, J. E.: Nephrotoxicity of paraquat in mice. *Toxicol. Appl. Pharmacol.,* 34:178–86, 1975.

Fowler, B. A.: Ultrastructural evidence for nephropathy induced by long-term exposure to small amounts of methyl mercury. *Science,* 175:780–81, 1972.

Fowler, B. A.; Brown, H. W.; Lucier, G. W.; and Krigman, M. R.: The effects of chronic oral methyl mercury exposure on the lysosome system of rat kidney. *Lab. Invest.,* 32:313–22, 1975.

Fowler, B. A.; Hook, G. E. R.; and Lucier, G. W.: Tetrachlorodibenzo-*p*-dioxin induction of renal microsomal enzyme systems: ultrastructural effects on pars recta (S_3) proximal tubule cells of the rat kidney. *J. Pharmacol. Exp. Ther.,* 203:712–21, 1977.

Gandolfi, A. J.; Nagle, R. B.; Soltis, J. J., and Plescia, F. H.: Nephrotoxicity of halogenated vinyl cysteine compounds. *Res. Commun. Chem. Pathol. Pharmacol.,* 33:249–61, 1981.

Ganote, C. E.; Reimer, K. A.; and Jennings, R. B.: Acute mercuric chloride nephrotoxicity: an electron microscopic and metabolic study. *Lab. Invest.,* 31:633–47, 1974.

Gardner, K. D., Jr.; Solomon, S.; Fitzgerrel, W. W.; and Evan, A. P.: Function and structure in the diphenylamine-exposed kidney. *J. Clin. Invest.,* 57:796–806, 1976.

Goldstein, R. S., and Mayor, G. H.: The nephrotoxicity of cisplatin. *Life Sci.,* 32:685–90, 1983.

Goyer, R. A.: Cadmium nephropathy. In G. A. Porter (ed.): *Nephrotoxic Mechanism of Drugs and Environmental Toxins.* Plenum Publishing Corp., New York, 1982, pp. 305–13.

Hall, P. W., III: Endemic Balkan Nephropathy. In Porter, G. A. (ed.). *Nephrotoxic Mechanisms of Drugs and Environmental Toxins.* Plenum Publishing Corp., New York, 1982, pp. 227–40.

Hassall, C. D.; Gandolfi, A. J.; and Brendel, L.: Effect of halogenated vinyl cysteine conjugates on renal tubular active transport. *Toxicology,* 26:285–94, 1983.

Hayes, A. W.: Mycotoxins: a review of biological effects and their role in human diseases. *Clin. Toxicol.,* 17:45–83, 1980.

Hinson, J. A.: Biochemical Toxicology of acetaminophen. In Hodgson, E.; Bend, J. R.; and Philpot, R. M., (eds.): *Review in Biochemical Toxicology,* Vol. 2. Elsevier/North-Holland, New York, 1980, pp. 103–29.

Hook, J. B., and Moore, K. E.: The renal handling of α-methyltyrosine. *J. Pharmacol. Exp. Ther.,* 168:310–14, 1969.

Hook, J. B.; Rose, M. S.; and Lock, E. A.: The nephrotoxicity of hexachloro-1:3-butadiene in the rat: studies of organic anion and cation transport in renal slices and the effect of monooxygenase inducers. *Toxicol. Appl. Pharmacol.,* 65:373–82, 1982.

Humes, H. D.; Weinberg, J. M.; and Knauss, T. C.: Clinical and pathophysiologic aspects of aminoglycoside nephrotoxicity. *Am. J. Kidney Dis.,* 11:5–29, 1982.

Kaloyanides, G. J.: Aminoglycoside-induced functional and biochemical defects in the renal cortex. *Fund. Appl. Toxicol.,* 4:930–43, 1984.

Kincaid-Smith, P.: Analgesic nephropathy. *Kidney Int.,* 13:1–4, 1978.

Kleinman, J. G.; Breitenfield, R. V.; and Roth, D. A.: Acute renal failure associated with acetaminophen injection: report of a case and review of the literature. *Clin. Nephrol.,* 14:201–205, 1980.

Kluwe, W. M.: The nephrotoxicity of low molecular weight halogenated alkane solvents, pesticides, and chemical intermediates. In Hook, J. B. (ed.): *Toxicology of the Kidney.* Raven Press, New York, 1981, pp. 179–226.

Kuo, C. H.; Braselton, W. E.; and Hook, J. B.: Effect of phenobarbital on cephaloridine toxicity and accumulation in rabbit and rat kidneys. *Toxicol. Appl. Pharmacol.*, **64**:244–54, 1982.

Kuo, C. H., and Hook, J. B.: Depletion of renal glutathione content and nephrotoxicity of cephaloridine in rabbits, rats, and mice. *Toxicol. Appl. Pharmacol.*, **63**:292–302, 1982.

Kuo, C. H.; Maita, K.; Sleight, S. D.; and Hook, J. B.: Lipid peroxidation: a possible mechanism of cephaloridine-induced nephrotoxicity. *Toxicol. Appl. Pharmacol.*, **67**:78–88, 1983.

Lau, S. S., and Zannoni, V. G.: Hepatic microsomal epoxidation of bromobenzene to phenols and its toxicological implication. *Toxicol. Appl. Pharmacol.*, **50**:309–18, 1979.

Lock, E. A., and Ishmael, J.: Hepatic and renal nonprotein sulfhydryl concentration following toxic doses of hexachloro-1,3-butadiene in the rat: the effect of Arclor 1254, phenobarbitone, or SKF 525A treatment. *Toxicol. Appl. Pharmacol.*, **57**:79–87, 1981.

Lock, E. A., and Ishmael, J.: The hepatotoxicity and nephrotoxicity of hexachlorobutadiene. In Yoshida, H.; Hagihara, Y.; and Ebashi, S. (eds.): *Advances in Pharmacology and Therapeutics II.* Vol. 5, *Toxicology and Experimental Models.* Pergamon Press, New York, 1982, pp. 87–96.

Lock, E. A.; Nash, J. A.; Green, T.; and Wold, R. C.: Hexachloro-1,3-butadiene mediated glutathione depletion: the role of rat liver microsomal and cytosolic S-transferase. *Pharmacologist*, **24**:136, 1982.

Luft, F. C.; Aronoff, G. R.; Evan, A. P.; and Connors, B. A.: The effect of aminoglycosides on glomerular endothelium: a comparative study. *Res. Commun. Chem. Pathol. Pharmacol.*, **34**:89–95, 1981.

Maher, J. F.: Toxic nephropathy. In Brenner, B. M., and Rector, F. C., Jr. (eds.): *The Kidney.* W. B. Saunders, Philadelphia, 1976.

Mazze, R. I.: Methoxyflurane nephropathy. In Hook, J. B., (ed.): *Toxicology of the Kidney.* Raven Press, New York, 1981, pp. 135–49.

McCormack, K. M.; Hook, J. B.; and Gibson, J. E.: Developmental anomalies of the kidney: a review of normal and aberrant renal development. In Hook, J. B. (ed.): *Toxicology of the Kidney.* Raven Press, New York, 1981, pp. 227–50.

McCormack, K. M.; Kluwe, W. M.; Rickert, D. E.; Sanger, U. L.; and Hook, J. B.: Renal and hepatic microsomal enzyme stimulation and renal function following three months of dietary exposure to polybrominated biphenyls. *Toxicol. Appl. Pharmacol.*, **44**:539–53, 1978.

McMurtry, R. J.; Snodgrass, W. R.; and Mitchell, J. R.: Renal necrosis, glutathione depletion and covalent binding after acetaminophen. *Toxicol. Appl. Pharmacol.*, **46**:87–100, 1978.

Mohandas, J.; Duggin, G. G.; Horvath, J. S.; and Tiller, D. J.: Metabolic oxidation of acetaminophen (paracetamol) mediated by cytochrome P-450 mixed function oxidase and protaglandin endoperoxidase synthetase in rabbit kidney. *Toxicol. Appl. Pharmacol.*, **61**:252–59, 1981.

Moldeus, P., and Rahimtula, A.: Metabolism of paracetamol to a glutathione conjugate catalyzed by prostaglandin synthetase. *Biochem. Biophys. Res. Commun.*, **96**:469–75, 1980.

Moldeus, P.; Andersson, B.; Rahimtula, A.; and Berggren, M.: Prostaglandin synthetase catalyzed activation of paracetamol. *Biochem. Pharmacol.*, **31**:1363–68, 1982.

Molland, E. A.: Experimental renal papillary necrosis. *Kidney Int.*, **13**:5–14, 1978.

Monks, T. J.; Hinson, J. A.; and Gillette, J. R.: Bromobenzene and p-bromophenol toxicity and covalent binding *in vivo. Life Sci.*, **30**:841–48, 1982.

Nanra, R. S.: Pathology, aetiology and pathogenesis of analgesic nephropathy. *Aust. N. Z. J. Med.*, **4**:602–603, 1974.

Nash, T., and Pattle, R. E.: The absorption of phosgene by aqueous solutions and its relation to toxicity. *Ann. Occup. Hyg.*, **14**:227–33, 1971.

Nelson, S. D.: Metabolic activation and drug toxicity. *J. Med. Chem.*, **25**:753–65, 1982.

Newton, J. F.; Braselton, W. E.; Kuo, C. H.; Kluwe, W. M.; Gemborys, M. W.; Mudge, G. H.; and Hook, J. B.: Metabolism of acetaminophen by the isolated perfused kidney. *J. Pharmacol. Exp. Ther.*, **221**:76–79, 1982a.

Newton, J. F.; Kuo, C. H.; Gemborys, M. W.; Mudge, G. H.; and Hook, J. B.: Nephrotoxicity of p-aminophenol, a metabolite of acetaminophen in the Fischer 344 rat. *Toxicol. Appl. Pharmacol.*, **65**:336–44, 1982b.

Newton, J. F.; Yoshimoto, M.; Bernstein, J.; Rush, G. F.; and Hook, J. B.: Acetaminophen nephrotoxicity in the rate. I. Strain differences in nephrotoxicity and metabolism. *Toxicol. Appl. Pharmacol.*, **69**:291–306, 1983a.

Newton, J. F.; Yoshimoto, M.; Bernstein, J.; Rush, G. F.; and Hook, J. B.: Acetaminophen nephrotoxicity in the rat. II. Strain differences in nephrotoxicity and metabolism of p-aminophenol, a metabolite of acetaminophen. *Toxicol. Appl. Pharmacol.*, **69**:307–18, 1983b.

Newton, J. F.; Bailie, M. B.; and Hook, J. B.: Acetaminophen nephrotoxicity in the rat. Renal metabolic activation *in vitro. Toxicol. Appl. Pharmacol.*, **70**:433–44, 1983c.

Nordberg, G. F.; Goyer, R.; and Nordberg, M.: Comparative toxicity of cadmium-metallothionein and cadmium chloride on mouse kidney. *Arch. Pathol.*, **99**:192–97, 1975.

Nordberg, G. F.: Metabolism of cadmium. In Porter, G. A. (ed): *Nephrotoxic Mechanisms of Drugs and Environmental Toxins.* Plenum Publishing Corp., New York, 1982, pp. 285–303.

Oken, D. E.: Acute renal failure caused by nephrotoxins. *Environ. Health Perspect.*, **15**:101–109, 1976.

Phillips, R.; Yamauchi, M.; Côté, M. G.; and Plaa, G. L.: Assessment of mercuric chloride-induced nephrotoxicity of p-aminohippuric acid uptake and the activity of four gluconeogenic enzymes in rat renal cortex. *Toxicol. Appl. Pharmacol.*, **41**:407–22, 1977.

Pohl, L. R.: Biochemical toxicology of chloroform. In Bend, J.; Philpot, R. M.; and Hodgson, F. (eds.). *Reviews of Biochemical Toxicology,* Vol. 1. Elsevier/North Holland, Amsterdam and New York, 1979, pp. 79–107.

Rush, G. F.; Maita, K.; Sleight, S. D.; Hook, J. B.: Induction of rabbit renal mixed function oxidases by phenobarbital: cell specific ultrastructural changes in the proximal tubule. *Proc. Soc. Exp. Biol. Med.*, **172**:430–39, 1983a.

Rush, G. F.; Wilson, D. M.; and Hook, J. B.: Selective induction of renal mixed function oxidases in the rat and rabbit. *Fund. Appl. Toxicol.*, **3**:161–68, 1983b.

Rush, G. F.; Smith, J. H.; Newton, J. F.; and Hook, J. B.: Chemically induced nephrotoxicity: role of metabolic activation. *CRC Crit. Rev. Toxicol.*, **13**:99–160, 1984a.

Rush, G. F.; Newton, J. F.; Maita, K.; Kuo, C. H.; and Hook, J. B.: Nephrotoxicity of phenolic bromobenzene metabolites in the mouse. *Toxicology*, **30**:259–72, 1984b.

Sabatini, S.: Pathophysiology of drug induced papillary necrosis. *Fund. Appl. Toxicol.*, **4**:909–21, 1984.

Segal, S., and Thier, S. O.: Renal handling of amino acids. In Orloff, J.; and Berliner, R. W. (eds.): *Handbook of Physiology.* Section 8, *Renal Physiology.* American Physiological Society, Washington, D.C., 1973.

Smith, J. H.; Maita, K.; Sleight, S. D.; and Hook, J. B.: Mechanism of chloroform nephrotoxicity. I. Time course of chloroform toxicity in male and female mice. *Toxicol. Appl. Pharmacol.*, **70**:467–79, 1983.

Smith, J. H., and Hook, J. B.: Mechanism of chloroform nephrotoxicity. II. *In vitro* evidence for renal metabolism of chloroform in mice. *Toxicol. Appl. Pharmacol.*, **70**:480–85, 1983.

Smith, J. H., and Hook, J. B.: Mechanism of chloroform nephrotoxicity. III. Renal and hepatic microsomal metabolism of chloroform in mice. *Toxicol. Appl. Pharmacol.*, **73**:511–24, 1984.

Striker, G. E.; Smuckler, E. A., Kohnen, P. W.; and Nagle, R. B.: Structural and functional changes in rat kidney during CCl$_4$ intoxication. *Am. J. Pathol.*, **53**:769–78, 1968.

Swann, P. F.; Magee, P. N.; Mohr, U.; Reznik, G.; Green, U.; and Kaufman, D. G.: Possible repair of carcinogenic damage caused by dimethylnitrosamine in rat kidney. *Nature (Lond.)*, **263**:134–36, 1976.

Tune, B. M.: Nephrotoxicity of cephalosporin antibiotics. Mechanisms and modifying factors. In Porter, G. A. (ed.): *Nephrotoxic Mechanisms of Drugs and Environmental Toxins*. Plenum Publishing Corp., New York, 1982, pp. 151–64.

Valtin, H.: *Renal Function: Mechanisms Preserving Fluid and Solute Balance in Health*. Little, Brown & Co., Boston, 1973.

Watrous, W. M., and Plaa, G. L.: Effect of halogenated hydrocarbons on organic ion accumulation by renal cortical slices of rats and mice. *Toxicol. Appl. Pharmacol.*, **22**:528–43, 1972.

Weiner, M. W., and Jacob, C.: Mechanism of cisplatin nephrotoxicity. *Fed. Proc.*, **42**:2974–78, 1983.

Wold, J. S.: Cephalosporin nephrotoxicity. In Hook, J. B. (ed.): *Toxicology of the Kidney*. Raven Press, New York, 1981, pp. 251–66.

Chapter 12

TOXIC RESPONSES OF THE RESPIRATORY SYSTEM

Daniel B. Menzel and *Mary O. Amdur*

INTRODUCTION

The primary function of the lung is to provide a means for the exchange of oxygen and carbon dioxide. To achieve this, the mammalian lung has evolved into a complex organ particularly suited for the uptake and excretion of volatile compounds in addition to oxygen and carbon dioxide. The large surface area, the airways, and the minute separation between the air space and capillary circulation make the lung an efficient organ for the absorption of nonvolatile toxicants as well. Toxicants can enter the respiratory system as gases, solids, or liquid aerosols and are readily taken up and transported to other organs. The lung receives all of the cardiac output, speeding distribution to other organs. Because of the vital nature of pulmonary function, direct action of toxicants on the lung can be acutely and chronically important to health. Respirable toxicants need not be absorbed to produce disease, as exemplified by fibrous minerals that produce pulmonary fibrosis and cancer.

Exposure to toxicants via inhalation occurs in all phases of human activity. Inhalation is the most important route of exposure in the workplace. Industrial atmospheres contain many gases and particles capable of producing pulmonary damage or damage to other organ systems when inhaled. The home is also contaminated with toxicants that can be inhaled. Gas cooking produces nitrogen dioxide and carbon monoxide, which may reach relatively high concentrations around the stove and in the kitchen. Formaldehyde is given off by particle board, carpet, upholstery materials, and foam insulation. The increase in air-tightness of homes and buildings in an effort to save energy has resulted in higher concentrations of indoor pollution. The air of most urban areas is contaminated with a myriad of air pollutants. Play and sports increase ventilation and result in exposure to higher doses of pollutants than occur at rest.

The reported incidence of pulmonary disease related to inhaled toxicants is increasing. This is because of better, more sensitive tests for the diagnosis of pulmonary disease and increased longevity of diseased patients. Individuals with chronic lung diseases such as asthma, bronchitis, emphysema, and pulmonary fibrosis constitute a large fraction of the population that may be especially at risk from inhaled toxicants.

As a further complication to the study of the toxicology of the lung, it has recently become apparent that the pulmonary capillary network has specialized functions to remove, metabolize, and excrete vasoactive hormones. The lung functions as an exocrine organ regulating angiotensin, biogenic amines, and prostaglandin concentrations in the circulation. Deterioration of these functions is likely to result in loss of local regulation of blood pressure and flow, potentially producing perfusion-ventilation abnormalities impairing gas exchange.

The lung also actively excretes toxicants either inhaled or absorbed through other routes. It possesses an active cytochrome P-450 system metabolizing many xenobiotic compounds. The excretion of these toxicants and the potential metabolism by the lung consequently may result in pulmonary toxicity. Clearance or removal is particularly important to proper pulmonary function. Electrolytes and nonionized compounds are rapidly cleared from the lung. Particles are removed by specialized mechanisms combining mucus secretion and ciliary action. The toxicity of the compound will increase in the pulmonary system as well as in other organ systems when diseases or other toxicants have impaired the clearance mechanisms of the lung. A common source of self-intoxication, tobacco smoking, is particularly important to these clearance mechanisms.

In this chapter, a general introduction to inhalation toxicology is presented. Some detail is provided on the structure of the lung, since structure is especially related to function in this organ. The complexity of the cell population of the lung is also emphasized, as specific functions are recognized for the different cell types. Pulmonary damage from a given toxicant may be localized in a specific cell type because of the particular sensitivity of that cell type. A general discussion is also provided on the specialized methodology of inhalation toxicology. A lack of sophistication in this aspect can lead to serious errors in estimating the toxicity of a compound to man or in the assessment of an inhalation hazard. Some specific toxicants are considered in a limited scope. Detailed descriptions of the toxicity of air pollutants appear in Chapter 25 and of inhaled radionuclides in Chapter 21. A basic understanding of pulmonary physiology is assumed in this discussion. Two excellent monographs by West (1974, 1977) provide this information and were used as the basic reference works for pulmonary physiology throughout.

STRUCTURE OF THE RESPIRATORY TRACT

The deposition and retention of inhaled gases and aerosols are influenced by many anatomic features of the respiratory tract, including lung volume, alveolar surface area, and structure and spatial relationships of conducting airways into alveoli. Distribution of deposited material as a function of time, in combination with the location of the over 40 cell types identified in the respiratory tract, determines the cells at risk for any inhaled material.

The respiratory tract may be considered as having three major regions: the *nasopharyngeal*, the *tracheobronchial*, and the *pulmonary*. The nasopharynx begins with the anterior nares and extends back and down to the level of the larynx. The nasal passages are lined with vascular mucous epithelium, which is characterized, except at the entrance, by ciliated columnar epithelium and scattered mucous glands. The nasopharynx filters out large inhaled particles and is the region in which the relative humidity is increased and the temperature of the air is moderated. The trachea, bronchi, and bronchioles serve as conducting airways between the nasopharynx and alveoli, where gas exchange occurs. The conducting airways are lined with ciliated epithelium and coated with a thin layer of mucus secreted by goblet cells and mucus-secreting cells. This mucous covering terminates at the film covering the alveolar membrane. The surface of the airways serves as a mucociliary escalator, moving particles from the deep lung to the oral cavities so they may be swallowed and excreted. The branching patterns and physical dimensions of the airways are critical in determining the deposition of particles and the absorption of gases by the respiratory tract.

Several mathematical models have been developed describing the physical dimensions of the airways (Weibel, 1963; Davies, 1961). The airways tend to be equally bifurcating in man, decreasing in diameter as they divide. The cross-sectional area, however, increases as bifurcation increases. In addition to the axial diffusion of gases along the streamline of the airways, the increase in cross-sectional area also produces a radial diffusion. Gases tend to be diluted by this anatomic feature of the lung, independent of mixing with other inspired gases. Rodent lungs are similar to man's, but have fewer divisions. Each division is sometimes referred to as a generation. The human airways have about 23 generations.

The *acinus* is the basic functional unit of the mammalian lung and is the primary location of gas exchange between the environment and blood. Anatomically, the acini consist of the structures distal to and including the first-order respiratory bronchiole, which is the first bronchiole with alveoli. The acini, of which there are about 200,000 in the adult human, include three or four orders of respiratory bronchioles, several orders of alveolar ducts and alveolar sacs, hundreds of alveoli and associated blood vessels, lymphatic tissues, supportive tissues, and nerve enervations. The anatomy of the acinus is described in detail by Pump (1964), Frasier and Pare (1971), Nagahi (1972), and Phalen *et al.* (1973). Quantitative anatomic information for these structures includes estimates of airway tube numbers, diameters, and lengths; alveolar numbers and diameters; surface areas; and mean thicknesses for the air-blood barrier (Weibel, 1963; Kliment, 1973).

Respiratory bronchioles are tubular structures with diameters of about 0.5 mm and lengths of about 1.0 mm in the adult human. Bronchioles are lined with low cuboidal epithelium and at times with ciliated epithelium. Their walls contain collagen, smooth muscle, and elastic fibers but no cartilage. This makes them quite distensible. The lumen is open along one side to alveoli; the other side is relatively smooth and in contact with branches of the pulmonary artery. Respiratory bronchioles occur in humans, dogs, and primates but not in rodents.

The *alveolar ducts and sacs* are thin-walled tubes, literally covered with alveoli on all sides. In adults their diameters are about 0.5 mm and lengths are about 0.7 mm. Alveolar sacs, which are clusters of two or more alveoli terminating in one or more alveoli, branch from alveolar ducts and are essentially closed-end versions of ducts. The total number of alveolar ducts and sacs in man is estimated to be about 10 to 25 million (Weibel, 1963).

Alveoli are thin-walled, polyhedral pouches

with one side open to either a respiratory bronchiole, an alveolar duct, or an alveolar sac. Thin, squamous pulmonary epithelial cells form most of the continuous inner lining of the alveolus. More rounded septal cells are also located within the walls, and free, motile phagocytic cells, pulmonary macrophages, often lie in contact with the inner surface of the alveolus. A dense capillary vascular plexus covers the alveolus. In man, the number of alveoli increases rapidly after birth until about eight years of age (Charnock and Doershuk, 1973), when approximately 300 million are present. The value of 300 million alveoli in the adult human is consistently reported, although recent estimates have ranged from 100 million (Kliment, 1973) to over 500 million (Davies, 1961). The alveolus of the adult human, though not strictly spheric, has an equivalent diameter of about 150 to 300 μm, but the range of 250 to 350 μm is probably more realistic (Weibel, 1963). Alveolar dimensions vary also with degree of lung inflation and with the vertical position within the thorax. The total alveolar surface area in the adult human is about 35 m^2 during expiration, 70 to 80 m^2 at three-fourths total lung capacity, and 100 m^2 during deep inspiration (von Hayek, 1960; Weibel, 1963). The thickness of the air-blood barrier is variable, even for a given alveolus. The air-blood barrier consists of endothelium, basement membrane, and alveolar epithelium, with a total thickness of 0.36 to 2.5 μm. The tissue thickness between adjacent alveoli is made up of the thickness of the alveolar wall, basement membrane, interstitium, and any interposed capillary. The capillary diameter is about 8 μm, and 90 to 95 percent of the alveolar surface is covered with capillaries. The mean tissue thickness between alveoli is then about 9 μm.

Well over 40 cell types are required to perform the diverse functions of the respiratory tract. These include 17 types of epithelium, nine types of unspecified connective tissue, two types of bone and cartilage, seven types of cells related to blood vessels, two distinctive types of muscle cells, and five types associated with the pleural or nervous tissue elements. The cells of greatest interest are those that are unique to the respiratory tract, such as ciliated bronchial epithelium, nonciliated bronchiolar epithelium (Clara cells), type I (squamous alveolar) pneumocytes, type II (great alveolar) pneumocytes, and alveolar macrophages. In addition, three other cell types are of special interest: endothelial cells and interstitial cells (fibroblasts and fibrocytes), which constitute the greatest percentage of total cells present; and lining cells of the trachea and bronchi, which account for only a small portion of the mass of the total respiratory tract. These latter three cell types are extremely susceptible to various types of injury.

The ciliated tracheobronchial epithelial cells are the predominant cells in the trachea, bronchi, and bronchioles of airways greater than 1 mm in diameter, where they outnumber goblet or mucus-secreting cells five to one. As the terminal bronchiole diminishes in diameter and terminates in the respiratory bronchiole, the cilia-bearing cells gradually disappear.

The ciliated epithelium functions to move a fluid film and particles deposited on it from the lung to the nasopharynx. Direct observations have shown that transport rates in the trachea or large bronchi in several species range from 1 to 3.5 cm/min. Mucociliary transport is capable of clearing inhaled particles from the conducting airways in a few hours and is a major detoxication mechanism.

Nonciliated bronchiolar cells (Clara cells) are present only in small bronchioles and can be identified by their bulging into the bronchiolar lumen, by the absence of cilia, and by the presence of apical cytoplasmic granules (Cutz and Conen, 1971). The ultrastructural characteristics reveal the presence of plasma membranes that form complex interdigitations, including desmosomes, with adjacent epithelial cells. The function of the Clara cells is not known, although ultrastructural and cytochemical evidence indicates that they are metabolically active, probably secretory, and have characteristics like merocrine-type secretory cells. Clara cells are major sites of lung injury from xenobiotic compounds which are metabolized to reactive intermediates by the lung cytochrome P-450 system (Boyd *et al.*, 1980). Depletion of glutathione enhances toxicity, which indicates the importance of glutathione in protecting the lung from injury by toxicants.

The surface of the pulmonary alveoli is largely covered by the continuous, exceedingly attenuated (0.1 to 0.2 μm) cytoplasm of the squamous epithelium, which has nuclei resembling those of capillary endothelium. This cell is located on the epithelial side of the basement membrane and, with the type II cells, completely lines the alveolus. The junction between the type I and type II cells is "tight," forming a *zonulae occludens*. The surface area of the type I cell has been calculated as 2,290 μm^2 and that of type II as 63 μm^2. Thus, even though the ratio of type I to type II cells in the alveolus is 2:3, the type I cell makes up most of the barrier of the blood-gas pathway. The cytoplasm of type I cells is barely visible with light microscopy and is equally unimpressive with electron microscopy because of its sparseness and the paucity of organelles. With the exception of pinocytotic vesicles, the cytoplasmic extensions of the type I cell are practically devoid of organelles. Some organelles are concentrated in the perinuclear cytoplasm.

With the light microscope, type II pulmonary epithelial cells are cuboidal. They are usually located in corners of the alveoli. The nucleus is spheric and the cytoplasm abundant with vacuoles. Type II cells from a number of species have basically similar ultrastructures (Sorokin, 1967). The cytoplasm has a loosely ordered granular endoplasmic reticulum, an extensive Golgi apparatus, numerous multivesicular bodies, and many large osmophilic multilamellated inclusions or cytosomes.

Type II cells are strongly implicated as the source of the pulmonary surfactant (Sorokin, 1967). Other functions of these cells have not been documented; however, the type II cells are frequently the proliferative cells in the repair of subtle diffuse injury to the squamous pulmonary epithelium, such as results from beryllium and oxygen toxicity (Kapanci et al., 1969; Carrington and Green, 1970; Bowden and Adamson, 1971). Type II cells have been classified as a renewing cell population by several investigators (Evans and Bils, 1969), with relatively long turnover times ranging from 20 to 84 days. Type II cells mature to type I cells with time.

The elaboration of the pulmonary surfactant by these cells is essential for proper ventilation. Surfactant consists mostly of dipalmitoyl lecithin and, as a thin film, has a very low surface tension characterized by unequal pathways of compression and relaxation. Surfactant lowers the surface tension in small alveoli so that inflation of small and large alveoli occurs at similar pressures. In the absence of surfactant, small alveoli coalesce into large alveoli, reducing the surface area available for gas exchange (respiratory distress syndrome of the premature infant).

Alveolar macrophages are the phagocytic cells of the lung and are found free in the alveoli. With light microscopy, alveolar macrophages in tissue sections are ovoid mononuclear cells, 7 to 10 μm in diameter. The nucleus is 5 to 6 μm in diameter and is round, oval, or kidney shaped. Macrophages washed from the lungs look similar, but they are larger (15 to 25 μm) and flatter and have more definitive cytologic detail.

The major function of alveolar macrophages is the ingestion of inhaled particulate material. Infectious particles are usually killed by the macrophages, except in some chronic bacterial and fungal infections, such as tuberculosis, and in some viral diseases where the virus actually replicates in the macrophage (Green, 1970; Green et al., 1977).

The endothelial cells form a continuous cytoplasmic tube lining the pulmonary vasculature. The adjoining cells become closely approximated or may interdigitate and overlap. The endothelium of the alveolar septa is separated from the epithelium by an interstitial space of variable thickness.

The pulmonary capillary endothelium functions to exchange gases and volatile metabolites between the blood and air. However, these cells may also interact with the blood that perfuses them and perform functions with significant implications. The pulmonary endothelial cells are stem cell, renewing-cell populations (Evans and Bils, 1969). The turnover time has not been determined but must be long, i.e., a matter of years.

The fibroblast is a cell of mesenchymal origin that is responsible for production of intercellular substances of connective tissues. These are relatively undifferentiated cells, and it is probable that the fibroblasts found in the lung are similar to those found elsewhere in the body.

The nasopharyngeal region has been largely ignored as a site of toxic action, with the exception of the perforated nasal septum produced by inhalation of certain chromium compounds. Recent evidence of tumors in the nares of rats and mice has focused interest in this area of the respiratory tract. Schreider and Raabe (1981) compared the anatomy of the airways of the head in the rat, rhesus monkey, and beagle dog. This comparison is illustrated in Figure 12–1. An active new area of research is investigation of the effect of these anatomic differences on the removal of gases and aerosols from inhaled air.

PULMONARY PHYSIOLOGY

Figure 12–2 is a very simplified diagram of the distribution of volumes and flows within the adult human lung. The role of each of these volumes in respiration can be seen in Figure 12–3 which represents the normal respiratory pattern at rest. The changes in volume and flow are recorded using a spirometer, a lightweight, gastight bell immersed in water. The movement of the bell is recorded with time as the subject breathes. Normally, only a small volume of the lung is ventilated, the tidal volume. The tidal volume of 500 ml inhaled over a minute at 15 breaths/min represents the minute volume of 7,500 ml/min. Maximal inspiration and expiration are shown and the total volume represents the vital capacity. Some gas remains in the lung following maximal expiration and amounts to about 150 ml. This is the residual volume. The difference between no gas in the lung and the minimum of the tidal volume represents the functional residual capacity.

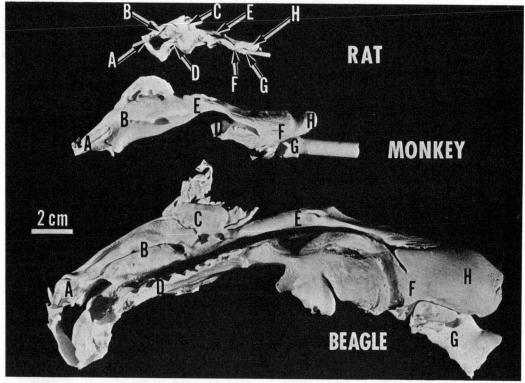

Figure 12–1. Comparison of silicone rubber casts of the respiratory airways of the head of the rat, rhesus monkey, and beagle showing (A) the external nares, (B) the maxilloturbinate region, (C) the ethmoturbinate region, (D) the mouth and oral pharynx, (E) the nasopharynx, (F) the larynx and laryngopharynx, (G) the trachea, and (H) the esophagus. (From Schreider, J. P., and Raabe, O. G.: Anatomy of the nasal-pharyngeal airway of experimental animals. *Anat. Rec.,* **200**:195–205, 1981.)

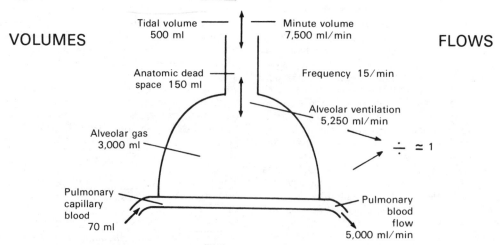

Figure 12–2. Diagram of a lung showing typical volumes and flows. There is considerable variation around these values. (From West, J. B.: *Respiratory Physiology—The Essentials.* © 1974 The Williams & Wilkins Co., Baltimore.)

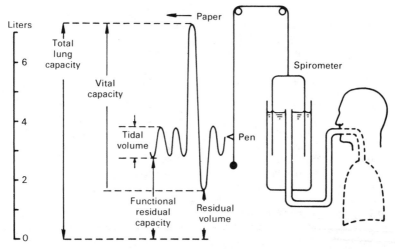

Figure 12–3. Lung volumes. Note that the functional residual capacity and residual volume cannot be measured with the spirometer. (From West, J. B.: *Respiratory Physiology—The Essentials.* © 1974 The Williams & Wilkins Co., Baltimore.)

The difference between the volume of gas entering the lung and the volume not exhaled during normal respiration is *alveolar ventilation,* or the volume of fresh gas available for exchange at the alveolus. In our example the alveolar ventilation is:

(Tidal volume − anatomic dead space) × breaths/min = (500 ml − 150 ml) × 15 breaths/min, or 5,250 ml/min

The pulmonary blood flow over the same minute is about 5,000 ml. The gas exchanged, or alveolar ventilation, is almost exactly the same volume as the blood perfusing the alveolus. The match of blood perfusion volume to alveolar ventilation is critical for proper gas exchange and oxygenation of the blood. A mismatch in either flow or ventilation actually decreases oxygenation (see West, 1974, for detailed explanation).

The amount of a gaseous toxicant delivered to the lung will be a function of its concentration in the incoming gas and the minute volume. The dose can be integrated over the time period of the exposure to give the total amount of toxicant to which the lung has been exposed. Alterations in the pattern of breathing, such as work or exercise, will alter the total dose received. Similarly, the deposition of aerosols will be a function of the tidal volume and respiratory rate, since these control the velocity of gas as it courses down the airway and the amount of aerosol reaching the lung. Because of the complex anatomy of the lung, flow rates are especially important in determining the rate and site of deposition of aerosols.

The flow of gas from the lung can be used to diagnose pathophysiologic changes in the lung. If the subject inhales and exhales maximally, *forced vital capacity* (FVC) and *forced expiratory volume at one second* ($FEV_{1.0}$) can be recorded. $FEV_{1.0}$ is a particularly reproducible and sensitive measure of obstructive or restrictive flows in the lung. Restrictive flows often result from exposure to inhaled toxicants. A detailed discussion of the pulmonary function tests used to discern pathophysiologic changes in the lung is provided in West (1977). Alterations in blood gases are particularly useful in determining perfusion-ventilation abnormalities. Chronic exposure to toxicants often results in either interstitial fibrosis or emphysema. Specific tests are available to determine these and other abnormalities. Similar tests can be conducted on experimental animals, although they are generally more difficult due to the lack of cooperation on the part of the animal in performing the maneuver. Anesthesia or other intervention is sometimes required.

Alterations in pulmonary mechanics produced by acute exposure to irritants or to pharmacologically active agents such as histamine or acetylcholine can be measured quantitatively in experimental animals and human subjects. Irritants that affect mainly the larger airways produce predominantly an increase in flow resistance. Irritants that have their action mainly in the peripheral portions of the lung produce predominantly a decrease in compliance. Response to specific irritant air pollutants is discussed in Chapter 25. Drazen (1976) presents an excellent discussion of the use of alterations in pulmonary mechanics to determine the site of toxic reaction. Kessler *et al.* (1973) demonstrated in dogs exposed to *Ascaris* that measurement of pulmonary mechanics to indicate site of action correlated well with localization of constriction demonstrated by tantalum bronchography. Properly interpreted, measurements of pulmonary mechanics are a useful tool of pulmonary toxicology.

Respiratory frequency is simple to measure and has been used to assess the response to irritants. As Drazen (1976) points out, however, a stimulus may have a profound effect upon the lung without altering the respiratory frequency. Given intravenously to guinea pigs, 10 mg/kg acetylcholine produced a response primarily in the small airways and parenchyma (decreased compliance). Increasing the dose to 30 mg/kg caused a response involving the entire lung (a further decrease in compliance and an increase in resistance). The frequency increased the same amount in response to both doses. Had frequency alone been measured, it would have been concluded that the pulmonary response was the same to both doses.

GASES AND VAPORS

Diffusion Dominates Toxicant Uptake

Unlike the exchange of oxygen and carbon dioxide, the uptake of toxic gases occurs throughout the respiratory system, starting with the nasopharyngeal cavity. The dominant driving force in the uptake of toxicants is diffusion. Since toxicants are present at very low concentrations in air, but vanishingly small concentrations in the tissue, the driving force for diffusion is essentially the concentration of the toxic gas in the inspired air. The solubility of the gas in water is generally the major characteristic determining the relative toxicities of gases. Unfortunately, there is no way, at present, by which toxicant concentrations can be measured directly in the airways at different points or within the tissues themselves during inhalation. Only a few attempts have been made to describe quantitatively by mathematical models the transport of inhaled toxicants (Miller *et al.*, 1978), and they are of such complexity as to be beyond the scope of this text. Generally, deposition of gases is much more poorly described than deposition of particles.

Henry's law describes the transfer of a solute from the gas to the liquid-solute phase. The flux or mass transfer is directly proportional to the concentration of the solute in the gas phase and inversely proportional to the diffusional radius of the solute in the liquid phase. The diffusion coefficient is generally not available for most toxicants of interest, but one can approximate it by the quotient of the solubility divided by the square root of the molecular weight. These considerations are of theoretic interest only until mathematical models accounting for the gas transport within the lung become more widely available. One should be aware of such models, as they represent the future predictive role of inhalation toxicology. As computer-based models become more popular and available, calculations of actual doses delivered to the lung will be possible by knowing the ambient concentration of the toxicant.

The airways are lined with protective and functional layers of fluids through which toxic gases must penetrate to reach the underlying lung tissue. The thickness of the liquid layer lining the airways varies from the mucus-secreting upper airway to the surfactant-lined alveolus. Most morphologists believe that mucus secretions are thickest in the upper airway and decrease in a linear manner down the airways toward the alveoli. As discussed above, the human airways are equally bifurcating and the diameter of the airway decreases exponentially with the bifurcations. The total surface area, however, increases due to the increasing number of airways. In rodents, the transitional generations of airways having both conducting and oxygen–carbon dioxide exchange function may be absent or much decreased compared to those present in man.

In laryngectomized patients, mucus production is about 10 ml/24 hr or about 6.9×10^{-3} ml/min. The velocity of transport of the mucus is about 0.02 cm/sec up and out of the airway to be swallowed or expectorated. Similar values have been reported for rats. Mucous layers can be calculated to range in thickness from 5 to 10 μm in man and animals according to these measurements.

The alveoli are lined with the pulmonary surfactant, which is a complex mixture predominantly composed of dipalmitoyl lecithin. Great debate centers around the presence of an aqueous layer between the lipid surfactant layer and the luminal surface of the alveolar cells. The thickness of this layer is estimated to be about 0.5 to 1 μm.

The diffusion of inhaled toxicants into these protective layers will also be a function of the radial and axial diffusion of the gas and its mixture with other nontoxic gases simultaneously inhaled, such as nitrogen, oxygen, carbon dioxide, and water vapor. Since several breaths are required before sufficient toxicant is absorbed, the transport of toxic gases can be treated as reaching a steady state. Naturally, steady state may not be achieved in the presence of very high concentrations of toxic gases such as hydrogen cyanide or hydrogen sulfide, which are lethal within minutes. Most toxicologic problems today, however, deal with chronic exposures and thus better fit the achievement of a steady state. Breath-by-breath models are needed to provide more quantitative estimates, however. Inhaled gases may react chemically with the components of the mucous or surfactant layer. Since the mucous layer is being constantly renewed and removed by ingestion or expectoration following the upward transport out of the airways by the cilia, dissolution in or reaction with the mucous layer is a mechanism of detoxication.

Other gases, such as anesthetic agents, diffuse through the lung and reach saturation in the blood. They are transported, dissolved in blood, to peripheral tissues where they diffuse into tissues. Concentration and local perfusion rates determine the speed of accumulation in peripheral tissues and their distribution. In these cases, direct effects of the toxicant do not occur in the lung but rather in other organs.

Inhaled toxicants can either react directly with the lung or be transported to other tissues in the blood. For example, nitrogen dioxide, ozone, and sulfur dioxide react directly with pulmonary tissue to produce major effects, whereas the anesthetic gases are readily absorbed and transported to bone marrow to where some may produce aplastic anemia.

When the concentration of the inhaled toxicant is sufficient to provide a measurable flux or mass transfer of toxicant across the protective mucous or surfactant layer to the surface of the pulmonary cells, toxicity to lung tissue will result. Highly reactive anhydrous acids or strong oxidants react directly with the pulmonary cells to cause changes in permeability or death. Less reactive gases such as nickel carbonyl may diffuse through the cells lining the lumen before causing toxic reactions with endothelial cells. Exposure may result in death of capillary endothelial cells without apparent damage to epithelial cells. This is confusing at first glance but only reflects the relative rate of reaction of the toxicant compared to its rate of diffusion.

Relative Permeability of the Lung to Solutes

Toxicants that do not exert immediate toxic effects on the lung may pass through the lung, reach the capillaries, and be transported to other tissues by the blood. The relative permeability of the respiratory tract to a number of solutes has been measured. The administration techniques used are such that it is difficult to determine the site of absorption, since a small volume of solution (either water, saline, or isotonic su-

crose) of the toxicant is instilled within the trachea, bathing the upper and lower airways. A number of lipid-insoluble neutral compounds, including urea, erythritol, mannitol, and sucrose, are removed at rates directly proportional to the concentration of the solute (Enna and Schanker, 1972). The relative rates of absorption are ranked in the same order as the diffusion coefficients of the solutes. Simple diffusion appears to account for removal of compounds of this nature. If one assumes diffusional absorption through pores or channels for such lipid-insoluble compounds, three classes of pores can be discerned: the smallest-diameter pores allow passage of urea and not the saccharides; a second allows passage of erythritol; and a third, all saccharides but not dextrans of 70,000 daltons. Organic cations and anions (sulfanilic acid, tetraethyl ammonium ion, p-aminohippuric acid, p-acetyl-hippuric acid, and procainamide ethobromide) are absorbed by diffusion, presumably through aqueous channels, since their rates of removal are not saturable with increasing concentration of solute and is roughly related to molecular size rather than to their lipid/aqueous partition coefficients. The main barrier for the diffusion of hydrophilic compounds appears to be the alveolar membrane, which has been calculated to have an equivalent pore radius of 8 to 10 Å in the dog (Taylor and Gaar, 1970).

Lipophilic compounds are also removed at diffusion-controlled rates. A number of antibiotics and corticosteroids were found to be removed rapidly, with $t_{1/2}$ of 1.9 to 33 minutes (Burton and Schanker, 1974a, 1974b). Highly lipophilic pesticides, such as DDT and leptophos, are removed at extremely slow rates, with $t_{1/2}$ of about 300 min in the rat. A comparison of the pulmonary absorption rate with the physical properties of the compound, such as the molecular weight and chloroform/water partition coefficient, suggests that partitioning into the lipid of the lung membrane is the rate-determining factor. The question is not closed and is in need of further investigation.

Specialized absorption systems probably exist in the lung and have been recognized for the absorption of phenol red (Enna and Schanker, 1973). Phenol red is partially absorbed by diffusion, but primarily by a carrier-mediated system. The system is saturated at high concentrations of phenol red and is inhibited by a number of closely related compounds. Organic anions such as benzylpenicillin and cephalothin are also competitors for the phenol red removal system.

A specialized storage or uptake mechanism also exists on the luminal surface of the lung. The herbicide paraquat is highly toxic to the lung and is stored within the lung on ingestion (Clark *et al.*, 1966; Rose *et al.*, 1976; Charles *et al.*, 1978). Paraquat is only poorly transported from the luminal surface of the lung, while the closely related and relatively nontoxic compound diquat is removed at much greater rates ($t_{1/2}$ 356 vs. 75 min). Unlike paraquat, diquat does not produce pulmonary toxicity. Paraquat uptake is both energy and concentration dependent. The site of paraquat storage may be the type II pneumocyte, which may also be the cell type most affected by paraquat poisoning.

Specialized sites of absorption and metabolism also exist in the pulmonary capillary bed. The lung functions in the removal and metabolism of a number of vasoactive hormones, and an appreciation of this nonrespiratory function has only recently become recognized.

The role of inhaled toxicants in the perturbation of this complex function has likewise only recently come to the fore and may be of importance in chronic lung diseases.

Nasopharyngeal Removal

Man is an obligatory mouth breather when exercising at work or play. Most experiments with animals, however, involve exposure to airborne toxicants under conditions in which the animals are obligatory nose breathers. This difference in respiratory pattern is particularly important, since the nasopharyngeal cavity can remove 50 percent or more of inhaled toxicants. The rate of removal of toxicants depends mostly on the water solubility of the toxicant. Anhydrous acid vapors such as SO_2 are more rapidly removed than relatively insoluble compounds such as O_3. The removal of organic vapors by the nasopharyngeal cavity has not been studied but, by analogy with the buccal absorption of drugs, is also likely to occur readily. The entrance of toxic gases into the nasopharyngeal cavity significantly reduces the final concentration to which the upper airways are exposed. The reduction in concentration of the inhaled toxicants is similar to the physiologic need for saturation of incoming air with water vapor prior to reaching the upper airways. While the inhaled vapor concentration is significantly reduced by this mechanism, entrance of toxicants into the body is not prevented. The nasopharynx provides little or no protection from toxicants that produce toxic effects in organs other than the lung. Generally, the lung is much more sensitive to toxic injury than distal organs and is thus protected by the scrubbing action of the nasopharynx.

Upper Airway Deposition

The upper airways are composed of several cell types, two of which, goblet and ciliated cells, are the predominant types lining the luminal side of the airway. The secretion of mucus by the goblet cells is stimulated by acetylcholine, presumably via cyclic GMP as the intracellular messenger. Cholinergic innervation has been suggested but not proven. The secretion of mucus is also a function of the prevalence of goblet cells. Dietary vitamin A determines the maximum number of goblet cells developed in the airways, since ciliated cells and squamous metaplastic cells dominate the upper airway population in vitamin A–deficient or marginally vitamin A–sufficient animals. The chemical composition of airway mucus is not known, but probably is similar to parotid gland mucus, which is highly glycosidated. The secretion of mucus may be influenced by the inhalation of toxicants, especially if the toxicant has cholinomimetic properties or if disruption of goblet cell integrity results on contact with the toxicant. In man, hyperplasia and probably altered molecular composition of the goblet cell mucus occurs in asthma, bronchitis, and cystic fibrosis. The exact effect of such chronic disease states on the absorption of toxicants from the upper airway is not known but might be greater, since these patients are more sensitive to NO_2, SO_2, and O_3. Bronchoconstriction evoked in bronchitic and asthmatic patients can be partially blocked by prior administration of atropine. Some of the atropine effect may be directly on the smooth muscles of the upper airways.

Bronchoconstriction is one of the most common immediate responses observed on the inhalation of a number of highly reactive gases. Inhalation of sulfuric acid or solid aerosols of soluble salts, such as some sulfate salts, also provokes constriction. Constriction may either be due to a direct action of the aerosol on the airway smooth muscles or occur indirectly through the release of histamine. Histamine release may not be the only factor involved.

After toxicants penetrate the mucous lining of the upper airway and come into contact with the goblet and ciliated cells, cytotoxicity is often observed. Ciliated cells are generally more sensitive to gaseous toxicants than are goblet cells. Cilia are often lost from the cell, and the entire cell may die and leave a denuded area. Fragments of ciliated cells can be found in the mucus as a result. Complex mixtures of gases and particles in cigarette smoke inhibit ciliary action without cytotoxicity.

As in the case of nasopharyngeal removal, gases can be classified as acting on either the upper or lower airways, depending on their relative solubility in water. Anhydrides of acids tend to produce bronchoconstriction and upper airway necrosis, while less water-soluble compounds reach the lower airway to produce alveolar damage.

Undoubtedly, chemical reaction with mucus is a highly important protective factor for the upper airway. An open question is the effect of chemical products of reaction with mucus on the airway itself.

The relative ventilation of different parts of the lung during breathing at rest versus exercise affects the distribution of toxicants within the airways as well. More extensive constriction occurs at exercise than at rest. Detailed studies of the airway response in man on exposure to O_3 and SO_2 have been undertaken, illustrating these effects. A review of the distribution of gases in the lung with exercise can be found in West (1974).

Lower Airway Deposition

The overall distribution of toxic effects of inhaled gases in the lower airways including the alveoli parallels the ventilation of that section of the lung. The lower lobes of the lung in man are more generally affected than the upper lobes, due to this differential ventilation. West (1974) describes the pulmonary mechanics responsible for these anomalies, which apply equally as well to toxic gases as to oxygen. As a result, from the top to the bottom of the lung, a pH gradient also exists that serves to accentuate differences in exposure to toxic gases and to exacerbate secondary infections resulting from toxic injury and inflammation. Ventilatory differences between the vertical lung of man and the horizontal lung of animals account for the differential effects seen in animals and man. In the interpretation of human effects on the basis of animal exposures, one must be careful to take these basic differences in pulmonary physiology into account. Similarly, the rat, a popular experimental animal, is highly susceptible to pneumonias that are often mistaken for toxic effects of inhaled gases.

Once the toxic gas has reached the level of the alveolus, the uptake of the gas can be treated essentially the same as that for oxygen. The lung is extremely well organized to promote diffusion across the very thin alveolar space into the blood. Figure 12–4 illustrates this intimate association of the airway with the capillary space. Diffusion again dominates the physical processes, accounting for uptake of the inhaled toxic gases. The alveolar region is essentially a sheet of blood interrupted in small regions by the connective tissue supporting the structure.

Certain regions of the lower airway are more affected by inhaled gases that act directly on the lung than others. The transitional region between the respiratory bronchiole and alveolus bounded by Clara cells is most susceptible to both ozone and nitrogen dioxide. The particular susceptibility can be accounted for on the basis of the total amount of these toxicants delivered to that region of the lung. The mass transfer of toxicant within the lung is a function of its axial and radial diffusion, solubility, and reactivity with upper air mucus and buccal cavity, and with the cyclic nature of respiration. These factors combine to deliver a greater dose of toxicant to the transitional region of the lower lung. This is the same region where pulmonary macrophages penetrate to the lumen to remove particles. Injury to the transitional region may have important consequences.

Another cell type exposed to inhaled toxicants in the alveolar region is the pulmonary macrophage. The macrophage acts mainly to remove from the alveolus particles such as bacteria, viruses, and inorganic and organic substances. The macrophage can be injured and die on exposure, releasing its cellular contents. Because of their phagocytic capacity, macrophages contain acid hydrolases that produce decompartmentalization of the alveolar sacs. The autolysis of the alveolar wall by proteases released from macrophages may be a contributor to emphysema.

The Lung as an Excretory Organ

The lung may be exposed to toxic gases and vapors through its function as an excretory organ. Volatile solvents, such as carbon tetrachloride and benzene, are excreted through the lung. Depending on the rate of metabolism of the compound to more polar, water-soluble substances of higher vapor pressure, excretion in the exhaled breath may be significant. Delayed pulmonary toxicity may occur following the ingestion of such toxicants as they are redistributed from the liver and exhaled. The lung has an active cytochrome P-450 system, capable of metabolizing many of these compounds to reactive intermediates that are bound to pulmonary macromolecules to promote necrosis in a fashion similar to that observed in the liver on metabolism of certain drugs.

The pulmonary capillaries are also specialized to take up amines, prostaglandins, and peptide hormones of angiotensin and the kinins. During redistribution of drugs or toxicants absorbed by other routes, the lung may accumulate high concentrations, resulting in pulmonary damage. Inhibition of the regulatory functions of the lung may be highly deleterious.

PARTICULATE MATERIAL

Classification of Particles

Many airborne materials of toxicologic importance can be considered under the generic term "aerosols." An aerosol is a relatively stable suspension of solid particles or liquid droplets in a

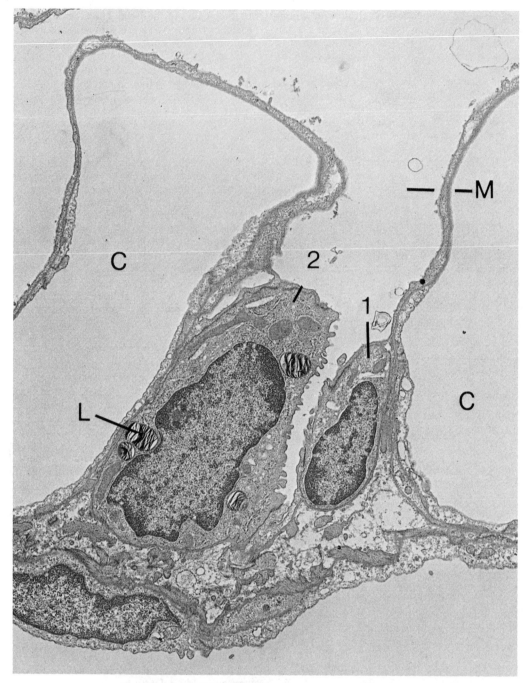

Figure 12–4. Electron micrograph of a rat lung. The alveolus is separated from the blood capillary (C) by a thin margin of the type I cell (1). Note the closeness of approach of these two compartments at M. A type II cell (2) can be seen containing lamelli bodies (L) presumed to be storage sites for the lung surfactant.

gaseous medium. Gases or vapors are frequently adsorbed on the surface or dissolved in aerosols. Traditionally, several terms have been used to describe aerosols.

Dusts arise from processes such as grinding, milling, or blasting. They are identical in chemical composition to the parent material. Depending on the process of generation, the size may vary from Ångstrom size to 100 μm in diameter. *Fumes* are formed by combustion, sublimation, or condensation. Usually the formation of fumes is accompanied by a chemical change. Many fumes of toxicologic importance are metal oxides. The particle size of fumes tends to be less than 0.1 μm and is often as small as 10 Å. Fumes have a marked tendency to flocculate and produce larger particles as the aerosol ages. *Smokes* are formed by combustion of organic materials. Particles are usually less than 0.5 μm in diameter and do not settle readily. *Mists* and *fogs* are liquid aerosols formed either by condensation of a liquid on particulate nuclei in air or by the uptake of liquid by hygroscopic particles. The term *smog* is applied to the complex mixture of particles and gases formed in the atmosphere by irradiation of automobile exhaust and other combustion products. The mixture contains photochemical oxidants and reduces visibility. (See Chapter 25.)

Aerosol Characterization and Behavior

The site of deposition of an aerosol in the respiratory tract is obviously of profound importance in assessing its toxicity. Particle size is usually the critical determining factor in regional deposition. Deposition of particles on the surface of the lung and airways is brought about by a combination of the morphometry and patterns of airflow in the respiratory system and the physical factors that lead to the removal of particles from the air. The toxicologist thus needs some knowledge of the terminology used to define particle size and of the physical behavior of aerosols. Space permits only a brief discussion here. More extensive discussions are readily available (Hatch and Gross, 1964; Mercer, 1973; Lippmann, 1970).

Particle Size. Except under controlled experimental conditions, inhaled particles are heterogeneous in size. It is, thus, necessary to define as precisely as possible the size distribution of an aerosol, which for most aerosols approximates a log-normal distribution. By assuming a log-normal function, the size distribution of particles may be described by the *median* or *geometric mean* and the *geometric standard deviation*. A plot of frequency of a given size against the log of the size produces a bell-shaped probability curve. Particle data are frequently handled by plotting the cumulative percentage of particles less than a stated size increment against the log of the stated size on log probability paper. This results in a straight line that may be fitted by eye or mathematically. Such a plot is shown in Figure 12–5. In actual practice it is not unusual to have some deviation from a straight line at the largest or smallest particle sizes measured. The geometric mean is the 50 percent size as the mean bisects the curve. The geometric standard deviation (σ_g) is calculated as:

$$\sigma_g = \frac{84.1\% \text{ size}}{50\% \text{ size}}$$

The σ_g of the particle size distribution is a measure of the heterogeneity of the aerosol. In the laboratory, values of σ_g of 1.8 to 3.0 are frequently encountered. In the field, values for ρ_g of 2.0 to 4.5 may be encountered. For some laboratory studies it is desirable to have aerosols that are uniform or nearly so in size (a monodisperse aerosol). For practical purposes, an aerosol with a σ_g of less than 1.2 may be considered as monodisperse.

The median diameter determined may reflect the number of particles as count median diameter (CMD) or reflect mass as mass median diameter (MMD). The latter is of particular significance in toxicology. The larger the mass of particles capable of penetrating the lung, the greater the probability of a toxic effect. The size distribution in relation to other factors, such as area, may also be of interest. Figures 12–5 and 12–6 show the interrelationship of these various factors. Surface area becomes of special importance when toxic materials are adsorbed on the surface of particles and thus carried to the lung.

Particles that are nonspheric in shape are frequently characterized in terms of equivalent spheres on the basis of equal mass, equal volume, or aerodynamic drag. The *aerodynamic diameter* takes into account both the density of the particle and aerodynamic drag. It represents the diameter of a unit density sphere having the same terminal settling velocity as the particle, whatever its size, shape, and density. Aerodynamic diameter is the proper measurement to consider for particles that are deposited by impaction and sedimentation. For very small particles, which are deposited primarily by diffusion, the critical factor is particle size, not density or shape. The aerodynamic diameter would underestimate diffusional deposition when real size is smaller than the aerodynamic diameter, i.e., the particles have a greater-than-unit density.

Another factor that must be kept in mind is that the size of the particles may increase in the respiratory tract. Materials that are hygro-

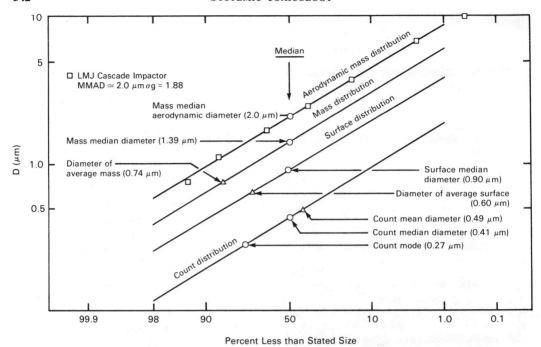

Figure 12–5. Plot of size distribution of an aerosol on log probability paper. Curves are shown which characterize aerosol size in regard to various parameters. See Raabe (1970).

scopic, such as sodium chloride, sulfuric acid, or glycerol, take on water and grow in size in the warm, saturated atmosphere of the respiratory tract.

Deposition Mechanisms. Deposition of particles may occur by *interception, impaction, sedimentation,* and *diffusion* (brownian movement). The last three are the most important.

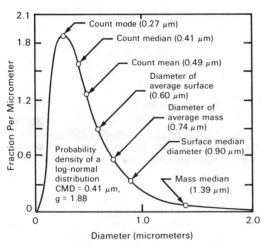

Figure 12–6. Data on the same aerosol as in Figure 12–5 plotted to show the probability density of a log—normal distribution. See Raabe (1970).

Interception occurs when the trajectory of a particle brings it near enough to a surface so that an edge of the particle contacts the surface. Interception is mainly important only for the deposition of fibers such as asbestos. Fiber diameter determines the probability of deposition by impaction and sedimentation. Interception depends on fiber length. Thus, a fiber with a diameter of 1 μm and a length of 200 μm would be deposited in the bronchial tree primarily by interception rather than by impaction.

Particles suspended in air, owing to inertia, tend to continue to travel along their original path. In a bending airstream, such as at an airway bifurcation, a particle may be impacted on the surface. Deposition rate is likely to be higher for particles moving in the center of the airway. Impaction probability is determined by a combination of air velocity and the square of the particle mass.

Sedimentation brings about deposition in the smaller bronchi, the bronchioles, and the alveolar spaces where the airways are small and the velocity of the airflow is low. As particles move downward through air, buoyancy and resistance of air act on the particles in an upward direction while the gravitational force acts on the particle in a downward direction. Eventually, the gravitational force equals the sum of the buoyancy and the air resistance, and the particle continues to settle with a constant velocity known as the terminal settling velocity. Quantitative discussions of the laws that govern this behavior may be found in the references cited at the start of this discussion as well as in the first edition of the present text. Sedimentation is no longer effective when the aerodynamic diameter reaches about 0.5 μm.

Diffusion is of importance in the deposition of submicron particles. A random motion is imparted to the particles by the impact of gas molecules. This brownian motion increases with decreasing particle size. Diffusion is an important deposition mechanism in small airways and alveoli for particles below about 0.5 μm.

Pulmonary Deposition

As was indicated above, the site of deposition of particles in the respiratory tract is determined by a combination of the physical forces that remove particles from an airstream and the anatomy of the respiratory tract. The measurement critical to assessment of toxicity is the regional deposition, rather than simply the total amount retained. The site of deposition affects (1) the severity of the consequences of tissue damage to the respiratory tract, (2) the degree of absorption of systemic toxicants, and (3) the clearance mechanisms available for the ultimate removal of the particles.

Factors Influencing Regional Deposition. Figure 12–7 illustrates schematically the nature of the interaction of physical and biologic factors leading to regional deposition. The size relationships shown for the various compartments are not quantitative. They are intended merely to indicate the increase in both size and surface area that occur with increasing depth in the respiratory tract. The directional changes imposed on the airflow become less abrupt and the velocity decreases as particles traverse the respiratory tract.

Particles having an aerodynamic diameter of 5 to 30 μm are largely deposited in the nasopharyngeal region by impaction. Because of their size, impaction is an important mechanism for their removal from an airstream. The high air velocity and the tortuous nature of the nasopharyngeal air passages, forcing many sharp changes in airflow direction, provide an ideal area for impaction. Particles having an aerodynamic diameter of 1 to 5 μm are deposited in the tracheobronchial regions by sedimentation. Such particles are of a size to be removed by sedimentation, and this mechanism of deposition is favored by the slower airflows, which allow time for deposition by gravitational forces. As the alveolar regions are approached, the velocity of the airflow decreases markedly, allow-

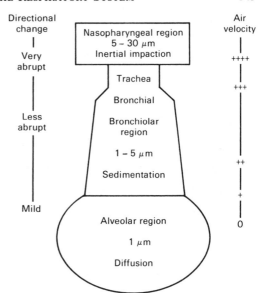

Figure 12–7. Parameters influencing particle deposition. (From Casarett, L. J.: The vital sacs: Alveolar clearance mechanisms in inhalation toxicology. In Blood, F. R. [ed.]: *Essays in Toxicology*, Vol. 3. Academic Press, Inc., New York, 1972.)

ing even more time for sedimentation. The small particles, generally less than 1 μm, that have penetrated to the alveoli are deposited primarily by diffusion. This is the principal mechanism by which submicron particles are deposited.

Additional physiologic or pathologic factors may act to influence particle deposition. One important factor is the pattern of breathing. During quiet breathing, in which the tidal volume is only two to three times the volume of the dead space, a large proportion of the inhaled particles may be exhaled. During exercise, where larger volumes are inhaled at higher velocities, impaction in the large airways and sedimentation and diffusion in the smaller airways and alveoli will increase. Breath holding also increases deposition from sedimentation and diffusion. This fact may be utilized in aerosol therapy by having the patient take a deep breath and hold it.

Factors that modify the diameter of the conducting airways can modify particle deposition. In patients with chronic bronchitis the mucous layer is much thickened and may partially block the airways in some areas. Jets formed by the air flowing through such partially occluded airways have the potential to increase deposition of particles by impaction and turbulent diffusion in the small airways. Irritant materials that produce bronchoconstriction would tend to increase tracheobronchial deposition of particles. Cigarette smoking has been shown experimentally to produce such an effect (Lippmann *et al.*, 1971).

Constraints of space have, of necessity, limited in scope the discussion of particle deposition. The serious student of inhalation toxicology will need additional information. There have been various models proposed to describe particle deposition in the different compartments of the respiratory tract. A variety of experimental techniques have been used to study deposition in both human subjects and experimental animals. An excellent review article (Lippmann, 1977) provides a critical discussion of the theoretical and experimental work in this area and cites references to the original literature.

Clearance of Particles

Particles that have been deposited on the surface of the respiratory tract are removed by mechanisms that vary, depending on the site of deposition. The speed and efficiency of clearance of deposited particles are obviously also critical factors in the assessment of their toxic potential. Rapid removal lessens the time available to cause critical damage to the pulmonary tissues and to permit systemic absorption of materials that have target organs other than the lung.

Respiratory tract clearance and its counterpart, retention of inhaled particles, are not completely understood. Perhaps, because of their relatively easier access and the extent to which changes take place rapidly, clearance from the ciliated surfaces of the tracheobronchial and nasopharyngeal regions has received much greater attention than has clearance from the pulmonary region. The brief discussion of clearance here is intended to supplement the simplified mathematical description of clearance developed by the Task Group on Lung Dynamics (TGLD) and given in Chapter 19. Detailed coverage of the subject may be found elsewhere (Hatch and Gross, 1964; Task Group on Lung Dynamics, 1966; Casarett, 1972; Green, 1973; Morrow, 1973; Kilburn, 1977).

Nasopharyngeal and Tracheobronchial Clearance

Clearance from the ciliated surfaces of the respiratory tract, which extend from the terminal bronchioles to the nose, is primarily by mucociliary transport. Goblet cells associated with the ciliated epithelial cells produce the mucous blanket that covers these surfaces. It has been suggested that the cilia beat in a serous fluid layer. The tips of the cilia contact the overlying sheet of mucus only when the movement of the ciliary tips is at the maximum forward velocity. Clearance rates from the ciliated surfaces have

been measured in man and laboratory animals using a variety of techniques. Radioactive particles have been inhaled, and radioactive or radiopaque substances have been insufflated, injected, or placed directly on the surfaces of interest and their rate of clearance observed by external monitoring of the radioactivity or by radiography.

Particles have been observed to move at about 7 mm/min in the human nose and trachea, at 1 mm/min in the upper bronchial tree, and at 0.4 to 0.6 mm/min in the lower bronchial tree (Quinlan *et al.*, 1969; Morrow *et al.*, 1967). The effect of these relatively high velocities is to clear the ciliated surfaces of particles in a matter of hours. It should be noted, however, that Patrick and Stirling (1977) have reported that about 1 percent of material deposited on the trachea is not cleared by 30 days. The cleared material is moved up to the oral cavity and ingested. Similar rates of clearance have been observed in other species.

Not all material deposited on the ciliated surfaces is cleared via the mucociliary process. The TGLD report includes constants for the absorption of materials from these surfaces into the bloodstream. Cuddihy and Ozog (1973) have reported the absorption of CsCl, $CeCl_3$, and $BaCl_2$, from the nasal cavity of the rat. Sorokin and Brain (1975) have reported the penetration of particles through the bronchial epithelium.

Pulmonary Clearance

There are three primary avenues by which particulate material is removed from the pulmonary region once it has been deposited: (1) particles may be phagocytized and cleared up the tracheobronchial tree via the mucociliary escalator; (2) particles may be phagocytized and removed via the lymphatic drainage; and (3) material may dissolve from the surfaces of particles and be removed via the bloodstream or lymphatics. Other particles, and perhaps some dissolved material, may be sequestered in the lung. The interaction of particles with the lung is very dynamic, with competition between each of the processes for removal, and perhaps with certain elements of lung tissue for retention of particles and complexed material.

The alveolar region of lung has a large population of macrophages, which is generally thought to originate from bone marrow. Within minutes after particles are inhaled they may be found within alveolar macrophages, and essentially all particles are engulfed within a matter of hours. Lavaging or washing the lung with physiologic saline solution removes many of the macrophages, including those laden with particles (Muggenburg *et al.*, 1977). This procedure has been advocated as a means of therapeutically removing inhaled particles in accidental exposure cases. Within a short time after lavage the alveoli are repopulated with macrophages, attesting to the dynamic state of macrophages within the lung. Many of the alveolar macrophages are ultimately transported to the mucociliary escalator. How they reach the ciliated surfaces is not clear. One of the most accepted theories is that the alveolar macrophages move via ameboid motion to the level of the respiratory bronchiole. It is also possible that the macrophages are carried to the bronchioles with alveolar fluid that contributes to the serous fluid layer in the airways.

Other macrophages with ingested particles are observed in the interstitial tissue spaces of the lung within hours after particles are inhaled. The lungs of beagle dogs have been lavaged immediately after inhalation of particles and at time intervals ranging up to 196 days (Felicetti *et al.,* 1975). At all time intervals, substantial numbers of particles have been removed in the lavage fluid. This suggests that macrophages, some of which contain particles, are continuously moving between the alveolar spaces and interstitium. The removal of particles by phagocytosis may be greatly influenced by the cytotoxicity of the particulate material. Macrophages also have an important bactericidal role that serves to protect the lung (Green, 1970).

Within a matter of days after particles have been inhaled, they are observed in the lymphatics and lymph nodes that drain the lung. For very insoluble material such as $^{239}PuO_2$, the amount of Pu in the tracheobronchial lymph nodes steadily increases and within one to two years exceeds the amount in the lung.

For most materials deposited in the alveoli, dissolution and removal of the solute are probably the most significant processes by which material is removed from the lung (Mercer, 1967; Kanapilly, 1977). The rate at which particles are dissolved is considered to depend primarily on their surface areas and the dissolution rates of the particular physicochemical form of the materials. Once material is dissolved it is available for removal in either a free or bound form. Kanapilly (1977) has also speculated on the possible binding of dissolved material within the lung.

Aerosol Characterization

A number of measurable characteristics of an aerosol may influence the deposition and retention within the respiratory tract, translocation within the respiratory tract and to other tissues, and ultimately the toxic effects of inhaled particles. The principal factors of concern are concentration, particle size and size distribution, surface area, chemical form, and dissolution properties. In the following paragraphs, key aspects of aerosol characterization will be briefly discussed. The reader interested in more detail is referred to several authoritative reviews or texts (Raabe, 1970; Drew and Lippmann, 1972; Mercer, 1973.)

Concentration. The most common means of determining the concentration of an aerosol is to collect a sample by drawing air through a suitable filter. Typically, filters are porous membranes or mats of fibers. Numerous different filters are available and vary in their efficiency for collection of particles, flow, and substrate characteristics. Lippmann (1972) and Mercer (1973) have compiled lists of available filters and their characteristics. The appropriate filter may be selected by knowing the material to be collected, the analytic method to be used, and the desired flow rate. The concentration of the aerosol may be determined by knowing the airflow through the filter and gravimetrically or chemically determining the mass of the material present. When the nature of the experiment permits, the use of a radioactive tracer can greatly facilitate the experimentation because of the ease with which the amount of radioactivity present can be determined. Light-scattering instruments may also be used to measure the concentration of aerosols; however, special care should be exercised in their calibration.

Particle Size and Size Distribution. The real size of particles may be determined by directly visualizing particles after collection on filters or electron microscopic grids. The larger respirable particles may be easily visualized by light microscopy; however, the smaller particles, which are of primary interest, may only be visualized using electron microscopic techniques. Electron microscope grids may be mounted in both thermal and electrostatic precipitators. In the thermal precipitator a heated surface is maintained on one side of the device and a cool surface on the other side, such that particles are attracted to the cool surface. In the electrostatic precipitator a corona discharge from a needle point on one side charges aerosol particles for collection on a grid that is grounded on the other side of the airstream. Care must be taken to assure that a representative sample is being evaluated. This may be done by scanning across a grid in the direction of the airflow.

As noted earlier, the aerodynamic diameter of particles is of special interest since this is the property that is primarily responsible for determining deposition of most respirable particles. A number of instruments have been built to sample particles according to their aerodynamic size.

Perhaps the most widely used in inhalation toxicity studies have been impactors of the type described by Andersen (1958), Lundgren (1967), and Mercer *et al.* (1970). In these devices air is drawn through a series of stages. The terminal stage is backed by a filter and the proximal stages by impaction plates, or in the Lundgren unit by a rotating drum, to minimize problems of overloading with use for long time periods. Each stage has successively smaller openings or jets such that the air exits at higher velocities. The air flows around the impaction plates. The particles that are aerodynamically the largest are unable to follow the airstream around the first impaction plate and are deposited. On each successive stage smaller particles are impacted, with the smallest particles being removed on the exit filter. With appropriate calibration the aerodynamic diameter distribution of the aerosol particles can be determined. Electron microscope grids can be mounted on the impaction plates so the particles can be visualized to determine their real size. With appropriate calibration and knowledge of the aerodynamic size, the density of the particles can be determined.

Diffusion Characteristics. At particle sizes of less than 0.5 μm the aerodynamic diameter becomes more difficult to measure and its usefulness in predicting deposition is lessened because deposition in this size range is largely determined by diffusion characteristics of the particles. The size properties of these very fine aerosol particles can be determined by using diffusion batteries (Sinclair and Hinchliffe, 1972).

Surface Area. Once particles are deposited in the pulmonary region of the respiratory tract the surface area of the particles becomes of major importance in determining the dissolution of the particles (Mercer, 1967). Perhaps the best approach to determining the surface area of particles is to measure the amount of material required to cover the particles with a single layer of molecules. This is called the BET (Brunauer-Emmett-Teller) method. This may be done using low-temperature adsorption of nitrogen or an inert gas from the vapor phase (Corn *et al.,* 1971).

Chemical Form and Dissolution Properties. The chemical form of particles is of obvious importance in determining the toxicity of a given aerosol. The techniques for chemically analyzing aerosol samples are too numerous to be summarized in this text. An important facet of the physicochemical nature of particles that determines toxicity is their dissolution characteristics. These characteristics will determine whether the specific element or compound of interest remains associated with the particle or is dissolved from the particle and is available for translocation. Although published values for the equilibrium (saturation) solubility of specific compounds in various solvents are a useful starting point in assessing the dissolution properties of particulate material in the lung, it must be emphasized that they are not wholly satisfactory for predicting the behavior in the dynamic environment of the lung. To provide information relevant to the lung environment, where dissolved material has the opportunity to be continuously removed from the solvent-solute interface, information is needed on dissolution rates. Several *in vitro* methods for obtaining dissolution rate data on aerosol samples have been reported and have yielded results that were usefully correlated with *in vivo* data (Kanapilly *et al.*, 1973).

Exposure Systems

Inhalation exposure poses a variety of specialized problems that are not encountered when other routes are used. Exposure systems vary in complexity from those required to expose one or two rodents for an hour or less to those used for continuous exposure of dogs or primates for periods of months or years. Chambers have also been designed for exposure of human subjects who may be exercising on a bicycle during portions of an exposure period of several hours. Several review articles set forth the principles of design criteria that are considered in construction and operation of exposure chambers (Drew and Laskin, 1973; Raabe *et al.,* 1973; Phalen, 1976; MacFarland, 1983).

Commonly used exposure chambers are so-called dynamic systems, which means that air flows continuously through the chamber and the toxic material being studied is added to this entering airstream. The main airstream is purified of extraneous contaminants and maintained at constant temperature and humidity. The chamber is usually operated at a slight negative pressure. This is a safety precaution to ensure that any leaks will let air enter the chamber rather than letting toxic material leak out to expose laboratory personnel.

Concentration of the toxic material in the chamber atmosphere is varied by altering the rate of addition of the substance to the main airstream and/or the rate of airflow through the chamber. From the respective flow rates it is possible to calculate the concentration. It is, however, necessary to measure the concentration by techniques of collection and analysis appropriate to the material being studied. Losses occur in duct work, on chamber walls, and on the fur of animals if it is a whole-body exposure. The actual concentration is thus always slightly lower than the calculated one. The concentration of importance is, of course, that in the breathing zone of the exposed animals: samples should therefore be taken that are representative of that concentration. It is necessary also to take samples from various locations in the chamber to be assured that uniform mixing has been achieved. Animals should be randomly assigned to positions within the chamber during exposures to guard against accidental bias of dose. Individual cages should be used within the exposure chamber to prevent animals from crowding together in one spot and reducing individual exposure. Groups of control animals are exposed for the same time periods to purified air alone in chambers of the same design as those used for exposure.

The method of generation of the material being tested varies with the nature of the material. Generation of gases or vapors is less complicated than generation of aerosols. The method chosen must be capable of generating a reproducible concentration of the material entering the airstream of the chambers over the time period of exposure. A most useful book by Nelson (1973) and an article by Rampe (1981) discuss the principles of generating experimental atmospheres of various types of materials.

More recently designed exposure systems for gas or vapor exposure incorporate computer-control using equations for feed-forward and feed-back control. Such systems also allow the accumulation of digitalized data for statistical analysis. Such interexposure analysis should be reported in publications to allow the reader to judge the contribution of variations in exposure to variations in experimental outcome rather than lumping these variables all together as the total experimental error.

Animals may be placed in the chamber or exposure may be with the nose or head only projecting into the chambers. Phalen (1976) gives a table summarizing the advantages, disadvantages, and special problems of these various modes of exposure. In whole-body exposure the animals are unrestrained, which has advantages for long-term experiments. The toxic material, especially if it is an aerosol, is deposited on the animals' fur; grooming leads to oral ingestion as well as inhalation. If the material is highly toxic or radioactive, such contamination can lead to exposure of personnel handling the animals. These problems are eliminated in nose or head-only systems. Restraint obviously adds some stress, but this can be minimized by appropriate design of the animal holders. The holder may be a body plethysmograph, which makes possible measures of pulmonary function during exposure.

Much useful information may be safely obtained by short-term exposures of human subjects especially when combined with toxicokinetic, physiologic, and biochemical measurements. Such data have been of particular value in assessing the response to low concentrations of air pollutants such as sulfur dioxide, ozone, or nitrogen dioxides. These exposures may be done in carefully designed chambers in which the subjects may freely move about or perform controlled exercises. They are more frequently done with the individual breathing through a mouthpiece or face mask connected to the contaminated atmosphere. The problems posed to extrapolation of such data to individuals breathing normally are discussed in Chapter 25.

PULMONARY RESPONSES TO SPECIFIC TOXICANTS

Despite the vast array of materials producing lung disease, the responses of the lung to toxic agents may be divided into the following general categories:

1. Irritation of the air passages, which results in constriction of the airways. Edema often occurs and secondary infection frequently compounds the damage.

2. Damage to the cells lining the airways, which results in necrosis, increased permeability, and edema. This edema is, in general, intraluminal (within the airways) rather than interstitial (within the cells of the airway).

3. Production of fibrosis, which may become massive and cause obliteration of the respiratory capacity of the lung. Local fibrosis of the pleura also occurs, restricting the movement of the lung and producing pain through the irritation of the pleural surfaces.

4. Constriction of the airways through allergic responses. Allergic alveolitis is a widespread response to the inhalation of some simple compounds, as well as of complex organic materials capable of producing specific antigenic responses.

5. Oncogenesis leading to primary lung tumors.

Examples of these categories of pulmonary response to toxic agents can be found in both occupational and environmental exposures. Table 12–1 lists the principal occupational exposures that are known to produce direct lung damage in workers. The chemical composition of the materials, the occupational source of exposure, the nature of the pulmonary injury, and the number of U.S. workers exposed are given. Dose-response relationships between exposure and development of disease are not easily deter-

Table 12–1. PRINCIPAL INDUSTRIAL TOXICANTS PRODUCING LUNG DISEASE THROUGH INHALATION

TOXICANT	CHEMICAL COMPOSITION	OCCUPATIONAL SOURCE	PULMONARY DAMAGE	NUMBER OF U.S. WORKERS EXPOSED
Asbestos	Fibrous silicates (Mg, Ca, and others)	Mining, construction, shipbuilding, manufacture of asbestos-containing materials	Asbestosis, lung cancer	250,000 in primary process, 3 million in secondary processes
Aluminum dust	Aluminum metal and small amount of Al_2O_3	Manufacture of aluminum products, fireworks, ceramics, paints, electrical goods, abrasives	Fibrosis	100,000
Aluminum	Al_2O_3	Manufacture of abrasives, smelting	Fibrosis initiated from short exposures	100,000
Ammonia	NH_3	Ammonia production, manufacture of fertilizers, chemical production, explosives	Irritation	500,000
Arsenic $Pb_3(AsO_4)_2$	As_2O_3, AsH_3(arsine) $Pb_3(AsO_4)_2$	Manufacture of pesticides, pigments, glass, alloys	Lung cancer, bronchitis, laryngitis	1.5 million
Beryllium	Be, $Be_2Al_2(SiO_3)_6$ (beryl, ore), Be(II) salts	Ore extraction, manufacture of alloys, ceramics	Dyspnea, interstitial granuloma, fibrosis, cor pulmonale, chronic disease	30,000
Boron	B_2H_6, B_4H_{10}, B_5H_9 (boron hydrides)	Chemical process	Acute CNS	
Cadmium oxide (fume dust)	CdO	Welding, manufacture of electrical equipment, alloys, pigments, smelting	Emphysema	2000
Carbides of tungsten titanium tantalum	WC TiC TaC	Manufacture of cutting edges on tools	Pulmonary fibrosis	15,000 50,000 2000
Chlorine	Cl_2	Manufacture of pulp and paper, plastics, chlorinated chemicals	Irritation	15,000
Chromium (IV)	Na_2CrO_4 and other chromate salts	Production of Cr compounds, paint pigments, reduction of chromite ore	Lung cancer	175,000
Coal dust	Coal plus SiO_2 and other minerals	Coal mining	Pulmonary fibrosis	200,000
Coke oven emissions	Polycyclic hydrocarbons, SO_x, NO_x, and particulate mixtures of heavy metals	Coke production	Lung cancer (9 times greater than other steelworkers)	10,000
Hydrogen fluoride	HF	Manufacture of chemicals, photographic film, solvents, plastics	Irritation, edema	70,000
Iron oxides	Fe_2O_3	Welding, foundry work, steel manufacture, hematite mining, jewelry making	Diffuse fibrosis	100,000
Kaolin	$Al_4Si_4O_{10}(OH)_8$ plus crystalline SiO_2	Pottery making	Fibrosis	10,000
Manganese	MnO, Mn(II) salts	Chemical and metal industries		9000
Nickel	NiCO (nickel carbonyl), Ni, Ni_2S_3 (nickel subsulfide), NiO	Nickel ore extraction, nickel smelting, electronic electroplating, fossil fuel	Nasal cancer, lung cancer, acute pulmonary edema (NiCO)	

TOXICANT	CHEMICAL COMPOSITION	OCCUPATIONAL SOURCE	PULMONARY DAMAGE	NUMBER OF U.S. WORKERS EXPOSED
Osmium tetraoxide	OsO_4	Chemical and metal industry	Irritation	3000
Oxides of nitrogen	NO, NO_2, HNO_3	Welding, silo filling, explosive manufacture	Emphysema	1.5 million direct or in direct
Ozone	O_3	Welding, bleaching flour, deodorizing	Emphysema	380,000
Phosgene	$COCl_3$	Production of plastics, pesticides, chemicals	Edema	10,000
Perchloro-ethylene	C_2Cl_4	Dry cleaning, metal de-greasing, grain fumigating	Edema	275,000
Silica	SiO_2	Mining, stone cutting construction, farming, quarrying	Silicosis (fibrosis)	1.2 million non-agricultural workers
Sulfur dioxide	SO_2	Manufacture of chemicals, refrigeration, bleaching, fumigation	Irritation	5 million
Talc	$Mg_6(SiO_2)OH_4$	Rubber industry, cosmetics	Fibrosis, pleural sclerosis	20,000
Tin	SnO_2	Mining, processing of tin	Benign pneumoconiosis	25,000
Toluene 2,4-diiso-cyanate	$CH_3\text{—}C_6H_3(\text{NCO})_2$	Manufacture of plastics	Decrement of pulmonary function (FEV_1)	40,000
Vanadium	VO_5	Steel manufacture	Irritation	10,000
Xylene	$C_6H_4(CH_3)_2$	Manufacture of resins, paints, varnishes, other chemicals, general solvent for adhesives	Edema	140,000

mined. Working conditions may vary sufficiently to produce different breathing patterns and, thus, different individual exposures to the same airborne concentration. Mouth breathing during heavy work reduces the protection provided by the upper respiratory tract and increases potential toxicity. Depth of respiration and minute volume will also influence the dose received by the lung. The added pulmonary stress of cigarette smoking increases the risk of serious disease from occupational exposure to these materials. Many of these agents are also present in polluted urban environments. The concentrations are much lower than in industrial environments, but the exposure may be more prolonged and the population exposed includes the infirm, the elderly, and sensitive individuals. Factors entering into considerations of risk assessment thus differ somewhat from those for occupational situations.

Table 12–2 provides additional information on the toxic action of these industrially important toxic materials. The common name of the resultant pulmonary disease and the site of toxic action within the respiratory system are given.

Many agents have an acute effect produced by initial exposure or by shorter exposure to high concentrations. These acute effects are listed, as are the chronic effects resulting from long-term exposure. Except in instances when the concentration is sufficient to threaten life or produce residual pulmonary damage, the chronic effects are the more significant clinically.

Direct Airway Irritation

The bronchial tone of the lung is influenced by many inhaled compounds. Cholinergic constriction is immediately induced by inhalation of pharmacologic agents such as aerosols of carbachol or acetylcholine. Bronchodilation is produced by inhalation of aerosols of isoproterenol, which acts on the β-adrenergic receptors of bronchial smooth muscle. The ready accessibility of the bronchial smooth muscles to inhaled agents is used extensively in asthma therapy, especially with isoproterenol.

Ammonia and chlorine are classic examples of irritant gases. Bronchoconstriction occurs immediately on inhalation. Dyspnea (the feeling of an inability to breathe) probably results from the

Table 12–2. SITE OF ACTION AND PULMONARY DISEASE PRODUCED BY SELECTED OCCUPATIONALLY INHALED TOXICANTS

TOXICANT	COMMON NAME OF DISEASE	SITE OF ACTION	ACUTE EFFECT	CHRONIC EFFECT
Asbestos	Asbestosis	Parenchyma		Pulmonary fibrosis, pleural calcification, lung cancer, pleural mesothelioma
Aluminum	Aluminosis	Upper airways, alveolar interstitium	Cough shortness of breath	Interstitial fibrosis
Aluminum abrasives	Shaver's disease, corundum smelter's lung, bauxite lung	Alveoli	Alveolar edema	Fibrotic thickening of alveolar walls, interstitial fibrosis and emphysema
Ammonia		Upper airway	Immediate upper and lower respiratory tract irritation, edema	Chronic bronchitis
Arsenic		Upper airways	Bronchitis	Lung cancer, bronchitis, laryngitis
Beryllium	Berylliosis	Alveoli	Severe pulmonary edema, pneumonia	Pulmonary fibrosis, progressive dyspnea, interstitial granulomatosis, cor pulmonale
Boron		Alveolus	Edema and hemorrhage	
Cadmium oxide		Alveolus	Cough, pneumonia	Emphysema, cor pulmonale
Carbides of tungsten, titanium, tantalium	Hard metal disease	Upper airway and lower airway	Hyperplasia and metaplasia of bronchial epithelium	Fibrosis, peribronchial and perivascular fibrosis
Chlorine		Upper airways	Cough, hemoptysis, dyspnea, tracheobronchitis, bronchopneumonia	
Chromium (VI)		Nasopharynx, upper airways	Nasal irritation, bronchitis	Lung tumors and cancers
Coal dust	Pneumoconiosis	Lung parenchyma, lymph nodes, hilus		Pulmonary fibrosis
Coke oven emissions		Upper airways		Tracheobronchial cancers
Cotton dust	Byssinosis	Upper airways	Tightness in chest, wheezing, dyspnea	Reduced pulmonary function, chronic bronchitis
Hydrogen fluoride		Upper airways	Respiratory irritation, hemorrhagic pulmonary edema	
Iron oxides	Siderotic lung disease: silver finisher's lung, hematite miner's lung, arc welder's lung	Silver finisher's: pulmonary vessels and alveolar walls; hematite miner's: upper lobes, bronchi and alveoli; arc welder's; bronchi	Cough	Silver finisher's: subpleural and perivascular aggregations of macrophages; hematite miner's: diffuse fibrosis-like pneumoconiosis; arc welder's: bronchitis
Kaolin	Kaolinosis	Lung parenchyma, lymph nodes, hilus		Pulmonary fibrosis
Manganese	Manganese pneumonia	Lower airways and alveoli	Acute pneumonia, often fatal	Recurrent pneumonia

TOXICANT	COMMON NAME OF DISEASE	SITE OF ACTION	ACUTE EFFECT	CHRONIC EFFECT
Nickel		Parenchyma (NiCO), nasal mucosa (Ni₂S₃), bronchi (NiO)	Pulmonary edema, delayed by 2 days (NiCO)	Squamous cell carcinoma of nasal cavity and lung
Osmium tetraoxide		Upper airways	Bronchitis, bronchopneumonia	
Oxides of nitrogen		Terminal respiratory bronchi and alveoli	Pulmonary congestion and edema	Emphysema
Ozone		Terminal respiratory bronchi and alveoli	Pulmonary edema	Emphysema
Phosgene		Alveoli	Edema	Bronchitis
Perchloroethylene			Pulmonary edema	
Silica	Silicosis, pneumoconiosis	Lung parenchyma, lymph nodes, hilus		Pulmonary fibrosis
Sulfur dioxide		Upper airways	Bronchoconstriction, cough, tightness in chest	
Talc	Talcosis	Lung parenchyma, lymph nodes		Pulmonary fibrosis
Tin	Stanosis	Bronchioles and pleura		Widespread mottling of x-ray without clinical signs
Toluene		Upper airways	Acute bronchitis, bronchospasm, pulmonary edema	
Vanadium		Upper and lower airways	Upper airway irritation and mucus production	Chronic bronchitis
Xylene		Lower airways	Pulmonary edema	

individual's inability to breathe rapidly and deeply enough to satisfy respiratory demands (West, 1977). Ammonia and chlorine are highly water soluble and are, therefore, primarily removed by the upper airways. Both gases are well tolerated in that, unless the concentration is sufficient to cause death, the acute effects do not result in chronic residual pulmonary damage (Weill *et al.*, 1969).

Arsenic compounds in industrial applications are usually of a sufficiently large particle size to be deposited in the nasopharyngeal region and the large airways. Irritation of the bronchi results in chronic cough and bronchitis, and laryngitis can result in chronic exposure. The lung also serves as a route of absorption for the more soluble arsenate salts. The toxicity of absorbed arsenic is discussed in Chapter 19.

Cellular Damage and Edema

A variety of materials produce damage to the cells of the airways and alveoli. The resulting increase in permeability leads to the release of edema fluid into the lumen of the airways and alveoli. The production of major edema may take several hours to develop so that seriously damaging or even fatal exposures may occur without the individual's being aware at the time of the extent of the potential damage. The cytotoxicity may be of a general nonspecific nature, but the effects may be localized in the lung and depend on the distribution of the toxic agent within the lung (Miller *et al.*, 1978). One major determinant of site of action is water solubility. As was indicated earlier, if the toxic agent is present as an aerosol, the prime determinant of site of action is the particle size.

Ozone and nitrogen dioxide are examples of toxic agents that produce cellular damage. The water solubility is sufficiently low that the main site of action is at the level of the respiratory bronchioles and alveoli. The most likely mode of action is through peroxidation of cellular membranes. The toxicity of these gases is discussed in detail in Chapter 25.

Phosgene is another irritant capable of producing delayed pulmonary edema. The moisture of the respiratory tract hydrolyzes phosgene to hydrochloric acid and carbon dioxide. A high concentration produces a burning sensation in the nose and upper respiratory passages. The gas that penetrates to the peripheral portions of the lung undergoes *in situ* hydrolysis, producing nascent hydrogen chloride, which destroys the permeability of the cells of the alveolar membranes. Clinically, a delay of approximately 24 hours lapses between exposure and symptomatology. Individuals exposed to phosgene should be under medical surveillance for at least 48 hours so that oxygen and other emergency measures are immediately at hand if major edema results.

Cadmium oxide is produced as a fume of extremely fine particle size that readily penetrates to the alveoli. Edema results and histopathology indicates an interstitial pneumonitis with a marked proliferation of the lining cells of the alveolar spaces. Chronic exposure results in emphysema, characterized by the loss of individual septa or decompartmentalization of the alveoli. The alveolar volume available for respiratory gas exchange is greatly reduced, and disparities between perfusion and ventilation arise in damaged segments. Perfusion-ventilation anomalies are serious impairments that can eventually result in almost total physical disability. The clinical features of emphysema, which is produced by a wide variety of toxic materials, are discussed by West (1977).

The toxicity of nickel compounds and nickel metal to the respiratory tract depends on the physical/chemical properties of the nickel (National Academy of Sciences, 1975). Nickel, nickel subsulfide, and nickel oxide are generated in relatively large particle sizes during the production and mining of nickel and are, thus, associated with damage to the nasal mucosa. Nickel carbonyl is a liquid with a high vapor pressure at room temperature. Exposure to vaporized nickel carbonyl occurs in electroplating, in nickel refining, and in the electronics industry. The highly insoluble vapor penetrates to the alveoli with resultant edema, which has a latent period of about two days. Nickel metal has been detected within alveolar cells following exposure to nickel carbonyl. This suggests that the nickel carbonyl has penetrated the cells, decomposed there to nickel metal, and produced cellular damage.

Paraquat is an example of a toxic agent that can produce direct damage to pulmonary cells when it enters the body by a route other than inhalation. Ingestion of paraquat produces a frothy exudate in the lungs and pulmonary edema (Clark *et al.*, 1966). It is only slowly removed from the lungs, where it appears to be concentrated in the type II cells. Paraquat may exert its toxic action through the generation of superoxide radical anions (O_2^-) or other free radicals. The closely related herbicide diquat is not toxic to the lung and is not retained by the lung (Charles *et al.*, 1978). Both paraquat and diquat are toxic to cultured lung cells. This suggests that the ability to be retained by type II cells is the critical difference in toxicity between the two compounds. The active transport system for paraquat in type II cells has not yet been fully elucidated.

Perchlorethylene and xylene produce effects on the lung typical of organic solvents. These solvents are sufficiently volatile and water insoluble that they reach the alveolar region of the lung. Much of the inhaled dose is removed readily and transported to other organs where it produces its toxic symptoms. Both compounds are acted upon by the cytochrome P-450 system of the liver and other organs. Oxygenated intermediaries may be produced in the lung leading to covalent binding. This covalent binding may be the mechanism that produces pulmonary edema through cellular necrosis.

Production of Fibrosis

The incidence of pulmonary fibrosis appears to be on the increase in the United States, but the cause of this increase is not known. This seriously debilitating disease was recognized as one of the earliest forms of occupational disease. Pneumoconiosis is the term applied to this general class of disease in which pulmonary fibrosis is the central factor. The widely publicized coal miner's pneumoconiosis is but one form of the disease. One of the most confusing aspects of pulmonary fibrosis initiated by dust inhalation is the difference in potency of different dusts. This has led to confusion regarding the hazards of dust inhalation and the mechanisms by which fibrosis is initiated. Originally, silica was thought to be the main responsible agent, but it is now recognized that fibrosis can be initiated by a wide variety of particles of different chemical composition. An excellent discussion of the occupational medical aspects of inhalation of dusts is given by Hunter (1969).

Silicosis. Silica (SiO_2) exists in several forms, but only the crystalline materials produce the chronic pulmonary condition termed specifically silicosis. Quartz is the most stable and common crystalline form of silica. Heating produces tridymite or cristobalite, both of which appear to have greater fibrogenic potency than quartz. These minerals occur naturally in some volcanic rock encountered in mining operations. They are also formed when quartz or amorphous silica is heated, for example, in the silica brick industry or in the calcining of diatomaceous earth.

Despite the fact that the incidence of silicosis dates from antiquity, current research still leaves many gaps in our knowledge relating to the precise manner in which the human pulmonary lesion develops, to the relationship of crystal structure and size of silica dust to the production of silicosis, and to the correlation between retained dust load and the degree of pulmonary tissue reaction. Numerous theories based on one or more characteristics of silica particles have been proposed. These have centered mainly on physical shape, solubility, crystalline structure, or cytotoxicity to macrophages. No single theory seems to provide a fully adequate explanation of the fibrotic lesions of silicosis.

The cytotoxic and fibrogenic activity appears related to the rupture of the lysosomal membrane of the macrophage and the release of lysosomal enzymes into the cytoplasm. The macrophage is, thus, digested by its own enzymes. Following lysis of the macrophage, the free silica particles are once again released to be ingested by fresh macrophages in which the cycle is repeated. Perivascular aggregation of lymphoid tissue and fibrosis follow, but the chain of events is not entirely clear. Heppleston (1969) has suggested that the damaged macrophages release factors capable of stimulating collagen formation. Phospholipids released from the dying macrophages cause stimulation of fibroblasts, which leads to collagen formation.

The so-called silicotic nodule is the typical pulmonary lesion that positively identifies silicosis. These are firm nodules of concentrically arranged bundles of collagen fibers, usually 1 to 10 mm in diameter. They appear in lymphatics around blood vessels, beneath the pleura in the lungs, and sometimes in mediastinal lymph nodes. The nodules may fuse, resulting in the condition known as progressive massive fibrosis. The blood vessels in the silicotic nodules become narrowed and blocked by fibrous tissue. Perifocal emphysema frequently occurs around the nodule, with destruction of alveolar walls and an increase in the size of the alveolar ducts and sacs. These changes further decrease the ventilation and blood flow in the lungs. Especially in the past, silicosis was frequently further complicated by tuberculosis.

Asbestosis. "Asbestos" is a general name for a large group of hydrated silicates that, when crushed or milled, separate into flexible fibers. The group is a continuous solid solution series of minerals that represents a small part of a larger mineral group of fibrous minerals, the amphiboles. Chrysotile is the most important commercially and represents some 90 percent of the total usage. Other minerals marketed as asbestos include amosite, crocidolite, anthophyllite, tremolite, and actinolite. Since this class of minerals is a solid solution series, the chemical composition varies considerably from locality to locality and from one class member to another. Tremolite occurs as a contaminant in talc, while others, and the amphiboles in general, occur in practically every other commercial mineral including coal. Use of asbestos is now extensive and is increasing with the development of greater technology.

Asbestosis was recognized as a respiratory disease very early and led to the development of some of the first standards regulating dust levels in the workplace. Asbestosis in man involves diffuse interstitial fibrosis, calcification and fibrosis of the pleura, bronchogenic carcinoma, and mesothelial tumors. There is some doubt about the relative potency of each mineral type of asbestos to produce all or some of these symptoms. All amphiboles, including those derived from nonasbestos sources, may be capable of initiating symptoms in man. The difficulty stems, in part, from the lack of knowledge of the mechanisms by which asbestos initiates these effects. The organization of the surface of the fibers, their lengths, and their diameters seems critical in the production of biologic effects in experimental animals. In man, bronchogenic carcinoma and mesothelial tumors rarely occur less than 30 years after exposure. Other environmental and personal habits exposing people to other carcinogens or potential carcinogens further complicate the interpretation of the incidence of cancer in man following asbestos exposure. Smoking clearly enhances cancer production. Also, the same mineral type of asbestos may be more or less carcinogenic, depending on the locality and population exposed.

Studies of the increase of asbestos fibers in the human lung indicate that all urban dwellers have retained large numbers of mineral fibers. The proportion of mineral fibers that are found in the lung on autopsy and are classified "asbestos" (e.g., chrysotile) cannot be easily determined. Minerals of a fibrous nature, aside from asbestos, will form "asbestos bodies" or protein-coated inclusions within the lung. This generalized type of reaction around a fibrous mineral particle is best referred to as a ferruginous body. These bodies can be identified with ease by both light and electron microscopy.

The production of interstitial fibrosis from asbestos inhalation is most common in the lower lobes of the lung. Bronchogenic carcinoma is widely distributed and derived from all cell types of the bronchial tree. There does not seem to be any localization within the lung. Mesothelial tumors in man are rare, but appear to be increasingly common. The ability of ingested asbestos to evoke mesothelial tumors is not resolved. Since asbestos fibers occur widely in food through the use of asbestos filters (fruit juices, beer, and wine, for example) and through the presence of asbestos and amphibole fibers in drinking water, the contribution of inhaled asbestos to the total incidence of mesothelial tumors is not clear. Similarly, the calcification of the pleura could be due to either ingested or inhaled fibers.

Exposure of experimental animals to asbestos and similar fibrous minerals generally produces fibrosis. Tumors occur at a low rate of incidence because only a short time period is possible between exposure and sacrifice. Rodent experiments in excess of two years are almost impossible to conduct. Tumor induction appears to require prolonged time periods and possibly multiple exposures, although single exposures at high levels have been reported to produce tumors after a long induction period. This is an example where rodents are not very useful as a model of human disease. Fiber migration clearly takes place by an unknown mechanism that removes inhaled fibers from the airways into the pleural cavity. Direct injection of fibers into the peritoneum evokes more rapid and frequent tumor response.

A critical problem is the relative potency of fibers of differing lengths and diameters. Generators producing experimental asbestos aerosols for animal studies are generally rather crude. The fibers are produced by some grinding process that tends to make a very disperse preparation with respect to both the chemical and physical properties of the fibers, but fibers of 5 μm in length and 0.3 μm in diameter seem to be the most active.

To date, no one has reported a mutagenic activity for these fibers in microbial or cell culture systems. The chemical mechanism (if one exists) for the induction of tumors is not known. The surfaces of these and other fibers are chemically very active, leading to the theory that these fibers produce mutagenesis and carcinogenesis by carrying sorbed chemical carcinogens into the lung. This suggestion is attractive, but still lacks direct evidence and does not explain the carcinogenesis observed with other inorganic compounds such as nickel salts.

The major concern with asbestos stems from the long period between exposure and malignancy as observed in U.S. shipworkers who were exposed, during World War II, to asbestos lagging applied to ship interiors. This group of workers has been identified as having a moderate exposure and has been found to have an increasing incidence of bronchogenic and mesothelial tumors now that 30 years have elapsed. The widespread use of asbestos in building materials, especially after 1940, for fireproofing has increased the total amount of this potential toxicant in the environment. As these buildings are demolished or renovated, much of this material is dispersed into the air, water, and soil. The nature of the dose-response curve in man is unknown. From the experience in occupational exposure of man, lowering the total fibers available for inhalation and decreasing the exposure frequency decrease the incidence of fibrosis and tumors. However, the quantitative relationship between the number and frequency of fibers inhaled and the risk of disease is not known.

Little is known about the basic pathogenic mechanisms that produce fibrotic lung disease following inhalation of asbestos or silica. Recent research (Brody et al., 1981; Brody and Hill, 1982) has elucidated initial patterns of deposition, translocation, and cellular response to chrysotile asbestos in rats following a one-hour exposure. Elegant use of electron microscopy shows the presence of asbestos fibers deposited at alveolar bifurcations; fibers were rarely seen in alveolar spaces or elsewhere on the alveolar duct surface. The heaviest deposits occurred on the bifurcations closest to a terminal bronchiole. There was less asbestos present five hours after exposure than was observed in animals killed immediately. Fibers were taken up by type I epithelial cells and by alveolar macrophages. By one month after exposure, numerous asbestos fibers were accumulated within the lung interstitium at alveolar bifurcations. Intracellular microcalcifications were found around many of these fibers. These probably resulted from membrane injury to the interstitial cells, perhaps the initial pathogenic event of asbestosis.

Induction of Allergic Response

Bronchoconstriction and chronic pulmonary disease can result from inhalation of a variety of materials that appear to act wholly or partly through an allergic response. This underlying mechanism is demonstrated by the presence of circulating or fixed antibodies to specific components of the inhaled materials. In some instances these reactions are caused by spores of molds or by bacterial contaminants. In other instances, as in the case of cotton dust, they appear to be related to components of the material itself.

Farmer's Lung. A classic example of a pulmonary disease related to inhalation of an organic dust is farmer's lung. The major cause of the disease is the inhalation of spores of thermophilic actinomycetes, organisms that flourish and produce vast numbers of spores when the temperature of damp hay rises to 40° to 60°C. The disease entity is characterized by extrinsic allergic alveolitis. A classic attack of farmer's lung may appear between five and six hours after exposure, but the disease also frequently develops insidiously with no consistent interval between exposure and appearance of symptoms. The disease is characterized by fever, malaise, chills with aches and pains, and weight loss. Severe dyspnea is a more common symptom than cough and is often out of proportion to the crepitant rales observed on examination. Radiologic findings in the chronic disease include evidence of fibrosis and "honeycomb" lung, especially in the upper lobes. Serologic, inhalation, and skin tests may provide a certain amount of valuable diagnostic information, especially when the clear-cut clinical picture of acute farmer's lung is no longer apparent.

Other Disorders. Other forms of extrinsic allergic alveolitis of a similar nature may be caused by microorganisms or fungi. Examples include mushroom picker's lung, maple bark stripper's disease due to a fungus, cheese washer's lung caused by *Penicillium* spores, and a disease resulting from inhalation of spores from moldy sawdust. A more complete discussion of these and other similar diseases is found in Hunter (1969) or in microbiologically oriented pathology texts.

Bagassosis occurs in workers exposed to the dust arising from handling of dried sugar cane that has been allowed to lie around following extraction of the sugar-containing juices. The disease does not arise from exposure to moist sugar cane, but only from the dried material known as bagasse. Signs and symptoms include shortness of breath, production of small amounts of black sputum, fever, chills, and weight loss. The onset may occur after one or two days to a month, depending in part on the dose inhaled. The termination of contact with bagasse dust results in reasonably complete recovery within weeks or months, although some patients may remain symptomatic for a year or longer. Once an individual has had the disease it is advisable to avoid all further contact with bagasse dust. Renewed contact almost invariably produces a relapse; each episode tends to be more severe and prolonged than the last. The cause is probably molds or fungi in the stored bagasse.

Byssinosis arises from the inhalation of cotton, flax, or hemp dusts. The symptoms, in the form of chest tightness and respiratory difficulty, frequently appear after a period of absence from work, either a weekend or a prolonged vacation. Unlike farmer's lung and bagassosis, byssinosis does not seem to result from bacterial or fungal action on the cotton since the disease occurs also in individuals who work with the cotton before it is brought to the factory. The bronchoconstriction results from an agent or agents contained in the fibers or dust of the cotton plant itself, especially the bracts. Agents have been found in cotton that promote the release of histamine and 5-hydroxytryptamine. Heat treatment of the cotton tends to decrease the potency of the dust, which suggests a heat-labile toxicant or allergen. Symptoms are reduced by prior treatment with drugs that prevent degranulation of pulmonary mast cells. Byssinosis and other respiratory problems of cotton workers are reviewed by Harris et al. (1972).

Toluene diisocyanate (TDI), widely used in the manufacture of polyurethane plastics, is an irritant material that also produced allergic-like symptoms on inhalation. Exposures to TDI produce a concentration-dependent immunologic response (Karol, 1983). Hyperresponsiveness of airways to acetylcholine challenge and an outpouring of inflammatory cells (polymorphonuclear leukocytes and eosinophils) were observed in guinea pigs 2 or 6 hours following a 1-hour exposure to 2ppm TDI (Gordon et al., 1985).

Some investigators have found a decrement in pulmonary function as assessed by measurement of 1 second forced expiratory volume ($FEV_{1.0}$). This is observed from Monday to Friday during a work week. The individuals who show the greatest reduction over the course of a week tend also to show a long-term reduction when measurements are repeated one to two years later. Whether this represents the response of sensitized individuals or merely the response of individuals most sensitive to the irritant action *per se* has been debated.

Methylisocyanate (MIC), used in the manufacture of the insecticide carbaryl, received world-wide attention when an accident in Bhopal, India in December, 1984 released 40 tons of the gas to the surrounding community. More than 2000 people died and over 100,000 were affected. Mammals of several species responded similarly, but birds and insects seemed unharmed. Examination of the victims (Kamat et al., 1985) indicated that initial symptoms were severe irritation of the eyes, nose, and throat; inability to open the eyes; irritating cough; chest pain; and a sensation of choking. Persistent symptoms in survivors included cough, throat irritation, dyspnea, chest pain, eye irritation, and blurred vision. Interstitial pneumonitis was notable and was corroborated by lung function and blood gas studies. Pulmonary function studies in 82 subjects indicated that a large majority showed a restrictive defect.

Methods used to evaluate sensory and pulmonary irritation in mice indicate that MIC is a potent sensory and pulmonary irritant (Ferguson *et al.,* 1986a). It is much more hazardous than other tested mono- or diisocyanates because of its potency as a pulmonary irritant and its high vapor pressure. Exposure of guinea pigs for 90 minutes to 2 to 35 ppm MIC (Ferguson *et al.,* 1986b) produced coughing in all animals that persisted for up to 5 days. Above 2 ppm, animals showed abnormal respiratiory patterns characteristic of airway obstruction. Flow-volume loops indicated diminished airflow and some flow interruption during expiration. Maximal response was observed within 7 days, and recovery from acute effects had occurred by 21 days.

An evaluation was made of the antibody response of individuals exposed in Bhopal and of guinea pigs exposed to MIC (Karol *et al.,* 1985). Antibodies to MIC were detected in exposed victims. Using inhibition assays, the specificity of antibodies for MIC was confirmed. The specificity of antibodies in the guinea pigs was identical to that observed in individuals exposed at Bhopal.

Production of Pulmonary Cancer

The high incidence of lung cancer in the United States has directed much attention to inhaled toxic materials that produce pulmonary cancer. Without much doubt, cigarette smoking is the main contributor to lung cancer in man. Cigarette smoke is composed of a myriad of compounds, which include recognized carcinogens as well as recognized irritants. The production of tracheobronchial cancer in experimental animals by cigarette smoke inhalation has been difficult. The self-exposure of man has provided sufficient data that demonstration of a similar response in experimental animals is certainly not needed to delineate the hazard of cigarette smoking. Epidemiologic data also indicate that cigarette smoking increases the incidence of cancer in asbestos workers.

Coke oven emissions contain benzo(a)pyrene and a number of other polycyclic aromatic hydrocarbons. These materials can be metabolized by the lung cytochrome P-450 system to reactive intermediaries capable of inducing mutations leading to malignant transformation. The action of chromate and nickel salts is less clearly understood. Nickel and nickel compounds produce mainly squamous cell carcinoma of the nasal cavity and the lung, suggesting that the mucus-secreting and cilia basal cells are most sensitive to transformation. Chromate and divalent nickel ions bind easily to DNA, but such binding is far removed from malignant transformation. These issues are discussed in more detail in Chapter 5.

REFERENCES

Anderson, A. A.: New sampler for the collection, sizing, and enumeration of viable airborne particles. *J. Bacteriol.,* **76**:471–84, 1958.

Bowden, D. H., and Adamson, I. Y. R.: Reparative changes following pulmonary cell injury. Ultrastructural, cytodynamic, and surfactant studies in mice after oxygen exposure. *Arch. Pathol.,* **92**:279–83, 1971.

Boyd, M. R.; Statham, C. M.; and Longo, N. S.: The pulmonary clara cells as a target for toxic chemicals requiring metabolic activation: studies with carbon tetrachloride. *J. Pharmacol. Exp. Ther.* **212**:109–14, 1980.

Brody, A. R.; Hill, L. H.; Adkins, B., Jr.; O'Conner, R. W.: Chrysotile asbestos inhalation in rats: deposition pattern and reaction of alveolar epithelium and pulmonary macrophages. *Am. Rev. Respir. Dis.,* **123**:670–79, 1981.

Brody, A. R. and Hill, L. H.: Interstitial accumulation of inhaled chrysotile asbestos fibers and consequent formation of microcalcifications. *Am. J. Pathol.,* **109**:107–14, 1982.

Burton, J. A., and Schanker, L. S.: Absorption of antibiotics from the rat lung. *Proc. Soc. Exp. Biol. Med.,* **145**:752–56, 1974a.

———: Absorption of corticosteroids from the rat lung. *Steroids,* **23**:617–24, 1974b.

Carrington, C. B., and Green, T. J.: Granular pneumocytes in early repair of diffuse alveolar injury. *Arch. Intern. Med.,* **126**:464–65, 1970.

Casarett, L. J.: The vital sacs: Alveolar clearance mechanisms in inhalation toxicology. In Hayes, W. J., Jr. (ed.): *Essays in Toxicology,* Vol. 3. Academic Press, Inc., New York, 1972, Vol. 3.

Charles, J. M.; Abou-Donia, M. B.; and Menzel, D. B.: Absorption of paraquat and diquat from the airways of the perfused rat lung. *Toxicology,* **9**:59–67, 1978.

Charnock, E. L., and Doershuk, C. F.: Development aspects of the human lung. *Pediatr. Clin. North Am.,* **20**(2):275–92, 1973.

Clark, D. G.; McElligott, T. F.; and Hurst, E. W.: The toxicity of paraquat. *Br. J. Ind. Med.,* **23**:126–32, 1966.

Corn, M.; Montgomery, T. L.; and Esmen, N. A.: Suspended particulate matter: seasonal variation in specific surface areas and densities. *Environ. Sci. Technol.,* **5**:155–58, 1971.

Cuddihy, R. G., and Ozog, J. A.: Nasal absorption of CsCl, SrCl₂, BaCl₂ and CeCl₃ in Syrian hamsters. *Health Phys.,* **25**:219–24, 1973.

Cutz, E., and Conen, P. E.: Ultrastructure and cytochemistry of Clara cells. *Am. J. Pathol.,* **62**:127–34, 1971.

Davies, C. N.: A formalized anatomy of the human respiratory tract. In Davies, C. N. (ed.): *Inhaled Particles and Vapours.* Pergamon Press, London, 1961, pp. 82–87.

Drazen, J. M: Physiologic basis and interpretation of common indices of respiratory mechanical function. *Environ. Health Perspect.,* **16**:11–16, 1976.

Drew, R. T., and Laskin, S.: Environmental inhalation chambers. In Gay, W. I. (ed.): *Methods of Animal Experimentation,* Vol. IV: *Environment and the Special Senses.* Academic Press., Inc., New York, 1973, pp. 1–41.

Drew, R. T., and Lippmann, M.: Calibration of Air Sampling Instruments - II. Production of Test Atmospheres for Instrument Calibration. *Air Sampling Instruments - 4th Edition,* American Conference of Governmental Industrial Hygienists (ACGIH), 1972.

Enna, S. J., and Schanker, L. S.: Absorption of saccharides and urea from the rat lung. *Am. J. Physiol.,* **222**:409–14, 1972.

————: Phenol red absorption from the rat lung: evidence of carrier transport. *Life Sci.*, 12:231–39, 1973.

Evans, M. J., and Bils, R. F.: Identification of cells labeled with tritiated thymidine in the pulmonary alveolar walls of the mouse. *Am. Rev. Respir. Dis.*, 100:372–78, 1969.

Felicetti, S. A.; Silbaugh, S. A.; Muggenburg, B. A.; and Hahn, F. F.: Effect of time post-exposure on the effectiveness of bronchopulmonary lavage in removing inhaled ^{144}Ce in fused clay from beagle dogs. *Health Phys.*, 29:89–96, 1975.

Ferguson, J. S.; Schaper, M.; Stock, M. F.; Weyl, D. A.; and Alarie, Y.: Sensory and pulmonary irritation with exposure to methyl isocyanate. *Toxicol. Appl. Pharmacol.* 82:329–35, 1986a.

Ferguson, J. S.; Stock, M. F.; and Alarie, Y.: Respiratory effects of methyl isocyanate vapor inhalation in guinea pigs. *Toxicologist*, 6:76, 1986b.

Frasier, R. G., and Pare, J. A. P.: *Structure and Function of the Lung.* W. B. Saunders Co., Philadelphia, 1971.

Gordon, T.; Sheppard, D.; McDonald, D. M.; Distefano, S.; and Scypinski, L: Airway hyperresponsiveness and inflammation induced by toluene diisocyanate in guinea pigs. *Am. Rev. Respir. Dis.*, 132:1106–12, 1985.

Green, G. M.: The J. Burns Amberson Lecture—in defense of the lung. *Am. Rev. Respir. Dis.*, 102:691–703, 1970.

————: Alveolobronchiolar transport mechanisms. *Arch. Intern. Med.*, 131:109–14, 1973.

Green, G. M.; Jakab, G. J.; Low, R. B.; and Davis, G. S.: Defense mechanisms of the respiratory membrane. *Am. Rev. Respir. Dis.*, 115:479–514, 1977.

Harris, T. R.; Merchant, J. A.; Kilburn, K. H.; and Hamilton, J. D.: Byssinosis and respiratory diseases of cotton mill workers. *J. Occup. Med.*, 14:199–206, 1972.

Hatch, T. F., and Gross, P.: *Pulmonary Deposition and Retention of Inhaled Aerosols.* Academic Press, Inc., New York, 1964.

Heppleston, A. G.: The fibrogenic action of silica. *Br. Med. Bull.*, 25:282–87, 1969.

Hunter, D.: *The Diseases of Occupations*, 4th ed. Little, Brown Co., Boston, 1969.

Kamat, S. R.; Mahashur, A. A.; Tiwari, A. K. B.; Potdar, P. V.; Gaur, M.; Kolhatkar, V. P.; Vaidya, P.; Parmar, D.; Rupwate, R.; Chatterjee, T. S.; Jain, K.; Kelkar, M. D.; and Kinare, S. G.: Early observations on pulmonary changes and clinical morbidity due to the isocyanate gas leak at Bhopal, *J. Postgrad. Med.*, 31:63–72, 1985.

Kanapilly, G. M.: Alveolar microenvironment and its relationship to the retention and transport into blood of aerosols deposited in the alveoli. *Health Phys.*, 32:89–100, 1977.

Kanapilly, G. M.; Raabe, O. G.; Goh, C. H. T.; and Chimenti, R. A.: Measurement of *in vitro* dissolution of aerosol particles for comparison to *in vivo* dissolution in the lower respiratory tract after inhalation. *Health Phys.*, 24:497–507, 1973.

Kapanci, Y.; Weibel, E. R.; Kaplan, H. P.; and Robinson, F. R.: Pathogenesis and reversibility of the pulmonary lesions of oxygen toxicity in monkeys. II. Ultrastructural and morphometric studies. *Lab. Invest.*, 20:101–18, 1969.

Karol, M. H.: Concentration-dependent immunologic response to toluene diisocyanate (TDI) following inhalation exposure. *Toxicol. Appl. Pharmacol.*, 68:229–41, 1983.

Karol, M. H.; Kamat, S. R.; Rubanoff, B.; Gangal, S.; and Taskar, S.: Immunologic investigation of methyl isocyanate antibodies in Bhopal victims. *Fifth Congress on Indian Respiratory Medicine,* Jaipur, India, 1985.

Kessler, G.-F.; Austin, J. H. M.; Graf, P. D.; Gamsu, G.; and Gold, W. M.: Airway constriction in experimental asthma in dogs: tantalum bronchographic studies. *J. Appl. Physiol.*, 35:703–708, 1973.

Kilburn, K. H.: Clearance mechanisms in the respiratory tract. In Lee, D. H. K.; Falk, H. L.; Murphy, S. D.; and Geiger, S. R. (eds.): *Handbook of Physiology, Section 9: Reactions to Environmental Agents.* American Physiological Society, Bethesda, Md., 1977, pp. 243–62.

Kliment, V.: Similarity and dimensional analysis. Evaluation of aerosol deposition in the lungs of laboratory animals and man. *Folia Morphol. (Warsaw)*, 21:59–69, 1973.

Lippmann, M.: "Respirable" dust sampling. *Am. Ind. Hyg. Assoc. J.*, 31:138–59, 1970.

————: Filter media for air sampling. In *Air Sampling Instruments for Evaluation of Atmospheric Contaminants*, 4th ed., pp. N2–N21. American Conference of Governmental Industrial Hygienists, 1972.

————: Regional deposition of particles in the human respiratory tract. In Lee, D. H. K.; Falk, H. L.; Murphy, S. D.; and Geiger, S. R. (eds.): *Handbook of Physiology. Section 9: Reactions to Environment Agents.* American Physiological Society, Bethesda, Md., 1977, pp. 213–32.

Lippmann, M.; Albert, R. E.; and Peterson, H. T.: Regional deposition of inhaled aerosols in man. In Walton, W. H. (ed.): *Inhaled Particles and Vapours.* Unwin, Old Woking, Surrey, England, 1971, pp. 105–20.

Lundgren, D. A.: An aerosol sampler for determination of particle concentration as a function of size and time. *J. Air Pollut. Control Assoc.*, 17:225–28, 1967.

MacFarland, H. N.: Design and operational characteristics of inhalation exposure equipment—a review. *Fund. Appl. Toxicol.*, 3:603–13, 1983.

Mercer, T. T.: On the role of particle size in the dissolution of lung burdens. *Health Phys.*, 13:1211–21, 1967.

————: *Aerosol Technology in Hazard Evaluation.* Academic Press, Inc., New York, 1973.

Mercer, T. T.; Tillery, M. I.; and Newton, G. J.: A multistage, low flow rate cascade impactor. *J. Aerosol Sci.*, 1:9–15, 1970.

Miller, F. J.; Menzel, D. B.; and Coffin, D. L.: Similarity between man and laboratory animals in regional pulmonary deposition of ozone. *Environ. Res.*, 17:84–101, 1978.

Morrow, P. E.: Alveolar clearance of aerosols. *Arch. Intern. Med.*, 131:101–108, 1973.

Morrow, P. E.; Gibb, F. R.; and Gazioglu, K. M.: A study of particulate clearance from the human lungs. *Am. Rev. Respir. Dis.*, 96:1209–21, 1967.

Muggenburg, B. A.; Felicetti, S. A.; and Silbaugh, S. A.: Removal of inhaled radioactive particles by lung lavage—a review. *Health Phys.*, 33:213–20, 1977.

Nagahi, C.: *Functional Anatomy and Histology of the Lung.* University Park Press, Baltimore, MD, 1972.

National Academy of Sciences: *Nickel.* Series: Medical and Biological Effects of Environmental Pollutants. NAS-NRC, Washington, D.C., 1975.

Nelson, G. O.: *Controlled Test Atmospheres: Principles and Techniques.* Ann Arbor Sci. Pub., Ann Arbor, Mich., 1971.

Patrick, G., and Stirling, C.: The retention of particles in large airways of the respiratory tract. *Proc. R. Soc. London Ser. B.*, 198:455–62, 1977.

Phalen, R. F.: Inhalation exposure of animals. *Environ. Health Perspect.*, 16:17–24, 1976.

Phalen, R. F.; Yeh, H.-C.; Raabe, O. G.; and Velasquez, D. J.: Casting the lungs *in-situ*. *Anat. Rec.*, 177:255–64, 1973.

Pump, K. K.: The morphology of the finer branches of the bronchial tree of the human lung. *Dis. Chest*, 46:379–98, 1964.

Quinlan, M. F.; Salman, S. D.; Swift, D. L.; Wagner, H. N., Jr.; and Proctor, D. F.: Measurement of mucociliary function in man. *Am. Rev. Respir. Dis.,* **99**:13–23, 1969.

Raabe, O. G.: Generation and characterization of aerosols. In Hanna, M. G., Jr.; Nettesheim, P.; and Gilbert, J. R. (eds): *Inhalation Carcinogenesis.* Proceedings of a Biology Division, Oak Ridge National Laboratory, Conference. U.S. Atomic Energy Commission, Oak Ridge, Tenn., 1970, pp. 123–72.

Raabe, O. G.; Bennick, J. E.; Light, M. E.; Hobbs, C. H.; Thomas, R. L.; and Tillery, M. I.: An improved apparatus for acute inhalation exposure of rodents to radioactive aerosols. *Toxicol. Appl. Pharmacol.,* **26**:264–73, 1973.

Rampe, L. W.: Generating and controlling atmospheres in inhalation chambers. In Gralla, E. J. (ed.): *Scientific Considerations in Monitoring and Evaluating Toxicological Research.* Hemisphere Publishing Corp., Washington, D.C., 1981, pp. 57–69.

Rose, M. S.; Lock, E. A.; Smith, L. L.; and Wyatt, I.: Paraquat accumulation: tissue and species specificity. *Biochem. Pharmacol.,* **25**:419–23, 1976.

Schreider, J. P., and Raabe, O. G.: Anatomy of the nasal-pharyngeal airway of experimental animals. *Anat. Rec.,* **200**:195–205, 1981.

Sinclair, D., and Hinchliffe, L.: Production and measurement of submicron aerosols. II. In Mercer, T. T.; Morrow, P. E.; and Stöber, W. (eds.): *Assessment of Airborne Particles.* Charles C Thomas Pub., Springfield, Ill., 1972.

Sorokin, S. P.: A morphologic and cytochemical study of the great alveolar cell. *J. Histochem. Cytochem.,* **14**:884–97, 1967.

Sorokin, S. P., and Brain, J. D.: Pathways of clearance in mouse lungs exposed to iron oxide aerosols. *Anat. Rec.,* **181**:581–626, 1975.

Task Group on Lung Dynamics, Committee II of the International Radiological Protection Commission: Deposition and retention models for internal dosimetry of the human respiratory tract. *Health Phys.,* **12**:173–207, 1966.

Taylor, A. E., and Gaar, K. A., Jr.: Estimation of equivalent pore radii of pulmonary capillary and alveolar membranes. *Am. J. Physiol.,* **218**:1133–40, 1970.

von Hayek, H.: *The Human Lung.* Hafner, New York, 1960.

Weibel, E. R.: *Morphometry of the Human Lung.* Academic Press, Inc., New York, 1963.

Weill, H.; George, R.; Schwarz, M.; and Ziskind, M.: Late evaluation of pulmonary function after acute exposure to chlorine gas. *Am. Rev. Respir. Dis.,* **99**:374–79, 1969.

West, J. B.: *Ventilation/Blood Flow and Gas Exchange.* Blackwell, Oxford, 1970.

———: *Respiratory Physiology—The Essentials.* Williams & Wilkins Co., Baltimore, 1974.

———: *Pulmonary Pathophysiology—The Essentials.* Williams & Wilkins Co., Baltimore, 1977.

Chapter 13

TOXIC RESPONSES OF THE CENTRAL NERVOUS SYSTEM

Stata Norton

INTRODUCTION

The central nervous system (CNS) is protected from toxicants by the blood-brain barrier. The "barrier" is a functional concept based on observations that some substances that enter and affect many of the soft tissues of the body, such as liver, kidney, and muscle, are excluded from the brain. Not all substances are preferentially excluded from the brain; for example, most anesthetics, analgesics, and tranquilizers penetrate readily. Nonpolar, lipid-soluble compounds usually penetrate the blood-brain barrier, while highly polar compounds tend to be excluded. In the immature brain, the barrier is generally not as effective, and toxic doses of some compounds, such as inorganic lead salts, may accumulate in the CNS of children, while the adult develops marked effects on the peripheral nervous system instead. Because of specificity of this kind in regard to uptake of substances in the brain, there is a considerable amount of research and speculation regarding the anatomic features that relate to the functional barrier.

Three concepts have received major consideration (Bondareff, 1965; Kuhlenbeck, 1970). One theory is that the blood-brain barrier may be due to the presence of glial cells. Much of the brain capillary endothelium is invested with astrocytic processes, and these present a barrier to free access of substances to the neurons in many places. In some brain areas, such as the median eminence of the hypothalamus and the area postrema of the fourth ventricle, the capillaries are not wrapped with glial processes and substances can reach the neurons more readily. Another theory is that unique properties of brain endothelial cells may constitute a barrier. Zonulae occludentes are structures joining blood capillary endothelial cells together to form tight junctions that are impermeable to many large molecules. However, small molecules may penetrate to the neuron through the junctions and through the cytoplasm of the endothelial cells and glia. In addition to the barrier presented by tight junctions, the endothelial cells in the CNS have other special properties. Normal endothelial cells lack pinocytotic vesicles in their cytoplasm and pores in the luminal endothelial membrane, which are present in capillaries in other tissues (Hirano *et al.*, 1978). These pinocytotic vesicles may appear in the endothelial cells of the CNS in various pathologic conditions in which the permeability of the blood-brain barrier is increased. The vesicles may transport some chemicals across the endothelial lining of small blood vessels in the CNS. When blood-brain barrier permeability is increased, some proteins (e.g., horseradish peroxidase) or chemicals combined with protein (e.g., Evans blue dye bound to albumin) may be observed in these intracellular vesicles (Westergaard *et al.*, 1977). Conditions that are known to increase vesicles are postirradiation brain edema (Cervós-Navarro and Rozas, 1978), ischemia (Welsh and O'Connor, 1978), and hypertension (Hazama, *et al.*, 1978).

The concept that the extracellular space may act as a barrier is also worthy of consideration. The extracellular basement membrane between the endothelial cells of the capillary and the glia and neurons is an ordered fibrillar mucoprotein structure and may have unique properties, as it does in the kidney, allowing it to serve as a "sieve" to transport molecules needed for cell nutrition and to regulate electro-osmotic flow of water while excluding other substances.

In the peripheral nervous system (PNS) the blood-neural barrier is present in some places and absent in others. The details of areas of the nervous system in which a barrier is absent are given in Table 13–1. In both the central and peripheral nervous system fenestrated epithelial cells have been found in areas that are permeable to large molecules such as horseradish peroxidase. The susceptibility of these barrier-free

Table 13–1. REGIONS OF THE NERVOUS SYSTEM THAT HAVE A DEFICIENT BARRIER AS MEASURED BY PENETRATION OF MACROMOLECULES

AREA	REFERENCES
Central Nervous System	
Median eminence with arcuate nucleus	Reese and Brightman, 1968
Median preoptic region	Brightman and Reese, 1969
Choroid plexus Area postrema	Olsson and Hossman, 1970
Peripheral Nervous System	
Dorsal root ganglia Autonomic ganglia	Brierley, 1955 Olsson, 1968 Jacobs *et al.*, 1976 Jacobs, 1977

areas to some toxic substances compared with the greater resistance of other areas of the central nervous system has been proposed to be due to differences in ease of penetration of the toxicant through the spaces between the epithelial cells (Jacobs *et al.*, 1976; Jacobs, 1977; Olney *et al.*, 1977).

Even those toxic substances which can penetrate brain tissue do not affect equally all of the cell types in the brain. Different brain areas usually have different sensitivities to toxicants, reflecting unique biochemistry of the cells as well as differences in degree of vascularization of brain areas. The three kinds of glial cells in the brain differ in their roles in the CNS and in their sensitivities to toxic agents. Astrocytes are closely associated with neurons in gray matter and have been called the nurse cells of neurons because they are thought to be essential in maintaining the stable microenvironment needed for neuronal function. The oligodendrocyte in the CNS has a role similar to that of the peripheral Schwann cell and invests neuronal axons with spiral wrappings of myelin. Microglia are phagocytic cells with primary functions resembling peripheral leukocytes. The role of the microglia in response to toxicants has not been widely investigated.

Although the brain is a highly vascularized organ, not all portions are equally supplied with blood. The variation in degree of vascularization accounts for some of the variation in sensitivity of brain areas to hypoxia. For example, the globus pallidus is more poorly vascularized than the cerebral cortex (hence the name, pallidus) but has about the same density of cell bodies in the tissue. In the adult brain, white matter is generally less vascularized than gray matter (Friede,

1966), but the lower oxygen requirement of the myelinated axons, which make up much of the white matter, makes white matter generally less sensitive than gray matter with its high cell body-to-neuropil ratio.

Apart from known differences in distribution of blood capillaries in the brain, there are other unique differences that account for variation in response of anatomic areas to toxicants. Some of these differences may be due to functional demands on cells. It has been proposed that excitatory amino acids may damage hypothalamic neurons by causing excessive stimulation and metabolic exhaustion of the cells (Olney, 1971). Quantitative differences in essential cell components may make one cell type more sensitive than another type. Small neurons, such as granule cells in the cerebellum and visual cortex, are preferentially killed when the whole brain is exposed to methyl mercury. The amount of cytoplasm and rough endoplasmic reticulum, which binds mercury, is less than in larger cells, and thus the small cells may be more likely to be overwhelmed by the effects of mercury (Jacobs *et al.*, 1977).

Studies of the microchemistry of the brain reinforce concepts of the diversity of structure of different areas. High concentrations of norepinephrine, serotonin, acetylcholine, and dopamine are found in various pathways of the phylogenetic "old brain," including the hypothalamus, reticular formation, basal ganglia, and limbic system. However, experimental techniques are not yet sophisticated enough to allow generalizations to be made regarding the role of brain structures and amine levels in specific functions.

Certain large cells in the central nervous system, such as cortical and hippocampal pyramidal cells, cerebellar Purkinje cells, and motor cells in the ventral horn of the spinal cord, have unusually large nuclei and the DNA is largely present as euchromatin, the form of chromatin most closely associated with transcription (Arrighi, 1974). These cells often have several nucleoli. All these structural differences point to high metabolic activity in these cells and thus increased susceptibility to anoxic damage. In fact, anoxia, in the presence of functional activity such as occurs in epileptic convulsions, is known to damage these cells (Chason, 1971).

The preceding considerations can be summarized to suggest the principle that governs responses of elements of the nervous system to toxicants: selective damage to one or more areas or components is achieved by selective exposure due to differences in ease of penetration to some cells through barriers, by selective anoxia via differences in blood flow and metabolic requirements of some elements, or by selective sensitivity resulting from qualitative or quantitative chemical differences in cell components. Identification of the selective nature of the damage from toxic agents is essential in determination of mechanism of action of toxicants but also has further value in analyzing the relation of brain structure to function.

STRUCTURAL TOXICITY

General Responses of Cells to Injury

When cells are damaged by exposure to toxic chemicals either by direct contact with the chemical or by secondary effects such as anoxia subsequent to diminished oxygen supply, some similar effects are observed. These effects are swelling of the cell and cytoplasmic organelles dispersion of the rough endoplasmic reticulum (RER), and swelling of the nucleolus. The changes are accompanied by decreases in cytoplasmic pH, in activity of oxidative enzyme systems, and in synthesis of protein and other cell components. Differences in response relate more to quantitative differences in amount and rate of change in organelles of different cell types than to qualitative differences. Thus, it has been pointed out (Scarpelli and Trump, 1971) that cells with little capacity for anaerobic metabolism but with rapid ionic shifts through the external membrane, such as myocardial cells and neurons, are susceptible during anoxia to rapid edema from the loss of integrity of the cell membrane. On the other hand, liver cells, exposed to carbon tetrachloride, will first show changes in the endoplasmic reticulum, diminished protein synthesis, and lipid accumulation. However, both the electrically excitable cells and liver cells will show both types of injury responses over a period of hours.

The neuron is a cell that has little capability for anaerobic metabolism and a high metabolic rate. The oxygen consumption of neurons is ten times higher than the oxygen consumption of glia (Ruščák et al., 1968). This combination of metabolic conditions puts the neuron at more risk than glial cells from anoxia. Neuronal damage starts within a few minutes after cessation of blood flow to the brain, and death of some neurons occurs before complete cessation of oxygen or glucose transport. Certain cells are more sensitive to anoxia than others. The sequence of vulnerability can be described in order of decreasing sensitivity: neurons, oligodendrocytes, astrocytes, microglia, and cells of the capillary endothelium.

Three types of anoxia are generally recognized: anoxic, ischemic, and cytotoxic.

Anoxic Anoxia. Primary oxygen lack (also called anoxic anoxia, which is a rather awkward term) is a term applied to inadequate oxygen supply in the presence of adequate blood flow. Such a primary condition can result from direct interference with respiration by toxic substances. For example, neuromuscular blocking agents, such as d-tubocurarine chloride, can cause respiratory paralysis by interference with the action of acetylcholine, the chemical transmitter at the neuromuscular junction. Respiratory paralysis can cause death of some neurons because of failure of oxygenation of blood. Circulation of blood to the brain is not prevented in respiratory failure, except as the eventual result of cardiac failure from continued anoxia. If respiration is restored before cardiovascular failure occurs, neurons in the CNS that are sensitive to anoxia may be destroyed without death of the organism. However, inadequate oxygen supply can also result from interference with the oxygen-carrying capacity of blood. Examples are the production of carboxyhemoglobin by carbon monoxide and methemoglobin by nitrites.

Ischemic Anoxia. This results from a decrease in arterial blood pressure to a level below that which supplies the brain adequately with oxygen. Ischemic anoxia differs from anoxic anoxia in that stagnation of the blood in the brain leads to an inadequate supply of needed substances and an accumulation of metabolic products such as lactic acid, ammonia, and inorganic phosphate. Cardiac arrest from toxic substances is one obvious cause of inadequate blood flow. Increased venous pressure in cardiac failure is an additional complication. Reduced cerebral blood flow, is, of course, not limited to cardiac failure. Extreme hypotension from vasodilation, particularly if the head is elevated, can also cause brain ischemia. Hemorrhage or thrombosis of cerebral vessels causes local ischemic anoxia of the brain areas supplied by these vessels and may further complicate the consequences of toxicants.

Cytotoxic Anoxia. Cytotoxic anoxia is a consequence of interference with cell metabolism in the presence of an adequate supply of both blood and oxygen. Cytotoxic anoxia may result from hypoglycemia, produced, for example, by an excess of insulin, or it may result from metabolic inhibitors such as cyanide, azide, dinitrophenol, malononitrile, and methionine sulfoximine. In contrast to the great susceptibility of the neurons of the adult brain to ischemic and anoxic anoxia, it is the oligodendroglia that are more susceptible to injury from repeated episodes of hypoglycemia or repeated toxic doses of metabolic inhibitors. In addition to producing cytotoxic anoxia, some of these agents may also produce ischemic anoxia; these combined effects are discussed later in more detail.

Effects of Anoxia. When a cell is damaged by acutely developing anoxia, a rapid sequence of changes is observed. The following description is characteristic of ischemic anoxia or the condition in which an aerobic cell with an electrically excitable membrane is deprived of glucose and oxygen and removal of metabolic products via blood flow is prevented. It is presumed that lesser degrees of anoxia and greater energy reserves in the cell would be reflected in variations in the intensity and type of change.

Early ischemic changes are seen in mitochondria and the cytoplasmic sap. These are related to the loss of oxidative enzyme activity with decreased ATP, decreased ATP synthesis, increased glycolysis, and decreased glycogen. As a consequence, the activity of the energy-dependent sodium pump in the cell membrane decreases and the neuron starts to pick up water. As intracellular lactate increases, the pH of the cell drops, resulting in clumping of nuclear chromatin. Loss of mitochondrial granules and slight clumping of the nuclear chromatin can be seen by the electron microscope in the first five minutes of ischemia (Trump and Arstila, 1975). The diminished activity in oxidative and phosphate-releasing enzymes can be attributed also to changes in cytoplasmic pH and ionic strength (Robinson *et al.*, 1975). The continual increase in intracellular sodium ion and influx of water results in swelling of the cell body, lysosomes, and mitochondria and dilation of the rough endoplasmic reticulum (Trump and Arstila, 1975). All of these rapid changes are diagrammed in Figure 13–1.

The second-phase changes in anoxic neurons have been known in detail for many years and have been called Spielmeyer's triad of late ischemic neuronal changes: (1) shrinkage of cell cytoplasm, (2) disappearance of Nissl substance, and (3) nuclear pyknosis with loss of nucleolar detail. These changes occur both *in vivo* (Brierley *et al.*, 1971) and in cell cultures *in vitro*. Vanderhaeghen and Logan (1971), on the basis of *in vitro* studies, have proposed that Spielmeyer's late ischemic changes accompany the development of an alkaline intracellular pH during recovery from anoxia. That is, the shift in pH from acidic, during the early phases of anoxia, to alkaline reflects a recovery from anaerobic glycolysis with its accumulation of lactic acid and other intermediary metabolites in the early phase, to a phase characterized by a pH of approximately 7.4 associated with adequate aerobic metabolism. This shift in pH can explain the characteristic disappearance of Nissl substance

in injured neurons. Nissl substance is composed of endoplasmic reticulum and fine granules containing ribonucleic acid (RNA) (Palay and Palade, 1955). Disappearance of RNA may be related to the activation of a polynucleotidase, alkaline ribonuclease type II, at the time of restoration of an alkaline pH, following an acidic pH phase during which some damage must have occurred.

There are two responses of cells in the CNS that result in brain edema. The acute, neuronal response to hypoxia has just been described. Although astrocytes are resistant cells, relative to neurons, cerebral edema resulting from swelling of astrocytes may occur as a response to brain hypoxia with accumulation of lactate, ammonia, and inorganic phosphate. The early hypoxic changes found in astrocytes have been proposed, as with neurons, to be a consequence of the acidosis resulting from anaerobic glycolysis. The astrocyte may respond in a manner similar to that of the extracellular space of other tissue (deRobertis, 1963). According to this theory, brain edema following hypoxia may be due to increased fluid accumulation inside the astrocytes rather than to accumulation of fluid in spaces between cells.

Although the changes described above refer to effects of anoxia, these changes have been dwelt on because the toxic responses of cells to chemical agents are often remarkably similar to responses to anoxia. This is not entirely unexpected since any toxic substance that interferes with glucose metabolism, ATP synthesis, or protein synthesis or that acts directly on cell membranes to affect permeability would be affecting cell metabolism at one or another place in the system that maintains the integrity of the cell.

Chronic Changes in Cell Organelles. Intracellular changes in response to toxic agents may be chronic rather than acute. For example, changes may slowly occur in the fibrous skeleton of the cell (the microtubules, about 240 Å in diameter, and neurofibrils, 40 to 100 Å in diameter). Both these structures are abundant in neurons and glia, and they may be functionally associated with transport of substances in axons and other cell processes (Schlaepfer, 1971). Toxic responses to some agents such as mitotic inhibitors result in development of intracellular neurofibrillar tangles. For example, intracisternal injection of vincristine or colchicine produces neurofibrillar tangles in neurons in experimental animals. Patients receiving the vinca alkaloids in leukemia therapy may also develop these changes (Shelanski and Wiśniewski, 1969). In some chronic disease states, such as Alzheimer's disease, the tangles consist primarily of double-stranded helices of 100-Å filaments

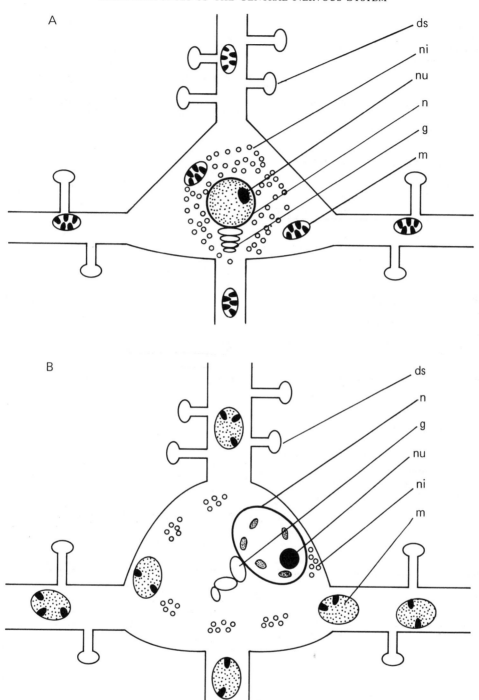

Figure 13–1. Anoxic changes in neurons. *A*. Normal neuron: *ds*, dendritic spine; *ni*, Nissl substance (RER); *nu*, nucleolus; *n*, nucleus; *g*, Golgi substance; *m*, mitochondrion. *B*. Anoxic neuron: swelling of dendritic spines, mitochondria, nucleus, nucleolus, and Golgi substance; clumping of chromatin in the nucleus (pyknosis) and dispersion of Nissl substance (chromatolysis). Lysosomes (not shown) also swell.

(Crapper *et al.*, 1976). The relationship of these cell inclusions to altered function is not known. Weakness and paralysis can develop in animals and patients treated with mitotic inhibitors, and it has been suggested that damage to these tubular cytoplasmic organelles may result in failure of protein synthesis or transport of essential substances to the terminals of cell axons in the peripheral nervous system (PNS).

Responses of the Immature and Mature Nervous System

In addition to the selective sensitivity of different cell types in the nervous system, certain anatomic areas are more prone to damage than other areas. Some of the sites that have been identified with damage from toxic substances are listed in Figures 13–2 and 13–3. Often when an anatomically delineated area is damaged, the location of the damage follows the anatomic boundaries so that it is appropriate to speak of damage to the globus pallidus, hippocampus, etc. For a description of the anatomic and functional relationship of defined areas in the brain, an extensive literature is available. General information can be found in reference texts such as the one by Crosby and coauthors (1962).

Two explanations have been suggested for the selective sensitivity of different brain areas to toxic substances. Spielmeyer in 1922 proposed that differences in vascular distribution are such that some areas of the brain are uniquely sensitive to altered blood flow. The Vogts, also in 1922, contended that there exist differences in neuronal composition, metabolism, or function that do not depend on differences in vascular supply and that determine sensitivity to toxic states. Although it is apparent that both concepts are involved in toxic reactions of the nervous system, there is convincing evidence that the response to many substances must depend on unique neuronal biochemistry and function apart from regional vascular patterns. A distinction must also be made in regard to the degree of maturity of the nervous system at the time of exposure. In some animals, humans included, where the young are born with a relatively immature nervous system, the pattern of neonatal toxic damage may differ from that of the mature nervous system. Major differences in cell structure and sensitivity are related to the degree of development of the blood-brain barrier, the degree of myelination of tracts (oligodendroglial or Schwann cell investiture of axonal processes), the degree of arborization of dendritic and axonal processes, and the extent of development of blood capillaries.

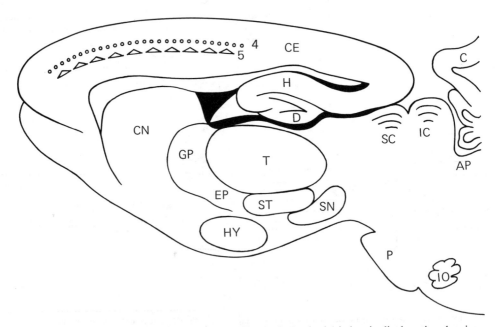

Figure 13–2. Diagram of representative mammalian brain (rat brain) in longitudinal section showing areas referred to in text. *CE*, cerebral cortex with layer 4 granule cells and layer 5 pyramidal cells; *C*, cerebellum; *H*, hippocampus with *D*, fascia dentata (dentate gyrus); basal ganglia (*CN*, caudate nucleus; *GP*, globus pallidus; and *EP*, entopeduncular nucleus); *T*, thalamus; *SC*, superior colliculus; *IC*, inferior colliculus; *AP*, area postrema; *ST*, subthalamus; *SN*, substantia nigra; *HY*, hypothalamus; *P*, pons; *IO*, inferior olivary nucleus.

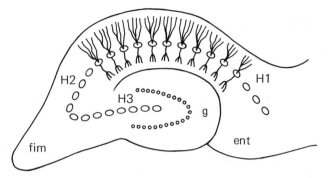

Figure 13–3. Diagram of representative mammalian hippocampus with pyramidal cell areas (*H1, H2, H3*) labeled with the terminology of Rose (1927) for human hippocampus. Comparable areas for the rodent brain are *H1* (*CA1*); *H2* (*CA3*); *H3* (*CA4*); *g*, granule cells; *fim*, fimbria; *ent*, entorhinal area.

Immature Nervous System. In the immature brain the pattern of lesions in anoxic anoxia differs from the lesions in metabolic disturbances (cytotoxic anoxia). The cerebral neocortex and the cerebellum are often unaffected in experimental neonatal anoxia under conditions when the neonatal somatic afferents and many diencephalic areas are severely affected. In the immature brain, anoxic encephalopathy may result in extensive damage to the brainstem as well as to sensory relay nuclei (lateral thalamic atrophy) but with apparent sparing of the neocortex. The basal ganglia and hippocampus commonly show damage (Windle, 1963). However, the neocortex can be damaged under conditions of partial asphyxia where blood supply is maintained in the presence of low oxygen (Myers, 1973). Results from several lines of investigation have led to the concept that the maintenance of some blood flow and a supply of glucose but with lack of oxygen may result in a lower pH than lack of oxygen and glucose (Ljunggren *et al.*, 1974). Under these conditions both the immature neocortex and basal ganglia may be damaged, the latter particularly when an episode of total ischemia follows partial ischemia (Myers, 1975).

As in the adult, interference with glucose metabolism affects the cerebral cortex, cerebellar folia, and hippocampus (especially area H_1). Bilirubin encephalopathy (kernicterus) affects areas that are often resistant to anoxic anoxia: globus pallidus, fascia dentata, and area H_2 of the hippocampus (Malamud, 1963). The subthalamus is also affected, and the superior olivary nucleus is often involved. A complex progression of behavioral effects has been described, related to some of these types of damage. (For a discussion of prenatal toxicity, see Chapter 7.)

Mature Nervous System. The mature nervous system can be distinguished from the immature nervous system in that the cells most sensitive to oxygen lack are neurons in the cerebral cortex, cerebellar cortex, and hippocampus. In the cerebral cortex, neurons of the fourth layer, which has major afferent connections from the sensory systems, are the ones commonly damaged in severe anoxia (Scholz, 1953). These sensitive neurons are small granule cells. Small cells in layer 5 may also be lost following anoxia. Large motor pyramidal cells are more resistant. In the cerebellar cortex the decreasing order of sensitivity is Purkinje cells, granule cells, and then Golgi cells (Scholz, 1959). In the hippocampus the pyramidal cells of field H_1 are most sensitive, followed by H_3 and the granular layer of the fascia dentata. In general, cells that are rich in cell processes with small cell bodies are especially vulnerable to anoxia, whereas motor cells with long axons and fewer processes are less sensitive (Jacob, 1963). With prolonged anoxia the adult may show damage to the basal ganglia and the associated subthalamic nucleus and substantia nigra. Ischemia with rapid cessation of blood flow is likely to result in a brainstem pattern of damage involving the inferior colliculus and inferior and superior olivary nuclei. Repeated episodes of anoxia usually result in damage to white matter. (See Figures 13–2 and 13–3 for general localization of the anatomic areas in the brain affected by anoxia.)

Reversibility of Damage

The principal event in irreversible damage to the nervous system can be described simply as neuronal death, since these differentiated cells cannot divide and be replaced. However, normal function may be restored for an individual even after considerable damage from exposure of the nervous system to toxic substances. Redundancy of function in a population of neurons and plasticity of organization are the methods by which restoration of function is presumed to occur after the death of some neurons. When some neurons die, other cells already having the same function may be adequate to maintain normal activity, or, failing this, other neurons may acquire the needed function. In situations where neither course is possible, for example in extensive damage to a specialized population of neurons or brain nucleus, then some loss of function must result.

Some degree of recovery of function usually occurs after nonfatal neurotoxic reactions. When cell death is not involved, the neurotoxic reaction lasts only until the toxic agent is removed or biotransformed or until cell constituents altered by the toxic event have regenerated. Reversible toxic reactions are often associated with toxicants but also occur after therapeutic administration of drugs. From this point of view, neurotoxicity could be considered to include all undesired nervous system effects of drugs or other chemicals. However, it is probable that many reversible toxic changes occurring in neurons or glial cells during therapeutic use of drugs may be closely related to the mechanisms of therapeutic activity. For example, the synaptic clefts between axons and dendrites of neurons are considered to be especially vulnerable to exogenous chemicals carried by the bloodstream, since the postsynaptic membrane is the site of receptors for chemical transmitters in the nervous system. Many psychoactive drugs are thought to cause psychic changes by altering neuronal transmission. This may involve blocking the access of normal chemical transmitters to postsynaptic receptors, acting as false transmitters, or affecting concentrations of transmitters through effects on synthesis, storage, release, reuptake, or enzymatic inactivation mechanisms. These effects are proposed to occur in areas of the CNS in which specific transmitter mechanisms are involved, that is, the anatomic areas in the brain that normally have high concentrations of some biogenic amines, particularly serotonin, norepinephrine, dopamine, acetylcholine, and gamma amino butyric acid. Examples of compounds presumed to act therapeutically by altering neurotransmitters are monoamine oxidase inhibitors, cholinesterase inhibitors, reserpine, phenothiazines, and L-DOPA. Other drugs, such as general anesthetics, appear to affect neurons generally, probably through a reversible effect on electrically excitable neuronal membranes.

The functional state of the CNS called "general depression" commonly results from overexposure to many solvents used in industrial operations. A state in which awareness or consciousness of workers is impaired is clearly a matter of concern, even though the effect may be completely reversible on removal of the worker from the exposure. Many fat solvents, like alcohol, either inhaled or ingested cause "general depression," characterized initially by drowsiness, difficulty in concentrating, and mood changes and progressing to slurred speech, ataxia, and disorientation followed by loss of consciousness. These effects mimic the effects of general anesthetics and may well have the same mechanism of action.

To the extent that reversible toxicity differs only quantitatively from therapeutic actions of drugs, these effects are appropriately discussed in numerous reviews and books on the subject of neuropharmacology.

FUNCTIONAL TOXICITY

The functioning of the nervous system in the presence of damage from toxic agents is obviously both of great importance and complexity. The nervous system possesses considerable redundancy of structure, which may mask functional change until the reserve capacity of the system is exceeded by the amount of damage. The nervous system is also capable of developing tolerance or adapting to some types of damage; hence function may return to normal during continuous exposure to a toxic substance. Thus damage may exist in the nervous system that can be detected by cytologic or neurochemical methods when functional damage is not detected. On the other hand, alterations in gait, visual-motor performance, emotional state, and many other behavioral parameters may, at times, be the earliest and most sensitive signs of nervous system toxicity. In the subsequent discussion the alterations in behavior that can occur as consequences of toxic damage to the nervous system are divided into alterations of the sensory, motor, and integrative functions of the nervous system.

Examples will be given in which motor functions are directly affected, such as peripheral neuropathies. Sensory functions, such as vision, may be damaged at various sites along the pathway from the sensory receptor to the cortex. Integrative processes, which are important and poorly understood functions of information processing by the brain, can be the functions primarily altered. Learning and memory are included in this group. Emotional components of behavior may be disturbed. It should be noted that when behavior is evaluated, it is difficult to examine the effects of toxicants on information processing apart from sensory and motor components since all behavioral tests must rely on evaluation of the output of the brain after information processing has taken place.

No analysis of the toxic effects of a chemical on the nervous system is complete without knowledge of effects on function. It might even be argued that without a functional change there is no toxicity to an organ. Such an argument ignores the equally valid concept that any irreversible change in an organ caused by an exogenous chemical is a toxic effect. The CNS differs from organs such as the liver in that neurons cannot divide once they have reached a mature state while hepatic cells retain the capacity to divide throughout the life of the organism. As an example, focal loss of a small number of granule cells in the cerebellum from a dose of methyl mercury will not be detected as locomotor changes or even as changes in fine movements. The nervous system not only has redundancy in this regard but also has the ability to compensate by adaptive mechanisms. Nevertheless, the loss of granule cells, in the above example, represents a reduction in the reserve capacity of the brain, which might well be detectable if additional demands were placed on the system.

As a generalization a distinction can be made between pharmacologic and toxicologic effects. Characteristically pharmacologic effects are short lasting and completely reversible while toxicologic effects often include irreversible damage. Because of this difference and the adaptability of the nervous system to damage,

mentioned above, histopathologic studies have a place in toxicology that they do not have in pharmacology. In spite of the limitations on functional tests, they are also an integral part of the study of toxicology of the nervous system.

Five categories of nervous system function are shown in Figure 13–4. These categoreis are: sensory, motor, two integrative functions (symbol formation and sensory-motor integration), and emotional states associated with any of the other four functions. Symbol formation, including language and visual symbols, incorporates learning and memory as the terms are commonly used in behavior studies. In a broader sense learning occurs in all integrative systems in Figure 13–4, perhaps to varying degrees. In this sense it could be said that the respiratory center "learns" tolerance to morphine-induced respiratory depression or that various complex visual-motor performances such as walking are "learned."

Sensory Functions

Damage to the senses of sight and hearing, alterations in the sensations of temperature, touch, and pain, and other paresthesias result from central demyelination and peripheral neuropathies. Neuronal atrophy in the cortical lay-

Peripheral Nervous System	Central Nervous System			Peripheral Nervous System
Anatomy	Function	Anatomy	Toxicity	Anatomy
	B. Symbol formation	Cerebral cortex Hippocampus Mammillary bodies	Impaired learning and memory Confusional states	
A. Sensory pathways	C. Sensory-motor integration			E. Motor pathways
	1. Life support systems	Hypothalamus Medulla	Impaired appetite reproduction, respiration	
	2. Voluntary and involuntary movement	Pyramidal motor system Basal ganglia system Cerebellum	Dyskinesias Activity changes Ataxias	
	D. Emotional overlay	Limbic lobe	Emotional instability Psychoses	

Figure 13–4. Types of functional changes resulting from effects on anatomic areas in the CNS.

ers in specific sensory receiving areas can cause loss of sensation, such as cortical blindness, even though the remainder of the sensory pathway is intact. Lead encephalopathy and severe poisoning in children from organic mercury compounds may result in marked sensory damage, including blindness and hearing loss.

Sensory neuropathies are commonly accompanied by numbness, tingling, and hypersensitivity to touch. The selective sensory fiber toxicity from organic mercury has already been mentioned. Inorganic lead salts and organophosphorus compounds, such as triorthocresyl phosphate, cause disturbances of both sensory and motor functions. Sensory damage alone can affect motor function since damage to muscle spindle afferents can be related to ataxia without direct damage to motor fibers.

Effective methods for detection of functional damage to senses, particularly vision and hearing, have been developed. Some of the most sensitive methods use operant conditioning techniques, which require discrimination of light intensity, tone intensity, or pitch. Examples of the use of these methods can be found in work of Stebbins and coworkers (Hawkins *et al.,* 1977) on damage to the cochlea of monkeys from dihydrostreptomycin and in the work of Luschei and coworkers (1977) on peripheral vision in monkeys intoxicated with methyl mercury. Generally these methods are time consuming and difficult to carry out successfully except in the hands of experienced investigators. Tests of motor function are used conjointly to establish the integrity of the motor system since the operant tests of sensory function rely on motor movements.

An interesting possibility for evaluation of sensory thresholds in humans as well as other animals is the startle response and comparable reflexes that involve the sensory and motor systems. Although the potential of these methods has been discussed (Reiter and Ison, 1977), very few data are available on the effects of toxic substances on reflex responses to stimuli.

Electrophysiologic methods have been used to monitor sensory pathways. For example, the visual-evoked potential, recorded from the surface of the cerebral cortex in the primary sensory receiving area, is a complex wave, and the components of this wave have been studied extensively. Damage to the visual pathway can be detected as alterations in the cortical wave form (Woolley, 1976).

Motor Functions

As with sensory systems, either demyelinating processes or neuronal damage can produce motor dysfunction. In addition to substances causing mixed motor and sensory neuropathy, motor fiber demyelination alone is the primary peripheral damage produced by compounds like isonicotinic hydrazide. The functional pathology seen with damage to motor nerve axons or terminals at skeletal muscle is weakness or paralysis of the involved muscles. Unsteadiness of gait may result from muscle weakness although ataxias may also result from damage to visual-motor integration without peripheral neuropathy. Several methods are available to monitor motor function. Direct functional tests of nerve-muscle function rely on physiologic methods of recording conduction velocity or the compound action potential of peripheral nerves. Tests of conduction velocity have not proved very sensitive in detection of peripheral nerve damage because not all axons in a nerve are damaged simultaneously by a toxic chemical and the undamaged axons conduct normally. The compound action potential, which records the summed amplitudes of action potentials of all conducting fibers, is more sensitive since it will be reduced proportionately to the number of damaged fibers. However, it is a more difficult technique and is subject to more variation. Behavioral tests of complex motor movements are used and do detect muscle weakness although involvement of higher control centers is difficult to eliminate. Appropriate methods for laboratory animals are performance on a rotating rod (Kinnard and Carr, 1957; Watzman and Barry, 1968), measurement of gait (Mullenix *et al.,* 1975), or performance on a treadmill (Gibbins *et al.,* 1968).

Integrative Functions

In Figure 13–4, three categories of central nervous system function are listed; symbol formation, sensory-motor integration, and emotional state. Learning, using the term in the broad sense of adaptation, is a characteristic of all three. Therefore, functional tests related to these categories reflect damage only after the adaptive capability of the CNS has been exceeded.

Symbol Formation. Methods of measurement of memory and learning, in the restricted sense of symbolic integration of information, are of great importance in evaluation of toxic effects of chemicals on subtle behavioral parameters. When memory or learning is severely impaired, the type of functional damage may be called confusional states.

Various tests have been described that are intended to detect impairment of memory and learning ability in humans, and these tests have counterparts in animal tests. Several tests of short-term memory in brain-damaged patients have been compared (Sterne, 1969). In clinical neurologic examinations a relation between lesion size and behavioral deficit has been reported (Boller *et al.*, 1970). Maze learning may also be compared in humans and animals, and performance in visual maze learning has been shown to be altered by some kinds of organic brain damage in humans (Milner, 1965) as well as by some brain lesions and toxic substances in experimental animals (Bullock *et al.*, 1966; Brown *et al.*, 1971).

One of the best localizations of cerebral function known is in regard to memory. It has been shown that memory deficit is produced by bilateral hippocampal resection. This effect has been further specified by Barbizet (1969): "The syndrome of normal capacity of immediate memory and gradual forgetting indicates a change in the hippocampomammillary system regardless of the nature of the underlying lesion. It is not observed in cortical lesions." The coordinated pathway of memory involves: hippocampus-fornix-hypothalamus-mammillary body-mammillothalamic tract-thalamus-cortex. In this system the mammillary body is the integrating center. Lesions of the mammillary body can be produced by thiamine deficiency, both experimentally by pyrithiamine administration and in thiamine-deficiency diseases such as Wernicke's encephalopathy and Korsakoff's syndrome. Memory is impaired in these conditions.

Although there is a good correlation between experiments in animals and clinical observations regarding the anatomic substrate for memory, the general problem of correlation of behavioral effects of toxic substances in animals and humans is difficult to resolve. Many studies on "memory" and "learning" have involved tests of function that have not been related to any anatomic damage. In animal tests, in particular, the failure of animals to perform a task may be related to many phenomena other than "memory" or "learning." Investigations in animals, including humans, must test comparable functions if meaningful correlations are to be made, and this may be experimentally hard to achieve.

Sensory-Motor Integration. There are obvious difficulties in comparisons of toxic brain damage in humans and other animals since the elaboration of language and the high level of concept formation and integration in humans tend to obscure whatever exist as generalizations of these functions in the mammalian brain. However, these fundamental difficulties in the study of toxic effects are compounded by the failure to consider that brain function in humans can be included in generalization of functions of other mammals. A start has been made in setting up tests for quantitative assessment of brain

damage in various mammals, including humans. These tests need to be compared for their predictive value in different kinds of brain damage. Some of the Halstead battery of tests, the Porteus maze, the Wisconsin card-sorting test, and reaction time tests appear to be useful predictors of the amount of general cortical impairment (Sterne, 1969; Strain and Kinzie, 1969; Vega, 1969).

Some fairly simple tests can be performed that correlate anatomic damage with functional damage. For example, finger-tapping speed and pegboard speed are measures of motor impersistence (Joynt *et al.*, 1962; Vega, 1969). Preservation has been measured using a card-sorting test (Milner, 1963). Careful studies using tests of reaction time in humans have shown a correlation between the size of brain lesions and the degree of slowing of reactions (Boller *et al.*, 1970). Not only localized lesions but also general cortical atrophy, measured by enlarged cerebral ventricles, correlates with impairment of function on tests requiring visual motor performance (Chapman and Wolff, 1959; Vega and Parsons, 1967).

In viscose rayon workers exposed chronically to 20 ppm or less of carbon disulfide during working hours for more than one year, there was a reduction in conduction velocity in motor and sensory nerve (Johnson *et al.*, 1983). In the same workers, no significant changes were detected using a set of psychomotor and visual function tests (Putz-Anderson *et al.*, 1983). More work is needed to determine the most useful functional tests to detect different types of nervous system damage. Very little is known of the presumed quantitative relationship between the amount of toxic agent and degree of functional brain damage in humans or animals.

Tests that measure sensori-motor performance can be studied in animals. Since results with tests of sensori-motor performance in humans appear to correlate well with some types of brain damage, such tests should be extensively employed in animals. A simple test is general activity, measured either in a home cage or in a special apparatus. Functional damage to the CNS from carbon monoxide has been demonstrated in this way (Culver *et al.*, 1975), and the alteration in activity correlates with morphologic changes in neurons (Norton and Culver, 1977). General activity, particularly circadian activity, is a measure of sensori-motor integration although many factors may modify it. Some other tests that can be used are measures of reaction times, such as shuttlebox avoidance tests, and the measurement of performance on a rotating rod, mentioned previously under motor function. Animals can be trained to exert a constant force on a lever and alterations in performance can be measured (Falk, 1969). The latter test requires extensive equipment and training of animals. Perhaps the simplest test is measurement of body weight in a chronic experiment. It should not be forgotten that the success of an animal in maintaining general body function is dependent on adequate CNS function. In a study of chronic administration of methyl mercury, Berthoud and coworkers (1976) found that body weight was altered at low doses and proposed that "defects in food and energy regulation may provide early indications of an incipient overt intoxication." Such a finding could result from a primary effect on any one of several major organs, including the CNS.

Emotional Responses. The limbic system, specifically the hippocampus, has a low seizure threshold, and some convulsions from toxic substances may result from effects on this system. In addition to being a focus for convulsant activity, the limbic system as defined by Papez (1937) may control "emotion" or emotional behavior. Although it is to be expected that lesions in the limbic system would alter emotional behavior, precise localization of the emotional components of behavior cannot be made. One of the most specific alterations of emotional behavior by toxic substances is caused in individuals chronically exposed to low levels of inorganic mercury. The earliest sign of toxicity commonly is a change in behavior called erethism, characterized by apprehension, emotional lability, and irritability. Early signs of involvement of motor and autonomic functions of the nervous system (fine tremor and salivation) may occur with erethism. Unfortunately, the involvement of any specific portion of the CNS, such as the limbic system, has not been established since erethism in the early stages of mercury toxicity is not associated with recognized alterations in neuronal structure.

Other examples can be given in which damage to the CNS by toxic substances results in emotional changes. Sequelae from acute exposure to carbon monoxide include loss of memory, depression, and emotional instability in the postanoxic period, which may persist for several weeks in those who survive the initial episode.

The problem of alterations in rat behavior induced by chronic exposure of rats to lead salts during the perinatal period presents a classic example of the difficulty of relating behavioral data from the laboratory to the consequences of comparable human exposure to the same chemical. It has been reported that exposure of the immature rat to lead results in hyperactivity, which may be a model for childhood hyperkinesis (Sauerhoff and Michaelson, 1973) al-though this finding has been challenged (Krehbiel et al., 1976).

Marked behavioral effects in rats, such as aggressiveness and irritability, which might be expected to correspond to behavioral instability in children exposed to excessive amounts of lead, have also been reported (Sauerhoff and Michaelson, 1973). A series of tests was employed by Overmann (1977) who again reported impressions of increased aggression and other behaviors that he suggested might be interpreted as a higher level of emotionality. Although changes have been observed in rats, no tests have been done that might measure emotional changes in lead-treated rats. Part of the problem resides in the uncertainty of making such evaluations in animals and translating the findings to human behavior. There is a real need for greater use of the few tests mentioned earlier that can be directly compared in humans and other animals. Also, sensitive new tests need to be developed that will allow comparisons to be drawn between behavioral effects in humans and other animals. When such correlative methodology is available, good use can be made of animal data in predicting and understanding responses of the nervous system of man to toxic substances.

TYPES OF NERVOUS SYSTEM TOXICANTS

The following discussion of substances toxic to the nervous system centers around the compounds for which the nervous system is a major target organ. The aim has been to provide a framework covering the types of effects rather than a complete catalog of toxic substances.

It is recognized that some neurotoxicants exert their effects by causing anoxia and others have a more direct affinity for specific structures. Various classifications have been proposed (Scholz, 1953; Malamud, 1963; Windle, 1963; Brucher, 1967; Brierley et al., 1971). As is to be expected, no one classification is ideal since a substance may have more than one effect and the susceptibility of the nervous system of different animal species or even individuals of the same species can hardly be considered identical. Furthermore, any classification is subject to some error since it depends on data that are sometimes fragmentary.

The neurotoxicants described below are classified, according to their primary toxic action, in the following types:

1. Anoxic damage to gray matter (neurons and astrocytes) with variation in pattern of damage depending on which of the three types of anoxia is produced.

2. Damage to myelin from substances affecting oligodendrocytes or Schwann cells, resulting in encephalopathy if central white matter is involved or polyneuritis if peripheral cells are damaged.

3. Substances with a predilection for causing damage to axons of peripheral neurons.

4. Agents causing primary damage to perikarya of peripheral neurons.

5. Neurotoxicants causing damage to synaptic junctions of the neuromuscular system.

6. Toxic substances causing lesions restricted to specialized CNS nuclear groups.

Type 1. Agents Causing Anoxia

Type 1 anoxias may occur as mixed encephalopathies. As might be expected, these patterns of neurotoxicity are associated not only with toxic effects of chemicals, but related pathology is seen in certain neurologic disorders occurring without exposure to toxicants. For example, a rare pathologic condition called familial holotopistic striatal necrosis, which has its onset in childhood, is characterized by bilateral symmetric necrosis of the caudate nucleus and putamen that resembles the toxicity from prolonged partial anoxia. The pathogenesis has been suggested to be vascular insufficiency of the affected areas (Miyoshi et al., 1969). More severe anoxic damage from partial anoxia followed by stasis can be compared to Leigh's disease (subacute necrotizing encephalomyelopathy) (Mettler, 1972), and damage to white matter can be compared to some demyelinating diseases. See Table 13-2.

Barbiturates. Usually recovery from barbiturate coma is without neurologic deficit even after severe poisoning. In the rare case in which the patient survives for several days in a coma there may be anoxic changes with laminar cortical necrosis, damage to field H_1 of the hippocampus, and loss of Purkinje cells from the cerebellum (Slager et al., 1966). The rarity of permanent damage after barbiturate coma contrasts with the not infrequent sequelae to carbon monoxide poisoning (see below). Either carbon monoxide has a toxic effect in addition to producing anoxia, as has been suggested, or barbiturates protect the cells during anoxia, possibly by stabilizing cell membranes or reducing cell metabolism.

Carbon Monoxide. Carbon monoxide produces both cytotoxic and ischemic damage to the CNS (see Chapter 8). By combining with hemoglobin to form carboxyhemoglobin, carbon monoxide causes anoxia without primary loss of blood circulation and initially differs from acute ischemic anoxia in that the supply of glucose is not immediately reduced and removal of metabolic products is not prevented. However, prolonged exposure to carbon monoxide results in ischemic anoxic damage. In this condition, the most sensitive brain areas are the basal ganglia and subthalamus.

Repeated anoxic episodes from any mechanism tend to damage the blood-brain barrier and to cause development of a pattern of diffuse sclerosis of white matter, or leukencephalopathy, as a consequence. Repeated exposure to cytotoxic anoxia combined with ischemia from metabolic inhibitors, which also depress cardiovascular function, are particularly likely to damage the white matter of the brain.

Leukencephalopathy may occur as an additional consequence of carbon monoxide coma. In persons recovering from carbon monoxide poisoning a relapse, or delayed toxicity, has been reported (Schwedenberg, 1959; Plum et al., 1962; Lapresle and Fardeau, 1967). This second toxicity occurs not earlier than five days after a severe acute exposure. Carbon monoxide leukencephalopathy has also been produced in dogs (Preziosi et al., 1970). A similar phenomenon has been noted in a report on rats subjected to anoxia. Levine (1960) reported that "repeated episodes of histotoxic anoxia damage the brain with sufficient predilection for white matter to invite comparison with demyelinating diseases."

Although the delayed toxicity from carbon monoxide has not been studied adequately under experimental conditions, the evidence is suggestive that enough damage to the blood-brain barrier may occur in prolonged carbon monoxide coma to allow the development of an autoimmune condition responsible for the delayed toxicity. The characteristic signs of delayed toxicity in humans are of sudden onset, after apparent recovery from poisoning, and consist of behavioral changes, confusion, disorientation, fever, and neurologic disturbances (especially ataxia, rigidity resembling parkinsonism, incoordination, and weakness). The condition is progressive, with death usually resulting within a few weeks. The primary finding, unlike the signs of acute toxicity, is generalized damage to the white matter with sparing of gray matter. This can be classified as severe status spongiosus with demyelination that spares the short fibers connecting the cortical columns. Axons of neurons are also relatively intact. Generally, sparing of the lower layers of cortical neurons accompanies the sparing of the cortical short association fibers in demyelinating conditions. The resemblance of delayed toxicity caused by carbon monoxide to "disseminated or

Table 13–2. PATTERNS OF DAMAGE AND ANATOMIC AREAS OF THE NERVOUS SYSTEM AFFECTED BY VARIOUS AGENTS

Agent	GRAY MATTER TYPE 1									WHITE MATTER TYPE 2				PERIPHERAL NEUROPATHY TYPES 3, 4, 5			LOCAL AREAS TYPE 6			
	ANOXIA					PROLONGED ANOXIA														
	Cortex IV	Cortex V	Hippocampus H_1	Caudate Nucleus	Putamen	Hippocampus H_2	Fascia Dentata	Globus Pallidus	Subthalamus	Internal Capsule	Corpus Callosum	Optic Chiasm	Schwann Cells	Sensory N. Thalamus	Anterior Horn Cells	Peripheral Axons	Hippocampus H_3	Hypothalamus Ventral N.	Mammillary Body	Tegmentum
Acetylpyridine						+								+			+			
Acrylamide													+							
Azide	+		+	+	+				+	+	+	+								+
Barbiturate	+	+																		
Carbon disulfide	+			+	+								+		+					
Carbon monoxide								+	+	+	+	+								
Cyanide	+		+	+	+				+			+	+	+						+
DDT														+	+					
Glutamate															+			+		
Gold thioglucose								+										+		
Hexachlorophene											+	+								
Iminodipropionitrile														+	+					
Isoniazid										+	+	+			+					
Lead (inorganic)																				
Adults													+		+					
Children	+	+								+	+	+			+					
Malononitrile				+	+						+	+								
Manganese				+	+			+	+											
Mercury (organic)	+											+				+				
Methyl bromide	+								+							+				
Nitrogen trichloride	+	+	+	+	+	+														
Pyrithiamine																			+	+
Triethyltin										+	+	+								
Triorthocresyl phosphate																+				
Vinca alkaloids														+	+					

diffuse sclerosis" has been pointed out (Schwedenberg, 1959). The condition also can be compared to acute hemorrhagic encephalopathy, a rare occurrence in man (see description by Paterson, 1971, for comparison).

Cyanide. The cortical gray matter, hippocampus (H_1), corpora striata, and substantia nigra are commonly affected (Hicks, 1950). This distribution of the effects of cyanide is like that associated with many other conditions causing cytotoxic anoxia. Cyanide also has a propensity for damaging white matter, particularly the corpus callosum (Levine, 1967; Bass, 1968).

Cyanide inhibits cytochrome oxidase and produces cytotoxic anoxia, but also causes hypotension through its effects on the heart. It has been proposed that the lower concentration of cytochrome oxidase in white matter renders it selectively sensitive to cyanide, but this hypothesis has not been verified as yet because of the difficulties of assigning *in vitro* results obtained for a single enzyme as a sole factor in view of the potential multiplicity of reactions occurring *in vivo*.

Experimentally, delayed toxicity has been produced with cyanide (Hurst, 1952), indicating that under appropriate conditions ischemic anoxia may be produced by cyanide.

Azide. Azide, like cyanide, inhibits cytochrome oxidase and produces similar lesions (Miyoshi, 1967). As with cyanide, it has not been established that inhibition of this enzyme by azide is solely responsible for the toxicity. There is good evidence that the pattern of damage is complicated as a result of hypotension from cardiac failure. Azide-induced lesions in most species of animals are similar. Hyperkinesis is a common behavioral result (Mettler, 1972).

Nitrogen Trichloride. This compound is of historic interest as a cause of the canine "hysteria" or "running fits" that occurred as a result of feeding wheat flour bleached with agene (containing nitrogen trichloride) to dogs. The toxicity results from the formation of methionine sulfoximine *in vivo*. A similar condition has been produced in rabbits but not in humans, monkeys, or cats. In dogs, changes in the hippocampus are marked, affecting both the pyramidal layer and the fascia dentata. There is also extensive neuronal loss in the lower layers of the cerebral cortex and the Purkinje cells of the cerebellum. In the cerebral cortex the short association fibers connecting the cortical columns also degenerate. Glial alterations are not marked. The extent to which the CNS damage is a primary effect of the nitrogen trichloride or secondary to the respiratory changes associated with convulsions is not known. The dogs suffer from repeated convulsions in a behavioral sequence consisting of sitting quietly followed by ataxic walking and running, and a convulsion during which the animal becomes anoxic (Lewey, 1950; Innes and Saunders, 1962).

Type 2. Agents Damaging Myelin

Since many axons in the nervous system are myelinated, agents that selectively damage the myelin-forming cells in the central and peripheral nervous system (oligodendroglia and Schwann cells, respectively) may cause both CNS damage, concentrated on the long axons, which are usually myelinated, and peripheral damage.

Isonicotinic Acid Hydrazide (INH, Isoniazid). This compound produces severe changes in the white matter of the CNS and also produces peripheral neuropathy. Dogs, rats, and Peking ducks show similar changes in response to INH. In humans, peripheral neuritis has been reported as the major effect involving the nervous system. The peripheral changes are inhibited by administration of pyridoxine but the central changes are not (Carlton and Kreutzberg, 1966). The central changes involve predominantly the white matter. The cerebellum shows extensive spongy degeneration with vacuoles present in smaller astrocytic processes, distended extracellular spaces, vacuolated oligodendrocytes, dilated axons, and splitting of myelin layers (Lampert and Schochet, 1968a). In addition to cerebellar damage, there may be some vacuolization of cerebral gray matter. In dogs the infe-

rior olivary nucleus sometimes shows damage (Worden *et al.*, 1967).

Triethyltin. Triethyltin causes severe damage to the white matter and peripheral neuropathy. The compound is highly toxic to oligodendroglia and considerably less toxic to the neurons. Extensive edema, vacuolization, and "spongy degeneration" are produced by triethyltin intoxication. Toxic doses of triethyltin cause intramyelinic splitting throughout the CNS, including the optic nerve. Capillary permeability to trypan blue is unchanged. The excess fluid in the cortical glia and in the clefts of myelin sheaths appears to be a serum ultrafiltrate containing sodium and chloride ions and relatively little protein (Aleu *et al.*, 1963). Triethyltin is thought to exert its effect by inhibiting the ATPase normally present in glial processes and axonal tubules (Torack, 1965).

Hexachlorophene. A condition resembling the central effect of triethyltin and INH has been reported in rats fed large doses of hexachlorophene (Kimbrough and Gaines, 1971). Hexachlorophene is widely used as an antibacterial agent in soaps and antiseptic solutions. Significant blood levels have been found in human infants bathed in 3 percent aqueous solution of hexachlorophene (Curley *et al.*, 1971). Dermal absorption has also been shown to occur in rats (Kennedy *et al.*, 1976a). Dietary administration of hexachlorophene to rats results in intramyelinic vacuoles in the peripheral nerves (Pleasure *et al.*, 1974) as well as in the CNS. The most severe vacuolization in the CNS is in the white matter of the cerebellum, less severe effect in the spinal cord, and least severe in the cerebrum and brainstem (Kennedy *et al.*, 1976b). Experimentally it has been shown that synthesis of myelin is inhibited in hexachlorophene-treated animals, possibly as a result of inhibition of oxidative phosphorylation (Pleasure *et al.*, 1974).

Lead. When peripheral myelin loss predominates with relative sparing of the axons, the condition is called segmental degeneration. This is characteristic of many pathologic neuropathies that are not thought to be induced chemically, such as the Guillain-Barré syndrome, as well as some chemically induced toxic conditions, such as chronic adult lead poisoning. This condition has been reproduced experimentally. When rats are fed lead in the diet for six to seven months, most axons appear normal in the sciatic nerves but demyelination is commonly found even in the presence of normal axons (Lampert and Schochet, 1968b). Sensory findings in humans are generally minimal and the upper extremities are affected more and earlier than the lower. In adult humans, rats, and guinea pigs the primary changes from lead salts are in the Schwann cells with segmental disintegration beginning at the nodes of Ranvier (Lampert and Schochet, 1968b; Schlaepfer, 1969). Some axons may show degeneration as in INH poisoning. In guinea pigs, however, it has been shown that the primary slowing of conduction velocity in lead neuropathy is related to segmental demyelination and not to axonal degeneration. The cause of conduction delay in humans has not been determined directly.

Children are particularly susceptible to lead encephalopathy, and severe cases result in permanent cerebral damage. Nonhuman primates have been reported to develop lead encephalopathy with the same symptoms: cerebral edema, laminar necrosis, and central demyelination (Sauer et al., 1970). Impaired myelin formation in the brain has also been found in lead intoxication in immature rats.

Lead exposure during late gestational development and the early postnatal period in the rat results in reduction in the size of the hippocampus (Petit et al., 1983) and decreased concentration of synapses in the mossy fibers of hippocampal pyramids (Campbell et al., 1982). Synaptic counts in the cerebral cortex are also reduced (Bull et al., 1983).

In many ways lead resembles the calcium ion, and it may not be surprising that application of lead salts can alter neuromuscular preparations in vitro. This effect is discussed below.

Thallium.   Acute thallium intoxication in humans is relatively rare but cases of poisoning have been reported. At one time thallium salts were used to produce depilation and such use resulted in paralysis of 10 to 15 percent of persons so treated (Cavanagh et al., 1974). Neurologic signs include ataxia and painful paresthesia. Leg weakness and diminished sensation develop in severe cases. Damage to ventral horn cells and dorsal root ganglion cells is found as well as to dorsal columns in the spinal cord (Kennedy and Cavanagh, 1976). However, the general appearance of the axons indicates secondary degeneration of axons, and the damage to myelin sheaths resembles lead neuropathy (Bank et al., 1972). There is no specific antidote to thallium. However, it has been proposed that some of the effects may be the result of ability of thallium ions to substitute for potassium ions, particularly by replacing potassium in potassium-activated ATPase (Inturrisi, 1969). Exchange of potassium for thallium in Prussian blue (potassium ferric cyano-ferrate) has been proposed as the mechanism of protection of rats by Prussian blue in experimental thallium poisoning (Heydlauf, 1969).

Tellurium.   The neurotoxicity of tellurium is dramatically affected by the age of the animal. As in the case of lead, the young animal is much more susceptible to tellurium. Low doses of tellurium localize in intracellular particles identified as lysosomes of glia and neurons. There is a high incidence of hydrocephalus in the offspring of pregnant rats fed low doses of tellurium even though no damage has been demonstrated in the mother at these doses (Duckett and Scott, 1971). Mild neurologic effects have been reported in humans, particularly in workers exposed in industrial manufacturing processes to tellurium salts. Chronic exposure of rats to tellurium salts has been reported to cause muscle weakness and behavioral deficits, including difficulty in discriminating visual patterns (Dru et al., 1972).

After prolonged administration to experimental animals, tellurium has been found to be distributed diffusely throughout the gray matter. Selective damage to cell groupings in the CNS has not been correlated with behavioral effects of the compound. Hindleg paralysis develops in young rats fed a diet containing tellurium. This paralysis has been interpreted to be a consequence of peripheral neuropathy characterized by segmental demyelination from damage to Schwann cells (Lampert et al., 1970).

Type 3. Agents Causing Peripheral Axonopathies

Four sites of damage to the peripheral motor nerves can be identified. Damage to the Schwann cell or demyelination has been described above as a consequence of exposure to some toxicants. Secondary degeneration of the axon may follow demyelination. Other types of damage to the motor nerve may result from a direct effect of a toxic substance on the perikaryon, axon, or termination of the nerve at the myoneural junction. Sensory neuropathies may also result and usually damage to cells in the dorsal root ganglion can be found in sensory neuropathies. The lack of a barrier in the dorsal root ganglion comparable to the blood-brain barrier has already been mentioned.

The following group of toxic compounds contains those causing "dying-back neuropathies" in which the primary lesion is observed in the axon and damage progresses in a cephalad direction from the most distal portions of the axons. These neuropathies may develop after a prolonged exposure, as with alcohol, or after a single acute exposure, as with triorthocresylphosphate. In either case the neuropathy has a delayed onset. Increasing the dose of the toxicant can shorten the onset of axonal degeneration to some extent, but even after a serious exposure to triorthocresyl phosphate and other neurotoxic organophosphates more than a week must elapse before the onset of signs of toxicity. When myelinated nerves are examined during the development of delayed neuropathies, the development of large blebs or swollen areas on the axons is the earliest sign of damage. However, the primary biochemical lesion may not be in the axon but could originate in the perikaryon or from trophic effects subsequent to synaptic damage.

As expected, exposure to neurotoxic chemicals resulting in axonal degeneration will cause secondary degenerative changes in skeletal muscle, including altered forms of acetylcholinesterase and increased creatine phosphokinase. Muscle fiber atrophy is also seen (Cisson and Wilson, 1982).

Alcohol. Chronic intake of ethyl alcohol can result in peripheral neuropathy with axonal degeneration of motor neurons primarily in the distal segments of nerves. Schwann cells are spared. Thiamine deficiency plays a role in the development of alcoholic neuropathy (Walsh and McLeod, 1970). Because distal axonal degeneration occurs from a variety of toxic substances, and also from thiamine deficiency, it has been proposed that the primary site of altered metabolic events may not be in the axon but in the nerve cell body, with subsequent failure of axonal transport (Bradley and Asbury, 1970).

Acrylamide. Acrylamide is a vinyl monomer with numerous industrial uses. Exposure occurs by dermal absorption, by inhalation, or by oral ingestion. Polymerized acrylamide is not toxic but the monomer can cause peripheral neuropathy. Acrylamide resembles triorthocresyl phosphate in its toxic effects (Fullerton and Barnes, 1966). Triorthocresyl phosphate is described below under the group of organophosphorus compounds. Chronic exposure to acrylamide results in polyneuritis in humans, with sensory changes in the limbs, weakness, and ataxia (Auld and Bedwell, 1967; Kesson et al., 1977). Similar changes are produced in animals given acrylamide chronically. Both sensory and motor axons are affected by acrylamide, and axonal transport may be blocked. Different mechanisms may be involved in production of neuropathy from acrylamide and triorthocresyl phosphate since the latter compound does not block axonal transport of protein (Pleasure et al., 1969) (see also Vinca Alkaloids below).

Bromophenylacetylurea. Both sensory and motor fibers are damaged by p-bromophenylacetylurea. Experiments in rats have shown that there is a characteristic delay in onset of neuropathy from this compound (Cavanagh and Chen, 1971a). By the seventh day after exposure to two oral doses of p-bromophenylacetyl-

urea, changes can be found in longer and larger axons in the hind limbs with gradual progression to the forelimbs and centrally from the peripheral parts of axons (Cavanagh et al., 1968). Young rats are less sensitive than adults, an age-linked pattern present in many "dying-back" neuropathies.

Carbon Disulfide. Most toxic exposures to carbon disulfide occur in the use of the solvent in the rayon and rubber industries. Predominant nervous system effects in humans are psychosis, tremor, and polyneuritis (Lewey, 1941a; Tiller et al., 1968). Chronic exposure has been reported to produce polyneuritis in 88 percent of intoxicated individuals, including lower-extremity weakness and paresthesias (Vigliani, 1950). The condition resembles thiamine deficiency and responds to thiamine injection (see also Alcohol, above). Experimentally in dogs similar signs are seen, and lesions of the corpora striata, Purkinje cells of the cerebellum, and loss of anterior horn cells of spinal cord have been demonstrated. Axons are more affected than myelin sheaths (Lewey, 1941b). Associated with a decrease in motor nerve conduction velocity there is an increased concentration of neurofilaments in the axons in peripheral nerve and spinal cord (Savolainen et al., 1977). It has been suggested that an increase in neurofilaments and decrease in axonal conduction velocity may be causally related (Saida et al., 1976a). Since a large amount of carbon disulfide is bound to neurofilament protein, such a mechanism might be involved here. Extrapyramidal signs, chorea, and athetosis occur in dogs as well as in humans and may be related to the lesions of the corpora striata, which involve the putamen, caudate nucleus, and globus pallidus. Behavioral changes also occur in both species: release from normal inhibitions, irritability, and psychosis occur in humans, while hyperreactivity, aggression, and apathy are seen in dogs. Some of these changes resemble the *type 1* anoxic changes resulting from methionine sulfoximine or azide.

Hexanedione. Two industrial solvents, both of which are biotransformed to 2,5-hexanedione, have been found to be responsible for neuropathy in chronically exposed industrial workers. The solvents, n-hexane and methyl n-butyl ketone, have been used in glues and cleaning fluids in the manufacture of shoes and printed fabrics. Serious exposures have occurred, notably in some factories in Italy and Japan.

A series of important papers has contributed to an understanding of this problem (Davenport et al., 1976; Saida et al., 1976; Spencer and Schaumburg, 1976). In 1975, Spencer and Schaumburg showed that 2,5-hexanedione had the same neurotoxic effect as methyl n-butyl ketone and in the following year DiVincenzo and co-workers showed that the neurotoxic chemicals, methyl n-butyl ketone and n-hexane, were metabolized to 2,5-hexanedione while the nontoxic compounds, methyl i-butyl ketone and methyl ethyl ketone, were not metabolized to 2,5-hexanedione thus establishing the parallel production of the active metabolite and neurotoxicity.

The potency of n-hexane, methyl-n-butyl-ketone, 2,5-hexanediol, and 2,5-hexanedione in causing delayed neurotoxicity is listed in order of decreasing dose required in hens following oral or intraperitoneal administration (Abou-Donia et al., 1982). Neurofilaments accumulate at nodes of myelinated fibers in hens exposed to 2,5-hexanedione and related chemicals. Axons in which these neurofilamentous masses do not disappear subsequently degenerate.

The primary toxic finding in humans, cats, rats, mice, and chickens, all of which show similar neuropathies from methyl n-butyl ketone, is the formation of large swellings in the axons of sensory and motor fibers and the axons of long ascending and descending pathways in the spinal cord. Larger doses are more likely to cause damage in the spinal pathway. With lower doses peripheral axons are selectively affected. With large doses or prolonged exposure some brainstem areas may show damage. The axonal enlargements contain accumulations of neurofilaments, which are seen initially in the distal portions of the axons. The increase in neurofilaments is one of the earliest changes. Giant axonal swelling is followed by thinning of the myelin sheath of myelinated fibers. The neuropathologic changes precede the observable paralysis by days or weeks. The axonal damage progresses from peripheral nerve endings up to the dorsal and ventral root bodies but rarely causes demonstrable changes in the cell bodies. It is proposed that disruption of fast and slow axonal transport results in loss of flow of nutrients down the axon, causing progressive degeneration of the axon (DeCaprio et al., 1983).

Organophosphorus Compounds. A series of organophosphorus compounds have been implicated in the production of delayed neurotoxicity. Attention was first drawn to the problem in 1930 by an outbreak of "ginger jake" paralysis caused by contamination of ginger extract by cresyl phosphates used in making the extract. Since then several serious episodes of poisoning have occurred from unintentional contamination of food by triorthocresyl phosphate (TOCP). Organophosphate esters have wide use as flame retardants and plasticizers for upholstery and wall coverings. In addition to TOCP two related esters, cresyldiphenyl phosphate and o-iso-propylphenyldiphenyl phosphate, are neurotoxic (Johannsen et al., 1977). Not all species of animal are equally affected. Like humans, the chicken and cat are sensitive to these compounds (Beresford and Glees, 1963). Adult animals are more sensitive than young. A second major class of organophosphorus compounds, the anticholinesterase insecticides, contains a few compounds that cause an identical delayed neuropathy. Delayed neurotoxicity has been reliably shown to occur in poisoning from DFP (diisopropyl fluorophosphate), leptofos (Abou-Donia and Preissig, 1976), and mipafox (Aldridge et al., 1969; Johnson, 1969). However, the action of the compounds causing delayed neuropathies is distinguished from the action on cholinesterase by the marked species dependency, relative insensitivity of young animals, delay in development of the lesion, and specificity of the type of neurologic damage. Although the young of many species are resistant to chemicals causing delayed neurotoxicity in adult animals, recent experiments suggest that the chick embryo is about as sensitive to tri-ortho-cresyl phosphate and leptofos as the adult hen (Sheets and Norton, 1982, 1983). Many related organophosphate insecticides, such as parathion and malathion, have not been shown to cause neuropathies in any species nor have the carbamate anticholinesterase insecticides.

After a single exposure of adequate magnitude to the neurotoxic organophosphorus compounds, axonal damage can be demonstrated after a delay of eight to ten days. In low-level exposures damage may appear only after chronic exposures of weeks or months. Axons are the primary target in both peripheral nerves and the long ascending and descending tracts of the spinal cord. The neuropathy is not reversed or prevented by thiamine. Originally it was proposed that the neurotoxic effects of organophosphorus insecticides might be due to cholinesterase inhibition. However, no good correlation was obtained between the inhibition of pseudo or true cholinesterase and the neurotoxic effect. Johnson and coworkers in a series of papers have proposed that the nervous system contains a neurotoxic esterase distinct from true or pseudocholinesterase. Phosphorylation of 80 percent or more of the neurotoxic protein by neurotoxic organophosphorus compounds reliably correlates with clinical neuropathy (Johnson, 1975).

Type 4. Agents Causing Primary Damage to Perikarya of Peripheral Neurons

The perikaryon (cell body) of a neuron is the main site of synthesis of protein that is essential for the normal function of the entire neuron including its long axon and multiply branched dendrites, which together may contain much more cytoplasm than the perikaryon. From the perikaryon many proteins and other cell constituents are transported centrifugally along the axon and dendrites. An extensive literature surrounding the phenomenon of axonal transport has developed (see, for example, Ochs, 1977), but the role of transport from the cell body in the development of axonal damage has yet to be clarified. The giant swellings that develop in some neuropathies are often associated with nodes of Ranvier in the Schwann cell and may represent areas where normal axon flow has ceased, with ballooning of the axons above the dammed-up areas. No matter where damage to a neuron occurs it can be difficult to identify the primary site. For example, in experimental axotomy Lieberman (1971) has proposed that "the nucleolus is perhaps the most sensitive indicator of changes in the functional state of the cell, and an increase in nucleolar volume is one of the earliest events of the axon reaction." The response to axotomy involves a burst of synthesis of ribosomal RNA in the nucleolus followed by an increase in cytoplasmic ribosomes and synthesis of structural proteins. Thus damage to the axon from any cause is unlikely to exist in the absence of perikaryal response. However, in only a few instances does it appear probable that the primary damage to the neuron is at the cell body and proceeds centrifugally rather than in the reverse direction. One of the aspects of neurotoxicity of organophosphorus compounds that has been stressed is the delayed appearance of the toxicity, the "silent phase" of 8 to 12 days before the onset of axonal or functional changes. Although compounds like the organomercurials affect the perikaryon, there is also a delay before the appearance of morphologic or functional changes.

Organomercury Compounds. The sensory cell bodies in the dorsal root ganglion of the spinal cord are more readily affected by organomercurials than other neurons, perhaps because of the lack of a blood barrier such as exists over much of the brain capillaries (Cavanagh, 1977). The earliest signs in experimental intoxication are in the cell bodies in which dispersion of the rough endoplasmic reticulum is seen in the electron microscope (Jacobs *et al.*, 1975). This dispersion of ribosomal material is equivalent to chromatolysis of Nissl substance observed in light microscopy. It should be noted, however, that chromatolysis is an early change after axotomy (Lieberman, 1971); so the presence of early effects on the cell body does not exclude a primary effect on peripheral portions of axons. Another early change is the diminished protein synthesis in these same cells as measured by incorporation of ^{14}C glycine (Cavanagh and Chen, 1971b). It has been proposed that organomercury compounds affect the entire neuron so that the whole fiber from the distal ending to the spinal root fragments at the same time (Cavanagh and Chen, 1971a).

The effects of organomercury compounds on central neurons are described below.

Vinca Alkaloids. Vincristine and vinblastine have been used therapeutically in the treatment of leukemia. Polyneuropathy, with sensory disturbances and motor nerve and muscle atrophy, is associated with their use (Shelanski and Wiśniewski, 1969). Aggregates of argentophilic filaments (100 Å) are found in the neurons of the brainstem, spinal cord, and dorsal root ganglia. The aggregates are localized primarily in the cytoplasm of the perikaryon, while the axons are less involved. In this, the effects of vinca alkaloids differ from the toxicity of iminodipropionitrile, the latter being associated primarily with axonal filament aggregates. The filaments in both conditions are not identical to the neurofibrillary degeneration associated with diseases such as Alzheimer's dementia or postencephalitic parkinsonism in which tangles of neurofibrils consist of double-stranded helices. The relationship of experimental and naturally occurring tangles to cell transport is a subject of considerable investigation since it is proposed that the neurofibrils normally transport substances from the perikaryon down the axon (Prineas, 1969; Johnson and Blum, 1970).

Iminodipropionitrile. The behavioral effect of this compound in mice and rats is to produce excitement and a "waltzing syndrome" associated with damage to axons in the spinal cord and brainstem. Although an increase in axoplasmic protein concentration and protein synthesis has been noted, Slagel and associates (1966) were unable to show a change in amount of RNA or base ratio of RNA in ventral horn cells and other brain areas. The toxic effects of this compound on axons thus appear to be independent of changes in RNA metabolism in the cell body. Mechanism of action of this chemical deserves further study.

Type 5. Neuromuscular Junction of Motor Nerve

Synaptic clefts and the terminals of myelinated axons are uniquely vulnerable to toxic chemicals. Since this location in the nervous system is designed to respond to chemical transmitters, it is not surprising that various exogenous chemicals may affect pre- and postsynaptic binding sites. The myelin sheath ends above the nerve terminal, and this area and the cleft between the motor nerve and muscle end plate are open to substances that can diffuse through the capillaries of skeletal muscle.

The pharmacology of the neuromuscular junction has been investigated in great detail, and extensive discussions of drug actions at the neuromuscular junction are available (e.g., Gilman *et al.*, 1985).

The effects of some toxic substances on the terminals of motor neurons are of unusual theoretic interest as well as being responsible for severe poisoning in humans.

Botulinum Toxin. When the depolarizing nerve action potential reaches the end of the axon, acetylcholine is released to cause an end-plate potential on the muscle side of the synapse. The end-plate potential, if of sufficient magnitude, will initiate the self-propagating muscle action potential. Botulinum toxin interferes with this sequence by preventing the release of acetylcholine from the axon terminal (Ambache, 1949). The binding of botulinum toxin to the terminal is irreversible and the muscle behaves as if denervated. The neuron responds as if the axon had been severed distally. After an early period of chromatolysis and swelling, there is an increase in nucleolar RNA followed by an increase in ribosomal RNA (Watson, 1969). Recovery from botulinum toxin involves sprouting of the nerve terminal and eventually formation of new contacts with the muscle (Duchen and Strich, 1968).

Tetrodotoxin. Tetrodotoxin has been responsible for deaths in humans as a result of consumption of improperly prepared puffer fish. Preparation of these fish as food by experienced handlers is required to prevent contamination of the flesh with the toxin from the liver. Death from tetrodotoxin results from skeletal muscle paralysis. However, sensory nerves are equally affected (Evans, 1969). The mechanism of action has been examined by various investigators, and it has been concluded that tetrodotoxin selectively blocks the sodium channels along the axon, preventing the inward sodium current of the action potential while leaving unaffected the outward potassium current (Kao, 1966).

Saxitoxin. Saxitoxin is the toxin produced by the dinoflagellate, *Gonylaulax*. When the toxin-containing plankton organism is ingested by shellfish, the mollusk becomes poisonous to humans. The action of saxitoxin on the sodium channel of the neuron resembles the effect of tetrodotoxin (Hille, 1968).

Batrachotoxin. Batrachotoxin is one of several related toxic steroidal compounds present in extracts of the skin of the South American frog *Phyllobates aurotaenia* and used as an arrow poison. The action of batrachotoxin is antagonistic to the effects on sodium flux of tetrodo-

toxin and saxitoxin. Batrachotoxin depolarizes the nerve membrane by increasing the permeability of the resting membrane to sodium ions. In the absence of sodium ions, batrachotoxin has no effect on the nerve. If tetrodotoxin is applied externally to an axon, the effect of batrachotoxin is blocked, showing the opposite effect these two toxins have on sodium channels (Narahashi *et al.*, 1971; Bartels-Bernal *et al.*, 1977).

Additional details of these toxins are to be found in Chapter 22 on toxins of animal origin.

DDT (Dichlorodiphenyltrichloroethane). Several insecticides cause repetitive firing of the motor end plate through repeated depolarizations of the presynaptic nerve terminal. Repetitive discharge occurs in sensory, central, and motor neurons in DDT-poisoned insects (Narahashi and Haas, 1968). The central effects of DDT are discussed below.

Pyrethrins. Pyrethrum is an insecticide extracted from species of *Chrysanthemum*. The toxic effects of the insecticide include various nervous system effects (see Chapter 18 on Pesticides). Over the past ten years several pyrethroid insecticides, derivatives of pyrethrum, have been developed. In this group of insecticides very active compounds are available, all of which are nonpersistent in the environment. The pyrethroids show a negative temperature coefficient; i.e., the compounds are more effective in biologic systems at lower temperatures. The relative sensitivity of the insect versus the mammal is proposed to be due to this negative temperature coefficient; thus, the warm-blooded mammal is less affected than the insect. The pyrethrins have been classified into two types, both of which include increased response to sensory stimuli. Type 1, exemplified by cismethrin and allethrin, causes intense tremor in mice and clonic seizures. Cockroaches show rapid, uncoordinated movements (Gammon *et al.*, 1982). The neurophysiologic action is to prolong the transient increase in sodium permeability during an action potential, resulting in repetitive firing. The prolonged permeability has been reported in both vertebrates and invertebrates (Wang *et al.*, 1972). Deltamethrin and fenvalerate are type 2 pyrethroids and cause unsteady gait with rigidity, followed by writhing spasms and hyperglycemia in rats (Cremer and Seville, 1982).

Lead. In addition to causing peripheral neuropathy, lead has been shown to have a direct synaptic action. Manalis and Cooper (1973) demonstrated that lead depresses the end-plate potential by presynaptic block. It is proposed that lead competitively inhibits calcium-mediated release of acetylcholine (Kober and

Cooper, 1976). The possible relation of these findings to lead neuropathies is unknown.

Type 6. Neurotoxicants Causing Localized CNS Lesions

The compounds in this group cause lesions restricted in distribution, affecting primarily localized anatomic areas in the CNS. Selective toxicity in the CNS may occur for several reasons. First, some areas are more exposed to substances present in blood. This has been discussed previously in the concept of the blood-brain barrier. Examples relating to areas lacking a blood-brain barrier are glutamic and kainic acids described below. Second, some areas have unique biochemical specialization for which the toxic substance has an affinity, such as pyrithiamine or mercury. Third, some areas in the CNS are affected indirectly as a result of changes elsewhere in the organism. One example of the response of the CNS to damage elsewhere is the specific condition in severe liver disease resulting in hepatic encephalopathy.

Hepatotoxicity. The neurologic syndrome that may occur as a result of alcoholic liver cirrhosis consists of ataxia, rigidity, tremor, facial grimacing, and mental changes such as emotional instability or dementia (Victor et al., 1965). The primary histologic finding is the presence of Alzheimer type II astrocytes in the basal ganglia, cerebral cortex, and cerebellum. These astrocytes have enlarged nuclei and perikarya. Some loss of neurons may occur in the areas where the large astrocytes are found. The condition has been reproduced experimentally in rats using a portocaval shunt and gavage with ammoniated cationic resin (Norenberg et al., 1974). In severe liver disease the ammonia concentration in the plasma may be increased several times above normal. It appears likely that the enlarged astrocytes are responding metabolically to the excess blood ammonia. Comparable changes in the CNS can be produced by chronic administration of carbon tetrachloride, which is a well-known hepatotoxic substance. After several weeks of dosing with carbon tetrachloride, astrocytes are enlarged and neurons are diminished in size in both the basal ganglia (Hasson and Leech, 1967; Diemer, 1976b) and cerebellum (Diemer, 1976a). This is particularly evident in the nuclei of these cells. The change in size of the nuclei may reflect altered metabolic activity in the cells (Diemer, 1976b).

Methione Sulfoximine. Although alterations in nuclear or perikaryal size may occur as an adaptive process during chronic treatment with a toxicant, there may be differences in acute and chronic changes with some toxic compounds. Prolonged administration of methionine sul-

foximine may cause damage to myelin (see Nitrogen Trioxide). Methionine sulfoximine inhibits glutamine synthetase, which is a key enzyme for handling ammonia in the brain. Large doses of methionine sulfoximine cause convulsions in rats after a delay of several hours. Prior to the onset of seizures, astrocytes in the cerebral cortex and basal ganglia enlarge and resemble the Alzheimer type II astrocytes seen in chronic hepatic encephalopathy (Guieterrez and Norenberg, 1975).

Glutamate. Large doses of monosodium L-glutamate produce hypothalamic and retinal lesions in newborn mice (Potts et al., 1960). The lateral geniculate nucleus also shows degeneration but this may be secondary to the retinal damage. The site of hypothalamic damage is the arcuate nucleus. The effect on this nucleus is probably not specific for monosodium glutamate since there is evidence that other acidic amino acids, such as aspartate and cysteine, produce the same changes, whereas neutral or basic amino acids do not (Olney, 1971). There is some controversy as to whether or not monosodium glutamate affects the hypothalamus in monkeys (Reynolds et al., 1971). The rat is affected like the mouse (Burde et al., 1971). Other areas that are damaged by large doses of the acidic amino acids are the areas in which the blood-brain barrier is deficient, including the area postrema (Olney et al., 1977). The mechanism of damage is proposed to be the sustained state of depolarization, energy depletion, and ionic imbalance produced by large doses of excitatory acidic amino acids. The neuronal sites sensitive to depolarization by these compounds are localized on the perikaryon and dendrites. Axons are unresponsive (Schwarcz and Coyle, 1977). Kainic acid is an analog of glutamic acid and, like glutamate, destroys the neurons it excites (Olney et al., 1974). Kainic acid has been used experimentally by injection as a tool to destroy neurons in selected brain areas while leaving axons from distant neurons intact (McGeer et al., 1976).

Gold Thioglucose. Neuropil dissolution in the ventromedial nucleus of the hypothalamus of mice has been reported following administration of gold thioglucose, but the lesion is not limited to this nucleus and may involve various brain areas in which the blood-brain barrier is normally reduced or absent (Perry and Liebelt, 1961). This lesion, like the lesion following monosodium glutamate, induces obesity in mice. Debons and co-workers (Debons et al., 1970) have shown that the gold localizes in oligodendroglia in the ventromedial nucleus. Presumably the heavy metal is toxic to cells and produces "scarring." This lesion does not occur in alloxan diabetic mice, implying that the presence of ''glucoreceptors'' in the hypothalamus is necessary for the deposition of gold in the ventromedial nucleus. No changes in the CNS of humans have been reported during use of gold thioglucose in arthritis.

Acetylpyridine. This compound is not of commercial importance but is an analog of nicotinic acid and may act as an antimetabolite for niacin. It causes highly selective damage limited to certain cells of the hippocampus (areas H_2 and H_3) in the mouse and in the squirrel monkey. In the squirrel monkey the lateral geniculate and inferior olivary nuclei are also damaged (Coggeshall and MacLean, 1958). MacLean (1963) has pointed out the uniqueness of this damage and its correlation with the high zinc concentration of areas H_2 and H_3, presumably associated with the high succinic dehydrogenase levels. Area H_1 (Sommer's sector), which does not contain high concentrations of zinc, is damaged by anoxic conditions but is not altered by 3-acetylpyridine. This chemical has been used experimentally to destroy the inferior olivary nucleus in the rat in investigations of the role of climbing fibers from neurons of the inferior olive. The Purkinje cells of the cerebellum have no contacts from climbing fibers in these animals and locomotion is seriously impaired (Sotelo et al., 1975). It has been proposed that the acute toxic effects are the result of synthesis of abnormal nucleotides in which pyridine is replaced by 3-acetylpyridine (Desclin and Escubi, 1974).

Trimethyltin. Organotin compounds have uses in both agriculture and industry. The toxicity of triethyltin and trimethyltin to the nervous system has been recognized for some years. Triethyltin damages myelin, as described above. The effects of trimethyltin are quite different: the primary target is the limbic system, specifically the neurons of the hippocampus and pyriform lobe (Brown et al., 1979). Damage to the developing brain is more widespread than to the adult brain. A single dose of trimethyltin to mouse pups on postnatal day 3 causes loss of hippocampal neurons, particularly area H-3, and also damage to cortical layers 2 and 3, basal ganglia, and cerebellar Purkinje and internal granule cells (Reuhl et al., 1983). The damage from trimethyltin on the developing brain resembles the effects of lead under similar exposure.

Pyrithiamine. Thiamine deficiency can be induced by administration of pyrithiamine, and the CNS lesions that result experimentally in mice from this compound closely resemble the lesions of thiamine deficiency (Wernicke's encephalopathy) in humans. Selective damage to the mammillary bodies from pyrithiamine has been shown to be associated with a decrease in transketolase activity (Collins, et al., 1970).

Other brain areas that are high in transketolase activity may also be damaged, for example, the tegmentum of the pons in the rat.

DDT (Dichlorodiphenyltrichloroethane). Repeated administration of DDT to animals results in tremor, incoordination, muscular twitching, and weakness. With chronic exposure these changes become irreversible. In dogs, changes are found in the anterior horn cells and in the cerebellum (loss of Purkinje cells) and neurons in the dentate nucleus (Haymaker et al., 1946). Glial changes have not been reported. In rabbits, the changes are confined to the anterior horn cells of the spinal cord (Cameron and Burgess, 1945). Single large doses of DDT produce convulsions in monkeys and rats (Woolley, 1970). These effects have not been reported for humans. The mechanism of the acute action of DDT on axonal firing has been elucidated in a series of papers by Narahashi and others (Narahashi and Haas, 1968). (See under Type 5 Neurotoxins.) The relation of the chronic effects to the acute toxicity of DDT is not known. Several related pesticides cause convulsions in acute overdose that resemble the effects of DDT. Experimentally chronic doses of chlordane cause hyperexcitability and tremors. Large doses cause convulsions (Hyde and Falkenberg, 1976). Endrin (Revzin, 1966) and lindane (Hanig et al., 1976) also cause convulsions. The latter compound is of interest in that this effect was produced by a single topical application of 1 percent lindane on weanling rabbits. Since topical lindane is used in treatment of scabies, the production of convulsions by this route of application is of significance.

Mercury. Chronic exposure to low levels of inorganic mercury or its compounds produces psychologic changes (erethismus mercurialis), presence of colored mercury compounds in the anterior lens capsule of the eye (mercurialentis), slight tremor, and signs of autonomic nervous system dysfunction (especially excess salivation). No CNS lesions have been found during ''micromercurialism,'' the stage of mercury poisoning with increased central and autonomic nervous system excitability.

The toxic signs of alkyl mercury compounds, such as methylmercury, show differences from inorganic mercurials. This may be due to greater penetration of organic mercury compounds into the brain. Localization of inorganic mercury in cerebellar Purkinje cells has been reported (Cassano et al., 1969), whereas methylmercury causes necrosis of the granule cell layer of the cerebellum (Hunter and Russell, 1954). The toxic effect of methylmercury on cerebellar granule cells is of interest since the granule cells are more resistant than Purkinje cells to anoxia but are vulnerable to disorders of kidney and carbohydrate metabolism (Olsen, 1959). Focal atrophy of the cortex with sensory disturbances, ataxia, and dysarthria is found after organic mercury intoxications. The emotional changes and autonomic nervous system involvement with inorganic mercury are not seen with organic mercury. Sensory nerve fibers are rather selectively damaged; motor fibers are much less involved (Miyakawa *et al.*, 1970, 1971). The primary mode of action of both kinds of mercury compounds may be interference with membrane permeability and enzyme reactions by binding of mercuric ion to sulfhydryl groups, but distribution of the organic and inorganic forms may differ. It has been pointed out that small neurons in the CNS are more likely to be damaged than large neurons in the same area by methylmercury. The greater sensitivity of small cells may be due to their greater amount of membrane for the amount of cytoplasm, and a greater ratio of membrane/cytoplasm may increase the likelihood of membrane damage from mercury (Jacobs *et al.*, 1977).

In recent years mercury compounds, especially organic mercury compounds, have been studied in great detail. Several reviews and detailed studies are available (Murakami, 1972; Shaw *et al.*, 1975; Jacobs *et al.*, 1977; Luschei *et al.*, 1977).

Manganese. The hazards of manganese have been known for a long time. Reports in the medical literature on manganese encephalopathy, in persons exposed to manganese dusts, date back to 1837. In monkeys injected with manganese compounds or exposed to manganese aerosols, neuronal degeneration has been found in the globus pallidus, subthalamic nuclei, caudate nucleus, putamen, and cerebellum. Some liver damage also occurs (Pentschew *et al.*, 1963). The functional disability in monkeys and humans closely resembles the extrapyramidal signs and symptoms of parkinsonism. Emotional changes may be present as an early symptom of toxicity. Cotzias (1958) has written an extensive review of the subject.

The description of toxic effects of the various agents listed above has been limited to the effects on the nervous system even when these compounds have distinct and sometimes dramatic effects on other organs in the body. For example, the interaction of compounds causing liver damage with CNS effects has been mentioned. The diverse somatic effects of substances such as isoniazid, lead, vincristine, and anticholinesterase compounds are also recognized, but are outside the scope of a general survey of nervous system toxicants.

REFERENCES

Abou-Donia, M. B., and Preissig, S. H.: Delayed neurotoxicity from continuous low dose and administration of leptofos to hens. *Toxicol. Appl. Pharmacol.*, **38**:595–608, 1976.

Abou-Donia, M. B.; Makkawy, H.-A. M.; and Graham, D. G.: The relative neurotoxicities of *n*-hexane, methyl *n*-butylketone, 2,5-hexanediol, and 2,5-hexanedione following oral or intraperitoneal administration in hens. *Toxicol. Appl. Pharmacol.*, **62**:369–89, 1982.

Aldridge, W. N.; Barnes, J. M.; and Johnson, M. K.: Studies on delayed neurotoxicity produced by some organophosphorus compounds. *Ann. N.Y. Acad. Sci.*, **160**:314–22, 1969.

Aleu, F. P.; Katzman, R.; and Terry, R. D.: Fine structure and electrolyte analysis of cerebral edema induced by alkyl tin intoxication. *J. Neuropathol. Exp. Neurol.*, **22**:403–13, 1963.

Ambache, N.: The peripheral action of *Cl. botulinum* toxin, *J. Physiol.*, **108**:127–41, 1949.

Arrighi, F. E.: Mammalian chromosomes. In Busch, H. (ed.): *The Cell Nucleus*, Vol. 2. Academic Press, Inc., New York, 1974, pp. 1–32.

Auld, R. B., and Bedwell, S. F.: Peripheral neuropathy with sympathetic over-activity from industrial contact with acrylamide. *Can. Med. Assoc. J.*, **96**:652–54, 1967.

Bank, W. J.; Pleasure, D. E.; Suzuki, K.; Nigro, M.; and Katz, R.: Thallium poisoning. *Arch. Neurol.*, **26**:456–64, 1972.

Barbizet, J.: Psychophysiological mechanisms of memory. In Vinken, P. J., and Bruyn, G. W. (eds.): *Handbook of Clinical Neurology*, Vol. 3. John Wiley & Sons, Inc., New York, 1969.

Bartels-Bernal, E.; Rosenberry, T. L.; and Daly, J. W.: Effect of batrachotoxin on the electroplax of electric eel: evidence for voltage-dependent interaction with sodium channels. *Proc. Natl Acad. Sci. USA*, **74**:951–55, 1977.

Bass, N. H.: Pathogenesis of myelin lesions in experimental cyanide encephalopathy. *Neurology*, **18**:167–77, 1968.

Beresford, W. A., and Glees, P.: Degeneration in the long tracts of the cords of the chicken and cat after triorthocresylphosphate poisoning. *Acta Neuropathol. (Berl.)*, **3**:108–18, 1963.

Berthound, H. R.; Garman, R. H.; and Weiss, B.: Food intake, body weight, and brain histopathology in mice following chronic methyl mercury treatment. *Toxicol. Appl. Pharmacol.*, **36**:19–30, 1976.

Boller, F.; Howes, D.; and Pattern, D. H.: A behavioral evaluation of brain-scan estimates of lesion size. *Neurology*, **20**:852–59, 1970.

Bondareff, W.: The extracellular compartment of the cerebral cortex. *Anat. Rec.*, **152**:119–27, 1965.

Bradley, W. G., and Asbury, A. K.: Radioautographic studies of Schwann cell behavior. I. Acrylamide neuropathy in the mouse. *J. Neuropathol. Exp. Neurol.*, **29**:500–506, 1970.

Brierley, J. B.: The sensory ganglia—recent anatomical, physiological and pathological contributions. *Acta Psychiat. Neurol. Scand.*, **30**:553–76, 1955.

Brierley, J. R.; Brown, A. W.; and Meldrum, B. S.: The nature and time course of the neuronal alterations resulting from oligaemia and hypoglycaemia in the brain of *Macaca mulatta*. *Brain Res.*, **25**:483–99, 1971.

Brightman, M. W., and Reese, T. S.: Junctions between intimately apposed cell membranes in the vertebrate brain. *J. Cell Biol.*, **40**:648–77, 1969.

Brown, A. W.; Aldridge, W. N.; Street, B. W.; and Verschoyle, R. D.: The behavioral and neuropathologic sequella of intoxication by trimethyltin compounds in the rat. *Am. J. Pathol.*, **97**:59–82, 1979.

Brown, S.; Dragann, N.; and Vogel, W. H.: Effects of lead acetate on learning and memory in rats. *Arch. Environ. Health*, **22**:370–72, 1971.

Brucher, J. M.: Neuropathological problems posed by carbon monoxide poisoning and anoxia. *Prog. Brain Res.*, **24**:75–100, 1967.

Bull, R. J.; McCauley, P. T.; Taylor, D. H.; and Croften, V. M.: The effects of lead on the developing central nervous system of the rat. *Neurotoxicology*, **4**:1–18, 1983.

Bullock, J. D.; Wey, R. J.; Zaia, J. A.; Zarembook, I.; and Schroeder, H. A.: Effects of tetraethyl lead on learning and memory in the rat. *Arch. Environ. Health*, **13**:21–22, 1966.

Burde, R. M.; Schainker, B.; and Kayes, J.: Acute effects of oral and subcutaneous administration of monosodium glutamate on the arcuate nucleus in mice and rats. *Nature*, **233**:58–60, 1971.

Cameron, G. R., and Burgess, F.: The toxicity of 2,2-bis(p-chlorphenyl) 1,1,1-trichlorethane (D.D.T.). *Br. Med. J.*, **1**:865–71, 1945.

Campbell, J. B.; Woolley, D. E.; Vijayan, V. K.; and Overmann, R.: Morphometric effects of postnatal lead exposure on hippocampal development of the 15 day old rat. *Dev. Brain Res.*, **3**:595–612, 1982.

Carlton, W. W., and Kreutzberg, G.: Isonicotinic acid hydrazide-induced spongy degeneration of the white matter in the brain of Pekin ducks. *Am. J. Pathol.*, **48**:91–106, 1966.

Cassano, G. G.; Viola, P. L.; Ghetti, B.; and Amaducci, L.: The distribution of inhaled mercury (Hg[203]) vapors in the brain of rats and mice. *J. Neuropathol. Exp. Neurol.*, **28**:308–20, 1969.

Cavanagh, J. B.: Metabolic mechanisms of neurotoxicity caused by mercury. In Roizin, L.; Shiraki, H.; and Grčevič, N. (eds.): *Neurotoxicology.* Raven Press, New York, 1977, pp. 283–88.

Cavanagh, J. B., and Chen, F. C. K.: The effects of methyl-mercury-dicyanidiamide on the peripheral nerves and spinal cord of rats. *Acta Neuropathol. (Berl.)*, **19**:208–15, 1971a.

——— : Amino acid incorporation of protein during the "silent phase" before organo-mercury and p-bromophenylacetylurea neuropathy in the rat. *Acta Neuropathol. (Berl.)*, **19**:216–24, 1971b.

Cavanagh, J. B.; Chen, F. C. K.; Kyu, M. H.; and Ridley, A.: The experimental neuropathy in rats caused by p-bromophenylacetylurea. *J. Neurol. Neurosurg. Psychiat.*, **31**:471–78, 1968.

Cavanagh, J. B.; Fuller, N. H.; Johnson, H. R. M.; and Rudge, P.: The effect of thallium salts, with particular reference to the nervous system changes. *Q. J. Med.*, **43**:293–319, 1974.

Cervós-Navarro, J., and Rozas, J. I.: The arteriole as a site of metabolic change. *Adv. Neurol.*, **20**:17–24, 1978.

Chapman, L. F., and Wolff, H. G.: The cerebral hemispheres and the highest integrative functions of man. *Arch. Neurol.*, **1**:357–424, 1959.

Chason, J. L.: Nervous system and skeletal muscle. In Anderson, W. A. D. (ed.): *Pathology*, Vol. 2, 6th ed. C. V. Mosby Co., St. Louis, 1971.

Cisson, C. M., and Wilson, B. W.: Degenerative changes in skeletal muscle of hens with tri-ortho-cresyl phosphate-induced delayed neurotoxicity: altered acetylcholinesterase molecular forms and increased plasma creatine phosphokinase activity. *Toxicol. Appl. Pharmacol.*, **64**:289–305, 1982.

Coggeshall, R. L., and MacLean, P. D.: Hippocampal lesions following administration of 3-acetylpyridine. *Proc. Soc. Exp. Biol. Med.*, **98**:687–89, 1958.

Collins, R. C.; Kirpatrick, J. B.; and McDougal, D. B., Jr.: Some regional pathologic and metabolic consequences in mouse brain of pyrithiamine-induced thiamine deficiency. *J. Neuropathol. Exp. Neurol.*, **29**:57–69, 1970.

Cotzias, G. C.: Manganese in health and disease. *Physiol. Rev.*, **38**:503–32, 1958.

Crapper, D. R.; Krishnan, S. S.; and Quittkat, S.: Aluminum, neurofibrillary degeneration and Alzheimer's disease. *Brain*, **99**:67–80, 1976.

Cremer, J. E., and Seville, M. P.: Comparative effects of two pyrethroids, deltamethrin and cismethrin, on plasma catecholamines and on blood glucose and lactate. *Toxicol. Appl. Pharmacol.*, **66**:124–33, 1982.

Crosby, E. C.; Humphrey, T.; and Lauer, E. W.: *Correlative Anatomy of the Nervous System.* Macmillan Publishing Co., New York, 1962.

Culver, B., and Norton, S.: Juvenile hyperactivity in rats after acute exposure to carbon monoxide. *Exp. Neurol.*, **50**:80–98, 1976.

Curley, A.; Kimbrough, R. D.; Hawk, R. E.; Nathenson, G.; and Finberg, L.: Dermal absorption of hexachlorophene in infants. *Lancet*, **2**:296–97, 1971.

Davenport, J. J.; Farrell, D. F.; and Sumi, S. M.: "Giant axonal neuropathy" caused by industrial chemicals. *Neurology*, **26**:919–23, 1976.

Debons, A. F.; Krimsky, I; From, A.; and Cloutier, R. J.: Gold thioglucose induction of obesity: Significance of focal gold deposits in hypothalamus. *Am. J. Physiol.*, **219**:1403–1408, 1970.

DeCaprio, A. P., Strominger, N. L., and Weber, P.: Neurotoxicity and protein binding of 2,5-hexanedione in the hen. *Toxicol. Appl. Pharmacol.*, **68**:297–307, 1983.

deRobertis, E.: Morphological aspects of water and ion shifts in the CNS. In Schadé, J. P., and McMenemey, W. H. (eds.): *Selective Vulnerability of the Brain in Hypoxaemia.* F. A. Davis Co., Philadelphia, 1963.

Desclin, J. C., and Escubi, J.: Effects of 3-acetylpyridine on the central nervous system of the rat, as demonstrated by silver methods. *Brain Res.*, **77**:349–64, 1974.

Diemer, N. H.: Number of Purkinje cells and Bergmann astrocytes in rats with CCl₄-induced liver disease. *Acta Neurol. Scand.*, **55**:1–15, 1976a.

——— : Glial and neuronal alterations in the corpus striatum of rats with CCl₄-induced liver disease. *Acta Neurol. Scand.*, **55**:16–32, 1976b.

DeVincenzo, G. D.; Kaplan, C. J.; and Dedinas, J.: Characterization of the metabolites of methyl n-butyl ketone, methyl iso-butyl ketone and methyl ethyl ketone in guinea pig serum and their clearance. *Toxicol. Appl. Pharmacol.*, **36**:511–22, 1976.

Dru, D.; Agnew, W. F.; and Greene, E.: Effects of tellurium ingestion on learning capacity of the rat. *Psychopharmacologia*, **24**:508–15, 1972.

Duchen, L. W., and Strich, S. J.: The effects of botulinum toxin on the pattern of innervation of skeletal muscle in the mouse. *Q. J. Exp. Physiol.*, **53**:84–89, 1968.

Duckett, S., and Scott, T.: The localization of tellurium in tellurium-induced hydrocephalus. *Experientia*, **27**:432–34, 1971.

Evans, M. H.: Mechanism of saxitoxin and tetrodotoxin poisoning. *Br. Med. Bull.*, **25**:263–67, 1969.

Falk, J. L.: Drug effect on discriminative motor control. *Physiol. Behav.*, **4**:421–27, 1969.

Friede, R. L.: *Topographic Brain Chemistry.* Academic Press, Inc., New York, 1966.

Fullerton, P. M., and Barnes, J. M.: Peripheral neuropathy in rats produced by acrylamide. *Br. J. Ind. Med.*, **23**:210–21, 1966.

Gammon, D. W.; Lawrence, L. J.; and Casida, J. E.: Pyrethroid toxicology: protective effects of diazepam and phenobarbital in the mouse and cockroach. *Toxicol. Appl. Pharmacol.*, **66**:290–96, 1982.

Gibbins, R. J.; Kalant, H.; and LeBlanc, A. E.: A technique for accurate measurement of moderate degrees of alcohol intoxication in small animals. *J. Pharmacol. Exp. Ther.*, **159**:236–42, 1968.

Gilman, A. G.; Goodman, L. S.; Rall, T. W.; and Murad,

F. (eds.): *Goodman and Gilman's The Pharmacological Basis of Therapeutics*, 7th ed. Macmillan Publishing Co., New York, 1985.

Gutierrez, J. A., and Norenberg, M. D.: Alzheimer II astrocytosis following methionine sulfoximine. *Arch. Neurol.*, 32:123–26, 1975.

Hanig, J. P.; and Yoder, P. D.; and Krop, S.: Convulsions in weanling rabbits after a single topical application of 1% lindane. *Toxicol. Appl. Pharmacol.*, 38:463–69, 1976.

Hasson, J., and Leech, R. W.: Experimental hepatocerebral disease. *Arch. Pathol.*, 84:286–89, 1967.

Hawkins, J. E., Jr.; Stebbins, W. C.; Johnsson, L.-G., Moody, D. B.; and Muraski, A.: The patas monkey as a model for dihydrostreptomycin ototoxicity. *Acta Otolaryngol.*, 83:123–29, 1977.

Haymaker, W.; Ginzler, A. M.; and Ferguson, R. L.: The toxic effects of prolonged ingestion of DDT on dogs with special reference to lesions in the brain. *Am. J. Med. Sci.*, 212:423–31, 1946.

Hazama, F.; Amano, S.; and Ozaki, T.: Pathological changes of cerebral vessel endothelial cells in spontaneously hypertensive rats with special reference to the role of these cells in the development of hypertensive cerebrovascular lesions. *Adv. Neurol.*, 20:359–69, 1978.

Heydlauf, H.: Ferric-cyanoferrate (II): An effective antidote in thallium poisoning. *Eur. J. Pharmacol.*, 6:340–44, 1969.

Hicks, S. P.: Brain metabolism *in vivo*. I. The distribution of lesions caused by cyanide poisoning, insulin hypoglycemia, asphyxia in nitrogen and fluoroacetate poisoning in rats. *Arch. Pathol.*, 49:111–37, 1950.

Hille, B.: Pharmacological modifications of the sodium channels of frog nerve. *J. Gen. Physiol.*, 51:199–219, 1968.

Hirano, A.; Ohsugi, T.; and Matsumura, H.: Pores and tubule-containing vacuoles in altered blood vessels of the central nervous system. *Adv. Neurol.*, 20:461–69, 1978.

Hunter, D., and Russell, D. S.: Focal cerebral and cerebellar atrophy in a human subject due to organic mercury compounds. *J. Neurol. Neurosurg. Psychiatr.*, 17:235–41, 1954.

Hurst, E. W.: Experimental demyelination in relation to human and animal disease. *Ann. J. Med.*, 12:547–60, 1952.

Hyde, K. M., and Falkenberg, R. L.: Neuroelectric disturbance as indicator of chronic chlordane toxicity. *Toxicol. Appl. Pharmacol.*, 37:499–515, 1976.

Innes, J. R. M., and Saunders, L. Z.: *Comparative Neuropathology*. Academic Press, Inc., New York, 1962.

Inturrisi, C. E.: Thallium-induced dephosphorylation of a phosphorylated intermediate of the (sodium + thallium-activated) ATPase. *Biochim. Biophys. Acta*, 178:630–33, 1969.

Jacob, H.: CNS tissue and cellular pathology in hypoxaemic states. In Schadé, J. F., and McMenemey W. H. (eds.): *Selective Vulnerability of the Central Nervous System in Hypoxaemia*. F. A. Davis Co., Philadelphia, 1963.

Jacobs, J. M.: Penetration of systemically injected horseradish peroxidase into ganglia and nerves of the autonomic nervous system. *J. Neurocytol.*, 6:607–18, 1977.

Jacobs, J. M.; Carmichael, N.; and Cavanagh, J. B.: Ultrastructural changes in the dorsal root and trigeminal ganglia of rats poisoned with methyl mercury. *Neuropathol. Appl. Neurobiol.*, 1:1–19, 1975.

——— : Ultrastructural changes in the nervous system of rabbits poisoned with methyl mercury. *Toxicol. Appl. Pharmacol.*, 39:249–61, 1977.

Jacobs, J. M.; MacFarlane, R. M.; and Cavanagh, J. B.: Vascular leakage in the dorsal root ganglia of the rat, studied with horseradish peroxidase. *J. Neurol. Sci.*, 29:95–107, 1976.

Johannsen, F. R.; Wright, P. L.; Gordon, D. E.; Levinskas, G. F.; Radue, R. W.; and Graham, P. R.: Evaluation of delayed neurotoxicity and dose-response relationships of phosphate esters in the adult hen. *Toxicol. Appl. Pharmacol.*, 41:291–304, 1977.

Johnson, A. B., and Blum, N. R.: Nucleoside phosphatase activities associated with the tangles and plaques of Alzheimer's disease. *J. Neuropathol. Exp. Neurol.*, 29:463–78, 1970.

Johnson, B. L.; Boyd, J.; Burg, J. R.; Lee, S. T.; Xintaras, C.; and Albright, B. E.: Effects on the peripheral nervous system of workers' exposure to carbon disulfide. *Neurotoxicology*, 4:53–66, 1983.

Johnson, M. K.: Delayed neurotoxic action of some organophosphorus compounds. *Br. Med. Bull.*, 25:231–35, 1969.

——— : The delayed neuropathy caused by some organophosphorus esters: mechanism and challenge. *CRC Crit. Rev. Toxicol.*, 3:289–316, 1975.

Joynt, R. J.; Benton, A. L.; and Fogel, M. L.: Behavioral and pathological correlates of motor impersistence. *Neurology*, 12:876–81, 1962.

Kao, C. Y.: Tetrodotoxin, saxitoxin and their significance in the study of excitation phenomena. *Pharmacol. Rev.*, 18:997–1049, 1966.

Kennedy, G. L.; Dressler, I. A.; and Keplinger, M. L.: The concentration of hexachlorphene in the blood of albino rats as a function of time postexposure, number of exposures, route of exposure, previous exposure and age. *Toxicol. Appl. Pharmacol.*, 37:425–31, 1976a.

Kennedy, G. L.; Dressler, I. A.; Richter, W. R.; Keplinger, M. L.; and Calandra, J. C.: Effects of hexachlorophene in the rat and their reversibility. *Toxicol. Appl. Pharmacol.*, 35:137–45, 1976b.

Kennedy, P., and Cavanagh, J. B.: Spinal changes in the neuropathy of thallium poisoning. *J. Neurol. Sci.*, 29:295–301, 1976.

Kesson, C. M.; Baird, A. W.; and Lawson, D. H.: Acrylamide poisoning. *Postgrad. Med. J.*, 53:16–17, 1977.

Kimbrough, R. D., and Gaines, T. B.: Hexachlorophene effects on the rat brain. *Arch. Environ. Health*, 23:114–18, 1971.

Kinnard, W. J., Jr., and Carr, C. J.: A preliminary procedure for the evaluation of central nervous system depressants. *J. Pharmacol. Exp. Ther.*, 121:354–61, 1957.

Kober, T. E., and Cooper, G. P.: Lead competitively inhibits calcium-dependent synaptic transmission in the bullfrog sympathetic ganglion. *Nature*, 262:704–705, 1976.

Krehbiel, D.; Davis, G. A.; LeRory, L. M.; and Bowman, R. E.: Absence of hyperactivity in lead-exposed developing rats. *Environ. Health Perspect.*, 18:147–57, 1976.

Kuhlenbeck, H.: *The Central Nervous System of Vertebrates*, Vol. 3, Part I. Academic Press, Inc., New York, 1970.

Lampert, P.; Garro, F.; and Pentshew, A.: Tellurium neuropathy. *Acta Neuropathol. (Berl.)*, 15:308–17, 1970.

Lampert, P. W., and Schochet, S. S.: Electron microscopic observations on experimental spongy degeneration of the cerebellar white matter. *J. Neuropathol. Exp. Neurol.*, 27:210–20, 1968a.

——— : Demyelination and remyelination in lead neuropathy. *J. Neuropathol. Exp. Neurol.*, 27:527–45, 1968b.

Lapresle, J., and Fardeau, M.: The central nervous system and carbon monoxide poisoning. II. Anatomical study of brain lesions following intoxication with carbon monoxide (22 cases). *Prog. Brain Res.*, 24:31–74, 1967.

Levine, S.: Anoxic-ischemic encephalopathy in rats. *Am. J. Pathol.*, 36:1–18, 1960.

——— : Experimental cyanide encephalopathy. *J. Neuropathol. Exp. Neurol.*, 26:214–22, 1967.

Lewey, F. H.: Neurological, medical and biochemical

signs and symptoms indicating chronic industrial carbon disulfide absorption. *Ann. Intern. Med.,* **15**:869–83, 1941a.

———— : Experimental chronic carbon disulfide poisoning in dogs. *J. Ind. Hyg. Toxicol.,* **23**:415–36, 1941b.

———— : Neuropathological changes in nitrogen trichloride intoxication of dogs. *J. Neuropathol. Exp. Neurol.,* **9**:396–405, 1950.

Lieberman, A. R.: The axon reaction: a review of the principal features of perikaryal responses to axon injury. *Int. Rev. Neurobiol.,* **14**:49–124, 1971.

Ljunggren, B.; Norberg, K.; and Siesjö; B. K.: Influence of tissue acidosis upon restitution of brain energy metabolism following total ischemia. *Brain Res.,* **77**:173–86, 1974.

Luschei, E.; Mottet, N. K.; and Shaw, C.-M.: Chronic methylmercury exposure in the monkey (*Macaca mulatta*): behavioral tests of peripheral vision, signs of neurotoxicity, and blood concentration in relation to dose and time. *Arch. Environ. Health,* **32**:126–31, 1977.

MacLean, P. D.: Comments on the selective vulnerability of the hippocampus. In Schadé, J. F., and McMenemey, W. H. (eds.): *Selective Vulnerability of the Central Nervous System in Hypoxaemia.* F. A. Davis Co., Philadelphia, 1963.

Malamud, N.: Patterns of CNS vulnerability in neonatal hyperemia. In Schadé, J. F., and McMenemey, W. H. (eds.): *Selective Vulnerability of the Central Nervous System in Hypoxaemia.* F. A. Davis Co., Philadelphia, 1963.

Manalis, R. S., and Cooper, G. P.: Presynaptic and postsynaptic effects of lead at the frog neuromuscular junction. *Nature,* **243**:354–55, 1973.

McGeer, E. G.; Innanen, V. T.; and McGeer, P. L.: Evidence on the cellular localization of adenylcylase in the neostriatum. *Brain Res.,* **118**:356–58, 1976.

Mettler, F. A.: Choreo-athetosis and striopallidonigral necrosis due to sodium azide. *Exp. Neurol.,* **34**:291–308, 1972.

Milner, B.: Effects of different brain lesions on card sorting. *Arch. Neurol.,* **9**:90–100, 1963.

———— : Visually-guided maze learning in man: effects of bilateral hippocampal, bilateral frontal, and unilateral cerebral lesions. *Neuropsychologia,* **3**:317–38, 1965.

Miyakawa, T.; Deshimaru, M.; Sumiyoshi, S.; Teraoka, A.; and Tatetsu, S.: Experimental organic mercury poisoning. Pathological changes in muscles. *Acta Neuropathol. (Berl.),* **17**:80–83, 1971.

Miyakawa, T.; Deshimaru, M.; Sumiyoshi, S.; Teraoka, A.; Udo, N.; Hattori, E.; and Tatetsu, S.: Experimental organic mercury poisoning—pathological changes in peripheral nerves. *Acta Neuropathol. (Berl.),* **15**:45–55, 1970.

Miyoshi, K.: Experimental striatal necrosis induced by sodium azide. A contribution to the problem of selective vulnerability and histochemical studies of enzymatic activity. *Acta Neuropathol. (Berl.),* **9**:199–216, 1967.

Miyoshi, K.; Matsuoka, T.; and Mizushima, S.: Familial holotopistic striatal necrosis. *Acta Neuropathol. (Berl.),* **13**:240–49, 1969.

Mullenix, P.; Norton, S.; and Culver, B.: Locomotor damage in rats after X-irradiation *in utero. Exp. Neurol.,* **48**:310–24, 1975.

Murakami, U.: The effect of organic mercury on intrauterine life. In Klingberg, M. A.; Abramovici, A.; and Chemke, J. (eds.): *Drugs and Fetal Development,* Advances in Experimented Medical Biology, Vol. 27. Plenum Press, New York, 1972, pp. 301–36.

Myers, R. E.: Two classes of dysergic brain abnormality and their conditions of occurrence. *Arch. Neurol.,* **29**:394–99, 1973.

———— : Fetal asphyxia due to umbilical cord compression. *Biol. Neonate,* **26**:21–43, 1975.

Narahashi, T.; Albuquerque, E. X.; and Deguchi, T.: Effects of batrachotoxin on membrane potential and conductance of squid giant axon. *J. Gen. Physiol.,* **58**:54–70, 1971.

Narahashi, T., and Haas, H. G.: Interaction of DDT with the components of lobster nerve membrane conductance. *J. Gen. Physiol.,* **51**:177–98, 1968.

Norenberg, M. D.; Lapham, L. W.; Nichols, L. W.; and May, A. G.: An experimental model for the study of hepatic encephalopathy. *Arch. Neurol.,* **31**:106–109, 1974.

Norton, S., and Culver, B.: A Golgi analysis of caudate neurons in rats exposed to carbon monoxide. *Brain Res.,* **132**:455–65, 1977.

Ochs, S.: Axoplasmic transport in peripheral nerve and hypothalamoneurohypophyseal systems. *Adv. Exp. Med. Biol.,* **87**:13–40, 1977.

Olney, J. W.: Glutamate-induced neuronal necrosis in the infant mouse hypothalamus. *J. Neuropathol. Exp. Neurol.,* **30**:75–90, 1971.

Olney, J. W.; Rhee, V.; and de Gubareff, T.: Neurotoxic effects of glutamate on mouse area postrema. *Brain Res.,* **120**:151–57, 1977.

Olney, J. W.; Rhee, V.; and Ho, O. L.: Kainic acid: a powerful neurotoxic analogue of glutamate. *Brain Res.,* **77**:507–12, 1974.

Olsen, S.: Acute selective necrosis of the granular layer of the cerebellar cortex. *J. Neuropathol. Exp. Neurol.,* **18**:609–19, 1959.

Olsson, Y.: Topographical differences in the vascular permeability of the peripheral nervous system. *Acta Neuropathol. (Berl.),* **10**:26–33, 1968.

Olsson, Y., and Hossman, K.-A.: Fine structural localization of exudated protein tracers in the brain. *Acta Neuropathol. (Berl.),* **16**:103–16, 1970.

Overmann, S. R.: Behavioral effects of asymptomatic lead exposure during neonatal development in rats. *Toxicol. Appl. Pharmacol.* **41**:459–71, 1977.

Palay, S. L., and Palade, G. E.: The fine structure of neurons. *J. Biophys. Biochem. Cytol.,* **1**:69–88, 1955.

Papez, J. W.: A proposed mechanism of emotion. *Arch. Neurol. Psychiatr.,* **38**:725–43, 1937.

Paterson, P. Y.: The demyelinating diseases: clinical and experimental correlates. In Samter, M. (ed.): *Immunological Disease,* Vol. 2. Little, Brown & Co., Boston, 1971.

Pentschew, A.; Ebner, F. F.; and Kovatch, R. M.: Experimental manganese encephalopathy in monkeys. *J. Neuropathol. Exp. Neurol.,* **22**:488–99, 1963.

Perry, J. H., and Liebelt, R. A.: Extra-hypothalamic lesions associated with gold-thioglucose induced obesity. *Proc. Soc. Exp. Biol. Med.,* **106**:55–57, 1961.

Petit, T. L.; Alfano, D. P.; and LeBoutillier, J. C.: Early lead exposure and the hippocampus: a review and recent advances. *Neurotoxicology,* **4**:79–94, 1983.

Pleasure, D.; Towfighi, J.; Silberg, D.; and Parris, J.: The pathogenesis of hexachlorophene neuropathy: *in vivo* and *in vitro* studies. *Neurology,* **24**:1068–75, 1974.

Pleasure, D. E.; Mishler, K. C.; and Engel, W. K.: Axonal transport of protein in experimental neuropathies. *Science,* **166**:524–25, 1969.

Plum, F.; Posner, J. B.; and Hain, R. F.: Delayed neurological deterioration after anoxia. *Arch. Intern. Med.,* **110**:18–25, 1962.

Potts, A. M.; Modrell, K. W.; and Kingsbury, C.: Permanent fractionation of the electroretinogram by sodium glutamate. *Am. J. Ophthalmol.,* **50**:900–907, 1960.

Preziosi, T. J.; Lindenberg, R.; Levy, D.; and Christenson, M.: An experimental investigation in animals of the functional and morphologic effects of single and repeated exposures to high and low concentrations of carbon monoxide. *Ann. N.Y. Acad. Sci.,* **174**:369–84, 1970.

Prineas, J.: The pathogenesis of dying-back polyneuropathies. I. An ultrastructural study of experimental tri-ortho-cresyl phosphate intoxication in the cat. *J. Neuropathol. Exp. Neurol.*, 28:571–97, 1969.

Putz-Anderson, U.; Albright, B. E.; Lee, S. T.; Johnson, B. L.; Chrislip, D. W.; Taylor, B. J.; Brightwell, W. S.; Dickerson, N.; Culver, M.; Zentmeyer, D.; and Smith, P.: A behavioral examination of workers exposed to carbon disulfide. *Neurotoxicology*, 4:67–78, 1983.

Reese, T. S., and Brightman, M. W.: Similarity in structure and permeability to peroxidase of epithelia overlying fenestrated cerebral capillaries. *Anat. Rec.*, 160:414, 1968.

Reiter, L. A., and Ison, J. R.: Inhibition of the human eyeblink reflex: an evaluation of the sensitivity of the Wendt-Yerkes method for threshold detection. *J. Exp. Psychol. Human Percept. Perform.*, 3:325–36, 1977.

Reuhl, K. R.; Smallridge, E. A.; Chang, L. W.; and Mackenzie, B. A.: Developmental effects of trimethyltin intoxication in the neonatal mouse. I. Light microscopic studies. *Neurotoxicology*, 4:19–28, 1983.

Revzin, A. M.: Effects of endrin on telencephalic function in the pigeon. *Toxicol. Appl. Pharmacol.*, 9:75–83, 1966.

Reynolds, W. A.; Lemkey-Johnson, N.; Filer, L. J., Jr.; and Pitkin, R. M.: Monosodium glutamate: absence of hypothalamic lesions after ingestion by newborn primates. *Science*, 172:1342–44, 1971.

Robinson, N.; Duncan, P.; Gehrt, M.; Sances, A.; and Evans, S.: Histochemistry of trauma after electrode implantation and stimulation in the hippocampus. *Arch. Neurol.*, 32:98–102, 1975.

Ruščák, M.; Ruščáková, D.; and Hager, H.: The role of the neuronal cell in the metabolism of the rat cerebral cortex. *Physiol. Bohemoslov.*, 17:113–21, 1968.

Saida, K.; Mendell, J. R.; and Weiss, H. S.: Peripheral nerve changes induced by methyl *n*-butyl ketone (MBk) and methyl ethyl ketone (MEK). *J. Neuropathol. Exp. Neurol.*, 35:113–1976a.

———: Peripheral nerve changes induced by methyl *n*-butyl ketone and potentiation by methyl ethyl ketone. *J. Neuropathol. Exp. Neurol.*, 35:207–25, 1976b.

Sauer, R. M.; Zook, B. C.; and Garner, F. M.: Demyelinating encephalomyelopathy associated with lead poisoning in nonhuman primates. *Science*, 169:1091–93, 1970.

Sauerhoff, M. W., and Michaelson, I. A.: Hyperactivity and brain catecholamines in lead-exposed developing rats. *Science*, 182:1023–24, 1973.

Savolainen, H.; Lehtonen, E.; and Vaino, H.: CS₂ binding to rat spinal neurofilaments. *Acta Neuropathol. (Berl.)*, 37:219–23, 1977.

Scarpelli, D. G., and Trump, B. F.: *Cell Injury.* University Association, Research in Educational Pathology. Upjohn Co., Kalamazoo, 1971.

Schlaepfer, W. W.: Experimental lead neuropathy: a disease of the supporting cells in the peripheral nervous system. *J. Neuropathol. Exp. Neurol.*, 28:401–18, 1969.

———: Vincristine-induced axonal alterations in rat peripheral nerve. *J. Neuropathol. Exp. Neurol.*, 30:488–505, 1971.

Scholz, W.: Selective neuronal necrosis and its topistic patterns in hypoxemia and oligenia. *J. Neuropathol. Exp. Neurol.*, 12:249–61, 1953.

———: The contribution of pathoanatomical research to the problem of epilepsy. *Epilepsia*, 1:36–55, 1959.

Schwarcz, R., and Coyle, J. T.: Striatal lesions with kainic acid: neurochemical characteristics. *Brain Res.*, 127:235–49, 1977.

Schwedenberg, T. H.: Leukoencephalopathy following carbon monoxide asphyxia. *J. Neuropathol. Exp. Neurol.*, 18:597–608, 1959.

Shaw, C.-M.; Mottet, N. K.; Body, R. L.; and Luschei, E. S.: Variability of neuropathologic lesions in experimental methyl mercurial encephalopathy in primates. *Am. J. Pathol.*, 80:451–70, 1975.

Sheets, L. P., and Norton, S.: Evidence for leptophos-induced neuropathy in chicks exposed on incubation day 14. *Toxicologist*, 2:149–50, 1982.

———: Functional and histological evidence of a peripheral neuropathy in chicks treated with TOCP as embryos. *Toxicologist*, 3:17, 1983.

Shelanski, M. L., and Wiśniewski, H.: Neurofibrillary degeneration induced by vincristine therapy. *Arch. Neurol.*, 20:199–206, 1969.

Slagel, D. E.; Hartmann, H. A.; and Edstrom, J. E.: The effect of iminodipropionitrile on the ribonucleic acid content and composition of mesencephalic V cells, anterior horn cells, glial cells, and axonal balloons. *J. Neuropathol. Exp. Neurol.*, 25:244–53, 1966.

Slager, U. T.; Reilly, E. B.; and Brandt, R. A.: The neuropathology of barbiturate intoxication. *J. Neuropathol. Exp. Neurol.*, 25:237–43, 1966.

Sotelo, C.; Hillman, D. E.; Zamora, A. J.; and Llinás, R.: Climbing fiber deafferentation: its action on Purkinje cell dendritic spines. *Brain Res.*, 98:574–81, 1975.

Spencer, P. S., and Schaumburg, H. H.: Experimental neuropathy produced by 2,5-hexanedione—a major metabolite of the neurotoxic industrial solvent methyl *n*-butyl ketone. *J. Neurol. Neurosurg. Psychiat.*, 38:771–75, 1975.

———: Feline nervous system response to chronic intoxication with commercial grades of methyl *n*-butyl ketone, methyl i-butyl ketone and methyl ethyl ketone. *Toxicol. Appl. Pharmacol.*, 37:301–11, 1976.

Spielmeyer, W.: *Histopathologie des Nervensystems.* Julius Springer, Berlin, 1922.

Sterne, D. M.: The Benton, Porteus and WAIS digit span tests with normal and brain-injured subjects. *J. Clin. Psychol.*, 25:173–77, 1969.

Strain, G. S., and Kinzie, W. B.: Reducing misdiagnosis of schizophrenic patients on a test for brain damage. *J. Clin. Psychol.*, 25:262–69, 1969.

Tiller, J. R.; Schilling, R. S. F.; and Morris, J. N.: Occupational toxic factor in mortality from coronary heart disease. *Br. Med. J.*, 4:407–11, 1968.

Torack, R. M.: The relationship between adenosine triphosphatase activity and triethyltin toxicity in the production of cerebral edema of the rat. *Am. J. Pathol.*, 46:245–62, 1965.

Trump, B. F., and Arstila, A. U.: Cell membranes and disease processes. In Trump, B. F., and Arstila, A. U. (eds.): *Pathobiology of Cell Membranes.* Academic Press, Inc., New York, 1975.

Vanderhaeghen, J. J., and Logan, W. J.: The effect of the pH on the *in vitro* development of Spielmeyer's ischemic neuronal changes. *J. Neuropathol. Exp. Neurol.*, 30:99–104, 1971.

Vega, A.: Use of Purdue Pegboard and finger tapping performance as a rapid screening test for brain damage. *J. Clin. Psychol.*, 25:255–58, 1969.

Vega, A., and Parsons, O. A.: Cross-validation of the Halstead-Reitan tests for brain damage. *J. Consult. Clin. Psychol.*, 31:619–25, 1967.

Victor, M.; Adams, R. D.; and Cole, M.: The acquired (non-Wilsonian) type of chronic hepatocerebral degeneration. *Medicine*, 44:345–96, 1965.

Vigliani, E. C.: Clinical observations on carbon disulfide intoxication in Italy. *Industr. Med. Surg.*, 19:240–42, 1950.

Vogt, C., and Vogt, O. (J. Psychol. Neurol., Lpz. 28, 1922), quoted by A. Meyer, Blackwood, W.; Meyer, A.; McMenemey, W. H.; Norman, R. M.; and Russell, D. S. (eds.): *Greenfields' Neuropathology*, 2nd ed. Edward Arnold, Ltd., London, 1963.

Walsh, J. C., and McLeod, J. J.: Alcoholic neuropathy. An electrophysiological and histological study. *J. Neurol. Sci.*, 10:457–65, 1970.

Wang, C. M.; Narahashi, T.; and Scuka, M.: Mechanism of negative temperature coefficient of nerve blocking action of allethrin. *J. Pharmacol. Exp. Ther.*, **182**:442–53, 1972.

Watson, W. E.: The response of motor neurons to intramuscular injection of botulinum toxin. *J. Physiol.*, **202**:611–30, 1969.

Watzman, N., and Barry, H., III: Drug effects on motor coordination. *Psychopharmacologia*, **12**:414–23, 1968.

Welsh, F. A., and O'Connor.: Patterns of microcirculatory failure during incomplete cerebral ischemia. *Adv. Neurol.*, **20**:133–149, 1978.

Westergaard, E.; van Deurs, B.; and Brondsted, H. E.: Increased vesicular transfer of horseradish peroxidase across cerebral endothelium evoked by acute hypertension. *Acta Neuropathol. (Berl.)*, **37**:141–52, 1977.

Windle, W. F.: Selective vulnerability of the central nervous system of rhesus monkeys to asphyxia during birth. In Schadé, J. F., and McMenemy, W. H. (eds.): *Selective Vulnerability of the Central Nervous System in Hypoxaemia*. F. A. Davis Co., Philadelphia, 1963.

Woolley, D. E.: Effects of DDT and of drug-DDT interactions of electroshock seizures in the rat. *Toxicol. Appl. Pharmacol.*, **16**:521–32, 1970.

———: Evaluation of behavioral and other neurological endpoints for assessing toxicity. In *Workshop on Behavioral Toxicology*. DHEW Publication No. NIH 76-1189, 1976, pp. 11–48.

Worden, A. N.; Palmer, A. C.; Noel, P. R. B.; and Mawdesley-Thomas, L. E.: Lesions in the brain of the dog induced by prolonged administration of monoamine oxidase inhibitors and isoniazid. *Proc. Eur. Soc. Study Drug Toxicol.*, **8**:149–61, 1967.

Wouters, W.; Van Den Bercken, J.; and Van Ginneken, A.: Presynaptic action of the pyrethroid insecticide allethrin in the frog motor end plate. *Eur. J. Pharmacol.*, **43**:163–71, 1977.

Chapter 14

TOXIC RESPONSES OF THE CARDIOVASCULAR SYSTEM

Tibor Balazs, Joseph P. Hanig, and Eugene H. Herman

INTRODUCTION

Chemicals can selectively affect the heart or the vasculature. The effect can be solely functional, lasting only during the exposure period, and its magnitude is usually dose-related. The risk of irreversibility of the effect increases with the dose or duration of exposure. Generally, after a functional change in the heart, the risk of lethality is greater than that which occurs after changes in other parenchymatous organs. Sudden death due to arrhythmia contributes to a major portion of the mortality caused by a drug overdose. Chemicals can also produce structural, i.e., degenerative and inflammatory, changes in the heart or blood vessels, and these in turn may lead to persistent functional changes. A structural change can develop even after a single exposure to drugs, e.g., the myocardial necrosis induced by a large dose of β-adrenergic agonist drugs.

Cardiovascular functional effects develop after administration of a lethal dose of most chemicals and are usually secondary to the changes in other organ systems. Primary cardiovascular toxicity is the most common consequence of an exaggerated pharmacologic effect after an overdose of cardiovascular drugs. Similarly, other organotropic drugs, e.g., those affecting the central nervous system (CNS) or the autonomic nervous system, may also affect the cardiovascular system; their toxicity can be unrelated to the therapeutic action and thus is a side effect.

Although cardiovascular diseases (hypertension, atherosclerosis, etc.) are the most prevalent chronic diseases of humans in industrialized societies today, the role of low-level chronic exposure to chemicals in the etiology of these conditions is unknown. A few chemicals such as lead, cadmium, and oral contraceptive steroids have been associated with the development of chronic cardiovascular disease in humans.

The mechanisms of selective, direct cardiovascular toxicity involve perturbations in membrane functions, particularly in ion transport and in the contractile or energy-supplying systems. Because of the great sensitivity of the heart to hypoxia and changes in acid-base balance and electrolytes, alterations via an effect of the chemical on other organs can indirectly lead to cardiovascular effects. It is conceivable that some of these conditions might play a role in the pathogenesis of insidiously developing cardiovascular diseases. For example, carbon monoxide reduces the amount of oxygen available to the heart, and tachycardia and electrocardiographic (ECG) changes suggestive of hypoxia can be the first sign of acute poisoning. Repeated long-term exposure to carbon monoxide can lead to structural damage of the blood vessels, which promotes the development of atherosclerosis. In addition to these toxicologic mechanisms, the immune system is involved in some of the cardiovascular reactions when the chemical acts as a hapten or directly affects the function of the immune system.

OVERVIEW OF CARDIOVASCULAR PATHOPHYSIOLOGIC AND PATHOLOGIC EFFECTS OF CHEMICALS

Cardiac Functions and Disorders

The most important manifestations of cardiac effects arise from alteration of electrical or contractile properties of the heart. Chemicals influence these properties by their actions on heart rate (chronotropic), conductivity (dromotropic), excitability (bathmotropic), or contractility (inotropic).

Arrhythmia. An arrhythmia can be caused by an alteration in the cardiac impulse rate, in the site of origin of the cardiac impulse, or in the velocity of cardiac impulse conduction. Arrhythmias are usually classified on the basis of

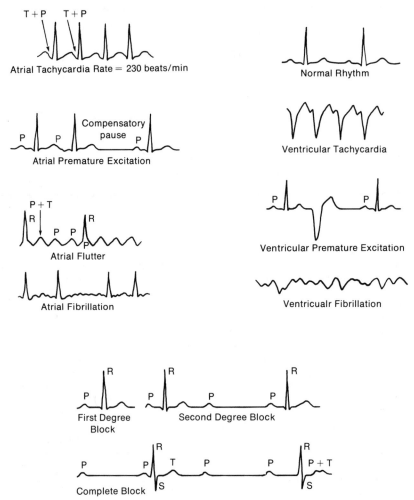

Figure 14–1. Electrocardiographic changes in various arrhythmias. (From Harvey, A. M., *et al.* [eds.]: *The Principles and Practice of Medicine,* 20th ed. Appleton-Century-Crofts, East Norwalk, Conn., 1980.)

ECG criteria (Figure 14–1). Some, such as sinus tachycardia or atrioventricular block, clearly result from disturbances of impulse formation or conduction, respectively. Others, such as ectopic beats arising in various parts of the heart, stem from excessive automaticity, from reentry excitation, or from impaired conduction, e.g., escape beats.

Disturbances of Impulse Formation. Under normal conditions, impulses originate in the heart by the spontaneous depolarization of specialized cells in the sinoatrial node (SA node). The rate of the depolarization can be altered by changes in autonomic nervous system activity. Increased vagal activity can slow or stop sinus nodal pacemakers, and increased sympathetic activity causes sinus tachycardia. Augmented automaticity in the His-Purkinje fibers of the

cardiac conducting system is a common cause of arrhythmias.

In contrast to normal mechanisms of automaticity, impulses arising from abnormal automatic mechanisms in the diseased or chemically altered heart can originate from atrial or ventricular working muscle cells as well as from the specialized conduction tissue. Normally the diastolic transmembrane potential of Purkinje fibers and ventricular cardiac cells is close to -90 mV and is largely the result of a potassium ion current in the resting cell. The action potential is initiated primarily by a rapid movement of sodium into the cell (fast current). However, when the diastolic transmembrane potential is reduced (shifted in the direction toward zero), depolarization can be mediated by the transport of other ions, particularly of calcium (slow current). Conditions predisposing to slow responses, such as regional acidosis or hyperkalemia accompanying ischemia, may result in an arrhythmia due to increased automaticity.

Chemicals can directly influence the initiation or propagation of the cardiac electrical impulse by altering the ionic gradients and fluxes that form the basis of these processes. For example, strontium and barium ions carry current through the slow channels in place of calcium ions, an action that initially stimulates the heart. However, they subsequently precipitate arrhythmias (ventricular extrasystoles and tachycardia leading to ventricular fibrillation) followed by cardiac standstill. These effects are thought to be due to impairment of the efflux of potassium ions from cardiac muscle cells.

If the action potential of a cardiac cell fails to return to the resting level along its normal time course so that repolarization is interrupted or delayed, a second action potential may arise (early afterdepolarization). Impulses can also arise by delayed afterdepolarization; in this instance, voltage swings to the resting diastolic level at the end of repolarization. However, rather than the voltage merely returning to the resting level, a secondary depolarization may occur in diastole. Delayed afterdepolarizations can cause either coupled extrasystoles or runs of tachyarrhythmias and can be triggered by premature systoles, by increases in spontaneous rate, calcium concentration, or sympathetic activity, and by agents such as the digitalis glycosides (Koch-Weser, 1979; Bigger and Hoffman, 1980).

Disturbances of Impulse Conduction. The two types of electrical activity (fast and slow responses) that have been detected either in anatomically different cardiac tissue or in chemically altered cardiac cells are recognized for their important role in the genesis of arrhythmias (Figure 14–2).

The action potential of fast-response cells is characterized by a large resting potential (-90 mV), a threshold potential of about -70 mV, a rapid influx of Na^+ (phase 0 of the action potential), and a large amplitude, all of which result in rapid conduction. Fast-response cells are located in the working atria and ventricles and in most portions of the conducting system except the SA and AV nodes. The fast-response fibers also possess a second slow inward current, carried by Ca^{2+} ions through separate, specific membrane channels. The slow response develops only when the fast Na^+ depolarizing current has decreased the transmembrane potential to about -55 mV. Sustained depolarization of the membrane to about -60 mV, by abnormal conditions such as increased extracellular K^+ or hypoxia, inactivates the fast Na^+ channel while leaving the slow calcium component functional. The ability of the slow-response action potential to propagate can be enhanced by catecholamines or phosphodiesterase inhibitors. The initiation and conduction of the slow-response action potentials in fibers that are partially depolarized by damage or hypoxia may initiate abnormalities of cardiac rhythm. Quinidine and other antiarrhythmic agents, paradoxically, may provoke rhythm dis-

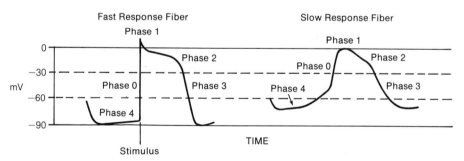

Figure 14–2. Action potential of cells of the cardiac conducting system. After depolarization during Phase 0, the cell slowly recovers and is fully repolarized by the end of Phase 3. A fast response fiber is illustrated on the left, and a slow response fiber on the right. Although the fast response fiber may have some spontaneous diastolic depolarization during Phase 4, most fibers are stimulated by an outside impulse, usually by propagation of an action potential from an adjacent cell in the conducting system. The slow response fiber, on the right, has a less negative maximum diastolic potential, a slower rate of rise of Phase 0, and has distinctly separated Phases 1, 2, and 3. Working muscle cells and cells in the conducting system outside the SA and AV nodes have action potentials more similar to the fast response fibers, with even less spontaneous diastolic depolarization. (From Harvey, A. M., *et al.* [eds.]: *The Principles and Practice of Medicine,* 20th ed. Appleton-Century-Crofts, East Norwalk, Conn., 1980.)

turbances as a result of an inhibiting effect on the fast inward Na^+ channel, thereby allowing development of slow responses.

In general, the most common site of conduction disturbance is the AV node, but similar disturbances may occur in branches of the bundle of His, or in the more peripheral Purkinje network. Agents that cause heart block do so by delaying propagation of electrical impulses in specialized myocardial conducting tissue. The digitalis glycosides increase the refractory period in the AV node and thus decrease impulse conduction velocity.

In certain situations, conduction delay and block paradoxically lead to tachyarrhythmias by the mechanism of reentry. Reentry consists of reexcitation caused by continuous propagation of the same impulse for one or more cycles. If the cardiac impulse enters a potentially reentrant pathway and conducts slowly through depolarized ischemic tissue in a circuitous pathway, it may reach normal myocardium, which has recovered its excitability. The SA and AV nodes are regions in which conduction is normally very slow, and further slowing by premature activation, disease, or certain agents leads to conditions that permit reentry. These factors also can create conditions that permit reentry in cells, such as the Purkinje fibers, that usually conduct cardiac impulses at very rapid rates. In most instances, marked slowing of conduction (the decrease of fast response or development of slow response) is the alteration that permits reentry.

Sensitization to Arrhythmias. The discovery that chloroform appeared to sensitize the heart to the effects of sympathomimetic amines was followed by the observation that a number of compounds, many of which are halogenated hydrocarbons, have the same property (Zakhari and Aviado, 1982; Reynolds, 1983). There are several actions by which the halogenated hydrocarbon chemicals can modify sensitivity of the cardiac pacemaking and conduction system to other agents. These include a marked suppression of SA nodal fibers with pacemaker migration to the AV junctional region and an enhanced propagation of premature beats due to a profound reduction of the refractory period of the Purkinje fibers. Some slowing of ventricular conduction may also contribute to enhanced arrhythmogenic activity by favoring reentry. Cardiac stimulation by catecholamines will result in a predictable sequence of events, regardless of the state of the organism. As the dose is increased, a sinus tachycardia followed by ventricular bigeminy, multifocal premature ventricular contractions, ventricular tachycardia, and finally ventricular fibrillation is a typical sequence. These effects will occur at lower doses when the heart has been exposed to halogenated hydrocarbon substances.

The increased myocardial sensitivity to the arrhythmogenic action of cardiac glycosides after potassium depletion by agents acting on the kidney is also well known. Digitalis glycosides produce a variety of cardiac arrhythmias by causing alterations in impulse formation, impulse conduction, or both. The cardiac arrhythmias that occur as part of digitalis toxicity appear to be due to an extension of the alteration of membrane Na^+-K^+-ATPase activity. Digitalis glycosides and extracellular K^+ have competitive affinities for Na^+-K^+-ATPase. K^+ may simultaneously stimulate enzyme activity and decrease the binding of glycosides to the ATPase. Cardiac glycosides will inhibit the exchange mechanism, resulting in a loss of intracellular K^+ and an increase in intracellular Na^+ concentration. A decrease in extracellular K^+ would enhance the inhibitory effect of the glycosides on the (Na^+-K^+-ATPase) system, allowing additional Na^+ to enter the cell. Under these conditions the magnitude of the membrane potential would approach the threshold for initiation of diastolic depolarization. This type of interaction can lead to sever arrhythmias, e.g., ventricular fibrillation (Deglin *et al.*, 1977; Bigger and Hoffman, 1980; Bowman and Rand, 1980).

Cardiac Contraction. Cardiac contraction is initiated by depolarization of the cardiac cell membrane, the sarcolemma (Figure 14–3). Immediately after the sudden surge of sodium into the cell, an equally rapid decrease in Na^+ membrane permeability toward the resting level occurs. In many mammals (e.g., humans, monkeys, dogs) the membrane remains depolarized at a relatively stable plateau before repolarization proceeds. The prolonged plateau phase of the action potential is due to a combination of a decrease in K^+ conductance and the activation of slow inward Ca^{2+} and Na^+ currents. Termination of the plateau phase and repolarization of the membrane follows as the conductance increases. As a consequence of these and other intracellular ionic events there is an increase in the intracellular free Ca^{2+} concentration obtained both from extracellular sources and by release of calcium stores loosely bound to sarcolemmal cisterns. The free calcium combines with one of the modulating myocardial proteins, troponin C, to alter the conformation of the troponin complex, releasing its inhibition on the myosin-ATPase contractile mechanism and thereby resulting in contraction. Relaxation follows as a result of active calcium uptake by the sarcoplasmic reticulum and possibly the sarcolemma and mitochondria (Bowman and Rand, 1980; Braunwald *et al.*, 1980a).

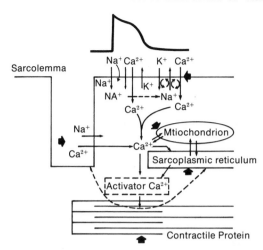

Figure 14–3. Schematic representation of organelles and molecular events of excitation-contraction coupling in the cardiac cell. Large shaded arrows indicate sites within the cardiac cell (sarcolemma, sarcoplasmic reticulum, mitochondria, and contactile proteins), where various agents, discussed in the text, may act to alter cardiac function and induce toxicity. (Reprinted with permission from Brody, T. M., and Chubb, J. M. In Balazs [ed.]: Cardiac Toxicology. Copyright 1981, CRC Press, Inc., Boca Raton, Fl.)

Effects of Chemicals on the Force of Contraction. Myocardial contraction is enhanced by an increase in availability of Ca^{2+} ions inside the cell. Catecholamines act through receptors located on the myocardial cell membrane that activate the adenyl cyclase system. The resulting increase in cyclic AMP ultimately affects membrane systems within the cells that deliver Ca^{2+} ions to the contractile proteins. Contraction is also increased to some degree by corticosteroids, angiotensin, serotonin, and glucagon. Myocardial contraction is decreased by hypoxia, by acidosis, and by many chemicals.

A decrease in force of contraction leading to acute heart failure may develop after an acute myocardial infarction or exposure to cardiodepressant substances. Certain conditions or substances (e.g., ethanol, haloalkanes, and cobalt) can also cause myocardial function to deteriorate slowly over many months or years. In this instance, cardiac output gradually becomes inadequate, and the overt signs of congestive heart failure develop.

Impaired cardiac contraction can result from interference with the autonomic nervous system control of the heart, from a decrease in cardiac energetics (availability of substrates for fuel, oxygen extraction, metabolic processes for energy production and/or utilization of energy), or from an alteration in the process of excitation contraction coupling.

Autonomic nervous system impulses reaching the heart result in the release of the neurochemical transmitters norepinephrine or acetylcholine. Sympathetic stimulation gives rise to an increased force of contraction. In contrast, interference with the release of norepinephrine attenuates sympathetic drive on the heart and decreases myocardial contractility.

Parasympathetic stimulation leads to a decrease in heart rate and force of contraction in the atria. Despite limited vagal innervation and muscarinic receptors in the ventricular muscle, vagal impulses or acetylcholine can also produce a negative inotropic effect in the ventricles of the intact heart.

Agents that interfere with the process of energy liberation and/or storage depress myocardial contractility (Merin, 1978; Van Stee, 1982). The energy contained in carbon-carbon and carbon-hydrogen bonds of substrates transported to the myocardial cells by blood in the coronary vascular bed is fundamental to the metabolic process. Cardiac muscle has the highest rate of oxygen consumption and the largest fractional extraction of arterial oxygen of any tissue. Oxygen availability becomes limited when coronary flow is reduced. When the coronary blood flow or oxygen extraction does not keep up with the demand, myocardial metabolism and function are disrupted.

Heart muscle can utilize energy from numerous fuel sources (Figure 14–4). Free fatty acids, ketone bodies, triglycerides, lactate, pyruvate, and glucose can all be extracted from the blood by the heart if the arterial concentrations are great enough. The energy available during oxidation of these substrates is conserved during oxidative phosphorylation and generation of adenosine triphosphate (ATP). Heart muscle obtains energy for contraction through hydrolysis of ATP. The heart stores this energy as both ATP and creatine phosphate (CP). CP is converted to ATP by reaction with adenosine diphosphate (ADP) under the influence of the enzyme creatine phosphokinase (CPK). Likely sites for chemical interference with energy metabolism would be the rate-limiting steps in the tricarboxylic acid cycle, electron transport systems, oxidative phosphorylation, and intracellular energy transport.

Energy utilization involves the conversion of chemical energy into mechanical energy, and into the energy necessary to drive ion pumps. Calcium ions provide a vital link in energy utilization. Catecholamines, by increasing cyclic AMP levels, regulate intracellular Ca^{2+} movements such as the entrance of Ca^{2+} during the cardiac action potential, the uptake of calcium into the sarcoplasmic reticulum, and phosphorylation of tropin. β-Adrenergic receptor block-

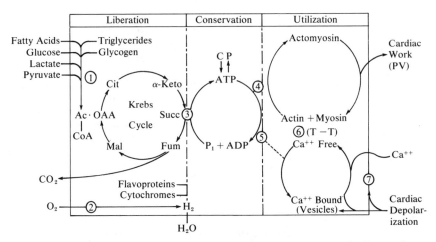

Figure 14–4. Schema of energetics in cardiac muscle. (From Olsen, R. E., *et al.*: Changes in energy stores in the hypoxic heart. *Cardiology*, **56**:114–24, 1971/72. Reprinted with permission of S. Karger AG, Basel.)

ing agents inhibit these actions and exert a negative inotropic effect. Interference with Ca^{2+} ion kinetics has been implicated as a locus of action of a number of substances that depress contractility (Braunwald, 1980; Braunwald *et al.*, 1980a, 1980b).

Chemicals can alter cardiac function by affecting any of the steps involved in the excitation-contraction coupling process (Brody and Chubb, 1981; Schlant and Sonnenblick, 1982).

Disturbances in the permeability of the cell membrane to ions or alterations in the activity of membrane-bound enzyme can change the shape and/or duration of the action potential and may influence myocardial contractile strength. Tetraethylammonium significantly alters the shape of the action potential and decreases the force of contraction by altering membrane potassium conductance. Inhibition of the cell membrane transport of calcium is yet another means by which drugs and chemicals can alter cardiac contractility and potentially cause cardiac toxicity. Verapamil blocks the slow inward calcium current, an action that decreases the concentration of intracellular calcium, and thus less calcium is available to interact with the contractile proteins and, as a result, contractile activity decreases. Alterations in membrane-bound enzyme activity can also affect cardiac function. For example, the ATP-dependent sodium pump (Na^+-K^+-ATPase), which maintains the normal transcellular gradient of Na^+ and K^+, is extremely sensitive to the cardiac glycosides, which inhibit its activity.

The smooth sarcoplasmic reticulum (SR) is involved in modulating calcium flux within the cell. The enzyme Ca^{2+}-Mg^{2+}-ATPase is embed-

ded within the SR membrane. Experimental evidence indicates that this enzyme (the "calcium pump") causes accumulation of intracellular free Ca^{2+} to an extent sufficient to effect complete relaxation of the myocardial muscles. The SR is also thought to release bound Ca^{2+} upon excitation of the muscle to effect contraction. Quinidine is known to have a depressant effect on cardiac contractility. *In vitro* studies, in which calcium uptake by partially purified SR vesicles was determined, indicated that quinidine exerted a dose-dependent inhibitory effect on this process. Thus, the mechanism by which quinidine inhibits calcium uptake may be mediated by a direct inhibitory effect on the SR "calcium pump."

Mitochondria have also been implicated as regulators of the cytosolic Ca^{2+} concentration. Drugs and chemicals that decrease the rate or extent of Ca^{2+} accumulation by the mitochondria may disrupt heart function. Lead concentrations at one-tenth of that required to inhibit heart mitochondrial oxidative phosphorylation significantly decreased the rate and extent of Ca^{2+} accumulation by mitochondria. If a significant impairment in mitochondrial Ca^{2+} accumulation occurs and if other organelles involved in the modulation of intracellular Ca^{2+} cannot remove the excess Ca^{2+}, cardiac structural alterations result.

The force that the muscle develops and the shortening that occurs is the result of the interaction of several protein molecules that make up the myofibrils of the myocardial cells. Myofibrils are divided into sarcomeres, which are composed of the proteins actin and myosin. Contraction occurs as a result of crossbridge formation between the actin and myosin molecules and subsequent lateral movement of the two proteins relative to each other. In order for crossbridges of the contractile proteins to form and lead to shortening or to force development, chemical energy must be supplied to the system in the form of ATP. ATPase activity is associated with the myosin protein, and the activity of this ATPase correlates with the ability of myosin to bind actin. Agents that alter the activity of myosin ATPase could conceivably affect cardiac performance. For example, the general anesthetic halothane depresses contractility, and this effect is mediated in part by the inhibition of myosin ATPase activity.

Circulatory Regulation and Disorders

For proper functioning of the cardiovascular system, at least two important parameters must be carefully regulated: mean arterial blood pressure and cardiac output. Mean arterial blood pressure (MABP) is controlled within fairly narrow limits while the cardiac output is regulated to match the work output or oxygen consumption of the organism and thus can vary over a wider range.

The short-term control of MABP is achieved through the arterial baroreceptors in the aortic arch and the carotid sinuses in conjunction with centers in the medulla, which have efferent connections to the heart, and to vascular smooth muscle in the arterioles and venules. The baroreceptors or pressoreceptors are maximally sensitive to arterial pressure changes near the normal range. Elevated arterial pressure increases the firing rate of the baroreceptor nerves and results in decreased output from the sympathetic regions and increased output from the parasympathetic regions of the brain. Decreased sympathetic discharge to the periphery decreases the heart rate and contractility in the heart, decreases arteriolar resistance, and increases venous capacitance. These effects combine to decrease peripheral resistance. A fall in MABP has the opposite effects.

The long-term regulation of MABP is primarily achieved by blood volume regulation and thus requires the integrity of kidney function along with the renin-angiotensin system, antidiuretic hormone, and aldosterone level. Maintenance of the MABP is important, since it is the driving force for blood flow through peripheral organs.

The cardiac output can vary over a five- to sixfold range. This variation is tightly linked to whole-body oxygen consumption. Of equal importance to the absolute level of the cardiac output is the distribution of the cardiac output to the vital organs. Important mechanisms that are responsible for the distribution of the cardiac output include neural control and local regulation. Neural control consists primarily of increasing or decreasing the level of sympathetic discharge to vascular smooth muscle in arterioles. The effects elicited by sympathetic stimulation are specific in each tissue and are largely dependent on the density and proportion of α- and β-adrenergic receptors. Stimulation of α receptors generally elicits vasoconstriction and stimulation of β receptors usually causes vasodilation. α-Adrenergic agonists increase Ca^{2+} influx via the slow inward current. Cytoplasmic bound Ca^{2+} activates an enzyme that phosphorylates myosin to interact with actin, leading to contraction of the vascular smooth muscle. β-Adrenergic agonists increase cyclic AMP, which, by activation of protein kinase, enhances the efflux of Ca^{2+} and results in relaxation of the vessel wall. Similarly, manganese, cobalt, and Ca^{2+} antagonists cause relaxation of the vascular smooth muscle.

In contrast to neural control is the local control of blood flow to certain tissues. The heart, brain, and skeletal muscles are very adept at regulating their own flow locally to match the metabolic needs of that particular tissue. The local control of blood flow, called autoregulation, is mediated by products of metabolism, so that increased work is accompanied by increased tissue metabolism along with an increased blood flow. Other organs of the body, such as the gastrointestinal tract and the skin, are more dependent on neural regulation of their flow and will exhibit an increase in blood flow with decreases in sympathetic discharge. This mechanism subserves GI function during digestion and also the important role of the skin in heat dissipation for temperature regulation.

The changes in cardiac output are the result of altered venous return from the periphery, along with changes in myocardial contractility and rate of contraction. The distribution of blood flow is primarily determined by neural mechanisms from the CNS as modified by local autoregulation in certain tissues. Thus, the cardiac output is generally distributed to organ systems in proportion to their activity, both mechanical and metabolic.

Hypotension, Shock. When cardiac output or the MABP falls to critically low levels, the perfusion of vital organs is reduced. Hypotension, a sustained reduction of systemic arterial pressure, is common in acute poisoning, e.g., with CNS depressants, in anaphylactic reactions, or with an overdose of certain antihypertensive agents (orthostatic hypotension). Circulatory insufficiency may not develop, since increased sympathoadrenal activity results in compensatory circulatory changes. However, in poisoning with cytotoxic chemicals, e.g., heavy metals, when a large amount of plasma is lost in the areas of inflammation and hemorrhage or when endotoxins from the gut flora enter the circulation, a state of circulatory insufficiency (shock) may develop. Inadequate blood volume in the absence of hemorrhage follows increased loss of body fluids brought about by persistent vomiting or diarrhea due to gastroenteritis, as occurs in poisoning with a variety of chemicals. Decreased intravascular volume leads to a decreased cardiac output. Other causes of shock include inadequate myocardial contraction resulting from severe arrhythmia, from cardiomyopathies, or inadequate peripheral circulation brought about by an altered vasomotor tone due to the effects of chemical mediators, e.g., histamine, leukotriene, and kinins. In shock, all physiologic parameters concerned with the perfusion of tissues are disturbed. The most critical effect involves the small blood vessels, the microcirculation, which is ultimately responsible for the exchange between blood and tissue. When compromised, signs of tissue death due to hypoxia and acidosis appear.

Hypertension. Chemicals can increase systemic arterial (systolic and/or diastolic) blood pressure as an acute event or can contribute to the development of its sustained increase by a variety of mechanisms.

Arterial hypertension may occur in the course of an overdose with sympathomimetic and anticholinergic drugs. Sudden drug-induced hypertension can cause cerebrovascular accidents when diseased blood vessels cannot adapt to high perfusion pressures. The sympathomimetic amines (norepinephrine, epinephrine, phenylephrine, etc.) elevate blood pressure by stimulating vascular α- receptors with or without increasing cardiac output. The administration of 10 percent phenylephrine, even as an eyedrop, may be followed by hypertension, especially in the neonate.

Mineralocorticoids, especially when administered with sodium chloride, cause sodium retention and elevate blood pressure via an increase in circulatory volume. Licorice, which contains glycyrrhizin, an aldosteronelike substance that exerts mineralocorticoid activity, can cause sustained hypertension. Agents that cause hyperreninemia, e.g., cadmium, raise blood pressure by the generation of angiotensinogen II, which acts directly on the vascular smooth muscle. Depletion of renomedullary vasodilator substances has been implicated in the hypertension associated with analgesic drug-induced nephropathy. Increased synthesis of angiotensinogen has been considered to be a factor in the hypertension produced by high dosages of estrogen-containing oral contraceptives.

Sustained hypertension is the most important risk factor predisposing to coronary and cerebral atherosclerosis. The mechanisms by which hypertension produces vascular degenerative lesions involve increased vascular permeability with entry of blood constituents into the vessel wall, activation of phospholipase, and release of free arachidonate. The role of oxygen-centered free radicals generated in the arachidonate-prostaglandin pathways has been implicated in the development of destructive lesions of endothelium and vascular smooth muscle (Kontos and Hess, 1983).

Hemorrhage. Although chemicals can affect the structure of large vessels, leading to hemorrhage, e.g., aneurysms produced by lathyrogens, the capillaries are more frequently affected, often by nonspecific mechanisms, e.g., anoxia. Capillaries are common targets of cytotoxic chemicals, and therefore petechial hemorrhages are common in several organs after acute poisonings. A chemically induced defect in the blood-clotting mechanism increases the probability that hemorrhage may occur after a trivial trauma. Several chemicals can decrease platelet count by either a toxic mechanism (certain antitumor drugs) or an immune system-mediated mechanism (antiplatelet antibodies). Chemicals can also inhibit the synthesis of clotting factors; e.g., coumarin inhibits the synthesis of prothrombin.

Thrombosis, Embolism. Thrombosis, the formation of a semisolid mass from blood constituents in the circulation, can occur both in arteries and in veins. Chemically induced predisposition to thrombosis most frequently occurs by induction of platelet aggregation, by an increase of their adhesiveness or by creation of a state of hypercoagulability via an increase or activation of clotting factors. Large doses of epinephrine can affect each of these events. Effects on the platelets play a role in the thrombogenic action of the azo dye Congo Red; when injected intravenously, the effect on coagulation is responsible for the thrombogenic effect of intravenously injected free fatty acids. Other sites of action of chemicals in predisposing to thrombosis include effects on antithrombin III (by oral contraceptive steroids) and inhibition of fibrinolysis (by corticosteroids, mercurials). Sudden changes in blood flow brought about by vasoconstriction (e.g., by ergotamine) or a decrease in peripheral resistance (e.g., by an autonomic blocking drug) can trigger arterial thrombosis. Venous stasis contributes to the development of venous thrombosis (Zbinden, 1976). Table 14-1 presents a list of thrombogenic agents and conditions.

Table 14–1. COMPOUNDS PRODUCING THROMBOSIS*

AGENT	SITE OF ACTION AND/OR MECHANISM
	Endothelial Damage
Homocystine	Deendothelialization
Endotoxin	Deendothelialization
Polyanethol sulfate	Deendothelialization
Sodium acetriozate (radiocontrast agent)	Disseminated thrombosis in capillaries and veins; formation of insoluble fibrinogen derivative due to extraction of glycoproteins
	Pathophysiologic Circulatory Dynamics
Ergotamine	Profound vasoconstriction in peripheral arteries
Pitressin	Profound vasoconstriction in coronary and mesenteric arteries
Oral contraceptives	Venous stasis in lower extremities
ACh and autonomic blockers	Hypovolemic hypotension and stasis
Sympathomimetic agents	Elevated blood pressure and turbulence at bifurcations; distensions of vessels to produce endothelial damage
	Effects on Platelets
Serotonin	Increase in platelet count (above
Progesterone	$10^6/mm^3$) symptomatic thrombocythemia
Testosterone	
Somatotropic hormone	
Vinblastine	
Vincristine	
Congo red	Increase in platelet aggregation
Ristocetin (antibiotic)	
Serotonin	
Thrombin	
Epinephrine	
Adenosine diphosphate	Increase in platelet adhesiveness
Epinephrine	
Thrombin	
Evans blue	
	Effects on Clotting Factors
Epinephrine	Increase in factors VIII and IX
Guanethidine	Secondary effects due to release of epinephrine
Debrisoquin	
Tyramine	
Lactic acid (iv infusion)	Activation of Hageman factor
Long-chain fatty acids (iv infusion)	Activation of Contact factors
Catecholamines	Elevation in circulating levels of fatty acids
ACTH	
Thymoleptics	
Nicotine	
Oral contraceptives	Decrease in antithrombin III levels
Mercuric chloride	Inhibition of fibrinolysis
Prednisolone (corticosteroids)	
ε-Aminocaproic acid	Plasminogen antiactivator
Tranexamic acid	
Aprotinine	Proteinase inhibitors
Iniprol	

*Data from Zbinden (1976).

Injury to the vessel wall by intravenous infusion of an irritating drug produces phlebitis, or by generalized endothelial damage (e.g., that caused by polyanethol sulfonate) produces thromboses at the sites of lesions. Portions of thrombi may break and travel in the vascular system until arrested—an embolus—in a vessel of smaller caliber than that of its origin. The consequence depends on the site of arrest. The most important drugs that produce thromboembolisms are the contraceptive steroids.

Chemically Induced Structural Changes in the Heart and in the Blood Vessels

Cardiac Changes. Chemically induced structural effects in the heart usually are manifested in the myocardium as focal or diffuse degenerative changes. A predilectional site is the left ventricular subendocardium because of its great sensitivity to hypoxia due to the lowest perfusion pressure of this area. Histologically, the muscle cells show increased eosinophilia, loss of striations, and granularity of the cytoplasm. Acute inflammatory signs, such as vascular dilation, tissue edema, and leukocytic infiltration, accompany the lesion (Figure 14–5). Lymphocytes, monocytes, macrophages, and fibroblasts are present in the subacute lesion and are gradually replaced by collagen. By electron microscopic examination the earliest change, observed two minutes after injection of a necrosis-inducing intraperitoneal dose of isoproterenol HCl to rats, consisted of hypercontraction of myofibrils in muscle cells in the apical subendocardium. Over the next few minutes "contraction bands" developed. This event was attributable to an excessive calcium influx. In two hours the bands disappeared, perhaps through the action of calcium-activated proteases. Doughnut-shaped granules then appeared in the mitochondria; they were identical to those observed when the mitochondria were calcium-loaded and are regarded as evidence of irreversible damage. Inflammatory cells appeared by eight hours. The lesion progressed to myocytolysis (Balazs and Bloom, 1982).

An increased Ca^{2+} contributes to ATP depletion by stimulating its hydrolysis and inhibiting mitochondrial ATP synthesis. As a result of ATP catabolism, hypoxanthine accumulates. Ca^{2+} activates neutral proteases, which convert xanthine dehydrogenase to xanthine oxidase, an enzyme that generates a superoxide radical from O_2 during hypoxia. The superoxide will react with itself and yields peroxide, which reacts with superoxide to yield oxygen, water, and the most reactive free OH radical (Titus, 1983).

In hypersensitivity myocarditis, focal or diffuse interstitial infiltrations with eosinophils, lymphocytes, and plasma cells are characteristic. Necrotic changes are usually absent. Vasculitis may be associated with this reaction, which heals without a scar after withdrawal of the chemical. Penicillin-, sulfonamide-, and methyldopa-induced myocarditis fit into this category (Billingham, 1980).

Slowly developing cardiomyopathies occur in chronic alcoholics and in patients treated with the antineoplastic anthracyclines. In these patients the heart fails progressively, and the clinical syndrome of congestive heart failure develops. Ventricular dilatation, diffuse myocardial cellular degeneration, and/or interstitial fibrosis are the main morphologic findings. Alcoholics have an accumulation of lipid droplets in the cardiac muscle cells. Anthracyclines produce myofibrillar loss and cytoplasmic vacuolization (Ferrans, 1982).

Prolonged administration of certain chemicals can lead to cardiac hypertrophy, an increase in the mass of the muscle due to the increase in size of the cells. In these cells the nuclei, mitochondria, and Golgi complexes are enlarged and the ribosomes are increased. Prolonged treatment with very high doses of sympathomimetics, such as isoproterenol or thyroid hormones, produce hypertrophy.

Inflammation of the serous membranes of the heart is most commonly a part of hypersensitivity reactions, e.g., a lupus erythematosus-like reaction induced by hydralazine or procainamide. Endocardial and valvular fibrosis has occurred in patients taking methysergide, a congener of LSD.

A few chemicals have produced tumors in the heart in rodents; e.g., 1,3-butadiene and nitrosamines caused sarcomas (Billingham, 1980).

Vascular Changes. Chemicals can produce degenerative and/or inflammatory changes in the blood vessels as a consequence of an excessive pharmacologic effect or by an interaction with a vascular structural or functional macromolecule. As a result of sustained arterial vasoconstriction, peripheral arterial lesions consisting of intimal proliferation and medial degenerative changes leading to gangrene develop with ergotamine intoxication. An example of a direct toxic mechanism is that produced by allylamine; when the compound was given orally to rats for a few weeks, it produced vascular smooth muscle hyperplasia that resulted in coronary artery and aortic lesions mimicking the arteriosclerotic process. The active metabolite is acrolein, which denatures protein and disrupts nucleic acid synthesis. Deposition of fibrinlike material in the ground substance of collagen leads to fi-

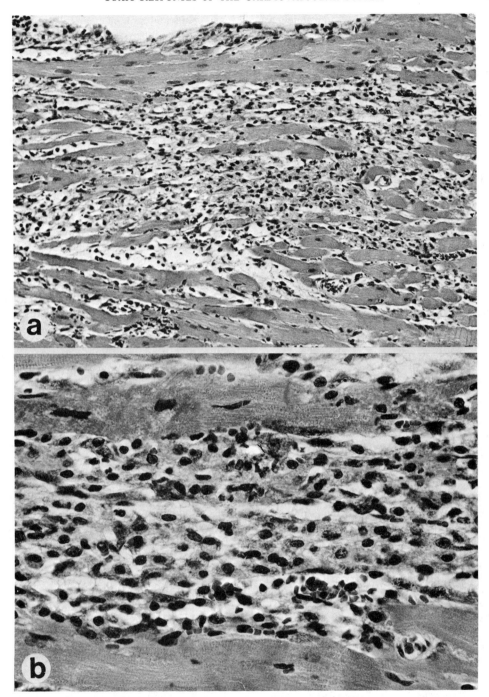

Figure 14–5. Hydralazine-induced lesions in a rat: (*a*) subendocardial region of left ventricular free wall, showing areas of necrosis and infiltrate of mononuclear cells; (*b*) high-power view shows fresh necrosis in some muscle cells at top, as evidenced by the loss of cross striations, presence of contraction bands, and apparent presence of mononuclear cells within the fibers. H&E 130X and 400X. (From Balazs, T., *et al.:* Study of the mechanism of hydralazine-induced myocardial necrosis in the rat. *Toxicol. Appl. Pharmacol.*, **59**:524–34, 1981.)

brinoid necrosis. It is an early consequence of hypertension due to the entry of fibrinogen into the wall of small arteries.

Changes in the collagen of the large arteries leading to localized dilatations (aneurysms) occur in lathyrism or are produced by β-aminopropionitrile in young rats and various avian species.

Atherosclerosis is a degenerative process occurring within arteries; plaques containing lipids, complex carbohydrates, blood products, and calcium accumulate in the intima and inner portion of the media. This lesion generally occurs in major blood vessels such as the aorta and coronary, carotid, and femoral arteries. Early experiments have shown that diets high in saturated fats and cholesterol produce atheromas; however, recently the low-density β-lipoproteins have been implicated along with stress and hypertension as predisposing factors. The principal consequence of atheroma is narrowing of an artery. If the narrowing occurs in a renal artery, a renal hypertension may develop. When this process occurs in the cerebral vessels, there is a potential for stroke; when it occurs in the coronary artery, myocardial ischemia can occur and may culminate in a myocardial infarction.

Chemicals can produce or enhance atheroma formation by several mechanisms. Carbon monoxide, which increases capillary permeability, accelerates plaque formation in animals on atherogenic, high-cholesterol diets. The effect of CO may actually be due, however, to a lack of oxygen, since atheroma formation is also enhanced in animals subjected to hypoxia. Another agent is carbon disulfide (CS_2), which has produced a two- to threefold increase in coronary heart disease in exposed industrial workers. In cholesterol-fed rabbits, CS_2 greatly accelerated the formation of atheroma. The mechanism for CS_2-atheroma production is thought to consist of direct injury to the endothelium coupled with changes in lipid metabolism associated with hypothyroidism, since thiocarbamate (thiourea), a potent antithyroid substance, is a principal urinary metabolite of CS_2. Homocysteine has direct effects on the arterial and venous walls. The process involves platelet adhesion, proliferation of smooth muscle cells, accumulation of lipid into these cells with their subsequent transformation into foam cells, and finally loss of the endothelial layer at the site of the atherogenic defect (Van Stee, 1982).

Hypersensitivity, immune system-mediated vasculitis, generally occurs in small vessels (arterioles, venules, capillaries), although the coronary arteries can be involved. The presence of eosinophils and mononuclear cells is characteristic. The pathogenesis is associated with the deposition of soluble immune complexes in the vessel wall and with the activation of the complement system. Gold salts, methyldopa, penicillin, sulfonamides, and several other drugs can produce this reaction in humans (Ferrans, 1982). Some of these drugs have also been suspected to exacerbate preexisting polyarteritis (a necrotizing vasculitis) or cause a syndrome like periarteritis nodosa, a vascular disease of unknown origin (Billingham, 1980).

Vascular Effects in Vital Organs

Brain. The integrity of the vascular components of the blood-brain barrier (BBB) relies on the metabolic status of the endothelial cells and the effectiveness of tight junctions between them.

Anoxia and ischemia of the brain will cause endothelial cells to swell and the junctions to widen, but it takes several hours for the barriers to break down, resulting in vascular disruption. In addition, hypercapnia (very high CO_2 concentrations) opens the BBB by abolishing autoregulation and producing brain edema. Cerebral blood flow is greatly increased, and hemorrhages may occur. Another process that increases cerebrovascular permeability is pinocytosis, and this is increased by agents such as divalent cations, high concentrations of norepinephrine and serotonin, and chemically induced convulsions (e.g., those caused by metrazol).

Lead is deleterious to sulfhydryl proteins that form structural units as well as biochemical enzyme systems. It produces encephalopathy with brain edema, and toxic effects on endothelial cells occur before those on the neurons and glia. Newborn rats exposed to lead showed separation at tight junctions, increase of permeability, and loss of a major portion of the BBB (Rapoport, 1976).

A variety of cytolytic agents break down the BBB by disruptive effects on cell membranes and capillaries. These agents include alcohols, other lipid solvents, cobra venom, surfactants, and high concentrations of sulfhydryl inhibitors (Bakay, 1956). Hypertonic solutions of NaCl, urea, mannitol, etc., cause reversible opening of the BBB due to shrinking of vascular endothelium and separation of tight junctions.

Lungs. Alveolar capillary fragility and permeability changes result in pulmonary edema and a serious decrease in oxygen exchange. This occurs often following inhalation of irritant gases. Excessive intravenous infusion of fluid is the most frequent cause of iatrogenic pulmonary edema, especially following replacement of blood loss by electrolyte solutions. Opiates (heroin, methadone) can produce delayed pulmonary edema after intravenous self-administration; neurogenic alterations of capillary permeability of central origin are implicated. Drug addicts who self-administer dissolved tablets intravenously develop pulmonary embolism and thrombosis because of the talc vehicle. Pulmonary thromboembolism has been associated with the use of high doses of oral contraceptive estrogens in women who are predisposed to thrombosis.

The pyrrolizidine alkaloid microcrotaline, at a single dose of 50 mg/kg in rats, produced pulmonary hypertension four weeks later. Ultrastructural changes consisted of evagination of vascular smooth muscle cells with loss of myofilament cells during the onset of hypertension (Smith and Heath, 1976). Pulmonary arterial hypertension often developed in obese patients taking large doses of an anorexic drug, aminorex fumarate. Histologically intimal and medial thickening was detected. These changes could not be reproduced in animal experiments.

Carbamylhydrazine HCl induced tumors in blood vessels of the lung after oral administration to mice (Toth *et al.*, 1975).

Liver. Hepatotoxins that produce hemorrhagic necrosis, e.g., dimethylnitrosamine, ultimately produce occlusion of veins. Pyrrolizidine alkaloids produce identical effects resulting in hepatic venoocclusive disease, which is not uncommon in children in South Asia. The initial lesion consists of a proliferation of the endothelium in the small efferent veins followed by a proliferation of the vascular connective tissue leading to an occlusion of these veins. This can result in early death.

Oral contraceptives have produced thrombosis in the portal circulation, involving proliferation and thickening of the intima. A rare condition, peliosis, is induced by estrogenic and androgenic steroids. This lesion consists of islands of dilated portal sinusoids, and fatal bleeding may occur from their rupture. Endotoxins produce swelling of Kupffer and endothelial cells, as well as adhesion of platelets to sinusoid walls, all of which affect the microcirculation.

Chronic hepatitis induced by oxyphenisatin or nitrofurantoin and cirrhosis induced by ethanol, arsenicals, or methotrexate, etc., lead to the development of portal hypertension. Tumors of the hepatic vasculature have been induced by thorium dioxide and vinyl chloride; hemangioendotheliomas and hemangiosarcomas, respectively, have been reported.

Kidney. Several nephrotoxins affect the renal blood vessels and can cause marked constriction of renal arteries. Preglomerular vasoconstriction and/or relaxation of the postglomerular vessels greatly depresses the glomerular filtration rate. A tubuloglomerular feedback control mediated by the vasoconstrictor effect of adenosine shuts down glomerular vessels following necrosis of the tubular epithelium. Nephropathies induced by cadmium, lead, and certain analgesics produce systemic arterial hypertension by affecting one or more components of the renal blood pressure regulatory systems. Structural changes of the renal vessels, consisting of diffuse fibrosis of the capillaries, have been reported after chronic exposure to cadmium in experimental animals.

Immune complex deposits on the basement membranes of glomerular capillaries are characteristic of hypersensitivity reactions induced by a large number of chemicals, e.g., gold salts, *d*-penicillamine in humans, and $HgCl_2$ in experimental animals.

Heart. A large number of endogenous substances, e.g., epinephrine, angiotensin, histamine, thromboxane, and leukotrienes, can cause marked constriction of the coronary arteries. Ergonovine and vasopressin are the most consistent provokers of coronary spasm in the clinical setting and also in experimental animals. Coronary constriction results in myocardial hypoxia with ECG signs such as ST segment deviation. It can precipitate death in patients with preexisting heart disease.

Withdrawal of coronary vasodilators such as nitroglycerin or nitroglycol caused sudden death in industrial workers who were exposed all week on the job and then abstained from the chemical on weekends. They were adapted and dependent on the continuous presence of these compounds to maintain a minimum level of coronary flow. A second mechanism for coronary artery toxicity due to nitrites and nitrates relates to the so-called aging of the coronary arteries due to repeated vasodilation and the metabolic sequelae of heme redox reactions. This toxicity is nonspecific, since it is also seen after prolonged exposure to CS_2 (Magos, 1981).

Structural changes consisting of intimal proliferation and vascular occulusion or atherosclerotic lesions have been produced by methysergide and cigarette smoke, respectively, in chronic animal experiments.

Teratogenic Effects

Cardiovascular teratologic changes have been produced by a variety of chemicals. In humans, the critical period for the cardiovascular teratogenesis is from the fifth to the eighth week after conception. Failures to form, to persist, or to involute a specific structure result in malformations. Ventricular or arterial septal defects, patent ductus arteriosus, and tetralogy of Fallot are the most common cardiovascular abnormalities that have been induced by chemicals. Trypan blue and bis(dichloroacetyl) diamine can produce changes in a high incidence (Jackson, 1981). Cardiovascular functional disturbances, e.g., systemic hypertension, can develop in the progeny after treatment with certain drugs (salicylate, indomethacin) during pregnancy (Balazs, 1982).

TOXICOLOGIC CLASSIFICATIONS OF CARDIOVASCULAR REACTIONS

Three mechanisms can be distinguished in the development of cardiovascular toxicity. The first is related to an exaggerated pharmacologic effect of a compound, e.g., to overdoses of cardiovascular drugs. Drugs increase or decrease the intensity of organ function; an effect beyond the physiologic limits represents a dysfunction. The cardiotoxicity of β-adrenergic agonists, e.g., isoproterenol, is an example of such a mechanism. This drug affects both the cardiac β_1 and vascular and bronchial β_2 receptors and produces tachycardia and hypotension in low multiples of the bronchodilator doses. Tachycardia increases the myocardial oxygen demand, which may not be met, and ECG signs of myocardial hypoxia, ST segment depression, and arrhythmia develop. The hypoxia is most marked in the least perfused left ventricular subendocardium, as evidenced by the greatest degree of ATP, phosphocreatine, and glycogen depletion and lactate accumulation. This is also the area where necrosis develops in experimental animals given a grossly very high dose of isoproterenol. β-Adrenergic-receptor blocking agents decrease both the pharmacologic and cardiotoxic effects of isoproterenol, indicating the role of the pharmacologic mechanism in the pathogenesis of the lesion (Balazs and Bloom, 1982).

Digitalis-, quinidine-, and procainamide-induced arrhythmias and antihypertensive-induced orthostatic hypotension are other examples of cardiovascular toxicities induced by exaggerated pharmacologic effects.

A second mechanism of cardiotoxicity involves an irreversible interaction of a chemical or its metabolite with a functional or structural molecule of vital significance. The binding is not a specific one, like that of a ligand to a receptor, but is nonspecific and covalent, like that of a free radical to a nucleophile. The development of the lesion depends on the rate of reactive metabolite formation and the concentration of protective substances in the cell. The protective mechanism against free radicals in the heart is at a lower level than that which exists in other parenchymatous organs, and therefore the heart is especially susceptible to the effects of these chemicals. A free-radical mechanism plays a role in the chronic cardiotoxicity of antineoplastic anthracyclines. These drugs are reducible to a semiquinone radical by flavin-dependent oxidoreductases. The semiquinone reacts with oxygen to produce a superoxide radical which, together with other reaction products, e.g., a free OH radical, initiates lipid peroxidation and thereby the lesion. The process leads to the development of a cardiomyopathy. Free-radical capturing agents ameliorate the cardiotoxicity of these drugs in experimental animals (Titus, 1983).

Another example of *in situ* formation of a reactive cardiotoxic metabolite is represented by acrolein, which is generated from allylamine by oxidative deamination. Oral administration of this compound to rats for a few weeks produces myocardial and vascular fibroses. Inhibition of the enzymatic transformation of allylamine to acrolein protects against the lesion (Boor, 1983). Acrolein conjugates with reduced glutathione and is excreted as mercapturic acid in the urine. Depletion of glutathione would be expected to enhance the toxicity.

A third mechanism of cardiovascular toxicity is represented by the immune system-mediated effects. In these "hypersensitivity" reactions, either the compound acts as a hapten that binds to an endogenous macromolecule, e.g., protein or nucleic acid, or the compound may act directly on the immune system, e.g., on helper or suppressor T cells. The cardiovascular system is affected in systemic anaphylaxis, where the protein-bound hapten binds to IgE on mast cells and basophils and elicits the release of histamine, serotonin, and leukotriene, the mediators of effects. The haptenic antigen may bind to the cell membrane and, combining with the antibody produced or via lymphocytes, triggers a cytotoxic reaction. Antigen-antibody complexes deposited in the tissue can initiate—via complement fixation—inflammatory reactions, often in the blood vessels. Although a large number of commonly used drugs, e.g., aspirin, sulfonamides, and penicillin, can produce a cardiovascular hypersensitivity reaction, the incidence is very low. It is likely, as with other hypersensitivity reactions, that immunogenetic determinants, coded by the genes of the major histocompatibility complex, predispose to their development. The gene products are extremely polymorphic. The presence of a set of specific alleles (haplotypes) is required to produce the determinant on which the susceptibility to the antigen and the development of the reaction depends (Balazs, 1983).

Cardiotoxic Chemicals

Aliphatic Alcohols, Aldehydes, and Glycols. Ethanol decreases the force of cardiac contraction at a blood concentration of 75 mg/100 ml in humans. Although a negative dromotropic effect and a decreased threshold for ventricular fibrillation have been shown to occur in dogs after a single intravenous administration of ethanol, arrhythmias are prominent only after long-term treatment. These effects also occur in chronic alcoholics and may result in ventricular fibrillation and sudden death. Chronic alcohol consumption (alcoholism) decreases myocardial capacity on increased demand, resulting in dyspnea due to pulmonary congestion. Cardiomegaly or dilation of the chambers with mural thrombi are the postmortem findings. Interstitial fibrosis and increased lipid in the muscle cells are seen histologically (Billingham, 1980).

Although the acute cardiotoxicity of methanol is comparable to that of ethanol, those of the longer-chain alcohols are geater on a molar basis (Rubin and Rubin, 1982).

Acetaldehyde, the hepatic metabolic product of ethanol oxidation, has negative inotropic effects at blood concentrations that occur after a moderate ethanol intake. At higher concentrations, acetaldehyde releases catecholamines; hence it produces sympathomimetic effects. Such an effect gradually decreases with aldehydes of increasing chain length.

Dihydroxyalcohols, e.g., propylene glycol and polyethylene glycol-500, have cardiac effects in some instances when they are used as a vehicle for drugs. The former enhances the arrhythmogenic effect of digitalis and the latter the pressor effect of epinephrine in experimental animals (Van Stee, 1982).

The mechanism of the acute cardiodepressant effects of alcohols and aldehydes is related to an inhibition of intracellular calcium transport. The mechanism of chronic cardiotoxicity of ethanol involves several metabolic changes, such as increased triglyceride and proteoglycan formations.

Halogenated Alkanes. The cardiotoxicity of low-molecular-weight halogenated hydrocarbons is greater than that of unsubstituted hydrocarbons. They depress the heart rate, contractility, and conduction. The number of halogen atoms and unsaturated bonds influences the relative potency; e.g., negative inotropism of the substituted ethanes increases with up to four

chlorines, and trichloroethylene is more potent than trichloroethanol. Some of these agents sensitize the heart to the arrhythmogenic effect of endogenous epinephrine or to β-adrenergic agonist drugs. Chloroform was one of the first agents to be recognized as having this sensitizing effect, and recently the low-pressure fluorocarbons, the Freons, have been reported to be sensitizing agents. Trichlorofluoromethane, one of the most toxic fluorocarbons, sensitized dogs to epinephrine at a concentration of 0.3 percent, and such an effect has also occurred in humans (Zakhari and Aviado, 1982).

Halogenated hydrocarbon anesthetics generally have effects similar to those described above. Halothane, methoxyflurane, and enflurane have negative chronotropic, inotropic, and dromotropic effects at the concentration used for anesthesia. Hence, they can produce myocardial depression and, although rarely, even cardiac arrest. Nevertheless, the stimulation of the sympathetic nervous system by respiratory acidosis, tracheal intubation, or surgical manipulation during an inadequate depth of anesthesia results in cardiac stimulation or even arrhythmia. The older and now obsolete anesthetics, e.g., cyclopropane and diethyl ether, were more potent sensitizers of the heart to epinephrine than are the modern anesthetics (Merin, 1981; Steffey, 1982).

The effects of the halogenated hydrocarbons are reversible, at least in patients without preexisting cardiovascular disease. Chronic exposure to certain haloalkanes has been surmised to produce degenerative cardiac changes in humans. In investigations of the cardiodepressant mechanisms of these agents, interference with energy production and utilization and in the transfer of intracellular calcium between subcellular compartments has been postulated.

Heavy Metals. Among heavy metals causally associated with cardiovascular disease, cadmium, lead, and cobalt have selective cardiotoxic effects. They are negative inotropics and dromotropics and can also produce structural changes in the heart. A single dose of cadmium at 3 mg/kg intraperitoneally or 6 months of oral treatment (130 mg/L in drinking water) in rats prolonged the P-R interval in the ECG. Chronic treatment also caused cardiac hypertrophy and vacuolation in the Purkinje cells. Lead given to rats for six weeks (100 mg/L) produced degenerative changes in the heart. Such changes have also been detected in humans, in "moonshine" drinkers, and in children exposed to high doses of lead. A delayed effect of prenatal exposure of rats to lead manifested itself as a sensitization to the arrhythmogenic effect of norepinephrine postnatally. Similar phenomena were observed in adult rats receiving lead as neonates. Arrhythmias also occur in children exposed to lead and disappear after chelation therapy.

Cobalt, given orally to rats for eight weeks at doses of 26 mg/kg after an initial 100 mg/kg dose, produced cardiomyopathy. Rats kept on a low-protein diet developed vacuolar hydropic lesions after two weeks of treatment with cobalt at 4 to 12.5 mg/kg. The lesions were similar to those observed in heavy beer drinkers consuming a specific brand of beer that contained cobalt as a foam stabilizer; these individuals developed heart failure within a few months. The cardiotoxic effects of these heavy metals is attributed to their antagonistic action toward Ca^{2+} as well as to their ability to form complexes with intracellular macromolecules.

Several other metals affect sarcolemmal ion channels. Manganese, nickel, and lanthanum block Ca^{2+} channels at a concentration similar to that of cobalt (1 mM). Barium is a potent arrhythmogen. $BaCl_2$ given intravenously at 5 mg/kg to rabbits produced ventricular tachycardia. This compound has been used as a model for screening antiarrhythmic agents. Traces of heavy metals are found in drinking water; however, calcium and magnesium in the water decrease their absorption (Revis, 1982).

Digitalis and Other Positive Inotropic Agents. Glycosides of digitalis, strophanthin, and oleandrin inhibit the sarcolemmal sodium pump, Na^+-K^+-ATPase, resulting in an increased intracellular Na^+ concentration, which in turn causes an elevation of intracellular Ca^{2+} concentration via Na^+/Ca^{2+} exchange. Consequently, cardiac contractility increases. However, the increased calcium enhances automaticity, which, along with other effects of digitalis, e.g., the increased vagal activity, and slowed A-V conduction, leads to arrhythmias. Premature ventricular contractions may lead to ventricular fibrillation. The slowed A-V conduction may progress to complete heart block.

Humans, dogs, and cats are the most sensitive species to digitalis, whereas rats are the least sensitive. Decreased concentration of potassium, brought about by certain diuretics, predisposes to the toxic effects. Decreased glomerular filtration rate prevalent in the elderly also predisposes to the toxicity of those glycosides that are eliminated by the kidney, e.g., digoxin. A moderately increased serum drug concentration (above the therapeutic level) can cause cardiotoxicity and, indeed, the incidence of these reactions has been as high as 20 percent in hospitalized patients (Cliff *et al.*, 1975; Akera and Brown, 1982).

Several structurally unrelated chemicals increase the resting Na^+ permeability or slow the inactivation of the Na^+ channel; hence they have digitalis-like cardiotoxic effects. Aconitine and *Veratrum* alkaloids and venoms secreted by lower animals, e.g., anemone toxins from coelenterata, palytoxin from corals, or batrachotoxin from the Columbian frog, produce arrhythmias and death by this mechanism. The extreme toxicity of palytoxin is shown by its intravenous LD50 value, which is 25 and 90 ng/kg in the rabbit and rat, respectively.

Other Cardiovascular Drugs and Biotoxins. Epinephrine and synthetic analogs, particularly the β-adrenergic-receptor agonists, e.g., isoproterenol, have positive chronotropic and inotropic effects, and the adverse reactions are related to these pharmacologic effects. In addition to tachycardia, ventricular arrhythmia can occur even at therapeutic doses on rare occasions. An overdose of these drugs can produce ECG signs of myocardial hypoxia (ST segment deviation and ectopic beats) and subendocardial necrosis. This lesion has been observed in several experimental animal species and has also been reported to occur in a few instances in humans. Myocardial hypoxia brought about by the increased oxygen demand that is not met and the consequent cellular calcium overloads has been a proposed mechanism for the observed toxicity (Balazs and Bloom, 1982).

Vasodilating antihypertensive drugs such as hydralazine can produce cardiotoxic effects similar to those mentioned above. These effects are elicited by a reflex tachycardia during hypotension.

The β-adrenergic-receptor blockers alone in overdose, as well as other antihypertensive drugs that inhibit adrenergic function (reserpine or guanethidine), decrease cardiac contractility and can cause AV block, and possibly precipitate heart failure. Adverse cardiac effects, e.g., angina and even myocardial infarction, can occur after sudden withdrawal of β blockers, due to receptor supersensitivity brought about by an increased number of the β-adrenergic receptors, which is an adaptive event during treatment.

Antiarrhythmic drugs decrease the conductivity and irritability of the myocardium, which is the basis of their therapeutic use. They block the sodium channel during its conducting state. Quinidine and procainamide prolong the QRS and Q-T intervals in low multiples of the therapeutic doses. This condition predisposes to arrhythmia, e.g., by the reentry mechanism. Lidocaine and phenytoin in overdoses produce sinus bradycardia and cardiac arrest. Local anesthetics of the amide type, after inadvertent intravenous injection, cause ventricular fibrillation and cardiac arrest.

A variety of venoms from marine species, e.g., saxitoxin or tetrodotoxin, decrease conduction in the sodium channel. Since the neurons are the most sensitive in poisoning, the nervous system symptoms are prominent.

Central Nervous System–Acting Drugs. Tricyclic antidepressants like imipramine and amitriptyline have quinidinelike effects on the heart. An overdose results in prolongation of the P-R, QRS, and Q-T intervals, in bundle branch block, and in supraventricular as well as ventricular arrhythmias.

Monoaminoxidase (MAO) inhibitor antidepressant drugs cause severe cardiovascular reactions (hypertensive crisis) when ingested with tyramine-containing foods or when used in combination with tricyclic antidepressants or sympathomimetic drugs. Tyramine is a sympathomimetic amine that is without effect when ingested in food because of its rapid biotransformation by MAO in the gut and liver. This reaction does not occur when MAO is inhibited.

Neuroleptic agents such as the phenothiazine and butyrophenone derivatives can produce dose-related tachyarrhythmias and other changes similar to those seen with the tricyclics, but the incidence is lower. In rare instances, sudden cardiac death preceded by ventricular fibrillation has been attributed to an overdose of these drugs. Aged patients with preexisting heart disease are at the greatest risk. Long-term or uncontrolled therapy with the antipsychotic drug lithium can produce ventricular arrhythmias and, rarely, myocardial lesions. Nonmedical use of psychoactive drugs, e.g., amphetamine, cocaine, and marijuana, can produce cardiovascular emergencies. These drugs increase the workload of the heart by increasing the heart rate and blood pressure and are particularly dangerous in individuals with angina, hypertension, coronary atherosclerosis, or cerebrovascular disease (Stimmel, 1979).

Chemotherapeutic Drugs. Among the antimicrobial antibiotics, the calcium antagonistic aminoglycosides, some of the macrolides, and chloroamphenicol have weak negative inotropic effects. An overdose can cause adverse effects in patients with preexisting heart disease. Certain antibiotics from *Streptomyces* that are used in veterinary medicine or as feed additives, e.g., monensin and lasalocid, increase sarcolemmal cationic transport and may cause cardiac effects (Akera and Brown, 1982). Emetine, an obsolete antiparasitic drug, causes arrhythmias and myocardial necrosis of dose-related severity.

Antineoplastic antibiotics such as the anthracyclines (daunorubicin and doxorubicin) are potent cardiotoxic agents. The first therapeutic doses can produce arrhythmia, possibly due to histamine release. Chronic treatment leads to congestive cardiomyopathy; its development is delayed for months after treatment and is related to the cumulative dose. Cardiac dilatation, atrophy, and degeneration of the myocytes, as well as interstitial edema and fibrosis, are the postmortem findings in humans and also in experimental animals. Generation of reactive oxygen, peroxidation of membrane lipids, and consequent changes in permeability and in cellular homeostasis have been considered in the pathogenesis of this injury (Balazs and Ferrans, 1978).

5-Fluorouracil, another antineoplastic drug, can produce signs of myocardial ischemia even during the early period of treatment and can ultimately precipitate cardiac arrest. Cyclophosphamide in large therapeutic doses can produce myocardial capillary microthrombosis, pericarditis, and cardiac failure. Radiation therapy combined with antineoplastic drugs produces capillary and pericardial lesions; e.g., anthracycline induces synergistic cardiotoxicity.

Table 14-2 presents the effects of selected chemicals on the heart.

Vasculotoxic Chemicals

Heavy Metals. In general, heavy metals produce their toxicity by destroying sulfhydryl proteins that comprise important structural components of vasculature.

Inorganic lead causes changes in arterial elasticity by specific effects upon the ground substance, and it has been shown to cause sclerosis of renal vessels. Severe lead intoxication has been linked with hypertension in humans, but lesser degrees of lead ingestion have not been implicated. Whereas pigeons have been shown to develop hypertension after exposure to 0.8 ppm Pb^{2+} for six months, a similar exposure in rats was without effect. Analysis of Pb^{2+} concentrations showed that the highest levels occurred in the aorta (Revis, 1982).

Cadmium is an insidiously acting compound on the vasculature, and it appears to play a role in the etiology of hypertension. Increased salt and water retention and hyperreninemia have been implicated in the mechanism. When Cd^{2+} is administered to rats in drinking water, hypertension results at exposure levels of 5 ppm, whereas hypotension occurs at levels of 50 ppm (Revis, 1982). Similarly, *in vitro*, low levels of Cd^{2+} (8.4 μg/L) stimulate vascular contraction, whereas high doses (840 μg/L) cause relaxation.

Table 14–2. CARDIOTOXIC EFFECTS*

	CHRONO- TROPIC	DROMO- TROPIC	BATHMO- TROPIC	INO- TROPIC	ARRHYTH- MOGENIC	STRUCTURAL
Ethanol		−	+	−	+	Chronic cardiomyopathy
Haloalkanes	−	−	+	−	+	Chronic degenerative changes
Heavy metals		−		−	+	Chronic degenerative changes
Digitalis	−	−	+	+	+	
Catecholamines	+	+	+	+	+	Acute focal necrosis cardiac hypertrophy
Antiarrhythmics	−	−		−	+	
Tricyclic antidepressants	+	−	+			
Neuroleptics		−		−	+	
Antineoplastic anthracyclines					+	Chronic cardiomyopathy

* Negative = decreased. Positive = increased.

In both rats and pigeons, the formation of atherosclerotic plaque has been enhanced by Cd^{2+} with a concomitant fall in serum high-density lipoproteins and cholesterol. In rats, chronic administration of Cd^{2+} caused renal arteriolar thickening as well as diffuse fibrosis of capillaries. Similar vascular changes are also responsible for development of testicular damage and atrophy. In the uterus, Cd^{2+} produces lesions in the endothelial clefts as well as having deleterious effects on the microcirculation. Destruction of the placenta in rats has also been reported. Many of the vascular effects may be reversed by either a Cd^{2+} chelator or zinc. There appears to be biologic antagonism between Cd^{2+} and Zn^{2+} and, in many instances, humans dying of hypertension have a higher ratio of Cd/Zn than normal, as well as a higher absolute level of Cd^{2+} (Schroeder, 1971).

Inorganic mercury produces vasoconstriction of the preglomerular vessels. In addition, the integrity of the blood-brain barrier may be disrupted by mercury. The opening of the BBB results in extravasation of plasma proteins across vascular walls into adjoining brain tissues.

Arsenic, in the form of the hydride arsine, affects the vasculature of the lungs leading to pulmonary edema. It has been proposed that the very high levels of As in soil and water of Taiwan is responsible for blackfoot disease, a severe form of arteriosclerosis. Arsenic has been reported to cause noncirrhotic portal hypertension in humans in India as a result of contamination of the water supply (Datta, 1976).

Chromium appears to play an important role in the maintenance of vascular integrity. A deficiency of this metal in animals results in elevated serum cholesterol levels and increased atherosclerotic aortic plaques. Autopsies of humans have revealed virtually no chromium in the aortas of individuals dying of atherosclerotic heart disease, in comparison with normal individuals dying of other causes (Schroeder, 1971).

Gases. Carbon monoxide exposure in rabbits, at 180 ppm exposure for four hours, results in focal intimal damage and edema. This is in the range of CO exposure that humans might experience from cigarette smoke (Thomsen and Kjeldsen, 1975). Atherogenesis may also be accelerated in rabbits exposed to CO while consuming an atherogenic diet. This phenomenon also occurred, however, during hypoxia in the absence of CO, so that the vascular wall deprived of oxygen, rather than being exposed to CO *per se,* may really be responsible for this effect. The conversion of more than 20 percent of the hemoglobin to carboxyhemoglobin increases the permeability of vascular walls to macromolecules, an incipient change in the pathogenesis of atherosclerosis.

Oxygen exposure causes toxicity primarily in the vasculature of the eye and the lungs. Administration of oxygen to the premature newborn can cause irreversible vasoconstriction and ultimate obliteration of retinal vasculature with resulting permanent blindness (Beehler, 1965). In the adult, high oxygen tension causes vascular effects that result in the shrinking of the visual field; however, these effects are reversible after cessation of exposure. In squirrel monkeys, exposure to 100 percent oxygen for 50 to 117 hours caused increases in vascular permeability with leakage and edema of the retina, as evidenced by fluorescein angiography. These effects are largely functional and reversible (Kinney *et al.,* 1977). In experimental studies in rats, exposure for two days to 60 percent O_2 did not produce tolerance, but in fact lowered survival time after 100 percent O_2 exposure. In the pulmonary capillary bed, the volume and thickness of capillary endothelium decreased, and perivascular edema was present (Hayatdavoudi *et al.,* 1981). Exposure to a high oxygen pressure of 1 to 4 atmospheres for two to four hours produced partial or total occlusion of capillaries and electron microscopic evidence of damaged endothelial cells in several species (Nasseri *et al.*, 1976). Ozone affects the pulmonary vasculature. The injuries usually take the form of pulmonary arterial lesions that lead to thickening of the artery walls, which is associated with increased levels of serum trypsin protein esterase. Ultrastructural alterations in the alveolar capillaries have also been demonstrated.

The complex gas mixture of automobile exhausts has been shown to cause structural changes in the myocardium and aorta of guinea pigs, as well as exaggeration of hemorrhage and infarct in the hemispheres and basal ganglia in spontaneously hypertensive rats (Roggendorf *et al.*, 1981). In addition, composition and deposition of lipids in the wall of the aorta of rats were affected, presumably owing to the known atherogenic effect of CO present in the gas mixture. Exposure of animals to cigarette smoke, which is known to contain CO, tars, nicotine, etc., has resulted in coronary artery disease.

Drugs and Other Medicinal Agents. Aspirin, the most widely consumed of all drugs, can produce endothelial damage as part of a pattern of gastric erosion. Studies in rats, utilizing transmission electron microscopy, have shown that there are very early changes in the basement membrane of the endothelial cell of the capillaries and postcapillary venules. This is the first step that may lead to obliteration of small vessels and ischemic infarcts in the gut (Robins, 1980).

The sympathomimetic amines cause damage to arterial vasculature. Amphetamine abuse caused damage to cerebral arteries, in an experimental animal model. Large doses of norepinephrine produced toxic effects on the endothelium of rabbit thoracic aorta (Christensen, 1974). Animal studies have demonstrated that nicotine is, upon chronic exposure, toxic to the aortic endothelium. Degenerative changes in the aortic arch have taken the form of increased numbers of microvilli and many focal areas of unusual endothelial cytoarchitecture (Booyse *et al.*, 1981). Degenerative changes of myocardial arterioles have been produced experimentally in dogs forced to smoke. Similar changes have also been detected in humans who were heavy smokers and died of noncardiac causes (Wald and Howard, 1975; Auerbach and Carter, 1980).

Anticoagulants can cause toxic vascular effects. Warfarin has been shown to cause subdural hematoma of the posterior fossa as well as spontaneous epidural spinal hematoma. Studies of warfarin in rats have revealed changes in capillary ultrastructure as well as evidence of cases of vasculitis in humans (Howitt *et al.*, 1982).

Oral contraceptive steroids can produce thromboembolic disorders. An increased incidence of deep-vein phlebitis, pulmonary embolism, and myocardial infarction has been associated with their use in young women (Stolley, 1980). They have been shown to cause intracranial venous thrombosis, which greatly increases the risk of stroke (Fairburn, 1981). Administration of 0.1 percent cholesterol or 0.05 percent dietary estrogen in the form of estradiol to experimental animals produced vascular lesions involving lipid vacuoles in the smooth muscle cells of the aorta. A combination of these two compounds produced severe degenerative atherosclerotic effects on coronary arteries as well as lipid deposition along the ascending aorta. A combination of testosterone and estradiol caused increased vascular smooth muscle cell mitosis and degeneration (Toda *et al.*, 1981).

Antineoplastic drugs cause a variety of effects on different vascular beds. For example, cyclophosphamide causes cerebrovascular and viscerovascular lesions, resulting in hemorrhages (Levine and Sowinski, 1974). In studies with 5-fluoro-2-deoxyuridine in dogs, chronic infusions into the hepatic artery resulted in GI hemorrhage and portal vein thrombosis.

Another category of agents that has been reported to produce vasculotoxic effects are the iodinated radio contrast dyes used for visualization of blood vessels in angiography. In addition to anaphylactic reactions, they can cause thrombophlebitis. The cyanoacrylate adhesives that have found use in repairing blood vessels and other tissues have produced degenerative changes in the arteries of dogs. Certain rapidly polymerizing polyurethane preparations used for transcatheter-embolization techniques in surgery have produced dissolution of arterial walls (Doppman *et al.*, 1978). Dermal microvascular lesions have been reported after plastic film wound dressings were applied in various animal species.

Toxins. Bacterial endotoxins produce a variety of toxic effects in many vascular beds. In the liver, they cause swelling of endothelial cells and adhesion of platelets to sinusoid walls, which affects the microcirculation (McCuskey *et al.*, 1982). In the lung, endotoxins produce increased vascular permeability and pulmonary hypertension. Infusion of endotoxin into experimental animals produces thickening of endothelial cells and formation of fibrin thrombi in small veins. These thrombi were soon lysed, and this process was followed by extravasation of erythrocytes. The excessive hydration of endothelial cells may play a role in these processes (Baris *et al.*, 1980). In piglets severe coronary artery damage was demonstrated. These changes included disappearance of microvilli from endothelial cells (exfoliation), followed by necrosis of medial smooth muscle cells. All these changes ultimately lead to stenosis of coronary arteries. The terminal phase of endotoxin effects on the systemic vasculature results in a marked hypotension (Personen *et al.,* 1981).

Staphylococcal α toxin in isolated mesenteric arteries caused delayed vasoconstriction and, when administered intravenously, caused hypertension in several experimental animal species. Lethal doses, however, caused hypotension and circulatory collapse (Svihovec and Raskova, 1967).

Vascular toxicities of selected chemicals are presented in Table 14–3.

DETECTION OF CARDIOVASCULAR TOXIC EFFECTS IN EXPERIMENTAL ANIMALS

The detectability of cardiovascular toxicities in animal experiments is a function of their mechanism. Although exaggerated pharmacologic effects are generally recognized, there are examples of species differences, as has already been mentioned for digitalis. Serotonin consistently increases the pulmonary blood pressure in dogs and cats but rarely in humans; L-dopa increases the systemic blood pressure in rats and cats but produces postural hypotension, at least with chronic administration, in humans; prostaglandin $F_2\alpha$ decreases the blood pressure in cats but increases it in humans (Brunner and Gross, 1979). Great differences in sensitivity of the contractile response to various agonists have been detected in the coronary arteries *in vitro* from the dog, pig, and cow (Ginsburg *et al.,* 1980). Some of these variations are most likely related to the differences in the distribution of subtypes of receptors that mediate different effects in the various species.

Since preclinical or premarketing toxicity studies of chemicals are done in healthy, well-nourished young adult animals, facultative toxicities, which require a predisposing condition, may be overlooked.

A preexisting cardiovascular disease can sensitize the cardiovascular system to toxicity. Patients with coronary artery disease have decreased exercise tolerance after the ingestion of 2 oz of ethanol; they may not tolerate the cardiovascular effects of inhalation anesthetics and may succumb with postsurgical myocardial infarction. Patients with valvular heart disease and congestive heart failure are at risk with respect to the slight negative inotropic effects of certain drugs, e.g., aminoglycoside antibiotics.

Obesity, poor nutritional status, or old age can contribute to cardiovascular toxicity. An example of the sensitizing role of overweight has been shown in animal experiments, e.g., with isoproterenol in rats. The subcutaneous LD50 is greatly reduced, and death is due to ventricular fibrillation (Balazs *et al.,* 1983). Poor nutritional status or deficiency of a specific vitamin (e.g., thiamine) predisposes to the cardiotoxicity of cobalt and of arsenic compounds. The adaptability of the cardiovascular system is reduced with age; this reduction and the large use of drugs in the elderly are responsible for the majority of adverse drug effects, especially those of the antidepressants, on this organ system.

Drug interactions play a major role in the development of severe acute cardiovascular toxicity. Diuretics that cause excess loss of K^+ and Mg^{2+} sensitize to the effects of digitalis and also to those of other cardiotoxic agents. Concurrent administration of cardiovascular drugs having similar effects, but which act by a different mechanism, results in potentiation of specific adverse effects, e.g., propranolol, a receptor blocker, with verapamil, a Ca^{2+} channel blocker, causes AV block and profound hypotension.

The detection of toxic effect is uncertain when the mechanism is not related to pharmacologic effect, i.e., when a reactive metabolite produces the injury. The biotransformation of the chemical as well as the rate of reactive metabolite formation varies between species. The most difficult is the detection of the hypersensitivity reactions, particularly the antibody- or lymphocyte-mediated cytotoxicity, and the immune complex-induced injuries. They are not likely to be detected, even in early clinical trials in humans, because of genetically controlled individual differences in susceptibility to the antigen.

Detection of cardiovascular toxicity requires a complete physical examination in both experimental animals and humans. The ECG is a generally applicable indicator of cardiac function, whereas the blood pressure is the circulatory indicator, for diagnostic purposes. A recent monograph deals with *in vivo* techniques as applied to toxicology in animal experiments (Brunner and Gross, 1979). Careful morphologic examinations should be conducted postmortem to detect and characterize the structural changes. In addition to *in vivo* pharmacologic measurements, *in vitro* electrophysiologic and biochemical methods are used to investigate the mechanism of action for various cardiovascular toxicities. These should be evaluated in relation to the desired pharmacologic effect in each tested species. Data obtained in experimental animals need to be studied further in humans; clinical pharmacologic and/or epidemiologic investigations should be performed to substantiate findings from animal experiments.

Table 14–3. VASCULOTOXIC AGENTS*

AGENT (CHEMICAL CLASS OR USE CATEGORY)	VASCULAR EFFECT AND/OR PRIMARY SITE	ASSOCIATED DISEASE STATE AND/OR MECHANISM
A. *Heavy Metals*		
Arsenic (arsine)	Arteriosclerosis Pulmonary vascular lesions	Peripheral vascular disease Noncirrhotic portal hypertension Pulmonary edema Occlusion of hepatic venous flow
Beryllium	Decreased hepatic flow; hemorrhage	Atherosclerosis
Cadmium	Aortic damage to endothelium allowing lipid deposition; lesions in uterine endothelial cleft; renal arteriolar thickening; effect on microcirculation	Hypertension
Chromium (deficiency)	Atherosclerotic aortic plaques	Atherosclerosis; elevated serum cholesterol
Copper (chronic)	Acceleration of atherosclerosis	
Copper (deficiency) (acute)	Hypotension Aortic aneurysms	
Germanium	Hemorrhage, edema in lungs and GI tract	
Indium	Hemorrhage and thrombosis in the kidney and liver	
Lead	Damage to endothelial cell with changes in blood-brain barrier permeability; changes in arterial elasticity; effects on ground substance; sclerosis of vessels in the kidney	Encephalopathy Hypertension
Mercury	Preglomerular vasoconstriction; glomerular immune complex deposits; lesions of the aorta; opening of blood-brain barrier	Glomerulonephritis; inhibition of amino acid uptake Atherosclerosis
Selenium	Atherosclerotic plaques	
Thallium	Perivascular cellular infiltration in the brain (cuffing)	
B. *Industrial and Environmental Agents*		
Allylamine	Renal artery lesion, intimal smooth muscle proliferation in coronary arteries	Endogenous formation of acrolein with destruction of vascular protein and nucleic acid components
β-Aminopropionitrile	Aortic lesions and atheroma formation	Damage to vascular connective tissue matrix; aneurysm
Boron	Hemorrhage; edema; increase in microvascular permeability in the lung	Pulmonary edema
Carbamylhydrazine HCl	Tumors of pulmonary blood vessels	Cancer
Carbon disulfide	Microvascular effect on ocular fundus and retina; direct injury to endothelial wall; promoter of atheroma formation	Coronary vascular disease Atherosclerosis Hypertension
Chlorophenoxy herbicides		Occlusion of veins
Dimethyl nitrosamine	Decreased hepatic flow; hemorrhage: necrosis	
4-Fluoro-10-methyl 12-benzyanthracene	Pulmonary artery lesions; coronary vessel lesion	

Table 14–3. VASCULOTOXIC AGENTS* *(continued)*

AGENT (CHEMICAL CLASS OR USE CATEGORY)	VASCULAR EFFECT AND/OR PRIMARY SITE	ASSOCIATED DISEASE STATE AND/OR MECHANISM
Glycerol	Strong renal vasoconstriction	Acute renal failure
Hydrochloric acid (aspiration of stomach contents)	Increased microvascular permeability	Pulmonary edema
Hydrogen fluoride	Hemorrhage; edema in the lung	Pulmonary edema
Paraquat	Vascular damage in lungs and brain	Cerebral purpura
Pyrrolizidine alkaloids	Pulmonary vasculitis; damage to vascular smooth muscle cells; proliferation of endothelium and vascular connective tissue in the liver	Pulmonary hypertension Hepatic venoocclusive disease
Organophosphate pesticides		Cerebral arteriosclerosis
Vinyl chloride	Portal hypertension; tumors of hepatic blood vessels	Cancer
C. Gases		
Auto exhaust	Hemorrhage and infarct in cerebral hemispheres; atheroma formation in aorta	Atherosclerosis due to CO content
Carbon monoxide	Damage to intimal layer; edema; atheroma formation	Atherosclerosis
Nitric oxide	Vacuolation of arteriolar endothelial cells; edema, thickening of alveolar-capillary membranes	Pulmonary edema
Oxygen	Vasoconstriction-retinal damage; increased retinal vascular permeability-edema; increased pulmonary vascular permeability-edema	Blindness in neonate; shrinking of visual field in adults; pulmonary edema
Ozone	Arterial lesions in the lung	Pulmonary edema
D. Drugs and Related Compounds *Antibiotic-Antimitotics*		
Cyclophosphamide	Lesions of pulmonary endothelial cells	
5-Fluorodeoxyuridine	GI tract hemorrhage, portal vein thrombosis	
Gentamicin	Long-lasting renal vasoconstriction	Renal failure
Vasoactive Agents		
Amphetamine	Cerebrovascular lesions secondary to drug abuse	Disseminated arterial lesions similar to periarteritis nodosa
Dihydroergotamine	Spasm of retinal vessels	
Ergonovine	Coronary artery spasm	Angina
Ergotamine	Vasospastic phenomena with and without thrombosis; medial atrophy	Gangrene of peripheral tissues
Epinephrine	Peripheral arterial thrombi in hyperlipemic rats	Participates in thrombogenesis

Histamine	Coronary spasm; damage to endothelial cells in hepatic portal vein	Coronary artery disease
Methysergide	Intimal proliferation: vascular occlusion of coronary arteries	
Nicotine	Alteration of cytoarchitecture of aortic endothelium; increase in microvilli	
Nitrites and nitrates	"Aging" of coronary arteries	Repeated vasodilation
Norepinephrine	Spasm of coronary artery; endothelial damage	
Metabolic Affectors		
Alloxan	Microvascular retinopathy	Diabetes; blindness
Chloroquine	Retinopathy	
Fructose	Microvascular lesions in retina	Diabetes-like condition
Iodoacetates	Vascular changes in retina	
Anticoagulants		
Sodium warfarin; warfarin	Spinal hematoma; subdural hematoma; vasculitis	Uncontrolled bleeding; hemorrhage
Radiocontrast Dyes		
Metrizamide; metrizoate	Coagulation, necrosis in celiac and renal vasculature	
Cyanoacrylate Adhesives		
2-Cyano-acrylate-n-butyl	Granulation of arteries with fibrous masses	
Ethyl-2 cyanoacrylate	Degeneration of vascular wall with thrombosis	
Methyl-2 cyanoacrylate	Vascular necrosis	
Miscellaneous Drugs and Compounds		
Aminorex fumarate	Intimal and medial thickening of pulmonary arteries	Pulmonary arterial hypertension
Aspirin	Endothelial damage; gastric erosion obliteration of small vessels; ischemic infarcts	Changes in the basement membrane of endothelial cells
Cholesterol: oxygenated derivatives of cholesterol; noncholesterol steroids	Atheroma formation; arterial damage	Atherosclerosis
Homocysteine	Increase of vascular fragility, loss of endothelium; proliferation of smooth muscle cells; promotion of atheroma formation	Atherosclerosis; effects on protein synthesis
Oral contraceptives	Thrombosis in cerebral and peripheral vasculature	Thromboembolic disorders
Penicillamine	Vascular lesion in connective tissue matrix of arterial wall; glomerular immune complex deposits	Glomerulonephritis; inhibits synthesis of vascular connective tissue
Talc and other silicates	Pulmonary arteriolar thrombosis, emboli	
Tetradecylsulfate Na	Sclerosis of veins (used as a sclerosing agent)	Cytotoxicity
Thromboxane A_2	Extreme cerebral vasoconstriction	Cerebrovascular ischemia

* Based on information gathered from sources listed in references.

REFERENCES

Akera, T., and Brown, B. S.: Cardiovascular toxicology of cardiotonic drugs and chemicals. In Van Stee, E. W. (ed.): *Cardiovascular Toxicology*. Raven Press, New York, 1982, pp. 109–35.

Auerbach, O., and Carter, H. W.: Smoking and the heart. In Bristow, M. R. (ed.): *Drug-induced Heart Disease*. Elsevier North-Holland Press, Amsterdam, 1980, pp. 359–76.

Bakay, L.: *The Blood Brain Barrier*. Charles C Thomas, Pub., Springfield, Ill., 1956, pp. 88–91.

Balazs, T.: An overview on delayed toxic effects of pre- and perinatal drug exposure. In Yoshida, H.; Hagrihara, Y.; and Ebashi, S. (eds.): *Advances in Pharmacology and Therapeutics II*. Pergamon Press, Ltd., Oxford, 1982, pp. 163–76.

_____: Detection of rare adverse reactions induced by chemicals. In Homburger, F. (ed): *Safety Evaluation and Regulation of Chemicals*. S. Karger, Basel, 1983, pp. 243–50.

Balazs, T.; Johnson, G.; Joseph, X.; Ehreich, S.; and Bloom, S.: Sensitivity and resistance of the myocardium to the toxicity of isoproterenol in rats. In Spitzer, J. (ed.): *Myocardial Injury*. Plenum Publishing Corp., New York, 1983, pp. 563–77.

Balazs, T., and Ferrans, V. J.: Cardiac lesions induced by chemicals. *Environ. Health Perspect.*, **26**:181–91, 1978.

Balazs, T., and Bloom, S.: Cardiotoxicity of adrenergic bronchodilator and vasodilating antihypertensive drugs. In Van Stee, E. W. (ed.): *Cardiovascular Toxicology*. Raven Press, New York, 1982, pp. 199–221.

Baris, C.; Guest, M. M.; and Frazer, M. E.: Direct effects of endotoxin on the microcirculation. *Adv. Shock Res.*, **4**:153–60, 1980.

Beehler, C. C.: Oxygen and the eye. *Surv. Ophthalmol.*, **9**:549–60, 1964.

Bigger, J. T., and Hoffman, B. F.: Antiarrhythmic drugs. In Gilman, A. G.; Goodman, L. S.; and Gilman, A. (eds.): *Goodman and Gilman's The Pharmacological Basis of Therapeutics*, 6th ed. Macmillan Publishing Co., New York, 1980, pp. 761–92.

Billingham, M. F.: Morphologic changes in drug-induced heart disease. In Bristow, M. R. (ed.): *Drug-induced Heart Disease*. Elsevier/North-Holland Press, Amsterdam, 1980, pp. 128–49.

Boor, P. J.: Allylamine cardiotoxicity: metabolism and mechanism. In Spitzer, J. (ed.): *Myocardial Injury*. Plenum Publishing Corp., New York, 1983, pp. 533–43.

Booyse, F. M.; Osikowicz, G.; and Quarfoot, A. J.: Effects of chronic oral consumption of nicotine on the rabbit aortic endothelium. *Am. J. Pathol.*, **102**:229–38, 1981.

Bowman, W. C., and Rand, M. J.: The heart and drugs affecting cardiac function. In Bowman, W. C., and Rand, M. J. (eds.): *Textbook of Pharmacology*. Blackwell Scientific Publications, Oxford; C. V. Mosby Co., St. Louis, 1980, pp. 22.10–22.75.

Braunwald, E.; Ross, J., Jr.; and Sonnerblick, E. H.: Disorders of myocardial function. In Isselbacher, K. J.; Adams, R. D.; Braunwald, E.; Petersdorf, R. G.; and Wilson, J. D. (eds.): *Harrison's Principles of Internal Medicine*, 9th ed. McGraw-Hill Book Co., New York, 1980a.

Braunwald, E.; Sonnerblick, E. H.; and Ross, J., Jr.: Contraction of the normal heart. In Braunwald, E. (ed.): *Heart Disease: A Textbook of Cardiovascular Medicine*. W. B. Saunders Co., Philadelphia, 1980b, pp. 413–52.

Braunwald, E.: Pathophysiology of heart failure. In Braunwald, E. (ed.): *Heart Disease: A Textbook of Cardiovascular Medicine*. W. B. Saunders Co., Philadelphia, 1980, pp. 453–71.

Brody, T. M., and Chubb, J. M.: Biochemical and ionic mechanisms of cardiotoxic agents. In Balazs, T. (ed.): *Cardiac Toxicology*, Vol. 1. CRC Press, Boca Raton, Fl., 1981, pp. 2–13.

Brunner, H., and Gross, F.: Cardiovascular pharmacology. In Zbinden, G., and Gross, F. (eds.): *Pharmacological Methods in Toxicology*. Pergamon Press, Ltd., Oxford, 1979, pp. 63–99.

Christensen, B. C.: Repair in arterial tissue. *Virchows Arch. Pathol. Anat.*, **363**:33–46, 1974.

Cliff, L. E.; Caranasos, G. J.; and Stewart, R. B.: Clinical problems with drugs. In Smith, L. H. (ed.): *Major Problems in Internal Medicine*. W. B. Saunders Co., Philadelphia, 1975, pp. 115–26.

Datta, D. J.: Letter: Arsenic and non-cirrhotic portal hypertension. *Lancet*, **21**:7956, 1976.

Deglin, S. M.; Deglin, J. M.; and Chung, E. K.: Drug-induced cardiovascular disease. *Drugs*, **14**:29–40, 1977.

Dontos, H. A., and Hess, M. L.: Oxygen radicals and vascular damage. In Spitzer, J. (ed.): *Myocardial Injury*. Plenum Publishing Corp., New York, 1983, pp. 365–77.

Doppman, J. L.; Aven, W.; Bowman, R. L.; Wood, L. L.; and Girton, M.: A rapidly polymerizing polyurethane for transcathetal embolization. *Cardiovasc. Radio.*, **1**:109–16, 1978.

Fairburn, B.: Intracranial venous thrombosis complicating oral contraceptive: treatment by anticoagulant drugs. *Br. Med. J.*, **2**:647, 1981.

Ferrans, V. J.: Overview of morphological reactions of the heart to toxic injury. In Balazs, T. (ed.): *Cardiac Toxicology III*. CRC Press Inc., Boca Raton, Fl., pp. 83–109.

Ginsburg, R.; Bristow, M. R.; Schroeder, J. S.; Harrison, D. C.; and Stinson, E. B.: Potential pharmacological mechanisms involved in coronary artery spasm. In Bristow, M. R. (ed.): *Drug-Induced Heart Disease*. Elsevier North-Holland Press, Amsterdam, 1980, pp. 457–65.

Hayatdavoudi, G.; O'Neal, J. J.; Barry, B. E.; Freeman, B. A.; and Crapo, J. D.: Pulmonary injury in rats following continuous exposure to 60% O_2 for 7 days. *J. Appl. Physiol.*, **51**:1220–31, 1981.

Howitt, A. J.; Williams, A. J.; and Skinner, C.: Warfarin induced vasculitis: a dose-related phenomena in susceptible individuals. *Postgrad. Med. J.*, **58**:233–34, 1982.

Jackson, B.: Developmental cardiotoxic effects of chemicals. In Balazs, T. (ed.): *Cardiac Toxicology III*. CRC Press, Inc., Boca Raton, Fl., 1981, pp. 163–77.

Kinney, J. A.; McKay, C. L.; and Gordon, R. A.: The use of fluoroscein angiography to study oxygen toxicity. *Ann. Ophthalmol.*, **9**:895–98, 1977.

Koch-Weser, J.: Drug-induced arrhythmias in man. *Pharmacol. Ther.*, **5**:125–31, 1979.

Levine, S., and Sowinski, R.: Cyclophosphamide induced cerebral and visceral lesions in rats. Enhancement by endotoxins. *Arch. Pathol.*, **98**:177–82, 1974.

Magos, L.: The effects of industrial chemicals on the heart. In Balazs, T. (ed.): *Cardiac Toxicology II*. CRC Press, Inc., Boca Raton, Fl., 1981, pp. 203–209.

McCuskey, R. S.; Urbaschek, R.; McCuskey, P. A.; and Urbaschek, B.: *In vivo* microscopic studies of responses of the liver to endotoxin. *Klin. Wochenschr.*, **60**:749–51, 1982.

Merin, R. G.: Myocardial metabolism for the toxicologist. *Environ. Health Perspect.*, **26**:169–74, 1978.

_____: Cardiac toxicology of inhalation anesthetics. In Balazs, T. (ed.): *Cardiac Toxicology II*. CRC Press, Inc., Boca Raton, Fl., 1981, pp. 1–15.

Nasseri, M.; Eisele, R.; Kotter, D.; Kirstaedter, H.; and Wolf, J.: Comparative studies on the effect of oxygen high pressure (OHP) on different species with special reference to organ preservation. *Respiration*, **33**:70–83, 1976.

Personen, E.; Kaprio, E.; Rapola, J.; Soveri, T.; and Okansen, H.: Endothelial cell damage in piglet coronary artery after i.v. administration of *E. coli* endotoxin. *Atherosclerosis*, **40**:65–73, 1981.

Rapoport, S.: *Blood-Brain Barrier in Physiology and Medicine*. Raven Press, New York, 1976, pp. 129–52.

Revis, N. W.: Relationship of vanadium, cadmium, lead, nickel, cobalt and soft water to myocardial and vascular toxicity and cardiovascular disease. In Van Stee, E. W. (ed.): *Cardiovascular Toxicology*. Raven Press, New York, 1982, pp. 365–77.

Reynolds, A. C.: Cardiac arrhythmias in sensitized hearts. *Res. Commun. Chem. Pathol. Pharmacol.*, **40**:3–14, 1983.

Robins, P. G.: Ultrastructural observations on the pathogenesis of aspirin-induced gastric erosions. *Br. J. Exp. Pathol.*, **61**:497–504, 1980.

Roggendorf, W.; Thron, N. L.; Ast, D.; and Kohler, P. R.: Effects of chronic exposure to auto exhaust gas on the CNS of normotensive and hypertensive rats. *Acta Neuropathol. (Suppl.) (Berl.)*, **7**:17–19, 1981.

Rubin, J. T., and Rubin, E.: Myocardial toxicity of alcohols, aldehydes and glycols, including alcoholic cardiomyopathy. In Van Stee, E. W. (ed.): *Cardiovascular Toxicology*. Raven Press, New York, 1982, pp. 353–63.

Schlant, R. C., and Sonnenblick, E. H.: Pathophysiology of heart failure. In Hurst, J. W. (ed.): *The Heart*. McGraw-Hill Book Co., New York, 1982, pp. 382–407.

Schroeder, H. A.: Trace elements in degenerative cardiovascular disease. In Conn, H. L., Jr., and Horwitz, O. (eds.): *Cardiac and Vascular Diseases*, Vol. II. Lea & Febiger, Philadelphia, 1971, pp. 973–77.

Smith, P., and Heath, D.: Evagination of vascular smooth muscle during early stages of crotalaria pulmonary hypertension. *J. Pathol.*, **124**:177–83, 1976.

Steffey, E. P.: Cardiovascular effects of inhalation anesthetics. In Van Stee, E. W. (ed.): *Cardiovascular Toxicology*. Raven Press, New York, 1982, pp. 259–81.

Stimmel, B.: *Cardiovascular Effects of Mood Altering Drugs*. Raven Press, New York, 1979.

Stolley, P. D.: Drug, thromboembolism and myocardial infarction. In Bristow, M. R. (ed.): *Drug-induced Heart Disease*. Elsevier/North-Holland Press, Amsterdam, 1980, pp. 313–21.

Svihovec, J., and Rashova, H.: Action of staphylococcal alpha toxin on arterial smooth muscle. *Toxicology*, **4**:269–74, 1967.

Thomsen, H. K., and Kjeldsen, K.: Aortic intimal injury in rabbit. An evaluation of a threshold limit. *Arch. Environ. Health*, **30**:604–607, 1975.

Titus, E. O.: A molecular biologic approach to cardiac toxicology. In Spitzer, J. (ed.): *Myocardial Injury*. Plenum Publishing Corp., New York, 1983, pp. 509–19.

Toda, J.; Leszozynski, D.; and Kummerow, F.: Vasculotoxic effects of dietary testosterone, estradiol and cholesterol on chick artery. *J. Pathol.*, **134**:219–31, 1981.

Toth, B.; Shimizeu, H.; and Erickson, J.: Carbamylhydrazine hydrochloride as a lung and blood vessel tumor inducer in Swiss mice. *Eur. J. Cancer*, **11**:17–22, 1975.

Van Stee, E. W.: Cardiovascular toxicology: foundation and scope. In Van Stee, E. W. (ed.): *Cardiovascular Toxicology*. Raven Press, New York, 1982, pp. 1–35.

Wald, N., and Howard, S.: Smoking, carbon monoxide and disease. *Ann. Occup. Hyg.*, **18**:1–14, 1975.

Zakhari, S., and Aviado, D. M.: Cardiovascular toxicology and aerosol propellants, refrigerants and related solvents. In Van Stee, E. W. (ed.): *Cardiovascular Toxicology*. Raven Press, New York, 1982, pp. 281–327.

Zbinden, G.: Evaluation of thrombogenic effects. In Elliott, H. W.; George, R.; and Okun, R. (eds.): *Annual Review of Pharmacology and Toxicology*, Vol. 16. Annual Review Inc., California, 1976, pp. 177–88.

Chapter 15

TOXIC RESPONSES OF THE SKIN

Edward A. Emmett

INTRODUCTION

In this chapter a survey of toxicologic principles related to the skin will be given. No attempt will be made to be exhaustive. There is a large amount of information available, especially with regard to the effects of specific materials for which more comprehensive works must be consulted. Several excellent recent sources are available (e.g., Foussereau *et al.*, 1982; Adams, 1983; Marzulli and Maibach, 1983). The discussion will generally be confined to the effects of chemical agents or to the combined effects of physical and chemical agents such as are responsible for photosensitization. The skin is, of course, vulnerable to the effects of physical agents; for example, both ionizing and nonionizing radiation have important and complex effects; and it is profoundly affected by heat, repeated trauma, cold, and humidity. However, these are not dealt with in this chapter.

The skin has great importance as an organ that interfaces with the external environment and constitutes a barrier and transition zone between the internal and external milieux. A major function of skin is to preserve the constituents and composition of the body contents—witness the massive and potentially lethal fluid losses in extensive burns.

The skin, and particularly the dead outer stratum corneum layer, is also an excellent barrier against certain external chemical agents, although others may penetrate readily. Indeed, there are many agents for which, under normal circumstances of exposure, the skin represents the major portal of entry. The subject of percutaneous absorption is thus of great importance both for general toxicology and for effects on the skin, since toxic reactions in the skin generally depend on interactions of toxicants with the less superficial, living layers of the skin.

The skin displays a limited, but fairly large, variety of toxic responses reflecting the major patterns of possible structural and functional changes. Because the surface of the skin is so readily visible, to a larger extent than for most other organs, toxic reactions have been described mainly on the basis of morphologic rather than functional changes. In the case of the skin the biochemical sequence of toxic events is often less well understood than for certain other organs. It is important to recognize that similar morphologic changes could result from widely differing toxicologic mechanisms. Although some efforts have been made, rigid standardization of morphologic criteria is not yet widely practiced.

In actual practice, chemical injury to the skin is influenced by a large number of environmental factors that alter the interface. These include variations in heat and humidity, friction, pressure, trauma, abrasion, wind, vibration, ultraviolet and visible radiations, electrical current, and coincident effects of infestations or infection. There are morphologic, physiologic and biochemical protective and homeostatic mechanisms in the skin; these include the epidermal barrier, eccrine sweating, phagocytic cells and processes, metabolic detoxication, specific immunologic processes, and protective mechanisms, such as melanin pigmentation, which protect against ultraviolet radiation. These may vary on a genetic or phenotypic basis and may be influenced by systemic or local disease or by the effects of other toxic substances. For example, individuals with atopy (characterized in part by infantile and adolescent eczema, hayfever, and asthma) seem particularly prone to develop irritant dermatitis. The actual expression or degree of expression of a toxic effect may thus be the end result of a markedly complex set of local and general factors. In experimental studies, these factors are also of crucial importance and may help to explain the rather poor concordance that has been reported between laboratories for assessment of effects such as irritation (Weil and Scala, 1971). Comparability of technique is of paramount importance in this field.

Although the actual burden of chemically induced human skin disease cannot be reliably computed from information currently available, it is clear that it is of significant proportions. Figures from the United States Department of Labor indicate that occupational skin disease, the vast majority of which is due to effects of toxic chemicals, is the most frequently reported occupational disease (Report to OSHA, 1978). In California, which has the most comprehensive occupational disease-reporting system, skin diseases accounted for 40 percent of reported diseases, eye conditions 29 percent, and chemical burns 9.7 percent. Thus, conditions primarily due to external contact comprised 79 percent of these diseases. By contrast, other conditions due to toxic materials accounted for 12.6 percent, namely, respiratory including pneumoconioses 5.5 percent, digestive and other symptoms 4.2 percent, and systemic effects 3 percent (Baginsky, 1982a). Furthermore, in 1977, of the occupational skin diseases in California, 92.5 percent were due to contact dermatitis, either irritant or allergic, 5.4 percent to primary or secondary infection, and 2.4 percent to other skin disorders (Baginsky, 1982b). In addition to occupational exposures from handling chemicals, there is a large variety of opportunities for potentially hazardous materials to contact the skin during the course of daily life, including contact with clothing, cosmetics, cleansing agents, contaminated surfaces, incompletely cured resins, plants, foods, jewelry, and a vast array of consumer products. Good epidemiologic data on the incidence of toxic cutaneous responses in nonoccupational settings are, however, sparse or nonexistent. The toxicity of agents contacting the skin is clearly of widespread interest and is vital to those interested in the safety of cosmetics, toiletries, and household products. A standard nomenclature and list of cosmetic ingredients has been established to assist in this task (CTFA, 1982).

The information available supports the conclusion that, other factors being equal, toxic effects on the skin are characterized by definable dose-response relationships, in which concentration, duration, extent of application, and the total dosage applied are important. However, in contrast to inhalation exposures to airborne substances other than in experimental circumstances, our ability to accurately assess cutaneous exposures is poorly developed. In order to estimate exposure, levels on contaminated surfaces have been measured, absorbant pads have been applied to the skin, skin surface wipings taken, and, for selected agents, quantitation of fluorescence or of indicator materials performed, but none of these is universally satisfactory. In the estimation of total dosage to the organism, biologic monitoring will satisfactorily measure total absorption by all routes including the percutaneous route. This is one of the reasons that it generally offers a better estimate of risk than ambient environmental monitoring (Lauwerys, 1983).

STRUCTURE AND FUNCTION

A diagrammatic representation of the structure of the skin is shown in Figure 15–1. The skin contains three main layers, an outer layer of epithelial tissue, the epidermis; a loose connective tissue layer, the dermis; and an inner layer of variable thickness containing adipose tissue and connective tissue, the hypodermis or panniculus adiposus (Montagna and Parakkal, 1974). The epidermis contains a number of cell types including keratinocytes, melanocytes, Langerhans cells, and Merkel cells. Most numerous are the kertinocytes, which serve to produce keratin in the process of keratinization or cornification.

The epidermis is divided into several layers based on the behavior of the keratinocytes. The basal layer consists of germinative cells, which are extremely active metabolically, divide rapidly, and display many mitotic figures as well as cells that label with thymidine. Above this layer are two differentiated layers of viable cells, the spinous or prickle cell layer and the granular cell layer. The outer layer, the stratum corneum, consists of a multicellular membrane of dried flattened keratinocytes, which have no metabolic activity and represent the nonviable end product of the synthetic activity of the lower layers. This layer is the main barrier site in the skin for water, electrolytes, most other chemicals, microorganisms, and electrical resistance. The epidermis also provides some mechanical resistance to stretching.

Keratinization begins with the synthesis of fibrous prekeratins in the basal layer; aggregated filaments run the length of the cell by the time it reaches the spinous layer. In the granular layer, protein granules are formed that contribute to the process. The stratum corneum contains keratin filaments that are lined parallel to the surface of the skin. Considerable lipid is present, and the water content varies from around 10 percent to 70 percent depending particularly on external environmental conditions. The chemical composition and structure is significantly different in certain skin diseases such as psoriasis. The complex chemical structure of the normal stratum corneum results in its effectiveness as a barrier (Scheuplein and Blank, 1971).

The epidermis contains a constantly renewing

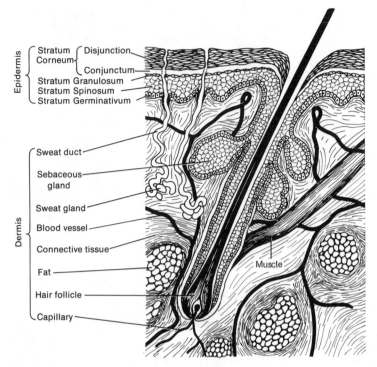

Figure 15–1. Diagram of a cross-section of human skin.

cell population. In the human, the transit time from mitosis within the viable epidermis is on the order of 12 to 14 days and within the stratum corneum about 15 days, for a total of about 28 days. In psoriasis, however, it may be as short as four days. These times are shorter for certain experimental species, most of which have a much thinner epidermis than humans.

Roughly 5 to 10 percent of the epidermal cells are Langerhans cells. These are mesenchyme-derived dendritic cells that form a network in the viable dermis. They are responsible for antigen recognition and processing. Melanocytes are dendritic cells derived from the neural crest that are responsible for the synthesis of melanin in a specialized organelle called the melanosome. These organelles are transferred to keratinocytes where they are aggregated and destroyed by phagolysosomes in Caucasians, but not in Negroids or Australoids. A number of morphologic differences exist between the races both in the production and lysis of melanosomes and in the degree and type of melanization. The role, if any, that pigmentation plays in modifying chemical damage in the skin is still contentious, although melanin has a major role in protection against ultraviolet radiation. The epidermis also contains specialized sensory cells, the Merkel cells, as well as free nerve endings. Inflammatory cells and lymphocytes may be seen in the epidermis from time to time.

The epidermis is separated from and attached to the dermis by a basal lamina. The epidermal-dermal junction has a characteristically ridged shape. The underlying dermis consists of loose connective tissue, which envelopes the body in a strong, flexible envelope. The dermis contains collagen, reticulin and elastin fibers, glycosaminoglycan ground substance, and a variety of scattered cells including the predominant fibroblast, as well as macrophages, mast cells, and lymphocytes. The dermis actively determines wound repair. The ground substance provides a slow diffusion medium for constituent fluids.

The dermis has substantial vascular plexuses, unlike the epidermis, which is avascular. Thus, if external bleeding is produced, the dermis must be penetrated. The dermal blood supply is substantially greater than required for its metabolic activity; thus dermal vessels can play an important role in thermoregulation by controlling the dissipation of heat to the surface. The dermis has a plexus of lymphatics, which drain to the regional lymph nodes and the thoracic duct. The dermis has abundant sensory and sensorimotor nerves.

There are a number of epithelial structures known collectively as the epidermal appendages, which are extensions of modified epidermal cells into the dermis. These include the eccrine sweat glands, apocrine sweat glands, hair follicles, and sebaceous glands. The eccrine sweat glands have a secretory portion located in the hypodermis immediately below the dermis and have a coiled duct leading to the epidermal surface. They are located over the entire body surface and produce sweat, a dilute aqueous solution whose function is evaporative cooling in thermoregulation. Eccrine sweating is produced by thermal, emotional, and gustatory stimuli, and the glands are under autonomic control. Apocrine glands, which have no known function, are confined to the axillary areas, genitalia, and nipples. Their secretion is emptied into the pilary (hair) canal. Initially odorless, it acquires odor through bacterial decomposition.

Hair follicles are located over the entire body surface. Each follicle appears to have the potential to be either a terminal hair, as in the scalp or the pubic region after puberty, a soft vellus hair, or fetal (lanugo) hair. The deepest portion of the hair follicle is the germinal matrix, one of the most metabolically active tissues in the body, which is surrounded by a highly vascularized connective tissue. The uppermost cells from the proliferating germinal follicle are pushed up into the external root sheath of the hair follicle, differentiate, become keratinized, and form the hair that protrudes from the canal. The keratin of hair and of nail, though similar, is immunologically distinct from that of the stratum corneum, has a higher cystine content, and may have an additional matrix protein with a high sulfur content that serves to cross-link filament bundles.

Sebaceous glands are associated with hair follicles except for the palms, soles, and dorsal of the foot. Sebaceous gland cells accumulate lipids, and as they break down they discharge a holocrine secretion, sebum, into the pilary canal. These glands are under hormonal control. Sebum is expelled partly by the contraction of the small arrectores pili muscles. Lipids on the surface of the skin vary in quantity depending on both the amount of sebum and the numbers of desquamating epidermal cells, which also contribute lipids. In areas where sebaceous glands are active and abundant, such as the scalp, forehead, and upper back, up to 90 percent of the surface lipids may originate from sebum.

There are substantial differences in the skin from one region of the body to another. The thickness of the epidermis varies greatly; whereas it is about 0.06 mm over much of the body, on the palms and soles the epidermis may be several millimeters thick. The distribution and activity of the appendages, the vascular and nerve supply, and other characteristics also vary markedly. These structural differences are matched by functional differences, for example, marked variations in percutaneous absorption as discussed in the following section.

The skin is one of the body's largest organs and represents about 10 percent of the body weight. It is an important contributor to the function, metabolism, and integrity of the whole organism.

PERCUTANEOUS ABSORPTION

Percutaneous absorption is both a critical determinant of the local effects of agents applied to the skin and a determinant of systemic toxicity. In general, the range of rates of percutaneous absorption is quite high. A number of materials, especially lipophilic substances, penetrate quite readily, such as organophosphate insecticides and polychlorinated biphenyls; for other substances, particularly those which are hydrophilic, penetration may be very slow.

The major barrier for almost all substances and particularly hydrophilic substances is the stratum corneum across which penetration occurs by passive absorption. It is felt that the major route for penetration is across the epidermis itself and that diffusion through the epidermal appendages plays relatively little role. This is based partly on stoichiometric considerations as the appendages such as hair follicles and sebaceous glands comprise only about 0.1 percent of the cross-sectional surface area presented to a potential penetrant. The appendages may be responsible for more rapid transient diffusion, particularly of lipophilic materials, before a steady state is established.

There appear to be different molecular pathways for the passage of polar and nonpolar materials. Polar substances may diffuse through the outer surface of protein filaments of the hydrated stratum corneum, while nonpolar molecules diffuse through nonaqueous lipid matrix (Blank and Scheuplein, 1969). It can be deduced from such observations that variations in the water content of the stratum corneum will have a profound effect on penetration, particularly of polar substances. Once through the epidermal barrier, substances must diffuse through the living layers of the epidermis and the dermis to reach the vessels of the systemic blood circulation and lymphatics, to reach targets in the underlying tissues of the skin, or to be biotransformed. Relatively little barrier to penetration is presented at these levels. The circulation is the limiting factor only for a few substances which either penetrate the stratum corneum very rapidly, such as helium (Scheuplein and Blank, 1971), or which severely damage the stratum corneum.

Information about percutaneous absorption comes from two major lines of investigation, the use of *in vitro* techniques and the use of *in vivo* techniques. Although the two approaches have to date produced somewhat different types of information, there appears to be fairly good agreement between results obtained from equivalent techniques when special care is given to duplicating experimental conditions (Franz, 1975; Bronaugh, 1982).

In Vitro *Studies*

In vitro techniques generally use diffusion cells in which excised skin is used as the membrane. The compound whose absorption is to be assessed is placed on one side in a suitable vehicle; this side may be open or closed. The compound is assayed in the fluid on the other side of the membrane, which is sampled regularly. This fluid is usually physiologic saline, and the experiment takes place at physiologic temperature. For these experiments, human or animal skin can be used, either epidermis separated by heat or chemically (using cantharadin) or surgical slices produced by a dermatome. Full-thickness skin from humans or animals with a thick dermis is technically unsatisfactory (Bronaugh and Maibach, 1983).

Studies with homologous groups of molecules and particularly with aliphatic alcohols (Scheuplein and Blank, 1971) have indicated that percutaneous absorption follows Fick's diffusion law, which can be expressed in integrated form as:

$$J_s = \frac{K_m D \, \Delta C_s}{\gamma}$$

and

$$K_p = \frac{K_m}{\gamma}$$

where J_s is the steady-state flux of solute (moles $\cdot$ cm^{-2} $\cdot$ hr^{-1}), K_m is the solute sorbed per milliliter of tissue or solute, D is the average membrane diffusion coefficient for solute (cm^2 $\cdot$ sec^{-1}), ΔC_s is the concentration difference of solute across membrane (moles $\cdot$ cm^{-3}), γ is the membrane thickness (cm), and K_p is the permeability constant for solute (cm hr^{-1}).

Thus the flux (J_s) is related particularly to the solvent-membrane distribution coefficient (K_m). K_m, in turn, is a major factor in determining the permeability constant (K_p). The solvent-membrane partition coefficient (K_m) can be readily determined for stratum corneum by mixing the substance and solvent in a cell with a small piece of accurately weighed dry stratum corneum followed by appropriate chemical analysis of the substance in the two phases.

Fick's law seems to hold fairly well for gases, ions, or nonelectrolytes; apparent exceptions occur when the applied substance damages tissue. Flux may be proportional to concentration for very dilute solutions of some substances such as butanol, but may increase at higher concentrations, apparently owing to the sorption of nonpolar molecules into the skin. Highly lipid soluble materials may be even more effective in this regard and when absorbed into the stratum corneum may increase the diffusivity of other test substances (Scheuplein and Ross, 1970; Scheuplein and Blank, 1971).

In Vivo *Studies*

In vivo studies of percutaneous absorption involve topical application of substances to the intact skin of whole animals for a defined time period. Radiolabeled tracers are generally used, especially as the levels of absorbed substances in blood or plasma are often very low, making chemical analysis difficult. The radiolabeled material may be measured in excreta so that the percentage absorbed is calculated. Alternatively, tracers can be given both topically and either intraperitoneally or intravenously. Radioactivity in excreta or elsewhere can be measured and percutaneous absorption measured by the ratio of the areas under the concentration versus time curves (AUC) for the two methods of administration (see Chapter 3). Such methods measure the percutaneous absorption of the substance to be assessed but, unless speciation of the radiolabeled material is performed, do not indicate the nature of the material absorbed. Methods comparing different routes of administration would be invalid if biotransformation of the chemical by skin was extensive and differed from that in other organs (Wester and Maibach, 1983).

Other approaches to *in vivo* measurement of absorption have been used. These include the use of a biologic response, such as cutaneous vasoconstriction, which has been used to detect absorption of topical corticosteroids, and remainder analysis, where the loss of radioactivity or substance from the skin surface is measured; however, the latter is less satisfactory both as the skin may act as a reservoir for unabsorbed material and as full recovery of radioactivity is never assured.

The rhesus monkey appears to produce results reasonably similar to those from humans (Wester and Maibach, 1976). Rodents appear to have higher permeability than man, with guinea pig, rat, and rabbit, in that order, showing increasingly greater penetrability (Tregear, 1966).

Factors Affecting Percutaneous Absorption

A considerable number of factors have been shown to affect percutaneous absorption. For convenience, these may be loosely classified as those associated with the skin, vehicle, or type of penetrant.

Skin. The amount absorbed is obviously dependent on the applied dose, the time before contact is terminated as by washing or removal, the concentration, and the surface area of application. The efficiency of absorption may change and can fall as the actual concentration increases although the total amount absorbed into the body seems always to increase (Wester and Maibach, 1976). The physical integrity of the stratum corneum is vital; partial or complete removal or changes in the composition and structure such as occur in certain diseases affect absorption. Important species differences exist, as previously indicated.

As with other cutaneous functions, there is a profound regional variation, as illustrated in Table 15–1, which shows relative permeability data for human skin regions (Feldman and Maibach, 1967).

Table 15–1. RELATIVE REGIONAL PERMEABILITY OF HUMAN SKIN TO TOPICAL ^{14}C HYDROCORTISONE*

Plantar foot arch	1
Lateral ankle	3
Palm	6
Ventral forearm	7
Dorsal forearm	8
Back	12
Scalp	25
Axilla	26
Forehead	43
Jaw angle	93
Scrotum	300

*Data from Feldmann and Maibach (1967).

The penetration of polar substances is increased by hydration of the stratum corneum. There is also a linear increase in the penetration of polar substances with temperature up to 50° C. With lipids, temperature dependence may be nonlinear, perhaps reflecting changes in viscosity. Both hydration and local skin temperature are increased by occlusion of the site of application using an impervious material such as a sheet of polyethylene. This has been taken advantage of in dermatologic therapy, particularly to increase the penetration of topically applied corticosteroids.

Vehicle. The vehicle or solvent has a profound effect on percutaneous absorption. The nature of the vehicle governs the vehicle/stratum corneum partition coefficient, which determines absorption. The vehicle may influence absorption in other ways. It may contain a damaging solvent or determine pH thus altering the ionization of electrolytes. The presence of anionic and cationic surfactants such as soaps and detergents, even in dilute concentration, will increase the permeability for water and for other polar substances by damaging the stratum corneum, although the precise mechanisms are incompletely understood. Nonionic surfactants are less active in this regard.

Substance. Although data are quite incomplete for many classes of compounds, some general principles can be derived (Scheuplein and Blank, 1971). The permeability of skin to water has been well studied. The stratum corneum is one of the most water impermeable of all biologic membranes. Simple polar nonelectrolytes appear to penetrate the stratum corneum at approximately the same rate as water. Water-miscible alcohols have similar permeability constants; adding additional polar groups drastically reduces the rate. Introducing methylene groups into a simple polar nonelectrolyte increases the membrane solubility resulting in a higher permeability. Electrolytes applied from aqueous solution penetrate poorly, and the ionization of a weak electrolyte radically reduces its permeability.

Organic liquids can be divided into those that are nondamaging to the membrane such as alcohols higher than C_2 and those that damage such as acetone, hexane, and other common solvents. Lipid solubility is an important determinant for nondamaging solvents; high permeability is guaranteed where the vehicle is polar. Damaging solvents delipidize the skin producing functional interstices in skin that serve as low-energy diffusion pathways. The result is a fairly porous nonselective membrane.

In general, true gases, as opposed to vapor phase concentrations of volatile liquids and solvents, penetrate the skin relatively well, although the diffusion coefficients are very small compared with those typical of gaseous diffusion.

Biotransformation

The skin and particularly the epidermis is an actively metabolizing organ that is capable of significant biotransformation of xenobiotics (Pannatier et al., 1978). A number of studies have addressed the presence of aryl hydrocarbon hydroxylase (AHH) activity in the skin; benzo[a]pyrene metabolites including epoxides may be formed in the skin (Pohl, 1976). This activity is inducible, and most of the enzymes are present in the lower epidermis rather than the dermis. The total AHH activity of skin toward benzo[a]pyrene is about 2 percent of that of liver.

Metabolic transformation may affect topically applied drugs. For example, it has been estimated that from 16 to 21 percent of a dose of glyceryl trinitrate applied to monkeys is biotransformed by the skin (Wester *et al.*, 1981).

In addition to metabolic transformation, substances in the superficial layers of the skin are subject to photochemical reactions if they absorb UV or visible radiation.

Biotransformation in other organs may also be important in the production of toxic effects in the skin. An example of how a number of processes may be involved is porphyria cutanea tarda, which is characterized by blistering and fragility of the skin, photosensitivity, pigmentary changes, and excessive hirsutism. An epidemic of this disease occurred among several thousand people in southeastern Turkey in the late 1950s when during a famine, wheat treated with hexachlorbenzene was eaten rather than planted (Schmid, 1960).

Hexachlorbenzene produces excessive accumulation of uroporphyrins and coprophyrins in liver as a result of interference with prophyrin metabolism (Goldstein, 1977). Consequently, porphyrins accumulate in various tissues including the skin. These substances render the skin photosensitive as a result of intense absorption of porphyrins in the 400-nm, SORET, band with subsequent photoactivation and damage to cell membranes and/or cell constituents (Goldstein and Harber, 1972).

Excretion from the Skin

Integumentary loss of body constituents including xenobiotics may occur with loss of desquamated cells, hair, or nails; in the eccrine or apocrine sweat; or in secretions such as tears and milk.

The average human adult scalp contains about 100,000 hairs with a growth rate of about 0.37 mm/day. Human hair grows in a cyclic manner, with a resting (telogen) phase lasting about three months and a growth phase (anagen) lasting for two to six years. There is also a brief involutional phase (catagen). Normally about 70 scalp hairs are lost daily. Certain metals are incorporated into the matrix of the growing hairs and remain in the hair tissue until it is eventually lost (Brown and Crounse, 1980). Measurement of the hair content of As, Cd, and Pb (after suitable washing to remove material externally deposited on hair) has been shown to reliably reflect exposures; however, this is not true for Zn and Cu (Hammer *et al.*, 1971).

There has been relatively little study of excretion in the eccrine sweat. Sweat volume varies from 250 ml to many liters per day. Sweat rates of greater than 1 liter per hour are seen in hot conditions or heavy work rates. Thus, the total amount of sweat loss is variable. Furthermore, acclimatization to heat is characterized both by decreased sweating and by decreased solute concentrations. Sodium and chloride are the main solutes in sweat, but many other substances are present. Substantial amounts of many metals are excreted in the sweat, including Cu, Zn, and Fe; concentrations of Pb, Cd, and Ni in sweat are equal to or higher than those in urine (Cohn and Emmett, 1978). Thus, the potential exists, depending on sweat rates and acclimatization, for substantial losses of these metals in sweat. A number of water-soluble drugs are excreted in sweat. The excretion of aminopyrine, antipyrene, sulfaguanidine, and sulfadiazine has been studied (Johnson and Maibach, 1971). These show a high sweat-to-plasma concentration, and their excretion behavior is consistent with partitioning between plasma of pH 7.4 and a fluid of pH near 5.

Animal models for eccrine sweating are sparse since apocrine glands predominate in other species.

Sweat can be obtained from collection in occlusive plastic bags applied to the skin, but use of this technique may alter sweat composition. The alternate approach of total-body washdown to collect human sweat is more accurate but tedious and cumbersome.

TOXIC SKIN REACTIONS

Irritant Responses

By the term cutaneous irritant, we generally refer to an agent that produces a local cutaneous inflammatory response (dermatitis) by direct action on skin without the involvement of an immunologic mechanism. In this sense irritation is not used to describe noninflammatory reactions such as subjective sensations (itch, burning, etc.) or more subtle biochemical or histologic changes such as epidermal thickening though these could represent variations of the same effect. Irritation of the skin is important and it is commonly thought to account for about 80 percent of the burden of clinically recognized human contact dermatitis, although this figure no doubt varies from location to location. Most of the remaining contact dermatitis represents allergic contact dermatitis. Contact dermatitis is manifest by signs of erythema and edema in experimental test animals. In humans more varied responses are seen, and erythema and edema frequently progress to vesiculation, scaling, and thickening of the epidermis. Histologically the hallmark is spongiosis or intracellular edema of the epidermis (Soter and Fitzpatrick, 1979).

It is useful to distinguish two reasonably distinct types of cutaneous irritation and two related conditions (NAS, 1977; McCreesh and Steinberg, 1983):

Acute irritation—a local reversible inflammatory response of normal living skin to direct injury caused by a single application of a toxic substance, without the involvement of an immunologic mechanism.

Cumulative irritation—reversible irritation resulting from repeated or continued exposures to materials that do not in themselves cause acute irritation.

Corrosion—direct chemical action on normal living skin that results in its disintegration and irreversible alteration at the site of contact. Corrosion is manifested by ulceration and necrosis with subsequent scar formation.

Phototoxicity (photoirritation)—irritation resulting from light-induced molecular changes in the structure of chemicals applied to the skin. Phototoxicity is dealt with elsewhere in this chapter.

Acute irritation is produced by a relatively large number of substances of varying chemical types many of which are highly chemically active such as relatively strong solvents, acids, bases, etc. However, no demonstrably reliable method for assessing irritancy based on chemical structure has been advanced.

In practice, a significant amount of irritant dermatitis appears to result from cumulative irritation resulting in so-called cumulative insult dermatitis. Substances that produce this type of reaction are termed marginal irritants. This type

of dermatitis is often multifactorial with both physical factors and multiple chemical exposures playing a role.

Figure 15–2 shows the results of the application of an aliquot of a concentrated synthetic laundry waste water to the same position on the backs of 20 human subjects under an occlusive patch for 21 consecutive days in a cumulative insult patch test. A response scored as 1+ indicates erythema with a definable margin, 2+ erythema with induration, and 3+ vesiculation or pustulation. Once a 3+ reaction was observed, the treatment was suspended. It is seen that no reactions were observed in any individual for the first several days; however, from day 4 to day 16 all subjects developed erythema, which progressed rapidly in virtually all individuals within a few days of its onset. It should be added that the rate of progression of cumulative irritation changes shows significant variation for different applied substances.

The biochemical mechanisms involved in irritation are not well characterized. Substances that are keratin solvents, dehydrating agents, oxidizing agents, reducing agents, and others may be irritants. To date there has not been a good correlation between measured biochemical changes in the skin and the development of irritation.

A large number of tests for predicting irritation have been proposed over recent years. Those in more widespread use fall into the general categories of single-application tests or cumulative-insult tests. The most widely used test is based on that described by Draize and colleagues in 1944.

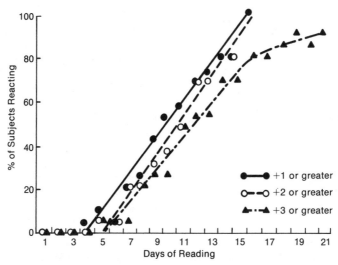

Figure 15–2. Cumulative percentage of subjects with grade 1, grade 2, or grade 3 reaction to repeated application of synthetic laundry waste water in cumulative insult patch test.

Substances are applied to abraded and intact skin of the albino rabbit, clipped free of hair. A minimum of six rabbits are used in abraded and intact skin tests. The substance is inserted under a square patch such as surgical gauze measuring 2.5 cm by 2.5 cm (1 in. by 1 in.) and two single layers thick, using 0.5 ml (in the case of liquids) or 0.5 g (in the case of solids and semisolids) of the test substance. Solids are dissolved in an appropriate solvent and the solution applied as for liquids. The animals are immobilized with patches secured in place by adhesive tape. The entire trunk of the animal is then wrapped with an impervious material such as rubberized cloth, for the 24-hour period of exposure. This material aids in maintaining the test patches in position and retards the evaporation of volatile substances. After 24 hours of exposure, the patches are removed and the resulting reactions are evaluated on the basis of certain designated values. Readings are made again at the end of 72 hours (CFR, 1980).

A number of modifications have been made in this test over the years by different authors. Although there is considerable dispute about a number of experimental details and its predictive competency, it is frequently a legal requirement (McCreesh and Steinberg, 1983). Different testing methods have been recommended depending on product usage, for example, shorter four-hour testing for certain household substances (NAS, 1977). Considerable variation in results obtained has been noted, particularly between laboratories (Weill and Scala, 1972). Nevertheless, the test is widely considered to be a relatively satisfactory method of identifying strong irritants.

For mild to moderate irritants, cumulative irritancy tests appear to give better predictive results (Phillips *et al.*, 1972). There is reasonable concordance between the results of such testing in albino rabbits and humans (Steinberg, 1975). All such test procedures are sensitive to methodologic variations including such factors as site of application, hair pattern, depilation technique, strain, species, occlusive technique, vehicle, size of application area, lighting, procedure for reading reactions, and others. In humans there are marked variations in the responses of different individuals to the same substance and of one individual to different substances, so that one is unable in any subject to predict the intensity of reaction to one irritant on the basis of the reaction to another.

Chemical Burns. Corrosive substances can cause severe ulceration in humans. Although terminology is not standardized, more severe corrosive changes are often designated as chemical burns.

Characteristics of these lesions vary depending on the nature of the toxic material. Severe burns from acids usually cause a dry crust from coagulation necrosis, the color varying with the anion. Alkalies produce softer burns, which may be extremely painful. Phenolics can result in local anesthesia so that pain will be absent after a short time. Some materials, such as nitrogen mustard and certain organotins, produce characteristically delayed reactions. The action of some corrosives differs from thermal burns in that toxic effects may continue indefinitely. In the case of alkyl mercury, it has been shown that evacuation of blister fluid containing the toxin helps prevent extension of the lesion.

A vital step in limiting tissue damage is rapid removal of the causal material. In practice this is almost always best done with copious soap and water. Among the few exceptions are quicklime (CaO), whose reaction with water is extremely exothermic, the solution of 1 g generating over 18,000 calories, and titanium tetrachloride and tin tetrachloride, which rapidly hydrolyze to form hydrochloric acid.

Specific therapeutic approaches are necessary with some substances including white phosphorus and hydrogen fluoride (Curreri *et al.*, 1970; Emmett, 1980). White phosphorus, which burns in air, can produce severe thermal and chemical injury. It may reignite as it dries. After washing, debridement is performed under water. Initial luminescence in the dark may help in particle identification. Treatment with 1 percent copper sulfate, sufficiently brief to avoid systemic absorption and copper poisoning, converts the phosphorus to copper phosphide, which is then removed. Hydrogen fluoride may produce extensive painful necrosis locally, which may progress over a few days. Hypocalcemia from the precipitation of calcium contributes to the local injury and may result in profound systemic hypocalcemia. Treatment with calcium gluconate locally and monitoring of serum calcium levels with calcium administration, as required, is necessary.

The effects of systemic absorption of toxic materials must always be considered.

Allergic Contact Responses

Allergic contact dermatitis occurs as a result of cell-mediated or type IV immune reactions (see Chapter 9; Dahl, 1981; Baer and Bickers, 1981). Allergic contact dermatitis is important because of both the specificity of the response and the quite low amounts of allergen that may elicit an inflammatory reaction.

Immunobiologic Process. A number of phases may be distinguished in the development of contact allergy. For a varying period of time, which may be a lifetime or only a few days, there is a *refractory period* during which sensitization does not take place. Sensitization develops in an *induction period,* which generally takes from 10 to 21 days. After the induction of sensitization is complete, reexposure to the antigen will result in *elicitation* of the reaction after a characteristic delay of usually 12 to 48 hours (hence the name delayed hypersensitivity). Once induced, the allergic sensitivity will persist for a varying period, possibly for a lifetime.

Why some exposures and not others initiate sensitization is not entirely clear, but appears to depend on the nature of the chemical, concentration, type of exposure, genetic susceptibility and nongenetic idiosyncrasies. It is clear that some allergens (e.g., poison ivy extract) are very potent sensitizers whereas others rarely sensitize despite extensive exposure.

Cutaneous antigens (haptens) are generally of low molecular weight. The first step in the allergic process appears to be absorption of the hapten into the skin and covalent binding to a carrier protein. The antigen is bound to cell surfaces especially of the epidermal Langerhans cell (Baer and Berman, 1981) or macrophages. These cells *process* the antigen by altering the configurational arrangement and *present* the antigen by holding it to the cell surface for subsequent interaction with histocompatible T lymphocytes. The T lymphocyte-macrophage interaction can occur in skin and does not appear to require cooperation of cells in the regional lymph node. Either Langerhans cells or T lymphocytes migrate from the skin to the regional lymph node. The antigen-bearing lymphocyte settles in the paracortical area of the lymph nodes. Following clonal proliferation to form immunoblasts in the paracortical areas, two populations of sensitized lymphocytes are formed, *effector* T lymphocytes, which travel to the skin surface in the peripheral blood, and long-lived *memory cells,* which will proliferate to form new populations of sensitized lymphocytes on recontact with the antigen.

The elicitation phase can take place once the sensitization phase has been completed and may occur as a result of reintroduction or persistence of the antigen. Effector T lymphocytes in the skin become activated as they recognize the hapten-protein complex, enlarge, and resemble lymphoblasts (blast transformation). The activated lymphocyte synthesizes a variety of substances called lymphokines which mediate the response. More than 30 lymphokines have been described, although it is not clear that they are all distinct substances. These include chemotactic, macrophage migration inhibition, macrophage-activating, leukocyte-inhibiting, and

lymph node permeability factors; lymphotoxins; transfer factors; and others. In addition to sensitized lymphocytes other lymphocytes not specifically sensitized to the antigen as well as monocytes and macrophages may be recruited to the reaction to contribute to the inflammatory response and to manufacture lymphokines. A variety of other cells including B lymphocytes and possibly cutaneous basophils may play a role in these responses.

Although it is considered prudent to assume that allergic contact sensitization persists indefinitely, it has been shown that the prevalence of positive patch tests to poison ivy extract declines with age, suggesting that some individuals may lose their sensitization. As memory cells appear to have a finite life, it is theoretically possible that sensitization could be lost.

Causes of Contact Allergy. Contact allergy may occur from a very large number of antigens; it seems possible that most substances may at least very rarely be antigens. A list of selected important allergens is seen in Table 15–2. However, there is a great range in antigenic potency, and a relatively small number of strong sensitizers have been identified experimentally or in humans. Strong allergens are often aromatic substances with molecular weights less than 500; they tend to be highly lipid soluble and quite reactive with protein, although exceptions occur.

Table 15–2. SELECTED IMPORTANT ALLERGIC CONTACT SENSITIZERS

Metals
  Nickel and nickel salts
  Chromium salts
  Cobalt salts
  Organomercurials
Plant sensitizers
  Toxicodendron genus: pentadecylcatechols and
    other catechols
  Primula obconica: α-methylene-γ-butyrolactone
  Compositae family: sesquiterpene lactones
Rubber additives
  Mercaptobenzthiazole
  Thiuram sulfides
  p-Phenylenediamine and derivatives
  Diphenylguanidine
  Resorcinol monobenzoate
Epoxy oligomer (M.W. 340)
Methyl methacrylate and other acrylic monomers
Pentaerythritol triacrylate and other multifunctional
    acrylates
Hexamethylenediisocyanate
p-Tertiary butyl phenol
Ethylenediamine, hexamethylenetetramine, and
    other aliphatic amines
Formaldehyde
Neomycin
Benzocaine
Captan

Two groups of dermatologists, the North American Contact Dermatitis Group (NACDG) and the International Contact Dermatitis Research Group (ICDRG), use a limited standard set of antigens for patch testing and centrally report and periodically publish results. The reported prevalence of contact allergic sensitivity on diagnostic patch testing in patients of both groups is shown in Table 15–3, taken from Rudner et al. (1973). It is seen that reactions to nickel were most frequent in each group. These statistics are an interesting guide to some of the more frequent antigens; they have important limitations, however, as they are not population based and do not necessarily contain all important antigens; for example, in the United States, because of ease of diagnosis poison ivy reactions are not included. The reported prevalence of sensitization in human populations is clearly a function of relative antigenic potency, extent of hazardous exposure, and the diagnostic test used. Figure 15–3 shows the structural formulae of a number of important contact allergens.

There is a wide number of situations in which sensitized subjects can contact antigens in a manner that will lead to development of contact dermatitis (Fregert, 1981; Foussereau et al., 1982; Adams, 1983). Common sources include, but are certainly not limited to, contact with metals (nickel); metal compounds (nickel, chromium, cobalt salts, and organomercurials); perfumes; preservations; hair dyes; colorants in cosmetics and toiletries; resins and dyes in clothing, additives, and adhesives in rubber and leather products; topical medicaments; many plants and plant products; pesticides; monomers used in plastics such as acrylates, polyurethanes, and epoxys; additives in coolants and cutting oils; photographic chemicals; and a wide variety of industrial chemicals. Fully cured plastics are usually not antigenic unless they release formaldehyde or contain leachable additives.

Either flareups of cutaneous reactions or possibly systemic symptoms may occur on ingestion of antigens to which contact allergic sensitization has been previously induced, although the frequency of such reactions is debated (Menne, 1983).

A number of terms are used in connection with allergic contact sensitivity. These include:

Sensitizing Potential. The relative capacity of a given agent to induce sensitization in a group of humans or animals.

Index of Sensitivity. The prevalence of sensitivity to a substance in a given population at a given time.

The removal of antigens from products, replacing them with substances of a lower sensitizing potential, is called *allergen replacement.*

Cross-Sensitization and Multiple Sensitization. Cross-sensitization may occur when two or more potential antigens share similar groups. This may depend on a particular chemical group, e.g., a primary para amine ($R-NH_2$) attached directly to an aromatic ring, or on structural similarity (e.g., some quinolines). The structural formulae for several substances with para amino groups that frequently appear to cross-react is shown in Figure 15–4. Cross-sensitization might be explained by the formation of similar reaction products *in vivo,* by the formation of common metabolites, or by the induction of similar

Table 15–3. REPORTED PREVALENCE OF SELECTED ALLERGIC SENSITIVITY REACTIONS ON DIAGNOSTIC PATCH TESTING WITH STANDARD SET OF ANTIGENS*

COMPOUND, TEST CONCENTRATION, AND VEHICLE		NORTH AMERICA ($n = 1200$), PERCENT POSITIVE REACTIONS	EUROPE† ($n = 4824$), PERCENT POSITIVE REACTIONS
Nickel sulfate	2.5% petrolatum	11	6.7
Potassium dichromate	0.5% petrolatum	8	
Thiomerosal	0.1% petrolatum	8	
p-Phenylenediamine	1% petrolatum	8	4.7
Ethylenediamine	1% petrolatum	7	
Neomycin sulfate	20% petrolatum	6	3.7
Benzocaine	5% petrolatum	5	4
Mercaptobenzothiazole	2% petrolatum	4	2
Formalin	2% aqueous	4	3.5
Tetramethylthiuram disulfide	2% petrolatum	4	2

* Modified from Rudner, E. F., et al.: Epidemiology of contact dermatitis in North America. *Arch. Dermatol.,* **108:**537–40, 1973.
† Data for Europe and North America are both given only where test concentration and vehicle were similar.

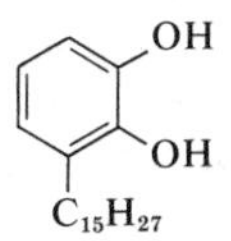

Pentadecylcatechol
Antigen in Toxicodendron
(poison ivy, oak, sumac, and others)

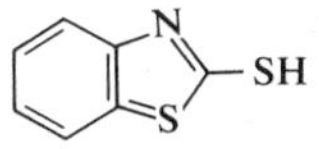

2-Mercaptobenzthiazole

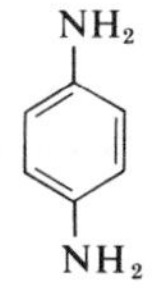

p-Phenylenediamine

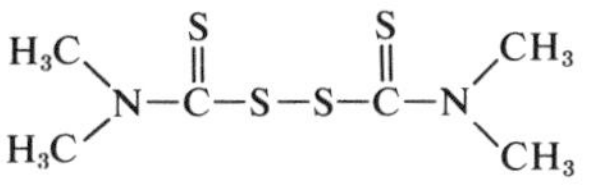

Tetramethylthiuram

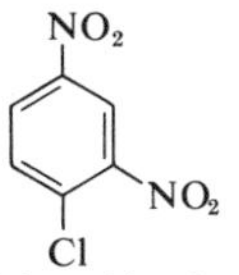

2,4-Dinitrochlorobenzene

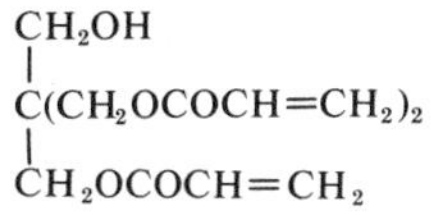

Pentaerythritol triacrylate

Figure 15–3. Structural formulae of some potent contact sensitizers.

changes in carrier proteins. Satisfactory explanations do not yet exist for all purported examples of cross-sensitization.

Terms used in connection with *multiple sensitization* include

Cross-sensitization. A is the *primary allergen* (antigen). Induction of sensitization to it is combined with the acquisition of sensitization to a chemically related molecule such as B, which is called a *secondary allergen* (antigen).

Concomitant Sensitization. This occurs when different substances A and B are present in the same product and sensitization to both takes place on the same occasion.

Simultaneous Sensitization. Simultaneous sensitization occurs when an individual is sensitized to different substances in different products.

False Cross-sensitivity. This occurs when the same antigen is present in different products (e.g., eugenol in perfumes, soft drinks, and underarm deodorants).

Diagnostic Patch Testing. The existence of allergic contact dermatitis is confirmed by diagnostic patch testing. The principle is simple: a concentration of the test substance that is known to be nonirritating and does not induce sensitization is applied to the skin in a suitable vehicle, commonly white petrolatum. It is also necessary that the application concentration be sufficient to elicit an allergic reaction in those sensitized. Nonirritancy is established by testing on a suitably large control population. In practice, suitable test concentrations have generally been established through trial and error, and the test is properly standardized and validated for only a limited number of substances. The material to be tested is applied to normal skin, usually on the back, and suitably occluded for 48 hours. Readings are generally made from 24 to 96 hours after removal of the patch. Adherence to exacting techniques in application and reading is very important (Cronin, 1980). In order to determine the relevance of positive patch test reactions to product exposure, usage testing with a product may be performed by daily application to skin such as at the elbow flexure. It has been possible to use *in vitro* tests such as lymphocyte transformation tests and macrophage migration inhibition tests to demonstrate type IV hypersensitivity in selected instances of allergic contact sensitization, but no *in vitro* test is yet sufficiently reliable for routine diagnostic use (Nordquist and Rosenthal, 1978).

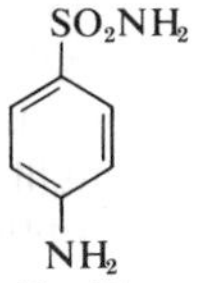

Sulfamide

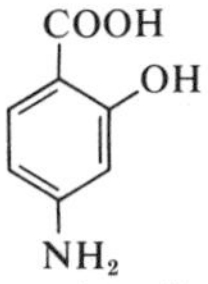

Para-aminosalicylic acid

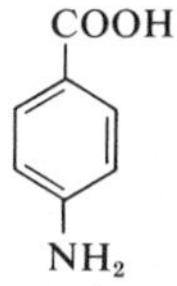

Para-aminobenzoic acid

Figure 15–4. Structural formulae of selected para-amino compounds that show cross-reactions in allergic contact sensitization.

A number of predictive tests have been developed to identify potential allergic contact sensitizers. To date no satisfactory *in vitro* tests are available, all tests require the use of intact mammals with functioning immunologic systems. Humans or guinea pigs of Hartley or Pinbright strains are generally used. In guinea pigs, the induction phase consists of a number of epicutaneous applications, intradermal injections, or both. Epicutaneous applications are generally considered most realistic and relevant to human exposure. Complete Freund's adjuvant may be administered to increase immunologic reactivity. After a rest period, a challenge test is performed by closed or open epicutaneous testing. An increase in reactivity compared with presensitization or control animals is considered to indicate sensitization. Compounds that induce a high incidence of contact sensitivity tend to be fairly well identified in currently available predictive tests, weak sensitizers less well. This creates a difficulty as the identification of relatively weak sensitizers may be very important for materials such as toiletries that will be used by millions of people. A number of different test variations are in current use (Klecak, 1983), and comparative studies are relatively limited. These tests are sensitive to variations in technique, and many experimental variables affecting the induction of sensitization in the guinea pig have been described (Magnusson and Kligman, 1970).

Test procedures in human volunteers generally follow a similar pattern with exposures to multiple occlusive patches followed by a rest period and challenge testing with nonirritant concentrations. Procedures to increase the yield of sensitization may be used; these include the use of local sodium lauryl sulfate applications and the use of high induction concentrations. Significant differences in results are seen from different techniques (Marzulli and Maibach, 1980). In these tests it is necessary to use a sufficiently large experimental sample to allow a reasonable extrapolation of results to exposed populations.

Photosensitization

A number of physiologic and pathologic changes occur in the skin as a result of exposure to the ultraviolet (UV) component of sunlight. These include erythema (sunburn); thickening of the epidermis; darkening of existing pigment (immediate pigment darkening); new pigment formation (delayed tanning); actinic elastosis (premature skin aging); proliferative and other changes in epidermal cells; suppression of T lymphocytes; actinic keratosis, a precancerous condition; and the development of squamous cell cancers, basal cell cancers, and probably some malignant melanomas (Parish et al., 1979; Kripke, 1980). These changes appear to occur as a result of the photochemical interaction of UV with normal components of the skin.

Foreign substances, either absorbed locally into the skin or reaching the skin through the systemic circulation, may be the subject of photochemical reactions within the skin, leading to either chemically induced photosensitivity reactions or altering the "normal" pathologic effects of light described above. Such reactions may augment pathologic changes like photocarcinogenesis or ameliorate them by absorbing potentially hazardous radiation or by scavenging potentially damaging excited molecular states. In recent times advantage has been taken of light as a therapeutic agent, for example, in the phototherapy of neonatal hyperbilirubinaemia.

Photobiologic Principles. Photochemical changes in the skin are important because humans have opportunities for extensive exposure both to sunlight and to a wide variety of artificial sources. That part of the solar spectrum of major toxicologic interest is from 290 to 700 nm. Shorter wavelengths are absorbed by the atmosphere, mostly by the ozone layer of the stratosphere, while longer wavelengths may cause tissue heating, but generally lack the energy to cause photochemical changes.

Electromagnetic radiation may be regarded as consisting of waves (characterized by their frequency, or wavelength in a particular medium) or photons (characterized by their energy). For photobiologic purposes, it is convenient to define particular wavebands that have certain physical or toxicologic characteristics. Currently accepted divisions of the spectrum are UV-C (germicidal UV), 220 to 280 nm; UV-B, 280 to 320 nm; UV-A, 320 to 400 nm; and visible, 400 to 760 nm. Progressively shorter than the UV-C are the vacuum UV and soft x-rays; longer than the visible is the infrared. UV-C is not present in sunlight received at the earth's surface, it is, however, capable of profound photochemical damage to DNA and proteins. UV-B is the main region of sunlight responsible for "normal" pathologic changes in skin, although increasingly the UV-A is felt to play an important role (Parrish et al., 1978). UV-A is responsible for most photosensitivity reactions. Visible radiations lack the energy to produce photochemical reactions in most proteins and in DNA, but are well absorbed by certain highly specialized molecules such as rhodopsin or chlorophyll and by colored substances in general.

The radiation actually delivered to any target in the skin will be dependent on skin optics (Anderson and Parrish, 1981). Skin is an optically inhomogeneous medium; reflection, refraction, scattering, and absorption all modify the radiation that reaches deeper structures. Important UV absorbers within the epidermis include melanin, which varies greatly in content and location between individuals and races; urocanic acid, a deamination product of histidine found in sweat; and for shorter wavelengths, proteins containing tryptophan and tyrosine. The net optical effect is that shorter wavelengths are selectively absorbed in the superficial layers, although a biologically significant amount of UV-B reaches the dermis. In addition, variations in epidermal thickness, water content of the skin, and the application of oils alter optical properties of skin.

The First Law of Photochemistry states that to produce an effect, radiation must be absorbed. Absorption of specific wavelengths of radiation by a chromophore results in electronically excited molecules. An excited singlet state has a lifetime of 10^{-8} seconds or less before either returning to the ground state or undergoing the process of intersystem crossing to a metastable triplet state with a lifetime in the range of 10^{-4} to 10^{-1} seconds. Triplet excited states may relax to the ground state by transfer of energy to another molecule, and both singlet and triplet excited states may return to the ground state by emission of light (fluorescence or phosphorescence); by emission of heat; or by undergoing photochemistry such as *cis-trans* isomerization, ionization, rearrangement, fragmentation, and intermolecular reactions. Through what is no doubt a complex series of events, initial almost instantaneous photochemical events lead to longer-term biologic effects. The entire sequence is not yet well understood for any particular effect.

A most important concept in photobiology is that of *action spectrum*, the relative response of a system to different wavelengths. In theory, the action spectrum should reflect the absorption spectrum of the responsible chromophore. In practice, the relationship appears less exact for one or more of several reasons. The *in vivo* absorption spectrum may differ from that determined in a solvent system *in vitro* (Cripps and Enta, 1970), and the wavelength distribution of radiation actually reaching the target molecules in tissue will be modified as a result of the optical properties of overlying layers.

Mechanisms of Chemically Induced Photosensitization. Photosensitization designates an abnormal adverse reaction to ultraviolet and/or visible radiation. Xenobiotics may produce such reactions in a number of ways (Emmett, 1979), as indicated in Table 15–4. Of these reactions the most important are phototoxicity and photoallergy. Phototoxicity designates a chemically induced increased reactivity of a target tissue to UV and/or visible radiation on a nonimmunologic basis. Each response is governed by a dose-response relationship between the intensity of the reaction and both the concentration of the inciting chemical in the target tissue and the amount of radiation of appropriate wavelengths (weighted for the action spectrum) to which that target tissue is exposed, provided that the time of administration is sufficiently short that photorecovery is not a factor.

Photoallergy designates an increased reactivity of the skin to UV and/or visible radiation produced by a chemical agent on an immunologic basis. This type of response can be elicited only in individuals who have been previously allergy sensitized by exposure to the chemical agent and appropriate radiation. Photoallergy is distinctly

Table 15–4. SELECTED MECHANISMS OF CHEMICALLY INDUCED PHOTOSENSITIZATION

Photoxicity
  e.g., 8-methoxypsoralen
Photoallergy
  e.g., tribromosalicylanilide
Depigmentation, with alteration in cutaneous optical properties
  e.g., p-tertiary-butylphenol
Induction of engenous photosensitizer
  e.g., hexachlorbenzene-induced porphyria cutanea tarda
Induction of disease characterized by photosensitivity
  Lupus erythematosus   e.g., procainamide
  Pellagra   e.g., INH
Undetermined mechanisms
  e.g., quinidine

less common than phototoxicity, although a few agents such as tetrachlorosalicylanilide are very potent photoallergens.

Phototoxicity.   Phototoxic reactions have been described after contact, ingestion, or injection of causal agents. In addition to reactions in humans, they are responsible for certain economically important diseases of domestic animals. The skin and eyes are the major organs affected. The actual skin changes vary with the agent and circumstances of exposure. Swelling and redness frequently occur, and blistering may be seen. Hyperpigmentation, associated with long-standing morphologic changes in melanosomes, may follow a reaction. Possible eye changes may include keratoconjunctivitis or corneal and lens opacities (Bernstein *et al.*, 1970; Emmett *el al.*, 1977).

Phototoxic reactions are broadly divided into those which are oxygen dependent (photodynamic action), and a lesser number which do not require oxygen. In photodynamic mechanisms, either the excited triplet state is reduced leading to the generation of highly reactive free radicals, which subsequently attach biological substrates (type I reaction), or the chromophore transfers its energy to O_2 generating singlet oxygen ($^1O_2$), an active oxidizing agent (type II reaction).

Nonphotodynamic compounds may in their excited state react directly with a target molecule. An example is the reaction of furocoumarins such as 8-methoxypsoralen with specific sites on DNA to form covalent bonds between the pyrimidine base and the furocoumarin (2 + 2 cycloaddition). Upon absorption of another photon, a second 2 + 2 cycloaddition reaction can take place resulting in a cross-linked DNA (Dall'Acqua, 1977). It is believed that these lesions are responsible for the major photosensitization effects of psoralens including photocarcinogenesis. Other substances such as chlorpromazine and protriptyline form stable toxic photoproducts after irradiation (Kochevar, 1981). Important subcellular targets for phototoxic reactions include nuclei, cytoplasmic organelles, and cell membranes.

A list of selected phototoxic agents is shown in Table 15–5.

Table 15–5. SELECTED PHOTOTOXIC CHEMICALS

Furocoumarins
  8-Methoxypsoralen
  5-Methoxypsoralen
Polycyclic aromatic hydrocarbons
  Anthracene
  Acridine
  Phenanthrene
Tetracyclines
Sulfonamides
Chlorpromazine
Nalidixic acid
Amyl o-dimethylaminobenzoic acid

Forbes et al. (1976) have nicely demonstrated that the phototoxic agent 8-methoxypsoralen is capable of markedly enhancing experimental UV carcinogenesis. Enhanced skin cancer formation has been described in humans treated with psoralens and UV-A for psoriasis (Stern et al., 1979).

A number of assay systems for phototoxic substances exist. They include the use of biochemical tests, anuclear cells, nucleated cells in suspension or culture, small organisms, nonhuman mammalian skin, and human skin (Emmett, 1979). This seems to be an area in which the use of alternative methods to whole-animal predictive testing may enjoy early success.

Photoallergy. Photoallergic reactions (Emmett, 1978; Harber and Bickers, 1981) result from type IV, cell-mediated immune reactions similar to allergic contact dermatitis although it remains possible that other immunologic pathways could be involved. In selected instances the immunologic nature of the reactions has been demonstrated by a variety of techniques, experimental induction of sensitization in guinea pigs and humans, passive transfer of sensitization, *in vitro* lymphocyte transformation, and macrophage migration inhibition tests. The vast majority of these reactions appear to be elicited by UV-A and to result from topical exposure. A number of reports have described apparent photoallergy resulting from systemically administered agents, but documentation is generally in-

complete. Clinical photoallergy is usually manifest as dermatitis on exposed areas, which may eventually spread to areas covered by clothes; lichenification and chronic pigmentary changes may also develop.

The main role of light in photoallergy appears to be in the conversion of the hapten to a complete allergen, although other roles are possible. The mechanisms may be complex and may differ depending on the allergen, but two types of reactions are thought to play a role. Radiation absorbed by the photosensitizer may result in its conversion to a photoproduct that is a more potent allergic sensitizer than the parent compound. For example, UV converts sulfanilamide to the potent allergic sensitizer p-hydroxylaminobenzene sulfonamide. Patients with sulfanilamide photoallergy have been shown to have an allergic reaction to the latter compound in the dark. Thus,

Sulfanilamide   p-Hydroxylaminobenzene sulfonamide

Alternatively, the short-lived, highly reactive, excited-state species formed on irradiation of a number of photoallergens may combine with proteins, forming light-induced hapten-protein complexes that could act as the complete allergens. The binding of a photoallergens such as the brominated salicylanilides to proteins upon irradiation has been shown to be quite complex (Alani and Dunne, 1973).

Table 15–6 lists some photoallergens. All are substances that absorb UV. They generally have a resonating structure and are at least weakly phototoxic in an appropriate experimental system. Photoallergy can be induced experimentally in the guinea pig, and human and predictive screening tests have been described, though their universality is open to question (Kochevar et al., 1979; Harber et al., 1982).

An important complication of photoallergy from some agents, such as halogenated salicylanilides and phenothiazines, is the development of *persistent light reaction.* In this condition, marked sensitivity to light persists despite the apparent removal of further exposure to the photoallergen, and the action spectrum broadens to include the UV-B as well as the UV-A. This condition may be very long lived and troublesome.

Table 15–6.   SELECTED REPORTED PHOTOALLERGENS

Halogenated salicylanilides and related agents
  3,3',4',5-Tetrachlorosalicylanilide
  Bithional
  3,4',5-Tribomosalicylanilide
  4',5-Dibromosalicylanilide
  4-Chloro-2-hydroxybenzoic acid *n*-butylamide
    (Jadit)
Sulfonamides
Phenothiazides
  Promethazine hydrochloride
4,6-Dichlorophenylphenol
Quinoxaline 1,4-di-*N*-oxide
Coumarin derivatives
  6-Methylcoumarin
  4-Methyl-7-ethoxycoumarin
  7-Methylcoumarin
Musk ambrette
Sunscreen components
  Glyceryl *p*-aminobenzoic acid
Plant products
  Compositae (ragweed, Australian bush dermatitis)

Chemical Acne, Including Chloracne

A number of agents produce acneiform lesions similar to those seen in acne vulgaris. These include greases and oils, coal tar pitch, creosote, a number of cosmetic preparations (acne cosmetica). These forms of acne typically start with comedones and inflammatory folliculitis on areas of the body contacted by the causal agent, which stimulates proliferation of the follicular epithelium of the sebaceous gland. The duct cells, which are usually lipid filled, keratinize, leading to the formation of keratin cysts and a sac filled with retained sebaceous lipid and keratin lamellae. A profollicular inflammatory response may be seen. Some systemically administered drugs, including iodides, bromides, and isoniazid, can also cause acne.

Chloracne is a somewhat more specific type of acneiform eruption due to poisoning by halogenated aromatic compounds with a specific molecular shape (Poland and Glover, 1977). A list of certain well-defined causal agents is given in Table 15–7. Structural formulae for TCDD, TCDF, and TCAB are shown in Figure 15–5. A number of these substances, including PCDDs, PCDFs, TCAB, and TCAOB, are formed as contaminants during the manufacture or use of other polychlorinated substances.

The chloracnegenicity as well as other toxic potentials of these substances depends on the lateral symmetry and position of the halogens. These substances compete for stereospecific binding sites in the hepatic cytosol that are thought to be receptor sites for a pleomorphic

Table 15–7.   CAUSES OF CHLORACNE

Polyhalogenated dibenzofurans
  Polychlorodibenzofurans (PCDF), especially tri-,
    tetra-, (TCDFs), penta- (PCDFs), and
    hexachlorodibenzofuran
  Polybromodibenzofurans (PBDFs), especially
    tetrabromodibenzofuran (TBDF)
Polychlorinated dibenzodioxins (PCDDs)
  2,3,7,8-Tetrachlorodibenzo-*p*-dioxin (TCDD)
  Hexachlorodibenzo-*p*-dioxin
Polychloronaphthalenes (PCNs)
Polyhalogenated biphenyls
  Polychlorobiphenyls (PCBs)
  Polybromobiphenyls (PBBs)
3,4,3',4'-Tetrachloroazoxybenzene (TCAOB)
3,4,3',4'-Tetrachloroazobenzene (TCAB)

response that includes the induction of hepatic aryl hydrocarbon hydroxylase (AHH) (Poland and Knudson, 1982). The ability to induce AHH correlates with chloracnegenecity.

Chloracne is characterized by small, straw-colored cysts and comedones (Taylor, 1979). Inflammatory pustules and abscesses may occur but are not prominent features except in severe cases where large cysts may be seen as well as follicular hyperkeratosis. The most sensitive areas of skin, which may be the only ones involved, are below and to the outer side of the eye (the malar crescent) and behind the ear. The eruption typically involves exposed areas but may also involve covered areas, particularly the scrotum. Chloracne may continue to appear after exposure to the chloracnegen has ceased, possibly as a result of its release from body stores. The clinical picture is distinctive but may not always be pathognomonic. Histologic

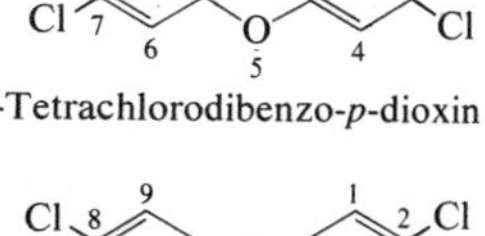

2,3,7,8-Tetrachlorodibenzo-*p*-dioxin (TCDD)

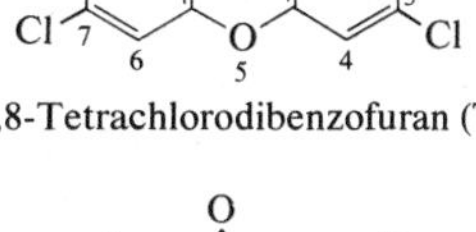

2,3,7,8-Tetrachlorodibenzofuran (TCDF)

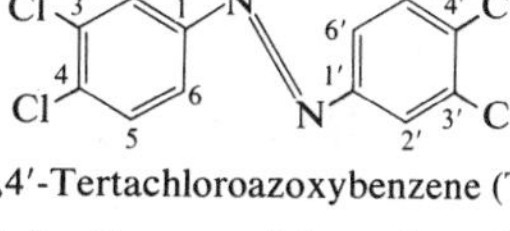

3,3'4,4'-Tertachloroazoxybenzene (TCAB)

Figure 15–5. Structural formulae of certain potent chloracnegens.

changes commence with keratinization of the epithelium of the sebaceous gland ducts and outer root sheath of the hair. The sebaceous gland becomes replaced by a keratinous cyst, which is always attached to the epidermis (Crow, 1983).

Chloracne is a symptom complex whose other features vary depending on the actual chloracnegen and the circumstances of exposure.

TCDD is the most potent chloracnegen. Over 20 serious accidents with TCDD overexposure have occurred worldwide. Acute effects of exposure may include nausea, vomiting, headache, mucosal irritation, and chemical burns of the skin, sometimes with blistering; the latter occur particularly from handling contaminated objects, or, as at Seveso, Italy, from being caught in the toxic cloud containing reactor contents following a reactor explosion. Chloracne is the first and most constant finding in the chronic stage. Other more variable findings have included: elevated porphyrin excretion, hyperpigmentation, hypertichosis, central and peripheral nervous system effects, changes in lipid metabolism, and hepatic effects. Experimental effects of TCDD include teratogenicity, immunosuppression, and tumor induction.

The effects of PCBs may depend largely on the contaminants and on the route of absorption. In industrially exposed populations where percutaneous absorption may be the main route of uptake, chloracne is uncommon. In these situations the serum levels of PCBs may be correlated with the levels of hepatic enzymes and serum lipids, particularly triglycerides, but other toxic effects are less prominent. In contrast are epidemics in both Japanese and Taiwanese populations who ingested rice oil contaminated with PCBs and developed Yusho show chloracne, a variety of other mucocutaneous symptoms including pigmentation, and meibomian gland metaplasia, as well as a number of systemic changes including increased porphyrin excretion and immunologic changes (Chang et al., 1982). This rather different clinical syndrome may be related to the high concentrations of TCDF, chlorinated terphenyls, and other contaminants present in the oil rather than to PCBs.

Chloracne may be produced experimentally in the rhesus monkey, which develops facial lesions similar to those in humans, and on the inner surface of the rabbit ear, but not elsewhere on rabbit skin.

Other Cutaneous Reaction Patterns

In addition to the conditions discussed to this point, a wide variety of other types of toxic reaction patterns is known. Because of the visibility of skin changes, these are best grouped accord-ing to the observed morphology. No exhaustive description is possible here.

Physical Dermatitis—Fiberglass. Fiberglass produces an intense pruritus (itching) of the skin in the presence or absence of pinpoint-sized papules, which are often excoriated and petechial. Urticaria and linear erosions are seen, generally secondary to scratching. The condition appears to be due to the physical properties of fiberglass. The likelihood of developing the condition appears directly related to the fiber diameter (which must be greater than 4.5 μm), and inversely to fiber length (Possick et al., 1970; Konzen, 1982).

Urticarial Reactions. Urticarial (wheal-and-flare) reactions may be produced after cutaneous exposure to a relatively large number of agents, usually within 30 to 60 minutes of contact (Odum and Maibach, 1976; VonKrogh and Maibach, 1983). Causal agents may directly release histamine and other vasoactive substances. Biogenic polymers released from plants (nettles), animals (caterpillars, jellyfish), and a number of other substances fall into this category. Alternatively, some reactions depend on immediate immunologic reactions, while for a number of substances the mechanism is uncertain. Severe reactions may involve other organs including angioedema, bronchial asthma, anaphylactoid reactions, rhinoconjunctivitis, and gastrointestinal dysfunction. Urticaria is a frequent component of immediate hypersensitivity reactions to ingested or parenterally administered agents.

Cutaneous Granulomas. Cutaneous granulomas are usually seen as slightly erythematous, more or less flesh-colored papules, which may be grouped and may be associated with inflammatory changes. They are generally localized to sites of contact and result from a dermal response of mononuclear cells to poorly soluble substances (Epstein, 1980). Granulomas may represent a purely foreign body reaction as to talc and silica, or an immunologic response as in the case of beryllium, zirconium, and, more rarely, chromium salts in tattoos. In the latter cases, appropriate immunologic testing may confirm sensitization.

Hair Damage and Loss. Hair is susceptible to damage both from agents contacting the hair externally and from those reaching the hair matrix through the dermis. Two major types of damage must be differentiated, keratolytic damage and matrix cell damage; the latter includes effluvium (hair loss) in the anagen or telogen phases.

Alkali, thioglycolates, and oxidizing agents such as peroxides and perborates produce keratolysis (dissolution of hair keratin) on local contact with the hair. Softening, matting, and increased fragility of hair ensues, which, depending on the extent of exposure, may involve local patches or the entire scalp. Regrowth of hair generally occurs as the dermal hair matrix cells are not damaged.

Agents that damage the hair matrix (Reeves and Maibach, 1983) may directly poison active cells in the anagen phase. This leads either to cessation of growth and the loss of the entire hair or to the later loss of excessively brittle hair at the site of a weak constricted area in the shaft. Hair loss (anagen effluvium) may occur within one to two weeks of exposure to the agent. Causes of anagen effluvium include antimitotic agents such as alkylating agents, antimetabolites, and colchicine.

A number of substances precipitate telogen effluvium by precipitating hairs into the telogen phase. Hair shedding in the telogen phase occurs two to four months after exposure. Causes include oral contraceptives, a number of anticoagulants, propranolol, and triparanol. Some agents such as thallium, phenyl glycidyl, and dixyrazine cause hair loss of a mixed type. Hair loss in anagen and telogen phases can be distinguished by examination of shed hairs or hairs plucked from the scalp. Other causes of hair loss must be distinguished from chemical hair loss.

Hair may be discolored by chemical exposure, for example, green hair from copper, blue from indigo or cobalt, yellow from picric acid.

Hypopigmentation. A number of substances produce localized pigmentary loss, particularly phenols and catechols including hydroquinone, monobenzyl ether of hydroquinone, monomethyl ether of hydroquinone (p-hydroxyanisole), p-tertiary butyl phenol, p-tertiary amyl phenol, and 4-tertiary butyl catecol. These agents appear to have selective melanotoxicity. As shown in Figure 15–6, they bear structural similarity to tyrosine, the major building block of melanin (Gellin et al., 1979).

The cosmetic disfiguration produced by these agents may be substantial, particularly in heavily pigmented individuals. Other agents such as arsenic can produce mixed pigmentary changes including circumscribed areas of pigment loss together with generalized increase in pigmentation.

As predictive skin testing is usually performed on albino animals in order that erythemia may be better detected, these tests are generally not sensitive to effects on the pigment system, so that a false sense of security may ensue.

Hyperpigmentation. A number of chemical agents have been described that produce localized or diffuse increases in pigmentation. Localized changes occur secondary to phototoxic re-

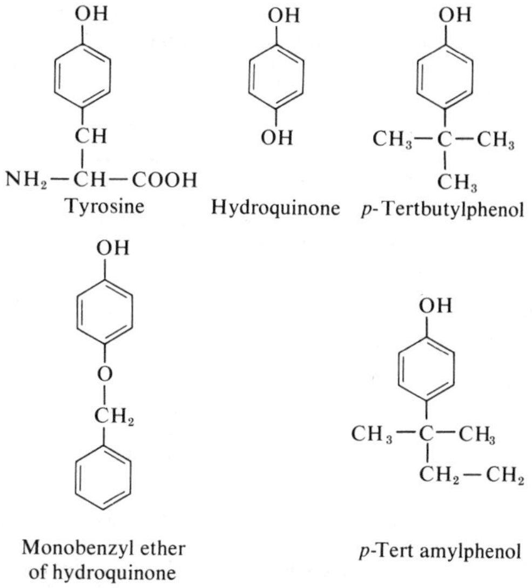

Figure 15–6. Chemical structure of tyrosine and of selected depigmenting agents.

sponses, especially with coal tar pitch and psoralens. Certain drugs including phenolphthalein and barbiturates produce a recurrent localized erythematous or dermatitic lesion that leaves a localized pigmented area, the so-called fixed drug eruption. These reactions recur at the same site on readministration of the agent; their pathogenesis is obscure. Large amounts of melanin-containing macrophages are found in the upper dermis.

Other causes of diffuse or local hyperpigmentation include heavy metals such as silver (argyria), bismuth, arsenic, and mercury; various acridines and 4-aminoquinolines used as antimalarials; phenothiazines; tetracyclines; busulfan; and other alkylating agents (Granstein and Sober, 1983). Color changes in the skin may occur from the accumulation of exogenous or endogenous pigments, for example, the yellow-orange color of carotenaemia from carotenoids.

Cancer of the Skin. Carcinogenesis is dealt with elsewhere in this book. Important causes of skin cancer in humans in addition to UV and ionizing radiation are polycyclic aromatic hydrocarbons, arsenic, and combined exposures to psoralens and UV radiation. It is clear that a number of chemical agents influence the carcinogenic effects of UV radiation (Emmett, 1973; Forbes et al., 1976).

REFERENCES

Adams, R. M.: *Occupational Skin Disease*. Grune & Stratton, Inc., New York, 1983.
Alani, M. D., and Dunne, J. H.: Effects of long wave ultraviolet radiation on photosensitizing and related

compounds. II. *In vitro* binding to soluble epidermal proteins. *Br. J. Dermatol.* **89**:367, 1973.

Anderson, R. R., and Parrish, J. A.: The optics of skin. *J. Invest. Dermatol.*, **77**:13–19, 1981.

Baer, R. L., and Berman, B.: Role of Langerhans cells in cutaneous immunological reactions. In Safai, B., and Good, R. A. (eds.): *Immunodermatology*. Plenum Publishing Corp., New York, 1981.

Baer, R. L., and Bickers, D. R.: Allergic contact dermatitis, photoallergic contact dermatitis and phototoxic dermatitis. In Safai, B., and Good, R. A. (eds.): *Immunodermatology*. Plenum Publishing Corp., New York, 1981.

Baginsky, E.: *Occupational Disease in California, 1978*. Division of Labor Statistics and Research, California Department of Industrial Relations, San Francisco, 1982.

———: *Occupational Skin Disease in California*. Division of Labor Statistics and Research, California Department of Industrial Relations, San Francisco, 1982.

Bernstein, H. N.; Curtis, J.; Earl, F. L; and Kuwzbara, T.: Phototoxic corneal and lens opacities in dogs receiving a fungicide: 2,6-dichloro-4-nitroaniline. *Arch. Ophthalmol.*, **83**:336–48, 1970.

Blank, I. H., and Scheuplein, R. J.: Transport into and within the skin. *Br. J. Dermatol.*, **81**(Suppl. 4):4–10, 1969.

Bronaugh, R. L., and Maibach, H. I.: *In vitro* percutaneous absorption. In Marzulli, F. N., and Maibach, H. I. (eds.): *Dermatotoxicology*, 2nd ed. Hemisphere Publishing Co., Washington, D.C., 1983.

Bronaugh, R. L.; Stewart, R. F.; Congdon, E. R.; and Giles, A. L.: Methods for *in vitro* percutaneous absorption studies. I. Comparison with *in vivo* results. *Toxicol. Appl. Pharmacol.*, **62**:474–80, 1982.

Brown, A. C., and Crounse, R. G.: *Hair, Trace Elements and Human Illness*. Praeger, New York, 1980.

CFR: United States, Code of Federal Regulations, Title 16, part 1500.41, 1980.

Chang, K. J.; Hsieh, K. H.; Lee, T. P.; and Tung, T. C.: Immunologic evaluation of patients with polychlorinated biphenyl poisoning: determination of phagocyte Fc and complement receptors. **28**:329–34, 1982.

Cohn, J. R., and Emmett, E. A.: The excretion of trace metals in human sweat. *Ann. Clin. Lab. Sci.*, **8**:270–75, 1978.

Cripps, D. J., and Enta, T.: Absorption and action spectra studies on bithional and halogenated salicylanilide photosensitivity. *Br. J. Dermatol.*, **82**:230–42, 1970.

Cronin, E.: *Contact Dermatitis*. Churchill-Livingstone, Edinburgh, 1980.

Crow, K. D.: Chloracne (halogen acne). In Marzulli, F. N., and Maibach, H. I. (eds.): *Dermatotoxicity*, 2nd ed. Hemisphere Publishing Co., Washington, D.C., 1983.

Curreri, W. P.; Asch, M. J.; and Pruitt, B. A.: The treatment of chemical burns: specialized diagnostic and prognostic considerations. *J. Trauma*, **10**:634–42, 1970.

CTFA: *Cosmetic Ingredient Dictionary*. Cosmetic, Toiletry, and Fragrance Association, Washington, D.C., 1982.

Dahl, M. V.: *Clinical Immunodermatology*. Year Book Medical Publishers, Chicago, 1981.

Dall'Acqua, F.: New chemical aspects of the photoreaction between psoralen and DNA. In Castellani, A. (ed.): *Research in Photobiology*. New York, Plenum Publishing Corp., 1977, pp. 245–55.

Emmett, E. A.: Ultraviolet radiation on a cause of skin tumors. *Crit. Rev. Toxicol.*, **2**:211–55, 1973.

———: Drug photoallergy. *Int. J. Dermatol.*, **17**:370–79, 1978.

———: Phototoxicity from endogenous agents. *Photochem. Photobiol.*, **40**:429–36, 1979.

———: Topical agents. In Hanenson, I. B. (ed.): *Quick Reference to Clinical Toxicology*. J. B. Lippincott Co., Philadelphia, 1980.

Emmett, E. A.; Stetzer, L.; and Taphorn, B.: Phototoxic keratoconjunctivitis from coal tar pitch volatiles. *Science*, **198**:841–42, 1977.

Epstein, W. L.: Foreign body granulomas. In Boros, D., and Yoshida, H. (eds.): *Basic and Clinical Aspects of Granulomatous Diseases*. Elselvier/North Holland, Amsterdam, 1980.

Feldmann, R. J., and Maibach, H. I.: Absorption of some organic compounds through the skin in man. *J. Invest. Dermatol.*, **54**:339–404, 1969.

Forbes, P. D.; Davies, R. E.; and Urbach, F.: Phototoxicity and photocarcinogenesis. Comparative effects of anthracene and 8 methoxypsoralen in the skin of mice. *Food Cosmet. Toxicol.*, **14**:303–306, 1976.

Foussereau, J.; Benezra, C.; and Maibach, H. I.: *Occupational Contact Dermatitis: Clinical and Chemical Aspects*. Munksgaard, Copenhagen, 1982.

Franz, T. J.: Percutaneous absorption. On the relevance of *in vitro* data. *J. Invest. Dermatol.*, **64**:190–95, 1975.

Fregert, S.: *Manual of Contact Dermatitis*, 2nd ed. Munksgaard, Copenhagen, 1981.

Gellin, G. A.; Maibach, H. I.; Misiaszek, M. H.; and Ring, M.: Detection of environmentally depigmenting substances. *Contact Dermatitis*, **5**:201–13, 1979.

Goldstein, B. D., and Harber, L. C.: Erythropoetic protoporphyria: lipid peroxidation and red cell membrane damage associated with photohemolysis. *J. Clin. Invest.*, **51**:892–902, 1972.

Goldstein, J. A., *et al.*: Effects of pentachlorphenol on hepatic drug-metabolizing enzymes and porphyria related to contamination with chlorinated dibenzo-*p*-dioxins and dibenzofurans. *Biochem. Pharmacol.*, **26**:1549–57, 1977.

Granstein, R. D., and Sober, A. J.: Drug and heavy metal induced hyperpigmentation. In Marzulli, F. N., and Maibach, H. I. (eds.): *Dermatotoxicology*, 2nd ed. Hemisphere Publishing Co., Washington, D.C., 1983.

Hammer, D. I.; Finklea, J. F.; Hendricks, R. H.; Shy, C. M.; and Horton, R. J. M.: Hair, trace metals and environmental exposure. *Am. J. Epidemiol.*, **69**:84, 1971.

Harber, L. C.; Armstrong, R. B.; Walther, R. R.; and Ichikawa, H.: Current status of predictive animals for drug photoallergy and the correlation with humans. In Kligman, A., and Leyden, J. (eds.): *Assessment of Safety and Efficacy of Topical Drugs and Cosmetics*. Grune & Stratton, New York, 1982.

Harber, L. C., and Bickers, D. R.: *Photosensitivity: Principles of Diagnosis and Treatment*. W. B. Saunders Co., Philadelphia, 1981.

Johnson, H. C., and Maibach, H. I.: Drug excretion in human eccrine sweat. *J. Invest. Dermatol.*, **56**:182–88, 1971.

Klecak, G.: Identification of contact allergens. In Marzulli, F. N., and Maibach, H. I. (eds.): *Dermatotoxicology*, 2nd ed. Hemisphere Publishing Co., Washington, D.C., 1983.

Kochevar, I.: Phototoxicity mechanisms: chlorpromazine photosensitized damage to DNA and cell membranes. *J. Invest. Dermatol.*, **77**:59–64, 1981.

Kochevar, I. E.; Zaler, G. L.; Embinder, J.; and Harber, L. C.: Assay of contact photosensitivity to musk ambrette in guinea pigs. *J. Invest. Dermatol.*, **73**:144–46, 1979.

Konzen, J. K.: Fiberglass and the skin. In Maibach, H. I., and Gellin, G. A. (eds.): *Occupational and Industrial Dermatology*. Year Book Medical Publishers, Chicago, 1982.

Kripke, M. L.: Immunologic effects of UV radiation and their role in photocarcinogenesis. *Photochem. Photobiol. Rev.*, **5**:257–92, 1980.

Lauwerys, R. R.: *Industrial Chemical Exposure: Guide-*

lines for Biological Monitoring. Biomedical Publications, Davis, Calif., 1983.

Magnusson, B., and Kligman, A. M.: *Allergic Contact Dermatitis in the Guinea Pig. Identification of Contact Allergens.* Charles C Thomas, Pub., Springfield, Ill., 1970.

Marzulli, F. N., and Maibach, H. I.: Contact allergy: predictive testing of fragrance ingredients in humans by Draize and maximization methods. *J. Environ. Path. Toxicol.,* 3:235–45, 1980.

Marzulli, F. N., and Maibach, H. I.: *Dermatotoxicology,* 2nd ed. Hemisphere Publishing Co., Washington, D.C., 1983.

McCreesh, A. H., and Steinberg, M.: Skin irritation testing in animals. In Marzulli, F. N., and Maibach, H. I. (eds.): *Dermatotoxicology,* 2nd ed., Hemisphere Publishing Co., Washington, D.C., 1983.

Menne, T.: Reactions to systemic exposure to contact allergies. In Marzulli, F. N., and Maibach, H. I. (eds.): *Dermatotoxicology,* 2nd ed. Hemisphere Publishing Co., Washington, D.C., 1983.

Montagna, W., and Parakkal, P. F.: *The Structure and Function of Skin.* Academic Press, Inc., New York, 1974.

NAS: *Principles and Procedures for Evaluating the Toxicity of Household Substances.* National Academy of Sciences, Washington, D.C., 1977.

Nordquist, B., and Rosenthal, S. A.: Studies on DNCB contact sensitivity in guinea pigs by the macrophage migration test. *Int. Arch. Allergy Appl. Immunol.* 56:73–78, 1978.

Odum, R. B., and Maibach, H. I.: Contact urticaria: a different contact dermatitis. *Cutis,* 18:672–676, 1976.

Pannatier, A.; Jenner, P.; *et al.:* The skin as a drug-metabolizing organ. *Drug Metab. Rev.,* 8:319–43, 1978.

Parrish, J. A.; Anderson, R. R.; Urbach, F.; *et al.: UV-A Biologic Effects of Ultraviolet Radiation with Emphasis on Human Responses to Longwave Ultraviolet.* Plenum Press, New York, 1978.

Parrish, J. A.; White, H A. D.; Pathak, M. A.: Photomedicine. In Fitzpatrick, T. B., *et al.,* (eds.): *Dermatology in General Medicine,* 2nd ed. McGraw-Hill Book Co., New York, 1979.

Phillips, L.; Steinberg, M.; Maibach, H. I.; and Akers, W. A.: A comparison of rabbit and human skin responses to certain irritants. *Toxicol. Appl. Pharmacol.,* 21:369–82, 1972.

Pohl, R.; Philpot, R.; and Fouts, J.: Cytochrome P-450 content and mixed-function-oxidase activity in microsomes isolated from mouse skin. *Drug Metab. Disp.,* 4:442–50, 1976.

Poland, A., and Glover, E.: Chlorinated biphenyl induction of amyl hydrocarbon hydroxylase activity: a study of the structure activity relationships. *Mol. Pharmacol.,* 13:924–38, 1977.

Poland, A., and Knutson, J. C.: 2,3,7,8-Tetrachlorodibenzo-*p*-dioxin and related halogenated aromatic hydrocarbons: examination of the mechanism of toxicity. *Annu. Rev. Pharmacol. Toxicol.,* 22:517–54, 1982.

Possick, P. A.; Gellin, G. A.; and Key, M. D.: Fibrous glass dermatitis. *Am. Ind. Hyg. Assoc. J.,* 31:12–15, 1970.

Reeves, J. R. T., and Maibach, H. I.: Drug and chemical-induced hair loss. In Marzulli, F. N., and Maibach, H. I. (eds.): *Dermatotoxicology,* 2nd ed. Hemisphere Publishing Co., Washington, D.C., 1983.

Report of the OSHA Advisory Committee on Cutaneous Hazards. Office of Consumer Affairs, U.S. Department of Labor, Washington, D.C., 1979.

Rudner, E. J., *et al.:* Epidemiology of contact dermatitis in North America. *Arch. Dermatol.,* 108:537–40, 1973.

Scheuplein, R. J., and Blank, I. H.: Permeability of the skin. *Physiol. Rev.,* 51:702–47, 1971.

Scheuplein, R. J., and Ross, L.: Effects of surfactants and solvents on the permeability of epidermis. *J. Soc. Cosmetic Chemists,* 21:853–73, 1970.

Schmid, R.: Cutaneous porphyria in Turkey. *N. Engl. J. Med.,* 263:397–98, 1960.

Soter, N. A., and Fitzpatrick, T. B.: Introduction and classification. In Fitzpatrick, T. B. (ed.): *Dermatology in General Medicine,* 2nd ed. McGraw-Hill Book Co., New York, 1979.

Steinberg, M.; Akers, W. A.; Weeks, M.: McCreesh, A. H.; and Maibach, H. I.: A comparison of test techniques. In Maibach, H. I. (ed.): *Animal Models in Dermatology.* Churchill Livingstone, New York, 1975.

Stern, R. S.; Thibodeu, L. A.; *et al.:* Risk of cutaneous carcinoma in patients treated with oral methoxsalen photochemotherapy for psoriasis. *N. Engl. J. Med.,* 300:809–13, 1979.

Taylor, J. S.: Environmental chloracne: Update and overview. *Ann. N.Y. Acad. Sci.,* 320:295–307, 1979.

Tregear, R. T.: *Physical Functions of the Skin.* Academic Press, Inc., New York, 1966.

vonKrogh, G., and Maibach, H. I.: The contact uticaria syndrome. *J. Am. Acad. Dermatol.,* 5(3):328–42, 1981.

Weil, C. S., and Scala, R. A.: Study of ultra- and interlaboratory variability in the results of rabbit eye and skin irritation tests. *Toxicol. Appl. Pharmacol.,* 19:276–360, 1971.

Wester, R. C., and Maibach, H. I.: Relationship of topical dose and percutaneous absorption in rhesus monkey and man. *J. Invest. Dermatol.,* 67:518–20, 1976.

Wester, R. C.; Noonan, P. K.; Smeach, S.; and Kosobud, L.: Estimate of nitroglycerin percutaneous first pass metabolism. *Pharmacologist,* 23:203, 1981.

Chapter 16

TOXIC RESPONSES OF THE REPRODUCTIVE SYSTEM

Robert L. Dixon

INTRODUCTION

Survival of any species depends on the integrity of its reproductive system. Genes located in the chromosomes of the germ cells transmit genetic information from previous generations and control cell differentiation and organogenesis. Under normal circumstances, germ cells ensure the maintenance of structures and functions in the organism in its own lifetime and from generation to generation. But human beings now live in an environment in which at least 10,000 chemicals are prevalent and to which some 700 to 1000 new compounds are added annually. It is the potential toxicity of these chemicals to human beings during their most vulnerable stages of development—gametogenesis to birth—that is among the least understood toxicologic phenomena. For the purposes of this chapter, reproductive toxicity will be defined as dysfunction induced by chemical (as well as physical and biologic) agents that affect the processes of gametogenesis from its earliest stage to implantation of the conceptus in the endometrium.

The toxic effects of drugs and environmental chemicals on the human reproductive system have become a major health concern; incidences of chemically induced germ cell damage and sterility appear to be on the increase. In the United States, male factory workers occupationally exposed to 1,2-dibromo-3-chloropropane (DBCP) became sterile, evidencing oligospermia, azoospermia, and germinal aplasia. Factory workers in battery plants in Bulgaria, lead mine workers in the state of Missouri, and workers in Sweden who handle organic solvents (toluene, benzene, and xylene) suffer from low sperm counts, abnormal sperm, and varying degrees of infertility. Diethylstilbestrol (DES), lead, kepone, methylmercury, and many cancer chemotherapeutic agents have been shown to be toxic to the male and female reproductive system and possibly capable of inflicting genetic damage to germ cells.

The potential hazard of chemicals to reproduction and the risks to humans from chemical exposure are difficult to assess because of the complexity of the reproductive process, the unreliability of laboratory tests, and the quality of human data. In the human, it is estimated that one in five couples are involuntarily sterile; over one-third of early embryos die, and about 15 percent of recognized pregnancies abort spontaneously. Among the surviving fetuses at birth, approximately 3 percent have developmental defects (not always anatomic), and with increasing age over twice that many become detectable.

For one to understand better the basis of reproductive toxicity, attention should be directed to the entire spectrum of reproductive processes and events that must function normally to produce a healthy offspring. Perturbation of any of these processes by environmental agents can result in reproductive dysfunction. Thus, each is a target for toxicity.

This chapter will consider how toxic agents affect reproductive processes to cause dysfunction, and how chemical hazards are identified in the laboratory. Pharmacokinetic and adaptive factors associated with gonadal toxicity will be discussed. In addition, chemicals known to affect the reproductive performance of laboratory animals and humans will be mentioned, and efforts to analyze human risk will be summarized.

GENERAL REPRODUCTIVE BIOLOGY

Because of the developing gonads' unique sensitivity to chemical insult and the reproductive organs' potential for teratogenic alterations, toxicologists should be generally familiar with the major aspects of urinary and genital organogenesis. During development, critical molecular and cellular processes must respond with integrity to a variety of hormones and other growth factors to ensure normal postnatal function. Thus, the potential for environmental chemicals to affect these processes is real. The development of normal reproductive capacity may offer particularly susceptible targets for toxins. Environmental factors might alter the genetic determinants of gonadal sex, the hormonal determinants of phenotypic sex, fetal gametogenesis, reproductive tract differentiation, as well as postnatal integration of endocrine functions and other processes essential for the propagation of the species. While the effects of environmental agents on sexual differentiation and the development of reproductive capacity are largely unstudied, a number of chemicals with diverse structures and actions have been shown to exert dramatic effects, especially on hormone synthesis and function. Dixon (1982) has recently reviewed this general area.

DEVELOPMENT OF REPRODUCTIVE CAPACITY

Gonadal Sex

A testis-determining gene on the Y chromosome apparently determines gonadal sex and converts the indifferent gonad to a testis. There is increasing experimental evidence that a plasma membrane protein, known as H-Y antigen, is this testis-determining gene product. The testis, in response to the H-Y antigen, then produces two kinds of hormones: the Mullerian inhibiting factor (MIF) and testosterone. Testosterone-induced masculine differentiation is mediated by androgen receptors controlled by genes on the X chromosome (Ohno, 1976). Alterations of the sex chromosomes may be transmitted by either one of the parents (gonadal dysgenesis) or may occur in the embryo itself. Failure of the sex chromosomes of either of the parents to separate during gametogenesis (nondisjunction) can lead to gonadal agenesis. Klinefelter's syndrome is characterized by testicular dysgenesis with male morphology and an XXY karyotype; Turner's syndrome includes ovarian agenesis with female morphology, a single X chromosome, and an XO karyotype.

True and pseudohermaphroditism have been observed in the human population secondary to nondisjunction of sex chromosomes during the first cleavage mitosis of the egg, which thereby results in sex mosaics of XY/XX or XY/XO. Pseudohermaphrodites are distinguished by secondary sex characteristics different from those predicted by genotype. Pseudohermaphroditism can be produced in rats.

With regard to chemical perturbation of the genetic determinants of sex, the chromosomes are the obvious targets, and nondisjunction is the most common genetic abnormality. Attempts have been made to monitor directly Y chromosomal nondisjunction in human male gametes by quantifying the number of spermatozoa with two fluorescent bodies (YFF). YFF sperm are increased in patients receiving antineoplastic and x-irradiation therapy. An increased incidence of YFF sperm has also been observed in dibromochloropropane (DBCP)-exposed workers (Hansmann and Probeck, 1979).

Single gene mutants that cause abnormal hormone synthesis or action and prevent normal sexual development have been identified. The tfm (Stanley-Gumbreck) pseudohermaphrodite strain is a testicular feminization model that demonstrates decreased Leydig cell responsiveness (Purvis et al., 1978). The role of chemical mutagens in the etiology of such conditions is unclear.

Sexual Differentiation

The gonads are formed from two types of cells. The reproductive germinal cells give rise to the primordial germ cells, and the nutrient supporting cells give rise to the Sertoli cells of the testis and the follicular cells of the ovary. This duality is explained by the different embryologic origin of these elements (Tuchmann-Duplessis and Haegel, 1974). The primitive germ cells migrate ameboidlike from the allantois to the germinal ridge where the primitive sexual cords, which eventually become the seminiferous tubules in the male and the medullary cords in the female, are formed. These germ cells, together with supporting cells, aggregate in cordlike strands in the center of the gonads. At this stage of development, the indifferent gonad is characterized by the primordial germ cells, which have migrated into the intermediate mesodermal ridge where they exist together with the primary sex cords. The ovaries can be identified only by the absence of testicular differentiation. Hoar's (1978) summary of the embryologic aspects of sexual differentiation is helpful.

Until about the eleventh day of gestation in the rat and at about the seventh week in the human, the undifferentiated gonads are indistinguishable as to sex. Gametogenesis takes place around gestational day 12 in the female rat and day 15 in the male and between weeks 8 and 10 in humans.

During development, sexual differences between the testis and ovary are referred to as primary while those related to the genital ducts, accessory glands, and the external genitalia (including the mammary glands) are referred to as secondary sex characteristics. Primary sex characteristics are determined genetically whereas development of secondary sex characteristics is dictated by the nature of the gonad itself.

The inborn sexual program is apparently female unless there is a testis secreting androgens or some other source of androgens. When genetic sex asserts itself, the duct system of the opposite sex disappears almost completely and the remaining system differentiates into its final form (Mittwoch, 1973; Gondos, 1979).

Gametogenesis

During early fetal gametogenesis, both ovarian and testicular germ cells derived from the yolk sac endoderm undergo a series of mitotic divisions. After numerous replications, testicular germ cells enter a period of mitotic arrest and ovarian germ cells shift from mitosis to meiosis. Male germ cells are arrested at the preleptotene (earliest stage of prophase in meiosis) stage; female gametes are arrested at the diplotene (late stage of prophase in meiosis) stage.

The characteristic ovarian differentiation, which consists of the formation of follicles and the delineation of the ovarian stroma, does not occur until later in life (Mossman and Duke, 1973). Oocytes and follicles first appear in the medullary portion of the gonad as derivatives of the primary gonadal cords during the latter half of fetal life, but follicular activity often persists into the juvenile period. Prior to the formation of ova, clusters of cells from the germinal epithelium invade the stroma. Each cluster forms a primary follicle. The innermost cell is the primary oocyte, which on maturation will become an ovum surrounded by follicular epithelial cells.

The prophase of the first meiotic division of ovarian development occurs very early in gestation. In most laboratory rodents, oogenesis occurs between days 10 to 14 of gestation and peaks on day 12. In rabbits, however, oocytes are formed during the neonatal period. Meiotic arrests are first seen at about 12 weeks of age in human embryos, and the entire complement of primary oocytes is formed by the seventh month of pregnancy. In contrast, sperm are formed shortly before puberty, and they continue to be produced throughout the reproductive lifespan.

Thus, since oocytes are produced prenatally and no new germ cells are formed after birth, the female fetus in most mammals is particularly vulnerable to chemicals affecting gametogenesis. Chemically induced damage to the fetal oocyte could result in decreased reproductive capacity, which would only be obvious later in the animal's life when sexual maturity was attained. For a chemical to exert a significant prenatal effect on the male gonads, all (or nearly all) of the gametes would have to be destroyed in order to prevent the remaining stem cells from repopulating the seminiferous tubules at puberty.

Chemicals which, when administered prenatally, affect reproductive capacity in the male or female offspring include those presented in Table 16–1. Antineoplastic agents, pesticides, synthetic nonsteroidal estrogen, pyrolysis products, and various environmental pollutants are included (McLachlan et al., 1981). With regard to mechanisms, chemicals that alter DNA structure or synthesis, such as alkylating agents, can be expected to interfere with germ cell replication and development. In both sexes, the toxic effects are focused directly on the immature germ cell during gestation and are manifested by reduced fertility in the mature mammal. As expected, the male is more resistant to such effects. Fewer chemicals have been identified as having effects on the male offspring. The male-germ-cell-damaging effects of prenatal exposure to procarbazine and DMBA have been described (MacKenzie et al., 1979).

Depletion of female germ cells in offspring of pregnant mice exposed to polycyclic aromatic hydrocarbons (MacKenzie et al., 1979; MacKenzie and Angevine, 1981), suggests that females born to women who smoke cigarettes or are exposed to certain pollutants may have compromised reproductive capacity.

Other chemicals may act by interfering with the normal hormonal function regulating spermatogenesis. For example, studies on male offspring of women treated with diethylstilbestrol (DES) during pregnancy indicate that the average values for sperm density and total motile spermatozoa ejaculated are less than one-half that of controls. Furthermore, the number of abnormal sperm in the DES-exposed offspring was significantly greater than in the control group (Bibbo et al., 1977). Similar results have been obtained with mice where 60 percent of offspring of DES-treated mothers were sterile. Gonadal abnormalities in the mouse included cryptorchid testes and a reduction in the number of spermatogonia in more than one-half of the males (McLachlan and Dixon, 1976; McLachlan et al., 1975).

Hormonal Determinants of Phenotypic Sex

The onset of testosterone synthesis by the testis is necessary for the initiation of male differentiation. While the testes are obligatory in male

**Table 16–1. SOME COMPOUNDS REPORTED TO ALTER
FERTILITY AFTER PRENATAL EXPOSURE***

COMPOUND GIVEN TO MOTHER	MAJOR EFFECTS IN OFFSPRING	SPECIES
Methoxychlor	Reduced fertility in males and females	Rat
Dimethylbenzanthracene (DMBA)	Gonadal dysplasia and reduced fertility in males and females	Mouse
Benzo[a]pyrene	Gonadal dysplasia and reduced fertility in males and females	Mouse
Diethylstilbestrol (DES)	Genital tract abnormalities and reduced fertility in females	Mouse
	Genital tract abnormalities and reduced fertility in females	Human
	Genital tract abnormalities and reduced fertility in males	Mouse
	Genital tract abnormalities including sperm	Human
Methyl methanesulfonate	Sterility in males	Rat
Procarbazine	Reduced fertility in females	Mouse
Cyclophosphamide	Reduced fertility in males and females	Mouse
Clomid	Reproductive tract	Rat
Busulfan	Gonadal dysplasia in males and females	Rat
Cyanoketone	Altered estrous cycles	Rat

* From McLachlan, J. A.; Newbold, R. R.; Korach, K. S.; Lamb, F. C., IV; and Suzuki, Y.: Transplacental toxicology: Prenatal factors influencing postnatal fertility. In Kimmel, C. A., and Buelke-Sam, F. (eds.): *Developmental Toxicology*. Raven Press, New York, 1981.

differentiation, the embryonic ovaries are not required to achieve the female phenotype. Female characteristics develop in the absence of androgen secretion. The fetal ovary is less actively involved in steroid synthesis than the testis during gestation and the early postnatal period. In the female rat, estrogens are detectable on postnatal day 10, and levels comparable to the adult are achieved by two weeks of age.

Two principal types of hormones are produced by the fetal testis, an androgenic steroid responsible for male reproductive tract development and a nonsteroid factor that causes regression of the Mullerian ducts. Sertoli cells are the likely source of the MIF. Leydig cell differentiation and regression correspond well with the onset and subsequent decline in testosterone synthesis by the fetal testis. Thus, the embryonic testis promotes the development of the Wolffian duct and its derivatives and suppresses the development of the Mullerian ducts, thereby imposing the male phenotype on the embryo. The rat's embryonic testis must remain functional until about gestational day 17 to ensure that the sex organs are completely established (Gondos, 1979).

Three critical periods for testosterone production have been described with regard to sexual differentiation. The first period occurs on days 14 to 17 of gestation in the rat and weeks 4 to 6 in the human. The second period occurs about day 17 of gestation to about two weeks postnatal age in the rat and from the fourth month of pregnancy to 1 to 3 months of postnatal age in man. The third period follows a long period of testicular inactivity in both species when testosterone production is reinitiated between 40 and 60 days of age in the rat and 12 to 14 years of age in man (Goldman, 1977).

Understanding the dynamics of testosterone production and cellular interactions is an important prerequisite to knowing which chemicals might affect sexual differentiation. Any factor that would reduce the ability of testosterone to be synthesized, activated, enter the cell, and/or affect the cell nucleus' ability to regulate the synthesis of androgen-dependent proteins would have a potential to alter sexual differentiation. Some of these are summarized in Table 16–2. A variety of endogenous and exogenous chemicals are capable of exerting a testosterone-depriving action on the developing systems. These include effects on the feedback regulation of gonadotropin secretion, gonadotropin effectiveness, testosterone and dihydrotestosterone synthesis, plasma binding, as well as cytoplasmic receptor and nuclear chromatin binding.

Insufficient amounts of androgens can feminize the male fetus with otherwise normal testes and an XY karyotype. Slight deficiencies

Table 16–2. FACTORS AFFECTING ANDROGEN EFFECTIVENESS*

TARGET	EFFECT	EXAMPLE
Hypothalamic-pituitary interaction	Feedback control of LHRH-mediated gonadotropin secretion	Estrogens, progestins
Gonadotropin action	Disrupt reproductive control processes involving gonadotropins	LH-FSH antibodies
Androgen synthesis	Inhibit key enzymes, e.g., cholesterol desmolase, 17α-hydroxylase, 3β-hydroxy-steroid oxidoreductase, C17-20 lyase, 17-keto reductase, 5α-reductase	Steroid analogs, diphenylmethylanes (amphenone B, DDD), pyridine derivatives (SU series), disubstituted glutartic acid imides (glutethimides), triazines, hydrazines, thiosemicarbazones
DHT synthesis	Inhibit 5α-reductase in target tissue	Androstene-17-carboxylic acid, progesterone
Plasma binding	Alter ratio of bound and free androgen in systemic circulation	Estrogens
Cytoplasmic receptors	Alter effect on target tissue by affecting binding to cytoplasmic receptors	Cyproterone acetate, 17α-methyl-β-testosterone, flutamide
DHT cellular binding	Block DHT effect on target tissue	Cyproterone acetate, spironolactone, dihydroprogesterone, RU-22930

* From Dixon, R. U.: Potential of environmental factors to affect development of reproductive systems. *Fund. Appl. Toxicol.,* **2**:5–12, 1982.

affect only the later stages of differentiation of the external genital organs and result in a small penis, hypospadia (urethra opens on under surface of penis), and vulviform appearance of the scrotum with masculine general morphology. However, a severe androgen deficiency allows the Mullerian system to persist and results in external genital organs of a female type (vagina and uterus) that coexist with ectopic testes and normal male efferent ducts.

A lack of androgen receptors can also lead to a testicular feminization-type syndrome, even when normal levels of testosterone are present.

Sexual behavior also appears to be "imprinted" in the central nervous system by the testis and could be affected by endogenous and exogenous chemicals.

Estrogens also have important developmental effects. The association between maternal treatment with the synthetic estrogen DES and vaginal adenocarcinoma in the female offspring was first reported a dozen years ago (Herbst, 1971). Other clinical reports have described alterations in reproductive tract function such as menstrual irregularities and subfertility in females exposed prenatally to DES.

The potential for environmental exposure to estrogens is real (Rall and McLachlan, 1980). The environmental estrogen burden is easily illustrated: 27,000 kg of DES has been used in the U.S. livestock industry; kepone and isomers and metabolites (DDE) of DDT are weakly estrogenic; the polychlorinated biphenyls (PCBs) are uterotropic in rats and have been found in mothers' milk; hydroxylated forms of some combustion-derived polycyclic aromatic hydrocarbons (PAHs) possess weak estrogen activity; zearalenone is a naturally occurring estrogenic mycotoxin; and more than 40 species of plants contain estrogenic substances such as coumestrol and genistein. The suggested hormonal activity of marijuana also deserves further study. The structural diversity of chemicals reported to have estrogenic activity have been summarized by Katzenellenbogen *et al.* (1980).

GONADAL FUNCTION

In both sexes, the gonads have a dual function: the production of germ cells (gametogenesis) and the secretion of sex hormones. The testes secrete androgens, principally testosterone, along with small amounts of estrogens. The ovaries secrete large amounts of estrogens and small amounts of androgens. The ovaries also secrete progesterone, a steroid that prepares the uterus for pregnancy.

The gametogenic and secretory functions of the gonads are both dependent on the secretion of the anterior pituitary gonadotropins, FSH and LH. The sex hormones (and inhibin) feedback through the hypothalamus to inhibit gonadotropin secretion. In males, gonadotropin secretion is noncyclic; in postpubertal females, an orderly cyclicity is required for menstruation, pregnancy, and lactation.

TESTICULAR FUNCTION

Spermatogenesis

The production of sperm, termed spermatogenesis, is a unique process in which the timing and stages of differentiation are known with a considerable degree of certainty.

The sperm is among the smallest cells in man. In humans, its length is about 50 μm or only about one-half the diameter of the ovum, the largest cell of the female organism. The relative volume of a sperm is about $\frac{1}{100,000}$ that of the egg. The sperm has a head, middle piece, and tail, which correspond, respectively, to the following functions: activation and genetics, metabolism, and motility.

Whereas only a few hundred human ova are released as cells ready for fertilization in a lifetime, millions of motile sperm are formed in the spermatogenic tubules each day. Oogenesis and spermatogenesis are compared in Figure 16–1.

Spermatogenesis starts at puberty and continues almost throughout life. The primitive male germ cells are spermatogonia, which are situated next to the basement membrane of the seminiferous tubules. Following birth, spermatogonia are dormant until puberty when proliferative activity begins again. The onset of spermatogenesis accompanies functional maturation of the

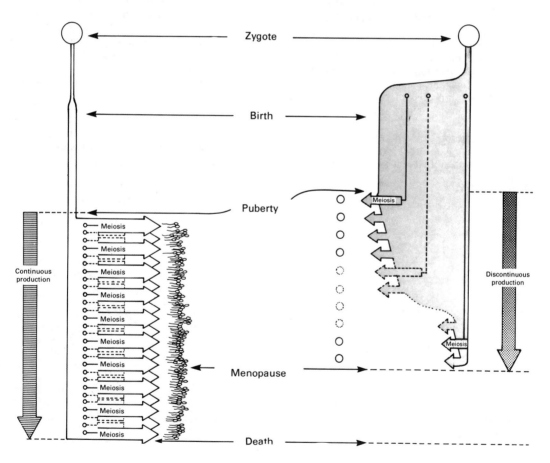

Figure 16–1. Chronology of gametogenesis. (Modified from Tuchmann-Duplessis H.; David, G.; and Haegel, P.: *Illustrated Human Embryology: Embryogenesis,* Vol. I. Springer-Verlag, New York, 1972.)

testes. Two major types of spermatogonia are present—type A, which generates other spermatogonia, and type B, which becomes mature sperm. The latter type develops into primary spermatocytes, which undergo meiotic divisions to become secondary spermatocytes. The process of meiosis results in the reduction of the normal complement of chromosomes (diploid) to half this number (haploid) (Figure 16–2). Meiosis ensures the biologic necessity of evolution through the introduction of controlled variability; although each gamete must receive one of each pair of chromosomes, whether it receives the maternal or paternal chromosome is a matter of chance. In the male, meiosis is completed within several days. In the female, meiotic division is begun during fetal life but then is suspended until puberty. Meiosis may be the most susceptible stage for chemical toxicity.

The secondary spermatocytes give rise to spermatids. Spermatids complete their development into sperm by undergoing a period of transformation (spermiogenesis) that involves extensive nuclear and cytoplasmic reorganization. The nucleus condenses and becomes the sperm head; the two centrioles give rise to the flagellum or axial filament; part of the Golgi apparatus becomes the acrosome; and the mitochondria concentrate into a sheath located between two centrioles.

The seminiferous tubules contain germ cells at different stages of differentiation and Sertoli cells. In a cyclical fashion, spermatogonia A of certain areas of a tubule become committed to divide synchronously, and the cohorts of the resulting cells differentiate in unison. Thus, a synchronous population of developing germ cells occupies a defined area within a seminiferous tubule. Cells within each cohort are connected by intercellular bridges.

In many laboratory species, a cross-section through a seminiferous tubule contains a single cellular association. However, this is not true for humans where different associations are intermingled in a mosaiclike fashion. Depending on the species and the observer, 6 to 14 cellular associations have been discerned. Each cellular association contains four or five types of germ cells organized in a specific, layered pattern. Each layer represents one cellular generation. Fourteen cellular associations are observed in the seminiferous epithelium in the rat (LeBlond and Clermont, 1952; Heller and Clermont, 1964).

If a fixed point within a seminiferous tubule could be viewed as the germ cells develop, it would sequentially acquire the appearance of each of the cellular associations characteristic of that species. This progression through the series of cellular associations would continue to repeat itself in a predictable fashion. The interval required for one complete series of cellular associations to appear at one point within a tubule is termed the duration of the cycle of the seminiferous epithelium. The duration of one cycle of the seminiferous epithelium depends on, and is thus equal to, the cell turnover rate of spermato-

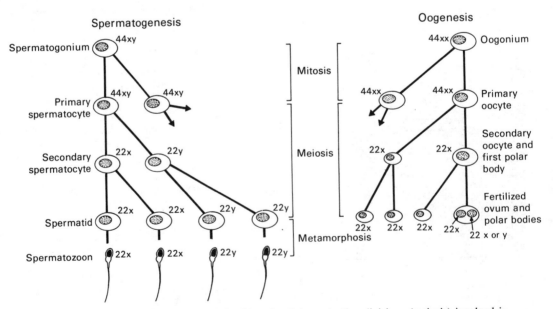

Figure 16–2. Cellular replication (mitosis) and cellular reductive divisions (meiosis) involved in spermatogenesis, oogenesis, and fertilization.

gonia. It takes approximately 13 days to complete one cycle in the rat; approximately 16 days in man. Spermatids, originating from spermatogonia committed to differentiate approximately 4.5 cycles earlier, are continuously released from the germinal epithelium. Table 16–3 compares the duration of the seminiferous epithelial cycle and other aspects of seminiferous tubule function for various species (Galbraith et al., 1982).

The physiologic changes that have been observed in sperm of various species as they pass along the tubules of the testes and epididymides of rodents include acquisition of the capacity for fertility, changes in motility, progressive dehydration of the cytoplasm, decreased resistance to cold shock, changes in metabolism, and variations in membrane permeability. Each ejaculate contains a spectrum of normal sperm as well as those which are either abnormal or immature.

Sertoli Cells

The Sertoli cell junctions form the blood-testis barrier that partitions the seminiferous epithelium into two compartments: a basal compartment containing spermatogonia and early sper-

matocytes; and an adluminal compartment containing the more fully developed spermatogenic cells. An ionic gradient is maintained between the two tubular compartments, and unique chemical milieus exist. Nutrients, hormones, and other chemicals must pass either between or through Sertoli cells in order to diffuse from one compartment to another. Germinal cells are found either between adjacent pairs of Sertoli cells or inside their luminal margin.

Sertoli cells secrete several products including androgen-binding protein (ABP), inhibin, Mullerian-inhibiting factor (MIF), and proteases. In rodents, ABP is thought to be a carrier of testosterone (or dihydrotesterone) transporting essential androgens from the testis to the epididymis. Inhibin appears to retard the release of FSH by the anterior pituitary. MIF suppresses the formation of the female internal genitalia during fetal development. Proteases may facilitate the passage of germ cells through the inter-Sertoli cell junctions during maturation. The Sertoli cells are also phagocytic.

The Sertoli cells are essential to normal spermatogenesis. Many chemicals affecting spermatogenesis may act indirectly via an effect on the

Table 16–3. CRITERIA FOR SPERMATOGENESIS IN LABORATORY ANIMALS AND MAN*

	MOUSE	RAT	RABBIT (New Zealand White)	DOG (beagle)	MONKEY (rhesus)	MAN
Duration of cycle of seminiferous epithelium (days)	8.6	12.9	10.7	13.6	9.5	16.0
Life-span of						
B-type spermatogonia (days)	1.5	2.0	1.3	4.0	2.9	6.3
L + Z† spermatocytes (days)	4.7	7.8	7.3	5.2	6.0	9.2
P + D† spermatocytes (days)	8.3	12.2	10.7	13.5	9.5	15.6
Golgi spermatids (days)	1.7	2.9	2.1	6.9	1.8	7.9
Cap spermatids (days)	3.5	5.0	5.2	3.0	3.7	1.6
Fraction of a life-span as						
B-type spermatogonia	0.11	0.10	0.08	0.19	0.19	0.25
Primary spermatocyte	1.00	1.00	1.00	1.00	1.00	1.00
Round spermatid	0.41	0.40	0.43	0.48	0.35	0.38
Testes wt (g)	0.2	3.7	6.4	12.0	49	34
Daily sperm production						
Per gram testis (10^6/g)	28	24	25	20	23	4.4
Per male (10^6)	5	86	160	300	1100	125
Sperm reserves in cauda (at sexual rest; 10^6)	49	440	1600	?‡	5700	420
Transit time (days) through (at sexual rest)						
Caput + corpus epididymides	3.1	3.0	3.0	?	4.9	1.8
Cauda epididymides	5.6	5.1	9.7	?	5.6	3.7

* From Galbraith, W. M.; Voytek, P.; and Ryon, M. G.: *Assessment of Risks to Human Reproduction and to Development of the Human Conceptus from Exposure to Environmental Substances.* Oak Ridge National Laboratory, U. S. Environmental Protection Agency, 1982. Available as order number DE82007897 from the National Technical Information Service, Springfield, Va.

† L = leptotene, Z = zygotene, P = pachytene, D = diplotene.

‡ A question mark indicates unclear or inadequate data.

Sertoli cells rather than directly on the germ cells. The Sertoli cells deserve more attention as a target for testicular toxicity.

Interstitium

The Leydig cells within the interstitium are the main site of testosterone synthesis and are closely associated with the testicular blood vessels and the lymphatic space, both of which facilitate androgen transport. The spermatic arteries to the testes are tortuous, and their blood flows parallel to, but in the opposite direction of, blood in the pampiniform plexus of the spermatic veins. This anatomic arrangement seems to facilitate a countercurrent exchange of heat, androgens, and other chemicals.

LH stimulates testicular steroidogenesis. Androgens are essential to spermatogenesis, epididymal sperm maturation, the growth and secretory activity of accessory sex organs, somatic masculinization, male behavior, and various metabolic processes.

POSTTESTICULAR PROCESSES

The product of testicular gametogenesis is immature sperm. Posttesticular processes involve ducts that move maturing sperm from the testis to storage sites where they await ejaculation. A number of secretory processes exist that control fluid production and ion composition; secretory organs contribute to the chemical composition (including specific proteins) of the semen.

Efferent Ducts

The fluid produced in the seminiferous tubules moves into a system of spaces called the rete testis, which is confluent with the efferent ducts. The chemical composition of the rete testis fluid is unique and has a total protein concentration much lower than that of the blood plasma. The efferent ducts open into the caput epididymis. At the point of entry into the epididymis, the testicular fluid is designated as testicular plasma.

Although the rete testis fluid normally contains inhibin, ABP, transferrin, myoinositol, steroid hormones, amino acids, and various enzymes, only ABP and inhibin appear to be specific products and useful indicators of the functional integrity of the seminiferous epithelium or Sertoli cells (Mann and Lutwak-Mann, 1981). However, relative concentrations of other constituents may indicate alterations in membrane barriers or active transport processes. The concentration of chemicals in the rete testis fluid relative to unbound plasma concentration has been used to estimate the permeability of the blood-testis barrier for selected chemicals (Okumura et al., 1975).

Epididymides

From the rete testis, testicular fluid first enters efferent ducts and then the epididymides. Here the sperm are subjected to a changing chemical environment as they move through the organ. The epididymis is conventionally and macroscopically divided into the head (caput), body (corpus), and tail (cauda); these three gross regions generally reflect the histologic variations of the organ.

The first two sections together (proximal part) are regarded as making up that part of the epididymis involved with sperm maturation, while the terminal (distal) segment is regarded as the site of sperm storage. There are, however, differences in the position and extent of the segments in various species of mammals.

In most species, from 1.8 to 4.9 days are required for sperm to move through the caput to the corpus epididymis where maturation takes place. In contrast, the transit time for sperm through the cauda epididymis in sexually rested males differs greatly among species and ranges from 3.7 to 9.7 days. Average transit time for a 21- to 30-year-old man is six days. The number of sperm in the caput and corpus epididymis is similar in sexually rested males and in males ejaculating daily. However, the number of sperm in the cauda epididymis is more variable, being lower in males ejaculating regularly.

Active transport processes are suggested by the fact that the amount of fluid flowing through the epididymis is only a small fraction of the volume obtained by cannulating the rete testis. Because much of the fluid produced by the testis is apparently absorbed in the epididymis, the relative concentration of sperm is increased.

Thus, important functions of the epididymis are reabsorption of rete testis fluid, metabolism, epithelial cell secretions, sperm maturation, and sperm storage. It is also likely that the chemical composition of the epididymal plasma plays an important role in both sperm maturation and sperm storage. It is possible that environmental chemicals might perturb these processes and produce adverse effects. However, even considering all of the potential sites for interference, few examples of chemicals that affect epididymal function are known.

Accessory Organs

The seminal plasma functions as a vehicle for conveying the ejaculated sperm from the male to the female reproductive tract. The seminal plasma is produced by the secretory organs of the male reproductive system which, along with the epididymides, include the prostate, seminal vesicles, bulbourethral (Cowper's) glands, and urethral (Littre's) glands. Any abnormal function of these organs can be reflected in altered seminal characteristics. Seminal plasma is normally an isotonic, neutral medium, which, in many species, contains sources of energy such as fructose and sorbitol that are directly available to sperm. The potential functions of the other constituents such as citric acid and inositol are not known. In general, the secretions from the prostate and seminal vesicles apparently contribute little to fertility (Mann and Lutwak-Mann, 1981).

Because all of the accessory organs are androgen dependent, they serve as indicators of the Leydig cell function and/or androgen action. The weights of the accessory sex glands are an indirect measure of circulating testosterone levels. The ventral prostate of rats has been used as a model to study the actions of testosterone and to investigate the molecular basis of androgen-regulated gene function.

It appears that human semen emission initially involves the urethral and Cowper's glands, with the prostatic secretion and sperm coming next and the seminal vesicle secretion delivered last. There is a considerable overlap between the presperm, sperm-rich, and postsperm fractions. Therefore, even if an ejaculate is collected in as many as six (split-ejaculate) fractions, it is rarely possible to obtain a sperm-free fraction consisting exclusively of prostatic or vesicular secretions.

Acid phosphatase and citric acid are markers for prostatic secretion, and fructose is an indicator for seminal vesicle secretion. It is estimated that about one-third of the entire human ejaculate is contributed by the prostate and about two-thirds by the seminal vesicles. Both the vas deferens and the seminal vesicles apparently synthesize prostaglandins. Semen varies both in volume and composition between species. Human, bovine, and canine species have a relatively small semen volume (1 to 10 ml); semen of stallions and boars is ejaculated in much larger quantities. Sperm move from the distal portion of the epididymis through the vas deferens (ductus deferens) to the urethra. Vasectomy is the surgical removal of the vas deferens or of a portion of it. The semen of some animals, including rodents and men, tends to coagulate on ejaculation. The clotting mechanism involves enzymes and substrates from different accessory organs.

Prostate. Although all male mammals have a prostate, the organ differs anatomically, physiologically, and chemically among species, and lobe differences in the same species may be pronounced. The rat prostate is noted for its complex structure and its prompt response to castration and androgen stimulation. The human prostate is a tubulalveolar gland made up of two prominent lateral lobes that contribute about a third of the ejaculate.

Prostate secretion in men and many laboratory species contains acid phosphatase, zinc, and citric acid. The prostatic secretion is the main source of acid phosphatase in human semen; its concentration provides a convenient method for assessing the functional state of the prostate. The human prostate also produces spermine. Certain proteins and enzymes (acid phosphatase, γ-glutamyl transpeptidase, glutamic-oxaloacetic transaminase), cholesterol, inositol, zinc, and magnesium have also been proposed as indicators of human prostatic secretory function.

Seminal Vesicle. As with the prostate, the structure of the seminal vesicle varies across animal species. The seminal vesicle is a compact glandular tissue arranged in the form of multiple lobes that surround secretory ducts. (Neither the dog nor the cat has a seminal vesicle.) Like the prostate, the seminal vesicle is responsive to androgens and is a useful indicator of Leydig cell function. The vesicular glands can be weighed as an indirect measure of circulating testosterone levels.

In man, the seminal vesicle contributes about 60 percent of the seminal fluid. The seminal vesicles also produce more than half of the seminal plasma in laboratory and domestic animals such as the rat, guinea pig, and bull. In man, bull, ram, and boar (but not rat), most of the seminal fructose is secreted by the seminal vesicles and consequently, in these species, the chemical assay of fructose in semen is a useful indicator of the relative contribution of the seminal vesicles toward whole semen. Seminal vesicle secretion is also characterized by the presence of proteins and enzymes, phosphorylcholine, and prostaglandins.

Erection and Ejaculation

Parasympathetic nerve stimulation results in dilatation of the arterioles of the penis, which initiates an erection. The erectile tissue of the penis fills with blood, veins are compressed to block outflow, and the turgor of the organ increases. In man, afferent impulses from the genitalia and descending tracts, which mediate erections in response to erotic psychic stimuli, reach the integrating centers in the lumbar segments of the spinal cord. The efferent fibers are located in the pelvic splanchnic nerves.

Ejaculation is a two-part spinal reflex that involves emission and ejaculation. Emission is the movement of the semen into the urethra; ejaculation is the propulsion of the semen out of the urethra at the time of orgasm. Afferent pathways involve fibers from receptors in the glans penis that reach the spinal cord through the internal pudendal nerves. Emission is a sympathetic response effected by contraction of the smooth muscle of the vas deferens and seminal vesicles. Semen is ejaculated out of the urethra by contraction of the bulbocavernosus muscle. The spinal reflex centers for this portion of the reflex are in the upper sacral and lowest lumbar segments of the spinal cord; the motor pathways traverse the first to third sacral roots of the internal pudendal nerves.

Since few laboratory and clinical studies are available, relatively little is known concerning the effects of chemicals on erection or ejaculation (Woods, 1984). However, many drugs act on the autonomic nervous system and affect potency. Impotence, the failure to obtain or sustain an erection, is rarely of endocrine origin; more often, the cause is psychologic. The occurrence of nocturnal or early-morning erections implies that the neurologic and circulatory pathways involved in attaining an erection are intact and suggests the possibility of a psychologic cause.

OVARIAN FUNCTION

Oogenesis

The ovarian germ cells with their follicles have a dual origin; the theca or stromal cells arise from fetal connective tissues of the ovarian medulla, the granulosa cells from the cortical mesenchyme. On the basis of their embryonic origin, the theca and granulosa cells in the female would be comparable, respectively, to the interstitial (Leydig) and nourishing (Sertoli) cells in the male. The theca and interstitial cells are endocrinologically active, while the granulosa and Sertoli cells apparently are endocrinologically less active.

In humans, between 300,000 and 400,000 follicles are present at birth in each ovary. After birth many of these die (atresia), and those that survive are continuously reduced in number. Any agent that damages the oocytes will accelerate the depletion of the pool and can lead to reduced fertility in females. About one-half of the number of oocytes present at birth remain at puberty; the number is reduced to about 25,000 by 30 years of age. About 400 primary follicles will yield mature ova during a woman's reproductive life-span (Figure 16–1). During the 30 years or more that constitute the reproductive period, follicles in various stages of growth can always be found. After menopause, follicles are no longer present in the ovary.

The follicles remain in a primary follicle stage following birth until puberty when a number of follicles start to grow during each ovarian cycle. However, most fail to achieve maturity. For the follicles that continue to grow, the first event is an increase in size of the primary oocytes. During this stage, fluid-filled spaces appear among the cells of the follicle, which unite to form a cavity or antrum. This is the graafian follicle.

The primary oocyte undergoes two specialized nuclear divisions, which result in the formation of four cells containing one-half of the number of chromosomes (Figure 16–2). The first meiotic division occurs within the ovary just before ovulation, and the second occurs just after the sperm fuses with the egg. In the first stage of meiosis the primary oocyte is actively synthesizing DNA and protein in preparation for entering prophase. The DNA content doubles as the prophase chromosomes each produce their mirror image. Each doubled chromosome is attracted to its homologous mate to form tetrads. The members of the tetrads synapse or come to lie side by side. Before separation, the homologous pairs of chromosomes exchange genetic material by a process known as crossing over. This accounts for most of the qualitative differences between the resulting gametes. The subsequent meiotic stages distribute the members of the tetrads to the daughter cells in such a way that each cell receives the haploid number of chromosomes. At telophase, one secondary oocyte and a polar body have been formed, which are no longer genetically identical.

The secondary oocyte enters the next cycle of division very rapidly; each chromosome splits longitudinally; the ovum and the three polar bodies now contain the haploid number of chromosomes and half the amount of genetic material. Although the nuclei of all four eggs are equivalent, the cytoplasm is divided unequally. The end products are one large ovum and three rudimentary ova known as polar bodies, which subsequently degenerate. The ovum is released from the ovary at the secondary oocyte stage; the second stage of meiotic division is triggered in the oviduct by the entry of the sperm.

Ovarian Cycle

Responding to pituitary gonadotropins, estrogens and progesterone are synthesized by the ovary. These female sex steroids determine ovulation and prepare the female accessory sex organs to receive the male sperm. Sperm, ejaculated in the vagina, must make their way through the cervix into the uterus where they are capacitated. Sperm then move into the oviducts where fertilization takes place. The conceptus then returns from the oviducts to the uterus and implants into the properly prepared endometrium.

POSTOVARIAN PROCESSES

The female accessory sex organs function to bring together the ovulated ovum and the ejaculated sperm. Chemical composition and viscosity of reproductive tract fluids, as well as the epithelial morphology of these organs, are controlled by ovarian (and trophoblastic) hormones.

Oviducts

Specialized functions of the oviducts include the taxis of the fimbria, which is under chemical and muscular control. The involvement of the autonomic nervous system in this process, as well as in oviductal transport of both the male and female gametes, raises the possibility that pharmacologic agents known to alter the autonomic nervous system may alter function and, therefore, fertility. Since oviductal fluid provides the environment for the gametes during fertilization, accumulation of xenobiotics may be deleterious.

Uterus

Uterine function depends on the endometrium and the myometrium. The endometrium reflects the cyclicity of the ovary as it is prepared to receive the conceptus. The myometrium's major role is contractile. In primates, at the end of menstruation, all but the deep layers of the endometrium have sloughed. Under the influence of estrogens from the developing follicle, the endometrium increases rapidly in thickness. The uterine glands increase in length but do not secrete to any degree. These endometrial changes are called proliferative. After ovulation, the endometrium becomes slightly edematous, and the actively secreting glands become tightly coiled and folded under the influence of estrogen and progesterone from the corpus luteum. These are secretory (progestational) changes.

From the point of view of endometrial function, the proliferative phase represents the restoration of the epithelium from the preceding menstruation; and the secretory phase, the preparation of the uterus for the implantation of the fertilized ovum. When fertilization fails to occur, the endometrium is shed, and a new cycle begins. Only primates menstruate. Other mammals have a sexual or estrus cycle. Female animals come into "heat" (estrus) at the time of ovulation. This is generally the only time during which the female is receptive to the male. In spontaneously ovulating species such as the rat, the underlying endocrine events are essentially the same as those in the menstrual cycle. In other species, such as the rabbit, ovulation is a reflex produced by copulation.

Cervix

The mucosa of the uterine cervix does not undergo cyclic desquamation, but there are regular changes in the cervical mucus. Estrogen, which makes the mucus thinner and more alkaline, promotes the survival and transport of sperm. Progesterone makes the mucus thick, tenacious, and cellular. The mucus is thinnest at the time of ovulation and dries in an arborizing, fernlike pattern on a slide. After ovulation and during pregnancy, it becomes thick and fails to form the fern pattern. Major functional disruptions of the cervix may be expressed as disorders of differentiation (including neoplasia), disturbed secretion, and incompetence. Exfoliative cytologic (Papanicolaou's stain) and histologic techniques are currently used to assess disorders of differentiation.

Vagina

Under the influence of estrogens, the vaginal epithelium becomes cornified, and these cells can be identified in the vaginal smear. Under the influence of progesterone, a thick mucus is secreted and the epithelium proliferates, becoming infiltrated with leukocytes. The cyclic changes in the vaginal smear in rats are easily recognized. The changes in humans and other species are similar but less apparent. Analysis of vaginal fluid or cytologic studies of desquamated vaginal cells (quantitative cytochemistry) reflect ovarian function. Vaginal sampling of cells and fluid might offer a reliable and easily available external monitor of internal function and dysfunction. Alteration in vaginal flora is a possible toxicologic problem, which was accentuated by the association of the toxic shock syndrome with the use of vaginal tampons.

FERTILIZATION

In the process of fertilization, the ovum contributes the maternal complement of genes to the nucleus of the fertilized egg and provides food reserves for the early embryo. The innermost envelope of the egg is the vitelline membrane. Outside the ovum proper lies a thick, tough, and highly refractile capsule termed the zona pellucida, which increases the total diameter of the human ovum to about 0.15 mm. Beyond the zona pellucida is the corona radiata derived from the follicle; it surrounds the ovum during its passage in the oviduct.

The formation, maturation, and meeting of a male and female germ cell are all preliminary to their actual union into a combined cell or zygote. Penetration of ovum by sperm and the coming together and pooling of their respective nuclei constitute the process of fertilization.

About ten minutes is required for the sperm to penetrate the zona pellucida after passing through the cumulus oophorus *in vitro* and probably sooner *in vivo*. The sperm makes its way along a curved oblique path. On entering the perivitelline space, the sperm head immediately lies flat on the vitellus; its plasma membrane fuses with that of the vitellus and then sinks into the ovum. The cortical granules of the egg disappear, the vitellus shrinks, and the second maturation division is reinitiated, which results in extrusion of the second polar body. A specific factor in the ovum appears to trigger the development of the male pronucleus; the chromatin of the ovum forms a female pronucleus. The male and female pronucleus develop synchronously, DNA is replicated, transcription of maternal and paternal genes begins, and protein synthesis occurs.

As syngamy approaches, the two pronuclei become intimately opposed but do not fuse. The nuclear envelopes of the pronuclei break up; nucleoli disappear and chromosomes condense and promptly aggregate. The chromosomes mingle to form the prometaphase of the first spindle, and the egg divides into two blastomeres. From sperm penetration to first cleavage usually requires about 12 hours in laboratory animals.

From the single fertilized cell (the zygote), cells proliferate and differentiate until more than a trillion cells of about 100 different types are present in the adult organism. Cell multiplication continues in most tissues throughout life replenishing the dying cells; every 24 hours almost 1 percent of the cells are discarded and renewed. Various tissues are characterized by their cell turnover rates.

IMPLANTATION

The developing embryo moves down the oviduct into the uterus. Once in contact with the endometrium, the blastocyst becomes surrounded by an outer layer or syncytiotrophoblast, a multinucleated mass of cells with no discernible boundaries, and an inner layer of individual cells, the cytotrophoblast. The syncytiotrophoblast erodes the endometrium, and the blastocyst implants. Placental circulation is then established and trophoblastic function continues. The blastocysts of most mammalian species implant about day 6 or 7 following fertilization. At this stage, the differentiation of the embryonic and extraembryonic (trophoblastic) tissues is apparent.

Trophoblastic tissue differentiates into cytotrophoblast and syncytiotrophoblast cells. The syncytiotrophoblast cells produce chorionic gonadotropin, chorionic growth hormones, placental lactogen, estrogen, and progesterone, which are needed to achieve independence from the ovary in maintaining the pregnancy. Rapid proliferation of the cytotrophoblast serves to anchor the growing placenta to the maternal tissue.

The early placenta consists of a mass of proliferating trophoblast, which expands rapidly and infiltrates the maternal vascular channels. Within hours of implantation, the syncytiotrophoblast is bathed by maternal venous blood, which supplies nutrients and permits an exchange of gases. Histiotrophic nutrition involves yolk sac circulation; hemotrophic nutrition involves the placenta. Placental circulation is established quite early in women and primates and, relatively, much later in rodents and rabbits. The invasive and metastatic character of placental tissue parallels two characteristics of malignant tumors.

INTEGRATIVE PROCESSES

Hypothalamo-Pituitary-Gonadal Axis

FSH and LH are glycoproteins synthesized and released from a subpopulation of the basophilic gonadotropic cells of the pituitary gland. Hypothalamic neuroendocrine neurones secrete specific releasing or release-inhibiting factors into the hypophyseal portal system, which carries them to the adenohypophysis where they act to stimulate or inhibit the release of anterior pituitary hormones. Luteinizing hormone-releasing hormone (LHRH) acts on gonadotropic cells, thereby stimulating the release of FSH and LH. LHRH and follicle-stimulating hormone-releasing hormone (FSHRH) appear to be the same substance. Native and synthetic forms of LHRH stimulate the release of both gonadotropic hormones; thus, it has been proposed to call this compound gonadotropin-releasing hormone (GnRH).

The neuroendocrine neurones have nerve terminals containing monoamines (norepinephrine, dopamine, serotonin) that impinge on them. The effects of reserpine or chloropromazine and other agents that alter or modify the content or actions of brain monoamines on reproductive function are well documented.

FSH probably acts primarily on the Sertoli cells, but it also appears to stimulate the mitotic activity of spermatogonia. LH stimulates steroidogenesis. A defect in the function of the testis (in the production of spermatozoa or testosterone) will tend to be reflected in increased levels of FSH and LH in serum because of the lack of the "negative feedback" effect of testicular hormones.

This sensitive and complex system presents several targets for environmental and industrial chemicals, and many drugs are thought to exert significant effects or to alter the normal functional state. It is clearly established that the effects of toxic agents on endocrine processes in the brain or pituitary gland may indirectly inhibit spermatogenesis, alter steroidogenesis, cause abnormal sexual development, and/or result in sterility. The gonadotropins are similarly important in the female.

Puberty

Puberty, strictly defined, is the period of growth and maturation when the endocrine and gametogenic functions of the gonads develop to the point where reproduction is possible. Following birth, the androgen-secreting Leydig cells in the mammalian fetal testes become quiescent, and a period follows in which the gonads of both sexes await final maturation of the reproductive system. A pituitary-inhibiting gonadal secretion has been suggested, but its existence is uncertain. Subtle mechanisms are responsible for the onset of puberty, and aberrations of puberty can be produced in laboratory animals with chemical treatment.

SEXUAL BEHAVIOR AND LIBIDO

The biologic processes that account for sexual behavior are not well understood. In any reproductive study, the investigator must determine whether or not the animals actually mate. In the rat, this can be determined by inspecting females each day for vaginal plugs. The number of mountings, thrusts, and ejaculations each can be quantified as indicators of reproductive behavior. It is also important to determine whether the male animal mounts females or other males. If the male copulates and is still sterile, one should look at the indicators of male fertility such as testicular function. If he does not copulate, then the emphasis of further investigation must be on neuromuscular and/or behavioral defects in the animal.

GENERAL PHARMACOLOGIC PRINCIPLES

The purpose of the toxicologic study of target organs is to define toxic effects of a chemical on target organs. The ultimate objective is to assess the toxic effects of a chemical in laboratory animals and to extrapolate the experimental data relevant to humans. To accomplish this, one must consider the main factors that may influence and modulate the toxic effects of chemicals in an organ. In gonads, for example, such modifying factors are the pharmacokinetic parameters that govern chemical absorption, distribution, activation, and detoxication; covalent bindings to macromolecules; and DNA damage and its repair in germ cells. A pharmacokinetic model of the testicular compartment is presented in Figure 16–3.

Most reproductive toxicologists attempt to determine the effects of chemicals or other factors on male and female reproductive function by using rather simple measures and observations. The design of such experiments is based on predetermined amounts and patterns of consumption (or exposure) of a substance, as well as on the chemical and physical properties that determine the pharmacokinetic variables for the chemical. The dose of the test chemical, selected with these pharmacokinetic factors in mind, must neither be so large that they overwhelm adaptive mechanisms nor be administered so often that they accumulate in the experimental animal in a manner contrary to the design of the experiment. The route of administration of the test chemical should parallel the human experience, and the purity of the test substance must be carefully determined and maintained. The value of simple pharmacokinetic parameters such as rate of absorption, volume of distribution, biologic half-life, and routes of biotransformation cannot be overstated. Generally, rodents are used for routine toxicity tests, but data obtained from larger laboratory animals (monkeys and dogs) are often of special value.

When assessing the reproductive and developmental toxicity of a chemical on gonads, phenomena such as biologic barriers, biotransformation mechanisms (which can decrease or increase the toxicity of a chemical), and the capacity of germ cells to repair DNA damage must receive attention. Although these processes are equally important in both the male and female gonads, much more information is available regarding the testis than the ovary (Dixon and Lee, 1980; Mattison *et al.*, 1983a).

BLOOD-TESTIS BARRIER

The blood-testis barrier (BTB) retards the passage of chemicals from the blood to the lumen of the seminiferous tubule. Setchell and co-workers (1969) first demonstrated that immunoglobulins and iodinated albumin, inulin, and a

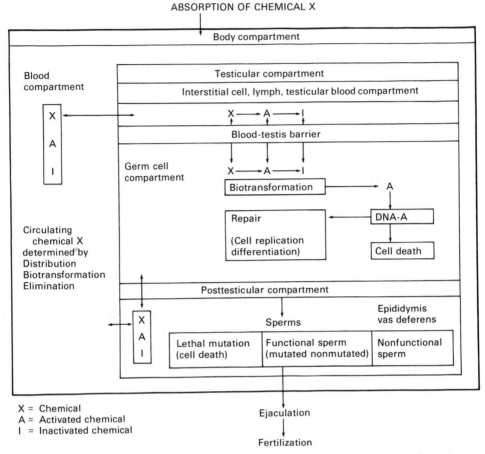

ABSORPTION OF CHEMICAL X

Figure 16–3. A model of pharmacokinetic, homeostatic, and adaptive factors involved in testicular toxicity. (From Lee, I. P., and Dixon, R. L.: Factors influencing reproduction and genetic toxic effects on male gonads. *Environ. Health Perspect.*, **24**:117–27, 1978.)

number of small molecules were excluded from the seminiferous tubules by the BTB. Dym and Fawcett (1970) suggested that the primary permeability barrier for the seminiferous tubules was composed of the surrounding layers of myoid cells while specialized Sertoli cell-to-Sertoli cell junctions within the seminiferous epithelium constituted a secondary cellular barrier. Okumura and co-workers (1975) quantified permeability rates for nonelectrolytes and selected drugs. Small molecules such as water and urea were transported readily across the BTB while larger molecules such as galactose and inulin moved much more slowly.

A positive correlation between the lipid solubilities of chemicals and their membrane penetrabilities was demonstrated. The rate-determining factors for transport of compounds across the BTB are molecular size, ionization, and lipid solubility at physiologic pH. The permeability characteristics of the BTB are similar to those of the membrane barriers that limit penetration of foreign chemicals into the central nervous system and aqueous humor of the eye. The ability of the BTB to control the entry of chemicals into the seminiferous tubules is affected by a number of physiologic, chemical, and pathologic factors (Dixon, 1981).

BIOTRANSFORMATION OF EXOGENOUS CHEMICALS

A number of investigators have reported on the capability of the testis to biotransform exogenous chemicals. Mukhtar, Bend, and Lee and their co-workers (1978a, 1978b) found appreciable activities of both mixed-function oxidases and epoxide-degrading enzymes, as well as cytochrome P-450, in testicular homogenates.

These and other studies have indicated that the enzymatic activity with respect to inactivating or detoxifying reactions is relatively greater in the testes and may serve a protective function. These include O-sulfotransferase (O-sulfation of DES, morphine, and estradiol) in the adult monkey testes (Namkung et al., 1977), epoxide hydratase in mouse testes (Oesch et al., 1977), and glutathione-S-transferase in the rat testes, ovaries, and adrenals (Mukhtar et al., 1978b).

Although aryl hydrocarbon hydroxylase (AHH) activity in testicular microsomes was only about 5 percent that of hepatic microsomes, the close proximity of activating enzymes to the germ cells may be important for enzyme-activated chemicals. Factors that affect enzyme activity and cytochrome P-450 levels are likely to play a significant role in germ cell toxicity. 2,3,7,8-Tetrachlorodibenzo-p-dioxin (TCDD) significantly induces testicular and prostate AHH activity and cytochrome P-448 (Lee et al., 1981). The biotransformation of benzo[a]pyrene by the isolated perfused testis has been contrasted to cell-free testicular systems such as homogenates (Nagayama and Lee, 1982). Qualitative and quantitative differences in the metabolites that were observed suggest that the perfused organ system is a better model for extrapolating data to the whole animal.

The ovary also seems to have the capability to biotransform certain exogenous substrates. However, the ovarian system has been studied less extensively than the testis. Mukhtar and co-workers (1978b) have compared the specific activities of AHH, epoxide hydrolase, glutathione transferase, and cytochrome P-450 in ovaries of 12-day-old and adult rats. Mattison and Thorgeirsson (1979) have reported basal as well as 3-methylcholanthrene-induced levels of AHH in two strains of mice. The treatment increased ovarian enzyme activity two to three times in one strain and had no effect on the other. The rate of primordial oocyte destruction after treatment with carcinogenic polycyclic aromatic hydrocarbons was faster in responsive mice than in nonresponsive animals. Primordial oocyte toxicity was blocked by simultaneous treatment with α-naphthoflavone, an inhibitor of polyaromatic hydrocarbon metabolism by induced forms of the cytochromes.

DNA REPAIR

Our laboratory and others have also been interested in the capacity of spermatogenic cells to repair DNA damaged as a consequence of exposure to environmental chemicals (Lee, 1983). It has been shown that both physical (ultraviolet and x-ray radiation) and chemical agents can cause damage to DNA molecules. Damage inflicted on the DNA templates, unless repaired, may interfere with transcription or cellular replication. Lethal mutations (cell death) and mutations that result in transformed cells or altered gene function may also occur. Testes of various mouse strains have been found to differ in their ability to repair DNA damage.

The velocity sedimentation cell separation technique has been used to identify spermatogenic cells capable of unscheduled DNA synthesis (Dixon and Lee, 1980). To study unscheduled DNA synthesis after methyl methanesulfonate (MMS) treatment, male mice were first treated with varying doses of MMS followed two hours later by the intratesticular administration of [³H] thymidine one hour before sacrifice. Spermatogenic cell types were then isolated. Control mice receiving saline followed by intratesticular injection of [³H] thymidine showed a single peak of radioactivity that identified spermatogonial cells passing through S phase. In contrast, the radioactive profiles obtained after MMS treatment demonstrated that thymidine incorporation now occurred not only in the spermatogonia but also in the leptotene, zygotene, pachytene, and diplotene cells in decreasing order. Normally no DNA synthesis occurs in these premeiotic cells; therefore, the thymidine incorporation in untreated cells is very low. These studies suggest that non-S-phase spermatogonial cells were also induced to undergo unscheduled DNA synthesis. In contrast, no thymidine radioactivity was present in spermatids or sperm (spermiogenic cells). Therefore, spermiogenic cells appear less able to repair DNA damage and, thus, may be more vulnerable to the effects of monofunctional alkylating agents such as MMS.

Because unscheduled DNA repair in spermatogenic cells appears to be dose and time dependent, the DNA repair systems might be saturated at high test doses or with repeated exposures to toxic chemicals. Overwhelming the repair system could result in a larger number of affected cells and increased toxicity. Thus, the DNA repair system is another protective mechanism with regard to toxic effects of environmental chemicals, as well as a sensitive indicator of chromosome damage. Sega and his colleagues have reviewed DNA repair in spermatocytes and spermatids and have commented on the potential of unscheduled DNA synthesis in testing for mutagens (Sega, 1982; Sega and Sotomayor, 1982).

Pedersen and Brandriff (1980) have reviewed studies showing that ultraviolet light or drug-induced unscheduled DNA synthesis in mammalian oocytes and embryos indicates that the female gamete has an excision repair capacity from the earliest stages of oocyte growth. In contrast to the mature sperm, the fully mature oocyte maintains a repair capacity and contributes this to the zygote. However, the oocyte's demonstrable excision repair capacity decreases at the time of meiotic maturation for unknown reasons.

TARGETS FOR CHEMICAL TOXICITY

There are numerous underlying biologic processes that environmental chemicals might alter to produce reproductive dysfunction. Research to identify the side effects of various therapeutic agents and to improve methods of contraception has revealed a number of vulnerable sites in the reproductive system. Chemicals can act as such, or they may require metabolic activation. Effects, likewise, can be due to the direct effect of a chemical on some subcellular molecule (the receptor for toxicity) that alters the ability of the cell to divide, differentiate, or otherwise function normally.

Toxicity may also result from an effect that is mediated indirectly, for instance, by altering the presence or effectiveness of a hormone. Laboratory prototypes for anatomic effects caused by agents acting indirectly can be produced centrally by hypophysectomy or by chemically blocking the gonadotropin-releasing hormones, or they can be produced peripherally by interrupting the synthesis of androgens or estrogens or by blocking their action with antihormones.

Our knowledge of mechanisms of toxicity is incomplete. The most thorough information available concerns those chemicals which are mutagens and carcinogens. It is generally agreed that their action involves a covalent interaction with cellular macromolecules such as DNA, RNA, and/or protein. However, the consequences of such a molecular interaction have not yet been clearly related to gene function and/or regulation or to the transformation of cells. Most carcinogens and mutagens require a bioactivation process to be effective. Many chemicals share the potential to cause mutagenic, carcinogenic, teratogenic, and reproductive toxicity. It is, thus, suggested that the toxicity of such chemicals lacks specificity and appears to have the potential to effect all replicating and differentiating cells.

A group of chemicals whose mechanisms of actions are generally well understood are those drugs developed to treat cancer. These antineoplastic agents are designed to be cytotoxic, and it is not surprising that most of them affect gametogenesis. The manner in which these chemicals act is fairly well documented, and interest in them extends beyond their toxicity to their use as tools in understanding basic toxicologic phenomena (Meistrich *et al.*, 1982).

On the other hand, little is known about environmental chemicals that might interact in more subtle ways to alter reproduction, and few laboratories are focusing on these areas. Figure 16–4 presents a number of processes that environmental chemicals might disrupt to cause reproductive dysfunction. Some of these mechanisms are highly specific and could alter reproduction

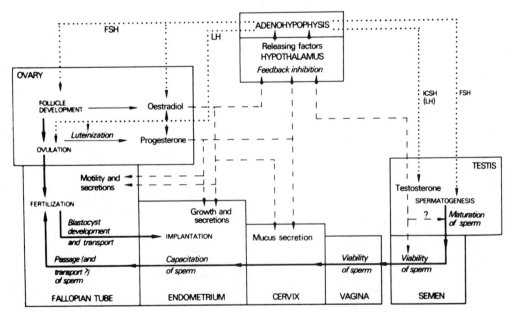

Figure 16–4. Schematic representation of the biologic processes that are essential for normal reproduction. (From Bowman, W. C., and Rand, M. J. [eds.]: *Textbook of Pharmacology,* 2nd ed. Blackwell Scientific Publications Ltd., London; C. V. Mosby Co, St. Louis, 1980.)

without producing general toxicity. This chart includes a number of mechanisms not yet directly associated with reproductive toxicity. Nevertheless, environmental chemicals, by acting in these ways, may be contributing both to the increasing rate of infertility and to the large number of conceptions that fail to implant and complete gestation successfully.

Cytotoxicity

It is obvious that cytotoxic chemical hazards capable of reducing the number of sperm or ova would have a high potential to produce infertility as well as other organ toxicity. Such chemicals are relatively easily identified in the laboratory. This group includes most of the anticancer drugs and many of the chemicals classified as mutagens.

Nerve Transmission

Many chemicals that affect the adrenergic and cholinergic branches of the autonomic nervous system are widely used clinically and have been associated with reproductive side effects. An even larger number of drugs is available that act on the central nervous system, including agents used as hypnotics and sedatives and to control anxiety and psychiatric disorders. A number of these drugs are known to disrupt reproductive function.

Hormone Action

The actions of both peptide and steroid hormones depend on a series of steps including synthesis, release, metabolism, transport, cytoplasmic receptors, nuclear translocation, and chromatin interactions. Analogous steps are involved in the synthesis, storage, release, and metabolism of the adrenergic transmitter norepinephrine (NE). The search for effective therapeutic agents to influence cardiovascular function and to control blood pressure has identified a wide variety of chemicals that affect the processes upon which neurotransmission depends.

Because a similar search directed, for instance, at steroid hormone action would likewise reveal numerous chemicals that would be of both therapeutic and toxicologic interest, it is useful to consider how chemicals can affect the adrenergic nervous system (Mayer, 1980). α-Methyl-p-tryosine interferes with adrenergic function by blocking the synthesis of norepinephrine (NE), which causes its depletion. A false and ineffective transmitter is produced when α-methyldopa is transformed metabolically as if it were the normal precursor of NE that competes for the receptor and displaces NE. Imipramine blocks the axonal membrane transport system for NE, and reserpine blocks NE uptake into the storage granule membrane allowing monoamine oxidase (MAO) to destroy NE and deplete it from the terminals. Guanethidine, by displacing NE from the axonal terminals, causes its destruction, while bretylium prevents the release of NE from the terminal. Phenylephrine and isoproterenol mimic NE at postsynaptic receptors to exert a sympathomimetic action; phenoxybenzamine blocks the endogenous transmitter at the postsynaptic receptors. Finally, MAO inhibitors such as pargyline inhibit the enzymatic breakdown of NE, which allows it to accumulate at certain sites. Drugs that affect the cholinergic nervous system in a like manner have also been developed.

Fluid Milieu

The volume and composition of the fluids in the gonads and accessory sex organs are critically regulated and essential to normal reproductive success. The fluid that carries the gametes from the testes through the epididymidis and eventually evolves into semen, as well as the luminal fluid of the oviduct, uterus, and vagina, are apparently all closely maintained and regulated by biologic barriers, active secretory mechanisms, and resorptive processes. Similar processes exist in a number of other organs, of which the kidney is the most familiar. Thus, one might expect diuretic drugs (and environmental chemicals) that disrupt fluid resorption and inhibit the transport of organic electrolytes to have an adverse effect on reproductive success. However, neither laboratory studies nor clinical reports have, as yet, clearly documented such effects.

Sertoli Cell Function

Too little attention has been directed to the role of Sertoli cell function in normal spermatogenesis and its potential as a target for drugs and other environmental chemicals. As mentioned, the Sertoli cells support the developing sperm, secrete fluids, produce an androgen-binding protein (ABP) in some species, and synthesize and release inhibin. They also contribute in a major way to the effectiveness of the blood-testis barrier. The essentiality of these processes, however, has not been well defined although general areas are under active investigation. Because Sertoli cells only replicate early in the life of a mammal, they are uniquely susceptible to chemicals that affect cellular replication early in life, and their susceptibility to such drugs decreases as the animal matures (Matter et al., 1983).

Epididymal Function

Resorption and metabolism of components entering the epididymis in rete testis fluid, secretion by the epithelium, sperm maturation, and maintenance of sperm fertility are important functions of the epididymis and perhaps targets for toxicity. Scientific inquiry over the past decade has more clearly revealed the role of the epididymis in sperm maturation and transport. However, a careful study of the effects of chemicals on these processes is still in its early phase. Sperm maturation apparently includes specific proteins synthesized by the epididymis that become part of the sperm surface.

Male Secretory Organ Function

From the epididymides, seminal fluid moves into the vas deferens where glandular secretions are added. Although it is well known that the male accessory sex organs are androgen dependent, their contribution to the sperm's fertilizing capacity is not well understood. However, dominant proteins in the semen arise specifically from the seminal vesicle, prostate, and other secretory organs. It is suggested that these proteins may stabilize sperm proteases and prevent capacitation. Because of the large incidence of prostatic disease in aging men, attention is focused mainly on the prostate and the role of environmental factors in benign and malignant prostatic disease. Semen "markers" for normal and abnormal prostatic tissue are being researched.

Sperm Capacitation

As the sperm move from the testis, the gametes mature and are stored to await ejaculation. But even ejaculated sperm are not yet functional. They still must undergo a series of changes, termed capacitation, before they can bind to, penetrate, and fertilize the ovum. This biochemical process prepares the sperm for morphologic changes that the acrosome undergoes when the sperm makes contact with the ovum. Capacitation destabilizes the sperm membrane and may also involve the removal of blocking agents (or decapacitation factors) and the activation of various sperm enzymes and receptor sites. Also included in capacitation are changes in membrane fluidity, changes in sperm ionic fluxes, and in acrosomal pH. Capacitated sperm have an increased oxygen uptake and more effective motility. In the rat uterus, capacitation can be depressed by a lack of estrogen or by the presence of progesterone. Sperm capacitation can be reversed in the presence of seminal plasma.

Sperm Enzymes

Impressive advances have been made in recent years in the understanding of sperm biochemistry and the role of various enzymes in maintaining their fertilizing capacity. Sperm possess two major enzyme systems. One is associated with the midpiece and tail and includes the enzymes involved in the membrane transport of chemicals, the maintenance of the citric acid cycle, oxidative phosphorylation, glycolysis, and other metabolic activities. These processes serve primarily to generate the energy required for sperm motility, and they are common to cells in general. Numerous compounds can inhibit these glycolytic and respiratory enzymes and, thus, immobilize sperm. However, most of these compounds are nonspecific and generally toxic. Lactate dehydrogenase (LDH) is one of the metabolic enzymes of the sperm midpiece. The sperm possess a form of this enzyme (LDH-X) specific to the genital tract. LDH-X antibodies have been used in attempts to identify variants of the isozyme in a population of sperm.

The second enzyme system is associated with the acrosome and includes mucolytic enzymes such as hyaluronidase, proteolytic enzymes such as acrosin, and various other enzymes. Hyaluronidase facilitates sperm passage through the follicular cell layer. Inhibitors of hyaluronidase specifically prevent the penetration of sperm through the follicular cell layer of mouse gametes. Acrosin, a proteinase, is also apparently involved in several aspects of the fertilization process. Acrosin inhibitors have been reported to prevent the sperm acrosome reaction, sperm binding to the zona pellucida, and sperm passage through the zona pellucida and vitellus. A naturally occurring acrosin inhibitor is present in seminal plasma. The acrosome reaction involves membrane changes that release the acrosome contents. These processes are also targets for chemical intervention.

A number of naturally occurring and synthetic sperm enzyme inhibitors have been shown to prevent fertilization, but only a few have been investigated in detail. The greatest attention has been directed to inhibitors of hyaluronidase and acrosin, yet none is available clinically. The only spermicides currently on the market are employed in vaginal contraceptives. The primary agent is nonoxynol-9, which immobilizes sperm because of a surfactant action. The development and clinical success of sperm enzyme inhibitors for contraception have been reviewed recently by Zaneveld (1982).

Oogenesis and Folliculogenesis

A variety of chemicals can affect oogenesis and formation of the follicles. Adverse effects may occur during the development of the ovary, primordial germ cell proliferation or migration, oogonial differentiation or proliferation, or formation of the primordial follicle. Chemicals may adversely affect the developed ovary through a direct effect on oocytes or follicles, disordered follicular growth, abnormal steroid hormone synthesis or action, disrupted hypothalamic-pituitary-ovarian interactions, inhibited oocyte release, or through altered corpus luteal function. A host of assay methods with varying degrees of specificity are available.

Ovulation

Ovulation involves the ovum in a complex differentiation process. Its stages include the oogonium, the primary oocytes, the fully grown primary oocyte in graafian follicle, and the ovulated secondary oocyte. Chemicals are known that disrupt this process (Mattison *et al.*, 1983b).

Corpus Luteal Function

The functional corpus luteum forms spontaneously after ovulation in the human and other animals. However, either LH or HCG will stimulate corpus luteum synthesis of hormones *in vivo* and *in vitro*. The corpus luteum synthesizes progesterone. Corpus luteal function is necessary for normal ovarian cyclicity and to support the early stages of pregnancy. Luteinization takes place in the follicle cells of graafian follicles that have matured and discharged their egg. The cells become hypertrophied and assume a yellow color as the follicles become the corpora lutea. The corpus luteal function is maintained during early pregnancy by the gonadotropins produced by the extraembryonic tissues of the conceptus. In women, the thermiogenic responses to progesterone production signal the development of a functional corpus luteum following ovulation. A luteal phase induced by means other than mating is known as pseudopregnancy.

Fertilization

The intricate biologic steps involved in fertilization seem to be a neglected area of toxicologic study that would most likely reveal not only subtle mechanisms of toxicity, but new approaches to contraception as well.

Variations and anomalies occur during fertilization. Aging of both sperm and ova may cause abnormal fertilization and lead to abnormal development. The most common errors of fertilization are polyspermy, polygyny, or digyny (failure of emission of first or second polar body) and immediate cleavage of the unfertilized egg followed by fertilization of both daughter cells. The first two errors lead to triploidy and the third to mosaic development. This area has been reviewed by Austin (1974).

Implantation

Implantation involves attachment of the conceptus to the endometrium and invasion of the cell layer. It is possible that drugs and other environmental agents might disrupt the biochemical interactions that must occur during the initial stages of attachment between the endometrium and the embryonic trophoblast. Only about one-half of human conceptuses implant successfully and complete their gestation.

Early Pregnancy

The search is underway for chemicals that could be ingested immediately after intercourse to prevent pregnancy or regularly on a once-a-month basis when a woman notices her period is late. Many organizations are active in this area of contraceptive development including the WHO Special Programme of Research Development and Research Training in Human Reproduction (WHO, 1982). One such group of chemicals that can terminate pregnancy are prostaglandins and prostaglandin analogs. The methyl ester of 15-methyl-PFG_{2a} has been studied extensively. The effectiveness of prostaglandin suppositories is being explored to induce menses when delayed by a few days. Methylsulfonylamide (Sulprostone) has been tried for interruption of early and second-trimester pregnancies. Anordrin and its derivatives are being tested for their efficacy as postcoital drugs. Derivatives of gonadotropins that would inhibit luteal function (luteolytic action) instead of stimulating it, thus disrupting the normal corpus luteum function needed for implantation to occur and pregnancy to be established, are also being sought. Such drugs administered at an appropriate time in the reproductive cycle could be expected to prevent the development and functioning of the corpus luteum and inhibit or disrupt implantation.

Because progesterone plays a fundamental role during implantation and early pregnancy in animals and women, progesterone antagonists or antiprogestins are being developed and tested as possible contraceptives. By binding to available endometrial progesterone receptors, such chemicals would prevent endogenous progesterone from promoting the development of the postovulatory secretory endometrium, which is necessary for implantation. A human progesterone receptor has been purified, and its structure is being mapped. New progesterone analogs are being synthesized and tested for receptor-binding activity as prototypes of new antiprogestins.

The WHO Programme has developed a vaccine against hCG to disrupt pregnancy. Vaccines for birth control are particularly attractive because they would be unlikely to disrupt menstrual cycles or to cause the metabolic disturbances associated with most current drugs. To avoid problems involving cross-reaction with other hormones and tissues, the research is being carried out with a unique fragment of the β-subunit of hCG.

GENERAL TOXICOLOGIC PRINCIPLES

The conventional chronic or long-term animal toxicity study is a key feature in assessing the safety of most chemicals. The duration of these tests is two to seven years depending on species. Like other areas of toxicology, reproductive toxicologists must develop more modern approaches to the assessment of toxicity that are more reliable, less expensive, and faster. Progress is being made by the National Toxicology Program and the U.S. Environmental Protection Agency in developing experimental approaches that are relatively simple and yield information regarding reproductive hazards and human health risks more quickly than current tests.

Aspects of reproductive toxicity are presented in a number of recent publications. The proceedings of the symposium on Target Organ Toxicity: Gonads (Reproductive and Genetic Toxicity) appeared in 1978 (Dixon, 1978). The March of Dimes Birth Defects Foundation published *Guidelines for Studies of Human Populations Exposed to Mutagenic and Reproductive Hazards* (Bloom, 1981), and *Assessment of Risks to Human Reproduction and to Development of the Human Conceptus from Exposure to Environmental Substances* is available (Galbraith *et al.*, 1982). *Methods for Assessing the Effects of Chemicals on Reproductive Functions* (Vouk and Sheehan, 1983), prepared by the Scientific Group on Methodologies for the Safety Evaluation of Chemicals (SGOMSEC), appeared most recently. Also, Mattison has recently edited *Reproductive Toxicology* (Mattison, 1983). There are many other references available. Concerning chemicals that affect reproduction, two recent reports are especially helpful: the Council of Environmental Quality's *Chemical Hazards to Human Reproduction* (Nisbet and Karch, 1983), and *Health Effects of Environmental Chemicals on the Adult Human Reproductive System* (Pruett and Winslow, 1982), prepared in cooperation with the National Library of Medicine for the Information Response to Chemical Crises Project by the Federation of American Societies for Experimental Biology. Also available are *Effects of Hormones, Drugs and Chemicals on Testicular Function* (Davies, 1980) and the text *Reproductive Hazards of Industrial Chemicals* (Barlow and Sullivan, 1982). Both are quality efforts that describe this area of concern.

Experimental results suggest that a large number of chemicals affect male and female reproduction. These are summarized in Tables 16–4 and 16–5. Although the extrapolation from laboratory animals to humans is inexact, a number of these chemicals do affect human reproduction; almost all require further study.

Testing Male Reproductive Capacity

Potential tests for evaluating male reproductive functions are listed in Table 16–6. As discussed previously, male fertility might be altered by a perturbation of any one of a number of processes. However, a relatively minor alteration in one or more of these might not be reflected in altered reproductive capacity. This table, which still lacks general scientific concurrence, was compiled and expanded from recent national (Dixon, 1980; Galbraith *et al.*, 1982) and international efforts (Vouk and Sheehan, 1983) to describe and assess laboratory and clinical approaches for reproductive toxicity testing. Most of the tests suggested fall into one of several categories: quantitative morphologic evaluations of reproductive tissues, analyses of hormone concentrations in blood or tissue, analyses of sperm production, examination of seminal characteristics, and examination of fertilization rates and litter size. A specific evaluation of sexual behavior and copulatory ability should also be considered.

A variety of morphologic, biochemical, and functional tests are used to assess toxic effects on male reproductive function. A brief discussion of some of these approaches follows.

Gross Pathology. A great deal of useful information can be obtained by measuring the weight and the volume of the testis, prostate, seminal vesicles, epididymis, and coagulating glands. Gross changes in the pituitary and adrenal glands are also useful parameters. When working with larger animals such as the beagle dog and rhesus monkey, it is important to realize that the dog does not reach puberty until one year of age and the monkey at about three years.

The external appearance of the genitalia is especially important in assessing the postnatal effects of gestational chemical exposure. For example, is the penis hypoplastic, is hypospadias evident? The genitoanal distance is useful in determining the sex of very young animals. The position of the testes should be determined. Are the testes scrotal or retained? Internal examination should concentrate on anatomic relationships noting retained testes, tumors, or "feminization" (the occurrence of vagina or uterus coexisting with male structures).

Histopathology. A histopathologic approach using light microscopy (LM) and electron mi-

Table 16–4. AGENTS REPORTED TO AFFECT MALE REPRODUCTIVE CAPACITY*

Steroids

Natural and synthetic androgens (antiandrogens), estrogens (antiestrogens) and progestins

Antineoplastic Agents

Alkaloids—vinca alkaloids (vinblastine, vincristine)

Alkylating agents—esters of methanesulfonic acid (MMS, EMS, busulfan); ethylenimines (TEM, TEPA); hydrazines (procarbazine); nitrogen mustards (chlorambucil, cyclophosphamide); nitrosoureas (CCNU, BCNU, MNU)

Antimetabolites—amino acid analogs [azaserine (DON)]; folic acid antagonists (methotrexate); nucleic acid analogs (azauridine, 5-bromodeoxyuridine, cytosine arabinoside, 5-fluorouracil, 6-mercaptopurine)

Antitumor antibotics—actinomycin D, adriamycin, bleomycin, daunomycin, mitomycin C

Drugs That Modify the Central Nervous System

Alcohols

Anesthetic gases and vapors—enflurane, halothane, methoxyflurane, nitrous oxide

Antiparkinsonism drugs—levodopa

Appetite suppressants

Narcotic and nonnarcotic analgesics—opioids

Neuroleptics (antidepressants, antimanic, and antipsychotic agents)—phenothiazines, imipramine, and amitriptyline

Tranquilizers—phenothiazines, reserpine, monoamine oxidase inhibitors

Drugs That Modify the Autonomic Nervous System

Antiadrenergic drugs (for hypertensive and cardiac disorders)—α- and β-blocking agents, clonidine, methyldopa, guanethidine, bretylium, reserpine

Other Therapeutic Agents

Alcoholism—tetraethylthiuram disulfide (antabuse)

Analgesics and antipyretics—phenacetin

Anticonvulsants—diphenylhydantoin (phenytoin)

Antiinfective agents—amphotericin B, hexachlorophene, hycanthone, nitrofuran derivatives (furacin, furadroxyl), sulfasalazine

Antischistosomal agents—niridazole, hycanthone

Antiparasitic drugs—quinine, quinacrine, chloroquine

Diuretics—aldactone, thiazides

Gout suppressants—colchicine

Histamines and histamine antagonists—chlorcyclizine, cimetidine

Oral hypoglycemic agents—chlorpropamide

Xanthines—caffeine, theobromine

Metals and Trace Elements

Aluminum, arsenic, boranes, boron, cadmium, cobalt, lead, mercury, methylmercury, molybdenum, nickel, silver, uranium

Insecticides

Benzene hexachlorides—lindane

Carbamates—carbaryl

Chlorobenzene derivatives—chlorophenothane (DDT), methoxychlor

Indane derivatives—aldrin, chlordane, dieldrin

Phosphate esters (cholinesterase inhibitors)—dichlorvos(DDVP), hexamethylphosphoramide

Miscellaneous—chlordecone (kepone)

Herbicides

Chlorinated phenoxyacetic acids—2,4-dichlorophenoxyacetic acid (2,4-D), 2,4,5-trichlorophenoxyacetic acid (2,4,5-T), yalane

Quaternary ammonium compounds—diquat, paraquat

Rodenticides

Metabolic inhibitors—fluoroacetate (fluoroacetamide)

Fungicides, Fumigants, and Sterilants

Apholate, captan, carbon disulfide, dibromochloropropane (DBCP), ethylene dibromide, ethylene oxide, thiocarbamates (cineb, maneb), triphenyltin

Table 16–4. (*continued*)

Food Additives and Contaminants

Aflatoxins, cyclamate, diethylstilbestrol (DES), dimethylnitrosamine, gossypol, metanil yellow, monosodium glutamate, nitrofuran derivatives

Industrial Chemicals

Chlorinated hydrocarbons—hexafluoroacetone, polybrominated biphenyls (PBBs) polychlorinated biphenyls (PCBs), 2,3,7,8-tetrachlorodibenzo-*p*-dioxin (TCDD)
Hydrazines—dithiocarbamoylhydrazine
Monomers—vinyl chloride, chloroprene
Polycyclic aromatic hydrocarbons (PAHs)—dimethylbenzanthracene (DMBA), benzo(a)pyrene
Solvents—benzene, carbon disulfide, glycolethers, hexane, thiophene, toluene, xylene
Miscellaneous—diethyl adipate, chloroprene, ethylene oxide cyclic tetramer

Consumer Products

Flame retardants—*tris*-(2,3-dibromopropyl) phosphate (TRIS)
Plasticizers—phthalate esters (DBP, DEHP)

Antispermatogenic Drugs (Investigational)

Derivatives of 1-benzylindazole-3-carboxylic acid, 1-*p*-chlorobenzyl-1H indazol-3-carboxylic acid, chlorohydrins, chlorosugars (6-chloroglucose), dichloracetyldiamines derivatives (Win 13,099, 17,416, 18,446), dihydronaphthalenes (nafoxidine), dinitropyrroles (ORF-1616), gossypol, 5-thioglucose, α-chlorohydrin, monothioglycerol

Miscellaneous

Personal habits—alcohol consumption, tobacco smoking
Agents of abuse—marijuana and other centrally acting drugs
Physical factors—heat, light, hypoxia
Radiation—α, β, and γ radiation; x-rays
Stable isotopes—deuterium oxide

* Both laboratory and clinical reports are included (Target Organ Toxicity Center Reproductive Toxicity Information File).

croscopy (EM) for detecting gonadal and accessory sex organ toxicity is essential to a better understanding of testicular toxicity. However, morphologic modifications are essentially limited to the assessment of rather obvious cytotoxic phenomena. Additional methods to detect more subtle effects are necessary to better understand mechanisms of reproductive toxicity and to interpret the etiology of chemically induced disease (Ettlin *et al.*, 1982).

The preparation of testicular tissue involves problems that generally are not thoroughly discussed in technical handbooks. Good tissue preservation and high resolution are essential for the early detection of subtle and specific cellular changes. The testis presents special challenges. Fixatives slowly penetrate the seminiferous tubules because the germ cells are protected by a complex system of membrane barriers. In addition, the connective tissue and tubules are too fragile to allow unfixed testicular tissue to be cut into thin sections to facilitate penetration by fixatives. Basic methods for histologic preparation of the testis have recently been summarized (Ettlin and Dixon, 1984). Because no fixative will penetrate more than a few millimeters of whole testis in a 24-hour period, optimal fixation is achieved only by delivering the fixative directly into the organ's vascular system. A retrograde perfusion method that delivers the fixative to the gonads via the lower abdominal aorta can be used (Vitale *et al.*, 1973).

A breakthrough regarding higher resolution for light microscopy was achieved by embedding samples of well-preserved perfused tissue in plastic materials. These materials polymerize and harden, thus providing thinner sections with less superposition of cellular details. Glycol methacrylate-embedded sections bind stains in much the same manner as tissue embedded in paraffin and are preferable to epoxy.

Testicular tissues routinely are stained with hematoxylin and eosin and PAS; the latter identifies the acrosomal system. Stains for connective tissue such as Masson's trichrome or van Gieson also may be useful. Histochemical investigations of gonadal tissue allow visualization of biochemical processes such as steroidogenesis.

Testicular Function. Spermatogenesis is considered to start when a spermatogonial stem cell commits itself to produce a cohort of spermatids. The duration of spermatogenesis is the interval from this point until that time when the resulting sperm are released from the Sertoli cells at spermiation. Because spermatogenesis requires about 4.5 cycles of the seminiferous epithelium, Amann (1982) recommends that a subchronic test of chemical effects on spermato-

Table 16–5.   AGENTS REPORTED TO AFFECT FEMALE REPRODUCTIVE CAPACITY*

Steroids

Natural and synthetic androgens (antiandrogens), estrogens (antiestrogens), and progestins

Antineoplastic Agents

Alkylating agents—cyclophosphamide, busulfan
Antimetabolites—folic acid antagonists (methotrexate)

Other Therapeutic Agents

Anesthetic gases and vapors—halothane, enflurane, methoxyflurane
Antiparkinsonism drugs—levodopa
Antiparasitic drugs—quinacrine
Appetite suppressants
Narcotic and nonnarcotic analgesics—opioids
Neuroleptics (antidepressants, antimanic, and antipsychotic agents)—phenothiazines, imipramine, and
    amitriptyline
Serotonin
Sympathomimetic amines—epinephrine, norepinephrine, amphetamines
Tranquilizers—phenothiazines, reserpine, monoamine oxidase inhibitors

Metals and Trace Elements

Arsenic, lead, lithium, mercury and methylmercury, molybdenum, nickel, selenium, thallium

Insecticides

Benzene hexachlorides—lindane
Carbamates—carbaryl
Chlorobenzene derivatives—chlorophenothane (DDT), methoxychlor
Indane derivatives—aldrin, chlordane, dieldrin
Phosphate esters (cholinesterase inhibitors)—parathion
Miscellaneous—chlordecone (kepone), mirex, hexachlorobenzene, ethylene oxide

Herbicides

Chlorinated phenoxyacetic acids—2,4,dichlorophenoxyacetic acid (2,4-D), 2,4,5-trichlorophenoxyacetic acid
    (2,4,5-T)

Food Additives and Contaminants

Cyclohexylamine, diethylstilbestrol (DES), dimethylnitrosamines, monosodium glutamate, nitrofuran derivatives
    (AF$_2$), nitrosamines, sodium nitrite

Industrial Chemicals and Processes

Building materials—formaldehyde
Chlorinated hydrocarbons—polychlorinated biphenyls (PCBs), chloroform, trichloroethylene
Paints and dyes—aniline
Plastic monomers—caprolactam, styrene, vinyl chloride
Polycyclic aromatic hydrocarbons (PAHs)—benzo(a)pyrene
Rubber manufacturing—chloroprene
Solvents—benzene, carbon disulfide, chloroform, ethanol, glycol ethers, hexane, toluene, trichloroethylene,
    xylene
Miscellaneous—cyanoketone, hydrazines

Consumer Products

Flame retardants—TRIS, polybrominated biphenyls (PBBs)
Plasticizers—phthalic acid esters (DEHP)

Miscellaneous

Personal habits—alcohol consumption, tobacco smoking
Agents of abuse—marijuana and other centrally acting drugs

* Both laboratory and clinical reports are included (Target Organ Toxicity Center Reproductive Toxicity Information File).

genesis should extend over 6.0 cycles of the seminiferous epithelium for the test species. This interval is based on the following considerations: (1) several days of administration may be required to attain a steady-state concentration of agent in the target organs; (2) an agent acting on the germinal epithelium may act on a specific type of somatic or germ cell and the affected

**Table 16–6. POTENTIALLY USEFUL TESTS
OF MALE REPRODUCTIVE TOXICITY
FOR LABORATORY ANIMALS AND/OR MAN***

Tests Accepted

Body weight

Testis

    Size *in situ*
    Weight
    Spermatid reserves
    Gross and histologic evaluation
    Nonfunctional tubules (%)
    Tubules with lumen sperm (%)
    Tubule diameter
    Counts of leptotene spermatocytes

Epidydimis

    Weight of distal half
    Number of sperm in distal half
    Motility of sperm, distal end (%)
    Gross sperm morphology, distal end (%)
    Detailed sperm morphology, distal end (%)
    Gross histology

Accessory Sex Glands

    Weight of vesicular glands
    Weight of accessory sex glands

Semen

    Total volume
    Gel-free volume
    Sperm concentration
    Total sperm/ejaculate
    Total sperm/day of abstinence
    Sperm motility, visual (%)
    Sperm motility, videotape (% and velocity)
    Gross sperm morphology
    Detailed sperm morphology
    Concentration of agent in sperm
    Concentration of agent in seminal plasma
    Concentration of agent in blood
    Biochemical analyses of sperm/seminal plasma

Endocrine

    Luteinizing hormone
    Follicle-stimulating hormone
    Testosterone
    Gonadotropin-releasing hormone

Fertility

    Ratio exposed: pregnant females
    Number embryos or young per pregnant female
    Ratio viable embryos: corpora lutea
    Ratio implantation: corpora lutea
    Number 2–8 cell eggs
    Number unfertilized eggs
    Number abnormal eggs
    Sperm per ovum
    Number of corpora lutea

In vitro

    Incubation of sperm in agent
    Hamster egg penetration test

Other Tests Considered

Tonometric measurement of testicular consistency
Qualitative testicular histology
Stage of cycle at which spermiation occurs
Quantitative testicular histology
    Counts of degenerating germ cells
    Complete germ cell counts
    Stem cell counts
    Relative frequency of stages of cycle
Epididymal histology
Biochemistry of epididymal fluids
Histology of accessory sex glands
Biochemical analysis of sperm
Sperm membrane characteristics
Evaluation of sperm metabolism
Fluorescent Y bodies in spermatozoa
Flow cytometry of spermatozoa
Karyotyping human sperm pronuclei
Cervical mucous penetration test
Studies on prepubertal animals

---

* See Galbraith *et al.* (1982) for complete table and discussion of the relative usefulness of these tests.

germ cells may be present for some time before they degenerate; (3) damage to the germinal epithelium is most evident by germ cells more mature than those being damaged from the germinal epithelium; (4) qualitative changes in germ cells may not be readily discernible until abnormal spermatozoa reach the epididymides or are ejaculated in semen.

It is desirable to allow six to eight days of sexual rest before test animals are killed to allow partial or complete restoration of the sperm reserves within the cauda epididymides. In studies evaluating the reversibility of damage to the germinal epithelium, the agent should be administered for approximately six cycles, and then 12 cycles without treatment should elapse to allow time for spermatogenesis to be reestablished. The interval of 12 cycles probably is sufficient to allow regeneration of the germinal epithelium in test animals, although a longer interval may be required in man.

Testicular Size. In normal males, the number of sperm produced per day by a testis (or the two testes) is largely determined by testicular size. In several species of laboratory and domesticated animals, testis size is highly correlated to daily sperm production and to sperm in semen of frequently ejaculated males. In a scrotal mammal, testicular size can be measured easily and precisely without damage to the animal. Although severe spermatogenic arrest ultimately will be accompanied by a reduction in testis size, this measurement is relatively insensitive.

At autopsy, the testis can be freed of both the epididymis and spermatic cord and weighed. Because testis weight and body weight are independent variables, absolute testis weight should be reported rather than weight per gram of body weight.

Spermatogenesis. Daily sperm production can be conveniently determined by counting spermatid nuclei in homogenates of testicular tissue in a salt solution containing Triton X-100 (Amann and Lambiase, 1969; Amann *et al.*, 1976). This procedure is simple, precise, and sensitive. Because the nucleoprotein in elongated spermatids is highly condensed and crosslinked, it resists disruption during homogenization. Thus, homogenization-resistant spermatid nuclei can be quantified and the actual daily sperm production estimated.

The clinical detection (semen analysis) of human reproductive capacity is generally unreliable. Therefore, a number of investigators have sought to develop a heterologous (interspecies) *in vitro* fertilization test system that utilizes human sperm and ova of laboratory animals. These techniques will be described later.

Epididymal Function. Although it may be useful to weigh the distal half of the epididymis, histologic examination of epididymal tissue usually contributes very little. The most meaningful determinations are the number of sperm stored within the cauda epididymis and a measure of their motility and morphology.

The motility and morphology of sperm in a small drop of plasma expressed from the distal cauda epididymis can be evaluated. This is the only practical way to evaluate qualitative changes in sperm when using laboratory animals because sperm from the caput epididymis are immotile. Sperm from the distal cauda epididymis should be progressively motile. The presence of a high percentage of immotile sperm is clear evidence of abnormal testicular or epididymal function.

Plant lectins interact with specific glycoproteins on the cell surface membranes and, therefore, may be useful probes for monitoring alterations in the number, distribution, and mobility of cell surface receptors associated with sperm maturation. In our NIEHS laboratory and others, fluorescence-conjugated lectins have been employed to determine modifications in rat sperm surface proteins during testicular and epididymal maturation that can be quantified visually. Lectins appear to have a potential for assessing sperm maturation and perhaps for identifying sperm rendered nonfunctional by exogenous chemicals.

The potential of using monoclonal antibodies to sperm surface proteins to determine sperm membrane alterations associated with sperm maturation or chemically induced toxicity is also being investigated in various laboratories. Monoclonal antibodies derived from hybrid cell lines provide highly specific probes that recognize unique determinants. Mice have been immunized with rat sperm obtained from the precaput, caput, and cauda epididymides. Splenocytes, obtained from minced spleen tissue, are fused with myeloma cells. After cell fusion, the hybridoma supernatant is screened for relevant antibodies. Positive wells are further cloned. These monoclonal antibodies bind to specific regions of the sperm surface and can be quantified by immunofluorescence. The potential for monoclonal antibodies to identify chemically induced sperm surface changes that might correlate with infertility remains to be defined.

Accessory Sex Organs. Because accessory sex organ function is dependent on the concentration of testosterone in peripheral blood and the availability of tissue receptors for this steroid, weighing the accessory sex glands is a crude bioassay of testosterone production and/or action.

Semen Analysis. Semen analysis is a reasonable predictor of testicular and posttesticular organ function. Semen can be collected from rabbits or dogs in chronic studies. Both quantitative and qualitative characteristics of more than one ejaculate must be evaluated to ensure that conclusions concerning testicular function are valid. Since semen represents contributions from the accessory sex glands as well as the testes and epididymides, only the total number of sperm in an ejaculate is a reliable estimate of sperm production. The number of sperm introduced into the pelvic urethra during emission and the volume of fluid from the accessory sex glands are independent. The potential sources of error in measuring ejaculate volume, concentration, and the seminal characteristics necessary to calculate total sperm per ejaculate must be considered (Amann, 1981).

The number of sperm in an ejaculate is influenced by many factors including age, season, testicular size, ejaculation frequency or interval since the preceding ejaculate and the degree of sexual arousal. Although ejaculation frequency or the interval since the last ejaculation alters the total number of sperm per ejaculate, ejaculation frequency does not influence daily sperm production. However, because of epididymal storage, frequent ejaculation is necessary if the number of sperm counted in ejaculated semen is to accurately reflect sperm production. If only one or two ejaculates are collected weekly, a 50 percent reduction in sperm production probably would remain undetected. Ejaculates should be collected daily (or every other day) over a period of time. The analysis of isolated ejaculates or even several ejaculates collected at irregular intervals cannot estimate daily sperm production or output. The first several ejaculates in each series contain more sperm than subsequent ejaculates because the number of sperm available for ejaculation is being reduced. In rabbits and dogs, seminal characteristics will usually stabilize after three to five ejaculates at one- to three-day intervals.

Semen collection should begin prior to exposure of the test animals to the agent in order to avoid the differences among males. Ejaculates should be collected at the same time of day. For rabbits, data collected 0 to 14 days after exposure would reflect alterations to sperm induced by the agent acting on them after they have left the testes. Changes that first appear between 15 and 35 days would reflect an alteration in the development of spermatids. Changes observed between 36 and 56 days after exposure would suggest an influence on primary spermatocytes or spermatogonia.

Analysis of sperm quality should include the percentage of progressively motile sperm and an evaluation of sperm morphology. Visual estimation of sperm motility is not ideal, but it can provide a useful estimate. Temperature must be carefully controlled (Amann, 1981).

Sperm morphology may be evaluated using either wet preparations or properly prepared, stained smears but requires an appropriate classification scheme (Wyrobek, 1983; Wyrobek *et al.*, 1983). Chromosomal analysis is used in the laboratory and clinic to diagnose genetic diseases.

Hormone Action. Cytoplasmic and nuclear androgen receptors in gonads and accessory sex organs are presently under study, and their toxicologic relevance is being investigated. The ability of chemicals to alter gonadotropin receptors or peptide hormone action also needs further study. Binding sites can be quantified, affinity constants can be estimated, and the effects of various exogenous chemicals on the hormone-receptor interaction and/or hormone action can be determined.

Testicular Enzymes. "Marker enzymes," indicative of normal or abnormal cellular differentiation of function, have been sought by many investigators (Hodgen, 1977). Shen and Lee (1977) studied eight enzymes: hyaluronidase (H); lactate dehydrogenase isoenzyme-X (LDH-X); and the dehydrogenases of sorbitol (SDH), A-glycerophosphate (GPDH), glucose-6-phosphate (G6PDH), malate (MDH), glyceraldehyde-3-phosphate (G3PDH), and isocitrate (ICDH). Because microscopically observed alterations correlated well with changes in enzyme activities, selected enzymes may be reliable indicators of chemically induced toxicity. Chapin *et al.* (1982) have also sought such markers.

Sexual Behavior. With both rats and rabbits, comprehensive evaluations of sexual behavior are possible, but the investigator must be experienced and special expertise is required. The number of mountings, thrusts, and ejaculations each can be quantified as indicators of reproductive behavior.

Male Reproductive Capacity. *Animal Models*. Evaluation of chemicals for potential hazard to humans requires one or more animal models. Rodents and rabbits offer several advantages in comparison to dogs and subhuman primates. Amann (1982) has summarized the reproductive characteristics of several potential models, but none has reproductive traits identical to those of humans. Sperm production is more efficient in all of these species than in the human male, and because the females are generally litter-bearing, a great range of responses is obtained.

Reproductive processes in humans, particularly in the male, are more vulnerable to deleterious events than in laboratory animals, assuming that a quantitatively similar response is induced in both species. Thus, fertility and fecundity of animal models are relatively insensitive criteria for identifying chemicals that are hazardous to reproduction.

Rats are preferable to mice or hamsters because of their convenient size, well-characterized reproductive processes, and general use in toxicologic studies. Rabbits are an ideal second species because they are the smallest common species from which semen can be quantitatively and conveniently collected in longitudinal studies. With both rats and rabbits, artificial insemination is practical. The dog is a widely used test species, but it is rarely used to evaluate reproductive performance. Use of subhuman primates for routine testing is unlikely because of cost and availability.

Use of an avian model, such as the chicken, has some advantages. Artificial insemination is possible, and fertilization and embryonic development can be monitored easily and relatively inexpensively.

As mentioned, mating rodents or rabbits are insensitive predictors of human toxic effects. These laboratory animals produce and ejaculate 10 to 100 times more sperm than are necessary for normal fertility and litter size (Aafjes *et al.*, 1980). A chemically induced reduction in daily sperm production or a functional alteration in 50 percent of the ejaculated sperm is unlikely to alter fecundity (Bechter *et al.*, 1982). However, when a number of sperm marginally adequate for normal fertility is artificially inseminated, a functional alteration of about 20 percent of the sperm will decrease the number of offspring produced. In order to more closely mimic the human capacity, strains of laboratory animals with less efficient reproductive capacity might be selected genetically or produced by radiation or chemical treatment during the perinatal period.

The technique of competitive fertilization is an intriguing attempt to increase the sensitivity of animal models. Sperm from a control and a treated male are placed in direct competition by simultaneously inseminating equal numbers of sperm from each of the two males into one female. Parentage can be determined by genetic markers or blood typing. It is also possible to distinguish the two populations of sperm in the recently fertilized ovum if the sperm are labeled with appropriate fluorochromes (Blazak and Fechheimer, 1980).

Any experiment to evaluate the effect of an agent on male reproductive function must include sufficient males per treatment group to detect a treatment effect. Amann (1982) presents the following analysis. For normal rabbits, a 25 percent decrease in testicular weight, determination of spermatid reserves per gram of testis, percentage of seminiferous tubules with sperm lining the tubule lumen, and seminiferous tubule diameter would have an 80 percent chance of being detected at the 5 percent level if 12 to 15 rabbits per test group were used. Variance associated with evaluations of seminal characteristics is larger. The coefficients of variance for ejaculate volume and sperm concentration typically exceed 50 percent. A reduction in daily sperm output of nearly one-half would have to occur to ensure an 80 percent chance of detection using 15 rabbits per group. Measurements of motile or morphologically normal sperm are more sensitive indicators of effect and thus require fewer animals.

Fertility Profiles. Serial mating assesses the biologic functioning of sperm cells and produces fertility patterns that are related inversely in time to the phase of spermatogenesis damaged by the treatment. The serial-mating technique using rodents is a useful test of both dominant lethal mutations (Epstein *et al.,* 1972) and male reproductive capacity (Lee and Dixon, 1972). After treatment with the selected chemical, each male is housed singly with a virgin female for five to seven days. This time period ensures that the female experiences one estrus cycle during the breeding period. During each mating period, female animals are examined daily for vaginal plugs to ensure that the treatment does not inter-fere with ejaculation and mating capability. After the mating period, the female is replaced with another. These breeding studies are usually continued for 70 days.

To construct a fertility profile (Lee and Dixon, 1972), the females are examined nine days after the breeding period when a female could be approximately 12.5 days pregnant. Uteri and fetuses are examined and the number of dead and viable fetuses are recorded. These data are graphed with the ordinate representing the percentage of fertile males as indicated by pregnant females and the abscissa representing days since treatment.

In order to relate the effect of a relationship between a drug or other environmental agent on fertility to the type of spermatogenic stage affected, as well as to suggest possible biochemical mechanisms, the timing of spermatogenesis should be recalled. The kinetics of the spermatogenic cycle are determined by following the development of [^{3}H] thymidine in pulse-labeled spermatogonia.

An example of a fertility profile is presented in Figure 16–5. It is apparent from the profile that the test chemical affected only spermatogonia and perhaps early primary spermatocytes in these mice. The major biochemical process unique to these cell types is DNA synthesis. In fact, the test chemical is an antineoplastic agent, cytosine arabinoside, which is an effective inhibitor of DNA synthesis. Similarly unique profiles are produced with chemicals that block cell division, such as vincristine, and with alkylating agents that affect both replicating and nonreplicating cells.

Testing Female Reproductive Capacity

The great complexity of the female mammalian reproduction system presents multiple targets for chemical injury and various end-points for detecting dysfunction. A single permanent set of oocytes formed during embryogenesis serves the entire reproductive lifetime, and the female mammalian reproductive system passes through periods of differential susceptibility during the prenatal period, at puberty, and during the reproductive years. Although relatively quiet during the late fetal and prepubertal periods, complex integrated reproductive circuits become active with puberty. Cyclic and dynamic changes occur in target organs that are controlled by pituitary and ovarian interactions.

Although less extensive than for the male, a number of functional, morphologic, and biochemical parameters are available to assess toxic effects on female reproductive function (Table 16–7). Female reproduction depends on oogenesis, ovulation, the development of sexual

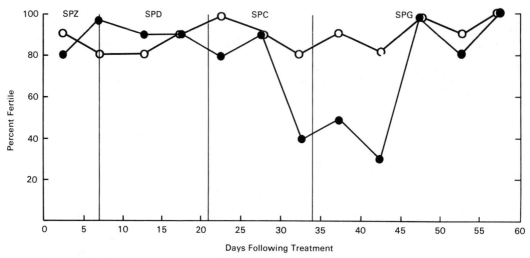

Figure 16–5. Fertility profiles expressing the percentages of males determined to be fertile as indicated by pregnant females (Lee and Dixon, 1972). Data indicate the spermatogenic cell types affected and suggest possible mechanisms of toxicity. These results demonstrate that spermatogonia (*SPG*) and perhaps early primary spermatocytes (*SPC*) were affected by a single injection of cytosine arabinoside at the time of treatment while this DNA synthesis inhibitor had no apparent effect on spermatids (*SPD*) or sperm (*SPZ*). Dysfunction was observed between days 30 and 45 after treatment.

receptivity, coitus, gamete and zygote transport, fertilization, and implantation of the conceptus. Maternal and fetal interactions support the intrauterine growth of the fetus to maturity and delivery of the offspring at term.

Female reproductive toxicity testing approaches overlap with some of the methods used in teratogenicity and mutagenicity testing. Endpoints such as preimplantation loss, spontaneous abortion, and reduced fetal growth may reflect genetic or nongenetic alterations of the gametes involved in producing the conceptus. A battery of screening tests if often employed to provide qualitative and quantitative assessment of chemically induced toxicity and to aid in the extrapolation of laboratory data to humans (Vouk and Sheehan, 1983).

Gross Pathology. Animals should be inspected for general appearance of the external genitalia. After sacrifice, the animals can be examined internally for conformity of anatomic relationships, cystic ovaries, and other gross abnormalities. Organ weights, especially of the ovaries and accessory sex organs, are useful.

Histopathology. Using light microscopy, all organs important to reproduction should be examined (Ettlin and Dixon, 1984). These include the vagina, cervix, uterus, oviducts, ovaries, adrenals, and pituitary. Periodic acid Schiff's (PAS) stain is used to identify mucus-secreting cells in the vagina and uterus. Transmission

electron microscopy (TEM) sometimes provides additional information especially with regard to the ovary and pituitary. Scanning electron microscopy (SEM) of luminal surfaces of the vagina, cervix, and uterus may reveal early anatomic changes.

Ovaries are fixed in Bouin's solution and serial sections prepared. Oocyte counts are generally made in every fifth section, and stages of follicular development are quantified and compared. A comparatively simple and sensitive quantitative method for estimating an increase in the normal rate of follicle atresia consists of using serial sections to count the number of the follicles and then to calculate the percent of atretic follicles.

Ovarian Function. *Oogenesis and Folliculogenesis.* Laboratory methods to directly assess the effects of test compounds on oogenesis and/or folliculogenesis include histologic determination of oocytes and/or follicle number (Dobson *et al.*, 1978). Chemical effects on oogenesis can be measured indirectly by determining fertility of the offspring (McLachlan *et al.*, 1981). Other indirect measures of ovarian toxicity in experimental animals include assessment of age at vaginal opening, onset of reproductive capacity, ovarian function, age at reproductive senescence, and total reproductive capacity (Gellert, 1978).

Morphologic techniques are available to quan-

**Table 16–7. POTENTIALLY USEFUL TESTS
OF FEMALE REPRODUCTIVE
TOXICITY FOR LABORATORY
ANIMALS AND/OR WOMEN**

Body weight
Ovary
  Organ weight
  Histology
  Number of oocytes
  Rate of follicular atresia
  Follicular steroidogenesis
  Follicular maturation
  Oocyte maturation
  Ovulation
  Luteal function
Hypothalamus
  Histology
  Altered synthesis and release of neurotransmitters,
    neuromodulators, and neurohormones
Pituitary
  Histology
  Altered synthesis and release of trophic hormones
Endocrine
  Gonadotropin releasing hormone levels
  LH, FSH, prolactin levels
  Chorionic gonadotropin levels
  Estrogen levels
  Progesterone levels
  Cyclicity of steroid hormone levels
Oviduct
  Histology
  Gamete transport
  Fertilization
  Transport of early embryo
Uterus
  Cytology
  Histology
  Luminal fluid analysis (xenobiotics, proteins)
  Decidual response
  Dysfunctional bleeding
Cervix
  Cytology
  Histology
  Mucus production
  Mucus quality (sperm penetration test)
Vulva/vagina
  Cytology
  Histology
  Virilization
  Adenosis
Fertility
  Ratio exposed: pregnant females
  Number of embryos or young per pregnant female
  Ratio viable embryos: corpora lutea
  Ratio implantation: corpora lutea
  Number 2–8 cell eggs
  Number of unfertilized eggs
  Number of abnormal eggs
  Number of corpora lutea
In vitro
  In vitro fertilization of superovulated eggs, either
    exposed to chemical in culture or from treated
    females

tify and assess primordial germ cell number, stem cell migration, oogonial proliferation, and urogenital ridge development. *In vitro* techniques can be used to evaluate primordial germ cell proliferation, migration, ovarian differentiation, and folliculogenesis (Ways *et al.,* 1980; Thompson, 1981).

Serial oocyte counts are used to monitor oocyte and/or follicle destruction in experimental animals (Pedersen and Peters, 1968). This approach is a reliable means of quantifying the effects of chemicals on oocytes and follicles.

Follicular growth may be assayed in experimental animals using [^{3}H] thymidine uptake, ovarian response to gonadotropins, and follicular kinetics (Hillier *et al.,* 1980). These approaches identify both direct and indirect effects on follicular growth and have been used by Mattison and co-workers to identify drugs and other environmental chemicals that are ovotoxic (Mattison and Nightingale, 1980).

Hormone Levels. Serum levels of estrogen or estrogenic effects on target tissues are indicators of normal follicular function. Tissue and organ responses include time of vaginal opening in immature rats, uterine weight, endometrial morphology, and/or serum levels of FSH and LH. Granulosa cell culture techniques are being developed as direct screens of the ability of test chemicals to inhibit cell proliferation and/or estrogen production (Hillier *et al.,* 1977; Zeleznik *et al.,* 1979). The biosynthesis of estradiol and its metabolism to estrone and estriol by the ovary is another indicator of the reproductive process. The peripheral catabolism of these steroids is principally a function of the liver and involves oxidative metabolism, as well as conjugation with glucuronic acid. These metabolic pathways are affected in various ways by exogenous chemicals.

The study of nuclear and cytoplasmic hormone receptors in target tissues is a rapidly developing field with important toxicologic applications. Estradiol and progesterone receptors are especially important, as are the chemicals that compete for these receptors and perhaps alter their molecular conformation. Steroid receptors may be relevant to the understanding of at least two aspects of reproductive toxicology. On one hand, the estrogen receptor may play a role in the initial toxicology of many environmental agents. For example, metabolites of DDT, DMBA, PCBs, and similar aromatic chemicals have been reported to bind to the cytoplasmic receptor for estrogen. Thus, interactions between apparently nonhormonal xenobiotics and cellular receptors may result in an inadvertent hormonal response (agonist), or they may block normal hormonal action (antagonist). In either case, abnormal responses by reproductive tissues can result. On the other hand, the number or availability of hormone receptors may be modified by exposure to foreign chemicals. Such quantitative changes in these cellular regulatory proteins could alter the response of the affected tissues to subsequent hormonal stimulation. Quantification of cytoplasmic estrogen receptors in human breast cancer is a useful adjunct to the therapy of this disease, and such measurements have helped to predict those mammary neoplasms which respond best to estrogen therapy.

Ovulation. Ovulation depends on the successful integration of the hypothalamic-pituitary-ovarian axis resulting in follicle growth, steroid hormone production, LH surge, follicle rupture, and oocyte release. Direct methods to assess ovulation in experimental animals include collection of oocytes from oviducts or uteri. This technique has been used extensively in reproductive biology to assay compounds, such as the prostaglandin synthetase inhibitors, which stop follicle rupture (Mori *et al.*, 1980), or other compounds, like phenobarbital or the cannabinoids, which block the LH surge (Barraclough and Sawyer, 1957; Cordova *et al.*, 1980; Kostellow *et al.*, 1980). Ovulation can also be monitored by techniques involving embryo flushing and quantifying implantation sites (Hammer and Mitchell, 1979; Shani *et al.*, 1979; Yoshinaga *et al.*, 1979), which measures both ovulation and fertilization. Implantation reflects the conceptus' ability to embed as well as the proper hormonal preparation of the endometrium that makes it receptive to the conceptus.

The estrus cycle of laboratory animals has been described by Perry (1971). Female rats, isolated from males, ovulate at intervals from four to five days. Ovulation occurs during estrus and is easily detected. The most commonly used method is vaginal cytology. Vaginal smears are obtained by inserting a spatula, a smooth rod, or a cotton swab into the vagina. These cells can also be sampled by washing the vagina with a small amount of saline. The cells are then smeared onto a microscope slide and air-dried; they may be stained, cleared, and permanently preserved under a cover glass. Simple staining that allows immediate examination is all that is required to follow the cycle. The cell sample must be collected carefully because pseudopregnancy can be induced by inadvertently stimulating the cervix while taking a vaginal smear or washing. A classical description of the rat's estrus cycle recognizes four stages: proestrus, estrus, metestrus, and diestrus. The number of cycles in the time period and the length of each stage of the cycle can be noted.

Postovarian Function. Female reproductive tract function depends on properly phased processes including motility (muscular or ciliary), secretion of luminal fluids, as well as adaptive cell growth and turnover, which mirror the ovarian cycle and are essential for pregnancy. Gamete transport, fertilization, zygote transport, and implantation are essential components of the reproductive process. Disruption of any one component will impair reproductive success. Exogenous chemicals may interfere directly or indirectly with one or more of these activities of the female genital tract. The function of each of these components can be assessed using laboratory animals. Relatively simple procedures exist for studying sperm and ovum transport, fertilization success, the rate of tubal transport of the zygote, early embryonic development, implantation, and the spacing of conceptuses along the uterine horns (West *et al.*, 1977).

Biochemical analysis, including electrophoresis, of vaginal and uterine luminal fluid is in many ways analogous to semen analysis in the male. In addition, in larger species like the rabbit, monkey, or dog, follicular fluid from the ovary can be analyzed for changes in certain components that indicate altered function.

Fertilization and Implantation. Many of the toxic influences on germ cells of both sexes manifest themselves in reduced rates of conception. The formation, maturation, and coming together of a male and female germ cell are all preliminary to their actual union into a combined cell or zygote.

In Vitro *Fertilization.* Fertilization can be achieved readily *in vitro* with sperm and ova from a variety of species including humans. Sperm must be capacitated and the sperm and ova incubated in a carefully defined medium with optimum salt concentrations, nutrients, osmolarity, and pH. Sperm concentrations are important, and the requirement for laboratory skill is obvious. Microdrops of medium under liquid paraffin or in tubes under special gas phases are used to achieve fertilization and cleavage. Early development of the conceptus can be supported *in vitro.*

Heterologous (human sperm/hamster egg) *in vitro* "fertilization" is being used to assess fertilizing capacity of human sperm. These studies, discussed in the following section, identify certain individuals as subfertile who have a routinely determined normal sperm number, motility, and morphology.

Methods of *in vitro* fertilization can be coupled with preimplantation embryo culture, transfer of blastocysts to pseudopregnant recipients, and evaluation of "pregnancy outcome" to identify critical early developmental targets of environmental chemicals. Male and female gametes can be exposed to environmental agents either *in vitro* or *in vivo* and then can be used for *in vitro* fertilization. The conceptus also can be recovered following the mating of treated animals. Subsequently, the zygote is cultured and the early embryo (blastocyst stage) is transferred to a pseudopregnant recipient. Using this approach, the following parameters can be monitored: sperm motility, *in vitro* fertilizing capacity, four- and eight-cell stage formation, morula and blastocyst development, implantation success (resorbed/dead/live fetuses), pregnancy rate, and malformations. Thus, studies of chemical effects on sperm and ova, early development, preimplantation and postimplantation embryos, and birth defects can be carried out (Schmid *et al.*, 1983).

Reproductive Performance. The success of pregnancy is the most efficient measure of the ability of the animal to produce gametes, to mate and conceive, and to produce viable offspring.

Assessing total reproductive capacity is especially suitable for studying chronic reproductive toxicity in female rodents. This procedure takes advantage of the fact that rodents experience a postpartum estrus. Females are caged with fertile males. Pregnant animals are removed immediately from the breeding cages. Following delivery, the female is returned to the male and can become pregnant again. This procedure provides information on whether the total reproductive capacity of the test animal is reduced by the selected treatment. This procedure can also be adapted to assess failures of fertilization, preimplantation embryo loss, and postimplantation dominant lethality in females. This approach has been used by McLachlan and co-workers to determine the effects of gestational exposure of DES on the reproductive capacity of female offspring (McLachlan *et al.*, 1982). Data for mice exposed prenatally to doses of 0, 0.1, 1, 10, and 100 μg/kg of DES on gestational days 9 to 16 are presented on Figure 16–6. The cumulative number of live young per mouse is recorded for a 35-week period of forced breeding.

Multigeneration Tests. Multigeneration studies are intended to provide data on gonadal function, estrus cycle, mating behavior, conception, implantation, abortion, fetal and embryonic development, parturition, postnatal survival, lactation, maternal behavior, and postpartum growth. The advantages of multigenerational tests include the wide range of reproductive processes that are assessed and the possibility of observing genetic and behavioral effects.

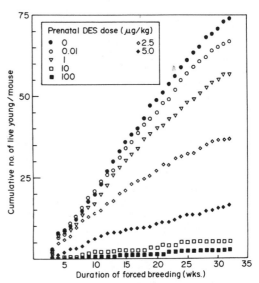

Figure 16–6. Total reproductive capacity of female mice exposed prenatally to DES. Timed pregnant CD-1 mice were treated subcutaneously with diethylstilbestrol from days 9 through 16 of gestation. Fertility was determined by repetitive force-breeding techniques and expressed as the total number of live young born per mouse over a 32-week interval. Each point on the figure represents a mean of 25 to 50 mice. (From McLachlan, J. A.; Newbold, R. R.; Shah, H. C.; Hogan, M. D.; and Dixon, R. L.: Reduced fertility in female mice exposed transplacentally to diethylstilbestrol (DES). *Fertil. Steril.*, 38:364, 1982. Reproduced with permission of the publisher, The American Fertility Society.)

The classic three-generation reproduction study requires continuous exposure of the parental generation (F_0) and the offspring of each succeeding generation to the test chemical (Collins, 1978). Mating indices can be calculated:

Mating index
$$= \frac{\text{Number of copulations}}{\text{Number of estrus cycles required}} \times 100$$

Fecundity index
$$= \frac{\text{Number of pregnancies}}{\text{Number of copulations}} \times 100$$

Male fertility index
$$= \frac{\begin{array}{c}\text{Number of males impregnating}\\ \text{females}\end{array}}{\begin{array}{c}\text{Number of males exposed to fertile}\\ \text{nonpregnant females}\end{array}} \times 100$$

Female fertility index
$$= \frac{\text{Number of females conceiving}}{\begin{array}{c}\text{Number of females exposed to fertile}\\ \text{males}\end{array}} \times 100$$

Incidence of parturition
$$= \frac{\text{Number of parturitions}}{\text{Number of pregnancies}} \times 100$$

Pups are examined for physical abnormalities at birth. The numbers of viable, stillborn, and cannibalized members of each litter are recorded. Observations for clinical signs are made daily. The number of survivors on days 1, 4, 12 and 21 postparturition is recorded. The following survival indices can be calculated:

Live birth index
$$= \frac{\text{Number of viable pups born}}{\text{Total number of pups born}} \times 100$$

24-hour survival index
$$= \frac{\text{Number of pups viable at lactation day 1}}{\text{Number of viable pups born}} \times 100$$

4-day survival index
$$= \frac{\text{Number of pups viable at lactation day 4}}{\text{Number of viable pups born}} \times 100$$

12-day survival index
$$= \frac{\text{Number of pups viable at lactation day 12}}{\text{Number of pups viable at lactation day 4}} \times 100$$

21-day survival index
$$= \frac{\text{Number of pups viable at lactation day 21}}{\text{Number of pups retained at lactation day 4}} \times 100$$

Data are compiled into tables presenting parental body weight, parental organ weight, food consumption (test compound intake), parental mortality, duration of gestation, reproductive data and indices, survival data and indices, progeny body weight, male/female ratio, and histopathologic findings (Committee to Revise NAS Publication 1138, 1977).

There are several variations on this classic scheme that are discussed later. Recently, others have suggested that no more than two generations are scientifically justified (Dixon and Hall, 1982).

REGULATORY REQUIREMENTS

Current test procedures for assessing reproductive function are used primarily to meet requirements of the various regulatory agencies. These reproduction studies classically utilize either rats or mice because of their early age of sexual maturity, their short gestational and lactational periods, and ease of handling. Tests are generally conducted to identify general reproductive failures; they usually do not seek information regarding the specific portions of the reproductive sequence involved. Other studies are done routinely for teratogenic or mutagenic effects.

Classically, two different kinds of tests are used: one for drugs, and the other for food additives or pesticides. The two test procedures differ with regard to the way in which either drugs or food additives come in contact with the consuming individual. Drugs are normally taken intentionally at levels that produce biologic effects; therefore, it is assumed their exposure can be controlled. On the other hand, food additives or other environmental contaminants are generally ingested continuously or intermittently at much lower levels—thus, not in a directly controllable manner.

Each of the U.S. agencies regulating toxic substances—Environmental Protection Agency (EPA), Food and Drug Administration (FDA), Occupational Safety and Health Administration (OSHA), and Consumer Products Safety Commission (CPSC)—has been actively developing protocols and approaches for detecting reproductive as well as other forms of toxicity. A more complete summary is available in Dixon and Hall (1982).

EPA Reproductive Hazard Evaluation

Mammalian Tests. The standards proposed by the EPA for the study of the effects of pesticides on reproduction represent a significant departure from traditional testing procedures (EPA, 1978). Instead of a three-generation study with two litters in each generation, EPA suggests a two-generation study with only one litter in each generation. The Agency believes that the proposed methodology is both more sensitive and considerably less expensive than the traditional test design.

Two litters per generation have been required because the first litters produced by adolescent mothers often show a great deal of variation. Thus, data based on the first litters are less useful than data from the second set of litter. While the EPA proposed guidelines require only one litter, the animals are not bred until they are fully mature.

The goal of multigeneration reproductive studies has been to detect genetic abnormalities. With these EPA guidelines, the potential for a chemical to cause genetic damage would be assessed in a battery of mutagenicity tests. Another reason for extending a reproduction study into the third generation is to detect cumulative effects. However, few (if any) toxic effects appear initially in the third generation of a reproductive study.

A properly designed test should satisfy the following standards: Testing should be performed with the technical grade of each active ingredient in the product. Testing is to be performed in at least one mammalian species, which may be the same as one of the two species used in the teratogenecity study; the rat is preferred. In testing with rodents, each dose and control group should contain enough females to produce approximately 20 litters (20 sampling units) at each breeding, assuming typical mating and fertility for the strain. At least ten fertile males per dose in the first mating of the F_0 generation are suggested. Subsequently, at least ten males per dose level are required. At least three dose level groups, in addition to the control group, should be tested. The highest dose level should produce an observable toxicologic or pharmacologic effect in the test animals, but not cause more than 10 percent fatalities. The lowest dose level should produce no observable adverse effects. Concurrent control groups are required. A vehicle control group is required if a vehicle is used in administering the test substance. The test substance should be administered by the route most closely equivalent to a typical route of human exposure, unless the chemical or physical characteristics or other properties suggest that another route of administration would be more appropriate.

The test substance should be administered to two generations of animals, F_0 and F_1. A third generation of animals, F_2, will be exposed to the test substance *in utero* and through nursing. Dosing of animals in the F_0 generation begins as soon as possible after weaning and acclimation, but in any case before the animals are six weeks old. The test substance is administered daily to the F_0 generation. Dosing shall continue until all F_1 generation animals have been weaned. Dosing of the animals selected from the F_1 generation for breeding begins as soon as the animals are weaned (approximately 30 days after birth). The test substance is administered daily to these animals with dosing continuing until 30 days after all F_2 animals have been weaned. Dosing of animals from the F_1 generation is not required if they have not been selected for breeding.

After the F_0 generation animals have received the test substance for at least 100 days, they are bred to produce the F_1 generation. Appropriate numbers of males and females are then selected at random from different litters of the F_1 generation for breeding. After the test substance has been administered to these animals for at least 120 days, they are bred to produce the F_2 generation. Figure 16–7 indicates the breeding and dosing schedule. The F_0 generation is dosed for a total of about 100 days; total exposure is about 160 days. The F_1 generation is dosed for about 210 days; total exposure is about 270 days. The

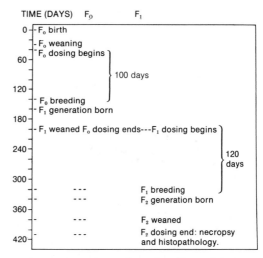

Figure 16–7. Approximate breeding and dosing schedule for EPA Reproduction Study. F_0 indicates parents; F_1, the first filial generation produced by crossing two individuals; F_2, the second filial generation produced by mating two members of the F_1 generation.

F_2 generation is not dosed; total exposure is about 60 days during gestation and nursing.

All litters should be examined as soon as possible after delivery, and the following parameters are recorded: litter size, number of stillborn, and number of live births. Viability counts and pup weights are recorded at birth, four days after birth, and at weaning. Additional viability counts between the fourth day and weaning are required for nonrodents. Any physical or behavioral abnormalities are noted.

In reporting the results, the following reproductive indices are used: "fertility index" (the percentage of matings resulting in pregnancy); "gestation index" (the percentage of pregnancies resulting in the birth of live litters); "viability index" (the percentage of animals born that survive four days or longer); "lactation index" (the percentage of animals alive at four days that survive the 21-day lactation period).

The relationships, if any, between exposures to the test substance and the incidence and severity of effects (including effects on reproduction, behavior, tumors and lesions, and mortality) is evaluated. The "no-effect" dosage level should also be determined. All data must be reported and evaluated statistically.

Nonmammalian Tests. The EPA also has proposed guidelines for reproductive studies using avian, fish, and aquatic invertebrate species for the registration of pesticides (EPA, 1979).

Avian Reproductive Assessment. An avian reproductive study is required to support the registration of a pesticide if any of the following conditions exist: the pesticide (or any of its major metabolites or degradation products) is persistent in the environment to the extent that toxic amounts could be expected in avian feed under normal use; the pesticide (or any of its major metabolites or degradation products) is stored or accumulated in plant or animal tissues; the product is intended for use where birds may be subjected to repeated or continued exposure, especially during the breeding season; or any test information indicates that reproduction of birds may be adversely affected by the pesticide. The technical grade of the active ingredient in the product is tested on bobwhite quail and mallard ducks approaching their first breeding season. The following observations are recorded: eggs laid, eggs cracked, eggs set (placed under incubation), viable embryos (fertility), live three-week embryos, hatchability, 14-day survivors, and eggshell thickness.

Fish and Aquatic Invertebrates. Embryolarvae and/or life-cycle tests of fish and aquatic invertebrates are required to support the registration of a formulated product if the pesticide product is used in or is expected to be transported to water from its intended use site.

Where appropriate, the following test data are gathered: reproductive effects; detailed records of spawning, egg numbers, fertility, and fecundity; estimated nondiscernible effect level and mortality data; statistical evaluation of effects; locomotion, behavioral, physiologic, and pathologic effects; definition of the criteria used to determine effects; summary of general observations of other effects or signs of intoxication and stage of life-cycle in which organisms were tested. References to detailed protocols can be found in the EPA guidelines published in the Federal Register (EPA, 1979).

Toxic Substances Control Act

As a consequence of the Toxic Substances Control Act (TSCA), the EPA has proposed a reproductive toxicity protocol that is essentially the same as that proposed by the EPA Pesticide Programs, (EPA, 1979).

Consumer Products Safety Commission

The Consumer Products Safety Commission (CPSC) sponsored a report describing toxicologic principles and procedures for evaluating the toxicity of household substances under the auspices of the Committee on Toxicology, Assembly of Life Sciences, National Research Council, (Committee to Revise NAS Publication 1138, 1977). They have suggested a multigeneration reproductive study that is adjusted specifically for the chemical to be tested on the basis of physical, chemical, and/or pharmacologic properties.

Food and Drug Administration

Although the FDA presently has no single set of toxicology guidelines that petitioners can use to submit data, the agency has made several attempts at providing such guidelines. In 1959, information concerning testing procedures was compiled by the FDA and published under the title *Appraisal of the Safety of Chemicals in Foods, Drugs, and Cosmetics, 1959* (Association of Food and Drug Officials of the United States, 1959).

In 1966, partly in response to the thalidomide crisis, guidelines for the three-segment study of drugs were issued (Goldenthal, 1966). A few years later, in 1970, the FDA published a report by the Panel on Reproduction (FDA, 1970). Test guidelines by the National Toxicology Advisory Committee's Reproduction Panel provide a review of the three-segment study (single-generation reproduction, teratology, and perinatal-postnatal studies) proposed in 1966 (Collins, 1978). The tests are organized according to segments or stages in the reproductive process, thus making it possible to evaluate the drugs' reproductive effects in a relatively brief time. The first segment provides information on fertility and general reproductive performance, particularly on gonadal function, estrus cycles, mating behavior, conception rates, and early stages of gestation. In the second segment, the embryotoxic or teratogenic potential of the drug is determined. In the final segment, studies are designed to determine the effects of the drug on late fetal development, labor and delivery, lactation, and newborn viability and growth (Collins, 1978).

Interagency Regulatory Liaison Group

The Interagency Regulatory Liaison Group (IRLG) consists of the heads of the five U.S. regulatory agencies concerned with toxic chemicals (EPA, CPSC, FDA, OSHA, and USDA) (IRLG, 1978). They recognized that although their agencies often regulate the same or similar chemicals, the toxicity-testing guidelines used by each agency are not always uniform— varying in the details of the methodology and not in fundamental toxicologic principles. The Testing Standards and Guidelines Work Group attempted to resolve these differences by developing guidelines for multigeneration reproductive tests in rodents. The design of subsequent tests was to be based on preliminary information about the effects of the test substance on neonatal morbidity, mortality, and teratogenesis.

The work of the IRLG was interrupted briefly with the change in administration in 1981. However, many of the IRLG activities have been recently reinitiated.

Canadian Health Protection Branch

The Canadian Health Protection Branch has published guidelines for the appraisal of the carcinogenic, mutagenic, and teratogenic potential of chemicals (Ministry of Health and Welfare, 1973). Their guidelines include a broad range of end-points to be assessed during reproductive toxicity tests. They include those used in standard toxicity tests such as food consumption and weight gain, as well as special parameters such as regularity of the estrus cycle, mating behavior, conception rates, fertility, embryotoxicity, fetotoxicity, weight of the newborn, sex distribution, and incidence of malformations. During the postnatal period, observations are made regarding the growth and survival of the offspring, suckling habits, toxicity during lactation, which may develop because of chemicals secreted into milk, and the reproductive performance of the offspring. Treatment is commonly continued for one or more generations.

National Academy of Sciences Committee

The National Academy of Sciences Committee for the Working Conference on Principles of Protocols for Evaluating Chemicals in the Environment published *Principles for Evaluating Chemicals in the Environment* (Committee for the Working Conference on Principles of Protocols for Evaluating Chemicals in the Environment, 1975). In their chapter on reproductive toxicity, the panel concluded that the three-generation test is probably the best measure available for assessing overall reproductive efficiency. They also suggested that the three-generation test could be made more powerful by observing the animals throughout their lifetimes for rate of growth and maturation, as well as for the appearance of tumors or chronic disease.

Pharmaceutical Manufacturer's Association

In 1977, the Pharmaceutical Manufacturers' Association (PMA) published toxicology guidelines to assess the safety of drugs and medical devices (PMA, 1977). Approaches to reproductive toxicity are currently being revised.

Good Laboratory Practice Regulations

Because of deficiencies in the design, conduct, and reporting of data in reports by both commercial and private laboratories, the FDA issued proposed regulations for Good Laboratory Practice Regulations (GLPs) for Nonclinical Laboratory Studies (FDA, 1976). The GLPs are a set of regulations on methods, facilities, and controls to better assure the quality and integrity of data.

The conduct of laboratory studies must comply with the Good Laboratory Practice Standards of the particular regulatory agency for which the tests are being conducted. These standards relate to the entire design and conduct of the toxicity test as well as the qualifications of the personnel involved with all aspects of the tests.

HUMAN RISK

Most humans are exposed to a vast number of chemicals that may be hazardous to their reproductive capacity. As mentioned, many chemicals have been identified as reproductive hazards in laboratory studies. Although the extrapolation of data from laboratory animals to humans is inexact, a number of these chemicals have also been shown to exert detrimental effects on human reproductive performance. The list includes drugs, especially steroid hormones and chemotherapeutic agents; metals and trace elements; pesticides; food additives and contaminants; industrial chemicals; and consumer products.

Reviews and textbooks are available concerning both male and female reproductive toxicity (Gomes, 1977; Lucier et al., 1977; Davies, 1980; Bingham, 1977; Walsh and Egdahl, 1980; and Hunt, 1979). Sieber and Adamson (1975) and Shalet (1980) have focused on the effects of cancer chemotherapeutic agents on reproduction. Spira and Jovannet (1982) have recently edited *Human Fertility Factors*. The Council on Environmental Quality (Nisbet and Karch, 1983) and Barlow and Sullivan (1982) treat the subject more broadly, while Schrag and Dixon (1985) have recently reviewed male reproductive dysfunction associated with industrial chemicals.

The fertility of humans is apparently more susceptible to alterations by environmental factors than is that of laboratory animals. One in five couples desiring children are unsuccessful in their attempts to become parents. Cause-and-effect relationships are particularly difficult to establish in the human population, which probably accounts for the fact that fewer than a dozen nontherapeutic environmental chemicals have been linked with reproductive effects on men (Table 16–8); fewer still have been shown to alter reproductive performance in women (Table 16–9). One reason for this is that methods to reliably estimate damage to human fertility are not readily available. Compounding the problem is the difficulty of measuring human exposure to

Table 16–8. ENVIRONMENTAL CHEMICAL EXPOSURE ASSOCIATED WITH REPRODUCTIVE DYSFUNCTION IN MEN*

Carbon disulfide
Chlordecone (Kepone)
Chloroprene
Dibromochloropropane (DBCP)
Ethylene dibromide
Ethylene oxide
Ethanol consumption
Glycol ethers
Hexane
Inorganic lead and other smelter emissions
Organic lead
Pesticides (occupational exposure)
Vinyl chloride

* Effects of nontherapeutic agents were selected from *Chemical Hazards to Human Reproduction* (Nisbet and Karch, 1983), *Reproductive Hazards of Industrial Chemicals* (Barlow and Sullivan, 1982), and *Industrial Chemicals Associated with Male Reproductive Dysfunction* (Schrag and Dixon, 1985).

chemicals, identifying situations where an exposure to only a single chemical exists, estimating dose-response relationships for chemicals affecting reproduction, and predicting human risk associated with levels of exposure. These areas have been recently considered by Wilcox (1983).

Indicators of Male Infertility

In the male, sterility may result from lack of or impairment of spermatogenesis due to testicular agenesis, hypogenesis, or cryptorchidism; to

Table 16–9. ENVIRONMENTAL CHEMICAL EXPOSURE ASSOCIATED WITH REPRODUCTIVE DYSFUNCTION IN WOMEN*

Anesthetic gases (operating room personnel)
Aniline
Benzene
Carbon disulfide
Chloroprene
Ethanol consumption
Ethylene oxide
Glycol ethers
Formaldehyde
Inorganic lead and other smelter emissions
Organic lead
Methylmercury
Pesticides (occupational exposure)
Phthalic acid esters (PAEs)
Polychlorinated biphenyls (PCBs)
Styrene
Tobacco smoking
Toluene
Vinyl chloride

* Effects of nontherapeutic agents were selected from *Chemical Hazards to Human Reproduction* (Nisbet and Karch, 1983) and *Reproductive Hazards of Industrial Chemicals* (Barlow and Sullivan, 1982).

castration or exposure to roentgen rays or toxic substances; to injury or inflammation; or to endocrine or nutritional disorders. Obstruction of the seminal vesicles and epididymis and pronounced deformity of the penis can interfere with the normal passage of the spermatozoa. Infection of the prostate or seminal vesicles may be injurious to the spermatozoa.

Routine Tests. Routine tests for male infertility include the following (Taymor, 1974):

1. Semen analysis. The semen is delivered into a clean glass container by withdrawal or masturbation. The following characteristics are considered normal:

a. Volume. Semen volume should be 3 to 5 ml.

b. Sperm count. Sixty million or more sperm per milliliter is unquestionably normal; below 30 million per milliliter unquestionably indicates reduced fertility. The significance of counts between 30 million and 60 million depends on the quality of motility and the degree of fertility in the female partner. A highly fertile female would be more susceptible to a count of borderline fertility.

c. Sperm motility. Forty percent or more of sperm should still be actively motile four to five hours after collection.

d. Sperm morphology. At least 60 percent of the spermatozoa should be of normal size and shape.

2. Prostatic secretion. Excess leukocytes in prostatic smears indicate that infection may play a contributory role.

Special Tests. These tests are used for males with reduced fertility as indicated by semen analysis.

1. Thyroid function is evaluated by basal metabolic rates, protein-bound iodine, or radioactive iodine uptake.

2. Testicular biopsy. A biopsy, in most cases, will result in a definitive diagnosis. However, because it is a surgical procedure, it is used very selectively.

3. Urinary gonadotropins. Gonadotropin levels may be low in pituitary deficiency and high in primary gonadal failure.

4. Sex chromatin determination.

5. Sperm penetration test.

Semen Analysis. Semen analysis is commonly used to predict infertility. Ejaculate volume, sperm number, sperm motility, and sperm morphology have been analyzed. Ejaculate volume and sperm morphology do not correlate well with the length of time required for a couple to achieve pregnancy. Sperm number is related to fertility only when the sperm count is less than 20 million per milliliter. The best predictor of fertility appears to be the fraction of motile sperm and the quality of their activity. However, even this variable is not highly correlated with time to pregnancy (Mann and Lutwak-Mann, 1981). Overstreet and co-workers (1981) have described the simultaneous assessment of human sperm motility and morphology by videomicrography.

More complex assays of sperm have been developed. Wyrobek and Bruce (1978) have proposed that abnormal sperm shapes indicate exposure to mutagens. A more direct indicator of fertilizing capacity is the heterologous interspecies *in vitro* fertilization test.

An evaluation of human semen and testicular function has led to the conclusion that human testes are often functioning at the threshold of pathology (Amann, 1981). For many men, the sperm ejaculated is less than twice the number required for fertility (Smith *et al.*, 1979; David *et al.*, 1979; MacLeod and Wang, 1979). Furthermore, the levels of progressively motile sperm and of morphologically normal sperm in human semen suggest that human sperm is of poorer quality than the semen produced by laboratory animals. Consequently, exposure of a population of human males to an environmental toxin that reduces sperm production by 60 percent could be expected to cause a demonstrable decline in fecundity, while a similar reduction of sperm count in animal models would not result in decreased fecundity (Amann 1982; Aafjes *et al.*, 1980).

The human male ejaculates 2.5 to 3.5 ml of semen after several days of continence. Semen volume and sperm count decrease rapidly with repeated ejaculations. Although there are normally about 100 million sperm per milliliter of semen, the count varies widely within a single individual (Belsey *et al.*, 1980). There are those who feel that sperm count and semen quality have been decreasing during the past decade (Dougherty *et al.*, 1981; James, 1980, James, 1982). James examined evidence related to changes in sperm count during the past 45 years and concluded that it seems likely that a secular decline has occurred. It is, however, very difficult to directly correlate sperm counts with fertility. Nevertheless, about 50 percent of men whose sperm count is between 20 and 40 million per milliliter and nearly all of those with counts below 20 million per milliliter are sterile. Another growing concern is the paternal role in the observed incidence of birth defects. Soyka and Joffe (1980) have described male-mediated effects of drugs on offspring.

Sperm Penetration Assay. Because the clinical detection (semen analysis) of human reproductive capacity is generally unreliable, a number of investigators have sought to develop a heterologous (interspecies) *in vitro* fertilization test system that utilizes human sperm and ova of laboratory animals. Ongoing research seeks to answer the question: Is the heterologous *in vitro* fertilization test system utilizing human sperm a reliable indicator of reproductive capacity? At the NIEHS (Hall, 1981), heterologous (human sperm/hamster ova) *in vitro* fertilization is being used to assess fertilizing capacity of human males. These studies have identified certain individuals as subfertile who have a routinely determined normal sperm number, motility, and morphology. This approach demonstrated that the usual parameters for semen analyses are unsure predictors of male subfertility; only the most extreme semen abnormalities reliably indicate subfertility. Thus, the *in vitro* penetration of laboratory animal ova by human sperm appears to be an improved technique to assess human fertilization potential.

The steps involved in the heterologous (interspecies) *in vitro* fertilization technique are presented in Figure 16–8. A human semen sample is obtained and a standard analysis is performed. The spermatozoa are washed in Tyrode's medium, centrifuged, and resuspended at a concentration of 4 to 8 million sperm per milliliter. Motility is assessed, and an aliquot of this stock solution, usually containing 1 million motile sperm per milliliter, is incubated under oil for 15 to 18 hours to capacitate the sperm. While the sperm are being prepared, ova are collected from the oviducts of superovulated female hamsters. This superovulation is induced by intraperitoneal injection of pregnant mares' serum gonadotropin followed by human chorionic gonadotropin two days later. Ova are recovered from the oviducts and placed in Tyrode's medium. The ova are treated with hyaluronidase to remove the cumulus cells and then washed. Trypsin treatment removes the zona pellucida. Zona pellucida-free hamster ova are added to the dish containing control or experimental sperm, and fertilizing capacity is assessed by measuring sperm binding to the ova, decondensed sperm heads, and/or the pronucleus with the corresponding sperm tail in the ovum's cytoplasm. Although termed "fertilization," the process under investigation is the penetration of the sperm into the ovum with subsequent decondensation of the sperm. Further parameters of normal fertilization, such as genetic union of the cells, do not occur under these controlled, artificial conditions. Without the normal process of genetic union, development of the hamster ovum penetrated by human sperm has never been observed.

Indicators of Female Infertility

In the female, sterility may result from impaired oogenesis as a consequence of deficient ovarian tissue (e.g., ovarian agenesis or hypo-

SPERM RECOVERY

Step (1) Perform standard semen analysis 1 hour after collection.

(2) Add semen aliquot to 15 ml centrifuge tube and wash sperm 3 times with Modified Tyrode's solution (centrifuge sperm suspension at 400 x g for 5 min.)

(3) Resuspend sperm at 4 to 8 x 10^6 sperm/ml and place under paraffin oil in petri dish.

(4) Evaluate motility, transfer 0.02 of this stock to a new dish and dilute with Tyrode's to 0.1 ml (10^6 motile sperm/ml) under oil and incubate at 37°C & 5% CO_2 in air for 15-18 h to capacitate sperm.

(5) Add zona pellucida-free hamster ova to dish containing control or experimental sperm for assessment of fertilizing capacity.

(6) Ova examined by phase contrast microscopy 3 h after transfer to sperm dish for evidence of fertilization.

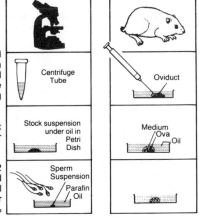

Centrifuge Tube

Stock suspension under oil in Petri Dish

Sperm Suspension / Parafin Oil

Oviduct

Medium / Ova / Oil

OVA RECOVERY

Step (1) Female hamsters are injected with 25 IU PMSG; 58 h later administered 25 IU HCG.

(2) Recover ova from oviducts into Tyrode's medium.

(3) Treat ova with hyaluronidase for 5 min. to remove cumulus cells and wash ova 5 times in culture medium (5 transfers).

(4) Treat ova with trypsin for 1-3 min. to remove zonae pellucidae and wash ova 5 times.

FERTILIZATION

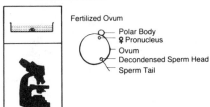

Fertilized Ovum

Polar Body
♀ Pronucleus
Ovum
Decondensed Sperm Head
Sperm Tail

Figure 16–8. Experimental steps involved in the heterologous sperm penetration test. Human sperm functionality apparently correlates with its ability to bind to or penetrate zona pellucida free-hamster ova. (From Hall, J. L.: Relationship between semen quality and human sperm penetration of zona-free hamster ova. *Fertil. Steril.*, **35**:457–63, 1981. Reproduced with permission of the publisher, The American Fertility Society.)

plasia, polycystic disease of the ovary with thickened capsule), the inability of the ovum to become impregnated owing to disease of the oviducts (such as infection and endometriosis), or uterine, cervical, or vaginal abnormalities in structure and function. In addition, debilitating diseases, endocrine abnormalities, and nutritional deficiencies may impair ovulation as well as fertilization and implantation of the ovum.

Routine Tests. Tests for female infertility include the following (Taymor, 1974):

1. Postcoital test. Cervical mucus is examined for its preovulatory qualities of clarity, spinnbarkeit (ability of the mucus to form a thread 5 to 10 cm in length when stretched between slide and cover slip), ferning (ability of the mucus to form fernlike pattern when dried and examined under low power of microscope), and for the number of viable spermatozoa 8 to 12 hours after coitus. More than 20 active sperm per high-power field are normally observed.

2. Tubal patency. Patency of the oviducts is evaluated initially by insufflation with carbon dioxide (Rubin test). Those patients who show failure of carbon dioxide to pass or who fail to conceive after an interval of time despite a normal Rubin test may be examined further with hysterosalpingography.

3. Ovulation and hormonal factors. These may be evaluated by measuring basal body temperature which characteristically shows a sustained rise after ovulation. The value of the temperature chart as an exact indicator of ovulation timing for purposes of timing coitus or insemination treatments can be overestimated. An endometrial biopsy that demonstrates a secretory change in the endometrium is a more valid indicator that ovulation has occurred. The presence of endometrium out of phase with the time of biopsy is evidence of a progestational deficiency.

4. Other tests. These include:
   a. Thyroid function.
   b. Hormone assays. Urinary gonadotropin and 17-ketosteroid may be determined in cases of anovulation or inadequate luteal function.
   c. Timing of ovulation. Vaginal or urinary smears and studies of cervical mucus may be utilized to time ovulation.

d. Culdoscopy. Culdoscopy may be used to detect early endometriosis, pelvic adhesions interfering with oviduct-ovarian function, or polycystic ovaries.

Menstrual Cycle. Ovarian cyclicity in women reflects the integrated functioning of the reproductive system. Serum estrogen and progesterone levels throughout the cycle correlate with follicular growth and steroid synthesis. Ovulation can be monitored indirectly by measuring progesterone production or by observing the effects of progesterone on responsive end organs. Changes in the fluidity, air-drying pattern, and elasticity of cervical mucus can be plotted to indicate ovulation and signal fertile and nonfertile periods (Billings *et al.,* 1977). Endometrial biopsies can be evaluated histologically for characteristic morphology (Noyes *et al.,* 1950). However, endometrial biopsy is not a common procedure. Endometrial aspiration techniques are also available (Smith, 1960).

The occurrence of anovulatory cycles is commonly observed among approximately one-third of infertile couples. Ovulation can be monitored easily using daily temperatures or urine assays of female hormones.

Human Chorionic Gonadotropin (hCG) Measurements. Human implantation failures or early pregnancy losses could be recognized if pregnancy tests are used routinely following ovulation. Pregnancy can now be detected as early as 10 days after conception by using radioimmunoassay (RIA) or radioreceptor assay (RRA) to detect the β subunit of human chorionic gonadotropin (hCG) in maternal serum or urine. Although large proportions of conceptuses are lost, little is known about the etiology of these early losses. The rate of spontaneous abortions (later than 28 days after conception) can be studied by examining hospital and other medical records, or by retrospective interviews. It is likely that the incidence of early spontaneous abortion has been significantly underestimated (Wilcox, 1983).

Fertility End-Points. Live births provide one obvious end-point for studying fertility, particularly the fertility of populations. Virtually all live births are routinely registered, so that data are easily obtainable. Still, live births do not represent all pregnancies. As mentioned, many pregnancies end with a miscarriage or stillbirth. Live births also do not separate infertility from preimplantation or early implantation failures. A large amount of fetal loss occurs very early after conception, before pregnancy is even recognized. More than one-third of the pregnancies diagnosed by urine assay terminated before they became clinically apparent (Miller, 1980).

The most precise end-point of fertility would be the incidence of conception. Human chorionic gonadotropin (hCG), produced by the conceptus, can be detected using radioimmunoassays seven to ten days following conception. A serum assay for an "early pregnancy factor," which detects changes in the maternal immune response shortly after conception, is also available for the early detection of conception (Morton *et al.,* 1977; Shaw and Morton, 1980).

The World Health Organization defines primary infertility as the failure of a couple to conceive their first pregnancy after two years without contraception. Secondary infertility occurs when a couple that has had one or more previous pregnancies fails to conceive another after two years without contraception. Primary infertility is as high as 30 percent in areas of the world where gonorrhea, genital tuberculosis, and other infections are prevalent.

Infertile couples are classified into clinical categories: men with abnormal semen analysis; and women with abnormal ovulation, endometriosis, obstructed tubes, and defects of the uterus or cervix. Other causative factors are radiation exposure, genetic disease, chromosomal anomalies, and severe malnutrition. When a large population displays a high degree of infertility with no readily apparent cause, concerns grow regarding the role of drugs and other environmental chemicals.

Extrapolation of Laboratory Data to Humans

The predictiveness of laboratory animal studies for humans is still not generally accepted. However, a great deal of species differences is being accounted for with our increased understanding of pharmacokinetics, especially biotransformation. In the past, there was too little reliance on animal studies to predict human effects. Yet, there are various examples in the literature where animal studies suggested toxic effects that become apparent in humans years later. Examples include the transplacental toxicity of diethylstilbestrol, the carcinogenic effect of the monomer vinyl chloride, and the reproductive toxicity of dibromochloropropane (DBCP). In more recent years, greater predictability has been achieved using well-validated animal models, although success is far from total. There has also been a beginning effort in developing mathematical models based on pharmacokinetic parameters and knowledge of mechanisms of action to aid extrapolation. In the future, computer models based on well-validated mechanisms, structure-activity relationships, pharmacokinetic data, *in vitro* data, and whole-animal models will greatly enhance the reliability of data extrapolation from the laboratory to humans.

Quantitative Assessment

Laboratory and clinical studies seek to identify chemical reproductive hazards and to estimate their human risk. As already discussed, in the laboratory, exposure levels can be regulated, and nearly all stages of the reproductive process can be carefully observed. However, these approaches are obviously limited to nonhuman species. For humans, chemical exposure and fertility effects are much harder to assess, and the results are less certain. Impotence and loss of libido are especially difficult to quantify.

When the chemical being studied is a prescribed drug, medical records may provide documentation of the dose although noncompliance is always a concern. It is even more difficult to estimate exposure to nonprescription drugs and other self-administered substances. Occupational exposures are also inexact, and environmental levels are even more difficult to document. All exposures usually involve mixtures of chemicals, and individuals may not be aware of all the chemicals with which they come into contact. For these reasons, the effect of individual chemicals is difficult to assess, and cause-and-effect relationships are nearly impossible to establish conclusively.

Epidemiologic Studies

Epidemiology is playing an ever-increasing role in evaluating the potential toxicity of environmental agents. Once defined only as that science dealing with the incidence, distribution, and control of epidemic disease, epidemiology has rapidly become an essential part of the process to ensure occupational and environmental safety.

Careful study of selected populations can support a variety of important areas. These include the ability to: validate laboratory studies and increase the reliability of extrapolating laboratory animal data to humans; monitor the effectiveness of established safety standards; warn of unexpected toxic effects associated with certain drugs, chemicals, or procedures; and analyze the natural experiments taking place in our population to help define the potential health hazards associated with such things as artificial sweeteners in soft drinks, preservatives in bacon, and residues of growth-promoting agents in meat. More sensitive indicators of chemical exposures that can provide an early warning of chemically induced disease must be assigned a high research priority.

In the past, epidemiologic studies have been primarily concerned with retrospective studies of disease incidence. Important efforts have been made recently to assess the association between disease incidence and occupational (or environmental) exposure to chemicals. In the future, the approach to epidemiology will be more prospective, looking ahead instead of behind, and the methods will incorporate sensitive early indicators of chemically induced disease to allow for the prediction of disease at its earliest and most readily reversible stage.

When exposure to a chemical has occurred in a human population, or when concern surrounds the use of a certain chemical, epidemiologic approaches may be used to identify effects on reproduction. Epidemiologic investigations are subject to many problems including low statistical power due to small population size, difficulties in defining exposure, bias in reporting, and the multiple end-points to be considered. The design of epidemiologic studies may involve either retrospective or prospective gathering of data. Statistical aspects to be considered in epidemiologic studies include power, sample size, significance level, and the magnitude of the effect.

A number of terms are commonly used in discussions of infertility. Infecundity is the inability to conceive or to impregnate. In medical literature the term infecundity often is synonymous with infertility. For instance, the World Health Organization (WHO) defines infertility as the inability to achieve conception within two years. Pregnancy wastage is the failure to carry a pregnancy to term, including both spontaneous abortion at any stage of pregnancy and stillbirth. Primary infertility means a couple has never achieved conception. Secondary infertility means at least one conception has occurred, but the couple is currently not able to achieve pregnancy. In popular use, the terms primary and secondary infertility also include the inability to carry a pregnancy to term. Sterility implies complete and permanent inability to conceive or impregnate, even after treatment. Childlessness—a common measure of infertility—means that a couple has not produced any children, whether due to infecundity, pregnancy wastage, contraception, or induced abortion. While demographers distinguish between fertility, as childbearing performance, and fecundity, as childbearing ability, medical and popular usage usually equates the two (Population Report, 1983).

Demographic Methods

The probability of pregnancy or birth occurring under defined conditions and within a fixed time can be determined using vital statistics. Efforts have been directed toward estimating fecundity for a population based on the pattern of live births and making some assumptions about fetal loss. The best estimates of fecundity are obtained from data that include either the time required for pregnancy to occur or the number of births within a certain time period. Others have proposed methods based on the intervals between live births or on the time required for conception to occur. These methods produce only rough estimates of fecundity.

The time required for pregnancy to occur can be measured more precisely by asking women the length of the noncontraceptive interval that precedes pregnancy. Nearly all women are able to specify the length of the preceding noncontraceptive interval. However, this approach excludes women who are unable to conceive and underrepresents women whose subfertility leads them to have fewer pregnancies than desired. To avoid this problem, women could be enrolled at the beginning of their noncontracepting interval and followed until they are pregnant.

The effect of selected occupational exposures on live births has been explored. Dobbins *et al.* (1978) have considered the interval between live births. Levine *et al.* (1980, 1981), by standardizing the occurrence of live births by year of birth, race, and maternal age, have estimated an "expected" fertility that is then compared with the test group.

Demographic methods usually necessitate large samples and involve the interpretation of patterns of live births. Their application in occupational settings is fairly recent, and their ability to identify chemicals that affect reproduction has not been clearly determined.

Other Studies

In case control studies, infertile couples can be compared with fertile couples to determine differences in chemical exposure. Particular classes of infertility, such as anovulatory women or men with abnormal semen analysis, may be studied.

The measurement of fertility for women who are being artificially inseminated by donor sperm is possible. Fertility could be estimated by the number of cycles of artificial insemination required before pregnancy occurs. In such a situation, it would be possible to monitor factors such as the times of ovulation and insemination. Wilcox (1983) has also proposed interesting new approaches to measure the capacity to conceive.

CONCLUSIONS

The complicated biologic interactions on which successful mammalian reproduction depend present many targets for toxic chemicals.

During the past decade, laboratory and clinical efforts directed toward identifying and describing those chemicals in our environment that perturb essential molecular and cellular processes and result in morphologic and functional alterations have increased greatly. However, our understanding of the underlying biologic mechanisms of reproductive toxicity remains incomplete, and the predictability of our current test approaches is unsure. But, advances have been made. We now have a clearer understanding of the biologic properties of the various cells and tissues that comprise the male (and female) reproductive systems. We also have a greater appreciation of their unique developmental and chemical susceptibilities. Likewise, our understanding of the events involved in fertilization and implantation phenomena continues to increase. We also know more about the pharmacokinetic factors that determine the amount of active chemical that reaches its site of toxicity, and we understand more about how the organism adapts to a chemical and recovers from damage. We are even beginning to understand the molecular dynamics of the toxic event and its direct and indirect consequences.

REFERENCES

Aafjes, J. H.; Vels, J. M.; and Schenck, E.: Fertility of rats with artificial oligozoospermia. *J. Reprod. Fertil.*, 58:345–51, 1980.

Amann, R. P.: A critical review of methods for evaluation of spermatogenesis from seminal characteristics. *J. Androl.*, 2:37–58, 1981.

Amann, R. P.: Use of animal models for detecting specific alterations in reproduction. *Fund. Appl. Toxicol.*, 2:13–26, 1982.

Amann, R. P.; Johnson, L.; Thompson, D. L., Jr.; and Pickett, B. W.: Daily spermatozoal production, epididymal spermatozoal reserves and transit time of spermatozoa through the epididymis of the rhesus monkey. *Biol. Reprod.*, 15:586–92, 1976.

Amann, R. P., and Lambiase, J. T., Jr.: The male rabbit. III. Determination of daily sperm production by means of testicular homogenates. *J. Anim. Sci.*, 28:369–74, 1969.

Association of Food and Drug Officials of the United States: *Appraisal of the Safety of Chemicals, Foods, Drugs and Cosmetics.* Association of Food and Drug Officials of the United States, Topeka, Kan., 1959.

Austin, C. R.: Recent progress in the study of eggs and spermatozoa: Insemination and ovulation to implantation. In Greep, R. O. (ed.): *Reproductive Physiology*, Vol. 8. University Park Press, Baltimore, 1974.

Barlow, S. M., and Sullivan, F. M.: *Reproductive Hazards of Industrial Chemicals.* Academic Press, London, 1982.

Barraclough, C. A., and Sawyer, C. H.: Blockade of the release of pituitary ovulating hormone in the rat by chlorpromazine and reserpine: Possible mechanisms of action. *Endocrinology*, 61:341–51, 1957.

Bechter, R.; Ettlin, R. A.; and Dixon, R. L.: Assessment of the testicular toxicity associated with anticancer agents. II. Sperm counts and serial mating. *Proc. West. Pharmacol. Soc.*, 25:385–87, 1982.

Belsey, M. A.; Eliasson, R.; Gallegos, A. J.; Moghissi, K. S.; Paulsen, C. A.; and Prasad, M. R. N. (eds.): *Laboratory Manual for the Examination of Human Semen and Semen-Cervical Mucus Interaction.* Press Concern, Singapore, 1980.

Bibbo, M.; Gill, W. B.; Azizi, F.; Blough, R.; Fang, V. S.; Rosenfield, R. L.; Schumacher, G. F. B.; Sleeper, K.; Sonek, M. G.; and Wied, G. L.: Follow-up study of male and female offspring of DES-exposed mothers. *Obstet. Gynecol.,* **49**:1–8, 1977.

Billings, E. L.; Billings, J. J.; and Catarinich, M.: *Atlas of the Ovulation Method,* 3rd ed. Advocate Press, Melbourne, 1977.

Bingham, E. (ed.): *Proceedings Conference on Women and the Workplace.* Society for Occupational and Environmental Health, Washington, D. C., 1977.

Blazak, W. F., and Fechheimer, N. S.: Gonosome-autosome translocations in fowl: Meiotic configurations and chiasma counts from singly and doubly heterozygous cockerels. *Can. J. Genet. Cytol.,* **22**:343–51, 1980.

Bloom, A. D. (ed.): *Guidelines for Studies of Human Populations Exposed to Mutagenic and Reproductive Hazards.* March of Dimes Birth Defects Foundation, White Plains, N.Y., 1981.

Bowman, W. C., and Rand, W. J. (eds.): *Textbook of Pharmacology,* 2nd ed. Blackwell Scientific Publications Ltd., London; C.V. Mosby Co., St. Louis, 1980.

Chapin, R. E.; Norton, R. M.; Popp, J. A.; and Bus, J. S.: The effects of 2,5-Hexanedione on reproductive hormones and testicular enzyme activities in the F-344 rat. *Toxicol. Appl. Pharmacol.,* **62**:262–72, 1982.

Collins, T. F. X.: Reproduction and teratology guidelines: Review of deliberations by the National Toxicology Advisory Committee's reproduction panel. *J. Environ. Pathol. Toxicol.,* **2**:141–47, 1978.

Committee to Revise NAS Publication 1138: *Principles and Procedures for Evaluating the Toxicity of Household Substances.* National Academy of Sciences, Washington, D.C., 1977.

Committee for the Working Conference on Principles of Protocols for Evaluating Chemicals in the Environment: *Principles for Evaluating Chemicals in the Environment.* National Academy of Sciences, Washington, D.C., 1975.

Cordova, T.; Ayalon, D.; Lander, N.; Mechoulam, R.; Nir, I.; Puder, M.; and Lindner, H. R.: The ovulation blocking effect of cannabinoids: structure-activity relationships. *Psychoneuroendocrinology,* **5**:53–62, 1980.

David, G.; Jouannet, P.; Martin-Boyce, A.; Spira, A.; and Schwartz, D.: Sperm counts in fertile and infertile men. *Fertil. Steril.,* **31**:453–55, 1979.

Davies, A. G.: *Effects of Hormones, Drugs and Chemicals on Testicular Function,* Vol. 1. Eden Press, St. Albans, Vt., 1980.

Dixon, R. L. (conf. chrm.): Symposium on target organ toxicity: gonads (reproductive and genetic toxicity). *Environ. Health Perspect.,* **24**:1–127, 1978.

Dixon, R. L.: *Workshop Recommendations: Reproductive Toxicology Workshop.* National Toxicology Program/National Institute of Environmental Health Sciences, Research Triangle Park, N.C., 1980.

——— : Potential of environmental factors to affect development of reproductive systems. *Fund. Appl. Toxicol.,* **2**:5–12, 1982.

Dixon, R. L., and Hall, J. L.: Reproductive toxicology. In Hayes, A. W. (ed.): *Principles and Methods of Toxicology.* Raven Press, New York, 1982.

Dixon, R. L., and Lee, I. P.: Pharmacokinetic and adaptation factors in testicular toxicity. *Fed. Proc.,* **39**:66–72, 1980.

Dixon, R. L., and Lee, I. P.: Pharmacokinetic and adaptive factors as modifiers of testicular toxicity and risk estimation. In Richmond, C. R.; Walsh, P. J.; and Co-

penhaver, E. D. (eds.): *Health Risk Analysis: Proceedings of the Third Life Science Symposium.* Franklin Institute Press, Philadelphia, 1981.

Dobbins, J. G.; Eifler, C. W.; and Buffler, P. A.: The use of parity survivorship analysis in the study of reproductive outcome. *Am. J. Epidemiol.,* **108**:245, 1978.

Dobson, R. L.; Koehler, C. G.; Felton, J. S.; Kwan, T. C.; Wuebbles, B. J.; and Jones, D. C. L.: Vulnerability of female germ cells in developing mice and monkeys to tritium, gamma rays, and polycyclic aromatic hydrocarbons. In Mahlum, D. D.; Sikor, M. R.; Hackett, P. L.; and Andrew, F. D. (eds.): *Developmental Toxicology of Energy-Related Pollutants.* Conference 771017, U.S. Department of Energy Technical Information Center, Washington, D.C., 1978.

Dougherty, R. C.; Whitaker, M. J.; Tang, S.-Y.; Bottcher, R.; Keller, M.; and Kuehl, D. W.: Sperm density and toxic substances: A potential key to environmental health hazards. In McKinney, J. D. (ed.): *Environmental Health Chemistry: Chemistry of Environmental Agents as Potential Human Hazards.* Ann Arbor Science Publishers, Inc., Ann Arbor, Mich., 1981.

Dym, M., and Fawcett, D. W.: The blood-testis barrier in the rat and the physiological compartmentation of the seminiferous epithelium. *Biol. Reprod.,* **3**:300–326, 1970.

Environmental Protection Agency: Proposed guidelines for registering pesticides in the United States; hazard evaluation: humans and domestic animals. *Federal Register,* **43**:(No. 163):37336–403, 1978.

——— : Proposed health effects test standards for Toxic Substances Control Act test rules. *Federal Register,* **44**:(No. 91):27334–75, 1979.

Epstein, S. S.; Arnold, E.; Andrea, J.; Bass, W.; and Bishop, Y.: Detection of chemical mutagens by the dominant lethal assay in mice. *Toxicol. Appl. Pharmacol.,* **23**:288–325, 1972.

Ettlin, R. A.; Bechter, R.; and Dixon, R. L.: Assessment of testicular toxicity associated with anticancer agents. I. Histopathology. *Proc. West. Pharmacol. Soc.,* **25**:381–84, 1982.

Ettlin, R. A., and Dixon, R. L.: Reproductive toxicology. In Mottet, N. K. (ed.): *Environmental Pathology. Chemicals.* Oxford University Press, New York, 1985.

Food and Drug Administration Advisory Committee on Protocols for Safety Evaluations, Panel on Reproduction: Report on reproduction studies in the safety evaluation of food additives and pesticide residues. *Toxicol. Appl. Pharmacol.,* **16**:264–96, 1970.

Food and Drug Administration: Good laboratory practice regulations: proposed rule. *Federal Register,* **49**(210):43530–37, 1984.

Galbraith, W. M.; Voytek, P.; and Ryon, M. G.: *Assessment of Risks to Human Reproduction and to Development of the Human Conceptus from Exposure to Environmental Substances.* National Technical Information Service, Springfield, Va., 1982.

Gellert, R. J.: Uterotrophic activity of polychlorinated biphenyls (PCB) and induction of precocious reproductive aging in neonatally treated female rats. *Environ. Res.,* **16**:123–30, 1978.

Goldenthal, E. I.: *Guidelines for Safety Evaluation of Drugs for Human Use.* Drug Review Branch, Division of Toxicological Evaluation, Bureau of Science, Food and Drug Administration, Washington, D.C., 1966.

Goldman, A. S.: Abnormal organogenesis in the reproductive system. In Wilson, J. G., and Fraser, F. C. (eds.): *Handbook of Teratology.* Vol. 2, *Mechanisms and Pathogenesis.* Plenum Press, New York, 1977.

Gomes, W. R.: Pharmacological agents and male fertility. In Johnson, A. D., and Gomes, W. R. (eds.): *The Testis.* Vol. IV; *Advances in Physiology, Biochemistry, and Function.* Academic Press, Inc., New York, 1977.

Gondos, B.: Development and differentiation of the testis and male reproductive tract. In Steinberger, A., and Steinberger, E. (eds.): *Testicular Development, Structure, and Testicular Function.* Raven Press, New York, 1979.

Hall, J. L.: Relationship between semen quality and human sperm penetration of zona-free hamster ova. *Fertil. Steril.,* **35**:457–63, 1981.

Hammer, R. E., and Mitchell, J. A.: Nicotine reduces embryo growth, delays implantation and retards parturition in rats. *Proc. Soc. Exp. Biol. Med.* **162**:333–36, 1979.

Hansmann, I., and Probeck, H. D.: Detection of nondisjunction in mammals. *Environ. Health Perspect.,* **31**:161–65, 1979.

Heller, C. G., and Clermont, Y.: Kinetics of the germinal epithelium in man. *Recent Prog. Horm. Res.,* **20**:545–75, 1964.

Herbst, A. L.; Ulfedler, H., and Poskanzer, D. C.: Adenocarcinoma of the vagina. Association of maternal stilbestrol therapy with tumor appearance in young women. *N. Engl. J. Med.,* **284**:878–81, 1971.

Hillier, S. G.; Zeleznik, A. J.; Knazek, R. A.; and Ross, G. T.: Hormonal regulation of preovulatory follicle maturation in the rat. *J. Reprod. Fertil.,* **60**:219–29, 1980.

Hoar, R. M.: Comparative female reproductive tract development and morphology. *Environ. Health Perspect.,* **24**:1–4, 1978.

Hodgen, G. D.: Enzyme markers of testicular function. In Johnson, A. D., and Gomes, W. R. (eds.): *The Testis.* Vol. IV, *Advances in Physiology, Biochemistry, and Function.* Academic Press, Inc., New York, 1977.

Hunt, V. R.: *Work and the Health of Women.* CRC Press, Boca Raton, Fl., 1979.

Interagency Regulatory Liaison Group: Notice of IRLG work plans and public meetings. *Federal Register,* **43**:(No. 34):7174–98, 1978.

James, W. H.: Secular trend in reported sperm counts. *Andrologia,* **12**:381–88, 1980.

———: Possible consequences of the hypothesized decline in sperm counts. In Spira, A., and Jouannet, P. (eds.): *Human Fertility Factors (with Emphasis on the Male).* INSERM, Paris, 1982.

Katzenellenbogen, J. A.; Katzenellenbogen, B. S.; Tatee, T.; Robertson, D. W.; and Landvatter, S. W.: The chemistry of estrogens and antiestrogens: relationships between structure, receptor binding, and biological activity. In McLachlan, J. A. (ed.): *Estrogens in the Environment.* Elsevier/North-Holland, New York, 1980.

Kostellow, A. B.; Ziegler, D.; Kunar, J.; Fujimoto, G. I.; and Morrill, G. A.: Effect of cannabinoids on estrous cycle, ovulation and reproductive capacity of female A/J mice. *Pharmacology,* **21**:68–75, 1980.

LeBlond, C. P., and Clermont, Y.: Definition of the stages of the cycle of the seminiferous epithelium of the rat. *Ann. N.Y. Acad. Sci.,* **55**:548–71, 1952.

Lee, I. P.: Adaptive biochemical repair response toward germ cell DNA damage. *Am. J. Industr. Med.,* **4**:135–47, 1983.

Lee, I. P., and Dixon, R. L.: Effects of procarbazine on spermatogenesis studied by velocity sedimentation cell separation and serial mating. *J. Pharmacol. Exp. Ther.,* **181**:219–26, 1972.

Lee, I. P.; Suzuki, K.; and Nagayama, J.: Metabolism of benzo(a)pyrene in rat prostate glands following 2,3,7,8-tetrachlorodibenzo-*p*-dioxin exposure. *Carcinogenesis,* **2**:823–31, 1981.

Levine, R. J.; Symons, M. J.; Balogh, S. A.; Arndt, D. M.; Kaswandik, N. T.; and Gentile, J. W.: A method for monitoring the fertility of workers I. Methods and pilot studies. *J. Occup. Med.,* **22**:781–91, 1980.

Levine, R. J.; Symons, M. J.; Balogh, S. A.; Milby,

T. H.; and Whorton, M. D.: A method for monitoring the fertility of workers. 2. Validation of the method among workers exposed to dibromochloropropane. *J. Occup. Med.,* **23**:183–88, 1981.

Lucier, G. W.; Lee, I. P.; and Dixon, R. L.: Effects of environmental agents on male reproduction. In Johnson, A. D., and Gomes, W. R. (eds.): *The Testis.* Vol. IV, *Advances in Physiology, Biochemistry, and Function.* Academic Press, Inc., New York, 1977.

MacKenzie, K. M.; Lucier, G. W.; and McLachlan, J. A.: Infertility in mice following prenatal exposure to 9,10-dimethyl-1,2-benzathracene (DMBA). *Proceedings of 12th Annual Meeting of the Society for the Study of Reproduction.* Quebec, Canada, 1979.

MacKenzie, K. M., and Angevine, D. M.: Infertility in mice exposed *in utero* to benzo(a)pyrene. *Biol. Reprod.,* **24**:183–91, 1981.

Macleod, J., and Wang, Y.: Male fertility potential in terms of semen quality: a review of the past, a study of the present. *Fertil. Steril.,* **31**:103–16, 1979.

Mann, T., and Lutwak-Mann, C.: *Male Reproductive Function and Semen: Themes and Trends in Physiology, Biochemistry and Investigative Andrology.* Springer-Verlag, New York, 1981.

Matter, R. H.; Bechter, R.; Weber, H.; Ettlin, R.; and Dixon, R.: Differential testicular toxicity associated with anticancer drugs administered during critical periods of postnatal development. *Toxicologist,* **3**:21, 1983.

Mattison, D. R. (ed.): *Reproductive Toxicology.* Progress in Clinical and Biological Research, Vol. 117. Alan R. Liss, Inc., New York, 1983.

Mattison, D. R., and Nightingale, M. S.: The biochemical and genetic characteristics of murine ovarian aryl hydrocarbon (benzo[a]pyrene) hydroxylase activity and its relationship to primordial oocyte destruction by polycyclic aromatic hydrocarbons. *Toxicol. Appl. Pharmacol.,* **56**:399–408, 1980.

Mattison, D. R.; Nightingale, M. S.; and Shiromizu, K.: Effects of toxic substances on female reproduction. *Environ. Health Perspect.,* **48**:43–52, 1983a.

Mattison, D. R.; Shiromizu, K.; and Nightingale, M. S.: Oocyte destruction by polycyclic aromatic hydrocarbons. *Am. J. Industr. Med.,* **41**:191–202, 1983b.

Mattison, D. R., and Thorgeirsson, S. S.: Ovarian aryl hydrocarbon hydroxylase activity and primordial oocyte toxicity of polycyclic aromatic hydrocarbons in mice. *Cancer Res.,* **39**:3471–75, 1979.

Mayer, S. E.: Neurohumoral transmission and the autonomic nervous system. In Gilman, A. G., Goodman, L. G., and Gilman, A. (eds.): *Goodman and Gilman's The Pharmacological Basis of Therapeutics,* 6th ed. Macmillan Publishing Co., Inc., New York, 1980.

McLachlan, J. A., and Dixon, R. L.: Transplacental toxicity of diethylstilbestrol: A special problem in safety evaluation. In Mehlman, M. A.; Shapiro, R. E.; and Blumenthal, H. (eds.): *New Concepts in Safety Evaluation. Advances in Modern Toxicology,* Vol. 1, Part 1. Hemisphere Publishing Co., Washington, D. C., 1976.

McLachlan, J. A.; Newbold, R.; and Bullock, B.: Reproductive tract lesions in male mice exposed prenatally to diethylstilbestrol. *Science,* **190**:991–92, 1975.

McLachlan, J. A.; Newbold, R. R.; Korach, K. S.; Lamb, J. C., IV; and Suzuki, Y.: Transplacental toxicology: prenatal factors influencing postnatal fertility. In Kimmel, C. A., and Buelke-Sam, J. (eds.): *Developmental Toxicology.* Raven Press, New York, 1981.

McLachlan, J. A.; Newbold, R. R.; Shah, H. C.; Hogan, M.; and Dixon, R. L.: Reduced fertility in female mice exposed transplacentally to diethylstilbestrol. *Fertil. Steril.,* **38**:364–71, 1982.

Meistrich, M. L.; Finch, M.; da Cunha, M. F.; Hacker, U.; and Au, W. W.: Damaging effects of fourteen chemotherapeutic drugs on mouse testis cells. *Cancer Res., 42*:122–31, 1982.

Miller, J. F.; Williamson, E; Glue, J.; Gordon, Y. B.; Grudzinskas, J. G.; and Sykes, A.: Fetal loss after implantation: a prospective study. *Lancet, 2*:554–56, 1980.

Ministry of Health and Welfare, Canada, Health Protection Branch: *The Testing of Chemicals for Carcinogenecity, Mutagenecity and Teratogenicity,* The Ministry, Ottawa, 1973.

Mittwoch, U.: *Genetics of Sex Differentiation.* Academic Press, Inc., New York, 1973.

Mori, T.; Kohda, H.; Kinoshita, Y.; Ezaki, Y.; Morimoto, N.; and Nishimura, T.: Inhibition by indomethacin of ovulation induced by human chorionic gonadotrophin in immature rats primed with pregnant mare serum gonadotrophin. *J. Endocrinol., 84*:333–41, 1980.

Morton, H.; Rolfe, B.; Clunie, G. J. A.; Anderson, J. M.; Morrison, J.: An early pregnancy factor detected in human serum by the rosette inhibition test. *Lancet,* 1:394–97, 1977.

Mossman, H. W., and Duke, K. L.: *Comparative Morphology of the Mammalian Ovary.* University of Wisconsin Press, Madison, 1973.

Mukhtar, H.; Lee, I. P.; Foureman, G. L.; and Bend, J. R.: Epoxide metabolizing enzyme activities in rat testes: postnatal development and relative activity in interstitial and spermatogenic cell compartments. *Chem. Biol. Interact., 22*:153–65, 1978a.

Mukhtar, H.; Philpot, R. M.; Lee, I. P.; and Bend, J. R.: Developmental aspects of epoxide-metabolizing enzyme activities in adrenals, ovaries, and testes of the rat. In Mahlum, D. D.; Sikor, M. R.; Hackett, P. L.; and Andrew, F.: *Developmental Toxicology of Energy-Related Pollutants.* Conference 771017, US Department of Energy, Technical Information Center, Washington, D.C., 1978b.

Munro, I. C., and Willes, R. F.: Reproductive toxicity and the problems of *in utero* exposure. In Galli, C. L.; Paoletti, R.; and Vettorazzi, G. (eds.): *Chemical Toxicology of Food.* Elsevier/North-Holland Biomedical Press, New York, 1978.

Nagayama, J., and Lee, I. P.: Comparison of benzo(a)pyrene metabolism by testicular homogenate and the isolated perfused testis of rat following 2,3,7,8-tetrachlorodibenzo-*p*-dioxin treatment. *Arch. Toxicol.,* 51:121–30, 1982.

Namkung, M. J.; Zachariah, P. K.; and Juchau, M. P.: *O*-Sulfation of *N*-hydroxy-2-fluorenylacetamide and 7-hydroxyl-*N*-2-fluorenylacetamide in fetal and placental tissues of humans and guinea pigs. *Drug Metab. Dispos.,* 5:288–94, 1977.

Nisbet, I. C., and Karch, N. J.: *Chemical Hazards to Human Reproduction.* Noyes Data, Park Ridge, N.J., 1983.

Noyes, R. W.,; Hertig, A. T.; and Roch, J.: Dating the endometrial biopsy. *Fertil. Steril., 1*:3–25, 1950.

Oesch, F.; Glatt, H.; and Schmassman, H.: The apparent ubiquity of epoxide hydratase in rat organs. *Biochem. Pharmacol., 26*:603–608, 1977.

Ohno, S.: Sexual differentiation and testosterone production. *N. Engl. J. Med., 295*:1011–12, 1976.

Okumura, K.; Lee, I. P.; and Dixon, R. L.: Permeability of selected drugs and chemicals across the blood-testis barrier of the rat. *J. Pharmacol. Exp. Ther., 194*:89–95, 1975.

Overstreet, J. W.; Price, M. J.; Blazak, W. F.; Lewis, E. L.; and Katz, D. F.: Simultaneous assessment of human sperm motility and morphology by videomicrography. *J. Urol., 126*:357–60, 1981.

Pedersen, R. A., and Brandriff, B.: Radiation- and drug-induced DNA repair in mammalian oocytes and embryos. In Generoso, W. M.; Shelby, M. D.; and

deSerres, F. J. (eds.): *DNA Repair and Mutagenesis in Eukaryotes.* Plenum Publishing Corp., New York, 1980.

Pedersen, T., and Peters, H.: Proposal for a classification of oocytes and follicles in the mouse ovary. *J. Reprod. Fertil., 17*:555–57, 1968.

Perry, J. S.: The ovarian cycle of mammals. In Treherne, J. E. (ed.): *University Reviews in Biology,* Vol. 13. Oliver & Boyd, Edinburgh, 1971.

Pharmaceutical Manufacturers' Association: *Guidelines for the Assessment of Drug and Medical Device Safety in Animals.* The Association, Washington, D.C., February, 1977.

Population Information Program Johns Hopkins University: Infertility and sexually transmitted disease: a public health challenge. *Popul. Rep., 11*:113–51, 1983.

Pruett, J. G., and Winslow, S. G.: *Health Effects of Environmental Chemicals on the Adult Human Reproductive System: A Selected Bibliography with Abstracts 1963–1981.* F.A.S.E.B., Special Publications, Bethesda, Md., 1982.

Purvis, K.; Clausen, O. P. F.; and Hansson, V.: Decreased Leydig cell responsiveness in the testicular feminized male rat. *Endocrinology, 102*:1053–60, 1978.

Rall, D. P., and McLachlan, J. A.: Potential for exposure to estrogens in the environment. In McLachlan, J. A. (ed.): *Estrogens in the Environment.* Elsevier/North-Holland, New York, 1980.

Schmid, B. P.; Hall, J. L.; Goulding, E.; Fabro, S.; and Dixon, R.: *In vitro* exposure of male and female mice gametes to cadmium chloride during the fertilization process, and its effects on pregnancy outcome. *Toxicol. Appl. Pharmacol., 69*:326–32, 1983.

Schrag, S. D., and Dixon, R. L.: Occupational exposure associated with male reproductive dysfunction. *Annu. Rev. Pharmacol. Toxicol., 25*:567–92, 1985.

Sega, G. A.: DNA repair in spermatocytes and spermatids of the mouse. In Bridges, B. A.; Butterworth, B. E.; and Weinstein, I. B. (eds.): *Indicators of Genotoxic Exposure: Banbury Report 13.* Cold Spring Harbor Laboratory, Cold Spring Harbor, N.Y., 1982.

Sega, G. A., and Sotomayor, R. E.: Unscheduled DNA synthesis in mammalian germ cells—its potential use in mutagenicity testing. In de Serres, F. J., and Hollaender, A. (eds.): *Chemical Mutagens—Principles and Methods for Their Detection,* Vol. 7. Plenum Press, New York, 1982.

Setchell, B. P.; Voglmayr, J. K.; and Waites, G. M. H.: A blood-testis barrier restricting passage from blood lymph into rete testis fluid but not into lymph. *J. Physiol., 200*:73–85, 1969.

Shalet, S. M.: Effects of cancer chemotherapy on gonadal function of patients. *Cancer Treat. Rev., 7*:141–52, 1980.

Shani, J.; Amit, M.; and Givant, Y.: Effect of the timing of perphenazine administration on pregnancy in the rat. *J. Endocrinol., 80*:409–11, 1979.

Shaw, F. D., and Morton, H.: The immunological approach to pregnancy diagnosis: A review. *Vet. Rec.,* 106:268–70, 1980.

Shen, R. S., and Lee, I. P.: Developmental patterns of enzymes in mouse testis. *J. Reprod. Fertil., 48*:301–305, 1977.

Sieber, S. M., and Adamson, R. H.: Toxicity of antineoplastic agents in man: chromosomal aberrations, antifertility effects, congenital malformations, and carcinogenic potential. *Adv. Cancer Res., 22*:57–155, 1975.

Smith, M. L.; Luqman, W. A.; and Rakoff, J. S.: Correlations between seminal radioimmunoreactive prolactin, sperm count and sperm motility in prevasectomy and infertility clinic patients. *Fertil. Steril., 32*:312–15, 1979.

Smith, S. E., Jr.: Plastic tube aspiration of the endometrium. *Obstet. Gynecol., 16*:375–76, 1960.

Soyka, L. F., and Joffe, J. M.: Male mediated drug effects on offspring. In Schwartz, R. H., and Yaffe, S. J. (eds.): *Drug and Chemical Risks to the Fetus and Newborn. Progress in Clinical and Biological Research,* Vol. 36. Alan R. Liss, Inc., New York, 1980.

Spira, A., and Jouannet, P. (eds.): *Human Fertility Factors (with Emphasis on the Male).* INSERM, Paris, 1982.

Takizawa, K., and Mattison, D. R.: Female reproduction. *Am. J. Industr. Med.,* 4:17–30, 1983.

Taymor, M. L.: Infertility. In Wintrobe, M. M.; Thorn, G. W.; Adams, R. D.; Braunwald, E.; Isselbacher, K. J.; Petersdorf, R. G. (eds.): *Harrison's Principles of Internal Medicine,* 7th ed. McGraw-Hill Book Co., New York, 1974.

Thompson, E. A., Jr.: The effects of estradiol upon the thymus of the sexually immature female mouse. *J. Steroid Biochem.,* 14:167–74, 1981.

Tuchmann-Duplessis, H., and Haegel, P.: *Illustrated Human Embryology.* Vol. 2, *Organogenesis.* Springer-Verlag, New York, 1974.

Vitale, R.; Fawcett, D. W.; and Dym, M.: The normal development of the blood-testis barrier and the effects of clomiphene and estrogen treatment. *Anat. Rec.,* 176:331–44, 1973.

Vouk, V. B., and Sheehan, P. J. (eds.): *Methods for Assessing the Effects of Chemicals on Reproductive Functions.* John Wiley & Sons, Inc., New York, 1983.

Walsh, D. C., and Egdahl, R. H. (eds.): *Women, Work and Health: Challenges to Corporate Policy.* Springer-Verlag, New York, 1980.

Ways, S. C.; Blair, P. B.; Bern, H. A.; and Staskawicz, M. O.: Immune responsiveness of adult mice exposed neonatally to diethylstilbestrol, steroid hormones, or vitamin A. *J. Environ. Pathol. Toxicol.,* 3:207–20, 1980.

West, J. D.; Frels, W. I.; Papaioannou, V. E.; Karr, J. P.; and Chapman, V. M.: Development of interspecific hybrids of *Mus. J. Embryol. Exp. Morph.,* 41:233–43, 1977.

Wilcox, A. J.: Surveillance of pregnancy loss in human populations. *Am. J. Industr. Med.,* 4:285–91, 1983.

WHO (World Health Organization): *Eleventh Annual Report: Special Programme of Research, Development and Research Training in Human Reproduction.* WHO, Geneva, 1982.

Woods, J. S.: Drug effects on human sexual behavior. In Woods, N. F. (ed.): *Human Sexuality in Health and Illness,* 3rd ed. C. V. Mosby Co., St. Louis, 1984.

Wyrobek, A. J.: Methods for evaluating the effects of environmental chemicals on human sperm production. *Environ. Health Perspect.,* 48:53–59, 1983.

Wyrobek, A. J., and Bruce, W. R.: The induction of sperm-shape abnormalities in mice and humans. In Hollaender, A., and deSerres, F. J. (eds.): *Chemical Mutagens,* Vol. 5. Plenum Press, New York, 1978.

Wyrobek, A. J.; Gordon, L. A.; Burkhart, J. G.; Francis, M. C.; Kapp, Jr., R. W.; Letz, G.; Malling, H. V.; Topham, J. C.; and Whorton, M. D.: An evaluation of the mouse sperm morphology test and other sperm tests in nonhuman mammals. A report of the U.S. Environmental Protection Agency Gene-Tox Program. *Mutat. Res.,* 115:1–72, 1983.

Yoshinaga, K.; Rice,C.; Krenn, J.; and Pilot, R. L.: Effects of nicotine on early pregnancy in the rat. *Biol. Reprod.,* 20:294–303, 1979.

Zaneveld, L. J. D.: Sperm enzyme inhibitors for vaginal and other contraception. *Res. Front. Fertil. Regul.,* 2(3), 1982.

Zeleznik, A. J.; Hillier, S. G.; Knazek, R. A.; Ross, G. T.; and Coon, H. G.: Production of long-term steroid producing granulosa cell cultures by cell hybridization. *Endocrinology,* 105:156–62, 1979.

ACKNOWLEDGMENT

The author acknowledges with sincere gratitude the help of Ms. Vickie Englebright and Ms. Susan Schrag in the preparation of this chapter. Their patience and good nature during the writing and repeated revisions of the manuscript are greatly appreciated. I know that they share with me a hope that those using this chapter will find the reading interesting and the information helpful.

Chapter 17

TOXIC RESPONSES OF THE EYE

Albert M. Potts

INTRODUCTION

To make this chapter both coherent and of moderate size, limits must be put on its scope. It is proposed to treat damage by chemical agents only. Structures dealt with are the globe and its contents, the adnexae, and CNS portions of the visual system only to the end of the retinal ganglion cell neuron in the lateral geniculate body. Major emphasis is on substances demonstrated to be harmful to humans. No distinction will be made between substances that have known therapeutic value and those that have none. It is axiomatic that a substance with pharmacologic activity can be toxic in high doses or when acting on a susceptible subject. Exceptions to these stipulations will be for good cause.

Treatment will emphasize varieties of toxic phenomena and mechanisms where known. Exhaustive treatment of ophthalmic toxicology requires volumes of text. Such texts exist and should be consulted for details on specific substances (see Galezowski, 1878; Uhthoff, 1911; Lewin and Guillery, 1913; Duke-Elder and Mac-Faul, 1972; Grant, 1974; Fraunfelder, 1982). References are also given on ocular anatomy and physiology (Duke-Elder and Wybar, 1961; Davson, 1972; Handbook, 1972–1977).

The eye, despite its small mass, contains derivatives of surface ectoderm (corneal epithelium and conjunctiva) and of mesoderm (choroid, iris, and ciliary body stroma). It contains true neural tissue (the inner retinal layer and optic nerve) and a highly specific light-sensitive modification of neural tissue (the photoreceptors). It contains two relatively large avascular areas (the lens and cornea), which are bounded by unique active transport systems responsible for maintaining a steady state of hydration and hence transparency. It contains a small private cerebrospinal fluid system (the aqueous system) where ciliary body processes are analogous to choroid plexus, where the barrier to circulating blood is as specific as that of the brain, and where the outflow system is so critical that loss of sight is the price of dysfunction. Unique chemical substances in significant concentration are the organ-specific lens proteins; the (at least) four photosensitive pigments; and the avid electron acceptor, melanin, present in ocular tissues at higher levels than anywhere else in the human body. These unique features in a small physical compass make for a multiplicity of types of reactions to injury and a potentially high sensitivity to toxic substances.

CORNEA, CONJUNCTIVA, AND NEIGHBORING TISSUES

Special Considerations

The cornea (Figure 17–1) and its neighboring partial analog, the conjunctiva, are the portions of the eye directly exposed to external insults. The cornea must maintain its transparency to remain functional. A scar, the normal body reparative process, with or without vascularization, is tolerated by other body structures with no adverse effects. In the case of the cornea a scar or vascularization can destroy function completely. Hence a very small amount of corrosive substance—an amount of no consequence elsewhere on the body—can be the cause of blindness if it reaches the cornea.

There is convincing evidence that corneal transparency is maintained by the boundary layers of epithelium and endothelium, which have small mass and relatively high metabolic activity (Maurice, 1969). Thus death of these boundary layers—20 to 25 mg of tissue in the adult eye—is responsible for imbibition of water and loss of transparency. The stoichiometric implications of these minute quantities is impressive.

External Contact Agents

Acids. A splash of acid in the eye is a medical emergency and offers a poor setting for gathering scientific data. We must rely on adequately controlled experimental studies for much of our knowledge of corneal burns. An excellent set of

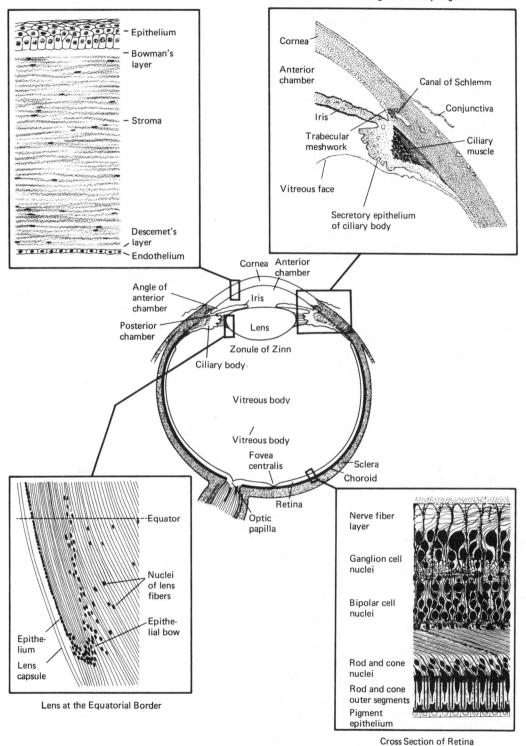

The Cornea

- Epithelium
- Bowman's layer
- Stroma
- Descemet's layer
- Endothelium

Chamber Angle and Ciliary Region

Cornea
Anterior chamber
Canal of Schlemm
Conjunctiva
Iris
Trabecular meshwork
Ciliary muscle
Vitreous face
Secretory epithelium of ciliary body

Cornea
Anterior chamber
Angle of anterior chamber
Iris
Lens
Posterior chamber
Zonule of Zinn
Ciliary body
Vitreous body
Vitreous body
Fovea centralis
Sclera
Choroid
Retina
Optic papilla

Lens at the Equatorial Border

Equator
Nuclei of lens fibers
Epithelial bow
Epithelium
Lens capsule

Cross Section of Retina

Nerve fiber layer
Ganglion cell nuclei
Bipolar cell nuclei
Rod and cone nuclei
Rod and cone outer segments
Pigment epithelium

Figure 17–1. Digrammatic horizontal cross-section of the eye, with medium-power enlargement of details in cornea, chamber angle, lens, and retina. (The enlarged retina diagram [lower right] is taken from Polyak, S.: *The Retina.* University of Chicago Press, Chicago, 1941. By permission of Mrs. Stephen Polyak.)

studies was performed during World War II under the auspices of the Office of Scientific Research and Development and was reported by Friedenwald and coworkers (Friedenwald *et al.*, 1944, 1946). These authors established standard techniques for applying acids (and bases) to the eye and set standards by which damage could be evaluated. Their results bore out the clinical impression that damage by acid was a dual function of pH and of the capacity of the anion in question to combine with protein. Acid burns vary in severity from those that heal completely to those that cause complete opacity or even perforation of the globe.

It has been assumed in the past that the degree of damage seen shortly after an acid burn is an accurate indicator of the eventual result to be expected. In view of some of the new developments in the treatment of alkali burns (see below), it may be that we will treat late acid effects with more success.

Special aspects of some acids complicate the picture. The dehydrating effect of concentrated sulfuric acid as well as the high heat of hydration adds to its acid properties in determining the severity of the burn. The affinity of the anion for the corneal tissue also plays a role in the severity of damage. Friedenwald and coworkers (1946) showed that buffered solutions of picric, tungstic, and tannic acids produced lesions of significant severity in the rabbit eye and with no great differences in severity from pH 1.5 to pH 9.

This effect was in sharp contrast to hydrochloric acid, which caused severe damage at pH 1 with virtually no effect at pH 3 and above. As the pH of buffered solutions applied to the human eye is decreased from 7.4, the onset of discomfort begins at about pH 4.5. Between pH 4.5. and 3.5 one creates punctate breaks in the corneal epithelium that are stainable with fluorescein but heal in a few hours' time.

Another special instance, more of a hazard in the past than in the present, is that of compressed sulfur dioxide. When many industrial refrigeration plants used SO_2 as the refrigerant, eye damage caused by a high-pressure jet of sulfur dioxide was not uncommon. The anhydrous liquid hitting the cornea under pressure not only combines with corneal water to form H_2SO_3 but because of its relative fat solubility it penetrates the cornea into the aqueous and hydrolyzes there causing deep keratitis and iritis. Studies on the mechanism of SO_2 injury were done by Grant (1947).

It is universally agreed that the one best treatment for acid burns is rapid irrigation with large volumes of water. The reduction of concentration, including hydrogen ion concentration, by dilution is most important. Mechanical removal from the site of injury by the stream of water is accomplished simultaneously. Attempts to obtain some special buffered solution or mildly alkaline wash only delay the start of treatment. Washing should begin as close in time and place to the site of the accident as possible. All industrial safety personnel should know this fact and be prepared to begin treatment by washing. Even in the case of concentrated sulfuric acid burns, where it is expected that the addition of water will generate heat, the water wash is best, using a large enough volume and a fast enough rate to dissipate heat as well as wash out acid.

Strong Alkalies—Ammonia, Collagenase. In addition to considerations of pH there are several factors specific to alkali burns. First, alkalies in concentrations that can cause serious eye burns exist in many homes. Household ammonia and sodium hydroxide-containing drain cleaners are the chief offenders. The second problem specific to alkalies is the serious late effects of alkali burns. Even burns that at the time of injury appear to be mild can go on to opacification, vascularization, ulceration, or perforation (Hughes, 1946a, 1946b). The photographs presented in Hughes' experimental paper (Hughes, 1946b) are eloquent on this subject. It should be noted that in experimental animals Hughes produced burns of all degrees of severity by exposure of the cornea to isotonic $N/20$ sodium hydroxide. Exposure for 30 seconds followed by washing caused signs that lasted for several weeks only and usually cleared with no residues. Exposure to the same agent for three minutes followed by washing caused severe early opacification, marked vascularization at three months, and residues of opacity, pigment, and vessels after ten months. Irrigation with $N/20$ NaOH for more than three minutes could cause catastrophic changes in the cornea and surrounding tissues leading to complete opacification and purulent infiltration within a week or ten days with ulceration and perforation.

One of the exceptions to the uniform behavior of alkali cations is that of ammonia. Of all the alkali cations measured, ammonium ion as ammonium hydroxide penetrates epithelium, stroma, and anterior chamber more rapidly than any other. Grant speculates on whether this is due to the fat solubility of nonionized NH_3, to rapid diffusion, or to the ability of NH_4OH to injure corneal epithelium (Grant, 1974). However this may be, it has been shown that ammonia is detectable in the anterior chamber 15 seconds after exposure of the cornea to concentrated NH_4OH (Siegrist, 1920). Uveitis may be an early manifestation in ammonia burns.

The Special Case of Lime Burns. The second

exception to the generalizations about cations is the case of calcium oxide, known popularly as unslaked lime. This substance, a component of Portland cement and of most commercial wall plasters, absorbs water to form calcium hydroxide with the liberation of heat. Calcium hydroxide is sparingly soluble in water, but in solution (saturated solution, 0.15 percent, pH = 12.4) causes the usual alkali burn. In addition to the generation of heat, the special problem in lime burns is that lime, plaster, or cement on reaching the eye tends to react with the moisture and protein found there and form clumps of moist compound, very difficult to remove by the usual irrigation. Such clumps tend to lodge deep in the cul-de-sacs inferiorly and superiorly and act as reservoirs for the liberation of $Ca(OH)_2$ over long periods of time. This is why physicians have been especially concerned about lime burns in the past and why special care must be taken in treatment of this condition. This treatment consists of (Grant, 1974) (1) rapid irrigation, to remove as much material as can be quickly washed away; (2) debridement, to remove physically whatever gross particles of lime can be seen on the cornea and in the cul-de-sacs; and (3) use of a complexing agent, preferably ethylenediaminetetraacetic acid disodium salt (EDTA), to remove the remainder of the $Ca(OH)_2$-generating material that cannot be handled grossly. With observation of these extra requirements lime burns can be made to follow the pattern of other alkali burns.

The Late Effects. The fact that early appearance of an alkali burn is not an adequate guide to prognosis and the possible appearance of infiltration, ulceration, and perforation about a week after the injury have caused much speculation about the mechanism of these late serious sequelae.

New reviews dealing with alkali burns are those of Pfister and Koski (1982) and Reim and Schmidt-Martens (1982). The first reviewers emphasize: (1) delayed epithelial repair after severe stromal burns; (2) rapid and prolonged rise of intraocular pressure secondary to prostaglandin release (Pfister and Burstein, 1976); (3) the release of lytic enzymes, particularly collagenase, from polymorphonuclear leukocytes presumably attracted to the site by the prostaglandins. This chain of events clarifies the finding by Slansky and co-workers (1968), confirmed by Brown et al. (1969), that significant amounts of collagenase are present in alkaliburned cornea. The amount is greater than that present in normal corneal epithelium and was correctly attributed by the Brown group to exogenous neutrophils (1970). The use of locally applied collagenase inhibitors improved the treatment of alkali burns measurably (Brown et al., 1972). (4) The observation that ascorbic acid in the aqueous humor falls to 30 percent of its normal value (normal = 15 to 20 times plasma) in alkali burns (Levinson et al., 1976) has led the Pfister group to postulate that the lower ascorbate causes localized scurvy of the cornea with inhibition of formation of repair collagen (Pfister and Paterson, 1977; Pfister et al., 1978). The two papers cited show significant reduction of corneal ulceration and perforation in alkali-burned rabbits when ascorbate is given subcutaneously or topically. A double-blind clinical trial of ascorbate is now under way.

Important aspects of the second review are: (1) an extended discussion of the appropriateness of anti-inflammatory steroids as therapy in alkali burns and the conclusion—based on Reim's work, and contrary to generally held opinion in the United States—that the use of steroids is indicated; (2) consideration not only of collagenase inhibitors but also of inhibitors of prostaglandin synthesis as therapeutic agents. This introduces the whole category of nonsteroidal antiinflammatory agents, but of these only topical indomethacin is mentioned as having clinical trial. Anderson and co-workers (1982) advocate such a trial for 2-(2-fluoro-4-biphenylyl)propionic acid, Flurbiprofen, on the basis of animal experiments.

An item of additional interest is the report of Nirankari et al. (1981) suggesting that the mechanism of action of ascorbate is as a superoxide radical scavenger and that both superoxide dismutase and ascorbate are effective in preventing ulceration after standard alkali burns.

Adding to the catalog of enzyme activities liberated from neutrophils in the alkali-burned cornea is the report of Chayakul and Reim (1982) on beta-N-acetylglucosaminidase.

Thus, renewed interest in the subject has revealed new mechanisms of injury, which, in turn, point to new therapeutic approaches.

Organic Solvents. Neutral organic solvents such as ethanol, acetone, ethyl ether, ethyl acetate, hexane, benzol, and toluene may contact the eye in industrial or laboratory accidents. These substances have in common their ability to dissolve fats. As a result, they cause pain on contacting the eye, and examination after a generous splash of solvent shows dulling of the cornea. The epithelium will show punctate staining with fluorescein. The damage appears to be scattered loss of epithelial cells due to solution of some of the fats that occur in these cells. The sensation is due to trauma of some of the populous and sensitive corneal nerve endings. Damage is never extensive or long lasting if the splash is at room temperature. Hot solvents of low volatility add the problem of thermal burn to that of solvent action, and the end result is potentially more serious and less predictable.

One must note an industrial hazard introduced by the needs of high technology. Trichlorosilane $(SiHCl_3)$ is used to clean the surface of silicon wafers in the manufacture of microcircuit chips. The solvent has a low flash point; the mixture of its vapors with air is highly explosive; it decomposes violently in contact with water, giving off voluminous HCl-containing vapors with eye burn capability. The report of Hübner and coworkers (1979) deals with a thermal burn plus chemical burn, but serves to underline the existence of the hazard.

Detergents. An increasing number of substances are used in technology as detergents, emulsifying agents, wetting agents, antifoaming agents, and solubilizers. They have the common property of lowering the surface tension of aqueous solutions and they possess discrete nonpolar and polar portions in the same molecule. The nonpolar portion is frequently a long aliphatic chain. The polar portion can be cationic, anionic, or nonionic.

Curiously, there appears to be no relation between surface tension-lowering ability and the amount of damage caused by any given detergent, and the mechanism of damage is not at all clear.

In general, cationic detergents are more damaging than anionic agents and both of these more than nonionics. For a rabbit eye test that has become the FDA standard and for a table of the maximum tolerated concentrations of 23 surface-active agents, see Draize and Kelley (1952). It is remarkable that such tolerated concentrations vary from 0.5 percent for the cationic lauryl dimethyl benzyl ammonium chloride through 20 percent for sodium lauryl sulfate to 100 percent for the nonionic sorbitan mono-laurate or mono-oleate. Note that one-third of the animals in the rabbit test have no washing of the eye after instillation of 0.1 ml of test substance, one-third have the eye washed after two seconds, and one-third have the eye washed after four seconds. A "tolerated concentration" is one in which there is no residual irritation after seven days.

Some of the surface-active agents, especially the cationic substances, in higher concentrations can cause severe burns with permanent opacity and vascularization. In human accidents the immediate severe pain leads to rapid washing out of the eye, and only in the most extreme circumstances will permanent damage result. One exceptional circumstance with hazard potential is that some nonionic detergents actually cause topical anesthesia of the cornea (Martin *et al.*, 1962). It is conceivable that if a formulation contains such a surfactant in combination with an anionic or a cationic detergent, the anesthetic surfactant might eliminate the pain warning and allow severe damage to occur.

Vesicant War Gases. A group of chemical substances have in common the property of causing severe skin burns on contact in very low concentrations. They have been used or their use has been considered as chemical warfare agents—thus the rubric for this section. All of these agents cause severe eye burns on contact with the liquid or vapor. The biochemistry of the "mustard" vesicants was reviewed by Gilman and Phillips (1946) and need not be repeated here. Lawley and Brookes (1965) presented evidence that these alkylating agents reacted selectively with the DNA synthesis mechanism.

Without reference to chemical warfare, a nitrogen mustard is an intermediate in the manufacture of meperidine (Pethidine, Demerol), and eye irritation has been reported among plant personnel (Minton, 1949). Furthermore, numerous variants on nitrogen mustards are now standard therapeutic agents for a number of neoplastic diseases, especially lymphomas and blood dyscrasias. The manufacture and utilization of these drugs will continue to present a finite eye hazard.

Lacrimators and Smog. A number of chemically reactive substances in very high dilution are able to stimulate corneal sensory endings and cause reflex tearing. These contrast sharply with the mustards, which show a long latent period for subjective symptoms and then cause severe damage. The lacrimators in threshold concentrations cause instant sensation and no tissue damage. However, in higher concentrations lacrimators can cause chemical burns with loss of corneal epithelium.

Typical lacrimators are as follows:

α-Chloroacetophenone   α-Brombenzyl cyanide

Ethyl iodoacetate

See Jacobs (1942).

Lacrimator eye damage is complicated by the method of delivery. The two most common forms of delivery are the pencil-like tear-gas gun, purchaseable by individuals in many states, and the aerosol can, used by law enforcement agencies under the trade name Mace. The pencil gun has a charge of powdered α-chloroacetophenone propelled by the equivalent of a 22-

caliber blank cartridge. When the gun is discharged near the eye, the force of the propellant can drive the powdered lacrimator deep into the cornea. The cartridge wadding can also strike the eye with force causing mechanical injury (Levine and Stahl, 1968). The chemical alone causes mechanical damage and its concentration in the eye exceeds the lacrimatory threshold by many, many times. This type of injury may lead to permanent corneal opacity. A similar but less severe injury can result if an aerosol can containing dissolved chloroacetophenone is discharged close to the eye instead of at a distance of several feet or more as recommended by the manufacturer (Thatcher *et al.*, 1971).

The mechanism of action of the lacrimators was investigated during World War II, notably by Dixon (1948) and Macworth (1948). Their investigations showed that whatever the chemical nature of the lacrimator, they all shared the property of inhibiting sulfhydryl enzymes. They had no effect on enzymes not dependent on SH groups for their activity.

There are a few incongruities not well explained by this theory. Iodoacetate is a sulfhydryl reagent but is not a lacrimator. Lewisite is a good sulfhydryl reagent; even under the conditions of the Dixon experiments it combines with 65 percent of the available SH groups; but it is not a lacrimator. The mustards react with SH groups. Whereas this reaction is a slow one and happens in minutes rather than seconds, the latent period for eye symptoms from the mustards is a matter of hours. Dixon himself pointed to another incongruity in the simple sulfhydryl reaction theory. The instant lacrimation on exposure to above-threshold concentration, the rapid cessation of effect on stopping exposure, the resumption of irritation on restoring the lacrimator, all speak against an irreversible combination of agent with critical tissue constituent. Dixon's suggestion that the nerve might respond to a *change* in -SH seems improbable. Recent publications on lacrimators have made no contribution to mechanism of action (Bleckmann and Sommer, 1981; Pfannkuch and Bleckmann, 1982). The whole subject of lacrimators is past due for reinvestigation.

The likely stimulus for such an investigation is the upsurge of an environmental lacrimator that must be dealt with expeditiously. This is photochemical smog. Not to be confused with industrial smog, this entity results from the interaction of automobile exhaust emissions and ultraviolet radiation from sunlight. It was first noticed in the Los Angeles area in the 1940s about the time when the last definitive work on chemical warfare lacrimators reached print.

It is now a major blight in every metropolitan area of the United States. We appear to be dealing with substances formed by ultraviolet-activated oxygen, with oxides of nitrogen, and the olefins, aromatics, and perhaps aliphatic hydrocarbons of automobile exhaust. Of the products the major identified component is the class of peroxyacyl nitrates, which have distinct lacrimator action. This is not the whole story, however, for artificially generated smog used in laboratory studies is several times more active a lacrimator than peroxyacetyl nitrate. For a competent review of this subject, see Jaffe (1967).

Despite increased emission control standards for new cars the smog problem will be with us in the foreseeable future. There will be intensified interest in the whole gamut of lacrimator substances in photochemical smog; how these substances work on the eye; and how the effects can be combatted or prevented. The beneficial fallout from the smog problem may be better understanding of the lacrimators.

Miscellaneous Substances. *Metallic Salts.* Heavy metal ions combine with protein functional groups. In high enough concentration metal salts cause tissue destruction. Thus workers with such materials have the hazard of corneal opacity and ulceration should a splash hit the eye. Adequate protection is indicated.

The more subtle deposition of metal components in the tissues of cornea, conjunctiva, and lids secondary to chronic overuse for therapeutic purposes is a phenomenon of the recent preantibiotic past when heavy-metal salts were the only available antibacterial agents. The tissue discoloration is a striking cosmetic defect. The chief offenders in the United States have been mild silver proteinate and yellow oxide of mercury (Wheeler, 1947; Wilkes, 1953). Outside of the United States there have been reports of argyrosis secondary to a silver-containing eyelash dye (Velhagen, 1953).

Hydroquinone. In many industries a fine dust of particles can be generated and in the absence of adequate exhaust velocity these particles can reach the eye. This set of events can occur in the manufacture of any noxious solid substance. A particularly striking report was that of Anderson (1947) on workers engaged in the manufacture of hydroquinone for many years. The colorless hydroquinone dust on reaching the eye (with a distribution corresponding to the palpebral fissure) oxidizes to brown benzoquinone. This material is stored in large granules in or near the basal layer of the corneal epithelium and in smaller granules in the more superficial epithelium. It is visible as a brown band keratopathy.

Dichloroethane. A remarkable note on species specificity is provided by the reaction of the dog cornea to the systemic administration of 1,2-dichloroethane. Milky-white opacity results after exposure to 1000 ppm for seven hours.

This appears not to be related to direct contact of the eye with the agent but is due to secondary action of the drug or a metabolic product on the corneal endothelium. Of many species of vertebrates tested, only the dog and the fox show the effect. For a report on a number of experiments see the review by Heppel and coworkers (1944).

Lash Lure. In the past when there were few restrictions on the composition of cosmetics in this country, hair dyes and eyelash dyes were sold whose principal ingredient was *p*-phenylenediamine. It was the severe reaction to such a preparation sold under the proprietary name Lash Lure that encouraged more stringent federal regulation. It appears that *p*-phenylenediamine and its analogs can easily sensitize the lid skin and external ocular structures. Continued application of the haptene can cause severe damage to the contacted tissues. Corneal ulceration with loss of vision and even a fatality have been reported. A concentration of papers appeared in the *Journal of the American Medical Association* in 1933 and 1934. For a review, see Linksz (1942).

Corneal Involvement by Internally Administed Substances

Uncommonly a systemic drug may affect the cornea selectively.

Quinacrine. The antimalarial quinacrine (Atabrine) is such a substance, and the effect is corneal edema. A typical report is that of Chamberlain and Boles (1946). This edema was a relatively rare occurrence in the Pacific theater during World War II where some 25 cases were recognized among many thousands of men taking the usual daily 100-mg prophylactic dose. The precise mechanism of action is unclear, though it is tempting to postulate a specific effect on the corneal endothelium.

Chloroquine. A second antimalarial substance affecting the cornea after oral administration is chloroquine. However, just as with the retinal lesions (see below), chloroquine keratopathy is seen chiefly in patients receiving 250 to 500 mg/day for rheumatoid arthritis or systemic lupus. The subjective symptoms are intolerance to glare and halos around lights. At ordinary levels of illumination vision is not impaired. Slit lamp examination shows grayish turbidity in the deep layers of the epithelium. Biopsy has shown that these particles fluoresce; so they are presumably chloroquine or a metabolic product. The involvement disappears on cessation of drug administration. For a good early report, see Calkins (1958). For retinal effects of chloroquine, see below.

Chlorpromazine. The eye effects of chlorpromazine are minimal, but in patients who have received daily doses of 500 mg or more for at least three years granular deposits have been noted on the corneal endothelium and the lens capsule. These findings were first reported by Greiner and Berry (1964) in 12 of 70 patients. DeLong and co-workers (1965) described an additional series of 49 involved patients in a series of 131. In this latter series only patients who received a cumulative dose of 1,000 g or more of the drug showed corneal changes.

Lids and Lacrimal Apparatus

As mentioned in a previous section, the lids are usually involved in heavy-metal pigmentation. Another function that may be disturbed by lid damage is the drainage of tears through the lacrimal puncta at the inner nasal margins of the upper and lower lids. The normal tear flow enters the lacrimal canaliculi in the lid margins via the puncta and continues on through common canaliculus, lacrimal sac, and nasolacrimal duct into the nasopharynx. Action of any of the corrosives discussed above can cause scarring shut of the puncta or canaliculi or both with obstruction of tear flow and annoying epiphora—tears running down the cheek. Indeed the scar need not even obstruct the drainage system. If it distorts lid position enough so that the lacrimal punctum is everted and no longer in contact with the tear film, this is enough to cause epiphora. Because the drainage system of the upper lid is often inefficient, sometimes involvement of the lower lid alone is enough to cause epiphora. Other effects of scarring can be turning in of the lids (entropion) with abrasion of the cornea by eyelashes. Turning out of the lids (ectropion) can cause desiccation of the cornea if it is exposed. The surgical correction of these scarring effects is difficult and not uniformly successful.

One medication that has the property of lowering intraocular pressure was found after ten years of general use to block the lacrimal drainage system. The structure of the drug, furfuryl trimethyl ammonium iodide (Furmethide), is as follows:

$$\text{O} \quad \text{CH}_2\text{N(CH}_3)_3\text{I}^-$$

It was introduced to ophthalmic practice by Meyerson and Thau (1940) and was used in 10 percent solution for cases of intractable glaucoma until the report of Shaffer and Ridgway in 1951 described numerous cases of lacrimal obstruction in patients who used the drug continuously for three months or more. The obstruction was caused by nonspecific inflammatory tissue. Biopsy showed such inflammation in conjunctiva and at multiple points in the lacrimal drainage system.

The toxicology of the sclera is peculiar in that for practical purposes it does not exist. Externally applied corrosives reach the cornea before the sclera. Since loss of transparency of the cornea is accomplished by relatively low concentrations of corrosives and since cornea and sclera are equally susceptible to extreme burns that might cause perforation, selective scleral damage by corrosives just does not happen. Similarly, when collagen synthesis is inhibited as in lathyrism, the greater exposure of the cornea makes it more susceptible to perforation, other things being equal.

The very real threat of cicatricial lid disease posed by the beta-adrenergic blocker Practolol has turned out to be a property of that drug and not of the group as a whole. In the United States propranolol has been used without reliably reported adverse ocular effects. Timolol (Timoptic), a topically applied beta blocker, has proved an effective antiglaucoma medication with minimal ocular side effects.

Practolol

Propranolol

Timolol

In a limited number of patients practolol causes an "oculocutaneous syndrome" with atrophy of the lacrimal gland, corneal ulceration, and even corneal perforation. Because of its appearance and immunologic behavior the syndrome has been called ocular cicatricial pemphigoid (Van Joost et al., 1976).

Elevated antinuclear antoantibodies have been demonstrated in two laboratories (Garner and Rahi, 1976; Jachuck et al., 1977).

Considering the structure of practolol versus that of innocuous propranolol, it would appear

that the β-blocking property is conferred by N-isopropyl propanolamine side chains, etherlinked to an aromatic nucleus. This suggests that the disease-producing property of practolol resides in the dissimilar portion of the molecule. The p-acetamidophenol of practolol suggests similarity to the sulfonamide moiety, which can cause the oculocutaneous syndrome Stevens-Johnson disease.

Apparently unrelated to hypersensitivity is the cicatricial ectropion reported to occur secondary to prolonged systemic 5-fluorouracil therapy (Straus et al., 1977). The condition is reversible on stopping the drug.

THE IRIS, AN INDICATOR OF AUTONOMIC ACTIVITY

Peripheral Effects

The special aspect of the iris (Figure 17-1) for pharmacology is its double innervation (sympathetic for dilator and parasympathetic for sphincter) and its being behind a transparent window, the cornea. Thus as one would expect, sympathomimetic and parasympatholytic substances dilate the pupil and parasympathomimetic and sympatholytic substances constrict the pupil—events easily observed in the intact subject. Allowing for the poor ocular penetration of very polar substances and for the coexistence of centrally initiated impulses, the pupil is an excellent indicator of autonomic activity of topically or systemically administered drugs and poisons.

The eye effects of extracts of mandragora and hyoscyamus were known to Galen in the second century A.D. These effects in sixteenth-century Venice gave rise to the plant name belladonna (Matthiolus, 1598). The early experiments of Thomas Fraser on physostigma (Fraser, 1863) and those of T. R. Elliott on epinephrine (Elliott, 1905) utilized observations of the iris in intact animals.

The greatest potential, happily unrealized, for observation of these types of effects in human toxicology is from the effects of so-called "nerve gases" in combat. All of these substances are so-called "irreversible" cholinesterase inhibitors. Diisopropyl fluorophosphate is an early synthesized example of such compounds. The acetylcholine constantly manufactured at cholinergic nerve endings and unhydrolyzed by normally present cholinesterase causes pupillary constriction in poisoning by these substances.

Since World War II, such cholinesterase inhibitors have been synthesized as insecticides. An occasional accidental toxic episode has been reported—usually concerning a worker standing in a field being dusted with insecticide from an airplane. Further, the pilot of such a plane may experience visual symptoms from the same cause (Upholt *et al.*, 1956).

A somewhat odd iris effect has been labeled "cornpicker's pupil." It is mydriasis caused by operating farm machinery in a cornfield containing jimson weed, *Datura stramonium*. Enough hyoscyamine and related parasympatholytic substances from the plant reach the eye to dilate the pupil over a period of days (Goldey *et al.*, 1966).

It is understood that accidental poisoning by any of the agents in the autonomic group will, if severe enough, cause pupillary signs that may be helpful in establishing a diagnosis.

Central Effects

Not all pupillary changes due to toxic substances are demonstrably direct effects on the iris. The markedly constricted pupil characteristic of morphine poisoning appears to be due to central reinforcement of the physiologic light reflex. Constriction of the pupil caused by morphine is abolished by section of the optic nerve. The consensual reflex caused in the optic nerve-sectioned eye by light stimulation of the intact eye is enhanced by systemic administration of morphine. There is a small residual pupillary constriction caused by morphine in the absence of light. This may be direct action on the pupillary constrictor center or on the muscle itself, but this effect is small in comparison to light reflex enhancement (McCrea *et al.*, 1942).

Similarly, any drug effects observed in the alert animal are algebraically additive with centrally originating reflexes such as sympathetic dilation in the startle reflex, or pupillary constriction that accompanies concentration on a near object. These tend to be transient and are able to be sorted out from toxic drug effects. Similarly, the effects of general anesthetics in first constricting, then dilating, the pupil are superimposed on other pharmacologic and toxicologic effects.

Inflammatory Iris Reactions

The highly vascular iris is quite sensitive to physical and chemical trauma. Its response to all types of insults is nonspecific and consists primarily of increase in vascular permeability. The result of this is, first, liberation of protein into the normally low-protein aqueous humor. Both serum proteins and fibrin can enter the anterior chamber, and fibrin coagulum can eventually cause blockage of outflow of the aqueous humor (see below). The second reaction to insult is

entry of leukocytes from inflamed iris vessels into the aqueous humor. Subsequent fibroblast metaplasia is again a threat to the aqueous outflow system.

Any of the corrosive substances discussed earlier can cause iritis if they reach the cornea in sufficient concentration to penetrate the anterior chamber or if they rapidly destroy the corneal epithelial barrier and then penetrate. In a special category are the relatively fat-soluble bases like ammonia and pyridine and acids or acid anhydrides such as sulfur dioxide, acetic acid, and acetic anhydride. These penetrate intact corneal epithelium rapidly and reach the iris in concentrations high enough to cause iritis.

The ciliary body (see below) is a pigmented vascular structure, protected by the iris from initial assault by harmful substances penetrating the cornea, but susceptible to leakage of protein and leukocytes if sufficient concentrations of noxious agent reach it. The vessels of iris plus ciliary body constitute the "blood-aqueous barrier." Evidence is adequate to implicate prostaglandins in the disruption of this barrier by corrosive substances or, more gently, by rapid lowering of the intraocular pressure. The latter experimental situation was used by VanHaeringen *et al.* (1982) to test the effectiveness of nonsteroidal anti-inflammatory agents, presumably in their role as inhibitors of prostaglandin synthesis.

Some insults to the iris are severe enough to cause loss of cellular integrity. This is most easily observable as liberation of melanin granules from the highly pigmented posterior iris epithelium into the aqueous humor. These granules may contribute to blockage of the aqueous outflow channels with consequent secondary glaucoma. The deposits on corneal endothelium and anterior lens capsule caused by high doses of phenothiazines resemble very tiny pigment granules. It seemed on personal observation that the white granules reported by others were diffraction halos around the tiny pigment particles as seen in the slit lamp. The remarkable storage of phenothiazines in the pigmented structures of the eye has already been reported (Potts, 1962). It seems highly probable, in view of this storage and in view of the fact that the chlorpromazine opacities are confined to surfaces bathed by the aqueous humor, that (1) the drug is responsible for very chronic and very low-grade loss of posterior pigment epithelial cells of the iris and (2) the pigment granules liberated from these cells accumulate on corneal endothelium and lens capsule and even may be eventually incorporated into these structures, giving rise to the clinical effects of chlorpromazine on the anterior segment.

THE AQUEOUS OUTFLOW SYSTEM

General Considerations

As was mentioned at the beginning of this chapter, the eye, a small segregated portion of the central nervous system, has its own equivalent of the cerebrospinal fluid system. Disturbances of this system are as disastrous to the eye as disturbances of the cerebrospinal fluid system are to the brain. The ocular equivalent of cerebrospinal fluid is the aqueous humor, which is actively secreted into the posterior chamber by the double epithelial layer covering the ciliary processes (Figure 17–1). The aqueous humor flows between the posterior surface of the iris and the anterior lens surface, enters the anterior chamber through the pupillary aperture, and leaves the eye at the anterior chamber angle via the trabecular meshwork, the canal of Schlemm, and the aqueous veins (Figure 17–1). Although pathways have not yet been worked out completely, there appears to be a homeostatic mechanism that maintains normal intraocular pressure within the physiologic limits of approximately 10 to 22 mm Hg. However, the mechanism does not have the capacity for 100 percent modulation, for when the aqueous outflow system becomes severely incompetent due to disease, aqueous secretion is not shut off and intraocular pressure rises. When this pressure exceeds 28 to 30 mm Hg, ischemic damage occurs to the optic nerve fibers just before they pierce the lamina cribrosa to exit from the eye. This damage due to increased intraocular pressure is glaucoma and may lead to complete blindness unless treated.

There are two major mechanisms by which glaucoma may originate. The first involves gradual diminution of the ability of the trabecular meshwork—canal of Schlemm system to pass fluid as with the inflammatory changes discussed in the previous section. This type of disease is characterized by insidious rise in pressure into the 30-to-40-mm-Hg range, absence of pain, and slow loss of peripheral visual field usually unnoticed by the patient. This type of disease is known as "chronic simple glaucoma" or "chronic open-angle glaucoma." When it follows an identifiable inflammatory episode such as a chemical burn it may be called "secondary" but it is still in the open-angle glaucoma category. The second mechanism is operative only in certain susceptible individuals who because of an inherited narrow chamber angle, or an angle narrowed by a swelling cataractous lens, can experience sudden and complete occlusion of the chamber angle filtration system by the most peripheral portion of the iris on iris dilation (cf. Figure 17–1). This type of disease is characterized by rapid rise in intraocular pressure to 60, 70, or even 100 mm Hg, severe pain, conjunctival and deep scleral injection, and rapid loss of vision. This type of disease is known as "acute congestive" or "angle-closure" glaucoma.

Open-Angle Glaucoma

Glaucoma of the first type, open-angle glaucoma, can occur secondary to any toxic inflammation. Burns by acid, alkali, and vesicant gases have been documented as initiators of open-angle disease (Duke-Elder, 1969). A more unusual cause of open-angle glaucoma is "epidemic dropsy" reported from India. Individuals show edema of the extremities, gastrointestinal disturbances, cardiac hypertrophy as well as glaucoma (Maynard, 1909). The occurrence has been attributed to contamination of cooking oil by oil from the seeds of Argemone mexicana and the offending agent has been said to be the alkaloid sanguinarine from the argemone oil (Sarkar, 1926; Sarkar, 1948). Claims have been made in the past that the disease could be reproduced in experimental animals by argemone oil and by sanguinarine administration (Hakim, 1954). A recent reevaluation of the problem suggests that administration of sanguinarine orally, intravenously, or by cardiac puncture to rabbits, cats, and chickens does not reproduce the effects of epidemic dropsy; however, administration of argemone oil to chickens does cause edema of wattles (Dobbie and Langham, 1961). There seems little question that the disease is attributable to contaminated cooking oil. One of the problems is that since the first reports of epidemic dropsy the term "sanguinarine" has changed its meaning from an impure mixture of substances obtained from Sanguinaria canadensis, the Canadian bloodroot (Dana, 1828), to a pure chemical substance—a naphthaphenanthridine alkaloid (Manske, 1954). It is by no means impossible that in this process the actual toxic agent of argemone oil has been lost and that we have been defeated by a change in semantics. Thus, although sanguinarine is probably not the toxic agent, some component of argemone oil is. This does not make the problem less real or less deserving of reinvestigation.

Another type of open-angle glaucoma that has been recognized only recently is that caused by long-term topical administration of anti-inflammatory corticosteroids for eye disease (François, 1961; Goldmann, 1962; Armaly, 1963). Armaly showed further that eyes already glaucomatous had greater rises in intraocular tension after corticoids than did normal eyes. Not only can steroid glaucoma be caused by topical application to the eye, but it may be caused by systemic administration as well (see Bernstein et *al.*, 1963a, for early literature references). The additional hazard with systemic administration is that therapy for allergic, rheumatic, and other disease will not be conducted by an ophthalmologist, and the idea of checking intraocular pressure or visual field may not occur to the physician until severe damage has occurred.

Angle-Closure Glaucoma

The second type of glaucoma, angle-closure glaucoma, can be induced in an individual who is susceptible because of a genetically narrow anterior chamber angle or who has an angle narrowed by intraocular changes. This disease is frequently iatrogenic and the precipitating event is often mydriasis for eye examination or for the treatment of iritis. The most commonly offending drug is atropine because of the effectiveness of its action and its difficult reversibility. However, any mydriatic can be the precipitating cause and all have been implicated at one time or another. For a partial list, see Duke-Elder (1969).

THE CILIARY BODY

The ciliary body, which lies just posterior to the root of the iris (Figure 17–1), is a structure with dual function. By means of the collagenous zonular fibers that stretch from lens to ciliary processes the ciliary body acts as the structure physically supporting the lens. Increase in tension of the radially directed and parasympathetically innervated ciliary muscle allows the tension on the zonular fibers to relax. This in turn allows the natural elasticity of the lens capsule to make the lens more spheric and to change the focus of the retinal image from distant to near objects. This is the mechanism of accommodation that is stimulated by parasympathomimetic agents and paralyzed by parasympatholytic agents. Thus in poisoning by cholinesterase inhibitors the small pupil caused by action of acetylcholine on the iris sphincter is accompanied by spasm of accommodation due to action on the ciliary muscle. This causes blurring of distant objects that were previously in focus. The converse is true in atropine poisoning. The pupil is wide and accommodation is paralyzed making it difficult to see near objects. When atropine or other parasympatholytics are used as medication in gastrointestinal disease, it is rare that the dose is high enough to cause measurable pupillary effects. However, it is not uncommon, particularly in a patient whose accommodation is already limited by presbyopia, that the medication will cause discomfort in near vision.

There are numerous medications said to cause blurring of vision where the mechanism of action is less understandable. One such instance is the blurring experienced from large doses of phenothiazines. It appears to be possible, at least, that the blurring described is due to ciliary muscle weakness secondary to very high concentrations of the drug in ciliary body due to storage of the polycyclic phenothiazine on melanin pigment in the ciliary body.

The second function of ciliary body depends on its vascularity and on the two specialized layers of epithelium that cover it. The epithelium secretes aqueous humor at the rate of approximately 1 μl/min. Although it is problematic whether any substance can increase aqueous secretion, there is evidence that both epinephrine and carbonic anhydrase inhibitors such as acetazolamide can decrease aqueous humor formation. Diuretics based on the property of carbonic anhydrase inhibition can lower intraocular pressure as a side effect, but there is no record of any of them causing serious difficulty such as phthisis bulbi.

THE LENS

Description

Normal Function and Composition. The lens (Figure 17–1) is an avascular, transparent tissue surrounded by an elastic, acellular, collagenous capsule. It has the property of acting with the transparent cornea as an essential element in the image-forming system of the eye.

The lens is composed of only a single cell type and continually grows throughout life without losing a single cell; growth rate is inversely related to age. The lens can be arbitrarily divided into its anterior and posterior parts with an equatorial region separating the two. On the anterior or corneal side, lying just beneath the capsule, is a layer of cuboidal epithelial cells: the only area where the cells possess the organelles typically found in all cells. The epithelial cells undergo mitosis and migrate toward the equatorial region where they elongate into fibers, become layered over older fibers, and continue migrating toward the anterior and posterior poles. Consequently, the major portion of the lens is composed of long, thin fibers that have a hexagonal cross-section and form closely packed, onion-like layers. The oldest fibers occupy the center of the lens or nucleus, while younger fibers surrounding the nucleus occupy the area known as the cortex. The most superficial cortical cells possess some cytoplasmic organelles, but as the cells continue to differentiate, these organelles gradually disappear, giving way to a low-density fibrillar material, which in turn allows greater transparency. The tips of the fibers differentiating from either side of the anterior pole eventually join and form a special arrangement called suture lines.

Water and protein are the primary chemical constituents of the lens (Paterson, 1972). The fibers are mostly composed of the soluble proteins α-, β-, and γ-crystallins and the insoluble protein albuminoid. These proteins are unique in being organ specific, not species specific, immunologically. With such a great proportion of protein, it is not surprising that the lens actively synthesizes proteins; in fact, lenticular growth and development depend on a continuous and abundant supply of biosynthetic proteins (Waley, 1969). Protein synthesis may also be the prime consumer of energy generated in the lens, which is necessary in the synthetic mechanics itself and in actively transporting amino acids against a concentration gradient from the aqueous humor into the epithelium (Kuck, 1970b).

Maintenance of an ionic equilibrium with a high intracellular K^+/Na^+ ratio through active transport of K^+ across the epithelium into the lens and Na^+ out of the lens expends a large quantity of energy. The flow of these ions through the lens has been attributed to the existence of a "pump-leak" mechanism (van Heyningen, 1969; Kuck, 1970b; Paterson, 1972). The high level of K^+ in the lenticular epithelium as a result of active transport from the aqueous humor favors diffusion of K^+ along a concentration gradient across the posterior capsule and into the vitreous. On the other hand, high vitreal content of Na^+ favors diffusion of Na^+ in the opposite direction proceeding toward the epithelial cell layer where it is actively transported out of the lens and into the aqueous humor. The enzyme presumed to be associated with active transport, Na^+- and K^+-activated adenosine triphosphatase, is almost exclusively located in the epithelium. The energy necessary to drive active transport and other endergonic reactions is derived from the metabolism of glucose and primarily from anaerobic glycolysis (van Heyningen, 1969; Kuck, 1970b). However, glucose degradation via the Krebs cycle with subsequent synthesis of ATP by the mitochondrial respiratory chain located solely in the anterior epithelium and superficial cortical fibers may possibly contribute as much as 30 percent to the total lenticular energy output (van Heyningen, 1969; Trayhurn and van Heyningen, 1971a, 1971b).

Other biochemical reactions important to lenticular metabolism include nucleic acid synthesis in areas undergoing mitosis, pentose shunt pathway supplying reduced nicotinamide adenine dinucleotide phosphate, sorbitol pathway, and the α-glycerophosphate cycle. Other cellular constituents include small amounts of lipids and glycoproteins, ophthalmic acid, and a relatively large quantity of reduced glutathione, whose role in lenticular metabolism has not been fully evaluated. Small amounts of Ca^{2+} are also necessary to maintain membrane integrity.

Cataract

Normal lenses are transparent permitting light to pass through and allowing it to be focused on the retina. Transparency is dependent not only on the highly ordered cellular arrangement, but also on fiber size, uniformity of dimension and shape, molecular structure, and regularity of packing (Kuck, 1970a, 1970c). In fact, the primary function of lenticular metabolism appears to be directed toward maintaining this organized structure and resulting transparency. Interference with normal lens metabolism, interference with active transport across the cell boundaries, breakage of the lens capsule, and many other types of insult cause alteration in optical properties. Such alterations take various morphologic appearances. Layers of cells in anterior or posterior cortex can change refractive index, the axial lens nucleus can change refractive index, or the anterior or posterior subcapsular layers can change refractive index. Although in medical jargon these changes are termed "opacities," they merely represent the change from perfect transparency to translucency. The result is that image quality in the optical system of the eye deteriorates and visual acuity falls. All such changes, whatever the cause, are lumped under the common term "cataract." Cataracts can be caused by a variety of unrelated circumstances (van Heyningen, 1969), for example, senile cataract due to age, congenital cataracts possibly related to immunologic or pathologic infections, inborn errors of metabolism such as in galactosemia, endocrine cataracts as in diabetes, and drug-induced cataracts. It is this latter category that will be described here, although similarities in mechanism may exist in all the above classes.

2,4-Dinitrophenol. In addition to a variety of toxic effects, systemic administration of 2,4-dinitrophenol (DNP) causes cataracts in some individuals. The classic instances of human dinitrophenol poisoning occurred during 1935 to 1937 when the substance was introduced as an antiobesity agent and was sold without prescription. Several hundred human cataracts resulted. For a review of these events, see Horner (1942). Lenticular opacity first develops in the anterior capsule and eventually spreads to include the cortex and the nucleus. Although cataracts may not develop until after months of treatment or until after drug withdrawal, the subcapsular and the posterior poles of the lens are the more severely affected. Vision is not immediately hindered but rapidly deteriorates as the cataract develops.

Experimental animals are insensitive to the cataractogenic activity of DNP, with the exception of young fowl and rabbits. A reversible cataract can be induced in chicks within one hour after systemic treatment. Analysis of aqueous humor, vitreous humor, and lens after a dose of DNP indicated a higher DNP concentration present in the young animal than in the adult, suggesting a possible explanation for both species and age sensitivity for DNP cataractogenic activity (Gehring and Buerge, 1969b). Within four to six hours after feeding a diet containing 0.25 percent DNP, vacuolization of the anterior lens can be induced in ducklings and chicks. *In vitro* incubation of lens with DNP forms cataracts (Gehring and Buerge, 1969a), with an increase in sodium influx and potassium efflux and swelling prior to cortical opacification (Ikemoto, 1971).

The cataractogenic activity of DNP may be related to its ability to uncouple oxidative phosphorylation, that is, inhibiting ATP synthesis without influencing electron transfer along the mitochondrial respiratory chain. Although experimental studies with other species indicate that lens metabolism is essentially anerobic, with ATP synthesis depending on glycolysis and therefore insensitive to DNP, mitochondrial oxidative phosphorylation in the epithelial cells may play a greater role in ATP synthesis in fowl and human lenses (Kuck, 1970b). As with any cell, removal of sodium ions from the lenticular cells may be the major energy utilizing reaction, in order to maintain proper ionic balances (Trayhurn and van Heyningen, 1971b). Other inhibitors of mitochondrial respiration, such as cyanide and amytal, also lead to increases in lenticular sodium content, which would be followed by decreases in ATP concentration, swelling, and opacification of the fibers.

Steroids. The first controlled study on the cataractogenic activity of corticosteroids was reported in 1960 (Black *et al.*, 1960). Thirty-nine percent of patients receiving prolonged therapy with either cortisone, prednisone, or dexamethasone for rheumatoid arthritis developed posterior subcapsular cataracts. A good correlation existed between cataract formation and dose and duration of therapy. No cataracts were observed in patients receiving low doses for a year or longer and medium or high doses for less than a year. In this study, there was no serious impairment of vision. Further investigation revealed that corticosteroid-induced cataracts could be distinguished by clinical morphology from cataracts caused by diabetes, 2,4-dinitrophenol, and trauma, but could not be distinguished from cataracts caused by intraocular disease and ionizing radiation (Oglesby *et al.*, 1961b). Later reports confirmed the etiology and morphology and a correlation was clearly established between the incidence of posterior subcapsular opacities and having received 15 mg of prednisone per day or equivalent for a year or longer (Oglesby *et al.*, 1961b; Crews, 1963; Williamson *et al.*, 1969; Williamson, 1970). In contrast, four children developed posterior subcapsular cataracts after receiving 1 to 3 mg of prednisolone or equivalent dose of paramethazone for only three to ten months, suggesting either a genetic or an age-dependent sensitivity (Loredo *et al.*, 1972). The clinical progression of the posterior subcapsular opacity has been graded I to IV by Williamson and co-workers (1969). Once vacuoles have formed, they are not reversible even if the drug is withdrawn during the early phases of opacification, although further progression to advanced stages will not occur (Lieberman, 1968). Grade III has been established as the point where visual difficulties become evident and vacuole extension into the cortex will progress in spite of drug withdrawal (Williamson, 1970). Similar findings have been reported after topical administration of corticosteroids (Becker, 1964). A useful review is that of Lubkin (1977).

Experimentally, steroidal cataracts were first observed in two out of four rabbits receiving 2 mg of betamethasone subconjunctivally for 41 weeks (Tarkkanen *et al.*, 1966). Long-term topical administration of several steroids also caused lenticular changes that were confined to the anterior subcapsular and cortical areas (Wood *et al.*, 1967) and therefore different from human cataracts. In contrast, short- or long-term systemic administration of prednisone or prednisolone did not result in cataracts when administered alone, although it did potentiate the cataractogenic activity of 2,4-dinitrophenol (Bettman *et al.*, 1964) and galactose (Bettman *et al.*, 1968), but not xylose, triparanol, or radiation. Betamethasome, applied topically, did enhance the formation of galactose cataracts (Cotlier and Becker, 1965).

The mechanism of steroid-induced cataracts has not been sufficiently investigated. *In vitro* studies (Ono *et al.*, 1971, 1972b) indicated that the lens can not only accumulate cortisol but also biotransform it to its sulfate and glucuronide conjugates. Cortisol also binds to the soluble proteins β-crystallin and α-crystallin (Ono *et al.*, 1972b). Alterations in Na^+ and K^+ ion transport have been reported resulting in increased hydration of the lens (Harris and Gruber, 1962). Inhibition of synthesis of lenticular proteins has been suggested as a possible mechanism of steroidal cataracts (Ono *et al.*, 1972a). It has been known since the work of Axelsson and Holmberg (1966) that long-acting cholinesterase inhibitors cause anterior and posterior subcapsular cataracts. This has been amply confirmed in humans and in monkeys (Shaffer and Hetherington, 1966; Kaufman *et al.*, 1977a). The mechanism of cataractogenesis is unknown. A new and curious finding is that topical application of atropine prevents the experimental cataract in monkeys (Kaufman *et al.*, 1977b).

Chlorpromazine. It was noted in the cornea section above that pigment granules appear on the anterior lens surface as well as the corneal endothelium in individuals who have received large doses of chlorpromazine over long periods of time. Although these granules are almost certainly exogenous to the lens in origin, they become incorporated into lens substance and cause loss of transparency. By these criteria this phenomenon is cataract and should be mentioned here.

Thallium. The soluble salts of thallium acetate and thallium sulfate have been used as insecticides, as rodenticides, and, at one time, as a systemic or topical depilatory agent. Thallous ion (Tl^+) is readily absorbed through the skin or gastrointestinal epithelium. Ingestion or application causes a variety of toxic symptoms, such as disturbances of the gastrointestinal tract, hair loss, polyneuritis of feet and legs, weakness or paralysis of the legs, psychic disturbances, neuritis of the optic nerve (described below), and, in rare instances, cataracts Duke-Elder, 1969; (Grant, 1974). Thallium acetate induces cataracts in rats within six weeks after initiating a daily dose of 0.1 mg, appearing first as radial striations in the anterior cortex between the sutures and the equator. While the early phases will remain stationary if thallium administration ceases, development of subcapsular opacities will occur if administration continues. Microscopic examination reveals areas of proliferation or deletion of subcapsular epithelium and accumulation of a homogeneous or granular material axially to the fibers (Duke-Elder, 1969). The nuclear region is spared.

Thallous ion rapidly accumulates in the lens both *in vivo* (Potts and Au, 1971) and *in vitro* (Kinsey *et al.*, 1971) possibly by an active transport mechanism dependent on the action of Na^+-K^+-ATPase. Thallium especially accumulates in those tissues with high K^+ levels, suggesting a competition for the same cellular transport mechanisms. In fact, thallium substitutes for potassium in many enzymes requiring K^+ for activity, but is effective at a concentration ten times lower than is needed for K^+. Examples of some enzymes studied are the following: (1)

brain K^+-activated phosphatases (Inturrisi, 1969a), (2) brain microsomal Na^+-K^+-ATPase (Inturrisi, 1969b), (3) muscle pyruvate kinase (Kayne, 1971), and (4) skin Na^+-K^+-ATPase (Maslova *et al.*, 1971). Whether any of the above reactions are affected in the lens has not been reported, but substitution for K^+ in the frog skin Na^+-K^+-ATPase results in inhibition of the Na^+-pump. Electron microscopic examination of the kidney, liver, and intestine from rats chronically receiving subacute doses (10 to 15 mg Tl^+ per kilogram) of thallium acetate reveals a possible primary lesion of the mitochondria, exhibiting swelling, loss of cristae, deposition of granular material, and aggregation of mitochondrial granules (Herman and Bensch, 1967). Additional morphologic changes include disruption of the endoplasmic reticulum and formation of autophagic vacuoles.

Busulfan. Busulfan (Myleran) is a 1,4-bis(methanesulphonyloxy)-butane alkyating agent used in treating chronic myeloid leukemia.

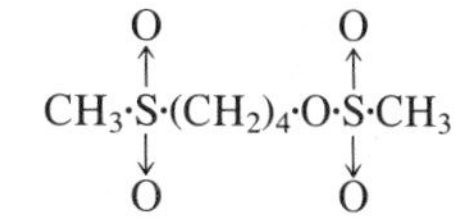

$$CH_3 \cdot \overset{\overset{O}{\uparrow}}{\underset{\downarrow}{S}} \cdot (CH_2)_4 \cdot O \cdot \overset{\overset{O}{\uparrow}}{\underset{\downarrow}{S}} \cdot CH_3$$

Busulfan (Myerlan)

Posterior subcapsular opacities or irregularities may result following chronic busulfan therapy (Podos and Canellos, 1969; Ravindranathan *et al.*, 1972; Grant, 1974; Hamming *et al.*, 1976), although the incidence or conditions surrounding these cataracts have not been fully investigated.

Experimentally induced cataracts can be obtained by feeding rats a diet containing 7.5 to 20.0 mg/kg of busulfan. An irreversible cataract is completely developed in five to seven weeks (Solomon *et al.*, 1955; von Sallmann, 1957). The earliest observation includes an increased mitotic activity of the epithelium primarily in the equatorial region, which eventually returns to and drops below normal levels. White dots or small vacuoles appear in the posterior and anterior lens, rapidly followed by opacification progressing from the equator to the posterior and anterior subcapsular zones. Similarities have been drawn between busulfan and ionizing radiation cataracts suggesting that those species with the slowest lens mitotic activity will develop cataracts more slowly (von Sallmann, 1957). The underlying mechanism may involve altered epithelial cell division. Injection of a single 12.5 mg/kg dose intraperitoneally reveals that busulfan acts during the relatively long G phase (Grimes *et al.*, 1964) of the cell cycle (Harding *et al.*, 1971), permitting normal synthesis of DNA but preventing subsequent mitosis. Consequently, the affected epithelial cells accumulate in preprophase, containing bizarre clumps of nuclear chromatin and twice the normal DNA content. Some of these cells undergo nuclear fragmentation and disintegration, while the remainder return to interphase with a tetraploid level of DNA. A similar mechanism occurs after chronic administration of busulfan (Grimes and von Sallmann, 1966). Following each cycle of DNA synthesis, mitosis is inhibited; and since the cells in the equatorial zone have the shortest intermitotic time (19 days), these are affected first. The cells in the equatorial zone normally migrate through the meridional rows and differentiate into lens fibers. However, death of these cells occurs after three days of busulfan treatment, leading to a decrease in cell density and disorganization of the meridional rows, and finally opacification. Continuous administration of this drug results in a depletion in the number of epithelial cells and complete disruption of the equatorial zone.

Triparanol. Triparanol (MER-29) was developed in the late 1950s as a blood cholesterol–lowering agent. Subsequent experiments in rats revealed decreased serum and tissue cholesterol levels and concomitant elevation in desmosterol levels. Triparanol inhibits cholesterol synthesis by inhibiting the $C_{24,25}$ double-bond reduction in desmosterol (Avigan et al., 1960; Steinberg and Avigan, 1960). Two reports published prior to the removal of triparanol from the market due to other toxicities confirmed the development of posterior and anterior subcapsular opacities following a dose of at least 250 mg per day for 15 to 18 months (Kirby et al., 1962; Laughlin and Carey, 1962).

Triparanol can induce cataracts in rats fed a diet containing 0.1 percent of the drug (von Sallmann et al., 1963). Small sudanophilic vesicles form on the fibers and eventually aggregate into large clusters. Prior to central and peripheral opacification, triparanol causes a tenfold increase in lens sodium content, causing hydration and swelling (Harris and Gruber, 1969, 1972). Upon returning to a normal diet, the cataracts are reversed as new fibers are laid down in the periphery, excess Na^+ and water are pumped out, and K^+ levels return to normal. Morphologic alterations have been observed under the electron microscope with other tissues sensitive to triparanol toxicity. Abnormalities consist of crystalloid and membranous intracytoplasmic inclusion bodies in neurons (Schutta and Neville, 1968), mitochondrial swelling, and rupture and fragmentation of the endoplasmic reticulum in the liver (Otto, 1971). Since cholesterol is an essential component of cellular membranes, inhibition of its synthesis could result in an overall inhibition of membrane synthesis (Rawlins and Uzman, 1970), involving all subcellular membranous structures, including mitochondria. Changes in mitochondrial oxidative metabolism (Otto, 1971) could conceivably result in deficiencies of the Na^+-pump mechanism in extruding intracellular Na^+ from the lens, and consequently lead to Na^+ accumulation in the lens. Further experimental evidence concerning the mechanism of triparanol cataracts is lacking.

Naphthalene. In addition to its retinotoxic action, systemic absorption of naphthalene vapor may result in cataracts (Grant, 1974). Oral administration of 1 g/kg/day to rabbits leads to lenticular changes, initially observed as a swelling in the peripheral portion of the lens. Vacuoles form between the epithelium cells within six hours after the first dose, spread toward the nucleus, and within two weeks the whole lens is affected with a mature cataract. Mitosis of the epithelial cells is inhibited after two or three doses, and the cells break down later. After one week, swelling and striations extend into the cortex and mitotic arrest is observed. Finally, after two weeks of naphthalene treatment, the epithelium shows areas of cell duplication, nuclear degeneration, and normal and abnormal mitosis. Since abnormal mitotic areas become partly denuded of cells, cells are irregularly arranged in the periphery (Pirie, 1968). The stages of naphthalene-induced cataract are similar to those that occur in the development of human senile cataract.

The biochemical basis for naphthalene cataract has been investigated (van Heyningen and Pirie, 1967) and shown to be related to the liver metabolite of naphthalene, 1,2-dihydro- 1,2-dihydroxynaphthalene. Lenticular catechol reductase biotransforms 1,2-dihydro-1,2-dihydroxynaphthalene to 1,2-dihydroxynaphthalene, which in turn is autooxidized in air at neutral pH to 1,2-naphthoquinone and hydrogen peroxide. Ascorbic acid reverses the latter reaction and forms dehydroascorbic acid, which can be reduced by glutathione. Since ascorbic acid diffuses out of the lens very slowly, it accumulates in the lens of the naphthalene-fed rabbit and in the lens incubated in vitro with 1,2-dihydro-1,2-dihydroxynaphthalene (van Heyningen, 1970a). The sequence of reactions involves reduction of ascorbic acid by 1,2-naphthoquinone in the aqueous humor to dehydroascorbic acid, which rapidly penetrates the lens and is reduced by glutathione. Oxidized glutathione and 1,2-naphthoquinone may compete for the enzyme glutathione reductase, which normally maintains high lenticular levels of reduced glutathione. A reduction in the concentration of these coupled with the removal of oxygen from the aqueous humor due to the autooxidation of 1,2-dihydroxynaphthalene may make the lens sensitive to naphthoquinone toxicity. Other diols that do not form quinones in similar *in vitro* experiments do not result in lenticular opacities or increased ascorbic acid levels (van Heyningen, 1970b).

In addition to the reduction of glutathione levels and aqueous humor oxygen content, 1,2-naphthoquinone is a very active compound and reacts with lenticular glutathione, amino acids, and proteins (Rees and Pirie, 1967). Interaction with the structural proteins results in the brown color of the lens characteristic of naphthalene cataracts and insoluble complexes of β- and γ-crystallins. However, combination with these proteins does not inhibit naphthoquinone oxidation of ascorbic acid. Reactions between coenzymes and enzymes and 1,2-naphthoquinone can cause changes in the oxidation/reduction potential of the lens and abnormal metabolic reactions, which either alone or in combination would lead to cellular disruption and, finally, cataracts.

Galactose. An unusual experimental cataract results from feeding animals a diet containing high levels of galactose. The morphologic changes in the lens during galactose feeding were photographed and described by Sippel (1966). Within two days after initiating a diet containing 50 percent galactose, rats showed water clefts situated between lenticular fibers in the anterior equatorial region. After ten days the cortex is almost completely liquefied and more transparent to light as a result of vacuole aggregation. Total lenticular opalescence is complete after 28 days of galactose feeding. Accompanying these changes is an increase in DNA synthesis (Weller and Green, 1969) and mitosis of the epithelial cells (Kuwabara *et al.*, 1969; van Heyningen, 1969) after three days of feeding. Eventually mitosis returns to and drops below normal activity as the cataract progresses.

The mechanism of galactose- and other sugar-related cataracts has been explained by excessive hydration of the lens observed as early as 12 hours after initiating a galactose-enriched diet. Galactose and other sugars are transported across the capsule and epithelial cell membrane by facilitated transport and diffusion (Elbrink and Bihler, 1972), and on entering the lens, galactose is either slowly phosphorylated to galactose-6-phosphate or reduced by the NADPH-dependent aldose reductase to dulcitol. While other sugar alcohols formed by aldose reductase are converted by polyol-NADP oxidoreductase to readily diffusible products, dulcitol is not further biotransformed. Since it diffuses out of the lens only very slowly, dulcitol accumulates to high levels and consequently exerts a strong osmotic force drawing water into the lens in order to maintain osmotic equilibrium. Therefore, increases in dulcitol levels are accompanied by a parallel increase in water content (Kinoshita, 1965; van Heyningen, 1971). If dulcitol synthesis is depressed by inhibiting aldose reductase with 3,3-tetramethyleneglutaric acid, water uptake and fiber vacuolization are prevented (van Heyningen, 1971). Furthermore, feeding young Carworth Farms Webster (CFW) mice a galactose-enriched diet does not produce cataracts, since lenses of this strain fail to biotransform galactose to dulcitol (Kuck, 1970c). Therefore, lenticular hydration resulting from the osmotic force due to dulcitol accumulation and retention explains fiber vacuolization and the initial structural alterations in galactose cataracts. Further investigations verified the lack of or very low activity of other lenticular enzymes that could biotransform dulcitol, e.g., galactokinase or 1-gulonate NADP oxidoreductase (van Heyningen, 1971).

Additional biochemical changes consist of a very early loss in amino acids due to a deficiency in the amino acid-concentrating mechanism and a marked drop in glutathione content (Kinoshita, 1965; Sippel, 1966a; Kinoshita *et al.*, 1969; van Heyningen, 1969, 1971). Both decreases are probably related to increased membrane permeability following swelling. Glycolysis and respiration decrease to 60 percent of normal after two days of galactose feeding but remain at this level of activity as the cataract progresses (Sippel, 1966b). Adenosine triphosphate levels decrease slightly during the early stages, but progressive vacuolization and opacification is accompanied by a 75 percent loss in ATP content. (Sippel, 1966b; Kuck, 1970c). Decreased aldolase activity correlates with progressive vacuolization of the cortex and glutathione loss during the first week of galactose diet; however, decreases in glucose-6-phosphate dehydrogenase, lactic acid dehydrogenase, and α-glycerophosphate dehydrogenase activity correlate with protein diminution occurring during the development of nuclear cataract (Sippel, 1967; Kuck, 1970c). Alterations in electrolyte balance do not occur until the late vacuolar stage. Surprisingly, the increased water uptake observed during the initial stages of cataract development is not accompanied by an increased Na^+ uptake and a loss of K^+ ions from the lens. In fact, Na^+ ion is pumped out of the lens during the initial development as effectively as from a normal lens, with only a slight loss in K^+. Only in the late vacuolar stage, with the development of nuclear opacification, does the lens fail to extrude Na^+, suggesting a second dramatic increase in membrane permeability to water during the terminal stages (Kinoshita, 1965). This is in the face of a still very much active cation pump mechanism. Decreases are observed in Mg^{2+}-dependent adenosine triphosphatase activity after six days of feeding a galactose-enriched diet, while Na^+-K^+-activated adenosine triphosphatase activity is markedly depressed after 15 days (Fournier and Patterson, 1971).

The lenticular opacities that develop on galactose feeding can be reversed if the sugar is withdrawn from the diet prior to nuclear involvement. After 10 to 12 days on the galactose diet, membrane permeability alters so that dulcitol leaks out as fast as it is formed. At this time, little if any protein is lost, but there is an increasing concentration of lens amino acids derived from protein, either from proteolysis or from inhibition of protein synthesis (Barber, 1972). As the cataract develops further, amino acids are suddenly reduced. Parallel accumulation of dulcitol and water in the lenticular fibers definitely causes the initial stages of cortical vacuolization and opacification. However, only failure of the lens to synthesize proteins or alterations in enzymic acticity essential in maintaining lens integrity could explain the irreversible nature of the mature nuclear cataract. The entire biochemistry of the lens would be deleteriously affected by the removal of reduced pyridine dinucleotide phosphate (NADPH) consumed during the reduction of galactose to dulcitol catalyzed by aldose reductase. Consequently, the reduced NADPH/NADP ratio alters the oxidation-reduction potential of the lens (Kuck, 1970b).

Experimentally induced galactose cataract has its counterpart in human physiology. Galactosemia is an autosomal recessive genetic deficiency in galactose metabolism. Affected infants on a milk diet show high blood and urine galactose levels, hepatomegaly, splenomegaly, eventual mental retardation, and cataracts. The genetic defect is deficiency in the enzymes galactose-1-phosphate-uridyl transferase or galactokinase (Kinoshita, 1965; Monteleone et al., 1971; Nordmann, 1971; Levy et al., 1972). These enzymes are necessary in transforming unusuable galactose into usable glucose-1-phosphate. Galactose or galactose-1-phosphate reaches excessive levels in the blood and aqueous humor triggering dulcitol synthesis in the lens and subsequent fibril vacuolization (van Heyningen, 1969). Removal of galactose from the diet can reverse the symptoms.

The multiple causes of cataract suggest multiple mechanisms rather than a final common pathway. This, in turn, suggests that we are not close to the multiple required solutions even though the sugar cataract problem appears to be solved brilliantly. Thus, new experimental test situations are to be welcomed. Merriam and Kinsey (1950) demonstrated that rabbit lenses could be maintained in organ culture for at least a week without loss of transparency, and this system has been exploited at various times. Mikuni et al. (1981) showed that microtubules disappear in cultured rat lenses in parallel with cataract formation. The size and orientability of microtubules suggest that they may well play a role in maintenance of lens transparency, and that this may be a profitable lead. Giblin et al. (1982), using cultured rabbit lenses, showed that glutathione and the hexose monophosphate shunt are vital in the detoxication of hydrogen peroxide in the culture medium. Since an early drop in glutathione level is characteristic in a number of cataracts including human ones, this lead, too, has promise. Sodium selenite injected into the intact rat causes large nuclear cataracts within 72 hours. Bunce and Hess (1981) showed that this event was also accompanied by a decrease in glutathione in lens. One is entitled to speculate whether this is a manifestation of selenium being an imperfect substitute for sulfur, or whether it has a more basic significance for chemical cataractogenesis.

THE RETINA AND CHOROID

The retina is the very compact and highly complex neural structure responsible for transducing the ocular light image and doing considerable preprocessing of the neural impulses before sending them toward the brain (Figure 17–1). The layer of rods and cones—modified neural structures containing photosensitive pigments—is the receptor of the light image. The receptor cells synapse with bipolar cells, which in turn synapse with ganglion cells. In addition, lateral synapses occur with horizontal cells and feedback synapses occur with amacrine cells. The Müller cells, the glia equivalent in retina, have nuclei near the center of the retinal thickness and long processes that extend through the whole retinal thickness. Finally, the single layer of retinal pigmented epithelium underlies the receptors and sends processes that envelop the receptor outer segments. It should be evident from these relationships—all of which exist in the 100- to 500-μm retinal thickness—that studies on the overall biochemistry and physiology of such a structure are likely to be confusing and misleading. To dispel any lingering hope that the retinal layers are uniform metabolically if not morphologically, one need only read below how specific toxic substances affect specific retinal layers. After one has recognized with Warburg (1926) that the retina as a whole is the most actively metabolizing structure in the normal body, one must view metabolic studies on whole retina with healthy skepticism. The extremely compact structure of the retina creates a real dilemma when one wishes to study a single cell type. One solution is that worked out by Lowry and coworkers (1956, 1961), who microdissected freeze-dried retina and picked out nuclei of each cell type for metabolic studies. Other approaches utilize histochemical techniques on retinas with individual cell layers destroyed by toxic substances. This subject is still very much open for definitive study and its incomplete state will hinder us greatly in reaching satisfying conclusions on the mechanism of action of retinotoxic substances.

The choroid is a vascular layer whose chief constituents in addition to the blood vessels are collagenous connective tissue and cells containing large numbers of melanin granules. The latter are important because of the affinity of melanin for polycyclic aromatic compounds. In primates, which have a well-established retinal blood supply, the choroid is responsible for nutrition of the receptor cell layer only. In lower vertebrates the choroidal vasculature supplies all of the retina.

Because of this dependence and because of physical proximity many diseases primary in the choroid cause retinal damage and some diseases primary in retina cause choroidal damage. Thus, chorioretinitis is a commonly encountered term. It is based on clinical observation and does not imply which structure is primary for the disease process.

Chloroquine

The 4-aminoquinoline chloroquine is effective as (1) an antimalarial, requiring doses of 500 mg

Chloroquine

per week for three to four weeks, with maintenance on 250 mg per week, and (2) an anti-inflammatory agent, requiring doses of at least 250 mg per day to be effective. The low-dose therapy used for malaria is essentially free from any toxic side effects; however, the chronic, high-dose therapy used for rheumatoid arthritis, discoid and systemic lupus erythematosus frequently causes a number of side effects, the most serious of which involves an irreversible loss of retinal functions. In 1959, the first cases of chloroquine-induced retinopathy were re-

ported (Hobbs *et al.*, 1959), but since then numerous reports have confirmed the etiology of similar observations as resulting from chloroquine therapy (see reviews by Nylander, 1967; Duke-Elder and MacFaul, 1972). Hydroxychloroquine has also been reported to cause a similar

Hydroxychloroquine

retinopathy (Crews, 1967; Shearer and Dubois, 1967), although the incidence of toxicity may be less (Shearer and Dubois, 1967; Sassaman *et al.*, 1970).

The clinical findings accompanying chloroquine retinopathy may generally be thought of in terms of early and late phenomena. Among the early findings are (1) a "bull's-eye retina," visualized as a dark, central pigmented area involving the macula, surrounded by a pale ring of depigmentation, which in turn is surrounded by another ring of pigmentation; (2) diminished electrooculogram; (3) possible granular pigmentation of the peripheral retina; and (4) subjective visual disturbances, observed as blurred vision and difficulty in reading, with words or letters missing in long sentences or long words. Late findings are (1) progressive scotoma, (2) constriction of the peripheral fields commencing in the upper temporal quadrant, (3) narrowing of the retinal arteries, (4) color and night blindness, (5) absence of a typical pigment pattern, and (6) abnormal electrooculograms and electroretinograms; these symptoms are irreversible. Indeed, there have been reports of irreversible chloroquine retinopathy where the entire development of the disease has occurred after cessation of the drug (R. P. Burns, 1966). It is generally recognized that the incidence of these chloroquine-induced toxic effects increases as the daily dose, total dose, and duration of therapy increase. The absence of permanent damage has been reported in patients receiving not more than 250 mg of chloroquine or 200 mg of hydroxychloroquine per day (Scherbel *et al.*, 1965). Nevertheless utilization of sensitive testing methods such as "macular dazzling" and retinal threshold tests has indicated some degree of retinal malfunction in all patients receiving even small doses of these drugs (Carr, 1968). Thus, there is a qualitative difference between the depression of visual function observed in all patients and the specific damage seen in relatively few individuals. Approximately 20 to 30 percent of the patients receiving higher doses of chloroquine will exhibit some type of retinal abnormality, while 5 to 10 percent show severe changes in retinal function (Butler, 1965; Crews, 1967; Nylander, 1967). One interesting paradox is worth noting. Despite severe retinopathy and "extinguished" ERG, normal or nearly normal dark adaptation performance is characteristic of chloroquine toxicity. This is in marked contrast to phenothiazine retinopathy (see below) (Krill *et al.*, 1971).

Experimentally induced chloroquine retinopathy was first produced in the cat after long-term, oral administration of subtoxic doses, 1.5 to 6.0 mg daily (Meier-Ruge, 1965a). A light pigmentation appeared in the cat's fundus four to seven weeks after the daily dosage schedule and the retinopathy was fully developed after eight weeks. Histologic and histochemical analysis revealed a thickening of the pigment epithelial cell layer, increases in the mucopolysaccharide and sulfhydryl group content, decreases in enzymatic activity of the pigment epithelium, migration of pigment into the outer nuclear layer, and finally total atrophy of the photoreceptors (Meier-Ruge, 1968). Similar findings were observed in rabbits (Dale *et al.*, 1965; Meier-Ruge, 1965b; François and Mandgal, 1967) and humans (Bernstein and Ginsberg, 1964; Wetterholm and Winter, 1964).

A report on miniature pigs fed chloroquine at 1000 times the human therapeutic level describes massive storage of gangliosides in the CNS and in retinal ganglion cells (Klinghardt *et al.*, 1981). Early in the 200-day feeding program epileptic and myoclonic fits were observed. Later "visual impairment" was observed. One wonders whether this finding is more related to the "myeloid bodies" seen in the retinal ganglion cells of experimental animals within a week of beginning chloroquine (e.g., Kolb *et al.*, 1972) than it is to the retinotoxicity of humans.

Because of its high affinity for melanin, the mechanism of chloroquine-induced retinopathy has been related to the extremely high concentrations that are attained in the pigmented eye and that remain at these high levels (Bernstein *et al.*, 1963b; Potts, 1964a, 1964b) long after other tissue levels have been depleted. Both hydroxychloroquine and desethylchloroquine, the major metabolite of chloroquine, behave similarly (McChesney *et al.*, 1965, 1967). Accumulation of chloroquine in the pigmented structures of the human choroid and pigmented epithelium has been reported and the amount depends on dosage and duration of drug therapy (Lawwill *et al.*, 1968). In addition, small amounts of chloroquine and its metabolites are excreted in the urine years after cessation of drug treatment (Bernstein, 1967). The prolonged exposure of the reti-

nal cell layers to chloroquine probably explains the irreversible nature of human retinopathy, which may not only progress (Okun *et al.*, 1963) but also develop after chloroquine has been withdrawn (R. P. Burns, 1966).

Investigations concerning the primary retinotoxic lesion caused by chloroquine have led to two schools of thought. Based on the histologic and histochemical findings and the melanin-binding property of chloroquine described above, one theory indicates a primary biochemical lesion in the pigmented epithelium cell layer of the retina. It is clear that storage in pigment in itself is not a sufficient cause for toxicity. It is simply that a toxic substance such as chloroquine like any other poison increases it effect as the concentration in tissue multiplied by time of exposure (C × T) increases. Storage on melanin causes enormous increases in this C × T factor for the melanin-containing tissue—in this case the retinal pigment epithelium.

Many biochemical reactions can be inhibited by chloroquine (reviewed by Bernstein, 1967; Sams, 1967; Mackenzie, 1970). Inhibition of protein metabolism of the pigment epithelium has been proposed as the primary cause for the retinotoxic effects of chloroquine (Meier-Ruge, 1968). *In vitro* experiments utilizing only whole-pigment epithelial cells have indicated that chloroquine and hydroxychloroquine markedly inhibit amino acid incorporation in protein (Gonasun and Potts, 1972).

Phenothiazines

The potency of phenothiazines as tranquilizers is related to the chemical constituent attached to the N-atom of the three-ring base: Group I compounds processing an aminopropyl side chain are least potent; group II compounds with a piperidine group in the side chain are more potent; and group III drugs composed of a piperazine group in the side chain are the most potent antipsychotic drugs (Boet, 1970). Successful remission of psychotic states requires persistent drug therapy at relatively high doses.

Chlorpromazine
(aminopropyl side chain)

Thioridazine
(piperidyl group in the side chain)

Prochlorperazine
(piperazinyl group in the side chain)

Therefore, it is not surprising that many side effects are associated with long-term high-dose phenothiazine therapy. Ocular complications may involve the cornea and the lens, described above, and the retina, described in this section.

The first phenothiazine derivative reported to alter retinal function belonged to group II: piperidylchlorophenothiazine (Sandoz NP-207). During clinical trials, the initial symptoms of visual disturbances were observed as impairment to adaptation in dim light. Further disturbances involved reduced visual acuity, constricted visual fields, and abnormal pigmentation of the retina, appearing in the periphery or macula as fine salt-and-pepper clumps of pigment (Kinross-Wright, 1956). Abnormalities in dark adaptation, color vision, and the ERG coupled with severe pigment clumping during the advanced stages indicated toxic effects in both rod and cone receptors. Disturbances of retinal function usually developed within two to three months after receiving 400 to 800 mg of the drug per day and a total of 20 to 30 g. Higher dosages required only 30 days to develop toxic symptoms. On withdrawal of the drug, some symptoms may be reversed although pigment clumping remains visible in the fundus. However, total reversal is not possible and in some cases severe visual loss

and blindness result. The strong evidence that NP-207 was the causative agent in these visual disturbances resulted in its removal from clinical study (Boet, 1970).

Replacement of the 2-chlorine of NP-207 with a methylmercapto group yields thioridazine, a phenothiazine derivative effective in treating schizophrenia and nonpsychotic severe anxiety without possessing some of the side effects common to the aminopropyl phenothiazines. Thioridazine also causes pigmentary and visual disturbances similar to those caused by NP-207 but dosages of over 1200 mg per day for 30 days are required to affect retinal function (Weekley *et al.*, 1960). Initially, a loss of visual acuity is observed, followed by night blindness, difficulty in adapting to average light conditions after being exposed to bright sunlight, and finally retinal pigmentary changes. In severe toxicity, excessive pigment deposition and an extinguished ERG are found. Usually, cessation of the medication is accompanied by complete or partial restoration of retinal function, although the pigmentary disturbances remain (Potts, 1968). Additional reports of thioridazine-induced retinopathy have been summarized (Siddall, 1966; Boet, 1970; Cameron *et al.*, 1972). The dosages required to produce these retinopathies are usually in excess of the recommended therapeutic levels. Normal dosages do not cause disturbances in retinal function even after years of treatment.

The group I phenothiazine chlorpromazine is generally free from retinotoxic effects. Rare cases have been reported (Siddall, 1965, 1966, 1968) of a reversible, fine granular pigmentation in the retinal background after 2.4 g of chlorpromazine per day for two years following 1 to 2 g per day for 6 to 28 months. Only one patient recorded heavy pigmentation.

The piperazine derivatives (group III) have not been reported to affect retinal function (Duke-Elder and MacFaul, 1972). Since these drugs are the most potent phenothiazine derivatives, less drug is needed to control the psychotic individual, resulting in a lessening of side effects.

Experimentally induced phenothiazine retinopathy was accomplished by orally administering NP-207 to cats; the initial dose of 10 mg/kg/day was slowly increased to 120 mg/kg/day (Meier-Ruge and Cerletti, 1966; Cerletti and Meier-Ruge, 1967). The first retinal changes appeared as fine grayish-blackish spots on the fundus after four to five weeks of treatment. These fine granules gradually coalesced and formed irregular patches of pigment as the retinopathy became fully developed after six to seven weeks of treatment. A partial explanation for the retinal changes was made by the finding that phenothiazine derivatives accumulate in very high concentrations in the uveal tract (Potts, 1962a, 1962b). Experiments utilizing labeled chlorpromazine, prochlorperazine, and NP-207 have indicated binding of these drugs to the melanin-containing tissues of the eye, allowing high concentrations to accumulate and remain in the eye for extended periods of time (Potts, 1962a, 1962b; Green and Ellison, 1966; Cerletti and Meier-Ruge, 1967). *In vitro* studies employing isolated choroidal melanin granules or synthetic melanin (Potts, 1964a, 1964b) have indicated that several phenothiazine derivatives bind to melanin, therefore verifying the result obtained *in vivo* that tissue melanin content is the essential component responsible for concentrating these N-substituted phenothiazines. As stated above for chloroquine, concentration on pigmented structures merely gets the phenothiazine to the tissue in high concentration. Both toxic and nontoxic phenothiazines participate in this effect. After storage the specific toxic activity (possibly one of the effects detailed below) must cause tissue damage.

Histologic examination of retinas from NP-207–treated cats has shown initial posterior vacuolization of outer segments one to two weeks after retinal pigmentation, followed by disorganization of the entire lamellar structure of the disk, and finally atrophy and disintegration of the rods and cones. Other cellular layers appear normal with the exception of a proliferative pigment epithelium (Cerletti and Meier-Ruge, 1967). Histochemical enzymic analysis of the same tissues revealed an increase in lactic acid dehydrogenase activity of the Müller cells, followed shortly by a decrease of this enzyme's activity in the rod and cone ellipsoids, both changes occurring prior to retinal pigmentation and structural changes. Similar but less marked alterations were noted for glutamic dehydrogenase, glucose-6-phosphate dehydrogenase, and 6-phosphogluconate dehydrogenase activities. Loss in enzymic activities of adenosine triphosphatase, succinic acid dehydrogenase, and DPN diaphorase paralleled the loss of rods and cones (Cerletti and Meier-Ruge, 1967). An increased amount of lipid-staining material in the pigment epithelium, due to the disintegration of outer segments, an increase of glycogen in the Müller cells, and a decreased amount of phospholipid-staining material were observed shortly before major morphologic changes.

Despite the plethora of metabolic activities attributable to phenothiazines (e.g., Guth and Spirtes, 1964), none have been identified that are restricted to the retinotoxic substances and are not shown by the innocuous ones. Thus a pathophysiologic mechanism for the toxic effect is not in hand.

Indomethacin

Administration of the anti-inflammatory drug, indomethacin, in dosages of 50 to 200 mg per day for one to two years may result in decrease of visual acuity, visual field changes, and abnormalities in dark adaptation, ERG, and the EOG (C. A. Burns, 1966, 1968; Henkes and van Lith, 1972; Henkes *et al.*, 1972). In one study of 34 patients (C. A. Burns, 1968), all exhibited a decreased retinal sensitivity, manifested as a lowered ERG or an altered threshold for dark adaptation. Ten of these patients had macular area disturbances, evidenced by paramacular depigmentation varying from mottled depigmentation to areas of pigment atrophy. Greater decreases in the scotopic component of the ERG than in the phototopic component have been reported

Indomethacin

(Palimeris *et al.*, 1972). However, except for the pigmentary disturbances, visual function improves upon cessation of drug treatment accompanied by a return to normal amplitudes in the a and b waves of the ERG.

Coupled to its anti-inflammatory properties, indomethacin prevents the release of lysosomal enzymes and stabilizes liver lysosomes when exposed to labilizing conditions (Ignarro, 1972). Inhibition of Ca^{2+} accumulation in injured tissue (Northover, 1972) and Ca^{2+} influx into stimulated smooth muscle by indomethacin (Northover, 1971) have been reported. However, the role of the metabolic reactions on indomethacin-induced retinopathy is unclear, since no experimental studies have been carried out involving indomethacin and the retina.

Oxygen

The therapeutic use of oxygen in concentrations greater than in ambient air has increased during the past several years. Healthy adults can usually tolerate breathing pure oxygen for up to three hours without exhibiting any uncomfortable symptoms; however, further inhalation at atmospheric pressure or short-term inhalation of high concentrations of oxygen at 2 to 3 atmospheres results in bilateral progressive constriction of the peripheral fields, impaired central vision, mydriasis, and constriction of the retinal vasculature (Grant, 1974; Nichols and Lambertsen, 1969; Mailer, 1970). All the symptoms are reversible upon inhalation of air. Although severe retinal damage in adults is rare during hyperoxia, one case was reported concerning an individual suffering from myasthenia gravis who developed irreversible retinal atrophy after breathing 80 percent oxygen for 150 days (Kobayashi and Murakami, 1972). The retinal vasculature was markedly constricted with no blood flowing through both eyes. The vascular disorder was limited only to retinal circulation.

Although there is a dose-dependent vasoconstriction of the retinal vessels and decrease in blood flow during hyperoxia, there is actually an increase in the oxygenation of the retina (Dollery *et al.*, 1969). Since the choriocapillaris can now supply the inner retinal layers with oxygen in addition to the supply from the retinal vessels, toxic levels of oxygen may accumulate and inhibit certain metabolic reactions essential for vision. More importantly, a decrease in the supply of nutrients, and especially glucose, to the visual cells results from the secondary decrease in blood flow, and only when the endogeneous supply of nutrients is metabolized and exhausted will deficiencies in vision be noticed (Nichols and Lambertsen, 1969).

A selective effect of hyperoxia on mature visual cells is exemplified by exposing adult rabbits to 100 percent oxygen for 48 hours. The result is loss of the ERG and visual cell death (Noell, 1955). Further experimentation with rabbits indicated that the centrally located rods, characterized by a low glycogen content and rich choroidal blood supply and therefore analogous to the human macula, are the most sensitive cells to oxygen toxicity (Bresnick, 1970). Peripheral rods and cones are less sensitive and spared from the toxic effects while other retinal layers—the inner nuclear layer, the ganglion cell layer, and the pigmented epithelial layer—appear normal. Rods containing a single synaptic ribbon appear to be more sensitive than rods with multisynaptic ribbons. The earliest morphologic changes in the outer nuclear layer include the formation of membrane-bound vesicles in the inner segment, swelling of the endoplasmic reticulum and Golgi apparatus followed by nuclear pyknosis, mitochondrial abnormalities, degeneration of the synaptic bodies, and vesiculation of the outer segment (Bresnick, 1970).

Although adults are not seriously affected by breathing high concentrations of oxygen, this is not true for premature infants. Frequently, premature infants are placed in incubators and breathe oxygen in concentrations greater than in air. On removal from hyperoxia, they develop an irreversible bilateral ocular disease known as retrolental fibroplasia. Critical in the development of this oxygen-induced disease is the embryologic nature of the human retinal vasculature. Beginning with the fourth month of gestation, the retinal vascular system develops from the hyaloid vascular stalk in the optic nerve, and by the eighth month, the retina is vascularized only in its nasal periphery. Development into the peripheral retina is not complete until after birth of a full-term infant (Patz, 1969–1970). Only the incompletely developed retinal circulation is susceptible to toxic levels of oxygen, whereas a mature retinal vascular system and other incompletely formed circulations are not sensitive to oxygen toxicity. Within six hours after an infant is placed in a high-oxygen-containing atmosphere, vasoconstriction of the immature vessels occurs, which is reversible if the child is immediately returned to air but is irreversible if hyperoxia therapy is continued (Beehler, 1964). Obliteration of the capillary lumen takes place as the vessel walls adhere to each other. This is followed by degeneration of the capillary endothelial cells and depression of the normal anterior forward growth of the retinal vessels. Immediately after returning to a normal oxygen atmosphere, vessels adjacent to the damaged area rapidly proliferate, invade the retina, penetrate the internal limiting membrane, and enter the vitreous. During the advanced stages, retinal fibrosis may cause retinal detachment. The opaque retrolental mass causes leukocoria (Beehler, 1964; Patz, 1969–1970).

Experimental investigations with kittens have indicated a similar and selective degeneration and proliferation of the developing retinal capillary endothelium. The vasoconstriction and lumen obliteration are directly related to the degree of immaturity of the retinal vascular system and to the concentration and duration of exposure to oxygen (Ashton and Pedler, 1962; Ashton, 1966, 1970; Patz, 1969–1970; Flower and Patz, 1971). While hyperoxia is selectively toxic to the immature retinal vascular system, no toxic effects are evident on the retina itself. Glycolytic and respiratory rates are unchanged (Graymore, 1970). These results contrast with the oxygen-induced photoreceptor atrophy observed in adult animals.

High concentrations of oxygen inhibit a number of enzymatic paths (Davies and Davies, 1965). Inhibition of respiration, electron transport, ATP synthesis, glycolysis, and a number of enzyme and coenzyme functions requiring free sulfhydryl groups for activity has been reported (reviewed by Haugaard, 1965, 1968; Menzel, 1970). The toxicity induced during maturation of the retinal vascular system, causing retrolental fibroplasia, may be explained by any of the above deficiencies, although no specific mechanism has been proposed. However, the toxicity on the mature photoreceptor cells may be explained by inhibition of glycolysis, which is essential for retinal function.

Epinephrine

In eyes that are aphakic, postcataract extraction cystoid macular edema has been described after the use of epinephrine (Kolker and Becker, 1968; Obstbaum et al., 1976). Recovery is expected but not invariable on cessation of use of the drug.

Iodate

In the preantibiotic era of the 1920s attempts were made to combat systemic septic disease, such as septicemia, by intravenous injection of inorganic antiseptics. It was found after the use of one of these—concentrated Pregl solution, known under the trade name of Septojod—that a number of individuals became blind (Riehm, 1927). It was demonstrated by Riehm (1929) that the primary retinal involvement was of the pigment epithelium and that this disease could be induced experimentally by injecting Septojod into pigmented rabbits. Vito (1935) was able to demonstrate that the actual toxic agent involved was sodium iodate. However, the exact way in which iodate causes degeneration and the reason for the particular susceptibility of the pigment epithelium have not been adequately worked out. Although iodate is known to be a relatively stable oxidizing agent, and though the probability of this mechanism of action is reinforced by the fact that the iodate effect can be completely neutralized by the reducing agent, cysteine (Sorsby and Harding, 1960), the effect has not been reproduced by other oxidizing agents, such as manganese dioxide, perborate, and persulfate (Sorsby, 1941). It is true, however, that none of these agents has the relative stability of iodate, and a dose comparable to that of iodate could not be given intravenously without killing the experimental animals.

Various experiments verified a primary effect of iodate on the pigment epithelium cell layer, followed by a secondary lesion and degeneration of the rod outer segments. Within hours after the administration of iodate, the thickness of the pigment epithelium layer is reduced, accompanied by loss of cellular limits, loss of definition, and formation of a granular cytoplasm (Graymore, 1970). Since the pigment epithelium cell layer lies between the choroidal vasculature and photoreceptors, it is responsible for exchange of nutrients and metabolites from the blood to the visual cells. Iodate-induced interruption in this flow of nutrients by possibly affecting the energy supply of the pigment epithelium or the rhodopsin cycle in the pigment epithelium would subsequently lead to photoreceptor degeneration.

Sparsomycin

The antibiotic sparsomycin, prepared from *Streptomyces sparsogenes,* is useful as an anticancer drug. One report (McFarlane et al., 1966) described two patients who received sparsomycin intravenously and developed pigmentary disturbances corresponding to bilateral ring scotomas. The total dose was 12 and 7.5 mg over a period of 13 to 15 days, respectively. Postmortem histologic examination of the eyes disclosed primary degeneration of the pigment epithelium and a closely associated secondary degeneration of the rods and cones, with a decrease in the acid mucopolysaccharide content of the damaged areas. As an inhibitor of protein synthesis, sparsomycin exerts its action by inhibiting peptide bond formation in both bacterial, mammalian (Trakatellis, 1968; Goldberg and Friedman, 1971), and human test systems (Neth and Winkler, 1972); but whether a similar effect occurs in the pigment epithelium as part of the sparsomycin-induced visual disturbances is not known.

Experimental Retinopathy

Iodoacetate. An important technique used in examining metabolic interrelationships between the different cell layers in the retina and also in determining which cells contribute to the components of the electroretinogram is to selectively destroy individual cell layers in experimental animals. A most potent tool for such studies is iodoacetate, which in carefully controlled doses rapidly and thoroughly obliterates receptor cells in rabbits (Schubert and Bornschein, 1951; Noell, 1952).

Graymore and Tansley (1959) were able to reproduce the effect in rats with the help of sodium malate in addition to the iodoacetate. Examination of the fundus of rabbits, cats, or monkeys indicates the development of a grayish retinal opacity after the first day of treatment, which persists for about a week. Retinal pigmentation, superficially similar to human retinitis pigmentosa, appears about a week following the initial dose. Electron microscopic examination of rabbit retinas indicates lesions in the rod and cone outer segments within three hours after treatment with iodoacetate in albino rabbits and within 12 hours after iodoacetate treatment in pigmented rabbits with marked disintegration of outer segments in albinos observed after 12 hours (Lasansky and de Robertis, 1959; Birrer, 1970). Disorganization of the outer segment through vesiculation and lysis of the membrane structure is accompanied by swelling and vacuolization of the endoplasmic reticulum and Golgi apparatus in the inner segment, by disintegration of mitochondria in the ellipsoid, by pyknosis of the nuclei, and by lysis of the synaptic vessicles. Widespread capillary closure rapidly follows destruction of the photoreceptor cell layer (Dantzker and Gerstein, 1969). Iodoacetate causes an irreversible decrease in the amplitudes of the a, b, and c-waves of the electroretinogram (Noell, 1959; François et al., 1969a). All the evidence indicates a selective retinotoxic effect of iodoacetate on the photoreceptor cells since even one week after a small dose, both the pigment epithelium and inner nuclear cell layers are intact (Dantzker and Gerstein, 1969).

The mechanism of iodoacetate-induced retinopathy may be twofold. Iodoacetate inhibits glyceraldehyde-3-phosphate dehydrogenase and therefore prevents the conversion of 1,3-diphosphoglyceraldehyde into 1,3-glyceric acid, a necessary reaction in pyruvate and lactate production during the glycolytic catabolism of glucose (Noell, 1959). Glycolysis provides the major source of energy to the photoreceptor cells, and inhibition of this reaction would necessarily lead to cell destruction. Moreover, anerobic glycolysis was inhibited 75 percent after ten minutes of treatment with iodoacetate in a dose that yielded visual cell damage (Graymore, 1970). However, this theory is inconsistent with other experimental observations. The ERG is diminished within minutes after infusion of iodoacetate (Noell, 1959), and decreases in enzyme activity do not always appear prior to morphologic and structural changes of these cells. Alteration in the free sulfhydryl group content of the visual cells has been reported (Reading and Sorsby, 1966) suggesting that damages to the membrane structure of the photoreceptor cells and outer segments may be the primary retinotoxic effect of iodoacetate. An additional effect on glycolysis may contribute to the irreversible nature of iodoacetate toxicity.

Dithizone. Administration of the diabetogenic (Kadota, 1950; Okamoto, 1955) chemical dithizone intravenously to rabbits in doses between 17.5 and 40 mg/kg causes retinal lesions (Grignolo et al., 1952; Weitzel et al., 1954; Sorsby and Harding, 1962). Ophthalmoscopic and histologic examination reveal severe retinal edema developing within 24 to 48 hours followed by the appearance of red islets indicating recovery from edema and pigmentary disturbances in the fundus. When the edema finally disappears, usually in six to eight days, the irregular pigmentation has spread throughout the retina (Sorsby and Harding, 1962). While the rabbit receptors appear to be the cell layer most sensitive to dithizone toxicity, there is swelling of the nerve fiber layer. The diffuseness of the lesion is reflected in the decreased amplitudes of the ERG and the EOG (Babel and Ziv, 1957, 1959; François et al., 1969a), initially observed as a suppression of the c-wave (Wirth et al., 1957) and b-wave amplitudes (Babel and Ziv, 1957). Eventually the entire ERG is completely obliterated. Finally, as the retina becomes disorganized, optic atrophy (François et al., 1969b) and proliferation of the pigment epithelium (Karli, 1963) are observed. Pretreatment of rabbits with cysteine does not protect against the retinotoxic action of dithizone as it does against iodate and iodoacetate poisoning (Sorsby and Harding, 1960, 1962). This suggests a difference in mechanisms between the three retinotoxic agents.

Dithizone-induced retinopathy appears to be species-specific, developing in those species possessing a tapetum, e.g., dogs and rabbits, but not developing in those species lacking a tapetum, e.g., rats, monkeys (Budinger, 1961; Delahunt et al., 1962), and man. A possible relationship, at least in the dog, has been suggested (Weitzel et al., 1954; Budinger, 1961; Delahunt et al., 1962) between the Zn^{2+}-chelating properties of dithizone and retinal degeneration. Dithizone depletes the canine tapetum of its rich supply of Zn^{2+}, leading to severe tapetal necrosis, retinal edema, and finally loss of retinal structure and function. On the other hand, in the rabbit, an early decrease of ERG amplitude and swelling of the neuroepithelium followed rapidly by complete retinal disorganization suggests that additional factors are involved in dithizone retinopathy. Experiments with ethambutol, another zinc chelator, show that tapetal zinc in dogs is lowered by an amount comparable to the lowering caused by dithizone. The green color of the tapetum is lost but no retinopathy results (Figueroa et al., 1971). Possible interference in the active transport of ions from the choriocapillaris through the pigment epithelium (François et al., 1969b) and alterations in the total and free sulfhydryl group content resulting from protein denaturation (Reading and Sorsby, 1966) have been reported. A similar compound, sodium di-

Dithizone (diphenylthiocarbazone)

ethyldithiocarbamate, not only causes tapetal necrosis in dogs but also inhibits oxygen consumption, pyruvate utilization, and citrate synthesis (DuBois *et al.*, 1961) in liver and kidney. Perhaps dithizone exerts a similar inhibitory effect on retinal metabolism.

Diaminodiphenoxyalkanes. A set of toxic substances that appear to be specific for pigment epithelium is the family of the diaminodiphenoxyalkanes.

$$H_2N-\langle\bigcirc\rangle-O-(CH_2)_n-O-\langle\bigcirc\rangle-NH_2$$

The series, in which $n = 5, 6$, and 7 are the most active, was originally synthesized for schistosomacidal properties. No human use was ever reported, but in susceptible animals—monkey, dog, and cat—a single oral or intravenous dose causes eventual pigmented retinopathy (Edge *et al.*, 1956; Sorsby and Nakajima, 1958) and complete loss of the electroretinogram within a few days (Nakajima, 1958). There is selective action on the pigmented epithelium, but when these cells are destroyed, the overlying receptor cells also degenerate (Ashton, 1957). This is like the iodate situation above.

An approach to the mechanism of toxic action was begun when Glocklin and Potts (1962) showed that uptake of ^{32}P into acid-soluble phosphorus fractions was inhibited by diaminodiphenoxyheptane in pigment epithelium *in vitro* but not in neuroretina.

THE GANGLION CELL LAYER AND OPTIC NERVE

General Considerations

The attribute that separates the ganglion cell (Figure 17–1) from the remainder of the retina is that it is the cell body of a neuron that extends into the depth of the central nervous system. The axons from the ganglion cell layer form the nerve fiber layer of the retina and exit from the eye at the optic papilla. Most of the fibers, carrying visual information, travel some 120 mm from the globe via optic nerve, optic chiasm, and optic tract to the point where they synapse in the lateral geniculate body of the midbrain. Like any other central nervous system neuron, the optic nerve fiber degenerates in both directions from a cut. Thus the ganglion cell of the retina may be damaged by direct action upon it, the cell body, or it may degenerate secondary to toxic destruction of the optic nerve. Instances of both types of damage will be cited below.

A second unique property of the ganglion cell-optic nerve is its behavior as a physiologically dual structure. The central 5 percent of the field of vision is the sole portion that possesses high visual acuity. This corresponds to an area of retinal receptors of 1.5-mm diameter centered on the fovea centralis. Although there is considerable preprocessing of visual information in the retina, there is still correspondence between receptor location and ganglion cell type or ganglion cell location or both. The result of this is that the information from that central most acute 5 percent of visual field runs in an identifiable bundle of fibers—the so-called papillomacular bundle—whose position can be identified by myelin degeneration stains at each position in the optic nerve and optic tract after damage to the central retina (Brouwer and Zeeman, 1926). Moreover, this fiber bundle acts as a separate entity in its behavior toward a number of toxic substances as well as toward some diseases.

It is not clear why this should be the case. We do know that papillomacular fibers are predominantly small fibers (Potts *et al.*, 1972). It is possible that these fibers with the greatest ratio of surface area to volume have the highest metabolic demand of all optic nerve fibers. However, in the case of some toxic substances the papillomacular bundle is spared and the peripheral fibers are hit. Thus it appears that specific chemical affinities may play a role. The opposite effect, the loss of the peripheral visual field to the action of a toxic substance, may not represent a case of selective affinity at all. If the substance has its primary action on the ganglion cell, and if there is uniform loss of absolute number of cells across the entire retinal area, the peripheral retina will be wiped out. The macular area will survive with at most a decrease in acuity, because there are so many more cells in the macular area. However this may be, some toxic substances affect the ganglion cell body; others affect the fibers of the papillomacular bundle; others affect peripheral fibers only. In each case, death of a portion of the neuron means death of the entire neuron and loss of that specific information transmission channel. To take cognizance of this attribute where damage to a retinal cell body can cause loss of function through an entire tract we will designate this section as dealing with the ganglion cell neuron (GCN).

One other special consideration deals with a clinical entity, pallor of the disk. When any considerable number of optic nerve fibers die, their lack of demand for nutrition is somehow conveyed to the surrounding capillaries. These disappear over a period of months. In the one place where optic nerve capillaries may be inspected with ease, the optic papilla, the nerve head becomes abnormally pale on ophthalmoscopic inspection, owing to loss of capillary supply.

There is a very good correlation between the pallor observed after the loss of a large number of fibers and optic atrophy. This has reached the point where many clinicians report "optic atrophy" on ophthalmoscopic examination when they mean "pale disk." Such an examination in marginal cases or done by a poor observer could lead to erroneous results. It is important for the reader of a report on toxicology to know whether the description of optic atrophy is a clinical or a histologic one.

Specific Substances

Methanol. A well-publicized and uniquely American poison affecting the GCN is methanol. The first practical distillation process that created a preparation potable by the unwary and the clinical report of the first 275 cases of methanol poisoning appeared in the United States (Wood and Buller, 1904). Whenever access to ethanol has been restricted, as in prohibition or in wartime, the incidence of methanol poisoning has risen, and epidemics centering on some local source of supply are reported in significant number. The characteristic results of an epidemic are that a third of those exposed to methanol recover with no residues, a third have severe visual loss or blindness, and a third die. Thus in sufficiently high doses methanol has profound systemic effects. Studies in the 1950s showed that methanol poisoning was a primate disease (Gilger and Potts, 1955) and that it was a palimpsest of three different diseases (Potts et al., 1955). Those diseases are (1) organic solvent poisoning (which is the only disease the subprimates show), (2) systemic acidosis, and (3) central nervous system effects, including changes in the eye and the basal ganglia. It was shown that the LD90 for primates gave only transient solvent toxicity signs and that a lucid interval set in, followed by systemic acidosis. Acidosis was enough to kill the animal unless it was combatted with base. If the acidosis was treated, the animal died later of the CNS disease. In many monkeys at the peak of the CNS signs, retinal edema was a common finding. In its most severe form it covered the entire retina and produced the rhesus equivalent of the cherry-red spot.

Because methanol poisoning in humans is a medical emergency and it is usually impossible to determine the dose ingested, this kind of unified picture is difficult to come by. However, all of the phases seen in the rhesus disease are seen in human disease even to the basal ganglion lesion (Orthner, 1950).

The specific eye effects are definite as far as they go. Everyone agrees that nerve head pallor is a constant finding in human cases who recover from methanol poisoning with permanent visual impairment. In monkeys marked demyelination of temporal retina has been demonstrated along with marginal loss of ganglion cells (Potts et al., 1955). Thus, optic atrophy is a definite finding in methanol poisoning but there is some question of whether the disease is primary in the ganglion cell layer. Arguments in favor are the observed retinal edema in the acute phase and the finding of loss of ganglion cells. Arguments against are lack of ganglion cell loss reported by McGregor (1943) and Orthner (1950).

The proximal toxic agent is generally accepted to be the methanol oxidation product formaldehyde (Potts, 1952; Cooper and Kini, 1962). It has now been established after some controversy that the mechanism of oxidation of methanol differs in primates and subprimates. In primates the principal metabolic pathway is via alcohol dehydrogenase (Kini and Cooper, 1961). In subprimates the favored pathway is via the catalase system (Tephly et al., 1963). It is tempting to attribute the primate nature of methanol poisoning to some difference in availability of formaldehyde from alcohol dehydrogenase oxidation. This does not seem to be the case. In unpublished results from our laboratory equal amounts of ^{14}C label from $^{14}CH_3OH$ are bound to eye and brain in rabbits and monkeys.

The report of Martin-Amat et al. (1978) that optic disk edema may be produced by infusions of formate in the monkey reopens the question of the proximal toxic agent in methanol poisoning. Since their experimental conditions require constant infusions of formate, it is difficult to design an experiment of long enough duration to determine whether the other criteria observed in human methanol poisoning can be met—i.e., death with destruction of the basal ganglia. Clearly, more work on the one-carbon metabolism of the primate is called for.

The treatment of methanol poisoning involves both combatting acidosis and preventing methanol oxidation. With the general availability of hemodialysis in the United States, prompt hemodialysis appears to be the method of choice in preventing methanol oxidation by removing it from the body. For a review of the literature on human cases treated by hemodialysis, see Gonda et al. (1978). Comparison of small groups of patients by Keyvan-Larijanari and Tannenberg (1974) appears to demonstrate that peritoneal dialysis is measurably less effective than hemodialysis.

Where dialysis is not available or is delayed, prevention of methanol oxidation may be achieved by administration of ethanol, which competes successfully for alcohol dehydrogenase. This allows time for methanol to be excreted unoxidized in urine and breath. The value of ethanol administration during dialysis is marginal because it is removed from blood at about the same rate as methanol. However, since dialysis requires a finite time for completion, there may be some benefit in attempting to maintain a blood ethanol level.

It was suggested by Gilger and coworkers (1956) that treatment for a 70-kg man be 4.5 oz of 50 percent ethanol initially, followed by 3.0 oz every four hours for 48 hours or until blood methanol reached negligible levels. In a number of sporadic cases this has appeared to be effective therapy.

Ethambutol. This substance was found by *in vivo* screening to be most effective against tu-

$$CH_2OH \diagdown \qquad \qquad C_2H_5 \\ \qquad HC—HN—(CH_2)_2—NH—CH \diagup \qquad \cdot 2HCl \\ C_2H_5 \diagup \qquad \qquad CH_2OH$$

d-2-2'-(Ethylenediimino)-di-1-butanol dihydrochloride

berculosis in mice (Thomas *et al.*, 1961). The drug, because of its relatively good tolerance and its efficacy against isoniazid-resistant tuberculosis, has become an established member of the antituberculosis armamentarium. In some 10 percent of patients receiving 25 to 50 mg/kg/day, loss of vision appears one to seven months after start of dosage (Carr and Henkind, 1962; Place and Thomas, 1963). (For a thorough review of human and animal toxicity, see Leibold, 1966; Place *et al.*, 1966; Schmidt, 1966.)

The typical toxic phenomenon is "retrobulbar neuritis" in the sense that there is visual field involvement without obvious swelling of the nerve head. However, in addition to central scotoma, which is thought of as the typical finding in retrobulbar neuritis, a smaller proportion of patients show loss of peripheral field with preservation of central vision (Leibold, 1966). All visual symptoms are dose-related. Figures collected from various sources in the literature by Citron (1969) suggest:

DOSAGE (mg/kg/day)	CASES	INCIDENCE OF COMPLICATIONS
50	60	15%
>35	59	18%
<30	59	5%
25	130	3%
15	—	Negligible

Visual disturbances appear to regress completely on cessation of drug administration.

The mechanism of therapeutic action and the mechanism of toxicity are far from clear. Ethambutol is a chelating agent that will remove zinc from the tapetum lucidum of dogs. However, it does not cause the pigmentary retinopathy that a chelating agent such as dithizone causes (Figueroa *et al.*, 1971). When *Mycobacterium smegmatis* is used as a model for *M. tuberculosis*, ethambutol-inhibited cells become deficient in RNA. As a consequence, protein synthesis is inhibited (Forbes *et al.*, 1965). A recent recommendation of substituting biweekly high-dose therapy for daily intermediate-dose therapy is said to eliminate visual system toxicity (Trumbull *et al.*, 1977).

Carbon Disulfide. This inflammable and volatile liquid (BP = 46.3°C) was important in the past as a solvent for sulfur in the rubber industry and as a solvent for alkali-treated cellulose in the viscose process for rayon and cellophane. Improved ventilation and substitution of other solvents has made classical carbon disulfide poisoning a thing of the past. The impressive complex of central scotoma, drop in visual acuity, widespread peripheral neuritis, personality changes, vascular encephalopathy, and generalized arteriosclerosis with cardiovascular and renal sequelae is not seen. However, there are recent disquieting reports from Japan and from Finland of subtle eye effects, seen at solvent levels which do not produce the classic symptoms, and which until now were thought to be safe (Sugimoto and Goto, 1980; Raitta and Tolonen, 1980).

Curiously, the retinopathy seen in Japan, which consists of microaneurysms and small hemorrhages, was not observed in Finnish workers to exceed the incidence in controls. In Finland the positive findings were delayed peripapillary filling on fluorescein angiography, widening of retinal arterioles, and lower peak to the ocular pulse wave. Clearly, carbon disulfide in industry needs another look.

A curious aspect of CS_2 poisoning is the lack of correspondence between anatomic and physiologic findings (Birch-Hirschfeld, 1900; Ide, 1958). One possible reason for this is restriction of the experimental situation to rodents, which do not appear to have a dual optic nerve. Much experimentation will be required to exploit the little we now know of carbon disulfide poisoning.

Thallium. Considerable clinical experience in thallium poisoning has arisen from use of thallous acetate in the 1920s as an epilating agent by dermatologists and its use as a rat poison (Celio Paste) with consequent accidental and intentional poisonings. For a short time in the early 1930s a cosmetic depilatory cream (Koremlu) caused additional chronic cases. (For reviews of this material, see Heyroth, 1947, and Prick *et al.*, 1955.) Systemic symptoms in thallium poisoning include gastroenteritis, polyneuritis, and allopecia. Ocular involvement is cataract, especially in rats, and optic neuritis in humans.

The unifying concept that made the behavior of lens and optic nerve understandable was developed in the 1960s when it became apparent that thallous ion is in many ways a stand-in for potassium ion. For a review of this, see Gehring and Hammond (1967). The University of Chicago laboratory was able to show that lens and optic nerve, two high-potassium tissues, were also able to store Tl^+ (Potts and Au, 1971). The ionic similarities are great enough that Tl^+ can activate (Na^+-K^+) activated ATPase (Britten and Blank, 1968). Kinsey and coworkers (1971) demonstrated that thallous ion accumulation in lens was by active transport and by the alkali metal-transporting system. An additional and unexpected finding was high storage of Tl^+ in melanin-containing eye structures (Potts and Au, 1971). Although Tl^+ can act for K^+ in many systems, it is clear that it cannot do so in every case. It seems logical that accumulation of thallium where potassium should normally be, without its being able to substitute for potassium in every enzyme system, is the basis for thallium toxicity. It is not clear which parts of the GCN are most affected.

Needless to say, prophylaxis is the only practical therapy in thallium poisoning.

Pentavalent Arsenic. Pentavalent arsenicals have been found in the past to be effective against trypanosomiasis (Thomas, 1905).

Sodium arsanilate (Atoxyl)

Sodium *N*-(carbamoylmethyl)-arsanilate (Tryparsamide)

The same ability to pass the blood-brain barrier that allowed effectiveness against trypanosomes also made possible treatment of neurosyphilis. Numerous derivatives of sodium arsanilate were synthesized by Ehrlich in his early investigations of trypanocidal and spirochetocidal activity. Tryparsamide, a substance of relatively low toxicity, was synthe-

sized at the Rockefeller Institute (Jacobs and Heidelberger, 1919) and introduced into tropical medicine shortly thereafter (Pearce, 1921). Tryparsamide was then found effective against neurosyphilis (Henrichsen, 1939).

Eye effects were a constant accompaniment of the use of pentavalent arsenicals and were a prime reason for their eventual abandonment. The clinical figures of Neujean and coworkers (1948) suggest that 3 to 4 percent of trypanosomiasis cases treated with tryparsamide show visual effects, and a third of these—i.e., 1 percent of all cases—show peripheral contraction of visual fields. There are anatomic findings to accompany the clinical symptoms, and here the peripheral area of the ganglion cell layer is most severely involved (Birch-Hirschfeld and Köster, 1910). There is considerable evidence that at the cellular level all of the arsenicals reach the same oxidation state, whatever their form at introduction (Ehrlich, 1909).

Interest has been maintained in organic arsenicals in recent years by the finding that when they are included in the feed of poultry and swine at an optimal level, the animals thrive and gain weight. Errors on the farm can expose animals and the growers to a toxic hazard. Studies like the thesis of Ledet (1979) should be extended.

Quinine. Although the massive use of quinine decreased abruptly with the advent of new synthetic antimalarials in the 1940s, plasmodia resistant to these new compounds appeared rapidly. Quinine is the drug of choice in these situations (Nieuwveld *et al.*, 1982). Thus, quinine has an established place in today's pharmacopoeia. An additional therapeutic effect is said to be relief of nocturnal recumbancy leg cramps. The availability of the drug allows ingestion in excessive doses for intended abortion and intended suicide as in the past. Hence quinine poisoning is still with us as are the poorly understood eye effects.

It is now clear that there are two dosage levels at which quinine (and its congeners) may be toxic. The first is a very low level caused by a single dose of as little as 12 mg (Belkin, 1967). The symptoms are those of thrombocytopenic purpura. The cause is an immune reaction in which the drug acts as a hapten. This phenomenon was treated exhaustively by Shulman (1958a, 1958b, 1958c, 1958d) where the offender was quinidine. The visual system is affected as much or as little as it would be in purpura caused by any other hapten. Its blood vessels are subject to hemorrhage secondary to thrombocytopenia as any set of vessels would be, but there is no specific selectivity for the eye.

The usual therapeutic regime for malaria is

1.3 g/day in four divided doses for seven days. Experiments on human volunteers have shown that eye effects of blurring, decrease of visual acuity, and loss of peripheral field occur with single doses of 2.5 to 4.0 g (Duke-Elder and MacFaul, 1972). A single dose of 8.0 g can be fatal. It is doses of 2.5 g and above that have specific eye effects. The eye effects have been attributed by some to arteriolar constriction, by others to direct action on the ganglion cell body, and by still others to effects on the whole retina. See the reports of Francois *et al.* (1967), Cibis *et al.* (1973), Brinton *et al.* (1980), and Gangitano *et al.* (1980) for the various arguments adduced and additional literature reviews. In a paper now in preparation, Potts and co-workers describe their results in cats given a sublethal dose of quinine sulfate. Early electroretinographic changes that show whole-retina involvement are transient. Early peripapillary and retinal edema, which suggests ganglion cell involvement, is also transient. The earliest anatomic changes that become permanent are pyknosis and then generalized loss of retinal ganglion cells. This is almost certainly the locus of high-dose specific eye effects.

Hemodialysis has been recommended as the treatment of choice, but some reservations are expressed by Dickinson *et al.* (1981).

Glutamate. An experimental entity involving the ganglion cell neuron is glutamate poisoning. Lucas and Newhouse (1957) reported that administration of high doses of sodium 1-glutamate to suckling mice caused degeneration of the retinal ganglion cell layer and failure of formation of the inner nuclear layer. Freedman and Potts (1962) were able to reproduce this phenomenon in newborn albino rats. They showed that glutaminase I was repressed in the retinas of these animals and postulated this as the mechanism of glutamate toxicity.

Later work has revealed an extensive series of compounds related to glutamate that have neuroexcitatory or neurotoxic properties or both. The term "excitotoxin," which implies that there is a relation between the two properties, has been coined. At all events, the entire subject area is in flux; some feel for this may be obtained from the review of Olney (1982).

Perhaps most important is the fact that whereas glutamate affects the developing retina only, some of the newer compounds cause selective cell loss when injected intravitreally in mature animals. This represents no human hazard, but promises to be a powerful experimental tool. DL-2-aminoadipic acid, the next higher homolog of glutamic, destroys Müller cells, and in high doses causes swelling of astrocytes and oligodendrocytes (Pedersen and Karlsen, 1979;

Ishikawa and Mine, 1983). Kainic acid, a sterically hindered analog of glutamic acid, destroys the "displaced amacrine cells" of the chicken retina (Ehrlich and Morgan, 1980). One anticipates more such findings to come.

In research performed during World War II on the vesicant methyl nitrosocarbamate (see section on vesicant gases, nitrosamines) it was found that there was selective chromatolysis and destruction of the retinal ganglion cell layer. The experiments were done in cats allowed to inhale

$$Cl-CH_2-CH_2-N-\overset{\displaystyle O}{\overset{\displaystyle \|}{C}}-OCH_3$$
$$|$$
$$N=O$$

Methyl *N*-β-chlorethyl-*N*-nitrosocarbamate

the vapor at a concentration of 50 μg/l for 10 minutes (Gates and Renshaw, 1946). The compound is an alkylating agent like the nitrogen mustards and its alkylates functional groups of proteins and nucleic acids in a more or less random manner. Unlike the amino acid series described above, this compound represents a hazard to its user during synthesis and during exposure of the test animal.

SMON. Special mention should be made of the optic nerve damage (accompanying widespread demyelination in the CNS) caused by 7-iodo-5-chloro-8-hydroxyquinoline, iodochlorhydroxyquin known as "Clioquinol," "EnteroVioform," and "Vioform."

The drug is an effective amebicide and is useful in the treatment of amebiasis when given at the level of 500 to 750 mg three times a day for ten days. An eight-day interval must be observed before a second ten-day course is given.

However, this drug has been available over the counter outside the United States principally to combat "traveler's diarrhea" where a specific diagnosis has not been made and where physician control of dosage is lacking. Particularly in Japan an entity has been recognized and labeled "subacute myelo-opticoneuropathy" (SMON) attributable to use of this substance. It is said that from 1955 to 1970, 10,000 cases of SMON were diagnosed in Japan. A national commission was formed by the Japanese government, and in 1970 the sale of the drug was prohibited. For a bibliography of the Japanese literature see Shigematsu (1975).

The entity is characterized clinically by paresthesias and numbness of the extremities, ataxia, and weakness in the legs. Twenty-seven percent of SMON patients have visual disturbances attributed to demyelination of the optic nerve (Sobue and Ando, 1971).

The extremely high incidence in Japan has not

been explained satisfactorily. High dosage levels, additive effects of environmental pollutants, and as-yet-unidentified factors have all been invoked. A representative of the manufacturer claims that since 1935 only 50 cases of SMON with a history of iodochlorhydroxyquin consumption have been identified in the rest of the world (Burley, 1977).

The disease can be reproduced in experimental animals by feeding the drug, and optic nerve demyelination is demonstrable in dogs and cats (Tateishi and Otsuki, 1975).

ORGANOMERCURIALS

Metallic mercury has been recognized to present a relatively low-level hazard to the individual and the eye. The eye does not appear to be involved in poisoning by inorganic salts of mercury. This is treated well by Grant (1974). The marked toxicity of organic compounds of mercury and their effect on vision have been known since the report of Edwards (1865), but this remained a laboratory caution until the multiple epidemics of the last decades. The presently accepted site of damage to the visual system puts the subject beyond the avowed scope of this chapter, but its importance requires that it be treated here.

Epidemics of organomercurial poisoning have originated in two major and diverse manners. The earliest cases of both series were found in 1956. The subtler, hence the more difficult, of the two to identify occurred in Japan, and in retrospect cases seen in 1951 were part of the epidemic. To summarize years of active research sponsored by the Japanese government, the hazard originated when metallic mercury, used as a catalyst in the acetaldehyde plant near Minamata Bay, was discharged into the bay as waste sludge. The aquatic plant life in the bay was able to convert elemental mercury to organomercurials, especially to methyl mercury. The fish and shellfish of the bay acquired methyl mercury from the plants and the contaminated water. The local inhabitants, many of whom were fishermen, were poisoned by the contaminated seafood and began to present with neurologic complaints at the local hospitals. In February 1963 the disease was identified as organomercurial poisoning. From 1965 to 1974 a series of 520 patients was seen in Nigata prefecture who were identified as having organomercurial poisoning. The source of the epidemic was a similar factory. The excellent account of the findings edited by Tsubaki and Irukayama (1977), entitled *Minamata Disease,* is a model of reporting.

The second type of epidemic arose in multiple sites and always with the same causation. Seed grain treated with an organomercurial antifungal agent was used by peasant farmers to make bread. Iraq had epidemics in 1956, 1960, and 1971–72 (Bakir *et al.,* 1973). The last caused 6530 cases admitted to hospitals, of whom 459 died. Similar but lesser outbreaks are recorded for Guatemala in 1963 to 1965, for Pakistan in 1961 and 1969, and Ghana in 1967.

The textbook description of organomercurial poisoning is that of Hunter, Bomford, and Russell (1940); the disease complex is often designated "Hunter-Russell syndrome." The components are: (1) ataxia, (2) impairment of speech, and (3) constriction of visual field. The Minimata cases also showed a high incidence of hearing loss and somatosensory change.

Histopathology was done on monkeys by Hunter *et al.* and by Shaw *et al.* (1975) and by Takeuchi and Ito (1977) (in Tsubaki, T., and Irukayama, K., eds., 1977) on the Minamata deaths. All of them agree that eye findings are negligible, and that the major and consistent finding is necrosis of neurons in the cerebral cortex, particularly in the depth of the sulci, and most particularly in the calcarine fissure of the visual cortex.

Clinically there is some description of disc hyperemia, and later disc pallor in Iraqi patients (Sabelaish and Hilmi, 1976). A curious and disturbing finding is the remarkable bilateral symmetry of the reported visual field defects, presumably caused by two parallel but separate pathologic events in the right and left calcarine cortex. One might expect some asymmetry and some difference in projection of the two hemifields to the right and left eye. This has not been reported.

REFERENCES

Anderson, B.: Corneal and conjunctival pigmentation among workers engaged in the manufacture of hydroquinone. *Arch. Ophthalmol.,* **38**:812–26, 1947.

Anderson, J. A.; Chen, C. C.; Vita, J. B.; and Shackleton, M.: Disposition of topical flurbiprofen in normal and aphakic rabbit eyes. *Arch. Ophthalmol.,* **100**:642–45, 1982.

Armaly, M.: Effect of corticosteroids on intraocular pressure and fluid dynamics. *Arch. Ophthalmol.,* **70**:482–91, 492–99, 1963.

Ashton, N.: Degeneration of the retina due to 1:5-di(*p*-aminophenoxy) pentane dihydrochloride. *J. Pathol. Bacteriol.,* **74**:103–12, 1957.

———: Oxygen and the growth and development of retinal vessels: *in vivo* and *in vitro* studies. *Am. J. Ophthalmol.,* **62**:412–35, 1966.

———: Some aspects of the comparative pathology of oxygen toxicity in the retina. *Ophthalmologica,* **160**:54–71, 1970.

Ashton, N., and Pedler, C.: Studies on developing retinal vessels. IX. Reaction of endothelial cells to oxygen. *Br. J. Ophthalmol.,* **46**:257–76, 1962.

Avigan, J.; Steinberg, D.; Vroman, H. E.; Thompson, M. J.; and Mosettig, E.: Studies on cholesterol biosynthesis. I. The identification of desmosterol in serum and tissues of animals and man treated with MER-29. *J. Biol. Chem.*, **235**:3123–26, 1960.

Axelsson, U., and Holmberg, A.: The frequency of cataract after miotic therapy. *Acta Ophthalmol.*, **44**:421–29, 1966.

Babel, J., and Ziv, B.: L'action du dithizone sur la rétine du lapin étude electrophysiológique. *Experientia*, **13**:122–23, 1957.

——— : L'action du métabolisme des hydrates de carbone sur l'électrorétinogramme du lapin. *Ophthalmologica*, **137**:270–81, 1959.

Bakir, F.; Damluji, S. F.; Amin-Zaki, L.; Murtadha, M.; Khalidi, A.; Al-Rawi, N. Y.; Tikriti, S.; Dhahir, H. I.; Clarkson, T. W.; Smith, J. C.; and Doherty, R. A.: Methylmercury poisoning in Iraq. *Science*, **181**:230–41, 1973.

Barber, G. W.: Physiological chemistry of the eye. *Arch. Ophthalmol.*, **87**:72–106, 1972.

Becker, B.: Cataracts and topical corticosteroids. *Am. J. Ophthalmol.*, **58**:872–73, 1964.

Beehler, C. C.: Oxygen and the eye. *Surv. Ophthalmol.*, **9**:549–60. 1964.

Belkin, G. A.: Cocktail purpura: an unusual case of quinine sensitivity. *Ann. Intern. Med.*, **66**:583–85, 1967.

Bernstein, H. N.: Chloroquine ocular toxicity. *Surv. Ophthalmol.*, **12**:415–77, 1967.

Bernstein, H. N., and Ginsberg, J.: The pathology of chloroquine retinopathy. *Arch. Ophthalmol.*, **71**:238–45, 1964.

Bernstein, H. N.; Mills, D. W.; and Becker, B.: Steroid-induced elevation of intraocular pressure. *Arch. Ophthalmol.*, **70**:15–18, 1963a.

Bernstein, H. N.; Zvaifler, N.; Rubin, M.; and Mansour, Sister A. M.: The ocular deposition of chloroquine. *Invest. Ophthalmol.*, **2**:384–92, 1963b.

Bettman, J. W.; Fung, W. E.; Webster, R. G.; Noyes, P. P.; and Vincent, N. J.: Cataractogenic effect of corticosteroids on animals. *Am. J. Ophthalmol.*, **65**:581–86, 1968.

Bettman, J. W.; Noyes, P.; and DeBoskey, R.: The potentiating action of steroids in cataractogenesis. *Invest. Ophthalmol.*, **3**:459, 1964.

Birch-Hirschfeld, A.: Beitrag zur Kenntnis der Netzhautganglienzellen unter physiologischen und pathologischen Verhältnissen. *Albrecht von Graefes Arch. Ophthalmol.*, **50**:166–246, 1900.

Birch-Hirschfeld, A., and Köster, G.: Die Schädigung des Auges durch Atoxyl. *Albrecht von Graefes Arch. Ophthalmol.*, **76**:403–63, 1910.

Black, R. L.; Oglesby, R. B.; von Sallmann, L.; and Bunim, J. J.: Posterior subcapsular cataracts induced by corticosteroids in patients with rheumatoid arthritis. *JAMA*, **174**:166–71, 1960.

Bleckmann, H., and Sommer, C.: Hornhauttrubungen durch chloracetophenon. *Graefes Arch. Clin. Exp. Ophthalmol.*, **216**:61–67, 1981.

Boet, D. J.: Toxic effects of phenothiazines on the eye. *Doc. Ophthalmol.*, **28**:1–69, 1970.

Bresnick, G. H.: Oxygen-induced visual cell degeneration in the rabbit. *Invest. Ophthalmol.*, **9**:372–87, 1970.

Brinton, G. S.; Norton, E. W. D.; Zahn, J. R.; and Knighton, R. W.: Ocular quinine toxicity. *Am. J. Ophthalmol.*, **90**:403–10, 1980.

Britten, J. S., and Blank, W.: Thallium activation of the $(Na^+-K^+$ activated ATPase of rabbit kidney. *Biochim. Biophys. Acta*, **159**:160–66, 1968.

Brouwer, B., and Zeeman, W. P. C.: The protection of the retina in the primary optic neuron in monkeys. *Brain*, **49**:1–35, 1926.

Brown, S. I.; Tragakis, M. P.; and Pearce, D. B.: Treatment of the alkali-burned cornea. *Am. J. Ophthalmol.*, **74**:316–20, 1972.

Brown, S. I.; Weller, C. A.; and Akiya, S.: Pathogenesis of ulcers of the alkali-burned cornea. *Arch. Ophthalmol.*, **83**:205–208, 1970.

Brown, S. I.; Weller, C. A.; and Wassermann, H. E.: Collagenolytic activity of alkali-burned corneas. *Arch. Ophthalmol.*, **81**:370–73, 1969.

Budinger, J. M.: Diphenylthiocarbazone blindness in dogs. *Arch. Pathol.*, **71**:304–10, 1961.

Bunce, G. E., and Hess, J. L.: Biochemical changes associated with selenite-induced cataract in the rat. *Exp. Eye Res.*, **33**:505–14, 1981.

Burley, D.: Clioquinol: Time to act. *Lancet*, **1**:1256, 1977.

Burns, C. A.: Ocular effects of Indomethacin. Slit lamp and electroretinographic (ERG) study. *Invest. Ophthalmol.*, **5**:325, 1966.

——— : Indomethacin, reduced retinal sensitivity and corneal deposits. *Am. J. Ophthalmol.*, **66**:825–35, 1968.

Burns, R. P.: Delayed onset of chloroquine retinopathy. *N. Engl. J. Med.*, **275**:693–96, 1966.

Butler, I.: Retinopathy following the use of chloroquine and allied substances. *Ophthalmologica*, **149**:204–208, 1965.

Calkins, L. L.: Corneal epithelial changes occurring during chloroquine (Aralen) therapy. *Arch. Ophthalmol.*, **60**:981–88, 1958.

Cameron, M. E.; Lawrence, J. M.; and Obrich, J. G.: Thioridazine (Mellaril) retinopathy. *Br. J. Ophthalmol.*, **56**:131–34, 1972.

Car, R. E.: Chloroquine and organic changes in the eye. *Dis. Nerv. Syst.*, **29** (Suppl.):36–39, 1968.

Carr, R. E., and Henkind, P.: Ocular manifestations of ethambutol. Toxic amblyopia after administration of an antituberculous drug. *Arch. Ophthalmol.*, **67**:566–71, 1962.

Cerletti, A., and Meier-Ruge, W.: Toxicological studies on phenothiazine induced retinopathy. In *Toxicity and Side Effects of Psychotropic Drugs. Proc. Eur. Soc. Drug Toxic.*, **9**:170–88, 1967.

Chamberlain, W. P., Jr., and Boles, D. J.: Edema of cornea precipitated by quinacrine (Atebrine). *Arch. Ophthalmol.*, **35**:120–34, 1946.

Chayakul, V., and Reim, M.: Enzymatic activity of beta-N-acetylglucosaminidase in the alkali-burned rabbit cornea. *Graefes Arch. Clin. Exp. Ophthalmol.*, **218**:149–52, 1982.

Cibis, G. W.; Burian, H. M., and Blodi, F. C.: Electroretinogram changes in acute quinine poisoning. *Arch. Ophthalmol.*, **90**:307, 1973.

Citron, K. M.: Ethambutol: a review with special reference to ocular toxicity. *Tubercle*, **50** (Suppl.):32–36, 1969.

Cooper, J. R., and Kini, M. M.: Biochemical aspects of methanol poisoning. *Biochem Pharmacol.*, **11**:405–16, 1962.

Cotlier, E., and Becker, B.: Topical steroids and galactose cataracts. *Invest. Ophthalmol.*, **4**:806–14, 1965.

Crews, S. J.: Posterior subcapsular lens opacities in patients on long-term corticosteroid therapy. *Br. Med. J.*, **1**:1644–46, 1963.

——— : The prevention of drug induced retinopathies. *Trans. Ophthalmol. Soc. U.K.*, **86**:63–76, 1967.

Dale, A. J.; Parkhill, E. M.; and Layton, D. D.: Studies on chloroquine retinopathy in rabbits. *JAMA*, **193**:241–43, 1965.

Dana: Sanguinarin, ein neues organisches Alkali in Sanguinaria. *Mag. Pharm.*, **23**:124, 1828.

Dantzker, D. R., and Gerstein, D. D.: Retinal vascular changes following toxic effects on visual cells and pigment epithelium. *Arch. Ophthalmol.*, **81**:106–14, 1969.

Davies, H. C., and Davies, R. E.: Biochemical aspects of oxygen poisoning. In Fenn, W. D., and Rahn, H. (eds.);

Handbook of Physiology, Vol. 2, Sect. 3, American Physiological Society, Washington, D.C., 1965.

Davson, H.: The Physiology of the Eye, 3rd ed. Academic Press, Inc., New York and London, 1972.

Delahunt, C. S.; Stebbins, R. B.; Anderson, J.; and Bailey, J.: The cause of blindness in dogs given hydroxypyridinethione. Toxicol. Appl. Pharmacol., 4:286–91, 1962.

DeLong, S. L.; Poley, B. J.; and McFarlane, J. R., Jr.: Ocular changes associated with long-term chloropromazine therapy. Arch. Ophthalmol., 73:611–17, 1965.

Dickinson, P.; Sabto, J.; and West, R. H.: Management of quinine toxicity. Trans. Ophth. Soc. N.Z., 3356–58, 1981.

Dixon, M.: Reactions of lachrymators with enzymes and proteins. Biochem. Soc. Symp., 2:39–49, 1948.

Dobbie, G. C., and Langham, M. E.: Reaction of animal eyes to sanguinarine argemone oil. Br. J. Ophthalmol., 45:81–95, 1961.

Dollery, C. T.; Bulpitt, D. J.; and Kohner, E. M.: Oxygen supply to the retina from the retinal and choroidal circulations at normal and increased arterial oxygen tensions. Invest. Ophthalmol., 8:588–94, 1969.

Draize, J. H., and Kelley, E. A.: Toxicity to eye mucosa of certain cosmetic preparations containing surface active agents. Proc. Sci. Sect. Toilet Goods Assoc., 17:1–4, 1952.

DuBois, K. P.; Raymund, A. B.; and Hietbrink, B. E.: Inhibitory action of dithiocarbomates on enzymes of animal tissues. Toxicol. Appl. Pharmocol., 3:236–55, 1961.

Duke-Elder, Sir S.: Cataract. In Duke-Elder, Sir S. (ed.): System of Ophthalmology. Vol. XI. Diseases of the lens and vitreous; Glaucoma and hypotony. Henry Kimpton, London, 1969.

Duke-Elder, Sir S., and Jay, B.: Diseases of the lens and vitreous; glaucoma and hypotony. In Duke-Elder, Sir S. (ed.): System of Ophthalmology, Vol. XI. Henry Kimpton, London, 1969.

Duke-Elder, Sir S., and MacFaul, P. A.: Injuries. In Duke-Elder, Sir S. (ed.): System of Ophthalmology, Vol. XIV, Part II, pp. 1011–1356. C. V. Mosby, St. Louis, 1972.

Duke-Elder, Sir S., and Wybar, K. C.: The anatomy of the visual systems. In Duke-Elder, Sir S. (ed.): System of Ophthalmology, Vol. II. C. V. Mosby, St. Louis, 1961.

Edge, N. D.; Mason, D. F. J.; Wein, R.; and Ashton, N.: Pharmacological effects of certain diaminodiphenoxy alkanes. Nature (Lond.), 178:806–807, 1956.

Edwards, G. N.: St. Barth. Hosp. Rep., i:141, 1865; ii:211, 1866.

Ehrlich, D., and Morgan, I. G.: Kainic acid destroys displaced amacrine cells in post-hatch chicken retina. Neurosci. Lett., 17:43–48, 1980.

Ehrlich, P.: Über den jetzigen stand der Chemotherapie. Ber. Dtsch. Chem. Ges., 42:17–47, 1909.

Elbrink, J., and Bihler, I.: Membrane transport of sugars in the rat lens. Can. J. Ophthalmol., 7:96–101, 1972.

Elliott, T. R.: The action of adrenalin. J. Physiol., 32:401–67, 1905.

Figueroa, R.; Weiss, H.; Smith, J. C., Jr.; Hackley, B. M.; McBean, L. D.; Swassing, C. R.; and Halstead, J. A.: Effect of ethambutol on the ocular zinc concentration in dogs. Am. Rev. Respir. Dis., 104:592–94, 1971.

Flower, R. W., and Patz, A.: Oxygen studies in retrolental fibroplasia. IX. The effects of elevated oxygen tension in retinal vascular dynamics in the kitten. Arch. Ophthalmol., 85:197–203, 1971.

Forbes, M.; Kuck, N. A.; and Peets, E. A.: Effect of ethambutol on nucleic acid metabolism in mycobacte-

rium smeginatis and its reversal by polyamines and divalent cations. J. Bacteriol., 89:1299–1305, 1965.

Fournier, D. J., and Patterson, J. W.: Variations in ATPase activity in the development of experimental cataracts. Proc. Soc. Exp. Biol. Med., 137:826–32, 1971.

François, J.: Glaucome apparement simple, secondaire à la cortisonothérapie locale. Ophthalmologica (Suppl.), 142:517–23, 1961.

François, J.; Jönsas, C.; and de Rouck, A.: Étude expérimentale sur l'effect de l'iodo-acétate de soude sur l'électro-rétinogramme et l'électro-oculogramme du lapin. Ann. Ocul. (Paris), 202:637–42, 1969a.

——— : Experimental studies on the effect of dithizone on the electro-retinogram and the electro-oculogram in rabbits. Ophthalmologica, 159:472–77, 1969b.

François, J., and Maudgal, M. C.: Experimentally induced chloroquine retinopathy in rabbits. Am. J. Ophthalmol., 64:886–93, 1967.

François, J.; Verriest, G.; and DeRouck, A.: Etude des fonctions visuelles dans deux cas d'intoxication par la quinine. Ophthalmologica, 153:324–35, 1967.

Fraser, T. R.: On the characters, actions and therapeutical sues of the ordeal bean of Calabar. Edinburgh Med. J., 9:36–56, 123–32, 235–48, 1863.

Fraunfelder, F. T.: Drug Induced Ocular Side Effects and Drug Interactions, 2nd ed. Lea & Febiger, Philadelphia, 1982.

Freedman, J. K., and Potts, A. M.: Repression of glutaminase I in the rat retina by administration of sodium-1-glutamate. Invest. Ophthalmol., 1:118–21, 1962.

Friedenwald, J. S.; Hughes, W. F.; and Herrmann, H.: Acid-base tolerance of the cornea. Arch. Ophthalmol., 31:279–83, 1944.

——— : Acid burns of the eye. Ibid., 35:98–108, 1946.

Galen: De Methodo Medendi. In Kuhn, C. G. (ed.): Opera Omnia, (Lib. III, Cap. 2) Vol. 10, p. 171. Knobloch, Leipzig, 1825.

Galezowski, X.: Des Amlyopies et des Amauroses Toxiques. P. Assaebin, Paris, 1878.

Gangitano, J. L., and Keltner, J. L.: Abnormalities of the pupil and visual-evoked potential in quinine amblyopia. Am. J. Ophthalmol., 89:425–30, 1980.

Garner, A., and Rahi, A. H. S.: Practolol and ocular toxicity. Br. J. Ophthalmol., 60:684–86, 1976.

Gates, M., and Renshaw, B.: Chemical warfare agents and related chemical problems. Sum. Tech. Rep. Div. 9. NDRC, Washington, D.C., 1946.

Gehring, P. J., and Buerge, J. F.: The cataractogenic activity of 2,4-dinitrophenol in ducks and rabbits. Toxicol. Appl. Pharmacol., 14:475–86, 1969a.

——— : The distribution of 2,4-dinitrophenol relative to its cataractogenic activity in ducklings and rabbits. Toxicol. Appl. Pharmacol., 15:574–92, 1969b.

Gehring, P. J., and Hammond, P. B.: The interrelationship between thallium and potassium in animals. J. Pharmacol. Exp. Ther., 155:187–201, 1967.

Giblin, F. J.; McCready, J. P.; and Reddy, V. N.: The role of glutathione metabolism in the detoxification of H_2O_2 in rabbit lens. Invest. Ophthalmol. Vis. Sci., 22:330–35, 1982.

Gilger, A. P., and Potts, A. M.: Studies on the visual toxicity of methanol. V. The role of acidosis in experimental methanol poisoning. Am. J. Ophthalmol., 39:63–86, 1955.

Gilger, A. P.; Potts, A. M.; and Farkas, I.: Studies on the visual toxicity of methanol. IX. The effect of ethanol on methanol poisoning in the rhesus monkey. Am. J. Ophthalmol., 42:244–52, 1956.

Gilman, A., and Philips, F. S.: The biological actions and therapeutic applications of the β-chlorethyl amines and sulfides. Science, 103:409–15, 1946.

Glocklin, V. C., and Potts, A. M.: The metabolism of

retinal pigment cell epithelium. I. The *in vitro* incorporation of P-32 and the effect of diamino-diphenoxyalkane. *Invest. Ophthalmol.*, **1**:111–17, 1962.

Goldberg, I. H., and Friedman, P. A.: Specificity in the mechanism of action of antibiotic inhibitors of protein and nucleic acid synthesis. *Pure Appl. Chem.*, **28**:499–524, 1971.

Goldey, J. A.; Dick, D. A.; and Porter, W. L.: Cornpicker's pupil: a clinical note regarding mydriasis from Jimson weed dust (Stramonium). *Ohio State Med. J.*, **62**:921, 1966.

Goldmann, H.: Cortisone glaucoma. *Arch. Ophthalmol.*, **68**:621–26, 1962.

Gonasun, L. M., and Potts, A. M.: *In vitro* inhibition of protein synthesis in the retinal pigment epithelium by chloroquine. *Invest. Ophthalmol. Visual Sci.*, **13**:107–15, 1974.

Gonasun, L. M., and Potts, A. M.: Possible mechanism of chloroquine induced retinopathy. Presented at the Fifth International Congress on Pharmacology, San Francisco, California, July 23–28, 1972.

Gonda, A.; Gault, H.; Churchill, D.; and Hollomby, D.: Hemodialysis for methanol intoxication. *Am. J. Med.*, **64**:749–58, 1978.

Grant, W. M.: Ocular injury due to sulfur dioxide. *Arch. Ophthalmol.*, **38**:755–61, 762–74, 1947.

——— : A new treatment for calcific corneal opacities. *Arch. Ophthalmol.*, **48**:681–85, 1952.

——— : *Toxicology of the Eye*, 2nd ed. Charles C Thomas Pub., Springfield, Ill., 1974.

Graymore, C. N.: Biochemistry of the retina. In Graymore, C. N. (ed.): *Biochemistry of the Eye*. Academic Press, Inc., New York, 1970.

Graymore, C. N., and Tansley, K.: Iodoacetate poisoning of the rat retina. I. Production of retinal degeneration. *Br. J. Ophthalmol.*, **43**:177–85, 1959.

Green, J., and Ellison, T.: Uptake and distribution of chlorpromazine in animal eyes. *Exp. Eye Res.*, **5**:191–97, 1966.

Greiner, A. C., and Berry, K.: Skin pigmentation and corneal and lens opacities with prolonged chlorpromazine therapy. *Can. Med. Assoc., J.*, **90**:663–65, 1964.

Grignolo, A.; Butturini, U.; and Baronchelli, A.: Ricerchi preliminari sul diabete sperimentale da ditizone. III. Manifestazioni oculari. *Boll. Soc. Ital. Biol. Sper.*, **28**:1416–18, 1952.

Grimes, P., and von Sallmann, L.: Interference with cell proliferation and induction of polyploidy in rat lens epithelium during prolonged myleran treatment. *Exp. Cell Res.*, **42**:265–73, 1966.

Grimes, P.; von Sallmann, L.; Frichette, A.: Influence of myleran on cell proliferation in the lens epithelium. *Invest. Ophthalmol.*, **3**:566–76, 1964.

Guth, P. S., and Spirtes, M. A.: The phenothiazine tranquilizers: biochemical and biophysical actions. *Int. Rev. Neurobiol.*, **7**:231–78, 1964.

Hakim, S. A. E.: Argemone oil, sanguinarine, and epidemic-dropsy glaucoma. *Br. J. Ophthalmol.*, **38**:193–216, 1954.

Hamming, N. A.; Apple, D. J.; and Goldberg, M. F.: Histopathology and ultrastructure of busulfan-induced cataract. *Albrecht von Graefes Arch. Ophthalmol.*, **200**:139–47, 1976.

Handbook of Sensory Physiology, Vol. VII. Autrum, H.; Jung, R.; Loewenstein, W. R.; MacKay, D. M.; and Teubner, H. L. (eds.). Springer-Verlag, Berlin, Heidelberg, New York, 1972–1977.

Harding, C. V.; Reddan, J. R.; Unakar, N. J.; and Bagchi, M.: The control of cell division in the ocular lens. *Int. Rev. Cytol.*, **31**:215–300, 1971.

Harris, J. E., and Gruber, L.: The electrolyte and water balance of the lens. *Exp. Eye Res.*, **1**:372–84, 1962.

——— : The reversal of triparanol induced cataracts in the rat. *Doc. Ophthalmol.*, **26**:324–33, 1969.

——— : Reversal of triparanol-induced cataracts in the rat. II. Exchange of ^{22}Na, ^{42}K, ^{86}Rb in cataractous and clearing lenses. *Invest. Ophthalmol.*, **11**:608–16, 1972.

Haugaard, N.: Poisoning of cellular reactions by oxygen. *Ann N.Y. Acad. Sci.*, **117**, Art. 2:736–44, 1965.

——— : Cellular mechanisms of oxygen toxicity. *Physiol. Rev.*, **48**:311–73, 1968.

Henkes, H. E., and van Lith, G. H. M.: Retinopathy due to indomethacin. *Ophthalmologica*, **164**:385–86, 1972.

Henkes, H. E.; van Lith, G. H. M.; and Canta, L. R.: Indomethacin retinopathy. *Am. J. Ophthalmol.*, **73**:846–56, 1972.

Henrichsen, J.: Tryparsamide in the treatment of syphilis—A review of the literature. *Venereal Dis. Inform.*, **20**:293–322, 1939.

Heppel,ˌL. A.; Neal, P. A.; Endicott, K. M.; and Porterfield, V. T.: Toxicology of dichloroethane. I. Effect on the cornea. *Arch. Ophthalmol.*, **32**:391–94, 1944.

Herman, M. M., and Bensch, K. G.: Light and electron microscopic studies of acute and chronic thallium intoxication in rats. *Toxicol. Appl. Pharmacol.*, **10**:199–222, 1967.

Heyroth, F. F.: Thallium, a review and summary of medical literature. *Public Health Service Reports* (Suppl.). Printing Office, U.S. Government, Washington, D.C., 1947.

Hobbs, H. E.; Sorsby, A.; and Friedman, A.: Retinopathy following chloroquine therapy. *Lancet*, **2**:478–80, 1959.

Horner, W. D.: Dinitrophenol and its relation to formation of cataract. *Arch. Ophthalmol.*, **27**:1097–1121, 1942.

Hübner, U.; Emmerlich, P.; and Heidenbluth, I.: Kandidose bei Explosionsverbrennung und Verätzung durch Trichlorsilan. *Dermatol. Monatsschr.*, **165**:795–98, 1979.

Hughes, W. F.: Alkali burns of the eye. I. Review of the literature and summary of present knowledge. *Arch. Ophthalmol.*, **35**:423–49, 1946a.

——— : Alkali burns of the eye. II. Clinical and pathological course. *Arch. Ophthalmol.*, **36**:189–214, 1946b.

Hunter, D.; Bomford, R. R.; and Russell, D. S.: Poisoning by methyl mercury compounds. *Q. J. Med. N.S.*, **9**:192–219, 1940.

Ide, T.: Histopathological studies on retina, optic nerve and arachnoidal membrane of mouse exposed to carbon disulfide poisoning. *Acta Soc. Ophthalmol. Jap.*, **62A**:85–108, 1958.

Ignarro, L. J.: Lysosome membrane stabilization *in vivo*. Effects of steroidal and nonsteroidal anti-inflammatory drugs on the integrity of rat liver lysosomes. *J. Pharmacol. Exp. Ther.*, **182**:179–88, 1972.

Ikemoto, K.: Effects of cataractogenic compounds, fatty acids and related compounds on cation transport of incubated lens. *Osaka City Med. J.*, **71**:1–18, 1971.

Inturrisi, C. E.: Thallium activation of K^+-activated phosphatases from beef brain. *Biochem. Biophys. Acta*, **173**:567–69, 1969a.

——— : Thallium-induced dephosphorylation of a phosphorylated intermediate of the (sodium and thallium-activated) ATPase. *Biochim. Biophys. Acta*, **178**:630–33, 1969b.

Ishikawa, Y., and Mine, S.: Aminoadipic acid toxic effects on retinal glial cells. *Jpn. J. Ophthalmol.*, **27**:107–18, 1983.

Jachuck, S. J.; Stephenson, J.; Bird, T.; Jackson, F. S.; and Clark, F.: Practolol induced autoantibodies and their relation to oculocutaneous complications. *Postgrad. Med. J.*, **53**:75–77, 1977.

Jacobs, M. B.: *War Gases.* Interscience, New York, 1942.

Jacobs, W. A., and Heidelberger, M.: Aromatic arsenic compounds. II. The amides and alkyl amides of N-arylglycine arsonic acids. *J. Am. Chem. Soc.,* **44:**1587–1600, 1919.

Jaffe, L. S.: Photochemical air pollutants and their effect on men and animals. I. General characteristics and community concentrations. *Arch. Environ. Health,* **15:**782–91, 1967.

Kadota, I.: Studies on experimental diabetes mellitus, as produced by organic reagents. Oxine diabetes and dithizone diabetes. *J. Lab. Clin. Med.,* **35:**568–91, 1950.

Karli, P.: Les dégénérescences rétiniennes spontanées et expérimentales chez l'animal. *Progr. Ophthalmol.,* **14:**51–89, 1963.

Kaufman, P. L.; Axelsson, U.; and Bárány, E. H.: Atropine inhibition of echothiophate cataractogenesis in monkeys. *Arch. Ophthalmol.,* **95:**1262–68, 1977.

——— : Induction of subcapsular cataracts in cynomolgus monkeys by echothiophate. *Arch. Ophthalmol.,* **95:**499–504, 1967.

Kayne, F. J.: Thallium (I) activation of pyruvate kinase. *Arch. Biochem. Biophys.,* **143:**232–39, 1971.

Keyvan-Larijarni, H., and Tannenberg, A. M.: Methanol intoxication, comparison of peritoneal dialysis and hemodialysis treatment. *Arch. Intern. Med.,* **134:**293–96, 1974.

Kini, M. M., and Cooper, J. R.: Biochemistry of methanol poisoning. III. The enzymatic pathway for the conversion of methanol to formaldehyde. *Biochem. Pharmacol.,* **8:**207–17, 1961.

Kinoshita, J. H.: Cataracts in galactosemia. *Invest. Ophthalmol.,* **4:**786–99, 1965.

Kinoshita, J. H.; Barber, G. W.; Merola, L. O.; and Fung, B.: Changes in the levels of free amino acids and myoinositol in the galactose-exposed lens. *Invest. Ophthalmol.,* **8:**625–32, 1969.

Kinross-Wright, V.: Clinical trial of a new phenothiazine compound NP-207. *Psychiatr. Res. Rep. Am. Psychiatr. Assoc.,* **4:**89–94, 1956.

Kinsey, V. E.; McLean, I. W.; and Parker, J.: Studies on the crystalline lens. XVIII. Kinetics of thallium (Tl⁺) transport in relation to that of the alkali metal cations. *Invest. Ophthalmol.,* **10:**932–42, 1971.

Kirby, T. J.; Achor, R. W. P.; Perry, H. O.; and Winkelmann, R. K.: Cataract formation after triparanol therapy. *Arch. Ophthalmol.,* **68:**486–89, 1962.

Klinghardt, G. W.; Fredman, P.; and Svennerholm, L.: Chloroquine intoxication induces ganglioside storage in nervous tissue: a chemical and histopathological study of brain, spinal cord, dorsal root ganglia, and retina in the miniature pig. *J. Neurochem.,* **37:**897–908, 1981.

Kobayashi, T., and Murakami, S.: Blindness of an adult caused by oxygen. *JAMA,* **219:**741–42, 1972.

Kolb, H.; Rosenthal, A. R.; Juxsoll, D.; and Bergsma, D.: Preliminary results on chloroquine induced damage to retina of rhesus monkey. Presented at Association for Research in Vision and Ophthalmology, Sarasota, Florida, Spring, 1972.

Kolker, A. E., and Becker, B.: Epinephrine maculopathy. *Arch. Ophthalmol.,* **79:**552–62, 1968.

Krill, A. E.; Potts, A. M.; and Johanson, C. E.: Chloroquine retinopathy. Investigation of discrepancy between dark adaptation and electroretinographic findings in advanced stages. *Am. J. Ophthalmol.,* **71:**530–43, 1971.

Kuck, J. F. R., Jr.: Chemical constituents of the lens. In Graymore, C. N. (ed.): *Biochemistry of the Eye.* Academic Press, Inc., New York, 1970a.

——— : Metabolism of the lens. In Graymore, C. N.

(ed.): *Biochemistry of the Eye.* Academic Press, Inc., New York, 1970b.

——— : Cataract formation. In Graymore, C. N. (ed.): *Biochemistry of the Eye.* Academic Press, Inc., New York, 1970c.

——— : Response of the mouse lens to high concentrations of glucose and galactose. *Ophthalmic Res.,* **1:**166–74, 1970d.

Kuwabara, T.; Kinoshita, J. H.; and Cogan, D. G.: Electron microscopic study of galactose-induced cataract. *Invest. Ophthalmol.,* **8:**133–49, 1969.

Lasansky, A., and de Robertis, E.: Submicroscopic changes in visual cells of the rabbit induced by iodoacetate. *J. Biophys. Biochem. Cytol.,* **5:**245–50, 1959.

Laughlin, R. C., and Carey, T. F.: Cataracts in patients treated with triparanol, *JAMA,* **181:**339–40, 1962.

Lawley, P. D., and Brookes, P.: Molecular mechanism of the cytotoxic action of difunctional alkylating agents and of resistance to this action. *Nature,* **206:**480–83, 1965.

Lawwill, T.; Appleton, B.; and Altstatt, L.: Chloroquine accumulation in human eyes. *Am. J. Ophthalmol.,* **65:**530–32, 1968.

Ledet, A. E.: Clinical, toxicological and pathological aspects of arsanilic acid poisoning in swine. Ph.D. thesis, Iowa State University, Ames, Iowa, 1970; University Microfilms, Ann Arbor, Mich., 1979.

Leibold, J. E.: The ocular toxicity of ethambutol and its relation to dose. *Ann. N.Y. Acad. Sci.,* **135:**904–909, 1966.

Levine, R. A., and Stahl, C. J.: Eye injury caused by tear-gas weapons. *Am. J. Ophthalmol.,* **65:**497–508, 1968.

Levinson, R. A.; Paterson, C. A.; and Pfister, R. R.: Ascorbic acid prevents corneal ulceration and perforation following experimental alkali burns. *Invest. Ophthalmol. Vis. Sci.,* **15:**986–93, 1976.

Levy, N. S.; Krill, A. E.; and Beutler, E.: Galactokinase deficiency and cataracts. *Am. J. Ophthalmol.,* **74:**41–48, 1972.

Lewin, L., and Guillery, H.: *Die Wirkung von Arzneimitteln und Giften auf das Auge,* Vols. 1 and 2. A. Hirshwald, Berlin, 1913.

Lieberman, T. W.: Prolonged pharmacology and the eye. Ocular effects of prolonged systemic drug administration. *Dis. Nerv. Syst.,* **29** (Suppl.):44–50, 1968.

Linksz, A.: Applied pharmacology of the skin in the ophthalmologists everyday practice. *Arch. Ophthalmol.,* **28:**959–82, 1942.

Loredo, A.; Rodriguez, R. S.; and Murillo, L.: Cataracts after short-term corticosteroid treatment. *N. Engl. J. Med.,* **286:**160, 1972.

Lowry, O. H.; Roberts, N. R.; and Lewis, C.: The quantitative histochemistry of the retina. *J. Biol. Chem.,* **220:**879–92, 1956.

Lowry, O. H.; Roberts, N. R.; Schulz, D. W.; Clow, J. E.; and Clark, J. R.: Quantitative histochemistry of retina. II. Enzymes of glucose metabolism. *J. Biol. Chem.,* **236:**2813–20, 1961.

Lubkin, V. L.: Steroid cataract—a review and a conclusion. *J. Asthma Res.,* **14:**55–59, 1977.

Lucas, D. R., and Newhouse, J. P.: The toxic effect of sodium l-glutamate on the inner layers of the retina. *Arch. Ophthalmol.,* **58:**193–201, 1957.

McChesney, E. W.; Banks, W. F., Jr.; and Fabian, R. J.: Tissue distribution of chloroquine, hydroxychloroquine and desethylchloroquine in the rat. *Toxicol. Appl. Pharmacol.,* **10:**501–13, 1967.

McChesney, E. W.; Banks, W. F., Jr.; and Sullivan, D. J.: Metabolism of chloroquine and hydroxychloroquine in albino and pigmented rats. *Toxicol. Appl. Pharmacol.,* **7:**627–36, 1965.

McCrea, F. D.; Eadie, G. S.; and Morgan, J. E.: The mechanism of morphine miosis. *J. Pharmacol. Exp. Ther.*, 74:239–46, 1942.

McFarlane, J. R.; Yanoff, M.; and Scheie, H. G.: Toxic retinopathy following sparsomycin therapy. *Arch. Ophthalmol.*, 76:532–40, 1966.

McGregor, I. S.: Study of histopathologic changes in the retina and late changes in the visual field in acute methanol poisoning. *Br. J. Ophthalmol.*, 27:523–43, 1943.

Mackenzie, A. H.: An appraisal of chloroquine. *Arthritis Rheum.*, 13:280–91, 1970.

Mackworth, J. F.: The inhibition of thiol enzymes by lachrymators. *Biochem. J.*, 42:82–90, 1948.

Mailer, C. M.: Paradoxical differences in retinal vessel diameters and the effect of inspired oxygen. *Can. J. Ophthalmol.*, 5:163–68, 1970.

Manske, R. H. F.: α-Napthaphenanthredine alkaloids. In Manske, R. H. F., and Holmes, H. L. (eds.): *The Alkaloids, Chemistry and Physiology*, Vol. IV. Academic Press, Inc., New York, 1954, pp. 253–63.

Martin, G.; Draize, J. H.; and Kelley, E. A.: Local anesthesia in eye mucosa produced by surfactants in cosmetic formulations. *Proc. Sci. Sect. Toilet Goods Assoc.*, 37:2–3, 1962.

Martin-Amat, G.; McMartin, K. E.; Hayreh, S. S.; Hayreh, M. S.; and Tephly, T. R.: Methanol poisoning: ocular toxicity produced by formate. *Toxicol. Appl. Pharmacol.*, 45:201–208, 1978.

Maslova, M. N.; Natochin, Y. V.; and Skulsky, I. A.: Inhibition of active sodium transport and activation of Na^+-K^+-ATPase by ions Tl^+ in frog skin. *Biokhimiia*, 36:867–69, 1971.

Matthiolus, P. A.: *Commentarius in sex libros super Dioscorides*. N. Baseus, 1598.

Maurice, D. M.: The cornea and the sclera. In Davson, H. (ed.): *The Eye*, Vol, I, 2nd ed. Academic Press, Inc., New York, 1969.

Maynard, F. P.: Preliminary note on increased intraocular tension met within cases of epidemic dropsy. *Indian Med. Gaz.*, 44:373–74, 1909.

Meier-Ruge, W.: Experimental investigation of the morphogenesis of chloroquine retinopathy. *Arch. Ophthalmol.*, 73:540–44, 1965a.

——— : Die Morphologie der experimentellen Chlorochinretinopathie des Kaninchens. *Ophthalmologica*, 150:127–37, 1965b.

——— : The pathophysiological morphology of the pigment epithelium and its importance for retinal structure and function. *Med. Probl. Ophthalmol.*, 8:32–48, 1968.

Meier-Ruge, W., and Cerletti, A.: Zur experimentellen Pathologie der Phenothiazin-Retinopathie. *Ophthalmologica*, 151:512–33, 1966.

Menzel, D. B.: Toxicity of ozone, oxygen, and radiation. *Annu. Rev. Pharmacol.*, 10:379–94, 1970.

Merriam, F. C., and Kinsey, V. E.: Studies on the crystalline lens. I. Technic for *in vitro* culture of crystalline lenses and observations on the metabolism of the lens. *Arch. Ophthalmol.*, 43:979–88, 1950.

Meyerson, A., and Thau, W.: Ocular pharmacology of furfuryl trimethyl ammonium iodide with special reference to intraocular tension. *Arch. Ophthalmol.*, 24:758–60, 1940.

Mikuni, I.; Fujiwara, T.; and Obazawa, H.: Microtubules in experimental cataracts: disappearance of microtubules of epithelial cells and lens fibers in colchicine-induced cataracts. *Tokai J. Exp. Clin. Med.*, 6:297–303, 1981.

Minton, J.: *Occupational Eye Diseases and Injuries*. Grune & Stratton, Inc., New York, 1949, p. 46.

Monteleone, J. A.; Beutler, E.; Monteleone, P. L.; Utz, C. L.; and Casey, E. C.: Cataracts, galactosuria and hypergalactosemia due to galactokinase deficiency in a child. *Am. J. Med.*, 50:403–407, 1971.

Nakajima, A.: The effect of amino-phenoxy-alkanes on rabbit ERG. *Ophthalmologica*, 136:332–44, 1958.

Neth, R., and Winkler, K.: Proteinsynthese in menschlichen Leukocyten. II. Wirkung einiger Antibiotica auf die Proteinsyntheseleistung von Zellsuspensionen und auf die Peptidyltransferase-Aktivität in zellfreien Systemen. *Klin. Wochenschr.*, 50:523–24, 1972.

Neujean, G.; Weyts, E.; Bacq, Z. M.: Action du B.A.L. sur les accidents ophthalmologiques de la thérapeutique à la tryparsamide. *Bull. Acad. R. Med. Belg.*, 13:341–50, 1948.

Nichols, C. W., and Lambertsen, C. J.: Effects of high oxygen pressures on the eye. *N. Engl. J. Med.*, 281:25–30, 1969.

Nieuwveld, R. W.; Halkett, J. A.; and Spracklen, F. H. N.: Drug resistant malaria in Africa: a case report and review of the problem and treatment. *South Afr. Med. J.*, 62:173–75, 1982.

Nirankari, V. S.; Varma, S. D.; Lakhanpal, V.; and Richards, R. D.: Superoxide radical scavenging agents in treatment of alkali burns. *Arch. Ophthalmol.*, 99:886–87, 1981.

Noell, W. K.: The impairment of visual cell structure by iodoacetate. *J. Cell Comp. Physiol.*, 40:25–45, 1952.

——— : Metabolic injuries of the visual cell. *Am. J. Ophthalmol.*, 40:60–70, 1955.

——— : The visual cell: electric and metabolic manifestations of its life processes. *Am. J. Ophthalmol.*, 48:347–70, 1959.

Nordmann, J.: L'oculiste et la detection preventive systematique de la galactosemie. *Ophthalmologica*, 163:129–35, 1971.

Northover, B. J.: Mechanism of the inhibitory action of indomethacin on smooth muscle. *Br. J. Pharmacol.*, 41:540–51, 1971.

——— : The effects of indomethacin in calcium, sodium, potassium and magnesium fluxes in various tissues of the guinea pig. *Br. J. Pharmacol.*, 45:651–59, 1972.

Nylander, U.: Ocular damage in chloroquine therapy. *Acta Ophthalmol.*, 92 (Suppl.):1–71, 1967.

Obstbaum, S. A.; Galin, M. A.; and Poole, T. A.: Topical epinephrine and cystoid macular edema. *Ann. Ophthalmol.*, 8:455–58, 1976.

Oglesby, R. B.; Black, R. L.; von Sallmann, L.; and Bunim, J. J.: Cataracts in rheumatoid arthritis patients treated with corticosteroids. *Arch. Ophthalmol.*, 66:519–23, 1961a.

——— : Cataracts in patients with rheumatic diseases treated with corticosteroids. *Arch. Ophthalmol.*, 66:625–630, 1961b.

Okamoto, K.: Experimental pathology of diabetes mellitus. (Report II) I. Experimental studies on production and progress of diabetes mellitus by zinc reagents. *Tohoku J. Exp. Med.*, 61 (Suppl. III):1–35, 1955.

Okun, E.; Gouras, P.; Bernstein, H.; and von Sallmann, L.: Chloroquine retinopathy. *Arch. Ophthalmol.*, 69:59–71, 1963.

Olney, J. W.: The toxic effects of glutamate and related compounds in the retina and the brain. *Retina*, 2:341–59, 1982.

Ono, S.; Hirano, H.; and Obara, K. O.: Absorption of cortisol-4-^{14}C into rat lens. *Jap. J. Exp. Med.*, 41:485–87, 1971.

——— : Presence of cortisol-binding protein in the lens. *Ophthalmic Res.*, 3:233–40, 1972a.

——— : Study on the conjugation of cortisol in the lens. *Ophthalmic Res.*, 3:307–10, 1972b.

Orthner, H.: *Methanol Poisoning*. Springer, Berlin, 1950.

Otto, H. F.: Tierexperimentelle Untersuchungen zur Hepato-Toxizität von Triparanol. *Beitr. Pathol.*, 142:177–93, 1971.

Palimeris, G.; Koliopoulos, J.; and Velissaropoulos, P.:

Ocular side effects of indomethacin. *Ophthalmologica,* **164**:339–53, 1972.

Paterson, C. A.: Distribution and movement of ions in the ocular lens. *Doc. Ophthalmol.,* **31**:1–28, 1972.

Patz, A.: Retrolental fibroplasia. *Surv. Ophthalmol.,* **14**:1–29, 1969–70.

Pearce, L.: Studies on the treatment of human trypanosomiasis with tryparsamide (the sodium salt of N-phenylglycineamide-*p*-arsonic acid). *J. Exp. Med.,* **34** (Suppl. 1):1–104, 1921.

Pedersen, O. O., and Karlsen, R. L.: Destruction of Müller cells in the adult rat by intravitreal injection of D,L-alpha-aminoadipic acid. An electron microscopic study. *Exp. Eye Res.,* **28**:569–75, 1979.

Pfannkuch, F., and Bleckmann, H.: Morphologische Befunde an der Kaninchencornea nach Tränengasverätzung. *Graefes Arch. Clin. Exp. Ophthalmol.,* **218**:177–84, 1982.

Pfister, R. R., and Burstein, N.: The alkali burned cornea. I. Epithelial and stromal repair. *Exp. Eye Res.,* **23**:519–35, 1976.

Pfister, R. R., and Koski, J.: Alkali burns of the eye: pathophysiology and treatment. *South. Med. J.,* **75**:417–22, 1982.

Pfister, R. R., and Paterson, C. A.: Ascorbic acid in the treatment of alkali burns of the eye. *Ophthalmology,* **87**:1050–57, 1980.

Pfister, R. R.; Paterson, C. A.; and Hayes, S. A.: Topical ascorbate decreases the incidence of corneal ulceration after experimental alkali burns. *Invest. Ophthalmol. Vis. Sci.,* **17**:1019–24, 1978.

Pirie, A.: Pathology in the eye of the naphthalene-fed rabbit. *Exp. Eye Res.,* **7**:354–57, 1968.

Place, V. A.; Peets, E. A.; Buyske, D. A.; and Little, R. R.: Metabolic and special studies of ethambutol in normal volunteers and tuberculous patients. *Ann. N.Y. Acad. Sci.,* **135**:775–95, 1966.

Place, V. A., and Thomas, J. P.: Clinical pharmacology of ethambutol. *Am. Rev. Respir. Dis.,* **87**:901–904, 1963.

Podos, S. M., and Canellos, G. P.: Lens changes in chronic granulocytic leukemia. *Am. J. Ophthalmol.,* **68**:500–504, 1969.

Potts, A. M.: Methyl alcohol poisoning. *ONR Resp. Rev.,* pp. 4–9, Nov., 1952.

——— : The concentration of phenothiazines in the eyes of experimental animals. *Invest. Ophthalmol.,* **1**:522–30, 1962a.

——— : Uveal pigment and phenothiazine compounds. *Trans. Am. Ophthalmol. Soc.,* **60**:517–52, 1962b.

——— : Further studies concerning the accumulation of polycyclic compounds on unveal melanin. *Invest. Ophthalmol.,* **3**:399–404, 1964a.

——— : The reaction of uveal pigment *in vitro* with polycyclic compounds. *Invest. Ophthalmol.,* **3**:405–16, 1964b.

——— : Agents which cause pigmentary retinopathy. *Dis. Nerv. Syst.,* **29** (Suppl.):16–18, 1968.

Potts, A. M., and Au, P. C.: Thallous ion and the eye. *Invest. Ophthalmol.,* **10**:925–31, 1971.

Potts, A. M.; Hodges, C. B.; Shelman, C. B.; Fritz, K. J.; Levy, N. S.; and Mangnall, Y.: Morphology of the primate optic nerve. III. Fiber characteristics of the foveal outflow. *Invest. Ophthalmol.,* **11**:1004–16, 1972.

Potts, A. M.; Praglin, J.; Farkas, I.; Orbison, L.; and Chickering, D.: Studies on the visual toxicity of methanol. VIII. Additional observations on methanol poisoning in the primate test object. *Am. J.Ophthalmol.,* **40**:76–82, 1955.

Prick, J. J. G.; Sillevis-Smitt, W. G.; and Muller, L.: *Thallium Poisoning.* Elsevier Publishing Co., New York, 1955.

Raitta, C., and Tolonen, M.: Microcirculation of the eye in workers exposed to carbon disulfide. In Merrigan, W. H., and Weiss, B. (eds.): *Neurotoxicity of the Visual System.* Raven Press, New York, 1980.

Ravindranathan, M. P.; Paul, V. J.; and Kuriakose, E. T.: Cataract after busulphan treatment. *Br. Med. J.,* **1**:218–19, 1972.

Rawlins, F. A., and Uzman, B. G.: Retardation of peripheral nerve myelination in mice treated with inhibitors of cholesterol biosynthesis. A quantitative electron microscopic study. *J. Cell Biol.,* **216**:505–17, 1970.

Reading, H. W., and Sorsby, A.: Retinal toxicity and tissue—SH levels. *Biochem. Pharmacol.,* **15**:1389–93, 1966.

Rees, J. R., and Pirie, A.: Possible reactions of 1,2-naphthaquinone in the eye. *Biochem. J.,* **102**:853–63, 1967.

Reim, M., and Schmidt-Martens, F. W.: Behandlung von Verätzungen. *Klin. Monatsbl. Augenheilkd.,* **181**:1–9, 1982.

Riehm, W.: Ueber Presojod-Schädigung des Auges. *Klin. Monatsbl. Augenheilkd.,* **78**:87, 1927.

——— : Akute Pigmentdegeneration der Netzhaut nach Intoxikation mit Septojod. *Arch. Augenheilkd.,* **100–101**:872–82, 1929.

Roe, O.: The ganglion cells of the retina in cases of methanol poisoning in human beings and experimental animals. *Acta Ophthalmol. Scand.,* **26**:169–82, 1948.

Rösner, H.: Untersuchungen zur Wirkung von Chlorpromazin im ZNS von Teleosteern. I. Einfluss auf das Normalverhalten sowie den Einbau von ^{3}H-Uridin und ^{3}H-Histidin. *Psychopharmacologia,* **23**:125–35, 1972.

Sabelaish, S., and Hilmi, G.: Ocular manifestations of mercury poisoning. *W.H.O. Reports,* **53** (Suppl.):83–86, 1976.

Sarkar, S. L.: Katakar oil poisoning. *Indian Med. Gaz.,* **61**:62–63, 1926.

Sarkar, S. N.: Isolation from argemone oil of dihydrosanguinarine and sanguinarine: toxicity of sanguinarine. *Nature (Lond.),* **162**:265–66, 1948.

Sassaman, F. W.; Cassidy, J. J.; Alpern, M.; and Maaseidvaag, F.: Electroretinography in patients with connective tissue diseases treated with hydroxychloroquine. *Am. J. Ophthalmol.,* **70**:515–23, 1970.

Scherbel, A. L.; Mackenzie, A. H.; Nousek, J. E.; and Atdjian, M.: Ocular lesions in rheumatoid arthritis and related disorders with particular reference to retinopathy. A study of 741 patients treated with and without chloroquinine drugs. *N. Engl. J. Med.,* **273**:360–66, 1965.

Schmidt, I. G.: Central nervous system effects of ethambutol in monkeys. *Ann. N.Y. Acad. Sci.,* **135**:759–74, 1966.

Schubert, G., and Bornschein, H.: Spezifische Schädigung von Netzhautelementen durch Jodazetat. *Experientia,* **7**:461–62, 1951.

Schutta, H. S., and Neville, H. E.: Effects of cholesterol synthesis inhibitors on the nervous system. A light and electron microscopic study. *Lab. Invest.,* **19**:487–93, 1968.

Shaffer, R. N., and Hetherington, J.: Anticholinesterase drugs and cataracts. *Am. J. Ophthalmol.,* **62**:613–28, 1966.

Shaffer, R. N., and Ridgway, W. L.: Furmethide iodide in the production of dacryostenosis. *Am. J. Ophthalmol.,* **34**:718–20, 1951.

Shaw, C.-M.; Mottet, N. K.; Body, R. L.; and Luschei, E. S.: Variability of neuropathologic lesions in experimental methylmercurial encephalopathy in primates. *Am. J. Pathol.,* **80**:451–70, 1975.

Shearer, R. V., and Dubois, E. L.: Ocular changes induced by long-term hydroxychloroquine (plaquenil) therapy. *Am. J. Ophthalmol.,* **64**:245–52, 1967.

Shigematsu, I.: Subacute myelo-optico-neuropathy (SMON) and clioquinol. *Jpn. J. Med. Sci. Biol.*, **28** (Suppl.):35–55, 1975.

Shulman, N. R.: Immunoreactions involving platelets. *J. Exper. Med.*, **107**:a. 665–90 b. 691–95 c. 679–710 d. 711–29, 1958.

Siddall, J. R.: The ocular toxic findings with prolonged and high dosage chlorpromazine intake. *Arch. Ophthalmol.*, **74**:460–64, 1965.

——— : Ocular toxic changes associated with chlorpromazine and thioridazine. *Can. J. Ophthalmol.*, **1**:190–98, 1966.

——— : Ocular complications related to phenothiazines. *Dis. Nerv. Syst.*, **29** (Suppl.):10–13, 1968.

Siegrist, A.: Konzentrierte Alkali-und Säurewirkung auf das Auge. *Z. Augenheilkd.*, **43**:176–94, 1920.

Sippel, T. O.: Changes in water, protein, and glutathione contents of the lens in the course of galactose cataract development in rats. *Invest. Ophthalmol.*, **5**:568–75, 1966a.

——— : Energy metabolism in the lens during development of galactose cataract in rats. *Invest. Ophthalmol.*, **5**:576–87, 1966b.

——— : Enzymes of carbohydrate metabolism in developing galactose cataracts of rats. *Invest. Ophthalmol.*, **6**:59–63, 1967.

Slansky, H. H.; Freeman, M. I.; and Itoi, M.: Collagenolytic activity in bovine corneal epithelium. *Arch. Ophthalmol.*, **80**:496–98, 1968.

Sobue, I., and Ando, K.: Myeloneuropathy with abdominal symptoms—5 clinical features and diagnostic criteria. *Clin. Neurol.*, **11**:244–48, 1971.

Solomon, C.; Light, A. E.; and De Beer, E. J.: Cataracts produced in rats by 1,4-dimethanesulfonoxybutane (myleran). *Arch. Ophthalmol.*, **54**:850–52, 1955.

Sorsby, A.: The nature of experimental degeneration of the retina. *Br. J. Ophthalmol.*, **25**:62–65, 1941.

Sorsby, A., and Harding, R.: Protective effect of cysteine against retinal degeneration induced by iodate and iodoacetate. *Nature (Lond.)*, **187**:608–609, 1960.

Sorsby, A., and Nakajima, A.: Experimental degeneration of the retina. IV. Diaminodiphenoxyalkanes as inducing agents. *Br. J. Ophthalmol.*, **42**:563–71, 1958.

Steinberg, D., and Avigan, J.: Studies on cholesterol biosynthesis. II. The role of desmosterol in the biosynthesis of cholesterol. *J. Biol. Chem.*, **235**:3127–29 1960.

Straus, D. J.; Mausolf, F. A.; Ellerby, R. A.; and McCracken, J. D.: Cicatricial ecotropion secondary to 5-fluorouracil therapy. *Med. Pediat. Oncol.*, **3**:15–19, 1977.

Sugimoto, K., and Goto, S.: Retinopathy in chronic carbon disulfide exposure. In Merrigan, W. H., and Weiss, B. (eds.): *Neurotoxicity of the Visual System.* Raven Press, New York, 1980.

Tarkkanen, A.; Esila, R.; and Liesmaa, M.: Experimental cataracts following long-term administration of corticosteroids. *Acta Ophthalmol.*, **44**:665–68, 1966.

Tateishi, J., andOtsuki, S.: Experimental reproduction of SMON in animals by prolonged administration of clioquinol: Clinico-pathological findings. *Jpn. J. Med. Sci. Biol.*, **28** (Suppl.):165–86, 1975.

Tephly, T. R.; Parks, R. E., Jr.; and Mannering, G. J.: Methanol metabolism in the rat. *J. Pharmacol. Exp. Ther.*, **143**:292–300, 1963.

Thatcher, D. B.; Blaug, S. M.; Hyndiuk, R. A.; and Watzke, R. C.: Ocular effects of chemical Mace in the rabbit. *Clin. Med.*, **78**:11–13, 1971.

Thomas, H. W.: Some experiments in the treatment of trypanosomiasis. *Br. Med. J.*, **1**:1140–43, 1905.

Thomas, J. P.; Baughn, C. O.; Wilkinson, R. G.; and Shepard, R. G.: A new synthetic compound with anti-tuberculous activity in mice: ethambutol dextro2,2′ ethylenediimino di-1-butanol. *Am. Rev. Respir. Dis.*, **83**:891–93, 1961.

Trakatellis, A. C.: Effect of sparsomycin on protein synthesis in the mouse liver. *Proc. Natl Acad. Sci. USA*, **59**:854–60, 1968.

Trayhurn, P., and van Heyningen, R.: The metabolism of glutamate, aspartate and alanine in the bovine lens. *Biochem. J.*, **124**:72P–73P, 1971a.

——— : Aerobic metabolism in the bovine lens. *Exp. Eye Res.*, **12**:315–27, 1971b.

Trumbull, G. C.; Sbarbaro, J. A.; and Iseman, M.: (Correspondence) High dose ethambutol. *Am. Rev. Respir. Dis.*, **115**:889–90, 1977.

Tsubaki, T., and Irukayama, K.: (eds.): *Minimata Disease.* Kodansha Ltd., Tokyo; Elsevier Scientific Pub. Co., Amsterdam, 1977.

Uhthoff, W.: Die Augenstörungen bei Vergiftungen. In Graefe-saemisch *Handbuch der Gesamten Augenheilkunde*, **11**:1–180, Engelmann, Leipzig, 1911.

Upholt, W. M.; Quinby, G. E.; Batchelor, G. S.; and Thompson, J. P.: Visual effects accompanying TEPP-induced miosis. *Arch. Ophthalmol.*, **56**:128–34, 1956.

van Haeringen, N. J.; Oosterhuis, J. A.; and van Delft, J. L.: A comparison of the effects of non-steroidal compounds on the disruption of the blood-aqueous barrier. *Exp. Eye Res.*, **35**:271–77, 1982.

van Heyningen, R.: The lens: Metabolism and cataract. In Davson, H. (ed.): *The Eye, Vegetative Physiology and Biochemistry*, Vol. 1, 2nd ed. Academic Press, Inc., New York, 1969.

——— : Ascorbic acid in the lens of the naphthalene-fed rabbit. *Exp. Eye Res.*, **9**:38–48, 1970a.

——— : Effect of some cyclic hydroxy compounds on the accumulation of ascorbic acid by the rabbit lens *in vitro*. *Exp. Eye Res.*, **9**:49–56, 1970b.

——— : Galactose cataract: a review. *Exp. Eye Res.*, **11**:415–28, 1971.

van Heyningen, R., and Pirie, A.: The metabolism of naphthalene and its toxic effect on the eye. *Biochem. J.*, **102**:842–52, 1967.

Van Joost, T. H.; Crone, R. A.; and Overdijk, A. D.: Ocular cicatricial pemphigoid associated with practolol therapy. *Br. J. Dermatol.*, **94**:447–50, 1976.

Velhagen, K.: Zur Hornhautargyrose. *Klin. Monatsbl. Augenheilkd.*, **122**:36–42, 1953.

Vito, P.: Contributo allo studio della degenerazione pigmentaria della retina indotta dalla soluzione iodica di Pregl. *Boll. Ocul.*, **11**:945–57, 1935.

von Sallmann, L.: The lens epithelium in the pathogenesis of cataract. *Am. J. Ophthalmol.*, **44**:159–70, 1957.

von Sallmann, L.; Grimes, P.; and Collins, E.: Triparanol induced cataract in rats. *Arch. Ophthalmol.*, **70**:522–30, 1963.

Waley, S. G.: The lens: function and macromolecular composition. In Davson, H. (ed.): *The Eye*, Vol. 1, 2nd ed. Academic Press, Inc., New York, 1969.

Warburg, O.: *Über den Stoffwechsel der Tumoren.* f. Springer, Berlin, 1926, p. 138.

Weekley, R. D.; Potts, A. M.; Reboton, J.; and May, R. H.: Pigmentary retinopathy in patients receiving high doses of a new phenothiazine. *Arch. Ophthalmol.*, **64**:65–74, 1960.

Weitzel, G.; Strecker, F. J.; Roester, U.; Buddecke, E.; and Fretzdorff, A. M.: Zinc im tapetum lucidum. *Hoppe Seylers Z. Physiol. Chem.*, **296**:19–30, 1954.

Weller, C. A., and Green, M.: Methionyl-tRNA synthetase detected by [76Se]-selenomethionine in lenses from normal and galactose-fed rats. *Exp. Eye Res.*, **8**:84–90, 1969.

Wetterholm. D. H., and Winter, F. C.: Histopathology of chloroquine retinal toxicity. *Arch. Ophthalmol.*, **71**:82–87, 1964.

Wheeler, M. C.: Discoloration of the eyelids from prolonged use of ointments containing mercury. *Trans. Am. Ophthalmol. Soc.*, **45**:74–80, 1947.

Wilkes, J. W.: Argyrosis of cornea and conjunctiva. *J. Tenn. Med. Assoc.*, **46**:11–13, 1953.

Williamson, J.: A new look at the ocular side-effects of long-term systemic corticosteroid and adenocorticotrophic therapy. *Proc. R. Soc. Med.*, **63**:791–92, 1970.

Williamson, J.; Paterson, R. W. W.; McGavin, D. D. N.; Jasani, M. K.; Boyle, J. A.; and Doig, W. M.: Posterior subcapsular cataracts and glaucoma associated with long-term oral corticosteroid therapy. In patients with rheumatoid arthritis and related conditions. *Br. J. Ophthalmol.*, **53**:361–72, 1969.

Wirth, A.; Quaranta, C. A.; and Chistoni, G.: The effect of dithizone on the electroretinogram of the rabbit. *Bibl. Ophthalmol.*, **48**:66–73, 1957.

Wood, C. A., and Buller, F.: Poisoning by wood alcohol. Cases of death and blindness from Columbian spirits and other methylated preparations. *JAMA*, **43**:972–77; 1058–62; 1117–23; 1213–21; 1289–96, 1904.

Wood, D. C.; Contaxis, I.; Sweet, D.; Smith, J. C., II; and Van Dolah, J.: Response of rabbits to corticosteroids. I. Influence on growth, intraocular pressure and lens transparency. *Am. J. Ophthalmol.*, **63**:841–49, 1967.

UNIT III
TOXIC AGENTS

Chapter 18

TOXIC EFFECTS OF PESTICIDES

Sheldon D. Murphy

INTRODUCTION

Pesticides occupy a rather unique position among the many chemicals that man encounters daily, in that they are deliberately added to the environment for the purpose of killing or injuring some form of life. Ideally their injurious action would be highly specific for undesirable target organisms and noninjurious to desirable, nontarget organisms. In fact, however, most of the chemicals that are used as pesticides are not highly selective but are generally toxic to many nontarget species, including humans, and other desirable forms of life that coinhabit the environment. Therefore, lacking highly selective pesticidal action, the application of pesticides must often be predicated on selecting quantities and manners of usage that will minimize the possibility of exposure of nontarget organisms to injurious quantities of these useful chemicals.

Toxicologic evaluations of the hazard of handling and use of pesticides have for many years focused primarily on preventing injury to humans, and common laboratory animals have served as the experimental models for humans' biochemical, physiologic, and pathologic responses to these chemicals. Problems of species differences in susceptibility have always left some doubt concerning assignment of safe dosages for humans on the basis of studies on common laboratory animals, but this approach appears to have been reasonably successful in protecting the *general population* in that there has not emerged any clear association between increasing use of pesticides and incidence of chronic diseases (Hayes, 1969). However, as discussed subsequently, occupational exposures have resulted in chronic or persistent neurologic disease states in the case of a few compounds.

Acute poisonings by pesticides do occur. They are usually the result of occupational exposures or of careless use, misuse, or mishandling the pesticides. The mortality rate attributed to poisoning by pesticides has been estimated at 0.65 per one million population in

the United States, but it has also been estimated that there are 100 nonfatal poisonings for each fatal one (Hayes, 1969). In spite of the fact that a clear association between chronic diseases and pesticide exposures is not apparent, new and sensitive toxicologic and analytic methods have raised many questions concerning the possibility of subtle effects that would be difficult to recognize unless one directed investigations specifically to reveal them. A review of the status of epidemiologic studies on pesticide toxicology pointed out design and interpretive pitfalls that give cause to question whether our knowledge is adequate to assess that degree of injury or lack of injury to human health resulting from past or current uses of pesticides (Secretary's Commission on Pesticides, 1969).

Furthermore, increased awareness and concern for ecologic implications of the use of pesticides have begun to direct the attention and research of toxicologists toward studies on wild species as well as on humans and domestic animals and laboratory animals that are selected as test models to represent humans. The toxicology of pesticides, therefore, must take into account problems relating to both their injurious effects directly upon humans and their effects on other species of animals in the environment from which humans derive pleasure as well as food or which are essential to maintain a proper ecologic balance.

It is not uncommon for people to equate *pesticides* with *insecticides*. This is erroneous since the term "pesticide" is a general classification and includes a variety of chemicals with different uses. Pesticidal chemicals have in common the capability of destroying life of some form and are classified as pesticides because the organisms against which they are directed are deemed to be undesirable by the person or society that applies them. Indeed, insecticides represent one group of pesticides that are used in large quantities and have a history of causing toxic effects in humans, but among the other types of pesticides one can find several potent, injurious agents. In terms of quantities used, the *herbicides,* chemicals used to destroy unwanted plants, rival the insecticides. Another common misconception is that pesticides imply a unity of action, that they all act similarly. This of course is not true. There is as great a diversity in their types of action and primary target tissues as there is diversity in their chemistry and physicochemical properties. There are a large number of pesticides whose acute toxicity is manifested through functional or biochemical action in the central and peripheral nervous systems, but there are others in which nervous system involvement does not occur or is merely secondary to primary effects in other organ systems. The literature on pesticides reveals great disparities in the extent of knowledge concerning specific mechanisms of action. For some groups of compounds the mechanism of toxic action is well understood at the molecular level. For others there is essentially no information concerning mechanisms of toxicity. Similarly the full gamut of toxic dose-response ranges is represented by pesticide chemicals. Even within a similar chemical class, individual compounds ranging from extremely toxic to practically nontoxic may be found. Obviously, therefore, one cannot generalize either qualitatively or quantitatively concerning the toxicity of pesticides.

ECONOMICS AND PUBLIC HEALTH: BENEFITS AND RISKS

As with the use of any potentially injurious chemical substance, the use of pesticides must take into consideration the balance of the benefits that may be expected versus the possible risk of injury to human health or to degradation of environmental quality. It is indeed extremely difficult to quantify the risk-benefit equation relating to the use of pesticides. In some cases the prospect of mass starvation due to destruction of food crops by insects and noxious weeds versus the question of possible injury to a few members of the population as a result of use of insecticides may clearly indicate an advantage of pesticide use in terms of numbers of people whose health and welfare are protected. Similarly where vector-borne diseases represent a major threat to the health of large populations of humans, and where the use of chemical pesticides to destroy the vectors of these diseases is a successful procedure, the application of these chemicals seems to be clearly indicated. On the other hand, widespread distribution of chemicals in the environment to control what may be primarily a nuisance situation raises questions as to whether the benefits to be achieved really justify any risk, however minimal, that human health may be jeopardized.

If one extends these considerations beyond purely a concern for human health and considers the question of ecologic balance, the risk-benefit equation takes on different proportions. In the first case, with the exception of possible exposures of the persons who handle the concentrated pesticides, the human population may not be exposed to any significant quantity of the chemical. However, when these chemicals are distributed over widespread areas of land and aquatic surfaces, there is a distinct possibility that desirable species in the environment, other than humans, will receive potentially toxic doses of the chemicals. This may not appear to have any direct effect on human health and welfare; however, if such effects lead to a serious ecologic imbalance, indirect effects on humans are possible. Perhaps the best known of all pesticides, DDT, exemplifies a situation of a product that when introduced as an insecticide in 1942 appeared to hold immense promise of benefit to agricultural economics and protection of public health against vector-borne disease. It was hailed as the miracle insecticide and for two decades was used with little concern for injury, and indeed little evidence that injury was produced. However, during the third decade of its use, effects on the environment, effects in nontarget species other than humans, began to raise serious doubts concerning its continued usefulness. Now, many countries of the world have greatly restricted the use of DDT because of evidence of environmental damage.

Control of Vector-Borne Disease

Pesticides of various types are used in the control of insects, rodents, and other pests that are involved in the life-cycle of vector-borne diseases such as malaria, filariasis, yellow fever, viral encephalitis, typhus, bubonic plague, Rocky Mountain spotted fever, rickettsialpox etc. The success of DDT in reducing the incidence of malaria in many parts of the world has been dramatic. To cite one example, in the Latina province of Italy in 1944 there were 175 new cases of malaria; in 1945 a DDT spray control program was initiated and by 1947 there were only five new cases of malaria, and by 1949 no new cases of malaria appeared.

This is only one example of a success story for DDT. The story has been repeated and continues to be repeated in some areas. Worldwide estimates of the lives saved by using DDT to destroy insects that transmit malaria and other diseases are numbered in the millions and the illnesses prevented are numbered in the hundreds of millions.

Agricultural Productivity

In many parts of the world excessive loss of food crops to insects and other destructive pests contribute to an obvious health problem—starvation. In these countries use of chemicals for controlling these pests clearly seems to have a favorable cost-benefit relationship. In lands of plenty such a clear health benefit may be less obvious. Then, attempts to evaluate the cost-benefit ratios are often reduced to economic considerations. It has been estimated that in 1963 the use of pesticides in the United States resulted in an increase in the value of farm production of about 1.8 billion dollars. This was achieved with an expenditure of about 0.44 billion dollars for control chemicals and procedures. Thus, one can estimate that the net economic benefit was an approximate 1.4-billion-dollar contribution to the gross national product (Headley and Kneese, 1969).

Urban Pest Control

Although the total usage of pesticides, in terms of pounds applied, is largest in those applications related to agriculture or forestry, these toxic chemicals are also used in urban areas. In addition to the use of pesticides by government service agencies, as in mosquito and rodent control programs and weed control on highways and utility rights of way, there is a rather large use of pesticides by individual home owners and gardeners. For example, during a one-year period in Salt Lake County, Utah, of the total of 200,865 lb of pesticides used, 102,490 lb were used for domestic or household applications. The balance was used by farmers, commercial applicators, fruit growers, and government agencies, and for mosquito abatement, and on livestock. There are, however, great contrasts in these proportions, as illustrated by the statistics for Arizona. The domestic usage for the state accounted for only about 0.6 percent of the total compared to over 50 percent of the total in Salt Lake County, Utah (Secretary's Commission on Pesticides, 1969).

A study of domestic use in South Carolina indicated that 89 percent of all families used pesticides in some form. In that study 50 percent of the pesticide purchases were made at the grocery store, the same source as the family's food. Lesser retail sources were feed and seed, drug, and general merchandise stores. Ninety percent of the families stored their pesticides in unlocked storage areas; 65 percent of these storage areas were within easy reach of children; about 50 percent of the families stored their pesticides near food or medicine. Moreover, 75 percent of the user families did not take simple precautions

such as washing or use of gloves when handling their pesticides. In spite of this almost flagrant violation of precautionary measures, it appeared there was no significant difference in the incidence of a variety of chronic diseases between pesticide user families and nonuser families (Kiel et al., 1969). In addition, there are a number of rather subtle possibilities for exposure to pesticides from a wide variety of sources. Pesticides have been incorporated into shelf papers. They are incorporated in some kinds of paints as antifungal agents, they are used in mixtures of swimming pool chemicals for algae control, in various types of automatic dispensers in public buildings and homes, and they have been used in dry-cleaning processes for rugs and other fabrics.

It is clear that the opportunities for exposure to pesticides are great. Because the use of pesticides is associated primarily with agricultural operations, major concern is usually for the food we eat. However, it is quite possible that less controlled and less regulated uses of pesticides may offer the greatest opportunity for exposure to toxicologically significant quantities.

Environmental Contamination

It is apparent that there are many sources of exposure of humans and other nontarget species to pesticides by direct contact with materials at the site of application. In recent years, however, it has become increasingly apparent that exposures to pesticides far from the source of application are also possible. This results from the translocation of the chemicals from their sites of application through the various media of the environment. The extent to which translocation within the environment occurs will depend to a large degree on the physicochemical properties of the pesticides. Perhaps one of the most important factors is the extent of and time required for degradation of chemicals to simpler nontoxic forms. Since several of the organochlorine insecticides and some of the heavy metals are the most persistent types of pesticides, these compounds have been the object of most concern for problems of translocation and biomagnification. For example, DDT is only slowly biotransformed by biologic systems. Some of the metabolites are extremely resistant to further degradation, but retain some of the biologic activities of the parent compound. In addition, the partition coefficient for DDT in fat-soluble substances, relative to aqueous media, is very high. Therefore, this chemical will be concentrated through a food chain since it tends to partition into lipoidal biological materials in increasing concentrations until, at the top of the food chain pyramid, a potentially hazardous concentration may exist.

DDT applied in a mosquito control program in a tropical or subtropical area may ultimately have adverse effects on species in Arctic regions. Thus, small quantities that may be present in mud and surface waters are taken up by plankton and other food sources for phytophagous fish. These fish ingest the plankton containing insecticide and its metabolites at a rate insufficient to poison them, but sufficient to allow storage and concentration in their fatty tissue. The phytophagous fish are eaten by carnivorous fish, again at a rate at which the dosage is not immediately harmful, but partitioning into the fat allows slow accumulation of a high concentration in fat. In turn, these fish may migrate and be ingested by birds in Arctic climates, such as falcons and eagles, in sufficient quantities to contribute doses of the insecticide or its metabolites that can affect avian reproduction (Secretary's Commission on Pesticides, 1969).

Other nonbiologic modes of translocation include vaporization and drift by airborne routes so that the materials are carried by prevailing wind patterns far remote from their site of application. Subsequently, they may be precipitated out by rainfall onto land and surface waters in areas in which the pesticides have not been applied directly. Application to the soil may result, ultimately, in suspension of the pesticides, which are adsorbed on soil particles, and their airborne translocation as dust. The extent to which pesticides will remain in soils after application depends upon a number of factors: such as soil type, moisture, temperature, pH, microorganism content, degradability of the pesticide itself, and the extent of cultivation and cover crops (Lichtenstein, 1966). In general, the organochlorine insecticides are most persistent in soils (with the exception of heavy metals, which of course are not further degraded), followed by certain of the herbicides and with the phosphate insecticides and carbamate insecticides and herbicides being the least persistent. An understanding of the potential for persistence and translocation, therefore, must take into consideration not only the biologic aspects of pesticides but also an analysis of their behavior under various physical and chemical characteristics of the environment. As will be pointed out subsequently, chemical changes of the parent insecticides that result from either physicochemical reactions in the environment or biologically catalyzed reactions may lead to products with either greater or lesser toxicity and with either greater or lesser potential for biotranslocation.

Production and Use Statistics

Before the mid-1940s the primary pesticides in use were botanical in origin and compounds of heavy metals. Subsequently, there has been a marked increase in total pesticide usage and a rapid proliferation of synthetic organic compounds. There are now approximately 900 chemicals that are registered for sale as pesticides against about 2,000 pest species (Secretary's Commission on Pesticides, 1969).

The estimated total pesticide purchases by farmers increased from 184 million dollars in 1955 to 1 billion dollars in 1968. This marked increase in sales of pesticides occurred in spite of the fact that the harvested acreage during this period declined from 335 million acres to 294 million acres. In recent years there have been rather dramatic shifts in the types of pesticides used by farmers. For example, until the mid-1960s insecticides were the leading class of pesticides used. Since then herbicides have begun to outpace insecticides. In 1971 the U.S. market for agricultural use of herbicides was estimated at 640 million dollars compared to $225 million for insecticides and $65 million for fungicides (NAS, 1976). The world market for herbicides, insecticides, and fungicides has been estimated will reach 4668, 3190, and 1761 million U.S. dollars, respectively, in 1984 (Ecobichon and Joy, 1982). In the mid-1960s there was a shift in the types of insecticides used, from the organochlorine to the less stable organophosphate and carbamate classes. In Europe, fungicide sales lead the pesticide market.

Shifts in uses of major classes reflect not only developments in agricultural practice but also the effect of regulatory restrictions and the development of resistance by the pests to certain classes of chemicals.

Human Poisonings

As stated initially, pesticides have a relatively good record in the United States in terms of fatalities resulting from exposure. The United States has escaped major incidents of mass acute fatal poisonings, but this is not the case when one considers the worldwide record (see Table 18–1). There have been several reports of various disease conditions or altered clinical test values resulting from chronic exposure to pesticides, but these conditions are generally reversible and thus cannot be classified as true chronic injury. The relatively small numbers of cases in which progressive chronic disease has been associated with pesticide exposure preclude establishment of cause-and-effect relationships and prevent the conclusion that the widespread use

Table 18–1. MASS POISONINGS BY PESTICIDES*

KIND OF ACCIDENT	PESTICIDE INVOLVED	MATERIAL CONTAMINATED	NUMBER AFFECTED	NUMBER DIED	LOCATION
Spillage during transport or storage	Endrin	Flour	159	0	Wales
	Endrin	Flour	691	24	Qatar
	Endrin	Flour	183	2	S. Arabia
	Dieldrin	Food	20	0	Shipboard
	Diazinon	Doughnut mix	20	0	U.S.A.
	Parathion	Wheat	360	102	India
	Parathion	Barley	38	9	Malaya
	Parathion	Flour	200	8	Egypt
	Parathion	Flour	600	88	Colombia
	Parathion	Sugar	300	17	Mexico
	Parathion	Sheets	3	0	Canada
	Mevinphos	Pants	6	0	U.S.A.
Eating formulation	Hexachlorobenzene	Seed grain	>3000	3–11%	Turkey
	Organic mercury	Seed grain	34	4	West Pakistan
	Organic mercury	Seed grain	321	35	Iraq
	Organic mercury	Seed grain	45	20	Guatemala
	Warfarin	Bait	14	2	Korea
Improper application	Toxaphene	Collards and chard	7	0	U.S.A.
	Nicotine	Mustard	11	0	U.S.A.
	Parathion	Used as treatment for body lice	>17	15	Iran
	Pentachlorophenol	Nursery linens	20	2	U.S.A.

* From Secretary's Commission on Pesticides, U.S. Department of Health, Education, and Welfare: *Report of the Secretary's Commission on Pesticides and Their Relationship to Environmental Health.* U.S. Governmental Printing Office, Washington, D.C., 1969.

of pesticides has contributed to an increasing incidence of chronic disease (Hayes, 1969). As new methods of toxicologic evaluation reveal subtle effects previously unknown and as this information is applied to well-designed epidemiologic studies, it may be found that pesticides have produced currently undetected effects on health. As discussed below, however, there is ample evidence that exposure to pesticides has resulted in acute fatal poisonings and reversible illnesses.

Statistical surveys of mortality and morbidity resulting from acute exposures to pesticides reveal that children are the victims of a high percentage of accidental fatal poisonings. Reich and coworkers (1968) reported that during the period of 1956 through 1967 there were 122 fatal cases of documented pesticide poisoning in Dade Country, Florida. Fifty-seven percent of these fatalities were suicidal, 29.8 percent were accidental, homicides accounted for 9.9 percent, and 2.5 percent were occupational. Twenty-seven percent of the fatalities were children under five years of age and the deaths were usually the result of accidental ingestions. Adults over 40 accounted for 48 percent of the cases (mostly suicides) and the route of exposure in 90 percent of these was also oral, with three cases of dermal exposure and five due to inhalation. Of the 122

cases, 65 involved organophosphate insecticides, with parathion as the agent in 53 of these 65. Heavy metals (with arsenic as the prime offender) and white phosphorus were responsible for 27 of the deaths. Succeeding these classes, in order of frequency, were nicotine, organochlorines, cyanide, strychnine, and miscellaneous.

From the period of 1964 to 1967 both mortality and morbidity data were available. Of the 133 cases of documented pesticide poisonings during this period, 47 (35 percent) were fatal. Of the 133 cases, 61 were the result of accidental poisonings with 11 of them fatal. The mean age for accidental poisoning was 8.6 years. There were 25 cases of occupational poisonings, but only one was fatal. There was a 70 percent case fatality rate when pesticides were ingested for suicidal purposes (in 37 of the total 133 poisonings). Of the occupational poisonings 24 of the 25 cases involved organophosphate insecticides. Parathion was the agent in one fatal case of occupational poisoning. Organophosphate insecticides accounted for 72 percent of the total accidental cases and 90 percent of the accidental fatalities, 60 percent of the total suicide attempts, and 51 percent of the successful suicides.

Death records of the California Department of Public Health (1969) for the period 1951 to 1969 revealed that, as in Florida, children accounted for over half (92) of the total (163) accidental deaths due to poisoning by agricultural chemicals, However, only 17 of the fatal childhood poisonings were due to organic phosphates, while arsenic compounds accounted for 48 of the deaths. There were 35 accidental nonoccupational, pesticide poisoning fatalities among adults during this period, 17 of them due to arsenic compounds. Occupational poisonings accounted for 36 of the 163 deaths. Eighteen of the occupational poisonings were due to organophosphate insecticides, seven to methyl bromide, and 13 to other agricultural chemicals. Thus, during the period of 1951 to 1969 arsenic-containing pesticides were involved most frequently in nonoccupational poisonings, while organophosphates were most frequently involved in occupational pesticide poisoning fatalities. It was concluded that organophosphates played a smaller role in fatal poisonings among children in California because state regulations made these agents less readily available for indiscriminate home use. Mortality attributed to accidental poisoning by pesticides in the United States appears to have been declining during the past two decades. Hayes and Vaughn (1977) report that in 1974 there were only 52 fatal accidental poisonings with pesticides, compared to 152 in 1956. During this period the proportion of fatal poisonings in children declined from 61 to 31 percent. This decline was attributed to an increased awareness on the part of poison control centers and pediatricians to the hazards of the pesticides to children.

Injuries from occupational exposures re-ported under the requirements of the State Workmen's Compensation Law in California have provided statistical compilations of the extent of injuries due to pesticides and other agricultural chemicals (California Department of Public Health, 1969). The rate for all occupational disease reports in agricultural workers in 1969 was 8.5 per 1000 workers, more than three times the rate for all industry (2.6 per 1000). There were 727 occupational disease reports attributed to agricultural chemicals in California in 1969. Thirty-two percent of these involved organic phosphate insecticides, 10 percent herbicides, 8 percent halogenated hydrocarbon insecticides, 6 percent fertilizers, and 44 percent miscellaneous or unidentified chemicals. Of the 175 cases diagnosed as systemic poisonings, organophosphate insecticides were responsible for 80 percent, and they were involved in 47 percent of another 160 reports of digestive and other nonlocalized symptoms of illness. This high contribution of systemic poisonings due to organic phosphates continued in the record of several years (from 1956 to 1969 from 125 to 407 reports of systemic occupational poisonings were reported annually in California). Parathion was the agent most frequently involved. Table 18–2 shows the types of disease conditions produced by various agricultural chemicals in California in 1969. Table 18–3 illustrates the industries and occupations in which poisonings by agricultural chemicals occurred. Clearly, workers involved in direct agricultural operations were a high-risk group, and clearly, organophosphorous insecticides were high-risk compounds. Although, as a class herbicides ranked second

Table 18–2.　TYPE OF OCCUPATIONAL DISEASE REPORTED CAUSED BY PESTICIDES AND OTHER AGRICULTURAL CHEMICALS IN CALIFORNIA IN 1969*

TYPE OF CHEMICAL	TYPE OF DISEASE				
	Systemic Poisoning	*Respiratory Condition*	*Skin Condition*	*Other and Unspecified*	TOTAL ALL TYPES
Organic phosphate pesticides	140	4	12	75	231
Halogenated hydrocarbon pesticides	9	7	19	22	57
Herbicides	3	9	50	14	76
Fertilizers	—	8	28	7	43
Fungicides	2	3	21	1	27
Phenolic compounds	2	1	10	2	15
Sulfur	1	2	25	3	31
Organomercury compounds	1	—	—	1	2
Lead or arsenic	2	—	2	5	9
Miscell.—specified	5	1	15	7	28
Unspecified	9	12	162	21	204
Total	175	47	345	160	727

* From California Department of Public Health: *Occupational Diseases in California Attributed to Pesticides and Other Agricultural Chemicals, 1969.* Bureau of Occupational Health and Environment Epidemiology, Sacramento, 1969.

Table 18–3. REPORTS OF OCCUPATIONAL DISEASE ATTRIBUTED TO PESTICIDES AND OTHER AGRICULTURAL CHEMICALS IN CALIFORNIA IN 1969*

TYPE OF CHEMICAL	TYPE OF INDUSTRY								
	Agriculture	Manufacturing	Construction	Transportation, Communication Utilities	Trade	Structural Pest Control	State and Local Government	Other	TOTAL ALL
Organic phosphate pesticides	162	40	1	12	1	1	11	3	231
Halogenated hydrocarbon pesticides	19	15	2	6	2	3	8	2	57
Herbicides	44	4	1	5	—	—	18	4	76
Fertilizers	23	7	1	—	2	—	3	7	43
Fungicides	18	3	1	—	2	—	1	2	27
Phenolic compounds	5	5	3	1	—	—	1	—	15
Sulfur	28	1	1	—	—	—	1	—	31
Organomercury compounds	—	—	—	—	—	—	1	1	2
Lead or arsenic	4	1	1	1	—	—	1	1	9
Carbamates	1	2	—	—	—	—	—	1	4
Miscell.—specified	13	5	1	1	1	1	4	2	28
Unspecified	137	19	1	7	12	3	15	10	204
Total	454	102	13	33	20	8	64	33	727

* Abstracted from California Department of Public Health: *Occupational Diseases in California Attributed to Pesticides and Other Agricultural Chemicals, 1969.* Bureau of Occupational Health and Environmental Epidemiology, Sacramento, 1969.

as a cause of occupational disease, less than 5 percent of these reports involved systemic poisoning.

Reports of studies on workers in the agricultural chemical industry indicate that acute poisonings do occur during the manufacture of insecticides. In a health survey of 300 workers in plants manufacturing toxic organochlorine pesticides (Aldrin, Dieldrin, and Endrin) over a nine-year period, no fatalities or permanent injuries were found but 17 of the workers had convulsive intoxications, and 5 of the 17 had more than one convulsion (Hoogendam et al., 1965). Moderate to severe chloracne was found in 18 percent of 73 employees engaged in manufacture of the herbicides 2,4-D and 2,4,5-T (Poland et al., 1971). Sixty-six percent of these workers had less severe degrees of acne. No systemic toxicity was found. In a more recent study, 41 workers had chloracne attributed to 3,4,3'4'-tetrachloroazoxybenzene present as a contaminant in the production synthesis of a new herbicide, 2-(3,4-dichlorophenyl)-4-methyl-1,2,4-oxodiazolidine-3,5-dione (Taylor et al., 1977). A five-year study of pesticide workers in a plant in Israel indicated that there was a higher incidence of complaints of symptoms referable to the respiratory, cardiovascular and nervous systems (Wasserman et al., 1970). In that study, 140 workers in the pesticide manufacturing plant were compared with 71 workers from a textile plant as the control group. In contrast to these reports of injury in the manufacture of pesticides, a study of 35 men with a work experience of 11 to 19 years in a plant producing DDT revealed no ill effects that could be attributed to exposure to the DDT, in spite of the fact that fat storage levels ranged from 38 to 647 ppm of DDT-derived material compared to 8 ppm for the general population (Laws et al., 1967).

Since 1949 there have been repeated cases of multiple poisonings among agricultural workers engaged in picking fruits sprayed with the highly toxic organophosphate insecticide parathion (Spear et al., 1975). These poisonings have been correlated with the "dislodgeable" residues of paraoxon, a toxic metabolite and/or weathering product of parathion, on the foliage of the parathion-sprayed fruit trees. An "epidemic" of poisoning due to malathion, an organophosphate that is generally considered safe, occurred among field workers in a malaria control program in Pakistan (Baker et al., 1978). Of 7500 workers involved in this mosquito control program, 2800 were estimated to have had at least one episode of malathion intoxication. Five of these were fatal cases. A combination of poor pesticide-handling techniques and the use of unusually toxic formulations (due to the presence of toxic by-products) contributed to this epidemic of poisonings.

Gross negligence in industrial hygiene resulted in poisoning of 76 of 148 exposed workers engaged in the manufacture of chlordecone (Kepone) (Taylor *et al.*, 1978). These workers suffered a syndrome of neurologic effects characterized by tremors, ocular flutter (opsoclonus), hepatomegaly/splenomegaly, rashes, mental changes, and widened gaits. Laboratory tests showed a reduced sperm count and reduced motility of sperm. Other complaints included headache, chest pain, arthralgia, and weight loss. The onset of signs in these workers varied from five days to eight months after the initial exposure to Kepone, and some signs and symptoms persisted for many months after cessation of exposure when the plant involved was closed down. Serious chronic neuropathy has also been reported among several workers involved in the manufacture of the insecticide leptophos (Xintaris *et al.*, 1978). The medical consultant to the company observed a cluster of three cases of suspected "multiple sclerosis," which suggested the possibility of pesticide poisoning. The possibility of concurrent exposure to *n*-hexane (also neurotoxic) complicated interpretation of these cases of occupational poisonings. From data collected in epidemiologic studies of morbidity and mortality in workers exposed occupationally to pesticides, Morgan *et al.* (1980) concluded that death by accidental trauma was unusually frequent among pesticide applicators. Mortalities from cancer and arteriosclerosis in the pesticide-exposed workers did not differ from controls, but dermatitis and skin cancer were "unusually common" in structural pest-control operators. There were apparent associations between high serum organochlorine pesticide levels and the subsequent appearance of hypertension and arteriosclerotic cardiovascular disease. Although there are numerous problems, pointed out by the investigators, in drawing definitive conclusions concerning the causal relationship of pesticide exposure to these conditions, it is noteworthy that Wang and MacMahon (1979) obtained essentially the same findings (i.e., no increased incidence of cancer but a statistically significant excess of deaths from cerebrovascular disease) in a retrospective mortality study of 1403 workers employed in the manufacture of chlordane and heptachlor. Wang and MacMahon concluded that the relationship of pesticide exposure to blood pressure and to cerebrovascular disease deserves more investigation. It is of interest that some ten years earlier, Radomski *et al.* (1968) reported that the organochlorine pesticide content in the body fat of persons who had died from hypertension was higher than in fat of victims of other diseases or of normal living subjects. Clearly, additional basic research will be required to establish whether, and by what mechanisms, these associations occur.

Routes of Exposure

Analysis of residues on masks or on pads placed on exposed skin surfaces of workers involved in pesticide applications indicated that the dermal route offers the greatest potential for occupational exposure (Wolfe *et al.*, 1967). The type of pesticide formulation applied was also a factor in the relative contribution of the respiratory route of exposure. When aerosols were used, an average of 2.87 percent of the total (dermal and respiratory) exposure was by the respiratory route, compared with 0.23 percent for dilute sprays and 0.94 percent for dusts. Different degrees of hazard were associated with different jobs. Thus, indoor house spraying was much more hazardous than outdoor spraying of several types. In an airplane spraying operation the relative hazard differed depending on the particular job. For example in the airplane spraying of a fruit orchard the loader received about three times as much as the pilot and 4½ times as much as the flagman. Of course, the hazard to applicators is dependent not only on the extent and route of exposure, but on several other factors such as the relative rates of absorption from the skin and lungs, particle sizes of dust and aerosols, and the inherent toxicity of the materials. Wolfe and coworkers (1967) found, in their studies of a wide variety of spraying operations involving 11 different pesticides, that the highest mean value for the percentage of toxic dose received per hour of work was 44.2 percent for workers who loaded airplanes with 1 percent TEPP (tetraethyl pyrophosphate) dust. Although there were several illnesses associated with this operation, these authors considered the incidence quite low in view of the relative hazard. They suggested that three factors might account for this: the number of hours per day (or week) that the worker is actually engaged in loading airplanes is low; knowledge of the high toxicity of TEPP may prompt more diligent use of protective clothing and respiratory protective devices; and only a small percentage of the dry dust impinging on exposed skin is likely to be absorbed.

Oral ingestion is the most frequent route of exposure in cases of nonoccupational poisonings. Dermal exposures have resulted in deaths of small children who come in contact with presumably empty containers for highly toxic pesticides. Respiratory exposure (as well as dermal) of the general population is possible as a result of drift from agricultural operations. Household use of pesticide aerosol "bombs," vaporizers, pest strips, and other aerosol or vapor-generating devices is a potential source of respiratory exposure in nonoccupational settings. Hayes (1969) reported that 19 different organophosphorous insecticides are known to have caused poisoning in humans. Of the other common types of insecticides that have resulted in human poisonings there were 20 compounds in the organochlorine class, five different carbamates, four botanicals, three inorganic elements, and six miscellaneous compounds for a total of 57 different insecticides. Eight herbicides were responsible for human poisonings, seven fungicides, six rodenticides, one molluscicide, and one nematocide for a total of 80 different compounds. References to the case reports of these poisonings are provided in Hayes's review.

As indicated in Table 18–1, numerous incidents of acute poisoning have resulted from eating food that had become grossly contaminated with pesticides during storage or shipping.

An interesting example is a case of poisoning of seven members of a single family who ingested tortillas prepared from flour that had been contaminated by carbophenothion, an organophosphate insecticide (Oldner and Hatcher, 1969). Although no fatalities resulted, six of the seven individuals required hospitalization and four advanced to coma. The severity of clinical signs and symptoms was related to the number of tortillas eaten. The contaminated food was not detected and discarded until two separate meals had been served (involving different members of the family). When the leftover food was finally discarded it was eaten by, and resulted in the deaths of, a dog, a cat, and eight chickens. The flour had become contaminated, apparently, as the result of carbophenothion contact at some point in storage or shipping. The insecticide had soaked through the paper flour sack. At least one other sack of flour had also been contaminated and was being used by a second family that had not (yet) been poisoned. The reason the first family was poisoned was apparently because they dumped their flour into a can and so had used the contents of the bottom of the sack (the most contaminated, 3220 ppm) first. The second family used their flour from the less-contaminated top of the sack. This case is one illustration of the insidious conditions under which acute pesticide poisonings have occurred.

INSECTICIDES

Only select examples of the various classes of insecticides will be discussed here. For additional discussion of their chemistry and biotransformation the reader should consult the extensive reports by Menzie (1969) and Aizawa (1982). Comprehensive compilations of chemical and common names, structures, and LD50 values in rats may be found in Gaines (1969), Frear (1969), and Worthing (1979). Acute toxicity data for fish and wildlife are available in several reports (Pickering et al., 1962; Tucker and Crabtree, 1970; Pimental, 1971). Summaries of results of subacute and chronic feeding studies for many compounds have been made available in the monograph by Lehman (1965) and in the series of annual monographs on pesticide residues in food published jointly by the Food and Agriculture Organization (FAO) of the United Nations and the World Health Organization (e.g., FAO, 1982). Several books and monographs (O'Brien, 1960, 1967, Heath, 1961; Chichester, 1965; Gould, 1966; Secretary's Commission on Pesticides, 1969; Matsumura, 1972; Hayes, 1975, 1982; Wilkinson, 1976) that are devoted exclusively to pesticides provide much more extensive coverage than is possible here. A handbook prepared by Morgan (1982) provides information on clinical toxicology and emergency treatment for many pesticides.

Organophosphorus Insecticides

As discussed earlier, insecticides (of the several classes of pesticides) have most frequently been involved in human poisonings and organophosphorous compounds have most frequently been the offending agents.

Historic Considerations. The first organophosphate insecticide was tetraethyl pyrophosphate (TEPP). It was developed in Germany as a substitute for nicotine, which was in short supply in that country during World War II. Related extremely toxic compounds such as ethyl N-dimethyl phosphoroamidocyanidate (tabun) and isopropyl methylphosphonofluoridate (sarin) were kept secret by the German government as potential chemical warfare agents. These, and other extremely toxic cmpounds, are the so-called nerve gas chemical warfare agents.

TEPP, although an effective insecticide, was highly toxic to mammals and was rapidly hydrolyzed in the presence of moisture. Further efforts to find more stable compounds for use in agriculture led to the synthesis by Schrader in 1944 of parathion (E605; O,O-diethyl O-p-nitrophenyl phosphorothioate) and its oxygen analog paraoxon (E600; O,O-diethyl O-p-nitrophenyl phosphate). Because it exhibited a wide range of insecticidal activity and suitable physical and chemical properties such as low volatility and sufficient stability in water and mild alkali, parathion became one of the most widely used organophosphorus insecticides. It continues to be used extensively in agriculture, but because of its high mammalian toxicity, by all routes of exposure, other less hazardous compounds have begun to take its place. Parathion has the dubious distinction of being the pesticide most frequently involved in fatal poisonings. During the last two decades the agricultural chemistry industry has developed many other organic triesters of phosphoric acid and phosphorothioic acid that have been registered for use as insecticides. Summaries of the toxicology of several of these are shown in Table 18–4.

Shortly after parathion became available for study, acute toxicity studies on experimental animals revealed signs of poisoning that resembled excessive stimulation of cholinergic nerves. These could be alleviated by atropine, a cholinergic blocking agent (DuBois *et al.*, 1948). This suggested inhibition of acetylcholinesterase of nerve tissues as the mechanism of toxic action, as had been demonstrated for related organophosphate triesters, and was confirmed by the finding that tissues of rats poisoned by parathion had markedly reduced cholinesterase activity and increased free acetylcholine in their brains (DuBois *et al.*, 1949). Thus, the biochemical basis for acute poisoning by parathion in mammals, i.e., inhibition of the acetylcholinesterase activity of nerve tissue, became known soon after its introduction as an insecticide. Subsequent development and research on other organophosphate insecticides have revealed that they all, in sufficient doses, inhibit acetylcholinesterase *in vivo* and thus share a common mechanism of acute toxic action. The chemical mechanism of cholinesterase inhibition is discussed in more detail later in this chapter and in several extensive reviews and monographs (Heath, 1961; Cohen and Oosterbaan, 1963; O'Brien, 1960, 1967, 1976).

Signs and Symptoms of Acute Poisoning. Signs and symptoms of acute systemic poisoning by organophosphate insecticides are predictable from their biochemical mechanism of action. Thus inhibition of acetylcholinesterase results in accumulation of endogenous acetylcholine in nerve tissue and effector organs with consequent signs and symptoms that mimic the muscarinic, nicotinic, and central nervous system actions of acetylcholine. Acetylcholine is the chemical transmitter of nerve impulses at endings of postganglionic parasympathetic nerve fibers, somatic motor nerves to skeletal muscle, preganglionic fibers of both parasympathetic and sympathetic nerves, and certain synapses in the central nervous system.

Muscarinic receptors for acetylcholine are found primarily in smooth muscles, the heart, and exocrine glands. Signs and symptoms of organophosphorus insecticide poisoning that result from stimulation of these receptors include tightness in the chest and wheezing expiration due to bronchoconstriction and increased bronchial secretions, increased salivation and lacrimation, increased sweating, increased gastrointestinal tone and peristalsis with consequent development of nausea, vomiting, abdominal cramps, diarrhea, tenesmus and involuntary defecation, bradycardia that can progress to heart block, frequent and involuntary urination due to contraction of smooth muscle of the bladder, and constriction of the pupils (miosis).

Nicotinic signs and symptoms result from accumulation of acetylcholine at the endings of motor nerves to skeletal muscle and autonomic ganglia. Muscular effects include easy fatigue and mild weakness followed by involuntary twitching, scattered fasciculations and cramps with progression to generalized fasciculations, and muscular weakness that affects the muscles of respiration and contributes to dyspnea and cyanosis. Nicotinic actions at autonomic ganglia may, in severe intoxication, mask some of the muscarinic effects. Thus tachycardia may result from stimulation of sympathetic ganglia to overcome the usual bradycardia due to muscarinic action on the heart. Pallor, elevation of blood pressure, and hyperglycemia also reflect nicotinic action at sympathetic ganglia.

Accumulation of acetylcholine in the central nervous system is believed to be responsible for the tension, anxiety, restlessness, insomnia, headache, emotional instability and neurosis, excessive dreaming and nightmares, apathy, and confusion that have been described after organophosphate poisoning. Slurred speech, tremor, generalized weakness, ataxia, convulsions, depression of respiratory and circulatory centers, and coma are other central nervous system effects.

The immediate cause of death in fatal organophosphate poisonings is asphyxia resulting from respiratory failure. Contributing factors are the muscarinic actions of bronchoconstriction and increased bronchial secretions, nicotinic action leading to paralysis of the respiratory muscles and the central nervous system action of depression and paralysis of the respiratory center.

Localized Effects. Localized effects at the site of exposure may be seen in the absence of obvious signs and symptoms of systemic absorption as described above. Exposure to vapors, dusts, or aerosols can exert local effects on the smooth muscles of the eyes and respiratory tract resulting in early miosis and blurred vision due to spasm of accommodation in the first case and bronchoconstriction in the case of respiratory exposure. Secretory glands of the respiratory

Table 18–4. TOXICOLOGY OF SOME ORGANOPHOSPHATE INSECTICIDES

COMPOUND	STRUCTURE	LD50 IN MALE RATS (mg/kg)* Oral	LD50 IN MALE RATS (mg/kg)* Dermal	"NO EFFECT LEVEL"† (mg/kg/day)	ADI‡ (mg/kg)
TEPP	$(C_2H_5O)_2$—P(=O)—O—P(=O)—$(OC_2H_5)_2$	1.1	2.4	—	—
Mevinphos	$(CH_3O)_2$—P(=O)—O—C(CH_3)=CHC(=O)—OCH_3	6.1	4.7	—	—
Disulfoton	$(C_2H_5O)_2$—P(=S)—S—CH_2CH_2—S—CH_2CH_3	6.8	15	—	—
Azinphosmethyl	$(CH_3O)_2$—P(=S)—S—CH_2—N(benzotriazinone ring)	13	220	Rat—0.125 Dog—0.125	0.0025
Parathion	$(C_2H_5O)_2$—P(=S)—O—C$_6$H$_4$—NO_2	13	21	Rat—0.05 Man—0.05	0.005
Methylparathion	$(CH_3O)_2$—P(=S)—O—C$_6$H$_4$—NO_2	14	67	—	—
Chlorfenvinphos	$(C_2H_5O)_2$—P(=O)—O—C(=CHCl)—C$_6$H$_3$Cl$_2$	15	31	Rat—0.05 Dog—0.05	0.002
Dichlorvos	$(CH_3O)_2$—P(=O)—O—CH=CCl_2	80	107	Rat—0.5 Dog—0.37 Man—0.033	0.004
Diazinon	$(C_2H_5O)_2$—P(=S)—O—C(pyrimidine ring)CHC$(CH_3)_2$; CH_3	108	200	Rat—0.1 Monkey—0.05 Dog—0.02 Man—0.02	0.002
Dimethoate	$(CH_3O)_2$—P(=S)—S—$CH_2CONHCH_3$	215	260	Rat—0.4 Man—0.04	0.02
Trichlorfon	$(CH_3O)_2$—P(=O)—CH(OH)CCl_3	630	>2000	Rat—2.5 Dog—1.25	0.01
Chlorothion	$(CH_3O)_2$—P(=S)—O—C$_6$H$_3$(Cl)—NO_2	880	1500—4500		

* Values obtained in standardized tests in the same laboratory (Gaines, 1969).

† Maximum rate of intake (usually for three-month to two-year feeding studies) that was tested and did *not* produce significant toxicologic effects (as listed in the monographs issued jointly by the Food and Agriculture Organization of the United Nations and the World Health Organization, as developed by joint meetings of expert panels on pesticide residues held annually, 1965–1972).

‡ Acceptable daily intake (ADI) = the daily intake of a chemical that, during a lifetime, appears to provide the practical certainty that injury will not result (in man) during a lifetime of exposure. Figures taken from World Health Organization (1973).

Table 18–4　(continued)

COMPOUND	STRUCTURE	LD50 IN MALE RATS (mg/kg)*		"NO EFFECT LEVEL"†	ADI‡
		Oral	Dermal	(mg/kg/day)	(mg/kg)
Malathion	(CH₃O)₂—P(=S)—S—CHCOOC₂H₅ / CH₂COOC₂H₅	1375	>4444	Rat—0.5 Man—0.02	0.02
Ronnel	(CH₃O)₂—P(=S)—O—C₆H₂Cl₃	1250	>5000	Rat—0.5 Dog—1.0	0.01
Abate	[(CH₃O)₂—P(=S)—O—C₆H₄—S—]₂	8000	>4000		

tract, as well as smooth muscles, may be affected by minimal inhalation exposure to the organophosphates leading to watery nasal discharge, nasal hyperemia, sensation of tightness in the chest, and prolonged wheezing respiration. Local effects of dermal exposure include localized sweating and fasciculations at the site of contact. Gastrointestinal manifestations are usually the first to appear after oral ingestion and some of them may be due to local anticholinesterase action in the gastrointestinal tract.

Systemic Effects. Systemic effects are, in general, similar irrespective of route of absorption, but the sequence and times may differ. Respiratory and ocular symptoms would be expected first after exposure to airborne organophosphates, while gastrointestinal symptoms and localized sweating would likely be first to appear after oral and dermal exposure, respectively. However, these generalizations may not hold for compounds that must be metabolically activated (see Figure 18–2). The onset of symptoms after exposure to organophosphate compounds is usually rapid, within a few minutes to two or three hours. The duration of symptoms is generally from one to five days. In fatal untreated poisonings, deaths usually occur within 24 hours. It should be recognized that, in addition to the usual factors of route of exposure, concentrations of active material, etc., the quality of signs and symptoms, their rate of onset, and their durations may differ markedly for different compounds by virtue of differences in rate of biotransformation, distribution, and affinities for acetylcholinesterase. For example, in five cases of attempted suicide by ingestion of

dichlofenthion, severe cholinergic crises did not appear until 40 to 48 hours but they persisted for five to 48 days in the three survivors (Davies et al., 1975). This extremely prolonged course was associated with persistent residues of this insecticide in the blood and fat of the patients. Dichlofenthion has a higher octanol/water partition coefficient than most organophosphorus insecticides, and the prolonged course of the poisonings was due to a slow release of the insecticide from adipose tissue reservoirs.

Organophosphate insecticides in common use are rapidly biotransformed and excreted, and subacute or chronic poisoning by virtue of accumulation of the compounds in the body does not occur. However, because several of the organophosphates produce slowly reversible inhibition of cholinesterase *accumulation of this effect* can occur. Signs and symptoms of poisoning that resemble those produced by a single high dose will occur when the accumulated inhibition of cholinesterase produced by smaller, repeated doses reaches a critical level. Cessation of exposure normally results in complete recovery. Chronic complaints associated with poisoning by organophosphates have been reported as due to sequelae of severe acute poisoning (Tabershaw and Cooper, 1966). A few compounds have produced delayed and persistent peripheral neuropathy, apparently unrelated to anticholinesterase action (see below). It has also been speculated that some of the effects of anticholinesterases may be mediated by biologically active peptides (e.g., endorphines, substance P) that are present in brain and other nerve tissue, and whose degradation by exo- and endopeptidases is inhibited by some organophosphates (O'Neill, 1981).

More detailed discussions of organophosphate insecticide poisoning in humans may be found in several reviews (Holmstedt, 1959; Grob, 1953; Hayes, 1975, 1982; Namba et al., 1971).

Delayed Neurotoxic Effects. These are produced by several phosphate triesters (Abou-Donia, 1981; Johnson, 1982). Although this can result from a single toxic dose, the neuropathology is generally delayed in onset. Most notorious of the compounds that produce this effect is triorthocresyl phosphate (TOCP). This compound is not a potent anticholinesterase, and it is not used as an insecticide. However, a number of compounds that are used as insecticides can produce this effect and it is common practice to screen for this action in safety evaluation tests. The functional disturbances associated with phosphate triester neuropathy begin in the distal parts of the lower limbs in both human and other sensitive animals. Mild sensory disturbances and motor weakness with ataxia occur, progressing in severity and extent to increased weakness and flaccidity of the legs and varying amounts of sensory disturbance. Upper limbs may also become involved. After several days to a few weeks the peak of the process is reached and thereafter improvement in the functional disturbance begins. Recovery is slow and not always complete.

Histopathologic studies of the peripheral nerves show that the distal fibers are affected earlier and more severely than proximal fibers. There is also a tendency of large-diameter fibers to be affected more than smaller-diameter fibers. The lesion has been described as a "dying-back" process, where the ends of the long nerves, distal to the nerve cell body, are affected first. Axonal degeneration followed by myelin degeneration is observed. These effects are believed to be due to a disturbed metabolism of the nerve cell body in spinal tracts with the consequence that nutrients are not synthesized and transported at a sufficient rate to maintain the long axons of the peripheral nerves (Cavanagh, 1969). Poisonings of this type have occurred in humans. Classic cases reported in the United States in the 1930s resulted from drinking ginger liquor that was contaminated with TOCP. The condition was popularly referred to as "ginger jake paralysis." Mass outbreaks of poisoning, again resulting from TOCP, have occurred in Morocco and other countries as a result of cooking with vegetable oil that had been contaminated with lubricating oil that contained some TOCP. An outbreak of 12 cases of serious peripheral neuropathy (Xintaras et al., 1978) among workers engaged in the manufacture

of leptophos, O-(4-bromo-2,5-dichlorophenyl) O-methyl phenylphosphorothioate, was felt to be due to its delayed neurotoxicity, which was demonstrated in hens given single large doses or repeated small doses of this compound (Abou-Donia and Preissig, 1976a, 1976b).

Although hens and humans seem to be the most sensitive species to the organic phosphate-triester neuropathy, studies on various compounds have shown that dogs, cats, calves, monkeys, sheep, pigs, horses, pheasants, ducks, and rats will also sustain this effect (Aldridge et al., 1969). For screening for possible production of this effect by pesticides, hens are usually used as the experimental animal. Because of potent anticholinesterase actions of many pesticides, it is often impossible to administer sufficient doses to the animal to produce the neuropathic effect. To overcome this and to screen for the neuropathy, a common procedure is to administer atropine to protect against the acute cholinergic action. Using this procedure Gaines (1969) found that 22 of 30 organophosphorus pesticides tested and three out of nine carbamate insecticides produced leg weakness in atropinized hens under sufficient time and dosage conditions. With all but three of the compounds, however, the onset of leg weakness occurred within 24 hours, and for most compounds the hens recovered within a month. Aldridge and Johnson (1971) consider this rapid onset and relatively rapid recovery to result from a different mechanism than for TOCP and other long-acting neurotoxins.

Although the precise mechanism that leads to the paralytic effect and axonal degeneration produced by organophosphorus triesters remains to be determined, Johnson (1982) has reviewed the considerable evidence that this involves the initial dialkyl phosphorylation and "aging" of a specific protein (see Figure 18–1) referred to as neurotoxic esterase.

For many years it was considered that the action was related to the antiesterase action of these compounds. Several studies, however, failed to establish an unequivocal correlation between the potency of various compounds to produce peripheral paralytic action and their capacity to inhibit acetylcholinesterase, butyrylcholinesterase, aliesterases, and several other hydrolytic enzymes. Subsequent studies, however, showed that paralytic compounds did have a common property of binding to a specific protein fraction in brains and spinal cords of hens. Although this protein fraction represented only a very small part of the total esterase activity of the nerve tissue, it did possess properties of an esterase and seemed to have a specificity for phenyl phenylacetate (Aldridge et al., 1969).

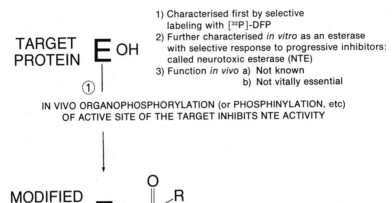

1) Characterised first by selective
   labeling with [³²P]-DFP
2) Further characterised *in vitro* as an esterase
   with selective response to progressive inhibitors:
   called neurotoxic esterase (NTE)
3) Function *in vivo* a) Not known
                     b) Not vitally essential

IN VIVO ORGANOPHOSPHORYLATION (or PHOSPHINYLATION, etc)
OF ACTIVE SITE OF THE TARGET INHIBITS NTE ACTIVITY

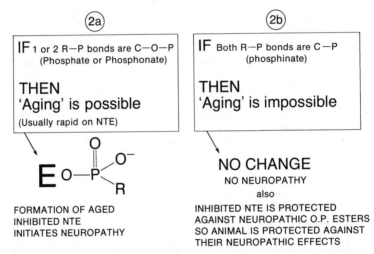

Figure 18–1. Proposed alternative chemical modifications of the target protein involved in organophosphate induced distal neuropathy (OPIDN). (From Johnson, M. K.: The target for initiation of delayed neurotoxicity by organophosphorus esters: Biochemical studies and toxicological applications. *Rev. Biochem. Toxicol.*, **4**:141–212, 1982.)

The physiologic role of this membrane-bound protein is unknown. Structure-activity studies with homologs of known paralytic compounds indicate that dimethyl derivatives are weak inhibitors of the ''neurotoxic'' esterases and have little or no neurotoxic action *in vivo* but that *in vivo* neurotoxicity and the specific antiesterase potency increased progressively with diethyl, dipropyl, and dibutyl derivatives of DFP and mipafox (Aldridge and Johnson, 1971). Refinement of a method for measuring the inhibition of hen's brain neurotoxic esterase has provided some further insight into the mechanism of delayed neurotoxicity and its structure-activity relationships (Johnson, 1975a, 1975b, 1975c). Phosphates, phosphoramidates, and phos-

phonates were capable of inhibiting neurotoxic esterase and were neurotoxic in intact hens, while phosphinates, sulfonates, and carbamates inhibited the enzyme but were not neurotoxic *in vivo*. In fact, when administered at appropriate times, the latter three types of compounds could prevent the neurotoxicity produced by the former three types. This protection is apparently due to competition for reaction at a critical target site. The determination of whether or not a compound that inhibited neurotoxic esterase would also be neurotoxic or protective appeared to depend on whether an ''aged'' inhibited neurotoxic esterase could be formed. This ''aging'' (loss of an alkyl group on the dialkyl phosphorylated enzyme) is believed to fix an extra charge to a protein whose function must be critical to normal function and integrity of neurons. The identity of the critical protein and its function have not yet been determined, but further research with neurotoxic organophosphate esters will likely provide insight into normal nerve physiology as well as elucidating the mechanism of delayed neurotoxicity of this class of insecticides. Studies with the insecticide EPN (ethyl *p*-nitrophenyl phenylphosphonothionate) demonstrate that optical isomerism may be a determinant of the nature of toxic action of these compounds (Ohkawa, 1977). The racemic (±), (+) isomer, and (−) isomer had equal acute toxicity to mice, the (+) isomer had three- to fourfold greater insecticidal activity than the (−) isomer, while the (−) isomer of EPN was the most active in producing delayed neurotoxicity in hens.

Altered neuromuscular function in pesticide workers who did not exhibit other detectable signs and symptoms of poisoning nor depressed blood cholinesterase activity has been detected using electromyographic methods to determine altered peripheral nerve and muscle function. Roberts (1976, 1977) reported on studies of workers in an organophosphorus pesticide factory that indicated that measurements of altered electromyograph patterns and nerve conduction velocities might provide a more sensitive and more meaningful index of excessive occupational exposure to these compounds than measurements of plasma or erythrocyte cholinesterase. Although deviations from "normal" could be detected by these neurophysiologic techniques, their physiologic significance and the mechanisms of their occurrence remain to be demonstrated. These changes most likely differ mechanistically from the severe delayed neuropathy caused by TOCP, leptophos, mipafox, and a few others.

Biotransformation-Toxicity Relationships. Several biotransformation reactions that organophosphorus insecticides undergo have been discussed in several reviews and monographs (O'Brien, 1960, 1967; Fukuto and Metcalf, 1969; Menzie, 1969; Dauterman, 1971; Eto, 1974; Kulkarni and Hodgson, 1979; Aizawa, 1982). In this section selected biotransformation reactions are discussed as illustrations of the development of knowledge that has led to an understanding of factors that affect the susceptibility of animals to poisoning by these compounds. The reactions shown in Figure 18–2 and the compounds shown in Table 18–4 can be used as reference models for this discussion.

Activation. The early organophosphorous anticholinesterases such as TEPP and DFP were phosphate triesters and were potent inhibitors of

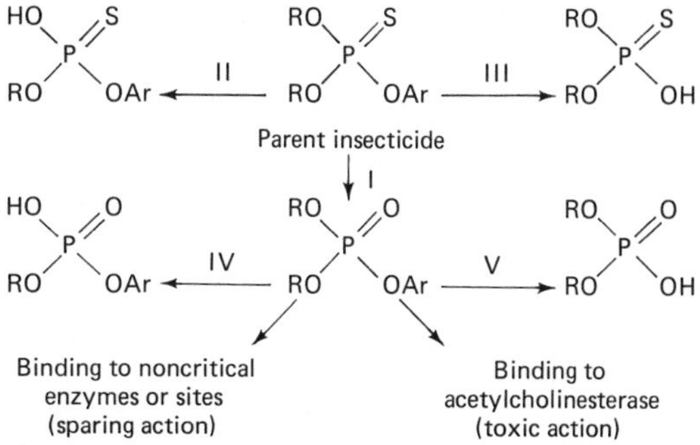

Figure 18–2. General scheme of biotransformation and action of dialkyl, aryl phosphorothioate insecticides.

cholinesterase both *in vivo* and *in vitro*. The development of parathion introduced the phosphorothionates. The majority of compounds now in use as insecticides contain the (=S) thiono moiety, and are either phosphorothionates (e.g., parathion, methyl parathion) or phosphorodithioates (e.g., azinphosmethyl, malathion). Early in research on parathion and its oxygen analog, paraoxon, it became apparent that in addition to conferring greater stability against nonenzymatic hydrolysis, substitution of =S for =O on the phosphorus compound altered its toxic properties. Parathion was less toxic to animals than paraoxon, and several factors that altered the toxicity of parathion in rats did not affect paraoxon's toxicity; although both compounds inhibited acetylcholinesterase and produced similar cholinergic signs of poisoning (DuBois *et al.,* 1949). Further studies showed that highly purified parathion did not inhibit cholinesterase *in vitro,* and that the inhibitory activity of less purified samples could be attributed to contamination with the S-ethyl and S-phenyl isomers of parathion or with its oxygen analog, paraoxon (Diggle and Gage, 1951). Subsequently it was demonstrated that paraoxon was the active anticholinesterase formed from parathion in intact rats.

Activation of parathion and other thionophosphorus insecticides that lacked direct (i.e., *in vitro*) anticholinesterase activity could be accomplished by incubating the compounds, aerobically, with liver slices (DuBois *et al.,* 1957). Further studies with a variety of compounds now have established that conversion of phosphorothionate and phosphorodithioate insecticides to their corresponding oxygen analogs is a necessary prerequisite for their action as cholinesterase inhibitors (reaction, I, Figure 18–2). The enzyme system(s) in liver that catalyzes this reaction belongs to the group of NADPH-dependent mixed-function oxidases of the microsomes (Murphy and DuBois, 1957, 1958; Nakatsugawa and Dahm, 1967; Neal, 1967, 1980; Kulkarni and Hodgson, 1979). Although the liver has by far the greatest capacity to catalyze this reaction *in vitro*, other tissues, including lung and brain, have some activity (Poore and Neal, 1972). Activation of phosphorothionates by extrahepatic tissues, even if only in minimal amounts, may be of great importance if these tissues are critical target organs for acetylcholinesterase inhibition.

There are other activation reactions, involving a few compounds, in which parent insecticides are converted to more potent anticholinesterase agents. They include oxidative *N*-demethylation of phosphoramidates, such as shradan,

$$[(CH_3)_2N]_2 \overset{O}{\underset{\|}{-}} P - O - \overset{O}{\underset{\|}{P}} - [N(CH_3)_2]_2,$$

and oxidation of the thioether linkage of some compounds, such as disulfoton (see Table 18–4) and its oxygen analog, to the corresponding sulfoxides and sulfones. (Kulkarni and Hodgson, 1979).

Inactivation. In addition to the requirement for an oxon (P = O) group to be present for anticholinesterase activity, metabolic modification of the alkyl and aryl substitutes can also influence activity. Reactions II, III, IV, and V (Figure 18–2) are enzymatic detoxication reactions that yield products that do not inhibit acetylcholinesterase. Largely as a result of *in vitro* studies, it was proposed that reaction V, catalyzed by paraoxonase (A-esterase), was the major pathway of detoxication of parathion. This enzyme is widely distributed among several tissues in rats and other mammals. It does not require addition of cofactors for measurements of activity *in vitro* and probably hydrolyzes several other organophosphates (P = O compounds), but apparently does not hydrolyze the P = S compounds directly. Thus, the proposed enzymatic mechanism of detoxication of parathion and other phosphorothionate insecticides was, for many years, based on the concept that hydrolytic detoxication (reaction V) followed the formation of the oxygen analogs (reaction I). However, studies using ^{32}P-labeled parathion have shown that the aryl-phosphorus bond can be cleaved (reaction III) without prior oxidation to paraoxon (Nakatsugawa and Dahm, 1967; Neal 1967; Poore and Neal, 1972).

This reaction is catalyzed by a microsomal enzyme that requires NADPH and oxygen, and was initially thought to be distinct from the enzyme that catalyzes reaction I (Neal, 1967). However, more recent evidence indicates that both microsomal cleavage and sulfur oxidation may pass through a common intermediate step (Ptashne *et al.*, 1971, Kamataki, *et al.*, 1976). The rate at which this oxidative cleavage or the combined oxidation-hydrolysis reaction was catalyzed by NADPH-fortified liver homogenates appeared to explain age and sex differences in susceptibility of rats to EPN, O-ethyl O-*p*-nitrophenyl phenylphosphorothioate. Adult females were more susceptible to poisoning and had less EPN detoxifying activity in their liver than adult males, and the greater susceptibility of young rats also corresponded to slower rates of enzymatic detoxification by their livers.

Dealkylation reactions II and IV apparently do not occur or occur to only a very minimal extent with parathion (Plapp and Casida, 1958). However, NADPH-dependent oxidative dealkylation has been demonstrated for other compounds. This appears to be a particularly important reaction for determining the toxicity of chlorfenvinphos (Donninger *et al.*, 1972. The relative rates of dealkylation by rat, mouse, rabbit, and dog livers were 1, 8, 24, and 88, respectively. Species with high rates were least susceptible with LD50 values of 10, 100, 500, and >1200 for rats, mice, rabbits, and dogs, respectively. Oxidative dealkylation also occurred with the dimethyl and diisopropyl analogs. However, the dimethyl compound, tetrachlorvinphos, was preferentially monodealkylated by another system, glutathione alkyltransferase (Hutson *et al.*, 1972). In contrast to the microsomal oxidative dealkylation, glutathione-dependent dealkylation occurred in the soluble fraction of the liver cells and did not show marked species differences in activity.

Glutathione-dependent demethylation yields S-methylglutathione and the corresponding desmethyl phosphate compound. The enzyme system that catalyzes this reaction has been termed *phosphoric acid triester-glutathione S-alkyltransferase* (Hutson *et al.*, 1972). There is considerable evidence that glutathione-dependent demethylation is an important pathway for several other O,O-dimethyl substituted organophosphorus insecticides, e.g., methyl parathion and azinphosmethyl (Plapp and Casida, 1958; Hollingworth, 1972; Benke *et al.*, 1974). It has been demonstrated, in mice, that pretreatment with diethyl maleate and methyl iodide, which reduce liver glutathione levels, potentiated the toxicity of organophosphorus insecticides that are demethylated by glutathione transferase (Hollingworth, 1970).

Another detoxication pathway (which is not represented in Figure 18–2) involves the hydrolysis of carboxyester or carboxyamide linkages in some insecticides by tissue or plasma carboxylesterases (sometimes called aliesterase).

Malathion and dimethoate are examples. Products of the hydrolysis of the carboxyester or amide groups do not inhibit cholinesterase, and enzymatic formation of these products has been demonstrated *in vivo* and in *in vitro* studies (Uchida *et al.*, 1964; Dauterman, 1971). In several species of mammals, this appears to be the major pathway of detoxication for these insecticides, and their selective insecticidal action is due to a relative lack of these hydrolytic enzymes in insects (Krueger *et al.*, 1960). The importance of this reaction in mammals as a detoxication pathway has been demonstrated in studies in which animals pretreated with other organophosphate compounds that strongly inhibit carboxylesterases became more susceptible to the acute toxicity and anticholinesterase action of malathion (DuBois, 1961; Murphy, 1969; Su *et al.*, 1971). Pretreatment with triorthocresyl phosphate (TOCP), a strong inhibitor of carboxylesterase but weak anticholinesterase, reduced the LD50 of malathion in rats from 1100 to 10 mg/kg, a 110-fold potentiation (Murphy *et al.*, 1959), and the normally very low dermal toxicity of malathion in rats could be markedly potentiated by pretreating the animals with TOCP (Murphy, 1980).

A "binding" type of inactivation by liver and other tissues has been demonstrated for the oxygen analogs of parathion and malathion, i.e., paraoxon and malaoxon (Lauwerys and Murphy, 1969a; Cohen and Murphy, 1972, 1974). This appears to represent a loss of the active cholinesterase inhibitors to noncritical tissue binding sites, thereby sparing the critical acetylcholinesterase of nerve tissue from inhibition. That this represents an important detoxication mechanism *in vivo* was demonstrated by showing that selective blocking of these binding sites with other compounds *in vivo* potentiated the toxicity of paraoxon (Lauwerys and Murphy, 1969b), and, conversely, that induction of increased binding sites reduced paraoxon's toxicity (Triolo *et al.*, 1970). Although these binding sites have not been identified, there is suggestive evidence, from the studies cited, that they may be nonspecific tissue esterases.

It is apparent from the above discussion that the relationships between biotransformation and toxicity of organophosphorus insecticides is extremely complex. The toxicity depends upon the net availability of active compound to inhibit acetylcholinesterase at critical sites in nerve tissue, and this in turn is dependent upon the dynamic relationships between activation and inactivation reactions. These are not always predictable from results of measurements of the relative rates of enzyme reactions under optimum conditions *in vitro*, particularly when both activation and inactivation reactions are catalyzed by enzyme systems with common cofactor requirements, tissue distribution, and intracellular location.

Acetylcholinesterase Inhibition and Reversal. There is abundant evidence that both the organophosphorus and carbamate insecticides (discussed subsequently) produce their acute toxic actions by inhibiting acetylcholinesterase. In addition to the fact that it has been demonstrated that many of these compounds are potent inhibitors *in vitro*, several lines of *in vivo* evidence support this mechanism. The consequence of acetylcholinesterase inhibition is accumulation of acetylcholine at effector sites, and the protection against acute poisoning offered by atropine and other cholinergic blocking agents supports the mechanism. Additionally, induced reversal of cholinesterase inhibition by chemical compounds, such as the oxime derivatives, results in alleviation of symptoms of poisoning. A combination of pharmacologic antidotes (atropine) and biochemical antidotes (oximes) is potentiative in its antidotal activity.

A scheme for substrate and inhibitor interactions with acetylcholinesterase is shown in Figure 18–3 for an organophosphorus insecticide, paraoxon, and a carbamate insecticide, carbaryl. The overall reaction can be illustrated by considering the insecticides as substrates:

$$\text{EOH} + \text{AX} \underset{k_{-1}}{\overset{k_1}{\rightleftharpoons}} \text{EOH} \cdot \text{AX} \overset{k_2}{\longrightarrow} \text{X}^- + \text{H}$$

$$\text{EOA} \xrightarrow[\text{H}_2\text{O}]{k_3} \text{EOH} + \text{A}^- + \text{H}^+$$

(Enzyme)   (Substrate or inhibitor)   (Reversible complex)

There are three important steps in the reaction: the first is complex formation and is governed by an affinity constant Ka (i.e., $k - 1/k_1$). This is quite small for the carbamate and phosphate insecticides as well as for the natural substrate acetylcholine; therefore, the enzyme substrate or enzyme inhibitor complex ($\text{EOH} \cdot \text{AX}$) is favored. With acetylcholine k_2 and k_3 are very fast so that the total reaction occurs rapidly and new enzyme is regenerated. With organic phosphates k_2 is moderately fast, but k_3 is extremely slow; so EOA accumulates while $\text{EOH} \cdot \text{AX}$ is minimal at any time. With carbamates, Ka is very low, k_2 is slower than for the phosphates; k_3 is slower than k_2 but still significant (and more rapid than for the phosphates). As a result, with carbamates, there are small levels of $\text{EOH} \cdot \text{AX}$ and large levels of carbamylated enzyme, EOA. If, however, carbamate is removed from the reaction (as by dilution or dialysis) the enzyme

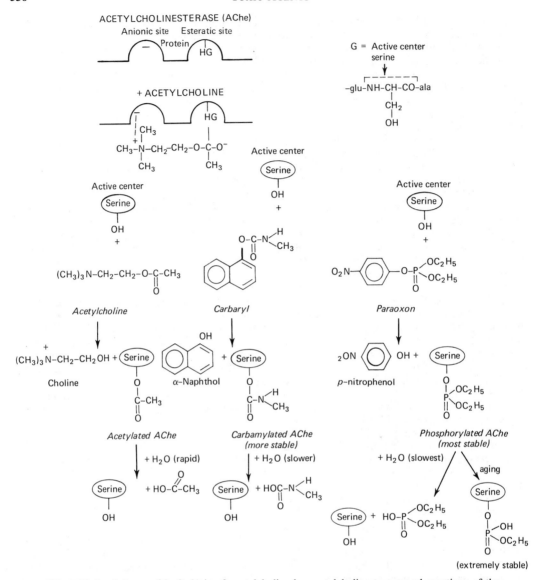

Figure 18–3. Scheme of hydrolysis of acetylcholine by acetylcholinesterase and reactions of the anticholinesterase insecticides carbaryl and paraoxon.

recovers rapidly, in part by reversal of the enzyme inhibitor complex and in part by decarbamylation, k_3. Of the three steps—(1) complex formation; (2) acetylation, phosphorylation, or carbamylation; and (3) deacetylation, dephosphorylation, or decarbamylation—the third (k_3) step is the most critical and slowest in each case. Calculated turnover numbers, the number of molecules hydrolyzed per minute by one molecule of enzyme, have been estimated as 300,000 for acetylcholine, 0.04 for methylcarbamates, and 0.008 for dimethyl phosphates. Therefore, the enzyme rapidly breaks down acetylcholine,

but is rather irreversibly inhibited by the organophosphates and markedly slowed by the carbamates (O'Brien, 1967, 1969; Aldridge, 1971).

The rate of recovery of free and active acetylcholinesterase following poisoning by organophosphorus and carbamate insecticides varies with different compounds. In general, the carbamates are usually considered reversible inhibitors of cholinesterase, and their duration of action is relatively short. In addition, because of the reversal of inhibition by dilution of the enzyme (as would occur if one sampled a tissue and diluted it with buffer during preparation for assay), determination of acetylcholinesterase inhibition by carbamates *in vivo* poses some technical difficulties. Unless care is taken, it is quite possible to observe the typical signs of anticholinesterase poisoning following carbamates; but by the time tissues are removed and prepared for assay, decarbamylation or reversal of enzyme-carbamate complex may have occurred and inhibition is undetectable. Therefore, in suspected cases of poisoning, where the history and signs and symptoms suggest a carbamate exposure, but clinical tests show a normal or nearly normal blood cholinesterase value, one must be guided by the history before concluding that the poisoning was not the result of a carbamate insecticide.

The case for organophosphate poisoning is somewhat different in that the compounds are in general much more slowly reversible inhibitors. However, even within this class there are marked differences in the persistence of inhibition following toxic doses of the compound (Table 18–5). Spontaneous reversal of enzyme inhibition (Figure 18–3) by organophosphates as well as carbamates can occur at varying rates, depending upon the insecticide, by hydrolysis of the phosphorylated cholinesterase (Reiner, 1971). The rate of reactivation *in vitro* of mouse brain and diaphragm acetylcholinesterase inhibited *in vivo* was five to ten times greater for azinphosmethyl and parathion-methyl than for azinphosethyl and parathion-ethyl (Levine and Murphy, 1977a).

With some compounds a phenomenon known as "aging" of the phosphorylated enzyme occurs. This represents a dealkylation of the dialkoxy phosphorylated enzyme. With some compounds dephosphorylation of the inhibited enzymes occurs extremely slowly or not at all. Diisopropyl fluorophosphate (DFP) is one such compound, and the rate of regeneration of the cholinesterase activity of a tissue of a poisoned animal coincides with the rate of resynthesis of new enzyme. For example, in animals poisoned with DFP, plasma cholinesterase activity returns to normal within several days to a few weeks, because it is relatively rapidly replaced by new enzyme synthesized in the liver. The

Table 18–5. VARIATION IN TIME TO ONSET AND DURATION OF INHIBITION OF CHOLINESTERASE BY SOME ORGANOPHOSPHATE INSECTICIDES IN RATS*

INSECTICIDE	TIME TO MAXIMUM INHIBITION	TIME FOR COMPLETE REVERSAL
Trichlorfon (Dipterex)	0.25 hours	6 hours
Azinphosmethyl (Guthion)	0.5 hours	24 hours
Disulfoton (Di-Syston)	3.0 hours	120 hours

* Selected from DuBois (1963). The compounds were given at dosages equivalent to ⅝ their LD50s, and all produced 50 percent or greater inhibition of brain or submaxillary cholinesterase activity.

acetylcholinesterase activity of the erythrocytes, however, remains depressed for the duration of the red cell's life. Erythrocyte cholinesterase activity inhibited by DFP only fully regenerates when there has been a full turnover and replacement of red cells.

Fortunately, there are available chemicals that will accelerate the hydrolysis of the phosphorylated enzyme, and hence accelerate regeneration of active acetylcholinesterase. The most successful compounds are oxime derivatives, and the best known of these is 2-pyridine aldoxime methiodide (2-PAM, pralidoxime), which is now a standard part of the therapy of organophosphorus poisoning. In addition to the capacity of 2-PAM to accelerate the dephosphorylation of acetylcholinesterase (Figure 18–4), it can also enhance the direct hydrolysis of the active inhibitor at physiologic pH. The effectiveness of 2-PAM in reversing cholinesterase inhibition *in vivo* is dependent upon its early administration following poisoning, because the "aged" phosphorylated enzyme is not reversible by the oximes. The rate of reactivation by oximes appears to vary with both the source of the cholinesterase and the substituents on the phosphorylating group. Diethoxy-phosphorylated enzyme appears to be most readily reactivated as compared with diisopropoxyphosphorylated and dimethoxy-phosphorylated enzymes. It is believed that the effectiveness of the oximes as dephosphorylating agents is in-

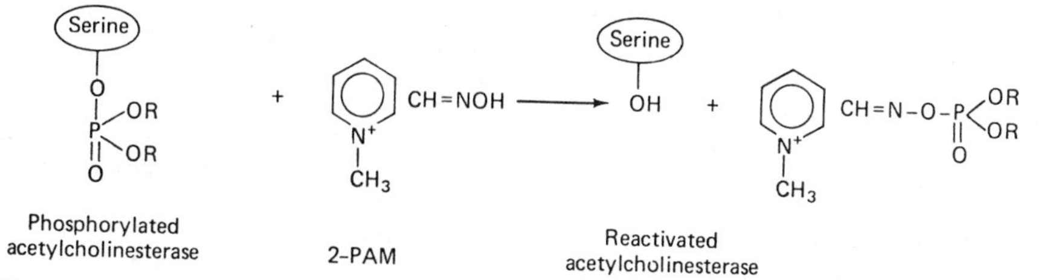

Phosphorylated acetylcholinesterase   2-PAM   Reactivated acetylcholinesterase

Figure 18–4. Reactivation of phosphorylated acetylcholinesterase by pralidoxime (2-PAM).

versely related to the rate of aging of the phosphorylated enzyme. Hence the dimethoxyphosphoryl enzyme and the diisopropoxy phosphoryl enzyme age more rapidly than the diethoxy phosphoryl enzyme (O'Brien, 1960, 1967; Hobbiger, 1963).

Although 2-PAM and other oximes are effective reversers of unaged phosphorylated acetylcholinesterase, their protective action against poisoning by organophosphates is limited when used alone. Treatment of mice with 2-PAM seldom protected against more than two times the lethal dose of potent inhibitors; however, treatment with both 2-PAM and atropine resulted in a synergistic protective action. For example, 2-PAM alone increased the lethal dose of paraoxon twofold to fourfold. Atropine alone increased the lethal dose by about twofold, but the combination of atropine and 2-PAM increased the lethal dose by 128-fold (O'Brien, 1960). The effectiveness of 2-PAM as an antidote for organophosphate poisoning is partly limited by its poor penetration into the central nervous system. Since it is a quaternary nitrogen derivative it will not readily penetrate the brain and is quite ineffective in reversing inhibition of brain acetylcholinesterase. Some newer bispyridinium oximes have been shown to penetrate the central nervous system, but the reversal of peripheral acetylcholinesterase inhibition by these compounds was more striking than for the enzyme in the central nervous system. Reversal of inhibited diaphragm and intercostal acetylcholinesterase by these compounds appeared to be quite effective in protecting against Soman poisoning (Clement, 1981). The aldoxime 2-PAM will inhibit cholinesterase at relatively high concentrations by binding to the anionic site of the enzyme. The use of 2-PAM is *contraindicated* in the case of poisoning by carbaryl, a carbamate cholinesterase inhibitor, probably because the reversal of the carbamate inhibited enzyme is so rapid that adding another short-acting though weak inhibitor adds insult to injury. More extensive discussions of the mechanism of inhibition of cholinesterase by organophosphates and carbamates and its reversal may be found in several reviews (O'Brien, 1960, 1969, 1976; Hobbiger, 1963; Aldridge, 1971; Wills, 1972).

Diagnosis and Treatment of Poisoning. As in any case of poisoning, careful taking of the history of events that led to signs and symptoms is essential. However, the organophosphate insecticides frequently produce poisoning rapidly and, if in sufficient doses, may have a rapid fatal outcome. It is important, therefore, to be guided by the characteristic signs and symptoms and take emergency action even though a complete history may not have been obtained.

In very severe cases the treatment should include (1) artificial respiration, preferably by mechanical means, and (2) atropine sulfate, 2 to 4 mg intravenously as soon as cyanosis is overcome. This may be repeated at five- to ten-minute intervals until signs of atropinization appear. Note that this dosage of atropine is greater than that usually used for other purposes, but because people poisoned by anticholinesterase compounds have increased tolerance for atropine, it is a safe dose, used carefully by an astute physician. (3) Following atropinization, administer 2-PAM, 1 g slowly, intravenously. In very severe cases, it may be necessary to begin treatment before time is spent in decontaminating the skin, stomach, or eyes as may be indicated; however, decontamination must be followed promptly. The skin should be washed with an alkaline soap, which will not only remove, but also help hydrolyze, the phosphate ester. Appropriate clinical procedures for evacuating the stomach and cleansing the eyes may be indicated. A case history of successful treatment of poisoning by dicrotophos, in which a total of 3911.5 mg of atropine and 92 g of pralidoxime chloride was given over a 23-day period, illustrates the importance of vigorous treatment in severe cases of poisoning (Warriner *et al.*, 1977).

In more usual and less severe cases the procedure should be as follows: Administer atropine SO_4, 1 to 2 mg, if symptoms appear. If excessive secretions occur, keep the patient fully atropinized by giving atropine sulfate every hour up to 25 to 50 mg in a day. Proceed with decontamination of the skin and removal of the poison from the stomach or eyes as the second step in this case. In these less severe poisonings, 2-PAM administration should be instituted if the patient fails to respond satisfactorily to atropine, followed, of course, by symptomatic treatment. The doses indicated above are those suggested for adults. Anyone expecting to face the possibility of dealing with severe poisoning by organophosphate insecticides should consult more detailed descriptions of diagnosis and therapy (Durham and Hayes, 1962; Doull, 1976; Hayes, 1982; Morgan, 1982).

Knowledge of the biochemical action of the organophosphate insecticides has provided a means for a relatively specific clinical test for diagnosis of excessive exposure to these compounds. Routine measurements of blood cholinesterase activity are frequently made in workers engaged in occupations where exposure to phosphate insecticides is a possibility. As discussed in several reports (Grob, 1963; Namba, *et al.*, 1971; Wills, 1972), the inhibition of the activity of plasma or red cell cholinesterase is reasonably well correlated with the severity of exposure and poisoning. Measurement of the cholinesterase activity of the blood only indirectly reflects the extent of biochemical lesion at critical sites in nerve tissues or effector organs, however. Depending upon the compound, the relative inhibition of plasma pseudocholinesterase and erythrocyte acetylcholinesterase may differ. Since the red cell enzyme is apparently identical to that in nerve tissue, assays on red cells are usually considered more reflective of nerve tissue activity. Rather marked inhibition of red cell and plasma cholinesterase may be present in the absence of symptoms. Total inhibition of plasma and 60 to 70 percent inhibition in red cell activity has been noted in the absence of overt signs of poisoning. However, the relationship between inhibition of blood cholinesterase activity and symptoms differs with different compounds and may reflect differences in distribution of the inhibitors. Relationships between blood and nerve tissue cholinesterase inhibition and signs of poisoning for various compounds in experimental animals have been reviewed by DuBois (1963) and Wills (1972).

Tolerance to Acute, Sublethal Effects of Some Organophosphates. This has been demonstrated in experimental animals (DuBois, 1965; Stavinoha, et al., 1969). In these experiments the phosphates were administered repeatedly or fed in the diet at sublethal doses for several days. Initially, acute cholinergic signs and symptoms were observed. In time, however, the animals no longer responded with obvious signs after each dose, and their general appearance, growth, and behavior appeared normal. However at sacrifice, these apparently normal animals had markedly inhibited blood and nervous tissue cholinesterase activity and elevated levels of acetylcholine in their brains. Adaptation or compensation to central nervous system and behavioral effects of anticholinesterase insecticides also occurs in rats in spite of continued brain acetylcholinesterase inhibition and elevated acetylcholine levels (Reiter et al., 1973; Bignami et al., 1975).

Experiments by Brodeur and DuBois (1964) suggested that the apparent tolerance involves development of a refractoriness of cholinergic receptor sites. Tolerant animals were resistant to the acute toxicity of carbachol, which has a direct effect on cholinergic receptors. More recently Schwab and Murphy (1981) demonstrated that rats could be made tolerant to carbachol by feeding the OP insecticide disulfoton for several weeks at a dietary concentration that did not produce signs of poisoning, even though acetylcholinesterase activity was markedly depressed. By using radiolabeled ligands that bind specifi-

cally to cholinergic receptor sites, several recent investigations have demonstrated that inhibition of acetylcholinesterase results in a reduction in the density of cholinergic receptors in several tissues. This corresponded in time of onset to the development of tolerance to the OPs or to direct cholinergic agonists (Costa et al., 1982; Murphy et al. 1983). Thus, current evidence suggests that the prolonged inhibition of acetylcholinesterase by OP compounds results in prolonged contact of the endogenous cholinergic agonist acetylcholine with the cholinergic receptors, which in turn leads to the inactivation or internalization of the receptors so that less agonist is bound, and, hence, less physiologic response is manifest in response to either exogenous or endogenous agonists. There are also reports that tolerance to reduced cholinesterase activity also occurs in humans (Johns and McQuillen, 1966).

Carbamate Insecticides

The acute toxicities of the carbamate insecticides also vary through a wide range as shown in Table 18–6. Unlike the organophosphates, most of the aromatic carbamate-ester insecticides have low dermal toxicities. However, one cannot generalize that carbamates are without dermal toxicity as illustrated by the extreme toxicity of aldicarb (Temik) by both the oral and dermal routes. This compound, because of its extreme toxicity, is recommended only for limited use in greenhouse operations. The carbamates are not broad-spectrum insecticides, and some of the common household insect pests such as the housefly and German cockroach are relatively immune (O'Brien, 1967); however, bees are extremely sensitive to these insecticides. For several of the compounds, the LD50 values for houseflies and German cockroaches are, on a body weight basis, greater than the LD50s for rats.

Action and Mechanism. The mode of action of the carbamates, like the organophosphates, is inhibition of acetylcholinesterase (Casida, 1963; O'Brien, 1967), and the signs and symptoms of poisoning are typically cholinergic with lacrimation, salivation, miosis, convulsion, and death. As indicated previously, however, the carbamates are relatively rapidly reversible inhibitors of cholinesterase. Atropine sulfate is the recommended antidote for poisoning by carbamate insecticides. Administration of 2-PAM is not recommended and, at least for some compounds, seems to be specifically contraindicated since there have been reports that it aggravates the toxicity of carbaryl (Carpenter et al., 1961).

Biotransformation-Toxicity Relationships. Studies of the correlation between toxicity and

Table 18–6. EXAMPLES OF RANGE OF ACUTE TOXICITIES OF SOME CARBAMATE INSECTICIDES

		LD50 IN MALE RATS* (mg/kg)	
		Oral	*Dermal*
Baygon (Propoxur)		83	>2400
Carbaryl		850	>4000
Mobam		150	>2000
Temik (Aldicarb)		0.8	3.0
Zectran		37	1500–2500

* Values obtained in standardized tests in the same laboratory (Gaines, 1969).

in vitro anticholinesterase activity of a series of monomethylcarbamates showed that there was good correlation between *in vitro* inhibition and intravenous LD50s in rats, but the *in vitro* anticholinesterase action was poorly correlated with oral LD50s (Vandekar *et al.,* 1971). The carbamate insecticides are direct inhibitors of acetylcholinesterase (i.e., they do not require metabolic activation), and the lack of correlation between the oral toxicity and *in vitro* anticholinesterase activity appeared to reflect differing rates of detoxication of the compounds. Hydrolysis of the carbamic acid ester linkage results in metabolites that lack anticholinesterase activity. The biotransformation pathways for typical carbamate insecticides are shown in Figure 18–5. Although hydrolysis occurs to some extent with all compounds, various oxidation steps that are catalyzed by mixed function oxidases also occur. The products formed by these reactions are not always less toxic than the parent compounds, but the parent compounds themselves, do have anticholinesterase action (Casida, 1963). The relative anticholinesterase activity of propoxur and four of its metabolites is shown in Figure 18–6.

Cholinesterase Inhibition and Symptoms. Studies of the relationship between cholinesterase inhibition and signs and symptoms of poisoning in rats showed that with dosages that did

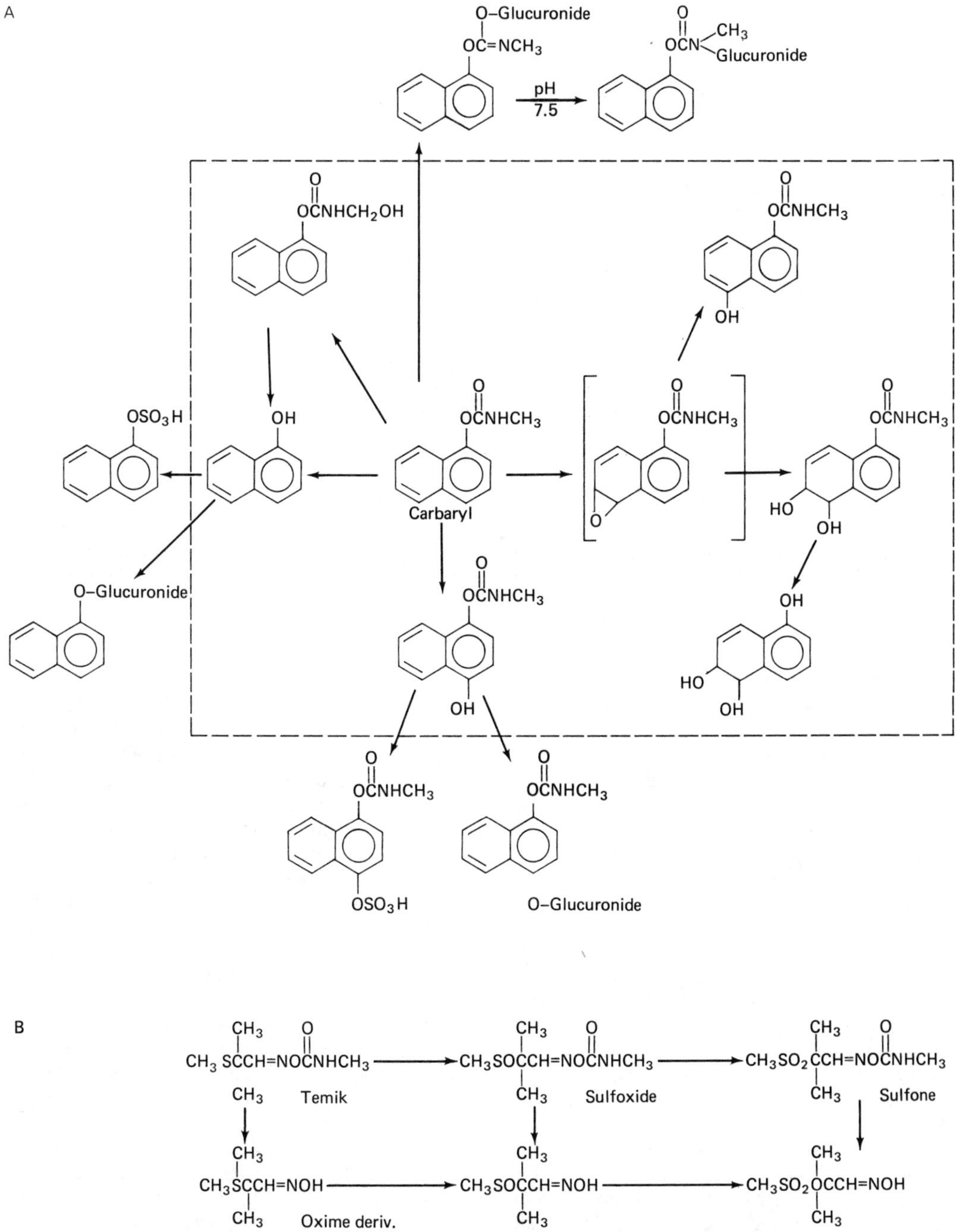

Figure 18–5. Examples of biotransformation of carbamate insecticides. *A*. Metabolism of carbaryl pathways within dashed rectangle demonstrated with liver microsomes *in vitro*. Compounds outside rectangle demonstrated urinary metabolites. *B*. Metabolism of Temik. Temik sulfoxide and sulfone are more potent anticholinesterases than the parent compound. Principal urinary metabolites in rats were Temik sulfoxide and the oxime sulfoxide. (Modified from Fukuto, T. R., and Metcalf, R. L.: Metabolism of insecticides in plants and animals. *Ann. N.Y. Acad. Sci.,* **160**:97–113, 1969.)

	CHEMICAL STRUCTURE		Relative antiAChE potency
⬡	$O-CO-NH-CH_3$ / $O-CH-[CH_3]_2$	propoxur	100
⬡	OH / $O-CH-[CH_3]_2$	2-isopropoxyphenol	1
⬡	$O-CO-NH-CH_3$ / OH	2-hydroxyphenyl methylcarbamate	17
⬡	$O-CO-NH-CH_2OH$ / $O-CH-[CH_3]_2$	2-isopropoxyphenyl N-hydroxy methyl carbamate	25
HO—⬡	$O-CO-NH-CH_3$ / $O-CH-[CH_3]_2$	2-isopropoxy-4-hydroxy phenyl methylcarbamate	300

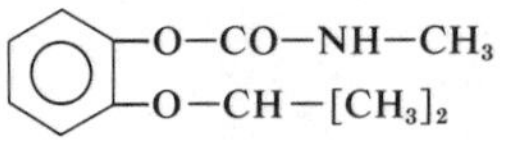

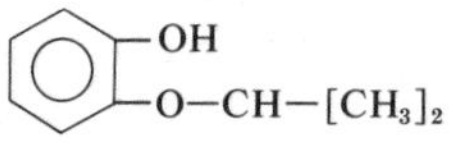

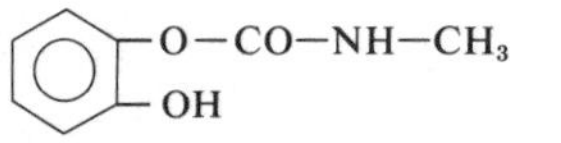

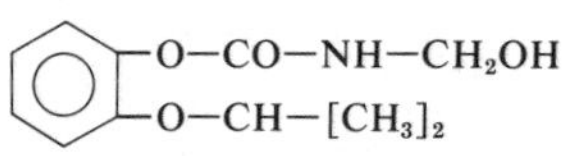

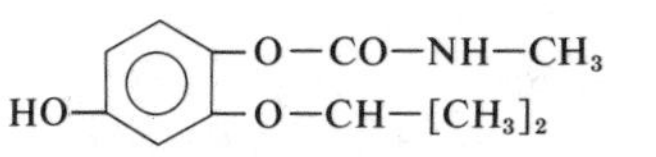

Figure 18–6. Propoxur(2-isopropoxyphenyl methylcarbamate), its principal identified metabolites, and their relative potency for inhibiting human plasma cholinesterase. (From Costa, L. G.; Hand, H.; Schwab, B. W.; and Murphy, S. D.: Tolerance to the carbamate insecticide propoxur. *Toxicology*, **21**:267–78, 1981. Data from Oonnithan and Casida, 1968.)

not produce any noticeable symptoms (0.25 to 1.0 mg/kg, intramuscularly, of propoxur) the activity of both brain and plasma cholinesterase was reduced as much as 40 percent. The dose at which a very slight tremor occurred (2 mg/kg) reduced the brain and plasma cholinesterase activities to 50 percent of normal level. At higher dosages (10 to 50 mg/kg) the degree of inhibition of both brain and plasma cholinesterase closely followed the severity of symptoms that were produced, with brain cholinesterase being slightly more inhibited than plasma (Vandekar *et al.*, 1971). Studies on human volunteers were also conducted to determine the relationship between the inhibition of erythrocyte cholinesterase and onset of signs of poisoning. The lowest erythrocyte cholinesterase activity (27 percent of normal) was observed at 15 minutes after ingestion of 1.5 mg/kg of propoxur in a 90-kg adult man. At this time no signs were observed, but moderate discomfort, that was described as pressure in the head was present. Blurred vision and nausea developed three minutes later, and 20 minutes after ingestion the man was pale and his face was sweating, pulse rate was 140 per minute compared to 76 before ingestion, and both systolic and diastolic blood pressures were increased. Following these symptoms, nausea, repeated vomiting, and profuse sweating developed. The symptoms lasted from about the thirtieth until the forty-fifth minute after ingestion, and during this period erythrocyte cholinester-ase activity recovered from a level of 50 to 55 percent of its normal value. Sixty minutes after ingestion the patient showed signs of improvement but felt nauseated and tired; pulse and blood pressure were normal. Two hours after ingestion the patient felt completely recovered. This rapid disappearance of symptoms was accompanied by further rapid recovery of erythrocyte cholinesterase activity. Studies on both rats and men indicated that the lethal dose of a carbamate insecticide is a considerably greater multiple of the dose causing the first signs of poisoning than for the organophosphorus insecticides. As a result, overexposure to carbamates might be expected to give early warning of poisoning in the form of appearance of slight symptoms, which, if heeded and exposure terminated, could prevent exposure to acutely dangerous quantities (Vandekar *et al.*, 1971).

Other Actions of Carbamates. One of the least acutely toxic carbamate insecticides, carbaryl, has reportedly produced teratogenic effects in experimental animals. Although in most species the doses for effects on fetuses were near the maternal toxic doses, in beagle dogs the teratogenic dose was found to be only about a tenth of the toxic dose to the mother (Smalley *et al.*, 1968), when given as single daily doses in gelatin capsules. Weil and co-workers (1972) reviewed the considerable literature on studies of reproductive and teratogenic action of carbaryl and concluded that the sensitivity of dogs to teratogenic action was related to the fact that dogs did not biotransform carbaryl to 1-naphthol, a major metabolic pathway in most other species including humans.

Cloudy swelling of cells in the proximal convoluted tubules of the kidneys was noted in rats and dogs fed 400 ppm of carbaryl in their diets for several months (Carpenter et al., 1961). Of related interest, it has been reported that the urinary amino acid-nitrogen: creatinine ratios were increased in a group of human volunteers who ingested daily doses of carbaryl of 0.12 mg/kg/day for several weeks (Wills et al., 1968). Although the exact relationships between the histologic changes in experimental animals and the biochemical changes in humans is not established, they would seem to be related effects.

Organochlorine Insecticides

The organochlorine insecticides include the chlorinated ethane derivatives, of which DDT is the best known example; the cyclodienes, which include chlordane, aldrin, dieldrin, hepatachlor, endrin, and toxaphene; and the hexachlorocyclohexanes, such as lindane. From the mid-1940s to the mid-1960s the organochlorine insecticides enjoyed wide use in agriculture, soil, and structure insect control, and in malaria control programs. However, they have, as a class, come into disfavor because they are very persistent in the environment and tend to accumulate in biologic as well as nonbiologic media. As a class, the organochlorine insecticides are often considered to be less acutely toxic, but of greater potential for chronic toxicity, than the organophosphate and carbamate insecticides. As shown in Table 18–7, however, there is a wide range of acute toxicities of individual compounds, from extremely toxic to slightly toxic. The organochlorine insecticides can also be classed as neuropoisons. However, their mechanism of action is not the same as that of the phosphates and carbamates. Indeed the precise mechanism is unknown for most of them.

DDT. DDT has been the best known, the cheapest, and probably one of the most effective of the synthetic insecticides. It was synthesized as early as 1874 but its insecticidal effectiveness was not discovered until 1939, and it was patented for this use in 1942. DDT was used extensively during World War II in control of lice and other insects by application directly to humans. There is no evidence that harm to these people resulted from this direct application. Indeed there seems to be no documented, unequivocal report of fatal human poisoning from DDT in spite of its widespread use and availability. Acute, nonfatal poisonings have occurred as a result of accidents or suicide attempts. Statistical associations between levels of storage of DDT and its metabolites and certain types of chronic disease in man have been reported (Casarett et al., 1968; Radomski et al., 1968); however, causal relationships have not been established and other reports indicate no association between tissue DDT levels and chronic disease (Hoffmann et al., 1967; Hayes et al., 1971). There is no question, however, that the general population has sustained exposure to DDT and derivatives, and as a result practically everyone born since the mid-1940s, when DDT was introduced into commerce, has had a lifetime of exposure and storage of some quantity of this insecticide in fatty tissues (Quimby et al., 1965; Hayes, 1966; Zavon et al., 1969). Thus chronic exposure to DDT has resulted in an accumulation of residues in humans and other animals, but the health significance of these residues is not currently apparent and remain to be further evaluated.

On the other hand, there is convincing evidence that DDT and metabolites accumulate in natural food chains by a process of biologic concentration in ecosystems (Dustman and Stickel, 1969; Edwards, 1970). As a result, organisms at the top of these natural food chains may sustain injury from DDT or its metabolites that are present as a result of gradual accumulations of residues in organisms that make up their food sources. Both field and laboratory studies have provided evidence that reproductive success in certain species of wild birds is adversely affected by exposure to DDT or its metabolites (Dustman and Stickel, 1969; Peakall, 1970; Longcore et al., 1971). Additionally, fish and some lower aquatic organisms are extremely sensitive to the acute toxicity of DDT (Pimental, 1971).

The prospect of possible ecologic imbalance from continued use of DDT, the uncertainty as to the effect, if any, of continued prolonged exposure and storage of low levels of DDT in humans, and the development of resistant strains of insects have prompted the Environmental Protection Agency to markedly restrict the use of DDT in the United States. Several other countries have taken similar actions. However, because of its relatively low cost, unavailability of substitutes that are both safe and effective, and its continuing presence as an environmental contaminant in spite of curtailed use, there continues to be interest in its toxicity.

Signs and Symptoms of Acute and Subacute Poisoning. Signs and symptoms of poisoning in humans and animals resulting from high doses of DDT include paresthesia of the tongue, lips, and face; apprehension; hypersusceptibility to stimuli; irritability; dizziness; disturbed equilibrium;

Table 18–7. TOXICOLOGY OF SOME ORGANOCHLORINE INSECTICIDES

COMPOUND	STRUCTURE	LD50 IN MALE RATS ORAL	DERMAL (mg/kg)*	"NO EFFECT LEVEL"† (mg/kg/day)	ADI‡ (mg/kg/day)
DDT	See Figure 18–7	113 (p,p'-DDT) 217 (technical)	— 2510	Rat—0.05	0.005¶
DDE§	See Figure 18–7	880	—	—	—
DDA§	See Figure 18–7	740	—	—	—
Methoxychlor	See Figure 18–7	5000–7000	—	Rat—10	0.1
Aldrin	(structure)	39	98	Rat—0.025 Dog—0.025	0.0001
Dieldrin	(structure)	46	90	Rat—0.025 Dog—0.025	0.0001
Endrin	(structure)	18	18	Rat—0.05 Dog—0.025	0.0002
Heptachlor	(structure)	100	195	Rat—0.25 Dog—0.06	0.0005

* Values obtained in standardized tests in the same laboratory (Gaines, 1969).

† Maximum rate of intake (usually for three-month to two-year feeding studies) that was tested and did *not* produce significant toxicologic effects (as listed in the monographs issued jointly by the Food and Agriculture Organization of the United Nations and the World Health Organization, as developed by joint meetings of expert panels on pesticide residues held annually, 1965–1972).

‡Acceptable daily intake (ADI) = the daily intake of a chemical that, during a lifetime, appears to provide the practical certainty that injury will not result (in man) during a lifetime of exposure. Figures taken from World Health Organization (1973).

¶ Metabolites of DDT.

§ Conditional ADI pending further evaluation.

tremor; and tonic and clonic convulsions. Motor unrest and fine tremors associated with voluntary movements progress to coarse tremors without interruption in moderate to severe poisoning. Symptoms appear several hours after large doses, and in animals poisoned with fatal doses death occurs in 24 to 72 hours. It has been estimated that a dose of 10 mg/kg will cause signs of poisoning in humans. Although there are rather marked species differences in susceptibility to acute poisoning by oral ingestion, when the compound is given by intravenous adminis-

Table 18–7. *(continued)*

COMPOUND	STRUCTURE	LD50 IN MALE RATS ORAL	DERMAL (mg/kg)*	"NO EFFECT LEVEL"† (mg/kg/day)	ADI‡ (mg/kg/day)
Chlordane		335	840	Rat—1.0 Dog—0.06	0.001
Lindane		88	1000	Rat—1.25	0.0125
Mirex		740	>2000	—	—

tration, the dose and time required for poisoning are quite similar for a wide variety of species including insects. Unlike most of the organophosphate insecticides, DDT is poorly absorbed after dermal exposure, especially when applied in the powder form. This poor absorption from the skin probably accounts for the rather good safety record of DDT in spite of its wide and sometimes careless use by applicators and formulators (Hayes, 1971).

Although the functional injury produced by high doses of DDT is referable to effects in the central nervous system, little pathologic change occurs there, and primary pathologic changes that result from exposure to high, but nonfatal, doses, or from subacute or chronic feeding, are observed in the liver. With large doses centrolobular necrosis of the liver has been reported. Smaller doses result in liver enlargement, which in rodents is somewhat characteristic in that the cells and mitochondria themselves are enlarged (Hayes, 1959). Histologic changes in the livers of male rats fed diets containing 5 to 15 ppm or more for six months include hypertrophy, inclusion bodies, and cytoplasmic granulation of a characteristic type in which the granules orient themselves around the periphery of the cell. DDT and related compounds induce mixed-function oxidase enzymes of the liver in several species, including humans (Hodgson

et al., 1980) and increases the incidence of liver tumors when fed in the diet of rodents (IARC, 1974a).

Cockerels given subcutaneous injections of DDT daily for 90 days had reduced testicular size (Hayes, 1959), and direct estrogenic effects have been observed in female rats given single doses of 50 mg/kg of DDT (Welch *et al.*, 1969). The compound *o,p'*-DDT occurs as a contaminant (ca. 15 percent) of technical grade *p,p'*-DDT. The *o,p'*-compound has been shown to compete with estradiol for binding the estrogen receptors in rat uterine cytosol (Kupfer and Bulger, 1976), 1982) and estrogen receptors in mammary tumors (Mason and Shulte, 1981). The affinity of *o,p'*-DDT for the estrogen receptor was much less than estradiol's affinity, but was capable of inducing the transfer of the receptor to the nucleus, which correlates with the estrogenic effects (Robison and Stancel, 1982).

Site and Mechanism of Toxic Action. The locus of primary toxic action of DDT is believed to be sensory and motor nerve fibers and the motor cortex. Narahashi (1969) studied the effect of DDT on giant nerve fibers of the squid and lobster by means of the voltage clamp technique. He concluded that DDT slows the turning-off process of sodium conductance across the nerve membrane and inhibits the turning-on process of the potassium conductance. A prolongation of negative afterpotential results in repetitive firing in the presynaptic nerve membrane, which is due primarily to the slowing of the falling phase of the sodium current and partly to the decrease in the steady-state potassium current. This action of DDT appears to be identical to that of certain pyrethroid insecticides (Narahashi, 1979, 1983). The involvement of other ion transport mechanisms for DDT's neurotoxicity has been suggested by Matsumura and Ghiasuddin (1979), who showed that a Ca^{2+}-ATPase formed in lobster nerve is highly sensitive to inhibition by DDT and other agents with neuroactivity similar to DDT.

Distribution and Storage. DDT and one of its major metabolic products DDE (Figure 18–7), have high fat:water partition coefficients and, therefore, tend to accumulate in adipose tissue. Studies in both humans and laboratory animals indicate there is a log-log relationship between the daily intake and the residues of DDT and DDT-derived material in adipose tissue. At a constant rate of intake, however, the concentration of the insecticide in adipose tissue reaches an equilibrium and remains relatively constant. Following cessation of exposure, DDT is slowly eliminated from the body. Elimination has been estimated at a rate of approximately 1 percent of stored DDT excreted per day (Hayes, 1971).

During the years of its most extensive use in the late 1950s and early 1960s, the average storage of DDT in fat was about 5 ppm. Total storage of DDT derived from material was about 15 ppm; this consisted primarily of DDT and its lipophilic metabolite, DDE. With declining use of DDT, there appears to have been a reduction in these levels so that the average adipose tissue level for humans in the late 1960s was 1 to 2 ppm of DDT and a total of about 9 ppm of total DDT-derived materials. Corresponding in time with these observations, analyses of whole meals indicated that the average amount of DDT that an adult in the United States obtained from food decreased from approximately 0.2 mg in 1958 to only about 0.04 mg per day in 1970 (Hayes, 1971).

Thus, in the general population there has been a gradual decline in body burden of DDT-derived materials since the marked curtailment of its use as an agricultural insecticide. However, human populations living in areas where there has been a high level of environmental contamination may still be at higher risk. Kreiss *et al.* (1981) determined blood levels of total DDT in 499 persons living downstream from a defunct DDT-manufacturing plant. The geometric mean blood concentration (mainly as DDE) was 76.2 ng/ml, more than five times the national geometric mean blood level. The high DDT levels were strongly associated with age

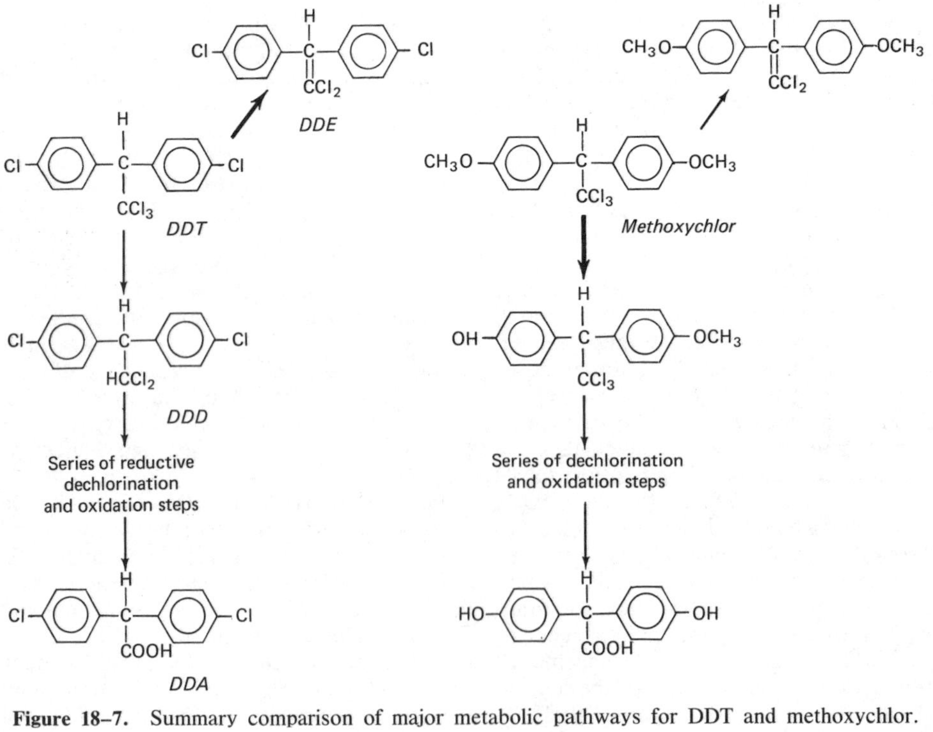

Figure 18–7. Summary comparison of major metabolic pathways for DDT and methoxychlor.

and with fish consumption, were not associated with specific illness or ill health, but were positively associated with levels of serum cholesterol, triglyceride, and γ-glutamyl transpeptidase.

There is evidence that, particularly in children, high body burdens may be derived from other than dietary sources of exposure such as the private use of DDT-containing insecticide preparations in and around the home and exposure to DDT-contaminated dust in agricultural communities (Davies *et al.,* 1969). The adipose tissue concentrations of DDT in heavily exposed workmen have achieved amazingly high concentrations (in the hundreds of parts per million) without clinical evidence of injury.

Because lipid storage of DDT is, in a sense, a detoxication mechanism (it removes the compound from sites of action in the nervous system) the insecticide can accumulate to relatively high concentration in adipose tissue when ingested by various species at low dosage rate over prolonged periods of time. This contributes to the so-called biomagnification of DDT in which a series of organisms in a food chain accumulate greater and greater quantities in their fat at each higher trophic level. Ultimately a species at the top of a food chain, e.g. carnivorous birds, may be adversely affected. Because of the nature of reproduction in birds, they may be considered a more susceptible species. Eggshell thinning has been demonstrated both in the field and in laboratory studies to result from ingestion of DDT and related chlorinated hydrocarbon insecticides. Increased breakage of thin-shelled eggs probably has contributed to population declines of these fish-eating birds.

Another action of DDT that may contribute to effects on wild bird populations is the capacity of DDT and related materials to enhance the metabolism of estrogens. This could create an endocrine imbalance that affects the egg-laying and nesting cycle in such a way that total reproductive success and survival of young during the nesting season may be reduced (Peakall, 1970).

An example of biomagnification related to human exposures was reported for nursing infants by Quimby and co-workers (1965). From an analysis of DDT content of typical meals, it was estimated that lactating women had an intake of 0.0005 mg/kg of DDT per day. Their milk contained 0.08 ppm of DDT. This would result in an infant dosage of .0112 mg/kg per day or approximately 20 times as much as the infants' mothers. Although this indicates the possibility of biomagnification involving humans there remains no evidence that infants have been harmed by these quantities.

Methoxychlor. Methoxychlor is a chlorinated ethane derivative that has enjoyed increasing use as an insecticide as the use of DDT has declined. The attractiveness of methoxychlor is that it is practically nontoxic to mammals and compared to DDT has relatively low persistence. Of course, it also has some less desirable insecticidal properties than DDT. Compared to oral LD50 values for rats in the range of 100 to 250 mg/kg for DDT, the LD50 for methoxychlor is 6000 mg/kg. While DDT has been estimated to be stored in fat at an average of 10 to 20 times its chronic rate of intake, methoxychlor has been estimated to be stored at only 0.01 to 0.1 times its chronic intake, and the half-life of stored methoxychlor in rats is one to two weeks compared with an estimated six months to a year for DDT. Although methoxychlor is slowly biotransformed to a small extent by pathways similar to those for DDT, (Figure 18–7), the major and much more rapid pathway of biotransformation is by O-demethylation and subsequent conjugation and excretion. These pathways are catalyzed by microsomal enzymes in mammals and by enzymes in soil organisms and other biota. Consequently, methoxychlor presents much reduced problems of persistence in the environment and biomagnification. Research by Metcalf (1972) on other analogs of DDT suggested the possibility of development of rapidly degradable compounds that have as effective insecticidal properties as DDT but with reduced persistence in the environment.

Chlorinated Cyclodiene Insecticides. These compounds are also neuropoisons, and many of the signs and symptoms of poisoning resemble those produced by DDT. Unlike DDT, however, these compounds tend to produce convulsions before other less serious signs of illness have appeared. Persons who have been poisoned by cyclodiene insecticides report headache and nausea, vomiting, dizziness, and mild chronic jerking. On the other hand, patients occasionally have convulsions with no warning symptoms (Hayes, 1963, 1971). Unlike the situation with DDT there have been a number of fatalities resulting from acute poisoning by the cyclodiene insecticides.

Davies and Lewis (1956) reported 14 case histories of acute endrin poisoning resulting from an incident in which at least 49 persons were made ill from eating bakery foods that had been prepared with endrin-contaminated flour. The source of the contamination was a railroad transport cart that had been used to transport bags of flour and that had, some two months previously, been used to transport a leaking container of a concentrated solution of endrin in xylene. The syndrome associated with these poisonings was referred to as fits and consisted of several, and in some cases sudden and unforewarned, convulsions.

Several human fatalities have resulted from drinking emulsions or solutions of dieldrin (Hayes, 1963). Garrettson and Curley (1969) described an incident in which a four-year-old boy and his two-year-old sister ingested a 5 percent solution of dieldrin. Generalized convulsions began within 15 minutes after ingestion and the younger child died before medical assistance could be obtained. At autopsy there were no gross abnormalities apparent. The older child sustained convulsive seizures for 7½ hours, but these were ultimately controlled with a high dose of anticonvulsants and he survived. Dieldrin distribution studies in this child showed that dieldrin strongly binds to serum proteins in a ratio of 440:1 (bound:unbound) plasma deildrin. Dieldrin partitioned into fat as fat biopsies showed ratios of fat to serum concentrations of 174:1 at three days after poisoning and 2200:1 at 179 days after poisoning. Liver function tests indicated some liver injury present for several months after the acute poisoning. Similar studies of a nonfatal case of acute chlordane poisoning in a child revealed signs of poisoning that were similar but the half-life of chlordane in the body appeared to be less than for dieldrin. Studies on persons exposed to dieldrin indicated that 20 mg/100 ml of blood is the approximate threshold at which symptoms of intoxication occur (Brown et al., 1964). Delayed and sudden appearance of symptoms of acute dieldrin poisoning several weeks or months after last exposure have been demonstrated in experimental animals and occupationally exposed men (Hayes, 1959b). Abnormal EEG recordings have been observed for months after exposure to dieldrin (Hoogendam et al., 1965).

Acute, subacute, and chronic toxicity studies of aldrin and dieldrin in experimental animals have been reviewed by Hodge and associates (1967). For 12 species of animals the acute lethal doses for both compounds ranged between 20 and 70 mg/kg. The lowest dietary levels that resulted in some mortality in short-term or chronic feeding studies in some common mammalian species were: monkeys, 5 ppm of dieldrin; mice, 10 ppm of aldrin or dieldrin; dogs, 10 ppm of aldrin, 25 ppm of dieldrin; rabbits, 80 ppm of aldrin, 20 ppm of dieldrin; rats, 100 to 150 ppm of aldrin or dieldrin. The most sensitive criteria of an effect appeared to be increased liver/body weight ratios and histologic changes in the liver, which consisted of large centrolobular hepatic cells and peripheral migration of basophilic granules that occurred at 0.5 ppm of dieldrin and 2 to 2.5 ppm of aldrin in rats.

Ingle (1965) reviewed toxicity studies on chlordane. Qualitatively the effects of chlordane are similar to those of aldrin and dieldrin; with the exception of alterations in hepatic histology, higher concentrations of chlordane were required to produce effects. The toxicology of heptachlor and its epoxide is similar to that for aldrin and its epoxide, dieldrin. Like DDT, all of the chlorinated cyclodiene insecticides are capable of inducing hepatic microsomal drug-metabolizing enzymes (Hodgson et al., 1980).

Increased incidence of liver tumors in mice fed dieldrin has been observed in chronic feeding studies. On the other hand, Deichmann and MacDonald (1971) found that overall tumor incidence in rats fed aldrin (20 to 50 ppm) or dieldrin (20 to 50 ppm) was lower than in controls and no different from controls in endrin-fed (2 to 12 ppm) rats. A panel review of several studies related to tumorigenicity of aldrin and dieldrin led to a conclusion that the available data did not meet criteria required to detect carcinogenic acitivity (Hodge et al., 1967). Another panel, however, concluded that aldrin, dieldrin, and heptachlor (as well as DDT) could be judged "positive" for tumor induction on the basis of adequate tests in one or more species of laboratory animal (Secretary's Commission on Pesticides, 1969). A working group of the International Agency for Research on Cancer (IARC, 1974a) concluded that dieldrin was hepatocarcinogenic in mice, but that conflicting reports prevented conclusion of carcinogenicity of aldrin and heptachlor. To a large extent, because of suspicion of carcinogenicity, the manufacture and use of these compounds have been severely curtailed. The subject of carcinogenic potential of the organochlorine insecticides remains an area of controversy and continued research (see Chapter 5).

Aldrin and dieldrin have been reported to produce various effects on reproduction in a variety of species, e.g., decreased fertility and decreased viability of the young, but the dietary concentrations required for these effects were as high as or higher than those that produced other effects such as histologic changes in livers of adult animals and were thought to be related to hormonal imbalance (Hodge et al., 1967; Deichmann and MacDonald, 1971).

Action Biotransformation, and Storage. Acute poisoning by the chlorinated cyclodienes can also be classified as neurotoxicity. Generally they are considered central nervous system stimulants; however, their precise site and mechanism of action are incompletely known. Biochemical studies have shown that in animals poisoned with dieldrin and other cyclodienes there was an alteration of brain amino acid ratios and an increased level of ammonia in the brain. These actions might explain the central nervous system effects; however, other convulsive agents produce similar effects, and it is not clear whether the biochemical changes in the brain were the cause or the result of convulsions produced by the insecticides. It has been reported that in brains of rats poisoned with dieldrin, gamma butyrobetaine and related compounds were released from brain mitochondria. It was suggested that they might be responsible for the effects of dieldrin, because intracranial injections of the betaine esters caused violent and fatal convulsions. Other treatments that produce convulsions also led to a release of betaine-coenzyme A esters. These treatments include electroshock, ammonium chloride, and camphor. Although the release of betaine esters as a common underlying mechanism for the convulsive effects of a variety of agents may be attractive, it also may be the result of postconvulsive action initiated by different mechanisms for different agents (O'Brien, 1967).

An important difference between DDT and the chlorinated cyclodienes that should be noted is that the cyclodienes are absorbed from the intact skin. As shown in Table 18–7, the difference between the oral and dermal LD50 values for the cyclodienes is much less than the difference for DDT. Whereas the cyclodienes may not pose any appreciably greater risk than DDT to the general population that might be exposed to small quantities of these materials in their food, from the standpoint of the occupational exposure, working with concentrated solutions of the cyclodienes would be more hazardous than working with concentrates of DDT.

Aldrin and heptachlor are biotransformed by microsomal enzymes to their corresponding epoxides (see Chapter 4). Because the epoxides are equally or more toxic by acute dosage than the corresponding parent compounds, it has been suggested that epoxide formation represents an activation reaction. However, it is also felt that the parent compounds are toxic in their own right (O'Brien, 1967). The epoxides of aldrin and heptachlor are lipid-soluble and it is the epoxides i.e., dieldrin and heptachlor epoxide, that are stored in the adipose tissue of humans and other animals (O'Brien, 1967). Evidence that epoxidation occurs readily in a variety of species is derived from the fact that analysis of residues in animals that have been exposed to the parent compounds aldrin and heptachlor reveals only storage of the epoxide forms. The epoxides of these compounds may be further biotransformed to more hydrophylic substances as the dihydrols, which can be conjugated and excreted in the urine. Biliary and fecal excretion

of the cyclodiene insecticides also occur (Cole et al., 1970).

Toxaphene. For several years this insecticide ranked first in quantity used in the United States with estimated annual production of the order of 75 to 95 million lb. Toxaphene is described as the mixed isomers of chlorinated camphene containing 67 to 69 percent chlorine. Thus, in spite of its commercial use as an insecticide for over 25 years, its exact chemical structure has been largely unknown, and it has been listed by the empiric formula $C_{10}H_{10}Cl_8$. Recently, the active ingredients of toxaphene have been the object of extensive investigation that has revealed that it includes more than 170 C_{10} compounds with six to ten chlorine atoms. Identified compounds include several endo-exo isomers of hexa-, hepta-, octa-, and nona- chlorobornanes and chlorobornenes of widely varying biologic activity (Turner et al., 1977; Saleh et al., 1977). Examples of the structure and comparative toxicities of a few of these compounds are shown in Table 18–8. In view of the extremely high toxicity of the 8-octachlorobornane, it is obvious that the proportion of this (and other highly toxic isomers) present in technical toxaphene could greatly influence the toxicity to both target and nontarget species. Piperonyl butoxide, an insecticide synergist and cytochrome P-450 mixed-function oxidase inhibitor, potentiated the toxicity of heptachlorobornane in both mice and houseflies. The other compounds were potentiated to a moderate degree in houseflies but not in mice. Heptachlorobornane undergoes reductive dechlorination by reduced microsomal cytochrome P-450 and in vivo in flies and rats. Enzymatic dehydrochlorination and oxidation of carbon substituents no doubt also help account for the extensive dechlorination that occurs in rats. Such extensive biotransformation probably also accounts for the relatively low persistence of toxaphene in comparison to other chlorinated hydrocarbon insecticides (Saleh et al., 1977).

Chronic exposure of laboratory animals to toxaphene in their diet resulted in degenerative or other changes in liver and kidneys, generally at concentrations in excess of 25 ppm. Terpene polychlorinates (Strobane ®), closely related to toxaphene, increased the incidence of hepatomas in one strain of mice (IARC, 1974a). Subsequently it was demonstrated that toxaphene itself produced liver tumors in mice and was mutagenic in tests with *Salmonella* (Hooper et al., 1979). As a result of these observations the uses of toxaphene have been drastically curtailed.

Lindane. The gamma isomer of hexachlorocyclohexane (HCH) (sometimes called benzene hexachloride [BHC]) produces signs

Table 18–8. COMPARATIVE ACUTE TOXICITY OF SOME COMPONENTS OF TOXAPHENE*

COMPOUND	LD50 24 HOURS		
	Mouse (mg/kg,ip)	Housefly (μg/g, topical)	Goldfish (PPb)
Toxaphene	47	18	20
Heptachlorobornane	75	11.5	2.9
3-exo-octachlorobornane	>100	18.5	43
8-Octachlorobornane	3.3	5.5	1.1
B-HCl(5,6) hexachlorobornene	65	225	>100

* Data derived from Turner *et al.* (1977).

of poisonings that resemble those produced by DDT, i.e., tremors, ataxia, convulsions, and prostration, with stimulated respiration. Violent tonic and clonic convulsions occur in severe cases of acute poisoning. Fatty changes in the liver and kidney tubule degeneration have been noted in fatal cases. Technical grades of HCH used in insecticidal preparations actually contain a mixture of isomers. The γ and α isomers are convulsant poisons, while the β and δ isomers are central nervous system depressants and the ϵ and η isomers appear to be inactive. The mechanism of neurotoxic action has not been demonstrated. One interesting but unproven hypothesis reviewed by O'Brien (1967) suggested that the differing actions of the isomers could be related to their binding and goodness-of-fit into pores of a "hypothetic" lattice in axonic membranes. Technical HCH and several of the isomers contained therein have been found to produce liver cell tumors in mice when fed in the diet at high concentrations for most of the animals' lifetime (IARC, 1974a).

Residues of HCH have been found in human fat and milk. Although the α, β, and γ isomers were all found as residues, the α and γ isomers are more rapidly biotransformed and the β isomer accounted for 90 percent of the total HCH isomer residue (Egan *et al.*, 1965; Hayes, 1966; Abbott *et al.*, 1968). Intraperitoneally administered HCH was eliminated in rats at a rate of 5 to 10 percent of the dose per day. Gamma HCH was biotransformed in rats by progressive dehydrochlorination, glutathione conjugation, and aromatic hydroxylation to yield 2,4-dichlorophenylmercapturic acid and conjugates of 2,3,5- and 2,4,5-trichlorophenols that are excreted in the urine (O'Brien, 1967).

Lindane has been directly or indirectly implicated as responsible for several cases of blood dyscrasias. Several cases of hypoplastic anemia that involved a history of lindane exposure were reported by the Council on Pharmacy and Chemistry of the American Medical Association as early as 1953. Of particular concern was the practice of using tablets of lindane in insecticide vaporizers, which posed the opportunity for acute accidental poisoning by ingestion of the vaporizer tablets as well as the possibility of repeated exposure to the vapors. Milby and Samuels (1971) found statistically significant, though not marked, differences in hematologic criteria in 40 people working in a lindane plant as compared to an equal number of unexposed controls. Because of the relatively few cases of lindane-associated blood dyscrasias and other complicating factors, the epidemiologic evidence for a causal relationship is not conclusive. Experimental animal studies have, apparently, failed to detect production of aplastic anemia; however, it is known that chemically induced aplastic anemia is not readily produced in animals even with drugs (e.g., chloramphenicol) for which evidence of this effect in sensitive humans is much more conclusive.

In a recent case control study involving 60 cases of aplastic anemia in North Carolina, Wang and Grufferman (1981) failed to find an association between the incidence of aplastic anemia and occupational pesticide exposures. They suggest, however, that the reported cases of aplastic anemia following pesticide exposure may be due to idiosyncratic bone marrow reactions in rare individuals.

Mirex and Chlordecone. Mirex has been used extensively in the southeastern United States for control of the fire ant. The acute toxicity of mirex to rats indicated that it was less toxic than DDT (Gaines, 1969; Gaines and Kimbrough, 1970). However, the chronicity factor (defined as the single dose LD50 in mg/kg divided by 90-dose LD50 in mg/kg per day [see Chapter 3; Hayes, 1967]), was much greater for mirex than for DDT (Gaines and Kimbrough, 1970). The respective chronicity factors for mirex, DDT, and dieldrin in rats were 60.8, 5.6, and 12.8. Rats fed mirex in the diet for 166 days had minimal pathologic changes in the liver with 5 ppm and definite enlargement of liver cells, cytoplasmic inclusions, and biliary stasis with 25 ppm. Female rats given 25 ppm of mirex in the diet gave birth to fewer and less viable offspring than control rats, and one-third or more of the offspring of mirex-fed rats developed cataracts (Gaines and Kimbrough, 1970). A total of 5 ppm in the diet had no effect on rats' reproduction. Mice given 1000 mg/kg mirex subcutaneously in a single dose developed tumors of various types, and oral administration of 10 mg/kg/day for three

weeks followed by feeding 26 ppm in the diet for 18 months resulted in a 40 percent incidence of hepatomas (Innes et al., 1969). Rats fed 50 or 100 ppm of mirex in their diet had a dose-dependent, increased incidence of hepatic megalocytosis, cellular alterations, and neoplastic nodules, with a significantly increased incidence of hepatocellular carcinoma only in males at the high dietary level (Waters et al., 1977).

Mirex stimulates hepatic microsomal cytochrome P-450 oxidative metabolism and causes proliferation of the smooth endoplasmic reticulum of the liver. There is little evidence of biotransformation of mirex in vivo and in vitro. It is excreted in the feces, and it is stored in adipose tissue. There is evidence for degradation of mirex to chlordecone (Kepone)

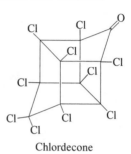

Chlordecone

in the environment (Carlson et al., 1976). Both mirex and chlordecone are highly persistent and have high lipid:water partition coefficients and have been shown to bioconcentrate several thousandfold in food chains (Waters et al., 1977).

The toxic effects of chlordecone, as seen in humans, were described earlier in this chapter (Taylor et al., 1978). These initial studies in occupationally poisoned workers stimulated considerable investigation of chlordecone's disposition and effects in humans and laboratory animals that has been recently reviewed (Guzelian, 1982). In humans and Mongolian gerbils chlordecone is reduced to chlordecone alcohol in the liver and is excreted in the bile as a glucuronide conjugate. Rats, guinea pigs, and hamsters do not form chlordecone alcohol. Both conjugated and unconjugated chlordecone and chlordecone alcohol are excreted in the feces. Chlordecone enters the intestine primarily from a nonbiliary source, probably by transmucosal transport in the gut, a process that is inhibited in humans, but not in the rat, by the presence of bile salts.

It is encouraging that a means for hastening the excretion of stored chlordecone has been developed. This involves the use of an anion-exchange resin, cholestyramine, which, when given orally to patients, enhanced fecal excretion of chlordecone by three- to eighteenfold, reduced the half-life of stored chlordecone dramatically, and enhanced the rate of recovery from the toxic manifestations, as judged by recovery toward normal sperm counts (Cohn et al., 1978). The rationale for the use of cholestyramine relates to the biliary-enterohepatic circulation, which cycles chlordecone; hence cholestyramine, by binding the insecticide, interrupts the reabsorption phase and shifts the equilibrium from reabsorption and storage to fecal excretion. In addition to binding the insecticide directly, cholestyramine may act to enhance fecal excretion of chlordecone by removing bile salts and thus releasing their inhibition of transluminal transport of chlordecone into the gut.

The toxic effects of chlordecone noted in excessively exposed workers, namely, tremor, liver injury, and altered reproductive potential, have been observed in laboratory animals (Huber, 1965; Good et al., 1965). Recent studies on the mechanisms of these effects in laboratory animals (Guzelian, 1982) indicate that the tremors are of central origin and may be the result of inhibition of mitochondrial and synaptosomal membrane-bound N_a^+-K^+-ATPases with consequent blocks of cellular uptake and storage of neurotransmitters. The liver enlargement in humans and animals exposed to chlordecone does not appear to result in a decrement of liver function, but there is an accumulation of smooth endoplasmic reticulum and an induction of cytochrome P-450 microsomal oxidases. The testicular atrophy and reduced sperm production and motility may be the result of a direct estrogenic action of chlordecone, which has been shown to be capable of binding to the estrogen receptor protein and affecting its transport into the nucleus. Chlordecone also produces a number of estrogenlike effects in the female reproductive system of rats and avian species. Studies at the National Cancer Institute (Cueto et al., 1976) revealed an increased incidence of hepatocellular carcinomas in mice and rats fed Kepone in the diet.

Treatment of Organochlorine Insecticide Poisoning. Treatment of acute poisoning by all of the organochlorine insecticides is largely symptomatic. Phenobarbital has been recommended as an antidote to control convulsions produced by DDT and other compounds. However, intravenous diazepam, because of its lesser respiratory depression, is recommended to sedate and control convulsions associated with most of the organochlorine insecticides (Doull, 1976; Morgan, 1982). Calcium gluconate has also been useful in controlling convulsions produced by DDT. As with all exposures, attention should be given

to removal of unabsorbed poison from the gastrointestinal tract and the skin. Oil-based cathartics should be avoided, however, as they may increase absorption. Also, do not give epinephrine or other adrenergic amines, because chlorinated hydrocarbons enhance myocardial irritability and sensitize the heart to catecholamines.

Botanical Insecticides

It is commonly felt that insecticides derived from natural products are less toxic to mammals than synthetic pesticides. The fallacy of this view, however, can be illustrated by the oral LD50s to rats of the three major products used as botanical insecticides: nicotine has an LD50 of 10 to 60 mg/kg, placing it amongst the most toxic insecticides; pyrethrum and rotenone have oral LD50s in the range of 100 to 300 mg/kg, comparable to several moderately toxic synthetics (O'Brien, 1967; Hayes, 1971).

Nicotine. Nicotine acts to stimulate nicotinic receptors in automic ganglia, at the neuromuscular junction, and in some pathways of the central nervous system. Its action at these sites mimics the normal transmitter acetylcholine. Poisoning in vertebrates is followed by symptoms of salivation and vomiting (from ganglionic stimulation), muscular weakness and fibrillation by stimulation at the neuromuscular junction, and ultimately, clonic convulsions and cessation of respiration (effects in the central nervous system). Treatment for nicotine poisoning is by use of anticonvulsants. Nicotine is oxidized and hydroxylated by microsomal oxidases, which yield less toxic metabolic products. Because it is the principal alkaloid in tobacco, nicotine has been studied extensively for its pharmacologic actions and detailed discussions of its pharmacology are available in textbooks of that science and in a comprehensive review on the effects of tobacco (Larson et al., 1961).

Rotenoids. A preparation extracted from tuber root, Derris elliptica, was used by primitive people to paralyze fish. It was from this use that its possibility for application as an insecticide developed. The active principle of the Derris species is the compound rotenone plus as many as 13 related derivatives. Poisoning by rotenone in man is rare, and it has been used by direct application for head lice, scabies, and other ectoparasites. Local effects include conjunctivitis, dermatitis, pharyngitis, and rhinitis. Orally, rotenone preparations produce gastrointestinal irritation, nausea, and vomiting. The estimated fatal oral dose for a 70-kg man is from 10 to 100 g. Inhalation of the dust is more hazardous, and it can cause respiratory stimulation followed by depression with fits and convulsions. A biochemical mode of action for rotenone in insect tissues, which also occurs in mammalian tissues, is the inhibition of the oxidation of reduced NAD (NADH$_2$ to NAD). The consequence of this blockage is that oxidation of substrates via the NAD system, such as glutamate, alphaketoglutarate, and pyruvate, are blocked by rotenone (O'Brien, 1967).

Pyrethrum. Pyrethrum is one of the oldest insecticides known, and the active principle of pyrethrum flowers are pyrethrin I and II and cinerin I and II. Pyrethrum extract is used in many household insecticides because of its rapid knock-down action. Signs and symptoms of poisoning by pyrethrum may take several forms. Contact dermatitis is the most common. Cases of asthmatic-like reactions have been reported in some individuals who had a previous history of asthma with a broad allergic background. Severe anaphylactic reactions with peripheral vascular collapse and respiratory difficulty are considered a rare accompaniment to the dermatologic reactions. With massive doses ingested orally, nervous system symptoms may occur, which include excitation and convulsions leading to paralysis and accompanied by muscular fibrillation and diarrhea. Death is due to respiratory failure (Hayes, 1971, 1982).

Synthetic Pyrethroids. In recent years synthetic pyrethroids have emerged as a potentially very useful class of insecticides with a high insect/mammal toxicity ratio, rapid detoxication in mammals, and lack of cumulative toxicity (Aldridge, 1983). Preparations containing synthetic pyrethroids are less likely to result in allergic reactions than preparations made from pyrethrum powder. The highly selective toxicity to insects versus mammals can be illustrated by comparing the ratios of rat LD50/insect LD50. When the adult desert locust was the test insect, this ratio was 1400 for the pyrethroid permethrin, compared to 1 for toxaphene, 11 for parathion, 45 for malathion, and 17 for carbaryl (Elliot, 1976). Two main toxic syndromes have been observed in acute toxicity studies in rats. These have been referred to as the T syndrome and the CS syndrome. The T syndrome in rats consists of aggressive sparring, sensitivity to external stimuli, and fine tremor (T) progressing to gross whole-body tremor and prostration. This syndrome is characteristic of permethrin, resmethrin, and bioresmethrin. The CS syndrome consists of pawing and burrowing behavior, salivation (S), course tremor progressing to choreoathetosis (C), a sinuous writhing, and clonic seizures. With repeated high doses, sufficient to kill some of the rats, Wallerian-type degenerative changes in sciatic and posterial tibial nerves have been observed. However, the occurrences of these lesions are sporadic and were not observed in one- and two-year feeding studies with cypermethrin at a dietary concentration nearly two-thirds that which was sufficient to kill some of the animals (Aldridge, 1983). The mechanism of action of the pyrethroids appears to be due to their rather specific effect on sodium channels in nerves (Narahashi, 1976, 1979, 1983). They prolong the membrane sodium current and thereby increase the depolarizing afterpotential, which causes repetitive discharges. Recent evidence suggests that the pyrethroids and DDT act at the sodium gate in the same manner, but the kinetics of the interactions with the sodium channels differ quantitatively with different compounds. These quantitative kinetic differences may help to explain the differences in toxic syndromes observed with different compounds (Narahashi, 1983; van den Bercken and Vijverberg, 1983). Abbassy et al. (1982) found that the pyrethroid allethrin had a high binding affinity for the channel sites of the nicotinic acetylcholine receptor of Torpedo ray electric organ, and they suggested this action may operate in concert with action on the sodium channel to explain pyrethroid toxicity. Soderland et al. (1983) found a particulate fraction of mouse brain that binds a potent pyrethroid insecticide stereospecifically and with high affinity, and which may represent the neural receptor involved in the stereospecific toxic action of pyrethroids.

The selective toxicity of pyrethroids to insects as compared to mammals appears to be largely due to their rapid biotransformation in mammals by way of ester hydrolysis and/or aromatic and methyl hydroxylation. However, this cannot explain some of the comparative toxicity differences, and it is felt that the rat's resistance to bioresmethrin (for example) is due to a lack of its affinity for target receptors in this species (Aldridge, 1983). Several pyrethroids were intermediate between parathion and DDT with respect to their persistence in soils, and the more persistent compounds, e.g., decamethrin and fenvalerate, were also the most resistant to degradation by esterase or oxidase activity. The pyrethroids are extremely toxic to aquatic organisms, unlike the case for mammals (Khan, 1983).

HERBICIDES

The production and use of chemicals for destruction of noxious weeds have increased markedly during the last 20 years. Herbicides now rival or exceed insecticides in quantity and value of sales. Because plants differ markedly from animals in their morphology and physiology, it might be expected that herbicides would present little hazard of chemical toxicity to vertebrates. Indeed some compounds have very low toxicity in mammals, but even among the herbicides there are highly toxic chemicals, and a number of these have caused fatal poisonings in man.

Chlorophenoxy Compounds

The compounds 2,4-dichlorophenoxyacetic acid (2,4-D) and 2,4,5-trichlorophenoxyacetic acid (2,4,5-T) as their salts and esters are probably the most familiar chemicals used as herbi-

2,4-d

(2,4-Dichlorophenoxy)acetic acid

2,4,5-T

(2,4,5-Trichlorophenoxy)acetic acid

cides. They are used in agriculture for control of broad-leaf weeds and in the control of woody plants along highways and utilities' rights of way. They exert their herbicidal action by acting as growth hormones in plants. They have no hormonal action in animals but their mechanism of toxic action is poorly understood. The acute toxicities of chlorophenoxy herbicides and various esters and salts have been summarized by Hayes, (1982). The LD50s ranged from 300 to >1000 mg/kg in several experimental species tested, with the exception that dogs were relatively more sensitive (LD50 of 100 mg/kg for 2,4,5-T isopropylester). Animals killed by massive doses of 2,4-D are believed to die of ventricular fibrillation. At lower doses, when death is delayed, various signs of muscular involvement are seen including stiffness of the extremities, ataxia, paralysis, and eventually coma. Sublethal doses, singly or repeated, lead to a general unkempt appearance without specific signs except a tenseness and muscular weakness. Feeding studies in animals indicate that repeated exposures to doses just slightly smaller than the single toxic dose are tolerated, indicating little cumulative effect. In a case of suicide, an oral dose of not less than 6500 mg led to death. It has been estimated that the oral dose required to produce symptoms in humans is probably about

3 to 4 g. Profound muscular weakness was noted in a patient recovering from an episode of acute poisoning by 2,4-D. Peripheral neuritis was reported for three men who had recent heavy occupational exposure to 2,4-D. Pathologic changes in experimental animals killed by the chlorophenoxy compounds are generally nonspecific with irritation of the stomach and some liver and kidney injury (Hayes, 1963).

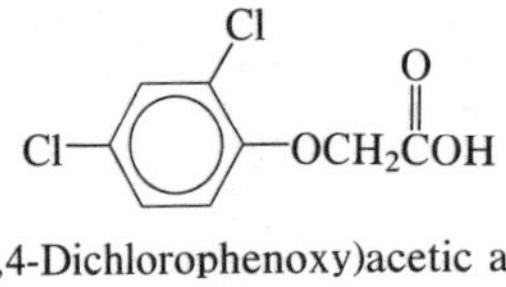

The chlorophenoxy herbicides have produced contact dermatitis in humans, and as mentioned earlier, a rather severe type of dermatitis, chloracne, has been observed in workmen involved in the manufacture 2,4,5-T (Poland *et al.*, 1971). This effect appears to be due primarily to the action of a contaminant, 2,3,7,8-tetrachlorodibenzo-ρ-dioxin.

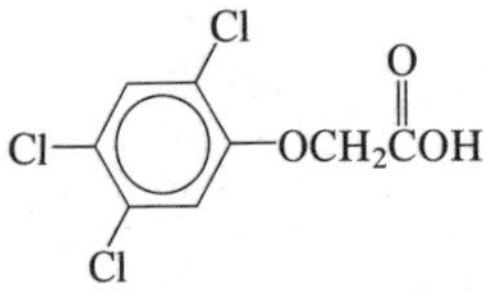

Concern about the toxicology of 2,4,5-T and related compounds centers primarily on teratogenic action in experimental animals (Moore and Courtney, 1971). The first studies to reveal this action were, it is now known, conducted with a sample of 2,4,5-T that contained a high level (about 30 ppm) of a contaminant, 2,3,7,8-tetrachlorodibenzo-ρ-dioxin. This contaminant is formed during the synthesis of the trichlorophenol precursor as shown below.

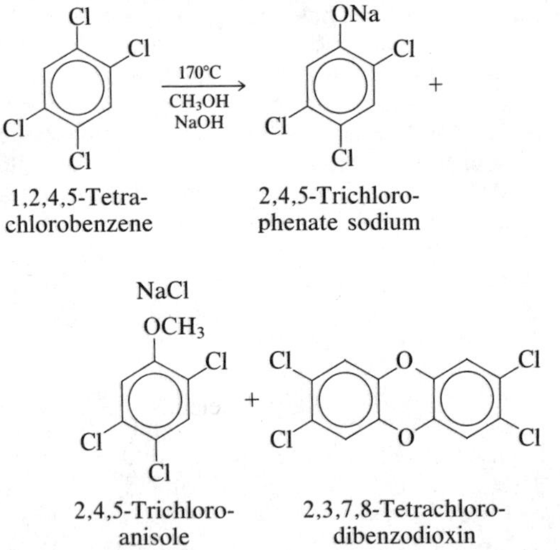

1,2,4,5-Tetra-   2,4,5-Trichloro-
chlorobenzene   phenate sodium

2,4,5-Trichloro-   2,3,7,8-Tetrachloro-
anisole   dibenzodioxin

Tetrachlorodioxin (TCDD) is an extremely toxic chemical with LD50s of 0.022 and 0.045 mg/kg for male and female rats and only 0.0006 mg/kg for female guinea pigs (Panel on Herbicides, 1971). For female guinea pigs, the ratio of the LD50 of 2,4,5-T to the LD50 of the dioxin is 630,000. For female rats the acute oral LD50 for tetrachlorodioxin is about 10,000 times less than the oral LD50 for 2,4,5-T. The daily dose of the dioxin given to pregnant rats during the gestational period that resulted in fetal toxicity was only about 1/400 of the maternal LD50 of dioxin, or about 1/4,000,000 of the single oral LD50 of 2,4,5-T to female rats. It would appear, then, that the concentration of dioxin as a contaminant in 2,4,5-T is a major factor in determining its teratogenicity.

These early experiments on the teratogenesis and fetotoxicity of 2,4,5-T illustrated an important principle for evaluation of the safety of commercial products; that is, one must be concerned not only with the major active component, but with minor contaminants that may be present as a result of their formation during manufacture or as the result of degradative reactions occurring in the environment. Presently, the TCDD content is regulated in 2,4,5-T at 0.1 ppm or less. Numerous experiments have now been conducted to test for a teratogenic action of relatively uncontaminated 2,4,5-T (i.e., less than 0.5 ppm TCDD). These experiments have demonstrated that in sufficient dosages (e.g., 15 to 100 mg/kg/day during organogenesis) the purified 2,4,5-T produced teratogenic (cleft palate and cystic kidney) and fetotoxic effects in mice and hamsters while rats and monkeys appeared resistant to the teratogenicity of 2,4,5-T itself (Hayes, 1982). Although there are a few reports that 2,4-D was teratogenic at high doses, most investigations have failed to find a teratogenic action for this compound. An epidemiologic investigation of aerial spraying of 2,4,5-T and human birth malformations in New Zealand (Hamify et al., 1981) found no association of spraying with the incidence of anencephaly, spina bifida, cleft lip, or cleft palate (the usual malformation seen in rodent studies), but there was a statistical association with exposure and congenital abnormalities of the foot (talipes) and the urethral opening (hypospadia and epispadia).

While a carcinogenic action of 2,4-D and 2,4,5-T has not been conclusively demonstrated experimentally, 2,3,7,8-TCDD has been demonstrated to produce an increased incidence of tumors, in multiple sites, in laboratory rodents fed concentrations in the diet in the parts-per-trillion to parts-per-billion range (van Miller et al., 1977; Kociba et al., 1978). The combined findings of several epidemiologic studies conducted on men occupationally exposed to chlorophenoxy herbicides in Sweden and the United States led Coggon and Acheson (1982) to conclude that there is suggestive evidence of a biologic association between phenoxy herbicides (or their contaminants) and soft tissue sarcomas. Evidence relating these products to the occurrence of lymphomas is weaker. Whether the apparent greater risk of soft tissue sarcomas was due to the herbicides themselves or contaminants (e.g., TCDD) could not be determined

from the epidemiologic studies. Indeed, further research and information is needed to confirm and quantify the increased risk of cancer from occupational exposures.

During the past 15 years a great deal of public attention has been focused on the herbicidal mixture known as "Agent Orange" that was used as a jungle defoliant during the Vietnam War in the mid 1960s. The active herbicidal ingredients of Agent Orange were equal quantities of 2,4-D and 2,4,5-T, but, in addition, some of the technical product also contained relatively high concentrations of the contaminant, TCDD. It has been estimated that 44 million pounds of 2,4,5-T (with varying contamination by TCDD, from less than 1 to 47 ppm) were sprayed in South Vietnam from 1962 through 1970 (Young et al., 1978). This has led to many claims and speculations of adverse health effects among veterans (of all involved countries) as well as among the civilian populations in the sprayed areas. Unfortunately epidemiologic studies to support or refute these claims are still fragmentary and inconclusive, although several are currently in progress. The complaints of ill health among veterans are diverse and often nonspecific, but then, so are the numerous effects of the toxic contaminant TCDD. These effects in man, based on occupational exposures and industrial accidents, include: chloracne (a characteristic dermatosis produced by TCDD at extremely low doses), porphyria, liver damage, polyneuropathies, and psychiatric disturbances. In laboratory animals TCDD is fatal in the order of 1 to 100 μg/kg. It produces in laboratory animals: liver damage, porphyria, microsomal enzyme induction, teratogenic, fetotoxic, and reproduction effects, immune suppression, tissue wasting and loss of body fat, and increased tumor incidence. A comprehensive review of the toxic effects of TCDD as well as the chlorophenoxy herbicides was published by IARC (1977).

Dinitrophenols

DNOC

OH
O$_2$N   CH$_3$
NO$_2$

4,6-Dinitro-o-cresol

DINOSEB

CH$_3$ OH
CH$_3$CH$_2$CH—   NO$_2$
NO$_2$

2-Sec-butyl-4,6-dinitrophenol

Several substituted dinitrophenols alone or as salts of aliphatic amines or alkalies are used in weed control. Human poisonings by dinitro orthocresol (DNOC) have been reported (Bidstrup and Payne, 1951). Signs and symptoms of acute poisoning in man include nausea, gastric upset, restlessness, sensation of heat, flushed skin, sweating, rapid respiration, tachycardia, fever, cyanosis, and finally collapse and coma. The illness runs a rapid course with death or recovery generally within 24 to 48 hours. These signs and symptoms reflect an increased metabolic rate, which may exceed several times normal values and is dose-dependent. If heat production exceeds the capacity for heat loss, fatal hyperthermia may result. Chronic exposure to dinitro-orthocresol may also produce fatigue, restlessness, anxiety, excessive sweating, unusual thirst, and loss of weight. A yellow staining of the conjunctiva has been noted, and cataract formation is another possible sequela of chronic dinitro-orthocresol exposure. Blood levels of DNOC below 10 ppm are considered of trivial importance; levels of 11 to 20 ppm indicate appreciable absorption; and above these blood levels toxic manifestations are likely. Levels greater than 50 ppm are critically dangerous. After removal of the poison from the skin or gastrointestinal tract, treatment consists of ice baths to reduce fever and administration of oxygen to assure maximal oxygenation of the blood. Fluid and electrolyte therapy may be necessary to replace loss by sweating. Atropine sulfate is absolutely contraindicated in cases of poisoning by dinitrophenolic compounds, and therefore care should be taken to avoid a misdiagnosis of organophosphate poisoning. Symptoms of poisoning and their severity are enhanced when the environmental temperature is high. In very cool weather blood levels as high as 50 ppm have been tolerated without symptoms. The oral LD50 of DNOC in rats is approximately 30 mg/kg (Hayes, 1971, 1982). Dinoseb (2,4-dinitro-6-sec-butylphenol) is also used as a herbicide and also has oral LD50 values of the order of 20 to 50 mg/kg in laboratory rodents.

It will be noted that the nitrocresol compounds produce symptoms of toxicity similar to those produced by dinitrophenol and therefore probably act by uncoupling of oxidative phosphorylation as has been proposed for dinitrophenol. Compounds that produce uncoupling of oxidative phosphorylation also have the peculiar property of rapidly producing rigor mortis after death. Studies on the toxicology of substituted nitrophenols used in agriculture may be found in a report by Spencer and coworkers (1948).

Bipyridyl Compounds

Paraquat is the best-known compound of this class of herbicides, which are increasing in use. Hundreds of cases of accidental or suicidal fatalities resulting from paraquat poisoning have

PARAQUAT

$$CH_3N^+ \langle \bigcirc \rangle - \langle \bigcirc \rangle N^+CH_3$$

1,1'Dimethyl-4,4'-bipyridylium ion

been reported during the past decade (Campbell, 1968; Davies *et al.*, 1977). Pathologic changes observed at autopsy in all of these fatal human poisonings showed evidence of lung, liver, and kidney damage. Some cases had myocarditis, and one case showed transient neurologic signs. The most striking pathologic change was a widespread cellular proliferation in the lungs. This pathology was also evident in a suicide case in which the paraquat was injected subcutaneously. In this case the victim died in respiratory distress, and the main pathologic findings at autopsy were in the lungs. Hence, paraquat produces lung damage even when administered by routes in which exposure of the lung is secondary. Although ingestion of paraquat results in gastrointestinal upset within a few hours after exposure, the onset of respiratory symptoms and eventual death by respiratory distress may be delayed for several days. One accidental case involved an individual who mistakenly took a mouthful of the herbicide from a "stout" bottle, and although he spat it out almost immediately, 14 days later cyanosis and severe dyspnea developed. A patient who administered paraquat by subcutaneous injection had chest radiograph changes three days after administration, but did not develop respiratory symptoms for an additional 11 days. Davies *et al.* (1977) suggest, on the basis of pharmacokinetic studies in dogs and humans, that because paraquat in the systemic circulation is rather rapidly cleared via the kidneys, accumulation of toxic amounts in the lung is secondary to kidney injury. They indicate that the presence of more than 0.2 μg/ml of paraquat in plasma, accompanied by impaired renal function in the first 24 hours after dosing, will usually result in fatal lung injury. On this basis, treatment of paraquat poisoning must be instituted early and involves (1) removal of paraquat from the alimentary tract by gastric lavage and use of cathartics; (2) prevention of further absorption by oral administration of Fuller's earth (30 percent w/v); and (3) removal of absorbed paraquat by hemodialysis or hemoperfusion. A very similar course of treatment was recommended by Cavalli and Fletcher (1977) who evaluated 96 published cases of paraquat poisoning, 70 of them fatal. They indicate that treatment, in order to be effective, should be initiated within ten hours of ingestion. Ten to fifteen milliliters of commercially prepared concentrate of paraquat is estimated as a lethal oral dose for adults, and massive overdoses of the order of 50 ml are very difficult to treat.

The toxicology of bipyridyl herbicides has been reviewed by Conning and associates (1969) and by Smith and Heath (1976). In animal studies all species examined showed the same response after a single large dose of paraquat given by mouth or by subcutaneous or intraperitoneal injection. There was an early onset of hyperexcitability, which in some cases led to convulsions or incoordination. The animals died over a period of ten days after administration. Early deaths were not associated with any specific systemic pathology. Later deaths that occurred at two to five days after administration usually were accompanied by severe pulmonary congestion and edema with hyaline membrane formation and inflammatory infiltrates. Animals that survive the pulmonary edema associated with a single dose occasionally show progression of lung lesions to fibrosis and eventual death from respiratory failure. As in humans, a single dose may produce pulmonary fibrosis in the dog. The feeding of 0.03 percent or more of paraquat in the diet of experimental animals led to the production of pulmonary fibrosis in most of the animals. Studies of organ cultures of lungs treated with paraquat revealed extensive necrosis of alveolar cells. Inhalation of paraquat aerosols for several hours produces severe congestion, alveolar edema, and bronchial irritation two to three days after the exposure. However, if the animal survives during this period there is, surprisingly, no further chronic fibrosis produced.

The LD50 for paraquat in guinea pigs, cats, and cows is in the range of 30 to 50 mg/kg. Rats appear to be somewhat more resistant with an LD50 of about 125 mg/kg. The LD50 for humans is estimated at about 40 mg/kg (Conning et al., 1969). Studies of several species indicate that absorption of paraquat from the gastrointestinal tract is relatively low, in no cases exceeding 20 percent of the administered dose. There is a rapid disappearance from the blood with 90 to 100 percent of the dose excreted in the urine within 48 hours. Since there is a long delay until onset of respiratory signs, this compound has been classified among the "hit-and-run" type of toxic agents. Exposure of the skin to solutions of dipyridyls results in erythemia and a mild reactive hyperkeratosis, which may be associated with pustule formation.

Diquat produces acute and chronic effects that differ from those produced by paraquat in that marked effects on the lung are not observed. This has been attributed to an energy-dependent system in the lung that selectively concentrates paraquat (Rose and Smith, 1977).

Oral doses near the LD50 produce hyperexcitability leading to convulsions and distention of the gastrointestinal tract with discoloration of intestinal fluids. The only pathology associated with long-term feeding of diquat at levels of 0.05 percent was the production of cataracts in about ten months.

DIQUAT

6,7-Dihydrodipyrido(1,2-α:2′,1′-c)pyrazidinium

There have been only a few cases of accidental or intentional human poisonings by diquat. As with orally dosed monkeys, the main target organs for diquat in humans were the gastrointestinal tract, liver, and kidney (Morgan, 1982; Hayes, 1983). Kidney lesions were also the only striking pathology noted in both acute and chronic studies.

It has been suggested that the mechanism of the herbicidal action of the dipyridyls is mediated by free radical reactions, and a similar mechanism has been proposed for the action in mammals. Gage (1968) showed that free radicals could be produced from paraquat and diquat incubated in the presence of reduced NADP and liver microsomes. Proposed biochemical mechanisms of paraquat toxicity are discussed in detail in the proceedings of a conference on this subject (Autor, 1977). The formation of free radicals via a cyclic single reduction-oxidation of paraquat predominates. Since initial reduction of oxidized paraquat uses NADPH, the possibility that paraquat competes for and deprives other systems (essential for cell integrity) of this biologic reducing agent is one aspect of the toxic mechanism (Smith, 1983). A more comprehensive mechanism that has been proposed involves the reoxidation of reduced paraquat by molecular oxygen with the concomitant production of superoxide radicals that dismutate nonenzymatically to singlet oxygen. These attack unsaturated lipids of cell membranes and produce lipid hydroperoxides, which may form lipid free radicals with consequent membrane damage or which may be reduced by GSH-dependent systems that depend on NADPH for GSH regeneration (Bus et al., 1976). The early event of paraquat-induced increased superoxide production is the underlying rationale for the proposal that administration of purified superoxide dismutase may be valuable in therapy of paraquat poisoning.

Carbamate Herbicides

PROPHAM

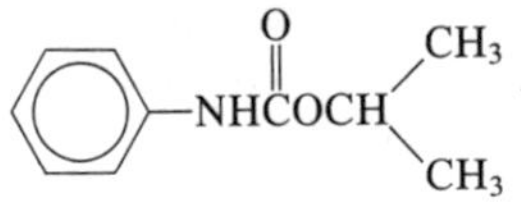

Isopropyl carbanilate

BARBAN

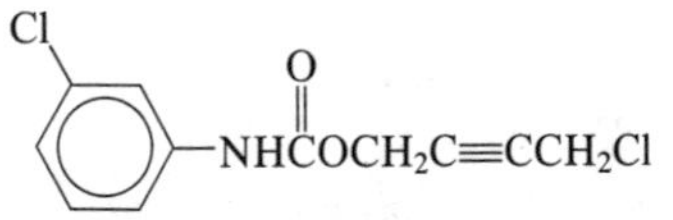

4-Chloro-2-butynyl *m*-chlorocarbanilate

This class of herbicides contains a large number of aromatic and aliphatic esters, which for the most part have relatively low acute toxicities (Dalgaard-Mikkelsen and Poulsen, 1962; Woodford and Evans, 1965). The compound propham is a typical example of this class of herbicides. Its LD50 by oral administration in rats and rabbits was of the order of 5000 mg/kg. Feeding rats dietary concentrations of 1000 ppm for three months produced no signs of effects on general condition and growth, fertility, or pathologic changes. Barban is somewhat more toxic than propham with an oral LD50 of 600 mg/kg for rats and rabbits and 24 mg/kg for guinea pigs. Daily oral administration of 75 mg/kg for 22 days produced some loss of weight, while half of this quantity produced no toxic action. Feeding experiments with rats showed no toxic action of 150 ppm in the diet for 18 months. Barban, however, is a potent skin-sensitizing agent in man, and allergic reactions and rash may develop on subsequent contact. Unlike the carbamates used as insecticides, the herbicidal carbamates do not possess strong anticholinesterase activity.

Substituted Ureas

MONURON

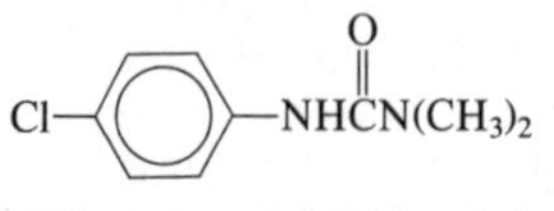

3-(*p*-Chlorophenyl)-1,1-dimethylurea

DIURON

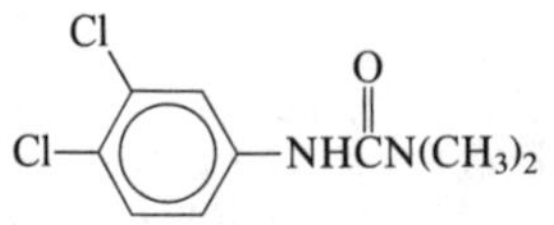

3-(3,4-Dichlorophenyl)-1,1-dimethylurea

Like the carbamate herbicides the substituted ureas are, as a class, rather nontoxic by acute oral administration. Monuron and diuron are typical examples, with LD50 values in rats of over 3000 mg/kg. Chronic toxicity studies suggest that monuron has carcinogenic potential (IARC, 1976). An increased incidence of lung tumors was observed in male mice of one of two strains tested by oral administration in one study. In another study an increased incidence of hepatomas was observed when mice were given 6 mg per animal weekly by gavage, but this study was subject to question as the survival of controls was not fully reported. In two separate studies, rats were fed monuron in their diets for 18 to 24 months. In one study no increased tumor rate over controls was observed, while in the second study 7 percent of monuron-fed rats developed tumors at various sites while control rats were reported to be tumor free.

Triazines

ATRAZINE

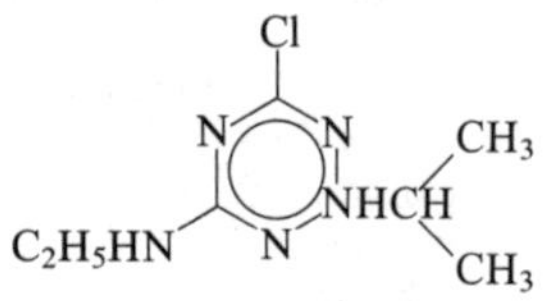

2-Chloro-4-(ethylamino)-6-
(isopropylamino)-*s*-triazine

SIMAZINE

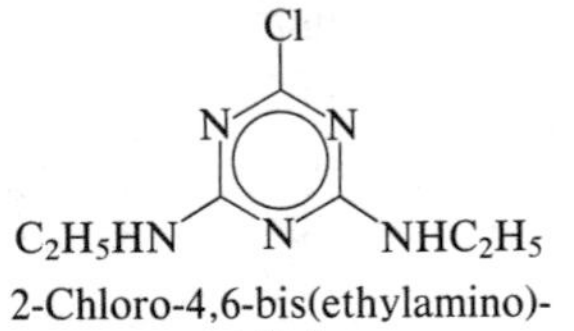

2-Chloro-4,6-bis(ethylamino)-
s-triazine

Most members of this class of herbicides also have low oral acute toxicities ranging above 1000 mg/kg. Simazine was nontoxic to a variety of animal species including mice, rats, rabbits, chickens, and pigeons. Rats survived daily doses of 2500 mg/kg for four weeks (Dalgaard-Mikkelsen and Poulsen, 1962). Simazine is, however, more toxic to sheep and cattle. Sheep were killed by three daily doses of 250 mg/kg, 14 daily doses of 100 mg/kg, or 31 daily doses of 50 mg/kg. Cattle were killed by three daily doses of 250 mg/kg (Palmer and Radeleff, 1964). The acute toxicity of atrazine to rats is greater than for simazine; however, cattle and sheep appear to be more resistant to atrazine than to simazine.

AMITROLE

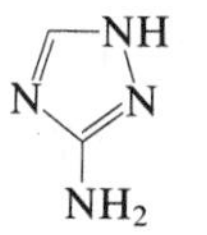

3-amino-1,2,4-triazole

The herbicide amitrole (3-amino-1H-1,2,4,-triazole), although not classified as a triazine, is structurally somewhat similar. This compound also has a very low acute oral toxicity to rats and mice (ranging from 15,000 to 25,000 mg/kg). However, amitrole is a rather potent antithyroid agent, and feeding levels of 2 ppm in the diet resulted in significant effects on thyroid function (Strum and Karnovsky, 1971). These functional changes occurred after only one week of feeding of amitrole, and goiters can be induced by amitrole with long continuous administration. Amitrole given to rats in the diet at 100 ppm for two years resulted in the development of thyroid adenomas and adenocarcinomas. This has resulted in prohibition of this compound for use as a herbicide where residues might occur on food crops. Amitrole inhibits peroxidase activity in livers and thyroids, and the mode of action in producing thyroid tumors appears to be related to the goitrogenic effect of amitrole with resultant increased TSH (thyroid-stimulating hormone) since other antithyroid agents that result in TSH stimulation also can produce thyroid tumors experimentally (Sinha *et al.*, 1965). The amitrole case illustrates an important principle in toxicology, that is, the fallacy of assuming safety purely on the basis of low acute toxicity. As is illustrated by this compound, which is practically nontoxic acutely, rather profound functional changes can occur that directly or indirectly may lead to irreversible pathology, e.g., cancer.

Amide Herbicides

Several aniline derivatives esterified with organic acids are currently used as herbicides. These compounds also have relatively high oral

PROPANIL

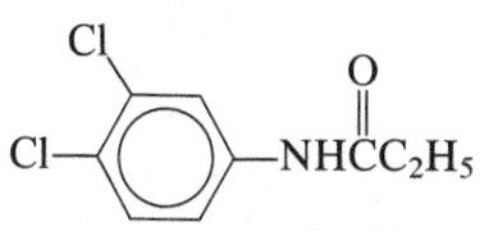

3′,4′-Dichloropropionanilide

LD50s for rats. A typical example is the herbicide propanil, which is used extensively to control noxious weeds in rice crops. The rice plant is selectively resistant to the herbicidal action of propanil because it contains an acylamidase that

hydrolyzes propanil to 3,4-dichloroaniline and propionic acid. An interesting case of herbicide potentiation was observed in field studies in which propanil was applied to rice following the application of organophosphate insecticides. This procedure resulted in damage to rice plants and was subsequently explained on the basis that the organophosphates inhibited the hydrolysis of propanil, and thus the parent compound was preserved and exerted its herbicidal action in the rice (Matsunaka, 1968). Williams and Jacobson (1966) demonstrated that mammalian livers also contained an amidase that hydrolyzed propanil, and they speculated that organophosphates and carbamates might potentiate the acute mammalian toxicity of this herbicide. Studies of interactions did not reveal a significant potentiation, however. Further investigation demonstrated that inhibition of liver acylamidase by triorthocresyl phosphate (TOCP) prevented the cyanosis that was observed when mice were given toxic doses of propanil (Singleton and Murphy, 1973). The cyanosis was due to methemoglobin formation following hydrolysis to 3,4-dichloroaniline. Other signs of poisoning, i.e., CNS depression and death, were not prevented by inhibiting the hydrolysis of the herbicide. It appears, therefore, that aromatic amides that are hydrolyzed to aniline derivatives may produce methemoglobin, but that the acute lethal action is due to a different mechanism.

Nitriles

DICHLOBENIL

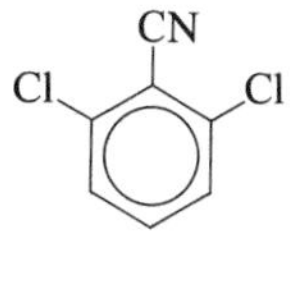

2,6-Dichlorobenzonitrile

IOXYNIL

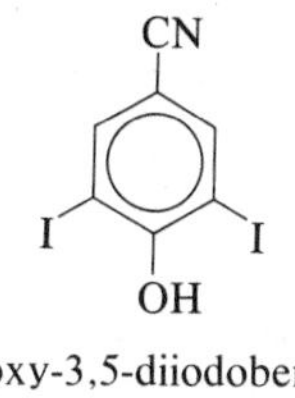

4-Hydroxy-3,5-diiodobenzonitrile

Dichlobenil and ioxynil are examples of herbicidal nitriles. The acute oral LD50s in rats are 270 and 110 mg/kg for diclobenil and ioxynil, respectively. These compounds uncouple oxidative phosphorylation. This mechanism corresponds to signs seen in occupational poisoning of four men involved in the manufacture of ioxynil and the related compound bromoxynil. They suffered from inordinate sweating and thirst, fever, headache, dizziness, vomiting, asthenia, weight loss, and myalgia of the legs. In 12-week feeding studies a no-effect level for rats was 50 ppm for dichlobenil and 110 ppm for ioxynil (Hayes, 1982).

Dinitroanilines

Trifluralin and Benefin are used as herbicides. It has been estimated that 17 million pounds of trifluralin were used in the United States in 1972. Their oral LD50 in rats exceeds 10,000 mg/kg for each, and rats and dogs showed no ill effects when fed 1000 ppm in the diet for two years (NAS, 1977; Hayes, 1983).

TRIFLURALIN

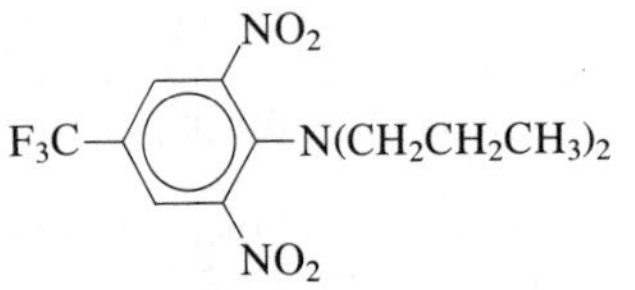

$$F_3C-C_6H_2(NO_2)_2-N(CH_2CH_2CH_3)_2$$

α,α,α-Trifluoro-2,6-dinitro-N,N-dipropyl-p-toluidine

BENEFIN

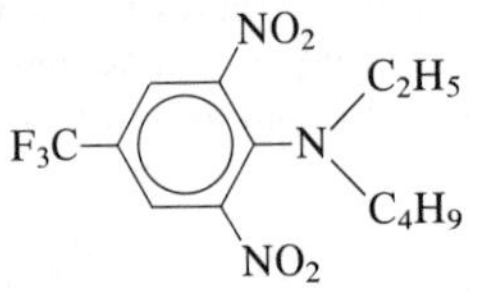

$$F_3C-C_6H_2(NO_2)_2-N(C_2H_5)(C_4H_9)$$

N-butyl-N-ethyl-α,α,α-trifluoro-
2,6-dinitro-p-toluidine

Arylaliphatic Acids

Dicamba and Chloramben are examples of this class of compounds that are used as pre-emergence herbicides. The acute oral toxicity of chloramben in rats ranges from 3500 to 5620 mg/kg and no-observed-adverse-effect doses were

DICAMBA

COOH, OCH₃, Cl, Cl

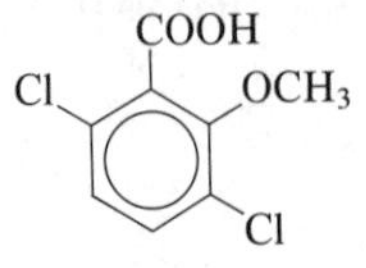

2-Methoxy-3,6-dichlorobenzoic acid

CHLORAMBEN

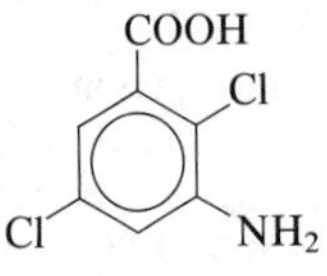

COOH, Cl, Cl, NH₂

3-Amino-2,5-dichlorobenzoic acid

250 and 500 mg/kg/day in dogs and rats, respectively. The reported oral LD50 values for dicamba ranged from 757 to 2900 mg/kg in rats. The no-adverse-effect doses were 19 to 25 mg/kg/day in rats and 1.25 mg/kg/day in dogs (NAS, 1977).

Organic Arsenicals

MSMA

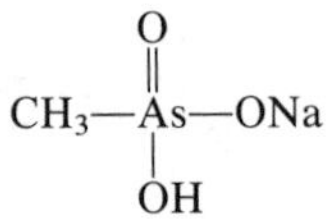

$$CH_3-\overset{\overset{\displaystyle O}{\|}}{\underset{\underset{\displaystyle OH}{|}}{As}}-ONa$$

Monosodium methanearsonate

CACODYLIC ACID

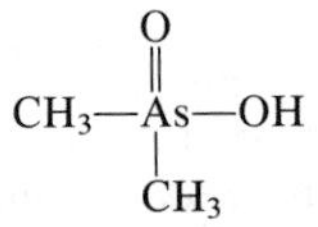

$$CH_3-\overset{\overset{\displaystyle O}{\|}}{\underset{\underset{\displaystyle CH_3}{|}}{As}}-OH$$

Hydroxydimethylarsine oxide

Cacodylic acid and mono- and disodium methyl arsenate are used as herbicides. Their toxic action resembles that of the trivalent or inorganic arsenicals, but they are generally less toxic. The signs and symptoms and treatment of poisoning by arsenicals is covered in detail in Chapter 19.

FUNGICIDES

Fungicides like other classes of pesticides comprise a heterogenous group of chemical compounds. With a few exceptions, the fungicides have not attracted the detailed toxicologic research as have insecticides. A detailed review of their action on the target organisms (fungitoxicity) has appeared (Lukens, 1971). Although many of the compounds used to control fungus diseases on plants, seeds, and produce are rather nontoxic acutely, there are some notable exceptions. The mercury-containing fungicides comprise the group that has been of greatest concern for hazard to health, and they have been responsible for many deaths or permanent neurologic disability resulting from the misdirection of mercury fungicide-treated seed grains into human and animal food (Haq, 1963). The toxicity of mercury and its compounds is discussed in Chapter 19.

Dicarboximides

CAPTAN

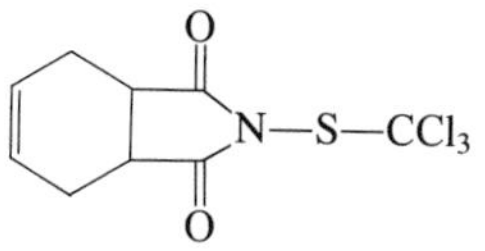

N-(trichloromethylthio)-4-cyclohexene-
1,2-dicarboximide

FOLPET

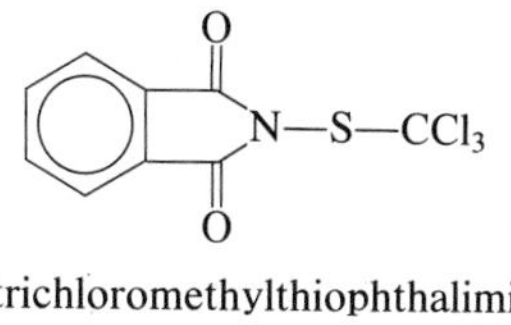

N-trichloromethylthiophthalimide

Captan and Folpet because of some structural
similarities to thalidomide were suspected as
being possible teratogens, and this effect was
confirmed in the developing chick embryo (Verrett et al., 1969). Robens (1970) reported teratogenic effects in hamsters with doses of 500 mg/
kg to pregnant females on days 7 and 8 of gestation. Other studies in rabbits, rats, and hamsters
failed to reveal teratogenic effects from folpet
(McLaughlin et al., 1969), but in one study nine
malformed offspring were observed out of 75
implantations in nine pregnant rabbits given
75 mg/kg/day of captan orally on days 6 through
16 of gestation. Rats fed a low-protein diet were
reported to be much more sensitive to the acute
oral toxicity (LD50, 480/mg/kg) of captan than
rats receiving a normoprotein diet (LD50,
12,500 mg/kg) Boyd and Krijnen, 1968). Most
chronic oral toxicity studies on captan and folpet
suggest a no-adverse-effect dosage of these
agents to be about 50 mg/kg/day; however, increased fetal mortality was reported in one study
in monkeys exposed to captan at 12.5 mg/kg/day
(NAS, 1977). Captan has also now been demonstrated to be mutagenic, carcinogenic, and immunotoxic as discussed later in this chapter.

Substituted Aromatics

PCP

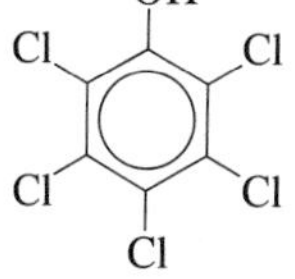

Pentachlorophenol

PCNB

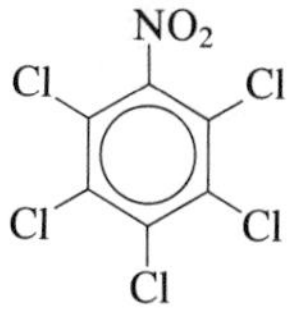

Pentachloronitrobenzene

HEXACHLOROBENZENE

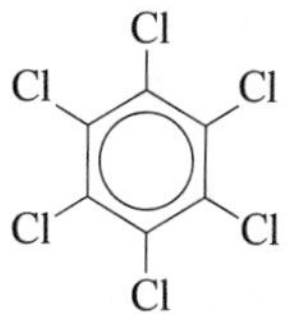

1,2,3,4,5,6-Hexachlorobenzene

Pentachlorophenol production and use are of
the order of 50 million lb per year. It is used as
an insecticide and herbicide as well as a fungicide, with major application as a wood preservative. Several cases of human poisonings have
resulted in association with these uses. Its acute
toxic action in humans and experimental animals
resembles that produced by the nitrophenolic
herbicides, i.e., marked increases in metabolic
rate as the result of uncoupling of oxidative
phosphorylation. It is readily absorbed through
the skin. Two cases of fatal poisonings and several nonfatal cases occurred in a hospital nursery in which pentachlorophenol had been used
as a fungicide in the laundry room (against the
labeled instructions) and ultimately contacted
infants through their diapers (Armstrong et al.,
1969). Several infants died before the cause and
source of poisoning were identified. The fatal
dose of pentachlorophenol for laboratory animals ranges from 30 to 100 mg/kg, and it is readily absorbed through the skin. In recent years it
has become apparent that many commercial
samples of pentachlorophenol are contaminated
with polychlorinated dibenzodioxins and dibenzofurans (Buser, 1975). These contaminants are
generally hexachlorinated or octachlorinated
dibenzodioxins or dibenzofurans, and they are
less toxic than the tetrachlorodioxin contaminant in 2,4,5-T. Nevertheless, some isomers of
hexachlorodibenzodioxin have LD50 values in
guinea pigs of the order of 60 to 100 μg/kg, ranking them as extremely toxic chemicals. The oc-
tachlorodioxins are much less acutely toxic, in
the order of 1 g/kg. Although pentachlorophenol
is highly toxic in its own right, some studies suggest that the contaminants may be responsible
for some of the toxic effects of the technical
grade. A comparison of effects of technical versus purified pentachlorophenol indicated that
only the technical grade produced chloracne,
chick edema, hepatic porphyria, and increased
relative liver weight (Johnson et al., 1973; Goldstein, 1976). Technical grade was also much
more active as a liver enzyme inducer.

Pentachloronitrobenzene (PCNB) is used as a
soil fungicide treatment. Its oral LD50 values in
rats range from 1200 to 1650 mg/kg. In two-year
feeding studies in rats and dogs, dietary no-

adverse-effect levels of 25 and 5 ppm, respectively, were observed. However, in mice fed 1206 ppm in the diet an increased incidence of hepatomas was observed. PCNB also produced cleft palate in offspring of pregnant mice treated with 500 mg/kg on days 7 to 11 of gestation. The possible carcinogenic action of PCNB requires additional investigation.

Dichloran (2,6-dichloro-4-nitroaniline), which is used as a protectant fungicide, has a rat oral LD50 of 8000 mg/kg, and 400 mg/kg/day could be tolerated for three months by rats. Dogs and monkeys were more susceptible to repeated dosing. In chronic feeding studies structural changes were seen in livers and kidneys of rats and monkeys. Dogs, but not pigs, developed corneal opacities when fed dichloran at a rate of 48 mg/kg/day. Opacities did not occur if the dogs were kept in the dark. Dichloran and one of its metabolites (3,5-dichloro-4-aminophenol) were potent uncouplers of oxidative phosphorylation *in vitro* (Hayes, 1982).

Another fungicide, *hexachlorobenzene* (note that this is distinct from hexachlorocyclohexane or lindane), produced more than 3000 cases of acquired toxic porphyria cutanea tarda, which was characterized by severe skin manifestations including photosensitivity, bulbae formation, deep scarring, permanent loss of hair and skin atrophy. The poisonings were traced to the consumption of wheat that had been prepared for planting by treating it with hexachlorobenzene for its fungicidal effects (Schmid, 1960).

Dithiocarbamates

Dithiocarbamate fungicides have enjoyed rather widespread use in agriculture. They have a low order of acute toxicity, with oral LD50 values in rats ranging from several hundred milligrams to several grams per kilogram. There is little evidence of human injuries from exposure to these compounds; however, some of these compounds have been reported to have teratogenic and/or carcinogenic potential (WHO, 1975). Two groups of dithiocarbamates have been used, the dimethyldithiocarbamates and the ethylenebisdithiocarbamates. Their respective general structures are as follows:

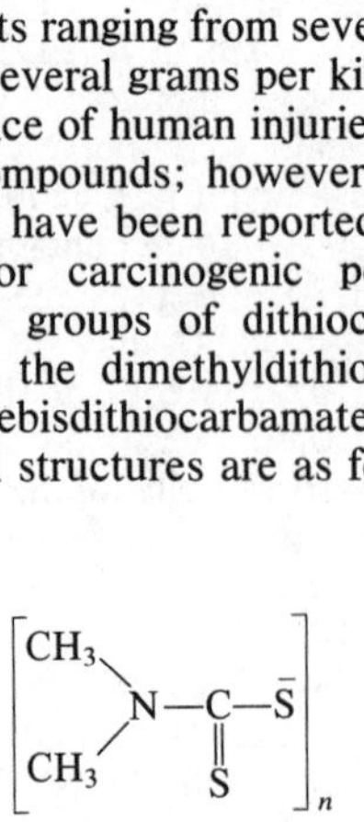

Dimethyldithiocarbamates

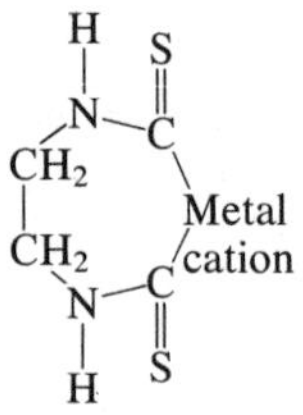

Diethyldithiocarbamates

The names of the fungicides are derived from the metallic cations. For example, when the cation is zinc or iron, the respective dimethyldithiocarbamates are ziram or ferbam. With manganese, zinc, or sodium as the cation in the diethyldithiocarbamates, the respective fungicide is maneb, zineb, or nabam. Some dimethyldithiocarbamates are reported to be teratogenic in animals, and they can be nitrosated to form nitrosamines *in vitro* and *in vivo* (WHO, 1975; IARC, 1974b). The ethylenebisdithiocarbamates maneb, nabam, and zineb are also reported to be teratogenic (Petrova-Vergieva and Ivanova-Chemishanska, 1973). Furthermore, this group of compounds breaks down to form ethylene thiourea (ETU) *in vivo*, in the environment, and during cooking of foods containing their residues. ETU is carcinogenic, mutagenic, and teratogenic as well as antithyroid (IARC, 1974b, 1976) A scheme (IARC, 1976) for the degradation of maneb is as follows:

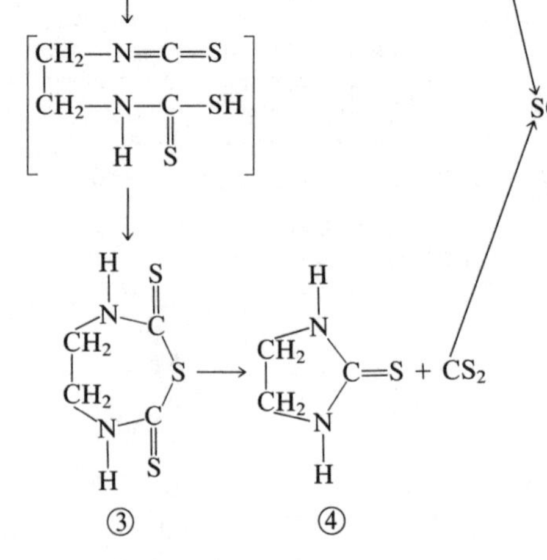

Maneb (1) is hydrolysed by acids to ethylene-diamine (2) and carbon disulfide. Carbon disulfide is also produced when ethylene bisthiuram monosulfide (3) is transformed into ETU (4). Maneb produced an increased incidence of lung tumors in only one of four strains of mice that have been tested and studies in rats were equivocal (IARC, 1976). However, because of its conversion to the much more active ETU, it and other fungicides of this class require further study and evaluation of hazard (WHO, 1975).

Nitrogen Heterocyclic fungicides

Benomyl and thiabendazole are examples of broad-spectrum systemic fungicides; i.e., they can translocate through the cuticle and across leaves of treated plants. The oral LD50 of benomyl in rats is greater than 10,000 mg/kg; however, when it was administered to rats during the first 20 days of pregnancy at dosages of 125 to 500 mg/kg/day, skull and central nervous system anomalies occurred in offspring at the rate of 4.6 to 100 percent. On the other hand, feeding pregnant rats as much as 5000 ppm in the diet did not adversely affect embryo development. Japanese workers, especially women, developed dermatitis associated with exposure to benomyl used in greenhouses.

BENOMYL

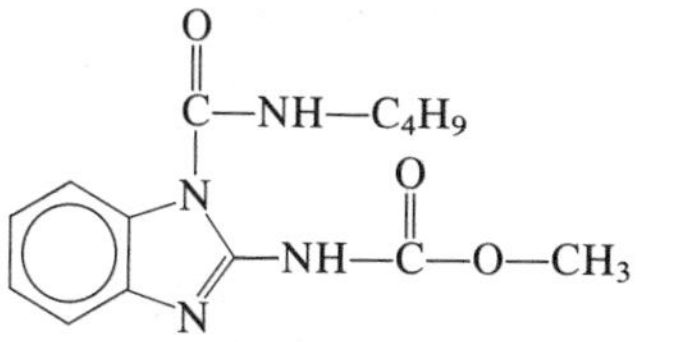

Methyl 1-(butylcarbamoyl)-2-benzimidazolecarbamate

THIABENDAZOLE

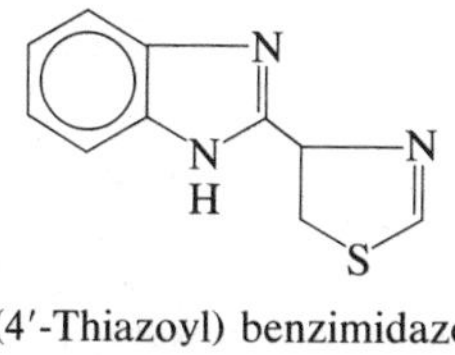

2-(4'-Thiazoyl) benzimidazole

Thiabendazole has an oral LD50 in rats of 3100 mg/kg. Rats tolerated repeated dosing with 200 mg/kg/day for six months. Dogs also tolerated this dosage except that it frequently produced vomiting. Hemosiderosis throughout much of the reticuloendothelial system was observed in both rats and dogs that received substantial doses (Hayes, 1982).

RODENTICIDES

A wide variety of chemicals, which defy classification, have been used in the control of rats and mice. Although they are used to kill mammals, which resemble humans in their physiology and biochemistry, there are wide differences in degree of hazard to humans. In some case the rodenticidal selectivity of these compounds is based on the peculiar physiology of rodents, which differs from that of primates and other desirable species, and in some cases it is merely a question of taking advantage of the habits of rodents as opposed to species that are to be protected. Four requirements for an ideal rodenticide are: (1) it must be effective in small quantities so it is not detected by rodents, (2) finished baits must not elicit bait shyness, (3) manner of death should be such that survivors do not become suspicious of its cause, and (4) the poison in the concentration used must be specific for the target species, unless its use can be made safe for humans and other animals by some other means. The anticoagulant rodenticides in general fulfill these requirements (Hayes, 1982).

In addition to potential widespread destruction of food and fiber by rodents, another primary reason for attempting their control is to eliminate intermediate hosts in the transmission of various vectorborne diseases, e.g., bubonic plague (Lisella *et al.*, 1971). Since rodenticides can be used in baits and placed in inaccessible places, their likelihood of becoming widespread contaminants of the environment is much less than that associated with the use of insecticides and herbicides. The toxicologic problem posed by rodenticides, therefore, is primarily acute accidental or suicidal ingestion.

Warfarin

WARFARIN

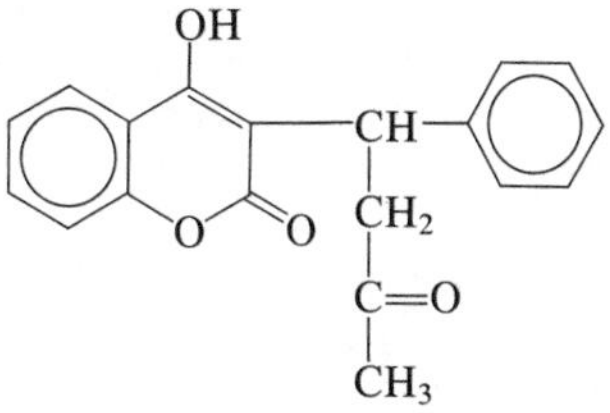

3-(α'-Acetonylbenzyl)-4-hydroxycoumarin

Warfarin, 3-(alpha-acetonylbenzyl)-4-hydroxy-coumarin, is one of the most widely used rodenticides. Its safe usage is based on the fact that it requires repeated dosing for toxicity to develop. Thus, placed in baits accessibe to rodents, repeated ingestion results in fatalities to rodents with little likelihood that pets or children would be repeatedly exposed.

The mechanism of action of warfarin is an anticoagulant. It is an antimetabolite of vitamin K, and hence it inhibits the synthesis of prothrombin. Multiple doses are usually required to maintain inhibition of synthesis until prothrombin levels are sufficiently depleted to result in hemorrhage throughout the whole body, which is the cause of death. In addition to its anticoagulant action, direct capillary damage has also been attributed to warfarin (Lisella *et al.*, 1971; Hayes, 1982). Single fatal doses in common laboratory animals range between 200 and 400 mg/kg. Basing estimates of toxicity to humans on values for single lethal doses for animals, it has been suggested that an adult human would have to eat 1.5 lb of a warfarin concentrate or about 30 lb of a strong rat bait to result in fatality. On the other hand, daily ingestion for six days of as little as 1 to 2 mg/kg has produced severe illness in an attempted suicide. Two members died of a Korean family of 14 persons who lived for 15 days on a diet of cornmeal containing warfarin that was intended as a rat bait. All became severely ill with hemorrhage. The estimated dosage was 1 to 2 mg/kg/day. Symptoms of poisoning, which begin after a few days or weeks of repeated ingestion, include epistaxis and bleeding gums, pallor, and sometimes petechial rash leading to hematomas around the joints and on the buttocks, ultimately blood in the urine and feces, and occasionally paralysis due to cerebral hemorrhage, and finally to hemorrhagic shock and death. The principal diagnostic test for excessive repeated exposure to warfarin is a markedly reduced prothrombin activity, and therapy is directed at correcting this by the administration of vitamin K. Additional details concerning the toxicity and treatment are given by Hayes (1982).

Related anticoagulants used as rodenticides are coumafuryl (3-[1-furyl-3-acetyl-ethyl]4-hydroxycoumarin), diphacinone (2-diphenylacetyl-1,3-indandione), and pindone (2-pivalyl-1,3-indandione). These have the advantage over warfarin of being more readily soluble in water.

Red Squill

The bulbs of red squill (*Urginen maritima*) have been used for many years as a relatively safe rodenticide. The active principles are glycosides scillaren-A and scillaren-B. These glycosides have cardiotonic actions like the digitalis glycosides. Crude red squill also contains a central-acting emetic, which causes vomiting in animals other than rodents. This emetic action is the main factor that contributes to the safety of

SCILLIROSIDE
(Active principle of Red Squill)

the rodenticide to humans. Symptoms that are associated with ingestion of large doses of red squill include vomiting and abdominal pain, blurred vision, cardiac irregularity, convulsions, and death from ventricular irregularities. Quinidine sulfate is used in treatment to reduce mild cardioirritability. The selective rodenticidal usefulness of squill, then, takes advantage of the physiologic peculiarity of the rat's inability to vomit (Lisella *et al.*, 1971).

Norbormide

NORBORMIDE

Norbormide is another rodenticide that takes advantage of a physiologic peculiarity of the rat for its selective toxicity. This compound acts directly on the smooth muscle of peripheral vessels causing them to constrict irreversibly resulting in widespread ischemia leading to death. The receptor sites for norbormide in the vascular smooth muscle apparently are different from the vasoconstrictive receptors for epinephrine. Since the compound is lethal to rats in dosages of 5 to 15 mg/kg and is essentially nontoxic for cats, dogs, chickens, ducks, primates, sheep, or swine, it must be assumed that the norbormide receptors in smooth muscle of peripheral vessels exist uniquely in the rat (Roszowski, 1965).

Sodium Fluoroacetate (Compound 1080) and Fluoroacetamide (Compound 1081)

SODIUM FLUOROACETATE (1080®)

$$F-CH_2-\overset{\overset{\displaystyle O}{\|}}{C}-O-Na$$

FLUOROACETAMIDE (1081, Fluorakil 100®)

$$F-CH_2-\overset{\overset{\displaystyle O}{\|}}{C}-O-NH_2$$

These rodenticides, whose use is largely restricted to licensed pest control operators, are among the most potent rodenticides known and are also highly toxic to other animals. Their mechanism of toxicity was well established by the work of Sir Rudolph Peters and fascinating accounts of that work are described in his book on biochemical lesions and lethal synthesis (Peters, 1963).

The oral LD50 for rats for fluoroacetate is 0.20 mg/kg, and for fluoroacetamide is 4 to 15 mg/kg (Autov and Mirkova, 1982; Hayes, 1982). Fluoroacetamide is metabolized to fluoroacetate, which produces its toxic action by inhibiting the citric acid cycle. The fluorine substituted acetate becomes incorporated, as normal acetate, into fluoroacetyl coenzyme A, which condenses with oxaloacetate to form fluorocitrate. Fluorocitrate inhibits the enzyme aconitase and thereby inhibits the conversion of citrate to isocitrate. As a result there is an accumulation of large quantities of citrate in the tissue, and the cycle is blocked. As might be expected, the heart and central nervous system are the most critical tissues involved in poisoning by a general inhibition of oxidative energy metabolism. Thus, the symptoms following fluoroacetate poisoning, in addition to nonspecific signs of nausea and vomiting, include cardiac irregularities, cyanosis, generalized convulsions, and death from ventricular fibrillation or respiratory failure.

Estimates of the mean lethal dose of fluoroacetate in humans range from 2 to 10 mg/kg, and there have been a number of human fatalities (Pattison, 1959). There are apparent species differences in the quality of symptoms that lead to death. Dogs die of convulsions or respiratory paralysis, but in humans, monkeys, horses, and rabbits central nervous system actions are usually incidental, and the dangerous fatal complication is ventricular fibrillation (Brockmann *et al.*, 1955). Provision of large quantities of acetate appears to antagonize fluoroacetate poisoning in a competitive manner in that monkeys have been successfully protected from fluoroacetate poisoning by the administration of glycerol monoacetate (Chenoweth *et al.*, 1951).

Alpha Naphthyl Thiourea (ANTU)

ANTU®

α-Naphthylthiourea

ANTU was developed as a rodenticide following the observation that phenylthiourea kills rats but is not toxic to humans. The thiourea derivative ANTU proved to be effective as a rodenticide because it lacked the bitter taste associated with phenylthiourea. However, some strains of rats are not sensitive to it, and others develop resistance. There is a wide range of susceptibility to the acute toxicity of ANTU among mammals. The LD50 to rats is a few milligrams, approximately 3 mg/kg. Dogs appear to be next most sensitive with LD50s of 10 mg/kg. Pigs, horses, and cows require 30 to 50 mg/kg for fatalities, and guinea pigs require 400 mg/kg. A mean lethal dose in monkeys was 4 g/kg, and it is assumed that humans would be similarly resistant. ANTU produces its principal toxic action in susceptible species by causing massive pulmonary edema and pleural effusion, apparently due to action on pulmonary capillaries. Resistant animals do not show pulmonary edema. Biochemical changes occurred in poisoned rats that suggested effects of ANTU on carbohydrate metabolism (DuBois, 1948); however, the altered carbohydrate metabolism may be secondary to adrenal stimulation since adrenal demedullation blocked these biochemical changes. Altered thyroid function also alters the toxicity of ANTU. Tolerance to the acute effects of ANTU in rats can be induced by administering progressively increasing doses, and pleural effusions are not present in tolerant animals that die from large doses. (McClosky and Smith, 1945). ANTU produces a cross-tolerance to several other edemagenic agents, including inhaled irritant gases such as ozone and NO_2 (Fairchild *et al.*, 1959). Reaction of ANTU with sulfhydryl groups may be a necessary part of the mechanism of toxic action, since it has been reported that sulfhydryl group blocking agents are effective antidotes in rats in some experimental conditions.

Strychnine

STRYCHNINE

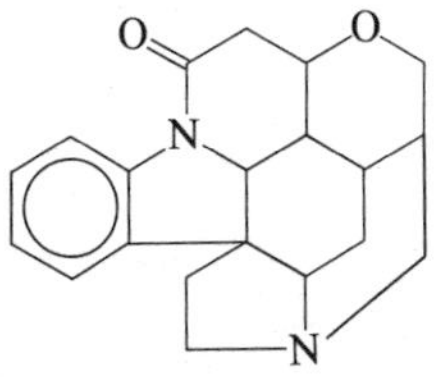

This alkaloid of the nux vomica plant is a potent convulsant poison with a lethal dose of a few milligrams per kilogram of body weight for most animals. It lowers the threshold for stimulation of spinal reflexes by blocking inhibitory pathways exerted by Renshaw cells over the motor cells in the spinal cord. As a result, poisoned animals go into tetanic convulsions in response to rather minimal sensory stimuli. Nux vomica was introduced into Germany in the sixteenth century for use as a rodenticide (Lisella *et al.*, 1971). Although its use has declined, it is still used in poisoned baits in control of vermin, and accidental poisonings in humans continue to occur. Strychnine nitrate has been used as a "bearicide" in Hokkaido, Japan. The minimal fatal dose for bears appears to be about 0.5 mg/kg.

Pyriminil (Vacor®)

VACOR®

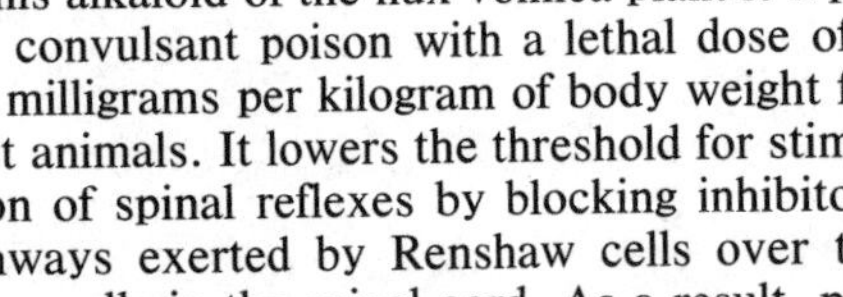

N-3-pyridylmethyl-N'-*p*-nitrophenyl urea

Pyriminil is a recently developed rodenticide that is effective against rats that have developed resistance to Warfarin. It is effective against rats in a single dose of as little as 5 mg/kg. The LD50 for dogs, monkeys, and chickens are all greater than 500 mg/kg. Pyriminil interferes with nicotinamide metabolism and rodents die from paralysis and respiratory arrest. Nicotinamide given intravenously or intramuscularly is recommended as an antidote. Pyriminil destroys the B cells of the pancreas and hence can cause a diabetic state. It also produces peripheral neuropathy and numerous CNS effects. In cases of human poisonings (by as little as 5.6 mg/kg) effects have often been prolonged for weeks or months and may require insulin treatment (Hayes, 1982).

Inorganic Rodenticides

A number of inorganic compounds are used in rodent control. Most of these are nonselective in their toxicity and are generally hazardous to humans and domestic animals so that their use has declined in favor of more selective or less hazardous organic compounds.

ZINC PHOSPHIDE

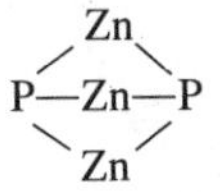

Zinc phosphide reacts with water and HCl in the gastrointestinal tract to produce the gas phosphine (PH_3), which causes severe gastrointestinal irritation (Antov and Mirkova, 1982; Hayes, 1982). Apparent insensitivity of dogs and cats has been attributed to the emetic qualities of zinc (Lisella *et al.*, 1971). Zinc phosphide, in the presence of moisture, may evolve phosphine, which inhaled in sufficient concentration can cause fatal pulmonary edema.

Thallium sulfate is lethal to most animals in doses of 10 to 20 mg/kg. It apparently acts by reacting with free sulfhydryl groups, but the precise mechanism of poisoning is uncertain. Acute poisoning is accompanied by gastrointestinal irritation, motor paralysis, and death from respiratory failure. Lower, sublethal doses taken over a period of time result in reddening of the skin and loss of hair. Pathologic changes include perivascular cuffing around blood vessels and degenerative changes in brain, liver, and kidney. Neurologic symptoms are prominent in repeated subacute poisoning and include tremors, leg pains, paresthesias of the hands and feet, and polyneuritis especially in the legs. Psychoses, delirium, convulsions, and other kinds of encephalopathy may also be noted. Dimercaprol (BAL) is of little benefit as a chelating agent in removal of absorbed thallium. Use of 1 percent thallium sulfate to control ground squirrels has resulted in outbreaks of thallotoxicosis in humans. In a 20-year period between 1935 to 1955, 778 persons were reported to have been poisoned by thallium-containing insecticides, rodenticides, and therapeutic chemicals, resulting in 46 fatalities (Grossman, 1955). Because of its high, cumulative toxicity the use of thallium has been restricted to applications by qualified personnel, with a resultant marked decline in its use as a rodenticide (Lisella *et al.*, 1971).

White or yellow elemental phosphorus has caused poisoning because of the practice of spreading pastes containing this element on bread as a rodenticide bait (Lisella *et al.*, 1971). A dose of 15 mg of phosphorus can cause severe poisonings in humans and as little as 50 mg may be fatal. Shortly after ingestion phosphorus produces severe gastrointestinal irritation, and if a sufficient dose is ingested, hemorrhage and cardiovascular failure may prove fatal within 24 hours. The vomitus after phosphorus ingestion is luminescent and has a characteristic garlic odor. If the patient survives the initial gastrointestinal irritation phase, secondary systemic poisoning due to liver necrosis may ensue. Severe acute yellow atrophy of the liver is one delayed sequela that may ultimately prove fatal.

Barium carbonate and arsenic trioxide have also been used as rodenticides, but currently have little application for this purpose. Barium produces severe colic, diarrhea, and hemorrhage. It has a direct action on smooth muscles of the arterioles and cardiac muscle, which can result in increased blood pressure, cardiac irregularities, and death.

A variety of other compounds have some occasional application in rodent control. Carbon monoxide, methyl bromide, and hydrogen cyanide have been used as fumigants to kill rodents in enclosed spaces. These chemicals are generally toxic to all species. DDT, commonly thought of as an insecticide, is used as a poison for the house mouse and for bats. The principle of this treatment is to treat inaccessible areas where mice travel so that they will pick up a sufficient amount of DDT on their feet and fur, and ultimately, in preening, ingest the DDT and become poisoned. At best this seems an inefficient means of rodent control Further discussion of action and therapy for poisoning by various rodenticides may be found in Hayes (1982) and Morgan (1982).

FUMIGANTS

Fumigants are used in the control of insects, rodents, and soil nematodes. They have in common the property of being in the gaseous form at the time they exert their pesticidal action and are used because they will penetrate to areas otherwise inaccessible for pesticide application (e.g., grain storage areas, rodent runways). Fumigants may be liquids that readily vaporize, solids that release a gas by chemical reaction (e.g., HCN from $Ca[CN]_2 + H_2O$), or gases contained in cylinders or ampuls (e.g., methyl bromide). Thus they provide a potential hazard from the standpoint of inhalation exposure as well as, in the case of solids and liquids, accidental ingestion or dermal exposure. Fumigants used in the protection of stored foodstuffs include acrylonitrile, carbon disulfide, carbon tetrachloride, chloropicrin, ethylene dibromide, ethylene oxide, hydrogen cyanide, methyl bromide, and phosphine. These chemicals have many other applications in industry and their toxicology has been discussed in other sections.

It is worthy of comment that *methyl bromide* is said to have been responsible for more deaths in recent years among occupationally exposed persons in California than all of the more publicized organophosphate group of insecticides (Hine, 1969). During the period of 1957 to 1964, 62 systemic poisonings with five deaths were reported. In the usual case the early symptoms are malaise, headache, visual disturbances, and nausea and vomiting. Pulmonary effects included acute pulmonary edema, and neurologic effects in fatal poisonings included clonic and toxic convulsions. Several nonfatal cases resulted in persistent neurologic and psychiatric complaints ranging from muscular soreness and headache through decreased libido, mental depression, phobias, and paranoia. Although the neurologic and psychiatric symptoms resemble chronic poisoning by inorganic bromides, the serum bromide levels achieved in serious cases of methyl bromide poisoning are considerably lower than those required for poisoning by inorganic bromides (Rathus and Landy, 1961; Collins, 1965). It has been suggested that this may be due to greater lipoid solubility of methyl bromide and hence greater penetration into the brain. However, since methyl chloride produces many of the same neurologic symptoms, it seems unlikely that the neurotoxicity of methyl bromide is due only to bromide ion. Methyl bromide methylates SH groups of cysteine, glutathione, and several SH-containing enzymes. Methylation of SH groups essential to cellular oxidation can be suggested as a possible mechanism for the neurologic effects of methyl bromide and methyl chloride, and therefore BAL has been considered of possible usefulness in therapy. BAL given before exposure protected against lethal exposures in animals, but had much less effect when given after exposure.

Phosphine (see Rodenticides), released from aluminum phosphide, although more acutely toxic than methyl bromide, is said to be safer for use as a grain fumigant under practical conditions (Hayes, 1971). Two children and 29 of 31 crew members aboard a grain freighter became acutely ill after inhaling phosphine, and one child died. More than half of the 3 crew members experienced shortness of breath, cough, nausea, jaundice, fatigue, and headache. Focal myocardial infiltration with necrosis, pulmonary edema, and widespread small-vessel injury were found at the autopsy of the child who died. The source of the phosphine was the result of fumigation of grain in the holds with aluminum phosphide. The gas is generated according to:

$$2AlP + 2H_2O \longrightarrow 2Al(OH)_3 + 2PH_3.$$

The gas leaked from the holds, and within four days the children were evacuated by helicopter and the rest of the crew was ill. This was the first voyage in which phosphine fumigation had been used on this particular ship. The highest concentrations of PH_3 (20 to 30 ppm) were measured in a void space of the main deck adjacent to the air intake system for ventilation amidships. Levels of 0.5 ppm phosphine were measured in some of the living quarters amidships (Wilson *et al.,* 1980).

Use of *acrylonitrile* as a fumigant is limited by its flammability and high cost. Its toxicity has been attributed to release of CN ion *in vivo,* however, differences in symptoms and CN blood levels associated with poisoning by inorganic cyanides and acrylonitrile have led to some question about that mechanism (Paulet and Desnos, 1961).

Chloropicrin (CCl_3NO_2) is a strong irritant, and sensory irritation gives early warning of its presence. It is, therefore, sometimes added in small amounts to other comparatively odorless fumigants to act as a warning agent. Ethylene oxide toxicity is also primarily due to its irritant actions in the lungs.

Ethylene dibromide in high concentrations (>200 ppm) produces primarily lung inflammation and edema in laboratory animals while repeated exposures to lower concentrations resulted in histopathologic changes in their livers and kidneys as well. No abnormal signs were observed in rats and guinea pigs given 40 to 50 mg/kg/day for four months. A dose of 2 mg/kg/day given to bulls was reported to have resulted in impaired spermatogenesis within two weeks. Ethylene dibromide residues in fumigated cereal grains have been observed for up to two months after fumigation, and laying hens fed diets containing 10 ppm (daily dose of 1 to 2 mg/kg) had a decrease in egg weights. Investigation of the possible mechanism of this effect led to observation of impaired follicle growth apparently arising from impaired permeability of the follicular membrane to protein transfer (Alumot, 1972). In a case of fatal human poisoning resulting from ingestion of 4.5 ml of ethylene dibromide, massive centrolobular necrosis of the liver and proximal tubular damage in the kidney were observed. Ethylene dibromide and 1,2-dibromo-3-chloropropane (DBCP), another nematocidal fumigant, were both found to rapidly produce highly malignant gastric squamous cell carcinoma in rats and mice (Olson *et al.,* 1973; Powers *et al.,* 1975; IARC, 1977).

DBCP also received considerable notoriety as a result of its being the probable cause of sterility and/or abnormally low sperm counts in workmen engaged in its manufacture. This resulted in a drastic reduction in its production and use (joint news release, OSHA, FDA, EPA, Sept. 8, 1977). Studies in laboratory animals 16 years earlier had suggested the potential for this toxic effect when it was observed that repeated inhalation exposure to as little as 5 ppm of DBCP has an adverse effect on the testes and on reproductive function of male rats (Torkelson *et al.,* 1961). Although the investigators, in that report, warned of the potential hazard, this warning was apparently not strong enough to prompt appropriate warnings to workers and/or improve industrial hygiene practice sufficiently to protect workers. The future use of both ethylene dibromide and DBCP as fumigants will likely be severely curtailed because of their strong carcinogenicity and their adverse action on reproductive function.

More extensive coverage of the toxicology and therapeutic management of poisonings by fumigants may be found in Hayes (1982) and Morgan (1982).

SPECIAL PROBLEMS

Interactions

Organophosphate Potentiation. For several years following the observation by Frawley and coworkers (1957) of marked synergism of the acute toxicity of EPN and malathion, the Food and Drug Administration required that all safety evaluations on anticholinesterase insecticides for which food residues were established should include tests of the toxicity of combinations. This led to routine tests for toxic interactions among this class of compounds. Most of these were acute toxicity tests using simultaneous administration. In 1961 DuBois reported studies in which the acute toxicity of various combinations of 13 different organophosphorus (OP) insecticides were tested in rats. Twenty-one pairs were additive in toxicity, 18 pairs less than additive, and four pairs synergistic. Since that time a few more pairs, involving new compounds, have been shown to be synergistic in acute toxicity tests. Combinations of several OP insecticides fed at recommended tolerance levels failed to produce significant synergistic toxicity in chronic feeding studies.

Malathion is one of the insecticides that has been observed most frequently as one constituent of a potentiating pair of organophosphorus insecticides. This, normally, relatively safe insecticide is detoxified by carboxylesterases that are inhibited by other OP insecticides. The mechanisms of synergism among OP insecticides have been reviewed by DuBois (1969) and Murphy (1969). Two major mechanisms appear to be involved: (1) inhibition of detoxication by tissue carboxylesterase (aliesterases) and amidases, and (2) competition for nonvital binding sites that normally act as a buffer system to spare the vital acetylcholinesterase enzyme (Murphy, 1969). Methods for screening for potentiating OP compounds by testing their potency as carboxylesterase inhibitors have been suggested as useful tests in acute studies and subacute feeding experiments. (Su *et al.*, 1971). Compounds that have a high potency as inhibitors of carboxylesterase relative to their anticholinesterase potency are likely to potentiate other OP insecticides or to alter the toxicity of other drugs and chemicals containing carboxylester or amide linkages. It has been demonstrated (Pellegrini and Santi, 1972; Umetsu *et al.*, 1977) that impurities present in technical grade samples of malathion and phenthoate potentiate the toxicity of these compounds, thus accounting for the greater toxicity of technical samples as compared to highly purified samples. Synergism of malathion toxicity by impurities was offered as a possible explanation for the poisonings of malathion spraymen in Pakistan (Baker *et al.*, 1978). Noninsecticidal organophosphorus esters such as triorthotolyl phosphate are also potentiators.

These mechanism studies have demonstrated that simultaneous administration of compounds may not be the most suitable method for testing for interactions among OP insecticides, that carboxylesterases are much more sensitive than cholinestrases to inhibition by some compounds and that tissue carboxylesterase essays are suitable for detecting this subtle action in relatively short-duration feeding studies. The mechanism of competition of OP insecticides for nonvital binding sites has received less attention and should be subjected to further investigation (Cohen and Murphy, 1972). Measurements of relative carboxylesterase/cholinesterase inhibitory potencies may be a useful method of predicting potentiators, but they should also be corroborated with some *in vivo* toxicity tests.

Organochlorine Insecticides. Tests of interactions among two or more pairs of organochlorine (OC) insecticides have usually involved measurements of the effects of one OC compound on the storage, excretion, and biotransformation of another. Street's work on rats suggests that the storage of DDT and dieldrin in adipose tissue is reduced when they are fed in combination (Street *et al.*, 1969). This was attributed to accelerated rates of biotransformation and excretion. Other indices of the toxicity of these compounds were not tested. A study by Diechmann and associates (1971) yielded the opposite effect with dogs; i.e., DDT fed with aldrin or dieldrin resulted in greater-than-expected residues of these compounds in fat and blood. Obviously additional work is required to determine whether these represent true species differences, or whether the discrepancies can be explained on the basis of differing experimental procedures.

Keplinger and Deichmann (1967) determined LD50s for over 100 mixtures containing two or three different insecticides. Most of the mixtures contained at least one OC insecticide. More than additive toxicities in mice were reported for endrin plus chlordane or aldrin, methoxychlor plus chlordane and dieldrin, and aldrin plus chlordane. Aldrin and chlordane were additive only in rats. Other potentiated mixtures included OC compounds with certain OP insecticides. The potentiations observed in this study were not striking (usually about twofold). It is possible that simultaneous administration of the compounds precluded the detection of some types of interactions.

Organochlorine insecticides protect against the acute toxicity of several OP insecticides. The mechanism of this protection appears to be due to the capacity of the OC insecticides to stimulate the enzymatic detoxication of OP compounds by liver microsomes or to increase noncatalytic binding sites for the OPs (DuBois, 1969; Murphy, 1969).

Other pesticides, drugs, and hydrocarbons that induce microsomal enzymes will, after an appropriate period of treatment, reduce the storage level of OC insecticides in rats (Street *et al.*, 1969) and protect rats against acute poisoning by OP insecticides. Microsomal enzymes catalyze both the activation and detoxication of OP insecticides. In most cases it appears that the dynamics of the enzyme reactions and inductions favor detoxication. However, at least a few OP insecticides are potentiated by pretreatment with certain microsomal enzyme inducers. Caution should be exercised, therefore, in making broad generalizations concerning the effects of microsomal enzyme inducers on the toxicity of various classes of pesticides. Additional research is necessary to determine the specificities of various inducers (or inhibitors) on the several alternate pathways of biotransformation of complex organic pesticides. Durham (1967) has reviewed many additional factors that may affect the toxicity of pesticides.

Pesticide-Drug Interactions. The capacity of organochlorine insecticides and certain herbicides to induce increased activity of liver microsomal cytochrome P-450 enzymes that biotransform a variety of drugs is well established (DuBois, 1969; Hodgson et al., 1980). However, attempts to correlate the increased capacity of tissues from pesticide-induced animals to biotransform drugs with effects of the pesticides on the intensity and duration of pharmacologic (or toxic) actions of the drugs are relatively few. Hexobarbital sleeping times or zoxazolamine paralysis times are often used as pharmacologic indices of altered drug metabolism in vivo, and in a few cases altered blood levels of drugs given to pesticide-treated animals have served as an in vivo index of pesticide-drug interactions. Conney and coworkers (1971) found that workers in a DDT factory had significantly higher excretion of 6-β-hydroxycortisol and a significantly reduced phenylbutazone half-life. This study suggests that at least occupational exposures can alter drug and steroid metabolism in man as well as experimental animals.

Pesticide "synergists" of the methylenedioxyphenyl type such as piperonyl butoxide have been shown to inhibit or induce microsomal drug-metabolizing enzymes and to prolong or reduce hexobarbital sleep time and to potentiate or antagonize phosphorothioate insecticides (Kamienski and Murphy, 1971) depending on the dose and time of pretreatment with the "synergist." When mice were pretreated with piperonyl butoxide, under conditions favorable to inhibition of cytochrome P-450 microsomal oxidases, they were slightly more susceptible to the diethyl-substituted phosphorothionates, parathion and azinphosethyl, but were markedly resistant to the corresponding dimethyl-substituted compounds. The mechanism for this appeared to be, in part, due to the fact that glutathione alkyl transferase could serve as an alternate (to oxidation) pathway of detoxication of the dimethyl but not the diethyl-substituted compounds. Additionally, a rapid rate of reversal of dimethylphosphorylated cholinesterase (as compared to the diethyl compounds) allowed for reversal of injury to keep pace with the piperonyl butoxide–induced oxidative production of the active anticholinesterase metabolites (Levine and Murphy, 1977a, 1977b).

The effect that microsomal enzyme induction or inhibition will have on the toxicity and action of a particular drug or chemical will depend not only upon the degree to which the enzyme activity is changed, but also upon the extent to which biotransformation of the drug is the limiting factor in determining its intensity and duration of action and the relative influence on possible alternate pathways of metabolism.

Carcinogenic, Teratogenic, and Mutagenic Properties of Pesticides

Since other chapters have been specifically devoted to these pathologic processes, they have not, with a few exceptions, been considered in detail in this chapter. The report of the Secretary's Commission on Pesticides (1969) contains discussion and summaries of data on carcinogenicity, mutagenicity, and teratogenicity of pesticides.

Pesticides that the Panel on Carcinogenesis of the Secretary's Commission on Pesticides (1969) considered "positive" for tumor induction on the basis of tests conducted adequately in one or more species, the results being significant at the 0.01 level, included aldrin, aramite, chlorbenzilate, p,p'-DDT, dieldrin, mirex, strobane, and heptachlor (all registered for use on food crops), and amitrole, avadex, bis(2-chloroethyl) ether, N-(2-hydroxyethyl)-hydrazine, and PCNB. The recommendation of the panel was that human exposures to these compounds be minimized and that their use be restricted to purposes for which there was a clear health benefit. Many other pesticides were given priorities for further testing because the panel felt that they had not been adequately evaluated in experimental animals. Only three pesticides were considered to have been proven negative to tumor induction on the basis of "adequate" tests in experimental animals. Obviously this report provoked much controversy. The situation for DDT is a case in point. The extensive use of this compound in industrial countries has not been associated with an increase in hepatic cancer in human populations, but many years ago Fitzhugh and Nelson (1947) reported that DDT fed in high doses to rats caused slight increases in hepatic cell tumors. Innes and associates (1969) reported a statistically significant increase in hepatomas in two strains of mice. Hepatic cell tumors in trout and tumors of several sites in F_2 and following generations of mice have followed DDT exposure (Halver, 1967; Tarjan and Kemény, 1969). Additional studies sponsored by the International Agency of Research in Cancer confirmed the hepatocarcinogenicity of DDT in mice (IARC, 1974a); hepatomas were also increased in mice fed 250 ppm of DDE or DDD. While some oncologists feel that hepatoma induction is indicative of carcinogenesis, others feel that hepatomas are reversible lesions. The daily dosages ingested by animals in the experimental demonstrations of hepatomas are considerably greater than the dosage rate that humans would receive, based on analyses of residues in typical meals. Epidemiologic studies have not demonstrated associations between DDT exposure and cancer in humans. Tomatis (1976) reviewed the program on the evaluation of the carcinogenic risk of chemicals to humans of the International Agency for Research on Cancer. There were no pesticides among the 17 chemicals that he listed as having been found to have carcinogenicity in humans or for which there was a strong suspicion of such action. Ten of the ninety-four chemicals, which the agency had determined to be carcinogenic in experimental animals only, were pesticides. These were amitrole, aramite, BHC, chlorobenzilate, DDD, DDE, DDT, dieldrin, lindane, and Mirex. Tomatis's review covered only compounds that IARC had reviewed by 1975.

Since then, additional pesticides that have been reported as being carcinogenic in at least one mammalian species include: aldrin, captan, chloramben, chlordane, chlordimeform, chlorothalonil, diallate, diaminazide, dicofol, ethylene dibromide, hepatachlor, hexachlorobenzene, nitrofen, pentachloronitrobenzene (quintozene), perthane, terpene polychlorinates (strobane), tetrachlorvinphos, toxaphene, and trifluralin (Weisburger, 1982; IARC, 1983). Many of the reported carcinogenic chlorinated pesticides are negative in *in vitro* mutagenicity tests. This has led to a proposal that they may exert their carcinogenic effect through an epigenetic tumor promotion mechanism, possibly as a result of their inhibiting cell-to-cell communication process (Williams, 1981, 1983). A review of the epidemiologic evidence for pesticide induced cancer among workers manufacturing, formulating, and using pesticides led an expert panel to conclude that: (a) for organic insecticides the available data from case reports and from epidemiologic studies provided inadequate evidence to evaluate their carcinogenicity as a broad class or as individual compounds, and (b) for herbicides the case reports and epidemiologic studies provide *limited* evidence for the carcinogenicity of phenoxy acids and chlorophenols, but do not allow unequivocal identification of the compounds involved (IARC, 1983).

Epstein and co-workers (1972) reported results of an extensive series of tests for mutagenic action of chemicals as determined by the dominant lethal assay in mice. Twenty-eight common pesticides were included in those tests. None of them was among the 16 chemical agents (out of a total of 174) that produced "unequivocal effects" on early fetal deaths and/or total implants, although TEPA (phosphine oxide, tris[1-aziridinyl]) and METEPA (phosphine oxide, tris[2-methyl-1-aziridyl]), which have been *proposed* as insect chemosterilants were positive. The results of a battery of six *in vitro* tests for

mutagenic and carcinogenic potential of several pesticides were reported by Waters *et al.* (1980). Of 38 compounds tested, 17 were positive in at least one test. Six compounds were positive in three or more of the six *in vitro* test systems: acephate, captan, demeton, folpet, trichlorphon, and monocrotophos (Waters *et al.*, 1980). For a review of the structural aspects of some mutagenic and teratogenic pesticides, including nitrogen-containing pesticides that may become mutagenic after reaction with NOx to form nitro derivatives, the reader is referred to Fishbein (1982). A comprehensive listing of the nitrosatable pesticides and the experimental evidence of their carcinogenic and mutagenic effects is contained in Volume 30 of the IARC monographs (IARC, 1983). Although, clearly, numerous pesticides can become nitrosated and mutagenic under certain extreme conditions, the health hazards from this reaction need further evaluation.

Durham and Williams (1972) reviewed studies in experimental animals in which at least some mammalian species at some testable dosage of the following pesticides were reported to have produced teratogenic effects: carbaryl, captan, folpet, difolatan, organomercury compounds, 2,3,4-T, pentachloronitrobenzene (PCNB), and paraquat.

Wilson (1977) summarized the literature concerning various embryotoxic effects of chemicals when given during pregnancy in animals. Table 18–9 lists those compounds that had been reported to produce malformations. In many cases other embryotoxic effects such as intrauterine death or growth retardation, stillbirth, and postnatal growth retardation were also reported. For this more detailed listing and the original references, Wilson's original review should be consulted.

Human consumption of organomercury compounds by pregnant women is known to have caused serious neurologic disorders in their offspring, which might be considered functional teratogenicity (or perhaps fetal toxicity). Other than this there is no confirmed relationship between exposure to pesticides and human terata. In the positive experimental studies the production of terata was usually demonstrated to be dose dependent, and the doses required were far in excess of what humans might be expected to receive under usual conditions. As with other toxic effects, pesticide teratogenicity and its relationship to human health must be considered from a dose-response standpoint and is subject to the same problems of interpretation and extrapolation as other dose-related effects, albeit a serious and tragic effect.

Table 18–9. PESTICIDES REPORTED TO PRODUCE MALFORMATIONS WHEN GIVEN DURING PREGNANCY IN MAMMALS*

AGENTS	SPECIES
Insecticides	
Aldrin	Hamsters, mouse
Carbaryl	Guinea pig, dog
Demeton	Mouse
Diazinon	±Rat, pig
Dichlorvos	Rat
Dieldrin	Hamster, mouse
Endrin	Hamster, mouse
Fenthein	Mouse
Kelthane	Mouse
Methyl parathion	Mouse
Herbicides	
2,4-D	±Rat
MCPA (ethyl ester)	Rat
Paraquat	±Rat
2,4,5-T	Mouse, hamster, rat
Fungicides	
Alkyldithiocarbamate salts	Rat
Captan	Hamster, rabbit, dog, ±Rat
Difolatan	Hamster
Folpet	Hamster
Griseofulvin	Rat, cat
Tetrachlorophenol	Rat
Thiram	Hamster

*Cited in Wilson (1977).

Perhaps as a result of the DBCP and kepone incidents in which temporary sterility occurred in occupationally exposed men, there has been increased concern about the influence of pesticides on human fertility. Table 18–10 lists some pesticides that have been reported to alter fertility when exposures occurred postnatally, as summarized by McLachlan *et al.* (1981), who cite the original reference sources. Of course, those effects must also be subjected to dose-response evaluation and compared with other toxic effects in order to put them into perspective. If the reproductive system is sensitive at chronic low dosages at which more immediately obvious types of effects do not occur, exposure to certain pesticides might have a subtle effect on human reproductive capacity.

Immunotoxicity

The effects of toxic chemicals on the immune system has recently emerged as an area of considerable concern. Vos *et al.* (1983) screened 17 pesticides in rats. They concluded that at least ten of these compounds had a "marked" effect on the immune system. These included atrazine, azinphosmethyl, captan, chlor IPC, dinitro or-

Table 18–10. SOME COMPOUNDS REPORTED TO ALTER FERTILITY*

COMPOUND	SEX	SPECIES
Herbicides		
Diquat	Male	Mouse
Paraquat	Male	Mouse
Polychlorinated biphenyls (PCB)	Female	Rat
Polychlorinated biphenyls (PCB)	Female	Rat, mouse
Polychlorinated biphenyls (PCB)	Male	Mouse
Yalane	Male	Rat
Fungicides		
Maneb	Male	Rat
Cineb	Male	Rat
Captan	Male	Mouse
Insecticides		
Mirex	Female	Rat
Aldrin	Male	Dog
Aldrin	Female	Rat
DDT	Male	Dog
DDT	Male	Mouse
DDT	Female	Rat
Chlordecone (Kepone®)	Female	Rat
Chlordane	Female	Mouse
Chlordane	Male	Rat
Dichlorvos (DDVP)	Male	Rat
Carbaryl	Both	Rat
Methyl parathione + DDT	Male	Rat
Lindane	Male	Rat
Polychloropinene	Male	Mouse, rat
Dieldrin	Female	Rat
Dieldrin	Male	Dog
1,2-Dibromo-3-chloropropane (DBCP)	Male	Human
Ethylene dibromide	Male	Bull

* Cited in McLachlan *et al.* (1981).

thocresol, hexachlorobenzene, lead arsenate, 2,4,5-T, triphenyltin hydroxide, quintozene, and zineb. Compounds that significantly altered an immunologic parameter as the most sensitive toxicologic criteria were atrazine, captan, lead arsenate, and triphenyltin hydroxide. In a review of the literature, Street (1981) cited 40 different pesticides that had been reported to alter, at some dosage regimen in some species, host defense mechanisms related to the functional immune system. These compounds are listed in Table 18–11. Both stimulation and suppression of a variety of immune responses were observed, often with the same agent during a single experiment. This mere listing of compounds that alter defense mechanisms does not, of course, indicate whether or not the immune system was affected directly or secondarily, e.g., secondary to stimulation of the adrenal cortex, or whether

Table 18–11. PESTICIDES REPORTED TO HAVE EFFECTS ON HOST DEFENSE MECHANISMS*

Chlorinated Insecticides	Organophosphate Insecticides
Dieldrin	Carbofenothion
DDT	Crufomate
Endrin	DEP
Heptachlor	Dichlorvos
Hexachlorobenzene	Dimethoate
Lindane	Leptophos
Mirex	Malathion
	Methylmercaptophos
	Methyl parathion
	Ronnel
Carbamate Insecticides	Triclorofon
Carbaryl	Triisopropyl phosphate
Carbofuron	
Dicresyl	*Fungicides*
	Eptom
	Maneb
Herbicides	Thiram
Barban	Zineb
Diquat	Ziram
Fluometuron	Triphenyl tin acetate
Linuron	
Molinate	
Monum	
Paraquat	*Miticides*
Propham	Chlorobenzilate
Tillam	Milbex

*Cited in Street (1981).

Table 18–12. RELATIVE TOXICITY OF VARIOUS INSECTICIDES TO RATS AND HOUSEFLIES*

CLASS	COMPOUND	MSR†
Organochlorines	DDT	59
	DDD	174
	Methoxychlor	668
	Chlordane	72
	Aldrin	27
	Dieldrin	24
	Endrin	2.4
	Heptachlor	72
	Lindane	107
Organophosphates	Parathion	4
	Methyl parathion	20
	Malathion	37.7
	Azinphosmethyl	4.1
	Chlorothion	85
	Dimethoate	390
	Ronnel	1315
Carbamates	Aldicarb	0.175
	Carbaryl	0.60
	Zectran	0.60
	Propoxur	4.5
	Mobam	10.0

* Data from Metcalf (1972).
† Mammalian selectivity ratio (MSR) is the ratio of the oral LD50 in rats to the topical LD50 in female houseflies in mg/kg for both species. Ratios of less than 1 indicate that per unit of body weight rats are more susceptible than houseflies.

the immunologic effects were highly sensitive or were accompanied by other toxic effects. The reader interested in these questions should consult the original references cited in Street's review. A different aspect of evidence of interaction with the immune system, allergic sensitization of human skin, was also reviewed by Street (1981). Fifty-one pesticides, including: many organophosphate and a few organochlorine insecticides, ten different fungicides, seven herbicides, and the rodenticide, phosphine, were cited as having been reported to cause human dermal sensitivity. The lung was seldom involved as there were few reports of asthma-like morbidity.

Comparative Toxicology

A high degree of selective toxicity to target organisms is a desirable goal in the development of useful pesticides. Metcalf (1972) has reviewed toxicity data for a large number of insecticides and calculated mammalian selectivity ratios, MSRs (mouse oral LD50/female housefly topical LD50). Several of these are shown in Table 18–12. Considering only these two species and only

acute toxicity it is apparent that there is an extremely wide range of relative toxicities. The situation becomes infinitely more complex when one considers a broader spectrum of nontarget species, as illustrated by only a few examples shown in Table 18–13.

There are indeed occasional marked differences in susceptibilities of common laboratory test animals, but even more striking are species differences noted among wild animals of the same vertebrate class. For example, Hayes (1967a) compared reported single-dose LD50 values for 20 pesticides in five mammalian species commonly used in safety evaluation studies. The range of susceptibilities generally varied within a factor of less than tenfold. All species were not compared for all 20 compounds, but in the majority of cases rats were more susceptible than mice, guinea pigs, rabbits, or dogs. Comparing the smallest single doses required to produce a serious effect in rats and humans, humans were more sensitive than rats (usually by factors of tenfold or less). In a similar comparison of reported acute insecticide toxicity values for five species of fish, Murphy (1972), calculated LD50 ratios of least to most sensitive of 2.7 for DDT, 4.7 for dieldrin, 246 for Guthion (azinphosmethyl), 49 for parathion, and 430 for mala-

Table 18–13. COMPARATIVE ACUTE TOXICITIES OF COMMON INSECTICIDES
IN VERTEBRATES*

PESTICIDES	MALE RATS—LD50 Oral (mg/kg)	MALE RATS—LD50 Dermal (mg/kg)	MALLARDS—LD50 Oral (mg/kg)	BLUEGILLS 96-HR TLM (μg/L)
DDT	113	>2510	>2240	16
Dieldrin	46	90	381	7.9
Methoxychlor	6000	—	>2000	62
Parathion	13	21	2.13	95
Methyl parathion	14	67	10	1900
Guthion	13	220	136	5.2
Malathion	1375	>4444	1485	90
Carbaryl	850	>4000	>2179	5300

* From Murphy, S. D.: The toxicity of pesticides and their metabolites. In *Degradation of Synthetic Organic Molecules in the Biosphere*. ISBN 0–309–02046–8, Proceedings of a Conference. National Academy of Sciences, Washington, DC., 1972.

thion. A similar calculation for ten avian species gave least to most sensitive species ratios of 45 for dieldrin and 192 for parathion. The mechanisms of these species differences have received relatively little research, but there is evidence that they include both differences in sensitivity of target enzymes as well as differences in rates of biotransformation to either more or less toxic metabolites. Certainly, for a class of toxic chemicals that become as widespread in the environment as pesticides, concern for effects on a broad spectrum of nontarget species is reasonable. Since it is clearly unrealistic to expect all pesticides to be tested for safety to all nontarget species that might be exposed, the only reasonable approach appears to be to attempt to understand basic mechanisms of species differences in susceptibility and, with this information base, to select or design compounds that will not only be safe for man but also be least likely to affect other nontarget organisms present in the specific areas in which they are applied. An impossible task? Perhaps. A worthwhile objective? Certainly.

REFERENCES

Abbassy, M. A.; Eldefrawi, M. E.; and Eldefrawi, A. T.: Allethrin interactions with the nicotinic acetylcholine receptor channel. *Life Sci.*, **31**:1547–52, 1982.
Abbott, D. C.; Goulding, R.; and Tatton, J. O'G.: Organochlorine pesticide residues in human fat in Great Britain. *Br. Med. J.*, **3**:146–49, 1968.
Abou-Donia, M. B.: Organophosphorus ester-induced delayed neurotoxicity. *Ann. Rev. Pharmacol. Toxicol.*, **21**:511–48, 1981.
Abou-Donia, M. B., and Preissig, S. H.: Delayed neurotoxicity of leptophos: Toxic effects on the nervous system of hens. *Toxicol. Appl. Pharmacol.*, **35**:269–82, 1976a.
Abou-Donia, M. B., and Preissig, S. H.: Delayed neurotoxicity from continuous low-dose oral administration of leptophos to hens. *Toxicol. Appl. Pharmacol.*, **38**:595–608, 1976b.
Aizwa, H.: *Metabolic Maps of Pesticides*. Academic Press, Inc., New York, 1982.

Aldridge, W. N.: The nature of the reaction of organophosphorus compounds and carbamates with esterases. *Bull. WHO*, **44**:25–30, 1971.
——— : Toxicology of pyrethiods. In Miyamoto, J. and Kearney, P. C. (eds.): *Pesticide Chemistry: Human Welfare and the Environment*. Vol. 3. *Mode of Action, Metabolism and Toxicology*. Pergamon Press, Oxford, 1983, pp. 485–90.
Aldridge, W. N.; Barnes, J. M.; and Johnson, M. K.: Studies on delayed neurotoxicity produced by some organophosphorus compounds. *Ann. N.Y. Acad. Sci.*, **160**:314–22, 1969.
Aldridge, W. N., and Johnson, M. K.: Side effects of organophosphorus compounds: delayed neurotoxicity. *Bull. WHO*, **44**:259–63, 1971.
Alumot, E.: The mechanism of ethylene dibromide action on laying hens. *Residue Rev.*, **41**:1–11, 1972.
Antov, G., and Mirkova E.: Rodenticides. In Kaloyanova, F., and Tarkowski, S. (eds.): *Toxicology of Pesticides*. World Health Organization, Regional Office for Europe, Copenhagen, 1982, pp. 170–94.
Armstrong, R. W.; Eichner, E. R.; Klein, D. E.; Barthel, W. F.; Bennett, J. V.; Jonsson, V.; Bruce, H.; and Loveless, L. E.: Pentachlorophenol poisoning in a nursery for newborn infants. II, Epidemiologic and toxicologic studies. *J. Pediatr.*, **75**:317–25, 1969.
Autor, A. P. (ed.): *Biochemical Mechanisms of Paraquat Toxicity*. Academic Press, Inc., New York, 1977.
Baker, E. L.; Zack, M.; Miles, J. W.; Alderman, L.; Warren, M.; Dobbin, R. D.; Miller, S.; and Teeters, W. R.: Epidemic malathion poisoning in Pakistan malaria workers. *Lancet*, **1**:31–34, 1978.
Benke, G. M.; Cheever, K. L.; Mirer, F. E.; and Murphy, S. D.: Comparative toxicity, anticholinesterase action and metabolism of methyl parathion and parathion in sunfish and mice. *Toxicol. Appl. Pharmacol.*, **28**:97–109, 1974.
Bidstrup, P. L., and Payne, D. J. H.: Poisoning by dinitro-*ortho*-cresol: report of eight fatal cases occurring in Great Britain. *Br. Med. J.*, **2**:16–19, 1951.
Bignami, G.; Rosic, N. Michalek, H.; Milošević, M.; and Gatti, G. L.: In Weiss, B., and Laties, V. (eds.): *Behavioral Toxicology*. Plenum Press, New York, 1975, pp. 155–209.
Boyd, E. M., and Krijnen, C. J.: Toxicity of captan and protein-deficient diet. *J. Clin. Pharmacol.*, **8**:225–34, 1968.
Brockmann, J. L.; McDowell, A. V.; and Leeds, W. G.: Fatal poisoning with sodium fluoroacetate. *J.A.M.A.*, **159**:1529–32, 1955.
Brodeur, J., and DuBois, K. P.: Studies on acquired tol-

erance by rats to 0,0-diethyl S-2-(Ethylthio) ethyl phosphorodithioate (Di-Syston). *Arch. Int. Pharmacodyn.,* **149**:560–70, 1964.

Brown, V. K. H.; Hunter, C. G.; and Richardson, A.: A blood test diagnostic of exposure to aldrin and dieldrin. *Br. J. Ind. Med.,* **21**:283–86, 1964.

Bus, J. S.; Cagen, S. Z.; Olgaard, M.; and Gibson, J. E.: A mechanism of paraquat toxicity in mice and rats. *Toxicol. Appl. Pharmacol.,* **35**:501–13, 1976.

Buser, H. R.: Analysis of polychlorinated dibenzo-*p*-dioxins and dibenzofurans in chlorinated phenols by mass fragmentography. *J. Chromatogr.,* **107**:295–310, 1975.

California Department of Public Health: *Occupational Disease in California Attributed to Pesticides and Other Agricultural Chemicals, 1969.* Bureau of Occupational Health and Environmental Epidemiology, Sacramento, 1969.

Campbell, S.: Paraquat poisoning. *Clin. Toxicol.,* **1**:245–49, 1968.

Carlson, D. A.; Konyha, K. D.; Wheeler, W. B.; Marshall, G. P.; and Zaylskie, R. G.: Mirex in the environment: its degradation to kepone and related compounds. *Science,* **194**:939–41, 1976.

Carpenter, C. P.; Weil, C. S.; Palm, P. E.; Woodside, M. W.; Nair, J. H., III; and Smyth, H. F., Jr.: Mammalian toxicity of 1-naphthyl-*N*-methylcarbamate (Sevin insecticide). *J. Agr. Food Chem.,* **9**:30–39, 1961.

Casarett, L. J.; Fryer, G. C.; Yauger, W. L., Jr.; and Klemmer, H. W.: Organochlorine pesticide residues in human tissue—Hawaii. *Arch. Environ. Health,* **17**:306–11, 1968.

Casida, J. E.: Mode of action of carbamates. *Annu. Rev. Entomol.,* **8**:39–58, 1963.

Cavalli, R. D., and Fletcher, K.: An effective treatment for paraquat poisoning. In Autor, A. P. (ed.): *Biochemical Mechanisms of Paraquat Toxicity.* Academic Press, Inc., New York, 1977, pp. 213–28.

Cavanaugh, J. B.: Toxic substances and the nervous system. *Br. Med. Bull.,* **25**:268–73, 1969.

Chenoweth, M. B.; Kandel, A.; Johnson, L. B.; and Bennett, D. R.: Factors influencing fluoroacetate poisoning: practical treatment with glyceryl monoacetate. *J. Pharmacol. Exp. Ther.,* **102**:31–49, 1951.

Chichester, C.O. (ed.): *Research in Pesticides.* Academic Press, Inc., New York, 1965.

Clement, J. G.: Toxicology and pharmacology of bispyridinium oximes—Insight into the mechanism of action vs Soman poisoning *in vivo. Fund. Appl. Toxicol.,* **1**:193–202, 1981.

Coggon, D., and Acheson, E. D.: Do phenoxy herbicides cause cancer in man? *Lancet,* **1**:1057–59, 1982.

Cohen, J. A., and Oosterbaan, R. A.: The active site of acetylcholinesterase and related esterases and its reactivity towards substrates and inhibitors. In Koelle, G. B. (ed.): *Handbuch der Experimentellen Pharmacologie,* XV, "Cholinesterases and Anticholinesterase Agents." Springer-Verlag, Berlin, 1963.

Cohen, S. D., and Murphy, S. D.: Inactivation of malaoxon by mouse liver, *Proc. Soc. Exp. Biol. Med.,* **139**:1385–89, 1972.

———: A simplified bioassay for organophosphate detoxification and interactions. *Toxicol. Appl. Pharmacol.,* **27**:537–50, 1974.

Cohn, W. J.; Boylan, J. J.; Blanke, R. V.; Fariss, M. W.; Howell, J. R.; and Guzelian, P. S.: Treatment of chlordecone (Kepone) toxicity with cholestyramine. *N. Engl. J. Med.,* **298**:243–48, 1978.

Cole, J. F.; Klevay, L. M.; and Zavon, M. R.: Endrin and dieldrin: a comparison of hepatic excretion in the rat. *Toxicol. Appl. Pharmacol.,* **16**:547–55, 1970.

Collins, R. P.: Methyl bromide poisoning: a bizarre neurological disorder. *Calif. Med.,* **103**:112–16, 1965.

Conney, A. H.; Welch, R. M.; Kuntzman, R.; Chang, R.; Jacobson, M.; Munro-Faure, A. D.; Peck, A. W.; Bye, A.; Poland, A.; Poppers, P. J.; Finster, M.; and Wolff, J. A.: Effects of environmental chemicals on the metabolism of drugs, carcinogens, and normal body constituents in man. *Ann. N.Y. Acad. Sci.,* **179**:155–72, 1971.

Conning, D. M.; Fletcher, K.; and Swan, A. A.: Paraquat and related bipyridyls. *Br. Med. Bull.,* **25**:245–49, 1969.

Costa, L. G.; Hand, H.; Schwab, B. W.; and Murphy, S. D.: Tolerance to the carbamate insecticide propoxur. *Toxicology,* **21**:267–78, 1981.

Costa, L. G.; Schwab, B. W.; and Murphy, S. D.: Tolerance to anticholinesterase compounds in mammals. *Toxicology,* **25**:79–97, 1982.

Cueto, C.; Page, N.; and Saffiotti, U.: *Report of Carcinogenesis Bioassay of Technical Grade Chlordecone (Kepone R).* National Cancer Institute, Bethesda, Md., 1976.

Dalgaard-Mikkelsen, S. and Poulsen, E.: Toxicology of herbicides. *Pharmacol. Rev.,* **14**:225–50, 1962.

Dauterman, W. C.: Biological and nonbiological modifications of organophosphorus compounds. *Bull. WHO,* **44**:133–50, 1971.

Davies, D. S.; Hawksworth, G. M.; and Bennett, P. N.: Paraquat poisoning. *Proc. Eur. Soc. Toxicol.,* **18**:21–26, 1977.

Davies, G. M., and Lewis, I.: Outbreak of food-poisoning from bread made of chemically contaminated flour. *Br. Med. J.,* **2**:393–98, 1956.

Davies, J. E.; Barquet, A.; Freed, V. H.; Haque, R.; Morgade, C.; Sonneborn, R. E.; and Vaclavek, C.: Human pesticide poisonings by a fat-soluble organophosphate insecticide. *Arch. Environ. Health,* **30**:608–13, 1975.

Davies, J. E.; Edmundson, W. F.; Maceo, A.; Baquet, A.; and Cassady, J.: An epidemiologic application of the study of DDE levels in whole blood. *Am. J. Public Health,* **59**:435–41, 1969.

Deichmann, W. B. (ed.): *Pesticides Symposia.* Halos and Associates, Inc., Miami, Fl., 1970.

Deichmann, W. B., and MacDonald, W. E.: Organochlorine pesticides and human health. *Food Cosmet. Toxicol.,* **9**:91–103, 1971.

Deichmann, W. B.; MacDonald, W. E.; and Cubit, D. A.: DDT tissue retention: sudden rise induced by the addition of aldrin to a fixed DDT intake. *Science,* **172**:275–76, 1971.

Diggle, W. M. and, Gage, J. C.: Cholinesterase inhibition *in vitro* by OO-diethyl O-*p*-nitrophenyl thiophosphate (Parathion, E605). *Biochem. J.,* **49**:491–94, 1951.

Donninger, C.; Hutson, D. H.; and Pickering, B. A.: The oxidative dealkylation of insecticidal phosphoric acid triesters by mammalian liver enzymes. *Biochem. J.* **126**:701–707, 1972.

Doull, J.: The treatment of insecticide poisoning. In Wilkinson, C. F. (ed.): *Insecticide Biochemistry and Physiology.* Plenum Press, New York, 1976, pp. 649–67.

DuBois, K. P.: New rodenticidal compounds. *J. Am. Pharm. Assoc.,* **37**:307–10, 1948.

———: Potentiation of the toxicity of organophosphorus compounds. *Adv. Pest Control Res.,* **4**:117–51, 1961.

———: Toxicological evaluation of the anticholinesterase agents. In Koelle, G. B. (ed.): *Handbuch der Experimentellen Pharmakologie,* XV. Springer-Verlag, Berlin, 1963.

———: Low level organophosphorus residues in the diet. *Arch. Environ. Health.* **10**:837–41, 1965.

———: Combined effects of pesticides. *Can. Med. Assoc. J.,* **100**:173–79, 1969.

DuBois, K. P.; Doull, J.; and Coon, J. M.: Toxicity and

mechanism of action of *p*-nitrophenyl diethyl thionophosphate (E605). *Fed. Proc.*, 7:216, 1948.

DuBois, K. P.; Doull, J.; Salerno, P. R.; and Coon, J. M.: Studies on the toxicity and mechanisms of action of *p*-nitrophenyl diethyl thionosphosphate (Parathion). *J. Pharmacol. Exp. Ther.*, **95**:79–91, 1949.

DuBois, K. P.; Thursh, D. R.; and Murphy, S. D.: Studies on the toxicity and pharmacologic action of the dimethoxy ester of benzotriazine dithiophosphoric acid to an anticholinesterase agent. *J. Pharmacol. Exp. Ther.*, **119**:572–83, 1957.

Durham, W. F.: The interaction of pesticides with other factors. *Residue Rev.*, 18:21–103, 1967.

Durham, W. F., and Hayes, W. J., Jr.: Organic phosphorus poisoning and its therapy. *Arch. Environ. Health*, 5:21–47, 1962.

Durham, W. F., and Williams, C. H.: Mutagenic teratogenic, and carcinogenic properties of pesticides. *Annu. Rev. Entomol.*, 17:123–48, 1972.

Dustman, E. H., and Stickel, L. F.: The occurrence and significance of pesticide residues in wild animals. *Ann. N. Y. Acad. Sci.*, 160:162–72, 1969.

Edwards, C. A.: *Persistent Pesticides in the Environment.* CRC Monoscience Series, Chemical Rubber Co., Cleveland, 1970.

Egan, H.; Goulding, R.; Roburn, J.; and Tatton, J. O'G: Organo-chlorine residues in human fat and human milk. *Br. Med. J.*, 2:66–69, 1965.

Elliott, M.: Properties and applications of pyrethroids. *Environ. Health Perspect.*, 14:3–13, 1976.

Epstein, S. S.; Arnold, E.; Andrea, J.; Bass, W.; and Bishop, Y.: Detection of chemical mutagens by the dominant lethal assay in the mouse. *Toxicol. Appl. Pharmacol.*, 23:288–325, 1972.

Eto, M.: *Organophosphorus Pesticides: Organic and Biological Chemistry.* CRC Press Inc., Cleveland, 1974.

Fairchild, E. J., II.; Murphy, S. D.; and Stokinger, H. E.: Protection by sulfur compounds against air pollutants, ozone and nitrogen dioxide. *Science,* 130:386–62, 1959.

FAO/WHO: *Evaluations of Pesticide Residues in Food—1979.* Food and Agriculture Organization of the United Nations, Rome, 1980.

——— : *Evaluations of Pesticide Residues in Food—1980.* Food and Agriculture Organization of the United Nations, Rome, 1981.

——— : *Evaluations of Pesticide Residues in Food—1981.* Food and Agriculture Organization of the United Nations, Rome, 1982.

Fishbein, L.: An overview of the structural features of some mutagenic and teratogenic pesticides. In Chambers, J. E., and Yarbrough, J. D. (eds.): *Effects of Chronic Exposures to Pesticides on Animal Systems.* Raven Press, New York, 1982, pp. 177–209.

Fitzhugh, O. G., and Nelson, A. A.: The chronic oral toxicity of DDT (2,2-bis(*p*-chorophenyl-1,1,1-trichloroethane). *J. Pharmacol. Exp. Ther.*, 89:18–30, 1947.

Frawley, J. P.; Fuyat, H. N.; Hagen, E. C.; Blake, J. R.; and Fitzhugh, O. G.: Marked potentiation in mammalian toxicity from simultaneous administration of two anticholinesterase compounds. *J. Pharmacol. Exp. Ther.*, 121:96–106, 1957.

Frear, D. E. H.: *Pesticide Index,* 4th ed. College Science Publishers, State College, Pa., 1969.

Fukuto, T. R.: Relationships between the structure of organophosphorus compounds and their activity as acetylcholinesterase inhibitors. *Bull. WHO*, 44:31–42, 1971.

Fukuto, T. R., and Metcalf, R. L.: Metabolism of insecticides in plants and animals. *Ann. N. Y. Acad. Sci.*, 160:97–113, 1969.

Gage, J. C.: The action of paraquat and diquat on the respiration of liver cell fractions. *Biochem. J.*, **109**:757–61, 1968.

Gaines, T. B.: Acute toxicity of pesticides. *Toxicol. Appl. Pharmacol.*, 14:515–34, 1969.

Gaines, T. B., and Kimbrough, R. D.: Oral toxicity of mirex in adult and suckling rats. *Arch. Environ. Health,* 21:7–14, 1970.

Garrettson, L. K., and Curley, A.: Dieldrin. Studies in a poisoned child. *Arch. Environ. Health,* 19:814–22, 1969.

Glaister, J.: *The Power of Poison.* Christopher Johnson Publishers, Ltd., London, 1954, pp. 78–86.

Goldstein, J. A.: Effects of pentachlorophenol on hepatic drug metabolizing enzymes and porphyria related to contamination with chlorinated dibenzo-*p*-dioxins and dibenzofurans. *Toxicol. Appl. Pharmacol.*, 37:145–46, 1976.

Good, E. E.; Ware, G. W.; and Miller, D. F.: Effects of insecticides on reproduction in the laboratory mouse: I. Kepone. *J. Econ. Entomol.*, 58:754–56, 1965.

Gould, R. F. (ed.): *Organic Pesticides in the environment.* Advances in Chemistry Series 60, American Chemical Society, Washington, D.C., 1966.

Grob, D.: Anticholinesterase intoxication in man and its treatment. In Koelle, G. B. (ed.): *Handbuch der Experimentellen Pharmakologie,* XV. Springer-Verlag, Berlin, 1963.

Grossman, H.: Thallotoxicosis: report of a case and a review. *Pediatrics,* 16:868–72, 1955.

Guzelian, P. S.: Comparative toxicology of chlordecone (Kepone) in humans and experimental animals. *Annu. Rev. Pharmacol. Toxicol.*, 28:89–113, 1982.

Halver, J. E.: Crystalline aflatoxin and other vectors for trout hepatoma. *Bur. Sport Fish. Wldl. Res. Rept.*, 70:78–102, 1967.

Hamify, J. A.; Metcalf, P.; Nobbs, C. L.; and Worsley, K. J.: Aerial spraying of 2,4,5-T and human birth malformations: an epidemiological investigation. *Science,* 212:349–51, 1981.

Haq, I. U.: Agrosan poisoning in man. *Br. Med. J.*, 1:1579–82, 1963.

Hayes, W. J., Jr.: The pharmacology and toxicity of DDT. In Muller, P. (ed.): *The Insecticide DDT and Its Importance.* Birkhäuser Verlag, Basel, 1959a.

——— : The toxicity of dieldrin to man: report on a survey. *Bull. WHO,* 20:891–912, 1959b.

——— : *Clinical Handbook on Economic Poisons.* Public Health Service Publication No. 476. U.S. Government Printing Office, Washington, D.C., 1963.

——— : Monitoring food and people for pesticide content. In *Scientific Aspects of Pest Control.* Pub. No. 1402, National Academy of Sciences. National Research Council, Washington, D.C., 1966, pp. 314–41.

——— : The 90-dose LD$_{50}$ and a chronicity factor as measures of toxicity. *Toxicol. Appl. Pharmacol.*, 11:327–35, 1967a.

——— : Toxicity of pesticides to man: risks from present levels. *Proc. Roy. Soc. (Biol.)*, 167:101–27, 1967b.

——— : Pesticides and human toxicity. *Ann. N. Y. Acad. Sci.*, 160:40–54, 1969.

——— : Insecticides, rodenticides and other economic poisons. In DiPalma, J. R. (ed.): *Drull's Pharmacology in Medicine,* 4th ed. McGraw-Hill Book Co., New York, 1971, pp. 1256–76.

——— : *Toxicology of Pesticides.* Waverly Press, Inc., Baltimore, 1975.

——— : *Pesticides Studied in Man.* Williams & Wilkins Co., Baltimore, 1982.

Hayes, W. J., Jr.; Dale, W. E.; and Pirkle, C. I.: Evidence of safety of long-term, high, oral doses of DDT for man. *Arch. Environ. Health,* 22:119–35, 1971.

Hayes, W. J., and Vaughn, W. K.: Mortality from pesticides in the United States in 1973 and 1974. *Toxicol. Appl. Pharmacol.*, 42:235–52, 1977.

Headley, J. C., and Kneese, A. V.: Economic implications of pesticide use. *Ann. N. Y. Acad. Sci.*, **160**:30–39, 1969.

Heath, D. F.: *Organophosphorus Poisons*. Pergamon Press, Oxford, 1961.

Hine, C. H.: Methyl bromide poisoning: a review of ten cases. *J. Occup. Med.*, **11**:1–10, 1969.

Hobbiger, F.: Reactivation of phosphorylated acetylcholinesterase. In Koelle, G. B. (ed.): *Handbuch der Experimentellen Pharmakologie*, XV. Springer-Verlag, Berlin, 1963, pp. 921–88.

Hodge, H. C.; Boyce, A. M.; Deichmann, W. B.; and Kraybill, H. F.: Toxicology and no-effect levels of aldrin and dieldrin. *Toxicol. Appl. Pharmacol.*, **10**:613–75, 1967.

Hodgson, E.; Kulkarni, A. P.; Fabacher D. L.; and Robacker, K. M.: Induction of hepatic drug metabolizing enzymes in mammals by pesticides: a review. *J. Environ. Sci. Health*, **15**(B):723–54, 1980.

Hoffman, W. S.; Adler, H.; Fishbein, W. I.; and Bauer, F. C.: Relation of pesticide concentrations in fat to pathological changes in tissue. *Arch. Environ. Health* **15**:758–65, 1967.

Hollingworth, R. M.: The dealkylation of organophosphorus triester by liver enzymes. In O'Brien, R. D., and Yamamoto, I. (eds.): *Biochemical Toxicology of Insecticides*. Academic Press, Inc., New York, 1972.

Holmstedt, B.: Pharmacology of organophosphorus cholinesterase inhibitors. *Pharmacol. Rev.*, **11**:567–688, 1959.

Hoogendam, I.; Versteeg, J. P. J.; and DeVlieger, M.: Nine years' toxicity control in insecticide plants. *Arch. Environ. Health*, **10**:441–48, 1965.

Hooper, N. K.; Ames, B. N.; Saleh, M. A.; and Casida, J. E.: Toxaphene, a complex mixture of polychloroterpenes and a major insecticide, is mutagenic. *Science*, **205**:591–93, 1979.

Huber, J. J.: Some physiological effects of the insecticide Kepone in the laboratory mouse. *Toxicol. Appl. Pharmacol.*, **7**:516–24, 1965.

Hutson, D. H.; Pickering, B. A.; and Donninger, C.: Phosphoric acid triester-glutathione alkyltransferase: a mechanism for the detoxification of dimethyl phosphase triesters. *Biochem. J.*, **127**:285–93, 1972.

IARC: *Monograph on the Evaluation of Carcinogenic Risk of Chemicals to Man:* Vol. 5, *Some Organochlorine Pesticides*. International Agency for Research on Cancer, Lyon, France, 1974a.

———: *Monographs on the Evaluation of Carcinogenic Risk of Chemicals to Man*. Vol. 7, *Some Antithyroid and Related Substances, Nitrofurans and Industrial Chemicals*. International Agency for Research on Cancer, Lyon, France, 1974b.

———: *Monographs on the Evaluation of Carcinogenic Risk of Chemicals to Man*. Vol. 12, *Some Carbamates, Thiocarbamates and Carbazines*. International Agency for Research on Cancer, Lyon, France, 1976.

———: *Monographs on the Evaluation of Carcinogenic Risk of Chemicals to Man*. Vol. 15, *Some Fumigants, the Herbicides 2,4,-D and 2,4,5-T, Chlorinated Dibenzodioxins and Miscellaneous Industrial Chemicals*. International Agency for Research on Cancer, Lyon, France, 1977.

———: *Monograph on the Evaluation of Carcinogenic Risk of Chemicals to Man*. Vol. 30, *Miscellaneous Pesticides*. International Agency for Research on Cancer, Lyon, France, 1983.

Ingle, L.: *A Monograph on Chlordane: Toxicology and Pharmacological Properties*. Library of Congress Card No. 65–28686, 1965.

Innes, J. R. M.; Ulland, B. M.; Valerio, M. G.; Petrucelli, L.; Fishbein, L.; Hart, E. R.; Pallotta, A. J.; Bates, R. R.; Falk, H. L.; Gart, J. J.; Klein, M.; Mitchell, I.; and Peters, J.: Bioassay of pesticides and industrial chemicals for tumorigenicity in mice: a preliminary note. *J. Natl. Cancer Inst.*, **42**:1101–14, 1969.

Johns, R. J., and McQuillen, M. P.: Syndrome simulating myasthenia gravis: asthenia with anticholinesterase tolerance. *Ann. N. Y. Acad. Sci.*, **135**:385–97, 1966.

Johnson, M. K.: The delayed neuropathy caused by some organophosphorus esters: mechanism and challenge. *CRC Crit. Rev. Toxicol.*, **3**:289–316, 1975a.

———: Organophosphorus esters causing delayed neurotoxic effects—mechanism of action and structure-activity studies. *Arch. Toxicol.*, **34**:259–88, 1975b.

———: Structure-activity relationships for substrates and inhibitors of hen brain neurotoxic esterase. *Biochem. Pharmacol.*, **24**:797–805, 1975c.

———: The target for initiation of delayed neurotoxicity by organophosphorus esters: biochemical studies and toxicological applications. *Rev. Biochem. Toxicol.*, **4**:141–212, 1982.

Johnson, R. L.; Gehring, P. J.; Kociba, R. J.; and Schwetz, B. A.: Chlorinated dibenzodioxins and pentachlorophenol. *Environ. Health Perspect.*, **5**:171–75, 1973.

Kamataki, T.; Leelin, M. C. M.; Belcher, D. H.; and Neal, R. A.: Studies of the metabolism of parathion with an apparently homogenous preparation of rabbit liver microsomal cytochrome P-450. *Drug Metab. Disp.*, **4**:180–89, 1976.

Kamienski, F. X., and Murphy, S. D.: Biphasic effects of methylenedioxyphenyl synergists on the action of hexobarbital and organophosphate insecticides in mice. *Toxicol. Appl. Pharmacol.*, **18**:883–94, 1971.

Keil, J. E.; Finklea, J. F.; Pietsch, R. L. and Gadsden, R. H.: A pesticide use survey of urban households. *Agricultural Chemicals*, **24**:10–12, 1969.

Keplinger, M. L., and Deichmann, W. B.: Acute toxicity of combinations of pesticides. *Toxicol. Appl. Pharmacol.*, **10**:586–95, 1967.

Khan, N. Y.: An assessment of the hazard of synthetic pyrethroid insecticides to fish and fish habitat. In Miyamoto, J., and Kearney, P. C. (eds.): *Pesticide Chemistry: Human Welfare and the Environment*. Vol. 3, *Mode of Active Metabolism and Toxicology*. Pergamon Press, Oxford, 1983, pp. 115–21.

Kociba, R. I.; Keyes, D. G.; and Beyer, J. E.: Results of a two year chronic toxicity and oncogenicity study of 2,3,7,8-tetrachlorodibenzo-*p*-dioxin in rats. *Toxicol. Appl. Pharmacol.*, **46**:279–303, 1978.

Kreiss, K.; Zack, M.; Kimbrough, R. D.; Needham, L. L.; Smreak, A. L.; and Jones, B. T.: Cross-sectional study of a community with exceptional exposure to DDT. *JAMA*, **245**:1926–30, 1981.

Krueger, H. R.; O'Brien, R. D.; and Dauterman, W. C.: Relationship between metabolism and differential toxicity in insects and mice of diazinon, dimethoate, parathion and acethion. *Econ. Entomol.*, **53**:25–31, 1960.

Kulkarni, A. P., and Hodgson, E.: Metabolism of insecticides by mixed function oxidase systems. *Pharmacol. Ther.*, **8**:379–475, 1979.

Kupfer, D., and Bulger, W. H.: Studies on the mechanism of estrogenic actions of *o,p'*-DDT: interactions with the estrogen receptor. *Pesticide Biochem. Physiol.*, **6**:461–570, 1976.

———: Estrogenic actions of chlorinated hydrocarbons. In Chambers, J. E., and Yarbrough, J. D. *Effects of Chronic Exposures to Pesticides on Animal Systems*. Raven Press, New York, 1982, pp. 121–46.

Larson, P. S.; Haag, H. B.; and Silvette, H.: *Tobacco: Experimental and Clinical Studies*. Williams & Wilkins Co., Baltimore, 1961.

Lauwerys, R. R., and Murphy, S. D.: Comparison of assay methods for studying O,O-diethyl, O-*p*-nitrophenyl phosphate (paraoxon) detoxication *in vitro*. *Biochem. Pharmacol.*, **18**:789–800, 1969a.

————: Interaction between paraoxon and tri-*o*-tolyl phosphate in rats. *Toxicol. Appl. Pharmacol.*, **14**:348–57, 1969b.

Laws, E. R., Jr.; Curley, A.; and Boris, F. J.: Men with intensive occupational exposure to DDT: a clinical and chemical study. *Arch. Environ. Health*, **15**:766–75, 1967.

Lehman, A. J.: *Summaries of pesticide Toxicity*. The Association of Food and Drug Officials of the United States, Topeka, 1965.

Levine, B. S., and Murphy, S. D.: Esterase inhibitions and reactivation in relation to piperonyl butoxide-phosphorothionate interactions. *Toxicol. Appl. Pharmacol.*, **40**:379–91, 1977a.

————: Effect of piperonyl butoxide on the metabolism of dimethyl and diethyl phosphorothionate insecticides. *Toxicol. Appl. Pharmacol.*, **40**:393–406, 1977b.

Lisella, F. S.; Long, K. R.; and Scott, H. G.: Toxicology of rodenticides and their relation to human health. *J. Environ. Health*, **33**:231–37, 361–65, 1971.

Longcore, J. R.; Samson, F. B.; Kreitzer, J. F.; and Spann, J. W.: Changes in mineral composition of eggshells from black ducks and mallards fed DDE in the diet. *Bull. Env. Contam. Toxicol.*, **6**:345–50, 1971.

Lukens, R. J.: *Chemistry of Fungicidal Action*. Springer-Verlag, New York, 1971.

McClosky, W. T., and Smith, M. I.: Studies of the pharmacologic action and the pathology of alphanaphthylthiourea. I. Pharmacology. *Public Health Rep.*, **60**:1101–1108, 1945.

McLaughlin, J., Jr.; Reynaldo, E. F.; Lamar, J. K.; and Marliac, J. P.: Teratology studies in rabbits with captan, folpet and thalidomide. *Toxicol. Appl. Pharmacol.*, **14**:641, 1969.

Mason, R. R., and Shulte, G. J.: Interaction of *o,p'*-DDT with the estrogen-binding protein (EPB) of DMBA-induced rat mammary tumors. *Res. Commun. Chem. Pathol. Pharmacol.*, **29**:281–90, 1981.

Matsumura, F.; Bousch, G. M.; and Misato, T. (eds.): *Environmental Toxicology of Pesticides*. Academic Press, Inc., New York, 1972.

Matsumura, F., and Ghiasuddin, S. M.: DDT-sensitive Ca-ATPase in the axonic membrane. In Narahashi, T. (ed.): *Neurotoxicology of Insecticides and Pheromones*. Plenum Publishing Corp. New York, 1979, pp. 245–57.

Matsunaka, S.: Propanil hydrolysis: inhibition in rice plants by insecticides. *Science*, **160**:1360–61, 1968.

McLachlan, J. A.; Newbold, R. R.; Korach, K. S.; Lamb, J. C.; and Suzuki, Y.: Transplacental toxicology: prenatal factors influencing postnatal fertility. In Kimmel, C. A., and Buelke-Sam, J. (eds.): *Developmental Toxicology*. Raven Press, New York, 1981, pp. 213–54.

Menzie, C. M.: *Metabolism of pesticides*. Bureau of Sport Fisheries and Wildlife Special Scientific Report, Wildlife No. 127, Washington, D.C., 1969.

Metcalf, R. L.: Development of selective and biogradable pesticides. In *Pest Control Strategies for the Future*. Agricultural Board, Division of Biology and Agriculture, National Research Council, National Academy of Science, Washington, D.C., 1972, pp. 137–56.

Milby, T. H., and Samuels, A. J.: Human exposure to lindane: comparison of an exposed and unexposed population. *J. Occup. Med.*, **13**:256–58, 1971.

Moore, J. A., and Courtney, K. D.: Tetratology studies with the trichlorophenoxyacid herbicides, 2,4,5-T and Silvex. *Teratology*, **4**:236, 1971.

Morgan, D. P.: *Recognition and Management of Pesticide Poisonings*, 3rd ed. Publication EPA-540/9-80-005, U.S. Environmental Protection Agency, 1982.

Morgan, D. P.; Lin, L. I.; and Saikaly, H. H.: Morbidity and mortality in workers occupationally exposed to pes-

ticides. *Arch. Environm. Contam. Toxicol.*, **9**:349–82, 1980.

Murphy, R. S.; Kutz, F. W.; and Strassman, S. C.: Selected pesticide residues or metabolites in blood and urine specimens from a general population survey. *Environ. Health Perspect.*, **48**:81–86, 1983.

Murphy, S. D.: Mechanisms of pesticide interactions in vertebrates. *Residue Rev.*, **25**:201–21, 1969.

————: The toxicity of pesticides and their metabolites. In *Degradation of Synthetic Organic Molecules in the Biosphere*. Proceedings of a Conference. National Academy of Sciences, Washington, D.C., 1972, pp. 313–35.

————: Toxic interactions with dermal exposure to organophosphate insecticides. In Holmstedt, B.; Lauwerys, R.; Mercier M.; and Roberfroid, M. (eds.): *Mechanisms of Toxicity and Hazard Evaluation*. Elsevier/North Holland Biomedical Press, Amsterdam, 1980, pp. 615–21.

Murphy, S. D.; Anderson, R. L.; and DuBois, K. P.: Potentiation of the toxicity of malathion by triorthototyl phosphate. *Proc. Soc. Exp. Biol. Med.*, **100**:483–87, 1959.

Murphy, S. D.; Costa, L. G.; and Schwab, B: Mechanisms of tolerance to anticholinesterase insecticide toxicity. In Miyamoto, J., and Kearney, P. C. (eds): *Pesticide Chemistry: Human Welfare and the Environment.*, Vol. 3, *Mode of Action, Metabolism and Toxicology*. Pergamon Press, Oxford, 1983, pp. 531–36.

Murphy, S. D., and DuBois, K. P.: Enzymatic conversion of the dimethoxy ester of benzotriazine dithiophosphoric acid to an anticholinesterase agent. *J. Pharmacol. Exp. Ther.*, **119**:572–83, 1957.

Murphy, S. D., and DuBois, K. P.: The influence of various factors on the enzymatic conversion of organic thiophosphate to anticholinesterase agents. *J. Pharmacol. Exp. Ther.*, **124**:194–202, 1958.

Nakatsugawa, T., and Dahm, P. A.: Microsomal metabolism of parathion. *Biochem. Pharmacol.*, **16**:25–38, 1967.

Namba, T.; Nolte, C. T.; Jackrel, J., and Grob, D.: Poisoning due to organophosphate insecticides: acute and chronic manifestations. *Am. J. Med.*, **50**:475–92, 1971.

Narahashi, T.: Effects of insecticides on nervous conduction and synaptic transmission. In Wilkinson, C. F. (ed.): *Insecticide Biochemistry and Physiology*. Plenum Press, New York, 1976, pp. 327–52.

————: Nerve membrane ionic channels as the target site of insecticides. In Narahashi, T. (ed.): *Neurotoxicology of Insecticides and Pheromones*. Plenum Publishing Corp, New York, 1979, pp. 211–43.

————: Interaction of pyrethroids and DDT-like compounds with the sodium channels in the nerve membrane. In Miyamoto, J., and Kearney, P. C. (eds.): *Pesticide Chemistry: Human Welfare and the Environment*, Vol. 3. Pergamon Press, Oxford, 1983, pp. 109–14.

NAS: *Pest Control: An Assessment of Present and Alternative Technologies*. Vol. V, *Pest Control and Public Health*. National Academy of Sciences, Washington, D.C., 1976.

————: *Drinking Water and Health*. National Academy of Sciences, Washington, D.C., 1977.

Neal, R. A.: Studies on the metabolism of diethyl 4-nitrophenyl phosphorothionate (parathion) *in vitro*. *Biochem. J.*, **103**:183–91, 1967.

————: Microsomal metabolism of thionosulfur compounds: Mechanisms and toxicological significance. *Rev. Biochem. Toxicol.*, **2**:131–71, 1980.

O'Brien, R. D.: *Toxic Phosphorus Esters: Chemistry, Metabolism and Biological Effects*. Academic Press, Inc., New York, 1960.

————: *Insecticides, Action and Metabolism*. Academic Press, Inc., New York, 1967.

———: V. Biochemical effects. Phosphorylation and carbamylation of cholinesterase. *Ann N. Y. Acad. Sci.,* **160:**204–14, 1969.

———: Acetylcholinesterase and its inhibition. In Wikinson, C. F. (ed.): *Insecticide Biochemistry and Physiology.* Plenum Press, New York, 1976, pp. 271–96.

Ohkawa, H.; Mikami, N.; Okuno, Y.; and Miyamoto, J.: Stereospecificity in toxicity of the optical isomers of EPN. *Bull. Env. Cont. Toxicol.,* **18:**534–40, 1977.

Oldner, J. J., and Hatcher, R. L.: Food poisoning caused by carbophenothion. *JAMA* **209:**1328–30, 1969.

Olson, W. A.; Habermann, R. T.; Weisburger, E. K.; Ward, J. M.; and Weisburger, J. H.: Induction of stomach cancer in rats and mice by halogenated aliphatic fumigants. *J. Natl. Cancer Inst.,* **51:**1993–95, 1973.

O'Neill, J. J.: Non-cholinesterase effects of anticholinesterases. *Fund. Appl. Toxicol.,* **1:**154–60, 1981.

Oonnithan, E. S., and Casida, J. E.: Oxidation of methyl and methylcarbamate insecticide chemicals by microsomal enzymes and anticholinesterase activity of metabolites. *J. Agric. Food Chem.,* **16:**28–44, 1968.

Palmer, J. S., and Radeleff, R. D.: The toxicologic effects of certain fungicides and herbicides on sheep and cattle. *Ann. N. Y. Acad. Sci.,* **111:**729–36, 1964.

Panel on Herbicides: *Report on 2,4,5,-T: A Report of the Panel on Herbicides of the President's Science Advisory Committee.* Executive Office of the President, Office of Science and Technology, U.S. Government Printing Office, Washington, D.C., 1971.

Pattison, F. L. M.: *Toxic Aliphatic Fluorine Compounds.* Elsevier Press, Inc., New York, 1959.

Paulet, G., and Desnos, J.: L'acrylonitrile: toxicite-mecanisme-d'action therapeutique. *Arch. Inst. Pharmacodyn.,* **131:**54–83, 1961.

Peakall, D. B.: Pesticides and the reproduction of birds. *Sci. Am.,* **222:**72–78, 1970.

Pellegrini, G., and Santi, R.: Potentiation of toxicity of organophosphorus compounds containing carboxylic ester functions toward warm-blooded animals by some organophosphorus impurities. *J. Agr. Food Chem.,* **20:**944–49, 1972.

Peters, R. A.: *Biochemical Lesions and Lethal Synthesis.* Macmillan Publishing Co., New York, 1963.

Petrova-Vergieva, T., and Ivanova-Chemishanska, L.: Assessment of the teratogenic activity of dithiocarbamate fungicides. *Food Cosmet. Toxicol.,* **11:**239–44, 1973.

Pickering, Q. H.; Henderson, C.; and Lemke, A. E.: The toxicity of organic phosphorus insecticides to different species of warmwater fishes. *Trans. Am. Fish. Soc.,* **91:**175–84, 1962.

Pimental, D.: *Ecologic Effects of Pesticides on Non-Target Species.* Report to Executive Office of the President, Office of Science and Technology, U.S. Government Printing Office, Washington, D.C., June 1971, pp. 20–23.

Plapp, F. W., and Casida, J. E.: Hydrolysis of the alkylphosphate bond in certain dialkyl aryl phosphorothioate insecticides by rats, cockroaches, and alkali. *J. Econ. Entomol.,* **51:**800–803, 1958.

Poland, A. P.; Smith, D.; Metter, G.; and Possick, P.: A health survey of workers in a 2,4-D and 2,4,5-T plant with special attention to chloracne, porphyria cutanea tarda, and psychologic parameters. *Arch. Environ. Health,* **22:**316–27, 1971.

Poore, R. E., and Neal, R. A.: Evidence for extrohepatic metabolism of parathion. *Toxicol. Appl. Pharmacol.,* **22:**68, 1972.

Powers, M. B.; Voelker, R. W.; Page, N. P.; Weisburger, E. K.; and Kraybill, H. F.: Carcinogenicity of ethylene dibromide (EDB) and 1,2-dibromo-3-chloropropane

(DBCP) after oral administration in rats and mice. *Toxicol. Appl. Pharmacol.,* **33:**171–72, 1975.

Ptashne, K. A.; Woolcott, R. M.; and Neal, R. A.: Oxygen-18 studies on the chemical mechanism of the mixed function oxidase catalyzed desulfuration and dearylation reaction of parathion. *J. Pharmacol. Exp. Ther.,* **179:**380–85, 1971.

Quimby, G. E.; Armstrong, J. F.; and Durham, W. F.: DDT in human milk. *Nature (Lond.),* **207:**726–28, 1965.

Radomski, J. L.; Deichmann, W. B.; and Clizer, E. E.: Pesticide concentrations in the liver, brain and adipose tissue of terminal hospital patients. *Food Cosmet. Toxicol.,* **6:**209–20, 1968.

Rathus, E. M., and Landy, P. J.: Methyl bromide poisoning. *Br. J. Ind. Med.,* **18:**53–57, 1971.

Reich, G. A.; Davis, J. H.; and Davies, J. E.: Pesticide poisoning in South Florida: an analysis of mortality and morbidity and a comparison of sources of incidence data. *Arch. Environ. Health,* **17:**768–75, 1968.

Reiner, E.: Spontaneous reactivation of phosphorylated and carbamylated cholinesterase. *Bull. WHO,* **44:**109–12, 1971.

Reiter, L.; Talens, G.; and Wooley, D.: Acute and subacute parathion treatment. Effects on cholinesterase activities and learning in mice. *Toxicol. Appl. Pharmacol.,* **25:**582–88, 1973.

Robens, J. F.: Teratogenic activity of several phthalimide derivatives in the golden hamster. *Toxicol. Appl. Pharmacol.,* **16:**24–34, 1970.

Roberts, D. V.: EMG voltage and motor nerve conduction velocity on organophosphorus pesticide factory workers. *Int. Arch. Occup. Environ. Health,* **36:**267–74, 1976.

Roberts, D. V.: A longitudinal electromyographic study of six men occupationally exposed to organophosphorus compounds. *Int. Arch. Occup. Environ. Health,* **38:**221–29, 1977.

Robison, A. K., and Stancel, G. M.: The estrogenic activity of DDT: correlation of estrogenic effect with nuclear level of estrogen receptor. *Life Sci.,* **31:**2479–84, 1982.

Rose, M. S., and Smith, L. L.: Tissue uptake of paraquat and diquat. *Gen. Pharmacol.,* **8:**173–76, 1977.

Roszowski, A. P.: The pharmacological properties of Norbormide, a selective rat toxicant. *J. Pharmacol. Exp. Ther.,* **149:**288–99, 1965.

Saleh, M. A.; Turner, W. V.; and Casida, J. E.: Polychlorobornane components of toxaphene: Structure-toxicity relations and metabolic reductive dechlorination. *Science,* **198:**1256–58, 1977.

Schmid, R.: Cutaneous porphyria in Turkey. *N. Engl. J. Med.,* **263:**397–98, 1960.

Schwab, B. W., and Murphy, S. D.: Induction of anticholinesterase tolerance in rats with doses of disulfoton that produce no cholinergic signs. *J. Toxicol. Environ. Health,* **8:**199–204, 1981.

Secretary's Commission on Pesticides, U.S. Department of Health, Education, and Welfare: *Report of the Secretary's Commission on Pesticides and Their Relationship to Environmental Health.* U.S. Government Printing Office, Washington, D.C., 1969.

Singleton, S. D., and Murphy, S. D.: Propanil(3,4-dichloropropionanilide) induced methemoglobin formation in mice in relation to acylamidase activity. *Toxicol. Appl. Pharmacol.,* **24:**20–29, 1973.

Sinha, D.; Pascal, R.; and Furth, J.: Transplantable thyroid carcinoma induced by thyrotropin: its similarity to human Hürtle cell tumors. *Arch. Pathol.,* **79:**192–98, 1965.

Smalley, H. E.; Curtis, J. M.; and Earl, F. L.: Teratogenic action of carbaryl in beagle dogs. *Toxicol. Appl. Pharmacol.,* **13:**392–403, 1968.

Smith, L. L.: Functional, morphologic and biochemical

correlates in pulmonary toxicity of paraquat. In Miyamoto, J., and Kearney, P. C. (eds.): *Pesticide Chemistry Human Welfare and the Environment.* Vol. 3, *Mode of Action, Metabolism and Toxicology.* Pergamon Press, Oxford, 1983, pp. 505–10.

Smith, P., and Heath, D.: Paraquat. *Crit. Rev. Toxicol.,* 4:411–45, 1976.

Smith, R. J.: Poisoned pot becomes burning issue in high places. *Sciences,* 200:417–18, 1978.

Soderland, D. M.; Ghiasuddin, S. M.; and Helmuth, D. W.: Receptor-like stereospecific binding of a pyrethroid insecticide to mouse brain membranes. *Life Sci.,* 33:261–67, 1983.

Spear, R. C.; Jenkins, D. L.; and Milby, T. H.: Pesticide residues and field workers. *Environ. Science Technol.,* 9:308–13, 1975.

Spencer, H. C.; Rowe, V. K.; Adams, E. M.; and Irish, D. D.: Toxicological studies on laboratory animals of certain alkyldinitrophenols used in agriculture. *J. Ind. Hyg. Toxicol.,* 30:10–25, 1948.

Stavinoha, W. B.; Ryan, L. C.; and Smith, P. W.: Biochemical effects of an organophosphorus cholinesterase inhibitor on the rat brain. *Ann. N. Y. Acad. Sci.,* 160:378–82, 1969.

Street, J. C.: Pesticides and the immune system. In Sharma, R. P. (ed.): *Immunologic Considerations in Toxicology,* Vol. I. CRC Press, Inc., Boca Raton, Fl., 1981, pp. 45–66.

Street, J. C.; Chadwick, R. W.; Wong, M.; and Phillips, R. L.: Insecticide interactions affecting residue storage in animal tissues. *J. Agr. Food Chem.,* 14:545, 1969.

Strum, J. M., and Karnovsky, M. J.: Aminotriazole goiter: fine structure and localization of thyroid peroxidase activity. *Lab. Invest.,* 24:1–2, 1971.

Su, M.; Kinoshita, F. K.; Frawley, J. P.; and DuBois, K. P.: Comparative inhibition of aliesterases and cholinesterase in rats fed eighteen organophosphorus insecticides. *Toxicol. Appl. Pharmacol.,* 20:241–49, 1971.

Tabershaw, I. R., and Cooper, W. C.: Sequelae of acute organic phosphate poisoning. *J. Occup. Med.,* 8:5–20, 1966.

Tarjan, R., and Kemény, T.: Multigeneration studies on DDT in mice. *Food Cosmet. Toxicol.,* 7:215–22, 1969.

Taylor, J. R.; Selhorst, J. B.; Houff, S. A.; and Martinez, A. J.: Chlordecone intoxication in man. 1. Clinical observations. *Neurology,* 28:626–35, 1978.

Taylor, J. S.; Wuthrich, R. C.; Lloyd, K. M.; and Poland, A.: Chloracne from manufacture of a new herbicide. *Arch. Dermatol.,* 113:616–19, 1977.

Tomatis, L.: The IARC program on the evaluation of the carcinogenic risk of chemicals to man. *Ann. N. Y. Acad. Sci.,* 271:396–409, 1976.

Torkelson, T. R.; Sadek, S. E.; Rowe, V. K.; Kodama, J. K.; Anderson, H. H.; Loquvam, G. S.; and Hine, C. H.: Toxicologic investigations of 1,2-dibromo-3-chloropropane. *Toxicol. Appl. Pharmacol.,* 3:545–59, 1961.

Triolo, A. J.; Mata, E.; and Coon, J. M.: Effect of organochlorine insecticides on the toxicity and *in vitro* plasma detoxication of paraxon. *Toxicol. Appl. Pharmacol.,* 17:174–80, 1970.

Tucker, R. K., and Crabtree, D. G.: *Handbook of Toxicity of Pesticides to Wildlife.* United States Department of Interior, Fish and Wildlife Service, Resource Publication No. 84. U.S. Government Printing Office, Washington, D.C., 1970.

Turner, W. A.; Engel, J. L.; and Casida, J. E.: Toxaphene components and related compounds: Preparation and toxicity of some hepta-, octa-, and nonachlorobornanes, hexa- and heptachlorobornenes, and a hexachlorobornadiene. *J. Agr. Food Chem.,* 25:1394–1401, 1977.

Uchida, T.; Dauterman, W. C.; and O'Brien, R. D.: The metabolism of dimethoate by vertebrate tissues. *J. Agr. Food Chem.,* 12:48–52, 1964.

Umetsu, N.; Grose, F. H.; Allahyari, R.; Abu-El-Haj, S.; and Fukuto, T. R.: Effect of impurities on the mammalian toxicity of technical malathion and acephate. *J. Agr. Food Chem.,* 25:946–53, 1977.

Van den Bercken, J., and Vijverberg, H. P. M.: Interaction of pyrethroids and DDT-like compounds with the sodium channels in the nerve membrane. In Miyamoto, J., and Kearney, P. C. (eds.): *Pesticide Chemistry: Human Welfare and the Environment.* Vol. 3, *Mode of Action, Metabolism and Toxicology.* Pergamon Press, Oxford, 1983, pp. 115–21.

Van Miller, J. P.; Lalich, J. J.; and Allen, J. R.: Increased incidence of neoplasm in rats exposed to low levels of 2,3,7,8-tetrachlorodibenzo-p-dioxin. *Chemosphere,* 6:537–44, 1977.

Vandekar, M.; Plestina, R.; and Wilhelm, K.: Toxicity of carbamates for mammals. *Bull. WHO,* 44:241–49, 1971.

Verrett, M. J.; Mutchler, M. K.; Scott, W. F.; Reynaldo, E. F.; and McLaughlin, J.: Teratogenic effects of captan and related compounds in the developing chicken embryo. *Ann. N. Y. Acad. Sci.,* 160:334–43, 1969.

Vos, J. G.; Krajnc, E. I.; Beekhof, P. K.; and van Logten, M. J.: Methods for testing immune effects of toxic chemicals: evaluation of the immunotoxicity of various pesticides in the rat. In Miyamoto, J. and Kearney, P. C. (eds.): *Pesticide Chemistry, Human Welfare and the Environment.* Vol. 3, *Mode of Action Metabolisms and Toxicology.* Pergamon Press, Oxford, 1983, pp. 497–504.

Wang, H. H., and Grufferman, S.: A plastic anemia and occupational pesticide exposure: a case-control study. *J. Occup. Med.,* 23:364–66, 1981.

Wang, H. H., and MacMahon, B.: Mortality of workers employed in the manufacture of chlordane and heptachlor. *J. Occup. Med.,* 21:745–48, 1979.

Warriner, R. A.; Nies, A. S.; and Hayes, W. J.: Severe organophosphate poisoning complicated by alcohol and turpentine ingestion. *Arch. Environ. Health,* 32:203–205, 1977.

Wassermann, W.; Wassermann, D.; Imanuel, V.; Israeli, R.; and Frydman, M.: Long term studies on body reactivity in a pesticides plant. *Ind. Med. Surg.,* 39:35–40, 1970.

Waters, E. M.; Huff, J. E.; and Gerstner, H. B.: Mirex. An overview. *Environ. Res.,* 14:212–22, 1977.

Waters, M. D.; Simon, V. F.; Mitchell, A. D.; Jorgenson, T. A.; and Valencia, R.: An overview of short-term tests for the mutagenic and carcinogenic potential of pesticides. *J. Environ. Sci. Health,* B15(6):867–906, 1980.

Weil, C. S.; Woodside, M. D.; Carpenter, C. P.; and Smyth, H. F., Jr.: Current status of tests of carbaryl for reproductive and teratogenic effects. *Toxicol. Appl. Pharmacol.,* 21:390–404, 1972.

Weisburger, E. K.: Carcinogenicity tests on pesticides. In Chambers, J. E., and Yarbrough, J. D. (eds.): *Effects of Chronic Exposures to Pesticides on Animal Systems.* Raven Press, New York, 1982, pp. 165–76.

Welch, R. M.; Levin, W.; and Conney, A. H.: Estrogenic action of DDT and its analogs. *Toxicol. Appl. Pharmacol.,* 14:358–67, 1969.

WHO: *1974 Evaluations of Some Pesticide Residues in Food.* World Health Organization Pesticide Residue Series, No. 4., pp. 261–263. Geneva, 1975.

Wilkinson, C. F. (ed.): *Insecticide Biochemistry and Physiology.* Plenum Press, New York, 1976.

Williams, C. H., and Jacobson, K. H.: An acylamidase in mammalian liver hydrolyzing the herbicide 3,4-dichloropropionanilide. *Toxicol. Appl. Pharmacol.,* 9:495–500, 1966.

Williams, G. M.: Epigenetic mechanisms of action of

carcinogenic organochlorine pesticides. In Bandal, S. K.; Marco, G. J.; Golberg, L.; and Leng, M. I. (eds.): *The Pesticide Chemist and Modern Toxicology: ACS Symposium Series No. 160,* American Chemical Society, New York, 1981.

———: Organochlorine pesticides and inhibition of intercellular communication as the mechanism for their liver tumor production. In Miyamoto, J. and Kearney, P. C. (eds.): *Pesticide Chemistry, Human Welfare and the Environment.* Vol. 3, *Mode of Action, Metabolism and Toxicology.* Pergamon Press, Oxford, 1983, pp. 475–528.

Wills, J. H.: The measurement and significance of changes in the cholinesterase of erythrocytes and plasma in man and animals. *CRC Crit. Rev. Toxicol.,* March:153–202, 1972.

Wills, J. H.; Jameson, E.; and Coulston, F.: Effects of oral doses of carbaryl on man. *Clin. Toxicol.,* 1:265–71, 1968.

Wilson, J. G.: Environmental chemicals. In Wilson, J. G., and Fraser, F. C. (eds.): *Handbook of Teratology.* Vol. 1, *General Principles and Etiology.* Plenum Press, New York, 1977, pp. 357–85.

Wilson, R.; Lovejoy, F. H.; Jaeger, R. J.; and Landrigan, P. L.: Acute phosphine poisoning aboard a grain freighter: epidemiologic, clinical and pathological findings. *JAMA,* 244:148–50, 1980.

Wolfe, H. R.; Durham, W. F.; and Armstrong, J. F.: Exposure of workers to pesticides. *Arch. Environ. Health,* 14:622–33, 1967.

Woodford, E. K., and Evans, S. A.: *Weed Control Handbook,* 4th ed. Blackwell Scientific Publications, Oxford, 1965.

World Health Organization: WHO Technical Report Series No. 525, Geneva, 1973.

Worthing, C. R. (ed.): The *Pesticide Manual.* British Corp Protection Council, Worcestershire, England, 1979.

Xintaris, C.; Burg, J. R.; Tanaka, S.; Lee, S. T.; Johnson, B. L.; Cottrill, C. A.; and Bender, J.: *Occupational Exposure to Leptophos and Other Chemicals.* DHEW (NIOSH) Publication No. 78–136. U.S. Government Printing Office, Washington, D.C., 1978.

Young, A. L.; Calcagni, J. A.; Thalken, C. E.; and Tromblay, J. W.: *The Toxicology, Environmental Fate and Human Risk of Herbicide Orange and Its Dioxin.* USAF OEHL Technical Report 78–92. National Technical Information Service (AD-A062-143), U.S. Department of Commerce, Springfield, Va., 1978.

Zavon, M. R.; Tye, R.; and Latorre, L.: Chlorinated hydrocarbon insecticide content of the neonate. *Ann. N. Y. Acad. Sci.,* 160:196–200, 1969.

Chapter 19

TOXIC EFFECTS OF METALS

Robert A. Goyer

INTRODUCTION

Metals differ from other toxic substances in that they are neither created or destroyed by humans. Nevertheless, utilization by humans influences the potential for health effects in at least two major ways: first, by environmental transport, that is, by human or anthropogenic contributions to air, water, soil, and food, and second, by altering the speciation or biochemical form of the element (Beijer and Jernelöv, 1979; Li, 1981).

Metals are redistributed naturally in the environment by both geologic and biologic cycles (Figure 19–1). Rainwater dissolves rocks and ores and physically transports material to streams and rivers, adding and deleting from adjacent soil, and eventually to the ocean to be precipitated as sediment or taken up in rainwater to be relocated elsewhere on earth. The biologic cycles include bioconcentration by plants and animals and incorporation into food cycles. Human industrial activity may greatly shorten the residence time of metals in ore, form new compounds, and greatly enhance worldwide distribution. These natural cycles may exceed the anthropogenic cycle, as is the case for mercury. However, the role of human activity in redistribution of metal is demonstrated by the 200-fold increase in lead content of Greenland ice beginning with a "natural" low level (about 800 B.C.) and a gradual rise in lead content of ice through the evolution of the industrial age, followed by a nearly precipitous rise in lead corresponding to the period when lead was added to gasoline in the 1920s (Ng and Patterson, 1981). Metal contamination of the environment, therefore, reflects both natural sources and contribution from industrial activity.

Metals emitted into the environment from combustion of fossil fuels in the United States are shown in Table 19–1. These include many of the metals most abundant in particulates in ambient air. The only metals or metallike elements that may be emitted in gaseous discharges in measurable concentrations are mercury or selenium. Metals in raw surface water reflect erosion from natural sources, fallout from the atmosphere, and additions from industrial activities. Metals in soil and water may enter the food chain. For persons in the general population, food sources probably represent the largest source of exposure to metals, with an additional contribution from air. Further potential sources of human exposure include consumer products and industrial wastes as well as the working environment.

Occupational exposure to metals is restricted to "safe" levels defined as the threshold limit value for an eight-hour day, five-day work week. These levels are intended to provide a margin of safety between maximum exposure and minimum levels that will produce illness. Permissible levels vary widely, and the differences reflect, in a sense, the toxicologic potency of the metal. As a general rule, the metals that are most abundant in the environment have lesser potential for toxicity as evidenced by the prevailing standard for permissible occupation exposure.

Metals are probably the oldest toxins known to humans. Lead usage may have begun prior to 2000 B.C. when abundant supplies were obtained from ores as a byproduct of smelting silver. Hippocrates is credited in 370 B.C. with the first description of abdominal colic in a man who extracted metals. Arsenic and mercury are cited by Theophrastus of Erebus (387–372 B.C.) and Pliny the Elder (A.D. 23–79). Arsenic was obtained during the melting of copper and tin, and an early use was for decoration in Egyptian tombs. On the other hand, many of the metals of toxicologic concern today are only recently known to humans. Cadmium was first recognized in ores containing zinc carbonate in 1817. About 80 of the 105 elements in the periodic table are regarded as metals, but less than 30 have compounds that have been reported to produce toxicity in humans. The importance of some of the rarer or lesser known metals such as indium or tantalum might increase with new

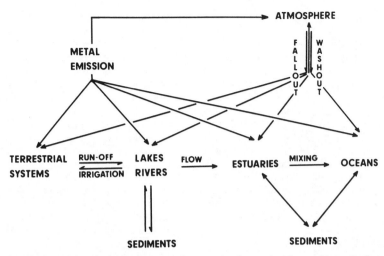

Figure 19–1. Routes for transport of trace elements in the environment. (From Beijer, K., and Jernelöv, A.: Sources, transport and transportation of metals in the environment. In Friberg, L.; Nordberg, G. F.; and Vouk, V. B. [eds.]: *Handbook of the Toxicology of Metals*. Elsevier, North-Holland, New York, 1979, pp. 47–63.)

Table 19–1. TOXICOLOGICALLY IMPORTANT METALS MOBILIZED BY COMBUSTION OF FOSSIL FUEL IN U.S. (COLUMN A), CONCENTRATIONS IN PARTICULATES IN AMBIENT AIR (COLUMN B) AND IN RAW SURFACE WATER (COLUMN C), AND BEST (WORLDWIDE) PREVAILING STANDARDS FOR THRESHOLD LIMIT VALUES (TLV) FOR EIGHT-HOUR OCCUPATIONAL EXPOSURE (COLUMN D)

A: FROM FOSSIL FUELS, U.S.* (10^3 tons)	B: IN PARTIC-ULATES IN AIR† TYPICAL (ng/m³)	C: IN WATER, μg/liter and FREQUENCY OF DETECTION‡			D: TLV$^\parallel$ mg/m³
		maximum	mean	%	
Al 6000	3080	2760	74	31	10
As 27	10	§			0.2
Ba 300	100	340	43	99	0.5
Be 15	0.2	1.22	0.19	5.4	0.002
Cd 1	1	120	10	2.5	0.02 dust
Co 15	5	48	17	2.8	0.05
Cr 0	20	112	10	25	0.05
Cu 9	500	280	15	75	0.1
Fe 6002	4000	4600	52	76	3.5
Li 39	4				0.025
Mg 1200	2000				5.0
Mn 33	100	3230	60	58	2.5
Mo 5	1	1500	68	38	10
Ni 11	20	30	19	16	0.1 sol.
Pb 126	2000	140	13	19	0.1
Sn	50				2.0 inorg.
Se 2	1				0.1
V 27	30	300	2	5	0.5
Zn 30	500	2010	79.2	80	1.0

* From Vouk and Piver, 1983, data from 1977 fuel consumption.
† From Thompson, 1979, ten-day period, six U.S. cities.
‡ From NAS, *Drinking Water and Health*, 1977.
§ Arsenic in water is extremely variable, 10 to 1100 μg/liter 728 samples surface water 22 percent in 10 to 20 μg range.
$^\parallel$ Levinson, 1972.

applications in microelectronics or other new technologies.

The conceptual boundaries of what is regarded as toxicology of metals continues to broaden. Historically, metal toxicology has largely concerned acute or overt effects, such as abdominal colic from lead toxicity or the bloody diarrhea and suppression of urine formation from ingestion of corrosive (mercury) sublimate. There must still be knowledge and understanding of such effects, but with present-day occupational and environmental standards, such effects are uncommon. Beyond this, however, is growing inquiry regarding subtle, chronic or long-term effects where cause-and-effect relationships are not obvious or may be subclinical. This might include a level of effect that causes a change that resides within the generally regarded norm of human performance, e.g., lower I.Q. and childhood lead exposure. Assigning responsibility for such toxicologic effects is extremely difficult and not always possible, particularly when the end-point in question lacks specificity in that it may be caused by a number of agents or even combinations of substances. The challenges, therefore, for the toxicologist are multiple. The major ones include the need for quantitative information regarding dose and tissue levels, greater understanding of the metabolism of metals particularly at the tissue and cellular level where effects that have specificity may occur, and finally, recognition of factors that influence toxicity of a particular level of exposure such as dietary factors or protein-complex formation that enhance or protect from toxicity. Treatment, particularly the administration of chelating agents remains an important topic particularly for those metals that are cumulative and persistent, e.g., Pb, Cd, Ni, etc. However, prevention of toxicity is the major objective of public health policies and occupational hygiene programs. There is increasing emphasis on the use of biologic indicators of toxicity such as heme enzymes in lead toxicity, renal tubular dysfunction in cadmium exposure, and neurologic effects in mercury toxicity to serve as guidelines for preventive or therapeutic intervention.

ESTIMATES OF DOSE-EFFECT RELATIONSHIPS

Estimates of the relationship of dose or level of exposure to a particular metal are, in many ways, a measure of dose-response relationships discussed in greater detail in Chapter 2. The conceptual background for this topic is also considered elsewhere (Friberg et al., 1979). Dose or estimate of exposure to a metal may be a multidimensional concept and is a function of time as well as concentration of metal. The most precise definition of dose is the amount of metal within cells of organs manifesting a toxicologic effect. Results from single measurements may reflect recent exposure or longer-term or past exposure, depending on retention time in the particular tissue. Blood, urine, and hair are the most accessible tissues in which to measure dose and are sometimes referred to as indicator tissues. In vivo, quantitation of metals within organs is not yet possible, although techniques such as neutron activation and fluorescence spectroscopy may hold promise for the future. Indirect estimates of quantities in specific organs may be calculated from metabolic models derived from autopsy data.

At the cellular level, toxicity is related to availability so that chemical form and ligand binding become critical factors. Alkyl compounds are lipid soluble and pass readily across biologic membranes unaltered by their surrounding medium. They are only slowly dealkylated or transformed to inorganic salts. Hence, their excretion tends to be slower than inorganic forms, and the pattern of organic toxicity differs. For example, alkyl mercury is primarily a neurotoxin versus the renal toxicity of mercuric chloride. Metals that have strong affinity for osseous tissue like lead and radium have a long retention time and tend to accumulate with age. Other metals are retained in soft tissues because of affinities for intracellular proteins, such as renal cadmium bound to metallothionein.

Blood and urine usually reflect recent exposure and correlate best with acute effects. An exception is urine cadmium where increased metal in urine reflects renal damage related to accumulation of cadmium in the kidney. Partitioning of metal between cells and plasma and between filtrable and nonfiltrable components of plasma should provide more precise information regarding the presence of biologically active forms of a particular metal. Such partitioning is now standard laboratory practice for blood calcium; ionic calcium is by far the most active form of the metal. Speciation of toxic metals in urine may also provide diagnostic insights. For example, cadmium metallothionein in urine may be of greater toxicologic significance than cadmium chloride.

Hair can be useful in assessing variations in exposure to metals over the long term. Analysis may be performed on segments so that metal content of the newest growth can be compared to past exposures. Correlation between blood levels of metal and concentration in hair is not expected because blood levels reflect only current exposures. Caution must be taken in washing hair prior to analysis to assure removal of metal deposits from external contamination (Laker, 1982).

FACTORS INFLUENCING TOXICITY OF METALS

There are only a few general principles available that contribute to understanding the pathophysiology of metal toxicity. Most metals affect multiple organ systems, and the targets for toxicity are specific biochemical processes (enzymes) and/or membranes of cells and organelles. The toxic effect of the metal usually involves an interaction between the free metal ion and the toxicologic target. There may be multiple reasons why a particular toxic effect occurs. For instance, the metabolism of the toxic metal may be similar to a metabolically related essential element. Such is the case for some of the effects of lead, e.g., lead and calcium in the central nervous system, lead, iron, and zinc in heme metabolism. Cells that are involved in the transport of metals, such as gastrointestinal, liver, or renal tubular cells, are particularly susceptible to toxicity. However, for many metals, these cells have protective mechanisms involving protein complex formation that permits intracellular accumulation of potentially toxic metals without causing cell injury.

Metal-protein complexes involved in detoxication or protection from toxicity have now been described for a few metals (Goyer, 1984). Morphologically discernible cellular inclusion bodies are present with exposures to lead, bismuth, and a mercury-selenate mixture. Metallothioneins form complexes with cadmium, zinc, copper, and other metals, and ferritin and hemosiderin are intracellular iron-protein complexes. The protein complexes formed by lead, bismuth, mercury-selenate, and iron, at least for hemosiderin, have attracted interest because these complexes are insoluble in tissues and can be observed histologically. However, it is this lack of solubility that has made detailed biochemical study very difficult. On the other hand, for those metal-protein complexes that are stable and soluble in aqueous media, such as metallothionein and ferritin, there is considerable biochemical information. More is known about ferritin than perhaps any of these protein complexes since it is soluble and at the same time it has a unique ultrastructural appearance so that it can be readily identified in cells and organelles. None of these proteins or metal protein complexes have

any known enzymatic activity. From these considerations it becomes clearer why speciation, that is, how much metal in a tissue that is in a particular biochemical form and what it is bound to, may be the ultimate determinant of toxicity.

Numerous exogenous factors influence the occurrence of toxicity in any particular subject (Nordberg et al., 1978). These include age, diet, and interactions and concurrent exposure with other toxic metals. Persons at either end of the life-span, young children or elderly, are believed to be more susceptible to toxicity from exposure to a particular level of metal than adults. Rapid growth and cell division represent opportunities for genotoxic effects. Intrauterine toxicity to methyl mercury is well documented. Lead crosses the placenta, and it is recommended that maternal blood lead levels be lower than those of persons in the general population.

The major pathway of exposure to many toxic metals in children is with food, and children consume more calories per body weight than adults. Moreover, children have higher gastrointestinal absorption of metals, particularly lead. Experimental studies have extended these observations to other metals, and milk diet, probably because of lipid content, seems to increase metal absorption.

Effects of some dietary factors on metal toxicity are at the level of absorption from the gastrointestinal tract. There is an inverse relationship between protein content of diet and cadmium and lead toxicity. Vitamin C reduces lead and cadmium absorption, probably because of increase absorption of ferrous ion. On the other hand, metabolically related essential metals may alter toxicity by interaction at the cellular level. Lead, calcium, and vitamin D have a complex relationship affecting mineralization of bone and more directly through impairment of 1–25-dihydroxy vitamin D synthesis in the kidney. Metal-metal interaction may have considerable influence on dose-effect relationships and are commented on in discussions of specific metals.

"Life-style" factors such as smoking or alcohol ingestion may have indirect influences on toxicity. Cigarette smoke in itself contains some toxic metals such as cadmium, and cigarette smoking may influence pulmonary effects. Alcohol ingestion may influence toxicity indirectly by altering diet and reducing essential mineral intake. For instance, a decrease in dietary calcium will influence toxicity of major toxic metals, including lead and cadmium.

Chemical form of the metal may be an important factor, not only for pulmonary and gastrointestinal absorption but in terms of body distribution and toxic effects. Dietary phosphate generally forms less soluble salts of metals than other anions. Alkyl compounds, such as tetraethyl lead and methyl mercury, are lipid soluble and more soluble in myelin than inorganic salts of these metals.

For metals that produce hypersensitivity reactions, the immune status of an individual becomes an additional toxicologic variable (Kazantzis, 1978). Metals that provoke immune reactions include mercury, gold, platinum, beryllium, chromium, and nickel. Clinical effects are varied but usually involve any of four types of immune responses. In anaphylactic or immediate hypersensitivity reactions, the antibody, IgE, reacts with the antigen on the surface of mast cells releasing vasoreactive amines. Clinical reactions include conjunctivitis, asthma, urticaria, or even systemic anaphylaxis. Cutaneous, mucosal, and bronchial reactions to platinum have been attributed to this type of hypersensitivity reaction. Cytotoxic hypersensitivity is the result of a complement-fixing reaction of IgG immunoglobulin with antigen or hapten bound to the cell surface. The thrombocytopenia sometimes occurring with exposure to organic gold salts may be brought about in this manner. Immune complex hypersensitivity occurs when soluble immune complex deposits (antigen, antibody, and complement) within tissues producing an acute inflammatory reaction. Immune complexes are typically deposited on the epithelial surface of glomerular basement membrane, resulting in proteinuria, and occur following exposure to mercury vapor or gold therapy. Cell-mediated hypersensitivity, also known as the delayed hypersensitivity reaction, is mediated by thymus-dependent lymphocytes and usually occurs 24 to 48 hours after exposure. The histologic reaction consists of mononuclear cells and is the typical reaction seen in the contact dermatitis following exposure to chromium or nickel. The granuloma formation occurring with beryllium and zirconium exposure may be a form of cell-mediated immune response.

CARCINOGENESIS

Given the long history of human exposure to metals, knowledge of the potential carcinogenicity of metal compounds has evolved slowly, and most of this information has only been obtained in recent years (IARC, 1980; Friberg and Nelson, 1981).

Furthermore, predictive *in vitro* methods using nonmammalian systems, such as the Ames test, do not seem as responsive as for organic compounds (Costa, 1980). Evidence of carcinogenicity for metals relates more precisely with specific compounds of metals than with the metal itself. That is, some forms of the metal seem to be carcinogenic; for example, nickel subsulfide (Ni_3S_2) is more carcinogenic than amorphorus nickel monosulfide (NiS); but such differences may be explained on the basis of cell uptake rates or solubility. Similar debates concern various compounds of chromium. Nevertheless, if any form of a metal is carcinogenic, the metal itself must be regarded as a carcinogen.

Although only a few metals show any evidence of carcinogenicity, this is an exceedingly important topic because of the ubiquity of most metals, their wide industrial use, and their persistence in the environment. Identification of metal carcinogens in industry is made even more perplexing because seldom is exposure to a single metal but it is usually to mixtures. And there is the added question of the role of metals as promoters or cocarcinogens with organic carcinogens because of their persistence in tissues, as may be the case for lead.

The chronology of observations on the carcinogenicity of metals is shown in Figure 19–2. Specific details pertaining to the carcinogenicity of each metal are discussed later in the chapter along with other toxicologic effects. However, the figure does provide an overview. Human case reports of skin cancer due to arsenic exposure were recognized in the nineteenth century, but epidemiologic support from case study observations did not occur until over 50 years later, and there has not yet been confirmation in experimental animals. On the other hand, lead is the only metal shown to be carcinogenic in animal models by oral administration. Yet, evidence in humans is limited to a couple of recent case reports. How much of what kind of evidence, animal and/or human, is required to label a metal as a carcinogen must be decided for each metal. Animal studies that use routes of administration different from those by which humans may be exposed, such as by injection, have limitations for extrapolation to humans.

CHELATION

Chelation is the formation of a metal ion complex in which the metal ion is associated with a charged or uncharged electron donor referred to a ligand. The ligand may be monodentate, bidentate, or multidentate; that is, it may attach or coordinate using one or two or more donor atoms. Bidentate ligands form ring structures that include the metal ion and the two ligand atoms attached to the metal (Williams and Halstead, 1982).

Chelating agents are generally nonspecific in regard to their affinity for metals. To varying

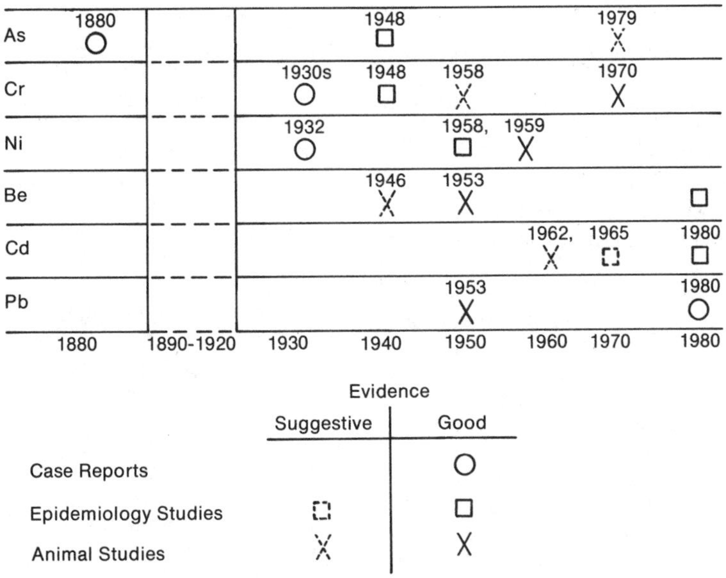

Figure 19–2. Chronology of observations on the carcinogenicity of metals. (Modified from Friberg, L., and Nelson, N.: Introduction, general findings and general recommendations. Workshop/Conference on the Role of Metals in Carcinogenesis. *Environ. Health Perspect.*, **40**:5–10, 1981.)

degrees, they will mobilize and enhance the excretion of a rather wide range of metals, including essential metals such as calcium and zinc (Table 19–2). Their efficacy depends not solely on their affinity for the metal of interest, but also on their affinity for endogenous metals, mainly Ca, which compete in accordance with their own affinities for the chelator. Properties of a few of the commonly used chelators will be described.

BAL

BAL (British Anti Lewisite) or 2,3-dimercaptopropanol was the first clinically useful chelating agent. It was developed during World War II as a specific antagonist to vesicant arsen-

ical war gases based on the observation that arsenic has an affinity for sulfhydryl-containing substances (Peters, 1965). BAL, a dithiol compound with two sulfur atoms on adjacent carbon atoms, competes with the critical binding sites responsible for the toxic effects. These observations led to the prediction that the "biochemical lesion" of arsenic poisoning would prove to be a thiol with sulfhydryl groups separated by one or more intervening carbon atoms. This prediction was borne out a few years later with the discovery that arsenic interferes with the function of 6,8-dithiooctanoic acid in biologic oxidation (Gunsalus, 1953).

BAL has been found to form stable chelates *in vivo* with many toxic metals including inorganic mercury, antimony, bismuth, cadmium, chromium, cobalt, gold, and nickel. However, it is not necessarily the treatment of choice for toxicity to these metals. BAL has been used as an adjunct in the treatment of the acute encephalopathy of lead toxicity. It is a potentially toxic drug, and its use may be accompanied by multiple side effects. Although BAL will increase the excretion of cadmium, there is a concomitant increase in renal cadmium concentration so that its use in cadmium toxicity is to be avoided. It does, however, remove inorganic mercury from kidneys but is not useful in treatment of alkyl or phenylmercury toxicity. BAL also enhances the toxicity of selenium and tellurium so it is not to be used to remove these metals.

Table 19–2. LIGANDS (CHELATING AGENTS) PREFERRED FOR REMOVAL OF TOXIC METALS

LIGAND	METAL
BAL	Arsenic, lead (with Ca-EDTA), mercury, inorganic
DMPS	Methyl mercury, inorganic mercury, cadmium, copper, and nickel
Calcium EDTA	Lead
Penicillamine	Copper, lead
Calcium DPTA	Cadmium (with BAL)
Desferrioxamine	Iron
Dithiocarb	Nickel carbonyl

DMPS

DMPS (2,3-dimercapto-1-propanesulfonic acid) is a water-soluble derivative of BAL developed to reduce the toxicity and unpleasant side effects of BAL. A recent study has found that DMPS reduces blood lead levels in children (Chisolm and Thomas, 1985). It has the advantage over EDTA in that it is administered orally and does not appear to have toxic side effects. It has been widely used in Russia to treat many different metal intoxications and even atherosclerosis by the adherents of the notion that this degenerative disorder of blood vessels is due to metal-ion accumulations in the blood vessel wall leading to inhibition of enzyme metabolism.

DMPS is effective in removal of both inorganic and methyl mercury, probably because it is not lipophilic like BAL and does not penetrate tissues but removes extracellular metal (Gabard, 1976). The important point is that it does not increase the concentration of metal in the brain and reduces organ concentration of metal including the kidney. It may also be effective in removal of copper, nickel, and cadmium immediately after exposure but not from tissue stores.

EDTA

Calcium EDTA is the calcium disodium salt of ethylene diamine tetraacetic acid. The calcium salt must be used clinically because the sodium salt has greater affinity for calcium and will produce hypocalcemic tetany. However, the calcium salt will bind lead with displacement of calcium from the chelate. It is poorly absorbed from the gastrointestinal tract so it must be given parenterally, and it becomes rapidly distributed in the body. It is the current method of choice for treatment of lead toxicity (Chisolm, 1974). The peak excretion is within the first 24 hours and represents excretion of lead from soft tissues. Removal from the skeletal system occurs more slowly with restoration of equilibrium with soft tissue compartments. Calcium EDTA does have the potential for nephrotoxicity, so it should be administered only when indicated clinically.

Penicillamine

Penicillamine (B,B[1]-dimethylcystein), a hydrolytic product of penicillin, is the choice for therapy of Wilson's disease (copper toxicity) and is effective in removal of lead, mercury, and iron (Walshe, 1964). It is also important to note that penicillamine removes other physiologically essential metals including zinc, cobalt, and manganese. It also has the risk of inducing a hypersensitivity reaction with a wide spectrum of undesired immunologic effects including skin rash, blood dyscrasias, and possibly proteinuria and the nephrotic syndrome. It has cross-sensitivity to penicillin so it should be avoided by persons with penicillin hypersensitivity. Recent studies have shown the effectiveness of a new orally active chelating agent, triethylene tetramine 2HCl (Trien) in Wilson's disease, particularly in those persons who have developed sensitivity to pencillamine (Walshe, 1983).

DTPA

DTPA or diethylenetriamine-pentaacetic acid has chelating properties similar to those of EDTA. The calcium salt (CaNA$_2$ DPTA) must be used clinically because of its high affinity for calcium. It has been used for chelation of plutonium and other radioactive metals but with mixed success. More recently there has been considerable experimental study of BAL for removal of cadmium alone, or DPTA in combination with BAL, but with limited success (Cherian, 1980).

Desferrioxamine

Desferrioxamine is a hydroxylamine isolated as the iron chelate of *Streptomyces pilosus* and is used clinically in the metal-free form (Keberle, 1964). It has a remarkable affinity for ferric iron and a low affinity for calcium and competes effectively for iron in ferritin and hemosiderin but not transferrin, or the iron in hemoglobin or heme-containing enzymes. It is poorly absorbed from the gastrointestinal tract so it must be given parenterally. Clinical usefulness is limited by a variety of toxic effects including hypotension, skin rashes, and possibly cataract formation. It seems to be more effective in hemosiderosis due to blood transfusion but is less effective in treatment of hemochromatosis.

Dithiocarb

Dithiocarb (diethyldithiocarbanate) or DDC has been recommended as the drug of choice in the treatment of acute nickel carbonyl poisoning. The drug may be administered orally for mild toxicity but parenterally for acute or severe poisoning (Sunderman, 1979).

MAJOR TOXIC METALS WITH MULTIPLE EFFECTS

Arsenic

Arsenic is particularly difficult to characterize as a single element because its chemistry is so complex and there are many different compounds of arsenic. It may be trivalent or pentavalent and is widely distributed in nature. The most common inorganic trivalent arsenic compounds are arsenic trioxide, sodium arsenite, and arsenic trichloride. Pentavalent inorganic compounds are arsenic pentoxide, arsenic acid, and arsenates, such as lead arsenate and calcium arsenate. Organic compounds may also be trivalent or pentavalent such as arsanilic acid, or even in methylated forms as a consequence of bimethylation by organisms in soil and fresh and seawaters. A summary of environmental sources of arsenic as well as potential health effects is contained in a WHO criteria document (WHO, 1981).

Arsenic is mainly transported in the environment by water, and airborne arsenic is generally due to contributions from industrial contamination and may range from a few nanograms to a few tenths of a microgram per cubic meter. The 133 stations of the National Air Sampling Network reported in 1964 that the average annual concentration of arsenic in air ranges from 0.01 μg/m^3 to 0.75 μg/m^3 in smelters. Near point emissions, concentrations may exceed 1 μg/m^3. Drinking water usually contains a few micrograms per liter or less. More than 18,000 community water supplies in the United States have concentrations less than 0.01 mg/liter, but levels exceeding 0.05 mg/liter have been found in Nova Scotia where arsenic content of bed rock is high. Even higher concentrations have been reported from various mineral springs, e.g., Japan—1.7 mg As/liter; Cordoba, Argentina—3.4 mg/liter; Taiwan (artesian well water)—1.8 mg/liter. Most foods (meat and vegetables) contain some level of arsenic, but the daily diet in the United States contains below 0.04 mg, but may contain 0.2 mg per day if the diet contains seafood. The total daily intake of arsenic by humans without industrial exposure, however, is usually less than 0.3 mg/day.

The major source of occupational exposure to arsenic in the United States is in the manufacture of pesticides, herbicides, and other agricultural products (Landrigan, 1981). High exposure to arsenic fumes and dust may occur in the smelting industries; the highest concentrations most likely occur among roaster workers.

Disposition. Airborne arsenic is largely trivalent arsenic oxide, but deposition in airways and absorption from lungs is dependent on particle size and chemical form.

Studies show that 6 to 9 percent of orally administered ^{74}As-labeled trivalent or pentavalent arsenic is eliminated in feces in mice (Vahter and Norin, 1980), indicating almost complete absorption from the gastrointestinal tract. Limited data also suggest nearly complete absorption of soluble forms of trivalent and pentavalent arsenic (Tam et al., 1979). Excretion of absorbed arsenic is mainly via urine. The biologic half-life

of ingested inorganic arsenic is about ten hours and 50 to 80 percent is excreted in about three days. The biologic half-life of methylated arsenic was found to be 30 hours in one study (Crecelius, 1977).

Arsenic has a predilection for skin and is excreted by desquamation of skin and in sweat, particularly during periods of perfuse sweating. It also concentrates in nails and hair. Arsenic in nails produces Mee's lines (transverse white bands across fingernails) appearing about six weeks after onset of symptoms of toxicity. Time of exposure may be estimated from measuring the distance of the line from the base of the nail and the rate of nail growth, which is about 0.3 cm/month or 0.1 mm/day. Arsenic in hair may also reflect past exposure, but intrinsic or systematically absorbed arsenic in hair must be distinguished from arsenic that is deposited from external sources. Human milk contains about 3 μg/liter of arsenic.

Placental transfer of arsenic has been shown in hamsters injected intravenously with high doses (20 mg/kg body weight) of sodium arsenate (Ferm, 1977) and studies of tissue levels of arsenic in fetuses and newborn babies in Japan show that the total amount of arsenic in the fetus tends to increase during gestation indicating placental transfer. A more recent study of women in the United States found cord blood levels of arsenic to be similar to maternal blood levels (Kagey et al., 1977).

Biotransformation. Biotransformation of arsenic has been difficult to study because of analytic problems. Pentavalent arsenic compounds are reduced in vivo to more toxic trivalent compounds (Johnstone, 1963). However, ingestion of trivalent arsenic by experimental animals and humans is followed by excretion of some percentage of administered dose as pentavalent arsenic (Bencko et al., 1976). The major form of arsenic in urine is dimethylarsinic acid, indicating in vivo methylation in humans.

Ingestion of arsenic-containing seafood does not result in increased excretion of inorganic arsenic and methyl- and dimethylarsinic acid, suggesting that the unknown organic compounds of arsenic are not converted to methylarsinic acid in vivo (Crecelius, 1977).

Cellular Effects. It has been known for some years that trivalent compounds of arsenic are the principal toxic forms, and pentavalent arsenic compounds have little effect on enzyme activity (Peters, 1965). A number of sulfhydryl-containing proteins and enzyme systems have been found to be altered by exposure to arsenic. Some of these can be reversed by addition of an excess of a monothiol such as glutathione; those enzymes containing two thiol groups can be reversed by dithiols such as 2,3-dimercapto-propanol (BAL) but not by monothiols.

Arsenic affects mitochondrial enzymes and impairs tissue respiration (Brown *et al.*, 1976), which seems to be related to the cellular toxicity of arsenic. Mitochondria accumulate arsenic, and respiration mediated by NAD-linked substrates is particularly sensitive to arsenic and is thought to result from reaction between arsenite ion and dihydrolipoic acid cofactor, necessary for oxidation of the substrate (Fluharty and Sanadi, 1961). Arsenite also inhibits succinic dehydrogenase activity and uncouples oxidative phosphorylation, which results in stimulation of mitochondrial ATPase activity. Mitchell *et al.*, (1971) proposed that arsenic inhibits energy-linked functions of mitochondria in two ways: competition with phosphate during oxidative phosphorylation and inhibition of energy-linked reduction of NAD.

Toxicology. Ingestion of large doses (70 to 180 mg) may be acutely fatal (Vallee *et al.*, 1960). Symptoms consist of fever, anorexia, hepatomegaly, melanosis, and cardiac arrhythmia with electrocardiograph changes that may be the prodroma of eventual cardiovascular failure. Other features include upper-respiratory-tract symptoms, peripheral neuropathy, and gastrointestinal, cardiovascular, and hematopoietic effects. Acute ingestion may be suspected from damage to mucous membranes such as irritation, vesicle formation, and even sloughing. Sensory loss in the peripheral nervous system is the most common neurologic effect, appearing one or two weeks after large exposures and consisting of Wallerian degeneration of axons, but is reversible if exposure is stopped. Anemia and leukopenia, particularly granulocytopenia, occur in a few days and are reversible.

Liver injury is characteristic of longer-term or chronic exposure, is initially reflected by jaundice, and may progress to cirrhosis and ascites. Toxicity to hepatic parenchymal cells results in elevations of liver enzymes in blood, and studies in experimental animals show granules and alterations in the ultrastructure of mitochondria, nonspecific manifestations of cell injury including loss of glycogen.

Peripheral vascular disease has been observed in persons with chronic exposure to arsenic in drinking water in Taiwan and Chile, is manifested by acrocyanosis and Raynaud's phenomenon, and may progress to endarteritis obliterans and gangrene of the lower extremities (blackfoot disease). This specific effect seems to be related to the cumulative dose of arsenic, but prevalence is uncertain because of difficulties in separating arsenic-induced peripheral vascular

disease from other causes of gangrene (Tseng, 1977).

Carcinogenicity. Arsenic has specific effects on the endothelial cells of the blood vessels in the liver, and hemangioendothelial tumors or angiosarcoma of the liver has been reported in vineyard workers following many years of exposure to arsenic-containing drinking water, Fowler's solution, wine, and arsenic-containing pesticides (Popper *et al.*, 1978).

The skin is the critical organ of arsenic toxicity, and a variety of skin lesions have been associated with arsenic intoxication, particularly from chronic exposure in drinking water and from certain occupational exposures. A characteristic finding is symmetric verrucous hyperkeratosis of the palms and soles. Hyperpigmentation or melanosis is also common. Cancer of the skin related to arsenic exposure was first reported by an English physician, Sir Jonathan Hutchinson, in persons with long-continued ingestion of Fowler's solution. Skin cancers from occupational exposures have since been well documented, particularly in the last 20 years. Available data suggest a dose-response relationship (Tseng, 1977).

Workers engaged in the production of arsenic-containing pesticides showed increased lung cancer mortality (Ott *et al.*, 1974), and workers involved in copper smelting, where arsenic exposure may be very high, are also reported to have an increased risk of dying from lung cancer (Lee and Fraumeni, 1969; Pinto *et al.*, 1978). Nonworker populations living near point emission sources of arsenic to air may have increases in lung cancer as well, but the studies to date are not definitive (Pershagan, 1981). Nevertheless, the relationship of ingestion of arsenic with skin cancer and angiosarcoma and inhalation of arsenic containing particulates and lung cancer establishes arsenic as a human carcinogen. However, in contrast to most other human carcinogens, it has been difficult to confirm in experimental animals. In one study, rats given a mixture of calcium arsenate, copper sulfate, and calcium oxide by intratracheal instillation developed lung tumors (Ivankovic *et al.*, 1979), but other studies testing trivalent and pentavalent arsenic compounds by oral administration or skin application have not shown potential for either promotion or initiation of carcinogenicity. Similarly, experimental studies for carcinogenicity of organic arsenic compounds have been negative.

Studies on mutagenic effects of arsenic have been generally negative. Inorganic arsenic compounds do interfere with DNA repair mechanisms in bacteria and dermal cell cultures. An increased frequency of chromosomal aberrations has been found among workers exposed to inorganic arsenic compounds and patients taking drugs containing arsenic (Lofroth and Ames, 1978).

Reproductive Effects and Teratogenicity. High doses of inorganic arsenic compounds to pregnant experimental animals produce various malformations somewhat dependent on time and route of administration. However, no such effects have been noted in people with excessive occupational exposures to arsenic compounds.

Arsine. Arsine gas is formed by the reaction of hydrogen with arsenic and is generated as a by-product in the refining of nonferrous metals. Arsine is a potent hemolytic agent, producing acute symptoms of nausea, vomiting, shortness of breath, and headache accompanying the hemolytic reaction. Exposure may be fatal and may be accompanied by hemoglobinuria and renal failure, and even jaundice and anemia in nonfatal cases where exposure persists (Fowler and Weissberg, 1974).

Biologic Indicators. Biologic indicators of arsenic exposure are blood, urine, and hair (Table 19–3). Because of the short half-life of arsenic, blood levels are only useful within a few days of acute exposure but are not useful to assess chronic exposure. Urine arsenic is the best indicator of current on recent exposure and has been noted to be several hundred micrograms per liter with occupational exposure. Hair or even fingernail concentration of arsenic may be helpful to evaluate past exposures, but interpretation is made difficult because of the problem of differentiating external contamination.

There are no specific biochemical parameters that reflect arsenic toxicity, but evaluation of clinical effects must be interpreted with knowledge of exposure history.

Treatment. BAL is used to treat acute dermatitis and pulmonary symptoms. BAL has also been used for the treatment of chronic arsenic poisoning, but there are no established biologic criteria or measures of effectiveness. BAL has been used most often in cases with dermatitis, but there is usually no change in the keratotic

Table 19–3. BIOLOGIC INDICATORS OF ARSENIC EXPOSURE

	NORMAL	EXCESSIVE EXPOSURE
Whole blood	< 10 μg/liter	Up to 50 μg/liter
Urine*	< 50 μg/liter	> 100 μg/liter
Hair	< 1 mug/kg	

* Best indicator of current or recent exposure.

lesions or influence on progression to skin cancer.

Arsine toxicity is best treated symptomatically. BAL is not considered helpful (Fowler and Weissberg, 1974).

Beryllium

The major toxicologic effects of beryllium are on the lung. It may produce an acute chemical pneumonitis, hypersensitivity, and chronic granulomatous pulmonary disease (berylliosis). A variety of beryllium compounds and some of its alloys have induced malignant tumors of the lung in rats and monkeys and osteogenic sarcoma in rabbits. Human epidemiologic studies are strongly suggestive of a carcinogenic effect in humans (Kuschner, 1981).

Beryllium in the environment largely results from coal combustion. Illinois and Appalachian coal contains an average of about 2.5 ppm; oil contains about 0.08 ppm. The combustion of coal and oil contributes about 1250 or more tons of beryllium to the environment each year (mostly from coal), which is about five times the annual production for industrial use. The major industrial processes that release beryllium into the environment are beryllium extraction plants, ceramic plants, and beryllium alloy manufacturers. These industries also provide the greatest potential for occupational exposure. A review published in 1959 states that inhalable beryllium in ore treatment rooms around baking furnaces or at the sites of fluorescent phosphor blending, milling, and salvaging must have been around 1 mg/m^3. The major current use is as an alloy, but about 20 percent of world production is for applications utilizing the free metal in nuclear reactions, x-ray windows, and other special applications related to space optics, missile fuel, and space vehicles.

Knowledge of the disposition of beryllium has largely been obtained from experimental animals, particularly the rat. Clearance of inhaled beryllium is multiphasic; half is cleared in about two weeks; the remainder is removed slowly, and a residuum becomes fixed in the tissues probably within fibrotic granulomata.

Absorption of ingested beryllium probably only occurs in the acidic milieu of the stomach, where it is in the ionized form, but passes through the intestinal tract as precipitated phosphate (Reeves, 1965). Transport in plasma is in the form of a colloidal phosphate probably bound to an α-globulin. Removal of radiolabeled beryllium chloride from rat blood is rapid, having a half-life of about three hours. It is distributed to all tissues, but most goes to the skeleton. High doses go predominantly to liver, but it is gradually transferred to bone. A variable fraction of the administered dose is excreted in urine, probably by way of transtubular secretion, rather than glomerular filtration.

Skin Effects. Contact dermatitis is the commonest beryllium-related toxic effect. Exposure to soluble beryllium compounds may result in papulovesicular lesions on the skin. It is a delayed-type allergic reaction. If contact is made with an insoluble beryllium compound, a chronic granulomatous lesion develops, which may be necrotizing or ulcerative. If insoluble beryllium-containing material becomes embedded under the skin, the lesion will not heal and may progress in severity. Use of a beryllium patch test to identify beryllium-sensitive individuals may in itself be sensitizing, and use of this procedure as a diagnostic test is discouraged.

Beryllium combines with proteins in the skin to act as the antigen in the hypersensitivity reaction. The hypersensitivity is cell mediated, and passive transfer with lymphoid cells has been accomplished in guinea pigs.

Pulmonary Effects. *Acute Chemical Pneumonitis.* Acute pulmonary disease from inhalation of beryllium is a fulminating inflammatory reaction of the entire respiratory tract, involving the nasal passages, pharynx, tracheobroncheal airways, and the alveoli, and in the most severe cases produces an acute fulminating pneumonitis. It occurs almost immediately following inhalation of aerosols of soluble beryllium compounds, particularly fluoride—an intermediate in the ore extraction process. Severity is dose related. Fatalities have occurred, although recovery is generally complete after a period of several weeks or even months.

Chronic Granulomatous Pulmonary Disease (Berylliosis). This syndrome was first described by Hardy and Tabershaw (1946) among fluorescent lamp workers exposed to insoluble beryllium compounds, particularly beryllium oxide. The major symptom is shortness of breath, but in severe cases may be accompanied by cyanosis and clubbing of fingers (hypertrophic osteoarthropathy—a characteristic manifestation of chronic pulmonary disease). Chest x-rays show miliary mottling. Histologically, the alveoli contain small interstitial granulomata, which resemble those seen in sarcoidosis. In the early stages, the lesions are composed of fluid, lymphocytes, and plasma cells. Multinucleated giant cells are common. Later, the granulomas become organized with proliferation of fibrosis tissue, eventually forming small, fibrous nodules. As the lesions progress, interstitial fibrosis increases with loss of functioning alveoli and effective air/capillary gas exchange and increasing respiratory dysfunction.

Beryllium is one metal in which evidence for carcinogenicity was observed in experimental studies, beginning in 1946, before the establishment of carcinogenicity in humans (Kuschner, 1981). Epidemiologic confirmation in humans has been evolving, so that there is increasing acceptance that beryllium is, in fact, a human carcinogen. Studies of humans with occupational exposure to beryllium prior to 1970 were negative. However, three recent reports of worker populations studied earlier show a small excess of lung cancer, but the total number of cases is small. It was the conclusion of a work group report in 1981 that beryllium is indeed "the cause of the excess mortality" in persons with excess occupational/environmental exposure to beryllium (Doll *et al.*, 1981).

In vitro studies of genotoxicity have shown that beryllium will induce morphlogic transformation in mammalian cells (DiPaolo and Casto, 1979). Beryllium will also decrease fidelity of DNA synthesis, but is negative when tested as a mutagen in bacterial systems (Rosenkrantz and Poirier, 1979).

Cadmium

Cadmium is a modern toxic metal. It was only discovered as an element in 1817, and industrial use was minor until about 50 years ago. But now it is a very important metal with many applications. The main use is electroplating or galvanizing because of its noncorrosive properties. It is also used as a color pigment for paints and plastics, and cathode material for nickel-cadmium batteries. Cadmium is a by-product of zinc and lead mining and smelting, which are important sources of environmental pollution.

Air concentrations as high as 4 to 5 mg/m^3 have been detected in certain workplace environments such as battery factories (Adams *et al.*, 1969), but airborne cadmium in the present-day workplace environment is generally less then 0.02 μg/m^3. Typical concentrations in ambient air in rural areas are 0.001 to 0.005 μg/m^3 and up to 0.050 or 0.060 μg/m^3 in urban areas (Kneip *et al.*, 1970).

Meat, fish, and fruit contain 1 to 50 μg/kg, grains contain 10 to 150 μg/kg, and the greatest concentrations are in liver and kidney of animals. Shellfish, such as mussels, scallops, and oysters, may be a major source of dietary cadmium and contain 100 to 1000 μg/kg. Shellfish accumulate cadmium from the water and then bind to cadmium-binding peptides (Frazier, 1979). Total daily intake from food in North America and Europe varies considerably but is generally less than 100 μg/day, whereas in heavily polluted areas as in parts of Japan, cadmium intake from food and water may be up to 150 μg/day (Underwood, 1977).

Rice grown in soil contaminated with cadmium and other grains contributes to dietary content. Cadmium is more readily taken up by plants than other metals such as lead (WHO, 1977a). Factors contributing to soil content of cadmium are fallout from air, cadmium content of water irrigating fields, and cadmium added with fertilizers. Commercial phosphate fertilizers usually contain less than 20 mg/kg, but Anderson and Hahlin (1981) found an annual increase in soil and barley grain from continued use of phosphate fertilizer over a 15-year period. Another concern is use of commercial sludge to fertilize agricultural fields (Pahren et al., 1979). Commercial sludge may contain up to 1500 mg of cadmium per kilogram of dry material.

Respiratory absorption of cadmium is about 15 to 30 percent. Workplace exposure to cadmium is particularly hazardous where there are cadmium fumes or airborne cadmium. Most airborne cadmium is respirable (Dorn, 1976). A major nonoccupational source of respirable cadmium is cigarettes. One cigarette contains 1 to 2 μg cadmium, and 10 percent of the cadmium in a cigarette is inhaled (0.1 to 0.2 μg) (Elinder et al., 1983). Smoking one pack or more packs of cigarettes a day may double the body burden of cadmium.

Disposition. Gastrointestinal absorption is less than respiratory absorption and is about 5 to 8 percent. It is enhanced by dietary deficiencies of calcium and iron, and diets low in protein. Low dietary calcium stimulates synthesis of calcium-binding protein, which enhances cadmium absorption. Women with low serum ferritin levels have been shown to have twice the normal absorption of cadmium (Flanagan et al., 1978). Zinc decreases cadmium absorption probably by stimulating production of metallothionein.

Cadmium is transported in blood bound to red blood cells and large-molecular-weight proteins in plasma, particularly albumin. A small fraction of blood cadmium may be transported by metallothionein. Blood cadmium levels in adults without excessive exposure is usually less than 1 μg/dl. Newborns have low body content of cadmium, usually less than 1 mg total body burden. The placenta synthesizes metallothionein and may serve as a barrier to maternal cadmium, but the fetus may be exposed with increased maternal exposure (Kowal et al., 1979). Breast milk and human milk are low in cadmium content, less than 1 μg/kg of milk (Schroeder and Balassa, 1961). About 50 to 75 percent of the body burden of cadmium is in liver and kidneys; half-life in the body is not exactly known, but is many years and may be as long as 30 years. With continued retention, there is progressive accumulation in soft tissues, particularly kidney, through ages 50 to 60 years when it begins to decline slowly. Because of the potential for accumulation in kidney, there is considerable concern for levels of dietary intake of cadmium by persons in the general population. Studies from Sweden have shown a slow but steady increase in cadmium content of vegetables over the years (Kjellstrom et al., 1975). Increase in body burden has been determined from an historic autopsy study (Elinder and Kjellstrom, 1977).

Toxicity. Acute toxicity may result from ingestion of relatively high concentrations of cadmium, as may occur in contaminated beverages or food. Nordberg (1972) relates an instance in which nausea, vomiting, and abdominal pain occurred from consumption of drinks containing approximately 16 mg/liter of cadmium. Recovery was rapid without apparent long-term effects. Inhalation of cadmium fumes or other heated cadmium-containing materials may produce an acute chemical pneumonitis and pulmonary edema.

The principal long-term effects of low-level exposure to cadmium are chronic obstructive pulmonary disease and emphysema and chronic renal tubular disease. There may also be effects on the cardiovascular and skeletal systems (Nomiyama, 1980; Friberg and Kjellstrom, 1981).

Chronic Pulmonary Disease. Toxicity to the respiratory system is proportional to the time and level of exposure. Obstructive lung disease results from chronic bronchitis, progressive fibrosis of the lower airways, and accompanying alveolar damage leading to emphysema. The lung disease is manifested by dypsnea, reduced vital capacity, and increased residual volume. The pathogenesis of the lung lesion is turnover and necrosis of alveolar macrophages. Released enzymes produce irreversible damage to alveolar basement membranes including rupture of septa and interstitial fibrosis. It has been found that cadmium reduces α-1-antitrypsin activity, perhaps enhancing pulmonary toxicity (Chowdbury and Louria, 1976). However, no difference in plasma α-1-antitrypsin activity could be found between cadmium-exposed workers with and without emphysema (Lauwerys et al., 1979).

Kidney. The effects of cadmium on proximal renal tubular function are manifested by increased cadmium in the urine, proteinuria, aminoaciduria, glucosuria, and decreased renal tubular reabsorption of phosphate. Morphologic changes are nonspecific and consist of tubular cell degeneration in the initial stages, progressing to an interstitial inflammatory reaction and fibrosis. The nephropathy occurs when cadmium concentration reaches a level in the kidney (200 μg/g) that has been widely referred to as the critical concentration of cadmium.

The proteinuria is principally tubular, consisting of low-molecular-weight proteins whose tubular reabsorption has been impaired by cadmium injury to proximal tubular lining cells. The predominant protein is a β_2 microglobulin, but a number of other low-molecular-weight proteins have been identified in the urine of workers with excessive cadmium exposure, such as retinol-binding protein, lysozyme, ribonuclease, and immunoglobulin light chains (Lauwerys et al., 1979). High-molecular-weight proteins in the urine, such as albumin and transferin, indicate that some workers may actually have a mixed proteinuria and suggesting a glomerular effect as well. The nature of the glomerular lesion in cadmium nephropathy has not been studied extensively, but circulating antiglomerular basement membrane antibodies have been identified in humans and rats chronically exposed to cadmium, suggesting the presence of immunologically induced glomerular disease in addition to the tubulonephropathy (Lauwerys et al., 1984).

Aminoaciduria in cadmium toxicity is generalized, reflecting increased excretion of amino acids normally reabsorbed by proximal tubular lining cells. The severity of the aminoaciduria is increased in cadmium workers with increasing levels of cadmium exposure. In addition, particularly large increases in proline and hydroxyproline excretion have been noted in patients with chronic cadmium toxicity with bone disease or Itai-Itai disease, but this probably reflects the changes in bone metabolism found in these people. Glucosuria and decreased tubular reabsorption of phosphate parallel the occurrence of low-molecular-weight proteinuria and aminoaciduria, reflecting the proximal tubular cell effect. Proximal tubular dysfunction may be symptom-free for a number of years, but tubular dysfunction may progress resulting in hypercalcuria, renal calculi, and rarely osteomalacia and evidence of distal tubular dysfunction (Kazantzis, 1979).

Although most of the data available to date related to cadmium exposure and cadmium nephropathy have been obtained from workers with occupational exposure, there is some evidence now that persons in the general population with nonoccupational exposure to cadmium may also have cadmium-related renal tubular dysfunction. Among inhabitants of cadmium-polluted areas of Japan where dietary content of cadmium is increased, the prevalence of proteinuria and glucosuria is higher than in control

areas, and there is some association between increased excretion of low-molecular-weight proteins in urine and level of cadmium pollution (Shigematsu et al., 1978). Also, Lauwerys et al. (1980) studied a group of Belgian women and found that a group of women living near a nonferrous metal smelter had a higher body burden as reflected by an increased excretion of cadmium in urine and a higher prevalence of signs of renal dysfunction than women from a control area.

Critical Concentration of Cadmium. With this awareness that cadmium-induced nephropathy may occur in persons in the general population, it becomes of major public health importance to know what is the maximum level of cadmium exposure that a person can be exposed to without risk of renal tubular dysfunction and cadmium nephropathy. Also, the concept of a critical concentration of cadmium has very important implications with regard to establishing maximum levels of cadmium that human populations may be exposed to with some margin of safety.

Kjellstrom et al. (1977), have established a metabolic model relating daily intake of cadmium and concentration of cadmium in renal cortex. The geometric average intake of cadmium was 14 μg cadmium per day, corresponding to a concentration of cadmium in the renal cortex at about age 50 of around 10 μg/g. The WHO Task Force estimated that daily ingestion of 200 to 300 μg cadmium per day would be required to reach the critical kidney cortex concentration of 200 μg cadmium per gram at age 50 for a 70-kg man. Rats given daily injections of cadmium also develop a nephropathy when renal cadmium concentration reaches about 200 μg/g kidney weight (Goyer, 1982).

Role of Metallothionein in Cadmium Toxicity. Accumulation of cadmium in the kidney without apparent toxic effect is possible because of formation of cadmium-thionein or metallothionein, a metal protein complex with a low molecular weight (about 6500 Daltons) (Suzuki, 1982).

The amino acid composition of metallothionein is characterized by approximately 30 percent cysteine and the absence of aromatic amino acids. Specific optical absorption is due to location of metal thiolate complexes in the protein. Metallothionein contains 61 amino acids and 20 are cysteine. Structural studies using nuclear magnetic resonance spectroscopy and electron spin resonance spectroscopy have identified two distinct metal clusters in mammalian metallothionein. The clusters seem to have significant differences in their affinity for different metal ions; one of the clusters has a high level of specificity for zinc. Metal binding is by trimer-captide bridges (Boulanger *et al.*, 1983). Metallothionein is primarily a tissue protein and is ubiquitous in most organs but is in highest concentration in liver, particularly following recent exposure, and in kidney where it accumulates with age in proportion to cadmium concentration.

A number of studies from experimental animals, as well as tissue culture models, confirm the protective role of metallothionein. It has been found that synthesis of metallothionein in tissues is directly related to exposure to metal and toxicity to kidney probably only occurs when exposure exceeds the ability of that organ to either synthesize metallothionein or store additional cadmium. Toxic cell injury is thought to be caused by unbound cadmium or free cadmium ion. Administration of metallothionein prepared with different ratios of cadmium and zinc to rats has demonstrated that renal tubular necrosis is related to the cadmium content, not the amount of metallothionein (Suzuki *et al.*, 1979; Suzuki, 1982).

Pretreatment of experimental animals with small doses of cadmium has been shown to prevent acute toxic effects of a large dose of cadmium. This property is not restricted to protection from cadmium toxicity alone. Pretreatment of experimental animals with small doses of cadmium or mercury salts can prevent the nephrotoxic effects of high doses of mercury chloride. There is also some experimental evidence that suggests that the teratogenic effects of cadmium in Golden hamsters is prevented by pretreatment with zinc salts of small amounts of metallothionein. Other studies have shown that certain sulfhydryl-requiring enzymes are inhibited *in vitro* by small amounts of cadmium but not affected *in vivo* where intracellular cadmium is bound to metallothionein. Human cells in tissue culture, in which metallothionein has been induced by pretreatment with cadmium, become resistant to previously lethal exposure to cadmium (Cherian and Nordberg, 1983).

Experimental studies have shown that cadmium administered parenterally as inorganic and cadmium bound to metallothionein has a different distribution in organs. Inorganic cadmium is largely recovered in liver whereas cadmium from cadmium metallothionein is preferentially taken up by kidney (Cherian *et al.*, 1976).

Skeletal System. Cadmium toxicity affects calcium metabolism, and individuals with severe cadmium nephropathy may have renal calculi and excess excretion of calcium, probably related to increased urinary loss, but with chronic exposure, urine calcium may be less than normal. Associated skeletal changes are probably related to calcium loss and include bone pain, osteomalacia, and/or osteoporosis. Bone changes are part of a syndrome recognized in postmenopausal multiparous women living the the Fuchu area of Japan prior to and during World War II. The syndrome consisted of severe bony deformities and chronic renal disease. Excess cadmium exposure has been implicated in the pathogenesis of the syndrome, but vitamin D and perhaps other nutritional deficiencies are thought to be cofactors. "Itai-Itai" translates to "ouch-ouch," reflecting the accompanying bone pain (Nomiyama, 1980).

Hypertension and Cardiovascular Disease. Schroeder and Balassa (1961) first reported that the chronic feeding of low levels (5 ppm) of cadmium in drinking water to rats could induce hypertension. These experimental results have been confirmed (Perry and Erlanger, 1974) and a number of mechanisms for the pathogenesis of the hypertension suggested, including increased sodium retention, direct vasoconstriction, hyperreninemia, and increased cardiac output. Recent studies from Japan found a twice-as-high cerebrovascular disease mortality rate among people who had cadmium-induced renal tubular proteinuria as among people in cadmium-polluted areas without proteinuria (Nogawa *et al.*, 1979).

Carcinogenicity. An increase in carcinoma of the prostate was first noted in a mortality study of battery workers in England in 1965, but this was not found in a study of a large worker population (Armstrong and Kazantzis, 1983). The problem of prostatic cancer is further complicated by the high incidence of latent *(in situ)* carcinoma of the prostate in elderly men in the general population and the implication of numerous other factors, such as marital status (singles), race (nonwhites), and even religion. There have been numerous experimental studies supporting the potential carcinogenicity of cadmium. Metallic cadmium or cadmium sulfide or sulfate given subcutaneously or intramuscularly will induce sarcomata at the site of injection in experimental animals. The tumors are truly malignant and have been found to metastasize to lymph nodes and lungs. Also, it was found many years ago that injection of several milligrams of cadmium per kilogram body weight to mice causes acute testicular necrosis followed by Leydig cell tumors. The pathogenesis of the Leydig cell tumors appears to be hormone dependent and is preceded by decreases in serum testosterone levels and stimulation of Leydig cell hyperplasia and tumors. Testicular necrosis as well as Leydig cell tumor formation is prevented by supplemental zinc (Piscator, 1981). Carcinoma of lungs has recently been produced by exposing rats to cadmium aerosols (Takenaka *et al.*, 1983).

Biologic Indicators. The most important measure of excessive cadmium exposure is increased cadmium excretion in urine. In persons in the general population, without excessive cadmium exposure, urine cadmium excretion is both small and constant. That is, it is usually in the order of only 1 or 2 μg/day, or less than 1 μg/g creatinine. With excessive exposure to cadmium as might occur in workers, increase in urine cadmium may not occur until all of the available cadmium binding sites are saturated. However, when binding sites (metallothionein) are saturated, increased urine cadmium reflects recent exposure and body burden and renal cadmium concentration so that urine cadmium measurement does provide a good index of excessive cadmium exposure. Nogawa *et al.* (1979), determined the urinary concentration of cadmium corresponding to a 1 percent prevalence rate of a number of abnormal urinary findings (Table 19–4). Tubular proteinuria, as indicated by measurable excretion of β_2-microglobulin, occurred at the 1 percent prevalence rate with a urinary cadmium concentration of 3.2 μg/g of creatinine. This was at a slightly lower urine cadmium level than other signs of renal tubular dysfunction. Retinol binding protein may be a more practical and reliable test of proximal tubular function than β_2 microglobulin because sensitive immunologic analytic methods are now available, and it is more stable in urine (Lauwerys *et al.*, 1984). Changes in urinary excretion of low-molecular-weight proteins are mainly observed in workers excreting more than 10 μg cadmium per gram creatinine (Buchet *et al.*, 1980).

Most of the cadmium in urine is bound to metallothionein, and there is good correlation between metallothionein and cadmium in urine in cadmium workers with normal or abnormal renal function (Shaikh and Hirayama, 1979). Therefore, measurement of metallothionein in urine provides the same toxicologic information as measurement of cadmium and, in addition, does not have the problem of external contamination. Radioimmunoassay techniques for measurement of metallothionein are evolving rapidly (Chang *et al.*, 1980; Tohyama and Shaikh, 1981).

Recently, *in vivo* neutron activation analysis has been used to measure cadmium in liver and kidney in exposed workers. The detection limits are at least 15 mg/kg in kidney cortex and 1.5 mg/kg in liver, so that the method is not suf-

Table 19–4. URINARY CADMIUM CONCENTRATION CORRESPONDING TO 1 PERCENT PREVALENCE RATE FOR PARAMETERS OF RENAL DYSFUNCTION*

URINARY FINDING	URINARY CADMIUM PER μg/g CREATININE	
	Male	*Female*
Tubular proteinuria		
β_2-microglobulin	3.2	5.2
Retinal binding protein	4.4	7.4
Aminoaciduria (proline)	10.4	5.1
Proteinuria with glucosuria	7.4	7.4

* Data from Nogawa *et al.* (1979).

ficiently sensitive to measure *in vivo* tissue levels in persons in the general population (Ellis *et al.*, 1981). Applying this technique to cadmium-exposed workers, Roels, Lawerys, and co-workers found a wide range of variability and overlap in kidney cadmium concentration associated with and without renal disease. On the basis of their study of 309 workers, the critical concentration of cadmium in renal cortex may range from 215 to 390 ppm (Roels *et al.*, 1983).

Treatment. Susceptibility to cadmium-induced toxicity is influenced by a number of factors, particularly ability of the body to provide binding sites on metallothionein. Protection is provided by dietary zinc, cobalt, or selenium. Treatment of the toxicity of cadmium on the kidney is to cease exposure to cadmium (Nordberg *et al.*, 1978). What severity of cadmium-induced tubular dysfunction is reversible is still not certain.

Chelation therapy is not available for cadmium toxicity in humans. Experimental studies have shown that the action of chelating agents on the pharmacokinetics of cadmium depends on the time of administration of the chelators after cadmium exposure. When the chelators are given shortly after cadmium exposure, when no new matallothionein has been synthesized, the thiol-containing chelators such as BAL and penicillamine increase the biliary excretion of cadmium while EDTA, DPTA, and related chelators increase urinary excretion (Cherian and Rodgers, 1982). For chronic cadmium exposure, when cadmium is bound to metallothionein, there is little effect from chelation therapy.

Chromium

Chromium is a generally abundant element in the earth's crust and occurs in oxidation states ranging from Cr^{2+} to Cr^{6+}, but only the trivalent and hexavalent forms are of biologic significance. The trivalent is the more common form. However, hexavalent forms of chromate compounds are of greater industrial importance. Sodium chromate and dichromate are the principal substances for the production of all chromium chemicals. Sodium dichromate is produced industrially by the reaction of sulfuric acid on sodium chromate. The major source of chromium is from chromite ore. Metallurgic-grade chromite is usually converted into one of several types of ferrochromium or other chromium alloys containing cobalt or nickel. Ferrochrome is used for the production of stainless steel. Chromates are produced by a smelting, roasting, and extraction process. The major uses of sodium dichromate are for the production of chrome pigments, for the production of chrome salts used for tanning leather, mordant dying, wood preservatives, and as an anticorrosive in cooking systems, boilers, and oil drilling muds (NAS, 1974; Fishbein, 1981).

Chromium in ambient air originates from industrial sources, particularly ferrochrome production, ore refining, chemical and refractory processing, and combustion of fossil fuels. In rural areas, chromium in air is usually less than 0.1 ng/m^3 and from 0.01 to 0.03 μg/m^3 in industrial cities. Particulates from coal-fired power plants may contain from 2.3 to 31 ppm, but this is reduced to 0.19 to 6.6 ppm by fly-ash collection. Cement-producing plants are another important potential source of atmospheric chromium. Chromium precipitates and fallout are deposited on land and water; land fallout is eventually carried to water by runoff, where it is deposited in sediments. A controllable source of chromium is waste water from chrome-plating and metal-finishing industries, textile plants, and tanneries. Chromium in food is low, and estimates of daily intake by humans is under 100 μg, mostly from food, with trivial quantities from most water supplies and ambient air.

Disposition. Trivalent chromium is the most common form found in nature, and chromium in biologic materials is probably always trivalent. There is no evidence that trivalent chromium is converted to hexavalent forms in biologic systems. However, hexavalent chromium readily crosses cell membranes and is reduced intracellularly to trivalent chromium.

The known harmful effects of chromium in humans have been attributed to the hexavalent form, and it has been speculated that the biologic effects of hexavalent chromium may be related to the reduction to trivalent chromium and the formation of complexes with intracellular macromolecules. High concentrations of chromium are normally found in RNA, but its role is

unknown. Trace quantities of trivalent chromium are essential for carbohydrate metabolism in mammals. It is a cofactor for insulin action and has a role in the peripheral activities of this hormone by forming a ternary complex with insulin receptors, facilitating the attachment of insulin to these sites. The most biologically active form of insulin appears to be a naturally occurring complex containing niacin as well as glycine, glutamic acid, and cysteine (Underwood, 1977).

Human chromium deficiency may be occurring in infants suffering from protein-caloric malnutrition and elderly people with impaired glucose tolerance, but this is not well documented. Prolonged use of a synthetic diet without chromium supplementation may lead to chromium deficiency, impaired glucose metabolism, and possibly effects on growth and on lipid and protein metabolism. Half-time for elimination of chromium from rats is 0.5, 5.9, and 83.4 days, according to a three-compartment model (Mertz, 1969).

Human kinetic studies have identified an erythrocyte chromium compartment that corresponds to the survival time of the red blood cell and is almost exclusively excreted in urine.

Toxicology. Systemic toxicity to chromium compounds occurs largely from accidental exposures, occasional attempts to use chromium as a suicidal agent, and previous therapeutic uses. The major acute effect from ingested chromium is acute renal tubular necrosis (Langard and Norseth, 1979).

Exposure to chromium, particularly in the chrome production and chrome pigment industries, is associated with cancer of the respiratory tract (Norseth, 1981). As early as 1936, German health authorities recognized cancer of the lung among workers exposed to chromium dust. In a review paper from 1950, Baetjer described 109 cases of cancer in the chromate-producing industry, 11 cases in the chrome pigment industry, and two cases in other industries. In a review of the histologic classification of 123 cases of lung cancer in chromate workers, Hueper (1966) found 46 squamous cell carcinomas, 66 anaplastic tumors, and 11 adenocarcinomas. The greatest risk to cancer is attributed to exposure to acid-soluble, water-insoluble hexavalent chromium as occurs in the roasting or refining processes. Other studies have supported the greater risk to cancer from exposure to slightly soluble, hexavalent compounds rather than trivalent chromium compounds. Hexavalent chromium is corrosive and causes chronic ulceration and perforation of the nasal septum. It also causes chronic ulceration of other skin surfaces, which is independent of hypersensitivity reactions on skin. Allergic chromium skin reactions readily occur with exposure and are independent of dose. Trivalent chromium compounds are considerably less toxic than the hexavalent compounds and are neither irritating nor corrosive. Nevertheless, nearly all workers in industries are exposed to both forms of chromium compounds, and at present, there is no information as to whether there is a gradient of risk from predominant exposure to hexavalent or insoluble forms of chromium to exposure to soluble trivalent forms. In a recent review, Norseth (1981) suggests that if there are similar increased risks in both groups, as estimated from the death rates, trivalent chromium should be considered as an equally potent carcinogen as are the hexavalent compounds.

Whether chromium compounds cause cancer at sites other than the respiratory tract is not clear. A slight increase in cancer of the gastrointestinal tract has been reported in other studies, but each involved only small groups of workers.

Animal studies support the notion that the most potent carcinogenic chromium compounds are the slightly soluble hexavalent compounds. Studies on *in vitro* bacterial systems, however, show no difference between soluble and slightly soluble compounds. Trivalent chromium salts have little or no mutagenic activity in bacterial systems. Since there is preferred uptake of the hexavalent form by cells and it is the trivalent form that is metabolically active and binds with nucleic acids within the cell, it has been suggested that the causative agent in chromium mutagenesis is trivalent chromium bound to genetic material after reduction of the hexavalent form (Norseth, 1981).

Human Body Burden. Tissue concentrations of chromium in the general population have considerable geographic variation, as high as 7 μg/kg in lungs of persons in New York or Chicago with lower concentrations in liver and kidney (Schroeder *et al.*, 1962a). In persons without excess exposure, blood chromium concentration is between 20 and 30 μg/liter and is evenly distributed between erythrocytes and plasma. With occupational exposure, increase in blood chromium is related to increase in chromium in red blood cells. Urinary excretion is generally less than 10 μg/day in the absence of excess exposure (Underwood, 1977).

Lead

If we were to judge of the interest excited by any medical subject by the number of writings to which it has given birth, we could not but regard the poisoning by lead as the most important to be known of all those that have been treated of, up to the present time.

ORFILA, 1817

Lead, the most ubiquitous toxic metal, is detectable in practically all phases of the inert environment and in all biologic systems. Because it is toxic to most living things at high exposures and there is no demonstrated biologic need, the major issue regarding lead is at what dose does it become toxic. Specific concerns vary with the age and circumstances of the host, and the major risk is toxicity to the nervous system. Several reviews and multiauthored books on the toxicology of lead are available (NAS, 1972; Goyer and Rhyne, 1973; WHO, 1977b; Nriagu, 1978; Singhal and Thomas, 1980; Needleman, 1980; Chisolm and O'Hara, 1982; Rutter and Jones, 1983).

Sources. The principal route of exposure is food, but it is usually environmental and presumably controllable sources that produce excess exposure and toxic effects. These sources include lead-based indoor paint in old dwellings, lead in air from combustion of lead-containing auto exhausts or industrial emissions, lead-based paint, hand-to-mouth activities of young children living in polluted environments, and, less commonly, lead dust brought home by industrial workers on their clothes and shoes, and lead-glazed earthen ware.

The total daily intake of lead for an adult in the United States varies from less than 0.1 mg/day to more than 2 mg/day (Kehoe, 1961; NAS, 1972). The major source of daily intake of lead in adults and children (without excess exposure) is food and beverages. Lead content of food is extremely variable, but there are practically no lead-free food items. The average adult diet contains from 150 μg/day, 0.75 to 120 μg/day for infants and small children. Most municipal water supplies measured at the tap contain less than the WHO-recommended limit of 0.05 μg/ml, so that daily intake from water is usually about 10 μg, and unlikely to be more than 20 μg.

Air is a third source of lead exposure for persons in the general population. Concentrations of lead in air vary widely and may be lower than 1.0 μg/m^3 in rural areas to 10 μg/m^3 in certain urban environments. For the contemporary urbanite, the magnitude of respired lead is about one-half the intake from the diet.

Disposition. The gastrointestinal absorption of lead is influenced by a large number of factors of which age and nutritional factors are of particular importance. Adults absorb 5 to 15 percent of ingested lead and usually retain less than 5 percent of what is absorbed. Children are known to have a greater absorption of lead than adults; one study found an average net absorption of 41.5 percent and 31.8 percent net retention in infants on regular diets.

Lead in the atmosphere exists either in solid

forms, dust or particulates of lead dioxide, or in the form of vapors, particularly alkyl lead that has escaped by evaporation from automobile fuel systems.

Lead absorption by the lungs also depends on a number of factors in addition to concentration. These include volume of air respired per day, whether the lead is in particle or vapor form, and size distribution of lead-containing particles. Only a very minor fraction of particles over 0.5 μm in mean maximal external diameter are retained in the lung but are cleared from the respiratory track and swallowed. However, the percentage of particles less than 0.5 μm retained in the lung increases with reduction in particle size. About 90 percent of lead particles in ambient air that are deposited in the lungs are small enough to be retained. Absorption of retained lead through alveoli is relatively efficient and complete.

More than 90 percent of lead in blood is in the red blood cells. There seem to be at least two major compartments for lead in the red blood cell, one associated with the membrane and the other with hemoglobin (Barltrop and Smith, 1971). Small fractions may be related to other red blood cell components. Plasma ligands are not well defined, but it has been suggested that plasma and serum may contain diffusible fractions of lead in equilibrium with soft tissue or end-organ binding sites for lead. This fraction is difficult to measure accurately, but there is an equilibrium between red cell and plasma lead.

Blood lead levels are a good indicator of recent exposure to lead and are influenced by inhalation and ingestion. A number of recent studies suggest that inhalation of air containing 1 μg/m^3 in respirable particles will increase blood lead concentrations by about 1 μg/dl when air lead concentrations are in the range of 1 to 5 μg/m^3 (WHO, 1977b).

Lead in blood varies with age (Figure 19-3) (Mahaffey et al., 1982). Children under seven years of age have significantly higher blood lead levels than older children, and there is no difference between boys and girls under age 12. Blood lead levels decline during adolescence probably related to bone growth and deposition of lead in bones with calcium. Blood lead levels are lower in adult females than adult males.

The total body burden of lead may be divided into at least two kinetic pools, which have different rates of turnover. The largest and kinetically slowest pool is the skeleton with a half-life of more than 20 years and a much more labile soft tissue pool. The total lifetime accumulation of lead may be about 200 mg and over 500 mg for an occupationally exposed worker. Kidney lead accumulates with age; lead in lung does not

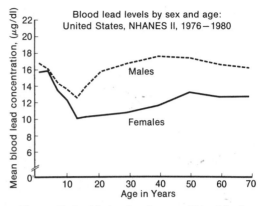

Figure 19-3. National estimates of blood lead levels in the United States. (From Mahaffey, K. R.; Annest, J. L.; Roberts, J.; and Murphy, R. S.: Estimates of blood lead levels: United States 1976-1980. Association with selected demographic and socioeconomic factors. *N. Engl. J. Med.*, **307**:573-79, 1982. Reprinted by permission of *The New England Journal of Medicine.*)

change. Lead in the central nervous system tends to concentrate in gray matter and certain nuclei. The highest concentrations are in the hippocampus, followed by cerebellum, cerebral cortex, and medulla. Cortical white matter seems to contain the least amount, but these comments are based on only a few reported human and animal studies.

Renal excretion of lead is usually with glomerular filtrate with some renal tubular resorption. With elevated blood lead levels, excretion may be augmented by transtubular transport.

Placental transfer of lead occurs. Cord blood generally correlates with maternal blood lead levels but is slightly lower. It is interesting that maternal blood lead decreases during pregnancy, suggesting that maternal lead is transferred to the fetus or excreted in some way.

Toxicity. The topic of greatest interest at the present time concerns the maximal level of lead exposure in the neonatal and young child that does not produce a cognitive or motor neurologic deficit. For the adult excess occupational exposure or even accidental exposure, the concerns are peripheral neuropathy and/or chronic nephropathy. Effects on the heme system provide biochemical indicators of lead exposure in the absence of chemically detectable effects, but anemia due to lead exposure is uncommon without other detectable effects or other synergistic factors. Other target organs are the gastrointestinal and reproductive systems.

Nearly all environmental exposure to lead is to inorganic compounds, even lead in food. Organolead exposures, including tetraethyl lead, have unique toxicologic patterns and will be discussed later.

Neurologic Effects. The central nervous system (CNS) effects of lead are the most significant in terms of human health and performance (Needleman, 1980; Rutter and Jones, 1983). Manifestations of CNS effects are encephalopathy and/or peripheral neuropathy. Symptomatic encephalopathy is almost always a disease of childhood and varies from ataxia to stupor, coma, and convulsions. This form of lead intoxication has decreased appreciably in North America over the past 20 years with better understanding of factors that contribute to lead toxicity, particularly reduction of lead exposure in children. Morphologic effects of lead on the brain are nonspecific. Lead encephalopathy is accompanied by severe cerebral edema, increase in cerebral spinal fluid pressure, proliferation and swelling of endothelial cells in capillaries and arterioles, proliferation of glial cells, neuronal degeneration, and areas of focal cortical necrosis in fatal cases.

The pathogenesis of neuronal damage in lead encephalopathy is not well understood. In severe cases, there are obvious changes in hemodynamics (cerebral edema) and cellular hypoxia, but it is now apparent that there is a direct effect of lead on neuronal and possibly synaptic transmission at levels of lead exposure that do not produce apparent symptoms of intoxication. These effects are termed "low-level lead toxicity" because they are believed to be associated with blood lead levels of approximately 30 to 50 μg/dl or possibly even lower bloodlead levels. These effects are also termed "subclinical lead toxicity" because they can only be detected by assessment of neuropsychologic behavior, such as hyperactivity, poor classroom behavior (decreased attention span), and even small decrements (point average in group studies) of four to five in I.Q. scores (Needleman *et al.*, 1979). Studies by others confirm the subclinical detrimental effects on I.Q., but possibly occurring at somewhat higher blood lead levels than found by Needleman (Ernhardt *et al.*, 1981). However, that low-level lead exposure (blood lead, 30 to 50 μg/dl) does, indeed, affect CNS function is further supported by the finding of changes in EEG brain wave patterns and CNS evoked potential responses in children displaying neuropsychologic deficits (Burchfield *et al.*, 1980). Neurochemical studies in experimental models have shown that lead in the absence of morphologic changes does produce deficits in neurotransmission through inhibition of cholinergic function, possibly by reduction of extracellular calcium. Other noted changes in neurotransmitter function include impairment of dopamine uptake by synaptosomes and impairment of the function of the inhibitory neurotransmitter γ-aminobutyric acid.

Peripheral neuropathy is a classic manifestation of lead toxicity, particularly the footdrop and wristdrop that characterized the house painter and other workers with excessive occupational exposure to lead more than a half-century ago (Thomas, 1904). Segmental demyelination and possibly axonal degeneration follow lead-induced Schwann cell degeneration (Lampert and Schochet, 1968). Wallerian degeneration of posterior roots of sciatic and tibial nerves is possible, but sensory nerves are less sensitive to lead than motor nerve structure and function (Schlaepfer, 1969). Motor nerve dysfunction, assessed clinically by electrophysiologic measurement of nerve conduction velocities, has been shown to occur with blood lead levels in the 50 to 70 μg/dl range or lower (Seppalainen *et al.*, 1975).

Hematologic Effects. Lead has multiple hematologic effects. In lead-induced anemia, the red blood cells are microcytic and hypochronic, as in iron deficiency, and usually there are increased numbers of reticulocytes with basophilic stippling. This morphologic characteristic has long been recognized as a feature of lead-induced anemia and in the past (pre–World War II), it was employed as a method of monitoring workers in the lead industry (McCord *et al.*, 1935).

The test is no longer useful because it is now known to be nonspecific and, most important, it is an uncommon occurrence with blood lead below 80 μg/dl, which is considerably above the present-day permissible industrial standard. Basophilic stippling results from inhibition of the enzyme pyrimidine-5-nucleotidase (Paglia *et al.*, 1975), which cleaves residual nucleotide chains remaining in erythrocytes after extrusion of the nucleus. The activity of this enzyme is decreased in persons with elevated blood lead levels even when stippling is not morphologically evident.

The anemia that occurs in lead poisoning results from two basic defects: shortened erythrocyte life-span and impairment of heme synthesis. Shortened life-span of the red blood cell is thought to be due to increased mechanical fragility of the cell membrane. The biochemical basis for this effect is not known but is accompanied by inhibition of sodium- and potassium-dependent ATPase's (Hernberg *et al.*, 1967).

A schematic presentation of effects of lead on heme synthesis is shown in Figure 19–4. Probably the sensitive effect is inhibition of δ-aminolevulinic acid dehydratase (ALA-D), resulting in a negative exponential relationship

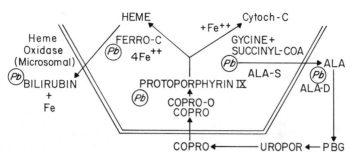

Figure 19–4. Scheme of heme synthesis showing sites where lead has an effect. *COA*, coenzyme A; *ALA-S*, aminolevulinic acid synthetase; *ALA*, *d*-aminolevulinic acid; *ALA-D*, aminoleuvulinic acid dehydratase; *PBG*, porphobilinogen; *UROPOR*, uroporphyrinogen; *COPRO*, coproporphyrinogen; *COPRO-O*, coproporphyrinogen oxidase; *FERRO-C*, Ferrochelatase; *CYTOCH-C*, cytochrome c; (Pb), site for lead effect.

between ALA-D and blood lead. There is also depression of coproporphyrinogen oxidase, resulting in increased coproporphyrin activity. Lead also decreases ferrochelatase activity. This enzyme catalyzes the incorporation of the ferrous ion into the porphyrin ring structure. Bessis and Jensen (1965) have shown that iron in the form of apoferritin and ferruginous micelles may accumulate in mitochondria of bone marrow reticulocytes from lead-poisoned rats. Failure to insert iron into protoporphyrin results in depressed heme formation. The excess protoporphyrin takes the place of heme in the hemoglobin molecule and, as the red blood cells containing protoporphyrin circulate, zinc is chelated at the center of the molecule at the site usually occupied by iron. Red blood cells containing zinc-protoporphyrin are intensely fluorescent and may be used to diagnose lead toxicity. Depressed heme synthesis is thought to be the stimulus for increasing the rate of activity of the first step in the heme synthetic pathway, δ-aminolevulinic acid synthetase, by virtue of negative feedback control as proposed by Granick and Levere (1964). As a consequence, the increased production of *d*-aminolevulinic acid and decreased activity of ALA-D result in a marked increase in circulating blood levels and urinary excretion of *d*-ALA. Prefeeding of lead to experimental animals also raises heme oxygenase activity, resulting in some increase in bilirubin formation. The change in rates of activity of these enzymes by lead produces a dose-related alteration in activity of affected enzymes, but anemia only occurs in very marked lead toxicity. The changes in enzyme activities, particularly ALA-D in peripheral blood and excretion of ALA in urine, correlate very closely with actual blood lead levels and serve as early biochemical indices of lead effect.

Renal Effects. Toxicologic effects of lead on the kidney divide into two major concerns: reversible renal tubular dysfunction that occurs mostly in children with acute exposure to lead, usually associated with overt central nervous system effects, and irreversible chronic interstitial nephropathy characterized by vascular sclerosis, tubular cell atrophy, interstitial fibrosis, and glomerular sclerosis (Goyer, 1971a). It is most often seen in workmen with years of exposure to lead. In the early stages of excess lead exposure, morphologic and functional changes in the kidney are confined to the renal tubules and are most pronounced in proximal tubular cells.

A pathognomonic feature of lead poisoning is the presence of characteristic nuclear inclusions bodies (Goyer, 1971b). By light microscopy the inclusions are dense, homogeneous eosinophilic bodies. They are acid-fast when stained with carbolfuchsin. Ultrastructurally the bodies have a dense central core and outer fibrillary region, as shown in Figure 19–5. The bodies are composed of a lead-protein complex (Moore *et al.*, 1973). The protein is acidic and contains large amounts of aspartic and glutamic acids and little cystine. It is suggested that lead binds loosely to the carboxyl groups of the acidic amino acids. Most of the lead in the tubular cell is bound to the inclusion body. The sequestering of lead in these complexes may protect more susceptible organelles like mitochondria and endoplasmic reticulum (Goyer, 1971b).

Experimental studies have shown that nuclear inclusion bodies are the earliest evidence of lead exposure and may be observed before any of the functional changes are detectable. Cells containing inclusion bodies are usually swollen and contain altered mitochondria. It has been shown that mitochondria isolated from kidneys of rats

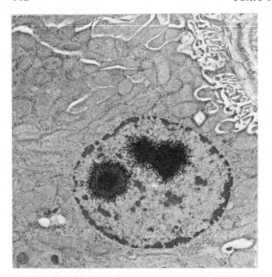

Figure 19–5. Lead-induced inclusion bodies in nucleus of renal tubular lining cell.

with lead toxicity have impaired oxidative and phosphorylative abilities. This may in part be responsible for the decrease in reabsorptive functions of proximal tubular cells. Experimental animals and people, that is, children and workmen with early exposure to lead, have a generalized amino aciduria, glycosuria, and hyperphosphaturia, and probably some impairment of sodium reabsorption. Some indirect evidence for an effect of lead on sodium transport is found in the clinical observation that the renin-aldosterone response to sodium deprivation is altered in people with lead intoxication (Sandstead *et al.,* 1970).

The pathogenesis of the inclusion bodies may be related to renal tubular cell transport and excretion of lead. Treatment of lead-exposed animals with chelating agents such as EDTA is accompanied by a sudden spike of urinary lead, which is maximum 12 to 24 hours after treatment (Goyer and Wilson, 1975). Also, no inclusion bodies can be found by morphologic study of renal tubular cells after EDTA therapy. The bodies may also be found intact in the urinary sediment of workmen with heavy exposure to lead (Schumann *et al.,* 1980). The bodies account for the major fraction of intracellular lead, and their loss in the urine may reflect a major pathway for lead excretion.

With continued exposure to lead there is a gradual change in morphology beginning with the appearance of peritubular and periglomerular fibrosis, particularly in the deep cortex of juxtamedullary zone (Goyer, 1971a). This is accompanied by atrophy of some tubules and hyperplasia of others. There are also fewer in-

clusion bodies present in the advanced stages of lead-induced nephrosclerosis, and it may be impossible to find any inclusion bodies in lead-induced nephrosclerosis. Recognition of interstitial fibrosis induced by lead, therefore, from any other forms of interstitial fibrosis is not possible morphologically, but must be made from history and knowledge of progression of the disease if this is available.

The most important feature of the changes associated with acute lead nephropathy is that they are reversible, either by reduction of lead exposure or by chelation therapy, but the progression into interstitial fibrosis is not reversible. It is very important, therefore, to diagnose this disorder as early as possible so that exposure to lead can be discontinued and decrease in function halted. At the present time there is no single definitive diagnostic test that will recognize lead-induced interstitial nephropathy except possibly renal biopsy, but this is not a practical measure. There have been several clinical studies in recent years of renal function in workmen with long-term occupational exposure to lead (Wedeen *et al.,* 1979; Lilis *et al.,* 1979; Hong *et al.,* 1980). If looked at together, the conclusion is reached that an early functional accompaniment of interstitial fibrosis is a reduction in glomerular filtration rate.

The relationship between chronic lead exposure and gouty nephropathy, suggested more than a hundred years ago by the English physician Garrod, has received recent support from studies showing that gout patients with renal disease have a greater chelate-provoked lead excretion than do renal patients without gout (Batuman *et al.,* 1981). Lead reduces uric acid excretion (Emerson, 1963). Elevated blood uric acid has been demonstrated in rats with chronic lead nephropathy (Goyer, 1971a).

The relationship between lead and hypertension is uncertain; it has been associated with lead poisoning in a number of studies but not in others. The second National Health and Nutrition Examination Survey (1976–1980) found a statistically significant relationship between blood pressure and blood lead levels in white males age 40–59 years (Pirkle *et al.* 1985). Hypertension may follow the vascular changes associated with lead-induced chronic renal disease, or changes in renin-angiotensin-aldosterone metabolism (Sandstead, 1970; Victery *et al.,* 1982).

Carcinogenesis. The possible carcinogenic effects of lead have been receiving increasing attention (IARC, 1980). It is clear that lead can induce cancer in kidneys of rodents fed high doses of lead (Moore and Meredith, 1979). On the other hand, the evidence that lead is carcinogenic to humans is very limited. A study of workmen in England many years ago with occupational exposure to lead did not show an increased incidence of cancer (Dingwall-Fordyce and Lane, 1963). A more recent study of causes of mortality in 7000 lead workers in the United States showed a slight excess of deaths from cancer (Cooper and Gaffey, 1975), but the statistical significance of these findings has been debated (Kang *et al.*, 1980; Cooper, 1980). The most common tumors found were of the respiratory and digestive systems, not the kidney. However, case reports of renal adenocarcinoma in workmen with prolonged occupational exposure to lead have appeared (Baker *et al.*, 1980; Lilis, 1981).

Other Effects. Severe lead toxicity has long been known to cause sterility, abortion, and neonatal mortality and morbidity. Studies have demonstrated gametotoxic effects in both male and female animals. However, the impact of levels of lead exposure occurring in today's society on reproductive effects is uncertain. The greatest concern is for intrauterine effects on the unborn fetus. Umbilical cord blood levels are the same as those of mother's blood, and because of the greater sensitivity of the fetus, pregnancy must be regarded as a period of increased susceptibility to lead.

A few clinical studies have found increased chromosomal defects in workers with blood lead levels above 60 μg/dl (Deknudt *et al.*, 1977). Experimental studies suggest that lead alters the humoral immune system and lead-induced immunosuppression occurs at low dosages in experimental animals in which there is no apparent evidence of toxicity (Koller *et al.*, 1983.) Also, children with asymptomatic increase in blood lead levels appear to have more frequent febrile illness (Perlstein and Attala, 1966).

Lead lines (Burton's lines) or purple-blue discoloration of gingiva is a classical feature of severe lead toxicity in children with lead encephalopathy. However, this feature of lead toxicity as well as the presence of lead lines at the epiphyseal margins of long bones seen on x-rays of children with severe lead exposure are uncommon today.

Interaction with Other Minerals. Lead toxicity is enhanced by dietary deficiencies in calcium and iron and possibly zinc (Mahaffey and Michaelson, 1980). The increased lead susceptibility found in animals on low calcium regimes is not a direct effect of calcium intake but of increased lead retention associated with decreased renal excretion of lead. In children, elevated blood lead is associated with decreased levels of 25-hydroxyvitamin D (synthesized in liver) and 1-to-25-dihydroxyvitamin D (synthesized in kid-

ney). Iron deficiency is thought to increase gastrointestinal absorption of lead but does not otherwise affect lead metabolism. Relationships between lead and zinc have been studies in experimental animals and veterinary practice. Animals fed diets low in zinc accumulate greater amounts of lead in bones. Extra zinc in the diet has been found to protect horses grazing on lead-contaminated pastures from clinical manifestations of lead toxicity.

Organolead Compounds. Alkyl lead compounds used as gasoline additives, tetraethyl and tetramethyl lead, are rapidly absorbed into the nervous system and are much more severe neurotoxins on an equivalent dose basis than inorganic lead. Although these compounds may be emitted in small amounts from automobile exhaust, they degrade rapidly in the atmosphere. However, the practice of young people sniffing gasoline for psychodelic effects is particularly hazardous. Experimental studies have shown that tetraethyl lead is converted to triethyl lead and inorganic lead. Triethyl lead is relatively stable and becomes rapidly distributed between brain, liver, kidney, and blood (Cremer, 1959).

Biologic Indicators of Lead Toxicity. The most serious effects of lead are related to the central nervous system, although other effects such as chronic nephropathy may be important in some individuals with chronic exposure to high lead levels. Effects on heme synthesis are less evident from a clinical viewpoint, but these are the effects that in biochemical terms are best understood. With continual improvement in industrial hygiene and consciousness and control of potential environmental exposures to lead, concern for recognition of lead poisoning, in terms of traditional clinical signs and symptoms, is less relevant now than the matter of interpretation of more subtle neurologic and biochemical effects. Table 19–5 shows blood lead levels below which various parameters of lead toxicity are not detected. Blood lead level greater than 80 μg/dl is usually associated with clinical symptoms. Persons with blood lead levels above 60 μg/dl may also have clinical manifestations of lead poisoning, particularly in terms of minimal brain dysfunction. For these reasons children with blood levels in this range are sometimes treated with chelating agents. However, effects of lead on heme synthesis, along with increased urinary excretion of δ-ALA, are associated with blood lead levels of 40 μg/dl.

Heme Metabolism. The ALA-D activity of peripheral red blood cells may currently be the most sensitive biochemical parameter affected by lead. Samples collected from both children and adults have shown a negative correlation

Table 19–5. BLOOD LEAD LEVELS BELOW WHICH THE
LISTED EFFECTS HAVE NOT BEEN DETECTED*

BLOOD LEVELS (μg pb/dl)	EFFECT	POPULATION
>10	Erythrocyte ALA-D inhibition	Adults, children
20–25	FEP†	Children
20–30	FEP	Adult, female
25–35	FEP	Adult, male
30–40	Erythrocyte ATPase inhibition	General
40	ALA excretion in urine	Adults, children
40	CP excretion in urine	Adults
40	Anemia	Children
40–50	Peripheral neuropathy	Adults
50	Anemia	Adults
50–60	Minimal brain dysfunction	Children
60–70	Minimal brain dysfunction	Adults
60–70	Encephalopathy	Children
>80	Encephalopathy	Adults

* From WHO Environmental Health Criteria 3. *Lead*. World Health Organization, Geneva, 1977.
† FEP, free erythrocyte protoporphyrin (see Figure 19–4).

between the log of ALA-D activity and the blood lead concentration over a range to below 20 μg/dl. At present they are considered chemical effects of lead rather than adverse health effects. However, children with blood lead levels less than 40 μg/dl exhibit behavioral and fine-motor changes. Therefore, the maximum blood lead level that is not associated with harmful effects is not known. It may, indeed, differ for different segments of the population. Furthermore, blood lead levels and alterations in heme metabolism are indicative of recent exposure but do not reflect past exposure or body burden and may not correlate with the appearance and persistence of chronic effects of lead that are due to tissue levels. This is particularly true of irreversible effects on the central nervous system and kidney.

Chelatable Lead. Urinary excretion of lead after chelation with EDTA or penicillamine reflects the mobilizable pool of lead located in soft tissue. Urinary excretion of lead in the 24-hour period after administration of the chelating agent correlates with blood lead levels for persons in the steady state, without unusual past or recent exposure to lead. However, for persons exposed to excess lead for one year or more, urinary excretion of lead is considerably greater. It has been estimated that nearly 20 percent of the body burden of lead is mobilized into the urine during the 24-hour period after an injection of 40 mg of $CaNa_2$ EDTA per kilogram body weight (Araki and Ushig, 1982).

Lead in Teeth. Lead concentration in circumpulpal dentine of deciduous teeth has been proposed as a method for estimating exposure to lead during childhood. It has been shown that dentine lead content is dose dependent and not reduced by chelation. The distribution of lead in various components of the tooth including enamel, root dentine, and coronal dentine is similar. However, lead content in secondary or circumpulpal dentine, the area of dentine adjacent to pulp and in immediate contact with blood, is higher than in other areas of the tooth and seems to reflect actual exposure to lead throughout the life of the tooth. Several studies now have found substantially higher dentine levels in teeth from urban children living in deteriorated housing or attending school in proximity to a major manufacturer of paint and lead products than in teeth from children considered to be at low risk for lead exposure (Shapiro *et al.*, 1975).

Treatment. Treatment of lead toxicity must go beyond medical care for specific tissue and organ effects and chelation of lead. For both asymptomatic excess exposure to lead as well as the symptomatic child or worker with occupational exposure the sources of lead must be identified and controlled. For the child, this might involve a review of life-style including diet, particularly iron deficiency, type of dwelling, play habits, and pica. Treatment might involve social services, modification of dwelling, and parent education. For the workman, industrial hygiene practices must be reviewed including appropriate environmental and biologic monitoring and deficiencies corrected. One must always be aware of the relationship between occupation and the home. Practices of changing or washing contaminated workclothes must be reviewed, and potential sources of transfer of metal and contamination need to be corrected.

Chelation usually has a role in the treatment of the symptomatic worker or child. Institution of chelation therapy is probably warranted in workmen with blood lead levels over 60 µg/100 ml, but this determination must be made after assessment of exposure factors including biologic estimates of clinical and biochemical parameters of toxicity.

For children, criteria have been established that may serve as guidelines to assist in evaluating the individual case (Chisolm and O'Hara, 1982). These include blood lead levels from 30 µg/dl up to 60 µg/dl depending on FEP levels, and results of a lead mobilization test.

Also, cautionary measures for the safe use of chelating agents have been expressed particularly for Ca EDTA (Lilis and Fischbein, 1976). Serum blood urea nitrogen and creatinine are followed as indicators of renal function, and serum calcium is measured to monitor untoward effects of EDTA. In children with severe lead poisoning including encephalopathy, the mortality rate may be 25 to 38 percent when EDTA or BAL is used singly; combination therapy of EDTA and BAL has been shown to be effective in reducing mortality.

Mercury

No other metal better illustrates the diversity of effects caused by different biochemical forms than does mercury. On the basis of toxicologic characteristics, there are three forms of mercury: elemental, inorganic, and organic compounds. The major source of mercury is the natural degassing of the earth's crust, including land areas, rivers, and the ocean, and is estimated to be in the order of 25,000 to 150,000 tons per year (WHO, 1976; Goldwater and Stopford, 1977; NRCC, 1979). Metallic mercury in the atmosphere represents the major pathway of global transport of mercury. Although anthropogenic sources of mercury have reached about 8000 to 10,000 tons per year since 1973, nonanthropogenic sources are the predominating factors. Nevertheless, mining, smelting, and industrial discharge have been factors in environmental contamination in the past. For instance, it is estimated that loss in water effluent from chloralkali plants, one of the largest users of mercury, has been reduced by 99 percent in recent years. Also, the use of mercury in the paper pulp industries has been reduced dramatically and has been banned in Sweden since 1966. Industrial activities not directly employing mercury or mercury products give rise to substantial quantities of this metal. Fossil fuel may contain as much as 1 ppm of mercury, and it is estimated that about 5000 tons of mercury per year may be emitted from burning coal, natural gas, and the refining of petroleum products. Calculations based on mercury content of the Greenland ice-cap show an increase from the year 1900 to the present day and suggest that the increment is related to increase in background levels in rainwater and is related to man-made release. As much as one-third of atmospheric mercury may be due to industrial release of organic or inorganic forms. Regardless of source, both organic and inorganic forms of mercury may undergo environmental transformation. Metallic mercury may be oxidized to inorganic divalent mercury, particularly in the presence of organic material such as in the aquatic environment. Divalent inorganic mercury may, in turn, be reduced to metallic mercury when conditions are appropriate for reducing reactions to occur. This is an important conversion in terms of the global cycle of mercury and a potential source of mercury vapor that may be released to the earth's atmosphere. A second potential conversion of divalent mercury is methylation to dimethyl mercury by anaerobic bacteria This may diffuse into the atmosphere and return to earth crust or bodies of water as methyl mercury in rainfall. If taken up by fish in the food chain, it may eventually cycle through humans.

Disposition. Toxicity of various forms or salts of mercury is related to cationic mercury *per se* whereas solubility, biotransformation, and tissue distribution are influenced by valence state and anionic component (Suzuki, 1977; Berlin, 1983; and Clarkson, 1983). Metallic or elemental mercury volatilizes to mercury vapor at ambient air temperatures, and most human exposure is by inhalation. Mercury vapor readily diffuses across the alveolar membrane and is lipid soluble so that it has an affinity for red blood cells and central nervous system. Metallic mercury, such as may be swallowed from a broken thermometer, is only slowly absorbed by the gastrointestinal tract (0.01 percent) at a rate related to the vaporization of the elemental mercury and is generally thought to be of no toxicologic consequence.

Inorganic mercury salts may be divalent (mercuric) or monovalent (mercurous). Gastrointestinal absorption of inorganic salts of mercury from food is less than 15 percent in mice and about 7 percent in a study of human volunteers, whereas absorption of methyl mercury is in the order of 90 to 95 percent. Distribution between red blood cells and plasma also differs. For inorganic mercury salts cell-plasma ratio ranges from a high of two with high exposure to less than one, but for methyl mercury it is about ten. The distribution ratio of the two forms of mercury between hair and blood also differs; for organic mercury it is about 250.

Kidneys contain the greatest concentrations of mercury following exposure to inorganic salts of mercury and mercury vapor, whereas organic mercury has a greater affinity for the brain, particularly the posterior cortex. However, mercury vapor has a greater predilection for the central nervous system than does inorganic mercury salts, but less than organic forms of mercury.

Excretion of mercury from the body is by way of urine and feces, again differing with the form of mercury, size of dose, and time after exposure. Exposure to mercury vapor is followed by exhalation of a small fraction, but fecal excretion is the major and is predominant initially after exposure to inorganic mercury. Renal excretion increases with time. About 90 percent of methyl mercury is excreted in feces after acute or chronic exposure and does not change with time (Miettinen, 1973).

All forms of mercury cross the placenta to the fetus, but most of what is known has been learned from experimental animals. Fetal uptake of elemental mercury in rats probably because of lipid solubility has been shown to be 10 to 40 times higher than uptake after exposure to inorganic salts. Concentrations of mercury in the fetus after exposure to alkylmercuric compounds are twice those found in maternal tissues, and methyl mercury levels in fetal red blood cells are 30 percent higher than in maternal red cells. The positive fetal-maternal gradient and increased concentration of mercury in fetal red blood cells enhance fetal toxicity to mercury particularly following exposure to alkylmercury. Although maternal milk may contain only 5 percent of the mercury concentration of maternal blood, neonatal exposure to mercury may be greatly augmented by nursing.

Metabolic Transformation and Excretion. Elemental or metallic mercury is oxidized to divalent mercury after absorption to tissues in the body and is probably mediated by catalases. Inhaled mercury vapor absorbed into red blood cells is transformed to divalent mercury, but a portion is also transported as metallic mercury to more distal tissues, particularly the brain where biotransformation may occur. Similarly, a fraction of absorbed metallic mercury may be carried across the placenta to the fetus. The oxidized divalent mercury is then accumulated by these tissues.

Alkylmercury also undergoes biotransformation to divalent mercuric compounds in tissues by cleavage of the carbon-mercury bond. There is no evidence of formation of any organic form of mercury by mammalian tissues. The aryl (phenyl) compounds are converted to inorganic mercury more rapidly than the shorter-chain alkyl (methyl) compounds. The relationship of these differences is rate of biotransformation versus rate of excretion and toxicity is not well

understood. In those instances where the organomercurial is more rapidly excreted than inorganic mercury, increasing the rate of biotransformation will decrease the rate of excretion. Phenyl and methoxyethylmercury are excreted at about the same rate as inorganic mercury whereas methyl mercury excretion is slower.

Biologic half-times are available for a limited number of mercury compounds. Biologic half-time for methyl mercury is about 70 days and is virtually linear, whereas the half-time for retained salts of inorganic mercury is about 40 days. There are few studies on biologic half-times for elemental mercury or mercury vapor, but it also appears to be linear with a range of values from 35 to 90 days.

Cellular Metabolism. Within cells, mercury may bind to a variety of enzyme systems including those of microsomes and mitochondria, producing nonspecific cell injury or cell death. It has a particular affinity for ligands containing sulfhydryl groups. In liver cells, methyl mercury forms soluble complexes with cysteine and glutathione, which are secreted in bile and reabsorbed from the gastrointestinal tract. Organomercurial diuretics are thought to be absorbed in the proximal-tubule-binding specific receptor sites that inhibit sodium transport. In general, however, organomercury compounds undergo cleavage of the carbon-mercury bond releasing ionic inorganic mercury.

Mercuric mercury, but not methyl mercury, induces synthesis of metallothionein probably only in kidney cells, but unlike cadmium-metallothionein it does not have a long half-life. Mercury within renal cells becomes localized in lysosomes (Madsen and Christensen, 1978).

Toxicology. *Mercury Vapor.* Inhalation of mercury vapor may produce an acute, corrosive bronchitis and interstitial pneumonitis and, if not fatal, may be associated with symptoms of central nervous system effects such as tremor or increased excitability.

With chronic exposure to mercury vapor the major effects are on the central nervous system (Friberg and Vostal, 1972). Early signs are nonspecific and have been termed the "asthenic-vegetative syndrome" or "micromercurialism." Identification of the syndrome requires neurasthenic symptoms and three or more of the following clinical findings: tremor, enlargement of the thyroid, increased uptake of radioiodine in the thyroid, labile pulse, tachycardia, dermographism, gingivitis, hematologic changes, or increased excretion of mercury in urine. With increasing exposure the symptoms become more characteristic beginning with intentional tremors of muscles that perform fine-motor functions (highly innervated), such as fingers, eyelids, and lips, and may progress to generalized trembling of the entire body and violent chronic spasms of the extremities. This is accompanied by changes in personality and behavior, with loss of memory, increased excitability (erethrism), severe depression, and even delirium and hallucination. Another characteristic feature of mercury toxicity is severe salivation and gingivitis.

The triad of increased excitability, tremors, and gingivitis has been recognized historically as the major manifestation of mercury poisoning from inhalation of mercury vapor and exposure in the fur, felt, and hat industry to mercury nitrate (Goldwater, 1972).

Sporadic instances of proteinuria and even nephrotic syndrome may occur in persons with exposure to mercury vapor, particularly with chronic occupational exposure. The pathogenesis is probably immunologic similar to that which may occur following exposure to inorganic mercury (see below).

Mercuric Mercury. Bichloride of mercury (corrosive sublimate) is the best-known inorganic salt of mercury, and the trivial name suggests its most apparent toxicologic effect when ingested in concentrations greater than 10 percent. A reference from the Middle Ages in Goldwater's book on mercury describes oral ingestion of mercury as causing severe abdominal cramps, bloody diarrhea, and suppression of urine (Goldwater, 1972). This is an accurate report of effects following accidental or suicidal ingestion of mercuric chloride or other mercuric salts. Corrosive ulceration, bleeding, and necrosis of the gastrointestinal tract are usually accompanied by shock and circulatory collapse. If the patient survives the gastrointestinal damage, renal failure occurs within 24 hours owing to necrosis of the proximal tubular epithelium followed by oliguria, anuria, and uremia. If the patient can be maintained by dialysis, regeneration of tubular lining cells is possible. These may be followed by ultrastructural changes consistent with irreversible cell injury including actual disruption of mitochondria, release of lysosomal enzymes, and rupture of cell membranes.

Injection of mercuric chloride produces necrosis of the epithelium of the pars recta kidney (Gritzka and Trump, 1968). Cellular changes include fragmentation and disruption of the plasma membrane and its appendages, vesiculation and disruption of the endoplasmic reticulum and other cytoplasmic membranes, dissociation of polysomes and loss of ribosomes, mitochondrial swelling with appearance of amorphous intramatrical deposits, and condensation of nuclear chromatin. These changes are common to renal cell necrosis due to various causes.

Although exposure to a high dose of mercuric chloride is directly toxic to renal tubular lining cells, chronic low-dose exposure to mercuric salts or even elemental mercury vapor levels may induce an immunologic glomerular disease. This form of chronic mercury injury to the kidney is clinically the most common form of mercury-induced nephropathy. Exposed persons may develop a proteinuria that is reversible after workers are removed from exposure. It has been stated that chronic mercury-induced nephropathy seldom occurs without sufficient exposure to also produce detectable neuropathy.

Experimental studies have shown that the pathogenesis of chronic mercury nephropathy has two phases: an early phase characterized by an antibasement membrane glomerulonephritis followed by a superimposed immune-complex glomerulonephritis (Roman-Franco et al., 1978). The pathogenesis of the nephropathy in humans appears similar although antigens have not been characterized. Also, the early glomerular nephritis may progress in humans to an interstitial immune-complex nephritis (Tubbs et al., 1982).

Mercurous Compounds. Mercurous compounds of mercury are less corrosive and less toxic than mercuric salts, presumably because they are less soluble. Calomel, a powder containing mercurous chloride, has a long history of use in medicine. Perhaps the most notable modern usage has been as teething powder for children and is now known to be responsible for acrodynia or "pink disease." This is most likely a hypersensitivity response to the mercury salts in skin producing vasodilation, hyperkeratosis, and hypersecretion of sweat glands. Children develop fever, a pink-colored rash, swelling of the spleen and lymph nodes, and hyperkeratosis and swelling of fingers. The effects are independent of dose and are thought to be a hypersensitivity reaction (Matheson et al., 1980).

Organic Mercury. Methyl mercury is the most important form of mercury in terms of toxicity, and health effects from environmental exposures and many of the effects produced by short-term alkyls are unique in terms of mercury toxicity but are nonspecific in that they may be found in other disease states. Most of what is known about methyl mercury toxicity is from detailed epidemiologic studies of exposed populations (WHO, 1976).

Two major epidemics of methyl mercury poisoning have occurred in Japan in Minamata Bay and in Niigata. Both were caused by industrial release of methyl and other mercury compounds into Minamata Bay and into the Agano River, followed by accumulation of the mercury by edible fish. The median level of total mercury in fish caught in Minamata Bay during the epidemic was estimated to be about 11 mg/kg fresh weight and less than 10 mg/kg in fish from the Agano River. The largest recorded epidemic of methyl mercury poisoning took place in the winter of 1971–1972 in Iraq, resulting in admission of over 6000 patients to hospitals and over 500 deaths in hospitals (Bakir *et al.,* 1973). Methyl mercury exposure was from bread containing wheat imported as seed grain and dressed with methyl mercury fungicide. The mean methyl mercury content of wheat flour samples was 0.1 mg/kg (range 4.8 to 14.6 mg). In one village the average daily intake of contaminated loaves was 3.2 loaves per person, but it varied. On this basis, average daily intake of methyl mercury was calculated to be about 80 μg/kg ranging up to 250 μg/kg/day.

Several previous epidemics occurred in Iraq in 1961, in Pakistan in 1963, in Guatamala in 1966, and in other countries, but on a more limited scale. From studies of these episodes, data have been obtained to relate clinical manifestations, organ pathology, and level of exposure. The major clinical features are neurologic, consisting of paresthesia, ataxia, dysarthria, and deafness, appearing in that order. The main pathologic features of methyl mercury toxicity include degeneration and necrosis of neurons in focal areas of the cerebral cortex, particularly in the visual areas of the occipital cortex and in the granular layer of the cerebellum. Experimental studies of both organic- and inorganic-mercury-related peripheral neuropathy show degeneration of primary sensory ganglion cells. The particular distribution of lesions in the central nervous system is thought to reflect a propensity of mercury to damage small nerve cells in cerebellum and visual cortex (Roizin *et al.,* 1977).

Biologic Indicators. *Metallic Mercury.* For persons in the general population, it is estimated that daily mercury exposure is about 1 μg/day from air, less than 2 μg/day from water, and about 20 μg/day from food, but may be up to 75 μg/day depending on the amount of fish in the diet. The recommended standard (time-weight average) for permissible exposure limits for inorganic mercury in air in the workplace is 0.05 mg Hg/m^3 (DHEW, 1977) and is equivalent to an ambient air level of 0.015 mg/m^3 for the general population (24-hour exposure).

The central nervous system is the major site of toxicity from exposure to elemental mercury. It is believed that a worker exposed to a constant average concentration of mercury vapor achieves a state of balance (steady state) after one year of exposure, and it can be expected that there is a consistent relationship between air levels and mercury content of blood or urine. Mercury content in blood and urine only reflects recent exposure to metallic mercury. Table 19–6 is an estimate of mercury concentration in blood and urine related to air concentration of elemental mercury vapor and earliest clinical effects (WHO, 1976). Urine mercury should be less than 100 μg/liter content.

Alkyl Mercury. The federal standard for alkyl mercury exposure in the workplace is 0.01 mg/m^3 as an eight-hour TWA with an acceptable ceiling of 0.04 mg/m^3. Although a precise correlation has not been found between exposure levels and mercury content of blood and urine, study of the Iraq epidemic has provided estimates of the lowest mercury levels of mercury in blood due to alkyl mercury exposure associated with mild symptoms (Figure 19–6). These studies do not indicate the percentage of people in the population who are sensitive at these levels, but other studies suggest that the frequency of paresthesia due to methyl mercury with these minimum mercury concentrations in blood and hair is 5 percent or less (WHO, 1976). However, studies reported from Minamata and elsewhere suggest that mothers with slight or no symptoms may have offspring who are retarded and have palsy. Mercury has been reported in breast milk of women exposed to methyl mercury from fish and from contaminated bread and averages about 5 percent of simultaneous concentrations in maternal blood. Figure 19–7 shows estimates of body burden of mercury onset and frequency of occurrence of these symptoms.

Mercury levels in hair may also be correlated with severity of clinical symptoms (WHO, 1976). Mild cases complained of numbness of extremities, slight tremors, and mild ataxia. Moderate cases had difficulty hearing, tunnel vision, and partial paralysis, and severe cases

Table 19–6. THE TIME-WEIGHTED AVERAGE AIR CONCENTRATIONS ASSOCIATED WITH THE EARLIEST EFFECTS IN THE MOST SENSITIVE ADULTS FOLLOWING LONG-TERM EXPOSURE TO ELEMENTAL MERCURY VAPOR. THE TABLE ALSO LISTS THE EQUIVALENT BLOOD AND URINE CONCENTRATIONS*†

AIR (mg/m^3)	BLOOD (μg/100 ml)	URINE (μg/liter)	EARLIEST EFFECTS
0.05	3.5	150	Nonspecific symptoms
0.1–0.2	7–14	300–600	Tremor

* Blood and urine values may be used only on a group basis owing to gross individual variations. Furthermore, these average values reflect exposure only after exposure for a year or more. After shorter periods of exposure, air concentrations would be associated with lower concentrations in blood and urine.
† From WHO Environmental Health Criteria 1. *Mercury.* World Health Organization, Geneva, 1976.

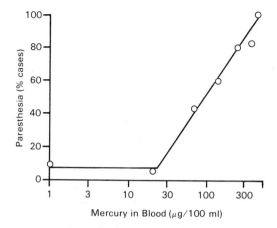

Figure 19–6. Dose-response relationship for methyl mercury using concentration of mercury in the blood as dose and paresthesia as response. (WHO, 1976. From Bakir, F. *et al:* Methylmercury poisoning in Iraq. *Science,* **181**:230–41, 1973. Copyright 1973 by the American Association for the Advancement of Science.)

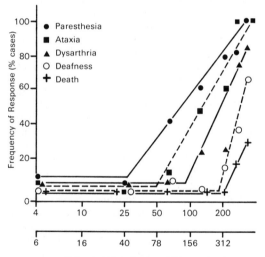

Figure 19–7. Dose-response relationships for methyl mercury. The upper scale of estimated body burden of mercury was based on the authors' actual estimate of intake. The lower scale is based on the body burden, which was calculated based on the concentration of mercury in the blood and its relationship to intake derived from radioisotopic studies of methyl mercury kinetics in human volunteers. (From Bakir, F., *et al.:* Methylmercury poisoning in Iraq. *Science,* **181**:230–41, 1973. Copyright 1973 by the American Association for the Advancement of Science.)

had some combination of complete paralysis, loss of vision, loss of hearing, loss of speech, and coma. Persons with no symtpoms might have mercury hair levels up to 300 mg/kg, the mildly affected group in the range of 120 to 600 mg/kg, the moderate group in the range of 200 to 600 mg/kg, and the severely affected from 400 to 1600 mg/kg. Total dose of mercury for this group is not known.

It is not really understood why exposure to methyl mercury has such selective effect on cerebellum and visual cortex. Concentration of mercury in these areas of the brain is not very different from that in areas of brain not affected by methyl mercury. Methyl mercury does inhibit protein synthesis in the brain before onset of signs of poisoning, and it has been found that recovery of protein synthesis does not occur in granular cells as it does in other types of neuronal cells (Clarkson, 1983).

Treatment. Therapy of mercury poisoning should be directed to lowering the concentration of mercury at the critical organ or site of injury. For the most severe cases, particularly with acute renal failure, hemodialysis may be the first measure along with infusion of chelating agents for mercury such as cysteine or penicillamine. For less severe cases of inorganic mercury poisoning, chelation with BAL may be effective. However, chelation therapy is not very helpful for alkyl mercury exposure. Biliary excretion and reabsorption by the intestine and the enterohepatic cycling of mercury may be interrupted by surgically establishing gallbladder drainage or by the oral administration of a nonabsorbable thiol resin that binds mercury and enhances intestinal excretion (Berlin, 1979).

Nickel

Nickel is a respiratory tract carcinogen in workmen in the nickel-refining industry. Other serious consequences of long-term exposure to nickel are not apparent, but severe acute and sometimes fatal toxicity may follow nickel carbonyl exposure. Allergic contact dermatitis is common among persons in the general population. Deficiency of nickel alters glucose metabolism and decreases tolerance to glucose. From studies on rats, there is growing evidence that nickel may be an essential trace metal for mammals (Sunderman, 1981a; Anke *et al.,* 1983).

Disposition. Nickel is only sparsely absorbed from the gastrointestinal tract. It is transported in the plasma bound to serum albumin and multiple small organic ligands, amino acids, or polypeptides. Excretion in the urine is nearly complete in four or five days. Kinetics have been described in rodents as a two-compartment model.

Dietary nickel intake by adults in the United States was estimated by Schroeder et al. (1962b), to be in the range of 300 to 600 μg/day. In a more recent study of nickel content of diets prepared in university or hospital kitchens in the United States, Myron et al. (1978) found nickel intake to average 165 (S.D. $\pm$ 11) μg/day or 75 $\pm$ 10 μg/1000 calories.

In one study, serum nickel was found to be 2.6 $\pm$ 0.9 μg/liter (range: 0.8 to 5.2) and mean excretion of nickel in urine of 2.6 $\pm$ 1.4 μg/day (range: 0.5 to 6.4) (McNeely et al., 1972). Serum nickel is influenced by environmental nickel or nickel concentration in the ambient air. Serum nickel measured in persons living in Sudbury, Ontario, which is in the vicinity of a large nickel mine, showed concentrations of 4.6 $\pm$ 1.4 μg/liter (range: 2.0 to 7.3) and urinary concentrations were 7.9 $\pm$ 3.7 μg/day (range: 2.3 to 15.7). Generally, fecal nickel is about 100 times urine nickel concentration.

Nickel administered parenterally to animals is rapidly distributed to kidney, pituitary, lung, skin, adrenal, and ovary and testis (Sunderman, 1981a).

The intracellular distribution and binding of nickel is not well understood. Ultrafiltrable ligands seem to be of major importance in transport in serum and bile and urinary excretion as well as intracellular binding. The ligands are not well characterized, but Sunderman (1981a) suggests that cysteine, histidine, and aspartic acid form nickel complexes either singly or as nickel-ligand species. In vivo binding with metallothionein has been demonstrated, but nickel at best induces metallothionein synthesis in liver or kidney only slightly.

A nickel-binding metalloprotein has also been identified in plasma with properties suggesting an α-1-glycoprotein with serum α-1-macroglobulin complex.

Evidence has accumulated over the past few years indicating that nickel is a nutritionally essential trace metal. Jackbean urease has been identified as a nickel metalloenzyme, and nickel is required for urea metabolism in cell cultures of soybean. However, a nickel-containing metalloenzyme has not yet been recovered from animal tissues. Nickel deficiency in rats is associated with retarded body growth and anemia, probably secondary to impaired absorption of iron from the gastrointestinal tract. In addition, there is significant reduction in serum glucose concentration. An interaction of nickel with copper and zinc is also suspected since anemia-induced nickel deficiency is only partially corrected with nickel supplementation in rats receiving low dietary copper and zinc (Spear, 1978).

Toxicology. *Carcinogenesis.* It has been known for 40 years that occupational exposure to nickel predisposes to lung and nasal cancer (Doll et al., 1977). Epidemiologic studies in 1958 showed that nickel refinery workers in Britain had a fivefold increase in risk to lung cancer and 150-times increase in risk to nasal cancers compared to people in the general population. More recently, increase in lung cancer among nickel workers has been reported from several different countries including suggestions of increased risks to laryngeal cancer in nickel refinery workers in Norway (Pedersen et al., 1978) and gastric carcinoma and soft tissue sarcomas from the Soviet Union. Six cases of renal cancer has been reported among Canadian and Norwegian workers employed in the electrolytic refining of nickel (Sunderman, 1981b). McEwan (1978) has been able to detect early cytologic changes in sputum of exposed workers prior to chest x-ray or clinical indicators of respiratory tract cancer.

Because the refining of nickel in the plants that were studied involved the Mond process with the formation of nickel carbonyl, it was believed for some time that nickel carbonyl was the principal carcinogen. However, additional epidemiologic studies of workers in refineries that do not use the Mond process also showed increased risk of respiratory cancer, suggesting that the source of the increased risk is the mixture of nickel sulfides present in molten ore. Indeed, studies with experimental animals have shown that the nickel subsulfide (Ni_3S_2) produces local tumors at injection sites and by inhalation in rats, and in vitro mammalian cell tests demonstrate that Ni_3S_2 and $NiSO_4$ compounds give rise to mammalian cell transformation (Costa, 1980).

Nickel Carbonyl Poisoning. Metallic nickel combines with carbon monoxide to form nickel carbonyl ($Ni[CO]_4$), which decomposes to pure nickel and carbon monoxide on heating to 200° C (Mond process). This reaction provides a convenient and efficient method for the refinement of nickel. However, nickel carbonyl is extremely toxic, and many cases of acute toxicity have been reported. The illness begins with headache, nausea, vomiting, and epigastric or chest pain, followed by cough, hyperpnea, cyanosis, gastrointestinal symptoms, and weakness. The symptoms may be accompanied by fever and leukocytosis, and the more severe cases progress to pneumonia, respiratory failure, and eventually cerebral edema and death. Autopsy studies show the largest concentrations of nickel in lungs with lesser amounts in kidneys, liver, and brain. (Sunderman, 1981a).

Dermatitis. Nickel dermatitis is one of the most common forms of allergic contact dermatitis; 4 to 9 percent of persons with contact dermatitis react positively to nickel patch tests. Sensitization might occur from any of the numerous metal products in common use, such as coins and jewelry. The notion that increased ingestion of nickel-containing food increases the probability of external sensitization to nickel is supported by finding increased urinary nickel excretion in association with episodes of acute nickel dermatitis (Menne and Thorboe, 1976).

Indicators of Nickel Toxicity. Blood nickel levels immediately following exposure to nickel carbonyl provide a guideline as to severity of exposure and indication for chelation therapy (Sunderman, 1981a). Sodium diethyldithiocarbamate is the preferred drug, but other chelating agents, such as *d*-penicillamine and triethylenetetraamine, provide some degree of protection from clinical effects.

ESSENTIAL METALS WITH POTENTIAL FOR TOXICITY

This group includes seven metals generally accepted as essential: cobalt, copper, iron, manganese, molybdenum, selenium, and zinc. Each of the seven essential metals has three levels of biologic activity, trace levels required for optimium growth and development, homeostatic levels (storage levels), and toxic levels. For these metals, environmental accumulations are generally less important routes of excess exposure than accidents or occupation.

Although chromium and arsenic are regarded as essential to humans and animals, respectively, the toxicologic significance of chromium and arsenic warrant their being discussed as major toxic metals in the context of this chapter. Tin and vanadium are also essential to animals but are of less importance toxicologically and are included in the group of minor toxic metals.

Cobalt

Cobalt is essential as a component of vitamin B_{12} required for the production of red blood cells and prevention of pernicious anemia. There is 0.0434 μg of cobalt per microgram of vitamin B_{12}. If other requirements for cobalt exist, they are not well understood. Deficiency diseases of cattle and sheep, caused by insufficient natural levels of cobalt, are characterized by anemia and loss of weight or retarded growth.

Cobalt is a relatively rare metal produced primarily as a by-product of other metals, chiefly copper. It is used in high-temperature alloys and in permanent magnets. Its salts are useful in paint driers, as catalysts, and in the production of numerous pigments.

Cobalt salts are generally well absorbed after oral ingestion, probably in the jejunum. Despite this fact, increased levels tend not to cause significant accumulation. About 80 percent of the ingested cobalt is excreted in the urine. Of the remaining, about 15 percent is excreted in the feces by an enterohepatic pathway, while the milk and sweat are other secondary routes of excretion. The total body burden has been estimated as 1.1 mg.

The muscle contains the largest total fraction, but the fat has the highest concentration. The liver, heart, and hair have significantly higher concentrations than other organs, but the concentration in these organs is relatively low. The normal levels in human urine and blood are about 98 and 0.18 μg/liter, respectively. The blood level is largely in association with the red cells.

Significant species differences have been observed in the excretion of radiocobalt. In rats and cattle, 80 percent is eliminated in the feces (Schroeder *et al.*, 1967b).

Polycythemia is the characteristic response of most mammals, including humans, to ingestion of excessive amounts of cobalt. Toxicity resulting from overzealous therapeutic administration has been reported to produce vomiting, diarrhea, and a sensation of warmth. Intravenous administration leads to flushing of the face, increased blood pressure, slowed respiration, giddiness, tinnitus, and deafness due to nerve damage (Browning, 1969).

High levels of chronic oral administration may result in the production of goiter. Epidemiologic studies suggest that the incidence of goiter is higher in regions containing increased levels of cobalt in the water and soil (Wills, 1966). The goitrogenic effect has been elicited by the oral administration of 3 to 4 mg/kg to children in the course of sickle cell anemia therapy (Browning, 1969).

Cardiomyopathy has been caused by excessive intake of cobalt, particularly from the drinking of beer to which 1 ppm cobalt was added to enhance its foaming qualities. Why such a low concentration should produce this effect in the absence of any similar change when cobalt is used therapeutically is unknown. The signs and symptoms were those of congestive heart failure. Autopsy findings revealed a tenfold increase in the cardiac levels of cobalt. Alcohol may have served to potentiate the effect of the cobalt (Morin and Daniel, 1967).

Hyperglycemia due to β-cell pancreatic damage has been reported after injection into rats. Reduction of blood pressure has also been observed in rats after injection and has led to some experimental use in humans (Schroeder *et al.*, 1967b).

Occupational inhalation of cobalt salts in the cemented carbide industry may cause respiratory symptoms probably as a result of irritation of the pulmonary tract. Allergic dermatitis of an erythematous papular type may also occur, and affected persons may have positive skin tests.

Single and repeated subcutaneous or intramuscular injection of cobalt powder and salts to rats may cause sarcomas at the site of injection, but there is no evidence of carcinogenicity from any other route of exposure (Gilman, 1962).

Copper

Copper is widely distributed in nature and is an essential element. Copper deficiency is characterized by hypochromic, microcytic anemia resulting from defective hemoglobin synthesis. Oxidative enzymes, such as catalase, peroxidase, cytochrome oxides, and others, also require copper. Medicinally, copper sulfate is used as an emetic. It has also been used for its astringent and caustic action and as an anthelmintic. Copper sulfate mixed with lime has been used as a fungicide.

Gastrointestinal absorption of copper is normally regulated by body stores (Aspin and Sass-Kortsak, 1981; Sarkar et al., 1983). It is transported in serum bound initially to albumin and later more firmly bound to α-ceruloplasmin where it is exchanged in the cupric form. The normal serum level of copper is 120 to 145 μg/liter. The bile is the normal excretory pathway and plays a primary role in copper homeostasis. Most copper is stored in liver and bone marrow where it may be bound to metallotheionein. The amount of copper in milk is not enough to maintain adequate copper levels in the liver, lung, and spleen of the newborn. Tissue levels gradually decline up to about ten years of age, remaining relatively constant thereafter. Brain levels, on the other hand, tend to almost double from infancy to adulthood. The ratios of newborn to adult liver copper levels show considerable species difference: human, 15:4; rat, 6:4; and rabbit, 1:6. Since urinary copper levels may be increased by soft water, under these conditions concentrations of approximately 60 μg/liter are not uncommon.

Copper is an essential part of several enzymes, including tyrosinase, involved in the formation of melanin pigments, cytochrome oxidase, superoxide dismutane, amine oxidases, and uricase. It is essential for the utilization of iron. Iron deficiency anemia in infancy is sometimes accompanied by copper deficiency as well. Molybdenum also influences tissue levels of copper.

There are two genetically inherited inborn errors of copper metabolism that are in a sense a form of copper toxicity (Sarkar et al., 1983). Wilson's disease is characterized by excessive accumulation of copper in liver, brain, kidneys, and cornea. Serum ceruloplasmin is low, and serum copper, not bound to ceruloplasmin, is elevated. Urinary excretion of copper is high. The disorder is sometimes referred to as hepatolenticular degeneration in reference to the major symptoms. Clinical abnormalities of the nervous system, liver, kidneys, and cornea are related to copper accumulation. Although the etiology of this disorder is genetic, the basic defect at the biochemical level is not known. Increased binding of copper to an abnormal intracellular thionein or altered tissue excretion has been proposed. Cultured fibroblasts from persons with Wilson's disease have increased intracellular copper when cultured in Eagle's minimum essential medium with fetal bovine serum (Chan et al., 1983). Clinical improvement can be achieved by chelation of copper with penicillamine (Walshe, 1964). Trien (triethylene tetramine, 2HCl) is also effective and has been used in patients with Wilson's disease who have toxic reactions to penicillamine (Walshe, 1983).

Menke's disease or Menke's "kinky-hair syndrome" is a sex-linked trait characterized by peculiar hair, failure to thrive, severe mental retardation, neurologic impairment, and death before three years of age. There is extensive degeneration of the cerebral cortex and of white matter. Again, the basic defect is not known. There are low levels of copper in liver and brain but high concentrations in other tissues. Even in cells with increased copper concentration there is a relative deficiency in activities of some copper-dependent enzymes. Some laboratories have reported that larger-than-normal quantities of copper-thionein accumulated in fibroblasts so that the basic defect may be in regulation of metallothionein synthesis. The finding of increased amounts of other metallothionein binding metals (zinc, cadmium, mercury) in kidneys of patients with this disease supports this hypothesis (Riordan, 1983).

Acute poisoning resulting from ingestion of excessive amounts of oral copper salts, most frequently copper sulfate, may produce death. The symptoms are vomiting, sometimes with a blue-green color observed in the vomitus, hematemesis, hypotension, melena, coma, and jaundice. Autopsy findings have revealed centrilobular hepatic necrosis (Chuttani et al., 1965). Few cases of copper intoxication as a result of burn treatment with copper compounds have resulted in hemolytic anemia. Copper poisoning producing hemolytic anemia has also been reported as the result of using copper-containing dialysis equipment (Manzler and Schreiner, 1970).

Iron

The major interest in iron is as an essential metal, but toxicologic considerations are important in terms of accidental acute exposures and chronic iron overload due to idiopathic hemochromatosis or as a consequence of excess dietary iron or frequent blood transfusions. The complex metabolism of iron and mechanisms of toxicity are detailed by Jacobs and Worwood, (1981).

Disposition. The disposition of iron is regulated by a complex mechanism to maintain homeostasis. Generally, about 2 to 15 percent is absorbed from the gastrointestinal tract, whereas elimination of absorbed iron is only about 0.01 percent per day (percent body burden or amount absorbed). During periods of increased iron need (childhood, pregnancy, blood loss) absorption of iron is greatly increased. Absorption occurs in two steps: absorption of ferrous ions from the intestinal lumen into the mucosal cells, and transfer from the mucosal cell to plasma where it is bound to transferrin for transfer to storage sites. Transferrin is a β_1-globulin with a molecular weight of 75,000 and is produced in the liver. As ferrous ion is released into plasma, it becomes oxidized by oxygen in the presence of ferroxidase I, which is identical to ceruloplasmin. There are 3 to 5 g of iron in the body. About two-thirds is bound to hemoglobin, 10 percent in myoglobin and iron-containing enzymes, and the remainder is bound to the iron storage proteins ferritin and hemosiderin. Exposure to iron induces synthesis of apoferritin, which then binds ferrous ions. The ferrous ion becomes oxidized, probably by histidine and cysteine residues and carbonyl groups. Iron may be released from ferritin by reducing agents; ascorbic acid, cysteine, and reduced glutathione release iron slowly. Normally, excess ingested iron is excreted, and some is contained within shed intestinal cells and in bile and urine and in even smaller amounts in sweat, nails, and hair. Total iron excretion is usually in the order of 0.5 mg/day.

With excess exposure to iron or iron overload, there may be a further increase in ferritin synthesis in hepatic parenchymal cells. In fact, the ability of the liver to synthesize ferritin exceeds the rate at which lysosomes can process iron for excretion. Lysosomes convert the protein from ferritin to hemosiderin, which then remains *in situ* (Trump *et al*, 1973). The formation of hemosiderin from ferritin is not well understood, but seems to involve denaturation of the apoferritin molecule. With increasing iron loading, ferritin concentration appears to reach a maximum and a greater portion of iron is found in hemosiderin. Both ferritin and hemosiderin are, in fact, storage sites for intracellular metal and are protective in that they maintain intracellular iron in bound form.

A portion of the iron taken up by cells of the reticuloendothelial system enters a labile iron pool available for erythropoiesis and part becomes stored as ferritin.

Toxicity. Acute iron toxicity is nearly always due to accidental ingestion of iron-containing medicines and most often occurs in children. As of 1970, there were about 2000 cases in the United States each year, generally among children aged one to five years, who eat ferrous sulfate tablets with candylike coatings. Decrease of this occurrence should follow use of "child-proof" lids on prescription medicines. Severe toxicity occurs after ingestion of more than 0.5 g of iron or 2.5 g of ferrous sulfate. Toxicity becomes manifest with vomiting, one to six hours after ingestion. The vomitus may be bloody owing to ulceration of the gastrointestinal tract; stools may be black. This is followed by signs of shock and metabolic acidosis, liver damage, and coagulation defects within the next couple of days. Late effects may include renal failure and hepatic cirrhosis. The mechanism of the toxicity is thought to begin with acute mucosal cell damage, absorption of ferrous ions directly into the circulation, which the cause capillary endothelial cell damage in liver.

Chronic iron toxicity or iron overload in adults is a more common problem. There are three basic ways in which excessive amounts of iron can accumulate in the body. The first circumstance is idiopathic hemochromotosis due to abnormal absorption of iron from the intestinal tract. The condition may be genetic. A second possible cause of iron overload is excess dietary iron. The African Bantu who prepares his daily food and brews fermented beverages in iron pots is the classic example of this form of iron overload. Sporadic other cases occur owing to excessive ingestion of iron-containing tonics or medicines. The third circumstance in which iron overload may occur is from the regular requirement for blood transfusion for some form of refractory anemias and is sometimes referred to as transfusional siderosis (Muller-Eberhard *et al.,* 1977).

The pathologic consequences of iron overload are similar regardless of basic cause. The body iron content is increased to between 20 and 40 g. Most of the extra iron is hemosiderin. Greatest concentrations are in parenchymal cells of liver and pancreas, as well as endocrine organs and heart. Iron in reticuloendothelial cells (spleen) is greatest in transfusional siderosis and in the Bantu. Further clinical effects may include disturbances in liver function, diabetes mellitus, and even endocrine disturbances and cardiovascular effects. At the cell level, increased lipid peroxidation occurs with consequent membrane damage to mitochondria, microsomes, and other cellular organelles (Jacobs, 1977).

Treatment of acute iron poisoning is directed toward removal of the ingested iron from the gastrointestinal tract by inducing vomiting or gastric lavage and providing corrective therapy for systemic effects such as acidosis and shock. Deferrioxamine is the chelating agent of choice for treatment of iron absorbed from acute exposure as well as for removal of tissue iron in hemosiderosis. Ascorbic acid will also increase iron excretion as much as twofold normal (Brown, 1983).

Inhalation of iron oxide fumes or dust by workers in metal industries may result in deposition of iron particles in lungs producing an x-ray appearance resembling silicosis. These effects are seen in hematite miners, iron and steel workers, and arc welders. Hematite is the most important iron ore (mainly Fe_2O_3). A report of autopsies of hematite miners noted an increase in lung cancer, as well as tuberculosis and interstitial fibrosis (Boyd et al., 1970). The etiology of the lung cancer may be related to concomitant factors such as cigarettes or other workplace carcinogens. Hematite miners are also exposed to silica and other minerals, as well as radioactive materials; other iron workers have exposures to polycyclic hydrocarbons (McLaughlin, 1956). Dose levels of iron among iron workers developing pneumoconiosis have been reported to exceed 10 mg Fe/m^3.

Manganese

Manganese is an essential element and is a cofactor for a number of enzymatic reactions particularly those involved in phosphorylation, cholesterol, and fatty acids synthesis. Manganese is present in all living organisms. While it is present in urban air and in most water supplies, the principal portion of the intake is derived from food. Vegetables, the germinal portions of grains, fruits, nuts, tea, and some spices are rich in manganese (NAS, 1973; Underwood, 1977).

Daily manganese intake ranges from 2 to 9 mg. Gastrointestinal absorption is less than 5 percent. It is transported in plasma bound to a β_1-globulin, thought to be transferrin, and is widely distributed in the body. Manganese concentrates in mitochondria so that tissues rich in these organelles have the highest concentrations of manganese including pancreas, liver, kidney, and intestines. Biologic half-life in the body is 37 days. It readily crosses the blood-brain barrier

and half-time in the brain is longer than in the whole body.

Manganese is eliminated in the bile and is reabsorbed in the intestine, but the principal route of excretion is with feces. This system apparently involves the liver, auxiliary gastrointestinal mechanisms for excreting excess manganese, and perhaps the adrenal cortex. This regulating mechanism, plus the tendency for extremely large doses of manganese salts to cause gastrointestinal irritation, accounts for the lack of systemic toxicity following oral administration or dermal application.

Manganese and its compounds are used in making steel alloys, dry-cell batteries, electrical coils, ceramics, matches, glass, dyes, in fertilizers, welding rods, as oxidizing agents, and as animal food additives.

Industrial toxicity from inhalation exposure, generally to manganese dioxide in mining or manufacturing, is of two types: The first, manganese pneumonitis, is the result of acute exposure. Men working in plants with high concentrations of manganese dust show an incidence of respiratory disease 30 times greater than normal. Pathologic changes include epithelial necrosis followed by mononuclear proliferation.

The second and more serious type of disease resulting from chronic inhalation exposure to manganese dioxide, generally over a period of more than two years, involves the central nervous system. In iron deficiency anemia, the oral absorption of manganese is increased, and it may be that variations in manganese transport related to iron deficiency account for individual susceptibility (Mena et al., 1969). Those who develop chronic manganese poisoning (manganism) exhibit a psychiatric disorder characterized by irritability, difficulty in walking, speech disturbances, and compulsive behavior that may include running, fighting, and singing. If the condition persists, a masklike face, retropulsion or propulsion, and a Parkinson-like syndrome develop (Mena et al., 1967). The outstanding feature of manganese encephalopathy has been classified as severe selective damage to the subthalamic nucleus and pallidum (Pentschew et al., 1963). These symptoms and the pathologic lesions, degenerative changes in the basal ganglia, make the analogy to Parkinson's disease feasible. In addition to the central nervous system changes, liver cirrhosis is frequently observed.

Victims of chronic manganese poisoning tend to recover slowly, even when removed from the excessive exposure. Metal-sequestering agents have not produced remarkable recovery; L-dopa, which is used in the treatment of Parkinson's disease, has been more consistently effective in the treatment of chronic manganese poisoning than in Parkinson's disease (Cotzias *et al.*, 1971).

The syndrome of chronic nervous system effects has not been successfully duplicated in any experimental animals except monkeys and then only by inhalation or intraperitoneal injection. After intraperitoneal administration of manganese to squirrel monkeys, dopamine and serotonin levels markedly decreased in the caudate nucleus regardless of whether or not behavioral effects were present. Manganese levels were increased in the basal ganglia and cerebellum. Histopathologic examination of animals did not reveal any morphologic changes (Neff *et al.*, 1969). Exposure of rats to manganese dioxide for 100 days does increase the brain manganese concentration but does not produce any hematologic, behavioral, or histologic effects.

Molybdenum

Molybdenum is an essential metal as a cofactor for the enzymes xanthine oxidase and aldehyde oxidase. In plants it is necessary for fixing of atmospheric nitrogen by bacteria at the start of protein synthesis. Because of these functions it is ubiquitous in food. Since plankton tend to concentrate molybdenum 25 times that of seawater, shellfish tend to have high concentrations of molybdenum. Molybdenum is added in trace amounts to fertilizers to stimulate plant growth. The average daily human intake in food is approximately 350 μg. The concentration of molybdenum in urban air is minimal, but it is present in more than one-third of fresh-water supplies (Table 19–1) and in certain areas the concentration may be near 1 μg/liter. Excess exposure can result in toxicity to animals and humans (Underwood, 1977; Winston, 1981).

The most important mineral source of molybdenum is molybdenite (MoS_2). The United States is the major world producer of molybdenum. The industrial uses of this metal include the manufacture of high-temperature resistant steel alloys for use in gas turbines and jet aircraft engines, production of catalysts, lubricants, and dyes.

Disposition. While molybdenum exists in various valence forms, biologic differences with respect to valence are not clear. The soluble hexavalent compounds are well absorbed from the gastrointestinal tract into the liver. It is a component of xanthine oxidase, which has a role in purine metabolism and has been shown to be a component of aldehyde oxidase and sulfite oxidase. Increased molybdenum intake in experimental animals has been shown to increase tissue levels of xanthine oxidase. In humans, molybdenum is contained principally in the liver, kidney, fat, and blood. Of the approximate total of 9 mg in the body, most is concentrated in the liver, kidney, adrenal, and omentum. More than 50 percent of molybdenum in the liver is contained in a nonprotein cofactor bound to the mitochondrial outer membrane and can be transferred to an apoenzyme transforming it into an active enzyme molecule (Johnson *et al.*, 1977). The molybdenum level is relatively low in the newborn and increases until age 20, declining in concentration thereafter. More than half of the molybdenum excreted is in the urine. The blood level, at least in sheep, is in association with the red blood cells. However, molybdenum has been detected in only about 25 percent of the blood samples of the human urban population. The excretion of molybdenum is rapid, mainly as molybdate. Excesses may be excreted also by the bile, particularly the hexavalent forms.

Inhalation of molybdenum by guinea pigs has resulted in increased bone levels. Injected radiomolybdenum increased liver and kidney levels, but the endocrine glands were also exceptionally high in content.

Toxicity. Pastures containing 20 to 100 ppm molybdenum may produce a disease referred to as "teart" in cattle and sheep. It is characterized by anemia, poor growth rate, and diarrhea. Copper or sulfate in the diet prevents the disease, and removal of the animals from pastures containing high levels of molybdenum facilitates their rapid recovery. Prolonged exposure has led to deformities of the joints. Experimental studies have revealed differences in toxicity of molybdenum salts. Molybdenum sulfide was well tolerated in rats at 500 mg/kg/day and was not injurious to guinea pigs at 28 mg/m^3. Hexavalent compounds were more toxic. In rats molybdenum trioxide at a dose of 100 mg/kg/day, by inhalation, was irritating to the eyes and mucous membranes and subsequently lethal. After repeated oral administration at sufficient levels, fatty degeneration of the liver and kidney was induced. In comparison with chromium and tungsten salts, sodium molybdate by intraperitoneal injection was less toxic in mice.

Interesting relationships of molybdenum with other metals with respect to toxicity in cattle and sheep have been documented. For example, copper prevents the accumulation of molybdenum in the liver and may antagonize the absorption of molybdenum from food. It is reported that by alternating the intake of copper and molybdenum at weekly intervals, black sheep can be made to grow striped wool. White wool in black sheep is a sign of copper deficiency. The antagonism of copper is dependent on sulfate in the diet. It has been suggested that sulfate may displace molybdate in the body. It may be that the anemia caused by molybdenum is due to the reduction of sulfide oxidase in the liver, resulting in the formation of copper sulfide, thereby inducing a functional copper deficiency. Feeding of tungstate has also been shown to displace molybdate. In addition, it has been reported that molybdenum may promote fluoride retention and thereby decrease dental caries (see Underwood), but the incidences of caries in children living in high molybdenum areas compared to children living in normal or low molybdenum areas do not differ (Curzan et al., 1970).

Selenium

The availability as well as the toxic potential for selenium and selenium compounds is related to chemical form and, most important, to solubility. Selenium occurs in nature and biologic systems as selenate (Se^{6+}), selenite (Se^{4+}), elemental selenium (Se^0), and selenide (Se^{2-}), and deficiency leads to a cardiomyopathy in mammals including humans (Underwood, 1977; Wilber, 1983).

Selenium in foodstuffs provides a daily source of selenium (NAS, 1975). Seafoods, especially shrimp, meat, milk products, and grains provide the largest amounts in the diet. River water levels of selenium vary depending on environmental and geologic factors; 0.02 ppm has been reported as a representative estimate. Selenium has also been detected in urban air, presumably from sulfur-containing materials.

Disposition. Selenates are relatively soluble compounds, similar to sulfates, and are readily taken up by biologic systems, whereas selenites and elemental selenium are virtually insoluble. Because of their insolubility, these forms may be regarded as a form of inert selenium sink. Selenides of heavy metals are also very insoluble compounds, in fact, so insoluble that the *in vivo* formation of mercury selenide by dietary administration of selenite has been proposed as a method for detoxication of methyl mercury. Other metallic selenides such as arsenic, cadmium, and copper also have low solubility affecting absorption, retention, and distribution within the body of selenium and heavy metal. Elemental selenium is probably not absorbed from the gastrointestinal tract. Absorption of selenite is from the duodenum. Monogastric animals have a higher intestinal absorption than ruminants, probably because selenite is reduced to an insoluble form in rumen. Over 90 percent of milligram doses of sodium selenite may be absorbed by man and widely distributed in organs, with highest accumulation initially in liver

and kidney, but appreciable levels remain in blood, brain, myocardium, and skeletal muscle and testis. Selenium is transferred through the placenta to the fetus and it also appears in milk. Levels in milk are dependent on dietary intake. Selenium in red cells is associated with glutathione peroxidase and is about three times more concentrated than in plasma (Burk, 1976).

Selenium compounds may be biotransformed in the body by incorporation into amino acids or proteins or by methylation (Diplock, 1976). Selenium amino acids, Se-cysteine, and Se-methionine are formed in plants and absorbed as free amino acid or from digested protein. Se-methionine can be directly incorporated into proteins in place of methionine (McConnell and Hoffman, 1972). It is also suggested that selenite may be converted to Se-cysteine and incorporated into protein. Dimethyl selenium is an intermediate in the formation of a urinary metabolite, trimethyl selenium. It may be exhaled during acute selenium toxicity when its formation exceeds the rate of further methylation and urinary excretion (Palmer et al., 1969).

The excretion pattern of a single exposure to selenite appears to have at least two phases: a rapid initial phase with as much as 15 to 40 percent of the absorbed dose excreted in the urine the first week. There is exponential excretion of the remainder of the dose with a half-life of 103 days. The half-life of Semethionine is 234 days. In the steady state, urine contains about twice as much as feces and increased urinary levels provide a measure of exposure. Urinary selenium is usually less than 100 μg/liter.

Excretory products appear in sweat and expired air. The latter may have a garlicky odor due to dimethyl selenide. Within certain physiologic limits, the body appears to have a homeostatic mechanism for retaining trace amounts of selenium and excreting the excess material. Selenium toxicity occurs when the intake exceeds the excretory capacity (McConnell and Portman, 1952; Schroeder and Mitchner, 1972).

Essentiality. A biologic role for selenium is attributed to its incorporation in Se-cysteine at each of the four catalytic sites of the enzyme glutathione peroxidase. This enzyme uses glutathione to reduce organic hydroperoxides and protects membrane lipids and possibly proteins and nucleic acids against oxidant damage (Sunde and Hoekstra, 1980). Selenium is also a component of heme oxidase. The antioxidant activity of selenium-containing enzymes suggests a close relationship to vitamin E, but it may have a more subtle effect not yet defined in that selenium is beneficial to animals adequately supplied with vitamin E.

Selenium-deficient diets cause liver necrosis

in rats and multiple organs (liver, heart, kidneys, skeletal muscle, and testes) in mice. In chicks, pancreatic fibrosis, exudative diathesis, and alopecia are responsive to selenium supplementation. Lambs and calves suffer from a muscle disease called stiff-lamb disease and white-muscle disease when raised in selenium ranges of selenium-deficient plants. Also, embryo mortality in ewes from selenium-deficient areas is reversed by supplementation. Liver necrosis and cardiac myopathy occur in young pigs on selenium-deficient diets and is prevented by the addition of selenium to the diet (Underwood, 1977). While the role of selenium as an essential mineral seems certain in animals, the requirement for humans has been more difficult to establish. However, there are now reports of the efficacy of oral sodium selenite in the prophylaxis and treatment of an endemic cardiomyopathy in the People's Republic of China (Keshan disease), (Chen *et al.*, 1980) and the alleviation by Se-methionine of muscle pain and tenderness in a New Zealand woman on intravenous feeding (Van Rij *et al.*, 1979). Both reports are from regions where, for geochemical reasons, the indigenous population has a low intake of selenium. Selenium depletion has also been reported in association with cardiovascular disease and other cardiomyopathies. Although these case reports and the Chinese study are not the rigorous criteria required to establish the essentiality of a trace metal, for many it does seem that certain clinical situations may be improved with the administration of selenium (Editorial, 1983).

Toxicity. Industrial exposure to hydrogen selenide, occurring as a result of a reaction to acid or water with metal selenides, produces "garlic" breath, nausea, dizziness, and lassitude. Eye and nasal irritation may occur. In experimental animals 10 ppm is fatal. Selenium oxychloride, a vesicant, presents an industrial hazard. In rabbits 0.01 ml applied dermally resulted in death. Percutaneous absorption increased blood and liver selenium concentrations.

Acute selenium poisoning produces central nervous system effects, which include nervousness, drowsiness, and sometimes convulsions. Symptoms of chronic inhalation exposure may include pallor, coated tongue, gastrointestinal disorders, nervousness, "garlic" breath, liver and spleen damage, anemia, mucosal irritation, and lumbar pain. It has been suggested that some of these symptoms are due to tellurium impurities (Patty, 1963).

"Blind stagger" caused by excess selenium in livestock consuming 100 to 1000 ppm is characterized by impairment of vision, weakness of limbs, and respiratory failure (Moxan and Rhian, 1943). Clear evidence of chronic selenium toxicity in humans occurs only in seleniferous areas when the local foods are processed. Signs of intoxication may include discolored or decayed teeth, skin eruptions, gastrointestinal distress, lassitude, and partial loss of hair and nails. Livestock foraging on plants containing about 25 ppm suffer from "alkali" disease, which is characterized by lack of vitality, loss of hair, sterility, atrophy of hooves, lameness, and anemia. Fatty necrosis of the liver is frequent. In rats given 3 ppm of the material in drinking water, selenite has been reported to be more toxic than selenate. Selenite produced increased numbers of aortic plaques and was found to be more toxic in female than male mice. Selenium has produced loss of fertility and congenital defects and is considered embryotoxic and teratogenic on the basis of animal experiments (Moxan and Rhian, 1943; Schroeder and Mitchner, 1972). Selenium sulfide produced an increase in hepatocellular carcinomas and adenomas, but selenium sulfide suspension and Selsun®, an antidandruff shampoo containing 2.5 percent selenium sulfide, applied to the skin of Swiss mice did not produce dermal tumors (NCI, 1980b, 1980c).

Epidemiologic investigations have indicated a decrease in human cancer death rates (age and sex adjusted) correlated with increasing selenium content of forage crops (Shamberger *et al.*, 1976). In addition, experimental evidence supports the antineoplastic effect of selenium with regard to benzo[a]pyrene- and benzanthracene-induced skin tumors in mice, N-2-fluorenylacetamide- and diethylaminoazobenzene-induced hepatic tumors in rats, and spontaneous mammary tumors in mice. A possible mechanism of the protective effects of selenium has been postulated to involve inhibition of the formation of malonaldehyde, a product of peroxidative tissue damage, which is carcinogenic.

In addition to the apparent protective effect against some carcinogenic agent, selenium is an antidote to the toxic effects of other metals, particularly arsenic, cadmium, mercury, copper, and thallium. The mechanism underlying these interactions is unknown (Howell and Hill, 1978).

Zinc

Zinc is a nutritionally essential metal, and deficiency results in severe health consequences. On the other hand, excessive exposure to zinc is relatively uncommon and requires heavy exposure. Zinc does not accumulate with continued exposure, but body content is modulated by homeostatic mechanisms that act principally on absorption and liver levels (Underwood, 1977; NRCC, 1981; Sandstead, 1981; Prasad, 1983).

Zinc is ubiquitous in the environment so that it is present in most foodstuffs, water, and air. Content may be increased in contact with galvanized copper or plastic pipes. Seafoods, meats, whole grains, dairy products, nuts, and legumes are high in zinc content. Vegetables are lower. Zinc applied to soil is taken up by growing vegetables. Zinc atmospheric levels are increased over industrial areas. The average American daily intake is approximately 12 to 15 mg, mostly from food.

Disposition. About 20 to 30 percent of ingested zinc is absorbed. The mechanism is thought to be homeostatically controlled and is probably a carrier-mediated process (Davies, 1980). It is influenced by prostaglandins E_2 and F_2 and is chelated by picolinic acid—a tryptophan derivative. Deficiency of pyridoxine or trypotophan depresses zinc absorption. Within the mucosal cell, zinc induces metallothionein synthesis and, when saturated, may depress zinc absorption. In the blood, about two-thirds of the zinc is bound to albumin and most of the remainder is complexed with β_2-macroglobin. Zinc enters the gastrointestinal tract as a component of metallothionein secreted by the salivary glands, intestinal mucosa, pancreas, and liver. About 2 g of zinc is filtered by the kidneys each day, and about 300 to 600 μg/day is actually excreted by normal adults. Renal tubular reabsorption is impaired by commonly prescribed drugs, such as thiazide diuretics, and is further influenced by dietary protein. There is good correlation between dietary zinc and urinary zinc excretion.

Zinc concentration in tissues varies widely. Liver receives up to about 40 percent of a tracer dose, declining to about 25 percent within five days. Liver concentration is influenced by humoral factors including adrenocorticotropic hormone, parathyroid hormone, and endotoxin. In the liver, as well as other tissues, zinc is bound to metallothionein. The greatest concentration of zinc in the body is in the prostate, probably related to the rich content of zinc-containing enzyme acid phosphatase.

Deficiency. More than 70 metalloenzymes require zinc as a cofactor, and deficiency results in a wide spectrum of clinical effects depending on age, stage of development, and deficiencies of related metals.

Zinc deficiency in humans was first characterized by Prasad and co-workers (1963) in adolescent Egyptian boys with growth failure and delayed sexual maturation and is accompanied by protein-caloric malnutrition, pellegra, iron, and folate deficiency. Zinc deficiency in the newborn may be manifested by dermatitis, loss of hair, impaired healing, susceptibility to infections, and neuropsychologic abnormalities. Dietary inadequacies coupled with liver disease from chronic alcoholism may be associated with dermatitis, night blindness, testicular atrophy, impotence, and poor wound healing. Other chronic clinical disorders, such as ulcerative colitis and the malabsorption syndromes, chronic renal disease, and the hemolytic anemias, are also prone to zinc deficiency. Many drugs affect zinc homeostasis particularly metal-chelating agents and some antibiotics, such as penicillin and isoniazid. Less common zinc deficiency may occur with myocardial infarction, arthritis, and even hypertension.

Biologic Indicators of Abnormal Zinc Homeostasis. The range of normal plasma zinc level is from 85 to 110 μg/dl. Severe deficiency may decrease plasma zinc to 40 to 60 μg/dl, accompanied by increased serum β_2-globulin and decreased α-globulin. Urine zinc excretion may decrease from over 300 μg/day to less than 100 μg/day. Zinc deficiency may exacerbate impaired copper nutrition and, of course, zinc interactions with cadmium and lead may modify the toxicity of these metals (Sandstead, 1981).

Toxicity. Zinc toxicity from excessive ingestion is uncommon, but gastrointestinal distress and diarrhea have been reported following ingestion of beverages standing in galvanized cans or from use of galvanized utensils. However, evidence of hematologic, hepatic, or renal toxicity has not been observed in individuals ingesting as much as 12 g of elemental zinc over a two-day period.

With regard to industrial exposure, metal fume fever resulting from inhalation of freshly formed fumes of zinc presents the most significant effect. The disorder has been most commonly associated with inhalation of zinc oxide fume, but it may be seen after inhalation of fumes of other metals, particularly magnesium, iron, and copper. Attacks usually begin after four to eight hours of exposure—chills and fever, profuse sweating, and weakness. Attacks usually last only 24 to 48 hours and are most common on Mondays or after holidays. The pathogenesis is not known, but is thought to be due to endogenous pyrogen released from cell lysis. Extracts prepared from tracheal mucosa and lungs of animals with experimentally induced metal fume fever produce similar symptoms when injected into other animals. Other aspects of zinc toxicity are not well established. Experimental animals have been given 100 times dietary requirements without discernible effects (Goyer *et al.*, 1979).

Exposure of guinea pigs three hours per day for six consecutive days to 5 mg/M^3 freshly formed ultrafine zinc oxide (the recommended TLV) produced decrements in lung volumes and carbon moxoxide diffusing capacity that persisted 72 hours after exposure. These functional changes were correlated with microscopic evidence of interstitial thickening and cellular infiltrate in alveolar ducts and alveoli (Lam *et al.*, 1985).

Testicular tumors have been produced by direct intratesticular injection in rats and chickens. This effect is probably related to the concentration of zinc normally in the gonads and may be hormonally dependent. Zinc salts have not produced carcinogenic effects when administered to animals by other routes (Furst, 1981).

METALS WITH TOXICITY RELATED TO MEDICAL THERAPY

Metals considered in this group include aluminum, bismuth, gold, lithium, and platinum. Metals at one time were used to treat a number of human ills, particularly heavy metals like mercury and arsenic. Gold salts are still useful for the treatment of forms of rheumatism, and organic bismuth compounds are used to treat gastrointestinal disturbances. Lithium has become an important aid in the treatment of depression. The toxicologic hazards from aluminum are not from its use as an antacid but rather the accumulations that occur in bone and other tissues in patients with chronic renal failure receiving hemodialysis therapy. Platinum is receiving attention as an antitumor agent. Barium and gallium are used as a radiopaque and radiotracer material, respectively, so they do have importance in medical therapy. Toxicologic effects are unlikely and seldom occur.

Aluminum

Aluminum is one of the most abundant metals in the earth's crust, and it is ubiquitous in air and water, as well as soil.

The toxicity of aluminum may be divided into three major categories: (1) the effect of aluminum compounds on the gastrointestinal tract; (2) the effect of inhalation of aluminum compounds; and (3) systemic toxicity of aluminum (Alfrey, 1981).

Aluminum compounds can affect absorption of other elements in the gastrointestinal tract and alter intestinal function. Aluminum inhibits fluoride absorption and may decrease the absorption of calcium and iron compounds (Spencer *et al.*, 1969, 1977) and possibly the absorption of cholesterol by forming an aluminum-pectin complex that binds fats to nondigestible vegetable fibers (Nagyvary and Bradbury, 1977). The binding of phosphorus in the intestinal tract can lead to phosphate depletion and osteomalacia (Lotz, 1968). Aluminum may alter gastrointestinal tract motility by inhibition of acetylcholine-induced contractions and may be the explanation of why aluminum-containing antacids often produce constipation.

Pulmonary effects of aluminum occur following inhalation of bauxite (Al_2O_3–$3H_2O$) fumes. The resultant pulmonary fibrosis produces both restrictive and obstructive pulmonary disease (Schaver, 1948). Interestingly, inhalation of aluminum mists was used in the 1930s to serve as prophylaxis of pulmonary fibrosis due to inhalation of silica particles. It is suggested that aluminum and silicic acid compete for a common reactive site in the oxidative phosphorylation pathway (Engelbrecht and Jordaan, 1972).

There has been increasing interest in the possible relationship of aluminum to dementia in humans (Wills and Savory, 1983). Intracerebral injection of aluminum phosphate or injection of aluminum powder in cerebrospinal fluid of animals has been noted to induce a progressive encephalopathy and neurofibrillary degeneration histologically comparable to the changes found in persons with senile and presenile dementia of the Alzheimer type (Deboni *et al.*, 1976). However, some morphologic differences have been noted at the ultrastructural level, and why specific individuals are affected by such a ubiquitous metal is an unresolved question.

A progressive fatal neurologic syndrome has also been reported in patients on long-term intermittent hemodialysis treatment for chronic renal failure (Alfrey *et al.*, 1972). The first symptom in these patients is a speech disorder followed by dementia, convulsions, and myoclonus. The disorder, which typically arises after three to seven years of dialysis treatment, may be due to aluminum intoxication. Aluminum content of brain, muscle, and bone tissues is increased in these patients. Crapper (1976) has shown that brain tissue of mammals normally contains 1 to 2 μg of aluminum per gram dry weight and that the toxic range is 4 to 8 μg/g dry weight of brain for the cat and rabbit.

Sources of the excess aluminum may be from oral aluminum hydroxide commonly given to these patients or from aluminum in dialysis fluid derived from tap water used to prepare the dialysate fluid. High serum and aluminum concentrations are generally present in these patients, and it is postulated that increased absorption may be related to increased parathyroid hormone due to low blood calcium and osteodystrophy common in patients with chronic renal disease. The syndrome may be prevented by avoidance of the use of aluminum-containing oral phosphate binders and monitoring of aluminum in the dialysate. Chelation of aluminum may be achieved with use of desferrioxamine, and progression of the dementia may be arrested or slowed (Crapper-McLachlan, 1983).

Bismuth

Bismuth has a long history of use in pharmaceuticals in Europe and North America. Both inorganic and organic salts have been used, depending on the specific application. There are three major categories of uses: antisyphylitic agents, topical creams, and antacids. Trivalent insoluble bismuth salts are used medicinally to control diarrhea and other types of gastorintestinal distress. Various bismuth salts have been used externally for their astringent and slight antiseptic property. Bismuth salts have also been used as radiocontrast agents. Further potential for exposure comes from the use of insoluble bismuth salts in cosmetics. Injections of soluble and insoluble salts, suspended in oil to maintain adequate blood levels, have been used to treat syphilis. Bismuth sodium thioglycollamate, a water-soluble salt, was injected intramuscularly for malaria (*Plasmodium vivax*). Bismuth glycolyarsanilate is one of the few pentavalent salts that have been used medicinally. This material was formerly used for treatment of amebiasis (Fowler and Vouk, 1977). Exposure to various bismuth salts for medicinal use has decreased with the advent of newer therapeutic agents. However, in the 1970s reports appeared from France and Australia of unique encephalopathy occurring in colostomy and ileostomy patients using bismuth subgallate, bismuth subnitrate, and tripotassium-dicitrate-bismuthate for control of fecal odor and consistency. The symptoms included progressive mental confusion, irregular myoclonic jerks, a distinctive pattern of disordered gait, and a variable degree of dysarthria. The disorder was fatal to patients who continued use of the bismuth compounds, but full recovery was rapid in those in whom therapy was discontinued. The severity of the disorder seemed to be independent of dose and duration of therapy (Thomas *et al.*, 1977).

Most bismuth compounds are insoluble and poorly absorbed from the gastrointestinal tracts, or when applied to the skin, even if the skin is abraded or burned. Symptomatic patients taking bismuth subgallate had an elevated median blood bismuth level of 14.6 μg Bi/dl, patients without clinical symptoms had a median blood level of 3 μg/dl, and colostomy patients not on bismuth therapy had a median bismuth blood level of 0.8 μg/dl. Health laboratory workers had a median bismuth blood level of 1.0 μg/dl. Binding in blood is thought to be largely to a plasma protein with a molecular weight greater than 50,000 daltons.

A diffusible equilibrium between tissues, blood, and urine is established. Tissue distribution, omitting injection depots, reveals the kidney as the site of the highest concentration. The liver concentration is considerably lower at therapeutic levels, but with massive doses in experimental animals (dogs), the kidney/liver ratio is decreased. Passage of bismuth into the amniotic fluid and into the fetus has been demonstrated. The urine is the major route of excretion. Traces of bismuth can be found in milk and saliva. The total elimination of bismuth after injection is slow and dependent on mobilization from the injection site.

Acute renal failure can occur following oral administration of such compounds as bismuth sodium triglycollamate or thioglycollate particularly in children (Urizar and Vernier, 1966). The tubular epithelium is the primary site of toxicity producing degeneration of renal tubular cells and nuclear inclusion bodies composed of a bismuth-protein complex analogous to those found in lead toxicity (Beaver and Burr, 1963; Fowler and Goyer, 1975).

The symptoms of chronic toxicity in humans consist of decreased appetite, weakness, rheumatic pain, diarrhea, fever, metal line on the gums, foul breath, gingivitis, and dermatitis. Jaundice and conjuctival hemorrhage are rare, but have been reported. Bismuth nephropathy with proteinuria may occur.

Chelation therapy using dimercaprol (BAL) is said to be helpful in removal of bismuth from children with acute toxicity (Arena, 1974).

Gallium

Gallium is of interest because of the use of radiogallium as a diagnostic tool for localization of bone lesions. It is obtained as a by-product of copper, zinc, lead, and aluminum refining and is used in high-temperature thermometers, as a substitute for mercury in arc lamps, as a component of metal alloys, and as a seal for vacuum equipment. It is only sparsely absorbed from the gastrointestinal tract, but concentrations of less than 1 ppm can be localized radiographically in bone lesions. Higher doses will visualize liver, spleen, and kidney as well.

Gallium is not readily absorbed by the oral route, but occurs in bone at concentrations less than 1 ppm. Increasing intake produces slight increases in gallium levels in the liver, spleen, kidney, and bone. The urine is the major route of excretion.

There are no reported adverse effects of gallium following industrial exposure. Therapeutic use of radiogallium produced some adverse effects, mild dermatitis, and gastrointestinal disturbances. Bone marrow depression has been reported and may be due largely to the radioactivity. In animals gallium acts as a neuromuscular poison and causes renal damage. Photophobia, blindness, and paralysis have been reported in rats. Renal damage ranging from cloudy swelling to tubular cell necrosis has been reported. Aplastic changes in the bone marrow have been observed in dogs (Browning, 1969).

Gold

Gold is widely distributed in small quantities but economically usable deposits occur as the free metal in quartz veins or alluvial gravel. Seawater contains 3 or 4 mg/ton and small amounts, 0.03 to 1 mg percent, have been reported in many foods. Gold has a number of industrial uses because of its electrical and thermal conductivity.

While gold and its salts have been used for a wide variety of medicinal purposes, their present uses are limited to the treatment of rheumatoid arthritis and rare skin diseases such as discoid lupus. Gold salts are poorly absorbed from the gastrointestinal tract. Normal urine and fecal excretions of 0.1 and 1 mg/day, respectively, have been reported. After injection of most of the soluble salts, gold is excreted via the urine, while the feces account for the major portion of insoluble compounds. Gold seems to have a long biologic half-life, and detectable blood levels can be demonstrated for ten months after cessation of treatment.

Dermatitis is the most frequently reported toxic reaction to gold and is sometimes accompanied by stomatitis. Use of gold in the form of organic salts to treat rheumatoid arthritis may be complicated by development of proteinuria and the nephrotic syndrome, which morphologically consists of an immune-complex glomerulonephritis with granular deposits along the glomerular basement membrane and in the mesangium. The pathogenesis of the immune-complex disease is not certain, but gold may behave as a hapten and generate the production of antibodies with subsequent disposition of gold protein-antibody complexes in the glomerular subepithelium. Another hypothesis is that antibodies are formed against damaged tubular structures, particularly mitochondria, providing immune complexes for the glomerular deposits (Voil *et al.*, 1977).

The pathogenesis of the renal lesions induced by gold therapy is probably initiated by the direct toxicity of gold with tubular cell components. From experimental studies it appears that gold salts have an affinity for mitochondria of proximal tubular lining cells, which is followed by autophagocytosis and accumulation of gold in amorphous phagolysosomes (Stuve and Galle,

1970), and gold particles can be identified in degenerating mitochondria in tubular lining cells and in glomerular epithelial cell by x-ray microanalysis (Ainsworth *et al.*, 1981).

Lithium

Lithium carbonate is an important aid in the treatment of depression. There must be careful monitoring of usage to provide optimal therapeutic value and not produce toxicity. Lithium is a common metal and present in many plant and animal tissues. Daily intake is about 2 mg. It is readily absorbed from the gastrointestinal tract. Distribution in the human organs is almost uniform. The normal plasma level is about 17 μg/liter. The red cells contain less. Excretion is chiefly through the kidneys, but some is eliminated in the feces. The greater part of lithium is contained in the cells, perhaps at the expense of potassium. In general, the body distribution of lithium is quite similar to that of sodium, and it may be competing with sodium at certain sites, for example, in renal tubular reabsorption.

Lithium has some industrial uses, in alloys, as a catalytic agent, and as a lubricant. Lithium hydride produces hydrogen on contact with water and is used in manufacturing electronic tubes, in ceramics, and in chemical synthesis. From the industrial point of view, except for lithium hydride, none of the other salts or the metal itself is hazardous. Lithium hydride is intensely corrosive and may produce burns on the skin because of the formation of hydroxides (Browning, 1969; Cox and Singer, 1981).

The therapeutic use of lithium carbonate may produce unusual toxic responses. These include neuromuscular changes (tremor, muscle hyperirritability, and ataxia), central nervous system changes (blackout spells, epileptic seizures, slurred speech, coma, psychosomatic retardation, and increased thirst), cardiovascular changes (cardiac arrhythmia, hypertension, and circulatory collapse), gastrointestinal changes (anorexia, nausea, and vomiting) and renal damage (albuminuria and glycosuria). The latter is believed to be due to temporary hypokalemic nephritis. These changes appear to be more frequent when the serum levels increase above 1.5 mEq/liter, suggesting that careful monitoring of this parameter is needed rather than reliance on the amount given.

Chronic lithium nephrotoxicity can occur with long-term exposure even when lithium levels remain within the therapeutic range. Tubular defects, particularly nephrogenic diabetes insipidus, may occur. There is more recent awareness of the possible development of chronic interstitial nephritis (Singer, 1981).

The cardiovascular and nervous system

changes may be due to the competitive relationship between lithium and potassium and may thus produce a disturbance in intracellular metabolism. Thyrotoxic reactions, including goiter formation, have also been suggested (Davis and Fann, 1971). While there has been some indication of adverse effects on fetuses following lithium treatment, none was observed in rats (4.05 mEq/kg), rabbits (1.08 mEq/kg), or primates (0.67 mEq/kg). This dose to rats was sufficient to produce maternal toxicity and effects on the pups of treated, lactating dams (Gralla and McIlhenny, 1972).

Lithium overdosage and toxicity may be treated by administration of diuretics and lowering of blood levels. Acetazolamide, a carbonic anhydrase inhibitor, has been used clinically. Animal studies have shown that urinary excretion of lithium can be further enhanced by the combined administration of acetazolamide and furosemide. Treatment with diuretics must be accompanied by replacement of water and electrolytes (Steele, 1977).

Platinum

Platinum-group metals include a relatively light triad of ruthenium, rhodium, and palladium and the heavy metals osmium, iridium, and platinum. They are found together in sparsely distributed mineral deposits or as a by-product of refining other metals, chiefly nickel and copper. Osmium and iridium are not important toxicologically. Osmium tetroxide, however, is a powerful eye irritant. The other metals are generally nontoxic in their metallic states but have been noted to have toxic effects in particular circumstances. Platinum is interesting because of its extensive industrial applications and use of certain complexes as antitumor agents.

Toxicological information for ruthenium is limited to references in the literature indicating that fumes may be injurious to eyes and lungs (Browning, 1969).

Rhodium trichloride produced death in rats and rabbits within 48 hours after intravenous administration at doses near the LD50 (approximately 200 mg/kg). It was suggested that death was attributable to central nervous system effects (Landolt et al., 1972). In a single study, incorporation of rhodium (rhodium chloride) or palladium (palladous chloride) into the drinking water of mice at a concentration of 5 ppm over the lifetime of the animals produced a minimally significant increase in malignant tumors. Most of these tumors were classified as of the lymphoma-leukemia type (Schroeder and Mitchener, 1971).

Palladium chloride is not readily absorbed from subcutaneous injection, and no adverse effects have been reported from industrial exposure. Colloid palladium (Pd[OH]$_2$) is reported to increase body temperature, produce discoloration and necrosis at the site of injection, decrease body weight, and cause slight hemolysis.

Platinum metal itself is generally harmless, but an allergic dermatitis can be produced in susceptible individuals. Skin changes are most common between the fingers and in the antecubital fossae. Symptoms of respiratory distress, ranging from irritation to an "asthmatic syndrome" with coughing, wheezing, and shortness of breath, have been reported following exposure to platinum dust. The skin and respiratory changes are termed platinosis. They are mainly confined to persons with a history of industrial exposure to soluble compounds such as sodium chloroplatinate, although cases resulting from wearing platinum jewelry have been reported.

The complex salts of platinum may act as powerful allergens, particularly ammonium hexachloroplatinate and hexachloroplatinic acid. The allergenicity appears to be related to the number of chlorine atoms present in the molecule, but other soluble nonchlorinated platinum compounds may also be allergenic. Biochemistry and antitumor activity of platinum complexes of major consideration for this group of metals are the potential antitumor and carcinogenic effects of certain neutral complexes of platinum such as cis-dichlorodiammine, platinum (II), and various analogs (Kazantzis, 1981). They can inhibit cell division and have antibacterial properties as well. These compounds can react selectively with specific chemical sites in proteins such as disulfide bonds and terminal-NH$_2$ groups, with functional groups in amino acids, and in particular with receptor sites in nucleic acids. These compounds also exhibit neuromuscular toxicity and nephrotoxicity.

For antitumor activity, the complexes should be neutral and should have a pair of cis-leaving groups. Other metals in the group give complexes that are inactive or less active than the platinum analog. At dosages that are therapeutically effective (antitumor), these complexes produce severe and persistent inhibition of DNA synthesis and little inhibition of RNA and protein synthesis. DNA polymerase activity and transport of DNA precursors through plasma membranes are not inhibited. The complexes are thought to react directly with DNA in regions that are rich in guanosine and cytosine.

Mutagenic and Carcinogenic Effects of Platinum Complexes. Cis-dichlordiamine platinum (cis-DDP) has been used clinically to treat some cancers of the head and neck, certain lymphomas, and testicular and ovarian tumors. Cis-DDP is a strong mutagen in bacterial systems and has been shown to form both intra- and interstrand cross-links probably involving the whole molecule with human DNA in HeLa cell cultures. There is also a correlation between antitumor activity of cis-DDP and its ability to bind DNA and induce phage from bacterial cells. It also causes chromosome aberration in cultured hamster cells and a dose-dependent increase in sister chromosome exchanges.

Although cis-DDP has antitumorigenic activity in experimental animals, it also seems to increase the frequency of lung adenomas and give rise to skin papillomas and carcinomas in mice. These observations are consistent with the activity of other alkylating agents used in cancer chemotherapy. There are no reports of increased risk to cancer from occupational exposure to platinum compounds.

Nephrotoxicity. Cis-DDP is a nephrotoxin. It produces compounds with antitumor activity and produces proximal and distal tubular cell injury mainly in the corticomedullary region where the concentration of platinum is highest (Madias and Harrington, 1978). Although 90 percent of administered cis-platinum becomes tightly bound to plasma proteins, only unbound platinum is rapidly filtered by the glomerulus and has a half-life of only 48 minutes. Within tissues, platinum is protein bound with largest concentrations in kidney, liver, and spleen, and has a half-life of two or three days. Tubular cell toxicity seems to be directly related to dose, and prolonged weekly injection in rats causes atrophy of cortical portions of nephrons and cystic dilatation of inner cortical or medullary tubules and chronic renal failure due to tubulointerstitial nephritis (Choie et al., 1981).

MINOR TOXIC METALS

Antimony

Antimony may have a tri- or pentavalance and it belongs to the same periodic group as arsenic. Its disposition metabolism is thought to resemble that of arsenic. It is absorbed slowly from the gastrointestinal tract, and many antimony compounds are gastrointestinal irritants. Antimony tartar has been used as an emetic. The disposition of the tri and penta forms differ. Trivalent antimony is concentrated in red blood cells and liver whereas the penta form is mostly in plasma. Both forms are excreted in feces and urine, but more trivalent antimony is excreted in urine whereas there is greater gastrointestinal excretion of pentavalent antimony. Antimony is a common air pollutant from industrial emmissions, but exposure for the general population is largely from food.

Antimony is included in alloys in the metals industry and is used for producing fireproofing chemicals, ceramics, glassware, and pigments. It has been used medicinally as an antiparasitic agent. Accidental poisonings can result in acute toxicity, which produces severe gastrointestinal symptoms including vomiting and diarrhea.

Most information about antimony toxicity has been obtained from industrial experiences. Occupational exposures are usually by inhalation of dust containing antimony compounds, antimony penta and trichloride, trioxide, and trisulfide. Effects may be acute, particularly from the penta and trichloride exposures, producing a rhinitis and even acute pulmonary edema. Chronic exposures by inhalation of other antimony compounds results in rhinitis, pharyngitis, tracheitis, and, over the longer term, bronchitis and eventually pneumoconiosis with obstructive lung disease and emphysema. Antimony does accumulate in lung tissue (Elinder and Friberg, 1977).

Oral feeding of antimony to rats has not produced an excess of tumors. However, increased chromosome defects occur when human lymphocytes are incubated with a soluble antimony salt (Paton and Allison, 1975), and Syrian hamster embryo cells show an undergo neoplastic transformation when treated with antimony acetate (Casto, et al., 1979). Transient skin eruptions, "antimony spots," may occur in workers with chronic exposure.

Antimony may also form an odorless toxic gas, stibine (H_3S_6), which, like arsine, causes hemolysis.

Barium

Barium is used in various alloys, in paints, soap, paper, and rubber, and in the manufacture of ceramics and glass. Barium fluorosilicate and carbonate have been used as insecticides. Barium sulfate, an insoluble compound, is used as a radiopaque aid to x-ray diagnosis. Barium is relatively abundant in nature and is found in plants and animal tissue. Plants accumulate barium from the soil. Brazil nuts have very high concentrations (3000 to 4000 ppm). Some water contains barium from natural deposits.

The toxicity of barium compounds depends on their solubility. The soluble compounds of barium are absorbed, and small amounts are accumulated in the skeleton. The lung has an average concentration of 1 ppm (dry weight). The kidney, spleen, muscle, heart, brain, and liver concentrations are 0.10, 0.08, 0.05, 0.05, and 0.03 ppm, respectively. Although some barium is excreted in urine, it is reabsorbed by the renal tubules. The major route of excretion is the feces. Occupational poisoning to barium is uncommon, but a benign pneumoconiosis (baritosis) may result from inhalation of barium sulfate (barite) dust and barium carbonate. It is not incapacitating and is usually reversible with cessation of exposure. Accidental poisoning from ingestion of soluble barium salts has resulted in gastroenteritis, muscular paralysis, decreased pulse rate, and ventricular fibrillation and extrasystoles. Potassium deficiency occurs in acute poisoning, and treatment with intravenous potassium appears beneficial. The digitalislike toxicity, muscle stimulation, and central nervous system effects have been confirmed by experimental investigation (Reeves, 1979).

Indium

Indium is a rare metal whose toxiocologic importance was related to its use in alloys, solders, and as a hardening agent for bearings. Use in the electronic industry for production of semiconductors and photovoltiac cells may greatly expand worker exposure. It is currently being used in medicine for scanning of organs and treatment of tumors. Indium is poorly absorbed from the gastrointestinal tract. It is excreted in the urine and feces. Its tissue distribution is relatively uniform. The kidney, liver, bone, and spleen have relatively high concentrations. Intratracheal injections produce similar concentrations, but the concentration in the tracheobronchial lymph nodes is increased.

There are no meaningful reports of human toxicity to indium. From animal experiments it is apparent that toxicity is related to the chemical form. Indium chloride given intravenously to mice produces renal toxicity and liver necrosis. These effects are accompanied by induction of P-450-dependent microsomal enzyme activity and decreased activity of heme-synthesizing enzymes (Woods et al., 1979). Hydrated indium oxide produces damage to phagocytic cells in liver and the reticuloendothelial system (Fowler, 1982).

Magnesium

Magnesium is used in lightweight alloys, as an electrical conductive material, and for incendiary devices such as flares. It is also an essential nutrient whose deficiency causes neuromuscular irritability, calcification, and cardiac and renal damage, which can be prevented by supplementation. The deficiency is called "grass staggers" in cattle and "magnesium tetany" in calves. Magnesium is a cofactor of many enzymes; it is apparently associated with phosphate in these functions.

Magnesium citrate, oxide, sulfate, hydroxide, and carbonate are widely taken as antacids or cathartics. The hydroxide, milk of magnesia, is one of the constituents of the universal antidote for poisoning. Topically, the sulfate is also used widely to relieve inflammation. Magnesium sulfate may be used as a parenterally administered central depressant. Its most frequent use for this purpose is in the treatment of seizures associated with eclampsia of pregnancy and acute nephritis.

Nuts, cereals, seafoods, and meats are high dietary sources of magnesium. The average city water contains about 6.5 ppm, but varies considerably, increasing with the hardness of the water (Schroeder et al., 1969).

Disposition. Magnesium salts are poorly absorbed from the intestine. In cases of overload this may be due in part to their dehydrating action. Magnesium is absorbed mainly in the small intestine. The colon also absorbs some. Calcium and magnesium are competitive with respect to their absorptive sites, and excess calcium may partially inhibit the absorption of magnesium.

Magnesium is excreted into the digestive tract by the bile and pancreatic and intestinal juices. A small amount of radiomagnesium given intravenously appears in the gastrointestinal tract. The serum levels are remarkably constant. There is an apparent obligatory urinary loss of magnesium, which amounts to about 12 mg/day, and the urine is the major route of excretion under normal conditions. Magnesium found in the stool is probably not absorbed. Magnesium is filtered by the glomeruli and reabsorbed by the renal tubules. In the blood plasma about 65 percent is in the ionic form, while the remainder is bound to protein. The former is that which appears in the glomerular filtrate. Mercurial diuretics cause excretion of magnesium as well as potassium, sodium, and calcium. Excretion also occurs in the sweat and milk. Endocrine activity, particularly of the adrenocortical hormones, aldosterone, and parathyroid hormone, has an effect on magnesium levels, although these effects may be related to the interaction of calcium and magnesium.

Tissue distribution studies indicate that of the 20-g body burden, the majority is intracellular in the bone and muscle. Bone concentration of magnesium decreases as calcium increases. Most of the remaining tissues have higher concentrations than blood, except for fat and omentum. With age, the aorta tends to accumulate magnesium along with calcium, perhaps as a function of atherosclerotic disease.

Toxicity. Freshly generated magnesium oxide can cause metal fume fever if inhaled in sufficient amounts, analogous to the effect caused by zinc oxide. Both zinc and magnesium exposure of animals produced similar effects. It is reported that particles of magnesium in the subcutaneous tissue produce lesions that resist healing. In animals, magnesium subcutaneously or intramuscularly administered produces gas gangrene as a result of interaction with the body fluids and subsequent generation of hydrogen and magnesium hydroxide. The tissue lesion is reversible.

Conjunctivitis, nasal catarrh, and coughing up of discolored sputum results from industrial inhalation exposure. With industrial exposures, increases of serum magnesium up to twice the normal levels failed to produce ill effects but were accompanied by calcium increases. Intoxication occurring after oral administration of magnesium salts is rare, but may be present in the face of renal impairment. The symptoms include a sharp drop in blood pressure and respiratory paralysis due to central nervous system depression (Browning, 1969).

Silver

The principal industrial use of silver is as silver halide in the manufacture of photographic plates. Other uses are for jewelry, coins, and eating utensils. Silver nitrate is used for making indelible inks and for medicinal purposes. The use of silver nitrate for prophylaxis of ophthalmia neonatorum is a legal requirement in some states. Other medicinal uses of silver salts are as a caustic, germicide, antiseptic, and astringent.

Silver does not occur regularly in animal or human tissue. The major effect of excessive absorption of silver is local or generalized impregnation of the tissues where it remains as silver sulfide, which forms an insoluble complex in elastic fibers resulting in argyria. Silver can be absorbed from the lungs and gastrointestinal tract. Complexes with serum albumin accumulate in the liver from which a fractional amount is excreted. Intravenous injection produces accumulation in the spleen, liver, bone marrow, lungs, muscle, and skin. The major route of excretion is via the gastrointestinal tract. Urinary excretion has not been reported to occur even after intravenous injection.

Industrial argyria, a chronic occupational disease, has two forms, local and generalized. The local form involves the formation of gray-blue patches on the skin or may manifest itself in the conjunctiva of the eye. In generalized argyria, the skin shows widespread pigmentation, often spreading from the face to most uncovered parts of the body. In some cases the skin may become black with a metallic luster. The eyes may be affected to such a point that the lens and vision are disturbed. The respiratory tract may also be affected in severe cases.

Large oral doses of silver nitrate cause severe gastrointestinal irritation due to its caustic action. Lesions of the kidneys and lungs and the possibility of arteriosclerosis have been attributed to both industrial and medicinal exposures. Large doses of colloidal silver administered intravenously to experimental animals produced death due to pulmonary edema and congestion. Hemolysis and resulting bone marrow hyperplasia have been reported. Chronic bronchitis has also been reported to result from medicinal use of colloidal silver (Browing, 1969; Luckey et al., 1975).

Tellurium

Tellurium is found in various sulfide ores along with selenium and is produced as a by-product of metal refineries. Its industrial uses include applications in the refining of copper and in the manufacture of rubber. Tellurium vapor is used in "daylight" lamps. It is used in various alloys as a catalyst and as a semiconductor.

Condiments, dairy products, nuts, and fish have high concentrations of tellurium. Food packaging contains some tellurium; higher concentrations are found in aluminum cans than tin cans. Some plants, such as garlic, accumulate tellurium from the soil. Potassium tellurate has been used to reduce sweating.

The average body burden in humans is about 600 mg; the majority is in bone. The kidney is the highest in content among the soft tissues. Some data suggest that tellurium also accumulates in liver (Schroeder et al., 1967a). Soluble tetravalent tellurities, absorbed into the body after oral administration, are reduced to tellurides, partly methylated, and then exhaled as dimethyl telluride. The latter is responsible for the garlic odor in persons exposed to tellurium compounds. Tellurium in the food is probably in the form of tellurates. The urine and bile are the principal routes of excretion. Sweat and milk are secondary routes of excretion.

Tellurates and tellurium are of low toxicity, but tellurites are generally more toxic. Acute inhalation exposure results in decreased sweating, nausea, a metallic taste, and sleeplessness. The typical garlic breath is a reasonable indicator of exposure to tellurium by the dermal inhalation, or oral route. Serious cases of tellurium intoxication from industrial exposure have not been reported. In rats, chronic exposure to high doses of tellurium dioxide has produced decreased growth and necrosis of the liver and kidney (Cerwenka and Cooper, 1961; Browning, 1969).

Sodium tellurite at 2 ppm in drinking water or potassium tellurate at 2 ppm of tellurium plus 0.16 μg/g in the diet of mice for their lifetime produced no effects in the tellurate group. The females of the tellurite (tetravalent) group did not live as long. In rats, 500 ppm in the diet of pregnant females induced hydrocephalus in the offspring. Abnormalities of and reduction in numbers of mitochondria were thought to be possible cellular causes of the transplacental effect.

One of the few serious recorded cases of tellurium toxicity resulted from accidental poisoning by injection of tellurium into the ureters during retrograde pyelography. Two of the three victims died. Stupor, cyanosis, vomiting, garlic breath, and loss of consciousness were observed in this unlikely incident.

Dimercaprol treatment for tellurium increases the renal damage. While ascorbic acid decreases the characteristic garlic odor, it may also adversely affect the kidneys in the presence of increased amounts of tellurium (Fishbein, 1977).

Thallium

Thallium is one of the more toxic metals and can cause neural, hepatic, and renal injury. It may also cause deafness and loss of vision. It is obtained as a by-product of the refining of iron, cadmium, and zinc. It is used as a catalyst, in certain alloys, optical lenses, jewelry, low-temperature thermometers, semiconductors, dyes and pigments, and scintillation counters. It has been used medicinally as a depilatory. Thallium compounds, chiefly thallous sulfate, have been used as rat poison and insecticides. This is one of the commonest sources of thallium poisoning.

Disposition. Thallium is not a normal constituent of animal tissues. It is absorbed through the skin and gastrointestinal tract. After parenteral administration a small amount can be identified in the urine within a few hours. The highest concentrations after poisoning are in the kidney and urine. The intestines, thyroids, testes, pancreas, skin, bone, and spleen have lesser amounts. The brain and liver concentrations are still lower. Following the initial exposure, large amounts are excreted in urine during the first 24 hours, but after that period excretion is slow and the feces may be an important route of excretion.

Toxicology. There are numerous acute clinical reports of acute thallium poisoning in humans characterized by gastrointestinal irritation, acute ascending paralysis, and psychic disturbances. Acute toxicity studies in rats have indicated that thallium is quite toxic. It has an oral LD_{50} of approximately 30 mg/kg. The estimated lethal dose in humans, however, is 8 to 12 mg/kg. Rat studies also indicate that thallium oxide, while relatively insoluble, is more toxic orally than by the intravenous or intraperitoneal route

(Downs *et al.*, 1960). The acute cardiovascular effects of thallium ions probably result from competition with potassium for membrane transport systems, inhibition of mitochondrial oxidative phosphorylation, and disruption of protein synthesis. It also alters heme metabolism.

The signs of subacute or chronic thallium poisoning in rats were hair loss, cataracts, and hindleg paralysis occurring with some delay after the initiation of dosing. Renal lesions were observed at gross necropsy. Histologic changes revealed damage of the proximal and distal renal tubules. The central nervous system changes were most severe in the mesencephalon where necrosis was observed. Perivascular cuffing was also reported in several other brain areas. Electron microscope examination indicated that the mitochondria in the kidney may have been the first organelles affected. Liver mitochondria also revealed degenerative changes. The livers of newborn rats whose dams had been treated throughout pregnancy showed these changes. Similar mitochondrial changes were observed in the intestine, brain, seminal vesicle, and pancreas. It has been suggested that thallium may combine with the sulfhydryl groups in the mitochondria and thereby interfere with oxidative phosphorylation (Herman and Bensch, 1967). A teratogenic response to thallium salts characterized as achondroplasia (dwarfism) has been described in rats (Nogami and Terashima, 1973).

In humans, fatty infiltration and necrosis of the liver, nephritis, gastroenteritis, pulmonary edema, degenerative changes in the adrenals, degeneration of peripheral and central nervous system, alopecia, and in some cases death have been reported as a result of long-term systemic thallium intake. These cases usually are caused by the contamination of food or the use of thallium as a depilatory. Industrial poisoning is a special risk in the manufacture of fused halides for the production of lenses and windows. Loss of vision plus the other signs of thallium poisoning have been related to industrial exposures (Browning, 1969; Fowler, 1982).

Tin

Tin is used in the manufacture of tinplate, in food packaging, and in solder, bronze, and brass. Stannous and stannic chlorides are used in dyeing textiles. Organic tin compounds have been used in fungicides, bactericides, and slimicides, as well as in plastics as stabilizers. The disposition and possible health effects of inorganic and organic tin compounds have been summarized in a WHO report (1980).

Disposition. There is only limited absorption

of even soluble tin salts such as sodium stannous tartrate after oral administration. Ninety percent of the tin administered in this manner is recovered in the feces. The small amounts absorbed are reflected by increases in the liver and kidneys. Injected tin is excreted by the kidneys, with smaller amounts in bile. A mean normal urine level of 16.6 μg/liter or 23.4 μg/day has been reported. The majority of inhaled tin or its salts remains in the lungs, most extracellularly, with some in the macrophages, in the form of SnO_2. The organic tins, particularly triethyltin, may be somewhat better absorbed. The tissue distribution of tin from this material shows highest concentrations in the blood and liver, with smaller amounts in the muscle, spleen, heart, or brain. Tetraethyltin is converted to triethyltin *in vivo*.

Chronic inhalation of tin in the form of dust or fumes leads to benign pneumoconiosis. Tin hydride (SnH_4) is more toxic to mice and guinea pigs than is arsine; however, its effects appear mainly in the central nervous system and no hemolysis is produced. Orally, tin or its inorganic compounds require relatively large doses (500 mg/kg for 14 months) to produce toxicity. The use of tin in food processing seems to demonstrate little hazard. The average U.S. daily intake, mostly from foods as a result of processing, is estimated at 17 mg. Inorganic tin salts given by injection produce diarrhea, muscle paralysis, and twitching.

Toxicology. Some organic tin compounds are highly toxic, particularly triethyl tin. Trialkyl compounds including triethyl tin cause an encephalopathy and cerebral edema. Toxicity declines as the number of carbon atoms in the chain increases. An outbreak of almost epidemic nature took place in France due to the oral ingestion of a preparation (Stalinon) containing diethyl tin diiodide for treatment of skin disorders (Barnes and Stoner, 1959).

Excessive industrial exposure to triethyltin has been reported to produce headaches, visual defects, and EEG changes that were very slowly reversed (Prull and Rompel, 1970). Experimentally, triethyltin produces depression and cerebral edema. The resulting hyperglycemia may be related to the centrally mediated depletion of catecholamines from the adrenals. Acute burns or subacute dermal irritation has been reported among workers as a result of tributyltin. Triphenyltin has been shown to be a potent immunosuppressant (Verschuuren *et al.,* 1970). Inhibition in the hydrolysis of adenosine triphosphate and uncoupling of oxidative phosphorylation taking place in the mitochondria have been suggested as the cellular mechanisms of tin toxicity (WHO, 1980).

Titanium

Most titanium compounds are in the oxidation state +4 (titanic), but oxidation state +3 (titanous) and oxidation state +2 compounds as well as several organometallic compounds do occur. Titanium dioxide, the most widely used compound, is a white pigment used in paints and plastics, as a food additive to whiten flour, dairy products, and confections, and as a whitener in cosmetic products. Because of its resistance to corrosion and inertness it has many metallurgical applications, particularly as a component of surgical implants and prostheses. It occurs widely in the environment; it is present in urban air, rivers, and drinking water and is detectable in many foods.

Disposition. Approximately 3 percent of an oral dose of titanium is absorbed. The majority of that absorbed is excreted in the urine. The normal urine concentration has been estimated at 10 μg/liter (Schroeder *et al.,* 1963; Kazantzis, 1981).

The estimated body burden of titanium is about 15 mg. Most of it is in the lungs, probably as a result of inhalation exposure. Inhaled titanium tends to remain in the lungs for long periods. It has been estimated that about one-third of the inhaled titanium is retained in the lungs. The geographic variation in lung burden is to some extent dependent on air concentration. For example, concentrations of 430, 1300, and 91 ppm in ashed lung tissue have been reported for the United States, Delhi, and Hong Kong, respectively. Mean concentrations of 8 and 6 ppm for the liver and kidney, respectively, were reported in the United States. Newborns have little titanium. Lung burdens tend to increase with age.

Toxicology. Occupational exposure to titanium may be heavy, and concentrations in air up to 50 mg/m³ have been recorded. Titanium dioxide has been classified as a nuisance particulate with a TLV of 10 mg/m³. Nevertheless, slight fibrosis of lung tissue has been reported following inhalation exposure to titanium dioxide pigment, but the injury was not disabling. Otherwise, titanium dioxide has been considered physiologically inert by all routes (ingestion, inhalation, dermal, and subcutaneous). The metal and other salts are also relatively nontoxic except for titanic acid, which, as might be expected, will product irritation (Berlin and Nordman, 1979).

A titanium coordination complex, titanocene, suspended in trioctanoin, administered by intramuscular injection to rats and mice, produced fibrosarcomas at the site of injection and hepatomas and malignant lymphomas (Furst and Haro, 1969). A titanocene is a sandwich arrangement of titanium between two cyclopentadiene molecules. Titanium dioxide was found not to be carcinogenic in a bioassay study in rats and mice (NCI, 1979).

Uranium

The chief raw material of uranium is pitchblende or carnotite ore. This element is largely limited to use as a nuclear fuel.

The uranyl ion is rapidly absorbed from the gastrointestinal tract. About 60 percent is carried as a soluble bicarbonate complex, while the remainder is bound to plasma protein. Sixty percent is excreted in the urine within 24 hours. About 25 percent may be fixed in the bone (Chen et al., 1961). Following inhalation of the insoluble salts, retention by the lungs is prolonged. Uranium tetrafluoride and uranyl fluoride can produce a typical toxicity because of hydrolysis to HF. Skin contact (burned skin) with uranyl nitrate has resulted in nephritis.

The soluble uranium compound (uranyl ion) and those that solubilize in the body by the formation of bicarbonate complex produce systemic toxicity in the form of acute renal damage and renal failure, which may be fatal. However, if exposure is not severe enough, the renal tubular epithelium is regenerated and recovery occurs. Renal toxicity with the classic signs of impairment, including albuminuria, elevated blood urea nitrogen, and loss of weight, is brought about by filtration of the bicarbonate complex through the glomerulus, reabsorption by the proximal tubule, liberation of uranyl ion, and subsequent damage to the proximal tubular cells. Uranyl ion is most likely concentrated intracellularly in lysosomes (Voegtlin and Hodge, 1949–1951; Passow et al., 1961; Ghadially et al., 1982).

Inhalation of uranium dioxide dust by rats, dogs, and monkeys at a concentration of 5 mg U/m^3 for up to five years produced accumulation in the lungs and tracheobronchial lymph nodes that accounted for 90 percent of the body burden. No evidence of toxicity was observed despite the long duration of observation (Leach et al., 1970).

Vanadium

Vanadium is a ubiquitous element. It is a byproduct of petroleum refining, and vanadium pentoxide is used as a catalyst in the various chemicals including sulfuric acid. It is used in the hardening of steel, in the manufacture of pigments, in photography, and in insecticides. It is common in many foods; significant amounts are found in milk, seafoods, cereals, and vegetables. Vanadium has a natural affinity for fats and oils;

food oils have high concentrations. Municipal water supplies may contain on the average about 1 to 6 ppb. Urban air contains some vanadium, perhaps due to the use of petroleum products or from refineries (Table 19–1), about 30 mg. The largest single compartment is the fat. Bone and teeth stores contribute to the body burden. It has been postulated that some homeostatic mechanism maintains the normal levels of vanadium in the face of excessive intake, since the element, in most forms, is moderately absorbed. The principal route of excretion of vanadium is the urine. The normal serum level is 35 to 48 $\mu g/100$ ml. When excess amounts of vanadium are in the diet, the concentration in the red cells tends to increase. Parenteral administration increases levels in the liver and kidney, but these increased amounts may only be transient. The lung tissue may contain some vanadium, depending on the exposure by that route, but normally the other organs contain negligible amounts.

The toxic action of vanadium is largely confined to the respiratory tract. Bronchitis and bronchopneumonia are more frequent in workers exposed to vanadium compounds. In industrial exposures to vanadium pentoxide dust a greenish-black discoloration of the tongue is characteristic. Irritant activity with respect to skin and eyes has also been ascribed to industrial exposure. Gastrointestinal distress, nausea, vomiting, abdominal pain, cardiac palpitation, tremor, nervous depression, and kidney damage, too, have been linked with industrial vanadium exposure.

Ingestion of vanadium compounds (V_2O_5) for medicinal purposes produced gastrointestinal disturbances, slight abnormalities of clinical chemistry related to renal function, and nervous system effects. Acute vanadium poisoning in animals is characterized by marked effects on the nervous system, hemorrhage, paralysis, convulsions, and respiratory depression. Short-term inhalation exposure of experimental animals tend to confirm the effects on the lungs as well as the effect on the kidney. In addition, experimental investigations have suggested that the liver, adrenals, and bone marrow may be adversely affected by subacute exposure at high levels (Waters, 1977).

REFERENCES

Adams, R. G.; Harrison, J. G.; and Scott, P.: The development of cadmium-induced proteinuria, impaired renal function and osteomalacia in alkaline battery workers. J. Med., **38**:425–43. 1969.
Ainsworth, S. K.; Swain, R. P.; Watabe, N.; Brackett, N. C.; Pilia, P.; and Hennigar, G. R.: Gold nephropathy, ultrastructural fluorescent, and energy-dispersive

x-ray microanalysis study. *Arch. Pathol. Lab. Med.,* **105**:373–78, 1981.

Alfrey, A. C.: Aluminum and Tin. In Bronner, F., and Coburn, J. W. (eds.): *Disorders of Mineral Metabolism.* Academic Press, Inc., New York, 1981, pp. 353–69.

Alfrey, A. C.; Mishell, J. M.; Burks, J.; Contiguglia, S. R.; Rudolph, H.; Lewin, E.; and Holmes, J. H.: Syndrome of dyspraxia and multifocal seizures associated with chronic hemodialysis. *Trans. Am. Soc. Artif. Intern. Organs.,* **18**:257–61, 1972.

Anderson, A., and Hahlin M.: Cadmium effects from phosphorus fertilization in field experiments. *Swedish J. Agric. Res.,* **11**:2, 1981.

Anke, M.; Grun, M.; Gropped, B.; and Kronemann, H.: Nutritional requirements of nickel. In Sarkar, B. (ed.): *Biologic Aspect of Metals and Metal-Related Diseases.* Raven Press, New York, 1983, pp. 89–105.

Araki, S., and Ushio, K.: Mechanism of increased osmotic resistance of red cells in workers exposed to lead. *Br. J. Industr. Med.,* **39**:157–60, 1982.

Arena, J. M.: Poisoning, 3rd ed. Charles C Thomas, Pub., Springfield, Ill., 1974, pp. 81–82.

Armstrong, B. G., and Kazantzis, G.: The mortality of cadmium workers. *Lancet,* **1**:1425–27, 1983.

Aspin, N., and Sass-Kortsak, A.: Copper. In Bronner, F., and Coburn, J. W. (eds.): *Disorders of Mineral Metabolism.* Vol. 1, Trace Minerals. Academic Press, Inc., New York, 1981, pp. 60–86.

Baetjer, A. M.: Pulmonary carcinoma in chromatic workers. *Arch. Industr. Hyg.,* **2**:487–93, 1950.

Baker, E. L.; Goyer, R. A.; Fowler, B. A.; Khettry, U.; Bernard, O. B.; Adler, S.; White, R.; Babayan, R.; and Feldman, R. G. Occupational lead exposure, nephropathy and renal cancer. *Am. J. Industr. Med.,* **1**:139–48, 1980.

Bakir, F.; Damluji, S. F.; Amin-Zaki, L.; Murtadha, M.; Khalidi, A.; Al-Rawi, N. Y.; Tikriti, S.; Dhahir, H. I.; Clarkson, T. W.; Smith, J. C.; and Doherty, R. A.: Methyl mercury poisoning in Iraq. *Science,* **181**:230–41, 1973.

Barltrop, D., and Smith, A.: Interaction of lead with erythrocytes. *Experientia,* **27**:92–93, 1971.

Barnes, J. M., and Stoner, H. B.: Toxicology of tin compounds. *Pharmacol. Rev.,* **11**:211–31, 1959.

Batuman, V.; Maesalsa, J. K.; Haddad, E.; Tepper, E.; Landry, E.; and Wedeen, R.: The role of lead in gout nephropathy. *N. Engl. J. Med.,* **304**:520–23, 1981.

Beijer, K., and Jernelöv, A.: Sources, transport and transformation of metals in the environment. In Friberg, L.; Nordberg, G. F.; and Vouk, V. B. (eds.): *Handbook on the Toxicology of Metals.* Elsevier/North-Holland, New York, 1979, pp. 47–63.

Bencko, V.; Benes, R.; and Cikrt, M.: Biotransformation of As(III) to As(V) and arsenic tolerance. *Arch. Toxicol.,* **36**:159–62, 1976.

Berlin, M.: Mercury. In Friberg, L.; Nordberg, G. F.; and Nordman, C. (eds.): *Handbook on the Toxicology of Metals.* Elsevier, Netherlands, 1979, pp. 503–30.

——: The toxicokinetics of mercury. In Schmidt, E. H. F., and Hildebrandt, A. G. (eds.): *Infant Formula and Junior Food.* Springer-Verlag, Berlin, 1983, pp. 147–60.

Berlin, M., and Nordman, C.: Titanium. In Friberg, L.; Nordberg, G. F.; and Vouk, V. B. (eds.): *Handbook on the Toxicology of Metals.* Elsevier/North-Holland, New York, 1979, pp. 627–36.

Bessis, M. D., and Jensen, W. N.: Sideroblastic anemia, mitochondria and erythroblastic iron. *Br. J. Haematol.,* **11**:49–51, 1965.

Boulanger, Y.; Goodman, C. M.; Forte, C. P.; Fesik, S. W.; and Armitage, I. M.: Model for mammalian metallothionein structure. *Proc. Natl Acad. Sci. USA,* **80**:1501–1505, 1983.

Boyd, J. T.; Doll, R.; Foulds, J. S.; and Leiper, J.: Cancer of the lung in iron ore (haematite) miners. *Br. J. Industr. Med.,* **27**:97–103, 1970.

Brown, E. B.: Therapy for disorders of iron excess. In Sarkar, B. (ed.): *Biological Aspects of Metal-Related Diseases.* Raven Press, New York, 1983, pp. 263–78.

Brown, M. M.; Rhyne, B. C.; Goyer, R. A.; and Fowler, B. A.: Intracellular effects of chronic arsenic administration on renal proximal tubule cells. *J. Toxicol. Environ. Health,* **1**:505–14, 1976.

Browning, E.: *Toxicity of Industrial Metals,* 2nd ed. Butterworths, London, 1969.

Buchet, J.-P.; Roels, H.; Bernard, A.; and Lauwerys, R.: Assessment of renal function of workers exposed to inorganic lead, cadmium, or mercury vapor. *J. Occup. Med.,* **22**:741–50, 1980.

Burchfiel, J. L.; Duffy, F. H.; Bartels, P. H.; and Needleman, H. L.: The combined discriminating power of quantitative electroencephalography and neuropsychologic measures in evaluating central nervous system effects of lead at low levels. In Needleman, H. C. (ed.): *Low Level Lead Exposures.* Raven Press, New York, 1980, pp. 75–90.

Burk, R. F.: Selenium in man. In Prasad, A. S., and Oberleas, D. (eds.): *Trace Elements in Human Health and Disease,* Vol. II. Academic Press, Inc., New York, 1976, pp. 105–34.

Casto, B. C.; Meyers, J.; and DiPaolo, J. A.: Enhancement of viral transformation for evaluation of the carcinogenic or mutagenic potential of inorganic metal salts. *Cancer Res.,* **39**:193–98, 1979.

Cerwenka, E. A., and Cooper, W. C.: Toxicology of selenium and tellurium and their compounds. *Arch. Environ. Health,* **3**:189–200, 1961.

Chan, W. Y.; Tease, L. A.; Liu, H. C.; and Rennert, O. M.: Cell culture studies in Wilson's disease. In Sarkar, D. (ed.): *Biological Aspects of Metals and Metal-Related Diseases.* Raven Press, New York, 1983, pp. 147–58.

Chang, C. C.; Vander Mallie, R. J.; and Garvey, J. S.: A radioimmunoassay for human metallothionein. *Toxicol. Appl. Pharmacol.,* **55**:94–102, 1980.

Chen, P. S.; Terepka, R.; and Hodge, H. C.: The pharmacology and toxicology of the bone seekers. *Annu. Rev. Pharmacol.,* **1**:369–93, 1961.

Chen, X.; Yang, G.; Chen, J.; Chen, X.; Wen, Z.; and Ge, K.: Studies on the relations of selenium and Keshan disease. *Biol. Trace Elem. Res.,* **2**:91–107, 1980.

Cherian, M. G.: Chelation of cadmium with BAL and DTPA in rats. *Nature,* **287**:871–72, 1980.

Cherian, M. G., and Nordberg, M.: Cellular adaptation in metal toxicology and metallothionein. *Toxicology,* **28**: 1–15, 1983.

Cherian, M. G., and Rodgers, K.: Chelation of cadmium from metallothionein *in vivo* and its excretion in rats repeatedly injected with cadmium chloride. *J. Pharmacol. Exp. Ther.,* **222**:699–704, 1982.

Cherian, M. G.; Goyer, R. A.; and Delaquerriere-Richardson, L.: Cadmium-metallothionein induced nephropathy. *Toxicol. Appl. Pharmacol.,* **38**:399–408, 1976.

Chisolm, J. J., Jr.: Chelation therapy in children with subclinical plumbism. *Pediatrics,* **53**:441–43, 1974.

Chisolm, J. J., Jr., and O'Hara (eds.): *Lead Absorption in Children. Management, Clinical and Environmental Aspects.* Urban & Schwarzenberg, Baltimore, 1982.

Chisholm, J. J., Jr., and Thomas, D.: Use of 2,3-dimercaptopropane-1-sulfonate in treatment of lead poisoning in children. *J. Pharmacol. Exp. Ther.,* **235**:665–69, 1985.

Choie, D. D.; Longenecker, D. S.; and Del Campo, A. A.: Acute and chronic cisplatin nephropathy in rats. *Lab. Invest.,* **44**: 397–402, 1981.

Chowdbury, P., and Louria, D. B.: Influence of cadmium and other trace elements on human α_1-antitrypsins: an *in vitro* study. *Science,* **191**:480–81, 1976.

Chuttani, H. K.; Gupti, P. S.; and Gultati, S.: Acute copper sulfate poisoning. *Am. J. Med.,* **39**:849–54, 1965.

Clarkson, T. W.: Methylmercury toxicity to the mature and developing nervous system: possible mechanisms. In Sarkar, D. (ed.): *Biological Aspects of Metals and Metal-Related Diseases.* Raven Press, New York, 1983, pp. 183–97.

Cooper, W. C.: Occupational lead exposure. What are the risks? *Science,* **180**:129, 1980.

Cooper, W. C., and Gaffey, W. R.: Mortality of lead workers. *J. Occup. Med.,* **17**:100–107, 1975.

Costa, M.: *Metal Carcinogenesis Testing, Principles and In Vitro Methods.* The Humana Press, Clifton, N. J., 1980, p. 71.

Cotzias, G. C.; Papavasiliou, P. S.; Ginos, J.; Stechk, A.; and Duby, S.: Metabolic modification of Parkinson's disease and of chronic manganese poisoning. *Annu. Rev. Med.,* **22**:305–26, 1971.

Cox, M., and Singer, I.: Lithium. In Bronner, F., and Coburn, J. W. (eds.): *Disorders of Mineral Metabolism.* Academic Press, Inc., New York, 1981, pp. 369–438.

Crapper, D. R.; Krishnan, S. S.; and Quittkat, S.: Aluminum, neurofibrillary degeneration and Alzheimer's disease. *Brain,* **99**:67–79, 1976.

Crapper-McLachlan, D. R.; Farnell, B.; Galin, H.; Kalik, S.; Eichhorn, G.; and DeBoni, U.: Aluminum in human brain disease. In Sarkar, B. (ed.): *Biological Aspects of Metals and Metal-Related Diseases.* Raven Press, New York, 1983, pp. 209–18.

Crecelius, E. A.: Changes in the chemical speciation of arsenic following ingestion by man. *Environ. Health Perspect.,* **19**:147–50, 1977.

Cremer, J. E.: Biochemical studies on the toxicity of triethyl lead and other organo-lead compounds. *Br. J. Industr. Med.,* **16**:191–99, 1959.

Curzon, M. E.; Adkins, B. L.; Bibby, B. G.; and Losee, F. L.: Combined effect of trace elements and fluorine on caries. *J. Dent. Res.,* **49**:526–28, 1970.

Davis, J. W., and Fann, W. E.: Lithium. *Annu. Rev. Pharmacol.,* **11**:285–98, 1971.

Davies, N. T.: Studies on the absorption of zinc by rat intestine. *Br. J. Nutr.,* **43**:189–203, 1980.

DeBoni, U.; Otvos, A.; Scott, J. W.; and Crapper, D. R.: Neurofibrillary degeneration induced by system aluminum. *Acta Neuropathol.,* **35**:285–94, 1976.

Deknudt, G.; Manuel, Y.; and Gerber, G. B.: Chromosomal aberration in workers professionally exposed to lead. *J. Toxicol. Environ. Health,* **3**:885–91, 1977.

DHEW: *Occupational Diseases: A Guide to Their Recognition.* U.S. Department of Health, Education and Welfare, Publication No. 77-1811, Washington, D.C., 1977, p. 305.

Dingwale-Fordyce, I., and Lane, R. E.: A follow-up study of lead workers. *Br. J. Industr. Med.,* **20**:313–15, 1963.

DiPaolo, J. A., and Casto, B. C.: Quantitative studies of *in vitro* morphologic transformation of Syrian hamster cells by inorganic metal salts. *Cancer Res.,* **39**:1008–19, 1979.

Diplock, A. T.: Metabolic aspects of selenium action and toxicity. *Crit. Rev. Toxicol.,* **4**:271–329, 1976.

Doll, R.; Fishbein, L.; Infante, P.; Landrigan, P.; Lloyd, J. W.; Mason, T. J.; Mastromalteo, E.; Norseth, T.; Pershagan, G.; Saffiotti, U.; and Saracci, R.: Problems of epidemiological evidence. *Environ. Health Perspect.,* **40**:11–20, 1981.

Doll, R.; Mathews, J. D.; and Morgan, L. G.: Cancers of the lung and nasal sinuses in nickel workers: reassessment of the period of risk. *Br. J. Industr. Med.,* **34**:102–106, 1977.

Dorn, C. R.; Pierce, J. O.; Phillips, P. E.; and Chases, C. R.: Airborne Pb, Cd, Zn, Cu concentration by particle size near a Pb smelter. *Atmos. Environ.,* **10**:443–46, 1976.

Downs, W. L.; Scott, J. K.; Steadman, L. T.; and Maynard, E. A.: Acute and subacute toxicity studies of thallium compounds. *Am. Ind. Hyg. Assoc. J.,* **21**:399–406, 1960.

Editorial. Selenium perspective. *Lancet,* **1**:685, 1983.

Elinder, C.-G., and Friberg, L.: Antimony. In Friberg, L.; Nordberg, G. F.; and Vouk, V. B. (eds.): *Handbook on the Toxicology of Metals.* Elsevier/North Holland, New York, 1977, pp. 283–92.

Elinder, C.-G., and Kjellstrom, T.: Cadmium concentration in samples of human kidney cortex from the 19th century. *Ambio,* **6**:270, 1977.

Elinder, C.-G.; Kjellstrom, T.; Lind, B.; Linnman, L.; Piscator, M.; and Sundstedt, K.: Cadmium exposure from smoking cigarettes. Variations with time and country where purchased. *Environ. Res.,* 1983 (in press).

Ellis, K. J.; Morgan, W. D.; Zanzi, I.; Yasumura, S.; Vartsky, D. D.; and Cohn, S. H.: Critical concentrations of cadmium in human renal cortex: dose-effect studies in cadmium smelter workers. *J. Toxicol. Environ. Health,* **7**:691–98, 1981.

Emmerson, B. T.: The clinical differentiation of lead gout from primary gout. *Arthritis Rheum.,* **11**:623–24, 1968.

Engelbrecht, F. M., and Jordaan, M. E.: The influence of silica and aluminum on the cytochrome c oxidase activity of rat lung homogenate. *S. Afr. Med. J.,* **46**:769–71, 1972.

Ernhardt, C. B.; Landa, B.; and Schnell, N. B.: Subclinical levels of lead and developmental deficit—a multivariate follow-up reassessment. *Pediatrics,* **67**:911–19, 1981.

Ferm, V. H.: Arsenic as a teratogenic agent. *Environ. Health Perspect.,* **19**:215–17, 1977.

Fishbein, L.: Sources, transport, and alteration of metal compounds: an overview. I. Arsenic, beryllium, cadmium, chromium, and nickel. *Environ. Health Perspect.,* **40**:43–64, 1981.

———: Toxicology of selenium and tellurium. In Goyer, R. A., and Mehlman, M. A. (eds.): *Toxicology of Trace Metals.* John Wiley & Sons, New York, 1977, pp. 191–240.

Flanagan, P. R.; McLellan, J.; Haist, J.; Cherian, M. G.; Chamberlain, M. J.; and Valberg, L. S.: Increased dietary cadmium absorption in mice and human subjects with iron deficiency. *Gastroenterology,* **74**:841–46, 1978.

Fluharty, A. L., and Sanadi, D. R.: On the mechanism of oxidative phosphorylation. II. Effects of arsenite alone and in combination with 2,3-dimercaptopropanol. *J. Biol. Chem.,* **236**:2772–78, 1961.

Fowler, B. A.: Indium and thallium in health. In Rose, J., (ed.): *Trace Metals in Human Health.* Butterworth, London, 1982.

Fowler, B. A., and Goyer, R. A.: Bismuth localization within nuclear inclusions by x-ray microanalysis. *J. Histochem. Cytochem.,* **23**:722–26, 1975.

Fowler, B. A., and Weissberg, J. B.: Arsine poisoning. *N. Engl. J. Med.,* **291**:1171–74, 1974.

Fowler, B. W., and Vouk, V.: Bismuth. In Friberg, L.; Nordberg, G. F.; and Vouk, V. B. (eds.): *Handbook on the Toxicology of the Metals.* Elsevier/North-Holland, New York, 1979, pp. 345–47.

Frazier, J. M.: Bioaccumulation of cadmium in marine organisms. *Environ. Health Perspect.,* **28**:75–79, 1979.

Friberg, L., and Kjellstrom, T.: Cadmium. In Bronner F., and Coburn, J. W. (eds.): *Disorders of Mineral Me-*

tabolism. Vol. 1, *Trace Minerals*. Academic Press, Inc., New York, 1981, pp. 318–34.

Friberg, L., and Nelson, N.: Introduction, general findings and general recommendations. Workshop/conference on the role of metals in carcinogenesis. *Environ. Health Perspect.*, **40**:5–10, 1981.

Friberg, L., and Vostal, J. (eds.): *Mercury in the Environment—Toxicological and Epidemiological Appraisal*. Chemical Rubber Co., Cleveland, 1972.

Friberg, L.; Nordberg, G. F.; and Vouk, V. B. (eds.): *Handbook on the Toxicology of Metals*. Elsevier/North-Holland, New York, 1979.

Furst, A.: Bioassay of metals for carcinogenesis: whole animals. *Environ. Health Perspect.*, **40**:83–91, 1981.

Furst, A., and Haro, R. T.: A survey of metal carcinogenesis. *Prog. Exp. Tumour Res.*, **12**:102–33, 1969.

Gabard, B.: Treatment of methyl mercury poisoning in the rat with sodium 2,3-dimercaptopropane-i-sulfonate: influence of dose and mode of administration. *Toxicol. Appl. Pharmacol.*, **38**:415–24, 1976.

Ghadially, F. N.; Lalonde, J. A.; and Yang-Steppuhn, S.: Uraniosomes produced in cultured rabbit kidney cells by uranyl acetate. *Virchows Arch. [Cell. Pathol.]*, **39**:21–30, 1982.

Gilman, W.: Metal carcinogenesis. II. Study on the carcinogenicity of cobalt, copper, iron, and nickel compounds. *Cancer Res.*, **22**:158–70, 1962.

Goldwater, L. J.: *Mercury: A History of Quicksilver*. York Press, Baltimore, 1972, pp. 270–77.

Goldwater, L. J., and Stopford, W.: Mercury. In Lenihan, J., and Fletcher, W. W. (eds.): *The Chemical Environment*. Blackie & Son, Ltd., London, 1977, pp. 38–63.

Goyer, R. A.: Cadmium nephropathy. In Porter, G. A. (ed.): *Nephrotoxic Mechanisms of Drugs and Environmental Toxins*. Plenum Medical Book Co., New York, 1982, pp. 305–13.

——: Lead and the kidney. *Curr. Topics Pathol.*, **55**:147–76, 1971a.

——: Lead toxicity: a problem in environmental pathology. *Am. J. Pathol.*, **64**:167–82, 1971b.

——: Metal-protein complexes in detoxification process. In Brown, S. S. (ed.): *Clinical Chemistry and Clinical Toxicology*, Vol. 2. Academic Press, Inc., London, 1984 (in press).

Goyer, R. A., and Rhyne, B.: Pathological effects of lead. *Int. Rev. Exp. Pathol.*, **12**:1–77, 1973.

Goyer, R. A., and Wilson, M. H.: Lead-induced inclusion bodies: results of EDTA treatment. *Lab. Invest.*, **32**:149–56, 1975.

Goyer, R. A.; Apgar, J.; and Piscator, M.: Toxicity of zinc. In Henkin, R. I., and Committee (eds.): *Zinc*. University Park Press, Baltimore, 1979, pp. 249–68.

Gralla, E. J., and McIlhenny, H. M.: Studies in pregnant rats, rabbits, and monkeys with lithium carbonate. *Toxicol. Appl. Pharmacol.*, **21**:428–33, 1972.

Granick, J. L., and Levere, R. D.: Hemesynthesis in erythroid cells. *Prog. Hematol.*, **4**:1–47, 1964.

Gritzka, T. L., and Trump, B. F.: Renal tubular lesions caused by mercuric chloride. *Am. J. Pathol.*, **52**:1225–77, 1968.

Gunsalus, I. C.: The chemistry and function of the pyruvate oxidation factor (lipoic acid). *J. Cell. Comp. Physiol.*, **41** (Suppl. 1):136–36, 1953.

Hardy, H. L., and Tabershaw, I. R.: Delayed chemical pneumonitis occurring in workers exposed to beryllium. *J. Industr. Hyg. Toxicol.*, **28**:197–216, 1946.

Herman, M. M., and Bensch, K. G.: Light and electron microscopic studies of acute and chronic thallium intoxication in rats. *Toxicol. Appl. Pharmacol.*, **10**:199–222, 1967.

Hernberg, S.; Nurminen, M.; and Hasan, H.: Non-

random shortening of red cell survival times in men exposed to lead. *Environ. Res.*, **1**:247–61, 1967.

Hong, C. D.; Hanenson, I. B.; Lerner, S.; Hammond, P. B.; Pesce, A. J.; and Pollack, V. E.: Occupational exposure to lead: effects on renal function. *Kidney Int.*, **18**:489–94, 1980.

Howell, G. O., and Hill, C. H.: Biological interactions of selenium with other trace elements in chicks. *Environ. Health Perspect.*, **25**:147–50, 1978.

Hueper, W. C.: *Occupational and Environmental Cancers of the Respiratory System*. Springer-Verlag, New York, 1966.

Hunter, D.: *The Diseases of Occupations*, 5th ed. Little, Brown & Co., Boston, 1975.

IARC Monograph on the Evaluation of the Carcinogenic Risk of Chemicals to Humans. Some Metals and Metallic Compounds. Vol. 23. World Health Organization, International Agency for Research on Cancer, Lyon, 1980.

Ivankovic, S.; Eisenbrandt, G.; and Preussmann, R.: Lung carcinoma induction in BD rats after single intratracheal instillation of an arsenic-containing pesticide mixture formerly used in vineyards. *Int. J. Cancer*, **24**:786–92, 1979.

Jacobs, A.: Iron overload—clinical and pathological aspects. *Semin. Hematol.*, **14**:89–113, 1977.

Jacobs, A., and Worwood, M.: Iron. In Bronner, F., and Coburn, J. W. (eds.): *Disorders of Mineral Metabolism*. Vol. 1, *Trace Minerals*. Academic Press, Inc., New York, 1981, pp. 2–59.

Johnson, J. L.; Jones, H. P.; and Rajagopalan, K. V.: *In vitro* reconstitution of demolybdosulfite oxidase by a molybdenum cofactor from rat liver and other sources. *J. Biol. Chem.*, **252**:4994–5003, 1977.

Johnstone, R. M.: Sulfhydryl agent: arsenicals. In Hochster, R. M., and Quasital, J. H. (eds.): *Metabolic Inhibitors: A Comprehensive Treatise*, Vol. 2. Academic Press, Inc., New York, 1963.

Kagey, B. T.; Bumgarner, J. E.; and Creason, J. P.: Arsenic levels in maternal-fetal tissue sets. In Hemphill, O. D. (ed.): *Trace Substances in Environmental Health XI*. University of Missouri Press, Columbia, 1977, pp. 252–56.

Kang, H. K.; Infante, P. F.; and Carra, J. S.: Occupational lead exposure and cancer. *Science*, **207**:935–36, 1980.

Kazantzis, G.: Renal tubular dysfunction and abnormalities of calcium metabolism in cadmium workers. *Environ. Health Perspect.*, **28**:155–60, 1979.

——: Role of cobalt, iron, lead, manganese, mercury, platinum, selenium and titanium in carcinogenesis. *Environ. Health Perspect.*, **40**:143–61, 1981.

——: The role of hypersensitivity and the immune response in influencing susceptibility to metal toxicity. *Environ. Health Perspect.*, **25**:111–18, 1978.

Keberle, H.: The biochemistry of desferrioxamine and its relation to iron metabolism. *Ann. NY Acad. Sci.*, **119**:758–68, 1964.

Kehoe, R. A.: The metabolism of lead in health and disease. The Harben Lectures. *J. R. Inst. Public Health Hyg.*, **24**:1–81, 1961.

Kjellstrom, T.; Ervin, P.-E.; and Rahnster, B.: Dose-response relationship of cadmium-induced tubular proteinuria. *Environ. Res.*, **13**:303–17, 1977.

Kjellstrom, T.; Lind, B.; Linnman, L.; and Elinder, C.-G.: Variation of cadmium concentration in Swedish wheat and barley. An indicator of changes in daily cadmium intake during the 20th century. *Arch. Environ. Health*, **30**:321–28, 1975.

Kneip, T. J.; Eisenbud, M.; Strehlow, C. D.; and Freudenthal, P. C.: Airborne particulates in New York City. *J. Air Pollut. Control Assoc.*, **20**:144–49, 1970.

Koller, L. D.; Exon, J. H.; Moore, S. A.; and Watanabe,

P. G.: Evaluation of ELISA for detecting *in vivo* chemical immunomodulation. *J. Toxicol. Environ. Health,* **11**:15–22, 1983.

Kowal, N. E.; Johnson, D. E.; Kaemer, D. F.; and Pahren, H. R.: Normal levels of cadmium in diet, urine, blood, and tissues of inhabitants of the United States. *J. Toxicol. Environ. Health,* **5**:995–1012, 1979.

Kuschner, M.: The carcinogenicity of beryllium. *Environ. Health Perspect.,* **40**:101–106, 1981.

Laker, M.: On determining trace element levels in man: the uses of blood and hair. *Lancet,* **1**:260–62, July 31, 1982.

Lam, H. F.; Conner, M. W.; Rogers, A. E.; Fitzgerald, S.; and Amdur, M. O.: Functional and morphological changes in the lungs of guinea pigs exposed to freshly generated ultrafine zinc oxide. *Toxicol. Appl. Pharmacol.,* **78**:29–38, 1985.

Lampert, P. W., and Schochet, S. S.: Demyelination and remyelination in lead neuropathy. *J. Neuropathol. Exp. Neurol.,* **27**:527–45, 1968.

Landoldt, R. R.; Berk, H. W.; and Russell, H. T.: Studies on the toxicity of rhodium trichloride in rats and rabbits. *Appl. Pharmacol.,* **21**:589–90, 1972.

Landrigan, P.: Arsenic—state of the art. *Am. J. Industr. Med.,* **2**:5–14, 1981.

Langard, S., and Norseth, T.: Chromium. In Friberg, L.; Nordberg, G. F.; and Vouk, V. B. (eds.): *Handbook on the Toxicology of Metals.* Elsevier/North Holland, New York, 1979.

Lauwerys, R. R.: *In vivo* tests to monitor body burdens of toxic metals in man. In Brown, S., and Savory, J. (eds.): *Clinical Toxicology and Clinical Chemistry of Metals.* Academic Press, Inc., New York, 1983, pp. 113–22.

Lauwerys, R. R.; Bernard, A.; Roels, H. A.; Buchet, J.-P.; and Viau, C.: Characterization of cadmium proteinuria in man and rat. *Environ. Health Perspect.,* **54**:147–52, 1984.

Lauwerys, R. R.; Roels, H. A.; Bernard, A.; and Buchet, J.-P.: Renal response to cadmium in a population living in a nonferrous smelter area in Belgium. *Int. Arch. Occup. Environ. Health,* **45**:271–74, 1980.

Lauwerys, R. R.; Roels, H. A.; Bucket, J.-P.; Bernard, A.; and Stanescu, D.: Investigations on the lung and kidney function in workers exposed to cadmium. *Environ. Health Perspect.,* **28**:137–46, 1979.

Leach, L. J.; Maynard, E. A.; Hodge, H. C.; Scott, J. K.; Yuile, C. L.; Sylvester, G. E.; and Wilson, H. B.: A five year inhalation study with uranium dioxide (UO₂) dust. I. Retention and biologic effect in the monkey, dog and rat. *Health Phys.,* **18**:599–612, 1970.

Lee, A. M., and Fraumeni, J. F., Jr.: Arsenic and respiratory cancer in man: an occupational study. *JNCI,* **42**:1945–2052, 1969.

Levinson, C.: *Threshold Limit Values, Best Prevailing Standards.* International Federation of Chemical, Energy and General Workers Unions, Geneva, 1982.

Li, Y.-H.: Geochemical cycles of elements and human perturbation. *Geochim. Cosmochim. Acta,* **45**:2073–84, 1981.

Lilis, R.: Long-term occupational lead exposure: Chronic nephropathy and renal cancer: a case report. *Am. J. Industr. Med.,* **2**:293–97, 1981.

Lilis, R., and Fishbein, A.: Chelation therapy in workers exposed to lead—a critical review. *JAMA,* **235**:2823–24, 1976.

Lilis, R.; Valciukas, J.; Fishbein, A.; Andrews, G.; and Selikoff, I. J.: Renal function impairment in secondary lead smelter workers: correlations with zinc protoporphyrin and blood lead levels. *J. Environ. Pathol. Toxicol.,* **2**:1447–74, 1979.

Lofroth, G., and Ames, B. N.: Mutagenicity of inorganic compounds in *Salmonella typhimurium:* arsenic, chromium and selenium. *Mutat. Res.,* **53**:65, 1978.

Lotz, M.; Zisman, E.; and Bartter, F. C.: Evidence for phosphorus-depletion syndrome in man. *N. Engl. J. Med.,* **278**:409–15, 1968.

Luckey, T. D.; Venugopal, B.; and Hutcheson, D.: *Heavy Metal Toxicity Safety and Hormonology.* Academic Press, Inc., New York, 1975.

Madias, N. E., and Harrington, J. T.: Platinum nephrotoxicity. *Am. J. Med.,* **65**:307–14, 1978.

Madsen, K. M., and Christensen, E. F.: Effects of mercury on lysosomal protein digestion in the kidney proximal tubule. *Lab. Invest.,* **38**:165–71, 1978.

Mahaffey, K. R., and Michaelson, J. A.: The interaction between lead and nutrition. In Needleman, H. E. (ed.): *Low Level Lead Exposure: The Clinical Implications of Current Research.* Raven Press, New York, 1980, pp. 159–200.

Mahaffey, K. R.; Annest, J. L.; Roberts, J.; and Murphy, R. S.: Estimates of blood lead levels: United States 1976–1980. Association with selected demographic and socioeconomic factors. *N. Engl. J. Med.,* **307**:573–79, 1982.

Manzler, A. D., and Schreiner, A. W.: Copper-induced acute hemolytic anemia. A new complication of hemodialysis. *Ann. Intern. Med.,* **73**:409–12, 1970.

Matheson, D. S.; Clarkson, T. W.; and Gelfand, E. W.: Mercury toxicity (acrodynia) induced by long-term injection of gamma globulin. *J. Pediatr.,* **97**:153–55, 1980.

McConnell, K. P., and Hoffman, J. G.: Methionine selenomethionine parallels in *E. coli* polypeptide chain initiation and synthesis. *Proc. Soc. Exp. Biol. Med.,* **140**:638–41, 1972.

McConnell, K. P., and Portman, O. W.: Toxicity of dimethyl selenide in the rat and mouse. *Proc. Soc. Exp. Biol. Med.,* **79**:230–31, 1952.

McCord, C. P.; Holden, F. R.; and Johnston, J.: Basophilic aggregation test in the lead poisoning epidemic of 1934–35. *Am. J. Public Health,* **25**:1089–96, 1935.

McEwan, J. C.: Five-year review of sputum cytology in workers at a nickel sinter plant. *Ann. Clin. Lab. Sci.,* **8**:503–509, 1978.

McLaughlin, A. I. G., and Harding, H. E.: Pneumoconiosis and other causes of death in iron and steel foundry workers. *Arch. Industr. Health,* **14**:350–62, 1956.

McNeely, M. D.; Nechay, M. W.; and Sunderman, F. W., Jr.: Measurements of nickel in serum and urine as indices of environmental exposure to nickel. *Clin. Chem.,* **18**:992–95, 1972.

Mena, I.; Meurin, O.; Feunzobda, S.; and Cotzias, G. C.: Chronic manganese poisoning. Clinical picture and manganese turnover. *Neurology,* **17**:128–36, 1967.

Mena, I.; Kazuko, H.; Burke, K.; and Cotzias, G. C.: Chronic manganese poisoning. Individual susceptibility and absorption of iron. *Neurology,* **19**:1000–1006, 1969.

Menne, T., and Thorboe, A.: Nickel dermatitis—nickel excretion. *Contact Dermatitis,* **2**:353–54, 1976.

Mertz, W.: Chromium occurrence and function in biological systems. *Physiol. Rev.,* **49**:163–239, 1969.

Miettenen, J. K.: Absorption and elimination of dietary mercury (Hg⁺⁺) and methyl mercury in man. In Miller, M. W., and Clarkson, T. W. (eds.): *Mercury Mercurials and Mercaptans.* Charles C Thomas, Pub., Springfield, Ill., 1973, p. 233.

Mitchell, R. A.; Change, B. F.; Huang, C. H.; and DeMaster, E. G. Inhibition of mitochondrial energy-linked functions by arsenate. *Biochemistry,* **10**:2049–54, 1971.

Moore, J. F.; Goyer, R. A.; and Wilson, M. H.: Lead-induced inclusion bodies, solubility amino acid content and relationship to residual acidic nuclear proteins. *Lab. Invest.,* **29**:488–94, 1973.

Moore, M. R., and Meredith, P. A.: The carcinogenicity of lead. *Arch. Toxicol.,* **42**:87–94, 1979.

Morin, Y., and Daniel, P.: Quebec beer-drinkers cardiomyopathy: etiological consideration. *J. Can. Med. Assoc.*, **97**:926–31, 1967.

Moxan, A. L., and Rhian, M.: Selenium poisoning. *Physiol. Rev.*, **203**:305–37, 1943.

Muller-Eberhard, U.; Miescher, P. A.; and Jaffe, E. R.: *Iron Excess. Aberrations of Iron and Porphyrin Metabolism.* Grune & Stratton, New York, 1977.

Myron, D. R.; Zimmerman, T. J.; Schuler, T. R.; Klevay, L. M.; Lee, D. E.; and Nielsen, F. H.: Intake of nickel and vanadium by humans. A survey of selected diet. *Am. J. Clin. Nutr.*, **31**:527–31, 1978.

Nagyvary, J., and Bradbury, E. L.: Hypocholesterolemic effects of Al^{3+} complexes. *Biochem. Res. Commun.*, **2**:592–98, 1977.

NAS Committee on Medical and Biological Effects of Atmospheric Pollutants: *Chromium.* National Academy of Sciences, Washington, D.C., 1974.

———: *Lead: Airborne Lead in Perspective.* National Academy of Sciences, Washington, D.C., 1972.

———: *Manganese.* National Academy of Sciences, Washington, D.C., 1973.

———: *Selenium.* National Academy of Sciences, Washington, D.C., 1975.

———: *Drinking Water and Health.* National Academy of Sciences, Washington, D.C., 1977.

NCI: *Bioassay of Titanium Dioxide for Possible Carcinogenicity.* National Cancer Institute Carcinogenesis Technical Report Series No. 97, Department of Health, Education and Welfare Publication No. (NIH) 79-1347, Washington, D.C., 1979.

———: *Bioassay of Selenium Sulfide (Gavage) for Possible Carcinogenicity.* National Cancer Institute Technical Report Series No. 194, NTP No. 80-17, Washington, D.C., 1980a.

———: *Bioassay of Selenium Sulfide (Dermal Study) for Possible Carcinogenicity.* National Cancer Institute Technical Report Series No. 197, NTP No. 80-18, Washington, D.C., 1980b.

———: *Bioassay of Selsun® for Possible Carcinogenicity.* National Cancer Institute Technical Report Series No. 199, NTP No. 80-19, Washington, D.C., 1980c.

Needleman, H.: *Low Level Lead Exposure, The Clinical Implications of Current Research.* Raven Press, New York, 1980.

Needleman, H. L.; Gunnoe, E. E.; Leviton, A.; Reed, R.; Peresie, H.; Maher, C.; and Barrett, P.: Deficits in psychologic and classroom performance of children with elevated blood lead levels. *N. Engl. J. Med.*, **300**:689–95, 1979.

Neff, N. H.; Barrett, R. E.; and Costa, E.: Selective depletion of caudate nucleus dopamine and serotonin during chronic manganese dioxide administration. *Experientia*, **25**:1140–41, 1969.

Ng, A., and Patterson, C.: Natural concentrations of lead in ancient Arctic and Antarctic ice. *Geochim Cosmochim. Acta*, **45**:2109–21, 1981.

Nogami, H., and Terashima, Y.: Thallium-induced achondroplasia in the rat. *Teratology*, **8**:101–102, 1973.

Nogawa, K.; Kobayashi, E.; and Honda, R.: A study of the relationship between cadmium concentrations in urine and renal effects of cadmium. *Environ. Health Perspect.*, **28**:161–68, 1979.

Nomiyama, K.: Recent progress and perspectives in cadmium health effects studies. *Sci. Total Environ.*, **14**:199–232, 1980.

Nordberg, G. F.: Cadmium metabolism and toxicity. *Environ. Physiol. Biochem.*, **2**:7–36, 1972.

Nordberg, G. F.; Fowler, B. A.; Friberg, L.; Jernelov, A.; Nelson, N.; Piscator, M.; Sandstead, H. H.; Vostal, J.; and Vouk, V. B.: Factors influencing metabolism and toxicity of metals: a consensus report. *Environ. Health Perspect.*, **25**:3–42, 1978.

Norseth, T.: The carcinogenicity of chromium. *Environ. Health Perspect.*, **40**:121–30, 1981.

NRCC: *Effects of Mercury in the Canadian Environment.* National Research Council of Canada Publication No. 16739, Ottawa, Canada, 1979.

———: *Zinc in the Aquatic Environment.* Chemistry, Distribution and Toxicology. National Research Council of Canada Publication No. 17589. Ottawa, Canada, 1981.

Nriagu, J.: *The Biogeochemistry of Lead.* Elsevier/North Holland Biomedical Press, Amsterdam, 1978.

Orfila, M. P.: *A General System of Toxicology.* M. Carey & Sons, Philadelphia, 1817, p. 184.

Ott, M. G.; Holder, B. B.; and Gordon, H. L.: Respiratory cancer and occupational exposure to arsenicals. *Arch. Environ. Health*, **29**:250–55, 1974.

Paglia, D. E.; Valentine, W. N.; and Dahlgner, J. G.: Effects of low level lead exposure on pyrimidine-5'-nucleotidase and other erythrocyte enzymes. *J. Clin. Invest.*, **56**:1164–69, 1975.

Pahren, H. R.; Lucas, J. B.; Ryan, J. A.; and Dotson, K. K.: Health risks associated with land application of municipal sludge. *J. Water Pollut. Control Fed.*, **51**:1588–98, 1979.

Palmer, I. S.; Fischer, D. D.; Halverson, A. W.; and Olson, O. E.: Identification of a major selenium excretory product in rat urine. *Biochim. Biophys. Acta*, **177**:336–42, 1969.

Passaw, H. A.; Rothstein, A.; and Clarkson, T. W.: The general pharmacology of the heavy metals. *Pharmacol. Rev.*, **13**:185–224, 1961.

Paton, F. R., and Allison, A. C.: Chromosome damage in human cell cultures induced by metal salts. *Mutat. Res.*, **16**:332–36, 1972.

Patty, F. A.: Arsenic, phosphorous, selenium, sulfur, and tellurium. In Fassett, D. W., and Irish, D. D. (eds.): *Industrial Hygiene and Toxicology*, 2nd ed., Interscience, New York, 1963, pp. 871–910.

Pederson, E.; Anderson, A.; and Hogetveit, A.: A second study of the incidence and mortality of cancer of respiratory organs among workers at a nickel refinery. *Ann. Clin. Lab. Sci.*, **8**:503–10, 1978.

Pentschew, W.; Ebner, F. F.; and Kovatch, R. M.: Experimental manganese encephalopathy in monkeys. *J. Neuropathol. Exp. Neurol.*, **22**:488–99, 1963.

Perlstein, M. A., and Attala, R.: Neurologic sequelae of plumbism in children. *Clin. Pediatr.*, **5**:292–98, 1966.

Perry, H. M., and Erlanger, M. W.: Metal-induced hypertension following chronic feeding of low doses of cadmium and mercury. *J. Lab. Clin. Med.*, **83**:541–47, 1974.

Pershagan, G.: Carcinogenicity of arsenic. *Environ. Health Perspect.*, **40**:93–100, 1981.

Peters, R. A.: *Biochemical Lesions and Lethal Synthesis.* Macmillan Publishing Co., New York, 1965, pp. 40–59.

Pinto, S. S.; Henderson, V.; and Enterline, P. E.: Mortality experience of arsenic-exposed workers. *Arch. Environ. Health*, **33**:325–31, 1978.

Pirkle, J. L.; Schwartz, J.; Landis, J. R.; and Harlan, W. R.: The relationship between blood lead levels and blood pressure and its cardiovascular risk implications. *Am. J. Epidemiol.*, **121**:246–58, 1985.

Piscator, M.: Role of cadmium in carcinogenesis with special reference to cancer of the prostate. *Environ. Health Perspect.*, **40**:107–20, 1981.

Popper, H.; Thomas, L. B.; Telles, N. C.; Falk, H.; and Selikoff, I. J.: Development of hepatic angiosarcoma in man induced by vinyl chloride thorotrast, and arsenic. *Am. J. Pathol.*, **92**:349–69, 1978.

Prasad, A. S.: Human zinc deficiency. In Sarkar, B (ed.): *Biological Aspects of Metals and Metal-Related Disease.* Raven Press, New York, 1983, pp. 107–19.

Prasad, A. S.; Miale, A., Jr.; Farid, Z.; Sandstead, H. H.; Schulert, A. R.; and Darby, W. J.: Biochemical studies on dwarfism, hypogonadism and anemia. *Arch. Intern. Med.,* **111:**407–28, 1963.

Prull, G., and Rompel, K.: EEG changes in acute poisoning with organic tin compounds. *Electroenceph. Clin. Neurophysiol.,* **29:**215–22, 1970.

Reeves, A. L.: Absorption of beryllium from the gastrointestinal tract. *Arch. Environ. Health,* **11:**209–14, 1965.

————: Barium. In Friberg, L.; Nordberg, G. F.; and Vouk, V. B. (eds.): *Handbook on the Toxicology of Metals.* Elsevier/North-Holland, New York, 1979, pp. 321–28.

Riordan, J. R.: Handling of heavy metals by cultured cells from patients with Menke's disease. In Sarkar, D. (ed.): *Biological Aspects of Metals and Metal-Related Diseases.* Raven Press, New York, 1983, pp. 159–70.

Roels, N. J.; Lauwerys, R.; and Dardenne, A. N.: The critical concentration of cadmium in human renal cortex: a reevaluation. *Toxicol. Lett.,* **15:**357–60, 1983.

Roizin, L.; Shiraki, H.; and Grceric, N.: *Neurotoxicology,* Vol. 1. Raven Press, New York, 1977, p. 658.

Roman-Franco, A. A.; Twirello, M.; Abini, B.; and Ossi, E.: Anti–basement membrane antibodies with antigen-antibody complexes in rabbits injected with mercuric chloride. *Clin. Immunol. Immunopathol.,* **9:**404–11, 1978.

Roman-Franco, A. A.; Twirello, M.; Abini, B.; and Ossi, E.: Anti–basement membrane antibodies with antigen-antibody complexes in rabbits injected with mercuric chloride. *Clin. Immunol. Immunopathol.,* **9:**404–11, 1978.

Rosenkrantz, H. S., and Poirier, L. A.: Evaluation of the mutagenicity and DNA-modifying activity of carcinogens and non-carcinogens in microbial systems. *JNCI,* **62:**873–82, 1979.

Rosenkrantz, H. S., and Poirier, L. A.: Evaluation of the mutagenicity and DNA-modifying activity of carcinogens and noncarcinogens in microbial systems. *JNCI,* **62:**873–92, 1979.

Rutter, M., and Jones, R. R. (eds.): *Lead Versus Health Sources and Effects of Low Level Lead Exposure.* John Wiley & Sons, New York, 1983.

Sanstead, H. H.: Zinc in human nutrition. In Bronner, F., and Coburn, J. W. (eds.): *Disorders of Mineral Metabolism.* Academic Press, Inc., New York, 1981, pp. 94–159.

Sanstead, H. H.; Michelakis, A. M.; and Temple, T. E.: Lead intoxication. Its effect on the renin-aldosterone response to sodium deprivation. *Arch. Environ. Health,* **20:**356–63, 1970.

Sarkar, B.; Laussac, J.-P.; and Lau, S.: Transport forms of copper in human serum. In Sarkar, D. (ed.): *Biological Aspects of Metals and Metal-Related Diseases.* Raven Press, New York, 1983, pp. 23–40.

Schlaepfer, W. W.: Experimental lead neuropathy. A disease of the supporting cells in the peripheral system. *J. Neuropathol. Exp. Neurol.,* **28:**401–18, 1968.

Schaver, C. G.: Pulmonary changes encountered in employees engaged in the manufacture of aluminum abrasives: clinical and roetgenologic aspects. *Occup. Med.,* **5:**718–28, 1948.

Schroeder, H. A., and Balassa, J. J.: Hypertension induced in rats by small doses of cadmium. *Am. J. Physiol.,* **202:**515–18, 1961.

Schroeder, H. A., and Mitchener, M.: Scandium, chromium (VI), gallium, yttrium, rhodium, palladium, indium in mice. Effects on growth and life span. *J. Nutr.,* **101:**1431–38, 1971.

Schroeder, H. A., and Mitchener, M.: Selenium and tellurium in mice. *Arch. Environ. Health,* **24:**66–71, 1972.

Schroeder, H. A.; Balassa, J. J.; and Tipton, I. H.: Abnormal trace metals in man: chromium. *J. Chronic Dis.,* **15:**941–64, 1962a.

Schroeder, H. A.; Balassa, J. J.; and Tipton, I. H.: Abnormal trace elements in man: nickel. *J. Chronic Dis.,* **15:**51–65, 1962b.

Schroeder, H. A.; Balassa, J. J.; and Tipton, I. H.: Abnormal trace metals in man: titanium. *J. Chronic Dis.,* **16:**55–69, 1963.

Schroeder, H. A.; Buckman, J.; and Balassa, J. J.: Abnormal trace elements in man: tellurium. *J. Chronic Dis.,* **20:**147–61, 1967a.

Schroeder, H. A.; Nason, A. P.; and Tipton, I. H.: Essential trace metals in man: cobalt. *J. Chronic Dis.,* **20:**869–90, 1967b.

Schroeder, H. A.; Nason, A. P.; and Tipton, I. H.: Essential trace metals in man: magnesium. *J. Chronic. Dis.,* **21:**815–41, 1969.

Schumann, G. B.; Lerner, S. I.; Weiss, M. A.; Gawronski, L.; and Lohiya, G. K.: Inclusion bearing cells in industrial workers exposed to lead. *Am. J. Clin. Pathol.,* **74:**192–96, 1980.

Seppalainen, A. M.; Tola, S.; Hernbrg, S.; and Kock, B.: Subclinical neuropathy at "safe" levels of lead exposure. *Arch. Environ. Health,* **30:**180–83, 1975.

Shaikh, Z. A., and Hirayama, K.: Metallothionein in the extracellular fluids as an index of cadmium toxicity. *Environ. Health Perspect.,* **28:**267–371, 1979.

Shamberger, R. J.; Tytko, S. A.; and Willis, C. E.: Antioxidants and cancer. Part VI. Selenium and age-adjusted human cancer mortality. *Arch. Environ. Health,* **31:**231–35, 1976.

Shapiro, I. M.; Mitchell, G.; Davidson, I.; and Katz, S. H.: Lead content of teeth. *Arch. Environ. Health,* **30:**483–86, 1975.

Shigamatsu, I.: Epidemiological studies on cadmium pollution in Japan. *Proceedings of First International Cadmium Conference.* San Francisco Metal Bulletin, Ltd., London, 1978.

Singer, I.: Lithium and the kidney. *Kidney Int.,* **19:**374–87, 1981.

Singhal, R. L., and Thomas, J. A. (eds.): *Lead Toxicity.* Urban & Schwarzenberg, Baltimore, 1980.

Spears, J. W.; Hatfield, E. E.; Forbes, R. M.; and Koenig, S. E.: Studies on the role of nickel in the ruminant. *J. Nutr.,* **108:**313–20, 1978.

Spencer, H.; Lewin, I.; Belcher, M. J.; and Samachson, J.: Inhibition of radiostrontium absorption by aluminum phosphate gel in man and its comparative effect on radiocalcium absorption. *Int. J. Appl. Radiat. Isot.,* **20:**507–16, 1969.

Steele, T. N.: Treatment of lithium intoxication with diuretics. In Brown, S. S. (ed.): *Clinical Chemistry and Chemical Toxicology of Metals.* Elsevier/North-Holland, New York, 1977, pp. 289–92.

Stuve, J., and Galle, P.: Role of Mitochondria in the renal handling of gold by the kidney. *J. Cell Biol.,* **44:**667–76, 1970.

Sunde, R. A., and Hoekstra, W. G.: Structure, synthesis, and function of glutathione peroxidase. *Nutr. Rev.,* **38:**265–73, 1980.

Sunderman, F. W., Jr.: Nickel. In Bronner, F., and Coburn, J. W. (eds.): *Disorders of Mineral Metabolism,* Vol. 1. Academic Press, Inc., New York, 1981a, pp. 201–32.

————: Recent research on nickel carcinogenesis. *Environ. Health Perspect.,* **40:**131–41, 1981b.

Sunderman, F. W., Sr.: Efficacy of sodium diethyldithiocarbamate (dithiocarb) in acute nickel carbonyl poisoning. *Ann. Clin. Lab. Sci.,* **9:**1–10, 1979.

Suzuki, K. T.: Induction and degradation of metallothioneins and their relation to the toxicity of cadmium. In Foulkes, E. C. (ed.): *Biological Roles of Metallothionein.* Elsevier, New York, 1982, pp. 215–35.

Suzuki, K. T.; Takenaka, S.; and Kubota, K.: Fate and

comparative toxicity of metallothionein with differing cadmium-zinc ratios in rat kidney. *Arch. Contemp. Toxicol.*, 8:85–90, 1979.

Suzuki, T.: Metabolism of mercurial compounds. In Goyer, R. A., and Mehlman, M. A. (eds.): *Toxicology of Trace Elements*. Hemisphere Publishing Co., Washington, D.C., 1977, pp. 1–39.

Takenaka, S.; Oldiges, H.; Konig, H.; Hochrainer, D.; and Oberdorster, G.: Carcinogenicity of cadmium chloride aerosols in W rats. *JNCI,* 70:367–73, 1983.

Tam, G. K. H.; Charbonneau, S. M.; Bryce, F.; Pomroy, C.; and Sandi, E.: Metabolism of inorganic arsenic ([74]As) in humans following oral ingestion. *Toxicol. Appl. Pharmacol.,* 50:319–22, 1979.

Thomas, D. W.; Hartley, T. F.; and Sobecki, S.: Clinical and laboratory investigations of the metabolism of bismuth containing pharmaceuticals by man and dogs. In Brown, S. S. (ed.): *Clinical Chemistry and Clinical Toxicology of Metals.* Elsevier/North-Holland, New York, 1977, pp. 293–96.

Thomas, H. M.: A case of generalized lead paralysis, a review of the cases of lead palsy seen in the hospital. *Bull. Johns Hopkins Hosp.,* 15:209–12, 1904.

Thompson, R. J.: Collection and analysis of airborne metallic elements. In Risby, T. H. (ed.): *Ultratrace Metal Analysis in Biological Sciences and Environment.* American Chemical Society, Washington, D.C., 1979, pp. 54–72.

Tohyama, C., and Shaikh, Z. A.: Metallothionein in plasma and urine of cadmium-exposed rats determined by a single-antibody radioimmunoassay. *Fund. Appl. Toxicol.,* 1:1–7, 1981.

Trump, B. F.; Valigersky, J. N.; Arstila, A. U.; Mergner, W. J.; and Kinney, T. D.: The relationship of intracellular pathways of iron metabolism to cellular iron overload and the iron storage diseases. *Am. J. Pathol.,* 72:295–324, 1973.

Tseng, W.-P.: Effects and dose-response relationships of skin cancer and blackfoot disease with arsenic. *Environ. Health Perspect.,* 19:109–19, 1977.

Tubbs, R. R.; Gephardt, G. N.; McMahon, J. T.,; Phol, M. C.; Vidt, D. G.; Barenberg, S. A.; and Valenzuela, R.: Membranous glomerulonephritis associated with industrial mercury exposure. *Am. J. Clin. Pathol.,* 77:409–13, 1982.

Underwood, E. J.: *Trace Elements in Human and Animal Nutrition,* 4th ed. Academic Press, Inc., New York, 1977.

Urizar, R., and Vernier, R. L.: Bismuth Nephropathy. *JAMA,* 198:187–89, 1966.

Vahter, M., and Norin, H.: Metabolism [74]As-labelled trivalent and pentavalent inorganic arsenic in mice. *Environ. Res.,* 21:446–57, 1980.

Vallee, B. L.; Ulmer, D. D.; and Wacker, W. E. C.: Arsenic toxicology and biochemistry. *AMA Arch. Industr. Health,* 21:132–51, 1960.

Van Rij, A. M.; Thomson, C. R.; McKenzie, J. M.; and Robinson, M. F.: Selenium deficiency in total parenteral nutrition. *Am. J. Clin. Nutr.,* 32:2076–85, 1979.

Vander, A. J.; Taylor, D. L.; Kalitis, K.; Mouw, D. R.; and Victery, W.: Renal handling of lead in dogs: clearance studies. *Am. J. Physiol.,* 233:F532–38, 1977.

Verschuuren, H. G.; Ruitenberg, E. J.; Peetoom, F.; Helleman, P. W.; and Van Esch, G. J.: Influence of triphenyltin acetate on lymphatic tissue and immune response in guinea pigs. *Toxicol. Appl. Pharmacol.,* 16:400–10, 1970.

Victery, W.; Vander, A. J.; and Mouw, D. R.: Renal handling of lead in dogs: stop-flow analysis. *Am. J. Physiol.,* 237:F408–14, 1979a.

Victery, W.; Vander, A. J.; and Mouw, D. R.: Effect of acid-base status on renal excretion and accumulation of lead in dogs and rats. *Am. J. Physiol.* 237:F398–F407, 1979b.

Victery, W.; Vander, A. J.; Shulak, J. M.; Schoeps, P.; and Julius, S.: Lead, hypertension and the renin-angiotensin system in rats. *J. Lab. Clin. Med.,* 99:354–62, 1982.

Voegtlin, C., and Hodge, H. C. (eds.): *The Pharmacology and Toxicology of Uranium Compounds,* Vols. 1–4. McGraw-Hill Book Co., New York, 1949–1951.

Voil, G. W.; Minielly, J. A.; and Bistricki, T.: Gold nephropathy tissue analysis by x-ray fluorescent spectroscopy. *Arch. Pathol. Lab. Med.,* 101:635–40, 1977.

Vostal, J., and Heller, J.: Renal excretory mechanisms of heavy metals. I. Transtubular transport of heavy metal ions in the avian kidney. *Environ. Res.,* 2:1–10, 1968.

Vouk, V. B., and Piver, W. T.: Metallic elements in fossil fuel combustion and products: amounts and form of emissions and evaluation of carcinogenicity and mutagenicity. *Environ. Health Perspect.,* 47:201–26, 1983.

Vouk, V. B., and Piver, W. T.: Metallic elements in fossil fuel combustion and products: amounts and form of emissions and evaluation of carcinogenicity and mutagenicity. *Environ. Health Perspect.,* 47:201–26, 1983.

Walshe, J. M.: Endogenous copper clearance in Wilson's disease: a study of the mode of action of penicillamine. *Clin. Sci.,* 26:461–69, 1964.

———: Assessment of treatment of Wilson's disease with triethylene tetramine 2HCl (Trien 2HCl). In Sarkar (ed.): *Biological Aspects of Metals and Metal Related Diseases.* Raven Press, New York, 1983, pp. 243–61.

Waters, M. D.: Toxicology of vanadium. In Goyer, R. A., and Mehlman, M. A. (eds.): *Toxicology of Trace Metals.* John Wiley & Sons, New York, 1977, pp. 147–89.

Wedeen, R. P.; Maesaka, J. K.; Weiner, B.; Lipat, E. A.; Lyons, M. M.; Vitale, L. F.; and Joselow, M. M.: Occupational lead nephropathy. *Am. J. Med.,* 59:630–41, 1975.

WHO Environmental Health Criteria 1. *Mercury.* World Health Organization, Geneva, 1976.

WHO Environmental Health Criteria for Cadmium. *Ambio,* 6:287–90, 1977a.

WHO Environmental Health Criteria 3. *Lead.* World Health Organization, Geneva, 1977b.

WHO Environmental Health Criteria 15. *Tin and Organotin Compounds: A Preliminary Review.* World Health Organization, Geneva, 1980.

WHO Environmental Health Criteria 18. *Arsenic.* World Health Organization, Geneva, 1981.

Wilber, C. G.: *Selenium: A Potential Environmental Poison and a Necessary Food Constituent.* Charles C Thomas, Pub., Springfield, Ill., 1983.

Williams, D. R., and Halstead, B. W.: Chelating agents in medicine. *Clin. Toxicol.,* 19:1081–1115, 1982–83.

Wills, J. H., Jr.: Goitrogens in foods. In Food Protection Committee: *Toxicants Occurring Naturally in Foods.* National Academy of Sciences Publication No. 1354, Washington, D.C., 1966, pp. 3–17.

Wills, M. R., and Savory, J.: Aluminum poisoning: Dialysis encephalopathy, osteomalacia, and anemia. *Lancet,* 2:29–33, 1983.

Winston, P. W.: Molybdenum. In Bonner, F., and Coburn, J. W. (eds.): *Disorders of Mineral Metabolism.* Vol. 1, *Trace Minerals.* Academic Press, Inc., New York, 1981, pp. 295–315.

Woods, J. S.; Carver, G. T.; and Fowler, B. A.: Altered regulation of hepatic heme metabolism by indium chloride. *Toxicol. Appl. Pharmacol.,* 49:455–61, 1979.

Chapter 20

TOXIC EFFECTS OF SOLVENTS AND VAPORS

Larry S. Andrews and *Robert Snyder*

INTRODUCTION

Nearly everyone is exposed to solvents. The utility of these fluids as solubilizers, dispersants, or diluents leads to the manufacture and use of billions of pounds each year. Occupational exposures can involve applications ranging from a secretary using correction fluid to a gas station attendant pumping gasoline. A refinery worker may be exposed to solvents on the job and upon returning home may paint a room, change the oil in the family car, or glue together an item in need of repair, thereby extending his exposure to solvents. Although the solvents, which are usually mixtures, have different trade names, they frequently contain similar chemicals. Clearly, exposure should not be equated with toxicity. The fundamental principle of toxicology, i.e., the does-response relationship, requires that there be (1) exposure and (2) a toxic effect. Nevertheless, the potential for toxicologic interaction increases as exposure increases, and exposure to mixtures leads to the possibility of unpredictable additivity, synergism, or potentiation of effects. Eventually, we must learn to understand the interactive effects because exposure of human populations in the environment is not usually to a single chemical. Until we have developed that needed body of knowledge, we must make use of the database available to us, which is the toxicology of individual solvents and the relationship between the structures of solvents and their toxicity within chemical classes.

PROPERTIES OF SOLVENTS

Exposure

Many solvents exhibit appreciable volatility under conditions of use, and consequently the worker is exposed to solvent vapors. Vapor concentrations are expressed as parts of vapor per million parts of contaminated air (ppm) by volume at room temperature and pressure. It is possible to relate ppm to mg of vapor/volume of air

by making use of the relationship that 1 mole of an ideal gas at 25° C and 760 mm Hg occupies 24.45 liters. The following equations define these relationships (Olishifski, 1979).

$$\text{mg vapor/m}^3 \text{ air} = \frac{\text{molecular weight}}{24.45} \text{ ppm}$$

$$\frac{\text{parts vapor}}{10^6 \text{ parts air}} \text{ (ppm)} = \frac{24.45}{\text{molecular weight}} \text{ mg/m}^3$$

The volatility of solvents indicates that a major route of exposure will be by the respiratory system. Once vapors enter the lungs, they may diffuse across respiratory membranes and enter the bloodstream. The ability of solvent vapors to enter the bloodstream depends on their lipid solubility since lipoprotein cell membranes must be traversed. Many solvents are quite lipid soluble and will enter the blood with ease. Since diffusion occurs from relatively high concentrations in lung air to low concentrations in blood and tissues, the driving force for the movement is the vapor concentration in inspired air.

Many factors including rate and depth of respiration will affect blood solvent concentrations. The rate at which the solvent distributes to the body organs through the blood is controlled by the cardiac output. The rate at which it leaves the blood to enter the organs is a function of the partition (Ostwald) coefficient. Thus, agents having a high blood/air partition coefficient, such as diethyl ether, leave the blood and enter the organs at a slow rate, whereas agents such as halothane have a low partition coefficient and thereby distribute more rapidly. An excellent description of processes involved in the uptake of vapors into the bloodstream is provided in Chapter 12 of this volume.

A second major route of exposure is the skin. The ubiquity of solvents and the casual approach to their use almost assure skin contact with liquid solvents. Frequent contact with lipid-soluble solvents can lead to a defatting of skin or to skin irritation. Of more importance for systemic toxicity is that some solvents may penetrate the skin (from both liquid and vapor phases) and enter the bloodstream (Rihimaki and Pfaffli, 1978). This observation has raised the possibility that toxic amounts of solvents may be absorbed through the skin as a result of occupational and consumer exposures. This question has not, as yet, been approached in a systematic fashion. However, it does not seem likely that the percutaneous route will be a major contributor to establishing a body burden of a solvent, since (1) the lung provides a much more efficient transfer of vapors to the bloodstream than does skin, and (2) the area of skin in contact with a liquid solvent often must be large for there to be absorption of appreciable amounts.

Another aspect of exposure to solvents is the frequency of exposure. Consumers, by virtue of the fact that they use small amounts of products, are generally not exposed to large amounts of solvents over long periods of time. Exposure to low levels with intermittent exposure to much higher levels is a likely exposure scenario in the consumer setting. For example, solvent from an opened can of paint stripper may evaporate into the garage over a period of time, but furniture refinishing is an infrequent activity. In the occupational setting, a similar situation exists, where there may be continuous exposure to low levels of solvent with brief exposure to high concentrations of solvents. It seems axiomatic that toxicity testing of solvents in experimental animals should incorporate these exposure realities into test protocols. However, little information is currently available on effects of intermittent exposure.

The American Conference of Governmental Industrial Hygienists (ACGIH, 1983–84) has recognized these aspects of solvent exposure in their program for establishing Threshold Limit Values (TLVs). ACGIH defines TLVs as airborne concentrations of substances that represent conditions under which it is believed that nearly all workers may be exposed day after day without adverse effect. TLVs are based on the best available information from industrial experience, and studies in animals and in human volunteers. This information is detailed in ACGIH's Documentation of Threshold Limit Values series. The ACGIH develops three categories of TLVs: (1) time-weighted average (TWA)—a value for a normal eight-hour workday and 40-hour workweek; (2) short-term exposure limit (STEL)—a value for a short period of time (usually 15 minutes); and (3) ceiling (TLV-C)—a value that should not be exceeded even briefly.

Toxicity

The toxic effects of solvents are both general and specific. The effect observed in studies in experimental animals or in the occupational exposure setting will depend on many factors including: solvent structure, exposure level, frequency and coexposure, and subject sensitivity. General sources on the toxicology of specific solvents and on solvents contained in trade name products are the texts by Browning (1953) and by Gosselin et al. (1976).

General. Many organic solvents, including hydrocarbons, chlorinated hydrocarbons, alcohols, ethers, esters, and ketones, have the potential upon acute high level vapor exposure to cause narcosis and death. A typical exposure scenario is the worker who enters a reaction vessel or holding tank without appropriate respiratory equipment. In such a confined space, solvent vapor concentrations may reach many hundreds or thousands of parts per million and workers may be quickly overcome. Of course, the experimental animal analogy is the acute inhalation toxicity study (LC50).

Workers exposed to solvents under these conditions will typically show signs of central nervous system disturbance. While there is some variation in signs and symptoms with solvent structure, results of high-level exposure are quite similar. Disorientation, euphoria, giddiness, confusion, progressing to unconsciousness, paralysis, convulsion, and death from respiratory or cardiovascular arrest is typically observed (Browning, 1965). The rapidity of the development of these symptoms almost ensures that the acute effects of solvents are due to the solvent itself and not the metabolites. In the majority of subjects, recovery from central nervous system effects is rapid and complete following removal from exposure. Less certain are the effects of acute high-level exposure on the extent and reversibility of specific toxicity discussed below.

The similarity of the narcosis produced by solvents of diverse structure suggests that these effects result from a physical interaction of a solvent with cells of the central nervous system. If a purely physical interaction is assumed, then the narcotic effect of the solvent will be dependent only on the molar concentration of the solvent in the central nervous system cell. Equimolar concentrations of different solvents will result in narcotic effects of equal intensity. A more detailed discussion of solvent-induced narcosis is found in the discussion of ethanol in this chapter. It is important to realize, however, that the ability of high-level exposure to solvents to cause these effects remains an important aspect of solvent toxicity.

Other effects of solvents that may be related to solvents in general and to relatively nonspecific actions on the central nervous system are those seen in behavioral toxicity tests. A list of such tests has been compiled from several recent reviews and is presented in Table 20–1 (Feldman *et al.,* 1980; Tilson and Cabe, 1978). A brief examination of the tests and symptomatology leads to the conclusion that most tests are not applicable for experimental animals. Thus, results in human studies cannot usually be correlated and explored in an animal model because we do not yet know how animals "think" or "feel" or "react." Of course, the inability to establish a closely related animal model is not a reason in and of itself to discount results of behavioral tests in humans. However, the inability to establish an animal model does make more critical problems generic to testing in humans. For example: What was the subject's baseline behavioral function prior to exposure? What is the degree of exposure? Is there coexposure to other materials? How does one match an exposed population with a control population to minimize confounding effects on behavior? An additional question that needs to be addressed is: Do behavioral effects precede in time or dose, coexist with or extend beyond demonstrable organic tissue damage? The study of a human population will make the answer to such a question very difficult to obtain.

Despite these obvious difficulties in study and interpretation, some recent studies on behavioral toxicity are of note. Behavioral toxicity studies on carbon disulfide (CS_2) are perhaps most conclusive of all solvents for which studies have been conducted.

Reaction time, psychomotor performance, and distractability are sensitive indicators of CS_2 exposure (Lillis, 1974; Hanninen *et al.,* 1978).

Lillis (1974) has concluded that behavioral effects precede obvious neurologic effects of CS_2.

A number of epidemiology studies on workers exposed to solvent mixtures have recently been reported (Elofsson *et al.,* 1980; Seppalainen *et al.,* 1980). These studies involved car painters and workers with a diagnosis of "solvent poisoning," respectively. While these studies report behavioral effects, they are especially subject to the difficulties of interpretation discussed above.

Specific. Distinct from acute central nervous system depressant actions of solvents are specific toxicities associated with them. Such effects include the hematopoietic toxicity of benzene, the CNS depressant effects of alkylbenzenes, hepatotoxicity of certain chlorinated hydrocarbons, the ocular toxicity of methanol, the hepatotoxicty and CNS depressant effects of ethanol, neurotoxicity of *n*-hexane and certain ketones, reproductive toxicity of ethylene glycol ethers, and the carcinogenicity of dioxane. Each of these effects will be discussed in more detail below, but first, two important aspects of evaluating solvents for specific adverse effects are discussed.

Exposure

In contrast to general effects of solvents, specific toxicity usually results from repeated exposure to tolerable levels of solvents rather than to acute exposure to very high levels. A typical exposure scenario is a worker who is exposed day after day to a material. The solvent, a toxic metabolite of the solvent, or tissue damage from either may accumulate until a worker develops a clinically recognizable illness. Good estimates of dose or time required to develop an illness are

Table 20–1.　SYMPTOMATOLOGY AND COMMONLY USED TESTS FOR BEHAVIORAL EFFECTS

SYMPTOMATOLOGY	TEST
Sensory—paresthesias, visual or auditory deficits	Neurologic, sight, and hearing examinations
Cognitive—memory (both short-term and long-term), confusion, disorientation	Wechsler memory scale Wechsler Adult Intelligence Scale (WAIS)
Affective—nervousness, irritability, depression, apathy, compulsive behavior	Eysenck Personality Inventory Rorschach Test Digit-symbol substitution Task Bourdon-Wiersma Vigilance Task
Motor—weakness in hands, incoordination, fatigue, tremor	Neurologic examination Santa Ana Dexterity Test Finger-tapping Test Simple or Choice Reaction Time

generally not available for solvents for which specific human toxicities are recognized.

Biotransformation

Specific toxicities of solvents, as distinct from general effects discussed above, are directly related to the biotransformation of the solvent. Thus, the hematopoietic toxicity of benzene, the neurotoxicity of n-hexane, and the reproductive toxicity of ethylene glycol ethers have all been attributed to toxic metabolites of these materials. This general phenomenon is termed bioactivation and is largely mediated by the family of enzymes termed cytochrome P-450-dependent mixed-function oxidases (see Chapter 4). Of course, not all biotransformation of a given solvent need result in bioactivation. Typically, one or more cytochrome P-450 mixed-function oxidases may mediate the conversion of a large percentage of the dose of solvent to a harmless metabolite, a process termed detoxication.

Mixed function oxidases are a family of enzymes, consisting primarily of the hemoprotein cytochrome P-450, and are located in the smooth endoplasmic reticulum of liver as well as most other tissues. These enzymes catalyze the oxidation or reduction of a wide variety of chemical structures. A postulated mechanism for mixed function oxidative reactions is visualized in Chapter 4.

Interactions. Since mixed-function oxidases have a broad specificity, it is not surprising that one solvent can compete with another for available catalytic sites. Thus, toluene has been shown to be a competitive inhibitor of the biotransformation of benzene (Andrews et al., 1977; Sato and Nakajima, 1979). This competitive interaction alleviates the metabolite-mediated toxicity of benzene as discussed below. Another example of biotransformation interactions among solvents is presented in Chapter 10 on toxic responses of the liver. Thus, prior exposure to a number of alcohols or ketones can potentiate the liver damage caused by chlorinated hydrocarbons.

Inducibility. The mixed function oxidase system contains a group of isozymes termed cytochromes P-450. Treatment of animals, and presumably humans, with any of a great number of chemicals leads to increases in the biotransformation of these and other chemicals because of elevations in the levels of the cytochromes P-450. The specificities of the induced enzymes vary. Some chemicals, such as benzene, are capable of increasing their own biotransformation and that of a few other chemicals (Snyder et al., 1967), whereas drugs like phenobarbital or environmental chemicals, such as polychlorinated biphenyls, can increase the biotransformation of a wide variety of chemicals.

The toxicity of a chemical may be dramatically altered as a result of enzyme induction. If metabolic activation of a solvent to its toxic metabolite is limited by the constitutive concentration of the specific species of cytochrome P-450 through which it is biotransformed, enzyme induction may lead to greater toxicity. Thus, bromobenzene, given to rats at doses that do not produce serious toxicity in uninduced animals, yields massive hepatic necrosis in animals pretreated with phenobarbital. Alternatively, toxicity of a given dose may be reduced by decreasing the fraction processed by the bioactivation pathway. Thus, treating rats with 3-methylcholanthrene prior to dosing with bromobenzene led to a reduction in expected hepatotoxicity because an alternative pathway leading to less toxic metabolites was induced, thereby reducing the fraction of the dose that passed through the bioactivation pathway.

Saturation. Implicit in the concept of enzyme-mediated detoxication or bioactivation is the phenomenon of enzymatic saturation (see Chapter 3). Exposure to massive amounts of a solvent may result in saturation of detoxication pathways resulting in a spillover into bioactivation pathways. Metabolic saturation has been demonstrated for a number of solvents including n-hexane, vinylidene chloride, methyl chloroform, perchloroethylene, and ethylene dichloride.

Saturation of biotransformation may have profound importance in the design and interpretation of safety evaluation studies employing maximum tolerated doses. Under these conditions, experimental animals may be exposed to doses that not only saturate detoxication pathways but are many times human exposure levels. Under conditions of high-level exposure, saturation of biotransformation pathways may prevail. When considering exposures at, or below, permissible standards however, saturation biotransformation may be less important in determining ultimate toxicity. Thus, Andersen et al. (1980) have found that at low vapor concentrations of several solvents, respiration and hepatic perfusion indices were rate-limiting factors in biotransformation and hence in the production of toxic metabolites.

Species, Genetics, and Age. Among many factors that can affect cytochrome P-450 mixed-function oxidase reactions are species, genetics, and age. Such confounding factors can greatly influence the metabolism and toxicity of solvents.

AROMATIC HYDROCARBONS

Benzene

Benzene has had a long history of extensive use in industry, first as a volatile solvent and later as a starting material for the synthesis of other chemicals. Thus, in the late nineteenth century benzene facilitated the rapid development of the rubber industry because of its ability to dissolve rubber latex and its ease of evaporation during the manufacture of formed or coated rubber products. It played a similar role in high-speed printing processes because it is an excellent solvent for inks that must dry rapidly. Many other industries also use benzene as a solvent or as starting material for chemical syntheses. The manufacturers of paints and plastics have been among the heaviest users. Today, because of its antiknock properties, a mixture of benzene-rich aromatics is added to gasoline as a replacement for alkyl lead compounds.

Because benzene has an appreciable vapor pressure at ambient temperatures, hazardous occupational exposure usually occurs via inhalation. Acute exposure to high concentrations of benzene may kill by depressing the central nervous system leading to unconsciousness and death or by producing fatal cardiac arrhythmias (Snyder and Kocsis, 1975).

The major toxic effect of benzene is hematopoietic toxicity, an effect unique to benzene among the simple aromatic hydrocarbons. Chronic exposure of humans to low levels of benzene in the workplace is associated with blood disorders including aplastic anemia and leukemia (Snyder and Kocsis, 1975). The bone marrow toxicity of benzene is characterized by a progressive decrease in each of the circulating formed elements of blood, i.e., erythrocytes, thrombocytes, and each of the various types of leukocytes. The extent to which each of the cell types is depleted varies with the individual and the degree of exposure to benzene. In both human and animal studies it appears that benzene-induced bone marrow depression is a dose dependent phenomenon. When all three cell types have been sufficiently depressed, the disease is called pancytopenia and results from benzene-induced damage leading to necrosis and fatty replacement of bone marrow. Pancytopenia in the absence of functional marrow is termed aplastic anemia.

In humans, signs of chronic benzene toxicity have been observed since the turn of the century. These studies generally show that a decreased level of circulating erythrocytes or leukocytes is a relatively good indication of early benzene toxicity; among leukocytes, granulocyte levels are usually depressed more than lymphocyte levels. Although individual workers vary in their reactions to benzene, the toxicity appears to be a function of both exposure level and duration of exposure. The present OSHA standard for occupational exposure to benzene is 10 ppm as a time-weighted average with a ceiling value of 25 ppm (RTECS, 1980). It is anticipated that the standard will soon be reduced. OSHA estimates that approximately 2 million workers are exposed to benzene.

In animals, benzene-induced bone marrow depression has been produced experimentally in a number of species. In each case exposure to benzene caused significant leukopenia, and in contrast to humans, lymphocytes were decreased in number more than were granulocytes. The production of anemia, first reported in 1897, has recently been studied using decreases in ^{59}Fe incorporation into red cell hemoglobin as a measure of benzene-induced depression of erythropoietic function (Lee et al., 1981; Bolscak and Nerland, 1983).

Leukemia is another type of blood dyscrasia associated with exposure to benzene. Leukemias are acute or chronic diseases that are further classified according to the cell type involved. The leukemia most commonly associated with benzene exposure is acute myelogenous leukemia. Acute myelogenous leukemia is characterized by an increased number of cells morphologically similar to the myeloblast. To date, benzene-induced leukemia has only been observed in humans, and no satisfactory animal model exists. However, recent reports have stressed the production of solid tumors in animals given benzene orally (Maltoni, 1983).

Evidence that benzene is a human leukemogen is primarily epidemiologic but is strongly supported by a large number of case control studies (IARC, 1982). In 1964, Vigliani reported several cases of leukemia in workers exposed to benzene (Vigliani and Saita, 1964). Aksoy and Erdem (1978) reported an increased incidence of leukemia in shoe workers occupationally exposed to benzene. McMichael et al. (1975) and Infante et al. (1977) reported cancers of the lymphatic and hematopoietic systems in worders in the U.S. rubber industry.

Exposure of experimental animals to benzene can result in cytogenetic aberrations in bone marrow and peripheral blood. These effects generally occur at high exposure levels and are largely limited to gaps and deletions. Abnormal forms are rare (Dean, 1978). Workers exposed to benzene in levels sufficient to disturb hematopoiesis display a greater incidence of chromosome aberrations in peripheral blood and bone marrow than do unexposed controls. The design of these studies in workers is such that it is not possible to estimate a minimum exposure level or exposure period needed to produce cytogenetic changes.

Morimoto and co-workers (Morimoto *et al.*, 1983) have shown that benzene biotransformation is necessary for benzene-induced sister chromatid exchanges (SCE). Working with whole blood cultures from human donors, they found that benzene could induce SCEs but only in the presence of microsomal enzymes. Addition of glutathione to blood cultures decreased benzene-induced SCEs. The benzene metabolites catechol and hydroquinone also induced SCEs. Significantly, addition of microsomal enzymes enhanced, and addition of glutathione inhibited, this response. Thus, the benzene metabolites catechol and hydroquinone and further metabolites of catechol and hydroquinone are implicated in DNA damage induced by benzene. The ability of glutathione to inhibit SCE induction suggests the electrophilic nature of the toxic metabolites. Tice *et al.* (1982) have shown that production of SCEs is directly related to benzene biotransformation *in vivo* since toluene, a competitive inhibitor of benzene biotransformation (Andrews *et al.*, 1977), protected against the benzene effect.

Tunek and co-workers (1982) have related benzene's ability to induce micronuclei in bone marrow cells with benzene biotransformation *in vivo*. Toft *et al.* (1982) exposed male mice to benzene vapors (1 to 200 ppm) for varying periods of time and reported that continuous exposure to 14 ppm benzene after one week resulted in a significant elevation in micronuclei. No effect was seen at the 1 to 10 ppm dose range but at higher doses the effect seemed to be related to a function of dose times time. Subcutaneous injection of hydroquinone induced micronuclei formation at doses above 20 mg/kg given repeatedly. Doses of catechol up to 42 mg/kg/day for six consecutive days did not induce micronuclei formation. Simultaneous injection of toluene (876 mg/kg) decreased the benzene- or hydroquinone-induced micronuclei formation. In related experiments benzene also produced micronuclei when administered parenterally.

Although these reports indicate a strong correlation between benzene exposure and leukemia, there are several reasons why a cause-and-effect relationship has not been universally accepted. Since all studies correlating exposure with effect are retrospective epidemiologic studies, data regarding duration and level of benzene exposure are usually deficient or cannot be obtained. Furthermore, there are no animal models for benzene-induced leukemia, and although there is evidence that benzene has caused chromosome damage, it has not been demonstrated

to be mutagenic using *in vitro* cell assays. As discussed above, benzene exposure in industry does not occur in total isolation from other solvents, and this is another complicating factor in trying to assign a cause-and-effect relationship between benzene exposure and leukemia. Nevertheless, on balance it must be accepted that benzene is a carcinogenic substance and is probably an important cause of acute myelogenous and perhaps others types of leukemia in humans.

In order to understand the mechanism of benzene toxicity it is essential to study its disposition. Parke and Williams (1953) were among the first to suggest that one of its metabolites might be responsible for benzene toxicity. Several studies have demonstrated that modification of benzene biotransformation leads to alterations in benzene toxicity. For example, Andrews *et al.* (1977) reported that toluene, a competitive inhibitor of benzene biotransformation, protected mice against benzene toxicity. Longacre *et al.* (1981) demonstrated that benzene metabolites were found at higher levels in bone marrow of DBA/2 mice, which were sensitive to benzene, than in C57B1/6 mice, which were relatively resistant to benzene. On the other hand, Ikeda and Ohtsuki (1971) reported that stimulation of detoxication processes by phenobarbital protected rats against benzene-induced leukopenia. On the basis of these and other studies it is well accepted that one or more of its metabolites are responsible for the production of the adverse hematologic effects of benzene.

Although the major route of human exposure is by inhalation, many animal studies have been performed in which benzene was administered by a parenteral route. There is no evidence to suggest that variations in the route of administration can qualitatively alter the toxicity of benzene. A significant portion of any dose of benzene is exhaled unchanged or stored in fat in both animals and humans. Rickert *et al.* (1979) reported that following inhalation of benzene in rats, excretion via the lung followed a biphasic pattern indicative of a two-compartment model.

The bulk of the evidence suggests that benzene toxicity is produced by one or more metabolites of benzene rather than by benzene itself (Snyder *et al.*, 1981). The broad outlines of benzene biotransformation were best established by Parke and Williams (1953) using ^{14}C-labeled benzene. Phenol, catechol, hydroquinone, and 1,2,4-trihydroxybenzene were recovered as ethereal sulfates and glucuronide conjugates in urine of treated animals. Other metabolites included *l*-phenylmercapturic acid and *trans-trans*-muconic acid.

The mechanism of benzene hydroxylation remains a matter of discussion. The metabolic

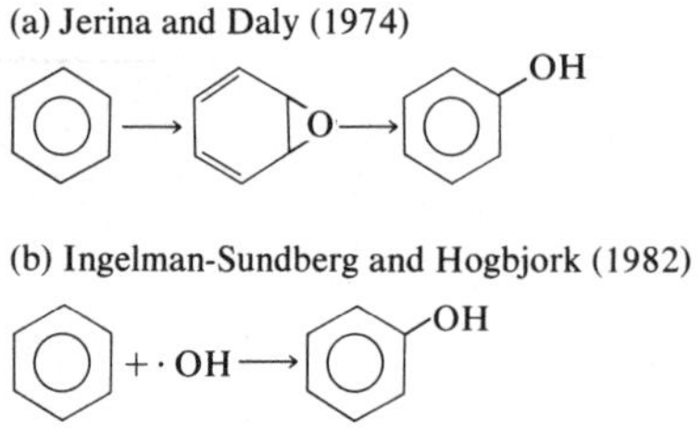

(a) Jerina and Daly (1974)

(b) Ingelman-Sundberg and Hogbjork (1982)

Figure 20–1. Mechanisms of benzene hydroxylation.

pathway (Snyder *et al.*, 1981) involves first the conversion of benzene to benzene oxide (Figure 20–1) (Jerina and Daly, 1974) by the hepatic microsomal mixed-function oxidase (Gonasun *et al.*, 1973). The oxide (Figure 20–2) may rearrange nonenzymatically to form phenol, may react with glutathione to form a premercapturic acid that is subsequently converted to *l*-phenyl-mercapturic acid, or may react with epoxide hydrolase, which converts it to benzene dihydrodiol. The mixed-function oxidase and epoxide hydrolase are microsomal enzymes, but the dihydrodiol is oxidized to catechol by a cytosolic dehydrogenase. Hydroquinone is the primary product of further hydroxylation of phenol.

Jerina and Daly (1974) suggest that the hydroxylation involves the intermediate formation of an epoxide, and much of the theory of carcinogenesis by bay region diol-epoxides is founded on this concept. Although the epoxide of benzene has never been isolated and identi-

fied during the enzymatic oxidation of benzene, Tunek *et al.* (1982) reported that the addition of an excess of purified epoxide hydrolase to a rat liver microsomal system during benzene biotransformation resulted in production of the dihydrodiol. This could only have been the result of the intermediate formation of the epoxide. However, Ingelman-Sundberg and Hagbjork (1982) suggested that hydroxylation could occur via the insertion of a hydroxyl free radical (Figure 20–1). They postulate that the free radicals are generated by an "iron-catalyzed cytochrome P-450-dependent Haber Weiss reaction," and their data are supported by the demonstration that several compounds that prevent free-radical formation or act as free-radical scavengers can inhibit the hydroxylation of benzene by an isolated, reconstituted rabbit liver microsomal mixed-function oxidase. These discrepancies could be reconciled if (1) there were two different cytochromes P-450 responsible for benzene hydroxylation, one of which generated free radicals which hydroxylated benzene and another which formed the epoxide, or (2) the cytochrome P-450 responsible for benzene oxide formation also functions as a NADPH oxidase, thereby producing H_2O_2 and subsequently hydroxyl radicals. In the former case, Post and Snyder (1983) recently demonstrated that there are at least two different rat liver mixed-function oxidases active in benzene hydroxylation, but their mechanisms of action have yet to be clarified. The latter alternative suggests that the mixed-function oxidase is inefficient and oxygen radical formation is an indication of uncoupling

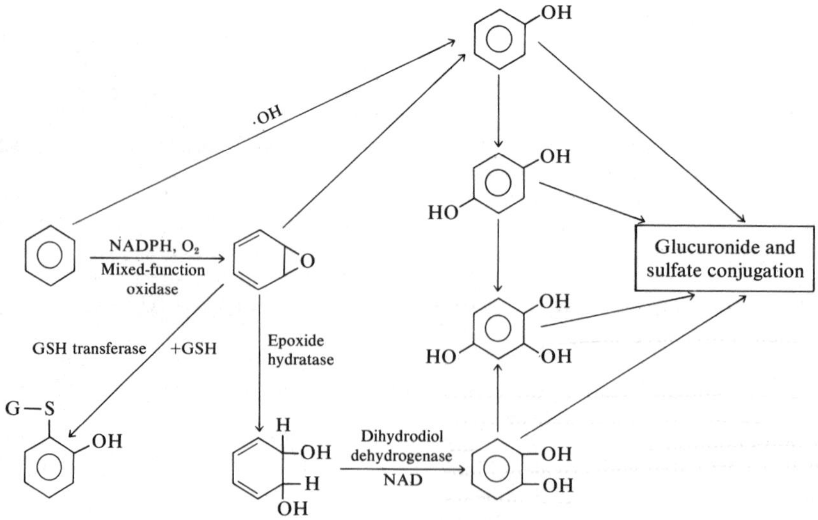

Figure 20–2. Biotransformation of benzene.

of NADPH oxidation from substrate oxidation.

The formation of the dihydroxylated metabolites, hydroquinone and catechol, seems to occur by different pathways. The dihydrodiol can be aromatized by a cytosolic dehydrogenase to yield catechol. Hydroquinone can be formed from phenol in a further hydroxylation step. Small amounts of catechol have also been observed arising from phenol (Sawahata and Neal, 1982). The formation of these compounds and possibly the trihydroxy compound have been postulated by Tunek *et al.* (1980) and by Irons *et al.* (1982) to occur via the intermediate formation of quinones and/or semiquinones (Figure 20–2). In each case of hydroxylation a free-radical insertion may be postulated as in Figure 20–1.

Still another mechanism must be developed to explain the formation of muconic acid (HOOCCH=CHCH=CHCOOH). Muconic acid was first identified as a metabolite of benzene produced by rabbits (Parke and Williams, 1953) and is also a known metabolite of catechol degradation by plant dioxygenases. Goldstein *et al.* (1982), however, have suggested that muconic dialdehyde might be the toxic metabolite that results from ring opening and is subsequently converted to muconic acid.

An alternative fate for benzene metabolites is covalent binding to cellular macromolecules, which many investigators believe is related to the mechanism of benzene toxicity and/or carcinogenicity. In these studies radiolabeled benzene must be used to detect covalent binding. Longacre *et al.* (1981) reported that benzene metabolites bind to proteins in mouse liver, bone marrow, kidney, spleen, blood, and muscle. Less covalent binding in bone marrow, blood, and spleen was observed in mice relatively resistant to benzene toxicity, i.e., C56B1/6, than in more sensitive mice, i.e., DBA2. Irons *et al.* (1980) found covalent binding to protein in perfused bone marrow preparations, and Lutz and Schlatter (1977) reported that in rats exposed to benzene vapor, liver DNA contained labeled benzene residues. Tunek *et al.* (1978) have argued that the covalent binding comes principally from a metabolite of phenol rather than from benzene oxide.

Gill and Ahmed (1981) have suggested that the mitochondria represent an important site of covalent binding for benzene. Kalf *et al.* (1982) have demonstrated that the inhibition of RNA synthesis in mitochondria from both liver and bone marrow was correlated with covalent binding of benzene metabolites to DNA. It appears that phenol, hydroquinone, catechol, benzoquinone, and 1,2,4-trihydroxy benzene can lead to adduct formation in bone marrow mitochondria. The significance of inhibited RNA synthesis in mitochondria relates to inhibition of the synthesis of critical mitochondrial proteins and the resulting impairment of mitochondrial function.

The search for the ultimate mechanism of benzene-induced bone marrow depression or leukemia is complicated by the fact that neither the specific target cell nor the intracellular location of the target has been clearly identified. The data suggest that benzene metabolites may damage both the pluripotential stem cell and/or the early proliferating committed cell in either the erythroid or myeloid line. Thus, Lee *et al.* (1974) suggested that early proliferating cells and maturing cells in marrow, such as the pronormoblast and the normoblast in the erythroid line, were most sensitive to benzene. Uyeki *et al.* (1977), who reported on the inhibition of spleen colony formation by cells from benzene-exposed animals, were the first to report effects of benzene on stem cells. Tunek *et al.* (1981) and Boyd *et al.* (1982) have reported on effects of benzene and its metabolites on colony-forming units for granulocytes. Studies underway currently in other laboratories support the concept that stem cells provide an important target for benzene. However, studies that have not been pursued, and which are required, are investigations into the effects of benzene on bone marrow microenvironmental factors.

In humans the adverse effects of benzene are variants of either aplastic anemia or leukemia. It is likely that in each case metabolites of benzene initiate the disease process and also appear to be implicated in mutational events such as increases in sister chromatid exchange and micronucleus formation. These effects could be produced as a result of any of several actions of benzene metabolites in bone marrow cells. Multiple sites have been identified as potential targets for benzene metabolites. Irons *et al.* (1982) and Irons and Neptun (1980) have shown that microtubule assembly, a critical process for cell replication, is inhibited by benzene metabolites. The data cited above demonstrate that benzene metabolites can covalently bind to DNA, RNA, and protein. Benzene metabolites may also inhibit specific enzymes. In each case an argument can be made that one of these events is responsible for the inhibition of cell replication. However, it may not be necessary to attempt to exclude any of these from consideration as a contributing event. The final disease process may be the result of the sum total of adverse effects of benzene metabolites on several events in the reproductive physiology of bone marrow cells.

Alkylbenzenes

The alkyl benzenes are single-ring aromatic compounds containing one or more aliphatic side chains. While there are theoretically thousands of alkylbenzenes, the major products of commerce and, therefore, those to which humans are most likely to be exposed include toluene (methylbenzene), ethylbenzene, cumene (isopropylbenzene), and the three xylenes (1,2-, 1,3-, and 1,4-dimethylbenzene). These compounds are primarily derived from petroleum distillation and coke oven effluents. The National Academy of Sciences (NAS/NRC, 1980) reported that the production of the alkylbenzenes in the United States, expressed in millions of metric tons, was toluene, 6.4, xylenes, 3.7, ethylbenzene, 3.9. and cumene, 1.8. It is clear that these compounds are major commodity chemicals, and there is a high potential for many workers to be exposed. It should also be recognized that mixtures of these compounds may account for levels as high as 38 percent of unleaded gasoline (NAS/NRC, 1980). The potential for human exposure, albeit often at low levels, is accordingly expanded beyond industrial workers to gasoline station workers and the general public at large. It is, therefore, necessary to have a full understanding of the potential effects of these compounds.

The acute toxicity of inhaled alkylbenzenes is best described as CNS depression. Inhaled alkylbenzene vapors cause death in animal models at air levels that are relatively similar. Thus, the LC50 for toluene in mice is 5320 ppm/eight hours, for mixed xylenes in rats the value is 6700 ppm/four hours, for cumene in rats the value is 8000 ppm/four hours, and the lowest dose of ethylbenzene reported to kill rats, i.e., LCLo, was 4000 ppm/four hours. It is likely that the mechanism of action of the alkylbenzenes under conditions of acute exposure resembles those of the general anesthetics.

With respect to longer-term exposure at lower doses, there is little information available for ethylbenzene or cumene, but it has been concluded that the major effects of toluene and the xylenes are on the CNS and as irritants to mucous membranes. No serious residual effects of the alkylbenzenes have been substantiated. It has been suggested, based on case reports, that some cases of "glue sniffers" who have abused glue solvents display acidosis, perhaps due to excessive production of acidic metabolites of toluene (NAS/NRC, 1980). Reports of hematologic effects or peripheral neuropathies are more likely due to use of glues containing benzene or hexane.

Studies of genetic toxicity with toluene, xylene, and cumene have shown that they do not produce mutations in the various salmonella strains used in the Ames test, with or without metabolic activation (NAS/NRC, 1980). Toluene and xylene are inactive as mutagens in the *Saccharomyces cerevisiae* D4 test for mitotic gene conversion and in the mouse lymphoma test. Although chromosome aberrations have been observed in rats exposed to toluene, they have not been seen in toluene-exposed humans.

Although it is important, with respect to the production of toxicity by most compounds, to ask why they are toxic, in the case of the alkylbenzenes, an important question may be why are they relatively nontoxic except during acute exposure to high concentrations. The toxicity of many chemicals requires metabolic activation to reactive species, which then cause adverse effects. In the case of the alkylbenzenes, however, the major metabolic pathways appear to be toward metabolites that have a low order of toxicity and are readily excreted. Thus, toluene is oxidized at the methyl group and a series of oxidations leads to benzoic acid, which is conjugated with glycine to form hippuric acid, which is then excreted. Hippuric acids are also metabolites of xylene and ethylbenzene. There is no evidence at present to indicate that these metabolic pathways can be saturated leading to the formation of toxic reactive intermediates and subsequent toxic or mutagenic effects.

CHLORINATED ALIPHATIC HYDROCARBONS

Chloroform

The primary effect of high-level exposure to chloroform ($CHCl_3$) is its effect on the central nervous system. Due to the use of chloroform as an anesthetic there is extensive information on effects in humans. Concentrations up to about 400 ppm can be endured for 30 minutes without complaint; 1000 pm exposure for seven minutes can cause dizziness and gastrointestinal upset; 14,000 ppm can cause narcosis.

Exposure to very high levels of $CHCl_3$ can cause liver and kidney damage as well as cardiac arrhythmias apparently due to sensitization of the myocardium to epinephrine. Orth (1965) has emphasized, however, that in human anesthesia, the major effect on the heart is more likely to be cardiac arrest secondary to vagal stimulation. He suggests that ventricular fibrillation occurs only after the heart has stopped, anoxia develops, and carbon dioxide levels are elevated. These effects can be prevented by adequate anticholinergic therapy. Nevertheless, the use of chloroform in anesthesia in this country has been discouraged since 1912 (Pohl, 1979.)

In humans who have developed liver failure following anesthesia, symptoms were observed within a few days following surgery. Nausea and vomiting were followed by jaundice and coma. Upon autopsy, evidence for central lobular necrosis extending into periportal areas was seen. The intermediate zones separating healthy and necrotic tissue contained ballooned and vacuolated cells laden with fat.

Repeated exposure to lower, subnarcotic levels of chloroform can cause liver and kidney toxicity. However, these effects have typically not been seen in workers, despite the extensive and long history of use of CHCl₃. Challen et al. (1958) reported on workers exposed in an industrial setting to 21 to 237 ppm CHCl₃. Worker complaints were of depression and gastrointestinal distress. Liver function tests did not reveal any evidence of liver damage.

Chloroform-induced liver damage is also well recognized in experimental animal models. Torkelson et al. (1976) exposed rabbits, rats, guinea pigs, and dogs to 25, 50, or 85 ppm CHCl₃, seven hours/day, five days/week for six months. Histopathologic evaluation of animals indicated centrilobular necrosis and cloudy swelling of kidneys. The effects of the 25-ppm dose were characterized as mild and reversible. Following oral administration of chloroform in a National Cancer Institute bioassay it was concluded that male rats developed an excess of renal epithelial cell tumors and mice developed liver tumors (Pohl, 1979).

The mechanism by which chloroform produces liver toxicity has been reviewed by Pohl (1979). Chloroform is biotransformed to reactive metabolites that covalently bind to hepatic proteins of the liver and deplete the liver of glutathione. The postulated toxic metabolite was phosgene. Dietz et al. (1982) have suggested that although reactive metabolites are formed from chloroform, the carcinogenic effect is not related to formation of a DNA adduct but to recurrent cytotoxicity with chronic tissue regeneration.

Carbon Tetrachloride

In recent years many studies on the mechanism of chemical-induced hepatic necrosis have focused on carbon tetrachloride (CCl₄), acetaminophen, or bromobenzene. Of these, the description of the series of events in the process of necrosis has been most completely described in the case of carbon tetrachloride. It is possible to outline a sequence of specific steps in morphologic and functional injury. The mechanism by which CCl₄ causes these injuries has been the subject of considerable disagreement, the end product of which has been the stimulation of much research.

Zimmerman (1978) has thoroughly reviewed the hepatoxicity of CCl₄. In humans, monkeys, rats, mice, rabbits, guinea pigs, hamsters, cats, dogs, sheep, and cattle, CCl₄ causes centrizonal necrosis and fat accumulation (see Chapter 10). The extent of injury may be modified by factors such as species differences, age, and sex. Less sensitive models include birds, fish, amphibians, and some types of monkeys, female rats, and newborn rats and dogs. It is likely that the differences in sensitivity are more closely related to the relative ability of the various models to metabolically activate CCl₄ to toxic species than to differences in sensitivity of target sites. This concept is supported by the observation of Rechnagel and Glende (1973) that administration of a small dose of CCl₄ to rats one day before administration of a large dose results in protection against the toxicity otherwise produced by the large dose. The reason is that the small dose was sufficient to inactivate the mixed-function oxidase and thereby prevent metabolic activation to toxic metabolites.

The effects of nutritional alterations have been difficult to interpret but appear to suggest that diets sufficiently low in protein to reduce mixed-function oxidase activity may be protective because of the reduced ability to yield metabolic activation of CCl₄. More prolonged protein deprivation, however, in the presence of residual mixed-function oxidase activity may lead to more severe liver damage because of the loss of protective sulfhydryl compounds such as glutathione.

The hepatic injury follows a well-studied course. After a single dose of CCl₄ given by gavage, or by most other routes, centrilobular necrosis begins to develop with evidence of the lesion by 12 hours and full-blown necrosis by 24 hours. However, evidence for the beginning of recovery, indicated by the appearance of mitotic figures, begins to appear within 24 hours, and the liver may be restored to normal within 14 days with removal of the residues of necrotic tissue (Smuckler, 1975). During the initial 48-hour period liver enzymes, such as aspartate aminotransferase (glutamic oxalacetic transaminase), alanine aminotransferase (glutamic pyruvic transaminase), and lactic dehydrogenase, etc., appear and then recede from the serum and can be used as a measure of the extent of liver damage.

Lipid accumulation develops early with the first drops of lipid seen under the electron microscope within the first hour, and these become observable under the light microscope within three hours. Single-cell necrosis is observable within five to six hours (Smuckler, 1975). Damage to mitochondria and the Golgi apparatus is evident. Other early signs of cell injury include disassociation of ribosomes from the rough endoplasmic reticulum to scattered sites in the cytoplasm and disarray of the smooth endoplasmic reticulum. This apparent membrane denaturing effect described by Reynolds (1972) probably reflects the loss of basophilia seen under the light microscope.

Although CCl₄-induced hepatotoxicity is dependent on its biotransformation, there is much discussion concerning the precise nature of the reactive metabolite. Biochemically, damage to the endoplasmic reticulum leads to the accumulation of lipid and to depression of protein synthesis and of mixed-function oxidase activity. The mechanism of impaired mixed-function oxidase activity is thought to be the irreversible binding of a CCl₄ metabolite to cytochrome P-450 thereby rendering it inactive. Eventually decreased mitochondrial function is also observed (Rechnagel and Glende, 1973).

Rechnagel and co-workers (1973) and Slater (1972) have argued that the mechanism of toxicity of CCl₄ involves the initial homolytic cleavage of a C—Cl bond by cytochrome P-450 to yield Cl₃C: and Cl· free radicals (Figure 20–3). The trichloromethyl free radical is then thought to attack enoic fatty acids in the membranes of the endoplasmic reticulum leading to secondary free radicals within the fatty acids. These are now subject to attack by oxygen, and the subsequent process, which is termed lipid peroxidation, produces damage to the membranes and the enzymes. Slater (1982) has suggested that the trichloromethyl free radical is less reactive than was once thought and that it is more likely that the reaction of O₂ with the trichloromethyl radical leads to a more reactive species, i.e., Cl₃COO:, the trichloromethylperoxy free radical. It would readily interact with unsaturated membrane lipids to produce lipid peroxidation. The net effect of lipid peroxidation is to set in motion the series of inevitable cellular degradations described above which follow upon this initial insult.

An alternative hypothesis has been the suggestion that covalent binding of CCl₄ metabolites to critical cellular macromolecules may lead to cell damage as in the case of acetaminophen and bromobenzene (Jollow and Smith, 1977). Mansuy *et al.* (1974) and Reiner and Uehleke (1971) have studied the splitting of carbon-halogen bonds under anerobic conditions to yield highly reactive metabolites having the general structure R₃C: and called carbenes. Uehleke (1977) reported on the covalent binding of ¹⁴C from CCl₄, CHCl₃, and halothane to macromolecules and suggested that under anerobic conditions covalent binding is probably mediated by the carbene metabolites. Sipes and Gandolfi (1982) showed that halothane-induced liver damage produced under relatively anerobic conditions is probably related to the formation of a carbene intermediate.

Thus, it appears that aerobically covalent binding and hepatotoxicity may be accounted for by the trichloromethyl free radical or the trichloromethyl peroxy free radical whereas carbenes may play a more important role when oxygen tension is low (Uehleke, 1977; Slater, 1982; Sipes and Gandolfi, 1982).

Other Haloalkanes and Haloalkenes

Many of the haloalkanes and haloalkenes are used as solvents and appear to have related mechanisms of toxic actions. Carbon tetrachloride is the prototype for these compounds, and its ability to cause both fatty infiltration and hepatic necrosis serves as the model for comparison. It should be stressed that although carbon tetrachloride, chloroform, and 1,1,2-trichloroethane also produce renal toxicity, there is no indication that this is a common property of other haloalkanes or haloalkenes (Plaa and Larson, 1965). Zimmerman (1978) has collected the data on the hepatotoxicity of the haloalkanes and haloalkenes and has classified them according to the severity of the hepatic effects. Thus, methyl-chloride, -bromide and -iodide, dichlordifluoromethane, trans-1,2-dichlorethylene, ethyl-chloride, -bromide, and -iodide, and *n*-butylchloride produce no liver damage and only slight fatty accumulation. Chlorobromomethane, dichloromethane, *cis*-1,2-dichloroethylene, tetrachloroethylene, and 2-chloro-*n*-butane produce fatty liver without necrosis. The following are characterized by the production of both fatty liver and necrosis:

(1) Rechnagel and Glende (1973)
$$CCl_4 \longrightarrow CCl_3 \cdot + Cl \cdot$$

(2) Slater (1982)
$$CCl_3 \cdot + O_2 \longrightarrow Cl_3COO \cdot$$

(3) Reiner and Uehleke (1971)
Mansby *et al.* (1974)
$$CCl_4 \longrightarrow Cl_3C:$$
(carbene)

Figure 20–3. Proposed reactive metabolites of CCl₄.

Carbon tetrachloride	1,1,2,2-tetrachloroethane
Carbon tetraiodide	1,2-dichloroethane
Carbon tetrabromide	1,2-dibromoethane
Bromotrichloromethane	1,1,1-trichloroethane
Chloroform	1,1,2-trichloroethylene
Iodoform	2-chloro-*n*-propane
Bromoform	1,2-dichloro-*n*-propane

The hepatotoxicity activity of these agents has been associated with the ease with which a halogen can be removed to produce a reactive metabolite. The factors associated with increasing toxicity are increasing numbers of halogens in the molecule, increasing size, i.e., atomic number or weight of the halogens, and increasing ease of homolytic cleavage. By the same token, there is an inverse relationship to the electronegativity of the halogens and the chain length.

The non-CNS-related toxic effects of the halocarbons are thought to require metabolic activation by the mixed-function oxidase, and the breakage of the C—H bond is usually the rate-limiting step. Biotransformation of the dihalomethanes leads to dehalogenation and the end product is carbon monoxide. In the case of dichloromethane the CO appears to arise from a formyl halide intermediate resulting from the loss of one halide. This intermediate, as an alternative to losing CO, can covalently bind to cellular protein or lipid. The involvement of nonmicrosomal enzymes in dihalomethane biotransformation leads to the production of formaldehyde and halide. A necessary step is the reaction of the dihalomethane with glutathione, which results in the loss of one halide. The resulting halomethylglutathione is postulated to undergo nonenzymatic hydrolytic dehalogenation leaving hydroxymethylglutathione. The next step would result in the release of the hydroxymethyl group as formaldehyde. Alternatively, it has been shown that in the presence of formaldehyde dehydrogenase and NAD, formic acid can be formed.

The biotransformation of the haloforms (trihalomethanes) also involves the mixed-function oxidase and initial step is the loss of a halide. Subsequent biotransformation may lead to CO production. Covalent binding to macromolecules resulting from the biotransformation of haloforms has been postulated to occur via the formation of phosgene, in the case of chloroform, and its analog dibromocarbonyl, in the case of bromoform.

The biotransformation and the production of reactive intermediates from the haloethylenes appear to proceed by a different mechanism. The first step in the biotransformation of vinyl chloride, trichloroethylene, perchloroethylene, vinyl bromide, vinyl fluoride, vinylidene chloride, and vinylidene fluoride has been proposed to involve microsomal oxidation leading to epoxide formation across the double bond (Figure 20–4) (Henschler and Hoos, 1982). These authors have suggested that the resulting oxiranes are highly reactive and therefore can covalently bind to nucleic acids with the eventual end result of mutations and cancer.

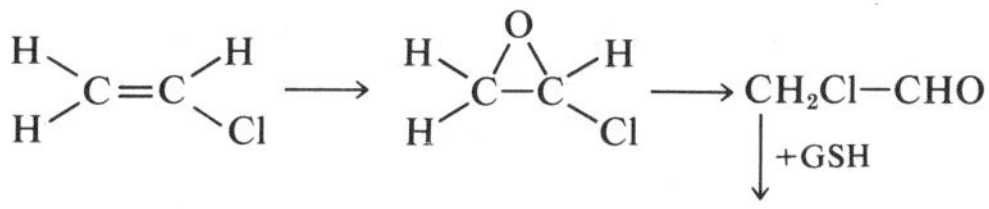

Figure 20–4. Biotransformation of vinyl chloride as an example of metabolism of haloalkenes.

Bolt *et al.* (1982) examined the covalent binding of ^{14}C to protein, both *in vivo* and *in vitro*, covalent binding to nucleic acids, mutagenicity in bacterial test systems, and carcinogenicity for these compounds. Although not all of these data points were available for each compound, some important comparisons resulted. Vinyl chloride and vinyl bromide exhibited positive responses in each category studied whereas trichloroethylene, which displayed some degree of positive response in each of the other categories, was not carcinogenic. Vinylidene chloride, which covalently bound to protein and nucleic acids and was mutagenic, was an equivocal carcinogen. They postulated that based on carcinogenic potency, the relative carcinogenicity of compounds that produced significant preneoplastic loci in livers of treated rats in this series was vinyl chloride > vinyl fluoride > vinyl bromide. Furthermore, a comparison of the monohaloethylenes and the 1,1-dihaloethylenes indicated that monohalo compounds were more carcinogenic.

The chemical reactivity of chlorinated ethylene epoxides was studied by Politzer *et al.* (1981), who compared the ease with which the two C—O bonds could be broken as a function of halogenated substituents on the carbons using ethylene oxide as the standard of reference. They showed that in a comparison of ethylene oxide, vinyl chloride (CH_2=CHCl), and vinylidene chloride (CH_2=CCl_2), with increasing chlorination of one carbon there is an increase in the bond strength of the chlorinated carbon to the oxygen and a decrease in the bond strength to the other, i.e., nonchlorinated carbon. When both carbons are substituted with single chloride, the C—O bonds are equal. When there are two chlorines on one carbon and one on the other, there is again weakening of the less chlorinated carbon to oxygen bond. These authors suggest that the unsymmetric chloroethylenes are more carcinogenic than the symmetric because the ease of bond breakage potentiates covalent binding to DNA.

While reactivity appears to be a fundamental principle of covalent binding, i.e., the toxic or carcinogenic metabolite must indeed be a highly reactive compound, Bolt *et al.* (1982) suggest that there are limits to the effectiveness of highly reactive species. For example, they suggest that a major reason for the weak activity of vinylidene chloride as a carcinogen may be related to the instability of its putative metabolite, 1,1-dichlorooxirane. It is likely to be largely degraded before it reaches its site of action. Thus, these authors suggest that there is an optimum degree of stability that allows the intermediate to be formed by the mixed-function oxidase, reach the DNA, and form the covalent bond. If the reactivity is too low, covalent binding may be poor. If the reactivity is too high, it may never reach the target.

Simple aliphatic halocarbons will continue to be an important area of research for some time to come. Some are found in drinking water as a result of chlorination procedures or because they enter ground water from leachates at chemical dump sites. Although some have been shown to be carcinogenic in long-term bioassays, it will be essential for us to accurately assess the risk of human exposure to these chemicals at the levels in which they are found in the environment.

ALIPHATIC ALCOHOLS

Ethyl Alcohol (Ethanol, Alcohol)

There is probably greater exposure to ethanol than to any other solvent with the exception of water. Not only is it used as a solvent in industry, but it is heavily consumed by large numbers of people as a component of potentially intoxicating beverages. As a result of the petroleum shortage, plans call for diluting gasoline with ethanol to form a combustible product termed "gasohol." At that point it is likely that we will experience universal exposure to ethanol. Nevertheless, historically, occupational exposure has been less important as a cause of injury than the fact that the worker may imbibe alcohol and thereby be rendered less likely to use safety precautions on the job. By the same token, the most important cause of death in auto accidents is drunken driving. Thus, most instances of death or injury related to ethanol come via abuse of ethanol as a beverage rather than to occupational exposure.

Blood Levels. Our information on the toxicity of ethanol comes from either clinical observations of human drinkers or controlled studies in animals and humans where ethanol has been administered either orally or parenterally. Although a TLV for ethanol at a level of 1000 ppm has been established (ACGIH, 1983–84), of greater concern has been the dose level likely to cause inebriation. As a practical matter the legal definition of intoxication has been set on the basis of the blood alcohol level detected in alleged drunken drivers. Thus, in many states the demonstration that the driver has a blood alcohol level of 100 mg/100 ml of blood (100 mg percent or 0.1 percent) is *prima facie* evidence of "driving under the influence of alcohol." In a 70-kg human it would require approximately 3 oz of pure alcohol to achieve a blood alcohol level in the range of 90 to 150 mg percent. In terms of intake of alcoholic beverages it would probably require that the individual would have to drink about 6 oz of 100-proof whiskey, 12 oz of fortified wine, i.e., sherry, or 8×12-oz bottles of beer to achieve that concentration, and people are inebriated under these conditions.

The blood level and the time necessary for it to be achieved are controlled largely by the quantity of food in the GI tract. Once absorbed the alcohol equilibrates with body water, and when drinking is complete, the blood alcohol level begins to drop to some extent because of excretion of alcohol in the breath and urine, but more important, because it is biotransformed in the liver. Ethanol is biotransformed at a rate sufficient to reduce the blood alcohol level linearly by approximately 15 to 20 mg percent per hour. Thus, if a blood alcohol concentration of 120 mg percent were detected, it could be assumed that it would require approximately six to eight hours for ethanol to reach negligible levels in the blood.

CNS Effects. The pharmacologic and toxicologic effects of alcohol relate to the fact that alcohol acts as both a general anesthetic and a nutrient. As a general anesthetic, ethanol causes a dose-dependent central nervous system depression. Although many people appear to be animated under the influence, it is likely that this is a manifestation of the release of inhibitions and is a mild form of the stage II excitement and delirium observed during anesthesia with diethyl ether.

The overt display of inebriation occurs at different blood alcohol levels depending on the extent to which the subject has had previous experience with alcohol. In heavy drinkers tolerance to the low-level effects of ethanol can be observed, and even social drinkers may not show obvious signs of intoxication at blood alcohol levels that would render novice drinkers clearly "under the influence." There are two reasons for these effects. In heavy drinkers they may actually demonstrate a greater rate of ethanol biotransformation. More important may be the fact that experienced drinkers have learned not to display their inebriation at the lower blood levels at which inexperienced drinkers clearly respond.

The literature on the biologic and medical effects of alcohol is the largest single literature in medical science. Ethanol is distributed with body water, and its adverse effects to most organs have been reported. For the purposes of this discussion some specific areas of the pharmacology and toxicology of ethanol will be discussed. These will include the effects of ethanol on the CNS, the fetal alcohol syndrome, the biotransformation of ethanol, and the effects of ethanol on the liver. For additional detailed reports on current trends in alcohol research the student is referred to compendia edited by Avogadro et al. (1979), Sherlock (1982), and Thurman and Hoffman (1983). Among the areas covered are interaction of ethanol with the endocrine system, interactions with xenobiotics, effects on renal, cardiovascular, and gastrointestinal systems, hematopoietic effects, enzymology, dependence and withdrawal, and other effects which indicate that alcoholism is a disease that encompasses the entire body.

The obvious behavioral effects of alcohol are well known. Loss of inhibitions has been eloquently described through several editions of a noted textbook of pharmacology: "Confidence abounds, the personality becomes expansive and vivacious, and speech may become eloquent and occasionally brilliant." Although some reflexes may be enhanced at low ethanol concentrations because of release of higher-center control, they soon deteriorate as the blood level increases. It can be demonstrated that contrary to what outer appearances may be, objective tests of manual dexterity and simple intellectual challenges demonstrate impairment at relatively low alcohol levels.

With increasing blood alcohol levels there is gradual reduction of visual acuity, decreased sense of smell and taste, increased pain threshold, impaired muscular coordination, and possibly nystagmus. As these worsen, a staggering gait becomes apparent. Eventually nausea and vomiting, diplopia, hypothermia, and loss of consciousness ensue. As an anesthetic, ethanol is thought to have a very low therapeutic index, and the subject is not far from death when anesthetic concentrations of ethanol are reached. While the level necessary to achieve loss of consciousness is not clearly defined, it is likely that at a blood alcohol level of 350 to 400 mg percent most people would be asleep.

The mechanism by which ethanol causes these effects is not known. By the same token, the mechanism of general anesthetics is not known. Because the structure of general anesthetics is so varied, theories of anesthesia have developed that consider generalized interactions with the central nervous system rather than effects at specific receptors. A number of physicochemical theories have been proposed to explain the mechanism of action of general anesthetics. For example, the Meyer-Overton theory (1937) suggested that the potency of a general anesthetic was directly related to its solubility in lipid membranes and was otherwise unrelated to its structure. Ferguson (1939) argued that the chemical potential or thermodynamic activity was more closely related to anesthetic activity, whereas Wulf and Featherstone (1957) argued that the critical property was the van der Waals constant. Pauling (1961) and Miller (1961) built their arguments around the effect of ethanol on water and suggested that clathrate formation in cells of the CNS created a structure for water that was conducive to anesthesia. The observation that elevation of ambient pressure caused experimental animals to awaken from anesthesia led Miller et al. (1973) to formulate a hypothesis that suggested that there was a linear relationship linking elevation of atmospheric pressure with decrease in anesthetic potency. It could then be suggested that the gas enters and distorts the membrane taking up a given volume of space. According to the thermodynamic gas laws, the volume of the gas must decrease as the pressure increases, suggesting that the volume of the anesthetic in the membranes of the CNS decreases with increasing pressure leading to reversal of anesthesia.

Singer and Nicolson (1972) have visualized the cell membrane as a two-dimensional solution of proteins and lipids. They visualize a bilayer composed largely of phospholipids in which the polar ends are in contact with water and the lipid ends meet in the membrane. The lipid bilayer is studded with proteins, which are partially embedded in the lipid and partially extend into the aqueous medium. It has been suggested that ethanol interacts with the bilayer to distort and expand the membrane thereby increasing its fluidity (Seeman, 1972; Rubin and Rottenberg, 1983). The result is displacement of critical membrane enzymes and alterations in membrane function. The outward signs of ethanol inebriation and anesthesia would then be a function of the significance of the role of the membranes of various cells in controlling these physiologic functions. It has been suggested that ethanol plays a role in depressing the activities of the reticular activating system in the CNS and thereby releases many functions from integrating control (Kalant, 1961). If that is true, the cell membranes of the reticular activating system may be especially sensitive to ethanol-induced changes in membrane fluidity or their activity is so critical that small alterations in their function lead rapidly to readily observed changes in behavior.

Fetal Alcohol Syndrome. One of the more serious consequences of ethanol consumption is the effect on the development of the embryo and fetus *in utero* (Pratt, 1982). The so-called fetal alcohol syndrome (FAS) is characterized by mental deficiency, microcephaly, and irritability. The infants are generally small and demonstrate poor muscular coordination. These children also exhibit a characteristic facies recognizable to the specialist (see Chapter 7). The severity appears to be related to the extent of alcohol consumption by the mother during pregnancy. In addition to the suggestion that ethanol may interfere with membrane function during development, other factors may be related to the cause of FAS. These include the possibility that acetaldehyde may escape the damaged liver of the alcoholic mother and reach the developing fetal brain, changes in the patterns of amino acids in the maternal circulation available to the fetus, and alcohol-induced hypoglycemia. These effects individually or in concert could cause damage to the developing brain and lead to FAS.

Biotransformation. It is recognized that the toxic effects of alcohol on the liver are directly related to the metabolism of alcohol, and it is therefore important to have a grasp of the pathways of alcohol biotransformation. In a large sense these have been well worked out over a considerable period of time. In recent years there has been considerable discussion over the relative toxicologic significance of the various enzymes capable of mediating the first step in alcohol biotransformation, namely, its oxidation to acetaldehyde. Alcohol dehydrogenase is a soluble enzyme found in high concentrations in liver which appears to play the major role in alcohol biotransformation. NAD is the coenzyme and the products are acetaldehyde and NADH. The reverse of the reaction, i.e., the conversion of acetaldehyde to ethanol, is favored, but during biotransformation the products are rapidly removed thereby preventing reversal of the reaction.

$$CH_3CH_2OH + NAD \xrightarrow{\text{Alcohol Dehydrogenase}} CH_3CHO + NADH$$

A second enzyme capable of converting ethanol to acetaldehyde is catalase, which by virtue of its peroxidative activity uses hydrogen peroxide to perform the oxidation. However, normally there is very little peroxide available to support the reaction in hepatocytes, and it is unlikely that catalase can account for more than 10 percent of ethanol biotransformation. This situation could change if peroxide levels in hepatocytes were elevated. For example, clofibrate, which stimulates peroxisomal fatty acid oxidation, increases peroxide levels and thereby en-

hances ethanol oxidation by catalase. However, it would only be under such unusual circumstances that catalase would be expected to play a significant role in ethanol biotransformation.

$$CH_3CH_2OH + H_2O_2 \xrightarrow{\text{Catalase}} CH_3CHO + H_2O$$

The third enzyme is located in the microsomes and has been termed by Lieber and DiCarli (1970) MEOS, i.e., microsomal ethanol oxidizing system, because it can be demonstrated that the addition of ethanol to isolated microsomes fortified with NADPH and oxygen results in the oxidation of ethanol to acetaldehyde.

$$CH_3CH_2OH + NADPH + O_2 \xrightarrow{\text{MEOS}} CH_3CHO + NADP + H_2O$$

Both the significance of this metabolic pathway in alcohol biotransformation and whether or not this is a unique enzyme system primarily devoted to the oxidation of ethanol have been the subject of considerable debate. Ohnishi and Lieber (1977) have reported the isolation of a cytochrome P-450 from rat liver that mediates this reaction. On the other hand, the uniqueness of the system has been questioned because of the ease with which ethanol can be oxidized by free-radical oxygen such as the hydroxyl free radical generated in microsomes by systems such as the flavoprotein reductase. Winston and Cederbaum (1983) have argued that both radical-mediated and non-radical-mediated microsomal oxidations of ethanol can be identified in rat liver microsomes. Morgan *et al.* (1982) have isolated a cytochrome P-450 from livers of ethanol-treated rabbit which they call LM 3a and which appears to oxidize ethanol at the active site of the enzyme. In contrast to ethanol oxidation by LM2, the phenobarbital-induced cytochrome P-450 appears to biotransform ethanol via generation of oxygen free radicals.

The contribution made by each of these enzymes to ethanol biotransformation has been estimated by various authorities. Damgaard (1982) and Havre *et al.* (1977) have argued that non-alcohol dehydrogenase-mediated biotransformation of ethanol accounts for no more than 10 percent of total ethanol metabolism. Vind and Grunnert (1983), on the other hand, estimate that nonalcohol dehydrogenase biotransformation of ethanol may account for as much as 20 percent and may increase to 30 percent or higher when substrates such as xylitol, which are capable of generating exceedingly high levels of NADH, are added. The argument is that at these high NADH levels electron transfer into the mixed-function oxidase pathway via cytochrome b5 is stimulated and, therefore, MEOS activity is enhanced. However, whether cytochrome b5 can function to stimulate MEOS activity in this manner has yet to be demonstrated. Nevertheless, regardless of which estimate more accurately reflects the percentage of non-alcohol dehydrogenase-mediated ethanol biotransformation, it appears that the major enzyme involved in ethanol oxidation is alcohol dehydrogenase. It is unlikely that catalase plays a significant role in ethanol biotransformation at concentrations of peroxide normally present in liver. The quantitative significance of the role of mixed-function oxidases in ethanol biotransformation has yet to be established.

The further metabolism of ethanol relates to the disposition of acetaldehyde. In the past the fate of acetaldehyde has been linked to several enzymes, located in various parts of the cell. In recent years, however, it has been postulated that acetaldehyde dehydrogenase, an NAD-requiring enzyme, plays the major role in its degradation, and this enzyme, although largely in mitochrondria in rat liver, is a cytosolic enzyme in humans.

$$CH_3CHO + NAD \xrightarrow{\text{Acetaldehyde Dehydrogenase}}$$
$$CH_3COO^- + NADH$$

The resulting acetate is released from the liver and oxidized peripherally probably because during ethanol oxidation there is an increase in the NADH/NAD ratio, which leads to decreased availability of oxaloacetate, decreased pyruvic dehydrogenase activity, and inhibition of citrate synthestase, which taken together inhibit the oxidation of acetate in the liver.

Liver Injury. The drinking of alcohol remains a leading cause of death due to liver cirrhosis. The diagnosis of early alcohol-induced liver disease involves recognition that the patient drinks alcohol to excess, that the patient may be experiencing social problems indicative of alcoholism, and that these are coupled with the finding of hepatomegaly, elevated serum transaminase, and possibly other clinical signs. At more advanced stages, patients may exhibit acute alcoholic hepatitis following heavy bouts of drinking. Signs include vomiting, diarrhea, jaundice, and psychiatric disturbances. The liver is enlarged and painful to palpation, whereas the spleen may be impalpable. The enlarged liver is due to fat accumulation as well as swelling of liver cells and accumulation of other components, such as proteins, which would otherwise be secreted. A wide variety of changes in serum enzymes and proteins can be determined that reflect impairment of hepatic function. Eventually, with continued heavy drinking frank hepatic cirrhosis, not unlike end-stage liver disease derived from other causes, will be observed and may be fatal.

The mechanism by which ethanol mediates liver damage has also generated much discussion. The underlying issue is whether alcoholic liver disease is the result of a direct toxic effect of ethanol on the liver or is the result of nutritional deficiencies that accompany excessive alcohol consumption. Alcohol provides 7.1 kcal/g. A pint of 100-proof whiskey would provide 1400 kcal, which is a significant portion of total caloric intake for most people. If alcoholics would maintain their normal diet plus large quantities of alcohol, they would gain weight at a rapid pace. Since obesity is not a usual corollary of alcoholism, it appears that alcohol replaces other sources of calories in the alcoholics' diet. Because alcohol contains no essential nutrients such as proteins, vitamins, or minerals and it replaces food that would contain these dietary components, it would be expected that alcoholics would develop nutritional deficiencies.

Clinical experience with alcoholics (Morgan, 1982) suggests that the stage of alcoholism in which the individual is viewed is critical to making nutritional judgments. Early clinical studies of patients with advanced alcohol-induced liver disease, especially involving patients from poor socioeconomic backgrounds, have reported that the patients exhibited weight loss and nutritional deficiencies. However, studies of alcoholics who did not display overt liver disease revealed normal nutrition. In another study where a segment of the alcoholic study group displayed liver disease and a segment were clinically malnourished, there did not appear to be a relationship between nutritional status and the severity of the disease. Morgan (1982) suggests that although the intake of nutrients in the diet in a controlled experiment may be similar between control and alcoholic groups, the greater percent of calories derived from alcohol led to significantly different nutritional status. Several factors that together can be considered as contributing to malabsorption may contribute to the development of malnourishment despite adequate intake of essential nutrients, and although they have been studied to some extent, further evaluation is needed of the effects of alcohol on gastric emptying time, physiology and morphology of the small intestine, secretion by the pancreas and biliary system, and splanchnic blood and lymph flow.

An alternative view offered by Lieber (1979) is that alcohol has a direct toxic effect on the liver that is not dependent on nutritional deficiency. The data come from studies in which humans given nutritional supplements while consuming excessive quantities of alcohol developed fatty livers. Furthermore, in a long-term study of 15 baboons fed alcohol and given nutritional supplements, all developed fatty liver, five developed hepatitis, and five cirrhosis (Lieber et al., 1975). It is significant, however, that in a similar study in rhesus monkeys, Rogers et al. (1981) were unable to demonstrate alcohol-induced liver disease.

Several questions remain to be answered before a conclusion can be reached on this issue. The central feature of the disease appears to be that the liver is unable to secrete lipid in the alcoholic, regardless of whether it is synthesized in the liver from ethanol or is taken in via the diet. Hence liver lipid accumulates and alcoholic liver disease ensues. The essence of the argument is that in humans and baboons these events proceeded despite nutritionally adequate diets. The definition of the nutritionally adequate diet is stated in terms of a diet sufficient to prevent liver disease in a nondrinking individual. The diets were then supplemented to ensure adequacy. Nevertheless, there is no yardstick for the nutritional requirements of the alcoholic. An increase in lipotrope content severalfold would represent excessive protection for the nondrinker but may not be adequate protection for the drinker. For example, Klatskin et al. (1954) reported on the increased choline requirement of the alcohol-fed rat, and Thompson and Reitz (1976) suggested that ethanol consumption led to an increase in choline oxidation in rats. It is not yet clear how these studies relate to the observations made in humans, the baboon, or the rhesus monkey in the studies cited above.

The conclusions that can be drawn at this time are that given the severe derangement of hepatic metabolism produced by chronic alcohol feeding, the effects of ethanol on the GI tract, and the frequency of malnourishment among alcoholics, it is likely that nutritional factors play a major role in the development of alcoholic liver disease. However, the challenging suggestion that there may be a direct effect of ethanol on the liver provides a stimulus for further research to segregate out the proposed direct effect from the nutritional effects. The development of a readily available animal model in which the disease can be accurately reproduced would help to settle the question because it would permit determination of the nutritional requirements of the alcoholic.

The toxicologic interaction of ethanol with other hepatotoxic agents is a well-recognized phenomenon (Zimmerman, 1978; Strubelt, 1980). The earliest indication of interaction between ethanol and CCl_4 came from clinical observations of hepatic injury associated with the use of CCl_4 as a vermifuge in the treatment of hookworm in humans who drank alcoholic beverages. The observation that ethanol potentiates CCl_4 toxicity has also been made in several species of laboratory animals (Zimmerman, 1978; Strubelt, 1980).

Pretreatment with ethanol also increases the hepatotoxicity of chloroform, trichloroethane, trichloroethylene, thioacetamide, dimethylnitrosamine, acetaminophen, and aflatoxin B_1. Ethanol was less effective against allyl alcohol and galactosamine and did not alter the effects of bromobenzene, phalloidin, or praseodymium. The toxic effects of α-amantidine were reduced by ethanol.

Methanol, 2-propanol, 2-butanol, and 2-methyl-propanol mimicked the effects of ethanol in increasing the hepatotoxicity of halogenated hydrocarbons and were more active. Whereas the ketone metabolites of the secondary alcohols, i.e., acetone and 2-butanone, increase the hepatotoxicity of CCl_4 and other halocarbons, acetaldehyde is lacking in this property and inhibition of ethanol biotransformation by pyrazole does not protect against the potentiating effect.

Although the mechanism of ethanol-enhanced hepatotoxicity is not fully understood, it may be a direct effect of ethanol rather than of a metabolite because of the lack of activity by acetaldehyde. Several possible mechanisms have been proposed to explain the effects of ethanol. These include attempts to demonstrate that ethanol acts by enhancing CCl_4 absorption, by inducing mixed-function oxidase, by depleting hepatic glutathione, by increasing lipid peroxidation, or by producing hypoxia. None has been successful and work in this field continues.

Methanol

Methanol, or wood alcohol, is another potential neurotoxin that finds extensive use in industry as a solvent. The proposal to add methanol to gasoline or to design automobiles that use neat methanol as a fuel will necessarily widen consumer exposure to the material.

Blindness. The target of methanol toxicity is the retina, a fact that has been documented in many case reports of unfortunate individuals who ingested large amounts of the solvent. At high doses, methanol can cause reversible or permanent blindness, and in severe cases, death. Intoxication is characterized by initial mild inebriation followed by an asymptomatic period of 12 to 24 hours. At this time, a marked metabolic acidosis develops, which, if not treated, can be fatal. Visual problems include eye pain, blurred vision, constriction of visual fields, and other visual complaints. Permanent blindness can develop after as little time as 48 hours. The pathology of the visual lesion has been described in some detail. A marked optic disc edema and dilated pupils with greatly reduced reaction to light are observed. Intraaxonal swelling in the areas of the optic disc and anterior optic nerve are observed with light microscopy (Benton and Calhoun, 1952).

This syndrome has not been described in most common laboratory species. Indeed, while metabolic acidosis and ocular toxicity are observed in humans and monkeys, rodents, dogs, and cats display only mild central nervous system depression following dosing with methanol (Tephly, 1977). A description of the species differences in methanol biotransformation has led to a better appreciation of the pathogenesis and treatment of methanol poisoning.

Biotransformation. Methanol is rapidly and well absorbed by inhalation, oral, and topical exposure routes (Dutkiewicz et al., 1980). Following absorption, the alcohol is rapidly distributed to organs according to the distribution of body water (Yant and Schrenk, 1937).

An abbreviated scheme for the biotransformation of methanol is presented below:

$$CH_3OH \longrightarrow HCHO \longrightarrow$$
Methanol   Formaldehyde

$$HCOOH \longrightarrow CO_2$$
Formic acid   Carbon dioxide

There are two pathways available in the mammalian organism for oxidation of methanol: a catalase peroxidative pathway and an alcohol dehydrogenase system. Studies by Mannering, Tephly, and their colleagues (Makar and Tephly, 1977; Mannering and Parks, 1975) have shown that in the rat, guinea pig, and rabbit the major route of methanol oxidation is through a catalase-dependent pathway, whereas in the monkey and in humans, an alcohol dehydrogenase system functions *in vivo*. Biotransformation to formic acid is quite rapid. Indeed, in monkeys or humans poisoned with very large amounts of methanol, formaldehyde is not detected even in very low levels in tissues at autopsy. Formic acid is further oxidized to carbon dioxide by an enzymatic pathway dependent on the presence of the cofactor, folic acid. The enzyme is active in both rodents and primates (Tephly et al., 1979).

The monkey appears to be an appropriate animal model for studying methanol poisoning since the resulting syndrome closely resembles that seen in humans. Using the primate as a model, Tephly and co-workers have elucidated in detail the relationship between methanol biotransformation and toxicity (McMartin et al., 1977, 1979, 1980). In rodents, a species that is not susceptible to methanol-induced ocular toxicity, methanol is rapidly biotransformed to CO_2. In contrast, in primates and humans, alcohol dehydrogenase- and folate-dependent pathways slowly biotransform methanol to CO_2. The kinetics of biotransformation and elimination of large doses of methanol in primates are such that formic acid accumulates in tissues including the eye (McMartin et al., 1977; Tephly et al., 1979; Noker and Tephly, 1980). A metabolic acidosis and the characteristic ocular toxicity of methanol exposure result. The ocular toxicity appears to be due to the presence of elevated levels of formic acid in blood (Tephly et al., 1979; Noker and Tephly, 1980).

Chronic Exposure. Much less information is available on the health effects of long-term exposure to low levels of methanol. The ACGIH presently recommends a TLV of (TWA— 200 ppm, STEL—250 ppm) for methanol vapors based on the irritancy of the solvent. Greenburg et al. (1938) reported on 19 workers exposed to a solvent consisting of three parts acetone and one part methanol in which the concentrations were 40 to 45 ppm of acetone and 22 to 25 ppm of methanol. Workers were evaluated by physical examination, neurologic tests, urinalysis, and hematology. No abnormal results were found. It is difficult to say with certainty that this exposure to methanol represents a no-observed-effect level since there was also concomitant exposure to acetone.

Office workers exposed to methanol in the vicinity of duplicating machines were studied by Kingsley and Hirsch (1954). The workers complained of frequent and recurrent headaches but no other symptoms. Methanol exposure levels were reported to range from 15 to 375 ppm, although most measurements fell in the 200 to 375-ppm range. Duplicating fluids were changed in favor of less methanol, but the authors fail to mention if there were any beneficial effects on worker headaches. It is unclear from this study if headaches were attributable to methanol or to other components of duplicating fluids.

Animal studies involving repeated long-term exposure to methanol are sparse. Indeed, it is debatable whether or not rodent studies would be meaningful because of the species differences in biotransformation described above. Primate studies could provide useful information, but are extremely expensive and time consuming. An intriguing alternative to primates may be the folate-deficient acatalasemic mouse (C_s^b-FAD). Smith and Taylor (1982) recently reported that this mouse attains high plasma formate levels and acidemia after dosing with methanol. Further work with the $C_s{}^b$-FAD mouse may lead to the development of an inexpensive small-animal model suitable for investigating effects of chronic exposure to methanol.

In the absence of well-designed epidemiologic studies and long-term animal studies, one may use pharmacokinetic principles to consider whether or not chronic exposure to low levels of methanol is likely to result in ocular toxicity. In poisoning cases in which humans consumed several ounces of methanol, blood concentrations in the hundreds of mg/100 ml of blood were noted (Gonda *et al.*, 1978). A review of these papers that have extensively considered methanol concentration in blood and the clinical outcome of poisonings indicates that an initial blood level in excess of 100 mg/100 ml would be required for irreversible effects, such as visual disturbances. In addition, a typical half-life for methanol in the blood following such massive doses was estimated to be in the range of 30 hours. While the half-life of blood methanol is quite long in poisoning cases, studies in human volunteers who ingested small amounts (1 to 5 ml) of methanol revealed that under these conditions the blood half-life is only about 3 hours (Dutkiewicz, 1980; Sedivec *et al.*, 1981). Under these conditions peak blood levels were in the range of 10 mg/100 ml.

If one considers the present ACGIH TLV of 200 ppm (261 mg/m^3) and assumes that there is 100 percent absorption of vapors and a respiratory volume of 10 m^3 in an eight-hour workday, then a total body burden may be calculated.

Body burden
= 261 mg/m^3 × 10 m^3 × 1.0 = 2610 mg

If one further assumes that this total body burden is absorbed within the first few minutes of the workshift and that the methanol distributes with total body water, a worst-case peak blood methanol level may be calculated.

Peak blood level = 2610 mg/49* liter
= 53 mg/liter = 5.3 mg/100 ml

This peak blood level is about ¹⁄₂₀ of a level that would be associated with acute irreversible toxic effects. Since the half-life of blood methanol in this blood concentration range is three hours, blood methanol concentrations would be at negligible levels by the time the next workshift began 24 hours later. Thus, it seems un-

likely that vapor exposure to methanol under ACGIH recommended exposures has any possibility of causing ocular toxicity. The possibility of achieving a high enough body burden under dermal exposure conditions seems even more remote.

GLYCOLS

In addition to their general use as heat exchangers, antifreeze formulations, hydraulic fluids, and chemical intermediates, glycols also have some use as industrial solvents for nitrocellulose and cellulose acetate and as a solvent for pharmaceuticals, food additives, cosmetics, inks, and lacquers. Due to their low volatility, the glycols in general produce little vapor hazard at ordinary temperatures. However, since they are used in antifreeze mixtures, as hydraulic fluids, and as heat exchangers they may be encountered in the vapor or mist form, particularly where the temperature is markedly elevated.

Ethylene Glycol (1,2-Ethanediol, $HOCH_2CH_2OH$)

When taken orally, ethylene glycol appears to be considerably more toxic to humans than to other animal species. The lethal oral dose in humans is approximately 1.4 ml/kg, which would be equivalent to approximately 100 ml for a 70-kg person. The acute oral LD50s reported for rats, guinea pigs, and mice ranged from approximately 5.5 to 13 ml/kg, indicating that on a weight basis, ethylene glycol appears to be less toxic in these animal species than in humans.

The species differences in toxicity noted above are consistent with a report of Gessner and coworkers (1961) where the minimum lethal dose is only 1 g/kg of body weight in cats, who excrete relatively large quantities of oxalates, compared with 7 g/kg in the dog (Kersting and Nielsen, 1966) and 9 g/kg in the rabbit (Gessner *et al.*, 1961).

Morris and associates (1942) studied the long-term ingestion of ethylene glycol in rats. Animals were maintained for two years on diets containing 1 and 2 percent ethylene glycol. The findings included shortened lifespan, calcium oxalate bladder stones, centrilobular liver degeneration, and severe injury to the renal tubules. The chronic toxicity of ethylene glycol has also been reported for the rat (Blood, 1965) and for the monkey (Blood *et al.*, 1962). In the rhesus monkey, no toxic effects were noted over a three-year period when ethylene glycol was given at levels ranging from 0.2 to 0.5 percent in the diet. Further studies on ethylene glycol toxicity in the monkey were reported by Roberts and Seibold (1969). The compound was adminis-

---

*Assumes a 70-kg person with 70 percent water content.

tered in drinking water at concentrations ranging from 0.25 to 10 percent. The renal histopathology, after 6 to 13 days, varied depending on the amount of ethylene glycol consumed. At high dose levels, deposition of calcium oxalate crystals occurred in the proximal renal tubules, and necrotic areas of tubular epithelium occurred adjacent to the crystals. In this study, it appeared that oxalate crystallization did not occur following doses less than 15 ml/kg. However, functional renal changes were present at dose levels above 1 ml/kg, suggesting that renal damage can occur in the absence of oxalate crystal formation. Gershoff and Andrus (1962) also found morphologic tubular changes in the rat given ethylene glycol when crystal formation was prevented by simultaneous ingestion of vitamin B_6

The only well-established metabolite of ethylene glycol in humans and other animals is oxalic acid, which usually accounts for less than 2 percent of the dose. Glycolic acid has also been reported to be a metabolite in rabbits, and unchanged ethylene glycol is excreted by dogs and humans.

The paper by Gessner and associates (1960) reported that in the rabbit, after a dose of 0.1 g/kg, about 40 percent of the glycol was eliminated as CO_2 in the expired air within 24 hours and as much as 60 percent excreted as CO_2 over a three-day period. The major compounds excreted in urine were unchanged ethylene glycol, with oxalic acid as a minor metabolite. In liver slice studies, glycolaldehyde and glyoxylic acid were detected as intermediates in the biotransformation of ethylene glycol.

Clay and Murphy (1977) have reported on the severe metabolic acidosis produced by ethylene glycol in the dog and pigtail monkey. This is consistent with clinical reports of human poisoning. The fact that inhibition of alcohol dehydrogenase by alcohol (Wacker *et al.,* 1965) or pyrazole (Mundy *et al.,* 1974) prevents the development of metabolic acidosis demonstrates the role of metabolites or the metabolic process in the acidosis. These studies demonstrate that the accumulation of the metabolite glycolic acid after ethylene glycol administration is sufficient to account for the metabolic acidosis that develops. The contribution of other possible metabolites was considered negligible.

Bove (1966) studied the renal pathology in a series of rats given ethylene glycol or its metabolites, including glycolaldehyde, glycolic acid, and glyoxylic acid. In animals given single large doses of ethylene glycol (9 to 12 g/kg), striking oxalate formation was present in renal tubules. Crystals appeared throughout the proximal and distal convoluted tubules and were less numerous in the collecting tubules. In only one rat, oxalate crystals were present in the brain, as has also been reported (Pons and Custer, 1946) in human poisoning. Oxalate crystals were also present in renal tubules of animals receiving glycoaldehyde, glycolic acid, and glyoxylic acid, although the renal oxalosis was less extensive with glycoaldehyde. The three proposed intermediates were all more toxic on an acute basis than was ethylene glycol since a number of animals died within eight hours of receiving 5 to 6 g/kg of body weight of the metabolites. Renal tubular pathology was not always accompanied by crystal formation, and the author concludes that cytotoxicity rather than simple mechanical obstruction is largely responsible for renal failure.

Studies by von Wartburg and co-workers (1964) demonstrated that human liver alcohol dehydrogenase biotransformed ethylene glycol as well as ethanol, methanol, and other alcohols. Ethanol, which is a much better substrate for alcohol dehydrogenase than is ethylene glycol, is thus a potent competitive inhibitor of ethylene glycol metabolism.

Experimental studies in animals have shown that ethanol markedly inhibits the biotransformation of ethylene glycol *in vivo* and protects against the acute toxicity resulting from its metabolism. The oral LD50 in rats was found to be 5.8 ml/kg for ethylene glycol and 10.5 ml/kg when animals received ethanol 15 minutes after the intraperitoneal injection of ethylene glycol.

With this information as background, clinical cases of ethylene glycol poisoning have been treated with ethanol. Wacker and associates (1965) reported two cases of individuals who had ingested 250 to 1000 ml of ethylene glycol antifreeze. Gastric lavage was not undertaken until admission to the hospital, some six to nine hours after the antifreeze was ingested; thus large quantities were presumably absorbed into the general circulation. Both patients were treated with ethanol infusion, which resulted in a prompt disappearance of oxaluria, and adequate urinary output was maintained. These individuals made uneventful recoveries from these rather massive ingestions of ethylene glycol. This treatment is, of course, consistent with the therapy proposed for methanol poisoning and is based on the same mechanism of substrate competition for alcohol dehydrogenase.

Diethylene Glycol ($HOCH_2CH_2OCH_2CH_2OH$)

Diethylene glycol is used in the lacquer industry, in cosmetics, in permanent antifreeze formulations, in lubricants, as a softening agent, and as a plasticizer. It presents little hazard during industrial handling at ordinary temperatures.

Where mists are generated or where operations are carried out at high temperatures, industrial hygiene control methods should be followed to eliminate repeated prolonged inhalation. The major hazard from diethylene glycol occurs following the ingestion of relatively large single doses. Impetus for the study of the toxicity of diethylene glycol was provided by 105 fatalities among 353 people who ingested a solution of sulfanilamide in an aqueous mixture containing 72 percent diethylene glycol (Ruprecht and Nelson, 1937; Smyth, 1952). The symptoms included nausea, dizziness, and pain in the kidney region. This was followed in a few days by oliguria and anuria with death resulting from uremic poisoning.

From the information provided in this episode of human poisoning, it has been estimated that the single oral dose lethal for humans is approximately 1 ml/kg.

A long-term rat-feeding study by Fitzhugh and Nelson (1946) showed that 1-percent diethylene glycol in the diet over a two-year period resulted in slight growth depression, a few calcium oxalate bladder stones, minimal kidney damage, and occasional liver damage. At the 4-percent dietary level, there was increased mortality, a marked depression of growth rate, bladder stones, severe kidney damage, and moderate liver damage. In addition, bladder tumors appeared rather frequently.

The authors concluded that bladder tumors never developed in the experimental rats without the preceding or concurrent presence of a foreign body. They suggest that diethylene glycol is not a primary carcinogen but, when fed in very high concentrations, does result in the formation of calcium oxalate bladder stones and subsequent rare bladder tumors.

Propylene Glycol (1,2-Propanediol, CH₃CHOHCH₂OH)

Propylene Glycol (1,2-Propanediol, CH$_3$CHOHCH$_2$OH)

Propylene glycol is used as a solvent in pharmaceuticals, cosmetics, and food materials, as a plasticizer, in antifreeze formulations, heat exchangers, and hydraulic fluids. Propylene glycol has a low order of toxicity and is used in food products, cosmetics, and pharmaceutical products with no apparent difficulty.

Acute oral LD50 values in rats, rabbits, and dogs are approximately 32, 18, and 9 ml/kg, respectively. Early studies demonstrated that the rat can tolerate 10 percent propylene glycol in drinking water without physiologic impairment. Robertson and coworkers (1947) exposed monkeys and rats to atmospheres saturated with propylene glycol vapor and found no adverse effects in animals after periods of 12 to 18 months.

Ruddick (1971) reported a low order of toxicity in the rat and chick with the major metabolic product being lactate and/or pyruvate. Dean and Stock (1974) found that two daily ip injections of 4 ml/kg body weight for three days resulted in an increased rate of liver microsomal metabolism of aniline and p-nitroanisole, a significant decrease in aminopyrine demethylation, and no change in cytochrome P-450 levels. Since propylene glycol has been suggested as a drug solvent in studies of the microsomal mixed-function oxidase system, these potential effects of the solvent should be recognized.

GLYCOL ETHERS

Glycol ethers (Figure 20–5) highlight another area of concern for solvent toxicity, the reproductive system. Ethylene glycol monomethyl ether (EM) and ethylene glycol monoethyl ether (EE) have recently been shown to have the potential to induce reproductive toxicity. In contrast, available information for the propylene series of glycol ethers does not identify these materials as reproductive toxins. Glycol ethers find extensive use in industry as solvents in the manufacture of lacquers, varnishes, resins, printing inks, textile dyes, anti-icing additives in brake fluids, and as gasoline additives. They find extensive use in consumer products such as latex paints and cleaners. The glycol ethers as a class of materials are not acutely hazardous by the oral route. The rabbit appears to be more sensitive than the rat with regard to acute oral toxicity. Glycol ethers, particularly the ethylene series, are well absorbed from the skin. Indeed, the dermal LD50 to oral LD50 ratio is approximately one. High vapor concentrations of the ethylene series are lethal, but saturation levels or levels approaching saturation of the propylene series are not lethal to rodents.

ETHYLENE GLYCOL ETHERS

$$R-OCH_2CH_2OH$$

$$R=CH_3-EM$$
$$CH_3CH_2-EE$$
$$CH_3CH_2CH_2CH_2-EB$$

METABOLITE

$$R-OCH_2COOH \qquad \text{Alkoxy acetic acid}$$

PROPYLENE GLYCOL ETHERS

$$\overset{\displaystyle CH_3}{\underset{\displaystyle |}{R-O-CH_2CHOH}}$$

$$R=CH_3-PM$$
$$CH_3CH_2-PE$$
$$CH_3CH_2CH_2CH_2-PB$$

METABOLITE

$$\overset{\displaystyle CH_3}{\underset{\displaystyle |}{HO-CH_2CHOH}} \qquad \text{Propylene glycol}$$

Figure 20–5. Glycol ethers and their metabolites.

Reproduction

The first report of the reproductive toxicity of ethylene glycol ethers was that of Nagano *et al.* (1979). In this study mice were given large amounts of EM, EE, or their respective acetic acid esters for five weeks. Each of these materials caused testicular atrophy and a decrease in white blood cells.

Studies more germane to the vapor exposure route were recently reported by Miller *et al.* (1983a) and Rao *et al.* (1983). Rabbits and rats were exposed to 0, 30, 100, or 300 ppm EM six hours/day, five days/week for 13 weeks. The male reproductive system was adversely affected in both rats and rabbits exposed to 300 ppm; every male exhibited degeneration of the testicular germinal epithelium. At the end of the exposure period, male rats were mated to unexposed females and found to be infertile. A second mating at 13 weeks postexposure revealed a partial recovery of fertility. Degenerative changes in testes of rabbits but not rats were also noted at 100 ppm, suggesting that for reproductive as well as acute effects, the rabbit is the more sensitive of the two species. A no-observed-effect level for the study was 30 ppm, which is quite close to the present recommended TLV for EM, which is 25 ppm as an eight-hour time-weighted average.

Teratology

The teratogenic potential of EM vapors has been reported by Nelson *et al.* (1984), who exposed pregnant rats to 0, 50, 100, or 200 ppm EE vapors, seven hours/day, during days 7 to 15 of gestation. Although there were no indications of maternal toxicity, 100 percent and 50 percent of fetuses died in the 200- and 100-ppm exposure groups, respectively. Cardiovascular and skeletal malformations were increased above unexposed control values in both 50-ppm and 100-ppm exposure groups.

The teratogenic potential of EE has also been reported. Andrew *et al.* (1981) exposed rabbits to EE vapors (160 or 617 ppm) seven hours/day during days 1 to 19 of gestation. At 617 ppm there was marked maternal toxicity and 100 percent embryo mortality. At the 160-ppm level, there was slight maternal toxicity, and no embryo mortality, but the incidence of major cardiovascular malformations was increased. In the same study, pregnant rats were exposed to either 200 ppm or 750 ppm EE vapors. The high exposure level caused maternal toxicity and embryo mortality. The 200-ppm exposure level caused an increased incidence of minor malformations. The teratogenicity of EE has also been demonstrated in rats by the dermal exposure route. Hardin *et al.* (1982) applied four times daily either 0.25 or 0.50 ml of EE to the skin of rats during days 7 to 15 of gestation. Maternal toxicity and embryo toxicity were seen. The fetuses that survived had an increased incidence of cardiovascular malformations.

In contrast to the adverse reproductive effects of EM and EE, propylene glycol monomethyl ether (PM) does not appear to be a reproductive toxin. Landry and Yano (1984) reported that exposure of rats and rabbits to 0, 300, 1000, or 3000 ppm PM six hours/day, five days/week for 13 weeks did not show any evidence of testicular effects. Central nervous system depression and increased absolute liver weights were noted at 3000 ppm. A no-observed-effect level was 1000 ppm. Nor does PM appear to have teratogenic potential in rats or rabbits. Exposure levels were 0, 500, 1500, or 3000 ppm PM six hours/day during days 6 to 15, 18, or gestation. The only effects noted in the study were transient decreases in body weight gain and central nervous system depression in rats exposed to 3000 ppm. There was no evidence of major malformations in rats or rabbits at any dose level. The 3000-ppm dose caused slight fetotoxicity in the rat as evidenced by delayed skeletal ossification. There was no evidence of fetotoxicity in rabbits at any dose. The no-observed-effect level for both rats and rabbits was 1500 ppm.

Biotransformation

These differences in reproductive toxicity between EM and PM may be explained by the biotransformation of the two materials. Miller *et al.* (1983b) administered a single oral dose of EM or PM, radiolabeled in the glycol carbons, to rats. The radioactivity appearing in the urine and expired air over the following 48 hours was quantitated and identified. Most of the administered PM is biotransformed to propylene glycol presumably by cytochrome P-450-dependent *O*-demethylation. Propylene glycol is further biotransformed to $^{14}CO_2$. In contrast, most of the administered dose of EM is biotransformed to methoxyacetic acid, presumably by liver alcohol dehydrogenase. Methoxyacetic acid is excreted in the urine.

Methyoxyacetic acid, the EM metabolite, has recently been shown to produce the same toxic effects of EM in tests on male rats (Miller *et al.*, 1982). Thus, it appears likely that methoxyacetic acid is responsible for the toxicity of EM. Furthermore, EE is biotransformed to an analogous metabolite, ethoxyacetic acid (Jonsson *et al.*, 1982). EB is biotransformed to butoxyacetic acid, and ethylene glycol isopropyl ether (EIP) is biotransformed to isopropoxyacetic acid (Jonsson *et al.*, 1982). It appears that the primary alcohol function on glycol ethers is easily oxidized to an alkoxyacid, probably by liver alcohol dehydrogenase. On the other hand, propylene glycol ethers have a secondary alcohol function, which is a much poorer substrate for alcohol dehydrogenase (Von Wartburg, 1964) and is a material that has not been shown to be a reproductive toxin.

Dioxane (1,4-Dioxane)

Dioxane ($C_4H_8O_2$) is a cyclic diether prepared either from reaction between two molecules of ethylene oxide or during the distillation of ethylene glycol in the presence of dilute sulfuric acid.

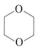

It is widely used in the chemical industry as a solvent and is one of the major commodity chemicals. As a result there is the potential for human exposure. Five cases of fatalities resulting from excessive exposure (Barber, 1934) revealed that the symptoms were irritation of upper respiratory passages, eye irritation, drowsiness, vertigo, headache, anorexia, stomach pains, nausea and vomiting, uremia, coma, and death. Johnstone (1959) has reported damage to kidneys, liver, and brain at autopsy following dioxane poisoning. Test subjects exposed to varying levels indicated that 200 ppm was the highest acceptable level before irritation became significant. Prolonged, repeated exposure of the skin to low levels has resulted in eczema.

In rodents oral LD50 values are relatively high. They range for rabbits, guinea pigs, rats, and mice from 2 to 6 g/kg. Chronic feeding studies using rats (Argus et al., 1965; Kociba et al., 1974; Hoch-Ligeti et al., 1970), guinea pigs (Hoch-Ligeti and Argus, 1970), and both rats and mice (IARC, 1976) demonstrated both toxic and carcinogenic effects of very large doses of dioxane. Principal sites of degeneration and necrosis were in renal, hepatic, and epithelial cells. Guinea pigs demonstrated liver tumors and hyperplasia of lung cells, as well as squamous cell carcinoma in the nasal cavity. In rats and mice, tumors were seen in liver and the nasal cavity. Using the inhalation route in rats, however, Torkelson et al. (1974) were unable to demonstrate carcinogenic effects of dioxane in males and females treated with 111 ppm chronically in an experimental design that encompassed two years.

Braun and Young (1977) identified β-hydroxyethoxyacetic acid (HEAA), a ring-opening product of dioxane, as the major metabolic product in the urine of rats. Young et al. (1976) reported that in humans exposed to dioxane at 1.6 ppm for 7.5 hours both dioxane and HEAA were recovered from the urine. Young et al. (1978) suggested that rats have a limited capacity to biotransform HEAA. Woo et al. (1977) reported the identification of p-dioxane-2-one, a carcinogenic metabolite of dioxane in the urine of dioxane-treated rats. Dioxane induces its own biotransformation, and the detoxication pathway is readily saturated (Young et al., 1978). Although a direct effect of dioxane has not yet been ruled out, further study is required of the metabolic pathways leading to the formation of HEAA and p-dioxane-2-one before we can understand the mechanism of the toxic and carcinogenic effects of dioxane.

ALIPHATIC HYDROCARBONS

The straight-chain hydrocarbons with less than four carbon atoms are gases and are present in natural gas (methane, ethane) and in bottled gas (propane, butane). Methane and ethane are simple asphyxiants and do not produce general systemic effects. The higher-molecular-weight aliphatic hydrocarbons are liquids, and inhalation of the vapor produces central nervous system depression resulting in dizziness and incoordination. Extremely high levels of C_5 to C_8 hydrocarbon vapor (pentane, hexane, heptane, octane) levels produce death in experimental animals.

Hexane

Until recently extensively used industrial hexacarbon solvents such as n-hexane and 2-hexanone (methyl n-butyl ketone) were thought to have little potential for hazard. It is now recognized that peripheral neuropathies can result from excessive exposure.

n-Hexane is produced during the cracking and fractional distillation of crude oil and is used in such applications as printing of laminated products, vegetable oil extraction, as a solvent in glues, paints, varnishes, and inks, as a diluent in the production of plastics and rubber, and as a minor component of gasoline. An estimated 2.5 million workers are occupationally exposed to n-hexane (Gonzalez and Downey, 1972; Paulson and Waylons 1976; Yamamura, 1969). 2-Hexanone has more limited use than n-hexane, but is used as a paint thinner, cleaning agent, solvent for dye printing, and in the lacquer industry. The National Institute for Occupational Safety and Health has estimated that nearly a quarter of a million workers have potential exposure to 2-hexanone (Couri and Milks, 1982).

It is not at all surprising that previous to the

discovery of their neurotoxic potential these two solvents were not regarded as industrial hazards since their acute toxicity is quite low. Vapor concentrations of many hundreds of parts per million are tolerated for several minutes without causing discomfort among workers. In recognition of the neurotoxic properties of *n*-hexane and 2-hexanone the ACGIH has recommended TLVs of 50 ppm and 5 ppm, expressed as eight-hour time-weighted averages, for the two solvents, respectively. STEL and ceiling values are not recommended (ACGIH, 1983–84).

Neurotoxicity. The first cases of *n*-hexane polyneuropathy were reported in 1964 in workers involved in laminating polyethylene products. In 1969 a major outbreak of disease was reported in a cottage industry in Japan that involved the use of an *n*-hexane-containing glue to assemble sandals. *n*-Hexane concentrations to which the workers were exposed were estimated to be 500 to 2500 ppm (Yamada, 1964; Yamamura, 1969; Sobue, 1968).

The neurotoxic syndrome is best described as a sensorimotor or motor polyneuropathy. The initial symptoms are symmetric sensory numbness and paresthesias of distal portions of the extremities. Sensory loss normally involves all modalities of the feet or hands. Motor weakness is typically observed in muscles of the toes and fingers but may also involve muscles of the arms, thighs, and forearms. The onset of these symptoms may be delayed for several months to a year after the beginning of exposure (Yamamura, 1969; Herskowitz *et al.*, 1971; Allen, 1979). The syndrome is characterized pathologically by axonal swelling on the proximal side of the node of Ranvier, demyelination, and nerve fiber degeneration resembling a dying-back neuropathy. Central and autonomic nervous systems are unaffected. The clinical course of disease is for complete recovery, but severe cases may retain distal sensorimotor deficits.

2-Hexanone was reported to cause neurotoxicity by several authors during the time frame of 1973–1977. Workers on rotogravure units in the printing industry, workers who spray painted in enclosed areas, and workers who used 2-hexanone-containing cleaners developed a neurotoxic syndrome strikingly similar to that seen for *n*-hexane (Allen *et al.*, 1975; Billmaier, 1974; McDonough, 1974). As described above, there may be a delay between exposure and the development of bilateral loss of sensorimotor of sensory modalities. Pathologic findings are also quite similar to those of *n*-hexane (Saida, 1976; Davenport, 1976).

Biotransformation. The rational basis for this similarity in neurotoxic action is contained in the biotransformation scheme presented in Figure 20–6. *n*-Hexane is biotransformed to 2-hexanol and further to 2,5-hexanediol by cytochrome P-450 mixed-function oxidases by omega-minus 1 oxidation. 2,5-Hexanediol may be further oxidized to 2,5-hexanedione, the major metabolite of *n*-hexane in humans. Through the omega-minus 1 oxidation process, 2-hexanone may also be biotransformed to 2,5-hexanedione. 2-Hexanol and 5-hydroxy-2-hexanone as well as 2,5-hexanedione are all common elements in the biotransformation of both *n*-hexane and 2-hexanone (Perbellini, 1980; Katz, 1980; DiVincenzo *et al.*, 1978; Krasavage *et al.*, 1980; Couri *et al.*, 1978).

Identification of 2,5-hexanedione as the major neurotoxic metabolite of *n*-hexane and 2-hexanone proceeded rapidly after its discovery as a urinary metabolite. 2,5-Hexanedione has been found to produce a polyneuropathy indistinguishable from *n*-hexane and 2-hexanone in experimental animals under a variety of exposure conditions (Spencer and Schaumburg, 1977; Krasavage *et al.*, 1980; O'Donoghue *et al.*, 1978; Couri and Nachtman, 1979). 2,5-Hexanedione is many times more potent that *n*-hexane or 2-hexanone in causing neurotoxicity in experimental animals (Krasavage *et al.*, 1980).

It appears that the neurotoxicity of 2,5-hexanedione resides in its γ-diketone structure, since 2,3-,2,4-hexanedione and 2,6-heptanedione are not neurotoxic, while 2,5-heptanedione and 3,6-octanedione and other γ diketones are neurotoxic (Spencer *et al.*, 1978; O'Donoghue and Krasavage, 1979a; O'Donoghue and Krasavage, 1979b).

A potentially important solvent interaction between 2-hexanone and 2-butanone (methyl ethyl ketone) has been reported (Abdel-Rahman *et al.*, 1976; Couri *et al.*, 1977). In these experiments rats were exposed to 2-hexanone alone or to a mixture of 2-hexanone and 2-butanone vapors. Animals exposed to the mixture showed an earlier onset and greater severity of neurotoxic signs, and produced dramatically higher concentrations of 2,5-hexanedione, than did animals exposed to 2-hexanone alone.

Gasoline and Kerosene

Gasoline and kerosene are primarily mixtures of hydrocarbons, including not only aliphatic hydrocarbon but, particularly in the case of gasoline, a variety of branched and unsaturated hydrocarbons, as well as aromatic hydrocarbons.

In spite of the widespread use of gasoline and the intermittent vapor exposure encountered by gas station attendants and the home auto mechanic, toxic effects do not normally occur

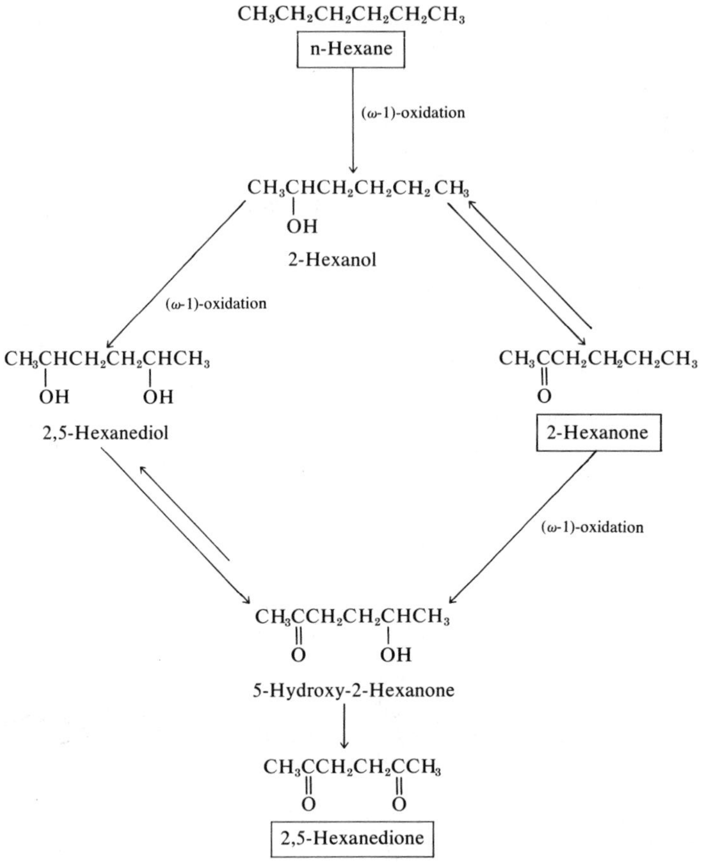

$$CH_3CH_2CH_2CH_2CH_2CH_3$$

| n-Hexane |

(ω-1)-oxidation

$$CH_3CHCH_2CH_2CH_2CH_3$$
$$\quad\ |$$
$$\quad OH$$

2-Hexanol

(ω-1)-oxidation

$$CH_3CHCH_2CH_2CHCH_3$$
$$\quad\ |\qquad\qquad |$$
$$\quad OH\qquad\ OH$$

2,5-Hexanediol

$$CH_3CCH_2CH_2CH_2CH_3$$
$$\quad\ ||$$
$$\quad O$$

| 2-Hexanone |

(ω-1)-oxidation

$$CH_3CCH_2CH_2CHCH_3$$
$$\quad\ ||\qquad\qquad |$$
$$\quad O\qquad\qquad OH$$

5-Hydroxy-2-Hexanone

$$CH_3CCH_2CH_2CCH_3$$
$$\quad\ ||\qquad\qquad ||$$
$$\quad O\qquad\qquad O$$

| 2,5-Hexanedione |

Figure 20–6. Biotransformation of *n*-hexane and 2-hexanone.

under these conditions. Some types of gasoline contain a considerable amount of benzene and could present a hazard that would be difficult to assess in the exposed population.

Extremely high-level exposures to gasoline vapor may result in dizziness, coma, collapse, and death. Exposure to high nonlethal levels is usually followed by complete recovery, although cases of permanent brain damage following massive exposure have been reported. At mospheric concentrations of approximately 2000 ppm are not safe to enter for even a brief time. No threshold limit value (TLV) has been set for gasoline since its composition varies widely. In general, the toxicity is related to the content of benzene and other aromatic hydrocarbons. Other additives could also alter the overall toxicity of gasoline.

CARBON DISULFIDE

Carbon disulfide (CS_2) is primarily used in the production of regenerated rayon and cellophane, and in the manufacture of carbon tetrachloride.

It is also used as a solvent for many applications including resins, rubber, and fats. Other applications include use as a pesticide, as a preservative for fresh fruit, and in the production of semiconductors. In 1978, approximately 200,000 tons of CS_2 were sold for these purposes. The ACGIH recommends a TLV of 10 ppm as an eight-hour time-weighted average for CS_2 (ACGIH, 1983–84).

Adverse effects of human exposure to CS_2 resulting from prolonged exposure to high levels of CS_2 have been extensively reported and documented. These include organic brain damage, peripheral nervous system decrements, neurobehavioral dysfunction, and ocular and auditory effects. In addition, adverse effects on the cardiovascular system are briefly discussed below. Excellent reviews of these effects were recently prepared by Coppack *et al.* (1981) and Beauchamp *et al.* (1983).

Severe CS_2 intoxication, which can lead to severe encephalopathies, was common in the early part of the twentieth century but is seldom encountered today. High-level exposures resulted in a syndrome of toxic psychoses, agitated delirium, seizures, and recurrent mental impairment (Gordy and Trumper, 1940). Most cases of CS_2-induced encephalopathy involve chronic exposure for a number of years to levels that exceed the current TLV. Symptoms typically include headaches, sleep disturbances, general fatigue, emotional lability, irritability, impairment of memory for recent events, and, commonly, loss of libido. A ''parkinsonian'' syndrome consisting of facial immobility, slurring of speech, impaired arm swing, and tremor, which is maximum at rest, was described for young subjects (Audo-Gianotti, 1932). More recent studies have investigated effects of CS_2 exposure on reduced performance in neurobehavioral tests (Horvath and Frantik, 1979).

Alpers and Lewey (1940) reported on the pathogenesis of CS_2 encephalopathy. Postmortem findings were neuronal degeneration with pallor, vacuolization, and cell loss diffusely distributed over the cerebral cortex, globus pallidus, and putamen. They report similar pathologic changes in cats and dogs exposed to 400 ppm CS_2 for two to six weeks.

CS_2 exposure also may cause a peripheral neuropathy, but this lesion, in contrast to central nervous system effects, is typically relatively mild. Knave et al. (1974) have described this syndrome as progressing from muscle cramps in the legs to muscle pain, paresthesias, and finally muscle weakness in the extremities. A prevalent finding was a fine-to-medium coarse tremor. Multifocal axonal swelling with neurofilament accumulation (Wallerian degeneration) has been reported as a pathologic finding in central and peripheral nervous system fibers of rats chronically exposed to CS_2 (Szendzikowski et al., 1974). There is no satisfactory treatment for the central or peripheral neural effects of CS_2, and prevention of excess exposure is necessary.

The mechanism by which CS_2 causes peripheral neuropathy is yet to be determined. Figure 20–7 represents an abbreviated scheme for the metabolism of CS_2 to highlight a prominent, if controversial, theory. Following exposure to CS_2 very little of the parent compound is excreted unchanged. Most of the absorbed dose is excreted as sulfur-containing urinary metabolites of CS_2, some of which are shown in Figure 20–7 (Pergal, 1972a; Pergal, 1972b; van Doorn et al., 1981a; van Doorn et al., 1981b). These reactions demonstrate the ability of CS_2 to react with amino acids in vivo. Dithiocarbamates and thiazolidines are known to chelate metal ions such as copper and zinc (Brieger, 1967), and it is proposed that dithiocarbamate metabolites of CS_2 may chelate metals necessary for proper enzyme function. In support of this theory, it has recently been shown that CS_2 exposure can

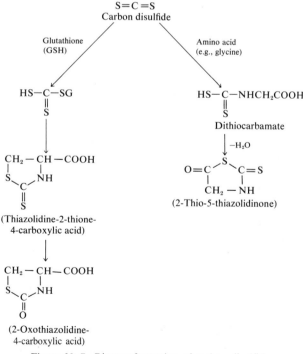

Figure 20–7 Biotransformation of carbon disulfide.

decrease the activity of the copper-requiring enzyme dopamine-β-hydroxylase (McKenna and DiStefano, 1977), that addition of copper and zinc to the diet exerted a protective effect for experimentally induced neurotoxicity in the rat (Lukas, 1979), and that copper levels in peripheral nerves were altered during intoxication of rats with CS_2 (Lukas, 1980). Animal models of CS_2 toxicity need to be further exploited to determine if this theory is indeed viable.

Another neurologic target of CS_2 is the eye. Over the years many changes of eye structure and function including fundal morphology, altered function, sensitivity, and motility have been described. Many of these findings were reported when typical exposures were in excess of 30 ppm (Beauchamp et al., 1983). In the past CS_2 retinopathy has been regarded by occupational physicians as an early indicator of intoxication. Many reports have described changes in the microcirculation of the eye, and some investigators feel that this finding is diagnostic of CS_2 overexposure (Tolonen, 1974). Other investigators have attributed vascular changes in the eye to the atherosclerotic effects of CS_2 described below (Gilioli et al., 1978). It seems clear that long-term exposure to CS_2 can cause eye damage including blind spots, narrowing of visual field, and a decreased ability to see in the dark. This effect has not been studied in experimental animals.

Yet another neurologic target of CS_2 is the auditory system. Hearing loss to high-frequency tones is a common feature of CS_2 intoxication (Zenk, 1970). This problem has not been successfully approached in an experimental animal model.

Exposure to CS_2 has been called a contributing factor in coronary heart disease (Tiller et al., 1968). This effect has been confirmed by Finnish epidemiologists studying an occupationally exposed cohort using a ten-year follow-up plan. While advanced age and hypertension were predominant factors in determining coronary heart disease, exposure to CS_2 alone contributed a statistically significant relative risk (Tolonen et al., 1975; Tolonen et al., 1979). It seems likely that occupational CS_2 exposure can be an important contributing factor to the development of coronary heart disease and that this issue should continue to be monitored in future epidemiology studies.

CONCLUSIONS

Solvents are a group of chemicals that have only two features in common: (1) they are liquid, and (2) because of their widespread use in commerce there is a potential for human exposure both during their use and after they have been discarded as chemical wastes.

It is not possible to predict the toxic effects of these chemicals merely because they share the term "solvent." Their toxic effects vary as widely as those of other chemicals. While there are groups of structurally related solvents, such as the haloalkanes and the haloalkenes, where the toxic effects may be related, among these there are both quantitative and qualitative differences in toxicity. Among single-ring aromatic compounds alkylbenzenes are dramatically different from benzene. Our ability to predict toxicity among solvents and perform accurate risk assessment depends on our knowledge of not only descriptive toxicology gained in acute and chronic treatment studies, but also on our understanding of the biotransformation and mechanism of action of these agents.

The major drawbacks to most studies on the toxicology of solvents is that actual occupational and environmental exposure is not to the pure compounds used in toxicologic research but to commercial mixtures of solvents. The need for the future is to develop strategies for studying the toxicology of mixtures. It is impractical to study interactions of more than three to four compounds at more than one dose level in a well-controlled study using procedures commonly employed in safety evaluation today. Yet in effluents from chemical waste sites there are frequently as many as 100 chemicals identified, some of which may be present at concentrations that pose a potential hazard for humans. Methods for studying these interactive effects have yet to be developed. Until that time risk assessment must depend on knowledge of the toxicity of the most toxic chemicals in the mixture modified with our understanding of interactions between chemicals in the mixture. For the most part, this information is currently insufficient for accurate predictions.

REFERENCES

Abdel-Rahman, M. S.; Hetland, L. B.; and Couri, D.: Toxicity and metabolism of methyl n-butyl ketone. Am. Ind. Hyg. Assoc. J., 37:95–102, 1976.
ACGIH: TLVs: Threshold Limit Values for Chemical Substances and Physical Agents in Work Environment with Intended Changes for 1983–84. American Conference of Governmental Industrial Hygienists, Cincinnati, 1983.
Aksoy, M., and Erdem, S.: Follow-up study on the mortality and the development of leukemia in 44 pancytopenic patients with chronic exposure to benzene. Blood, 52:285–93, 1978.
Allen, N.; Mendell, J. R.; Billmaier, D. J.; Fontaine, R. E.; and O'Neill, J.: Toxic polyneuropathy due to methyl n-butyl ketone. Arch. Neurol., 32:209–18, 1975.
Allen, N.: Solvents and other industrial organic compounds. In Vinken, P. J., and Bruyn, G. W. (eds.):

Handbook of Clinical Neurology: Intoxications of the Nervous System, Vol. 36 (Part 1). Elsevier/North-Holland, New York, 1979, pp. 361–89.

Alpers, B. J., and Lewey, F. H.: Changes in the nervous system following disulfide poisoning in animals and in man. *Arch. Neurol. Psychiatry,* **44**:725–39, 1940.

Andersen, M. E.; Gargas, M. L.; Jones, R. A.; and Jenkins, L. J., Jr.: Determination of the kinetic constants for metabolism of inhaled toxicants *in vivo* using gas uptake measurements. *Toxicol. Appl. Pharmacol.,* **54**:100–16, 1980.

Andrew, F. D.; Buschbom, R. L.; Cannon, W. C.; Miller, R. A.; Montgomery, L. F.; Phelps, D. W.; and Sikev, M. R.: *Teratologic Assessment of Ethylbenzene and 2-Ethoxyethanol.* Battelle Pacific Northwest Laboratories Report to NIOSH, 1981.

Andrews, L. S.; Lee, E. W.; Witmer, C. M.; Kocsis, J. J.; and Snyder, R.: Effects of toluene on metabolism, disposition, and hematopoietic toxicity of (^{3}H) benzene. *Biochem. Pharmacol.,* **26**:293–300, 1977.

Argus, M. F.; Argus, J. C.; and Hoch-Ligeti, C.: Studies on the carcinogenicity of protein-denaturing agents—hepatotoxicity of dioxane. *J. Natl. Cancer Inst.,* **35**:949–58, 1965.

Audo-Gianotti, G. B.: Le parkinsonisme—sulfo-carbone professionnel. *Presse Méd.,* **40**:1289–91, 1932.

Avogadro, P.; Sirtori, C. R.; and Tremoli, E. (eds.): *Metabolic Effects of Ethanol.* Elsevier, Amsterdam, 1979, 430 pp.

Barber, H.: Haemorrhagic nephritis and necrosis of the liver from dioxane poisoning. *Guy's Hosp. Rep.,* **84**:267–80, 1934.

Beauchamp, R. O., Jr.; Bus, J. S.; Popp, J. A.; Boreiko, C. J.; and Goldberg, L.: A critical review of the literature on carbon disulfide toxicity. *CRC Crit. Rev. Toxicol.,* **11**:169–278, 1983.

Benton, C. D., and Calhoun, F. P.: The Ocular effect of methyl alcohol poisoning. *Trans. Am. Acad. Ophthalmol. Laryngol.* **56**:874–85, 1952.

Billmaier, D.; Yee, H. T.; Allen, N.; Craft, B.; Williams, N.; Epstein, S.; and Fontaine, R.: Peripheral neuropathy in a coated fabrics plant. *J. Occup. Med.,* **16**:665–71, 1974.

Blood, F. R.: Chronic toxicity of ethylene glycol in the rat. *Food Cosmet. Toxicol.,* **3**:229–34, 1965.

Blood, F. R.; Elliot, G. A.; and Wright, M. S.: Chronic toxicity of ethylene glycol in the monkey. *Toxicol. Appl. Pharmacol.,* **4**:489–91, 1962.

Bolcsak, L. E., and Nerland, D. E.: Inhibition of erythropoiesis by benzene and benzene metabolites. *Toxicol. Appl. Pharmacol.,* **69**:363–68, 1983.

Bolt, H. M.; Filser, J. G.; and Laib, R. J.: Covalent binding of haloethylenes. In Snyder, R.; Parke, D. V.; Kocsis, J. J.; Jollow, D. J.; Gibson, G. G.; and Witmer, C. M. (eds.): *Biological Reactive Intermediates—II: Chemical Mechanisms and Biological Effects.* Plenum Press, New York, 1982, pp. 667–83.

Bove, K. E.: Ethylene glycol toxicity. *Am. J. Clin. Pathol.,* **45**:46–50, 1966.

Boyd, R.; Griffiths, J.; Kindt, V.; Snyder, R.; Caro, J.; and Erslev, A.: Relative toxicity of five benzene metabolites on CFU-GM cultures. *Toxicologist,* **2**:121, 1982.

Brieger, H.: Carbon disulfide in living organisms—retention, biotransformation and patho-physiologic effects. In Brieger, H. (ed.): *Toxicology of Carbon Disulfide.* Excerpta Medica, Amsterdam, 1967.

Braun, W. H., and Young, J. D.: Identification of hydroxyethoxyacetic acid as the major urinary metabolite of 1,4-dioxane in the rat. *Toxicol. Appl. Pharmacol.,* **39**:33–38, 1977.

Browning, E.: *Toxicity of Industrial Organic Solvents.* Her Majesty's Stationery Office, London, 1953.

———: *Toxicity and Metabolism of Industrial Solvents.* Elsevier Publishing Co., New York, 1965.

Challen, P. J. R.; Hickish, D. E.; and Bedford, J.: Chronic chloroform intoxication. *Br. J. Ind. Med.,* **15**:243–49, 1958.

Clay, K.; Murphy, R.; and Watkins, W. D.: Experimental methanol toxicity in the primate. Analysis of metabolic acidosis. *Toxicol. Appl. Pharmacol.,* **34**:49–61, 1975.

Coppack, R. W.; Buck, W. B.; and Mabee, R. L.: Toxicology of carbon disulfide: a review. *Vet. Hum. Toxicol.,* **23**:331–36, 1981.

Couri, D.; Hetland, L. B.; Abdel-Rahman, M. S.; and Weiss, H.: The influence of inhaled ketone solvent vapors on hepatic microsomal biotransformation activities. *Toxicol. Appl. Pharmacol.,* **41**:285–89, 1977.

Couri, D.; Abdel-Rahman M. S.; and Hetland, L. B.: Biotransformation of *n*-hexane and methyl *n*-butyl ketone in guinea pigs and mice. *Am. Ind. Hyg. Assoc. J.,* **39**:295–300, 1978.

Couri, D., and Nachtman, J. P.: Biochemical and biophysical studies of 2,5-hexanedione neuropathy. *Neurotoxicology,* **1**:269–83, 1979.

Couri, D., and Milks, M.: Toxicity and metabolism of the neurotoxic hexacarbons *n*-hexane, 2-hexanone, and 2,5-hexanedione. *Annu. Rev. Pharmacol. Toxicol.,* **22**:145–66, 1982.

Damgaard, S. E.: The ^{D}(VK) isotope effect of the cytochrome P-450-mediated oxidation of ethanol and its biological applications. *Eur. J. Biochem.,* **125**:593–603, 1982.

Davenport, J. G.; Farrell, D. F.; and Sumi, S. M.: Giant axonal neuropathy caused by industrial chemicals. *Neurology,* **26**:919–23, 1976.

Dean, B. J.: Genetic toxicology of benzene, toluene, xylenes and phenols. *Mutat. Res.,* **47**:75–97, 1978.

Dean, M. E., and Stock, B. H.: Propylene glycol as a drug solvent in the study of hepatic microsomal metabolism in the rat. *Toxicol. Appl. Pharmacol.,* **28**:44–52, 1974.

Dietz, F. K.; Reitz, R. H.; Watanabe, P. G.; and Gehring, P. J.: Translation of pharmacokinetic/biochemical data into risk assessment. In Snyder, R.; Parke, D. V.; Kocsis, J. J.; Jollow, D. J., Gibson, G. G.; and Witmer, C. M. (eds.): *Biological Reactive Intermediates—II: Chemical Mechanisms and Biological Effects.* Plenum Press, New York, 1982, pp. 1399–1424.

DiVincenzo, G. D.; Hamilton, M. L.; Kaplan, C. J.; Krasavage, W. J.; and O'Donoghue, J. L.: Studies on the respiratory uptake and excretion and the skin absorption of methyl *n*-butyl ketone in humans and dogs. *Toxicol. Appl. Pharmacol.,* **44**:593–604, 1978.

Dutkiewicz, B.; Konczalik, J.; and Karwacki, W.: Skin absorption and *per os* administration of methanol. *Int. Arch. Occup. Environ. Health,* **47**:81–88, 1980.

Elofsson, S. A.; Gamberale, F.; Hindmarsch, T.; Iregren, A.; Isaksson, A.; Johnsson, I.; Knave, B.; Zydahl, E.; Mindus, P.; Persson, H. E.; Phillipson, B.; Steby, M.; Struwe, G.; Soderman, E.; Wennberg, A.; and Widen, L.: Exposure to organic solvents. *Scand. J. Work Environ. Health,* **6**:239–73, 1980.

Feldman, R. G.; Ricks, N. L.; and Baker, E. L.: Neuropsychological effects of industrial neurotoxins: a review. *Am. J. Ind. Med.* **1**:211–27, 1980.

Ferguson, J.: The use of chemical potentials as indices of toxicity. *Proc. Roy. Soc.* **127** (Series B):387–404, 1939.

Fitzhugh, O. G., and Nelson, A. A.: Comparison of the chronic toxicity of triethylene glycol with that of diethylene glycol. *J. Ind. Hyg. Toxicol.,* **28**:40–43, 1946.

Gershoff, S. N., and Andrus, S. B.: Effect of vitamin B_6 and magnesium on renal deposition of calcium oxalate by ethylene glycol administration. *Proc. Soc. Exp. Biol. Med.,* **109**:99–102, 1962.

Gessner, P. K.; Parke, D. V.; and Williams, R. T.: Studies in detoxication. *Biochem. J.*, **74**:1–5, 1960.
———: Studies in detoxication. *Biochem. J.*, **79**:482–89, 1961.
Gilioli, R.; Bulgheroni, C.; Bertazzi, P. A.; Cirla, A. M.; Tomasini, M.; Cassitto, M. G.; and Jacovone, M. T.: Study of neurological and neurophysiological impairment of carbon disulfide workers. *Med. Lav.*, **69**:130–43, 1978.
Gill, G. F., and Ahmed, A.: Covalent binding of [^{14}C]benzene to cellular organelles and bone marrow nucleic acids. *Biochem. Pharmacol.*, **30**:1127–31, 1981.
Goldstein, B. D.: Hematotoxicity in man. In Laskin, S., and Goldstein, B. D. (eds.): *A Critical Evaluation of Benzene Toxicity. J. Toxicol. Environ. Health*, (Suppl. 2):69–105, 1977.
Goldstein, B. D.; Witz, G.; Javid, J.; Amoruso, M. A.; Rossman, T.; and Wolder, B.: Muconaldehyde, a potential toxic intermediate of benzene. In Snyder, R.; Parke, D. V.; Kocsis, J. J.; Jollow, D. J.; Gibson, G. G.; and Witmer, C. M. (eds.): *Biological Reactive Intermediates—II: Chemical Mechanisms and Biological Effects*. Plenum Press, New York, 1982, pp. 331–39.
Gonda, A.; Gault, H.; Churchill, D.; and Hollomby, D.: Hemodialysis for methanol intoxication. *Am. J. Med.*, **64**:749–58, 1978.
Gonzalez, E. G., and Downey, J. A.: Polyneuropathy in a glue sniffer. *Arch. Physiol. Med.*, **53**:333–37, 1972.
Gordy, S. T., and Trumper, M.: Carbon disulfide poisoning. *Industr. Med.*, **9**:231–34, 1940.
Gosselin, R. E.; Hodge, H.E.; Smith, R. P.; and Gleason, M. N.: *Clinical Toxicology of Commercial Products*, 4th ed. Williams & Williams Co., Baltimore, 1976.
Greenburg, L.; Mayers, M. R.; Goldwater, L. J.; and Burke, W. J.: Health hazards in the manufacture of "fused collars." II. Exposure to acetone-methanol. *J. Ind. Hyg. Toxicol.*, **20**:148–54, 1938.
Hanninen, H.; Nurminen, M.; Tolonen, M.; and Martelin, T.: Psychological tests as indicators of excessive exposure to carbon disulphide. *Scand. J. Work Environ. Health*, **19**:163–74, 1978.
Hardin, B. D.; Niemir, R. W.; Smith, R. J.; Kuczuk, M. H.; Mathinos, P. R.; and Weaver, T. E.: Teratogenicity of 2-ethoxyethanol by dermal application. *Drug Chem. Toxicol.*, **5**:277–94, 1982.
Havre, P.; Abrams, M. A.; Corall, R. J. M.; Ling, C. Y.; Szczepanik, P. A.; Feldman, H. B.; Klein, P.; Kong, M. S.; Margolis, J. M.; and Landau, B. R.: Quantitation of pathways of ethanol metabolism. *Arch. Biochem. Biophys.*, **182**:14–23, 1977.
Henschler, D., and Hoos, R.: Metabolic activation and deactivation mechanisms of di, tri-, and tetrachloroethylenes. In Snyder, R., Parke, D. V., Kocsis, J. J., Jollow, D. J., Gibson, G. G., and Witmer, C. M. (eds.): *Biological Reactive Intermediates—II: Chemical Mechanisms and Biological Effects*. Plenum Press, New York, 1982, pp. 55–66.
Herskowitz, A.; Ishii, N.; and Schaumburg, H.: *n*-Hexane neuropathy. *N. Engl. J. Med.*, **285**:82–85, 1971.
Hoch-Ligeti, C., and Argus, M. F.: Effects of carcinogens on the lungs of guinea pigs. Nettesheim, P.; Hanna, M. G., Jr.; and Deatherage, J. W., Jr. (eds.): *Morphology of Experimental Respiratory Carcinogenesis*. Atomic Energy Commission, Office of Information Services, 1970, pp. 267–79.
Hoch-Legeti, C; Argus, M. F.; and Argus, J. C.: Induction of carcinomas in the nasal cavity of rats. *Br. J. Cancer*, **24**:164–67, 1970.
Horvath, M. and Frantik, E.: Industrial chemicals and drugs lowering central nervous activation level. Quantitative assessment in man and animals. *Act. Nerv. Super.*, **21**:269, 1979.
IARC: Benzene. In: *Monographs on the Evaluation of the Carcinogenic Risk of Chemicals to Humans*. Vol. 29, *Some Industrial Chemicals and Dyestuffs*. International Agency for Research on Cancer, Lyons, France, 1982, pp. 93–148.
———: 1,4-Dioxane. In: *Monographs on the Evaluation of the Carcinogenic Risk of Chemicals to Man*. Vol. 11, *Cadmium, Nickel, Some Epoxides, Miscellaneous Industrial Chemicals, and General Considerations on Volatile Anesthetics*. International Agency for Research on Cancer, Lyons, France, 1976, pp. 247–56.
Ikeda, M., and Ohtsuki, H.: Phenobarbital-induced protection against toxicity of toluene and benzene in rats. *Toxicol. Appl. Pharmacol.*, **20**:30–43, 1971.
Infante, P. F.; Rinsky, R. A.; Wagoner, J. K.; and Young, R. J.: Benzene and leukemia. *Lancet*, **2**:868–69, 1977.
Ingelman-Sundberg, M., and Hagbjork, A. L.: On the significance of the cytochrome P-450-dependent hydroxyl radical-mediated oxygenation mechanism. *Xenobiotica*, **12**:673–86, 1982.
Irons, R. D.; Dent, J. G.; Baker, T. S.; and Richert, D. E.: Benzene is metabolized and covalently bound in bone marrow *in situ*. *Chem.-Biol. Interactions*, **30**:241–45, 1980.
Irons, R. D.; Greenlee, W. F.; Wierda, D.; and Bus, J. S.: Relationship between benzene metabolism and toxicity: a proposed mechanism for the formation of reactive intermediates from polyphenol metabolites. In Snyder, R.; Parke, D. V.; Kocsis, J. J.; Jollow, D. J.; Gibson, G. G.; and Witmer, C. M. (eds.): *Biological Reactive Intermediates—II: Chemical Mechanisms and Biological Effects*. Plenum Press, New York, 1982, pp. 229–43.
Jerina, D., and Daly, J. W.: Arene oxides: a new aspect of drug metabolism. *Science*, **185**:573–82, 1974.
Johnstone, R. T.: Death due to dioxane? *AMA Arch. Ind. Health*, **20**:445–47, 1959.
Jollow, D. J., and Smith, C.: Biochemical aspects of toxic metabolites: Formation, detoxication and covalent binding. In Jollow, D. J., Kocsis, J. J., Snyder, R., and Vainio, H. (eds.): *Biological Reactive Intermediates: Formation, Toxicity, and Inactivation*. Plenum Press, New York, 1977, pp. 42–59.
Jonsson, A. K.; Pederson, J.; and Steen, G.: Ethoxyacetic acid and *N*-ethoxyacetylglycine: metabolites of ethoxyethanol (Ethylcellosolve) in rats. *Acta Pharmacol. Toxicol.*, **50**:358–62, 1982.
Kalant, H.: The pharmacology of alcohol intoxication. *Qu. J. Stud. Alcohol*, **22**(Suppl.):1–23, 1961.
Kalf, G. F.; Rushmore, T.; and Snyder, R.: Benzene inhibits RNA synthesis in mitochondria from liver and bone marrow. *Chem.-Biol. Interactions*, **42**:353–70, 1982.
Katz, G. V.; O'Donoghue, J. L.; DiVincenzo, G. D.; and Terhaar, C. J.: Comparative neurotoxicity and metabolism of ethyl *n*-butyl ketone and methyl *n*-butyl ketone in rats. *Toxicol. Appl. Pharmacol.*, **52**:153–58, 1980.
Kersting, E. J., and Nielsen, S. W.: Experimental ethylene glycol poisoning in the dog. *Am. J. Vet. Res.*, **27**:574–82, 1966.
Kingsley, W. H., and Hirsch, F. G.: Toxicologic considerations in direct process spirit duplicating machines. *Compen. Med.*, **40**:7–8, 1954–55.
Klatskin, G.; Krahl, W. A.; and Conn, H. O.: The effect of alcohol on the choline requirement. I. Changes in rat liver following prolonged ingestion of alcohol. *J. Exp. Med.*, **100**:605–14, 1954.
Knave, B.; Kolmodin-Hedman, B.; Persson, H. E.; and Goldberg, J. M.: Chronic exposure to Carbon disulfide. Effects on occupationally exposed workers with special reference to the nervous system. *Work Environ. Health*, **11**:49–58, 1974.
Kociba, R. J.; McCollister, S. B.; Park, S.; Torkelson, T. R.; and Gehring, P. J.: 1,4-Dioxane. I. Results of a

two year ingestion study in rats. *Toxicol. Appl. Pharmacol.*, **30**:275–86, 1974.

Krasavage, W. J.; O'Donoghue, J. L.; DiVincenzo, G. D.; and Terhaar, C. J.: The relative neurotoxicity of methyl *n*-butyl ketone, *n*-hexane and their metabolites. *Toxicol. Appl. Pharmacol.*, **52**:433–41, 1980.

Landry, T. D., and Yano, B. L.: Dipropylene glycol monomethylether: a 13-week inhalation toxicity study in rats and rabbits. *Fund. Appl. Toxicol.*, **4**:612–17, 1984.

Lee, E. W.; Kocsis, J. J.; and Snyder, R.: The use of ferrokinetics in the study of experimental anemia. *Environ. Health. Perspect.*, **39**:29–37, 1981.

———: Benzene: acute effect on ^{59}Fe incorporation into circulating erythrocytes. *Toxicol. Appl. Pharmacol.*, **27**:431–36, 1974.

Lieber, C. S.: Pathogenesis and diagnosis of alcoholic liver injury. In Avogadro, P.; Sirtori, C. R.; and Tremoli, E. (eds.): *Metabolic Effects of Alcohol.* Elsevier, Amsterdam, 1979, pp. 237–58.

Lieber, C. S.; DeCarli, L. M.; and Rubin, E.: Sequential production of fatty liver, hepatitis, and cirrhosis in subhuman primates fed ethanol with adequate diets. *Proc. Natl Acad. Sci. USA*, **72**:437–41, 1975.

Lieber, C. S., and DeCarli, L. M.: Hepatic microsomal ethanol oxidizing system: *in vitro* characteristics and adaptive properties *in vivo*. *J. Biol. Chem.*, **245**:2505–12, 1970.

Lillis, R.: Behavioral effects of occupational carbon disulfide exposure. In: Behavioral toxicology: early detection of occupational hazards. *Natl Inst. Occup. Safety Health*, **74–126**:51–59, 1974.

Longacre, S. L.; Kocsis, J. J.; and Snyder, R.: Influence of strain differences in mice on the metabolism and toxicity of benzene. *Toxicol. Appl. Pharmacol.*, **60**:398–409, 1981.

Lukas, E.: Eight years experience with experimental CS$_2$ polyneuropathy in rats. *G. Ital. Med. Lav.*, **1**:7–17, 1979.

Lukas, E.; Kujalova, V.; and Sperlingova, I.: The role of copper metabolism in the development of carbon disulfide polyneuropathy in rats. In Manzo, L.; Lery, N.; Lacasse, Y.; and Roche, E. (eds.): *Adv. Neurotoxicol., Proc. Int. Congr.* Pergamon Press, Oxford, 1980, pp. 181–85.

Lutz, W. K., and Schlatter, C.: Mechanism of the carcinogenic action of benzene: irreversible binding to rat liver DNA. *Chem.-Biol. Interactions*, **18**:241–45, 1977.

Makar, A. B., and Tephly, T. R.: Methanol poisoning. VI. Role of folic acid in the production of methanol poisoning in the rat. *J. Toxicol. Environ. Health*, **2**:1201–1209, 1977.

Maltoni, C.; Conti, B.; and Cotti, G.: Benzene: a multipotential carcinogen. Results of long-term bioassays performed at the Bologna Institute of Oncology. *Am. J. Ind. Med.*, **4**:589–630, 1983.

Mannering, G. J., and Parks, R. E., Jr.: Inhibition of methanol metabolism with 3-amino-1,2,4-triazole. *Science*, **126**:1241–42, 1975.

Mansuy, D.; Nastainczyk, W.; and Ullrich, V.: The mechanism of halothane binding to microsomal cytochrome P-450. *Naunyn-Schmiedebergs Arch. Pharmakol.*, **285**:315–24, 1974.

McDonough, J. R.: Possible neuropathy from methyl *n*-butyl ketone. *N. Engl. J. Med.*, **290**:695, 1974.

McKenna, M. J., and DiStefano, V.: Carbon disulfide. II. A proposed mechanism for the action of carbon disulfide on dopamine beta-hydroxylase. *J. Pharmacol. Exp. Ther.*, **202**:253–66, 1977.

McMartin, K. E.; Martin-Amat, G.; Makar, A. B.; and Tephly, T. R.: Methanol poisoning. V. Role of formate metabolism in the monkey. *J. Pharmacol. Exp. Ther.*, **201**:564–72, 1977.

McMartin, K. E.; Martin-Amat, G.; Noker, P. E.; and Tephly, T. R.: Lack of a role for formaldehyde in methanol poisoning in the monkey. *Biochem. Pharmacol.*, **28**:645–49, 1979.

McMartin, K. E.; Ambre, J. J.; and Tephly, T. R.: Methanol poisoning in human subjects—role for formic acid accumulation in the metabolic acidosis. *Am. J. Med.*, **68**:414–18, 1980.

McMichael, A. J.; Spirtas, R.; Kupper, L. L.; and Gamble, J. F.: Solvent exposure and leukemia among rubber workers: an epidemiologic study, *J. Occup. Med.*, **17**:234–39, 1975.

Meyer, K. H.: Contributions to the theory of narcosis. *Faraday Soc. Trans.*, **33**:1062–64, 1937.

Miller, K. W.; Paton, W. D. M.; Smith, R. A.; and Smith, E. B.: The pressure reversal of general anesthesia and the critical volume hypothesis. *Mol. Pharmacol.*, **9**:131–43, 1973.

Miller, R. R.; Carreon, R. E.; Young, J. T.; and McKenna, M. J.: Toxicity of methoxyacetic acid in rats. *Fund. Appl. Toxicol.*, **2**:158–60, 1982.

Miller, R. R.; Ayres, J. A.; Young, J. T.; and McKenna, M. J.: Ethylene glycol monoethyl ether. I. Subchronic vapor inhalation study with rats and rabbits. *Fund. Appl. Toxicol.*, **3**:49–54, 1983a.

Miller, R. R.; Hermann, E. A.; Langvardt, P. W.; McKenna, M. J.; and Schwetz, B. A.: Comparative metabolism and disposition of ethylene glycol monomethyl ether and propylene glycol monomethyl ether in male rats. *Toxicol. Appl. Pharmacol.*, **67**:229–37, 1983b.

Miller, S. L.: A theory of gaseous anesthetics. *Proc. Natl Acad. Sci. USA*, **47**:1515–24, 1961.

Morgan, E. T.; Koop, D. R.; and Coon, M. J.: Catalytic activity of cytochrome P-450 isozyme 3a isolated from microsomes of ethanol-treated rabbits. *J. Biol. Chem.*, **257**:13951–57, 1982.

Morgan, M. Y.: Alcohol and nutrition. *Br. Med. Bull.*, **38**:21–29, 1982.

Morimoto, K.; Wolff, S.; and Koizumi, A.: Induction of sister chromatid exchanges in human lymphocytes by microsomal activation of benzene metabolites. *Mutat. Res.*, **119**:355–60, 1983.

Morris, H. J.; Nelson, A. A.; and Calvery, H. O.: Observations on the chronic toxicities of propylene glycol, ethylene glycol, diethylene glycol, ethylene glycol monoethylether, and diethylene glycol monoethylether. *J. Pharmacol. Exp. Ther.*, **74**:266–73, 1942.

Mundy, R. L.; Hall, L. M.; and Teague, R. S.: Pyrazole as an antidote for ethylene glycol poisoning. *Toxicol. Appl. Pharmacol.*, **28**:320–22, 1974.

Nagano, K.; Nakayama, E.; Koyano, M.; Dobayaski, H.; Adachi, H.; and Yamada, T.: Testicular atrophy of mice induced by ethylene glycol monoalkyl ethers. *Jpn. J. Ind. Health*, **21**:29–35, 1979.

NAS/NRC: *The Alkyl Benzenes.* Committee on Alkyl Benzene Derivatives, Board on Toxicology and Environmental Health Hazards, Assembly of Life Sciences, National Research Council, National Academy of Sciences. National Academy Press, Washington, D.C., 1980.

Nelson, B. K.; Setzer, J. V.; Brightwell, W. S.; Mathinos, P. R.; Kuczuk, M. H.; Weaver, T. E.; and Good, P. T.: Comparative inhalation teratogenicity of four glycol ether solvents and an amino derivative in rats. *Environ. Health Perspect.*, **57**:261–71, 1984.

Noker, P. E., and Tephly, T. R.: The role of folates in methanol toxicity. *Adv. Exp. Med. Biol.*, **132**:305–15, 1980.

O'Donoghue, J. L.; Krasavage, W. J.; and Terhaar, C. J.: Toxic effects of 2,5-hexanedione. *Toxicol. Appl. Pharmacol.*, **45**:269, 1978.

O'Donoghue, J. L., and Krasavage, W. J.: Hexacarbon

neuropathy: a gamma-diketone neuropathy? *J. Neuropathol. Exp. Neurol.* 38:333, 1979a.

O'Donoghue, J. L., and Krasavage, W. J.: The structure-activity relationship of aliphatic diketones and their potential neurotoxicity. *Toxicol. Appl. Pharmacol.,* 48:A55, 1979b.

Ohnishi, K., and Lieber, C. S.: Reconstitution of the microsomal ethanol oxidizing system (MEOS): qualitative and quantitative changes of cytochrome p-450 after chronic ethanol consumption. *J. Biol. Chem.,* 252:7124–131, 1977.

Olishifski, J. B.: *Fundamentals of Industrial Hygiene,* 2nd ed. National Safety Council, Chicago, 1979, pp. 540–48.

Orth, O. S.: General anesthesia. I. Volatile agents. In DiPalma, J. R. (ed.): *Drill's Pharmacology in Medicine.* McGraw-Hill Book Co., New York, 1965, pp. 100–15.

Parke, D. V., and Williams, R. T.: Studies in detoxication. The metabolism of benzene containing ^{14}C benzene. *Biochem. J.,* 54:231–38, 1953.

Pauling, L.: A molecular theory of general anesthesia. *Science,* 134:15–21, 1961.

Paulson, G. W., and Waylons, G. W.: Polyneuropathy due to n-hexane. *Arch. Intern. Med.,* 136:880–82, 1976.

Perbellini, L.; Brugnone, F.; and Pavan, I.: Identification of the metabolites of n-hexane, cyclohexane, and their isomers in men's urine. *Toxicol. Appl. Pharmacol.,* 53:220–29, 1980.

Pergal, M.; Vukojevic, N.; Cirin-Popov, N.; Djuric, D.; and Bojovic, T.: Carbon disulfide metabolites excreted in the urine of exposed workers. *Arch. Environ. Health,* 25:38–41, 1972a.

Pergal, M.; Vukojevic, N.; and Djuric, D.: a. II. Isolation and identification of thiocarbamide. *Arch. Environ. Health,* 25:42–44, 1972b.

Plaa, G. L., and Larson, R. E.: Relative nephrotoxic properties of chlorinated methane, ethane, and ethylene derivatives in mice. *Toxicol. Appl. Pharmacol.,* 7:37–44, 1965.

Pohl, L. R.: Biochemical toxicology of chloroform. In Hodgson, E.; Bend, J. R.; and Philpot, R. M. (eds.): *Reviews in Biochemical Toxicology,* Vol. 1. Elsevier/North Holland, New York, 1979, pp. 79–107.

Politzer, P.; Trfonas, P.; and Politzer, I. R.: Molecular properties of the chlorinated ethylenes and their epoxide metabolites. *Ann. N.Y. Acad. Sci.,* 367:478–92, 1981.

Pons, C. A., and Custer, R. P.: Acute ethylene glycol poisoning. *Am. J. Med. Sci.,* 211:544–52, 1946.

Post, G. G., and Snyder, R.: Effects of enzyme induction on microsomal benzene metabolism. *J. Toxicol. Environ. Health,* 11:811–25, 1983.

Pratt, O. E.: Alcohol and the developing fetus. *Br. Med. Bull,* 38:48–53, 1982.

Rao, K. S.; Cobel-Geard, S. R.; Young, J. T.; Hanley, T. R., Jr.; Hayes, W. C.; John, J. A.; and Miller, R. R.: Ethylene glycol monomethyl ether II. Reproductive and dominant lethal studies in rats. *Fund. Appl. Toxicol.,* 3:80–85, 1983.

Recknagel, R. O., and Glende, E. A.; Jr.: Carbon tetrachloride toxicity: an example of lethal cleavage. *CRC Crit. Rev. Toxicol.,* 2:263–97, 1973.

Reiner, O., and Uehleke, H.: Bindung von Tetrachlokohlenstoff und reduziertes mikrosomales Cytochrom P-450 und an Haem. *Hoppe-Zeyler's Z. Physiol. Chem.,* 352:1048–52, 1971.

Reynolds, E. S.: Comparison of early injury to liver endoplasmic reticulum by halomethanes, hexachloroethane, benzene, toluene, bromobenzene, ethionine, thioacetamide, and dimethylnitrosamine. *Biochem. Pharmacol.* 21:2555–61, 1972.

Rickert, D. E.; Baker, T. S.; Bus, J. S.; Barrow, C. S.; and Irons, R. D.: Benzene disposition in the rat after

exposure by inhalation. *Toxicol. Appl. Pharmacol.,* 49:417–23, 1979.

Rihimaki, V., and Pfaffli, P.: Percutaneous absorption of solvent vapors in man. *Scand. J. Work Environ. Health,* 4:73–85, 1978.

Rinsky, R. A.; Young, R. J.; and Smith, A. B.: Leukemia in benzene workers. *Am. J. Industr. Med.,* 2:217–45, 1981.

Roberts, J. A., and Seibold, H. R.: Ethylene glycol toxicity in the monkey. *Toxicol. Appl. Pharmacol.,* 15:624–31, 1969.

Robertson, O. H.; Loosli, C. G.; Puck, T. T.; Wise, H.; Lemon, H. M.; and Lester, W., Jr.: Tests for the chronic toxicity of propylene glycol and triethylene glycol on monkeys and rats by vapor inhalation and oral administration. *J. Pharmacol. Exp. Ther.,* 91:52–76, 1947.

Rogers, A. E.; Fox, J. G.; and Murphy, J. C.: Ethanol and diet interactions in male rhesus monkeys. *Drug-Nutr. Interactions,* 1:3–14, 1981.

RTECS: *Registry of Toxic Effects of Chemical Substances.* U.S. Department of Health and Human Services, Public Health Service, Center for Disease Control, National Institute for Occupational Safety and Health, Cincinnati, 1980.

Rubin, A., and Rottenberg, H.: Ethanol and biological membranes: Injury and adaptation. *Pharmacol. Biochem. Behav.* 18(suppl. 1):7–13, 1983.

Ruddick, J. A.: Toxicology, metabolism, and biochemistry of 1,2-propanediol. *Toxicol. Appl. Pharmacol.,* 21:102–11, 1971.

Ruprecht, H. A., and Nelson, I. A.: Preliminary toxicity reports on diethylene glycol and sulfanilamide. V. Clinical and pathologic observations. *JAMA,* 109(2):1537, 1937.

Saida, K.; Mendell, J. R.; and Weiss, H. S.: Peripheral nerve changes induced by methyl n-butyl ketone and potentiation by methyl ethyl ketone. *J. Neuropathol. Exp. Neurol.,* 35:207–23, 1976.

Sato, A., and Nakajima, T.: Dose-dependent metabolic interaction between benzene and toluene *in vivo* and *in vitro. Toxicol. Appl. Pharmacol.,* 48:249–56, 1979.

Sawahata, T., and Neal, R. A.: Horse radish peroxidase-mediated oxidation of phenol. *Biochem. Biophys. Res. Commun.,* 109:988–94, 1982.

Sedivec, V.; Mraz, M.; and Flek, J.: Biological monitoring of persons exposed to methanol vapours. *Int. Arch. Occup. Environ. Health,* 48:257–71, 1981.

Seeman, P.: The membrane action of anesthetics and tranquilizers. *Pharmacol. Rev.,* 24:583–655, 1972.

Seppalainen, A. M.; Lindstrom, K.; and Martelin, T.: Neurophysiological and psychological picture of solvent poisoning. *Am. J. Ind. Med.,* 1:31–42, 1980.

Sherlock, S.; (ed.): Alcohol and disease. *Br. Med. Bull.,* 38:1–113, 1982.

Singer, S. J., and Nicolson, G. L.: The fluid mosaic model of the structure of cell membranes. *Science,* 175:720–31, 1972.

Sipes, I. G., and Gandolfi, A. J.: Role of reactive intermediates in halothane associated liver injury. In Snyder, R.; Parke, D. V.; Kocsis, J. J.; Jollow, D. J.; Gibson, G. G.; and Witmer, C. M. (eds.): *Biological Reactive Intermediates—II: Chemical Mechanisms and Biological Effects.* Plenum Press, New York, 1982, pp. 603–18.

Slater, T. F.: *Free Radical Mechanisms in Tissue Injury.* J. W. Arrowsmith, Ltd., Bristol, 1972, pp. 118–63.

———— : Free radicals as reactive intermediates in tissue injury. In Snyder, R.; Parke, D. V.; Kocsis, J. J.; Jollow, D. J.; Gibson, G. G.; and Witmer, C. M. (eds.): *Biological Reactive Intermediates—II: Chemical Mechanisms and Biological Effects.* Plenum Press, New York, 1982, pp. 575–89.

Smith, E. N., and Taylor, R. T.: Acute toxicity of methanol in the folate-deficient acatalasemic mouse. *Toxicology*, 25:271–87, 1982.

Smuckler, E. A.: The molecular basis of acute liver cell injury. In: Good, R. A., Day, S. B., and Yunes, J. J. (eds.): *Molecular Pathology*. Charles C Thomas, Pub., Springfield, Ill., 1975, pp. 490–510.

Smyth, H. F., Jr.: Physiological aspects of glycols and related compounds. In Curme, G. O., Jr., and Johnston, F. (eds.): *Glycols*. Reinhold Publishing Co., New York, 1952.

Snyder, C. A.; Goldstein, B. D.; Sellakumar, A.; Wolman, S. R.; Bromberg, I.; Erlichman, M. N.; and Laskin, S.: Hematotoxicity of inhaled benzene to Sprague Dawley rats and AKR mice at 300 ppm. *J. Toxicol. Environ. Health*, 4:605–18, 1978.

Snyder, R.; Uzuki, F.; Gonasun, L.; Bromfeld, E.; and Wells, A.: The metabolism of benzene *in vitro*. *Toxicol. Appl. Pharmacol.*, 11:346–60, 1967.

Snyder, R., and Kocsis, J. J.: Current concepts of chronic benzene toxicity. *CRC Crit. Rev. Toxicol.*, 3:265–88, 1975.

Snyder, R.; Longacre, S. L.; Witmer, C. M.; Kocsis, J. J.; Andrews, L. S.; and Lee, E. W.: Biochemical toxicology of benzene. In: *Reviews in Biochemical Toxicology*, Vol. 3. Elsevier/North Holland, New York, 1981, pp. 123–53.

Sobue, I.; Yamamura, Y.; Ando, K.; Iida, M.; and Takayanagi, T.: *N*-hexane polyneuropathy. *Clin. Neurol. (Jpn.)*, 8:393–403, 1968.

Spencer, P. S., and Schaumburg, H. H.: Ultrastructural studies of the dying-back process. IV. Differential vulnerability of PNS and CNS fibers in experimental central-peripheral distal axonopathies. *J. Neuropathol. Exp. Neurol.*, 36:300–320, 1977.

Spencer, P. S.; Bischoff, M. C.; and Schaumburg, H. H.: On the specific molecular configuration of neurotoxic aliphatic hexacarbon compounds causing central peripheral distal axonopathy. *Toxicol. Appl. Pharmacol.*, 44:17–28, 1978.

Strubelt, O.: Interactions between ethanol and other hepatotoxic agents. *Biochem. Pharmacol.*, 29:1445–49, 1980.

Szendzikowski, S.; Stetkiewicz, J.; Wronska-Nofer, T.; and Karasek, M.: Pathomorphology of the experimental lesion of the peripheral nervous system in white rats chronically exposed to carbon disulphide. In Hausmanowa-Petrusewicz, I., and Vedrzejowska, H. (eds.): *Structure and Function of Normal and Diseased Muscle and Peripheral Nerve*. Polish Medical Publishers, Warsaw, 1974, pp. 319–26.

Tephly, T. R.: Introduction, factors in responses to the environment. *Fed. Proc.*, 36(5):1627–28, 1977.

Tephly, T. R.; Makar, A. B.; McMartin, K. E.; Hayreh, S. S.; and Martin-Amat, G.: Methanol—its metabolism and toxicity. *Biochem. Pharmacol. Methanol*, 1:145–64, 1979.

Thompson, J. A., and Reitz, R. C.: Studies on the acute and chronic effects of ethanol on choline oxidation. *Ann. NY Acad. Sci.*, 272:194–204, 1976.

Thurman, R. G., and Hoffman, P. L. (eds.): First Congress of the International Society for Biomedical Research on Alcoholism. *Pharmacol. Biochem. Behav.*, 18(Suppl. 1):593, 1983.

Tice, R. R.; Vogt, T. F.; and Costa, D. L.: Cytogenetic effects of inhaled benzene on murine bone marrow. In Tice, R. R.; Costa, D. L.; and Schaich, K.M. (eds.): *Genotoxic Effects of Airborne Agents*. Plenum Press, New York, 1982, pp. 257–75.

Tiller, J. R.; Schilling, R. S. F.; and Morris, J. W.: Occupational toxic factor in mortality from coronary heart disease. *Br. Med. J.*, 4:407–11, 1968.

Tilson, H. A., and Cabe, P. A.: Strategy for the assessment of neurobehavioural consequences of environmental factors. *Environ. Health Perspect.*, 26:287–99, 1978.

Toft, K.; Oloffson, T.; Tunek, A.; and Berlin, M.: Toxic effects on mouse bone marrow caused by inhalation of benzene. *Arch. Toxicol.*, 51:295–302, 1982.

Tolonen, M.: Chronic subclinical carbon disulfide poisoning. *Work Environ. Health*, 11:154–61, 1974.

Tolonen, M.; Hernberg, S.; Nuriminen, M.; and Tiitola, K.: A follow-up study of coronary heart disease in viscose rayon workers exposed to carbon disulfide. *Br. J. Ind. Med.*, 32:1–10, 1975.

Tolonen, M.; Nurminen, M.; and Hernberg, S.: Ten-year coronary mortality of workers exposed to carbon disulfide. *Scand. J. Work Environ. Health*, 5:109–14, 1979.

Torkelson, T. R.; Leong, B. J.; Kociba, R. J.; Richter, W. A.; and Gehring, P. J.: 1,4-Dioxane II. Results of a 2-year inhalation study in rats. *Toxicol. Appl. Pharmacol.*, 30:287–98, 1974.

Torkelson, T. R.; Oyen, F.; and Rowe, V. K.: *Am Ind. Hyg. Assoc. J.*, 37:697–705, 1976.

Tunek, A.; Platt, K. L.; Bentley, P.; and Oesch, F.: Microsomal metabolism of benzene to species irreversibly binding to microsomal protein and effects of modification of this metabolism. *Mol. Pharmacol.*, 14:920–29, 1978.

Tunek, A.; Platt, K. L.; Przybylski, M.; and Oesch, F.: Multi-step metabolic activation of benzene. Effect of superoxide dismutase on covalent binding to microsomal macromolecules, and indentification of glutathione conjugates using high pressure liquid chromatography and field desorption mass spectrometry. *Chem.-Biol. Interactions*, 33:1–17, 1980.

Tunek, A.; Hogstedt, B.; and Oloffson, T.: Mechanism of benzene toxicity. Effects of benzene and benzene metabolites on bone marrow cellularity, number of granulopoietic stem cells and frequency of micronuclei in mice. *Chem. Biol. Interact.*, 3:129–38, 1982.

Uehleke, H.: Binding of haloalkanes to liver microsomes. In Jollow, D. J.; Kocsis, J. J.; Snyder, R.; and Vainio, H. (eds.): *Biological Reactive Intermediates: Formation, Toxicity, and Inactivation*. Plenum Press, New York, 1977, pp. 431–45.

Uyeki, E. M.; Ashkar, A. E.; Shoeman, D. W.; and Bisel, T. U.: Acute toxicity of benzene inhalation to hemopoietic precursor cells. *Toxicol. Appl. Pharmacol.*, 40:49–57, 1977.

van Doorn, R.; Leijdekkers, C. P. M. J.; Henderson, P. T.; Vanhoorne, M.; and Vertin, P. G.: Determination of thio compounds in urine of workers exposed to carbon disulfide. *Arch. Environ. Health*, 36:289–97, 1981a.

van Doorn, R.; Delbressine, L. P. C.; Leijdekkers, Ch.-M.; Vertin, P. G.; and Henderson, P. Th.: Indentification and determination of 2-thiothiazolidine-4-carboxylic acid in the urine of workers exposed to carbon disulfide. *Arch. Toxicol.*, 47:51–58, 1981b.

Vigliani, E. C., and Saita, G.: Benzene and leukemia. *N. Engl. J. Med.*, 27:872–76, 1964.

Vind, C., and Grunnet, N.: Interaction of cytoplasmic dehydrogenases: quantitation of pathways of ethanol metabolism. *Pharmacol. Biochem. Behav.*, 18(Suppl. 1):209–13, 1983.

von Wartburg, J. P.; Bethune, J. L.; and Vallee, B. L.: Human liver-alcohol dehydrogenase. Kinetic and physiochemical properties. *Biochemistry*, 3:1775–82, 1964.

Wacker, E. C.; Haynes, H.; Druyan, R.; Fischer, W.; and Coleman, J.: Treatment of ethylene glycol poisoning with ethyl alcohol. *JAMA*, 194:1231–33, 1965.

Winston, G. W., and Cederbaum, A. I.: NADPH-dependent production of oxy radicals by purified components of the rat liver mixed function oxidase system.

II. Role in microsomal oxidation of ethanol. *J. Biol. Chem.*, **258**:1514–19, 1983.

Woo, Y.; Arcos, J. C.; Argus, M. F.; Griffin, G. W.; and Nishiyama, K.: Structural identification of *p*-dioxane-2-one as the major urinary metabolite of *p*-dioxane. *Arch. Pharmacol.*, **299**:283–87, 1977.

Wulf, B. S., and Featherstone, R. M.: A correlation of van der Waals constants with anesthetic potency. *Anesthesiology*, **18**:97–105, 1957.

Yamada, S.: An occurrence of polyneuritis by *n*-hexane in the polyethylene laminating plants. *Jpn. J. Industr. Health*, **6**:192–94, 1964.

Yamamura, Y.: *N*-hexane polyneuropathy. *Folia Psychiatr. Neurol. Jpn.*, **23**:45–47, 1969.

Yant, W. P., and Schrenk, H. H.: Distribution of methanol in dogs after inhalation and administration by stomach tube and subcutaneously. *J. Ind. Hyg. Toxicol.*, **19**(7):337–45, 1937.

Young, J. D.; Braun, W. H.; Gehring, P. J.; Horvath, B. S.; and Daniel, R. L.: 1,4-Dioxane and beta-hydroxyethoxyacetic acid excretion in humans exposed to dioxane vapors. *Toxicol. Appl. Pharmacol.*, **38**:643–46, 1976.

Young, J. D.; Braun, W. H.; and Gehring, P. J.: Dose-dependent date of 1,4-dioxane in rats. *J. Toxicol. Environ. Health*, **4**:709–26, 1978.

Zenk, H.: CS_2 effects upon olfactory and auditory functions of employees in the synthetic-fiber industry. *Int. Arch. Arbeitsmed.*, **27**:210, 1970.

Zimmerman, H. J.: *Hepatotoxicity: The Adverse Effects of Drugs and Other Chemicals on the Liver.* Appleton-Century-Crofts, New York, 1978.

Chapter 21

TOXIC EFFECTS OF
RADIATION AND RADIOACTIVE MATERIALS

Charles H. Hobbs and *Roger O. McClellan*

INTRODUCTION

Radiation toxicology is a specialized area of toxicology of considerable breadth and depth. Obviously it cannot be covered in great detail in a book such as this. Nonetheless, its importance related to the increasing use of radiation in the modern world dictates that certain basic elements of radiation toxicology be presented in this chapter. The manner of presentation then is of a survey nature with emphasis on providing both specific and general references that will assist the interested reader in obtaining a more detailed understanding of the subject.

BASIC PHYSICAL CONCEPTS

Ionizing radiation is a term applied to radiations that give rise, directly or indirectly, to ionizations when they interact with matter. Ionizing radiations comprise electromagnetic radiation, such as gamma and x-rays, and particulate or corpuscular radiation, such as alpha particles, beta particles, electrons, positrons, neutrons, and protons. The absorption of the energy of ionizing radiations in cells involves ionization of atoms and the production of ions within the cells. Although the exact mechanism of action of ionizing radiation is not known, radiation injury is considered to be related in some way to the production of ions within the cell.

The electromagnetic ionizing radiations, gamma and x-rays, are part of the electromagnetic spectrum with characteristic wavelengths and photon energies as illustrated in Figure 21–1. These rays have penetrating power that is generally directly related to the energy of the photon. For example, gamma or x-rays with energies of 300 Kev would be more penetrating than those with energies of 50 Kev.

X-rays originate outside the nucleus of atoms. In x-ray machines, they are produced by applying a high positive voltage between the source of electrons and a collecting terminal within a vacuum tube. When the electrons strike a suitable target, such as tungsten, their energy is partly converted into x-ray photons.

Gamma rays originate from unstable atomic nuclei releasing energy to gain stability. They have definite energies, characteristic of the nuclide from which they are emitted. Gamma and x-rays ionize materials largely indirectly through a variety of mechanisms that involve ejection of high-speed electrons from the atoms by which they are absorbed. The three primary types of interactions of gamma and x-rays following absorption by matter are photoelectric effect, Compton scattering, and pair production.

The alpha particle (α) is identical to a helium nucleus consisting of two neutrons and two protons. It results from the radioactive decay of heavy elements such as uranium, plutonium, radium, and thorium. Alpha particles have a large mass as compared to most other types of particulate radiations, such as neutrons and electrons. Decay of alpha-emitting radionuclides may result in the emission of several different alpha particles, each with its own discrete energy rather than a continuous distribution of energies. Because of their double positive charge, α particles have great ionizing power but their large size results in very little penetrating power. Their range in tissues is measured in micrometers.

Beta particles (β^-) are electrons resulting from the conversion of a neutron to a proton in the nucleus of an atom. They are identical to electrons from other sources such as those from tubes and heated filaments. Electrons that arise from outside the nucleus by internal conversion and the so-called Auger electrons are also identical but usually are designated by "C" rather than "B." Beta particles are not emitted with discrete energy levels, but rather a continuous spectrum of energy levels from a maximum value characteristic of each beta emitter down to

669

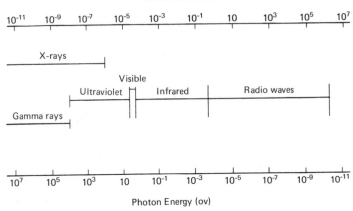

Figure 21–1. Approximate wavelengths and photon energies of major types of electromagnetic radiation. (From Casarett, A. P.: *Radiation Biology*. © 1968 by U.S. Atomic Energy Commission, Washington, D.C. Reprinted by permission of Prentice-Hall, Inc., Englewood Cliffs, N.J.)

zero. The decay emission of a beta particle generally results from atoms with large values of the ratio of neutrons to protons in the nucleus. Electrons have a greater range and penetrating power but much less ionizing power than alpha particles.

The positron (β^+) is a particle with the same mass as an electron but possesses a single positive charge. The emission of a positron from the nucleus is equivalent to converting a proton to a neutron and is the preferred mode of decay of unstable atoms with a small ratio of neutrons to protons in the nucleus. Electron capture is another way in which electron-deficient nuclei convert protons to neutrons by capturing orbital electrons into the nucleus. An annihilation reaction results when positrons and electrons interact resulting in the formation of two photons each with an energy of 511 Kev.

The neutron is a particle consisting of an electron and a proton. Neutrons may be released from elements that decay by spontaneous fission and from those fission products that possess metastable states with respect to neutron emission. The process of fission results in the release of from one to three neutrons. Due to their mass, neutrons have great kinetic energy, and because they have no charge, they penetrate readily. Neutrons produce ionization indirectly. In biologic materials this usually results from the ejection of protons from the nuclei of hydrogen atoms. These recoil nuclei are charged and are directly ionizing. Neutrons also activate hydrogen and other elements by neutron capture, which results in the release of gamma rays. Free neutrons are unstable and will undergo beta decay with half-lives of about 9 to 30 minutes if uncaptured.

Protons are identical to hydrogen nuclei and

are produced in tissues by the interactions of neutrons. Their charge and mass make them potent ionizers.

The radiations discussed above all produce ionizations. The directly ionizing particles are charged and, by virtue of their mass and motion, possess the energy to produce ionizations along their path as a result of impulses imparted to orbital electrons via electrical forces between the charged particles and orbital electrons. Indirectly ionizing radiations are not charged and penetrate through a medium with no interaction with electrons until they collide with elements of the atom and liberate energetically charged particles that are ionizing.

Radioactive decay occurs from unstable natural and artificially produced isotopes of elements decaying by the emission of subatomic particles and gamma or x-ray photons. In the case of very heavy elements, there is a pronounced tendency to decay by the emission of alpha particles. In the case of lighter elements, beta emission is the most frequent decay process. As discussed previously, beta decay occurs when there is an excess in the neutron-to-proton ratio. A less frequent mode of decay is by positron emission, which is favored by a small neutron-to-proton ratio in the nucleus. Gamma rays often accompany the emission of alpha and beta particles from a nucleus due to an excess in energy in the daughter nucleus following the alpha or beta decay.

The half-life of a radionuclide is the time required for the number of atoms present to decrease by one-half. The disintegration of radioactive nuclei is a random process and the rate of disintegration is directly proportional to the number of radioactive atoms present. Thus, when half the atoms in a sample have decayed, the rate of decay will have decreased by 2. The mathematical expression of radioactive decay is the exponential equation

$$N_t = N_0 e^{-\lambda t} \tag{1}$$

where

N_t = number of nuclei present at any time (t)
N_0 = number of nuclei present initially
λ = the radioactive decay constant
e = base of natural logarithms

The half-life of a radionuclide is then represented by

$$\frac{N_0}{2} = N_0 e^{-\lambda t_{1/2}} \tag{2}$$

which can be solved to give

$$T_{1/2} = \frac{\ln 2}{\lambda} = \frac{0.693}{\lambda} \tag{3}$$

The unit used to express radioactivity is the curie (Ci). The curie was originally related to the activity of 1 g of radium but is now defined as 3.7×10^{10} nuclear disintegrations per second or 2.22×10^{12} disintegrations per minute. A millicurie (mCi), microcurie (μCi), nanocurie (nCi), and picocurie (pCi) are $\frac{1}{10}^3$, $\frac{1}{10}^6$, $\frac{1}{10}^9$, and $\frac{1}{10}^{12}$ curies, respectively. The specific activity is the activity per unit weight of radioactive material. This activity is usually expressed in curies per gram and may be calculated by

$$\text{Curies per gram} = \frac{1.3 \times 10^8}{(T_{1/2})(\text{atomic weight})}$$

where

$T_{1/2}$ is the half-life in days (Schleien and Terpilak, 1984)

The roentgen (R) is a unit of exposure related to the amount of ionization caused in air by gamma or x-radiation. One roentgen equals 2.58×10^{-4} coulomb per kilogram of air. In the case of gamma radiation over the commonly encountered range of photon energy, the energy deposition in tissue for a dose of 1 R is about 0.0096 joules/kg.

The rad is the unit of radiation-absorbed dose and is a measurement of energy deposition in any medium by all types of ionizing radiation. One rad is equal to 100 ergs/g or 0.01 J/kg in any medium. The rad has more application than the R and should be used whenever the absorbed dose is known.

The dose equivalent, expressed as rem, takes into consideration such modifying factors of dose (in rads) as the quality of the radiation. The rem is the product of the absorbed dose in rads times the unitless quantities of radiation quality and any other factors such as dose distribution within the target tissue. In practice the latter factors are still so uncertain that they are generally assigned a value of 1 so that the dose equivalent in rems is equal to the rad dose times the quality factor. The terms of the dose equivalent and qualifications of its use have been defined and discussed (ICRU, 1980).

The quality factor for the various types of ionizing radiation is based on the linear energy transfer (LET) of the type of radiation. The LET is the rate at which charged particles transfer their energies to the atoms in a medium and is a function of the energy and velocity of the charged particle. For example, alpha particles with their large mass, +2 charge, and slow speed impart much more energy over their path than do electrons. The damage produced in tissue by absorption of a given amount of energy is generally greater as the distance over which this energy is imparted decreases, that is, the LET increases. In general, the higher the LET of the radiation, the greater the injury for a given absorbed dose. Values of the quality factor for various types of ionizing radiation are given in Table 21–1.

The term relative biologic effectiveness (RBE) is used to denote the experimentally determined ratio of the absorbed dose from one radiation type to the absorbed dose of a reference radiation required to produce an identical biologic effect under the same conditions. Gamma rays of ^{60}Co and 200 to 250 Kev x-rays have been used as reference standards. The term RBE has been restricted to experimental radiobiology and the term quality factor for use in calculations of dose equivalents for radiation protection purposes (NCRP, 1971b; ICRP, 1977).

It should be noted that the question of the appropriate quality factor for neutrons and alpha particles is under question. The ICRP has recommended the use of a quality factor of 20 for alpha particles and uncharged particles. Rossi (1975) in postulating a theory of dual radiation action has suggested that the relative biologic effectiveness for neutrons may approach 100 in some cases. Thus, there is also the need to reexamine the appropriate quality factor for use with neutrons. It was anticipated that the most useful human data in this regard would be derived from studies of the Japanese atomic bomb survivors since it was originally thought that individuals exposed in Hiroshima received relatively more neutron exposure than did the survivors in Nagasaki. Unfortunately, recent work suggests that the neutron exposures in both cities may have

Table 21–1.   QUALITY FACTORS*†

1. X-rays, electrons, and positrons of any specific ionization

$$QF = 1$$

2. Heavy ionizing particles

AVERAGE LET IN WATER (Mev/cm)	QF
35 or less	1
35 to 70	1 to 2
70 to 230	2 to 5
230 to 530	5 to 10
530 to 1750	10 to 20

For practical purposes, a QF of 10 is often used for alpha particles‡ and fast neutrons and protons up to 10 Mev. A QF of 20 is used for heavy recoil nuclei.

The following values for quality factors may be used for neutrons when the neutron energy spectrum is known:

NEUTRON ENERGY (*Mev*)	QF
Thermal	2
0.0001	2
0.001	2.5
0.1	7.5
0.5	11
1.0	11
10	6.5

* From Shapiro, J.: *Radiation Protection.* Harvard University Press, Cambridge, Mass., 1972, p. 52.
† Data from ICRP, 1963; NCRP, 1971a; NCRP, 1971b.
‡ The ICRP (ICRP, 1977) recommended a quality factor of 20 for alpha particles.

been smaller than originally projected (Marshall, 1981). Thus, although Japanese atomic bomb survivor data are still extremely valuable in estimating human health risks of external radiation exposure, the data may not be very useful for estimating the RBE of neutrons.

In order to conform to the International System of Units (SI) most of the currently used radiation units are being changed. The ICRU (1980), ICRP (1984), and NCRP (1985b) now recom-

mend that the rad, the roentgen, the curie and the rem be replaced by the SI units the gray (Gy), the Coulomb per kilogram (C/kg), the becquerel (Bq), and the sievert (Sv), respectively. Unfortunately, the old and new units may not be used interchangeably as explained below.

The SI unit, the joule per kilogram when used for ionizing radiation, is the gray with the symbol Gy; 1 Gy = 100 rad = 1 J/kg. The SI unit of one per second (reciprocal second) for activity is the becquerel with the symbol Bq; 1 Bq = 1/sec ~ 2.703×10^{-11} Ci. The SI unit proposed by ICRU for the rem is the sievert (Sv). As the dose equivalent is the product of the absorbed dose in grays times the unitless modifying factors such as the quality factor

$$1 \text{ Sv} = 1 \text{ J/kg} (= 100 \text{ rem})$$

For a more complete discussion of the above concepts the reader should refer to texts on radiation protection, radiation physics, and radiobiology (Casarett, 1968; Hall, 1976; Groseh and Hopwood, 1979; Lovell, 1979; Fullerton *et al.*, 1980; Mettler and Moseley, 1985). For a review of radioactivity measurements, procedures, and radiation-monitoring methods the reader is referred to publications of the National Council on Radiation Protection and Measurements (NCRP, 1978a, 1978b, 1978c) and the International Commission on Radiological Protection (ICRP, 1979, 1982).

SOURCES OF IONIZING RADIATION EXPOSURE

The sources for exposure of humans and animals to ionizing radiation can be broken down into four major groups: (1) natural sources of irradiation, both external and internal; (2) medical sources, such as diagnostic or therapeutic x-irradiation, and radiopharmaceuticals; (3) nuclear reactions, such as nuclear power reactors and nuclear weapons; and (4) other sources, such as industrial x-ray machines. Exposure to natural sources of irradiation is unavoidable for the most part, but the degree of exposure to man-made sources is subject to change, depending on intelligent and judicial use of such sources.

Natural Background Radiation

Exposure to natural sources of external ionizing radiation results from the levels of cosmic and terrestrial x-irradiation present in the environment. Cosmic irradiation at the earth's surface is affected by altitude, geomagnetic latitude, and solar modulation. For example, the dose rate at 1800 m is about double that at sea level. Within the United States, the effect of latitude and solar modulation on the dose rate from cosmic radiation dose rate is less than 10 percent. Because the components of cosmic radiation are highly penetrating, they result in whole-body irradiation. The average dose rate from cosmic radiation to the U.S. population has been estimated to be about 31 mrem/year disregarding structural shielding, which reduces the dose about 10 percent (BEIR, 1980 NCRP, 1975a). Humans are also exposed to external gamma radiation from concentrations of radioactive materials in soils and rocks. The dose level for this source of radiation varies markedly depending on the mineral content of the area and other factors such as the types of building materials used. Estimates of the annual dose for this type of exposure vary from about 15 to 140 mrem/year for various parts of the United States with an average of about 40 mrem/year disregarding shielding (BEIR, 1980). When the effect of shielding by structures and other parts of the body is considered, this is reduced to about 28 mrem/year (NCRP, 1975a; BEIR, 1980).

Internally deposited, naturally occurring radioactive materials also contribute to the natural radiation dose from inhalation and ingestion of these materials in air, food, and water. Included are the radionuclides of lead, polonium, bismuth, radium, radon, potassium, carbon, hydrogen, uranium, and thorium. Potassium-40 is the most prominent radionuclide of normal foods and human tissues. The dose to whole body (i.e., bone marrow) from these internally deposited radionuclides has been estimated to be about 24 mrem/year (NCRP, 1975a; BEIR, 1980).

It should be noted that the dose to the organs from these sources is not uniform. The dose to the lung from natural sources has been estimated to be 180 to 450 mrem/year and that to bone surfaces about 120 mrem/year compared to a dose for the bone marrow (whole body) of 80 mrem/year (BEIR, 1980; NCRP, 1975a). Most of the larger dose to the lung is attributable to the inhalation of the alpha-emitting daughters of the naturally occurring radionuclide ^{222}Rn. Also, the dose-equivalent rates to the lungs of smokers may be up to three times higher than for non-smokers owing to inhalation of ^{210}Po and ^{210}Pb from the cigarette. Some of the lung dose is also received from radionuclides released during combustion of fossil fuels, which contain small quantities of naturally occurring radionuclides (NCRP, 1977d).

Health Science Applications

Use of x-rays by the healing arts represents the largest source of exposure of the United States population to man-made radiation. An estimated average absorbed-dose rate for bone marrow from this source is 103 mrad/year (BEIR, 1980). In the case of this type of exposure, however, the average dose to the population may have little meaning as the dose is not equally distributed among the population (Mettler and Moseley, 1985). For example, the average vertebral marrow dose for a diagnostic upper gastrointestinal examination on a patient was reported to be 1.6 rads at midfield (Margulis, 1973). Substantial reductions in the dose to individuals and the population could be made by restricting the radiographic examinations to those in which a high yield of diagnostic information is obtained and by the use of the best available equipment and techniques (Margulis, 1973).

It has been estimated that some 10 to 12 million doses of radiopharmaceuticals are administered for diagnostic purposes each year by the over 10,000 physicians licensed to administer them in the United States. The rate of growth of the use of nuclear medicine procedures has also been increasing. It has been estimated that whole-body patient doses from the diagnostic use of radiopharmaceuticals represented about 20 percent of the patient doses resulting from medical diagnostic radiology (BEIR, 1980). A series of reports by the Medical Internal Radiation Dose Committee (MIRD) of the Society of Nuclear Medicine has detailed the physical, chemical, and biochemical characteristics, the biologic distribution, and absorbed-dose calculations for various radiopharmaceuticals (MIRD 1968, 1969a, 1969b, 1971, 1975a, 1975b). The International Commission on Radiation Units and Measurements has also recently reviewed the assessment of absorbed dose from radiopharmaceuticals (ICRU, 1979).

Nuclear Reactions

After the discovery of nuclear fission, the first nuclear reactor was developed toward the end of 1942 by Fermi and associates. This was followed by the Manhattan Project, which developed the first atomic weapons by the end of World War II. Nuclear fission follows the capture of a single neutron by the nucleus of a fissionable material such as ^{235}U or ^{239}Pu. The fission releases one to three neutrons and, if additional fissionable material is present in sufficient quantity and in the right configuration, a chain reaction results and the reaction is said to be critical. Slow or thermal neutrons are the most efficient for the production of nuclear fission from ^{235}U and ^{238}U mixtures. Thus, materials such as graphite, heavy water, beryllium, and organic chemicals are used as moderators to slow the neutrons. The enrichment of natural uranium with ^{235}U has lessened the need to slow the neutrons, and the operation of reactors with ordinary water as the moderator or with no moderator is now possible. Control rods of neutron-absorbing materials such as cadmium and boron control the chain reaction in many types of nuclear reactors. The process of nuclear fission, in addition to the liberation of from one to three neutrons from the nucleus, produces fission fragments or products with atomic mass numbers of 72 to 160. These fission products have unstable nuclei and decay by beta decay often with gamma emission. In the process of nuclear fission, there is a decrease in total mass, which results in a corresponding gain in energy that is released in a nuclear weapon detonation or is harnessed in a reactor for the production of power.

Most of the world's present-day supply of uranium contains only about 0.7 percent ^{235}U and about 99 percent ^{238}U. ^{238}U as well as ^{232}Th is said to be a fertile substance in that it cannot itself sustain a chain reaction but can be converted into fissionable material following neutron capture. One possible breeding reaction is represented by the following equation:

$$^{238}_{92}U + ^{1}_{0}N \longrightarrow ^{239}_{93}U \xrightarrow[23\ min]{\beta^-} ^{239}_{93}Np \xrightarrow[23\ min]{\beta^-} ^{239}_{94}Pu$$

Nuclear reactors in which the ratio of conversion to fission is greater than 1 are said to be breeder reactors. The breeder reactors now in the most advanced stages of development use ^{238}U as the fertile material. In addition, ^{239}Pu will be used as fuel. Thorium, which is estimated to be more abundant in the earth's crust than uranium, could also be used as a fertile material in breeder reactors.

After the initial development of isotopic separation techniques and nuclear reactors, ^{235}U and ^{239}Pu were obtained in sufficient quantities to construct bombs. When these fissionable materials are assembled into critical masses under properly controlled conditions, an uncontrolled, but of course self-depleting, chain reaction results that releases tremendous quantities of energy. The fissioning of each ^{235}U nucleus releases about 200 Mev of energy. In theory, it is possible for about 5 lb of ^{235}U to release energy with an expansive pressure equal to 20,000 tons of TNT (Behrens, 1969).

Nuclear energy can also be released by fusion of smaller nuclei into larger nuclei if during the process there is a decrease in mass. For fusion to take place, the interacting nuclei must have sufficient kinetic energy to overcome the repulsive force of like electrostatic charges. One method by which a fusion process can be ac-

complished is at extremely high temperatures ($\sim 10^8$ °K) such as occur following the explosion of fission-type nuclear weapons. These reactions are termed thermonuclear and generally involve isotopes of hydrogen. Thermonuclear or fusion-type weapons have been tested. Fusion reactors for the production of heat and power offer the potential for essentially unlimited power.

Since fusion technology is still unproven and, therefore, undergoing development, it is not possible to accurately estimate potential environmental and health risks associated with its use. At this time, it appears that it may pose less risk to human health than do fission reactors because fission products will not be present. The primary environmental and health concerns will likely be related to the quantities of tritium to be handled and activation products such as ^{60}Co, ^{59}Fe, and ^{95}Zr encountered in maintenance activities.

Nuclear Weapons

The first nuclear weapon test explosion took place in 1945 and from then until 1963 large-scale nuclear weapon testing in the atmosphere was conducted by the United States, Russia, and the United Kingdom. In 1963, a ban on atmospheric testing was agreed on by these major powers but limited atmospheric testing has been conducted periodically by France and China. A number of other countries are also thought to have the capability of producing nuclear weapons. Underground nuclear testing allowed by the treaty has continued and contributes comparatively little to global fallout of radioactive materials (Eisenbud, 1973). After the explosion of atomic weapons, fission products and products of neutron activation from materials used for bomb construction and in the area of the explosion are released as radioactive fallout. The effects of nuclear weapons have been reviewed (Glasstone and Dolan, 1977).

Of the many radionuclides produced in nuclear and thermonuclear explosions, the primary contributors to exposure of humans are ^{89}Sr, ^{90}Sr, ^{95}Zr, ^{193}Ru, ^{106}Ru, ^{131}I, ^{137}Cs, ^{141}Ce, and ^{144}Ce. Although ^{239}Pu is present in considerable quantity, its solubility characteristics prevent it from becoming a significant contributor to the dose from fallout. The significance of these and other internally deposited radionuclides is discussed further under Internal Emitters in this chapter. The primary dose from fallout radiation is through external gamma doses, assimilation through the food chain, or beta dose to the skin. The projected annual average whole-body dose rate from global atmospheric weapons testing is projected to be 4 to 5 mrem/year through the year 2000 for the United States population (BEIR, 1980).

Nuclear Power Production

The production of power by nuclear reactors could increase considerably over the next 50 years. The extent to which this increase occurs will depend largely on technology development, the establishment of the environmental and health costs of nuclear reactors compared to those from conventional sources, and their public and political acceptance. Although dose estimates of potential exposures from the use of nuclear power reactors for power production appear to be reasonable from an environmental standpoint, the impact of catastrophic accidents, however unlikely they are to occur, is more difficult to assess. For the production of power from nuclear reactors, there are a number of areas such as uranium mining, fuel fabrication, the reactor itself, fuel reprocessing, and storage of radioactive wastes that may result in the exposure of humans and the environment to radiation. Most of these are discussed below.

Although uranium mining increases the amount of uranium and its decay products accessible to humans, the process has not been associated with measurable increases in environmental radioactivity outside the immediate vicinity of the mines. The serious health problems in uranium miners associated with ^{222}Rn and the attachment of its short-lived daughters to dust particles are discussed elsewhere. The same considerations exist for uranium mills and fuel fabrication plants in that proper location and appropriate control of tailings and liquid wastes can prevent significant population exposures from these sources. Previously, failure to control these processes resulted in increased ^{226}Ra in water near plants and its subsequent deposition in crops from irrigation water. Also, the use of tailings in home construction resulted in increased gamma ray and radon exposure of the occupants of the houses (Eisenbud, 1973; NCRP, 1975b).

The quantity and availability of radionuclides for release vary considerably with the type and design of the reactor. The current nuclear power reactors are almost all either boiling-water and pressurized-water types of light water or reactors in which water is utilized as both coolant and moderator. A few gas (helium)-cooled reactors are also in operation, primarily in Great Britain. As light-water reactors are relatively inefficient and convert only about 1 to 2 percent of the potentially available energy into heat, there is currently a large international research effort under way to produce practical fast-breeder reactors that can use up to about 75 per-

cent of the energy in uranium (Eisenbud, 1973). Of the various possibilities for this reactor type, the so-called liquid metal-cooled fast-breeder reactor (LMFBR) appears to be the first type that will be developed, and commercially used, most likely in Europe.

In the current light-water-cooled reactors, the principal radionuclides present in reactor effluents under normal operations are ^{3}H, ^{58}Co, ^{60}Co, ^{95}Kr, ^{85}Sr, ^{90}Sr, ^{130}I, ^{131}I, ^{131}Xe, ^{133}Xe, ^{134}Cs, ^{137}Cs, and ^{140}Ba (Eisenbud, 1973). Gaseous and volatile radionuclides such as ^{85}Kr, ^{131}Xe, and ^{133}Xe contribute to the external gamma dose while the others contribute to the dose externally by surface deposition and internally by way of the food chain. Currently, the dose rate for the average person in the United States from environmental releases of all radionuclides from nuclear operations is less than 1 mrem/year (BEIR Report, 1980).

Under catastrophic accident conditions, radionuclides that may escape from nuclear reactors can be classified as volatile or nonvolatile. The volatile radionuclides of importance include iodine, tritium, and noble gases such as krypton and xenon. The nonvolatile radionuclides include all fission products, many activation products, and fuel components. Under accident situations, the most likely route of exposure is inhalation rather than environment contamination (BEIR Report, 1972). In any accidents involving the LMFBR, there exists the potential for inhalation of particles of plutonium and other transuranic radionuclides as well as ^{22}Na.

Nuclear reactor design has placed considerable emphasis on safeguards against complete failure of containment systems under accident situations. With light-water thermal reactors, the event that could conceivably result in the most catastrophic situation would be a complete failure of the coolant systems including failure of the emergency core cooling systems. This would result in a melting of the core with subsequent rupture of the containment vessel. The subsequent release of volatile and nonvolatile fission products in the form of a cloud would create a potential for exposure of a large number of people downwind from the reactor. For LMFBR, concern for population safety has been expressed because of the use of plutonium, the opportunity for sodium-water reactions, and the risk of accidental changes in core configuration resulting in prompt criticality (Eisenbud, 1973).

Catastrophic accidents, however unlikely, probably represent the most difficult risk-versus-benefit judgments concerning the increased use of nuclear reactors for the production of power. On March 28, 1979, the United States experienced the worst accident in the history of commercial nuclear power generation at a nuclear power facility on Three Mile Island in Pennsylvania (Kemeny, 1979; Moss and Sills, 1981). In spite of serious damage to the plant, most of the radiation was contained, and the actual release of radioactivity was so low that there is little chance that physical health effects (cancer) can be detected in the population exposed (Kemeny, 1979; Upton, 1981). A committee investigating the accident also concluded that even if the accident had resulted in a meltdown, there was a high probability that the reactor containment would have prevented the escape of a large amount of radioactivity (Kemeny, 1979). However, the public reaction to the accident illustrates the concern that is associated with nuclear power production.

A major study that assessed the accident risks in United States nuclear power plants was conducted (WASH-1400, 1975a). The study considered the risks and consequences from accidents involving large nuclear power reactors of the pressurized-water and boiling-water types that are now being used in the United States. The results of this study suggest that the risk to the public from accidents involving nuclear power reactors are relatively small as the consequences of reactor accidents were predicted to be no larger and in many cases smaller than those of nonnuclear accidents and as accidents involving nuclear reactors were predicted to be much less likely than many nonnuclear accidents having similar consequences. They estimated that the likelihood of an individual being killed in any one year in a reactor accident is one chance in 5 billion for each 100 operating reactors. This was in contrast to a chance in 4,000 for being killed in an automobile accident and a chance in 2 million of being killed by lightning. The early somatic effects, the late somatic effects, and the genetic effects in humans likely to be associated with a nuclear reactor accident were extensively reviewed in this study (WASH-1400, 1975b).

After reaching the end of its useful life, the reactor core could be reprocessed to convert the fission products to a form suitable for long-term storage and to recover the remaining uranium and the transuranic elements, which could then be used to fuel other reactors. After a period of storage to allow time for decay of the short-lived fission products, the spent cores would then be transported to plants for chemical reprocessing. No reprocessing is now being done in the United States. In fact, the United States is currently actively attempting to discourage reprocessing by other nations due to concerns for nuclear weapon proliferation. Although this temporarily eliminates any problems associated with reprocessing, it creates problems in the storage of unprocessed fuel. If reprocessing plants become operational, the quantities, the types of materials, and the chemical processes used require safety precautions to prevent inhalation and other types of exposures of workers and contamination of the environment by volatile and nonvolatile fission products as well as plutonium.

A very significant problem of the nuclear fuel cycle that has not been adequately resolved is the long-term storage of high-level nuclear wastes. At the present time these wastes are being stored in an aqueous form in large underground tanks ranging in capacity from about 15,000 gallons to 1 million gallons. These tanks have a finite lifetime of about 15 to 40 years. Thus, it will be necessary to store these wastes in some other fashion in the future. The major methods being considered for disposal or long-term storage of these wastes are disposal of solids in salt mines, storage as solids in deep underground caverns, storage as solids in man-made vaults at or near the earth's surface, disposal as solids in the deep ocean, disposal as solids in ice sheet areas, disposal as liquids in deep wells, perpetual storage as liquids in deep wells, perpetual storage as liquids in deep underground caverns, and perpetual storage as liquids in tanks (Eisenbud, 1973; Schneider, 1974; NAS, 1983).

Other Radiation Sources

Several consumer and industrial products, such as television sets, luminous-dial watches, airport luggage inspection systems, smoke detectors, electron microscopes, and building materials, yield ionizing radiation or contain radioactive material and can therefore cause radiation exposure to the general population. The estimated average whole-body dose rate to the U.S. population from these sources has been estimated to be about 4 to 5 mrem/year. Most of this exposure is due to naturally occurring radionuclides in building material (BEIR, 1980; NCRP, 1977d). Air travel also increases the radiation exposure of travelers owing to increased exposure to cosmic radiation and to a lesser extent from radionuclides transported by air (BEIR, 1980).

The extent to which the population is exposed to ^{222}Rn and its daughters in the air, especially indoors, has recently received increased attention (BEIR Report, 1980; NAS, 1981; Nero and Lowder, 1983; NCRP, 1984a). Levels of indoor ^{222}Rn and daughter concentrations arise from several sources in addition to entering from the outside air. They include building materials, the soil and rock underlying the building, and water supplies to the building. The level in homes may also be affected by the ventilation rate, which, due to energy conservation measures, is generally being decreased in houses in the United States (Nero, 1983). The extent to which these exposures to ^{222}Rn and its daughters in the indoor environment may contribute to the overall incidence of lung cancer is of concern (BEIR, 1980; Evans *et al.*, 1981; NAS, 1981; Nero and Lowder, 1983; NCRP, 1984b). See Table 21-2.

BASIC RADIOBIOLOGIC CONCEPTS

The basic reaction of ionizing radiation with molecules is either ionization or excitation. In ionization, an orbital electron is ejected from the molecule resulting in the formation of an ion pair. In excitation, an electron is raised to a higher energy level. Molecules may receive energy directly from the incident radiation such as when ionization results from interaction of the radiation and an orbital electron. This may be termed a direct effect of radiation. On the other hand, a molecule may receive energy from the molecule originally ionized and become ionized or excited itself, which constitutes an indirect effect of the irradiation. The latter effect is particularly important in aqueous biologic systems. Thus, one of the most fundamental effects of ionizing radiation on biologic systems is the ionization of water with resulting free radical formation, although hydrogen bonds, double bonds, and the sulfhydryl groups of other molecules may be split, also resulting in the formation of free radicals.

The initial process leading to radiation in a cell is dissipation of the physical energy of the radiation. This occurs within a short time period ($\sim10^{-6}$ sec) and results in ionization or excitation of molecules within the cell. The process of ionization of water may be written as follows:

$$H_2O \xrightarrow{\text{radiation}} HOH^+ + e^-$$

This results in the production of an ion pair. The energy lost in air by a charged particle is about 34 electron volts for every ion pair produced. The energy gained by tissue per ion pair formed is often assumed to be the same as that observed in air (34 ev). The linear energy transfer or the energy transferred per unit length of tract of the primary ionizing particle in tissue is related to the number of ionizations that may occur within the tissues.

Following energy deposition, ionization, and excitation, there is a period ($\sim10^{-6}$ sec) in which physicochemical reactions between the ions and other molecules occur. For water this can be written as follows:

$$H_2O + e^- \longrightarrow HOH^-$$

Thus, from the ionization of water both H_2O^+ and H_2O^- result. These then dissociate into free radicals (electrically neutral molecules having an unpaired electron, i.e., H· or OH·). For water the process may be written as follows:

$$\text{Radiation} \rightsquigarrow HOH \xrightarrow{e^-} HOH^+$$
$$HOH^+ \longrightarrow H^+ + OH·$$
$$e^- + HOH \longrightarrow HOH^- \longrightarrow H· + OH^-$$

Table 21-2. SUMMARY OF MAJOR SOURCES OF ANNUAL DOSE RATES OF IONIZING RADIATION IN THE UNITED STATES*

SOURCE	EXPOSED GROUP	BODY PORTION EXPOSED	AVERAGE DOSE RATE, mrem/yr†
Natural background			
Cosmic radiation	Total population	Whole body	28
Terrestrial radiation	Total population	Whole body	28
Internal sources	Total population	Bone marrow	24
Medical and dental			
X-rays	Patients	Bone marrow	78
Radiopharmaceuticals	Patients	Bone marrow	14
Atmospheric weapons tests	Total population	Whole body	4–5
Nuclear industry	Total population	Whole body	<1
Building materials	Population in brick and masonry buildings	Whole body	3–4

* Condensed and adapted from *Biological Effects of Ionizing Radiations Committee, National Academy of Science/National Research Council Report: The Effects on Populations of Exposure to Low Levels of Ionizing Radiation, 1980.* National Academy Press, Washington, D.C., 1980.

† The numbers shown are average values only and in some cases represent a proration of the dose received by a subpopulation over the total population. Also, for given segments of the exposed population dose rates considerably greater than these may be experienced.

Or the overall reaction as

$$H_2O \xrightarrow{\text{radiation}} H\cdot + OH\cdot$$

An alternate theory is

Radiation $\rightsquigarrow$ HOH $\longrightarrow$ HOH$^+$ + e^-

HOH* (excited)

H·   OH·

In any case, the extremely reactive radicals H· and OH· are formed. These can exist only a minute fraction of a second before undergoing a chemical reaction. A portion of these interact with one another resulting in H_2O, H_2, or H_2O_2 (hydrogen peroxide). The remainder of the free radicals diffuse into solution where they may interact with biologically important molecules.

As oxygen is present in most biologic systems, another free radical HO_2 may be formed by the reaction of the H· radical with oxygen. The HO_2 radical is then reduced to the oxidizing agent H_2O_2. The formation of the HO_2 radical and the increased amounts of H_2O_2 may account for the increased radiosensitivity of cells in the presence of oxygen. The oxygen effect is important for low LET radiations but not for high LET radiations probably because of the high ionization density of high LET radiations.

As was mentioned previously, molecules may be either ionized or excited by radiation. At one time, it was assumed that excited molecules had received energy transfer insufficient for ionization and would lose that energy through such processes as oscillation. However, it is now thought that an excited molecule with energy that exceeds that required for ionization may lose energy through such processes as dissociating into free radicals without passing through the stage of ionization.

The free radicals and other reactive molecules that are formed from the above processes may then react with biologically important molecules within the cell. These reactions (indirect) or the same type of reactions resulting directly from radiation on these biologically important molecules may have a profound effect on the cell when the chemical alterations involve molecules or structures (i.e., chromosomes) of great importance to cell function and viability. Radiation effects have been shown to occur with proteins, enzymes, nucleic acids, lipids, and carbohydrates, all of which may have marked effects on the cell.

The cytopathologic changes observed in cells following radiation are numerous, varied, and complex and are similar to those seen after other types of cellular injury. The response of individual cells and types of cells to radiation is variable depending on such things as the cell cycle and the oxygenation status of the cell. The response of cells and their various components to radiation has been reviewed by several authors (Rubin and Casarett, 1968; Casarett, 1980; ICRP, 1984; Mettler and Moseley, 1985). Many of these responses may result in cell death, which, if extensive, may result in death of the organism. Other cells may undergo either total or partial repair. These changes may also be expressed at later times by tumors or mutations.

For purposes of radiation protection, the effects of radiation have been categorized as being of two types, nonstochastic or stochastic (ICRP, 1984). Nonstochastic effects are those for which both the probability and severity of the effect vary with dose and a threshold for the effect exists. Examples are pancytopenia following irradiation of bone marrow and pneumonitis and pulmonary fibrosis following irradiation of the lung. Stochastic effects are those for which the probability of the occurrence of effect, and not its severity, varies as a function of dose in the absence of a threshold. The major stochastic effects are heritable effects and cancer.

EXTERNAL RADIATION EXPOSURE

General Considerations. The usual exposure of humans or animals to external ionizing radiation is to either natural or man-made sources of x-ray or gamma irradiation. Under certain conditions, however, such as in radiotherapy, space flight, and accident situations, other types of radiation such as neutrons, protons, and beta particles may also be sources of external irradiation.

Many factors, both extrinsic and intrinsic, may modify the response of a living organism to a given dose of radiation. The former include external factors such as dose rate, the quality of radiation, the geometry of the exposure, and the portion of the body exposed, and, the latter, biologic factors such as species, age, sex, oxygen tension, and metabolic status of the organism.

Early to Intermediate Effects

Early to intermediate effects can be taken to include the somatic effects of exposure to irradiation excluding life-span shortening and carcinogenesis. These relatively early effects, seen only after exposures to relatively high doses (>50 rads), include such diverse effects as acute radiation sickness and pulmonary fibrosis. These nonstochastic responses of different organs and tissues have been reviewed by the ICRP (1984).

Probably the most sensitive indicator of irradiation is the use of the frequency of chromosome aberrations in the lymphocytes of human peripheral blood (Bender and Gooch, 1962; Brewen and Preston, 1975). This method is useful when either the whole body or a substantial part of it has been exposed to a dose of 25 rads or more of penetrating radiation. It should be recognized that many other agents are also capable of causing chromosome aberrations in peripheral lymphocytes.

The early effects of exposure to ionizing radiation result primarily from cell death. The radiosensitivity of cells is generally considered to be related to how often they undergo mitosis. Cells that frequently undergo mitosis are the most radiosensitive, whereas those with no mitosis are the most radioresistant. This principle was recognized as early as 1904 by Bergonie and Tribondeau, who stated in their first "law" of irradiation that the radiosensitivity of cells is related directly to their reproductive capacity and indirectly to their degree of differentiation.

Other investigators (Rubin and Casarett, 1968) have extended the working classification of cells to include five classes of radiosensitivity based on the above principles. The first class is termed vegetative intermitotic cells, which are the most radiosensitive. These cells are characterized as short-lived individual cells, primitive and dividing regularly to produce daughter cells. Included in this class are hematopoietic stem cells, dividing cells in the intestinal glands, type A spermatogonia, granulosa cells of ovarian follicles, germinal cells of the epidermis, gastric and holocrine glands, and large- and medium-sized lymphocytes. Small lymphocytes are also very radiosensitive, but they divide infrequently and are an exception to the relationship.

The second class is termed differentiating intermitotic cells. These cells are not quite as sensitive as vegetative intermitotic cells. This class includes such cells as the differentiating hematopoietic series in the intermediate stages of differentiation in bone marrow, the more differentiated spermatogonia and spermatocytes, and oocytes. The third class is termed multipotential connective tissue cells and is intermediate in radiosensitivity. These cells typically divide irregularly or sporadically and in response to special stimuli. This class includes such cells as endothelial cells, fibroblasts, and mesenchymal cells.

The remaining two classifications include the relatively radioresistant cells. The first of these, reverting postmitotic cells, have long lives and do not divide at a high rate except under conditions of special stimuli. The class includes such cells as epithelial parenchymal cells, duct cells of salivary glands, liver, kidney, and pancreas, cells of the adrenal, thyroid, parathyroid, and pituitary gland, and many other cells. The last class, termed fixed postmitotic cells, includes the most radioresistant cells. These cells, which normally do not divide or have lost completely the ability to divide, are well differentiated and specialized in function. Cells of this type are long-lived neurons, perhaps some muscle cells, neutrophils, erythrocytes, spermatids, spermatozoa, superficial cells of the alimentary tract, and epithelial cells of sebaceous glands.

If the above classification of the relative radiosensitivity of cells is applied to the various organs and systems of the body, the dose-response relationships of radiation injury are more easily understood. For example, if entire populations of essential stem cells are destroyed, such as the hematopoietic stem cells, survival of an individual is virtually impossible, but destruction of the germ cells of the testes would play no role in early lethality even though sterility would result.

Acute Whole-Body Radiation Exposure. Exposure of the whole body or a substantial portion of it to penetrating radiation of various types is likely to occur only under accident situations, nuclear warfare, or possibly during manned space flights (Langham, 1967). Manifestations of early effects occur only after relatively high doses (above about 50 rads) delivered at relatively high dose rates (several rads per hour). Normally these acute early effects, which appear to be threshold phenomena, are dose-rate dependent and their incidence and severity increase nonlinearly with increasing dose.

About one or two hours after an acute whole-body exposure to penetrating ionizing radiation, a combination of gastrointestinal and neuromuscular symptoms, known as the prodromal syndrome, is likely to appear. Anorexia, nausea, vomiting, and diarrhea are the more common symptoms observed, but apathy, tachycardia, fever, and headaches are also likely to occur. Although the time of onset and severity of the symptoms are largely a function of the total absorbed dose, they vary widely among individuals. Lushbaugh (1981), from a review of available human data, estimated the following approximate doses required to produce these symptoms in 50 percent of the individuals exposed: anorexia, 100 rads; nausea, 120 rads; vomiting, 180 rads; and diarrhea, 230 rads. At very high doses (~1000 to ~5000 rads), the prodromal response merges with the fatal gastroenteric syndrome, whereas at lower doses there is a latent period before the hematologic syndrome. The pathogenesis of the prodromal syndrome is not known.

Depending on the size and distribution of the absorbed dose, the clinical manifestations of the acute radiation syndrome can be divided into three forms: the central nervous system (CNS), the gastrointestinal, and the hematopoietic (Figure 21–2). At higher doses, however, damage to all tissues and organs may cause the symptoms and effects of one form to blend into the others. With whole-body doses approaching 5000 rads or more, death apparently results from neurologic and cardiovascular degeneration and usually occurs within minutes to 48 hours, depending on the dose. This has typically been termed the CNS syndrome.

When total-body exposure dose is between 1000 and 5000 rads, the survival time may be from five to ten days and death is associated with bloody diarrhea and destruction of the gastrointestinal mucosa, particularly that of the small intestine (gastrointestinal syndrome). The epithelial cells lining the small intestine have a short life and need to be renewed every few days (Patt and Quastler, 1963). Large doses of irradia-

tion cause cell death of the relatively radiosensitive crypt cells, which produce the cells that eventually migrate to replenish the epithelial lining cells. Thus, without continual replacement of the cells, ulceration and hemorrhage develop. These changes develop throughout the gastrointestinal tract but are more pronounced in the small intestine owing to the lack of cell renewal. Gastrointestinal changes are complicated by changes in many other tissues, particularly the bone marrow where depression also occurs from these doses. At the lower end of the dose range for the gastrointestinal syndrome, animals may be kept alive with the use of large amounts of fluids and antibiotics, and regeneration of intestinal epithelium is quite rapid (Bond *et al.*, 1969). Animals treated in this manner, however, usually die later from the bone marrow syndrome, which is extremely difficult to treat following doses high enough to produce the gastrointestinal syndrome.

Penetrating whole-body doses from about 50 to 1000 rads cause symptoms related primarily to injury of the bone marrow (hematopoietic syndrome). Damage to the bone marrow cells is reflected by changes in the circulating blood. The severity of bone marrow depression and the latent period between exposure and appearance

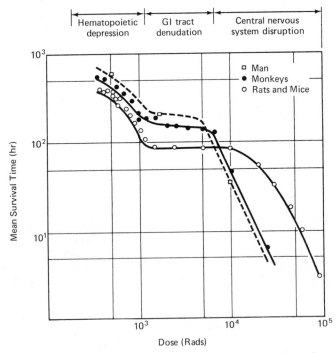

Figure 21–2. Survival time and associated mode of death in relation to dose of acute whole-body irradiation. (From Langham, W. H.; Brooks, P. M.; and Grahn, D.: Biological effects of ionizing radiation. *Aerospace Med.*, **36**:1–55, 1965.)

of the symptoms are related to the magnitude of dose. The changes in the peripheral blood are largely the result of damage to lymphocytes and the precursor stem cells of the bone marrow. The earliest and one of the more dramatic changes in the peripheral blood is a drastic fall in the number of circulating lymphocytes. This is apparent within one to two days after exposure to doses as low as 50 to 100 rads. The circulating lymphocyte count may approach zero at doses in the lethal range. The return to normal of the lymphocyte count is slow and may be depressed months to years after exposure (Langham, 1967).

The total white cell count may be maintained for a few days despite the rapid fall in the lymphocyte count due to a temporary increase in the neutrophil count. However, the neutrophil count soon begins a steady decline followed by a period of leveling off or an "abortive rise." Lack of this abortive rise has been associated with a poor prognosis at doses near the lethal range (Langham, 1967). Following this the neutrophil count again declines, reaching a low at about four to six weeks in humans. If death does not occur, the count will increase slowly to normal in a few months. The danger of infection in this stage of the syndrome is closely associated with the level of neutrophils in the peripheral blood.

The platelet count in the peripheral blood decreases similarly to the neutrophil count. When the platelets reach a critical level, hemorrhage is likely to occur and may result in the death of the individual.

Because of the radioresistance and long lifespan of mature erythrocytes, red blood cell levels fall slowly if at all in the absence of complicating hemorrhage. Normally, anemia is not an urgently severe consequence of acute exposure to ionizing radiation.

The treatment of acute radiation exposure is very similar to that for any pancytopenia. A complete discussion of the treatment of the acute radiation syndrome has been published (Cronkite et al., 1969). Procedures have also been published for the management of persons accidentally contaminated with radionuclides (NCRP, 1980).

For acute, high-dose-rate exposure to ionizing radiation, the lethal dose for most species is usually presented as the LD50/30 days. The LD50/30 of various species of animals varies markedly as illustrated in Table 21–3 (Bond et al., 1969). The distribution of deaths at doses near the LD50 as a function of time also varies significantly with species. In rodents most post-exposure deaths occur between 9 and 14 days, in dogs between 10 and 25 days, and in humans and most species of monkeys within a range of about 20 to 60 days.

A precise LD50 for acute exposure of humans to irradiation is not known. From a review of the data available, Lushbaugh (1982) has estimated an LD50/60 days for humans of about 300 rads and has proposed a broad basis for relating the dose to survival for man. Survival is almost certain at doses less than 100 rads, probable at 100 to 200 rads, possible at 200 to 500 rads, and not probable at larger doses. Survivors of the acute

Table 21–3. REPRESENTATIVE LD50/30 DAY VALUES FOR VARIOUS MAMMALIAN SPECIES*

SPECIES	TYPE OF RADIATION	LD50/30 DAY Exposure in Air (R)	LD50/30 DAY Absorbed Dose at Midcenter (rads)
Mouse	250 KVP x-ray	443	538
Rat	200 KVP x-ray	640	796
Guinea pig	200 KVP x-ray	337	400
Rabbit	250 KVP x-ray	805	751
Monkey	250 KVP x-ray	760	546
Dog	250 KVP x-ray	281	244
Swine	1000 KVP x-ray	510	247
Sheep	Gamma approx. 0.7 Mev	524	205
Goat	200 KVP x-ray	350	237
Burro	Gamma approx. 1.1 Mev	651	256

* From Bond, V. P.; Cronkite, E. P.; and Conrad, R. A.: Acute whole body radiation injury: Pathogenesis, pre- and post-radiation protection. In Behrens, C. F.; King, E. R.; and Carpender, J. W. J. (eds.): *Atomic Medicine*, 5th ed. Williams & Wilkins Co., Baltimore, © 1969.

radiation syndrome will be at high risk of developing late effects of irradiation such as leukemia.

Acute Partial-Body Radiation Exposure. The effects of acute exposure to penetrating ionizing radiation of a portion of the body are usually seen in patients undergoing radiotherapy for the treatment of cancer. In essence, early to intermediate effects can be produced by irradiation of any tissues and organs of the body. There are several textbooks with complete discussions of the response of various organs and systems to irradiation (Rubin and Casarett, 1968; Casarett, 1981; Mettler and Moseley, 1985). The effects usually result in atrophy and fibrosis with a disorder in the architectural pattern of some organs and late necrosis of individual cells in others. Also typical is the presence of foamy, bizarre, or giant cells in some organs and various degrees of cellular proliferation or differentiation, or both, in others. Whether these changes are related to the eventual development of neoplasia is not known, and many of them are similar to those that develop after other types of injury to the same organ.

With partial-body irradiation at doses less than 500 to 1000 rads, serious effects are not immediately apparent except in the skin, gonads, or eyes unless a substantial portion of the body is irradiated and significant bone marrow depression occurs. At doses of about 500 rads, many individuals will show skin changes initially as erythema, progressing to dry desquamation and eventually to a dry, hairless skin (McLean, 1973). More dramatic skin changes such as ulceration develop at higher doses. The reaction of skin to ionizing radiation has been reviewed (Goldschmidt and Sherwin, 1980).

The germ cells of both males and females are radiosensitive. In males, acute doses of 10 to 100 rads will cause a dose-related depression of the sperm count, which recovers slowly. With doses in the range of 500 rads, permanent sterility is likely. In females, destruction of oocytes results in permanent sterility due to a lack of stem cells in the adult ovary. Also, destruction of germinal epithelium of the ovary involves interruption of the production of the sex hormones (McLean, 1973).

Exposure of the lens of the eye to ionizing radiation such as x-rays, gamma rays, beta particles, and neutrons may cause cataracts. The latent period in humans between exposure and cataract formation is dose related and may vary from months to as long as five years or more. Cataracts have not been observed in humans from irradiation of gamma or x-rays at doses less than about 600 R, but cataracts have been found in mice exposed to doses as low as 100 rads of x-rays. Neutron doses as low as 1 rad have produced cataracts in mice.

Factors That Modify the Response to Irradiation. Dose rate and dose fractionation both influence the total dose required to produce all of the acute effects of low linear energy transfer (LET) radiation in experimental animals. Dose rate and dose fractionation both influence the total dose to produce the acute effects of low-linear-energy-transfer (LET) radiation (NCRP, 1980). Figure 21–3 illustrates the effect of dose rate on the LD50 values for exposure to ^{60}Co gamma rays. As can be seen, the lower the dose rate (R/day), the higher the LD50 dose (rads). In all cases, the predominant cause of death was hematopoietic damage. However, as the dose rate was decreased, the mean time to death increased from 20 days in the case of dogs given an acute high-dose-rate exposure (15 R/minute or 21,600 R/day) to a mean of 1865 days at a much lower dose rate (0.0034 R/min or 5 R/day). Over the same range of dose rates, the LD50 total dose increased from 258 rads at the high dose rate to about 7000 rads at the 5 R/day dose rate (Fritz et al., 1978).

Similar data on the effect of lowered dose rates on hematologic effects in humans are not available, but in one accident case, a man with evidence of severe hematologic depression survived a dose of ^{60}Co gamma irradiation of about

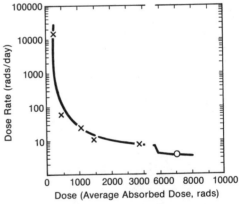

Figure 21–3. LD50 dose for beagle dogs given whole-body gamma irradiation at various dose rates. The point at 3.75 RE/day (O) is for a continuous exposure to death. The other dose rates (×) of 21,600 R/day, 61 R/day, 35 R/day, 24.8 R/day, 17 R/day, 10 R/day, and 5 R/day were terminated at the end of a predetermined total dose. As discussed in the text, the time to death also varied markedly. (From Fritz, T. E., et al.: Relationship of dose rate and total dose to responses of continuously irradiated beagles. In *Late Biological Effects of Ionizing Radiation*, Vol. II. IAEA-SM-224/206, Vienna, 1978, pp. 71–82.)

1000 rads protracted over 119 days (Martinee *et al.*, 1964, *Rev. Med. Inst. Mex. Seguro Social*, 3:14–68, cited in Langham, 1967).

Normally, there is much less dose rate effect from high LET radiation than from low LET radiation. A possible explanation for this is that most cells are incapable of repairing damage caused by high LET radiations.

Dose fractionation, where doses are delivered at high dose rates but split into various fractions, is a technique that has been used for many years to alter the therapeutic ratios in tumor therapy. Depending on the schedules used and the tissues irradiated, fractionation can either decrease or increase the effect of a given dose on a given population of cells. Usually, tissues tolerate larger total doses when the dose is fractionated (Rubin and Casarett, 1968; Casarett, 1981; Mettler and Moseley, 1985).

The age of an animal at the time of exposure may also affect its radiosensitivity. Radiation received by the embryo and fetus during early gestation is likely to cause developmental abnormalities particularly microencephaly or impaired body growth (NCRP, 1977b). The data from studies on Hiroshima survivors showed that microencephaly was induced by relatively low doses of mixed gamma and neutron radiation (average fetal dose, 5.3 rads gamma plus 0.4 rad neutrons) (BEIR, 1980). Because of the uncertainties over the dose response, therapeutic abortions have been advised by some authors (Rubin and Casarett, 1968) following abdominal exposures of 5 to 10 rads during early pregnancy. Very young animals are also consistently more radiosensitive than adults (Bond *et al.*, 1969). Increased radiosensitivity of aged animals has been observed in only a few of the systems studied (Bond *et al.*, 1969).

Although it is probably of little practical significance except for radiotherapeutic applications, the oxygen tension of cells at the time of irradiation has a marked effect on cellular radiosensitivity. Decreasing the oxygen tension of the cells (hypoxia) decreases their radiosensitivity.

Late Somatic Effects

Within the past few years, there has been increased focus on the potential for even very low doses of irradiation to produce deleterious biologic effects in the human population. Experimental animal data and observations of groups of humans have clearly established that ionizing radiation is carcinogenic and mutagenic at relatively high doses usually delivered at high dose rates. However, owing to uncertainties as to the shape of the dose-response curves, concern exists for the effects of irradiation at doses and

dose rates that extend down to doses that may be received from the environment and diagnostic radiography. Furthermore, there is the apparent need for risk-versus-benefit judgments for all of the varied uses and proposed uses of radiation. Animal experiments may provide a sound scientific basis for risk estimates, but the estimation of benefits and the balance between the two remain largely subjective.

The most important late somatic effect of ionizing radiation is cancer induction (BEIR, 1980). The scope of this discussion is necessarily limited; however, comprehensive discussions of the late somatic effects of exposure to ionizing radiation have recently been published (BEIR, 1980; UNSCEAR, 1982). Several recent reviews also specifically consider the subject of radiation carcinogenesis (Upton, 1973, 1982; Yuhas *et al.*, 1976; Beebe, 1982).

Laboratory animals, exposed to single or divided doses of radiation in the sublethal range, have demonstrated a shortened life-span (Lindop and Sacher, 1966; Grahn, 1969). Examination of data from many of these experiments has revealed that not all of the excess mortality was due to cancer, but extended over the spectrum of diseases usually observed in the animals. However, analysis of data from various groups of humans exposed to doses of irradiation has not consistently shown any nonspecific life-shortening effects due to exposure (BEIR Report, 1980). The most detailed human study is that of the Japanese atomic bomb survivors in which detailed evaluation through October 1, 1974, of over 14,000 deaths from natural causes other than cancer provided no evidence that diseases other than cancer were involved in the late radiation mortality, the total effect on excess mortality was attributed to neoplasia (Beebe *et al.*, 1978). There has been established, however, a clear relationship between radiation dose and excess risk of cancer in these irradiated human populations and in animal experiments. Thus, carcinogenesis appears to be the primary late somatic effect of ionizing radiation.

A detailed discussion of the dose-response relationship of carcinogenesis following exposure to ionizing radiation is beyond the scope of this discussion. However, the pertinent questions that remain to be resolved along these lines are (1) whether the dose-response curve is linear or nonlinear and/or whether it has a threshold, and (2) the effect of lowering the radiation dose rate or protracting the dose on the dose-response relationship.

Based on current information, a linear dose-response curve probably overestimates the risk for low-LET radiation (BEIR, 1980; NCRP, 1980). For high-LET radiation, the application of a linear estimate is less likely to overestimate the risk and could lead to underestimates (BEIR, 1980). Also, most data in experimental animals indicate that for low-LET radiation, the response at low dose rates will be less than estimated from doses received at high dose rates (NCRP, 1980; Beebe, 1982). For a recent more complete discussion of the shape of the dose-response curves and the models used to predict human health effects from radiation, the reader is referred to recent reviews (BEIR, 1980; Land, 1980; NCRP, 1980; UNSCEAR, 1982) of this subject. Table 21–4 presents a summary of the excess cancer risk from exposure to low-LET radiation as projected in the recent BEIR Committee Report (1980) and compares them to others that have been made (BEIR, 1972; UNSCEAR, 1977). For risk factors for individual cancer sites (i.e., leukemia and breast cancer), the reader is referred to discussions in the above documents (UNSCEAR, 1977; BEIR, 1980). It should be noted that the 1980 BEIR Committee favored the use of a linear quadratic model to predict these risks (BEIR, 1980). This represented a departure from the past use of a pure linear model (BEIR, 1972; UNSCEAR, 1977). Also, this report was published about the time the contribution of the neutron dose to the Japanese atomic blast survivors was questioned (Marshall, 1981). These points led to the dissention of some committee members from the 1980 report (BEIR, 1980). The reader should refer to the original reports (BEIR Reports, 1972, 1980; UNSCEAR, 1977, 1982) for a more complete discussion of the derivation and use of risk estimates. It should also be noted that some authors (i.e., Gofman, 1981) would place the risk much higher than those generally utilized (i.e., BEIR, 1980).

The induction of leukemia in experimental animals and humans by exposure to external ionizing radiation is well documented (NCRP, 1980; Beebe, 1982; Upton, 1982). The epidemiologic studies by the Atomic Bomb Casualty Commission (ABCC), now called the Radiation Effects Research Foundation, on the A-bomb survivors of Hiroshima and Nagasaki provide the largest set of data from more nearly uniform conditions of exposure on the effect of ionizing radiation on the production of leukemia and other cancers in humans. In these studies, age at exposure was an important factor in the susceptibility of atomic bomb survivors to the development of leukemia. Children less than ten years old at exposure were most susceptible to the induction of leukemia. The susceptibility appeared to decrease between 10 and 19 years, then increased slowly after 20 years, and became relatively high in persons over 50 years (Jablon and Kato, 1972; Beebe et al., 1978). The types of leukemias induced by radiation depend on the age at exposure and such conditions of exposure as dose and dose rate. The incidence of chronic lymphatic leukemia does not appear to be affected by radiation. A review of all available information from human radiation exposure, including the ABCC data available to that time, information from patients who received partial-body x-irradiation for ankylosing spondylitis, and other sources, has provided the following risk estimates for leukemia for large population groups (BEIR Report, 1972): a percentage increase in relative risk per rem of 0 to 3 for adults and from 5 to 10 for children and an absolute risk (cases/10^6 persons/year/rad) of from 1 to 2 for adults and from 2 to 3 for children.

Animal experiments have shown that the leu-

Table 21–4. COMPARATIVE ESTIMATES FOR LIFETIME EXCESS CANCER MORTALITY RISK FOR LOW-LET RADIATION*
(Average Value per Rad per Million Population Exposed)

SOURCE	DOSE-RESPONSE MODEL[†]	SINGLE EXPOSURE TO 10 RADS		CONTINUOUS LIFETIME EXPOSURE TO 1 RAD/YR	
		Absolute[†]	Relative	Absolute[†]	Relative[†]
BEIR, 1980‡	Linear quadratic	66	226	67	169
	Linear	167	501	158	403
	Quadratic	10	28	—	—
BEIR, 1972 factors§	Linear	117	621	115	568
UNSCEAR, 1977‖	Linear			75–175	

* Modified from *The Effects on Populations of Exposure to Low Levels of Ionizing Radiation: 1980,* Committee on the Biological Effects of Ionizing Radiations. National Academy Press, Washington, D.C., 1980. The reader is cautioned to consult that report for a complete discussion of the models and sources used to make these estimates.

† See BEIR, 1980, for discussion of models and their application to the available data.

‡ The values are average values per rad, and are not to be taken as estimates at only 1 rad of dose.

§ As applied in BEIR, 1980.

‖ As cited in BEIR, 1980.

kemogenic effect of ionizing radiation varies with the quality of radiation, LET, dose rate, and total accumulated dose. Studies in which mice were exposed to either gamma rays or neutrons have shown a marked dose-rate dependence for gamma rays but none for neutrons for the development of myelogenous leukemia in the mouse (Upton et al., 1970). These results illustrate the influence of dose rate on the effectiveness of low-LET and high-LET radiations as observed for most effects of ionizing radiation in that for high-LET radiation there appears to be no dose-rate dependence, whereas for low-LET radiation lower dose rates are generally less effective (Upton, 1968b). The data from humans exposed to ionizing radiation are insufficient to show whether or not there is a dose-rate dependence for leukemia in humans as is apparently the case for the mouse.

Most, but not all, types of cancer can be increased in frequency by exposure to radiation. However, radiation-induced cancers have no distinguishing features by which they can be recognized as being caused by radiation (Upton, 1982). Typically, following exposures of the total body or a significant portion of the bone marrow to ionizing radiation leukemia is the cancer with the shortest latent period and other cancers appear at later times. Myeloid leukemia and the acute leukemias are perhaps the most readily induced of the radiation-induced neoplasms. The studies of the ABCC have shown a higher incidence for leukemia than for other cancers prior to 1960. At that time, the incidence of leukemia appeared to decrease, while that of other cancers started to increase. Evaluation of the Japanese atomic bomb survivors through October 1, 1974 (Beebe et al., 1978), indicate that excess incidence of myelogenous leukemia, lymphomas, and cancer of thyroid, breast, lung, esophagus, stomach, and urinary organs have been induced by the radiation exposure. The minimal latent period for most of the carcinogenic effects was under 15 years and depended on age at exposure and site of cancer. Twenty-five years after receiving the high dose-rate exposures the leukemogenic effect is reduced, although still present, and the average absolute risk for other malignant cancers exceeds that for leukemia (BEIR, 1980). The studies of Stewart (1971) and MacMahon (1962) on children irradiated *in utero* have also shown a shorter latent period for leukemia than for other cancers.

Numerous studies have reported an increased incidence of thyroid nodules, both benign and malignant, following radiation exposure (WASH-1400, 1975; NCRP, 1977c; BEIR, 1980). Tumors of the thyroid following exposure to ^{131}I are discussed elsewhere in the chapter. Below doses of 1500 rem of external radiation the incidence of nodules appears to be linearly related to dose. From studies on persons exposed to mixed internal (radioiodine) and external radiation exposure and children who received radioiodine therapy, it appears that children are about two times as susceptible as adults to the induction of benign neoplasms of the thyroid. Children and adults appear to be equally susceptible to the induction of cancer from ^{131}I, mixed radioiodines, and external radiation. Using the above assumption, the absolute individual risk for adults exposed to external radiation has been reported to be 4.4 and 8.4 per million persons per rem per year for cancer and for total nodules, respectively. The absolute risk for children has been reported as 4.3 and 12.4 per million persons per rem per year for thyroid cancer and for total nodules, respectively (WASH-1400, 1975b; NCRP, 1977c). The NCRP (1985a) has projected for external radiation an overall lifetime incidence of fatal thyroid cancer of 7.5 cases per rad for a general population of one million persons.

Skeletal tumors have been reported at the sites of therapeutic external irradiation in some instances (BEIR, 1980). The tumors have been of both bone and cartilage. Osteosarcomas have been observed in patients 10 to 60 years of age who had received doses to bone greater than 3000 rads. The latent period following irradiation has averaged about nine years. Some fibrosarcomas and chondrosarcomas have also been observed in these patients. Other radiation-induced bone neoplasms and risk estimates are discussed more fully under the heading Internal Emitters in this chapter.

Increased incidence of mammary tumors has been observed in (1) female A-bomb survivors, (2) women who received multiple fluoroscopic examinations while receiving treatment for tuberculosis with artificial pneumothorax, and (3) women who received radiation therapy for acute postpartum mastitis. The dose to the mammary gland was estimated to be very high (>1000 rads) for those who received the fluoroscopic examination, about 200 rads for the postpartum mastitis group, and greater than 90 rem for those exposed from the atomic attack. A risk estimate of an 0.83 percent increase in the spontaneous incidence per rad has been made (BEIR Report, 1972).

An increased incidence of lung tumors has been reported in survivors of the A-bomb explosions and in the ankylosing spondylitis patients treated by radiotherapy (BEIR Report, 1972). Most of the data on radiation-induced lung cancer, however, have been accumulated from uranium miners and studies in which the radiation has been from internally deposited radionuclides rather than from exposure to external irradiation.

Epidemiologic studies have demonstrated a correlation between very low doses of x-irradiation received *in utero* and cancer incidence (MacMahon, 1962; Stewart and Kneale, 1970a, 1970b; Stewart, 1973). The studies of Mac-Mahon demonstrated an approximately 50 percent increase of all cancers in children exposed to irradiation *in utero* and that this increased incidence was present from birth to about eight years of age. In the studies of Stewart and Kneale, the effect appeared to last through the ten years of observation. The data from these studies have been disputed on various grounds and appear to be in contrast to the ABCC studies in which no excess cancers in children exposed *in utero* have been observed (BEIR Report, 1972; NCRP, 1977b).

Contradictory reports have been published on the effects of radiation on a large population of individuals who were employed at a major facility of the U.S. Atomic Energy Commission (later to become the U.S. Energy Research and Development Administration and yet later the U.S. Department of Energy). Mancuso *et al.* (1977) and Kneale *et al.* (1981, 1982) reported an excess of cancer associated with low-level irradiation of workers. They noted cancer of bone marrow, pancreas, and lung as being definitely radiation associated. An independent analysis of data on workers at the same plant was reported by Marks *et al.* (1978). They concluded that cancer mortality rates at the plant were well below natural rates and that overall cancer mortality was not correlated with the level of worker exposure to radiation. A significant correlation with level of exposure was demonstrated for only two cancer types, multiple myeloma and cancer of the pancreas, but the authors were reserved in the interpretation of those results because of the few deaths involved and the failure to demonstrate a similar relationship for myelogenous leukemia in this population (Marks *et al.*, 1978; Gilbert and Marks, 1979; Hutchinson *et al.*, 1979; Mole, 1982).

In summary, there is no reason to doubt that irradiation is carcinogenic. There is still a great deal of controversy on the magnitude of the risk following exposure to low and very low doses of irradiation.

Genetic Effects

Ionizing radiation produces gene mutations and chromosome aberrations. Mutated germ cells (genetic mutation) involved in the production of new organisms have been shown to result in offspring that may be abnormal in various ways and to various degrees.

Mutations from ionizing radiation are not different from "spontaneous" mutations or those produced by other mutagens. Most evidence indicates, however, that any increase in the genetic mutation rate will be harmful on a long-term basis, thereby causing a concern for any agent that will increase the spontaneous mutation rate (BEIR, 1980). Owing to the complexity of genetic damage and the time necessary for expression of the eventual genetic effect on future generations, little is known about the induction of genetic mutations by radiation in humans. Most of the information on the genetic effects of irradiation is derived from experiments with the fruit fly (*Drosophila melanogaster*) and mouse.

Point or gene mutations are those produced without visible changes in the chromosomes and which behave as changes in a single gene. They involve changes in the molecular structure of the gene. These mutations may be dominant, recessive, or sex-linked recessive. Recessive mutations may require numerous generations prior to their expression. Most of the conclusions regarding radiation-induced mutations of this type are based on the studies of Russell (1971) in mice using the specific locus method.

In a large series of experiments, Russell examined the effect of the radiation dose rate by the specific locus method by exposing large groups of mice to 90, 9, 0.8, 0.009, and 0.001 R/min for prolonged periods. The data from these studies suggest that in the mouse spermatogonia mutations increase essentially linearly with dose and with no threshold for mutation. Dose rates of 0.8 and 0.009 R/min, however, showed significantly fewer specific locus mutations in spermatogonia than a dose rate of 90 R/min, but a dose rate of 0.001 R/min did not reduce the mutational frequency significantly from that observed at 0.009 R/min. A dose rate of 9 R/min was intermediate between 90 and 0.8 R/min (Russell, 1971). The slope of the response for the low dose-rate exposures was about 0.3 of that for the high dose-rate exposures. For females, the effect of dose rate was even more dramatic with no leveling out of the dose-rate effect as was observed in males. Russell has hypothesized that these results can be explained by the repair of mutational or premutational damage, but the repair process is either damaged or saturated at high doses and high dose rates.

As indicated previously, ionizing radiation can produce chromosome aberrations in both somatic and germ cells. These aberrations are produced by the breakage of chromosomes.

Many of these will rejoin leaving no visible effect in the cell. Others may fail to rejoin or rejoin in abnormal configurations leaving deletions, duplications, inversions, or translocations. Many of these chromosome aberrations result in cell death at the time of cell division. In the case of germ cells, some of these chromosome aberrations may be passed to offspring. Errors in chromosome distribution may result in individuals with too many or too few chromosomes, producing such abnormalities as mongolism, a condition in which individuals have an extra representative of a specific chromosome. This type of genetic error has not been associated with radiation exposure. The most frequent radiation-induced chromosomal aberration in the mouse is constituted by reciprocal translocations. These result in excess or deficiency in genetic material, which results in early embryonic death (abortions) or physical and mental abnormalities. Radiation-induced chromosome aberrations and point mutations have been extensively reviewed in recent reports (BEIR, 1980; UNSCEAR, 1982). The estimated risk to humans from chronic radiation exposure at low doses is a doubling dose between 50 and 250 rem (BEIR Report, 1980).

INTERNAL EMITTERS

Radioactive materials that gain entry to the body are typically called "internal emitters." Their toxicity depends on the temporal and spatial dimensions of the radiation dose pattern that results from their internal deposition. The temporal and spatial aspects of the radiation dose pattern are governed by both the physical and chemical characteristics of the element, which influence its distribution within the body and its retention. In addition, the temporal dimensions of the radiation dose pattern are influenced by the physical half-life of the radioactive material as contrasted to the biologic half-life, which is the retention half-time corrected for physical decay. The retention half-time, which includes both physical and biologic half-times, is referred to as the effective half-life. Besides the retention and distribution kinetics of the radioactive material, the radiation dose pattern is a function of the radiation emissions of the material, i.e., alpha or beta particles or gamma rays.

The basic concepts related to the temporal aspects of the radiation dose pattern are illustrated in Figure 21–4. Curve A represents the physical decay of a radioactive source similar to the material injected into the subject. Note that when plotted on a logarithmic scale as a function of time, a straight line is obtained indicating that

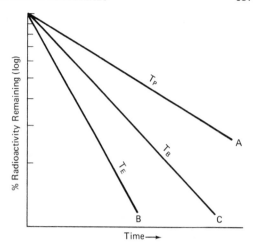

Figure 21–4. Idealized curves illustrating the relationships between physical decay (T_P), effective half-life (T_E), and biological half-life (T_B) of an internally deposited radionuclide.

the fraction of material decaying per unit time is constant, i.e., an exponential rate of loss. This rate of loss is characteristic of the radionuclide and is called the physical half-life. Curve B represents an idealized, single-component, exponential function for whole-body retention of a radionuclide following intravenous injection. Under these conditions, it is also represented as a straight line on semilogarithmic paper. Note that the slope is steeper and thus the rate of loss greater for curve B than curve A. This occurs because the overall rate of loss from the body is a function of both the physical half-life of the radionuclide (illustrated in curve A) and the biologic half-life of the element and is referred to as the effective half-life. If the effective half-life (illustrated by curve B) is corrected for the physical rate of decay, the remaining rate of loss reflects biologic loss and the resultant curve (curve C) is the biologic half-life of the element. The physical, biologic, and effective half-lives are related by the following equation:

$$T_B = \frac{T_E T_P}{T_E + T_P}$$

The basic concepts related to the spatial dimension of radiation dose can be illustrated by considering a radionuclide such as ^{131}I that deposits primarily in thyroid and ^{137}Cs that distributes throughout the body. Obviously decay of ^{131}I results in energy deposition in the thyroid with minimal radiation exposure of other tissues, whereas decay of the ^{137}Cs results in energy deposition throughout the body.

The average alpha or beta radiation dose and rate at any time (t) in days following internal deposition of a radionuclide with a known initial concentration of Co (μCi/g) in the specific tissue may be calculated as follows:

$$\begin{aligned}\text{Dose rate} \atop \text{(rads/day)} &= C(t)\,\frac{\mu\text{Ci}}{g} \times \overline{E}\,\frac{\text{Mev}}{\text{dis}} \times \frac{2.2 \times 10^6 \text{ dis}}{\text{min } \mu\text{Ci}} \\ &\times \frac{60 \text{ min}}{\text{hr}} \times \frac{24 \text{ hr}}{\text{day}} \times \frac{10^6 \text{ ev}}{\text{MeV}} \\ &\times \frac{1.6 \times 10^{-12} \text{ ergs}}{\text{ev}} \times \frac{1 \text{ g rad}}{10^2 \text{ ergs}} \times f\end{aligned}$$

or

$$\frac{\text{Dose rate}}{\text{(rads/day)}} = 51.2 C(t)\overline{E}f$$

and

$$\text{Cumulative dose} = 51.2\overline{E}f \int_0^t C(t)\,dt$$

where

$C(t) = \text{Co } e^{-0.693/T_E}$
$\overline{E}$ = average beta energy or E = alpha energy (Mev)
f = fraction of emitted energy deposited in tissue of interest
T_E = effective half-life in days for the radionuclide in the tissue of interest

Complete discussions of radiation dosimetry are available (Hine and Brownell, 1956; Attix and Roesch, 1966, 1968; Lovell, 1979). It should be noted that in most cases the quantity of radioactivity present, the tissue weight, and the absorbed fraction of the beta energy are the main uncertainties in the calculation of the dose. For gamma-emitting radionuclides, the quantity of radioactivity present can frequently be measured externally with appropriate detectors and calibration or by removal and radioactive counting of individual tissues. The situation is more complex for beta- and alpha-emitting radionuclides where the amount of radioactivity can be estimated by external counting only with sophisticated techniques that measure low-energy secondary emissions of photons. Typically, accurate tissue burden measurements of alpha- and beta-emitting radionuclides can be made by radioanalysis of the specific tissues frequently after chemical separation of the radioactive element of interest. Estimation of tissue weight is often uncertain at best. An extensive compilation of data on the mass, dimensions, and elemental composition as well as other key biologic data on humans has been published (ICRP, 1975). For gamma-emitting radionuclides the situation is considerably more complex since radioactivity deposited in one tissue serves as a source of radiation not only for that tissue but to a varying degree for other tissues dependent upon the spatial relationships of the tissues and the gamma energy of the photons. The subject has been covered in very understandable fashion in the MIRD handbooks (1968; 1969a; 1969b; 1971; 1975a; 1975b).

From the equation above it is seen that the radiation dose is a function of (1) the effective retention half-time, (2) the energy released in the tissue, (3) the amount of radioactivity initially introduced, and (4) the mass of the organ. A lower radiation dose will result if the effective retention half-life is shorter, the energy released in the tissue is lower, the amount introduced is smaller, or the mass of the tissue is larger, all other factors being equal. Although these considerations are straightforward, they may be overlooked, for example, in the case of the individual who argues that the effect of 10 μCi of ^{131}I in the rat and human must be similar, neglecting the large difference in the mass of the thyroid in the rat and human and thus differences in radiation dose from identical amounts of radioactivity in the two species.

The dose pattern for radioactive materials in the body may be strongly influenced by the route of entry of the material. For industrial workers, inhalation of radioactive particles with pulmonary deposition and puncture wounds with subcutaneous deposition have been the most frequent. The general population has been exposed via ingestion of low levels of naturally occurring radionuclides as well as man-produced radionuclides from nuclear weapons testing and nuclear power operations. Further, the potential exists for catastrophic nuclear accident situations in which members of the general population might be exposed by inhalation.

Routes of Entry

Since there are certain features common to the various modes of entry, irrespective of the radionuclide, the two most important routes of entry, ingestion and inhalation, will be considered in some detail.

Ingestion. Ingestion of radioactive materials is most likely to occur with contaminated foodstuff or water. Ingestion of radioactive material may result in toxic effects as a result of either absorption of the radionuclide or irradiation of the gastrointestinal tract during passage through the tract, or a combination of both. The fraction of a radioactive material absorbed from the gastrointestinal tract is variable, depending on the specific element, the physical and chemical form of the material ingested, and the diet. For example, ^{137}Cs is almost totally absorbed from the gastrointestinal tract (Furchner *et al.,* 1964) whereas [144]Ce is very poorly absorbed (McClellan *et al.,* 1965). The absorption of some elements is influenced by age with higher absorption in the very young. Ballou and coworkers (1962) noted this for [239]Pu and McClellan (1964) observed this for both [45]Ca and [90]Sr. The influence of diet is particularly apparent for essential minerals, trace elements, and related elements. For example, ^{90}Sr and [45]Ca fractional absorption was decreased in the presence of increased levels of Ca and PO_4 in the diet (Thompson and Palmer, 1960; Palmer and Thompson, 1964).

Most studies of radionuclide uptake from the gastrointestinal tract have utilized "spiked" food or relatively pure chemical forms given by gavage. The applicability of such studies may be questioned based on studies of radionuclide uptake from "spiked" diets compared to studies utilizing diets formulated with plants that had incorporated radionuclides. For ^{99m}Tc, plant incorporation reduced gastrointestinal uptake by a factor of 3 to 5, while for [239]Pu it increased uptake by two- to fourfold (Sullivan *et al.,* 1979).

Eve (1966) has reviewed the physiology of the gastrointestinal tract in relation to radiation doses from radioactive materials. The gastrointestinal tract is viewed as four compartments with the characteristics noted in Table 21–5.

Eve defined the occupancy factor as the fraction of 24 hours during which a section of the gastrointestinal tract is full of food residue. Based on Eve's review, Dolphin and Eve (1966) derived equations for the dosimetry of the gastrointestinal tract following oral intake of radioactive material. Beyond having utility for calculating the radiation dose to the gastrointestinal tract from ingested radionuclides, their work is useful in considering the "dose" to the gastrointestinal tract from ingested nonradioactive toxic materials. Such an approach may be of assistance in relating the pathogenesis of certain diseases of the gastrointestinal tract, such as cancer of the colon, to poorly absorbed toxic materials ingested in small quantities.

Early studies indicated that the damage to

crypt cells of the intestine was responsible for early "gastrointestinal" deaths. The critical importance of such information was emphasized by the Rasmussen (WASH-1400, 1975) Study Report on the consequences of reactor accidents, which indicated the importance of ingestion and gastrointestinal tract irradiation in determining early morbidity and mortality following a catastrophic accident with release of massive quantities of fission products. Stimulated by the Rasmussen study, Sullivan *et al.* (1978) critically examined the dosimetry and effects of ingestion of fission products, radionuclides of varied beta decay energy, by rats or dogs. Their studies verified that damage to the crypt cells was responsible for death. Their work emphasized the importance of estimating the radiation dose to the crypt cells.

Inhalation. The inhalation mode of exposure has long been recognized as being of major importance for both nonradioactive and radioactive materials. This recognition has led to substantial research on the toxicity of inhaled radionuclides, research that has already yielded significant improvement in our general understanding of inhalation toxicology. A report from a Task Group of the International Commission on Radiological Protection (ICRP, 1966a) provides an excellent overview of our understanding of the deposition and retention of inhaled particles in the respiratory tract. An updated view of this report and other more recent work in the area is presented in a report by the International Atomic Energy Agency Panel on "Inhalation Hazards from Radioactive Contaminants" (IAEA, 1973). In both reports, the respiratory tract is viewed as consisting of three basic compartments: (1) the nasopharynx, (2) the tracheobronchial compartment, and (3) the pulmonary compartment (Figure 21–5). The nasopharynx (NP) begins with the anterior nares and extends to the level of the larynx or epiglottis. The tracheobronchial (TB) compartment consists of the trachea and bronchial tree including terminal bronchioles. The pulmonary compartment (P) consists of the more distal portions

Table 21–5. CHARACTERISTICS OF THE GASTROINTESTINAL TRACT OF HUMANS*

PORTION	MASS OF CONTENTS (g)	TIME FOOD REMAINS (hr)	OCCUPANCY FACTOR	EFFECTIVE RADIUS (cm)
Stomach	250	1	6/24	10
Small intestine	400	4	14/24	10
Upper large intestine	220	13	18/24	5
Lower large intestine	135	24	22/24	5

* From Eve, I. S.: A review of the physiology of the gastrointestinal tract in relation to radiation doses from radioactive materials. *Health Phys.,* **12**:131–61, 1966.

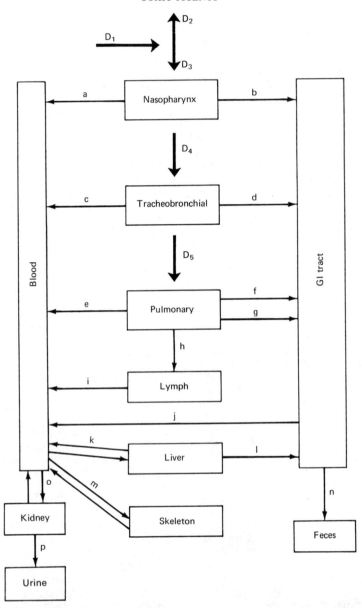

Figure 21–5. Schematic portrayal of deposition sites and clearance processes of the respiratory tract. D_1, total activity inhaled; D_2, the activity in the exhaled air; D_3, activity deposited in nasopharynx as a percentage of D_1; D_4, activity deposited in the tracheobronchial compartment as a percentage of D_1; and D_5, activity deposited in the pulmonary compartment as a percentage of D_1; a through i represent specific clearance and translocation processes (see text). (From International Commission on Radiological Protection [Task Group on Lung Dynamics]: Deposition and retention models for internal dosimetry of the human respiratory tract. *Health Phys.*, **12**:173–207, 1966.)

of the lung, which are involved in functional gas exchange. To consider the toxicity of inhaled materials in the context of the total animal, other compartments should be included: pulmonary lymph nodes, gastrointestinal tract, blood, and tissue compartments such as skeleton, liver, and kidneys.

Using Figure 21–5 as a guide, it is appropriate to consider in some detail the deposition of inhaled particles. The Task Group used the notations D_1 through D_5, where D_1 was the activity inhaled, D_2 the activity in the exhaled air, D_3 the activity deposited in NP as a percentage of D_1, D_4 the activity deposited in TB as a percentage of D_1, and D_5 the activity deposited in P as a percentage of D_1. Deposition, defined as the process that accounts for the amount of inhaled or inspired material that remains after expiration, is accomplished by (1) inertial impaction, (2) gravitational settling, and (3) diffusion by brownian movement. Inertial impaction is greatest for particles 5 μm and larger in diameter and occurs primarily in the NP and TB compartments. Gravitational settling, involving particles in the range of 0.5 to 5 μm, is of some significance in the NP and TB compartments but is even more significant in the P compartment. Diffusion, involving particles smaller than about 0.5 μm, is of great significance for deposition in the P compartment and, for very small particles, may be the process by which large quantities of activity are deposited in the NP compartment.

In recent years, increased use has been made of the concept of "equivalent aerodynamic diameter" in considering the deposition of inhaled particles. This parameter may be defined as the diameter of a unit density sphere having the same settling velocity as the particle in question regardless of shape (but crudely spheric) and density (IAEA, 1973). This approach is realistic when considering deposition in that it recognizes that the aerodynamic size of the particle is more significant than the real size. Adoption of this concept, in its fullest sense, requires one to use inertial air-sampling devices such as the cascade impacter to separate particles according to their aerodynamic size as contrasted to many sampling devices such as large filters that collect all of the particles in the air irrespective of particle size.

Figure 21–5 may again be used in considering the retention of inhaled material remaining in the respiratory tract at any time. Retention is a function of clearance and translocation, clearance being the transport of material out of the respiratory tract, and translocation, the absorption and movement of material to other tissues. The letters (a) through (i) in Figure 21–5 represent specific clearance and translocation processes associated with clearance of various compartments as established by the ICRP Task Group. Specifically*

(a) represents the rapid uptake of material deposited in the nasopharynx directly into the systemic blood;
(b) represents the rapid clearance of all dusts

from the nasopharynx by ciliary-mucus transport;

(c) represents the rapid absorption of dust deposited in the TB compartment into the systemic circulation;

(d) is analogous to (b) and represents the rapid ciliary clearance of TB; the dust cleared by (d) goes quantitatively to the GI tract;

(e) represents the direct translocation of dust from the pulmonary region to the blood;

(f) represents the relatively rapid clearance of the pulmonary region, which presumably depends on recruitable macrophages, and this, in turn, is coupled to the ciliary-mucus transport process. Therefore, the dust cleared by (f) goes to the GI tract via the tracheobronchial tree;

(g) is a secondary pulmonary clearance process, which is typically much slower than (f) but still depends on endocytosis and ciliary-mucus transport and the cleared dust goes via TB to the GI tract; the important distinction is that the clearance is apparently rate limited in the pulmonary region by the nature of the deposited dust, per se;

(h) is a process describing the slow removal of dust from the pulmonary compartment via the lymphatic system; we can regard this process as qualitatively similar to (g) with the exception that lymph transport replaces the ciliary-mucus transport;

(i) represents a secondary pathway in which dust cleared by the lymphatic system (h) is introduced into the systemic blood; this pathway obviously depends on the ability of the cleared material to penetrate the lymph tissue, especially the lymph nodes; this implies dissolution of the dust particles, partially or completely, but the turnover of lymphocytes may contribute (Stohlman, 1959);

(j) represents the process by which material in the gastrointestinal tract from processes (b), (d), (f), and (g) reaches the bloodstream. This process is closely related to the gastrointestinal tract considerations of Eve (1966) and Dolphin and Eve (1966) noted earlier.

In considering the clearance of materials from the respiratory tract, the ICRP Task Group found it appropriate to group elements into three categories; class D, expected to exhibit maximal clearance half-times of less than one day; class W, representing material with maximal clearance half-times of a few days to a few months; and class Y, for materials expected to manifest maximal biologic half-times to six months to several years. The following examples serve to illustrate this classification: class D, cesium chloride; class W, lanthanide carbonates, calcium sulfate; and class Y, lanthanide and acti-

---

* International Commission on Radiological Protection (Task Group on Lung Dynamics); Deposition and retention models for internal dosimetry of the human respiratory tract. *Health Phys.*, **12**:173–207, 1966.

nide oxides. For each class, the Task Group suggested constants for use in the clearance model (Table 21–6).

The Task Group report established the importance of particle solubility in determining long-term pulmonary retention, a concept that was emphasized by Mercer (1967). More recent research (Kanapilly, 1977) has indicated the complex nature of particle dissolution phenomena with differences in dissolution rate ascribed to the chemical and physical characteristics of the particles. The surface area of the particles is of special importance.

The biologic effects of inhaled radionuclides have been reviewed by the ICRP (1980). In the following section the effects of inhalation of several important radionuclides will be discussed.

Specific Radionuclides

Because the toxicity of internally deposited radionuclides is very radionuclide specific, it is appropriate to provide a limited summary on several of the more significant radionuclides. The presentation will be directed toward covering the more important aspects of the radionuclide, element, or group of elements, hopefully providing a base for the interested reader to explore other more detailed references (Stannard, 1973; ICRP, 1979; McClellan, 1982).

Alkaline Earth Elements. The metabolic behavior of the alkaline earth elements has recently been reviewed (Marshall *et al.*, 1973). Two alkaline earth elements are of particular interest: radium and strontium. Probably more is known about the late effects in humans of ^{226}Ra

than any other radionuclide. This large body of knowledge has been and is still being derived from the study of individuals (radium dial painters and chemists) involved in the luminous dial industry that flourished in the early 1900s as well as individuals that received radium as therapeutic nostrums. The radium dial painters were largely young women who used luminous paints containing ^{226}Ra and, as a consequence of an early industrial practice of "tipping" the brush on their lips, ingested significant quantities of ^{226}Ra (Cloutier, 1980). Because radium is a metabolic analog of calcium it is deposited in the skeleton. Within the skeleton, a portion is deposited uniformly in the mineral while the remainder is deposited in "hot spots" corresponding to the areas of very active mineral accretion at the time of radium intake. The ^{226}Ra retained in the skeleton serves as a source of alpha radiation of bone and contiguous tissues at a dose rate that decreases slowly with time.

Pioneering studies at Massachusetts Institute of Technology under the leadership of R. D. Evans and at Argonne Cancer Research Hospital and Argonne National Laboratory by A. J. Finkel, R. J. Hasterlik, and C. E. Miller have clearly established that radium induces osteosarcomas of the skeleton and carcinomas of the mastoid and paranasal air sinuses (Evans, 1981). In general, the lower the burden of radium, the later and less frequent the appearance of a malignant tumor and subsequent death of the subject. These results led Evans and his associates (1969) to suggest the existence of a "practical threshold" of dose, below which the

**Table 21–6.   AMENDED CONSTANTS FOR USE WITH
CLEARANCE MODEL*†**

		CLASS (D)	CLASS (W)	CLASS (Y)
N-P	(a)	0.01 d/0.5‡	0.01 d/0.10	0.01 d/0.01
	(b)	0.01 d/0.5	0.40 d/0.90	0.40 d/0.99
T-B	(c)	0.01 d/0.95	0.01 d/0.50	0.01 d/0.01
	(d)	0.20 d/0.05	0.20 d/0.50	0.2 d/0.99
P	(e)	0.5 d/0.80	50 d/0.15	500 d/0.05
	(f)	n.a.	1 d/0.40	1 d/0.40
	(g)	n.a.	50 d/0.40	500 d/0.40
	(h)	0.5 d/0.20	50 d/0.05	500 d/0.15
Lymph	(i)	0.5 d/1.00	50 d/1.00	1000 d/0.90

* From International Commission on Radiological Protection: *The Metabolism of Compounds of Plutonium and Other Actinides.* ICRP Publication No. 19, Pergamon Press, Oxford, 1972, as amended from the International Commission on Radiological Protection (Task Group on Lung Dynamics): Deposition and retention models for internal dosimetry of the human respiratory tract. *Health Phys.,* **12**:173–207, 1966.

† For pulmonary clearance purposes, the radionuclides are classified into three classes: Y for avid retention, W for moderate retention, and D for minimal retention.

‡ The first value is the biologic half-life; the second is the regional fraction. The lymphatic clearance for class Y compounds indicates that a 90 percent regional fraction follows a 1000-day biologic half-life. The remaining 10 percent is presumed to be permanently retained in the nodes and is subject only to radioactive decay.

required tumor appearance time generally exceeds the life-span, and hence radiation-induced tumors appear with negligible frequency.

The follow-up of over 3000 radium-exposed individuals has now been consolidated at the Argonne National Laboratory and we hope it will be continued through the lifetime of the exposed individuals.

Rowland *et al.* (1983) have recently summarized the incidence of bone sarcoma among 3055 female radium-dial workers who entered the industry before 1950. They analyzed two subpopulations. The first included all cases that survived five years after the start of employment. It contained 1468 women who experienced 42 bone sarcomas compared to 0.4 expected. The second subpopulation included all cases who survived at least two years after measurement of their body burden. It contained 1257 women who experienced 13 bone sarcomas compared to 0.2 expected.

A linear-quadratic-exponential (LQE) dose-response function, $I = (C + \alpha D + \beta D^2)e^{-\gamma D}$, and simplifications of this general form were fit to the data. The incidence (I) is in units of bone sarcoma per person-year of risk, C is the expected number of naturally occurring bone sarcoma cases per person-year in the group, and D is a measure of intake, the quantity of radium in μCi that entered the blood during the exposure period. Two functions, $I = (C + \alpha D + \beta D^2)e^{-\gamma D}$ and $I = (C + \beta D^2)e^{-\gamma D}$ fit the data for the year of entry subpopulation ($p \geq 0.05$). Both these functions and $I = C + \alpha D$ fit the data for the first measurement subpopulation.

At high levels of intake, radium induced an excess incidence of bone sarcomas with the minimum induction period appearing to be independent of intake level and an inverse relationship existing between the maximum induction period and systemic intake. No bone sarcomas were observed among 1680 measured cases with systemic intakes less than 50 μCi indicating the low probability of bone sarcoma induction with small to moderate intakes of radium. The analysis based on first exposure to radium could only be fit with a linear relationship between intake and effect when the intake ranges were appropriately selected.

A dose-squared exponential function appeared to be the best dose-response function. An LQE function was a valid description of the actual relationship between dose and response; however, the data set only provided an upper limit for the coefficient of the linear term with $\alpha = 1.3 \times 10^{-5}$ bone sarcoma per person-year μCi. The analysis based on symptom-free first analysis also suggested a dose-squared exponential relationship between intake and effect, but it

did not eliminate the possibility of a linear relationship.

Rowland *et al.* (1983) note the markedly different results obtained at low intakes for the dose-squared and LQE functions. They use as an example an intake equal to the 5 pci/l standard or 843 pci of ^{226}Ra per year, proposed by the U.S. Environmental Protection Agency. The LQE function after a one-year intake with $\alpha = 0$ would predict a lifetime risk from radium of 5×10^{14} bone sarcomas/person-year, which with $\alpha = 1.3 \times 10^{-5}$ the prediction is 1×10^{-8} bone sarcomas/person-year, a factor of 2×10^5 greater. Even if the population at risk were equal to the U.S. population, neither of the induced rates could be distinguished from the natural incidence, which for adults is about 10^{-5} bone sarcomas/person-year.

A second nuclide of radium, ^{224}Ra, which is an alpha emitter with a half life of 3.6 days, has been used in Europe since 1946 to treat various disorders such as ankylosing spondylitis. An excess of malignant bone cancer has been observed in the ^{224}Ra-treated individuals (Wick and Gössner, 1983). The ^{224}Ra deposits primarily on bone surfaces and, because of its short half-life, decays there. Thus, these cases are of particular interest since it is felt they may give some insight into the dose-response relationships for ^{239}Pu, which deposits primarily on bone surfaces as will be discussed later.

The extensive body of data available on radium toxicity in humans is one of the major sources of information for developing radiation protection standards for irradiation of the skeleton. To extend this database to other radionuclides that may be encountered by humans, numerous laboratory animal studies have been conducted comparing the disposition, dosimetry, and effects of radium and other radionuclides. The results of these studies are summarized in several symposia (Jee, 1976; NCRP, 1982; Rundo *et al.*, 1983; Gössner *et al.*, 1986).

A second alkaline earth element, strontium, is of major interest related to the abundance of ^{90}Sr in the fission products of nuclear weapon detonations and in the fuel cycle of nuclear power reactors. Because of early concern related to its presence in nuclear weapons fallout, the toxicity of ^{90}Sr has been extensively studied in mice, rats, beagle dogs, and miniature swine with much of the resultant information summarized at several symposia (McClellan and Jones, 1969; Lenihan *et al.*, 1967; Goldman and Bustad, 1972). The basic findings have been that strontium, as a metabolic analog of calcium, is readily absorbed from the gastrointestinal tract or the lung into the bloodstream and is subsequently deposited in bone. A single brief intake orally, intravenously, or by inhalation results in a high incidence of neoplasia of bone and bone-related tissues. The most frequently observed neoplasms have been osteosarcoma, hemangiosarcoma, fibrosarcoma, and epidermoid carcinomas. Chronic ingestion of ^{90}Sr in beagle dogs and miniature swine produced a high incidence of myeloproliferative disease, including frank leukemia, at the highest levels of ^{90}Sr intake, a finding that contrasts sharply with a lack of a similar high incidence with single acute intake of ^{90}Sr. Chronic ^{90}Sr intake resulted in only a few bone tumors in miniature swine while a high incidence was observed in beagle dogs. Mays and Lloyd (1972a) have reviewed ^{90}Sr experimental animal and ^{226}Ra human data and developed estimates of the human bone sarcoma risk from ^{90}Sr. They found that the data did not support a linear dose-response relationship over a wide dose range and that at low levels the data were fit well by practical threshold or sigmoid dose-response relationships. Their best cumulative 50-year risks below 1000 rads from ^{90}Sr were 1 ± 1 sarcomas/10^6 person rads for a low-dose linear model and 4 ± 4 sarcomas/10^{10} person rads^2 for a dose-squared model.

Iodine. The toxicity of radioiodine, particularly ^{131}I, has received considerable attention related to its widespread use in nuclear medicine applications and its abundance in the inventory of an operating reactor and in nuclear weapons fallout (Book *et al.*, 1986). Radioiodine, irrespective of the route of administration, is rapidly absorbed into the bloodstream and concentrated in the thyroid. High levels of ^{131}I result in virtually complete destruction of the thyroid with an associated decrease in thyroid hormone production. Levels of ^{131}I that damage thyroid but leave some tissue capable of proliferative response lead to hyperplasia, adenomas, and thyroid carcinomas.

The subject of the risk of thyroid neoplasia from radioiodine has been reviewed (WASH-1400, 1975; NCRP, 1977c; NCRP, 1985). The risk of both benign and malignant nodules of the thyroid following ^{131}I exposure appears to be $\frac{1}{10}$ to $\frac{1}{60}$ on a per rad basis of that from external radiation based on the results of both human epidemiologic studies and animal studies. This difference may be related to the low-energy beta emission of ^{131}I and its nonuniform distribution in the gland. Based on the human epidemiologic data, the estimated absolute risks for children for thyroid nodules is 0.064 and 0.023 per million persons per rem per year for thyroid cancers and total nodules, respectively. Based on the results of the Marshall Islanders exposed to mixed external radiation and radioiodine and on children who received ^{131}I therapy, children appear to be

about twice as susceptible as adults to the induction of benign neoplasms, but about equal to adults in the susceptibility to the induction of cancer.

The National Council on Radiation Protection and Measurements has recently provided guidance on the protection of the thyroid gland in the event of release of radioiodine (NCRP, 1977c). For situations that might result in exposures above 10 rads to the thyroid, consideration should be given to the use of potassium iodide as a blocking agent to minimize the dose to the thyroid.

Alkali Metals. Of the alkali metal elements, ^{137}Cs is of greatest interest because of its long physical half-life, 30 years, and its abundance as a fission product in nuclear weapons fallout and in the inventory of a nuclear reactor or a fuel-reprocessing plant. Dispositionally, ^{137}Cs behaves as an analog of potassium. Irrespective of the mode of administration, it is rapidly absorbed into the bloodstream and distributes throughout the active tissues of the body. Its distribution throughout the body and the energetic beta and gamma radiation from the decay of ^{137}Cs and its daughter, ^{137}Ba, result in essentially whole-body irradiation (Boecker, 1972). Thus, when large quantities of ^{137}Cs are injected, it is not surprising that acute toxicity with death related primarily to bone marrow destruction is observed, similar to the effects of exposure to high doses of gamma or x-irradiation (Redman *et al.*, 1972). Single acute intakes of lower levels of ^{137}Cs in beagle dogs appear to result in life shortening related to development of neoplasia late in life (Norris *et al.*, 1966). A recent report provides detailed information on the disposition and dosimetry of ^{137}Cs (NCRP, 1977a).

Lanthanides. A number of lanthanide elements have radionuclides that are produced abundantly in nuclear reactors or in the detonation of nuclear weapons. ^{144}Ce is of particular interest because of its relatively long physical half-life, 285 days, and the energetic beta emissions from it and its daughter, ^{144}Pr. The physical, chemical, and biologic properties of radiocerium relative to radiation protection guidelines have recently been summarized (NCRP, 1978d). ^{144}Ce is poorly absorbed from the gastrointestinal tract. Its toxicity following inhalation is of special interest since it may be considered as typical of beta-emitting radionuclides. When inhaled as ^{144}CeCl$_3$ by beagle dogs, ^{144}Ce has an effective retention half-time in lung measured in days and weeks with translocation to liver and skeleton such that, by 64 days after a single brief inhalation exposure, liver and skeleton retain 47 and 37 percent, respectively, of the total ^{144}Ce retained in the body (Boecker and Cuddihy, 1974). The morbidity and mortality from ^{144}CeCl$_3$ inhaled in graded activity levels by beagle dogs have been well characterized to over 2000 days after ^{144}Ce exposure (Benjamin et al., 1973, 1975; Jones et al., 1974). At the highest activity levels, deaths were observed in less than 40 days due to bone marrow aplasia. At slightly lower levels, with survival times of less than 1000 days, the primary causes of death were radiation pneumonitis, hepatic necrosis, and bone marrow aplasia. At generally lower levels and at 799 days or more after ^{144}Ce exposure, deaths were primarily due to myelogenous leukemia or neoplasms of the liver or skeleton.

When ^{144}Ce is inhaled in a more insoluble form, in fused clay particles, it is tenaciously retained in the lung with an effective half-life of approximately 170 days. Small quantities of the cerium, apparently still in particles, are translocated to the tracheobronchial lymph nodes while other ^{144}Ce apparently released from the particles is translocated to liver and skeleton.

Hahn et al. (1983) have reported on the effects of a single brief exposure of beagle dogs to this relatively insoluble form of ^{144}Ce, which results in chronic beta irradiation of the lung. At the highest exposure levels, dogs died within 1.5 years with radiation pneumonitis and pulmonary fibrosis. At lower levels, lung cancers were observed and the risk of lung cancer to 10 years after exposure was estimated to be 5 tumors/10^6 rads to lung. In a companion study in which beagle dogs were exposed to ^{91}Y in fused aluminosilicate particles with an effective half-life in lung of 50 days, the beta irradiation was about eight times as effective in producing lung cancer per rad to the lung. The lesser effectiveness of the ^{144}Ce was attributed to the greater protraction of the radiation dose compared to the ^{91}Y. The protracted beta irradiation of lung from ^{144}Ce was about one-twentieth as effective as alpha irradiation from ^{239}Pu in causing lung cancer. The lower carcinogenic efficiency of beta irradiation of the lung is well established and is in accord with basic radiobiologic principles (ICRP, 1980).

Other lanthanide elements have been observed to distribute similarly to cerium with deposition primarily in liver and skeleton. Durbin (1962) has reviewed the tissue distribution of the actinide and lanthanide elements and its relationship to the ionic radius of the elements. A good correlation was obtained with decreasing skeletal burden and increasing liver burden with increasing ionic radius.

Actinides. All of the actinide elements are of interest from a radiation toxicity viewpoint because they are all radioactive; however, several are of special interest in view of their abundance. The disposition of the actinides has been reviewed (ICRP, 1972; Nenot and Stather, 1979). Natural uranium (^{238}U plus small amounts of ^{235}U and ^{234}U) has been studied extensively because of its importance as the starting point for the uranium fuel cycle for nuclear reactors. In soluble forms, it is largely nephrotoxic with the effects of this very low-specific-activity material thought to be due to chemical rather than radiation effects. Long-term (5 mg U/M^3 for five days per week for five years) inhalation exposures to an insoluble form with subsequent follow-up for 6.5 years resulted in major biologic effects in the lung; in monkeys this was manifest as extensive fibrosis and in beagle dogs with epithelial proliferation, metaplasia, and pulmonary neoplasms (Leach et al., 1970).

Although the toxicity of plutonium has been of interest since its discovery, mostly because of its use in nuclear weapons, there is recent intensified interest in its toxicity as well as that of transplutonium elements such as americium and curium. This intensified interest is multifold and is related to (1) several major incidents involving nuclear weapons or nuclear weapons-related facilities, (2) the use of large quantities of ^{238}Pu as fuel in space electric power systems, and (3) the anticipated development of breeder-reactor systems that will have large inventories of plutonium and transplutonium radionuclides. A number of excellent symposia proceedings and reviews are available on the toxicity of plutonium (Mays et al., 1969; Stover and Jee, 1972; Thompson et al., 1972; Hodge et al., 1973; Bair and Thompson, 1974; Healy, 1975; Jee, 1976; Rundo et al., 1983).

When inhaled, plutonium is retained in the lung with an effective half-life that varies from hundreds of days for plutonium oxides to tens of days for more soluble forms. A significant portion of the plutonium oxide that leaves the lung is translocated to the tracheobronchial lymph nodes. Plutonium apparently solubilized within the lung is translocated to the liver and skeleton where it is very tenaciously retained (Bair et al., 1973). A classic long-term toxicity study has been performed by Bair and his associates in which the effects of inhaled plutonium oxide were studied in beagle dogs for up to ten years following inhalation exposure. At the highest levels of deposited activity, the dogs died within several hundred days with radiation pneumonitis and pulmonary fibrosis; at later times death was related to severe pulmonary fibrosis, and beyond 1000 days, although pulmonary fibrosis was still prominent, death was due to primary pulmonary neoplasia. The most common neoplasm was bronchioloalveolar carcinoma. Hahn *et al.* (1983), using data reported by Bair and Thomas (1976), calculated the risk factor for [239]Pu alpha irradiation of lung to be 600 lung tumors/10^6 rads to lung or, assuming an RBE of 20, 30 lung tumors/10^6 rem to lung.

During the 1970s public interest in the toxicity of inhaled plutonium has been aroused by concern for its continued use in nuclear weapons and the potential for use of large quantities in breeder reactors. Using current standards, the present allowable dose for lung from deposited [239]Pu is 15 rem/year. Tamplin and Cochran (1974) claimed that this was too high by a factor of 115,000 times; later they reduced this to about 1000. Their contention was based on the hypothesis that a "hot" particle of plutonium in the lung containing just an appropriate amount of radioactivity to intensely irradiate a local volume of lung tissue would be extraordinarily toxic as compared to the same amount of radioactivity distributed more uniformly throughout the lung. The contention of Tamplin and Cochran has been reviewed extensively by a number of groups (NAS, 1976; MRC, 1975; NCRP, 1975b). All have reached the conclusion that there is no unique hazard associated with inhalation of "hot" particles and that standards directed at protection against more uniform irradiation of the lungs are appropriate for use with "hot" particles.

Plutonium ([239]Pu) citrate injected intravenously deposits primarily in the skeleton, on bone surfaces, and in the liver resulting in numerous osteosarcomas and a few liver cancers. With injections as low as 0.016 μCi/kg in the beagle dog, 29 percent of the dogs developed bone cancer, with the average life-span shortened by about one year. The calculated dose to the skeleton was 55 rad to one year prior to death. Using the dog data and data from people injected with [224]Ra, Mays *et al.* (1976) estimated the cumulative risk to people for [239]Pu to be 200 bone cancers/10^6 person-rad (average skeletal dose). This was derived from a linear dose-response model; thus, it may be estimated that about 200 bone cancers would result in a population of 1,000,000 persons each receiving 1 rad to the skeleton from [239]Pu.

Several publications concerning plutonium in humans are of special interest. One by Durbin (1971) critically reviews data collected in 1945 and 1946 on humans who were injected with tracer doses of [239]Pu and compares the results with those obtained in experimental animals. Others by Hempelmann and co-workers (1973) and Voelz (1975) review the follow-up experience on humans who were accidentally exposed in World War II and had estimated burdens of 0.005 to 0.42 μCi, exclusive of lung. To date,

there have been no medical findings that can definitely be attributed to the individual's plutonium burdens.

Fewer toxicity data are available on transplutonium radionuclides such as americium and curium; however, the data that are available indicate a qualitative similarity to the toxicity of plutonium (Hodge *et al.*, 1973). McClellan and associates (1972) noted that inhaled americium and curium, even as oxides, appear more soluble than inhaled plutonium and rapidly translocated to liver and skeleton.

Radon and Radon Daughters. An occupational exposure problem of substantial magnitude that has caused problems on two continents involves miners who work underground in uranium mines. This problem was recognized many years ago in the miners in the Erz Mountains of Central Europe who had an excessive incidence of disease of the respiratory system including lung cancer. More recently, the problem has been evident in miners of the Colorado plateau region of the United States. The problem is basically related to the emanation of radon into the mines and decay of the radon with its short-lived radioactive daughters ([216]Po, [214]Pb, [214]Bi, [214]Po) attaching to dust particles, which are inhaled and result in alpha radiation exposure of the respiratory airways. A high incidence of small-cell undifferentiated type of bronchial carcinoma has been observed in the miners. The situation is complicated by recognition that most of the miners are heavy smokers, a factor whose role is uncertain (BEIR, 1980).

The BEIR Committee evaluated the risk for the uranium workers and obtained a value of 22 to 45 excess cases per million person-years per rad to the bronchial epithelium for white miners (BEIR, 1982). The U.S. population of uranium miners is still being studied very intensively and should yield additional valuable data before the lung disease incidence hopefully returns to normal in association with improved working conditions in the mines.

Although the original concern for radon and its daughters focused on uranium miners, concern has developed in the 1970s for low-level emanations from uranium mine tailings either from tailing piles or when the tailings have been inappropriately used for fill around dwellings. This latter practice has been discontinued and in some cases tailings used as fill around houses have been removed. Increased attention is being given to the maintenance of tailing piles and consideration is being given to remedial treatment of abandoned tailing piles.

Tritium. Tritium, a radioactive isotope of hydrogen (^{3}H), is formed in the upper atmosphere by interactions of cosmic rays with gases.

It is also formed in large quantities in both fission and fusion reactions and is present in effluents from nuclear reactors and weapons. Currently, the tritium present in the environment and the relative contribution of the sources have been estimated to be about 0.5 to 1 megacurie from nuclear reactors, 10 to 10^2 megacuries from natural sources, and about 10^3 megacuries from nuclear explosions (BEIR, 1972). Tritium, as tritiated water, is readily absorbed into the bloodstream from the gastrointestinal tract, skin, and lungs and distributes as body water. Any radiation effects are comparable to whole-body irradiation (Osborne, 1972; Stannard, 1973). When tritium enters the body in organic form, particularly as a label for nucleic acids, concern has been expressed over its concentration into vital structures such as DNA. Several reviews on the radiotoxicology of tritium have concluded that the use of a quality factor of 1 for tritium is justified, that for chronic environmental exposures to tritium concentration effects and transmutation effects are unimportant, and that the use of body water as the critical organ is conservative since no tissue has a higher proportion of hydrogen (Vennart, 1969; Osborne, 1972). Techniques for measurements of tritium are well developed and documented (NCRP, 1976a). Information on tritium relevant to considering its radiological implications have recently been reviewed (NCRP, 1979).

RADIATION PROTECTION STANDARDS

Biologic injury resulting from exposure to ionizing radiation was observed very soon after the discovery of radiation. Because many of the first applications of radiation were in the medical field, it is not surprising that, in at least qualitative terms, a cause-effect relationship was accepted for radiation and effects such as dermatitis. The establishment of a quantitative relationship, however, was handicapped by a lack of accurate radiation dose measurements. Nonetheless, the observed qualitative cause-effect or dose-response relationship provided a basis for instituting control procedures to limit exposure both to the field of interest of the patient and to the radiologist through the use of protective devices such as gloves and aprons and later through protection built into the x-ray machines.

The first organized step toward radiation protection occurred in 1915 at a meeting of the British Roentgen Society when a resolution was introduced calling for stringent rules to assure the personal safety of operators conducting x-ray examinations. Unfortunately, no further organized action was taken until World War I, action that was aided in part by extensive publicity associated with deaths due to aplastic anemia of individuals who had been exposed while working in the military medical corps. The activity that occurred after that war led to the organization of a number of different committees primarily under the aegis of medical and radiologic societies. The work of one of these committees led to publication of the first general set of radiation protection recommendations in the *Journal of the Roentgen Society* in 1921. Later at the First International Congress of Radiology in London in 1925 and the Second International Congress of Radiology in Stockholm in 1928, there was considerable interest in radiation protection, which led to creation of what is now the International Commission on Radiation Units (ICRU) and the International x-ray and Radium Protection Committee, the forerunner of the present-day International Commission on Radiological Protection(ICRP). As a prelude to the Second International Congress and organization of the ICRP, the Advisory Committee on x-ray and Radium Protection, later to become the National Council on Radiation Protection and Measurements (NCRP), was organized in the United States with its "home" to be the National Bureau of Standards.

During the 1920s, the concept of a tolerance dose, the amount of radiation the tissue of concern was able to tolerate, emerged. This concept centered on concern for immediate observable alterations in structure and function of the body, such as erythema of the skin. The importance of dose rate (i.e., variations in units of radiation dose per unit time) and dose fractionation (the delivery of a given radiation dose in several fractions at different times) was recognized and incorporated in the tolerance dose of 0.1 R per day adopted by the NRCP and 0.2 R per day adopted by the ICRP in 1934.

During the late 1930s, several reports were prepared by the NCRP. One of the most significant, NCRP Report No. 5 (1941), concerned the safe handling of radioactive luminous compounds. The impetus for this report derived from the growing body of information on severe or even fatal injury to radium dial painters. This report recommended that any worker who showed a deposit of more than 0.1 μg of radium change his occupation immediately. Later, this recommendation was to be a keystone in the development of standards for other radioactive materials that might be internally deposited. This value and the value of 0.1 R per day for external exposure were to provide the basis for the radiation protection practices used in the World War II Manhattan Project directed toward developing a nuclear weapon.

Within the Manhattan Project, extensive biomedical investigations on the effects of radiation from both external and internal sources were initiated and the body of knowledge on biologic effects of radiation began to increase markedly. After the conclusion of World War II, this extensive research program was continued by the newly created U.S. Atomic Energy Commission. In the years immediately after World War II the ICRP and ICRU were reactivated, their activities having understandably been interrupted by the war. At the same time, the NCRP activities were expanded and accelerated. In each case this led to a number of reports too numerous for individual citation. One of these on external exposure, NCRP Report No. 17 (1954) issued in preliminary form in 1949 and as a final report in 1954, reduced the basic Maximum Permissible Dose for radiation workers to 0.3 rem per week, a value later adopted by the ICRP (ICRP, 1959).

In the early 1950s, concern over the effects of fallout from nuclear weapons stimulated a wave of concern over radiation effects and radiation protection standards. This concern directed attention to a number of important issues including the adequacy of existing standards, their appropriateness for limiting exposure of the general population, and the adequacy of our knowledge of radiation effects especially as embodied in dose-response relationships. Not surprisingly, one response was the organization of several new committees. One of the new organizations was the United Nations Scientific Committee on the Effects of Atomic Radiation (UNSCEAR) organized in 1956, which has issued seven reports (UNSCEAR, 1958, 1962, 1964, 1966, 1972; 1977, 1982). These reports provide excellent bibliographies to the literature. Within the United States several committees on the Biological Effects of Atomic Radiation (BEAR) were organized under the aegis of the National Academy of Sciences (BEAR, 1956). A recommendation of the latter committees was a further reduction in the basic maximum permissible dose from 15 to 5 rem per year for radiation workers, a reduction stimulated by concern for genetic hazards. To provide latitude for small overdose the concept of age proration was introduced whereby the individual's total exposure was limited to 5 $(n - 18)$ rem at a given time where n is the individual's age in years (NCRP, 1957, 1958). At the same time, the principle was enunciated that radiation exposure to persons outside of a controlled area from operations within a controlled area should not exceed one-tenth the value of that for radiation workers.

In 1957, in response to public concern the Joint Committee on Atomic Energy (JCAE) of the U.S. Congress began a series of hearings addressing the question of radiation hazards. These hearings were noteworthy in calling public attention to the problem and emphasizing that radiation standards are inexact: "safe" and "unsafe" have only relative meaning and the meaning may be interpreted differently by different individuals including scientists. A question inherent in this discussion was, and continues to be, the shape of the dose-response curve; i.e., is it linear or curvilinear?

An outgrowth of the JCAE hearing was recognition that the U.S. government had no official standard-setting organization and that in fact it was, by and large, using the standards established by the NCRP and ICRP. Recognizing that there were some desirable features of having a single government agency responsible for establishing radiation standards, an Executive Order was issued in 1959 creating such an agency, the Federal Radiation Council (FRC). Within a short period of time, the FRC arrived at a set of standards essentially identical to those of the NCRP. In 1970, with organization of the Environmental Protection Agency (EPA) the activities and functions of the FRC were transferred to the EPA.

A second outgrowth of the JCAE hearing was the initiation of action to formally sever the relationships between the National Bureau of Standards and NCRP, resulting in establishment of the NCRP as an independent body. This was accomplished in 1964 when the NCRP was issued a federal charter.

During the late 1950s and the 1960s, additional reports of both a general and a specific nature were issued by the ICRP and NCRP. The most significant of these were Reports 1 and 2 of the ICRP (1959, 1960), the first covering both external and internal radiation and the second specifically considering internal radiation. Since ICRP Report No. 2 was prepared under the leadership of individuals also responsible for NCRP activities, a portion of it appeared as NCRP Report No. 22 (1959). ICRP Publication No. 9 (1966c) represents an updated and revised version of ICRP Publication No. 1 and included a discussion of the concept of risk based in large part on ICRP Publication No. 8 (1966b), which specifically addressed the evaluation of risks from radiation. ICRP Publication No. 26 (1977) provides the latest recommendations of the ICRP, recommendations that have not yet been fully adopted within the United States.

The ICRP (1977) system of radiation protection is strongly risk oriented (Lindell, 1982). It considers both stochastic and nonstochastic effects. The stochastic effects are those such as cancer and genetic damage for which no threshold has been established and the occurrence of which, in the population, although related to individual doses, is randomly distributed at equal doses. The severity of the effect is independent of dose. In contrast, nonstochastic effects are viewed as having a threshold dose, and above the threshold the disease severity such as altered function (i.e., hypothyroidism) increases with increasing dose. The ICRP system assumes proportionality between dose and the probability of stochastic effects over the dose range of interest. The ICRP uses a concept of effective dose equivalent to weigh the dose received by individual organs and assess the overall effect. To limit nonstochastic effects, the ICRP recommends an organ equivalent dose limit of 500 mSv (50 rem) in any one year for workers and one-tenth of this for the general population. An exception is the lens of the eye of workers, for which the dose limit is 150 mSv (15 rem). To limit stochastic effects in the individual, the ICRP recommends an effective dose limit of 50 mSv (5 rem) in any one year and one-tenth this level for members of the public.

The most recent major publication of the NCRP on radiation protection standards is Report No. 39 (1971)—*Basic Radiation Protection Criteria*, which updates the Council's position on basic standards. Because of their importance, the primary recommendations contained in the report are presented in Table 21–7 (NCRP (1975c) states the position of the NCRP on issues concerning basic standards that were raised by the BEIR report (1972), discussed below, and the 1972 UNSCEAR report. The NCRP (1985c) has presented general concepts and guidance for dealing with the special issue of the dosimetry and standards for internally deposited radionuclides. The NCRP has published a number of other reports generally of a more specific nature, some of which have been referenced in this chapter. One additional general report (NCRP,

Table 21–7. DOSE-LIMITING RECOMMENDATIONS OF THE NCRP*†

Maximum Permissible Dose Equivalent for Occupational Exposure

Combined whole-body occupational exposure	
Prospective annual limit—paragraphs 229, 233	5 rems in any one year
Retrospective annual limit—paragraphs 230, 233	10–15 rems in any one year
Long-term accumulation to age N years—paragraph 231	$(N - 18) \times 5$ rems
Skin—paragraphs 234, 235	15 rems in any one year
Hands—paragraphs 236, 237	75 rems in any one year (25/qtr)
Forearms—paragraphs 236, 237	30 rems in any one year (10 qtr)
Other organs, tissues, and organ systems—paragraphs 238, 239	15 rems in any one year (5 qtr)
Fertile women (with respect to fetus)—paragraphs 240, 241	0.5 rem in gestation period

Dose Limits for the Public or Occasionally Exposed Individuals

Individual or occasional—paragraphs 245, 246, 253, 254	0.5 rem in one year
Students—paragraphs 255, 256	0.1 rem in any one year

Population Dose Limits

Genetic—paragraphs 247, 248	0.17 rem average per year
Somatic—paragraphs 250, 251	0.17 rem average per year

Emergency Dose Limits—Life Saving

Individual (older than 45 years if possible)—paragraph 258	100 rems
Hands and forearms—paragraph 258	200 rems, additional (300 rems, total)

Emergency Dose Limits—Less Urgent

Individual—paragraph 259	25 rems
Hands and forearms—paragraph 259	100 rems, total

Family of Radioactive Patients

Individual (under age 45)—paragraphs 267, 268	0.5 rem in any one year
Individual (over age 45)—paragraphs 267, 268	5 rems in any one year

* From National Council on Radiation Protection and Measurements: *Basic Radiation Protection Criteria*. NCRP Report No. 39. National Council on Radiation Protection and Measurements, Washington, D.C., 1971.
† The paragraph numbers in the table refer to the text of the complete NCRP report. It is important to recognize that many of the recommendations or numbers are qualified by the information in the text, and the reader is referred to the complete report.

1976b) providing guidance for personnel working with radiation or radioactive materials will be of interest to some readers.

Before leaving the subject of radiation standards it is important to note some recent events in the area. In early 1970, a major challenge to existing standards, especially as utilized by the U.S. Atomic Energy Commission, was raised by Gofman and Tamplin who made several calculations of cancer mortality at exposure levels on the order of existing standards. A basic assumption of their calculations is that the dose-response relationship is linear at all dose levels; hence, even at very small doses, if large populations are exposed, a number of deaths may be estimated (Gofman and Tamplin, 1970; Tamplin and Gofman, 1970a, 1970b). Their charges were challenged by U.S. Atomic Energy Commission officials (Thompson and Bibb, 1970) and ultimately provided the major stimulus for an independent evaluation of the question of the effects of low levels of ionizing radiation by a committee of the NAS-NRC. That committee's report (BEIR Report, 1972) provides a valuable and well-documented review of the literature on radiation effects. The committee in 1972 specifically considered the effects of exposure of the total United States population at 5 rem per 30 years and estimated that such exposures by virtue of genetic risk would lead to an increase of 5 percent in the ill health of the population and that the somatic risk would lead to an increase of about 2 percent in the spontaneous cancer death risk, which is an increase of about 0.3 percent in the overall death rate from all causes. The committee suggested that a radiation protection guide of 0.17 rem per year was unnecessarily high.

In estimating the risk at low levels of exposure, the committee endorsed the use of a linear dose-response model for standard setting purposes. It should be kept in mind that this endorsement does not represent scientific proof of the linear model; indeed the committee noted that such scientific proof was unlikely: "Some human populations are so large that even very small linear estimates of risk, in the region of dose prescribed by current guidelines, yield finite estimates of induced cancers, i.e., deaths. These estimates of risk are beyond empirical demonstration. It is unlikely that the presence or absence of a true threshold for cancer in human populations can be proved. If the intent of authorities is to minimize the loss of life that radiation exposures may entail, they must indeed, be guided by such estimates, and will not rely on notions of a threshold" (BEIR Report, 1972). The above quote is worthy of careful consideration relative not only to radiation but to other physical and chemical agents introduced into the environment. It is obvious that the quantification of societal risks such as those made by the BEIR Committee also demands quantification of societal benefits if critical risk-benefits analyses and judgments are to be made. A recent report specifically addresses considerations in making health benefit-cost analyses for activities involving radiation exposure and alternative activities that may also have associated risks (NAS, 1977). It is likely that future standards for radiation, as well as other toxicants, will explicitly state the risk associated with the standard and approaches to balancing risk versus benefit.

REFERENCES

Attix, F. H., and Roesch, W. C.: *Radiation Dosimetry,* 2nd ed. Vol. I, *Fundamentals.* Academic Press, Inc., New York, 1968.
———: *Radiation Dosimetry,* 2nd ed. Vol. II, *Instrumentation.* Academic Press, Inc., New York, 1966.
Attix, F. H., and Tochilin, E.: *Radiation Dosimetry,* 2nd ed. Vol. III, *Sources, Fields, Measurements, and Applications.* Academic Press, Inc., New York, 1969.
Bair, W. J.; Ballou, J. E.; Park, J.; and Sanders, C. L.: Plutonium in soft tissues with emphasis on the respiratory tract. In Hodge, H. C.; Hursch, J. B.; and Stannard, J. N. (eds.): *Uranium, Plutonium and the Transuranic Elements,* Handbook of Experimental Pharmacology, Vol. 36. Springer-Verlag, New York, 1973, Chap. 11.
Bair, W. J., and Thomas, J. M.: Prediction of the health effects of inhaled transuranic elements from experimental animal data. In *Transuranium Nuclides in the Environment.* International Atomic Energy Agency, Vienna, 1976, pp. 569–85.
Bair, W. J., and Thompson, R. C.: Plutonium: biomedical research. *Science,* 183:715–22, 1974.
Ballou, J. E.; George, L. A., II; and Thompson, R. C.: The combined toxic effects of plutonium plus x-ray in rats. *Health Phys.,* 8:581–87, 1962.
Beebe, G. W.: Ionizing radiation and health. *Am. Sci.,* 70:35–44, 1982.
Beebe, G. W.; Kato, H.; and Land, C. E.: Studies of the mortality of A-bomb survivors. *Radiat. Res.,* 75:138–201, 1978.
Behrens, C. F.: Nuclear reactors and bombs: some basic considerations. In Behrens, C. F.; King, E. R.; and Carpender, J. W. J. (eds.): *Atomic Medicine,* 5th ed. Williams & Wilkins Co., Baltimore, 1969.
Behrens, C. F.; King, E. R.; and Carpender, J. W. J. (eds.): *Atomic Medicine,* 5th ed. Williams & Wilkins Co., Baltimore, 1969.
Benjamin, S. A.; Hahn, F. F.; Chiffelle, T. L.; Boecker, B. B.; Hobbs, C. H.; Jones, R. K.; McClellan, R. O.; Pickrell, J. A.; and Redman, H. C.: Neoplasia in beagle dogs after inhalation of $^{144}CeCl_3$. In Sanders, C. L., et al. (eds.): *Radionuclide Carcinogenesis.* AEC Symposium Series 29. U.S. Atomic Energy Commission, Office of Information Services, Springfield, Va., 1973.
Benjamin, S. A.; Hahn, F. F.; Chiffelle, T. L.; Boecker, B. B.; Hobbs, C. H.; Jones, R. K.; McClellan, R. O.; and Snipes, M. B.: Occurrence of hemangiosarcomas in beagles with internally deposited radionuclides. *Cancer Res.,* 35:1745–55, 1975.
Bender, M. A., and Gooch, P. C.: Types and rates of x-ray-induced chromosome aberrations in human blood

irradiated *in vitro. Proc. Natl Acad. Sci. USA*, **48**:522–32, 1962.

Biological Effects of Atomic Radiation (BEAR): *Summary Reports*. National Academy of Sciences, National Research Council, Washington, D.C., 1956.

Biological Effects of Ionizing Radiation (BEIR) Advisory Committee: *Report: The Effects of Populations of Exposure to Low Levels of Ionizing Radiation*. National Academy of Sciences, National Research Council, Washington, D.C., 1972.

Biological Effects of Ionizing Radiations (BEIR) Committee, National Academy of Science/National Research Council Report: *The Effects on Populations of Exposure to Low Levels of Ionizing Radiation*. National Academy Press, Washington, D.C., 1980.

Boecker, B. B.: Toxicity of ^{137}CsCl in the beagle: metabolism and dosimetry. *Radiat. Res.*, **50**:556–73, 1972.

Boecker, B. B., and Cuddihy, R. G.: Toxicity of ^{144}Ce inhaled as ^{144}CeCl$_3$ by the beagle dog: metabolism and dosimetry. *Radiat. Res.*, **60**:133–54, 1974.

Bond, V. P.; Cronkite, E. P.; and Conard, R. A.: Acute whole body radiation injury: pathogenesis, pre- and postradiation protection. In Behrens, C. F.; King, E. R.; and Carpender, J. W. J. (eds.): *Atomic Medicine*, 5th ed. Williams & Wilkins Co., Baltimore, 1969.

Book, S. A.; Bustad, L. K.; Soldat, J. K.; and Voilleque, P. G.: *Radioiodine: Its Industrial Hygiene and Biological Aspects*. 1986.

Brewen, J. G., and Preston, R. J.: The use of chromosome aberrations for predicting genetic hazards to man. In Nygaard, O. F.; Adler, H. I.; and Sinclair, W. K. (eds.): *Radiation Research: Biomedical, Chemical, and Physical Perspectives*. Academic Press, Inc., New York, 1975, pp. 926–36.

Casarett, A. P.: *Radiation Biology*. Prentice-Hall, Inc., Englewood Cliffs, NJ, 1968.

Casarett, G. W.: *Radiation Histopathology*, Vols. I and II. CRC Press, Boca Raton, Fl., 1980.

Cloutier, R. J.: Florence Kelley and the radium dial painters. *Health Phys.*, **39**:711–16, 1980.

Cronkite, E. P.; Bond, V. P.; and Conard, R. A.: Diagnosis and therapy of acute radiation injury. In *Atomic Medicine*, 5th ed. Williams & Wilkins Co., Baltimore, 1969.

Dolphin, G. W., and Eve, I. S.: Dosimetry of the gastrointestinal tract. *Health Phys.*, **12**:163–72, 1966.

Durbin, P. W.: Distribution of the transuranic elements in mammals. *Health Phys.*, **8**:665–71, 1962.

————: Plutonium in man: a twenty-five year review. University of California, Lawrence Radiation Laboratory Report, UCRL-20850, 1971.

Eisenbud, M.: *Environmental Radioactivity*, 2nd ed. Academic Press, Inc., New York, 1973.

Evans, R. D.: Inception of standards for internal emitters, radon and radium. *Health Phys.*, **41**:437–48, 1981.

Evans, R. D.; Harley, J. H.; Jacobi, W.; McLean, A. S.; Mills, W. A.; and Stewart, C. G.: Estimate of risk from environmental exposure to radon-222 and its decay products. *Nature*, **290**:98–100, 1981.

Eve, I. S.: A review of the physiology of the gastrointestinal tract in relation to radiation doses from radioactive materials. *Health Phys.*, **12**:131–61, 1966.

Fritz, T. E.; Norris, W. P.; Tolle, D. V.; Seed, T. M.; Poole, C. M.; Lombard, L. S.; and Doyle, D. E.: Relationship of dose rate and total dose to responses of continuously irradiated beagles. In *Late Biological Effects of Ionizing Radiation*, Vol. II. IAEA-SM-224/206, Vienna, 1978, pp. 71–82.

Fullerton, G. D.; Waggener, R. A.; Kott, D. T.; and Webster, E. W. (eds.): *Biological Risks of Medical Irradiations*. Monograph No. 5, American Institute of Physics, New York, 1980.

Furchner, J. E.; Trafton, G. A.; and Richmond, C. R.: Distribution of cesium-137 after chronic exposure in dogs and mice. *Proc. Soc. Exp. Biol. Med.*, **116**:375–78, 1964.

Garner, R. J.: *Transfer of Radioactive Materials from the Terrestrial Environment to Animals and Man*. CRC Press, Cleveland, 1972.

Gilbert, E. S., and Marks, S.: An analysis of the mortality of workers in a nuclear facility. *Radiat. Res.*, **79**:122–48, 1979.

Gladstone, S., and Dolan, P. J.: *The Effects of Nuclear Weapons*, 3rd ed. U.S. Department of Defense, U.S. Department of Energy, Washington, D.C., 1977.

Gofman, J. W.: *Radiation and Human Health*. Sierra Club Books, San Francisco, 1981.

Gofman, J. W.; Gofman, J. D.; Tamplin, A. R.; and Kovich, E.: Radiation as an environmental hazard. In *Environment and Cancer*. Williams & Wilkins Co., Baltimore, 1972.

Gofman, J. W., and Tamplin, A. R.: Low dose radiation and cancer, IEEE (Inst. Elec. Electron Eng.). Transaction on Nuclear Science, Part I, NS-17, 1970, pp. 1–9.

Goldman, M., and Bustad, L. K. (eds.): *Biomedical Implications and Radiostrontium Exposure*. AEC Symposium Series 25. U.S. Atomic Energy Commission Office of Information Services, Springfield, Va., 1972.

Goldschmidt, H., and Sherwin, W. K.: Reactions to ionizing radiation. *J. Am. Acad. Dermatol.*, **3**:551–79, 1980.

Gössner, W.; Gerber, G. B.; Hagen, U.; and Luz, A. (eds.): *The Radiobiology of Radium and Thorotrast*. Urban & Schwarzenberg, Baltimore, 1986.

Grahn, D.: Biological effects of protracted low dose radiation exposure of man and animals. In Fry, R. J. M.; Grahn, D.; Griem, M. L.; and Rust, J. H. (eds.): *Late Effects of Radiation*. Proceedings of a Colloquium held in the Center for Continuing Education, University of Chicago, May 15–17, 1969. Taylor and Francis, Ltd., London, 1970. Chap. V.

Grosch, D. S., and Hopwood, L. E. (eds.): *Biological Effects of Radiations*. Academic Press, Inc., New York, 1979.

Hahn, F. F.; Boecker, B. B.; Cuddihy, R. G.; Hobbs, C. H.; McClellan, R. O.; and Snipes, M. B.: Influence of radiation dose patterns on lung tumor incidence in dogs that inhaled beta emitters: a preliminary report. *Radiat. Res.*, **96**:505–17, 1983.

Hall, E. J.: *Radiation and Life*. Pergamon Press, New York, 1976.

Healy, J. W. (ed.): *Plutonium; Health Implications for Man*. Proceedings of the Second Los Alamos Life Sciences Symposium held in Los Alamos, New Mexico, May 22–24, 1974. *Health Phys.*, **29**(4):489–94, 1975.

Hempelmann, L. H.; Langham, W. H.; Richmond, C. R.; and Voelz, G. L.: Manhattan project plutonium workers: a twenty-seven year follow-up study of selected cases. *Health Phys.*, **25**:461–79, 1973.

Hine, G. J., and Brownell, G. L.: *Radiation Dosimetry*. Academic Press, Inc., New York, 1956.

Hodge, H. C.; Hursh, J. B.; and Stannard, J. N. (eds.): *Handbook of Experimental Pharmacology*. Vol. 36, Uranium, Plutonium and the Transplutonic Elements. Springer-Verlag, New York, 1973.

Hutchison, G. B., and MacMahon, B.: Review of report by Mancuso, Stewart and Kneale of radiation exposure of Hanford workers. *Health Phys.*, **37**:207–20, 1979.

International Atomic Energy Agency: *Inhalation Risks from Radioactive Contaminants*. Technical Report Series No. 142. International Atomic Energy Agency, Vienna, 1973.

International Commission on Radiation Units and Measurements: *Methods of Assessment of Absorbed Dose in Clinical Use of Radionuclides*. ICRU Report 32, International Commission on Radiation Units and Measurements, Washington, D.C., 1979.

——— : *Radiation Quantities and Units*. ICRU Report 33, International Commission on Radiation Units and Measurements, Washington, D.C., 1980.

International Commission on Radiological Protection: *Recommendations of the International Commission on Radiological Protection* (Adopted September 9, 1958). ICRP Publication No. 1. Pergamon Press, Oxford, 1959.

——— : *Recommendations of the International Commission on Radiological Protection Report of Committee II on Permissible Dose for Internal Radiation* (1959). ICRP Publication No. 2, *Health Phys.*, 3:1–380, 1960.

——— : *Recommendations of the International Commission on Radiological Protection Report of Committee IV on Protection Against Electromagnetic Radiation Above 3 MeV and Electrons, Neutrons and Protons* (Adopted 1962; with revisions adopted 1963). ICRP Publication No. 4, Pergamon Press, Oxford, 1963.

——— : (Task Group on Lung Dynamics): *Deposition and Retention Models for Internal Dosimetry of the Human Respiratory Tract*. *Health Phys.*, 12:173–207, 1966a.

——— : *Recommendations of the International Commission on Radiological Protection* (Adopted September 17, 1965). ICRP Publication No. 9, Pergamon Press, Oxford, 1966b.

——— : (Task Group of Committee 2): *The Metabolism of Compounds of Plutonium and Other Actinides*. ICRP Publication No. 19, Pergamon Press, Oxford, 1972.

——— : *Report of the Task Group on Reference Man*. ICRP Publication No. 23, Pergamon Press, Oxford, 1975.

——— : *Recommendations of the International Commission on Radiological Protection*. ICRP Publication 26. Annals of the ICRP 1 (3), 1977. International Commission on Radiation Units and Measurements, Washington, D.C., 1977.

——— : *Radionuclide Release into the Environment: Assessment of Doses to Man*. ICRP Publication No. 29, Pergamon Press, Oxford, 1979.

——— : *Biological Effects of Inhaled Radionuclides*. ICRP Publication No. 31, *Annals of ICRP*, Vol. 4, Issue 1/2, 1980.

——— : *General Principles of Monitoring for Radiation Protection of Workers*. ICRP Publication No. 35, *Annals of ICRP*, Vol. 9, Issue 4, 1982.

——— : *Nonstochastic Effects of Ionizing Radiation*. ICRP Publication No. 41, *Annals of ICRP*, Vol. 14, Issue 3, 1984.

Jablon, S., and Kato, H.: Studies of the mortality of A-bomb survivors. 5. Radiation dose and mortality 1950–1970. *Radiat. Res.*, 50:649–98, 1972.

Jee, W. S. S. (ed.): *The Health Effects of Plutonium and Radium*. J. W. Press, Salt Lake City, 1976.

Jones, R. K.; Hahn, F. F.; Hobbs, C. H.; Benjamin, S. A.; Boecker, B. B.; McClellan, R. O.; and Slauson, D. O.: Pulmonary carcinogenesis and chronic beta irradiation of lung. In Karbe, E., and Park, J. F. (eds.): *Experimental Lung Cancer; Carcinogenesis and Bioassays*. Springer-Verlag, Berlin, 1974, pp. 454–67.

Kanapilly, G. M.: Alveolar microenvironment and its relationship to the retention and transport into blood of aerosols deposited in the alveoli. *Health Phys.*, 32:89–100, 1977.

Kemeny, J. G. (chairman): *The President's Commission on the Accident at TMI*. Pergamon Press, New York, 1979.

Kneale, G. W.; Mancuso, T. F.; and Stewart, A. M.: Hanford radiation study III: a cohort study of the cancer risks from radiation to workers at Hanford (1944–77

deaths) by the method of regression models in life-tables. *Br. J. Indust. Med.*, 38:156–66, 1981.

Kneale, G. W., and Stewart, A.: Hanford radiation study. *Br. J. Indust. Med.*, 39:201–202, 1982.

Land, C. E.: Estimating cancer risks from low doses of ionizing radiation. *Science*, 209:1197–1203, 1980.

Langham, W. H. (ed.): *Radiobiological Factors in Manned Space Flight*. National Academy of Sciences, National Research Council, Washington, D.C., 1967.

Leach, L. J.; Maynard, E. A.; Hodge, C. H.; Scott, J. K.; Yuile, C. L.; Sylvester, G. E.; and Wilson, H. B.: A five-year inhalation study with natural uranium dioxide (UO_2) dust. I. Retention and biologic effect in the monkey, dog and rat. *Health Phys.*, 18:599–612, 1970.

Lenihan, J. M. A.; Loutit, J. F.; and Martin, J. H. (eds.): *Strontium Metabolism*. Academic Press, Inc., London and New York, 1967.

Lindell, B.: A risk system for setting radiation dose limits. In *Critical Issues in Setting Radiation Dose Limits*. National Council on Radiation Protection and Measurements, Bethesda, Md., 1982.

Linden, K.: The new special names of SI units in the field of ionizing radiations. *Health Phys.*, 30:417–18, 1976.

Lindop, P. J., and Sacher, G. A. (eds.): *Radiation and Ageing*. Proceedings of a Colloquium held in Semmering, Austria, June 23–24, 1966. Taylor and Francis, Ltd., London, 1966.

Lovell, S.: *Introduction to Radiation Dosimetry*. Cambridge University Press, Cambridge, 1979.

Lushbaugh, C. C.: The impact of estimates of human radiation tolerance upon radiation emergency management. In *The Control of Exposure of the Public to Ionizing Radiation in the Event of Accident or Attack*. National Council on Radiation Protection and Measurements Report, Bethesda, Md., 1982.

McClellan, R. O.: Calcium-strontium discrimination in miniature pigs as related to age. *Nature* (Lond.), 202:104–106, 1964.

——— : Health effects from internally deposited radionuclides released in nuclear disasters. In *The Control of Exposure of the Public to Ionizing Radiation in the Event of Accident or Attack*. National Council on Radiation Protection and Measurements, Washington, D.C., 1982.

McClellan, R. O.; Boyd, H. A.; Gallegos, A. F.; and Thomas, R. G.: Retention and distribution of ^{244}Cm following inhalation of $^{244}CmCl_3$ and $^{244}CmO \cdot$ by beagle dogs. *Health Phys.*, 22:877–85, 1972b.

McClellan, R. O.; Bustad, L. K.; and Keough, R. F.: Metabolism of some SNAP radionuclides in miniature swine. *Aerospace Med.*, 36:16–20, 1965.

McClellan, R. O., and Jones, R. K.: ^{90}Sr-induced neoplasia: A selective review. In Mays, C. W., *et al.* (eds.): *Delayed Effects of Bone-Seeking Radionuclides*. University of Utah Press, Salt Lake City, 1969.

McLean, A. S.: Early adverse effects of radiation. *Br. Med. Bull.*, 29:69–73, 1973.

MacMahon, B.: Prenatal x-ray exposure and childhood cancer. *J. Natl. Cancer Inst.*, 28:1173–91, 1962.

Mancuso, T. F.; Stewart, A.; and Kneale, G.: Radiation exposures of Hanford workers dying from cancer and other causes. *Health Phys.*, 33:369–85, 1977.

Margulis, A. R.: The lessons of radiobiology for diagnostic radiology. *Am. J. Roentgenol. Radium Ther. Nucl. Med.*, 117:741–56, 1973.

Marks, S.; Gilbert, E. S.; and Breitenstein, B. D.: Cancer mortality in Hanford workers. In *Late Biological Effects of Ionizing Radiation*, Vol. I, 1978, pp. 369–86.

Marshall, E.: New A-bomb studies alter radiation estimates. *Science*, 212:900–903, 1981.

Marshall, J. H.; Lloyd, E. L.; Rundo, J.; Liniecki, J.; Marotti, G.; Mays, C. W.; Sissons, H. A.; and Snyder,

W. S.: Alkaline earth metabolism in adult man. *Health Phys.*, **24**:125–222, 1973 (ICRP Report 20).

Mays, C. W.; Jee, W. S. S.; Lloyd, R. D.; Stover, B. J.; Dougherty, J. H.; and Taylor, G. C. (eds.): *Delayed Effects of Bone-Seeking Radionuclides.* University of Utah Press, Salt Lake City, 1969.

Mays, C. W., and Lloyd, R. D.: Bone sarcoma risk from ^{90}Sr. In Goldman, M., and Bustad, L. K. (eds.): *Biomedical Implications of Radiostrontium Exposure.* AEC Symposium Series 25, CONF-710201, National Technical Information Service, Springfield, VA, 1972a.

Mays, C. W.; Spiess, H.; Taylor, G. N.; Lloyd, R. D.; Jee, W. S. S.; McFarland, S. S.; Taysum, D. H.; Brammer, T. W.; and Pollard, T. A.: Estimated risk to human bone from ^{239}Pu. In Jee, W. S. S. (ed.): *The Health Effects of Plutonium and Radium.* J. W. Press, Salt Lake City, 1976, pp. 343–62.

Medical Internal Radiation Dose Committee: MIRD, *Journal of Nuclear Medicine,* Supplement No. 1, Pamphlets 1–3. Society of Nuclear Medicine, Inc., New York, 1968.

——— : MIRD, *Journal of Nuclear Medicine,* Supplement No. 2, Pamphlet 4. Society of Nuclear Medicine, Inc., New York, 1969a.

——— : MIRD, *Journal of Nuclear Medicine,* Supplement No. 3, Pamphlet 5. Society of Nuclear Medicine, Inc., New York, 1969b.

——— : MIRD, *Journal of Nuclear Medicine,* Supplement No. 5, Pamphlet 7–8. Society of Nuclear Medicine, Inc., New York, 1971.

——— : MIRD, *Journal of Nuclear Medicine,* Supplement, Pamphlet 10. Society of Nuclear Medicine, Inc., New York, 1975.

——— : MIRD, *Journal of Nuclear Medicine,* Supplement, Pamphlet 11. Society of Nuclear Medicine, Inc., New York, 1975b.

Medical Research Council. *The toxicity of Plutonium.* Her Majesty's Stationery Office, London, 1975.

Mercer, T. T.: On the role of particular size in the dissolution of lung burdens. *Health Phys.,* **13**:1211–21, 1967.

Mettler, Jr., F. A., and Moseley, Jr., R. D. (eds.): *Medical Effects of Ionizing Radiation.* Grune & Stratton, Inc., Orlando, Fl., 1985.

Mole, R. H.: Hanford radiation study. *Br. J. Indust. Med.,* **39**:200–201. 1982.

Moss, T. H., and Sills, D. L. (eds.): *Three Mile Island Nuclear Accident: Lessons and Implications.* The New York Academy of Sciences, New York, 1981.

National Academy of Sciences Advisory Committee on the Biological Effects of Ionizing Radiations (the BEIR Committee): *Considerations of Health Benefit-Cost Analysis for Activities Involving Ionizing Radiation Exposure and Alternatives.* EPA 5201/4-77-003. National Academy of Sciences, National Research Council, Washington, D.C., 1977.

National Academy of Sciences, National Research Council: *Health Effects of Alpha-Emitting Particles in the Respiratory Tract.* EPA 520/4-76-013, Washington, D.C., 1976.

——— : Adverse effects of classes of pollutants: Radon and radon progeny. In *Indoor Pollutants.* National Academy of Sciences, Washington, D.C., 1981.

——— : *A Study of the Isolation System for Geologic Disposal of Radioactive Wastes.* Waste Isolation Systems Panel, Board on Radioactive Waste Management, National Academy Press, Washington, D.C., 1983.

National Council on Radiation Protection and Measurements: *Safety Handling of Radioactive Luminous Compounds.* NCRP Report No. 5. National Council of Radiation Protection and Measurements, Washington, D.C., 1941.

——— : *Permissible Dose from External Sources of Ionizing Radiation.* NCRP Report No. 17. National Council on Radiation Protection and Measurements, Washington, D.C., 1954.

——— : *Maximum permissible radiation exposure to man: A preliminary statement of the National Commission on Radiation Protection and Measurements* (January 8, 1957). *Radiology,* **18**:260, 1957.

——— : *Maximum permissible radiation exposures to man* (April 16, 1958): Addendum to NCRP Report No. 17. *Radiology,* **71**:263, 1958.

——— : *Maximum Permissible Body Burdens and Maximum Permissible Concentrations of Radionuclides in Air and Water for Occupational Exposure.* NCRP Report No. 22. National Council on Radiation Protection, Washington, D.C., 1959.

——— : *Protection Against Neutron Radiation.* NCRP Report No. 38. National Council on Radiation Protection and Measurements, Washington, D.C., 1971a.

——— : *Basic Radiation Protection Criteria.* NCRP Report No. 39. National Council on Radiation Protection and Measurements, Washington, D.C., 1971b.

——— : *Natural Background Radiation in the United States.* NCRP Report No. 45. National Council on Radiation Protection and Measurements, Washington, D.C., 1975a.

——— : *Alpha-Emitting Particles in Lungs.* NCRP Report No. 46. National Council on Radiation Protection and Measurements, Washington, D.C., 1975b.

——— : *Tritium Measurement Techniques.* NCRP Report No. 47. National Council on Radiation Protection and Measurements, Washington, D.C., 1976a.

——— : *Radiation Protection for Medical and Allied Health Personnel.* NCRP Report No. 48. National Council on Radiation Protection and Measurements, Washington, D.C., 1976b.

——— : *Cesium-137 from the Environment to Man: Metabolism and Dose.* NCRP Report No. 52. National Council on Radiation Protection and Measurements, Washington, D.C., 1977a.

——— : *Review of NCRP Radiation Dose Limit for Embryo and Fetus in Occupationally-Exposed Women.* NCRP Report No. 53. National Council on Radiation Protection and Measurements, Washington, D.C., 1977b.

——— : *Protection of the Thyroid Gland in the Event of Releases of Radioiodine.* NCRP Report No. 55. National Council on Radiation Protection and Measurements, Washington, D.C., 1977c.

——— : *Radiation Exposure from Consumer Products and Miscellaneous Sources.* NCRP Report No. 56. National Council on Radiation Protection and Measurements, Washington, D.C., 1977d.

——— : *Instrumentation and Monitoring Methods for Radiation Protection.* NCRP Report No. 57. National Council on Radiation Protection and Measurements, Washington, D.C., 1978a.

——— : *A Handbook of Radioactivity Measurements Procedures.* NCRP Report No. 58. National Council on Radiation Protection and Measurements, Washington, D.C., 1978b.

——— : *Operational Radiation Safety Program.* NCRP Report No. 59. National Council on Radiation Protection and Measurements, Washington, D.C., 1978c.

——— : *Physical, Chemical and Biological Properties of Radiocerium Relevant to Radiation Protection guidelines.* NCRP Report No. 60. National Council on Radiation and Measurements, Washington, D.C., 1978d.

——— : *Review of the Current State of Radiation Protection Philosophy.* NCRP Report No. 43, National Council on Radiation Protection and Measurements, Washington, D.C., 1975.

——— : *Tritium and Other Radionuclide Labeled Organic Compounds Incorporated in Genetic Material.* NCRP Report No. 63, National Council on Radiation

Protection and Measurements, Washington, D.C., 1979.

——— : *Influence of Dose and Its Distribution in Time on Dose-Response Relationships for Low-LET Radiations.* NCRP Report No. 64. National Council on Radiation Protection and Measurements, Washington, D.C., 1980.

——— : *Exposure from the Uranium Series with Emphasis on Radon and Its Daughters.* NCRP Report No. 77, National Council on Radiation Protection and Measurements, Washington, D.C., 1984a.

——— : *Evaluation of Occupational and Environmental Exposures to Radon and Radon Daughters in the United States.* NCRP Report No. 78, National Council on Radiation Protection and Measurements, Washington, D.C., 1984b.

——— : *Induction of Thyroid Cancer by Ionizing Radiation.* NCRP Report No. 80, National Council on Radiation Protection and Measurements, Washington, D.C., 1985a.

——— : *SI Units in Radiation Protection and Measurements.* NCRP Report No. 82, National Council on Radiation Protection and Measurements, Washington, D.C., 1985b.

——— : *General Concepts for the Dosimetry of Internally Deposited Radionuclides.* NCRP Report No. 84, National Council on Radiation Protection and Measurements, Washington, D.C., 1985c.

National Council on Radiation Protection and Measurements: *The Control of Exposure of the Public to Ionizing Radiation in the Event of Accident or Attack.* The Council, Bethesda, Md., 1982.

Nenot, G. C., and Stather, J. W.: The toxicology of plutonium, americum, and curium. Commission of European Communities, 1979.

Nero, A. V.: Airborne radionuclides and radiation in buildings: a review. *Health Phys., 45*:303–22, 1983.

Nero, A. V., and Lowder, W. M. (eds.): *Indoor Radon. Health Physics 45.* Pergamon Press, New York, 1983.

Norris, W. P.; Poole, C. M.; and Rehfeld, C. E.: Cesium-137: current status and late effects. USAEC Report ANL-7278, 1966.

Osborne, R. V.: Permissible levels of tritium in man and the environment. *Radiat. Res., 50*:197–211, 1972.

Palmer, R. F., and Thompson, R. C.: Strontium-calcium interrelationships in the growing rat. *Am. J. Physiol., 207*:561–66, 1964.

Patt, H. M., and Quastler, H.: Radiation effects on cell renewal and related systems. *Physiol. Rev., 43*:357–93, 1963.

Redman, H. C.; McClellan, R. O.; Jones, R. K.; Boecker, B. B.; Chiffelle, T. L.; Pickrell, J. A.; and Rypka, E. W.: Toxicity of $^{137}CsCl$ in the beagle: early biological effects. *Radiat. Res., 50*:629–48, 1972.

Rossi, H. H.: Biophysical implications of radiation quality. In Nygaard, O. F.; Adler, H. I.; and Sinclair, W. K. (eds.): *Radiation Research: Biomedical, Chemical, and Physical Perspectives.* Academic Press, Inc., New York, 1975, pp. 994–97.

Rowland, R. E.; Stehney, A. F.; and Lucas, H. F.: Dose-response relationships for radium-induced bone sarcomas. *Health Phys., 44*:15–31, 1983.

Rubin, P., and Casarett, G. W.: *Clinical Radiation Pathology.* W. B. Saunders Co., Philadelphia, 1968, chap. 1, p. 33.

Rundo, J.; Failla, P.; and Schlenker, R. A. (eds.): *Radiobiology of radium and the actinides in man. Health Phys., 44*, Suppl. 1, 1983.

Russell, W. L.: The genetic effects of radiation. In *Peaceful Uses of Atomic Energy.* Proceedings of the Fourth International Conference on the Peaceful Uses of Atomic Energy held jointly by the United Nations and the International Atomic Energy Commission, in Geneva, 6–16, Sept. 1971.

Saccomanno, G.; Archer, V. E.; Auerbach, O.; Kuschner, M.; Saunders, R. P.; and Klein, M. G.: Histologic types of lung cancer among uranium miners. *Cancer, 27*:515–23, 1971.

Schneider, K. J.: High Level Waste. In Sagan, L. A. (ed.): *Human and Ecologic Effects of Nuclear Power Plants.* Charles C Thomas Pub., Springfield, Ill, 1974, Chap. 8.

Shapiro, J.: *Radiation Protection.* Harvard University Press, Cambridge, Mass., 1972.

Shleien, B., and Terpilak, M. S. (eds.): *The Health Physics and Radiological Health Handbook.* Nucleon Lectern Associates, Inc., Olney, Md., 1984.

Stannard, J. N.: Toxicology of radionuclides. *Annu. Rev. Pharmacol., 13*:325–57, 1973.

——— : Some historical highlights and portents for the future of biomedical research on radium and the actinides. *Health Phys., 44*:3–14, 1983.

Stewart, A.: Low dose radiation cancers in man. In *Advances in Cancer Research,* Vol. 14. Academic Press, Inc., New York, 1971, pp. 359–90.

——— : The carcinogenic effects of low level radiation. A re-appraisal of epidemiological methods and observations. *Health Phys., 24*:223–40, 1973.

Stewart, A., and Kneale, G. W.: Radiation dose effects in relation to obstetric x-rays and childhood cancers. *Lancet, 1*:1185–88, 1970a.

——— : Age-distribution of cancers caused by obstetric x-rays and their relevance to cancer latent periods. *Lancet, 2*:4–8, 1970b.

Stohlman, F., Jr. (ed.): *The Kinetics of Cellular Proliferation.* Grune & Stratton, Inc., New York, 1959.

Stover, B. J., and Jee, W. S. S. (eds.): *Radiobiology of Plutonium.* The J. W. Press, University of Utah, Salt Lake City, 1972.

Sullivan, M. F.; Garland, T. R.; Cataldo, D. A.; and Schreckhise, R. G.: Absorption of plant-incorporated nuclear fuel cycle elements from the gastrointestinal tract. In *Biological Implications of Radionuclides Released from Nuclear Industries,* Vol. I. IAEA-SM-237/58, CONF-790325, 1979, pp. 447–456.

Sullivan, M. F.; Ruemmler, P. S.; Beamer, J. L.; Mahoney, T. D.; and Cross, F. T.: Acute toxicity of beta-emitting radionuclides that may be released in a reactor accident and related effects. *Radiat. Res., 73*:21–36, 1978.

Tamplin, A. R., and Gofman, J. W.: *Population Control Through Nuclear Pollution.* Nelson-Hall Co., Chicago, 1970a.

——— : The radiations effects controversy. *Bull. Atomic Scientists; Science Public Affairs, 26*(7):2, 1970b.

Tamplin, A. R., and Cochran, T. B.: *Radiation Standards for Hot Particles: A Report on the Inadequacy of Existing Radiation Protection Standards Related to Internal Exposure to Man to Insoluble Particles of Plutonium and Other Alpha-Emitting Hot Particles.* Natural Resources Defense Council, Washington, D.C., 1974.

Thompson, R. C., and Palmer, R. F.: Strontium-calcium interrelationships in the mature rat. *Am. J. Physiol., 199*:94–102, 1960.

Thompson, R. C.; Park, J. F.; and Bair, W. J.: Some speculative extensions to man of animal risk data on plutonium. In Stover, Betsy J., and Jee, W. S. S. (Eds.): *Radiobiology of Plutonium.* J. W. Press, University of Utah, Salt Lake City, 1972.

Thompson, T. J., and Bibb, W. R.: Response to Gofman and Tamplin: The AEC position. *Bull. Atomic Scientists; Science Public Affairs, 26*:9–12, 1970.

United Nations: Report of the United Nations Scientific Committee on the Effects of Atomic Radiation, 1958, 1962, 1964, 1966, 1972, 1977, and 1982. United Nations, New York.

United Nations Scientific Committee on the Effects of

Atomic Radiation: *Ionizing Radiation: Levels and Effects*. Vol. I, Levels. Publication No. E.72.IX.17. United Nations, New York, 1972a.

———— : *Ionizing Radiation: Levels and Effects*. Vol. II, Effects. Publication No. E.72.IX.18. United Nations, New York, 1972b.

Upton, A. C.: The influence of dose rate in mammalian radiation biology. Quality effects. In Brown, D. G., *et al.* (eds.): *Dose Rate in Mammalian Biology*, CONF-680410, U.S. Atomic Energy Commission, Division of Technical Information, Oak Ridge, 1968b.

———— : Radiation. In *Cancer Medicine*. Lea & Febiger, Philadelphia, 1973. Chaps. 1–5.

———— : Health impact of the Three Mile Island accident. *Ann. N.Y. Acad. Sci., 365*:63–75, 1981.

———— : The biological effects of low-level ionizing radiation. *Sci. Am., 246*:41–49, 1982.

Upton, A. C.; Randolph, M. L.; and Conklin, J. W.: Late effects of fast neutrons and gamma rays in mice as influenced by the dose rate of irradiation: induction of neoplasma. *Radiat. Res.., 41*:467–91, 1970.

Vennart, Radiotoxicology of tritium and ^{14}C compounds. *Health Phys., 16*:429–40, 1969.

Voelz, G. L.: What we have learned about plutonium from human data. *Health Phys., 29*(4):551–61, 1975.

WASH-1400 (NUREG-75/014). United States Nuclear Regulatory Commission: *Reactor Safety Study, An Assessment of Accident Risks in U.S. Commercial Nuclear Power Plants*. United States Nuclear Regulatory Commission, Oct. 1975.

Wick, R. R., and Gossner, W.: Follow-up study of late effects in ^{224}Ra treated ankylosing spondylitis patients. *Health Phys., 44*:187–196, 1983.

Yuhas, J. M.; Tennant, R. W.; and Regan, J. D.: *Biology of Radiation Carcinogenesis*. Raven Press, New York, 1976.

Chapter 22

TOXIC EFFECTS OF ANIMAL TOXINS

Findlay E. Russell

INTRODUCTION

Venomous or poisonous animals are found in all the animal classes with the exception of the birds. For the most part they are widely distributed throughout the animal kingdom from the unicellular protistan *Gonyaulax* to certain of the chordates, the platypus, and the short-tailed shrew. Venomous animals are found in almost all seas and oceans of the world and on all continents. Although there are no exact figures on the numbers of such animals, there are approximately 1200 species of venomous or poisonous marine animals (Russell, 1984a), the number of venomous arthropods is countless, and there are some 375 species of snakes considered dangerous to humans.

The term *venomous animal* is usually applied to those creatures which are capable of producing a poison in a highly developed secretory gland or group of cells and which can deliver this toxin during a biting or stinging act. *Poisonous animals,* on the other hand, are generally regarded to be those whose tissues, either in part or in their entirety, are toxic. These animals have no mechanism or structure for the delivery of their poisons. Poisoning by these forms usually takes place through ingestion (Russell, 1965). In reality, all venomous animals are poisonous but not all poisonous animals are venomous.

A venom may have one or several functions in an animal's armament. It may play a role in offense, as in the capture and digestion of food, or may contribute to the animal's defense, as in protection against predators or aggressors. It may also serve both functions. The principal biologic property of the venom of the snake is its food-securing potential. In this respect venom is a superior modification to speed, size, strength, or better concealment, as well as other characteristics that many of the nonvenomous snakes have developed. In addition, the venom plays a role in the digestion of the prey. Finally, the venom can play a role in the snake's defensive posture, as in the spitting cobra and ringhals, or

in kills or underkills in a defensive situation (Russell, 1984b). The venomous snakes are considered to be the most successful of all the reptiles. This supposition is based on their survival in both numbers and species, which for the most part reflects the deployment of their venom.

The black widow spider and many other species of spiders use their venom to paralyze their prey before extracting hemolymph and body fluids. The venom is not primarily designed to kill the prey, only to immobilize it. Were it to cause immediate death, removing the hemolymph and body fluids would be made much more difficult and would seem inconsistent with the evolution of the function. The venom apparatus of the stingray is used in defense. It is not employed in getting food, and for the most part its defensive posture appears to have been spent eons ago. The lionfishes, stonefishes, and weeverfishes also use their venomous spines in defense, never in offense. Scorpions, on the other hand, use their venom in both offense and defense.

Most venoms used in an offensive posture are associated with the oral pole of the host animal, obviously the most functional place for their dispense. Defensively designed venoms are usually associated with the aboral pole, as in the stingrays, or with dermal tissues, as is the case with the scorpionfishes and certain other fishes (Russell, 1965; Halstead, 1970). Evidence at the present time seems to indicate that the primary function of a defensive venom is related to its pain-producing property.

In poisonous animals the poison or toxin may play little, if any, role in either the animal's offensive or defensive statures. The poison may be a product or by-product of metabolism that just happens to be toxic. Tetrodotoxin plays no offensive or defensive role in the tetrodotoxic fishes. It would hardly seem reasonable to evolve toxicity in the gonads of a fish, as either an offensive or defensive weapon and then only during certain periods of a cycle. Poisonousness can also come about through the ingestion of certain toxic organisms, as in the case of ciguatera. Ciguateric fishes feed on smaller toxic fishes or other toxic marine animals which, in turn, have fed on smaller toxic organisms. As each step in the feeding process progresses more toxin is accumulated, so that while poisoning in humans may not occur on eating the smaller toxic fishes or marine organisms, by the time a large grouper, barracuda, snapper, or other toxic fish that has fed on smaller toxic organisms is eaten, poisoning occurs. This sequence of events is known as the "food-chain phenomena," most eloquently described by Halstead (1967).

In considering the venomousness or poisonousness of an animal it is wise to consider the use to which that animal puts its toxin. Among other things, this provides a clue as to the possible chemistry and pharmacology of the poison. In addition, a knowledge of the biology of the animal is a valuable asset to the physician treating a case of venom poisoning. It is also well to remember that transposition of data from a simple isolated tissue preparation to the human must be carried out with great care. Errors in clinical judgment have been perpetrated by the overzealous application of *in vitro* data from laboratory experiments. In the intact animal, bioavailability, membrane transport, site accumulation, metabolism, and excretion have values that often cannot be evaluated in a single cell or single fiber preparation (Russell, 1980a).

PROPERTIES OF ANIMAL TOXINS

As one might expect from the uses to which animals put their poisons, these toxins vary considerably in their chemistry and toxicology. Venoms, for instance, may be composed of proteins of both large and small molecular weight, including polypeptides and enzymes. They may be amines, lipids, steroids, aminopolysaccharides, quinones, 5-HT, glycosides, or other substances. The biologic properties of snake venoms have been reviewed by Zeller (1948), Russell (1967), Dowling, Minton and Russell (1968), Minton and Minton (1969), Elliott (1978), Lee (1979), Habermehl (1981), and Russell (1983). With respect to the venoms of spiders, the text of Maretić and Lebez (1979) provides a good discourse and ample references. Keegan's (1980) work on the scorpions is a fine basic text that provides a good overview on the venom of this arthropod. The toxins of marine animals have been thoroughly described by Halstead (1965–1970) and by Russell (1965, 1971). The series of texts by Scheuer (1973, 1978–1981) provides additional data on some marine animal toxins, as does the excellent work of Southcott (1979). The interested reader will find the book by Hashimoto (1979) a most useful source

on the biochemistry of marine toxins. I have recently updated the biology, chemistry, and toxicology of marine invertebrate toxins (Russell, 1984a).

One of the unfortunate facts in the study of the chemistry and pharmacology of venoms is that their structure and function are most easily studied by taking them apart. This has two shortcomings: first, a destructive process is used in an attempt to understand a progressive and integrative one; and second, the essential quality of the venom is often destroyed before we have made suitable acquaintance with it. Often, the process of examination becomes so exacting that the end is lost sight of in our preoccupation with the means, so much so that in some cases the means becomes a substitute for the end.

Another shortcoming in the study of venoms has been the naive and oversimplified habit of classifying the whole poison or even its component parts as "neurotoxins," "cardiotoxins," "hemotoxins," "myotoxins," and other loosely articulated synonyms. Most venoms probably exert their effects on almost all cells or tissues, and their pharmacologic properties are determined by how much of a specific biologically active component accumulates at an activity site where it is capable of producing a change. That change probably has a common chemical basis in most tissues, not only specific to the component but to the alteration in ion exchange it perpetuates at the cell or tissue site. It is true, of course, that most venoms have a more particular effect on one or several tissue sites, but more recent experimental work demonstrates the wide scope of the toxicologic effects that a venom or venom fraction can precipitate. For instance, it has been shown that "cardiotoxin," a component isolated from a snake venom, also causes a neuromuscular block, a block in axonal conduction, membrane depolarization, anticholinesterase activity, local tissue effects, hemolysis, vasoconstriction, cytotoxic action, skeletal and smooth muscle contractions, and cardiac arrest. Other studies have also shown that some of the so-called neurotoxins have myotoxic activities, and "myotoxin" seems to provoke tissue changes in a variety of tissues.

In understanding the actions of a venom neither the toxicologist nor the clinician should lose sight of the fact that an envenomation represents a complex poisoning and that no biologic activity of a venom can afford to be overlooked. This has been noted elsewhere (Russell, 1963):

"The clinician must never slight any symptom or sign his patient presents, or minimize any manifestation on the naive assumption that the venom has to be either a 'neurotoxin,' 'cardiotoxin,' 'hemotoxin,' or 'myotoxin' and its activity limited to one organ or system. While the patient may have respiratory distress from a 'neurotoxic venom' he can also have changes in cardiac dynamics or vascular permeability and these can become far more life-threatening situations, particularly if the physician centers his attention and therapy on the so-called neurotoxin of the venom (an effect that can often be adequately treated by simple positive pressure respiration). The physician must guard his knowledge and experience zealously and be aware of the limits of application of pharmacologic data based on animal experimentation. On the other hand, he must explore, carefully, the pharmacologic literature on venoms for those data that give him a greater knowledge of the mechanisms involved in venom poisoning and, hopefully, provide him with better methods of therapy."

Venoms have other important properties aside from those of their component parts. Important synergisms that are not obvious from the study of individual fractions become apparent in the activity of the whole venom. In addition, the crude venom may precipitate autopharmacologic reactions that are not produced by individual fractions. Finally, the problem of the formation of metabolites in the envenomated organism has not been explored to any degree and this might be an important consideration in clinical cases.

The action of a venom or venom component in an organism is dependent on a number of variables, including its route of administration, absorption, distribution, passage across a succession of membranes, accumulation and action at the receptor site, and its metabolism and excretion. All these factors play some role in determining the action of a venom or venom component. During the past two decades it has become increasingly clear that there are very significant variations in the roles of these factors for different venoms and in different species of experimental animals. In some cases the variations in different kinds of animals are more important than the difference usually attributed solely to the weight of the animal. Studies carried out in pigs, opossums, certain species of rats, and other animals purport to show that these animals are more "immune" to a toxin than mice. Such investigations fail to take into account the dependent physiologic variables involved in processing a toxin in different kinds of animals, influences that are not related to any principle of immunity. It is a fallacious assumption to treat the LD50 of mice and the opossum or another animal as a direct product of the differences in their weights. In this respect the toxicologist must always be concerned with the question of whether or not a particular difference in various kinds of animals is caused by variables in the effectiveness of the toxin at the receptor site or in its absorption, distribution, metabolism, or excretion. The fate of a venom or venom fraction, as its activities are spent in the animal, has been discussed elsewhere (Russell, 1980a, 1980b, 1983).

REPTILES

From the very beginnings of human record few subjects have stimulated the minds and imagination of humans more than the study of snakes and snake venoms. No animal has been more worshipped yet more cast out, more loved yet more despised, and more collected yet more trampled upon than the snake. The essence of the fascination and fear of snakes has been with their venom. In times past the consequences of bites by venomous snakes were often attributed to forces beyond nature, sometimes to vengeful deities thought to be embodied in the serpents. To early peoples the effects of snakebites were so surprising and so violent that snakes and their poisons were usually shrouded with much myth and superstition.

Snakes have been used in man's worship, magic, entertainment, science, food, sport, medicine, commerce, witchcraft, war, and even in tortures on his fellow man. They have been the symbol of love, hate, procreation, health, disease, immortality, sin, death, temptation, riches, poverty, and even wisdom. The Morrises have put it aptly: "It is a paradox. It is both sides of the coin, and mankind has seldom ignored it" (Morris and Morris, 1965).

Of the more than 3500 species of snakes, approximately 375 are considered sufficiently venomous to be of a danger to humans (Dowling, Minton and Russell, 1968; Minton and Minton, 1969; Harding and Welch, 1980; Russell, 1980b, 1983). Venomous species can be divided into the Elapidae—the cobras, kraits, mambas, and coral snakes; Hydrophidae—the true sea snakes; Laticaudae—the sea kraits; Viperidae—the Old World vipers and adders; Crotalidae—the rattlesnakes, water moccasins, and copperheads of North America, and the fer-de-lance and bushmaster; and certain Colubridae, of which the clinically most important are the boomslang and bird snake of Africa, and the red-necked keelback of Asia. However, several other colubrids must be viewed with concern (Mebs, 1977; Minton and Minton, 1969; Minton, 1976). The death adder and copperhead of Australia are elapids, as is the African garter snake. There are no poisonous snakes in New Zealand, Ireland, or in many other islands of the world. The Gila monster, *Heloderma suspectum*, and the beaded lizard or escorpion, *H. horridum*, are the only venomous lizards and are confined to the southwestern United States and Mexico.

Some of the medically more important venomous snakes of the world and their general distribution are shown in Table 22–1.

Table 22–1. SOME MEDICALLY IMPORTANT SNAKES OF THE WORLD*

SCIENTIFIC AND COMMON NAMES	DISTRIBUTION
Crotalids	
Agkistrodon bilineatus—Common coontail	Mexico south to Guatemala and Nicaragua
Agkistrodon contortrix—Copperhead	New York south to Florida and west to Nebraska and Texas
Agkistrodon halys—Mamushi	Caspian Sea to Japan
Agkistrodon rhodostoma—Malayan pit viper	Much of Southeast Asia
Bothrops asper and/or *atrox*—Fer-de-lance —Barba amarilla —Terciopelo	Southern Sonora to Peru and northern Brazil
Bothrops jararaca—Jararaca	Brazil, Paraguay and Argentina
Bothrops jararacussu—Jararacussu	Brazil, Bolivia, Paraguay, and Argentina
Bothrops neuwiedi—Jararaca pintada	Brazil, Bolivia, Paraguay, northern Argentina
Crotalus adamanteus—Eastern diamondback rattlesnake	Southeastern United States
Crotalus atrox—Western diamondback rattlesnake	Southwestern United States to central Mexico
Crotalus basiliscus—Mexican west-coast rattlesnake	Oaxaca and west coast of Mexico
Trimeresurus flavoviridis—Habu	Amami and Okinawa islands
Trimeresurus mucrosquamatus—Chinese habu	Taiwan and southern China west through Vietnam and Laos to India
Viperids	
Atractaspis sp.—Mole or burrowing vipers	Lebanon south through part of Arabian Peninsula, Africa
Bitis arietans—Puff adder	Morocco and western Arabia through much of Africa
Bitis caudalis—Horned puff adder	Angola south through Nambia into central and part of south Africa
Causus sp.—Night adders	Most of Africa south of the Sahara
Cerastes cerastes—Horned viper	Sahara, Arabian Peninsula to Lebanon
Cerastes vipera—Sahara sand viper	Central Sahara to Lebanon
Echis carinatus—Saw-scaled viper	Bengal to Senegal and Ghana
Echis coloratus—Saw-scaled viper	Eastern Egypt, western Arabian Peninsula north to Israel
Vipera ammodytes—Long-nosed viper	Italy through southeast Europe, Turkey, Jordan to northwest Iran
Vipera berus—European viper	British Isles through Europe, northern Asia to Korea
Vipera lebetina—Levantine viper	Cyprus through Middle East to Kashmir
Vipera russelli—Russell's viper	Indian subcontinent, southeast China to Taiwan and parts of Indonesia
Vipera xanthina—Near East viper	European Turkey and Asia Minor
Elapids	
Coral Snakes (c.s.)	
Calliophis species—Oriental c.s.	Southeast Asia, Orient
Micrurus alleni—Allen's c.s.	Atlantic Nicaragua to Panama
Micrurus corallinus—c.s.	Southern Brazil to Uruguay, northern Argentina
Micrurus frontalis—Southern c.s.	Southwestern Brazil, northern Argentina, Uruguay, Paraguay, and Boliva

* The common names in this table are those generally employed as literature identifications for the snakes. However, these names may not be the ones used by the people in the specific area where the snake abounds.

Table 22–1. (*continued*)

SCIENTIFIC AND COMMON NAMES	DISTRIBUTION
Micrurus fulvius fulvius—Eastern c.s.	Southeastern, southern U.S.A. and north central Mexico
Micrurus mipartitus—Black-ringed c.s.	Venezuela and Peru to Nicaragua
Micrurus nigrocinctus—Black-banded c.s.	Southern Mexico to northwest Columbia
Cobras	
Hemachatus haemachatus—Ringhals cobra	Southeast and southern Africa
Naja haje—Egyptian or brown cobra	Northern Africa and part of Arabian peninsula
Naja naja atra—Chinese cobra	Thailand and South China to Taiwan
Naja naja naja—Indian cobra	Most of Indian subcontinent
Naja nigricollis—Spitting cobra	West Africa and southern Egypt to near the Cape
Naja naja oxiana—Central Asian cobra	Northern West Pakistan to Iran, southern Russia
Naja naja philippinensis—Philippine cobra	Philippines
Naja naja sputatrix—Malayan cobra	Malayan peninsula and Indonesia
Naja nivea—Cape or yellow cobra	Nambia, Botswana south to the Cape
Ophiophagus hannah—King cobra	Indian subcontinent and Philippines
Walterinnesia aegyptia—Desert blacksnake or desert cobra	Egypt to Iran
Kraits and Mambas	
Bungarus caeruleus—Indian or blue krait	India, Pakistan, Sri Lanka, Bangladesh
Bungarus candidus—Malayan krait	Thailand, Malaysia, Indonesia
Bungarus multicinctus—Many-banded krait	Burma, southern China to Hainan, Taiwan
Dendroaspis polylepsis—Black mamba	Ethiopia and Somalia to Angola, Zambia, Nambia, southwest Africa
Australian Elapids	
Acanthophis antarcticus—Common death adder	Most of Australia, Moluccas, New Guinea
Notechis scutatus—Tiger snake	Southeastern Australia
Oxyuranus scutellatus—Taipan	Northern coastal Australia, parts of New Guinea
Pseudechis australis—Mulga	Most of Australia except southeast and southern coast, New Guinea
Pseudonaja nuchalis—Western brown snake	Most of Australia except east and southeast coast
Pseudonaja textilis—Eastern brown snake	Eastern Australia

Snake Venoms

The venoms of snakes are complex mixtures, chiefly proteins, a number of which have enzymatic activities. In some species the most lethal component of the venom is a peptide or polypeptide. In addition, snake venoms contain inorganic substances—sodium, calcium, potassium, magnesium, and small amounts of metals—zinc, iron, cobalt, manganese, and nickel. The importance of the metals in snake venoms is not known, although in the case of some elapid venoms the zinc ions are necessary for anticholinesterase activity, and it has been suggested that calcium may play a role in the activation of phospholipase A_2 and the direct lytic factor. Some of the proteases appear to be metalloproteins. Some snake venoms also contain carbohydrates (glycoproteins), lipids, and biogenic amines, while others contain free amino acids (Russell, 1967; Elliott, 1978; Tu, 1977; Lee, 1979; Habermehl, 1981; Russell, 1980b, 1983).

Enzymes. The venoms of snakes contain at least 25 enzymes, although no single snake venom contains all of these. Enzymes are the proteins responsible for the catalysis of numerous specific biochemical reactions that occur in living matter. They are the agents upon which cellular metabolism depends. Enzymes are universally accepted as proteins, although a few have crucial dependencies on certain nonprotein prosthetic groups, or cofactors. All living cells contain enzymes. Some of the more important snake venom enzymes are shown in Table 22–2.

Proteolytic enzymes catalyze the breakdown of tissue proteins and peptides. These are known variously as proteolytic enzymes, peptide hy-

Table 22–2. ENZYMES OF SNAKE VENOMS*

Proteolytic enzymes	Phosphomonoesterase
Arginine ester hydrolase	Phosphodiesterase
Thrombin-like enzyme	Acetylcholinesterase
Collagenase	RNase
Hyaluronidase	DNase
Phospholipase A_2 (A)	5'-Nucleotidase
Phospholipase B	NAD-nucleotidase
Phospholipase C	L-Amino acid oxidase
Lactate dehydrogenase	

* From Russell, F. E.: *Snake Venom Poisoning*. F. B. Lippincott Co., Philadelphia, 1980; Scholium International, Great Neck, N.Y., 1983.

drolases, proteases, endopeptidases, peptidases, and proteinases. There may be several proteolytic enzymes in a single venom; at least five have been found in one venom. It must be admitted, however, that most of the proteases have not been characterized, either biochemically or pharmacologically. The proteolytic enzymes have molecular weights between 20,000 and 95,000. Some are inactivated by EDTA and certain reducing agents. The role of metal ions in catalysis was demonstrated by Wagner and Prescott in 1966. The removal of zinc ions by *o*-phenanthroline in the presence of calcium ions inhibited the action of *Agkistrodon piscivorus* peptidase A (Wagner *et al.*, 1968). Reactivity was initiated by the addition of zinc ions. Zinc appears to be the catalytically necessary metal. Metals appear to be intrinsically involved in the activity of certain venom proteases and phospholipases.

All crotalid venoms so far examined appear to be rich in proteolytic enzyme activity. Viperid venoms have lesser amounts, while elapid and sea snake venoms either have no proteolytic activity or very little. Venoms that are rich in proteinase activity are associated with marked tissue destruction. The lethal effect of proteolytic enzymes has been studied but the data are difficult to evaluate, in view of the fact that investigators have used different assay parameters. Maeno *et al.* (1959) demonstrated that proteinase isolated from *Trimeresurus flavoviridis* venom produced hemorrhagic necrosis with severe lysis of muscles, but other workers have reported that the proteases and hemorrhagic factors were separable. Hemorrhagic activity may be associated with some proteases but not with others.

Arginine ester hydrolase is one of a number of noncholinesterases found in snake venoms. The substrate specificities are directed to the hydrolysis of the ester or peptide linkage to which an argine residue contributes the carboxyl group. This activity is found in many crotalid and viperid venoms and some sea snake venoms, but is lacking in elapid venoms, with the possible exception of *Ophiophagus hannah*. It was first demonstrated by Deutsch and Diniz (1955) in 15 snake venoms and has subsequently been identified in many others. Some crotalid venoms contain at least three chromatographically separable arginine ester hydrolases. The pharmacologic activities of the arginine ester hydrolases have not been classified. The bradykinin-releasing and perhaps clotting activities of some crotalid venoms may be related to esterase activity.

Thrombin-like enzymes are found in significant amounts in the venoms of the Crotalidae and Viperidae while those of Elapidae and Hydrophiidae contain little or none. The mechanism of fibrinogen clot formation by snake venom thrombin-like enzymes invokes the preferential release of fibrinopeptide A (or B); thrombin releases both fibrinopeptides A and B. Paradoxically, the thrombin-like enzymes have been shown to act as defribinogenating anticoagulants *in vivo*, whereas *in vitro* they clot plasma, citrated or heparinized plasma, or purified fibrinogen. Because of the obvious clinical potential of these enzymes as defibrinating agents more attention has been directed toward the characterization and study of the thrombin-like enzymes than of the other venom procoagulant or anticoagulant enzymes (see Russell, 1983). The proteolytic action of thrombin and thrombin-like snake venom enzymes is shown in Table 22–3.

Thrombin-like enzymes have been purified from the venoms of *Crotalus adamanteus* (Crotalase), *C. horridus horridus*, *Agkistrodon rhodostoma* (Ancrod), *A. contortrix contortrix*, *A. acutus*, *Bothrops atrox* (Batroxobin), *B. marajoensis*, *B. moojeni*, *Trimeresurus gramineus*, *T. okinavensis*, and *Bitis gabonica*. In Table 22–4 are shown some of the physical and chemical properties of the thrombinlike enzymes. All of these enzymes appear to be glycoproteins, and with the exception of two all appear to have molecular weights in the range of 29,000 to 35,000.

Thrombin-like enzymes have been used clinically and in animals for therapeutic and investigative studies. In experimentally induced venous thrombosis in dogs, treatment with Ancrod prior to the formation of the thrombus prevents thrombosis and assures vessel patency. However, Ancrod has no thrombolytic effect when administered after thrombus formation. Trials of Ancrod versus heparin and Ancrod versus streptokinase in the treatment of deep venous thromboses of the lower leg have been made. It appears that neither heparin nor Ancrod has a significant effect on thrombus resolution, whereas streptokinase produces more lysis of thrombi than Ancrod. Crotalase is being employed to evaluate the role of fibrin deposition in burns in animals (Bajwa and Markland, 1978). The role of fibrin deposition is also being evaluated in tumor metastasis, in which fibrinogen is removed by treatment with Ancrod or Batroxobin. Ancrod has also been used to prevent the deposition of fibrin on prosthetic heart valves that have been implanted in calves (see Russell, 1980b, 1983).

Collagenase is a specific kind of proteinase that digests collagen. This activity has been demonstrated in the venoms of a number of species of crotalids and viperids. The venom of

Table 22-3. PROTEOLYTIC ACTION OF THROMBIN AND THROMBIN-LIKE SNAKE VENOM ENZYMES*

ENZYME	ACTION ON HUMAN FIBRINOGEN		ACTIVATION OF FACTOR XIII	PROTHROMBIN FRAGMENT CLEAVAGE	PLATELET AGGREGATION AND RELEASE	ACTIVATION OF FACTOR VIII	ACTIVATION OF FACTOR V
	Fibrinopeptides Released	*Chain Degradation*					
Thrombin	A + B	α(A)	Yes	Yes	Yes	Yes	Yes
Thrombin-like enzymes	A†	α(A)‡ or β(B)§	No	Yes or no"	No	No	No
Agkistrodon c. contortrix venom	B	n.d.#	Incomplete	n.d.	No	n.d.	n.d.
Bitis gabonica venom	A + B	n.d.	Yes	n.d.	n.d.	n.d.	n.d.

* From Russell, F. E.: *Snake Venom Poisoning*. J. B. Lippincott Co., Philadelphia, 1980; Scholium International, Great Neck, N.Y., 1983.
† Includes ancrod, batroxobin, crotalase, and the enzyme from *T. okinavensis*
‡ Ancrod (batroxobin degrades α(A) chain of bovine, but not human fibrinogen)
§ Crotalase
" Fragment 1 released by crotalase and *Agkistrodon controtrix* venom but not by ancrod or batroxobin
n.d.: not determined.

Table 22–4. COMPARISON OF SNAKE VENOM THROMBIN-LIKE ENZYMES*

VENOM ENZYME	MOLECULAR WEIGHT	CARBOHYDRATE CONTENT (%)	NH$_2$-TERMINAL RESIDUE	ACTIVE SITE SERINE	ACTIVE SITE HISTIDINE
Agkistrodon rhodostoma	35,400	36.0	Val	+	+
Crotalus adamanteus	33,700	5.4	Val	+	+
Bothrops marajoensis	31,400	high	Val	+	n.d.†
Bothrops moojeni	29,100	26.7	Val	+	n.d.
Crotalus horridus horridus	19,400	Very low	n.d.	n.d.	n.d.
Agkistrodon acutus	33,500	13.0	n.d.	+	+
Trimeresurus gramineus	29,500	25.0	n.d.	+	n.d.
Trimeresurus okinavensis	34,000	6.0	n.d.	+	n.d.
Agkistrodon contortrix contortrix	100,000	n.d.	n.d.	+	n.d.
Bitis gabonica	32,500	n.d.	n.d.	n.d.	n.d.

* From Russell, F. E.: *Snake Venom Poisoning.* J. B. Lippincott Co., Philadelphia, 1980; Scholium International, Great Neck, N.Y. 1983.

† n.d.: not determined.

Crotalus atrox digests mesenteric collagen fibers but not protein. EDTA inhibits the collagenolytic effect but not the argine esterase effect.

Hyaluronidase catalyzes the cleavage of internal glycoside bonds of certain acid mucopolysaccharides. This results in a decrease in the viscosity of connective tissues. The breakdown in the hyaluronic barrier allows other fractions of the venom to penetrate the tissues. The enzyme is thought to be related to the extent of the edema produced by the whole venom but to what degree it contributes to clinical swelling and edema is not known. The enzyme has also been referred to as the "spreading factor."

Phospholipase A (phospholipase A$_2$, PhA$_2$) has been found in the venoms of more than 20 species of snakes and appears to be widely distributed throughout the venoms of elapids, vipers, crotalids, sea snakes, and even colubrids. It catalyzes the hydrolysis of one of the fatty ester linkages in diacyl phosphatides, forming lysophosphatides and releasing both saturated and unsaturated fatty acids. As has been noted by several workers, data from many studies on PhA$_2$ must be evaluated with care, principally because impure preparations of the enzyme have often been employed. The molecular weights of this enzyme differ considerably. However, the molecular weight for the dimer of PhA$_2$ in *Crotalus atrox* venom is 29,500 that of *C. adamanteus* venom (PA$_2$—α), 29,500 to 29,900, and that of *C. viridis helleri* venom, approximately 29,500 to 30,000. There appears to be a considerable similarity in the positions of the sulfur atoms in many of the PhA$_2$ enzymes, and there are a number of other similarities, but there are also a number of important differences. The interested reader should consult the excellent review by Rosenberg (1979) for a more thorough understanding of the activities of the enzyme. Although generalizations concerning the pharmacologic activities of PhA$_2$ must be viewed with caution, some tentative assumptions might be noted. Contrary to earlier reports, the enzyme is not nearly as lethal as was suspected. In mice, the intravenous LD50 for the basic PhA$_2$ for *Naja nigricollis* venom is 0.25 mg/kg body weight, while that of the acidic PhA$_2$ is approximately 0.8 mg/kg. The two proteins with PhA$_2$ activity of *Vipera ammodytes* venom have been found to have intraperitoneal LD50 values of 0.19 and 0.64 mg/kg, respectively. The intravenous LD50 for the basic PhA$_2$ of *Crotalus durissus terrificus* is 0.54 mg/kg, and its lethal activity descends in the following order: chick, mouse, rabbit, rat. The results to date indicate that the basic PhA$_2$ enzymes are more lethal than the acidic PhA$_2$ enzymes, but there are variations in the lethal indices of both groups (see Russell, 1980b, 1983c).

Phosphomonoesterase (phosphatase) is widely distributed in the venoms of all families of snakes except the colubrids. It has properties of an orthophosphoric monoester phosphohydrolase. There are two nonspecific phosphomonoesterases, and they have optimal pH at 5.0 and 8.5. Many venoms contain both acid and alkaline phosphatases, while others contain only one or the other.

Phosphodiesterase has now been found in the venoms of all five families of poisonous snakes. It is an orthophosphoric diester phosphohydrolase that releases 5-mononucleotide from the polynucleotide chain and thus acts as an exonucleotidase, attacking DNA and RNA. More recently, it has been found that it also attacks derivatives of arabinose.

Acetylcholinesterase was first demonstrated

in cobra venom and is widely distributed throughout the elapid venoms. It is also found in sea snake venoms but is totally lacking in the viperid and crotalid venoms. It catalyzes the hydrolysis of acetylcholine to choline and acetic acid. The role of the enzyme in snake venoms is not clear. Its so-called effect on ganglionic and neuromuscular transmission as a venom constituent is highly questionable.

RNase is present in some snake venoms in small amounts as the endopolynucleotidase RNase. It appears to have specificity toward pyrmidine containing pyrimidyladenyl bonds in DNA. The optimum pH is 7 to 9, when ribosomal RNA is used as the substrate. This enzyme in *Naja oxiana* venom has a molecular weight of 15,900.

DNase acts on DNA and gives predominantly tri or higher oligonucleotides that terminate in 3′ monoesterified phosphate. *Crotalus adamanteus* venom contains two DNases, with optimum pH at 5 and 9.

5′-Nucleotidase is a common constituent of all snake venom and in most instances it is the most active phosphatase in snake venoms. It specifically hydrolyzes phosphate monoesters, which links with a 5′ position of DNA and RNA. It is found in greater amounts in crotalid and viper venoms than elapid venoms. The molecular weight as determined from amino acid composition and gel filtration with *Naja naja atra* venom has been estimated at 10,000. The enzyme from *N. naja* venom was enhanced by Mg^{2+}, inhibited by Zn^{2+}, inactivated at 75°C at pH 7.0 or 8.4, and has an isoelectric point of about 8.6. That from *Agkistrodon halys blomhoffii* showed a pH optimum of 6.8 to 6.9, with activity being enhanced by Mg^{2+}, and Mn^{2+}, and inhibited by Zn^{2+}. The enzyme has a low order of lethality and its pharmacologic role in the venom is not understood (see Russell, 1980b, 1983).

NAD nucleotidase has been found in the venoms of 9 of 37 species examined. The enzyme catalyzes the hydrolysis of the nicotinamide N-ribosidic linkage of NAD, yielding nicotinamide and adenosine diphosphate riboside. Its optimum pH is 6.5 to 8.5; it is heat labile, losing activity at 60°C. Its toxicologic contribution to snake venoms is not known.

L-Amino acid oxidase has been found in all snake venoms so far examined. It gives a yellow color to the venom. The enzyme catalyzes the oxidation of L-α-amino and α-hydroxy acids. This activity results from a group of homologous enzymes, showing molecular weights from 85,000 to 150,000. It has a high content of acidic amino acids. We found that the mouse intravenous LD50 of the enzyme from *Crotalus*

adamanteus venom was 9.13 mg/kg body weight, approximately four times less than the lethal value for the crude venom, and it had no effect on nerve, muscle, or neuromuscular transmission (see Russell, 1980b, 1983).

Lactate dehydrogenase reversibly catalyzes the conversion of lactic acid to pyruvic acid and has been reported to have been found in nine elapid venoms but was not found in three others.

Polypeptides. The snake venom polypeptides are low-molecular-weight proteins that do not have enzymatic activity. They are often logged under "neurotoxins," unfortunately, and this practice is not likely to change. As Will Rogers once said, "It is more difficult to change the label than the stuff in the bottle."

In 1938, Slotta and Fraenkel-Conrat isolated a crystalline protein from the venom of the tropical rattlesnake *Crotalus durissus terrificus*. The protein exhibited most of the toxic properties of the crude venom and was named *crotoxin*. In addition to the toxic nonenzymatic protein portion, it was found to contain the enzymes hyaluronidase, phospholipase, and possibly several others. It did not appear to have proteolytic or coagulant properties, or 5′-nucleotidase activity, but it had neurotoxic, indirect hemolytic, and smooth muscle–stimulating properties. Following removal of phospholipase A, crotoxin was further separated into a general toxic principle known as *crotactin*, which was found to have a greater lethal index than crotoxin, and a second component that may have been *crotamine*. The word crotoxin has been retained in one form or another in the literature as an identification for 17 different components of the venom of *Crotalus durissus terrificus* over the past 30 years. This has resulted in considerable confusion and more than once has led to disputes on research techniques, which could be more easily resolved on the basis of a difference in interpretation of what the investigator meant by crotoxin.

During the past 15 years various peptides of snake venoms have been characterized. In 1965 the first amino acid composition of a snake venom peptide was published (Yang, 1965), and at the First International Symposium on Animal Toxins in 1966 Professor Nobuo Tamiya presented a paper on the chromatography, crystallization, electrophoresis, ultracentrifugation, and amino acid composition of the venom of the sea snake *Laticauda semifasciata*. Almost all the lethal activity of the poison was recovered as two toxins, *erabutoxin a* and *b*, using carboxymethylcellulose chromatography, and 30 percent of the proteins were erabutoxins. The homogeneity of the crystalline toxins was demonstrated by rechromatography, disc electrophoresis, and ultracentrifugation (Tamiya *et al.,* 1967).

At the same meeting in 1966, Su and colleagues reported on the isolation of a cobra "neurotoxin." The toxin was separated by repeated fractionation with ammonium sulfate. The final product was a polypeptide and was approximately seven times more lethal than the crude venom. A product said to be identical to this in its lethal index and certain other pharmacologic characteristics was also obtained by starch gel electrophoresis. When the ammonium sulfate fraction was subjected to the same electrophoretic procedure, it concentrated as a single peak, with but little increase in its lethal property (Su *et al.,* 1967). Since 1966, more than 60 polypeptides having pharmacologic activities have been isolated from snake venoms. The interested reader will find definitive reviews on these peptides in the excellent work of Elliott (1978) and the book by Tu (1977). The texts edited by Rosenberg (1978), Lee (1979), and Eaker and Wadström (1980) contain other good papers on venom polypeptides.

Toxicology

It is not within the confines of this review to discuss all the pharmacologic activities of snake venoms. The interested reader is referred to Russell (1967), Mebs (1978), Russell (1983), and to articles in the compendiums noted above for a more thorough consideration of the specific toxicologic effects of these poisons and their components. However, some remarks will be made about the venoms of the North American crotalids, particularly the rattlesnake. The LD50's of some North American snake venoms are shown in Table 22–5.

In general, the venoms of the rattlesnakes and other New World crotalids produce alterations in the resistances (and often the integrity) of the blood vessels, changes in the blood cells and

blood coagulation mechanisms, direct or indirect changes in cardiac and pulmonary dynamics, alterations in the nervous system, and changes in respiration. Experimentally, these changes can be produced by varying the dose and kind of crotalid venom, the route and speed of administration, and the choice of the test animal. In humans, the course of the poisoning is determined by the kind and amount of venom injected, where it is deposited, the general health, size, and age of the patient, and the kind of treatment. Clinical experience indicates that death in humans occurs between less than one hour to several days, with most deaths occurring between 18 and 32 hours. Hypotension or shock is the major therapeutic problem. In some cases the hypotension is associated with acute blood loss secondary to bleeding and/or hemolysis but in most patients the shock is associated with a decrease in circulating fluid volume, with varying degrees of blood cell loss. It is not surprising, therefore, to find that numerous studies have been directed at determining the mechanisms responsible for snake venom poisoning, hypotension, and shock. These have been reviewed in some thoroughness elsewhere (Russell, 1983).

In 1962 it was found that an intravenous bolus injection of *Crotalus* venom caused an immediate fall in blood pressure and varying degrees of shock, which were associated with an initial hemoconcentration followed by a decrease in hematocrit values. There was an increased blood volume in the lungs, an increase in pulmonary artery pressure with a concomitant decrease in pulmonary artery flow, and a relatively stable heart stroke volume (Russell *et al.,* 1962). Other workers, using a 30-minute perfusion of *Crotalus* venom, concluded that the hypotension was related to the formation of pulmonary thromboemboli in the pulmonary vascular bed (Halmagyi *et al.,* 1965). Multiple pulmonary emboli may be found in animals receiving a fatal rattlesnake bite; however, the production of

Table 22–5.   LD50 BY DIFFERENT ROUTES OF INJECTION*†

VENOM	INTRAVENOUS	INTRAPERITONEAL	SUBCUTANEOUS
Crotalus viridis helleri	1.29	1.60	3.65
Crotalus adamanteus	1.68	1.90	13.73
Crotalus atrox	2.18	3.71	17.75
Crotalus scutulatus	0.21	0.23	0.31
Agkistrodon piscivorus	4.17	5.10	25.10
Agkistrodon contortrix	10.92	10.50	26.10
Sistrurus miliarius	2.91	6.89	25.10

* All determinations in 20-g. female mice of the same group. All mice were injected within a 1-hour period and were observed for 48 hours.

† From Russell, F. E.: *Snake Venom Poisoning.* J. B. Lippincott Co., Philadelphia, 1980; Scholium International, Great Neck, N.Y., 1983.

thromboembolism within one minute after administration of a bolus injection or even after a 30-minute infusion of the venom might be a difficult explanation for the rapid onset of pulmonary hypertension and the precipitous fall in systemic arterial pressure seen in experimental animals. Clumping of blood cells in the lungs, thrombosis, or even multiple pulmonary emboli might conceivably cause pulmonary hypertension within this short period, but it seems unlikely that thromboembolism is responsible for the immediate circulatory failure. There is another finding that adds to the unlikelihood of this proposed mechanism. In postmortem reports on victims who survived less than three hours after a rattlesnake bite, there is no evidence of pulmonary thromboembolism (Russell, 1983).

Crotalus venom appears to produce a pooling of blood in the hepatosplanchnic bed in the dog (Vick *et al.,* 1967). However, the hepatosplanchnic bed in the cat and human is known to be a lesser target area in most shock states than in the dog, and it seems unlikely that this explanation for the hypertension is consistent with snake venom poisoning in humans. Again, postmortem examinations in humans have not shown remarkable involvement of the hepatosplanchnic bed. More recently, Carlson and his colleagues have observed that when *Crotalus* venom is given intravenously and slowly over a 30-minute period, there is hypovolemia secondary to an increase in capillary permeability to protein and red blood cells. The laboratory findings showed initial hemoconcentration, lactacidemia, and hypoproteinemia (Carlson *et al.,* 1975). In cats, the same findings are seen, followed by a fall in hematocrit and, in some cases, hemolysis which is related to the dose of venom. During this period the cat may be in shock or at near-shock levels, depending on the amount of venom injected or perfused. Respirations become labored, and if the period is prolonged the animal becomes oliguric, rales develop, and the animal dies.

There appears to be no doubt that the shock or hypotension is caused by a decrease in circulating blood volume secondary to an increase in capillary permeability leading to the loss of fluid, protein, and, to some extent, erythrocytes. The severity of the hypotension is dose related, and restoration of circulating fluid volume can be achieved with intravenous fluids. In patients with venom shock, steroids are of no value, but the use of isoproterenol hydrochloride may be indicated. Antivenin in itself may not reverse a deep shock state, but a combination of parenteral fluids or plasma expanders, isoproterenol hydrochloride, and antivenin is of definite value.

Although the lung may suffer the most delete-rious changes in crotalid venom poisoning shock, almost all organs and tissues can be involved. Certainly, the venom can cause severe changes in blood coagulation, in erythrocyte integrity, or in other mechanisms. Although the action on the heart and kidneys is usually secondary to changes in the lung, blood, or blood dynamics, the crotalid venoms can affect these structures directly. The only organ that appears to be relatively unaffected by crotalid venoms is the brain, although several workers have indicated some electroencephalographic changes associated with crotalid venom injections. However, these changes are more easily explained on the basis of a decreased blood supply to the brain, resulting in cerebral anoxemia secondary to ischemic anemia.

Evidence to the present time indicates that the most probable fraction of the venom responsible for the circulatory failure is a peptide. In 1970, Dubnoff and Russell reported on the presence of two biologically active peptides in the venom of the rattlesnake *Crotalus viridis helleri.* Ion exchange chromatography on carboxymethyl-cellulose and on IRC-50 indicated molecular weights of approximately 6000 each. The peptides moved as cations on cellulose acetate at pH 8.6. Peptide I was identified as the major peak (Dubnoff and Russell, 1970). Subsequently, Bonilla and Fiero isolated highly basic proteins from the venoms of three species of rattlesnakes: *Crotalus viridis viridis, C. horridus horridus,* and *C. h. atricaudatus.* The proteins were separated by recycling adsorption chromatography using Bio-Gel P-2 and by ion-exchange chromatography on carboxymethylcellulose. These fractions were of low molecular weight, had isoelectric points above pH 6.8 (Bonilla and Fiero, 1971), and showed pharmacologic properties similar to those of the *C. v. helleri* isolated by Dubnoff and Russell.

Toxicologic studies have been carried out on the various fractions of *C. v. helleri* venom. One peptide, *C. v. helleri* Peptide 1, which moved as a cation on strip and gel electrophoresis and on ion-exchange chromatography, was resolved into three lethal peaks. The major fraction (*C. v. h.* Peptide Ic) was a basic polypeptide containing 43 amino acid residues with six half-cystine and had a molecular weight of 4490, as calculated from its sequence. Analysis showed that the peptide contained almost 20 percent lysine (Maeda *et al.,* 1978). The peptide was found to be responsible for hypotension or shock produced by the crude venom. When injected into rats, this peptide produced shock characterized by hypotension, lactacidemia, hemoconcentration, hypoproteinemia, and metabolic acidosis. Death occurred in some rats and respiratory distress was observed just prior to death. Hemolysis did not occur, but hemolysis and hematuria were observed in rats given the nonpeptide fractions (Schaeffer *et al.*, 1978).

The primary action of the peptide on the cardiovascular system involves its ability to produce a transient increase in vascular permeability to plasma protein, which, eventually, with certain other proteins, causes the loss of red blood cells. The peptide appears to alter the endothelial cells of the vascular wall, giving rise to the escape of plasma protein and some red blood cells. This finding for rattlesnake venom appears to differ from that presented for elapid venoms in that *C. viridis helleri* Peptide I is capable of producing rapid endothelial changes without enzyme involvement. Other protein components of the venom, some of which are enzymes, appear to have little effect on the vascular membrane but, rather, induce red blood cell changes or lysis. There may be some synergistic action but for the most part vascular properties are rather distinct.

Lizard Venoms

The Gila monster, *Heloderma suspectum,* and the beaded lizard, *H. horridum,* are divided into five subspecies. These large, corpulent, relatively slow-moving, and largely nocturnal reptiles have few enemies other than humans. They are far less dangerous than generally believed. Their venom is transferred from the venom glands in the lower jaw through ducts that discharge their contents near the base of the larger teeth of the lower jaw. The venom is then drawn up along grooves in the teeth by capillary action. The venom of this lizard has serotonin, amine oxidase, phospholipase A, proteolytic, and hyaluronidase activities but lacks phosphomono- and diesterase, acetylcholinesterase, nucleotidase, ATPase, DNase, RNase, amino acid oxidase, and fibrinogenocoagulase activities. The high hyaluronidase content seems to be consistent with the tissue edema seen in many clinical cases, and the low proteolytic activity is also consistent with the minimal tissue breakdown in clinical cases. Injection of large doses of *Heloderma* venom produces a fall in systemic arterial pressure with a decrease in circulating blood volume, tachycardia, and respiratory distress, and in lethal doses a loss of ventricular contractility (Russell and Bogert, 1981).

Clinical Problem

Snake venom poisoning is a medical emergency requiring immediate attention and the exercise of considerable judgment. Delayed or inadequate treatment may result in tragic consequences. However, before any treatment is instituted it is essential that a working diagnosis be established. In making a diagnosis it must be remembered that being bitten by a venomous snake does not necessarily mean being envenomated by that snake. A venomous snake may bite a person and not inject venom. Also, in treating snake venom poisoning one should keep in mind that he is faced with a case of multiple and complex poisoning. There is no single therapeutic measure other than antivenin which can effectively neutralize all of the physiopharmacologic activities of the venom.

Symptoms and signs of pit viper envenomation include the presence of fang marks, swelling, pain, ecchymosis, weakness, various paresthesia, faintness, nausea and vomiting, alterations in temperature, pulse, and blood pressure, fasciculations, urinary changes, early hemoconcentration followed by a decreased hematocrit, decreased platelets, petechiae, and shock. The most diagnostic sign of snakebite is rapid, progressive swelling. In most patients there is some swelling around the bite areas within 5 to 10 minutes, and often the swelling involves the entire finger, hand, toe, or foot, depending on the severity. A common symptom following the bites by many rattlesnakes is paresthesia about the mouth, often the forehead and scalp, and sometimes of the fingers and toes. This is usually present following the bites of the eastern diamondback rattlesnake (*Crotalus adamanteus*), the Pacific rattlesnakes (*C. viridis helleri* and *C. viridis oreganus*), most other *viridis* species, and some other species. The venom of some rattlesnake species, however, does not cause this complaint.

The degree of poisoning should be determined. A bite may appear minor at one hour but prove serious or even fatal at three hours. Most of the suggested grading systems for crotalid bites are precarious, for they usually depend on a few selected symptoms or signs and these are often stipulated for a specific time, for instance, 12 hours.

It is far more simple and practical to grade envenomations as minimal, moderate, or severe based on *all* clinical findings, including the laboratory data. One must then remember that the grading may need to be changed as the course of the poisoning or treatment progresses.

A determination should be made as to whether or not antivenin is necessary. It need not be given in trivial bites. The antivenin should be put in 250 to 1000 ml of an appropriate vehicle. Antivenin is compatible with commonly used dextrose and electrolyte solutions. The best results are obtained when it is administered during the first four hours following the bite, but its efficacy seems apparent for at least 24 hours after the bite, and perhaps longer. Antivenin has corrected blood clotting deficits even after 24 hours. In most cases, antivenin is not needed for copperhead bites but it may be indicated in water moccasin bites. A skin test should always be administered before giving antivenin. The patient should be slightly sedated, if not contraindicated, and put to bed with the injured part lightly immobilized in a functional position, and slightly below heart level. Medication for tetanus, pain, sleep, and anxiety should be given, if necessary. In moderate or severe envenomations, laboratory work should be done at least twice a day. Food should be avoided during the first 24 hours. Detailed clinical reports on bites by American species will be found in Russell (1980b, 1983) and Parrish (1980).

AMPHIBIA

The class Amphibia contains approximately 2600 species and is divided into the Anura, the toads and frogs, and the Urodela, the salamanders and newts. Although there are a number of amphibians known to be poisonous, very few of these are of a danger to humans. The most important toxic Anura are toads of the family Bufonidae; frogs of the families Atelopodidae, Dendrobatidae, Discoglossidae, Hylidae, Phyllomedusae, Pipidae, and Ranidae; newts of the genera *Taricha* and *Triturus;* and certain salamanders of the genus *Salamandra* (Kaiser and Michl, 1958; Habermehl, 1981; Daly, 1982).

Amphibian Toxins

The poisons of amphibians are produced in certain highly developed secretory glands in the skin. These secretions are generally excreted in a steady state, although there may be increased elaboration under duress or other conditions. Although it is commonly believed that their only function is related to a deterrent posture, that is, defense against predators, it has been shown that in some amphibians another important function is their role in protecting the host against microorganisms in the environment. When the skin is freed of the secretions of these particular glands, infection occurs and death often results. The secretions have been shown to inhibit the growth of bacteria and fungi in concentrations as low as 10^{-3} to 10^{-5} moles/liter (Habermehl, 1981).

The chemical composition of amphibian secretions are highly diversified. In the toads, biogenic amines, including adrenaline, noradrenaline, dopamine, and epinine are sometimes found, while among the indoalkylamines, the bases bufotenin, bufotenidin, and bufoviridin have been noted.

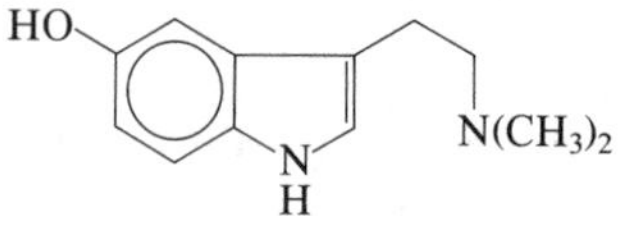

Bufotenin

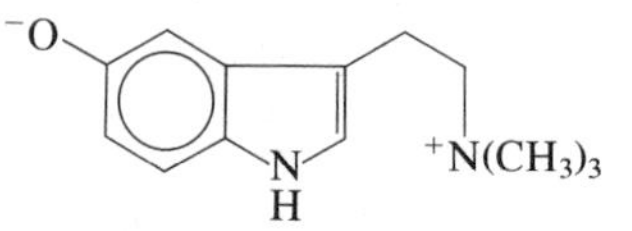

Bufotenidin

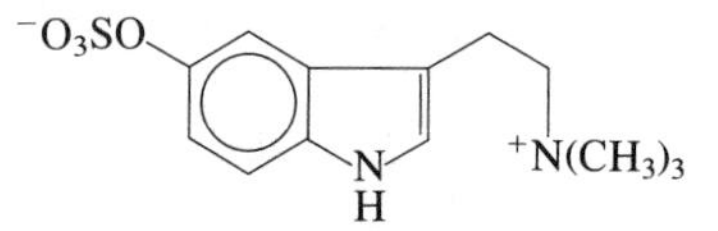

Bufoviridin

These substances have been described as causing vasoconstriciton, hypotension, and hallucinations. However, their specific toxicologic properties are poorly understood. A second group of toxic secretions in the toads is the bufogenines, presented as a formula by Meyer (1949), of which bufotalin is representative.

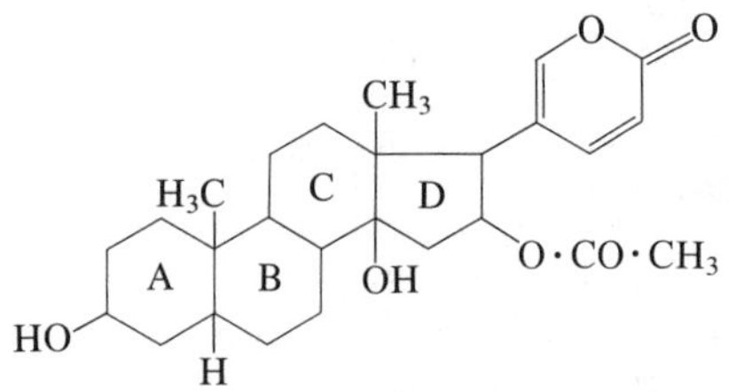

Bufotalin

The overall toxicologic properties of this group of secretions is not known but they appear to have a marked effect on smooth muscle, including the heart.

The frog toxins are even more diversified than the toad poisons. In the Atelopodidae, *Atelopus* species, a group of toxins known as *zetekitoxins* are found. The poison from the golden arrow frogs of Costa Rica, Panama, and Columbia has long been used on hunting darts by the Indians in those areas. The structure of these toxins is not clear, although a guanidine group has been described, and the poison contains no peptides, carbohydrates, or steroids. The subcutaneous "lethal dose" in mice for zetekitoxin AB is 11 μg/kg, for zetekitoxin C, 80 μg/kg body weight. Their toxicologic properties are not known. *Tetrodotoxin* has been isolated from the skin and egg clusters of *A. varius,* while both tetrodotoxin and *chiriquitoxin* have been found in the skin and eggs of *A. chiriquensis*. In the Dendrobatidae, particularly *Phyllobates* and *Dendrobates,* more than 100 toxic skin secretions have been identified (Daly, 1982). Most of these are alkaloids, and their use as dart or arrow poisons by certain South Central American Indians is well known (Marki and Witkop, 1963). Among the steroid alkaloids are *batrachotoxin, batrachotoxin A, homobatrachotoxin, dihydrobatrachotoxin,* and *3-0-methylbatrachotoxin,* all found in certain *Phyllobates* species.

Batrachotoxin

Batrachotoxin is one of the most toxic substances known, the subcutaneous lethal dose in mice being 100 nanograms; the estimated lethal dose for humans is less than 200 μg. Although generally classified as a "neurotoxin," the alkaloid has a marked effect on the heart, first evident as arrythmias and then by changes leading to cardiac arrest. It has a direct effect on the peripheral nervous system, producing membrane depolarization, which is probably due to an increase in cell membrane permeability by sodium, without changes in the potassium or calcium ions. Both tetrodotoxin and saxitoxin prevent and even reverse the depolarization caused by batrachotoxin. Certain anesthetics antagonize the action of the alkaloid, while certain local anesthetics block its action. Batrachotoxin also causes a massive release of acetylcholine in nerve-muscle preparations. The ultrastructure changes in nerve and muscle precipitated by this toxin are due to osmotic alterations produced by the massive influx of sodium ions. These various activities are time and stimulus dependent, suggesting that activity requires prior activation or opening of the sodium channel. It has been suggested that batrachotoxin also has a central nervous system effect (Daly, 1982).

From the skin secretions of *Dendrobates pumilio* and *D. auratus,* three alkaloids have been isolated, *pumiliotoxin A* ($C_{19}H_{33}NO_2$), *B* ($C_{19}H_{33}NO_3$), and *C* ($D_{13}H_{25}N$). The skin secretions from the latter frog have also yielded

other alkaloids, while spiropiperidine alkaloids have been identified in the skin secretions of *D. histrionicus.* The subcutaneous "minimal lethal dose" in mice for pumiliotoxin A is 2.5 mg/kg body weight; for pumiliotoxin B, 1.5 mg/kg; and for pumiliotoxin C, 20 mg/kg. These doses produce ataxia, "clonic convulsions," and death within 20 minutes. Pumiliotoxin B potentiates both direct and indirect evoked contractions of striated muscle, which is thought to be due to mechanism-related facilitation of calcium influx of the muscle fiber and/or a facilitation of release of calcium from the sarcoplasmic reticulum. It does not appear to have an effect on sodium, potassium, or chloride conductances, or on the resting membrane potential (Albuquerque *et al.,* 1981). The poisons of the Disoglossidae, or the disc tongue frogs, have been the object of extended study by Michl and his colleagues in Vienna (see Kaiser and Michl, 1958). The skin secretions of *Bombina bombina* have yielded large amounts of serotonin, free amino acids, and basic peptides. In *B. variegata,* 12 α-amino acids, γ-amino-butyric acid, and serotonin, two nonapeptides, and a hemolytic polypeptide of 87,000 daltons have been demonstrated (Habermehl, 1981).

The poisons of the newts and salamanders have undergone considerable study. Tarichatoxin has been isolated from three species of newts, *Taricha torosa, T. rivularis,* and *T. granulosa.* It is, of course, the same toxin found in the pufferfish *Sphoeroides* species, and known as tetrodotoxin. Tarichatoxin, or tetrodotoxin, is also found in some species of frogs, and at least one octopus, as well as a number of other fishes beside the puffers. Among the steroid alkaloids found in the salamanders are *samanin, samandenon, cycloneosamandaridin, cycloneosamandion, samandarin,* and *samandaridin.* Samandarin is a very potent toxin, which is said to act on the central nervous system and has hypertensive and anesthetic properties.

MARINE ANIMALS

Like the snakes, the venomous and poisonous marine animals have enjoyed a fascinating history, including sea serpents that crawled ashore and copulated with vipers, others that sprayed their venom onto unassuming seamen on sailing ships, thus paralyzing them on the spot, and stingrays that stung and killed trees. These are only a few of the numerous bits of folklore recorded in the literature. The interested reader should consult the compendium of Halstead (1965–70), and the works of Phillips and Brady (1953), Kaiser and Michl (1958), Russell (1965),

Baslow (1969), Russell (1971), Martin and Padilla (1973), Scheuer (1973, 1978–1981), Halstead (1978), Southcott (1979), and Russell (1984a) for the more historical accounts on venomous marine animals.

There are approximately 1200 species of marine organisms known to be venomous or poisonous (Russell, 1983a). For the most part these animals are widely distributed throughout the marine fauna from the unicellular protistan *Gonyaulax* to certain of the chordates. They are found in almost all seas and oceans of the world. In most areas they do not constitute a medical or socioeconomic problem. However, in a few scattered regions, such as the South Pacific, where ciguatera poisoning sometimes gives rise to serious public health and economic problems, and in the case of paralytic shellfish poisoning, the poisonous marine animals have presented a threat to our health and economy.

Marine Toxins

While the marine toxins as a whole are far more varied in their chemical composition than those from terrestrial animals, there is some degree of component consistence within a particular genus or species of each group. However, there are some notable exceptions. Some organisms, such as the clams and mussels, may be toxic only during one period, or a particular period, or in one place and not elsewhere, while the toxicity in tetraodons varies with the species of fish, the organs studied, and other factors. Toxicity in ciguateric fishes is, at the present time, and for all practical purposes, almost unpredictable with respect to the species involved, location, and time of year.

Some marine toxins are proteins of low molecular weight, while others are of high molecular weight. Some marine venoms or poisons are composed of lipids, amines, quinones, quaternary ammonium compounds, alkaloids, guanidine bases, phenols, steroids, mucopolysaccharides, or halogenated compounds. The fish venoms are unstable but most of the other toxins, including the fish poisons, are relatively stable, particularly in the dried or lyophilized form. In some marine organisms there are several toxins present, and in some instances two organisms are necessary to produce one toxin. Finally, it is known that the venom of one species or genus within one phylum may be similar or even identical to that found in an animal of an entirely different phylum. The newt poison, tarichatoxin, and the pufferfish poison, tetrodotoxin, are one and the same.

As would be expected, the pharmacologic or toxicologic activities of marine toxins vary as remarkably as do their chemical properties.

Some marine toxins provoke rather simple effects, such as transient vasoconstriction or dilatation, pain, or localized erythema, while others produce more complex responses, such as parasympathetic dysfunction or multiple concomitant changes in cardiovascular or blood dynamics. And there is no doubt that in the evolution of marine toxins, as in snake and other terrestrial venoms (Russell, 1980a), synergistic and possibly antagonistic reactions may occur as the result of interactions between individual venom components.

Protista

Among the protistan are the various protozoans, algae, diatoms, bacteria, yeasts, and fungi. The marine protista are widely distributed throughout neritic waters and in the high seas from the polar oceans to the tropics. There are at least 80 species that are known to be toxic to humans and other animals. A listing of these will be found in Russell (1984a). Most of the toxic organisms are of the order Dinoflagellata, of which there are more than 1200 species. Protistan have been shown to contain or release a toxin that (1) gives rise to paralytic shellfish poisoning through the food chain, (2) produces respiratory or gastrointestinal distress or dermatitis in humans, (3) causes mass mortality of marine animals, or (4) has been implicated by laboratory experiments as being toxic. Blooms of protistan sometimes occur and result in the phenomenon frequently referred to as "red tide," or "red water." However, the bloom may appear yellowish, brownish, greenish, bluish, or even milky in color, depending on the organism involved and other factors. Such blooms usually become visible when 20,000 or more of the organisms are present in 1 ml of water. However, some blooms may contain 50,000 or more organisms. The red color in red tides is probably due to peridinin, a xanthophyll.

Paralytic shellfish poison (PSP), variously known as *saxitoxin, Gonyaulax toxin, dinoflagellate poison, mussel or clam poison,* or *mytilotoxin,* is a toxin or group of toxins found in certain molluscs, arthropods, echinoderms, and some other marine animals that have ingested toxic protistan and have become "poisonous." PSP through the food chain is well known in animals and humans. Although the relationship between blooms of plankton and shellfish poisoning was first noted by Lamouroux (cited by Chevallier and Duchesne, 1851), it was not until 1937 that Sommer and Meyer published the results of their intensive investigation on paralytic shellfish poisoning. They demonstrated a direct relationship between the number of *Gonyaulax catenella* in seawater and toxicity in the mussel

Mytilus californianus. They also established methods for extracting and assaying the poison.

The amount of poison in the shellfish or other organism is dependent on the number of toxic protistan filtered by the host animal. Off California, mussels become dangerous for human consumption when 200/ml or more protistan are found in the coastal waters. As the count rises, the mussels become more toxic. Within a week or two, in the absence of the toxic protistan, the mussels become relatively free of the poison. The toxin has been studied by extractions from shellfish, from dinoflagellates secured from natural blooms and, more recently, from laboratory cultures. PSP can be obtained from all three sources in like form. Burke *et al.* (1960), Schantz *et al.* (1966), and Proctor *et al.* (1975) have grown *Gonyaulax catenella* in axenic cultures in cell densities equal to those occurring during natural blooms, and Schantz (1960) showed that the chromatographic properties of the toxin from the cultured organisms appear identical to those of the toxin found in natural blooms and mussels. It was not until 1975 that Schantz *et al.* presented the absolute configuration:

There is some question as to how many toxins exist in the complex of PSP. In the earlier works it was considered as a single poison but it must now be thought of as a complex of toxins. In the case of toxins from *Gymnodinium breve,* there appears to be several if not a number of toxins, but at this point in time it has not been established that the toxins reflect differences in the techniques employed in isolation procedures or are the result of distinct differences in the toxin(s). In the dinoflagellate *Gonyaulax tamarensis* there are several other toxins in addition to saxitoxin and these differ from saxitoxin only in their weak binding ability on carboxylate resins. Further studies on organisms isolated from red tides along the New England coast have resulted in the isolation of two other toxins, *gonyautoxin II* (GTX₂) and *gonyautoxin III* (GTX₃) (Shimizu, 1978). Another toxin, *neosaxitoxin,* has also been isolated from *G. tamarensis.*

While a number of pharmacologic and toxicologic studies on shellfish poisons were carried out before the turn of this century, it was not until Meyer *et al.* (1928), Prinzmetal *et al.*

(1932), and Sommer and Meyer (1937) that the more definitive work was reported. Prinzmetal *et al.* (1932) showed that the poison from the mussel *Mytilus californianus* was slowly absorbed from the gastrointestinal tract and rapidly excreted by the kidneys. It was said to depress respiration, the cardioinhibitory and vasomotor centers, and conduction in the myocardium. Subsequent studies showed that saxitoxin had a marked effect on peripheral nerve and skeletal muscle in the frog. The "curarelike" action was attributed to some mechanism that prevented the muscle from responding to acetylcholine. The toxin produced progressive diminution in the amplitude of the end-plate potential in the frog nerve-muscle preparation. It also depressed mammalian phrenic nerve potentials, suppressed the indirectly elicited contractions of the diaphragm, and often reduced the directly stimulated contractions. It was concluded that the effect of the poison was greater on reflex transmission than on the nerve. Contraction of isolated muscle fibers in the presence of ATP and magnesium ions was not inhibited by the poison, nor did the toxin alter the rate of oxygen consumption in the respiring diaphragm of the mouse. With respect to the cardiovascular system, the toxin was shown to have a direct effect on the heart and its conduction system. It produced changes that ranged from a slight decrease in heart rate and contractile force, with simple P-R interval prolongation or S-T segment changes, to severe bradycardia and bundle-branch block, or complete cardiac failure. The poison provoked a prompt but reversible depression in the contractility of isolated cat papillary muscle (see Russell, 1983a, for references).

In 1967, Kao demonstrated that the toxin blocks action potentials in nerves and muscles by preventing, in a very specific manner, an increase in the ionic permeability that is normally associated with the inward flow of sodium. It appears to do this without altering potassium or chloride conductances. Evans (1967) showed that in cats, mussel poison blocks transmission between the peripheral nerves and the spinal roots. The large myelinated sensory fibers are blocked by intravenous doses of 4.5 to 13 μg/kg, while the large motor fibers are not blocked until this dose is increased by approximately 30 to 40 percent. He also observed that when dilute solutions of saxitoxin were applied locally to thin peripheral nerve branches in cats, conduction was not blocked. However, conduction was blocked in dorsal and ventral spinal root fibers following the topical application of far smaller concentrations. He suggests that one of the layers in the connective tissue sheath of peripheral nerve is impermeable to saxitoxin, while the leptomeninges covering the spinal roots are either deficient in or lack this layer.

Sommer and Meyer (1937) found that 3000 *Gonyaulax* weighed 100 μg (wet weight) and that this number yielded 15 μg of the dry extract, which in turn gave 1 μg of pure poison, or 1 mouse unit. A mouse unit, or average lethal dose, was defined as the amount of toxin that would kill a 20-g mouse in 15 min (Prinzmetal *et al.*, 1932; Sommer and Meyer, 1937). Thus, the amount of toxin contained in a single *Gonyaulax* was taken as $\frac{1}{3000}$ of a mouse unit. McFarren and associates (1956) found the oral LD50s per kg body weight to vary considerably with the animal used and with its strain and weight. Their figures would indicate that the human is twice as susceptible to the poison as the dog and approximately four times more susceptible than the mouse.

During the 1950s the Canadian–United States Conference on Shellfish Toxicology adopted a bioassay based on the use of the purified toxin isolated by Schantz and his colleagues (1958). The intraperitoneal minimal lethal dose of the toxin for the mouse was approximately 9.0 μg/kg body weight. The intravenous minimal lethal dose for the rabbit was 3.0 to 4.0 μg/kg of body weight, while the minimal lethal oral dose for humans was thought to be between 1.0 and 4.0 mg. Wiberg and Stephenson (1960) demonstrated that the LD50 of the then purified toxin in mice was:

Oral route	263 (251–267) μg/kg
Intravenous route	3.4 (3.2–3.6) μg/kg
Intraperitoneal route	10.0 (9.7–10.5) μg/kg

More recently, various figures on the toxic and lethal doses for humans have been presented by various workers. The figures presented by Prakash *et al.* (1971) seem consistent with our own calculations; that is, a mild case of poisoning can be caused by ingesting 1 mg of toxin, which might be the amount found in one to five poisonous mussels or clams weighing about 150 g each. A moderate case of poisoning can be caused by ingesting 2 mg of the poison, while a serious poisoning would be caused by 3 mg. One would expect that 4 mg of the toxin would be lethal to humans if vigorous treatment was not instituted.

The latest standards for toxicity are those set by the Association of Official Analytical Chemists (A.O.A.C.) (1975). However, this standard, like others, has several shortcomings. A number of assays have been proposed to circumvent these deficiencies. For example, an immunochemical technique has been suggested while another method employs an analysis based on the oxidation of saxitoxin to a fluorescent derivative. Spectrophotometric analysis has been proposed and a unique cockroach bioassay has been described. One of the most promising assays incorporates flow cytometric analysis of cellular saxitoxin, dependent on mithramycin fluorescent staining (see Russell, 1983, for references). With the advent of the enzyme-linked immunosorbent assay (ELISA) and radioimmunology, new and improved techniques for determining toxicities should appear within the next few years.

Porifera (Sponges)

Sponges are among the simplest of animals. They are highly organized colonies of unicellular nomads composed of loosely integrated cells covered by a skin and, with few exceptions, supported internally by a skeleton of silica, calcite, or spongin. There are more than 5000 species and they are found in almost every sea from midtide levels to the deepest parts of the oceans. Some sponges release a toxic substance into their environment. De Laubenfels (1932) observed that when *Tedania toxicalis* was placed in a bucket with fishes, crabs, molluscs, and worms, in an hour or perhaps less these animals will be found dead. Although this phenomenon has usually been considered as a purely defensive reaction initiated when the sponge becomes endangered, Green (1977) suggested that the toxic material may be released as a continuous product into the surrounding water, and thus serve as a warning or deterrent to an approaching predator.

Many sponges have an offensive odor and taste, but what part these qualities play in defense or in poisoning is not known. Although some studies on the chemistry of sponges have progressed with great rapidity during recent years, specific chemical and toxicologic investigations on the toxic components have lagged far behind. The more important marine sponges of biologic importance are described elsewhere (Russell, 1983). The interested reader should also consult Halstead (1965), Jakowska and Nigrelli (1970), Stempien *et al.* (1970), Green (1977), and Bakus and Thun (1979) for more detailed data on the toxicity of these species. It should be noted that some sponges of the same genus as those found to be toxic to fishes have also been found to be nontoxic. The family Haliclonidae appears to have the most consistently toxic species.

Perhaps the most extensive studies of toxic observations on fishes have been those by Bakus and his colleagues. Essentially, their shipboard preliminary assay method involves grinding 5 g of the sponge in 10 ml of seawater, centrifuging, pouring the supernatant into a bowl with 300 ml of seawater, and then placing a 1.5- to 5-g sargent major (*Abudefduf saxatilis*) into the water and observing the fish's behavior over a designated period of time. After preliminary testing serial dilutions of the crude extract are prepared, starting with 0.1 g crude material/ml tapwater; an alcohol extract is used for comparison and the LC50 (lethal concentration for 50 percent of the animals) determinations are done for the more highly toxic sponges. Toxicity is determined on the basis of the fishes swallowing air, blowing bubbles, being bitten by normal fish, equilibrium loss, erratic swimming behavior, slow swimming movements, escape responses, thrashing behavior, extreme lethargy or stupor, failure to recover when put in fresh water, and death (Bakus and Thun, 1979).

In 1906, Richet precipitated a substance from extracts of the siliceous sponge *Suberites domunculus,* which when injected into the dog produced vomiting, diarrhea, and dyspnea, and caused hemorrhages in the gastric and intestinal mucosa, peritoneum, and endocardium. The lethal dose in dogs was 10 mg/kg and the toxic substance was found to be nontoxic when administered orally. The poison was called "suberitine" (Richet, 1906; Lassabliere, 1906). Arndt (1928) demonstrated that extracts from certain fresh-water sponges produced diarrhea, dyspnea, prostration, and death when injected into homoiothermic animals. These same extracts had some hemolytic effect on sheep and pig erythrocytes and blocked cardiac function in the isolated frog heart preparation. The extracts were heat stable and produced no deleterious effects when taken orally. Das *et al.* (1971) found that extracts of *S. inconstans* produced a histamine-like effect on the guinea pig intestine and attributed this to histamine, which they found in the sponge. On paper chromatography they detected five other amines, three having phenolic groups. Dried specimens of *Fasciospongia cavernosa* yielded crystals of *N*-acyl-2-methylene-β-alanine methyl esters. In mice, the subcutaneous lethal dose of the crystals was approximately 120 mg/kg body weight (Kashman *et al.,* 1973), obviously not very toxic. Algelasine from *Agelas dispar* has activities of a saponin. A unique sesquiterpene, 9-isocyanopupukeanane, has been isolated from the nudibranch *Phyllidia varicosa* and has been found to be present in the sponge *Hymeniacidon* sp., on which the nudibranch feeds (Burreson *et al.*, 1975).

Cariello *et al.* (1980) isolated and characterized Richet's suberitine. The toxin, which had an approximate molecular weight of 28,000 produced a marked hemolytic effect on human erythrocytes and showed some ATPase activity. Studies on the giant axon of the abdominal nerve of the crayfish indicated in a concentration of 4.4 mg/ml there was depolarization, followed by an irreversible block in the indirectly stimulated action potential. The authors speculated that this irreversible block may explain the flaccid paralysis seen in crabs following injection of suberitine into the arthropod's hemolymph. Wang *et al.* (1973) demonstrated that a preparation of an extract of *Haliclona rubens* exerted a depolarizing action on the end-plate membrane of the frog skeletal muscle and that a lesser depolarization occurred in the membrane elsewhere than at the end plate. This activity differed from that caused by *batrachotoxin* and *grayanotoxin* (a toxin from the plant Ericaceae).

Clinical Problem. With respect to humans, poisoning probably occurs through deposit of the toxin(s) in the superficial abrasions produced by the fine, sharp spicules of the sponge. It is known that traumatic injury to the human skin can be produced by the spicules, particularly those of the hexactinellids, and it is believed that in many cases of poisoning this occurs prior to the deposit of the poison on the skin. Certainly, an abraded skin is more likely to absorb a toxin than an uninjured one (Russell, 1965). The most frequently offending sponges are *Tedania nigrescens, T. inconstans,* and *Neofibularia nolitangere.* Symptoms and signs consist of a burning or irritating sensation over the hands or other part contacted by the sponge, subsequent mild pain, sometimes confined to the joints of the hand, pruritus, often severe, and malaise. The contact areas are warm to touch and there may be mild edema. Systemic manifestations and infections are rare. Treatment consists of thoroughly washing the hands with soapy water and applying "Russell's balm" (Land/sea balm®; hydrocortisone, tetracaine, and diphenhydramine hydrochloride) four times a day (Maretić and Russell, 1983).

Cnidaria (Coelenterates)

The phylum Cnidaria (hydroids, jellyfish, sea anemones, and corals) are simple metazoans that possess the two basic tissues found in all higher animals, a layer of jellylike material with supporting elastic fibres between the ectoderm and endoderm known as "mesoglea," a gastrovascular cavity that opens only through its mouth, radial symmetry, and tentacles bearing abundant nematocysts. In the Portuguese man-of-war, *Physalia,* and in many other cnidarians the tentacles contain long muscle strands which can be contracted to bring the animal's prey to the feeding polyps below the umbrella. These polyps engulf the prey and digest it. Venomous forms are found in all three classes of living cnidarians: Hydrozoa, or hydroids, hydromedusae, and fire corals; Scyphozoa, or true jellyfish; Anthozoa, or sea anemones, sea feathers, and corals. The Hydrozoa are branched or simple polyps, some having budded medusae. The order Siphonophora includes the Portuguese man-of-war, *Physalia*. The Scyphozoa, true medusae or jellyfish, are typified by a body, umbrella, or bell, which is usually convex above and concave below. The Cubomedusae or sea wasps are the most dangerous of all the cnidarians, particularly *Chironex fleckeri* and *Chiropsalmus quadrigatus* of Australia. Finally, the class Anthozoa contains the corals, sea anemones, and alcyonarians. The anemones are sedentary, flowerlike structures. The alcyonarians include the stony, soft, horny, and black corals, as well as colonial sea pens and sea pansies. The cnidarians of particular importance because of their stings on humans or their unusual toxicologic properties are listed elsewhere (Russell, 1984a).

The stinging unit of the cnidarians is the nematocysts. I might be venturist to say that all 9000 species of cnidarians have nematocysts (Russell, 1984a). Nematocysts have been classified on the basis of their structure, function, and taxonomy. Weill (1934) described 17 categories of nematocysts, and while these have been qualified with the passing of time, in general, this approach still offers a basis for common communication. The nematocyst, which is a capsulated, ovoid cell varying in size from 4 to 225 μm, contains an operculum, a long coiled tube or hollow thread, matrix, and venom. The nematocyst is formed as "metaplasmic organelle" within an interstitial cell, the cnidoblast. These cnidoblasts are distributed throughout the epidermis, except on the basal disk. The coiled tubule in the undischarged nematocyst varies in length from 50 μm to over 1 mm, depending on the species of cnidarian. When discharged the operculum is released and the everted tubule explodes, remaining attached at the original site of the operculum. The nature of nematocyst discharge and the localized fashion in which these cells respond to stimuli, whether chemical, mechanical, or electrical, have been the object of extensive study (see Russell, 1984a, for references).

As in many of the earlier studies on marine venoms, the chemical and toxicologic properties of the cnidarian toxins were carried out with crude saline or water extracts prepared from the whole animal or from one or several of its parts. It is apparent that some early workers were studying normal constituents of the animal's tissues, several of which appear to be limited to tissues in the lower phyla. When these substances were injected into higher animals, they produced deleterious reactions. These reactions then became aligned with clinical findings and, unfortunately, led to misunderstandings and questionable therapeutic advice (Russell, 1965). Such substances as *thalassin, congestin,* and the *Cyanea principle* were probably derived from tentacular tissues rather than venom-bearing nematocysts.

The modern period of fire coral toxicology began with the work of Wittle *et al.* (1971) and Middlebrook *et al.* (1971). These investigators studied nematocyst toxin from *Millepora alcicornis.* They obtained a product with a molecular weight of approximately 100,000 and an intravenous mouse LD50 of 0.04 mg/kg body weight. The toxin had hemolytic and dermonecrotic activities and was antigenic with cross-protection against *M. alcicornis* toxin. They also obtained an electrophoretically pure toxin from the fire coral, *Millepora dichotoma.* The LD50 was 0.038 mg/kg body weight, quite similar to that found for *M. alcicornis.* The signs in mice were also similar. The sea whip *Lophogorgia rigida* contains a toxin known as *lophotoxin.* Its formula is $C_{22}H_{24}O_8$. The toxin has a subcutaneous LD50 in mice of 8.9 mg/kg body weight and was found to block the indirectly elicited contractions in a mammalian nerve-muscle preparation, while not affecting the directly elicited contractions. It was concluded that lophotoxin produces an irreversible postsynaptic block, although the possibility of a presynaptic function could not be excluded (Culver and Jacobs, 1981).

While techniques for separating nematocysts are not new, the initial studies on a nematocyst preparation from *Physalia physalis* were performed by Lane and Dodge (1958). They found their nematocyst preparation to be a highly labile protein complex, rich in glutamic acid and having an approximate intraperitoneal lethal dose in mice of 0.037 ml/kg body weight of a preparation containing 0.02 percent total nitrogen. The toxin produced paralysis in fish, frogs, and mice. Animals killed following stingings by *Physalia* exhibited marked pulmonary edema, right cardiac dilatation, with venous congestion of the larger vessels of the chest and portal circulations. Since the original work of Lane and Dodge a number of advances in the preparation of nematocyst toxins from *P. physalis* have been made. These and the toxicologic studies have been reviewed elsewhere (Russell, 1984a). Various investigations on crabs, rats, dogs, and a nerve-muscle preparation of the frog indicated that the toxin produced changes in the Na-K pump, resulting in depolarization of the cell membranes. In the rat, where the LD50 was approximately 100 μg/kg body weight, low doses of the toxin caused an increase in the Q-T interval, a decrease in the P-R interval, and P-wave inversion. Large doses produced marked ECG changes leading to cardiac failure. Subsequent studies showed that the ability of skeletal muscles sarcoplasmic reticulum to bind ionic calcium and nuclear alterations and dissolution of intercellular collagen in cultured hamster ovary K-1 cells are important properties of the toxin (Calton *et al.*, 1973; Neeman *et al.*, 1981).

Tamkun and Hessinger (1981) obtained a hemolytic protein from *P. physalis*. This protein, *physalitoxin*, was also lethal to mice at the 0.20 mg protein/kg body weight level, while the LD50 for the crude venom was 0.14 mg/kg. A molecular weight of 212,000 was calculated. The authors suggested that the toxin was composed of three subunits of unequal size, each of which is glycoylated. Physalitoxin was about 28 percent of the total nematocyst venom protein. Its carbohydrate content was 10.6 percent and represented the major glycoprotein of the crude venom. This hemolytic and lethal toxin was inactivated by concanavalin A.

Initial studies of extracts of the frozen tentacles of the sea wasp, *Chironex fleckeri*, indicated that the extracts had lethal, necrotizing, and hemolytic properties (Southcott and Kingston, 1959). Barnes (1967) isolated a *Chironex* nematocyst crude toxin by employing human amnion membrane and electrically stimulating the tentacles. In his initial study, Barnes found that the undiluted toxin was lethal to mice at the 0.005 ml/kg body weight level but it was not known what this might be in dry weight, mg protein, or protein nitrogen. Endean *et al.* (1969) found proteins, carbohydrates, cystine-containing compounds, and 3-indolyl derivatives in the nematocysts of the tentacles of *C. fleckeri*. Saline extracts of the contents of the nematocysts were highly toxic to prawn and fish, and were lethal to mice and rats. In mice, the intravenous LD50 was between 20,000 and 25,000 nematocysts, while in rats the LD50 was approximately 150,000 nematocysts. Using partially purified extracts of the tentacles, Freeman and Turner (1969) found that extracts produced respiratory arrest, which they attributed to a central origin. They also implicated deleterious cardiac changes leading to an atrioventricular block. Blood pressure and chemistry changes were consistent with a reduced circulating blood volume and hypoxia. The toxins had a nonspecific lytic effect on cells and no particular differential effect on the guinea pig diaphragm preparation. It was found that 0.1 ml of a 5000-fold dilution of the tentacle extract would kill a 20-g mouse in

less than 2 minutes and that the toxin was hemolytic. The fraction was nondialyzable and an estimated molecular weight of 8000 was suggested.

Crone and Keen (1969) obtained two toxic proteins using tentacle extracts. The hemolytic activity was related to a protein component with a molecular weight of approximately 70,000. The second toxin had a molecular weight of about 150,000, and while both components had cardiotoxic activity, the larger fraction had considerably more than the smaller fraction. Two *Chironex* tentacle extracts were studied by Freeman and Turner (1971), who found that both the fractions produced an initial increase in systemic arterial pressure followed by a fall in pressure, bradycardia, and cardiac arrythmia. In the perfused guinea pig heart, both toxins caused a reduction in rate, amplitude of contraction, and coronary flow. The authors concluded that the cardiovascular effects were due "direct vasoconstriction, cardiotoxicity, a baroreceptor stimulation and possible depression of the vasomotor center."

These various data have been controversial. It appears that the toxin(s) derived from tentacles is quite different from that obtained from discharged or undischarged nematocysts. An attempt to resolve the discrepancies was made by Endean and Nobel (1971). Using methods previously described by their group, they separated material within the nematocysts from the residual tentacular material. The two products were studied by injection into mice and rats, on the barnacle muscle preparation, the rat phrenic nerve-diaphragm preparation, the toad sciatic nerve-gastrocnemius and sciatic nerve conduction preparations, rat ilea and heart preparations, and certain other isolated tissue preparations. It was found that following removal of the nematocysts from the tentacles, the remaining product possessed quite different biologic activities from that extracted from the nematocysts. Although the work of Endean and Noble indicates certain differences, it is difficult to define these accurately in the absence of a standard tissue weight or solution. Furthermore, some of the differences demonstrated by the various investigators for *Chironex* toxins, as well as several other cnidarian toxins, might be due to the dose relationships rather than the toxins employed. This is particularly true for the rat or guinea pig diaphragm-phrenic nerve preparation. Changes in the dose of toxins cause not only quantitative changes but qualitative ones. Furthermore, when the muscle of a mammalian nerve-muscle preparation is shortened, it is most difficult to determine the effect on the indirectly elicited contraction. In fact, in a shortened muscle it is even difficult to determine the significance of the direct effect. Obviously, a substance that is highly irritating to an entire muscle membrane presents a problem when one hopes to define its action on the nerve, or even on the activity of a single muscle fiber.

Baxter and his colleagues at the Commonwealth Serum Laboratories in Australia, using saline extracts of nematocysts obtained after the method of Barnes (1967), or as described by Endean *et al.* (1969), demonstrated that the biologically active fractions causing lethal, hemolytic, and dermonecrotizing reactions were in the 10,000 to 30,000 molecular-weight range. In rabbits, a lethal intravenous dose of the venom caused labored and deep respirations followed within several minutes by prostration, hyperextension of the head, "spasms," and respiratory and cardiac arrest. In sheep, a similar respiratory deficit was seen, followed by unsteadiness, muscle tremors, and "spasms." The head drooped to one side, prostration occurred, and the tongue was said to be paralyzed and cyanotic. In primates, the animal became inactive, "dull," confused, and exhibited slight ataxia and incoordination. The eyelids drooped, the mouth was open, and the head "weaved." Heart rate was irregular, and breathing became labored, deep, and irregular. Within a few minutes the animal collapsed, the heart rate deteriorated, and cyanosis developed just prior to death. Postmortem examination revealed marked congestion of the vessels of the lungs, pulmonary edema, the right ventricle was engorged, the kidneys and liver were congested, and the vessels of the menenges of the cerebrum were engorged (Baxter *et al.*, 1972).

Considerable study has been done on the nematocyst toxin of the sea nettle *Chrysaore quinquecirrha* by Burnett and his group at the University of Maryland School of Medicine. Blanquet (1972) found that the toxin was contained within the nematocyst and that the discharged nematocyst capsules and threads were free of toxin. Further studies showed that the toxic material was associated with a protein fraction having a molecular weight greater than 100,000 which could be separated into two major fractions. The more toxic of these two proteins was found to be rich in aspartic and glutamic acids, which composed approximately 27 percent of the total detectable amino acid content. Burnett and Calton (1977) reviewed the cardiotoxic, dermonecrotic, musculotoxic, and neurotoxic properties of the venom. Subsequently, it has been demonstrated that the toxin produced striking cytologic changes, including nuclear alterations and dissolution of intercellular collagen. The lethal property is thought to exert its effect by altering the transport of calcium across the conduction system of the heart. From experiments on rat and frog nerve and muscle, and on the neurons of *Aplysia californica,* it was concluded that the toxin appeared to induce a nonspecific membrane depolarization by a sodium-dependent tetrodotoxin-insensitive mechanism which secondarily increases Ca influx.

The collagenase from *C. quinquecirrha* has been isolated and purified 237-fold. A monoclonal antibody to the lethal factor of the venom has also been prepared. Ascites fluid from a cloned hybridoma-breeding mouse showed an ELISA titer of 12,800 and neutralized an intravenous $2 \times LD50$ injection of the crude venom.

Among the sea anemones, *Anemonia sulcata* is of particular interest, since it is of considerable medical importance in the Adriatic Sea where it inflicts numerous stings on bathers (Maretić and Russell, 1983). In 1973, a partially purified, toxic, basic polypeptide from *A. sulcata* was isolated. Its molecular weight was estimated to be 6000 and its LD100 in rats was 6 mg/kg body weight. In 1975, three toxic polypeptides were isolated from *A. sulcata.* Toxin I contained 45 amino acid residues, toxin II, 44, and toxin III, 24. Toxins I and II had similar toxicologic properties. When injected into a crustacean, fish, or mammal these toxins produced paralysis and cardiovascular changes. When injected into crabs the toxins caused convulsions and paralysis, and were lethal at 2.0 g/kg. They also caused paralysis and death in fishes. Toxin III caused neurotransmitter release from rat synaptosomes. Toxin II was far more toxic than toxin I and produced a positive inotropic effect on isolated electrically driven atria of the guinea pig. At high concentrations it caused contracture and arrhythmia. On the Langendorff heart preparation, low concentrations enhanced the contractile force of the atrium and ventricle, while high concentrations caused contracture and arrhythmia, which appeared to be limited to the atrium. Ferlan and Lebez (1974) isolated a highly basic protein toxin, *equinatoxin,* from the sea anemone, *Actinia equina.* It had a molecular weight of 20,000, with an isoelectric point of 12.5 and 147 amino acid residues. In rats, equinatoxin had an intravenous LD50 of 33 μg/kg body weight and was found to have hemolytic, antigenic, cardiotropic, and certain other activities. Subsequently, it was found that equinatoxin, *in vitro,* exhibited strong lytic action on erythrocytes and that it did not have phospholipase activity. A cytolytic toxin, *metridiolysin,* from the anemone *Medtridium senile* showed similar hemolytic activity. Like equinatoxin, the hemolytic activity was restricted to a relatively narrow pH range (see Russell, 1984a, for references).

Shapiro and his colleagues at Harvard carried out a series of chemical and pharmacologic studies on a stable acetone powder from tentacle homogenates of the large Caribbean anemone *Condylactis gigantea*. A toxin was obtained which acted as a basic protein and had an approximate molecular weight of 10,000 to 15,000. Assays on crayfish caused a paralysis characterized by an initial or spastic phase, followed by a flaccid phase. The immobilization dose was about 1 μg/kg body weight and the yield from a 70-g anemone with 23 g of tentacles was 1 g of the acetone powder, or a sufficient amount to paralyze approximately 2100-kg crayfish. Further studies on a crayfish preparation showed that the toxin had a direct effect on the crustacean nerve but not on the muscle membrane. No evidence for a truly synaptic effect was observed. Using the lobster giant axon and crayfish slow-adapting preparations it was found that the toxin transformed action potentials into prolonged plateau potential of up to several seconds duration, and that the eventual conduction block was not due solely to depolarization (Shapiro and Lilleheil, 1969).

A central nervous system stimulant in the form of a basic polypeptide has been isolated from homogenized tissues of the anemone *Stoichactis kenti*. The stimulation was described as "fighting episodes." A partially purified toxin from *S. helianthus*, with a mouse intraperitoneal LD50 of 0.25 mg/kg and hemolytic properties inhibited by sphingomyelin, has been reported (Bernheimer and Avigad, 1976). A cytotoxic poison from the anemone *Stoichactis helianthus* acts on black lipid membranes and liposomes by channel formation and detergent action. This mechanism is also suspected for the hemolytic activity of some of the other sea anemone "cytolytic" toxins. However, there appears to be a considerable number of different cytolytic toxins in the sea anemones and the mechanisms by which they damage membranes may be quite different. Hessinger and Lenhoff (1976), for instance, demonstrated that the toxin of *Aiptasia pallida* caused lysis through the action of phospholipase A on membrane phospholipids, while other workers suspect ionic or nonenzymatic roles. Several other Actiniidae species have been shown to contain toxins. A polypeptide, termed *anthopleurin-A*, from *Anthopleura xanthogrammica* that closely resembles toxin II from *A. sulcata* in its amino acid sequence has been described. In mice, *anthopleurin A* had an LD50 of 0.3 to 0.4 mg/kg body weight and was said to stimulate cardiac activity. A second polypeptide toxin, *anthopleurin B*, has also been identified in the same anemone (see Russell, 1984a, for references).

In 1967, Hashimoto and colleagues collected specimens of the file fish, *Alutera scripta,* from the Ryuku Islands following a report that several pigs had died after eating the viscera of this fish. On examining the gut contents of the fish the investigators found polyps of the zoanthid *Palythoa tuberculosa*. About the same time, Scheuer and his group were investigating the toxin from *Palythoa toxica*, found at Hana off the island of Maui and called *lima-make-O-Hana* (death seaweed of Hana). Palythoa toxin, *palytoxin*, was found to be a most potent poison, having a mouse intravenous LD50 of 0.15 μ/kg body weight. It has an approximate molecular weight of 3000 and appears to have a unique structure which, as yet, is undetermined.

Clinical Problem. As pointed out by Halstead (1965), it has long been known that the nematocysts of certain cnidarians can penetrate the human skin. In 1965, approximately 70 of the 9000 species of cnidarians were noted to have been involved in injuries to humans (Russell, 1965). More recent clinical records would indicate that about 78 species have been implicated in such injuries. While most nematocysts are capable of piercing only the thin membranes of the mouth or conjunctiva, some possess sufficient force to pierce the skin of the inner sides of the arms, legs, and more tender areas of the body. Still others can penetrate the thicker skin of the hands, arms, and feet (Russell, 1965). Swallowing the tentacles or even the umbrella can cause epigastric pain and discomfort (Maretić and Russell, 1983).

The cutaneous lesions, as well as other clinical manifestations produced by the various cnidarians, vary considerably, depending on the species involved and the number of fired nematocysts. Contrary to common belief, the stings of many cnidarians produce little or no immediate pain. Sometimes, itching is the first complaint that calls the victim's attention to the injured area, and this may not be for hours following the initial contact. In the author's experience, stings by hydroids usually do not produce pain, although there may be subsequent localized discomfort. In most cases, the lesions produced by hydroids are minimal. The fire or stinging corals, *Millepora*, produce small reddened, somewhat papular eruptions, which appear one to ten hours following contact and usually subside within 24 to 96 hours. In severe cases the papules may proceed to pustular lesions and subsequent desquamation. The stinging is usually associated with some localized, prickinglike pain, generally of short duration, and with some subsequent pruritus and minimal swelling (Russell, 1984a).

Contact with the Portuguese man-of-war,

Physalia, causes immediate pain, sometimes severe, and the early appearance of small reddened, linear, papular eruptions. At first the papules are surrounded by an erythematous zone, but as their size increases the area takes on the appearance of an inflammatory reaction with small periodic, demarcated, hemorrhagic papules. In some cases these papules are very close together, indicating multiple discharge of nematocysts as the tentacle passed over the injured part. The papules develop rapidly and often increase in size during the first hour. The affected area becomes painful and severe pruritus is not uncommon. Pain may spread to the larger muscle masses in the involved extremity or even to the whole body. Pain sometimes involves the regional lymph nodes. In some cases the papules proceed to vesiculation, pustulation, and desquamation. I have seen several cases in which hyperpigmentation of the lesions was obvious for years following a stinging (Russell, 1966). General systemic manifestations may also develop following *Physalia physalis* envenomation. Weakness, nausea, anxiety, headache, spasms in the large muscle masses of the abdomen and back, vascular spasms, lacrimation and nasal discharge, increased perspiration, vertigo, hemolysis, difficulty and pain on respiration, described as being unable to "catch one's breath," cyanosis, renal failure, and shock have all been reported.

Contact with most of the true jellyfishes gives rise, in the less severe cases, to manifestations similar to those noted for *Physalia,* with symptoms sometimes disappearing within ten hours. In the more severe cases there is immediate, intense, burning pain, with contact areas appearing as swollen wheals, sometimes purplish, and often bearing hemorrhagic papules. The areas may proceed to vesiculation ad necrosis. Localized edema is common, and in the more severe cases muscle mass pain, difficulties in respiration, and severe spasms of the back and abdomen with vomiting are reported. Vertigo, mental confusion, changes in heart rate, and shock are sometimes seen (Barnes, 1960; Russell, 1965; 1984a; Halstead, 1965).

The sea wasps, *Chironex fleckeri* Southcott and *Chiropsalmus quadrigatus* Haeckel and certain other species, are extremely dangerous Cubomedusae responsible for a number of deaths, particularly in Australian waters. Although systemic effects usually develop within 5 to 150 minutes following envenomation, some deaths occur in less than five minutes. Stings by these Cubomedusae cause a sharp prickling or burning sensation with the appearance of a wheal, which at first appears like a "rounded area of gooseflesh." An erythematous wheal soon develops and may become considerably larger than the area of contact. At first, it may show little pattern to suggest whether the stinging had been by tentacles or by the animal's umbrella. The wheals may either disappear, as when the stinging is minimal, or after an hour or so become enlarged as the nematocyst punctures become more apparent and appear as very small hemorrhagic vesicles surrounded by inflammation. A stinging pain develops and may persist for one to three hours. In linear lesions the nematocyst injuries may be no more than 5 mm wide but extend for 10 cm or more. Vesiculation and pustular formation may occur and full-thickness skin necrosis is not uncommon. Edema about the area may persist for ten or more days. Stingings by the anemones are usually of lesser consequence than those inflicted by the jellyfishes and rarely are they painful or disabling. The lesion area takes on a reddened and slightly raised appearance, bearing irregularly scattered pinhead-sized vesicles or hemorrhagic blebs. The area becomes painful, particularly to touch or heat. In stings by *Anemonia sulcata* seen by the author there has been some diffuse edema around the injured site. Residual hyperpigmentation or hypopigmentation is unusual following anemone stings. Stings by the stony corals (*Acropora*) are said to give rise to some minor pain often followed by itching and the development of small diffuse wheals, which may progress to vesiculation but rarely necrosis. "Sponge fisherman's disease" is due to the actinian *Sarortia elegans.* Troublesome are small spicules of coral that sometimes break off and become embedded in the skin, occasionally giving rise to infection.

Treatment consists of removing the tentacles, preferably with gloves, washing the affected area with seawater, immersing the part in vinegar or Burow's solution for 10 to 15 minutes and, in the case of *Chironex* stings, applying a dry powder or shaving soap and scraping the area with a sharp knife to remove any nematocysts embedded in the skin, washing the area thoroughly with soapy water, and then applying a corticosteroid-analgesic-antihistamine ointment ("Russell's Balm"). Systemic manifestations are best treated symptomatically.

Chills and fever have been reported after grinding dried specimens of *P. caribaeorum,* which were being studied for the presence of wax esters. Toxic zoanthids have also been found in various parts of the Pacific. Accidental contact with the mucus of *Palythoa* through the abraded skin is said to produce weakness and malaise, as well as localized irritation.

On some Pacific islands, as well as elsewhere in the world, sea anemones are eaten following cooking but some are apparently poisonous whether uncooked or cooked. *Rhodactis howesi* and *Physobrachia douglasi* are poisonous when eaten raw but said to be safe when cooked. *Radianthus paumotensis* and another *Radianthus* species are said to be poisonous, whether raw or cooked. Intoxication is typified by nausea, vomiting, abdominal pain, and hypoactive reflexes. In severe cases, marked weakness, malaise, cyanosis, stupor, and death have occurred.

Echinodermata

In most cases echinoderms are characterized by radial or meridional symmetry, a calcareous endoskeleton made up of separate plates or ossicles that often bear external spines, a well-developed coelom, a water-vascular system, and a nervous system, but no special excretory system. Approximately 85 of the 6000 species composing the four classes (Asteroidea, Ophiuroidea, Echinoidea, Holothuroidea) are known to be venomous or poisonous. Some of the more important toxic starfishes, sea urchins, and sea cucumbers have been described elsewhere (Russell, 1984a). Asteroids, starfishes, or sea stars have a central disk and five or more tapering rays or arms. On the upper surface are many thorny spines of calcium carbonate in the form of calcite intermingled with organic materials. The calcite spines are covered by a thin integument composed of an epidermis and a dermis. Within the epidermis is an acidophilic cell thought to release a toxin. The toxin is discharged into the water or, as in the case of humans, directly onto the skin. In addition, sea stars have pedicellariae, which contain poison glands in the concave cavity of their valves. Some sea stars produce poisoning following ingestion.

The regular sea urchins have rounded radially symmetric bodies, which are enclosed in a hard calcite shell from which calcareous spines and the venomous pedicellariae arise. The spines may be straight and pointed, curved, flat-topped, club-shaped, oar-shaped, umbrella-shaped, thorny, fan-shaped, or hooked. They may vary in length from less than 1 mm to over 30 cm. The spines serve in locomotion, protection, digging, feeding, and producing currents; certain of the primary and secondary spines bear poison glands.

The principal venom apparatus in the sea urchin, heart urchin, or sand dollar is the pedicellaria. In essence, pedicellariae are modified spines with flexible heads. There are four primary kinds and some urchins possess all four kinds. The pedicellariae function in food getting, grooming, and self-defense. The glandular, gemmiform, or globiferous type pedicellaria serves as a venom organ. In most echinoids the so-called "head" of the pedicellaria is composed of three calcareous jaws or valves, each having a rounded, toothlike fang. The jaws are usually invested in a globose, fleshy, and somewhat muscular sac, which possesses a single or double gland over each valve. A second trilobed gland system, anatomically and histologically distinct from the head gland, is present in some urchins. The primary and secondary spines of some urchins have specialized organs containing a gland, which is said to empty its contents through the hollow-spine tip under certain conditions. Our group found a toxin in the secondary spines of *Echinothrix calamaris* and *E. diadema* but not in their primary spines. The secondary spines of *Asthenosoma varium* Grube and *Araesoma thetidis* contain a venom. According to Halstead (1978), the spine venom glands are best developed in the secondary aboral spines of *A. varium*.

The sea cucumbers, *Holothuroidea*, are soft-bodied animals covered by a leathery skin that contains only microscopic calcareous plates. According to Nigrelli and Jakowska (1960), at least 30 species belonging to four of the five orders are toxic. Some members possess special defense organs known as Cuvierian tubules. When these animals are irritated they emit these organs through the anus. The tubules become elongated by hydrostatic pressure so that once through the anus they become extremely sticky threads in which the attacking animal becomes ensnared. The process of elongation may split the outer layer of covering cells, thereby releasing a proteinaceous material that forms an amorphous mass having strong adhesive properties. In some sea cucumbers, however, as in *Actinopyga agassizi,* the tubules do not become sticky, nor do they elongate, but they are eviscerated in a somewhat similar manner and they discharge a toxin from certain highly developed structures filled with granules. The toxin is capable of killing fishes and other animals. In *Holothuria atra,* which does not possess Cuvierian tubules, the toxin may be discharged through the body wall. In Guam, natives cut up the common black sea cucumbers and squeeze the contents of the animal into crevices and pools to deactivate fish.

Many echinoderms secrete a mucus or liquid from their integument that appears to play a role in their defensive armament. The viscous discharge from the massive multicellular integumentary glands of the brittle star, *Ophiocomina nigra,* is characterized as a highly sulfated acid mucopolysaccharide, containing amino sugars, sulfate esters, and other substances complexed to proteins. The pH of this discharge is approximately 1, which probably makes it very offensive to other marine animals that might seek to prey upon it. Among other substances isolated from the echinoderms is a quaternary ammonium base ($C_7H_7NO_2$, picolinic acid methyl betaine) known as *homarine,* several phosphagens (phosphoarginine and phosphocreatine), sterols, saponins, and other compounds (Hashimoto, 1979). Perhaps, one of the difficulties, again, in determining the toxic substance(s) in the echinoderms is related to the differences in the origin of the test material, that is, not only the chemical variations in different species but the differences in the kind of product extracted from the animals. Pharmacologically, the task is even more difficult, not only because of the differences in products but also because of the differences in the bioassays that have been employed. Some investigators use the toxicity to fish assay, while others use a hemolytic test, an oral or parenteral mammalian assay, and still other researchers use an intact mollusc or other invertebrate and measure the withdrawal response or lethality. Finally, a few investigators use specific marine isolated tissue preparations. Hashimoto (1979) has done an excellent job of reviewing the chemistry and pharmacology of echinoderm toxins, and he has been wise enough to avoid attempting to interpret unrelated and sometimes confusing data.

When the pedicellariae of *Toxopneustes pileolus* were allowed to sting the shaved abdomen of a mouse, the animal developed respiratory distress and exhibited a decrease in body temperature. The injection of thermostable extracts from the macerated pedicellariae of *Sphaerechinus granularis,* and certain other species, has been found to be lethal to isopods, crabs, octopods, sea stars, lizards, and rabbits. While the presence of a dialyzable, acetylcholinelike substance in the pedicellariae of *Lytechinus variegatus* has been reported, it was not until 1965 that the protein nature of pedicellarial toxin was first described. This protein had an intravenous LD50 in mice, based on the quantity of precipitable protein nitrogen, of 1.59×10^{-2} mg/kg body weight for the crude material and 1.16×10^{-2} mg/kg for the protein (Alender and Russell, 1966). It possessed hemolytic activity against human type A and B, rabbit, guinea pig, beef, sheep, and fish erythrocytes. Intravenously, it produced a dose-related hypotension that was responsive to adrenalin. It had a deleterious effect on the isolated heart and guinea pig ileum. In both these preparations the toxin caused the release of histamine and serotonin. It seems to have little effect on isolated toad nerve. However, Parnas and Russell

(1967), using the deep extension abdominal muscle of the crayfish, showed that the toxin produced a rapid block in the response of the indirectly stimulated muscle. Even with low concentrations there was an irreversible block in the muscle's response to intracellular stimulation. The compound action potential of the crayfish limb nerve was also blocked by the toxin, but this potential reappeared on washing. The toxin caused considerable damage to the muscle fibers. These findings seemed to indicate that pedicellariae toxin blocks the response from both nerve and muscle and is cytolytic.

Subsequently, it was observed that pedicellarial toxin from *T. gratilla* elicited prolonged contractions of isolated guinea pig ileum. Chemical evidence was obtained for the release of histamine from ileal, cardiac, and pulmonary tissues, as well as from the colonic and pulmonary tissues of the rat. The histamine release was quantitatively dependent on the concentration of the toxin acting on the tissue. The active material obtained from the reaction between crude sea urchin toxin and heated plasma was a mixture of pharmacologically active peptides, one of which was bradykinin (see Russell, 1984a, for references). Fleming and Howden (1974) obtained a partly purified toxin from the pedicellariae of *T. gratilla.* The toxin, as established by intraperitoneal injection in mice, was at the 5.0 to 5.1 isoelectric point. When this fraction was chromatographed, a molecular weight of $78,000 \pm 8000$ was found. This seems consistent with the sediment coefficient of 4.7 (67,000) previously reported.

It has been known since 1880 that the discharged tenacious filaments of sea cucumbers can produce wounds in humans and that eating the sea cucumber *Stichopus variegatus* can cause death. According to Halstead (1965), the initial studies of the poisonousness of sea cucumbers were carried out by Yamanouchi, who observed that when fish were placed in the aquarium to which aqueous extracts of *Holothuria vagabunda* were added, the fish died. Subsequently, he obtained a toxic crystalline product, termed *holothurin,* and found it present in 24 of 27 species of sea cucumbers examined. More recently, Bakus and Green (1974) have found that the more tropical the locality, the greater the probability that the holothurin will be toxic to fishes. The toxic substance (holothurin) extracted from the Bahamian sea cucumber *Actinopyga agassizi* was found to be composed of 60 percent glycosides and pigments, 30 percent salts, polypeptides, and free amino acids, 5 to 10 percent insoluble protein, and 1 percent cholesterol. The cholesterol-precipitated fraction, known as *holothurin A,* represented 60 percent of the crude holothurin and was given the empirical formula $C_{50-52}H_{81}O_{25-26}SNa$. Its provisional structure is (Friess *et al.*, 1967):

Compound	R
Holothurin	$-OSO_3^-Na^+$
DeH	$-H$

SUGAR	SYMBOL
D-GLUCOSE	G
D-XYLOSE	X
D-QUINOVOSE	Q
3-O-METHYLGLUCOSE	G – OMe

In 10 ppm, holothurin was found to be lethal to *Hydra,* the mollusc *Planorbis,* and the annelid *Tubifex tubifex.* It has slightly greater hemolytic action than saponin and stimulated hematopoiesis in the bone marrow of winterized frogs. It also appears to have some antimetabolic activity. In the mammalian phrenic nerve-diaphragm preparation, holothurin A produces contracture of the muscle, followed by some relaxation and a gradual decrease in the recorded amplitude of both the directly and indirectly elicited contractions, the latter decreasing at a slightly greater rate than the former. The intravenous LD50 in mice was approximately 9 mg/kg body weight. In frogs, holothurin A produced an irreversible block and destruction of excitability on the single node of Ranvier in the sciatic nerve. The toxin did not produce any observable damage to the axonal walls or sheath (see Russell, 1984a, for references).

A major aglycone from the holothurin A of *H. vagabunda* was named *holothurigenin* ($C_{30}H_{44}O_5$). It contained three hydroxyls, a five-membered lactone, and a heteroannular diene. The toxins from the Cuvierian organ and body wall of a number of species have been summarized by Habermehl and Volkwein (1971). According to the authors, these compounds are glycosides of tetracyclic triterpenes, which are derivatives of lanosterol and were the first glycoside triterpenes derived from animals.

Holothurin has been shown to have hemolytic and cytolytic properties. It is considered to be one of the most potent saponin hemolysins known. In some concentrations it is lethal to animals and plants, inhibits the growth of certain protozoa, modifies the normal development of sea urchin eggs, possesses antimicrobial and antitumoral properties, retards pupation in the fruit fly, and inhibits regeneration processes in planariae. The effects of various preparations of holothurin on the peripheral nervous system have been the object of a number of studies by Friess and his group at the Naval Medical Research Institute in Bethesda, Maryland. Holothurin in concentrations of 9.8×10^{-3} M causes a decrease in the height of the propagated potential without reduction of the conduction velocity in the desheathed sciatic nerve of the frog. This change is concentration dependent and independent of pH and is completely irreversible. A similar change is produced in the single fiber-single node of Ranvier preparation. In concentrations of 2.5×10^{-5} to 1.0×10^{-3} M, the toxin produced a diminuition of the action current with a concomitant rise in the stimulation threshold. However, in approximately 80 percent of the preparations studied the loss of nodal excitation caused by this same concentration was accompanied by a loss in basophilic, macromolecular material from the axoplasm in and near the node of Ranvier (see Russell, 1983a, for references). In summarizing various of their studies, Friess *et al.* (1970) note that the most obvious functional similarity from data with the cervical ganglia of the cat, the peripheral neuromuscular junction of the rat, and the medullated nerve nodes of the frog was the possession of cholinergic subsystems at some anatomic level, chiefly within the excitable membranes of conducting and junctional structures. They felt that a common target for holothurin A action was "the cholinergic receptor population triggered by acetylcholine ion (ACh+) in the associated hydrolase enzyme AChE, or in the enzyme choline acetylase responsible for resynthesis of ACh+."

Clinical Problem. In 1965, I treated a student working with *Acanthaster planci,* who had inadvertently slipped and fallen, landing forcibly with his left hand impaled on the sea star. Twenty minutes after the injury the patient had intense pain over the palm of the left hand, "shooting pains" up the volar aspect of the forearm, weakness, nausea, vertigo, and tingling in the fingertips. There were at least ten puncture wounds over the hand and some of them were bleeding freely. I suggested that the patient put his hand in cold vinegar/water and be admitted to the hospital emergency room. On arrival there

15 minutes later, the pain was less intense and the nausea had somewhat subsided. Unfortunately, the patient was given 100 mg meperidine hydrochloride and five minutes later he was vomiting. (In my opinion the vomiting was due to the medication and most of the other symptoms to hyperventilation.) The patient was placed on cold vinegar/water and occasional aluminum acetate soaks over the next two days and all symptoms and signs, including the mild edema, slowly resolved. Several broken spines were removed from the puncture wounds. Four days following the accident the patient complained of burning and itching over the left palm. Examination revealed a scaly, erythematous dermatitis. Topical corticosteriods were used, but two days later the patient had to be placed on systemic corticosteroid therapy for the dermatitis. It cleared in six days.

A second episode involving *A. planci* was related to me by Dr. W. L. Orris in 1974. The patient had immediate, severe, burning pain and localized edema. These responded to aluminum acetate soaks and corticosteroids. According to Endean (1964), the puncture wounds produced by *Asthenosoma periculosum* give rise to immediate and sometimes acute pain but few other symptoms or signs. The discharge from *Marthasterias glacialis* is said to cause edema of the lips. It is known that allergic dermatitis can occur following extensive contact with these animals.

Stings by the pedicellariae of certain sea urchins are well documented (Russell, 1965; Halstead, 1965; Cleland and Southcott, 1965). One investigator experienced severe pain, syncope, respiratory distress, partial paralysis of the lips, tongue, and eyelids, and weakness of the muscles of phonation and of the extremities following a stinging by seven or eight pedicellariae from *Toxopneustes pileolus*. Another biologist experienced severe pain of several hours' duration at the site of a stinging by *Tripneustes gratilla*. The sting of a single globiferous pedicellaria from *T. gratilla* was found to be equal in pain severity to that experienced following a bee sting. Swelling appeared around the puncture wounds within minutes of the stinging and a red wheal 1 cm in diameter soon developed. Subsequent stingings during the following two-year period resulted in a more severe reaction. In one instance the wheal was 12 cm in diameter and persisted for eight hours. In none of these experiences were there any systemic manifestations (Alender and Russell, 1966; Russell, 1971). It might be concluded that pedicellariae stings give rise to immediate pain, localized swelling and redness, and an aching sensation in the involved part. Other findings might include those reviewed by Halstead (1965).

As previously noted, the secondary spines of *E. calamaris*, *E. diadema*, *A. varium*, *A. thetidis*, and the primary oral spines of *P. bursarium* are said to have a venom gland and are capable of envenomation (Alender and Russell, 1966). However, case reports on verified stingings are almost nonexistent, and in the several known to the author it is not possible to decide whether the pain, "dizziness," and minimal localized swelling were due to a venom or to the effects of a simple puncture wound complicated by hyperventilation. The primary spines of almost 50 species of sea urchins have been implicated in injuries to humans. Urchins of the family Diadematidae are particularly troublesome because of their long length and fragility. When these break off in a puncture wound, they can be difficult to find and remove. I have attended injuries in which I have had to remove more than a dozen broken spine tips. With some species there is no giveaway dark color around the puncture wound, and finding the broken spines is not easy. Although the fragments of some spines will dissolve in tissue and cause no difficulties, others can give rise to granulomatous reactions, some of which may need to be removed surgically. Still others may migrate through the foot or hand without causing complications. Occasionally, spines will lodge against a nerve or bone and cause complications requiring surgical intervention. Secondary infections from spine injuries are relatively rare.

It has long been known that the ovaries of sea urchins were toxic, and perhaps lethal. Halstead (1980) notes that the gonads of *Paracentrotus lividus*, *Tripneustes ventricosus*, and *Centrechinus antillarium* are poisonous. Poisonings by following the ingestion of certain sea cucumbers, however, are not uncommon and have occurred frequently in the South Pacific, Philippines, Japan, China, and Southeast Asia. The most frequently implicated holothurian species are *Holothuria atra*, *H. axiologa*, *Stichopus variegatus*, and *Thelenota ananas*. The symptoms and signs are usually of short duration and without serious sequelae. Pruritus with mild swelling and redness of the hands has been reported following the handling of some sea cucumbers. Acute conjunctivitis has been observed in persons who have swum in waters polluted with the tissue discharge of sea cucumber Cuvierian organs.

Mollusca

Molluscs are unsegmented invertebrates having a mantle that often secretes a calcareous shell, a ventral muscular foot used for locomotion, a reduced coelom, an open circulatory system, and a raula or tonguelike organ (absent only in the bivalves). Jaws are present in some species. There are approximately 80,000 species of molluscs, of which about 85 have been implicated in poisoning to humans or are known to be toxic under certain conditions. The majority of the venomous or poisonous species are found in three of the five classes of molluscs: Gastropoda, Pelecypoda, and Cephalopoda. In the class Gastropoda, the univalve snails and slugs, the most dangerous members are of the genus *Conus*, of which there are perhaps 400 species. The cone shells are confined almost exclusively to tropical and subtropical seas and oceans and are usually found in shallow waters along reefs, although some of the more dangerous species are found on sandy bottoms. They range in length up to approximately 25 cm. The venom apparatus of *Conus* serves as an offensive weapon for the gaining of food and, to a much lesser extent, as a defensive weapon against predators. It consists of a muscular bulb, a long coiled venom duct, the radula (the radula sheath), and the radular teeth. The venom is thought to be secreted in the venom duct and forced under pressure exerted by the duct and the venom bulb into the radula and thus into the lumen of the radular teeth. The radular teeth are passed from the radula into the pharynx and then into the proboscis. They are then thrust by the proboscis into the prey during the stinging act. The radular teeth are needlelike, from 1 to 10 mm in length, and almost transparent. The reader is referred elsewhere for a more complete review of the structure of the venom apparatus of *Conus* (Russell, 1984a).

The various species of Conidae have been divided into those that were vermivorous, molluscivorous, or piscivorous. Endean *et al.* (1967) demonstrated that of 37 species studied the paralytic effects of the venoms were indeed directly related to the prey hunted. They concluded that only the piscivorous Conidae were capable of serious injuries to humans.

Initial studies indicated that the venom was white, gray, yellow, or black, depending on the species involved, was viscous, and had a pH range of 7.6 to 8.2. The active principle was nondialyzable, and its toxicity was reduced by heating or incubation with trypsin. The lethal fraction was thought to be a protein or bound to a protein. It was found that the amount of venom in the ducts of *C. striatus* was sufficient to immobilize the small fish on which it preys but not of sufficient quantity to cause serious injury to a human. A toxin, having a molecular weight of over 10,000, with a low lethal index as compared with other *Conus* species, caused ataxia, depressed respirations leading to apnea and cardiac arrest in mammals, precipitated a block in the compound action potential of the isolated toad sciatic nerve, blocked both the directly and indirectly elicited contractions of a mammalian nerve-muscle preparation, and markedly depressed the amplitude of intracellular recorded action potentials in the rat diaphragm. The chemical nature of the toxic fraction of *Conus* venom is not known. Various authors have reported that the active fraction is a protein, or a poison with a molecular weight of about 10,000, or a peptide (see Russell, 1984a, for references).

Some abalone, such as *Haliotis*, are toxic to eat. The toxin is concentrated in the digestive gland or liver and can be distinguished by its blue-green pigment. It is thought that the pigment, pyropheophorbide *a*, originates from chlorophyll in the seaweed on which the abalone feeds. Hashimoto (1979) noted that ingestion of the viscera of *Haliotis* caused dermatitis in cats and humans. On the basis of this observation he carried out experiments demonstrating the importance of photosensitization in the development of the dermatitis and suggested an assay method. He also suggested that the use of fluorescent pigments should be prohibited from foods and that care should be taken to see that drugs are not transformed into fluorescent substances in the body. In the hypobranchial gland of *Murex* there is a secretion that at first is colorless or yellow but on exposure to sunlight becomes brilliant violet and gives off a strong fetid odor. The gland also produces a toxic secretion. Subsequent studies indicated that two pharmacologically active substances were present. One of these was enteramine or 5-hydroxytryptamine and the other was murexine ($C_{11}H_{18}O_3N_3$). Further investigations showed that murexine had the structure of β-[imidazolyl-(4)]-acrylcholine. It was thus called urocanylcholine. Murexine has also been found in the midgut of the sea hare *Aplysia californica*, senecioylcholine has been identified in the hypobranchial gland of *Thais floridana*, and acrylylcholine in *Buccinum undatum*. The amount of these cholinesters in the hypobranchial gland was approximately 1 to 5 mg/g tissue. They exhibited muscarinelike and nicotinelike activity, and they caused cardiovascular changes with hypotension, increased respirations, gastric motility and secretions, and some contraction of the frog rectus muscle and guinea pig ileum. The intravenous LD50 of murexine in mice was 8.1 to 8.7 mg/kg. Dihydromurexine has been isolated from the hypobranchial gland of *T. haemastoma*, and the muricacean gastropod *Acanthina spirata* produces a paralytic substance with high acetylcholine content in both its hypobranchial and salivary-accessory gland complex. The toxin is thought to be a carboxylic ester of choline (see Russell, 1984a, for references).

A vasodilator and hypotensive agent has been described from the salivary gland extract of the gastropod *T. haemastoma* (Clench). The extract produced behavioral changes in mice, followed by lethargy. When lethal doses were given, respirations first increased and then decreased and became shallow and death ensued. The toxin produced bradycardia and a fall in blood pressure, which was partly blocked by atropine. In the isolated rabbit heart the extract produced a decrease in rate and contraction, with a fall in heart output. It also produced contractions of the isolated guinea pig ileum and rabbit duodenum. The salivary poison of the gastropod *Neptunea arthritica* is thought to be tetramine ($C_4H_{12}N$). It has been suggested that histamine, choline, and choline ester, also found in the salivary glands of this mollusc, act synergistically with the tetramine in producing the poisoning. In *N. antiqua* the tetramine is probably responsible for almost all of the biologic activity of the salivary gland extract. In the viscera of the ivory shell, *Babylonia japonica*, a water-soluble toxin, has been found, which is slightly methanol and ethanol soluble, heat labile, dialyzable, ninhydrin positive, and Dragendorff and biuret negative. It has a potent mydriatic activity. The toxin is said to be a complex bromo compound, having the formula, $C_{25}H_{26}N_{50}O_{13}Br \cdot 7H_2O$, with a molecular weight of 810.53. It has been named *surugatoxin* (SGTX) after Suruga Bay, where the molluscs were taken (see Hashimoto, 1979, for references).

In the sea hare, *A. californica*, acetone extracts of the digestive glands had an intraperitoneal LD50 of approximately 30 mg sea hare tissue per kilogram mouse body weight. Signs in mammals included increased respiration, blanching and drooping of the ears, increased salivation, muscle fasciculations, agonal signs, ataxia, prostration, and death. The extract was also found to be lethal when given orally at approximately 12 times the intraperitoneal dose. A partially purified toxin, called *aplysin*, had an immediate but transient hypotensive effect in the dog. There was some initial arrythmia followed by a slower but regular rate. In the isolated heart of the frog, aplysin caused cardiac standstill. The anterior cervical sympathetic ganglion of the cat was stimulated initially and then reversibly blocked. The frog rectus abdominis muscle responded by contracture, and in the rat diaphragm-phrenic nerve the neuromuscular junction was blocked. In another sea hare, two bromine-containing sesquiterpenes were isolated. These were named *aplysin* and *aplysinol*. A debromo derivative, debromoaplysin, and subsequently a third bromo compound, diterpene aplysin-20, have also been isolated. Observation of a sea hare feeding on the alga *Laurencia nipponica* led to several experiments that indicated that steam distillates of the alga were toxic to worms and carp. Based on this observation, Irie *et al.* (1969) extracted aplysin, debromoaplysin, and aplysinol from the red alga *Laurencia okamurai*, while Waraszkiewicz and Erickson (1974) obtained aplysin from *L. nidifica*. From these observations it is suggested that the bromo toxins originate in algae. Two lethal extracts, one ether soluble and the other water soluble, have been separated from the digestive glands of the Hawaiian sea hares *Dolabella auriculasia*, *A. pulmonica*, *Stytocheilus longicauda*, and *Dolabrifera dolabriefa*. In mice the ether-soluble toxin caused irritability, viciousness, and severe flaccid paralysis. The water-soluble toxin, in contrast, caused "convulsions" and respiratory distress. Sublethal doses of the ether-soluble residue produced hypertension when injected intravenously into rats, whereas the crude water-soluble residue produced a transient hypotension, bradycardia, and apnea. The hypertension produced by the ether-soluble toxin was resistant to both α- and β-adrenergic blocking agents. The hypotensive effect of the water-soluble extract was not abolished by vagotomy or pretreatment with either atropine or Benadryl. It was concluded that both extracts may have direct effects on the contractility of vascular smooth muscle that are not mediated by α-adrenergic or cholinergic mechanisms. Choline esters were found in the aqueous fraction of the digestive gland of *A. californica*. Both acetylcholine and urocanylcholine were identified. The latter accounted for the cholinesterase-resistant cholinomimetic activity of extracts of the gland. An "antifeedant" has been observed in *A. brasiliana*. It is the aromatic bromoallene panacene. It is suggested that the panacene is biosynthesized from a C_{15} algal precursor (see Russell, 1984a, for references).

In the Cephalopods, the cuttlefishes, squids, nautilis, and octopuses are the venomous octopods and possible several venomous and poisonous squid. The venom apparatus of the octopus is an integrated part of the animal's digestive system. The secretions serve in prey capture and digestive function, in some ways similar to the venom glands of snakes. The apparatus consists of paired posterior salivary glands, two short (salivary) ducts that join them with the common salivary duct, paired anterior salivary glands and their ducts, the buccal mass and the mandibles, or beak. An impressive number of substances have been isolated from or identified in the salivary glands of various cephalopods. Many of these substances have been shown to have biologic activities, although these activities were not always apparent in the physiopharmacologic effect of the whole toxin, and some substances either do not have a significant biologic activity or the state of knowledge does not indicate what activity is present. It now appears that many of the substances reported in the literature were actually normal constituents of the salivary glands of cephalopods and not necessarily venom constituents. Some of the substances found in the salivary glands are tyramine, octopine, agmatine, adrenaline, noradrenaline, 5-hydroxytryptamine, L-*p*-hydroxyphenylethanolamine, histamine, dopamine, tryptophan, and certain of the 11-hydroxysteroids, polyphenols, phenolamines, indoleamines, and guanidine bases.

The posterior salivary glands of *O. apollyon* or *O. bimaculatus* have been shown to contain decarboxylate L-3,4-dihydroxyphenalalanine (DOPA), DL-5-hydroxytryptophan, DL-*erythro*-3,4-dihydroxyphenylserine, and DL-*erythro-p*-hydroxyphenylserine, as well as DL-*m*-tyrosine, DL-*erythro-m*-hydroxyphenylserine, histidine, L-histidine, DL-*erythro*-phenylserine, 3,4-dihydroxyphenylserine, tyrosine, and *m*-tyrosine. In general, the salivary glands of cephalopods contain little or no proteolytic enzymes, amylases, or lipases. A protein, *cephalotoxin,* from the posterior salivary glands of *Sepia officinalis* has been suggested as the biologically active component of the animal's toxin. The toxin contained no cholinesterase or aminoxidase activity. Analysis of cephalotoxin from the posterior salivary gland of *Octopus vulgaris* showed: protein 74.05 percent (N determination), 64.25 percent (biuret reaction); carbohydrates, 4.17 percent, and hexosamines, 5.80 percent.

The posterior salivary glands of *Eledone moschata* and *E. aldrovandi* contained a substance that, when injected into mammals, caused marked vasodilation and produced hypotension and stimulation of certain extravascular smooth muscles. The substance was first called *moschatin* but was later renamed *eledoisin*. It was an endecapeptide. It was found that eledoisin was 50 times more potent than acetylcholine, histamine, or bradykinin in its ability to provoke hypotension in the dog. It produced an increase in the permeability of the peripheral vessels, stimulated the smooth muscles of the gastrointestinal tract, and caused an increase, which was atropine resistant, in salivary secretions. In spite of its marked pharmacologic activities, the role and significance of this substance in the salivary glands of *Eledone* are not clear. It is not found in the salivary glands of *O. vulgaris* or *O. macropus,* indicating that it is not a necessary component of cephalopod toxin. It appears that eledoisin plays some part in protein synthesis in the salivary gland.

Reports of envenomation by Australian octopuses, some of which were fatal, stimulated renewed interest in the venom of cephalopods. A saline extract of homogenized glands of *H. maculosa* was found to be a dialyzable, heat-stable product that resisted mild acid hydrolysis. When studied on a number of pharmacologic preparations, it was concluded that animals died in respiratory failure, due to a phrenic nerve block and/or to deleterious changes at the neuromuscular junction. The product also produced bradycardia and hypotension, without remarkable changes in the electrocardiogram. It was found that within four minutes of placing a live *H. maculosa* on the back of a rabbit a small bleeding puncture wound surrounded by a blanched area could be seen, the rabbit became restless, and there was some exophalmos and "one slight convulsion" with cessation of all muscular activity, other than cardiac. Cyanosis developed and death followed at 19 minutes. It was concluded that a young octopus has sufficient venom in its posterior salivary glands to cause paralysis in 750-kg rabbits, that the gland extracts have a high concentration of hyaluronidase, and that neostigmine does not reverse or reduce the toxic effects of the venom.

Further investigations yielded an extract of gland tissue partially purified by filtration that was given the name *maculotoxin*. On the basis of lethality determinations, there appeared to be a close similarity between the toxin and tetrodotoxin, and it was concluded that maculotoxin appeared to resemble tetrodotoxin more closely than it did saxitoxin. Saline and water extracts of the homogenized whole glands of *H. maculosa* produced paralysis and death at the 1 mg gland/2 kg rabbit level. Antibodies were produced to a nontoxic high-molecular-weight component but not for the toxic low-molecular-weight component. It was suggested that the molecular weight below 540 accounted for the lack of antigenicity. Maculotoxin was found to block neuromuscular transmission in the isolated sciatic-sartorius nerve-muscle preparation of the toad by inhibiting the action potential in the motor nerve terminals, and it had no postsynaptic effect. It was suggested that the toxin may block action potentials by displacing sodium ions from negatively charged sites in the membrane. One major toxin, maculotoxin, and a minor one having similar chemical properties were found in the venom of *H. maculosa.* The maculotoxin behaved as a cation of low molecular weight (<700), and it was felt that it was chemically different from tetrodotoxin. In 1978, the previous observations on the likeness of maculotoxin to tetrodotoxin were confirmed. Direct spectral and chromatographic comparisons showed these two toxins to be indistinguishable. This is of particular interest because here we have a poison (tetrodotoxin) that is also a venom (maculotoxin). In the former the presence of the poison is thought to be a product of metabolism, while in the latter the venom is used to immobilize and perhaps kill the prey (see Russell, 1984a, for references).

The Pelecypoda, scallops, oysters, clams, and mussels, are the principal transvectors of paralytic shellfish poisoning. The genera most often involved with PSP are *Mya, Mytilus, Modiolus, Protothaca, Spisula,* and *Saxidomus,* according to Halstead (1978). The eating of the ovaries of the Japanese callista, *Callista brevisphonata,* has resulted in numerous cases of illness. The ovaries contain large amounts of choline but no histamine. Cats fed the shellfish showed few signs, other than hypoactivity and some loss of coordination. Three of nine human volunteers who ate the ovaries developed urticaria and very mild symptoms. *Venerupin* poisoning is caused by ingestion of the oyster *Crassostrea gigas.* In one series of 81 persons poisoned, 54 died (Halstead, 1965). In a second outbreak in 1941, of six patients, five died, and from 1942 to 1950 there were 455 additional cases involving the eating of oysters and the short-necked clam *Tapes japonica* (Hashimoto, 1979). The toxin causes hemorrhage in the heart, lungs, and viscera, with diffuse hemorrhage, necrosis, and fatty degeneration of the liver.

Clinical Problem. A number of cones have been implicated in injuries to humans, including *Conus geographus, C. aulicus, C. gloria-maris, C. marmoreus, C. textilis, C. tulipa, C. striatus, C. omaria, C. catus, C. obscurus, C. imperialis, C. pulicarius, C. quercinus, C. litteratus, C. lividus,* and *C. sponsalis.* The first six would seem the most dangerous, since they are said to have the highest developed venom apparatus (Halstead, 1978).

The sting often gives rise to immediate, sometimes intense, localized pain at the site of the injury. Within five minutes the victim usually notes some numbness and ischemia about the wound, although in a case seen by the author the affected area was red and tender rather than ischemic. A tingling or numbing sensation may develop about the mouth, lips, and tongue, and over the peripheral parts of the extremities. Other symptoms and signs during the first 30 minutes following the injury include: hypertonicity, tremor, muscle fasciculations, nausea and vomiting, dizziness, increased lacrimation and salivation, weakness, and pain in the chest, which increases with deep inspiration. The numbness about the wound may spread to involve a good part of the extremity or injured part. In the more severe cases, respiratory distress with chest pain, difficulties in swallowing and phonation, marked dizziness, blurring of vision and an inability to focus, ataxia, and generalized pruritus have been reported. In fatal cases, "respiratory paralysis" precedes death (Russell, 1965).

Poisoning following the ingestion of the whelk, *Neptunea arthritica,* is characterized by dizziness, nausea, vomiting, weakness, ataxia, photophobia, external ocular weakness, dryness of the mouth, and, on occasion, urticaria. Ingestion of the toxic abalone produces erythema, swelling, and pain over the face and neck, and sometimes the extremities, and in the more severe cases a fulminating dermatitis. Latin and medieval writers from the time of Pliny considered the sea hare *Aplysia* to be very poisonous, and although Halstead (1965) notes that extracts of *Aplysia* were "frequently employed to dispatch political enemies," there are no recent reports of death from the eating of sea hares. Tasting them produces a burning sensation in the mouth and slight irritation of the oral mucosa. Handling the animals is not likely to be dangerous. However, I suspect that it would not be safe to rub one's eyes after handling these animals. A number of poisonings occurred in Hokkaido, Japan, from the ingestion of *Calista brevisiphonata* in the early 1950s. These poisonings necessitated prohibiting the sale of the shellfish in the marketplace. The illness was a rapid onset, often occurring while the patient is still dining. It has been characterized as an "allergic-like" reaction, which is thought to be due to the presence of excessive choline in the ovaries. The most common findings are flushing, urticaria, wheezing, and gastrointestinal upset. It is self-limiting (Russell, 1971). Hashimoto (1979) notes a total of 542 cases of venerupin poisoning in Japan with 185 deaths. Fortunately, there have been no reported cases since 1950. It was observed following the eating of the oyster, *Crassostrea gigas,* or the asari, *Tapes japonica.* The poisoning is characterized by a long incubation period (24 to 48 hours, and sometimes longer), anorexia, halitosis, nausea, vomiting, gastric pain, constipation, headache, and malaise. These findings may be followed by increased nervousness, hematemesis, and bleeding from the mucous membranes of the nose, mouth, and gums. In serious cases, jaundice may be present, and petechial hemorrhages and ecchymosis may appear over the chest, neck, and arms. Leukocytosis, anemia, and a prolonged blood-clotting time are sometimes observed. The liver is usually enlarged. In fatal poisonings, extreme excitation, delirium, and coma occur.

The more common types of shellfish poisoning are recognized as gastrointestinal, allergic, and paralytic. Gastrointestinal shellfish poisoning is characterized by nausea, vomiting, abdominal pain, weakness, and diarrhea. The onset of symptoms generally occurs 8 to 12 hours following ingestion of the offending mollusc. This type of intoxication is caused by bacterial pathogens and is usually limited to gastrointestinal signs and symptoms. It rarely persists for more than 48 hours.

Allergic or erythematous shellfish poisoning is characterized by an allergic response, which may vary from one individual to another. The onset of symptoms and signs occurs 30 minutes to six hours after ingestion of the mollusc to which the individual is sensitive. The usual presenting signs and symptoms are diffuse erythema, swelling, urticaria, and pruritus involving the head and neck and then spreading to the body. Headache, flushing, epigastric distress, and nausea are occasional complaints. In the more severe cases, generalized edema, severe pruritus, swelling of the tongue and throat, respiratory distress, and vomiting sometimes occur. Death is rare, but persons with a known sensitivity to shellfish should avoid eating all molluscs. The sensitizing material appears more capable of provoking a serious autopharmacologic response than most known sensitizing proteins.

Paralytic shellfish poisoning is known variously as gonyaulax poisoning, paresthetic shellfish poisoning, mussel poisoning, or mytilointoxication. Pathognomonic symptoms develop within the first 30 minutes following ingestion of the offending mollusc. Paresthesia, described as tingling, burning, or numbness, is noted first about the mouth, lips, and tongue; it then spreads over the face, scalp, and neck, and to the fingertips and toes. Sensory perception and proprioception are affected to the point that the individual moves incoordinately and in a manner similar to that seen in another, more common form of intoxication. Ataxia, incoherent speech, and/or aphonia are prominent signs in severe poisonings. The patient complains of dizziness, tightness of the throat and chest, and some pain on deep inspiration. Weakness, malaise, headache, increased salivation and perspiration, thirst, and nausea and vomiting may be present. The pulse is usually thready and rapid; the superficial reflexes are often absent and the deep reflexes may be hypoactive. If muscular weakness and respiratory distress grow progressively more severe during the first eight hours, death may ensue. If the victim survives the first ten to twelve hours, the prognosis is good. Death is usually attributed to "respiratory paralysis" (Russell, 1965, 1971).

Among the cephalopods that have been implicated in bites on humans are *Hapalochaena*

(= *Octopus*) *maculosa, Octopus australis, O. lunulatus, O. doefleini, O. vulgaris, O. apollyon, O. bimaculatus, O. macropus, O. rubescens, O. fitchi, O. flindersi, Ommastrephes sloani pacificus, Eledone moschata, E. aldrovandi,* and *Sepia officinalis*. The bite of most octopuses result in a small puncture wound; it appears to bleed more freely than one would expect from a similar nonenvenomized, traumatic wound. Pain is minimal, and in the two cases seen by the author it was described as no greater than that which would have been produced by a sharp pin. The area around the wound is first blanched but then becomes erythematous and in severe envenomations may become hemorrhagic. Tingling and numbness about the wound site are not uncommon complaints. Swelling is usually minimal immediately following the injury but may develop 6 to 12 hours later. Muscle fasciculations have been noted following *H. maculosa* bites (Sutherland and Lane, 1969). Localized pruritus sometimes occurs over the edematous area. "Lightheadedness" of several hours' duration and weakness where reported in both cases observed by us; there were no other systemic symptoms or signs, although the wounds healed without complications (Russell, 1965). In the case reported by Flecker and Cotton (1955), bitten by *H. maculosa*, the patient complained of dryness in the mouth and difficulty in breathing following the bite, but no localized or generalized pain. Subsequently, breathing became more labored, swallowing became difficult, and the patient began to vomit. Severe respiratory distress and cyanosis developed, and the victim expired. The findings at autopsy were negative. Subsequently, Cleland and Southcott (1965) reviewed the literature on cephalopod bites and noted several unreported bites on humans.

Fishes

Poisonous Fishes. Approximately 700 species of marine fishes are known to be toxic or may on ingestion be poisonous to man. This number does not include those fishes which have caused a poisoning traceable to bacterial pathogens. Most, but by no means all, of these species are found in the coral reef belt. As a whole their distribution is spotty, even in a particular part of the ocean or around an island. They tend to occur in greater numbers around islands than along continental shores. Most species are nonmigratory. They may be either herbivores or carnivores. Some poisonous species have tissues that are toxic at all times; other species are poisonous only at certain periods, or in certain areas, while still others have only specific organs that are toxic, and the toxicity of these tissues may vary with time and location.

Fish poisoning is synonymous with *ich-thyotoxism*. Halstead (1964) divided the ich-thyotoxic fishes into three subdivisions: (1) *Ich-thyosarcotoxic*—those fishes which contain a toxin within their musculature, viscera, or skin, which when ingested produces deleterious effects; (2) *Ichthyootoxic*—those fishes which produce a toxin that is related to gonadal activity; most members of this subdivision are freshwater species; this group includes those fishes whose roe is poisonous; and (3) *Icthyohemotoxic*—those fishes which have a toxin in their blood. Some freshwater eels and several marine fishes make up this group. The word *ichthyocrinotoxic* is sometimes used for those fishes which produce a poison through glandular secretions not associated with a venom apparatus. This word might be used for the soapfishes, certain gobies, some cyclostomes, boxfishes, toadfishes, lampreys, and hagfishes, which may release toxic skin secretions into the water, perhaps under stressful conditions, or as repellants, or in defense.

Ichthyosarcotoxism. This type of poisoning is generally identified with the kind of fish involved: elasmobranch, chimaeroid, clupeoid, ciguatera, tetraodon, scombroid, etc.; it also includes hallucinatory fish poisoning.

Ciguatera. The word ciguatera was perhaps first applied to a poisoning caused by the ingestion of the marine snail *Livona pica* (''cigua''), a staple seafood found throughout the Caribbean. The word is now commonly used to indicate that type of fish poisoning characterized by certain gastrointestinal-neurologic, and sometimes cardiovascular, manifestations. It may occur following the ingestion of certain tropical reef and semipelagic marine species, such as the barracudas, groupers, sea basses, snappers, surgeonfishes, parrotfishes, jacks, wrasses, eels, as well as certain gastropods. A listing of the ciguateric fishes has been provided by Russell (1965), Halstead (1967), and Bagnis *et al.* (1970). Elsewhere I have noted that approximately 300 species of fish have been implicated in ciguatera poisoning but Bagnis *et al.* (1970) note approximately 400 species. Since almost all of these fishes are normally edible, and some are valuable food fishes in some parts of the world, ciguatera poisoning is not only the most common but also the most treacherous form of ichthyotoxism.

This form of fish poisoning is associated with the food chain or food web (Russell, 1952, 1965; Dawson *et al.*, 1955; Randall, 1958; Halstead, 1965; Banner, 1976; Southcott, 1979). It has been shown to exist in both the South Pacific and the Caribbean. The responsible organism is a photosynthetic benthic dinoflagellate, *Gambierdiscus toxicus*, but the poison found in most ciguateric fishes is probably a combination of several toxins, the principal one being *ciguatoxin* and, in some cases, lesser ones being *maitotoxin* and *scaritoxin*. The chemical structure has not yet been elicited. The toxin is a colorless, heat-stable, hydroxylated lipid molecule, with a molecular weight of about 1100, and it shows little olefinic character and no observable proton signals below 6. The toxin increases membrane permeability to sodium, causing depolarization, and in different doses produces changes in the rate and force of contraction of the heart. Large doses precipitate more severe cardiac changes. Contrary to published reports that it is an anticholinesterase, it has been found to be antagonized by physostigmine.

Signs of poisoning in animals include increased salivation and lacrimation, miosis, respiratory difficulties, cyanosis, decreased body temperature, ataxia and loss of reflexes, and prostration. In humans, symptoms and signs include perioral parasthesia, often with a feeling of loose teeth in the lower jaw, nausea and vomiting, abdominal pain, changes in sensory perception, pruritus, diarrhea, hypoactive reflexes, and bradycardia. The patient often complains of dizziness, marked weakness, and, on occasion, some myalgia and joint pain. Paresis, particularly of the legs, is a common finding in severe poisonings. Presence of the toxin can be demonstrated by ELISA and RIA.

Tetrodotoxin. Tetrodotoxin, puffer or fugu poison, is found in certain puffers, ocean sunfishes, and porcupinefishes. Tetrodotoxin (tarichatoxin) is also found in certain amphibian species of the family Salamandridae and the blue-ringed octopus. The puffers or pufferlike fishes appear to be the only fishes universally regarded as poisonous. Of the approximately 100 species of these fishes, over 50 have been involved in poisonings to humans or are known to be toxic under certain conditions. Some of the more important of the toxic species have been noted by Russell (1965), Kao (1966), Halstead (1967), and Hashimoto (1979). Table 22–6 shows the concentration of tetrodotoxin for various tissues of Tetraodontidae species and for the amphibian *Taricha torosa*. It can be seen that in most causes the toxin is concentrated in the ovaries and liver, with lesser amounts being found in the intestines and skin, and very small amounts in the body musculature and blood. In almost all fish species so far studied the concentration in the ovaries has been considerably higher than in the corresponding male tissues. The appearance and amount of toxin in the fish are related to the reproductive cycle and appear to be greatest just prior to spawning, which varies with the species involved and the locale. The

Table 22–6. CONCENTRATIONS OF TETRODOTOXIN IN TETRAODONTIDAE FISHES AND A NEWT*

SPECIES	OVARY	LIVER	SKIN	INTESTINES	MUSCLE	BLOOD
Sphaeroides niphobles	400	1000	40	400	4	1
Sphaeroides alboplumbeus	200	1000	20	40	4	
Sphaeroides pardalis	200	1000	100	40	1	1
Sphaeroides vermicularis	400	200	100	40	4	
Sphaeroides porphyreus	400	200	20	40	1	
Sphaeroides oscellatus	1000	40	20	40	<0.2	
Sphaeroides basilewskianus	100	40	4	40	<0.2	
Sphaeroides chrysops	40	40	20	4	<0.2	<0.2
Sphaeroides pseudommus	100	10	4	2	<0.2	
Sphaeroides rubripes	100	100	1	2	<0.2	<0.2
Sphaeroides xanthopterus	100	40	1	4	<0.2	
Sphaeroides stictonotus	20	<0.2	2	1	<0.2	
Lagocephalus inermis	0.4	1	<0.2	0.4	0.4	
Canthigaster rivulatus	<2	2	40	4	<0.2	
Taricha torosa ♂	25	<0.1	25	(0.1)†	2	1
Taricha torosa ♂	<0.1‡	<0.1	80	(0.5)†	8	21

* From Kao, C. Y.: Tetrodotoxin, saxitoxin, and their significance in the study of the excitation phenomena. *Pharmacol. Rev.*, **18**:997, 1966. © by Williams & Wilkins, 1966. Amounts expressed in mcg toxin/g fresh tissue of female specimens.
† Visceral organ.
‡ Testis.

chemistry of tetrodotoxin up until 1970 has been reviewed elsewhere (Russell, 1971). Its structure is:

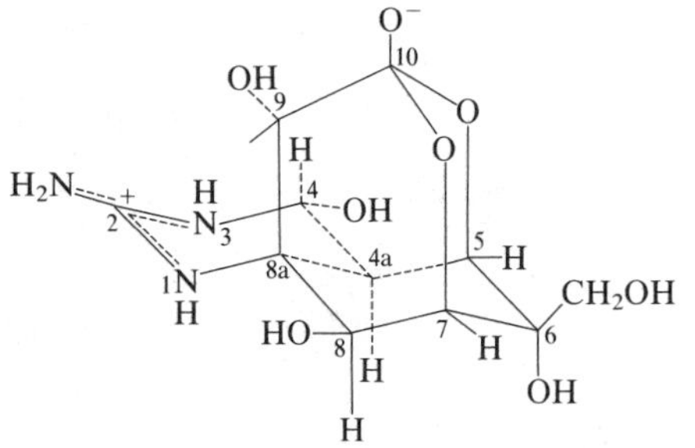

The lethal dose-response curve of tetrodotoxin is characteristically steep. The intraperitoneal minimal lethal dose in mice in 8 μg/kg, while the LD99 is 12 μg/kg, and the intraperitoneal LD50 is approximately 10 μg/kg (Kao and Fuhrman, 1963). The oral LD50 in mice is 322 μg/kg, while that in cats is in excess of 0.20 mg/kg. The toxin prevents the increase in the early transient ionic permeability of the nerve normally associated with the inward movement of sodium during excitation. This can be seen in the classic nerve preparations as a conduction block, and in the voltage-clamp axon preparations as a decrease in the peak current of the inward sodium. The subsequent outward movement of potassium is unaffected by the toxin. It is also capable of blocking the inward movement of all substituted cations that could account, under experimental conditions, for the early current change. In blocking this early cur-

rent, the toxin prevents both the inward and outward movement of ions. The mode of the block is not ion specificity but changes provoked in the membrane of the nerve.

To a lesser extent tetrodotoxin blocks the skeletal muscle membrane. It has no direct effect on the junction, exclusive of that on the nerve ending and the muscle membrane. It provokes hypotension and has a deleterious effect on respiration. It has some effects on the central nervous system but little on the autonomic nervous system. Tetrodotoxin has pharmacologic and toxicologic properties similar in many ways to those of saxitoxin, but the two are chemically distinct. The proposed "cork-in-a-bottle" hypothesis for tetrodotoxin seems highly questionable at this time. Recent studies have shown that binding of tetrodotoxin, like saxitoxin, is a function separate from that of cation selectivity, which has been the basis of the cork-in-a-bottle model (Kao, 1981).

While less than 75 people now die from tetraodon poisoning in Japan each year, many of those using the poison in suicide, and additional deaths are reported from elsewhere in the Orient and Pacific, the total number of deaths worldwide is probably less than 125. At one time the mortality rate was 80 percent, but through the years it has been reduced, due in part to the fine work of Hashimoto and his colleagues in licensing fugu restaurants in Japan. At the present time about 40 percent of those developing significant symptoms and signs subsequently die. The clinical case is characterized by the rapid onset (5 to 30 minutes) of weakness, dizziness, pallor, and paresthesia about the lips, tongue, and throat. The paresthesia is usually described as "tingling or pricking sensations" and is often noted in the limbs, particularly the fingers and toes, as the illness develops. Weakness is a common complaint. Increased salivation and diaphoresis are often present, and the patient may become hypotensive. Changes in heart rate are common. There may be vomiting and sometimes it is severe and frequent. Bradycardia, dyspnea, cyanosis, and shock may develop, and generalized flaccidity may ensue. Treatment consists of oxygen, intravenous fluids, atropine, and, if appropriate, activated charcoal, saline catharses, and nasoepigastric suctioning. Calcium, naloxone, and sedatives are contraindicated. The poison can be detected from autopsy material by gas chromatography.

Scrombroid Poisoning. Certain of the mackerellike fishes (tunas, skipjacks, and bonitos) are occasionally involved in human poisonings. The clinical manifestations of these poisonings are quite different from that provoked by ciguatera toxin, although some of these same fishes may also be implicated in ciguatera poisoning. Although more than 50 papers on this subject have been written during the past decade, they have added little to that reported by Halstead (1967). A notable exception is the review by Arnold and Brown (1978). If scombroids are inadequately preserved, a toxic substance is formed within the body musculature. This substance was once thought to be histamine, formed by the action of enzymes and bacteria or released by bacterial action on the death of the fish. However, more recent evidence seems to indicate that the toxic component is not histamine alone, although histamine is involved in the reaction. The toxic factor has been given the name "saurine" by some investigators. Following ingestion of the offending fish, the victim usually complains of nausea, vomiting, diarrhea, and epigastric distress, flushing of the face, headache, and burning of the throat, sometimes followed by numbness, thirst, and generalized urticaria. These signs and symptoms usually appear within two hours of the meal and subside within 16 hours. In the more severe cases there may be some muscular weakness. The poisoning is rarely serious. The offending fish is often said to have a "peppery taste" (Russell, 1971).

Cyclostome Poisoning. The slime and flesh of certain lampreys and hagfishes appear to contain a toxin that may produce gastrointestinal signs and symptoms. The chemical, pharmacologic, and toxicologic nature of the toxin is not known.

Elasmobranch Poisoning. Consumption of the musculature of the Greenland shark, *Somniosus microcephalus,* has caused poisonings in both humans and dogs, while the livers of several species of tropical sharks have caused severe poisonings and even deaths. Species reported to be poisonous at times include: *Carcharhinus melanopterus, Heptranchias perlo, Hexanchus grisseus, Carcharodon carcharias,* and *Sphyrna zygaena.* In some cases the poisoning appears to be ciguateric in nature. The eating of shark livers has been known to cause another kind of poisoning, which appears to be due to hypervitaminosis A. Hypervitaminosis A is well known following the consumption of the lives of some polar bears, seals, and halibut (Russell, 1967; Halstead, 1970).

Hallucinatory Fish Poisoning. This type of poisoning is characterized by central nervous system signs and symptoms, and by the lack of gastrointestinal manifestations. It has occurred following the ingestion of certain mullet and surmullet (goatfish). Among the species reported to have caused this poisoning are: *Mugil cephalus, Neomyxus chaptalli, Paraupeneus chryserydros,* and *Upeneus arge.* Reports of poisoning have been filed in the tropical Pacific and Hawaii. Nothing is known of the chemistry or toxicology of this poison. However, the findings in human cases seem to indicate that the offending substance is different from that responsible for ciguatera poisoning. The onset of symptoms occurs 10 to 90 minutes following ingestion of the toxic fish. The victim complains of light-headedness or dizziness, weakness, muscular incoordination, and sometimes ataxia, hallucinations, and depression. In the severe cases, there may be paresthesia about the mouth, and some muscular paralysis and dyspnea. The agonal period is usually of short duration, 1 to 24 hours, and few cases are serious enough to bring the victim to the doctor. If the victim goes to sleep immediately following the poisoning he is said to have violent nightmares. This complaint accounts for the term "nightmare weke" being given to the causative fish *U. arge* (Helfrich and Banner, 1960).

Ichthyootoxic Fishes. A number of freshwater fishes and a few marine species produce a toxin that appears to be restricted to their gonads. In these fishes the body musculature and even the gastrointestinal organs are edible. Poisoning occurs following ingestion of the roe, or gonads and roe. The eggs of *Scorpaenichthys marmoratus* appear to be avoided by fish-eating and scavenging birds, as well as by mink and racoon, while the roe of the alligator gar is known to produce cardiovascular changes. An excellent review of this problem will be found in Fuhrman (1974). The poisoning is characterized by the rapid onset of nausea, vomiting, and epigastric distress. Diarrhea, dryness in the mouth, thirst, tinnitus, and malaise sometimes occur. In the more severe cases, syncope, respiratory distress, chest pain, convulsions, and coma may ensue. Complete recovery usually occurs within a few days.

Ichthyohemotoxic Fishes. A toxic substance has been found in the blood of many species of fishes, although the principal contributions to our knowledge of the toxin have come to us through studies on the blood of the eels *Anguilla* and *Muraena*. Poisonings from the ingestion of fresh blood are extremely rare. The few cases reported have occurred in persons who of their own volition have drunk quantities sufficient to cause symptoms; most of these have occurred following the ingestion of blood from the European freshwater eels, or *M. helena*.

Crinotoxic Fishes. Halstead (1970) has recorded approximately 50 teleost species as being crinotoxic. Hashimoto has added a few additional, and with the study of Cameron *et al.* (1981), and others, the total number must now approach 65. These fishes are known to release a toxic substance from the skin that is capable of killing other fishes and perhaps other marine animals. This toxin appears to be part of the animal's defensive armament and is probably released as an alarm substance to deter predators. Cameron *et al.* (1981) suggest that in the case of the stonefish the toxin liberated from the tubercle glands might be antibiotic in nature, protecting the fish against the plethora of potential harmful organisms that occur in the immediate environment of the virtually scaleless integument of the fish.

A toxic factor has been separated from the skin secretions of the boxfish, or trunkfish, *Ostracion lentiginosis*. The toxin is heat stable, nondialyzable, and soluble in water, methanol, ethanol, acetone, and chloroform, but insoluble in diethyl ether and benzene. Repeated extractions of residues obtained from drying the skin secretions with acetone or chloroform and diethyl ether give a particulate substance that forms stable foams in aqueous solutions and is toxic to fish at concentrations of 1:1,000,000. Approximately 50 to 100 mg of the crude dried toxin could be obtained at one time from a single adult boxfish. The toxin was called "ostracitoxin." Further studies showed that when a crude solution was extracted into 1-butanol, a 20-fold purification of the toxin could be obtained. The product was called "pahutoxin." Spectroscopic data, hydrolytic degradations, and synthesis gave the formula $C_{23}H_{46}NO_4Cl$ and the structure:

$$CH_3-(CH_2)_{12}-\overset{\overset{\displaystyle H}{|}}{\underset{\underset{\displaystyle OCOCH_3}{|}}{C}}-CH_2-CO_2-(CH_2)_2-\overset{+}{N}(CH_3)_3Cl^-$$

Pahutoxin is thus the choline chloride ester of 3-acetoxyhexadecanoic acid. It and its C_{14} and C_{12} homologs have been synthesized as the racemates. When ostracitoxin was added to an aquarium containing other reef fishes, these fishes exhibited "irritability," gasping, then activity with a decrease in opercular movements, loss of equilibrium and locomotion, and finally, sporadic convulsions, and death. When the skin mucus was injected into the boxfish the fish immediately lost its balance, and death occurred within a few minutes. When injected into mice, ostracitoxin produced ataxia, labored respirations, coma, and death. The MLD was 200 mg/kg body weight. Ostracitoxin caused hemolysis of vertebrate erythrocytes *in vitro*. Pahutoxin was quantitated for its hemolytic property, which correlated with its lethal property. The minimum lethal concentration for fish was found to be 0.176 µg/ml, when death was measured at one hour (see Russell, 1971, for references).

The Red Sea flatfish, *Pardachirus marmoratus,* has 212 to 235 secretory glands along its dorsal and anal fins. Its secretions are toxic to fishes and the toxic factor, pardaxin, is a protein having a molecular weight of approximately 15,000, with a single chain and four disulfide bridges. The toxin has an intraperitoneal LD50 in mice of 24.6 mg/kg and inhibits Na^+-K^+ − ATPase but enhances esterase activity. It causes hemolysis in dog red blood cells, which lack ATPase, but the toxin-induced hemolysis is not caused by ATPase inhibition. It was suggested that the different responses to the poison, with respect to esterase and ATPase, could be due to differences in the way these enzymes are anchored in the plasma membrane (Primor and Lazarovici, 1981).

Venomous Fishes

More than 200 species of marine fishes, including stingrays, scorpionfishes, zebrafishes, stonefishes, weevers, toadfishes, stargazers, and certain of the sharks, ratfishes, catfishes, and surgeonfishes are known or thought to be venomous. The great majority of venomous piscines are nonmigratory and slow swimming. They tend to live in protected habitats, or around rocks, corals, or kelp beds. Stingrays spend much of their time buried in sand. Most species use their venom apparatus as a defensive weapon. The toxins of the venomous fishes differ markedly in their chemical, pharmacologic, and toxicologic properties from the toxins of the poisonous fishes, as well as from the toxins of the other venomous animals. A common characteristic of the toxins of the venomous fishes is their relative instability. Few of them are stable at room temperatures, and toxicity appears to be lost or markedly reduced even on lyophilization of freshly prepared crude extracts. No basic structure for the toxin of any venomous fishes has yet been established, or even proposed with any degree of fervor. The reader is referred to the works of Russell (1965, 1969, 1971; 1984a) and Halstead (1970, 1978) for a review of the toxins of the venomous fishes.

Stingrays. The stingrays include the families Dasyatidae, the whiprays; Urolophidae, the round stingrays; Myliobatioidae, the bat- or eagle-rays; Gymnuridae, the butterfly rays; and the Potamotrygonidae or river rays. These elasmobranches range in size from several inches in diameter to over 14 feet in length. For the most part, they are nonmigratory, shallow-water fishes. The venom apparatus of the stingray consists of a bilaterally serrated, dentinal caudal spine located on the dorsum of the animal's tail. The spine is encased in an integumentary sheath. The venom is contained with certain highly specialized secretory cells within this sheath. These cells and the supporting structures have been described in detail (see Russell, 1965; Halstead, 1970; Smith *et al.*, 1978). Unlike most venomous animals the stingray has no true venom gland. The venom is contained in the secretory cells within the grooves of the caudal spine, and these cells and their supporting tissues must be ruptured in order to release the toxin, as in the traumatic act of stinging.

Stingray venom is known to exert a deleterious effect on the mammalian cardiovascular system. Low concentrations of the venom give rise to either vasodilatation or vasoconstriction, with mild bradycardia and an increase in the P-R interval. Cats receiving larger amounts of the venom show, in addition to the P-R interval change, almost immediate ST, T-wave change indicative of ischemia and, in some animals, true heart muscle injury. High concentrations cause vasoconstriction and produce marked changes in heart rate and amplitude of systole, and may often cause complete, irreversible, cardiac standstill (Russell and van Harreveld, 1954). While small doses of the venom may cause some increase in the respiratory rate, large doses depress respiration. Part of this depression is secondary to the cardiovascular changes, but the venom may provoke changes in behavior. The venom has little or no effect or neuromuscular transmission.

Mice injected with a lethal dose of stingray venom develop hyperkinesis, prostration, marked dyspnea, blanching of the ears and retina, and exophthalmos. These are followed by complete atonia, cyanosis, gasping respiratory movements, coma, and death. In cats and monkeys a similar pattern has been observed. The LD99 in mice has been calculated as 28.0 mg/kg

for crude extracts of the tissues from the ventrolateral grooves of the sting. However, we have found that the peak II portion of a Spehadex G-200 fraction has an intravenous LD50 in mice of approximately 2.9 mg protein/per kilogram body weight (see Russell, 1971, for references).

Scorpionfishes. The family Scorpaenidae, the scorpionfishes or rockfishes, contains approximately 80 species that have been implicated in poisonings to humans, or whose venom has been studied by chemists and toxinologists. Included in this group are the sculpins, zebrafishes, stonefishes, bullrout, and waspfish. They are widely distributed throughout all tropical and the more temperate seas. A few are found in Arctic waters. The venom apparatus of these fishes has been described in considerable detail. In most species it consists of a number of dorsal, several anal, and two pelvic spines. The spines differ considerably in their size and structure. The enveloping integumentary sheath and the glandular complex lying within the anterolateral grooves make up the remaining components of the venom apparatus. The venom apparatuses of these fishes have been divided into three types. A more thorough review of the variations in the venom gland structures, the chemistry, and the toxicology of the venom has been reviewed by Halstead (1970) and Russell (1971). The pharmacologic properties are summarized in Table 22–7.

Weeverfishes. The weevers, member of the piscine family Trachinidae, are small marine fishes that are confined to the eastern Atlantic and Mediterranean coasts. The name "weever" is probably derived from a corruption of the Anglo-Saxon "wivre," meaning viper. These fish are found in large numbers in the shallow waters of certain offshore sandy grounds along the southeast English coast, in the continental southern North Sea, and along the coasts of the English Channel and Mediterranean and Adriatic seas. The venom apparatus of the weeverfishes consists of two opercular spines, five to eight dorsal spines, and the tissues contained within the integumentary sheaths surrounding the spines. The two dentinal opercular spines extend caudally and very slightly downward from near the superior margin of each operculum. The five to eight dorsal spines are enclosed within individual integumentary sheaths connected by their interspinous membranes. The venom is contained within the various grooves of the spines. These spines and the venom have been described elsewhere (Russell and Emery, 1960; Halstead, 1978; Russell, 1971, 1984a).

Clinical Problem. Stings by venomous marine fishes are common in many areas of the world. Approximately 750 people have been

Table 22-7. SOME PROPERTIES OF SCORPAENIDAE VENOMS*

	pterosis	SYNANCEJA	SCORPAENA
Small dose	Decreased arterial pressure Minimal ECG changes Increased respiratory rate Muscular weakness in mice	Decreased arterial pressure Minimal ECG changes Increased respiratory rate Tremor	Slight decrease in arterial pressure Increased then decreased venous pressure Minimal ECG changes Increased respiratory rate with decreased respiratory excursions
Medium dose	Marked fall in arterial pressure Myocardial ischemia, injury or conduction defects Increased respiratory rate Partial paralysis of legs in mice	Marked fall in arterial pressure Myocardial ischemia, injury or conduction defects Increased respiratory rate Muscular weakness in mice Tremor	Fall in arterial pressure Myocardial ischemia, injury or conduction defects Changes in venous and CSF pressures Increased respiratory rate with decreased respiratory excursions Muscular weakness in mice
Lethal dose	Precipitous, irreversible fall in systemic arterial pressure Extensive ECG changes Markedly decreased respiratory rate → cessation Complete paralysis of legs in mice Intravenous LD50 mice, 1.1 mg protein/kg body weight	Precipitous, irreversible fall in systemic arterial pressure Extensive ECG changes Markedly decreased respiratory rate → cessation Some paralysis of legs in mice Possible neuromuscular junction changes Produces tremors, convulsions, marked muscular weakness, coma; myotoxic Intravenous LD50 mice, 200 µg protein/kg body weight	Precipitous, irreversible fall in arterial pressure Extensive ECG changes Markedly decreased respiratory rate → cessation Some paralysis of legs in mice Intravenous LD50 mice, in excess 2.0 mg protein kg body weight

* From Russell, F.E.: Pharmacology of toxins of marine origin. In Raskova, H. (ed.): *International Encyclopedia of Pharmacology and Therapeutics*. Pergamon Press, Ltd., Oxford, 1971, Sec. 71, Vol. 2, pp. 3–114.

reported stung by stingrays along the North American coasts in a single year. Fortunately, deaths from the effects of the venom are very rare. Stings by other *Scorpaena* are very common. Approximately 300 persons in the United States are stung by *S. guttata* or related species each year (see Russell, 1971, for references). Envenomations by the lionfishes or zebrafishes were once quite rare, but with the importation of lionfishes for tropical sea aquaria more than 50 cases of stings by these fish were reported in 1978–79. Injuries inflicted by weeverfishes are also common in certain coastal areas of Europe. However, no deaths attributable to the stings of these fishes have been reported in recent years.

Of 1097 stingray injuries reported over a six-year period in North America from 1952 to 1959, 232 patients were seen by a physician at some time during the course of their recovery. That is not true today. Only about 5 percent are now seen by physicians due to the effective first aid

provided by the lifeguard services. Unlike the injuries inflicted by many venomous animals, wounds produced by the stingray may be large and severely lacerated, requiring extensive debridement and surgical closure. A sting no wider than 5 mm may produce a wound 3.5 cm long, and larger stings may produce wounds 17.5 cm long. The sting itself is rarely broken off in the wound. The stinging is followed by the immediate onset of intense pain, out of proportion to that which might be produced by a similar nonvenomous injury. While the onset of pain is usually limited to the area of injury, it rapidly spreads, though gradually diminishing in severity over 6 to 48 hours.

For the most part the symptoms and signs of the poisoning are limited to the injured area. However, syncope, weakness, nausea, and anxiety are common complaints and may be attributed in part to peripheral vasodilatation and in part to the reflex phenomenon precipitated by the severe pain. Vomiting, diarrhea, sweating, fasciculations in the muscles of the affected extremity, generalized cramps, inguinal or axillary pain, and respiratory distress are infrequently reported. True paralysis is extremely rare, if it occurs at all. Examination reveals either a puncture or a lacerating wound, usually the latter, jagged, bleeding freely, and often contaminated with parts of the stingray's integumentary sheath. The edges of the wound may be discolored. However, within two hours the discoloration may extend several centimeters from the wound. Subsequent necrosis of this area occasionally occurs in untreated cases.

Treatment, to be successful, must be instituted early. The standard procedure for treatment of fish stings is well established. Injuries to an extremity should be irrigated with the salt water at hand. An attempt should be made to remove the integumentary sheath, if present in the wound. The extremity should then be submerged in hot water at as high a temperature as the patient can tolerate without injury for 30 to 90 minutes. The addition of sodium chloride or magnesium sulfate to the hot water is optional. The wound should then be further cleaned, debrided, and sutured, if necessary. The appropriate antitetanus agent should be administered. Infections of these wounds are rare in properly treated cases. Elevation of the injured extremity is advised.

Envenomation by *Scorpaena,* such as the California sculpin, *S. guttata,* is followed almost immediately by intense, sometimes pulsating pain in the area of the injury. Almost all stings are inflicted on the hands of fishermen while they are attempting to dislodge the fish from their hooks. The area around the wound may appear ischemic at first, but in time the injured part becomes red and swollen. The pain may extend up the forearm and into the axilla within 15 minutes of the injury. Nausea, vomiting, weakness, pallor, syncope, and an urgency to urinate are frequent complaints. Increased perspiration, headache, conjunctivitis, and diarrhea are sometimes reported. Paresthesia about the injured part and even up the forearm is not uncommon. Swelling and tenderness of the axillary nodes occurred in at least 30 percent of one series of untreated cases. The pain subsides in three to eight hours, although the swelling and tenderness may persist for several days. In severe stingings the pain may be excruciating. Primary shock may occur, and in several cases seen by the author the patients were brought to the hospital under oxygen. Respirations may become labored and painful. Pulmonary edema has been reported and abnormal electrocardiograms demonstrated. In one case known to the author the patient had a pulmonary embolism

and was hospitalized for 24 days. The standard treatment for *S. guttata* stings had been to soak the injured part in hot water for 30 minutes. In many cases the fisherman adds household ammonia.

Envenomation by the lionfish gives rise to immediate intense, sometimes burning pain, which often radiates within minutes from the wounded area. The tissues about the wound may appear blanched, and the victim may complain of numbness, weakness, and paresthesia about the injury or even over the entire affected part. Weakness, dizziness, and shock may ensue but are not common. In cases of shock there is bradycardia, hypothermia, and respiratory distress. The wound site is sometimes discolored, edematous, and tender. Necrosis may occur about the wound. The pain often persists for 8 to 12 hours, and the injured part may be sore and edematous for several weeks. First-aid treatment is the same as for stingray injuries. Meperidine hydrochloride has been used to control pain. Intravenous calcium gluconate has been said to afford some relief. Cardiovascular tone should be maintained with intravenous fluids and vasopressor agents.

Stingings by the stonefishes *Synanceja horrida* and *S. tractanis* are usually more serious than those inflicted by any other of the venomous fishes. The clinical course following poisoning by a stonefish is similar to, although considerably more severe than, that previously described for the stingrays and lionfishes. Necrosis of tissues at the site of the injury, and the subsequent sloughing of these tissues, are more common following stings by *Synanceja* than following injuries by the other venomous fishes. Treatment of wounds produced by stonefishes must be instituted immediately following envenomation. Immersion of the injured part in hot water, as described for stingray wounds, should be tried. Injection of emetine hydrocloride directly into the wound has been tried, with indifferent results. In one case seen by the author, a soap solution was injected directly into the wound area 15 minutes after the hot-water treatment had been initiated. There were no untoward effects and no local tissue changes developed. An antivenin is now prepared by the Commonwealth Serum Laboratories of Australia and should be used when the seriousness of the poisoning warrants.

The weeverfishes, *Trachinus,* may inflict either a single or a multiple puncture-type wound. Persons stung by these fishes report having received a sharp, immediately painful stab. It increases in severity during the first 20 to 50 minutes following the injury and may persist for 16 to 24 hours if treatment is not undertaken. As noted by Halstead (1957), the pain can be so severe that a victim stung by one of these fishes while in the water may experience difficulty in reaching shore. I have obtained similar reports from bathers along the Devon and Cornwall coasts of England. It seems unlikely that it is the excruciating pain rather than true muscular paralysis that is responsible for the victim's motor incapacity. The degree of swelling about the wound varies, although some swelling appears to be a constant finding. The tissues adjacent to the wound often appear discolored; the surrounding area may be somewhat blanched. Localized necrosis at the wound site may occur, and sloughing of these tissues has been reported. It is possible that repeated stings, and the effects of the venom and low-grade infection, are contributing factors in cases of arthritis seen in fishermen on trawlers in the North Sea (see Russell, 1971, for references).

In severe cases of envenomation by weevers there may be weakness, dizziness, nausea, primary shock, and respiratory distress. Fisherman at Ijmuiden, Holland, told me that there was often an urgency to urinate, and that in severe stings there was axillary and chest pain, as well as changes in pulse rate and respiration.

A few thoughts on the treatment of weeverfish stings seem indicated, and perhaps this is an appropriate place to present an additional reflection or so on the therapeutics of the injuries produced by venomous fishes in general. After having seen and treated a good many such injuries during the past three decades, I have been impressed with the differences between the advice found in medical texts and that suggested and used by fishermen or lifeguards, or persons familiar with envenomations by fishes. I am distressed to note that in most cases the nonprofessional advice has not only proved to be more effective, but often more rational. Much of the advice given in texts devoted to tropical medicine, where the problem of venomous animal injury is most often discussed, stems from the false and antiquated idea that all venoms are related chemically and thus all respond to similar therapeutic measures. From the early studies on snake venoms a number of remedies found their way into the therapeutics for venomous fish injuries. Among these were acetic acid, alcohol, formaldehyde, urine, potassium permanganate, ink, gold salts, carbolic acid, cassava bread, and cauterization. While all these measures have been found to be ineffective, some are still advised in an occasional medical text. The more recent therapeutic fads for antihistamines, corticosteroids, and ice water as "shotgun" therapeutic methods are slowly waning, fortunately for the patient.

It is refreshing to find that a review of the literature for the past several centuries reveals a highly effective method of treatment, based on trial and error. When I suggested (Russell and Emery, 1960) that the use of hot water in weeverfish stings might be effective, I did so on the basis of its very effective use in stingray and scorpionfish injuries, and on the basis of a limited number of case histories and observations on weeverfish stings that I studied in England, France, and Holland during 1958. Subsequently, I reviewed the quite extensive earlier literature on this problem and found a great number of statements concerning the effectiveness of heat, in one form or another, in the treatment of weeverfish poisonings (see Russell, 1965). In a controlled experiment in humans we found that the methods suggested for the treatment of stingray, scorpionfish, and catfish injuries are equally effective in alleviating the severe pain and other symptoms provoked by the venom of the weeverfishes. Maretić (1957) has used intravenous calcium gluconate with good success for relieving the pain of the injury. Local injections of procaine may be of some value in less severe poisonings, and intramuscular or intravenous meperidine is of definite value in those cases in which there is severe pain after the first hour following the injury. An experimental antivenin has been developed at the Institute of Immunology in Zagreb, and in a limited number of clinical tests it has been shown to be effective (Maretić, personal communication, 1981). However, its use should probably be limited to the more serious stings where there are significant manifestations.

ARTHROPODS

Only a relatively small number of arthropods are sufficiently venomous to be of potential danger to humans. Nevertheless, arthropods are implicated in far more poisonings on humans than all the other phyla combined. Almost all of the 30,000 species of spiders are venomous, but luckily for humans only a relatively small number have fangs long and strong enough to penetrate the human skin (Gertsch, 1979). There are some 500 species of scorpions and all are venomous, although only a small number are sufficiently dangerous to be of a problem to humans. In the order Hymenoptera, the bees, wasps, yellow jackets, and ants, there are numerous species of medical importance, particularly because of the anaphylactic problems they precipitate. Among the ticks, caterpillars, kissing bugs, water bugs, moths, butterflies, grasshoppers, centipedes, and millipedes are additional arthropods of medical importance. The venoms of arthropods are highly diversified, and if the spider venoms so far studied are an indication, these poisons may prove to be more complex than originally suspected. Like the snake venoms, the arthropod poisons exert their deleterious effects at the cellular level. The arthropod venoms have been reviewed in detail by Bettini (1978).

The number of deaths from arthropod stings and bites is not known, nor do most countries keep records ot the incidence of such injuries. In Mexico, parts of Central and South America, and North Africa, deaths from scorpion stings may exceed several thousand a year. Spider bites probably do not account for more than 200 deaths a year, worldwide. The number of deaths from arthropod bites or stings in the temperate countries is far greater than the number of deaths from snakebite. However, most of these deaths are anaphylactic in nature. In the underdeveloped countries of the tropics a far greater number of deaths from arthropods are due to the direct effects of the venom. A common problem in suspected arthropod bites or stings relates to the differential diagnosis. Of approximately 600 suspected spider bites seen in one series of cases, 80 percent were found to be caused by arthropods other than spiders, or by other disease states (Russell and Gertsch, 1983). The arthropods most frequently involved in the misdiagnoses were ticks (including their embedded mouth parts), mites, bedbugs, fleas (infected flea bites), lepidopterous insects, flies, vesicating beetles, water bugs, and various stinging Hymenoptera. Among the disease states that have been confused with spider bites or arthropod bites or stings are erythema chronicum migrans, Stevens-Johnson syndrome, toxic epidermal necrolysis, erytherma nodosum, herpes simplex, purpura fulminans, diabetic ulcer, poison oak, and gonococcal arthritic dermatitis. As with the snake, a spider or other arthropod may bite or sting and not eject venom, but this must be a rare rather than a common event.

Anaphylactic reactions and anaphylaxis are sometimes encountered following arthropod injuries and become medical emergencies. More common are other autopharmacologic reactions, which may mistakenly be attributed to the direct action of the venom. The author has seen many unusual responses, varying from mild agitation to a vesicle-pustule-ulcer-eschar lesion following the sting of a bee. Also, the development of a lesion or lesions at a previous sting may follow a new sting and present difficulties in differential diagnosis, unless a careful history is taken. Finally, some arthropod venom poisonings give rise to symptoms and signs of a previously undiagnosed, subclinical disease. The problem of diverse disease states following the bites or stings of various venomous animals is recognized (Russell, 1977), and when a case of venom poisoning persists, or develops into a new syndrome, the patient should be reexamined for the possible presence of an undiagnosed disease. In some cases stings or bites may induce stress reactions and the patient may present a more complex and distressing problem.

Spiders

There are at least 200 species of spiders that have been implicated in significant bites on humans. Some of the more important of these are noted in Table 22–8. A more complete review of the problem of spider bites will be found in the excellent work by Maretić and Lebez (1979), and the lesser contributions of Southcott (1976) and Russell and Gertsch (1983).

Latrodectus Species (Widow Spiders). These spiders are commonly known as the black widow, brown widow, or red-legged spider in the United States. They have many other common names in English: hourglass, poison lady, deadly spider, red-bottom spider, T-spider, gray lady spider, or shoe-button spider. The widow spiders are found almost circumglobally, in all continents having temperate or tropical climates. In the United States, there are four species of widow spiders, with the possibility of a fifth species from the Pacific northwest. Although both the male and female widow spiders are venomous, only the latter has fangs large and strong enough to penetrate the human skin. Mature females range in body length from 10 to 18 mm, while males range from 3 to 5 mm. These spiders have a globose abdomen, varying in color from gray to brown to black, depending on the species. In the black widow the abdomen is shiny black with a red hourglass or red spots, and sometimes white ones, on the venter.

The chemistry of the venom has been reviewed by Bettini and Maroli (1978) and by Maretić and Lebez (1979). The difficulties with many of the biochemical and toxicologic studies on this spider's venom have related to the nature of the starting material. Most studies have been done on extracts of homogenized glands rather than the venom itself. Thus, the chemical nature of the venom cannot be separated or determined from the normal constituents of the venom gland. The pharmacologic properties reported in the literature also reflect the activities of the whole gland, and since some of the reported properties carried out on definitive preparations are not consistent with human experiences, their chemical applied validity is open to question.

Most workers have isolated five or six proteins from the venom or venom glands (see Bettini and Maroli, 1978, for references). The so-called neurotoxin appears to have a high content of isoleucine and leucine and a low content of tyrosine. The fraction has a suspected molecular

**Table 22–8. GENERA OF SPIDERS FOR WHICH SIGNIFICANT BITES
ON HUMANS ARE KNOWN**

GENUS	FAMILY	COMMON NAME	DISTRIBUTION
Aganippe species	Ctenizidae	Trap-door spider	Australia
Aphonopelma species	Theraphosidiae	Tarantula	North America
Araneus species	Araneidae	Orbweaver	Worldwide
Arbanitis species	Ctenizidae	Trap-door spider	Australia, East Indies
Argiope species	Araneidae	Argiope	Worldwide
Atrax species	Macrothelinae	Funnel-web spider	Australia
Bothriocyrtum species	Ctenizidae	Trap-door spider	California
Chiracanthium species	Clubionidae	Running spider	Europe, North Africa, Orient, North America
Cupiennius species	Ctenidae	Banana spider	Central America
Drassodes species	Gnaphosidae	Running spider	Worldwide
Dyarcyops species	Ctenizidae	Trap-door spider	Australia
Dysdera species	Dysderidae	Dysderid	Eastern Hemisphere, Americas
Elassoctenus species	Ctenidae	Ctenid	Australia
Filistata species	Filistatidae	Hackled-band spider	Temperate and tropical worldwide
Harpactirella species	Barychelidae	Trap-door spider	South Africa
Heteropoda species	Sparassidae	Giant crab spider	East Indies, tropical Asia, south Florida
Isopoda species	Sparassidae	Giant crab spider	Australia, East Indies
Ixeuticus species	Amaurobiidae	Amaurobiid	New Zealand, S. California
Lampona species	Gnaphosidae	Running spider	Australia, New Zealand
Latrodectus species	Theridiiae	Widow spider	Temperate and tropical regions worldwide
Liocranoides species	Clubionidae	Running spider	Appalachia and California
Lithyphantes species (=*Steatoda* species)	Theridiiae	Sheet-web weaver	Worldwide
Loxosceles species	Loxoscelidae	Brown or violin spider	Americas, Africa, Europe, Eastern Asia, Pacific Islands
Lycosa species	Lycosoidae	Wolf spider	Worldwide
Missulena species	Actinopodidae	Trap-door spider	Australia
Misumenoides species	Thomisidae	Crab spider	North and South America
Miturga species	Theraphosidae	Running spider	Australia
Mopsus species	Salticidae	Jumping spider	Australia
Neoscona species	Araneidae	Orbweaver	Worldwide
Olios species	Sparassidae	Giant crab spider	North and South America
Pamphobeteus species	Theraphosidae	Tarantula	South America
Peucetia species	Oxyopidae	Green lynx spider	Worldwide
Phidippus species	Salticidae	Jumping spider	North and South America
Phoneutria species	Ctenidae	Hunting spider	Central and South America

Table 22–8. (*continued*)

GENUS	FAMILY	COMMON NAME	DISTRIBUTION
Selenocosmia species	Theraphosidae	Tarantula	East Indies, India, Australia, tropical Africa
Steatoda species	Theridiidae	False black widow	Worldwide
Thiodina species	Salticidae	Jumping spider	North and South America
Trechona species	Dipluridae	Funnel-web	West Indies, South America
Ummidia species	Ctnizidae	Trap-door spider	North and South America

weight of 130,000. It affects the frog neuromuscular junction and is active on rat brain synaptosomes. Lipoproteins are also present. A proteolytic enzyme was absent from extracts of the venom glands, while venom taken from the fangs possessed the activity. The presence of hyaluronidase is also dependent on the original material. In our own studies we were able to demonstrate 15 or more bands in the crude venom by gel electrophoresis. The average amount of venom from each spider was 0.22 mg and the intravenous LD50 in mice was 0.55 mg/kg body weight (Russell and Buess, 1970).

Clinical Problem. In most patients there is a history of having received a sharp, pinprick-like bite, but in some cases the bite is so minor that it goes unnoticed. The initial pain is sometimes followed by a dull, occasionally numbing pain in the affected extremity, and by pain and some cramps in one or several of the large muscle masses. Rarely is there any local skin reaction, but piloerection in the bite area is sometimes seen. Muscle fasciculations can frequently be seen within 30 minutes of the bite. Sweating is common, and the patient may complain of weakness and pain in the regional lymph nodes, which are often tender on palpation and may be enlarged; lymphadenitis is frequently observed. Pain in the low back, thighs, or abdomen is a common complaint, and rigidity of the abdominal muscles is seen in most cases in which envenomation has been severe. Severe paroxysmal muscle cramps may occur, and arthralgia has been reported. "Fascies latrodectisimica" is rare in bites by American species.

In bites on the upper extremities, and sometimes on the lower extremities, there is rigidity of the muscles of the shoulders and back, sometimes accompanied by pain on inspiration and varying degrees of headache, dizziness, and ptosis. Edema of the eyelids, conjunctivitis, skin rash, hyperemia, and pruritus are sometimes

observed. The patient may become very restless and find difficulty in sitting or standing still. Reflexes are usually accentuated. There may be a fine body tremor, and nausea and vomiting are not uncommon. The patient sometimes gropes along slowly when attempting to walk. Hypertension is a common finding in moderate to severe envenomations. Blood studies are usually normal.

There is no effective first-aid treatment. In most cases, intravenous calcium gluconate, 10 ml of 10 percent, will often relieve muscle pain, but this may need to be repeated at four- to six-hour intervals for optimum effect. Muscle relaxants, such as methocarbanol, 10 ml by slow push, as directed, or diazepam, 5 to 10 mg t.i.d. (three times a day), can be used. Meperidine hydrochloride, 50 to 100 mg, has been used when respiratory deficits were not a problem. Acute hypertensive crises may require intravenous diazoxide, 5 mg/kg. The use of antivenin (Antivenin *Latrodectus mactans*) should be restricted to the more severe cases and where the above measures have been unsuccessful. One ampule, intravenously, is usually sufficient. In patients under 16 or over 60 years, or with any history of hypertension or hypertensive heart disease, and who show significant symptoms and signs, the use of antivenin seems warranted.

Loxosceles **Species (Brown or Violin Spiders).** These primitive spiders are variously known in North America as the fiddle-back or violin spider, or the brown recluse. There are over 100 species of *Loxosceles*. Twenty of these species range from temperate South Africa northward through the tropics into the Mediterranean region and southern Europe. Another 84 species are known from North, Central, and South America, and the West Indies. The most widely distributed is *L. rufescens,* the so-called "cosmopolitan" species. It is found in the Mediterranean area, southern Russia, most of North Africa including the Azores, Madagascar, Near East, the Orient from India to southern China and Japan, parts of Malaysia and Australia, some islands of the Pacific, and North America. *Loxosceles laeta* is mostly South American, but it has been introduced into Central America and small areas in Cambridge, Massachusetts, Sierra Madre and Alhambra, California, and the Zoology Building of the University of Helsinki. The abdomen of these spiders varies in color from grayish through orange and reddish-brown to dark brown. The "violin" on the carapace is brown to blackish and distinct from the pale yellow to reddish-brown background of the cephalothorax. This spider has six eyes grouped in three diads, forming a recurved row. Females average 8 to 12 mm in body length while males average 6 to 10 mm. Both males and females are venomous. The most important species in the United States are *L. reclusa* (brown recluse spider), *L. deserta* (desert violin spider), and *L. arizonica* (Arizona violin spider).

The chemistry and toxicology of *Loxoceles* venom has been reviewed by Schenone and Suarez (1978). The venom is composed of approximately 26 percent protein, and the average amount of venom protein per spider in *L. reclusa* is about 68 μg. The necrotizing activity of the venom is associated with the protein portion, and it has been suggested that the fraction is a glycoprotein. On fractionation of the venom, two major components have been separated. The high-molecular-weight fraction, (1), is lethal to mice, while the low-molecular-weight fraction is nonlethal. On further separation of (1), two toxins have been isolated. Their molecular weight is about 24,000. One of these was responsible for the lesions produced in rabbits and was shown to be lethal to mice and rabbits. The venom contains a considerable number of enzymes. Injection of the venom in mammals produces, in addition to the local tissue reaction, varying degrees of thrombocytopenia, some intravascular hemolysis, and hemolytic anemia. The venom also appears to have some coagulating activity. Neither the enzymes nor their amounts can explain the development of the unusual lesion. A potent, nondialyzable inhibitor of hemolytic complement activity has been demonstrated in the venom of *L. reclusa*. It has been suggested that this factor might interfere with the function of the fifth component of human blood. It seems that *Loxosceles* venom interferes with receptor sites for complement fractions located at the membrane surface (see Schenone and Suarez, 1978, for references).

Clinical Manifestations. The bite of this spider produces about the same degree of pain as the sting of an ant, but sometimes the patient is completely unaware of the bite. In most cases a local burning sensation develops about the injury. This may last for 30 to 60 minutes. Pruritus over the area often occurs and the area becomes red, with a small blanched area around the immediate bite site. Skin temperature is usually elevated over the lesion area. The reddened area enlarges and becomes purplish during the subsequent one to eight hours. It often becomes irregular in shape, and as time passes, hemorrhages may develop throughout the area. A small bleb or vesicle forms at the bite site and increases in size. It subsequently ruptures and a pustule forms. The red, hemorrhagic area continues to enlarge, as does the pustule. The whole area may become swollen and painful, and lymphadenopathy is common. During the early stages the lesion often takes on a bull's-eye appearance, with a central white vesicle surrounded by the reddened area, ringed by a whitish or bluish border. The central pustule ruptures, and necrosis to various depths can be visualized. The necrosis can invade the underlying muscle.

In serious bites the lesion can measure 8 × 10 cm with severe necrosis invading muscle tissue. On the face, large lesions resulting in extensive tissue destruction and requiring subsequent plastic surgery are sometimes seen following bites by *L. laeta* in South America. Systemic symptoms and signs include fever, malaise, stomach cramps, nausea and vomiting, jaundice, spleen enlargement, hemolysis, hematuria, and thrombocytopenia. Fatal cases, while rare, are usually preceded by intravascular hemolysis, hemolytic anemia, thrombocytopenia, hemoglobinuria, and renal failure.

There are no first-aid measures of value. In fact, all first-aid procedures should be avoided as the natural appearance of the lesion is most important in determining the diagnosis. A cube of ice may be placed on the wound. At one time, excision of the bite area with ample margins was advised, when this could be done within an hour or so of the bite, and when *Loxosceles* was definitely implicated. This practice is no longer favored. The value of steroids has also been questioned. This writer, however, has had seemingly good results by placing the patient on a corticosteroid, such as intramuscular dexamethasone, 4 mg every six hours during the acute phase. If the poisoning is severe, hydrocortisone should be given intravenously 300 to 500 mg in divided doses daily, until the patient begins to improve. Subsequent doses should then be determined by clinical judgment, followed by decremental doses over a four-day period. Antihistamines are of questionable value during the acute period. The use of Dapsone has been suggested (King and Rees, 1983) and seems encouraging, but further evaluation is necessary. Ulcerating lesions should be cleansed with peroxide and soaked in 1:20 Burow's solution t.i.d. (three times a day) for at least 15 minutes. Three times a week, if indicated, the lesions can be painted with an aqueous solution of brilliant green 1:400, gentian violet 1:400, and acriflavin 1:1000. At night the lesion should be covered with polymyxin-bacitracin-neomycin ointment. Oxygen to the wound through an improvised plastic bag is helpful. If skin grafting becomes necessary, the procedure is best deferred for four to six weeks after the injury. Systemic manifestations should be treated symptomatically (Russell, 1982).

Steatoda Species (Cobweb Spiders). These small spiders, variously called the false black-widow, combfooted, or cupboard spiders, are abundant in the Old World and reached the Americas through trading sources. According to Gertsch (personal correspondence, 1983), they are gaining such a wide range they deserve to be called cosmopolitan. These spiders are often mistaken for black-widow spiders and, indeed, the first clinical case of *Steatoda grossa* envenomation directed to the author in 1961 was thought to be caused by *L. mactans,* owing to misidentification of the spider. The female of *S. grossa* differs from *L. mactans* and *L. hesperus* in having a purplish-brown abdomen rather than a black one; it is less shiny and its abdomen is more oval than round, as in *Latrodectus.* It may have pale yellow or whitish markings on the dorsum of the abdomen and no markings on the ventra. The abdomen of some species is orange, brown, or chestnut in color and often bears a light band across the front dorsum.

The literature on poisoning by these species is scanty, and little is known about the chemistry of the venom. According to Maretić and Lebez (1979), *S. paykulliana* gives rise to "strong motor unrest, clonic cramps, exhaustion, ataxia and then paralysis in guinea pigs." However, this writer has never seen such a syndrome following the bites of *S. grossa* or *S. fulva* in humans. Instead, bites have been followed by local pain, induration, pruritus, and the occasional breakdown of tissue at the bite site. The wound should be debrided and covered with a sterile dressing. A steriod-antihistamine cream can be applied to the wound.

Phidippus Species (Jumping Spiders). These spiders, variously known as crab spiders or eyebrow spiders, are large-eyed jumping spiders, usually less than 20 mm in length and have a somewhat elevated, rectangular cephalothorax that tends to be blunt anteriorly. The abdomen is often oval or elongated. There is a great deal of variation in the color of these spiders. In the

female the cephalothorax may be black, brown, red, orange, or yellowish-orange, and the abdomen tends to be slightly lighter in color. In most species there are various white, yellow, orange, or red spots or markings on the dorsum of the abdomen. The bite of this spider produces a sharp pinprick pain, and the area immediately around the wound may become painful and tender. The pain usually lasts five to ten minutes. An erythematous wheal slowly develops. In the cases seen by the author the wheal measured 2 to 5 cm in diameter. A dull, sometimes throbbing pain may subsequently develop over the injured part, but it rarely requires attention. A small vesicle may form at the bite site. Around this is an irregular, slightly hyperemic area, which in turn may be surrounded by a blanched area tender to touch and pressure, Generally, there is only mild lymphadenitis. Swelling of the part may be diffuse and is often accompanied by some pruritus. The symptoms and signs usually abate within 48 hours. There is no specific treatment for the bite of this spider Methdilazine HCl, 8 mg three times a day, is often effective.

Chiricanthium Species (Running Spiders). The 160 species of this genus enjoy an almost circumglobal distribution, although only four or five species have been implicated in bites on humans. Maretić and Lebez (1979) name *C. punctorium, C. inclusum, C. mildei,* and *C. diversum* as the spiders most often implicated in envenomations. The abdomen is convex and egg-shaped and varies in color from yellow, green, or greenish-white to reddish-brown, and the cephalothorax is usually slightly darker than the abdomen. The chelicerae are strong, and the legs are long, hairy, and delicate. The spider ranges in length from 7 to 16 mm. The author's experiences with nine bites by *C. inclusum* have been very similar and the following description is based on these experiences. Like *Phidippus,* but even more so, *Chiracanthium* tends to be tenacious and must sometimes be removed from the bite area. For that reason there is a high degree of identification of these spiders. The patient usually describes the bite as sharp and painful, with the pain increasing during the first 30 to 45 minutes. The patient complains of some restlessness, a dull pain over the injured part. A reddened wheal with a hyperemic border develops. Small petechiae may appear near the center of the wheal. Skin temperature over the lesion is often elevated, but body temperature is usually normal. Lymphadenitis and lymphadenopathy may develop. Five cases of necrotic arachnadism have been attributed to *C. mildei,* but the status of this finding remains circumstantial (see Russell, 1984, for references).

Scorpions

Approximately 75 of the 800 species of scorpions can be considered of sufficient importance to warrant medical attention. Some of the more important of these are noted in Table 22–9. In addition, members of the genus *Pandinus*, *Hadrurus*, *Vejovis*, *Nebo*, and some of the others are capable of inflicting a painful and oftentimes erythematous lesion. The problem of scorpion stings has been reviewed by Keegan (1980).

Centruroides Species. There are approximately 30 species of this genus confined in distribution to the New World. Of these, about seven species are of considerable medical importance and most of these are found in Mexico. In the United States they are commonly referred to as "bark scorpions" because of the preference for hiding under the loose bark of trees or in dead trees or logs. They often frequent human dwellings. Their general color is straw to yellowish-brown, or reddish-brown, and they are often easily distinguishable from other scorpions in the same habitat by their long, thin telson, or tail, and the pedipalps, or pincerlike claws. Adults of this genus show a considerable difference in length. *C. sculpturatus* in the southwestern United States and adjacent Mexico reaches a length of approximately 5.5 cm, while *C. vittatus* of the Gulf States and adjacent Mexico are generally slightly larger. *C. suffusus*, a particularly dangerous Mexican species, may attain a length of 9 cm, but *C. noxious*, another important species, seldom exceeds 5 cm in length. In Mexico between 1940–1949 and 1950–1957 there were 20,352 deaths from scorpion envenomation. Most of these deaths were in children less than three years of age. Various estimates of the total number of stings per year in Mexico range

Table 22–9. MEDICALLY IMPORTANT SCORPIONS

GENUS	DISTRIBUTION
Androctonus species	North Africa, Middle East, and Turkey
Buthus species	France and Spain to Middle East and North Africa, Mongolia, China
Buthotus species	Africa, Middle East, and Central Asia
Centruroides species	North, Central and South America
Heterometrus species	Central and Southeast Asia
Leiurus species	North Africa, Middle East, and Turkey
Mesobuthus species	Turkey
Parabuthus species	Southern Africa
Tityus species	Central and South America

from 20,000 to 70,000. Working in Mexico in 1953, the writer estimates that there were over 40,000 stings that year of which 10,000 were treated. The total number of deaths, usually in infants, appeared slightly less than 1500. As with the other scorpion stings, envenomation by this genus appears to vary with the species concerned.

In children, stings by *C. exilicauda* (= *sculpturatus*) produce initial pain, although it rarely is severe. However, some children do not complain of pain and are unaware of the injury. The area becomes sensitive to touch, and merely pressing lightly over the injury will elicit immediate retraction. Usually, there is little or no local swelling or erythema. The child becomes tense and restless and shows abnormal and random head and neck movements. Often, the child will display roving eye movements. In their excellent review of *C. sculpturatus* stings, Rimsza *et al.* (1980) noted visual signs including roving eye movements, nystagmus, and oculogyric movements in 12 of their 24 patients stung by this scorpion. Loud noises, such as banging the examination table behind the child's back, will often cause the patient to jump. Tachycardia will usually be evident within 45 minutes, and hypertension, although it is not seen in children as early or as severe as in adults, may often be present one hour following the sting. Respiratory and heart rates are increased, and by 90 minutes postbite the child may appear quite ill. Fasciculations may be seen over the face or large muscle masses, and the child may complain of generalized weakness and display some ataxia or motor weakness. The respiratory distress may proceed to respiratory paralysis. Excessive salivation is often present and may further embarrass respiratory function. Slurring of speech may be present and convulsions may occur. If death does not occur, the child usually becomes asymptomatic within 36 hours.

In adults the clinical picture is somewhat similar, but there are some differences. Almost all adults complain of immediate and sometimes severe pain following the sting, regardless of the *Centruroides* species involved. Adults do not show the restlessness seen in children. Rather, they are tense and anxious. They develop tachycardia and hypertension, and respirations are increased. They may complain of difficulties in focusing and swallowing, as may children. In some cases there is some general weakness, and pain on moving the injured extremity. Convulsions are very rare, but ataxia and muscle incoordination may occur. Most adults are asymptomatic within 12 hours but may complain of generalized weakness for 24 or more hours.

A review of the therapy for scorpion stings

will provide the reader with a fascinating dash of mythology, folklore, hunches (educated and otherwise), and a listing of all sorts of therapeutic devices from electroshock to mechanical compression bandages. The list of drugs that have been tried includes atropine, barium, digitalis, epinephrine, heparin, hyoscyamine, iodine, procaine, morphine, physostigmine, reserpine, steroids, snake, spider and scorpion antivenins, and vitamin C, to mention only a few. Other than scorpion antivenin, there is no evidence that any of these drugs are of specific value. There are no first-aid measures of value. In any severe scorpion envenomation by one of the known dangerous species, or in infants or children, the specific or suggested polyvalent scorpion antivenin should be used. The author generally gives twice the recommended dose, and gives it intravenously, unless indicated otherwise. The antivenin should be diluted with 100 to 200 ml of 5 percent dextrose in water or physiologic saline and given in a drip. Mild sedation is often indicated. If convulsions occur, intravenous phenobarbital is suggested, but great care must be used with respect to the dose. Valium may be of value. Assisted ventilation is sometimes necessary, particularly in children. Hypertension that does not respond to antivenin may need to be treated with the appropriate antihypertensive drugs. Inderal has been used for tachycardia. In those patients who decompensate, digitalis and diuretics may be of value. The role of corticosteroids and atropine in severe poisonings is questionable. The stings by species of *Vejovis* and *Hadrurus,* though far more common in the United States than those by *Centruroides,* rarely require more than minor treatment for the local pain. However, it is wise to put any person stung by a scorpion, particularly children, at bed rest for several hours following the accident.

Centipedes and Millipedes

Some of the larger centipedes of the genus *Scolopendra* can inflict a painful bite, with some localized swelling and erythema. Lymphangitis and lymphadenitis are not uncommon. Necrosis is rare and infection almost unknown. Symptoms and signs seldom persist for more than 48 hours. Millipedes do not bite but when handled may discharge a toxic secretion that can cause local skin irritation and, in severe cases, some necrosis. Some non-United States species can spray a highly irritating repugnant secretion that may cause conjunctival reactions. An ice cube will control the pain of most centipede bites. Corticosteroids have been used as anti-inflammatory agents. The toxic secretions of millipedes should be washed from the skin with copious amounts of soap and water. Cleansing with alcohol should be avoided. A corticosteroid lotion or cream should be applied if a skin reaction develops. Eye injuries require immediate irrigation and the application of a corticosteroid-analgesic ointment.

Hymenoptera (Ants, Bees, Wasps, and Hornets)

The stings of these animals are responsible for more deaths in the United States than the bites and stings of all other venomous creatures. This is due to sensitization to the venom from repeated stings, resulting in anaphylactic reactions, including acute anaphylaxis. The number of acute anaphylactic reactions involving cardiovascular, respiratory, or nervous system changes may number over 200,000 per year in the United States. Those not sensitive to bee venom may tolerate up to 100 simultaneous stings, but any number over this can be fatal. The venom of these insects contains peptides, nonenzymatic proteins, such as apamin and melettin or kinins; enzymes, such as phospholipase A and B and hyaluronidase; and amines, such as histamine and 5-hydroxytryptamine. The sting of many *Hymenoptera* may remain in the skin and should be removed by teasing or scraping rather than pulling. An ice cube placed over the sting will reduce pain; an analgesic-corticosteroid lotion is often useful. Persons with known hypersensitivity to such stings should carry a kit containing an antihistamine and epinephrine when in endemic areas. Desensitization can be carried out using insect whole-body antigen or, preferably, whole-venom antigens (Russell, 1982).

Ticks and Mites

Ticks are vectors of many diseases. In addition to these disorders, ticks are also involved in poisonings. In North America, some species of *Dermacentor* and *Amblyomma* cause tick paralysis. Symptoms and signs include anorexia, lethargy, muscle weakness, incoordination, nystagmus, and ascending flaccid paralysis. Bulbar or respiratory paralysis may develop. The bites of some *Ornithodorus* ticks ("pajaroello") found in Mexico and southwestern United States cause a local vesiculation, pustulation, rupture, ulceration, and eschar, with varying degrees of local swelling and pain, often resembling those of *Loxosceles,* although the development of the lesion is slower. Mite infestations are quite common and are responsible for "chiggers" (intensely pruritic dermatitis caused by the mite larva, or chigger), various forms of scabies, demodicidosis, and a number of other diseases. The bites produce varying degrees of local tissue reactions, with or without sensitization. Ticks are best removed by applying gasoline, or by slowly withdrawing the arthropod with flat-tip forceps. Care should be taken not to leave the capitulum in the wound, as it may induce chronic inflammation or may migrate into deeper tissues and give rise to a granuloma. The bite should be cleansed and a corticosteroid lotion applied. Treatment of tick paralysis is symptomatic. Oxygen and respiratory assistance may be needed. An antitoxin is presently under study. Pajaroello tick lesions should be cleansed, soaked in 1:20 Burow's solution, and debrided. Corticosteroids are of value in severe reactions. Infections are not uncommon during the ulcer stage but rarely require more than local antiseptic measures.

Other Biting Arthropods

In the United States, a number of biting arthropods possess salivary secretions that can produce various reactions and lesions. Among the more common biting and sometimes blood-sucking arthropods are the ticks and mites; sand-, horse-, and deerflies; mosquitoes; fleas; lice; bedbugs; kissing bugs; and certain water bugs. The composition of the saliva of these arthropods varies considerably, and the lesion produced by their bites can vary from a small papule to a large, ulcerating wound with swelling and acute pain. Dermatitis may also occur. Most serious bites are complicated by sensitivity reactions or infection. In hypersensitive persons, the bites of some of these arthropods can be fatal.

REFERENCES

Albuquerque, E. X.; Warnick, J. E.; Maleque, M. A.; Kauffman, F. C.; Tamburini, R.; Nimit, Y.; and Daly, J. W.: The pharmacology of pumilitoxin-B. I. Interaction with calcium sites in the sarcoplasmic reticulum of skeletal muscle. *Mol. Pharmacol.*, 19:411–24, 1981.

Alender, C. B., and Russell, F. E.: Pharmacology. In Boolootin, R. A. (ed.): *Physiology of Echinodermata.* Interscience, New York, 1966, p. 529.

Arndt, W.: Die Spongern als kryptotoxische Tiere. *Zool. Jahrb.*, 45:343, 1928.

Arnold, S. H., and Brown, W. D.: Histamine toxicity from fish products. *Adv. Food Res.*, 24:113, 1978.

Association of Official Analytical Chemists: Paralytic shellfish poison biological method. In *Official Methods of Analysis*, 12th ed. Association of Official Analytical Chemists, Washington, D.C., 1975, p. 319.

Bagnis, R.; Berglund, F.; Elias, P. S.; VanEsch, G. J.; Halstead, B. W.; and Kojima, K.: Problems of toxicants in marine food products. *Bull. WHO*, 42:69, 1970.

Bajwa, S. S., and Markland, F. S.: Defibrinogenation studies with crotalase: possible clinical applications. *Proc. West. Pharmacol. Soc.*, 21:755, 1976.

Bakus, G. J., and Green, G.: Toxicity in sponges and holothurians: a geographic pattern. *Science*, 185:951, 1974.

Bakus, G. J., and Thun, M.: Bioassays on the toxicity of Caribbean sponges. *Biol. Spongiaries*, 291:417, 1979.

Banner, A. H.: Ciguatera: a disease from coral reef fish. In Jones, O. E., and Endean, R. (eds.): *Biology and Geology of Coral Reefs*, Vol. III. Academic Press, Inc., New York, 1976, p. 177.

Barnes, J. H.: Observations of jellyfish stingings in North Queensland. *Med. J. Aust.*, (2):993, 1960.

———: Extraction of cnidarian venom from living tentacle. In Russell, F. E., and Saunders, P. R. (eds.): *Animal Toxins*. Pergamon Press, Oxford, 1967, pp. 115–29; see also *Toxicon*, 4:292, 1967 (abstr.).

Baslow, M. H.: *Marine Pharmacology*. Williams & Wilkins Co., Baltimore, 1969.

Baxter, E. H.; Walden, N. B.; and Marr, A. G.: Fatal intoxication of rabbits, sheep and monkeys by the venom of the sea wasp *(Chironex fleckeri)*. *Toxicon*, 10:653, 1972.

Bernheimer, A. W., and Avigad, L. S.: Properties of a toxin from the sea anemone *Stoichactis helianthus*, including specific binding to sphingomyelin. *Proc. Natl. Acad. Sci. USA*, 73:467, 1976.

Bettini, S.: *Arthropod Venoms*. Springer-Verlag, New York, 1978.

Bettini, S., and Maroli, M.: Venoms of Theridiidae, genus *Latrodectus*. In Bettini, S. (ed.): *Arthropod Venoms*. Springer-Verlag, New York, 1978, pp. 149–85.

Blanquet, R. S.: A toxic protein from the nematocysts of the scyphozoan medusa *Chrysaora quinquecirrha*. *Toxicon*, 10:103, 1972.

Bonilla, C. A., and Fiero, M. K.: Comparative biochemistry and pharmacology of salivary gland secretions. II. Chromatographic separation of the basic proteins from North American rattlesnake venoms. *J. Chromatogr.*, 56:253, 1971.

Burke, J. M.; Marichisotto, J.; McLaughlin, J. J. A.; and Provasoli, L.: Analysis of the toxin produced by *Gonyaulax catenella* in axenic culture. *Ann. Rev. N.Y. Acad. Sci.*, 90:837, 1960.

Burnett, J. W., and Calton, H. J.: The chemistry and toxicology of some venomous pelagic coelenterates. *Toxicon*, 15:177, 1977.

Burreson, B. J.; Christophersen, C.; and Scheuer, P. J.: Coocurrence of a terpenoid isocyanide-formamide pair in the marine sponge *Halichondria* sp. *J. Am. Chem. Soc.*, 97:201, 1975.

Calton, G. J.; Burnett, J. W.; Rubenstein, H.; and Heard, J.: The effect of two jellyfish toxins on calcium ion transport. *Toxicon*, 11:357, 1973.

Cameron, A. M.; Surridge, J.; Stablum, W.; and Lewis, R. J.: A crinotoxin from the skin tubercle glands of a stonefish *(Synanceia trachynis)*. *Toxicon*, 19:159, 1981.

Cariello, L.; Zanetti, L.; and Rathmayer, W.: Isolation, purification and some properties of subertine, the toxic protein from the marine sponge *Suberites domuncula*. In Eaker, D., and Wadström, T. (eds.): *Natural Toxins*. Pergamon Press, Oxford, 1980, pp. 631–36.

Carlson, R. W.; Schaeffer, R. C.; Russell, F. E.; and Weil, M. H.: A comparison of corticosteroid and fluid treatment after rattlesnake venom shock in rats. *Physiologist*, 18:160, 1975.

Chevallier, A., and Duchesne, E. A.: Mémoire sur les empoisonnements par les huitres, les moules, les crabes, et par certains poissons de mer et de rivière. *Ann Hyg. pub.*, 46:108, 1851.

Cleland, J. B., and Southcott, R. V.: Injuries to Man from Marine Invertebrates in the Australian Region. Commonwealth of Australia, Canberra, 1965, p. 195.

Crone, H. D., and Keen, T. E. B.: Chromatographic properties of the hemolysin from the cnidarian *Chironex fleckeri*. *Toxicon*, 7:79, 1969.

Culver, P., and Jacobs, R. S.: Lophotoxin: a neuromuscular acting toxin from the sea whip *(Lophogorgia rigida)*. *Toxicon*, 19:825, 1981.

Daly, J. W.: Biologically active alkaloids from poison frogs (Dendrobatidae). *Toxin Rev.*, 1:33, 1982.

Das, N. P.; Lim, H. S.; and Teh, Y. F.: Histamine and histamine-like substances in the marine sponge *Suberites inconstans*. *Comp. Gen. Pharmacol.*, 2:473, 1971.

Dawson, E. Y.; Aleem, A. A.; and Halstead, B. W.: Marine algae from Palmyra Island with special reference to the feeding habits and toxicology of reef fishes. *Occ. Pap. Allan Hancock Fdn.*, 17:1, 1955.

De Laubenfels, M. W.: The marine and freshwater sponges of California. *Proc. U.S. Natn. Mus.*, 81:1, 1932 (Publ. No. 2927).

Deutsch, H. F., and Diniz, C. R.: Some proteolytic activities of snake venoms. *J. Biol. Chem.*, 216:17, 1955.

Dowling, H. G.; Minton, S. A.; and Russell, F. E.: *Poisonous Snakes of the World*. U.S. Government Printing Office, Washington, D.C., 1968.

Dubnoff, J. W., and Russell, F. E.: Isolation of lethal protein and peptide from *Crotalus viridis helleri* venom. *Proc. West. Pharm. Soc.*, 13:98, 1970.

Eaker, D., and Wadström, T. (eds.).: *Natural Toxins*. Pergamon Press, Elmsford, N.Y., 1980.

Elliott, W. B.: Chemistry and immunology of reptilian venoms. In Gans, C. (ed.).: *Biology of the Reptilia*, Vol. 8. Academic Press, London, 1978, pp. 163–436.

Endean, R.: A new species of venomous echinoid from Queensland waters. *Mem. Queensland Mus.*, 14:95, 1964.

Endean, R.; Izatt, J.; and McColm, D.: The venom of the piscivorous gastropod *Conus striatus*. In Russell, F. E., and Saunders, P. R. (eds.): *Animal Toxins*. Pergamon Press, Oxford, 1967, p. 137.

Endean, R.; Duchemin, C.; McColm, D.; and Fraser, E. H.: A study of the biological activity of toxic material derived from nematocysts of the cubomedusan *Chironex fleckeri*. *Toxicon*, 6:179, 1969.

Endean, R., and Noble, M.: Toxic material from the tentacles of the cubomedusan *Chironex fleckeri*. *Toxicon*, 9:255, 1971.

Evans, M. H.: Block of sensory nerve conduction in the cat by mussel poison and tetrodotoxin. In Russell, F. E., and Saunders, P. R. (eds.): *Animal Toxins*. Pergamon Press, Oxford, 1967, p. 97; see also *Toxicon*, 5:289, 1967.

Ferlan, I., and Lebez, D.: Equinatoxin, a lethal protein from *Actinia equina*. I. Purification and characterization. *Toxicon*, 12:57, 1974.

Flecker, H., and Cotton, B. C.: Fatal bites from octopus. *Med. J. Aust.*, (2):329, 1955.

Fleming, W. J., and Howden, M. E. H.: Partial purification and characterization of steroid glycosides from the starfish *Acanthaster planci*. *Comp. Biochem. Physiol.*, 53b:267, 1974.

Freeman, S. E., and Turner, R. J.: A pharmacological study of the toxin of a cnidarian *Chironex fleckeri* Southcott. *Br. J. Pharmacol.* 35:510, 1969.

Freeman, S. E., and Turner, R. J.: Cardiovascular effects of toxins isolated from the cnidarian *Chironex fleckeri* Southcott. *Br. J. Pharmacol.* 41:154, 1971.

Friess, S. L.; Durant, R. C.; Chanley, J. D.; and Fash, F. J.: Role of the sulphate charge center in irreversible interactions of holothurin A with chemoreceptors. *Biochem. Pharmacol.*, 16:617, 1967.

Friess, S. L.; Chanley, J. D.; Hudak, W. V.; and Weems, H. B.: Interactions of the echinoderm toxin holothurin A and its desulfated derivative with the cat superior cervical ganglion preparation. *Toxicon*, 8:211, 1970.

Fuhrman, F. A.: Fish eggs. In Liener, I. E. (ed.): *Toxic Constituents of Animal Foodstuffs*. Academic Press, Inc., New York, 1974, p. 73.

Gertsch, W. J.: *American Spiders*, 2nd ed. Van Nostrand Reinhold, New York, 1979.

Green, G.: Ecology of toxicity in marine sponges. *Mar. Biol.*, 40:207, 1977.

Habermehl, G. G.: *Venomous Animals and Their Toxins*. Springer-Verlag, Berlin, 1981.

Habermehl, G. G., and Volkwein, G.: Aglycones of the toxins from the cuvierian organs of *Holothuria forskali* and a new nomenclature for the aglycones from Holothurioideae. *Toxicon*, 9:319, 1971.

Halmagyi, D. F. J.; Starzecki, B.; and Horner, G. J.: Mechanism and pharmacology of shock due to rattlesnake venom in sheep. *J. Appl. Physiol.*, 20:709, 1965.

Halstead, B. W.: Weever stings and their medical management. *U.S. Armed Forces Med. J.*, 8:1441, 1957.

———: Fish poisonings—Their diagnosis, pharmacology and treatment. *Clin. Pharmacol. Ther.*, 5:615, 1964.

———: *Poisonous and Venomous Marine Animals of the World*. U.S. Government Printing Office, Washington, D.C. Vol. I, 1965; Vol. II, 1967; Vol. III, 1970.

———: *Poisonous and Venomous Marine Animals of the World*, rev. ed. Darwin Press, Princeton, N.J., 1978.

———: *Dangerous Marine Animals*, 2nd ed. Cornell Maritime Press, Centreville, Md., 1980, p. 77.

Harding, K. A., and Welch, K. R. G.: *Venomous Snakes of the World: A Checklist*. Pergamon Press, Elmsford, N.Y., 1980.

Hashimoto, Y.: *Marine Toxins and Other Bioactive Metabolites*. Japan Scientific Society, Tokyo, 1979.

Hashimoto, Y.; Konosu, S.; Yasumoto, T.; Iomie, A.; and Noguchi, T.: Occurrence of toxic crabs in Ryukyu and Amami Islands. *Toxicon*, 5:85, 1967.

Helfrich, P., and Banner, A. H.: Hallucinatory mullet poisoning. *J. Trop. Med. Hyg.*, 63:86, 1960.

Hessinger, D. A., and Lenhoff, H. M.: Membrane structure and function. Mechanism of hemolysis induced by nematocyst venom: roles of phospholipase and direct lytic factor. *Arch. Biochem. Biophys.*, 173:603, 1976.

Irie, T.; Suzuki, M.; and Hayakawa, Y.: Isolation of aplysin, debromoaplysin, and aplysinol from *Laurencia okamurai* Yamada. *Bull. Chem. Soc. Jpn.*, 42:843, 1969.

Jakowska, S., and Nigrelli, R. F.: Antimicrobial substances from sponges. *Ann. N.Y. Acad. Sci.*, 90:913, 1970.

Kaiser, E., and Michl, H.: *Die Biochemie der tierischen Gifte*. Franz Deuticke; Wien, 1958.

Kao, C. Y.: Tetrodotoxin, saxitoxin, and their significance in the study of the excitation phenomena. *Pharmacol. Rev.*, 18:997, 1966.

———: Comparison of the biological actions of tetrodotoxin and saxitoxin. In Russell, F. E., and Saunders, P. R. (eds.): *Animal Toxins*. Pergamon Press, Oxford, 1967, p. 109–14.

———: New perspectives on the tetrodotoxin and saxitoxin receptors. In Singer and Ondarza (eds.): *Molecular Basis of Drug Action*. Elsevier/North-Holland, New York, 1981.

Kao, C. Y., and Fuhrman, F. A.: Pharmacological studies on tarichatoxin, a potent neurotoxin. *J. Pharmacol. Exp. Ther.* 140:31, 1963.

Kashman, Y.; Fishelson, L.; and Neeman, I.: N-acyl-2-methylene-β-alanine methyl esters from the sponge *Fasciospongia cavernosa*. *Tetrahedron*, 29:3655, 1973.

Keegan, H. L.: *Scorpions of Medical Importance*. University Press of Mississippi, Jackson, Miss., 1980.

King, L. E., and Rees, R. S.: Dapsone treatment of a brown recluse bite. *JAMA*, 250:648, 1983.

Lane, C. E., and Dodge, E.: The toxicity of *Physalia* nematocysts. *Biol. Bull.*, 115:219, 1958.

Lassabliere, M. P.: Influences des injections intraveineuses de suberitine sur la resistance globulaire. *C. R. Seanc. Soc. Biol.*, 61:600, 1906.

Lee, C.-Y. (ed.): *Snake Venoms*. Springer-Verlag, New York, 1979.

Maeda, N.; Tamiya, N.; Pattabhiraman, T. K.; and Russell, F. E.: Some chemical properties of the venom of the rattlesnake *Crotalus viridis helleri*. *Toxicon*, 16:431, 1978.

Maeno, H.; Morimura, M.; Mitsuhashi, S.; Sawai, Y.; and Okonogi, T.: Studies on habu snake venom. 2b. Further purification and enzymic and biological activities of Ha-proteinase. *Jpn. J. Mikrobiol.*, **3**:277, 1959.

Maretić, Z.: Erfahrungen mit Stichen von Giftfischen. *Acta Tropica*, **14**:157, 1957.

Maretić, Z., and Lebez, D.: *Araneism*. Nolit, Belgrade, Yugoslavia, 1979.

Maretić, Z., and Russell, F. E.: Stings by the sea anemone *Anemonia sulcata* in the Adriatic Sea. *Am. J. Trop. Med. Hyg.*, **32**:891, 1983.

Marki, F., and Witkop, B.: The venom of the Columbian arrow poison frog *Phyllobates bicolor*. *Experientia*, **19**:329, 1963.

Martin, D. F., and Padilla, G. M. (eds.): *Marine Pharmacognosy*. Academic Press, Inc., New York, 1973.

McFarren, E. F.; Schafer, M. L.; Campbell, J. F.; Lewis, K. H.; Jensen, E. T.; and Schantz, E. J.: Public health significance of paralytic shellfish poison. A review of literature and unpublished research. *Proc. Natl Shellfish Assoc.*, **47**:114, 1956.

Mebs, D.: Bi Bverletzungen durch "ungiftige" Schlangen. *Deutsche Med. Wochensc.*, **40**:1, 1977.

———: Pharmacology of reptilian venoms. In Gans, C. (ed.): *Biology of the Reptilia*, Vol. 8. Academic Press, London, 1978, pp. 437–560.

Meyer, K.: Über herzaktive krötengifte. *Pharm. Acta Helvetiae*, **24**:222, 1949.

Meyer, K. F.; Sommer, H.; and Schoenholz, P.: Mussel poisoning. *J. Prev. Med.*, **2**:365, 1928.

Middlebrook, R. E.; Wittle, L. W.; Scura, E. D.; and Lane, C. E.: Isolation and purification of a toxin from *Millepora dichotoma*. *Toxicon*, **9**:333, 1971.

Minton, S. A., Jr.: A list of colubrid envenomations. *Kentucky Herp.*, **7**:4, 1976.

Minton, S. A., Jr., and Minton, M. G.: *Venomous Reptiles*. Charles Scribner's Son, New York, 1969.

Morris, R., and Morris, D.: *Men and Snakes*. McGraw-Hill, New York, 1965.

Neeman, I.; Calton, G. J.; and Burnett, J. W.: Purification of an endonuclease present in *Chrysaora quinquecirrha* venom. *Proc. Soc. Exp. Biol. Med.*, **166**:374, 1981.

Nigrelli, R. F., and Jakowska, S.: Effects of holothurin, a steroid saponin from the Bahamian sea cucumber (*Actinopyga agassizi*) on various biological systems. *Ann. N.Y. Acad. Sci.*, **90**:884, 1960.

Parnas, I., and Russell, F. E.: Effects of venoms on nerve, muscle and neuromuscular junction. In Russell, F. E., and Saunders, P. R. (eds.): *Animal Toxins*. Pergamon Press, Oxford, 1967, pp. 401–15.

Parrish, H. M.: *Poisonous Snakebites in the United States*. Vantage Press, New York, 1980.

Phillips, C., and Brady, W. H.: *Sea Pests: Poisonous or Harmful Sea Life of Florida and the West Indies*. University of Miami Press, Miami, 1953.

Prakash, A.; Medcof, J. C.; and Tennant, A. D.: Paralytic shellfish poisoning in eastern Canada. *Bull. Fish. Res. Bd. Can.*, **177**:1, 1971.

Primor, N., and Lazarovici, P.: *Pardachirus marmoratus* (Red Sea flatfish) secretion and its isolated toxic fraction pardaxin: the relationship between hemolysis and ATPase inhibition. *Toxicon*, **19**:573, 1981.

Prinzmetal, M.; Sommer, H.; and Leake, C. D.: The pharmacological action of "mussel poison." *J. Pharmacol. Exp. Ther.*, **46**:63, 1932.

Proctor, N. H.; Chan, S. L.; and Taylor, A. J.: Production of saxitoxin by cultures of *Gonyaulax catenella*. *Toxicon*, **13**:1, 1975.

Randall, J. E.: A review of ciguatera, tropical fish poisoning, with a tentative explanation of its cause. *Bull. Mar. Sci. Gulf Caribb.*, **8**:236, 1958.

Richet, C.: De la variabilité de la dose toxique de subéritine. *C.R. Soc. Biol.*, **61**:686, 1906.

Rimsza, M. E.; Zimmerman, D. R.; and Bergeson, P. S.: Scorpion envenomation. *Pediatrics*, **66**:298, 1980.

Rosenberg, P. (ed.): *Toxins: Animal, Plant and Microbial*. Pergamon Press, Elmsford, N.Y., 1978.

Rosenberg, P.: Pharmacology of phospholipase A$_2$ from snake venoms. In Lee, C.-Y. (ed.): *Snake Venoms*. Vol. 52, Handbook of Experimental Pharmacology. Springer-Verlag, Berlin, 1979, p. 11.

Russell, F. E.: Poisonous fishes. *Engineer. Sci.*, **15**:11, 1952.

———: Venomous animals and their toxins. *London Times Sci. Rev.*, **49**:10, 1963.

———: Marine toxins and venomous and poisonous marine animals. In Russell, F. S. (ed.): *Advances in Marine Biology*, Vol. III. Academic Press, London, 1965, pp. 255–384.

———: Physalia stings—A report of two cases. *Toxicon*, **4**:65, 1966.

———: Comparative pharmacology of some animal toxins. *Fed. Proc.*, **26**:1206, 1967.

———: Poisons and venoms. In Hoar, W. S., and Randall, D. J. (eds.): *Fish Physiology*, Vol. III. Academic Press, Inc., New York, 1969, pp. 401–49.

———: Pharmacology of toxins in marine origin. In Raskova, H. (ed.): *International Encyclopedia of Pharmacology and Therapeutics*, Sec. 71, Vol. 2. Pergamon Press, Oxford, 1971, pp. 3–114.

———: Envenomation and diverse disease states (letter). *JAMA*, **238**:581, 1977.

———: Pharmacology of venoms. In Eaker, D., and Wadström, T. (eds.): *Natural Toxins*. Pergamon Press, Elmsford, N.Y., 1980, p. 13.

———: Venomous bites and stings. In Berkow, R. (ed.): *The Merck Manual*, 14th ed. Merck, Sharp & Dohme, Res. Lab., Rahway, N.J., 1982, pp. 2451–62.

———: *Snake Venom Poisoning*. J. B. Lippincott Co., Philadelphia, 1980b; Scholium International, Great Neck, N.Y., 1983.

———: Marine toxins and venomous and poisonous marine animals. In Blaxter, J. H. S.; Russell, F. S.; and Yonge, C. M. (eds.): *Advances in Marine Biology*. Academic Press, London, 1984a.

———: Snake venoms. In Ferguson, M. W. J. (ed.): *The Structure, Development, and Evolution of Reptiles* (Symposia of the Zoological Society of London). Academic Press, London, 1984b.

———: Poisoning caused by venomous and poisonous animals. In Goldsmith, R. S., and Heyneman, D. (eds.): *Tropical Medicine and Medical Parasitology*. Lange Medical Publications, Los Altos, Cal., 1986 (in press).

Russell, F. E., and Van Harreveld, A.: Cardiovascular effects of the venom of the round stingray, *Urobatis halleri*. *Arch. Intern. Physiol.*, **62**:322, 1954.

Russell, F. E., and Emery, J. A.: Venom of the weevers *Trachinus draco* and *Trachinus vipera*. *Ann. N.Y. Acad. Sci.*, **90**:805, 1960.

Russell, F. E.; Buess, F. W.; and Strassburg, J.: Cardiovascular response to *Crotalus* venom. *Toxicon*, **1**:5, 1962.

Russell, F. E., and Buess, F. W.: Gel electrophoresis: a tool in systematics. Studies with *Latrodectus mactans* venom. *Toxicon*, **8**:81, 1970.

Russell, F. E., and Bogert, C. M.: Gila monster: its biology, venom and bite—a review. *Toxicon*, **19**:341, 1981.

Russell, F. E., and Gertsch, W. J.: Letter to the editor (arthropod bites). *Toxicon*, **21**:337, 1983.

Schaeffer, R. C., Jr.; Carlson, R. W.; Whigham, H.; Weil, M. H.; and Russell, F. E.: Acute hemodynamic effects of rattlesnake, *Crotalus viridis helleri*, venom. In Rosenberg, P. (ed.): *Toxins: Animal, Plant and Microbial*. Pergamon Press, Oxford, 1978, p. 383.

Schantz, E. J.: Biochemical studies on paralytic shellfish poisons. *Ann. N.Y. Acad. Sci.*, **90**:843, 1960.

Schantz, E. J.; McFarren, E. F.; Schaffer, M. L.; and

Lewis, K. H.: Purified shellfish poison for bioassay standardization. *J. Assoc. Off. Agric. Chem.*, **41**:160, 1958.

Schantz, E. J.; Lynch, J. M.; Vayvada, G.; Matsumoto, K.; and Rappoport, H.: The purification and characterization of the poison produced by *Gonyaulax catenella* in axenic culture. *Biochemistry*, **5**:1191, 1966.

Schantz, E. J.; Ghazarossian, V. E.; Schnoes, H. K.; Strong, F. M.; Springer, J. P.; Pezzanie, J. D.; and Clardy, J.: The structure of saxitoxin. *J. Am. Chem. Soc.*, **97**:1238, 1975.

Schenone, H., and Suarez, G.: Venoms of Scytodidae. Genus *Loxosceles*. In Bettini, S. (ed.): *Arthropod Venoms*. Springer-Verlag, New York, 1978, pp. 247–75.

Scheuer, P. J.: *Chemistry of Marine Natural Products*. Academic Press, Inc., New York, 1973.

Scheuer, P. J. (ed.): *Marine Natural Products: Chemical and Biological Perspectives*. Academic Press, Inc., New York. Vols. 1 and 2, 1978; Vol. 3, 1980; Vol. 4, 1981.

Shapiro, B. I., and Lilleheil, G.: The action of anemone toxin on crustacean neurons. *Comp. Biochem. Physiol.*, **28**:1225, 1969.

Shimizu, Y.: Dinoflagellate toxins. In Scheuer, P. J. (ed.): *Marine Natural Products: Chemical and Biological Perspectives*, Vol. I. Academic Press, Inc., New York, 1978, pp. 1–42.

Slotta, K., and Fraenkel-Conrat, H.: Two active proteins from rattlesnake venom. *Nature*, **142**:213, 1938.

Smith, D. S.; Cayer, M. L.; Russell, F. E.; and Rubin, R. W.: Fine structure of stingray spine epidermis with special reference to a unique microtubular component of venom secreting cells. In Rosenberg, P. (ed.): *Toxins: Animal, Plant and Microbial*. Pergamon Press, Oxford, 1978, p. 565.

Sommer, A., and Meyer, K. F.: Paralytic shellfish poisoning. *Arch. Pathol.*, **24**:560, 1937.

Southcott, R. V.: Arachnidism and allied syndromes in the Australian region. *Rec. Adelaide Children's Hosp.*, **1**:97; 1976.

————: Marine toxins. In Cohen, M. H., and Klawars, H. L. (eds.): *Handbook of Clinical Neurology*, Vol. 37. North-Holland Publ. Co., Amsterdam, 1979, pp. 27–106.

Southcott, R. V., and Kingston, C. W.: Lethal jellyfish stings: a study in sea-wasps. *Med. J. Aust.*, (1):443, 1959.

Stempien, M. F.; Ruggieri, G. D.; Nigrelli, R. F.; and Cecil, J. T.: Physiologically active substances from extracts of marine sponges. In Youngken, H. W. (ed.): *Food-Drugs from the Sea Conference*. Marine Tech. Society, Washington, D.C., 1970, p. 295.

Su, C., Chang, C., and Lee, C.-Y.: Pharmacological properties of the neurotoxin of cobra venom. In Russell, F. E., and Saunders, P. R. (eds.): *Animal Toxins*. Pergamon Press, Oxford, 1967, pp. 259–67.

Sutherland, S. K., and Lane, W. R.: Toxins and mode of envenomation of the common ringed or blue-banded octopus. *Med. J. Aust.*, **1**:893, 1969.

Tamiya, N.; Arai, H.; and Sato, S.: Studies on sea snake venoms: crystallization of "erabutoxins" a and b from *Laticauda semifasiata* venom, and of "laticotoxin" a from *Laticauda laticauda* venom. In Russell, F. E., and Saunders, P. R. (eds.): *Animal Toxins*. Pergamon Press, Oxford, 1967, pp. 249–58.

Tamkun, M. M., and Hessinger, D. A.: Isolation and partial characterization of a hemolytic and toxic protein from the nematocyst venom of the Portuguese man-of-war, *Physalia physalis*. *Biochem. Biophys. Acta*, **667**:87, 1981; see also *Fed. Proc.*, **38**:824, 1979 (abstr.).

Tu, A. T.: *Chemistry and Molecular Biology*. John Wiley & Sons, New York, 1977.

Vick, J. A.; Ciuchta, H. P.; and Manthei, J. H.: Pathophysiological studies on ten snake venoms. In Russell, F. E., and Saunders, P. R. (eds.): *Animal Toxins*. Pergamon Press, Oxford, 1967, p. 269.

Wagner, F. W.; Spiekerman, A. M.; and Prescott, J. M.: Leucostoma peptidase A. Isolation and physical properties. *J. Biol. Chem.*, **243**:4486, 1968.

Wang, C. M.; Narahashi, T.; and Mendi, T. J.: Depolarizing action of *Haliclona* toxin on end-plate and muscle membranes. *Toxicon*, **11**:499, 1973.

Waraszkiewicz, S. M., and Erickson, K. L.: Halogenated sesquiterpenoids from the Hawaiian marine alga *Laurencia nidifica*: nidificene and nidifidiene. *Tetrahedron Lett.*, **23**:2003, 1974.

Weill, R.: *Contributions a l'etude des Cnidaires et de leur Nematocystes*, Tome 10 11. Trav. Stat. Zool. Wimiereux, Paris, 1934.

Wiberg, G. S., and Stephenson, N. R.: Toxicologic studies on paralytic shellfish poison. *Toxicol. Appl. Pharmacol.*, **2**:607, 1960.

Wittle, L. W.; Middlebrook, R. E.; and Lane, C. E.: Isolation partial purification of a toxin from *Millepora alcicornis*. *Toxicon*, **9**:327, 1971.

Yang, C. C.: Crystallization and properties of cobrotoxin and their relationship to lethality. *Biochim. Biophys. Acta*, **133**:346, 1965.

Zeller, E. A.: Enzymes of snake venoms and their biological significance. In *Advances in Enzymology*, Vol. 8. Interscience, New York, 1948, p. 459.

Chapter 23

TOXIC EFFECTS OF PLANT TOXINS

Kenneth F. Lampe

INTRODUCTION

The emphasis of this chapter will be on plants injurious to man. The poisoning of grazing animals also is important because it represents an enormous economic loss. Useful information on this aspect is contained in the previous editions of this text.

Inquiries concerning plant ingestions constitute about 10 percent of calls to Poison Control Centers, but only a small fraction of these are associated with symptomatic poisoning. The majority concern children three years of age and younger. The age of the victim often determines the plants that are involved. Infants are exposed primarily to plants in the home. The list of houseplants encountered is remarkably constant regardless of geography (Table 23–1). Symptomatic poisoning in this age group almost invariably results from chewing the leaves of dumbcane (*Dieffenbachia* spp.) or one of the philodendrons, generally *Philodendron scandens* ssp. *oxycardium*. Older preschool-age children also are exposed to yard plants (Table 23–2). They seek colorful berries or plants to serve as food while "playing house." These plants are more geographically distinctive. Adolescents and adults may experiment with plants and mushrooms thought to have hallucinogenic properties, although this rarely results in serious poisoning. More severe intoxications result from consumption of large quantities of wild plants inappropriately selected for food. Plants occasionally are consumed for abortifacient (now uncommon) or suicidal purposes.

A new potential source of toxic plant material is the health food store, where such items as raw apricot pits, tansy, and pennyroyal may be purchased. The ingredients may be mislabeled or may contain more than one plant. Plant medicinals obtained outside the United States often contain drugs, such as phenylbutazone, that are not listed on the label.

One must be aware that many so-called plant poisonings involve harmless species that have been treated with insecticides, weed killers, or fertilizers.

RESEARCH ON PLANTS INJURIOUS TO HUMANS

Although research on plants that poison animals has been pursued actively for many years by the USDA and schools of veterinary medicine, an equivalent interest in plants injurious to humans (except those producing dermatitis) has not been forthcoming. It is important, therefore, that research papers on this subject be free from defects that would diminish their value. The following are examples of recurring problems.

Failure to Document the Plant

Identification of the plant only by its trivial (common) name occurs frequently in clinical case reporting. Unfortunately, many plants of diverse botanical relationship share the same trivial name, even in the same locality. See the previous edition for a more detailed discussion.

Failure to place a voucher specimen of the plant in an herbarium with reference to such placement in the publication is primarily a prob-

Table 23–1. FREQUENCY OF PLANT SPECIES INVOLVED IN INQUIRIES TO THE ROCHESTER, NEW YORK, POISON CONTROL CENTER INVOLVING INGESTIONS BY CHILDREN ONE YEAR OF AGE OR LESS*

1. Philodendron
2. Jade plant
3. Wandering Jew
4. Swedish ivy
5. Spider plant
6. Dieffenbachia and rubber plant
7. Asparagus fern
8. Aloe
9. String-of-pearls
10. Pothos

* From Lawrence, R.A.: *Proceedings, Ann. Mtg. Am. Acad. Clin. Toxicol/Am. Assoc. Poison Control Centers/Can. Acad. Clin. Anal. Toxicol.* Chicago, Oct. 18–20, 1978.

Table 23–2. INQUIRIES CONCERNING PLANT INGESTIONS TO POISON CONTROL
CENTERS SHOWING THE MOST FREQUENTLY INVOLVED SPECIES

AAPCC Annual Report* (data from all reporting centers)	Salt Lake City, Utah[†]	Rochester, New York[‡]	Miami, Florida[§]
1. Philodendron	1. Philodendron	1. Yew	1. Brazilian pepper
2. Dieffenbachia	2. Pyracantha	3. Nightshade	2. Dieffenbachia
3. Poinsettia	3. Apricot and other pits	3. Honeysuckle	3. Rosary pea
4. Jade plant	4. Dieffenbachia	4. Philodendron	4. Pencil tree cactus
5. Schefflera	5. Poinsettia	5. Poinsettia	5. Ficus
6. Holly	6. Honeysuckle	6. Pokeweed	6. Oleander, Philodendron
7. Pyracantha	7. Wandering Jew	7. Wandering Jew	7. Ixora, Allamanda
8. Pokeweed	8. Horse chestnut	8. Dieffenbachia	8. Poinsettia
9. Yew	9. Sweet pea	9. Jade plant	9. Coral plant
10. Rhododendron, Azalea	10. Creeping Charlie	10. Coleus	10. Balsam pear, Angel's trumpet, Bischofia
11. Spider plant, Pothos	11. Jimson weed, Schefflera		11. Hibiscus, Sea grape, Crown-of-thorns, "Croton," Bottle brush
12. Ornamental pepper, Mountain ash, Honeysuckle	12. Oregon grape, Tulip		

* Litovitz, T., and Veltri, J. C.: *Am. J. Emerg. Med.* 3:423–50, 1985.
† Spoerke, D. G. and Temple, A. R.: *Vet. Human Toxicol.*, **20**:85–90, 1978.
‡ Lawrence, R. A., and Schneider, M. F.: *Proceedings, Ann. Mtg. Am. Acad. Clin. Toxicol./Am. Assoc. Poison Control Centers/Can. Acad. Clin. Anal. Toxicol.*, Ste.-Adele, P.O., Canada, Aug. 2–5, 1977.
§ Fawcett, N. P.: *J. Fla. Med. Assoc.*, **65**: 199–204, 1978.

lem in research. The important studies of phenolics in *Toxicodendron* by the late Dr. C. R. Dawson are diminished in value, because it is now impossible to determine what species and varieties of the plant were examined.

Failure To Use Appropriate Route of Administration

Parenteral administration, particularly in small animals, is technically easier than oral administration, but can lead to spurious results. Plants containing more than one toxin may exhibit different biologic activities, depending on the route of administration. Some plants contain lectins that cause erythrocyte agglutination and hemolysis, in addition to an orally active toxin. Lectins are not absorbed from the intestine and do not affect erythrocytes unless given intravenously. Many publications on poisonous plants improperly describe hemolysis as the major mechanism of toxicity for mushrooms and the castor bean, since each contains such lectins. Thus, alkalinization of the urine to protect the kidneys against hemoglobinuria has been recommended in some protocols for castor bean poisoning, and for a number of years the Pasteur Institute in Paris prepared a serum against the parenterally toxic lysin in *Amanita phalloides* in the mistaken belief that it was an antidote. Some toxins are active only orally, for example, amygdalin, which must be hydrolyzed in the stomach to release cyanide, or macroazamin, which must be acted upon by the β-glucosidases of intestinal bacteria to release methylazoxymethanol. When screening for biologic activity, however, both oral and parenteral administration should be employed.

Failure To Use an Appropriate Assay

Various screening tests are employed to study the biologic activity of plants; these are limited only by the amount of plant material available, length of time, amount of money, and particular interests of the investigator. It is not practical to perform an assay for every conceivable type of pharmacologic activity. On the other hand, if a specific end-point has been determined, it is important to select an assay method or species sensitive to that end-point. For example, the chemists who fractionated tremetol, the crude extract from *Eupatorium rugosum*, used lethality in fish as an assay. *E. rugosum* causes a condition called trembles in cows and a potentially fatal syndrome, milksickness, in people who ingest the milk. The fractions of the extract from tremetol were given to fish, which are convenient test animals since the material can be added to the water and only small amounts of material are required. Unfortunately, it was not determined in advance that fish show the same biochemical alterations as cows or humans; thus, the end result was the isolation of a toxic material to which fish were exquisitely sensitive, but which was inactive as a cause of trembles in mammals.

Failure To Provide Standard Medical Care

When studying the value of treatments of plant poisoning in animals, particularly with drugs, there is a tendency to divide the animals into two groups, poison all of them, give the proposed treatment to half, and, after an appropriate time, count the survivors in each group. Little or no attempt is made to correct dehydration, provide respiratory support, monitor and correct electrolyte and glucose deficiencies, or provide other standard care as for an actual patient. Such care should be given and should be extended equally to each group. This failure to provide standard care lends an element of uncertainty to the value of a proposed "antidote," which may persist in a half-accepted twilight zone for years. A current example is the place of thioctic acid in the management of *Amanita phalloides* intoxication.

Interpretation of the Literature

Considerable care must be exercised in evaluating the literature on toxic plants. In some cases, results of animal toxicity studies have been extrapolated inappropriately to humans. In many cases, plant lore has been passed uncritically through generations of textbooks. For example, it was observed around 1900 that nettle stings were not unlike the stings of ants. From that time, with no experimental study, the statement that nettles, like ants, contain formic acid is often encountered.

On the other hand, specific case reports may be very useful. Many plants with physiologic activity were used as medicinals during the nineteenth century, and numerous cases of overdosage were reported, which provide valuable starting points for research on human pharmacology.

SYSTEMIC POISONING FROM VASCULAR PLANTS

General Principles

In any inquiry concerning plant ingestion, an attempt should be made to identify the plant, the part(s) ingested, and the approximate quantity. As in any poisoning, this information often will be incomplete or incorrect. With the exception of ingested plants known to be hazardous or patients who are already symptomatic, observa-

tion at home with instructions to call if there is a change in condition is usually recommended by the Poison Center. Routine follow-up calls are often made by the Center. Following ingestion of mushrooms or known toxic plants (other than those causing oral irritation only), and in symptomatic cases, emptying of the stomach is recommended. Considering the size of plant particles, vomiting induced by syrup of ipecac and water is probably more effective than gastric lavage. This should be followed by instillation of activated charcoal.

As in most cases of poisoning, care is usually symptomatic. Special monitoring and specific drug therapy are indicated in some instances. Because life-threatening intoxications are exceptionally rare, little experience may be available among local hospital staff for an appropriate management protocol. In this event, help should be solicited from a regional Poison Control Center, which maintains a nationwide roster of consultants available to share their expertise.

A cardinal rule in the management of pediatric intoxications is to provide adequate hydration. Most poisonous plants, regardless of their ultimate toxicologic effect, induce fluid loss through vomiting and/or diarrhea. Children have a limited buffer capacity for such loss and have died from eating plants causing simple gastroenteric irritation.

Another easily missed effect of plant poisoning is diminished tidal volume. Respiratory rate may appear to be unchanged, but a toxin acting as a muscle relaxant may severely reduce the tidal volume, which, if uncorrected, can proceed to sudden respiratory failure and cardiac arrest.

The diagnosis of plant poisoning, in the absence of a history of plant ingestion, is probably impossible, unless the vomitus or stool can be seen to contain plant fragments. When wild plants are prepared as food, the differential diagnosis should include bacterial toxins, contamination with pesticides or weed killers, and individual food idiosyncrasy.

The toxicity of plants varies with plant part, maturity, growing condition, and genetic variation. Plants grown in some parts of the country or in some years may be toxic, but can be eaten with impunity at other times or places. The age of the patient is also a factor; solanine-containing plants, for example, are far more dangerous to children than to adults. Children less than one year old tend to texture plant parts in their mouths rather than swallowing; thus, ingestion is minimal. The seed coats of the castor bean (*Ricinus communis*) and rosary pea (*Abrus precatorius*) are very hard, and unless broken, the seeds of these exceedingly toxic plants will pass harmlessly through the intestine. Other factors influencing toxicity could be cited. Obviously, it is impossible to determine prognosis simply on the basis that there has been an exposure. It is possible only to consider some plants more hazardous than others.

The following discussion of systemic poisoning by plants and mushrooms is not complete. It includes more common or interesting species. Information on additional plants may be found in the references at the end of this chapter.

Plants Producing Irritation of the Oral Cavity

The dumbcane (*Dieffenbachia* spp.) is so named because biting into a leaf causes immediate burning pain and swelling of oral tissues that may result in a transient loss of the ability to speak. The pain and edema do not require medical treatment, but may be relieved by holding cool liquid or ice cream in the mouth. Obstruction of the airway is a rare complication. This response is produced to a greater or lesser degree by all members of the botanical family Araceae, which includes the cultivated houseplants (outdoors in Florida and Hawaii), *Philodendron* spp., *Caladium* spp., and the calla lily (*Zantedeschia aethiopica*); plants cultivated for edible parts, the ceriman (*Monstera deliciosa*) and malanga (*Xanthosoma violaceum*); and woodland species, the skunk cabbage (*Symplocarpus foetidus*), Jack-in-the-pulpit (*Arisaema triphyllum*), and green dragon (*Arisaema dracontium*).

When the plant cells are ruptured by chewing, bundles of long, needle-shaped crystals (raphides) of calcium oxalate are driven into the oral tissue. The mechanism of the production of pain is controversial. Based on work on an unrelated raphide-containing fishtail palm (*Caroyta mitis*) that causes a similar response when its fruit is bitten, it was proposed that mechanical injury from the calcium oxalate needle alone was responsible. Others maintain that the mechanical injury provides a pathway for injection of pain-inducing protein material. This might be resolved by using fruit from one of the Araceae, since raphides are easier to isolate from the fruit than from the leaf of *Dieffenbachia* on which all work has been done.

Plants Producing Emesis Not Associated with Diarrhea

The bulbs of the family Amaryllidaceae, whose resemblance to onions makes them ready objects for accidental poisoning, elicit vomiting not associated with diarrhea. This family contains various *Narcissus* spp. (narcissus, jonquil, daffodil) and species of *Amaryllis*. Despite the apparent severity of the intoxication, which is characterized by repeated episodes of vomiting, recovery essentially is complete within 24 hours. Treatment is symptomatic, although there have been no clinical reports on whether phenothiazine antiemetics are useful.

The intoxication results from the action of the alkaloid lycorine on emetic receptors in the central nervous system. The emetic toxins in *Wisteria* species produce a similar, but longer-lasting, response. The emetic toxins in *Wisteria* apparently have not been identified, although various lectins from this plant have been studied.

Plants Producing Diarrhea That May Be Associated with Emesis

Outside of a few medically useful cathartic-containing plants, those containing anthraquinone derivatives for example, the active substances in these plants have received scant attention. Even the actions of our cathartic drugs are poorly understood and controversial. Two representative toxins will be discussed.

The saponins are steroidal glycosides widely distributed throughout the plant kingdom, although they are not always present in concentrations sufficient to induce a symptomatic response. Within a species, the concentration depends on the maturity of the plant and the conditions of growth. Absorption of saponins is poor, and severe gastroenteritis is usually the only consequence of ingestion. The most important saponin-containing plant in eastern North America is the pokeweed (*Phytolacca americana*). Intoxications result from the misidentification of its root as horseradish and the use of uncooked mature leaves in salads. The mature berries are usually harmless. There is usually a latent period of two to three hours prior to the onset of symptoms during which the saponins are hydrolyzed to their active triterpene components. There is an initial prodroma of warmth in the throat and stomach and a scratchy feeling in the throat, which may be accompanied by coughing. This is followed by severe gastritis with frequent episodes of vomiting, which may continue at intervals for ten hours, and diarrhea, which may persist for 48 hours. Intoxications with similar symptoms have been produced by consumption of the nuts of the horse chestnut (*Aesculus hippocastanum*), fruit from the blue cohosh (*Caulophyllum thalictroides*), pigeon berry (*Duranta repens*), the fruit or leaf of English ivy (*Hedera helix*), and the yam bean (*Pachyrhizus erosus*).

Members of the buttercup family, Ranunculaceae, contain a glycoside that yields the irritant protoanemonin on enzymatic hydrolysis. The plants associated with intoxications are the buttercups (*Ranunculus* spp.), baneberry (*Ac-*

taea pachypoda), marsh marigold (*Caltha palustris*), pasque flower (*Anemone* spp.), and *Clematis* spp. Protoanemonin produces a burning sensation in the oropharynx, profuse salivation, emesis, colicky gastroenteritis, and diarrhea. A portion of the toxin may be absorbed and excreted unchanged by the kidney; hematuria, polyuria, and, sometimes, painful urination may occur. Adequate hydration to maintain a dilute urine is indicated to reduce renal damage. Conventionally, these patients have been given demulcents orally (egg white and milk), but no study has been made to determine if this is helpful or if simple dilution would be equally satisfactory.

Plants Producing Gastroenteritis After a Latent Period of Several Hours

Poisoning with colchicine-containing plants occurs after a partially dose-dependent latent period (usually of many hours) and has resulted from ingestion of leaves, seeds, bulbs, or flowers of the crocus or meadow saffron (*Colchicum* spp.). The plant has even been used successfully for suicide. Less commonly, poisonings have followed the ingestion of tubers from the glory lily (*Gloriosa superba* and *G. rothschildiana*), which have been mistaken for sweet potatoes. The gastroenteric effects resemble those encountered with colchicine during treatment of gout. Colchicine is a mitotic poison. Massive overdose may result in vascular damage, thrombocytopenia, bone marrow depression, hypothermia, muscle weakness, and, in survivors, alopecia.

Solanine alkaloids is the general name for the steroidal glycoalkaloids found in nightshades (*Solanum* spp.), immature fruit of some groundcherries (*Physalis* spp.), the jessamines (*Cestrum* spp.), and many other plants. Fatalities have resulted from the ingestion of fruit from the European bittersweet (*Solanum dulcamara*) and the horse nettle (*Solanum carolinense*). Children seem to be especially sensitive, but this may represent a dose-response effect rather than greater intestinal absorption. The symptoms are those of an infectious gastroenteritis: temperature is elevated, headache is common, and, after a prodromal scratchy feeling in the oropharynx, there is anorexia, nausea, vomiting, and diarrhea. Management is symptomatic.

The most toxic flowering plants are the castor bean (*Ricinus communis*) and the rosary pea (*Abrus precatorius*). The toxins of these plants, formerly called toxalbumins, are nearly identical lectins composed of two polypeptide chains connected by a disulfide bridge. One of these chains binds to the intestinal cell wall permitting entry of the other chain into the cytoplasm. The toxin inhibits ribosomal protein synthesis. A single molecule of toxin is sufficient to kill the cell. The castor bean also contains the harmless cathartic castor oil, and both species contain an orally inactive (nontoxic) agglutinin.

If seeds with broken seed coats are swallowed, persistent diarrhea, often with bloody mucus, begins after a latent period of up to three days. Death may occur two to three days later of complications related to loss of intestinal function. Autopsy reveals hemorrhagic gastric mucosa and cecum. The gut-associated lymphoid tissue (Peyer's patches) in the ileum are severely inflamed and edematous. Intravenous fluids and parenteral alimentation should be provided, but cerebral edema, oliguria, and cardiac arrhythmias secondary to changes in plasma composition usually prove to be unmanageable.

The mistletoe (*Phoradendron serotinum*) is often named as one of the hazards in the home in newspaper lists appearing about Christmas time. In the 1920s, it was shown that the fruit contains tyramine, and textbooks ever since have listed this as the toxic ingredient with headache and hypertension as symptoms, although neither has appeared in a case history. It is hard to imagine the tyramine in even a handful of fruit surviving a first pass through the portal circulation in a patient with intact monoamine oxidase activity. Recently, it was demonstrated that the European mistletoe (*Viscum album*) contains a lectin with activity similar to that in the castor bean but with only about ⅟₃₀th the activity. This lectin was isolated from the leaves, and although not specified, the article suggested that the lectin is either not present or present in low concentration in the fruit. According to European reports, children who swallow the fruit experience only mild gastroenteritis. Although toxic proteins are known to be present in American mistletoe, they have been studied only after parenteral administration, and neither their pathology nor mechanism of action has been described.

Plants Containing Convulsants

Although there are a number of plants in North America containing convulsant toxins, actual clinical cases have involved only the water hemlocks (*Cicuta* spp.). These plants have a distinct odor of raw parsnip and may be mistaken for that vegetable. Treatment requires management of the airway, relief of convulsions if persistent, and respiratory support. Acute renal failure secondary to convulsion-induced rhabdomyolysis is an infrequent complication. One of the most toxic plants in Great Britain, the water dropwort (*Oenanthe crocata*), has a similar toxin and is a rare introduced species in the

United States in the Washington, D.C. area. A related species, *Oenanthe sarmentosa*, is common along the West Coast but has not been associated with poisoning. It would be of interest to determine if it is devoid of the convulsant toxin.

Plants Containing Belladonna Alkaloids

All species of *Datura*, particularly the jimson weed (*Datura stramonium*) and the angel trumpets (*Brugmansia* spp.), contain the belladonna alkaloids. The entire plant is toxic, including the nectar, but the seeds are encountered most commonly in accidental poisoning. Both seeds and dried leaves are used for their deliriant effect. Although physostigmine may be employed to antagonize the atropinic effects (dry mouth with dysphonia and dysphagia, tachycardia, dry skin, elevated body temperature, which may be accompanied by rash, blurred vision, occasional mydriasis, delirium, and excitement), therapeutic intervention is not necessary except in the presence of severe delirium or hyperthermia. Topical application to the eye, an occupational hazard among farmers, may cause unilateral mydriasis; in the absence of suspicion as to the cause, this may lead to unneeded neurologic investigation.

Plants Primarily Affecting the Cardiovascular System

The foxglove (*Digitalis purpurea*), lily-of-the-valley (*Convallaria majalis*), oleander (*Nerium oleander*), and yellow oleander or lucky nut (*Thevetia peruviana*) all contain digitalislike glycosides. The entire plant is toxic, including smoke from burning foliage and water in which the flowers have been placed. Acute digitalis poisoning differs from digitalis overdosage as seen in a patient with congestive failure. It is expressed usually as conduction defects and sinus bradycardia. Hyperkalemia may be present. Rhythm disturbances, other than escape beats, are not necessarily exhibited. Intoxications require serial monitoring of the electrocardiogram and serum potassium. Conduction defects may be relieved by atropine or transvenous pacing. Dialysis and forced diuresis are not useful.

Monkshood (*Aconitum* spp.) produces a tingling, burning sensation on the lips, tongue, mouth, and throat almost immediately after ingestion. This is followed by numbness and a feeling of constriction in the throat. The toxic alkaloid, aconitine, causes reflex bradycardia, slows conductions, and induces arrhythmias. Other symptoms are nausea, vomiting, and muscular weakness. Aconitine acts on nerve axons by opening sodium channels. On myocardial tissue, it inhibits complete repolarization of the

excitable membrane causing repetitive firing. In isolated tissue preparations, this action can be antagonized by procaine; an infusion of 0.1 percent procaine was effective in one report of human intoxication but has not been examined in laboratory preparations. The green hellebores (*Veratrum* spp.) and the death camas (*Zigadenus* spp.) contain veratridine. Plants in the botanical family Ericaceae (*Rhododendron* spp., *Kalmia* spp., *Pieris* spp., and others) contain the nonnitrogenous grayanotoxins (formerly called andromedotoxins). Both veratridine, the most potent of the veratrum alkaloids, and the grayanotoxins have a physiologic action identical to that of aconitine, although intoxication from these plants appears to be associated more with bradycardia and hypotension than with rhythm disturbances. This may, however, be a dose artifact, and if equivalent quantities were ingested and retained (early and profuse emesis usually removes much swallowed material), the clinical picture with all three types of poisoning might be indistinguishable. Honey made from the nectar of Ericaceae contains toxic concentrations of grayanotoxins.

All parts of the yew tree (*Taxus* spp.), except the bright-red, fleshy aril that cups the seed, contain the complex taxine alkaloids. Onset of intoxication occurs after a latent period of one to three hours. Nausea, diffuse abdominal pain, shallow respiration, and cardiac conduction disturbances resembling hyperkalemia occur. The atrial P waves may be absent. The syndrome complex suggests the need for temporary transvenous pacing, but human intoxications are so rare that there is little clinical experience. The pharmacology of the taxine alkaloids has not been examined since the early 1930s; thus, no conclusions may be drawn regarding mechanism.

Plants That Affect Skeletal Muscle Tone

Of the toxic species that may affect skeletal muscle tone, those most frequently encountered clinically contain nicotine or anabasine, particularly the tree tobacco (*Nicotiana glauca*), which contains the latter. Similar poisoning is produced by coniine found in poison hemlock (*Conium maculatum*); or cytisine, found in laburnum (*Cytisus laburnum*) and the mescal or burning bean (*Sophora secundiflora*); and lobeline, which is present in cardinal flowers (*Lobelia* spp.). Poisoning causes nausea and emesis, a sensation of sweating, dizziness, and, sometimes, clonic convulsions. Death is due to paralysis of respiratory muscles. An older investigation, by visual observation, described the action at the myoneural junction as succinylcholinelike rather than curarelike. Patients can be maintained with controlled respiration. It would be interesting to verify the neuromuscular action by electrophysiologic studies and to see if neostigmine antagonizes the blockade. There is a great need for some basic pharmacokinetic data on humans on nicotine and anabasine.

Most intoxications involving the Carolina yellow jessamine (*Gelsemium sempervirens*) have resulted from children sucking the nectar from the flowers, but all parts of this vine contains the toxins gelsemine, gelsemicine, and related alkaloids. Ingestions produce headache, dizziness, visual disturbances, pronounced ptosis, and dry mouth with dysphonia and dysphagia. In severe cases, muscular weakness becomes pronounced. There are coexistent signs of a weak strychninelike action with tetanic contractions and extensor spasms following tendon taps. Convulsions, however, are unusual. Little is known of the pharmacology of the alkaloids although a tincture of gelsemium was used extensively in medicine and a number of intoxications are reported in the nineteenth-century medical literature. Minor intoxications may be managed with respiratory support.

Karwinskia humboldtiana is best known by its Mexican names, coyotillo or tullidora, in the American Southwest, but is sometimes called (inappropriately) buckthorn in the American literature. The fruit contains a number of toxic anthracenones. Several weeks after consumption, the muscles become increasingly weak, beginning with the lower extremities. Full paralysis may develop over another month. Fatalities are due to failure of the respiratory muscles. The initial defect is segmental loss in myelin of the peripheral motor nerves followed by fragmentation and disappearance of the axon itself in a Wallerian-like fashion. These toxins are currently under study. No specific management of the poisoning can be suggested.

SYSTEMIC POISONING FROM MUSHROOMS

It has been a particular pleasure to watch the development of our knowledge of the chemistry and clinical toxicology of poisonous mushrooms during the past two decades. Not only has the management of patients been simplified and made more specific as the underlying pathophysiology was clarified, but some of the mushroom toxins have evolved into powerful evaluative tools in biochemical and neurologic research.

Unlike vascular plant poisoning, facility for mushroom identification during an emergency may be difficult or impractical. Fortunately, there are relatively limited varieties of toxins, which permits differential diagnosis on the basis of history and symptoms. Mushrooms that produce a response within two hours of ingestion or shortly after the ingestion of an alcoholic beverage rarely are considered of serious consequence and require only conservative symptomatic management. They may be subdivided into: (1) mushrooms whose response is primarily gastroenteric symptoms, with nausea, abdominal discomfort, and sometimes vomiting and/or diarrhea; (2) mushrooms evoking sweating; (3) mushrooms inducing inebriation or hallucinations without drowsiness or sleep; (4) mushrooms producing delirium associated with sleep or coma; and (5) mushrooms eliciting a disulfiramlike response to alcohol.

Intoxications characterized by a latent period of six hours or more are associated with serious, sometimes life-threatening symptoms. These may be subdivided into: (1) those producing severe headache and a feeling of abdominal fullness about six hours after ingestion; (2) those provoking emesis and profuse diarrhea about 12 hours after ingestion; and (3) those producing polydipsia and polyuria about three days after ingestion.

Mushrooms Producing Gastroenteric Discomfort of Rapid Onset

Many species of mushrooms produce varying degrees of abdominal discomfort within three hours of ingestion. Some may cause persistent emesis and/or diarrhea, which may produce severe dehydration and hypovolemic shock, particularly in children. The irritant mushroom need not be identified. Treatment is entirely symptomatic as for gastroenteritis of any other etiology. Replacement of fluids and electrolytes and support of circulation may be required.

Mushrooms Evoking Sweating

These mushrooms contain clinically significant concentrations of muscarine, which is not affected by cooking. There is a dose-response relationship in symptoms, the most sensitive indicator being profuse sweating. More severe intoxications produce nausea, emesis, abdominal pain, and, occasionally, blurred vision and other parasympathetic effects. Symptoms usually subside without treatment within two hours. In uncomfortable patients, atropine may be given until symptoms are abolished or until dryness of the mouth is produced.

Mushrooms Evoking Inebriations or Hallucinations

These mushrooms contain psilocybin. The clinical response is determined by the dose, setting, psychoactive substance, and sophistication, mood, and personality of the patient. The usual duration is two hours. In accidental poisoning in adults, the response resembles alcohol intoxication. In young children exposed to large doses, the hallucinations are accompanied by hyperthermia, loss of consciousness, and tonic-clonic convulsions. Adults do not require treatment. Young children exhibiting neurologic involvement require external cooling and respiratory management as indicated. There have been a few recorded fatalities in this age group.

Mushrooms Producing Delirium Associated with Sleep or Coma

The toxins involved are muscimol and ibotenic acid, which are components of *Amanita muscaria* and *A. pantherina*. Muscimol is a conformationally restricted analog of GABA with potent activity on bicuculline-reactive postsynaptic receptors. Symptoms of poisoning normally appear in 20 to 90 minutes. There may be an initial gastroenteritis, but this is often minimal or absent. After about one hour, drowsiness and dizziness develop, which may be accompanied by sleep. This may be followed by elation, increased motor activity, tremors, illusions, and even manic excitement. This may alternate with periods of drowsiness or sleep. Poisoning in adults is rarely severe, but may require protective action to prevent injury if manic excitement appears. In children, complex neurologic signs may persist for up to 12 hours and include coma and convulsions. Usually no therapy is necessary other than respiratory support, if indicated.

Mushrooms Exhibiting a Disulfiramlike Effect

Coprinus atramentarius, although edible, elicits a disulfiramlike response to alcohol consumption for up to three days after eating the mushroom. The active component is cyclopropanone hydrate, a metabolite of the mushroom toxin, 1-cyclopropanol-1-N^5-glutamine (coprine). Other mushrooms with a similar alcohol-sensitizing action include *Clitocybe clavipes*, *Boletus luridus*, and *Verpa bohemica*. None of these contain coprine, and their activity in this regard needs investigation.

Mushrooms Inducing Headache About Six Hours After Ingestion

This intoxication is associated most often with *Gyromitra exculenta*, which may be mistaken for the edible morel by inexperienced collectors. The toxin is monomethylhydrazine, which antagonizes pyridoxine. The toxin is volatile, and the mushroom may be made edible by air drying or by extraction of the toxin with boiling water, which is then discarded.

Onset of symptoms is sudden, usually about six to eight hours after ingestion or inhalation of the vapor from cooking mushrooms. It is characterized by headache, malaise, abdominal fullness, and emesis (but *not* diarrhea). Generally, the patient recovers completely within two to six days. However, fatal hepatic necrosis has developed. Treatment is the same as for isoniazid overdosage and consists of administration of pyridoxine and correction of systemic acidosis.

Mushrooms Causing Emesis and Profuse Diarrhea About 12 Hours After Ingestion

Almost all fatalities caused by mushroom poisoning in North America are caused by *Amanita phalloides* and its relatives. The toxins are a family of thermostable, cyclic octapeptides, known collectively as amatoxins. They bind to and inhibit RNA polymerase II, preventing the elongation of messenger RNA, and thereby disrupting the continuous maintenance of the cell. Clinically, the intoxication resembles acute hepatitis, although there have been cases, particularly minimal intoxications without a fulminant course, in which renal damage of very late onset (over one week) becomes evident. It is presumed that their selective action on the liver and kidney results from inability to enter other cell types freely.

Approximately one-half of a mature mushroom cap of *Amanita phalloides* is the lethal dose for an adult. Symptoms usually occur only after a period of 12 hours, and begin with nausea, vomiting, profuse diarrhea, and abdominal pain. This may be followed by a symptom-free period, succeeded by rapidly developing hepatic insufficiency indistinguishable from acute viral hepatitis. The increase in serum transaminase factors is the most sensitive indicator of the extent of hepatocellular damage. Blood glucose and clotting factors of hepatic origin are decreased. Jaundice is an inconsistent finding. Even with intensive, symptomatic care, the fatality rate is about 10 percent. In the early phase, fluids should be replaced and, when tolerated, activated charcoal given orally in serial boluses. Otherwise, the management is as for acute, fulminant hepatitis. A return toward normal of Factor V and fibrinogen is a prognostic feature for recovery.

Since *Amanita phalloides*-type mushroom poisoning is associated with high mortality, a large number of agents have been tried in human intoxications without previous research investigation. These include high-dose vitamin therapy, corticosteroids, sex hormones, and glucose loading. Two such agents, thioctic acid (α-lipoic acid) and high-dose penicillin G, have been used extensively in Europe and are included in some management protocols in the United States. It would be highly desirable if experimental animals, preferably the dog, which resembles man closely in *Amanita* poisoning, were given minimally toxic doses (to minimize the need for critical care) of mushroom extract (or a pure amatoxin, such as α-amanitin) and the influence of each of these proposed agents on hepatic transaminase changes with time was determined.

Mushrooms Causing Polydipsia and Polyuria Three or More Days After Ingestion

These poisonings are caused by *Cortinarius* species and have not been reported in the United States, although some species occur in California that are reported as toxic in Europe. There is a latent period of 3 to 17 days between ingestion and the appearance of symptoms. The first effect is severe polydipsia, during which the patient may drink several liters a day. This is followed by nausea, headaches, muscular pains, and chills. In severe cases, there is an initial polyuria succeeded by oliguria or anuria. Postmortem examination shows renal tubular necrosis, fatty degeneration of the liver, and severe inflammatory changes in the intestine. Management is symptomatic as for renal failure. There is still controversy surrounding the chemistry of the toxic component.

Unclassified Toxic Mushrooms

There are isolated reports on mushrooms producing unique actions that suggest interesting research projects. Examples are: the puffball, *Scleroderma aurantium,* causes tetany and paresthesias; *Verpa bohemica,* usually associated with mild gastroenteritis, produces significant motor incoordination in others; *Omphalotous olearius* (syn. *Clitocybe illudens*), whose chemistry has been investigated extensively, can produce gastroenteritis, sensory disturbances, and marked muscle relaxation; and *Stropharia coronilla* produced intense "bone pain" in two adolescents seeking hallucinogenic activity.

PLANTS CAUSING SKIN INJURY

In contrast to the rather low morbidity associated with systemic plant poisoning, plant dermatitis is a problem of enormous magnitude. Approximately one-half of the workmen's compensation claims filed annually in California are for poison oak (*Toxicodendron diversilobum*) dermatitis. With the exception of photoallergy (probably only because it is yet to be recognized), all forms of contact dermatitis are produced by plants. These include mechanical injury, delayed contact sensitivity, contact urticaria, phototoxicity, primary chemical irritation, or some combination of these.

Plants Causing Mechanical Injury

Injuries produced by splinters, thorns, awns, and sharp leaf edges are mechanisms for the introduction of fungi and bacteria through the skin or into the eye. Various noninfectious skin lesions caused by plant fragments include folliculitis, soft tissue granulomas, synovitis, and osteoblastic and osteolytic responses.

Plants Causing Delayed Contact Sensitivity (Allergic Contact Dermatitis)

Sensitivity to a substance must be developed after cutaneous contact. Once sensitized, subsequent exposure will elicit a response. Usually, five days to three weeks is needed after the sensitizing exposure for development of an immunologically reactive skin. The chemistry of the sensitizing chemicals is known for most commonly offending plants. They are low-molecular-weight compounds (haptens) that react with cutaneous protein to form antigens. More than one contact may be required to induce sensitization. With less potent haptens, sensitization occurs more readily if the plant is applied to damaged skin. Some haptens induce only transient sensitivity, but that caused by poison ivy and poison oak persists for decades and possibly for life.

Once sensitization develops, the whole body surface becomes reactive, but only areas that actually touch the plant exhibit a clinical response. Reactions are seen rarely on the palms, soles, and hairy scalp because of the greater physical barrier there present. The severity of response to an equivalent amount of hapten among previously sensitized patients varies greatly, but in a given individual, the degree of response depends on the dose.

Poison ivy (*Toxicodendron radicans*) and Western poison oak (*T. diversilobum*) cause more cases of delayed contact sensitivity than all other known sensitizers combined. Probably 50 percent of the North American population has been sensitized to *Toxicodendron* and another 20 percent may be sensitized. The remaining 30 percent seem to possess genetic, antigen-specific tolerance. Age, sex, and race seem to have little role in the ability to become sensitized to *Toxicodendron,* but certain pathologic conditions (lymphoma, sarcoidosis, atopy) impair sensitization.

After a sensitized individual is reexposed to the hapten, 12 to 48 hours, or more, is required to develop a visible cutaneous response. This delay is an essential element in differential diagnosis. It represents a cell-mediated immune reaction affected by thymus-derived lymphocytes (T cells). The latent period can be shortened by exposure to greater concentrations of hatpen. Erythema and edema appear initially. Pruritus is always present and may be intense. Vesicles form during the subsequent 24 hours; serous fluid in the vesicles does not contain antigen and cannot spread the rash to other parts of the body or to other individuals. There may be marked exudation, but crusting and scaling begin to develop within a few days. In the absence of complications due to excoriation and infection or continued exposure, healing is complete in about ten days.

Toxicodendron dermatitis is managed effectively with corticosteroids. Prevention, however, is an active area for research. Oral hyposensitization is troublesome, affords only partial protection, and is effective for only six months. Two investigational approaches are studies on ring-substituted derivatives of pentadecylcatechol, which may block the immune responses, and induction of tolerance in patients not yet sensitized by intramuscular administration of *Toxicodendron* extracts. The study of delayed contact sensitivity and the role of Langerhans cells in antigen transport and of bone marrow–derived lymphocytes (B-cells) and basophils in the modulation of immune response is being performed currently.

Plants Causing Contact Urticaria

This reaction may be immunologic or nonimmunologic in nature. The latter is more common, but plants have produced both forms. Cutaneous contact induces a transient urticarial or, less frequently, a wheal-and-flare response.

Nettles are an example of plants that cause nonimmunologic contact urticaria. These plants have hollow stinging hairs that inject a chemical after penetration of the skin; a burning sensation and pruritus occur almost immediately. The injected material of the North American nettles, *Urtica urens* and *U. dioica,* has been identified as a mixture of acetylcholine, histamine, and serotonin on the basis of the response of smooth muscle to nettle extract alone and in the presence of antagonists to these substances. The Australian nettle, *Dendrocnide moroides,* also contains these substances, but its activity has been attributed to a thermostable, nondialyzable carbohydrate. Interdermal injection of this material produced piloerection, local vasodilation, sweating, and pain resembling that produced by the nettle. This or a similar material should be sought in the North American species, since injection of an artificial mixture of the known components does not simulate the response to the nettle exactly.

Some individuals develop contact urticaria of the immunologic type after contact with a number of edible vegetables. Scraping the peel from new potatoes, for example, elicits various noncutaneous allergic responses, such as sneezing or wheezing. Other possible reactions are rhinoconjunctivitis, angioedema, gastroenteric disturbances, and anaphylaxis. Although the immunologic basis for this form of contact urticaria can be demonstrated by the Prausnitz-Küstner test (passive serum transfer), little is known of the essential features of sensitization or the chemistry of the antigens.

Plants Causing Phototoxicity

A number of cultivated plants of the carrot family (Umbelliferae), such as parsnips, caraway, dill, and parsley, and the rue family (Rutaceae), which includes the citrus plants, sensitize the skin to long-wave ultraviolet light (UV-A). These plants contain furocoumarins (psoralens), which can penetrate moist skin. Within 6 to 24 hours of contact with the plant and exposure to sunlight or fluorescent light, the area of contact will selectively burn. The reaction ranges from mild erythema to severe damage with bullae, and hyperpigmentation ensues that may persist for several months. Pruritus is minimal. Inflammation can be ameliorated by prostaglandin inhibitors, such as aspirin, or by systemic corticosteroids in severe cases.

The mechanism of phototoxicity is not completely understood. The psoralens are intercalated into DNA, followed by UVA-induced covalent bonding. Hyperpigmentation results from proliferation of functional melanocytes and altered distribution of melanosomes from a nonaggregated to an aggregated state.

Plants Causing Primary Chemical Irritation

These plants contain substances that produce skin damage resembling that from contact with a corrosive acid. The degree of damage depends on the potency of the irritant, its concentration, and exposure time. The reaction varies according to the area of the body exposed and the age of the patient. Genetic factors influence vulnerability, but sex and race appear to have little consistent effect. Physical factors, particularly temperature and humidity, also affect the severity of response.

The spurges, in the family Euphorbiaceae, the buttercups (*Ranunculus* spp.), daphne (*Daphne mezereum*), and wild pepper (*Capsicum frutescens*) are most frequently involved. The most serious reactions involve the eye; severe keratoconjunctivitis with transient blindness may occur. The eye should be irrigated immediately, the pupil should be dilated, and artificial tears instilled. Steroids should be avoided because of the danger of encouraging a fungal infection.

SUMMARY

Many types of plants causing injury have not been discussed, such as those producing hayfever, food allergy, allergic alveolitis, Bud-Chiari syndrome. There also are carcinogenic plants, teratogenic plants, and those that contain estrogen, thyroid-blocking substances, toxic amino acids, or hypoglycemic substances.

A great deal remains to be learned even about the plants that have been summarized. In addition to the research suggested, mechanisms of action should be investigated further. In the past, it was sufficient to identify a toxic plant because it caused hypoglycemia or arrhythmia. How much better it would be if one could identify the biochemical changes that induce the hypoglycemia or the membrane effects that cause the arrhythmia. Such studies will lead to better management of intoxications and, perhaps, to the development of new research tools and therapeutic agents.

ANNOTATED BIBLIOGRAPHY

Human Poisoning by Plants

Common Poisonous and Injurious Plants. HHS Pub. No. (FDA) 81-7006, U.S. Govt. Printing Office, Washington, D.C. This is an inexpensive, color-illustrated bulletin of the most common poisonous and injurious plants in the United States and Canada. It is written primarily for lay readers.

Hardin J. W., and Arena J. M.: *Human Poisoning from Native and Cultivated Plants*, 2nd ed. Duke University Press, Durham, N.C., 1974. This book is intended primarily for parents, camp and school counselors, and scout leaders.

Lampe, K. F., and McCann, M. A.: *AMA Handbook of Poisonous and Injurious Plants*. Chicago Review Press, Chicago, 1985. Although intended to provide physicians and other health professionals with an easily used reference for the management of plant intoxications, the format and color photographs make it a useful field guide for the recognition of dangerous and injurious plants.

Pammel, L. H.: *Manual of Poisonous Plants*. Torch Press, Cedar Rapids Iowa, 1910; a Xerox reproduction is available from University Microfilms, Ann Arbor, Mich. This encyclopedic work is a frequent help concerning an inquiry about a plant not discussed in more recent, but slimmer, compilations.

Veterinary Plant Poisoning

Kingsbury, J. M.: *Poisonous Plants of the United States and Canada*. Prentice-Hall, New York, 1964. This is the standard textbook for veterinary students.

Poisonous Mushrooms

Lampe, K. F.: Toxic fungi. *Annu. Rev. Pharmacol. Toxicol.*, **19**:85–104, 1979.

Lincoff, G., and Mitchel, D. H.: *Toxic and Hallucinogenic Mushroom Poisoning*. Van Nostrand Reinhold, New York, 1977.

Rumack, B. H., and Salzman, E. (eds): *Mushroom Poisoning Diagnosis and Treatment*. CRC Press, Boca Raton, Fl., 1978.

Plant Dermatitis

Fisher, A. A.: *Contact Dermatitis*, 2nd ed. Lea & Febiger, Philadelphia, 1973. This is the best introduction to the subject. A third edition is in production (1986).

Mitchell, J., and Rook, A.: *Botanical Dermatology: Plants and Plant Products Injurious to the Skin*. Greengrass, Vancouver, 1979. This is a worldwide encyclopedia with a bibliography provided individually for each species.

Stoner, J. G., and Rasmussen, J. E.: Plant dermatitis. *J. Am. Acad. Dermatol.*, **9**:1–15, 1983.

Hallucinogenic Plant Poisoning

Schultes, R. E., and Hofmann, A: *Botany and Chemistry of Hallucinogens*, 2nd ed. Charles C Thomas, Pub., Springfield, Ill., 1980. This is a definitive treatment of this selected subject.

Chronic Plant Poisoning

Liener, I. E. (ed.): *Toxic Constituents of Plants Foodstuffs*. Academic Press, Inc., New York, 1980.

Rechcigl, M. Jr. Inc., (ed.): *Handbook of Naturally Occurring Food Toxicants*. CRC Press, Boca Raton, Fl., 1983.

Toxicants Occuring Naturally in Foods, 2nd ed. National Academy of Sciences, Washington, D.C., 1973.

Important Foreign Sources on Plant Toxicology

Chopra, R. N.; Badhwar, R. L.; and Ghosh, S.: *Poisonous Plants of India*, 2 vols. Indian Council of Agricultural Research, New Delhi, 1965.

Connor, H. E.: *Poisonous Plants in New Zealand*, 2nd ed. E. C. Keating, Wellington, 1977.

Everist, S. L.: *Poisonous Plants of Australia*. Angus & Robertson, Sydney, 1974.

Frohne, D., and Pfänder, H. J.: *A Color Atlas of Poisonous Plants: A Handbook for Pharmacists, Doctors, Toxicologists, and Biologists*. Wolfe House, London, 1983.

Watt, J. M., and Breyer-Brandwijk, M. G.: *Medicinal and Poisonous Plants of Southern and Eastern Africa*. E. & S. Livingstone, Edinburgh, 1962.

UNIT IV
ENVIRONMENTAL TOXICOLOGY

Chapter 24

FOOD ADDITIVES AND CONTAMINANTS

Johnnie R. Hayes and *T. Colin Campbell*

INTRODUCTION

A major concern of individual humans and human societies has been and is the attainment of sufficient quantities of food to provide a healthful and productive life. Historically, the major expenditure of time and effort, on both an individual and a societal basis, has been the pursuit of an adequate food supply. It is only after significant progress toward the attainment of this goal is realized that the energies of societies can be devoted to progress in other areas. In fact, a major impetus to the formation of groups and societies with individual interactivity has been the division of labor to allow certain segments of the population to pursue nonfood production tasks. As agricultural methodology developed and food-producing animals were domesticated, a smaller number of individuals within the population needed to be engaged in direct food production, allowing not only the number of individuals within the group to increase, but also a diversification of skills within the group.

Seasonal climatic conditions resulted in an abundance of food during the harvest period, but inadequate food supplies during the remainder of the year. This placed a limit on the number of individuals that a particular territory could support. To ensure an adequate food supply during nonagriculturally productive periods, it was necessary to find methods to preserve the abundant food available at harvest time and the game collected during the peak hunting periods. To meet this requirement, methods employing the addition of various substances to food were developed. Among the first substances added to food as preservatives were sodium chloride, which is still a major preservative, and smoke. Processes were developed by which various spices could be used not only to aid in the preservation of food but also to disguise the unacceptable flavor of inadequately preserved foods. The search for chemicals useful in preserving foods and increasing the palatability of preserved foods continues today. This practice has become more important as the percentage of the population in the United States involved in agricultural production has decreased to the present level of 5 percent, particularly when this division of labor is compared with the increases in population and the trend toward the development of large population centers.

Cultural mores also affect the types and amounts of various substances to be found in foods. A food that is considered a delicacy in one culture may be taboo in another. The accepted appearance, color, texture, and flavor of a food are often defined by both experience and cultural tastes. The utilization of various substances during processing to maintain these organoleptic characteristics is therefore important in maintaining an acceptable food supply, even, perhaps, at the expense of a portion of the nutritional value.

Over the last several decades, developed societies have undergone many life-style changes that have led to an increase in the addition of various substances to food for technologic purposes. Processed foods now represent over 50 percent of the American diet. For instance, the annual per capita consumption of fresh citrus fruits decreased from 32 to 28 lb between 1960 and 1976, whereas consumption of processed fruit increased from 50 to 90 lb. Soft-drink consumption more than doubled during the same time period (National Academy of Sciences, 1978). Several trends, such as the increased demand for "ready-to-eat" and snack foods, the population shift from rural to urban areas, the interest in ethnic foods, the demand for a constant, year-round supply of seasonal foods, and the demand for stable and low food prices, have increased the utilization and need for the addition of various substances to food (President's Science Advisory Committee, 1973). The trend toward the increased use of various substances added for technologic purposes, coupled with the public demand for an essentially risk-free food supply, has increased both the scientific and public debate over the safety of these materials added to food. In addition, the development of toxicologic methodology with increased sensitivity has further emphasized the concern over these substances. These factors have emphasized the necessity for a logical, rational, and scientific approach to the regulation of these materials in the food supply. Decisions in this area not only impact on public health but also have economic impact on both the food industry and the consumer.

Any restricted discussion of food additives and contaminants must be limited in scope by time and length. Therefore, the authors have attempted to present a general discussion, emphasizing areas that they feel are important. We realize that we have inadequately covered certain areas and have not discussed certain controversies and controversial chemicals in detail. It has been our goal to introduce the student to the basic concepts associated with food additives and contaminants with the hope that the student will pursue the area in more depth by consideration of other sources.

DEFINITIONS OF FOOD ADDITIVES

Chemicals that are added to food are generally termed "food additives." However, exactly what is meant by this term is a source of some controversy. Food additives may be defined in legalistic terms, in terms associated with their technical use, and in terms associated with consumer understanding. Therefore, it is important for the toxicologist to understand the meaning of these definitions in order to aid in the resolution of these controversies and to aid in consumer understanding of the benefits and risks associated with food additives.

Legal Definition of Food Additives

In the United States at the turn of the twentieth century, laws concerning the sanitary aspects and adulteration of foods were under the control of the individual states. Such laws lacked uniformity in context and enforcement. Therefore, in the early 1900s Dr. Harvey W. Wiley led a campaign for the passage and enforcement of uniform laws concerned with food safety. His various interests included the control of chemicals such as boric acid, salicyclic acid, and formaldehyde utilized as food preservatives. His efforts led to the congressional passage of the original Food and Drug Act of 1906, along with the Meat Inspection Act. Generally, this Act prohibited the addition of poisonous preservatives and dyes to food and prohibited misbranded and adulterated foods and drinks in interstate commerce. Since the original 1906 Food

and Drug Act, the legislation has been expanded and ammended several times, most notably in 1938, 1958, and 1962. The current legal definition of food additives may be found within this legislation. The Federal Food, Drug and Cosmetic Act, as amended in October 1976, Sec. 201(s) states:

"The term "food additive' means any substance the intended use of which results or may reasonably be expected to result, directly or indirectly, in its becoming a component or otherwise affecting the characteristics of any food (including any substance intended for use in producing, manufacturing, packing, processing, preparing, treating, packaging, transporting, or holding food; and including any source of radiation intended for any such use), if such substance is not generally recognized, among experts qualified by scientific training and experience to evaluate its safety, as having been adequately shown through scientific procedures (or, in the case of a substance used in food prior to January 1, 1958, through either scientific procedures or experience based on common use in food) to be safe under the conditions of its intended use; except that such term does not include:
(1) a pesticide chemical in or on a raw agricultural commodity; or
(2) a pesticide chemical to the extent that it is intended for use or is used in the production, storage, or transportation of any raw agricultural commodity; or
(3) a color additive; or
(4) any substance used in accordance with a sanction or approval granted prior to the enactment of this paragraph . . . pursuant to this Act, the Poultry Products Inspection Act . . . or the Meat Inspection Act; or
(5) a new animal drug."

As can be seen, the legal definition of food additives is initiated with a comprehensive statement concerning "any substance" that by its "intended use" could become "a component or otherwise affecting the characteristics of any food." However, what follows confuses the issue by exempting (1) pesticides, (2) color additives, (3) prior-sanctioned substances approved before the 1958 Food, Drug and Cosmetic Act, (4) new animal drugs, and (5) substances "generally regarded as safe" (GRAS). The exemptions to the legal definition are covered by specific sections of the law and will be discussed below. The legal definition of food additives can be confusing and lead to misunderstandings without complete consideration for the various laws that are concerned with food safety.

Technical Definition of Food Additives

The technical definition of food additives is generally more broad than the legal definition and can be exemplified by the definition utilized by the Food Protection Committee of the Food and Nutrition Board of the National Academy of Sciences: "A substance or mixture of substances other than a basic foodstuff which is present in a food as a result of any aspect of production, processing, storage or packaging" (National Academy of Sciences, 1979). Technically, food additives are divided into two major categories based on the terminology used in the legal definition. Those substances that are intentionally added to a food directly during production, etc., for a functional purpose are termed "direct or intentional food additives." The second category consists of the "indirect or nonintentional food additives" that are not intentionally added to food, but result from either the environment of food production or processing and storage. According to this definition, a pesticide used during the agricultural production of food, a machine oil from a processing machine, and a plasticizer that leaches from a package would all be considered indirect food additives. The concept of food contaminants is somewhat different from that of indirect additives. Although indirect additives may be considered as contaminants, thus blurring the dividing line between these two groups, a category of contaminants is nonetheless important from the aspect of food safety. Contaminants consist of those substances which may become a part of food during production, processing, and storage owing generally to natural processes. They include such substances as nitrate, selenium, and lead, which may be incorporated into plants grown in soil with unusually high levels of these chemicals, fungal metabolites produced from mold growth during production, processing, and storage, and bacteria and bacterial products. The products of food chemical reactions, such as oxidized lipids contained in cooking oil, may also be included in this category. Contaminants may be considered as a "catchall" category containing miscellaneous substances that are not included as direct and indirect additives.

Consumer Perceptions of Food Additives

The consuming public does not appear to have a precise definition of food additives because of their changing perceptions about these substances. Concern about food additives can be unpredictable and illogical. For instance, when the artificial sweetener saccharin was to be banned because of its potential carcinogenicity, there was a public outcry for its continued use in soft drinks and other foods in order to decrease caloric intake (Anonymous, 1978). In contrast, there appears to be a general fear of low levels of noncarcinogenic pesticide residues in food, even though through the use of pesticides there may be a greater availability of food at lower cost. Public attitudes appear to shift between concern and apathy about food additives depending on the activity of consumer activist groups and the media. Other factors contributing to public concern about food additives include the expanded labeling information on food products, governmental action in this area, and continuing scientific controversies concerning specific additives such as nitrite and saccharin. Adding additional weight to these concerns are the "back-to-nature" groups, which exhort the benefits of natural foods grown with organic fertilizers and containing no "additives" and their claims of the adverse effects of foods containing additives and "artificial" nutritional supplements. The public concern about food additives is continuing as evidenced by discussions in the popular press and other communication media. Recently, computer programs have become available that allow the comsumer not only to undertake nutrient analyses, but also to estimate the contents of food additives. It is obviously important that the public receives adequate information on the benefits as well as the risks from food additives.

Utilization of Direct (Intentional) Food Additives

As previously discussed, the use of direct food additives predates recorded history when meats and fish were smoked and salted for preservation. The Romans made extensive use of salt as a preservative and, until recently, the use of potassium nitrate (saltpeter) was widespread. Also, during the Middle Ages spices from the Orient became an important category of food additives and were used not only to alter and enhance the flavor of certain foods, but to preserve food and disguise the flavor of spoiled foods (Tannahill, 1973).

As part of the industrial revolution in the latter half of the nineteenth century, the fledgling food industry developed. The availability of roads and improved transportation and the development of highly populated industrial centers were as important to the development of the food industry as was the development of processing equipment. The development of the food industry brought along with it the increased adulteration of food and an increase in the use of various food additives. Certain of these food additives, such as acorns in coffee and brick dust in cocoa, were added as filler to increase profits. Others represented significant health risk, such as the use of copper and lead salts to color foods such as candy and cheeses (Tannahill, 1973). The development of laboratory analysis of foods emphasized the need for food regulation and aided in the passage of the Food and Drug Act of 1906.

Currently there may be as many as 2800 substances used as direct food additives (Lehmann, 1974). The vast majority of these additives are used in trace amounts and only a few represent those used in large quantities. The FDA has estimated that sucrose, corn syrup, dextrose, and salt represent 93 percent, by weight, of the total food additives used. The inclusions of black pepper, caramel, carbon dioxide, citric acid, modified starch, sodium bicarbonate, yeasts, and yellow mustard brings this figure up to 95 percent (Larkin, 1976).

Main Groups

The direct food additives are utilized by the food industry for a variety of technical effects. Below are listed the five main groups of direct food additives and the various categories of additives within each major group:

Processing Aids. These additives are intended to aid in the processing of foods during production and after purchase by the consumer and are exemplified by—anticaking agents, dough conditioners, drying agents, emulsifiers, various enzymes, flour-treating agents, formulation aids, humectants, leavening agents, lubricants, pH control agents, solvents and vehicles, surface-active agents, and various synergists.

Texturing Agents. These additives are provided in order to give specific foods a desirable consistency and texture—various enzymes, firming agents, formulation aids and binders, stabilizers and thickeners, aerating agents, and texturizers.

Preservatives. These additives are utilized to decrease the rate of degradation of foods during processing and storage—antioxidants, curing and pickling agents, antibacterials, gases, and sequestrants that react with various food components, i.e., metals that promote instability.

Flavoring and Appearance Agents. These additives are used either to enhance existing flavors or to add flavor to foods, and to improve the appearance—flavor enhancers, flavoring agents, nonnutritive sweeteners, and surface-finishing agents such as waxes.

Nutritional Supplements. These additives include the required nutrients and are added either to replace those lost during processing or to supplement existing levels of nutrients. They may consist of varied analogs of macronutrients and micronutrients, including vitamins and trace minerals.

The colors have been purposefully excluded from this listing since they are regulated as a separate group and will be discussed later.

The various additives within these major groups and categories vary from simple salts, such as sodium chloride, to complex biologic polymers, such as starches, and various synthetic chemicals, such as ethyl vanillin. A partial listing of some of these agents is given in Table 24–1 to illustrate the diversity of chemicals utilized as food additives.

Standardization

As can be seen, the direct food additives consist of a diverse grouping of chemical substances. One of the first problems encountered in a discussion of specific additives, especially the natural products of biologic origin, is exactly what are we talking about? This may seem like a simple question, but when one considers the potential composition of a complex biologic product such as gum arabic, which may contain various biologic molecules that coextract with the desired product and the variable composition of a particular additive as the source and manufacturer of the additive varies, the question becomes quite complex. This can be a problem with the synthetic additives also, which may contain variable impurities depending on the manufacturing process. To overcome these problems and to introduce specific specifications to ensure the purity and uniformity of food additives, the U.S. Food and Drug Administration requires information on the physical, chemical, biologic, and purity characteristics as well as the source and method of manufacture. As standards for food grade additives, the FDA relies on either specifications written into its own regulations or those present in the Food Chemicals Codex. The Food Chemicals Codex is a compilation of specifications for food-grade products used as food additives compiled by the Committee on Food Protection of the National Academy of Sciences (National Academy of Sciences, 1972). These specifications ensure uniform standardization of food additives manufactured and utilized by different food processors, thus providing some measure of assurance of food quality and safety.

UTILIZATION OF INDIRECT (NONINTENTIONAL) FOOD ADDITIVES

Indirect food additives consist of the class of substances that are not natural constituents of food and have not been added to food for a tech-

Table 24–1.   SELECTED FOOD ADDITIVES*

Anticaking Agents

Aluminum calcium silicate
Sodium aluminosilicate
Sodium calcium aluminosilicate

Chemical Preservatives

Ascorbic acid
Ascorbyl palmitate
Butylated hydroxyanisole
Calcium propionate
Dilauryl thiodipropionate
Erythorbic acid
Methylparaben
Potassium sorbate
Propionic acid
Propylparaben
Sodium bisulfite
Sodium metabisulfite
Sodium sulfite
Stannous chloride
Sulfur dioxide
Tocopherols

Emulsifying Agents

Cholic acid
Desoxycholic acid
Glycocholic acid
Mono- and diglycerides
Propylene glycol
Ox bile extract

Nutrients and Dietary Supplements

Alanine
Arginine
Aspartic acid
Biotin
Calcium citrate
Calcium pantothenate
Carotene
Choline chloride
Copper gluconate
Cysteine
Cystine
Ferric pyrophosphate
Ferrous lactate
Histidine
Inositol
Isoleucine
Leucine
Lysine
Magnesium oxide
Manganese gluconate
Manganous oxide
Methionine
Niacinamide
d-Pantothenyl alcohol
Potassium glycerophosphate
Proline
Pyridoxine hydrochloride

Riboflavin-5-phosphate
Serine
Sorbitol
Thiamine mononitrate
Threonine
Tocopherol acetate
Tryptophane
Valine
Vitamin A
Vitamin B_{12}
Vitamin D_3
Zinc sulfate

Sequestrants

Calcium acetate
Calcium gluconate
Calcium phytate
Dipotassium phosphate
Disodium phosphate
Monoisopyropyl citrate
Potassium citrate
Sodium diacetate
Sodium hexametaphosphate
Sodium metaphosphate
Sodium potassium tartrate
Sodium pyrophosphate
Sodium tartrate
Sodium thiosulfate
Stearyl citrate
Tartaric acid

Stabilizers

Acacia (gum arabic)
Agar-agar
Calcium alginate
Carob bean gum
Ghatti gum
Guar gum
Sterculia (or Karaya) gum

Miscellaneous Additives

Acetic acid
Adipic acid
Aluminum potassium sulfate
Ammonium bicarbonate
Bentonite
Butane
Calcium gluconate
Calcium hydroxide
Calcium phosphate
Carnauba wax
Dextrans
Ethyl formate
Glutamic acid hydrochloride
Glycerin
Helium
Hydrochloric acid
Lactic acid
Lecithin

* Modified from Kilgore, W. W., and Li, M. Y.: Food additives and contaminants. In Doull, F.; Klaassen, C. D.; and Amdur, M. O. (eds.): *Casarett and Doull's Toxicology: The Basic Science of Poisons.* Macmillan Publishing Co., Inc., New York, 1980, pp. 593–607.

Table 24–1.   (*continued*)

Magnesium hydroxide	Triacetine
Malic acid	Triethyl citrate
Methylcellulose	
Monopotassium glutamate	*Synthetic Flavoring Substances*
Nitrogen	Acetaldehyde
Papain	Acetoin
Phosphoric acid	Benzaldehyde
Potassium hydroxide	*d*- or *l*-carvone
Propylene glycol	Cinnamaldehyde
Rennet	Decanal
Sodium acid pyrophosphate	Ethyl butyrate
Sodium carboxymethylcellulose	Geraniol
Sodium caseinate	Geranyl acetate
Sodium hydroxide	Limonene
Sodium pectinate	Linalool
Sodium sesquicarbonate	Methylanthranilate
Succinic acid	Piperonal
Sulfuric acid	Vanillin

nological purpose. These substances may become a constituent of food from a variety of sources, including the environment in which the food is produced, during processing and storage at manufacturing sites, and during subsequent packaging and storage. The total number of individual substances is unknown and may rapidly change as processing technologies change. The National Science Foundation (1973) has estimated that food packaging may contribute close to 3000 substances to the indirect additive category. A major aim of both the food production industry and the regulatory agencies is to decrease the number of indirect additives that occur in food and to ensure that those which cannot currently be eliminated are present at levels that do not represent a risk to consumers.

Table 24–2 lists potential sources of indirect food additives and examples of the categories of substances found at each source. Several of these categories are discussed in other chapters of this text, whereas other categories, such as processing aids, are well known only by food technologists and packaging experts.

UTILIZATION OF ANIMAL DRUGS

Drugs are employed in food-producing animals for two major purposes: veterinary pharmaceuticals and feed additives. These compounds represent a wide diversity in chemical structure and biologic activity. They differ from food additives in that they are designed to be pharmaceutically active in the consuming animal. Both types of drugs have the potential to become incorporated into animal products and tissues destined for human consumption. Thus

their risk to human health must be evaluated (Committee on Animal Health, 1980).

With respect to potential exposure to consumers, the veterinary pharmaceuticals used to treat specific animal diseases generally represent a lower potential for exposure than do the feed additives. These agents are normally used

Table 24–2. SOURCES OF NONINTENTIONAL ADDITIVES OF POSSIBLE TOXICOLOGIC SIGNIFICANCE*

During Production

1. Antibiotics and other agents used for prevention and control of disease
2. Growth-promoting substances
3. Microorganisms of toxicologic significance
4. Parasitic organisms
5. Pesticides residues (insecticides, fungicides, herbicides, etc.)
6. Toxic metals and metallic compounds
7. Radioactive compounds

During Processing

1. Microorganisms and their toxic metabolites
2. Processing residues and miscellaneous foreign objects
3. Radionuclides

During Packaging and Storage

1. Labeling and stamping materials
2. Microorganisms and their toxic metabolites
3. Migrants from packaging materials
4. Toxic chemicals from external sources

* Modified from Kilgore, W. W., and Li, M. Y.: Food additives and contaminants. In Doull, J.; Klaassen, C. D.; and Amdur, M. O. (eds.): *Casarett and Doull's Toxicology: The Basic Science of Poisons.* Macmillan Publishing Co., Inc., New York, 1980, pp. 593–607.

for specific animals, and their use is sporadic. This increases the opportunity for clearance from the animal before marketing. Although products produced by animals undergoing treatment may contain drug residues, it is generally simple and of little economic loss to withhold these products during the treatment period. In terms of total usage, veterinary pharmaceuticals are not used as frequently as the feed additives, thereby presenting less potential for routine human exposure.

The case is quite different with respect to drugs utilized as feed additives. It has been estimated that nearly 100 percent of poultry, 90 percent of swine and veal calves, and 60 percent of cattle receive feed supplemented with antibacterials, and 70 percent of the beef cattle produced in the United States have received growth-promoting drugs to increase weight gain (Office of Technology Assessment, 1979). At least 80 percent of the animal protein consumed in the American diet comes from animals exposed to medicated feeds for at least part of their lives (President's Science Advisory Committee, 1973). These drugs are important in maintaining the production levels of animal products and tissues at a cost that ensures their availability to the consumer and also in maintaining the quality of these products. Along with the benefits afforded by animal drugs comes the risk of potential toxicity associated with consumption of drug residues in animal products and tissue.

A unique problem in the determination of the potential human health hazards associated with animal drugs is the probability that animal metabolism will modify the molecular structure and toxicity of the drug (Hayes and Borzelleca, 1982). As previously discussed in Chapter 4, animals have the capacity to biotransform drugs to a large number of metabolites with diverse molecular structures and toxicity. The cytochrome P-450-dependent monooxygenase systems generally convert drugs to oxidized products, which may demonstrate decreased toxicity by their increased water solubility. The transferase enzymes conjugate the drug and/or its metabolites with endogenous molecules and increase their excretability and modify their structure to produce products that are generally less toxic. However, these same enzymes may convert drugs and other xenobiotics to products that demonstrate increased biologic activity and toxicity. In some instances products of these reactions possess sufficient reactivity to covalently bind to tissue macromolecules. Animal products and tissues may therefore contain not only the parent drug, but also metabolites including both conjugated and nonconjugated forms and resi-

dues that are either tightly bound or covalently bound to tissue macromolecules. Although it might be assumed that the animal acts as a "predetoxication" system for these drug residues, this is not always the case. These drug metabolites, after consumption, may still be converted into more toxic products. For example, if a drug is present as the detoxified glucuronide conjugate in the animal product, it may subsequently be hydrolyzed by the consumer's intestinal microflora β-glucuronidase, thus freeing the original drug metabolite for absorption. The quantity of drug residues in a particular product or tissue will depend on their pharmacokinetic characteristics within the consuming animal. The absorption and retention of these residues in the tissues of consumers will subsequently be dependent on their pharmacokinetic characteristics within the consuming human.

Most mutagenicity and carcinogenicity is thought to result from highly reactive electrophilic metabolites of less biologically active parent compounds. It might be assumed that these activated metabolites would be a serious threat as tissue residues. However, this is probably not the case. The high reactivity and short half-lives of these metabolites would result in little chance of encountering them in animal products owing to their rapid covalent binding to tissue macromolecules. Even if they existed in the animal at the time of sacrifice, they would either spontaneously decompose or interact with nucleophilic sites during processing and storage. Activated metabolites that have become covalently bound to tissue macromolecules would, in most instances, represent little human health hazard since the covalent binding alters their structure and subsequent digestion of the macromolecular fractions would not release these compounds in an activated form. For example, the feeding of hepatic macromolecule fractions obtained from rats fed aflatoxin B_1 and containing covalent adducts of aflatoxin B_1 to rats produced no evidence of the production of adducts in the second set of rats (Jaggi et al., 1980).

It would be extremely rare to encounter drug residues in animal products and tissues at concentrations that are high enough to elicit acutely toxic symptoms in the consumer. However, residue levels sufficient to produce chronic toxicity could be encountered. Because carcinogenicity is the type of chronic toxicity of most concern, the section of the Food, Drug and Cosmetic Act concerning animal feed additives contains its own "Delaney Clause." This prohibits approval of a new animal drug if it "induces cancer when ingested by man or animal." The act continues by adding "unless no residue of such drug will be found (by methods of examination prescribed or approved by the Secretary . . .), in any edible portion of such animals after slaughter or in any food yielded by or derived from the living animals." Therefore, it is possible to use drugs in animals that have been shown to be carcinogenic as long as no detectable residues occur in animal products or tissues. Withholding animals and animal products from market for specific periods during and after drug treatment to allow for dissipation of the drug from the animal body appeared to solve the problem encountered with certain drugs, such as the growth promoter diethylstilbesterol. However, recent improvements in analytic methodology have allowed for the detection of smaller quantities of drug residues in animal tissues. In 1973 the FDA proposed regulations further defining the no-residue requirement, which was, of course, based on the existing methodology at that time. This proposal has now been replaced by a new proposal which was issued in 1979 and which interprets the regulation according to the "sensitivity of method." This proposal is based on the more realistic concept that, since absolute food safety is impossible, the determination of allowable residue levels should be based on an estimate of a negligible lifetime risk of cancer in humans as, for example, with an estimate of one chance in a million. The methodology is then selected in order to estimate drug residues associated with this negligible risk level. As analytic methods are improved to detect still lower residue levels, it is therefore not necessary to alter the regulations concerning specific drug residues. This argument ignores the controversy of what type benefit is acceptable. That would require a much more extensive discussion, which is not appropriate for this chapter. A discussion of benefit-risk analysis associated with food chemicals can be found in the article by Campbell (1980).

The use of antibiotics as animal feed additives involves a new concern not related to toxicologic response. Antibiotics are added to animal food as a prophylaxis against disease and, as such, appear to promote the growth of animals. Almost all poultry in the United States and a large percentage of cattle and swine are fed feeds containing antibiotics. These antibiotics may become residues in animal products and tissues. The concern expressed by some is the possibility that their use will lead to the development of antibiotic-resistant strains of bacteria, thus eroding the ability of specific antibiotics to be of use in the treatment of human disease (National Academy of Sciences, 1980). The FDA has proposed that the prophylactic use of the penicillins in animal feeds be stopped and the tetracyclines be used only where there are no substitutes.

UTILIZATION OF FOOD COLORS

Nature abounds in color and, as a result, human foods generally are colorful. Certain foods are recognized not only by their shape and texture, but also by their color. In many instances the quality and acceptability of a food are judged not only by texture, taste, and smell but also by color. If a food that society and experience have defined as having a particular color, hue, and intensity lacks these characteristics, it will be unacceptable, even if wholesome. Colors also make food more interesting and appealing, as evidenced by colored confections and drinks.

The use of both natural and synthetic colors to enhance, alter, and produce expected and appealing colors in foods dates far back in history. The Egyptians utilized colors in candy, and Pliny the elder discussed artificially colored wines around 400 B.C. Historically, the major problem associated with food colors has been their use to deceive potential consumers as to the quality of the food and the toxic nature of certain of the color agents. For instance, in the eighteenth century copper sulfate was used to color pickles green, cheeses were colored with vermillion (HgS) and red lead, used tea leaves were dyed for resale with agents such as copper arsenite, lead chromate, and indigo, and candies were dyed with lead chromate and carbamate as well as red lead and vermillion. At the turn of the century in England milk was tinted yellow to prevent the detection of skimming and watering. The practice was so widespread that the public refused to purchase untinted milk for fear that it was adulterated. In 1925 the tinting of milk was made illegal in Britain, long after the 1396 edict in Paris banning the tinting of butter. The major sources of dyes for food coloring were natural biologic pigments and various-colored mineral salts until the advent of synthetic dyes in the mideighteenth century. At the turn of the century many of the synthetic dyes were being used in a large number of foods to produce the desired color. These dyes were blended in various ways to produce assorted hues and intensities. Various dyes of the same hue were employed because a single dye does not always produce the same effect in different foods.

Although the use of colors in food had been sporadically regulated, the first attempt at developing systematic regulations on the use of dyes in food was initiated by the U.S. Department of Agriculture. The responsibility for determining the usage and public health risk of the synthetic dyes was given to Dr. Bernhard C. Hesse. He found that, of the 695 coal-tar dyes on the market at that time, only 80 were used as food colors. After consideration of the available literature on the toxicity of the compounds and the needs of the food industry, Hesse selected the following seven dyes for food use: amarath (red 2), erythrosine (red 3), indigo disulfonic acid (blue 2), light green SF yellowish (green 2), naphthol yellow S (yellow 1), poceau 3R (red 1), and orange 1 (red 1). (The notations following the dyes are the FDA denotations given the dyes in 1938.) Other colors and various hues and intensities were obtained by combinations of these seven compounds. These dyes were recognized under the Pure Food and Drug Act of 1906, and dyes could be certified (chemically tested) by the Secretary of Agriculture on a voluntary basis. Between 1916 and 1929 ten additional colors were added to the approved list. The Federal Food, Drug and Cosmetic Act of 1938 required that all food colors be "harmless" and listed those coal-tar derived colors approved for food use as well as specifications as to manufacture, certification, and sale. In the early 1950s the FDA initiated a series of toxicity studies and the term "harmless" was refined to mean the color would produce no "harm" to test animals *in any quantity* and under *any conditions*. This led to the banning of eight FDC colors between 1956 and 1960 and the realization that this interpretation would result in the banning of all food colors and was toxicologically unsound. Passage of the Color Additive Amendments of 1960 to the Food and Drug Act allowed the FDA to overcome this problem by setting safe levels or tolerances on the quantity of color used in foods. The amendments also brought all synthetic colors under the provisions of the law, not just the coal-tar-derived colors. They required that all new colors undergo premarketing toxicity testing and allowed the FDA to require new testing of previously approved colors if any questions concerning their safety arose. A safety factor of 100 to 1 was suggested in extrapolating no-adverse-effects levels obtained in animal studies to humans. Provisional certification was given to those colors in use pending more comprehensive toxicity testing. More recently, the FDA has determined that the provisional-listing status of the food colors is to be eliminated. This means that a color must either be permanently listed or prohibited from use. The FDA has asked industry to retest all the approved food colors. These studies are currently nearing completion and should clarify the future use of food colors and will result in the colors being the most intensely tested group of additives.

Utilization of food colors is still controversial with certain groups claiming that synthetic colors should not be added to foods since they serve no purpose other than aesthetic and increase the human xenobiotic burden. On the other hand, others feel that the aesthetic values they serve far outweigh any supposed risk. For instance, a colorless grape-flavored drink would lose much of its appeal, and margarine the color of lard would be less appetizing. There is little question that the use of colors increases the appeal of certain foods, and as long as food is judged visually, the use of colors will be important.

Although the synthetic food colors have received the majority of public, scientific, and regulatory attention, the natural color agents are receiving increased attention. Currently, approximately 25 color additives have been given exemption from certification in Part 73 of the Code of Federal Regulations. These agents consist of a variety of natural and a few synthetic compounds generally obtained by various extraction and treatment technologies and in a few cases by chemical synthesis. Comprising this group of colors are preparations such as dried algae meal, beet powder, grape skin extract, fruit juice, paprika, caramel, carrot oil, cochineal extract, ferrous gluconate, and iron oxide. A problem encountered in attempts to regulate these additives is the lack of a precise chemical definition of many of these preparations. For instance, cochineal extract is defined as the aqueous-alcoholic extract of the scale insect *Dactylopius coccus costa*. The females of this species contain a bright-red body fluid containing high levels of carminic acid. With a few exceptions, such as caramel, actually the most widely used color, the natural colors have not been heavily used. In part, this may be due to economic reasons, but these colors generally do not have the intensity of color characteristic of the synthetic colors, therefore necessitating higher concentrations to obtain a specific color intensity. They also lack the chemical and color stability of the synthetic colors and have a tendency to fade with time.

Colors are added to foods during processing for several reasons including (1) to add color when the food has no color of its own, such as gelatins, candies, and certain beverages; (2) when the natural color of a food is lost during processing and storage; (3) when the natural color of a food varies with respect to season and geography, such as dairy products and oranges; and (4) to correlate foods with certain flavors and increase their attractiveness, thereby increasing their aesthetic value.

Although intake varies among individuals, the

maximal intake of food colors is estimated to be approximately 53.5 mg/day, whereas the *average* intake per day is approximately 15 mg (Committee on Food Protection, 1971). Only about 10 percent of food consumed in the United States contains food colors. Those foods which utilize food colors in order of quality of color utilized are: (1) beverages; (2) candy and confections; (3) dessert powders; (4) bakery goods; (5) sausage (casing only); (6) cereals; (7) ice cream; (8) snack foods; and (9) gravies, jams, jellies, etc. (Committee on Food Protection, 1971). Controversies over the utilization of food colors will continue, even if toxicologic studies prove as conclusively as currently possible that they have little potential for harm when utilized according to good manufacturing practices. With the exception of certain dairy products, the inclusion of artificial colors in foods must be listed on the label, giving the consumer the option of either using or not using the food product.

OCCURRENCE OF PESTICIDES IN FOODS

Pesticides are not added directly to foods, but may indirectly become components of food. The use of pesticides is said to be an important contributing factor to the agricultural revolution, resulting in an increased quantity and quality of food. Associated with the benefits from their use are the risk of adverse health effects from residues that become components of the food supply. Pesticides can occur not only in plant materials destined for human and animal consumption, but also in animal products and tissues. Major sources of pesticides in the food supply are derived from their use in protecting plants from pest damage during both growth and storage. Residues may also appear in animal products and tissues from animals fed feeds contaminated with pesticides. A more extensive discussion of pesticides can be found in Chapter 18.

Section 408 of the Food, Drug and Cosmetic Act sets forth regulations for "tolerances for pesticide chemicals in or on raw agricultural commodities." Pesticides can be regulated in one of three ways: (1) a total ban on the use of a particular pesticide and zero residue levels in foods; (2) tolerances that are acceptable in foods; and (3) action levels stipulating the maximal level that can occur in food. Since tolerances are generally given only to substances whose allowable levels will probably not be changed in the near future, pesticides are generally regulated as action levels. To set action levels, regulators must consider not only the quantities of a specific pesticide that may occur in food, but also the quantities that may come from other environmental sources. A benefit-risk analysis is also required for the determination of action levels.

As with animal drugs, the major consideration in the regulation of pesticides is their potential carcinogenicity. That concern is relevant because, as with many carcinogens, a regular low level of consumption is the usual manner in which chemical carcinogens elicit their effects. Acute toxicity from the consumption of food contaminated with pesticides is rare. Such effects are produced primarily from the careless or accidental use of pesticides.

REGULATION OF FOOD ADDITIVES

A comprehensive discussion of the regulations involved with the use of food additives is well beyond the scope of this chapter. Only a minimal discussion of the regulations is therefore provided.

As previously mentioned, the first national law concerning food safety was provided by the Pure Food and Drug Act of 1906. In 1938, the Act was revamped by Congress as the Food, Drug and Cosmetic Act. In 1954, the Miller Pesticides Amendment, which controlled the requirements for setting safety limits for pesticide residues on raw agricultural commodities, was passed. In 1958, the Food Additive Amendment (Public Law 85-929) was added. This new amendment forbade the utilization of a substance as a food additive until the petitioner, or sponsor, provided evidence for its safety and the FDA specified the conditions for use of the substance as a food additive. This amendment also states that only the minimal quantity of a food additive that is needed to produce the desired technologic effect can be added to food and no additive that could result in consumer deception can be added.

Another clause of the 1958 Amendment (often called the Delaney Amendment) deals with food additives that may be carcinogenic. The so-called Delaney Clause states: "That no additive shall be deemed to be safe if it is found to induce cancer when ingested by man or animal, or if it is found, after tests which are appropriate for the evaluation of the safety of food additives, to induce cancer in man or animal . . . " (Federal Food, Drug and Cosmetic Act, Section 409[c][3][A]). As the molecular mechanisms associated with chemical carcinogenesis have begun to be uncovered, it has now become clear that the clause is oversimplistic. Criticisms have been heard from both the scientific and regulatory communities. The controversial aspects of this clause will be discussed in a later section of this chapter.

As can be seen by referring to the quotation from the Act on page 4, not only are pesticides excluded from this regulation but so also are color additives. Colors are regulated under the Color Additives Amendment enacted in 1960. The regulation of color additives in foods, drugs, and cosmetics has been discussed in a separate section. Another exemption is "new animal drugs," as previously discussed.

An extremely important aspect of the 1958 Food, Drug and Cosmetic Act was the "grandfather clause," which exempted the vast majority of food additives in use at that time. Unlike food additives proposed after the 1958 Act wherein safety must be proven by toxicologic testing (substances can still be added to the GRAS category with FDA approval), those compounds in use before the passage of the Act could be used based on: (1) "experience based on common use in food"; (2) "having been shown through scientific procedures" (to be nonhazardous); and (3) if a substance has been deemed "generally recognized, among experts qualified by scientific training and experience to evaluate its safety . . . to be safe under the conditions of its intended use." The substances that were "grandfathered" have been placed in a category referred to as "generally regarded as safe," and are generally referred to as GRAS. GRAS substances were collectively approved and approval could only be disallowed if the FDA *itself* demonstrated that they had the potential to be hazardous in their intended use as food additives. The impetus thus fell on the FDA to prove the compounds were hazardous as opposed to the requirement that the sponsor or manufacturer prove them nonhazardous. This is an important distinction and can be responsible for considerable misunderstanding. The FDA published a list of over 600 substances considered GRAS and noted that this list was not exhaustive. Owing to the importance of the category from the aspects of both quantity used and total number of substances, the GRAS category will be discussed in a separate section.

As food has assumed an ever-increasing importance in world trade, food additive problems have arisen. Additives that may be permissible in one country may be banned in another. Most countries now have laws governing food safety, which are often based on, but not identical to, those of the United States and Great Britain. To assist and encourage food trade among nations, several international agencies are involved in the complex task of reconciling the laws associated with food additives among international trading partners. A Joint Expert Committee on Food Additives has been formed under the auspices of the Food and Agriculture Organization (FAO) and the World Health Organization (WHO) with assistance from the United Nations. The joint FAO/WHO committee has used the approach of determining an accepted daily intake (ADI) for food additives. The ADI represents a level of daily intake that should result in no health hazard from a particular food additive. Because of differences in food habits and availability of specific foods in different countries, the intake of a specific food may vary significantly from nation to nation, making an assessment of total intake difficult. To assist in the determination of potential dietary intake of food additives in various nations, the FAO/WHO Codex Alimentarus Commission attempts to determine the national intake of foods containing additives. A particular food may be assigned either an unconditional ADI, a conditional ADI, or a temporary ADI, depending on the quality of the data supporting its degree of hazard when used as intended. The decisions of the FAO/WHO Commission are not legally binding to the member nations and therefore compliance is not mandatory, but is only recommended. Smaller groups of nations have joined together in attempts to unify the food additive legislation of member nations. For instance, the Council of Europe makes recommendations to its member nations on food additives. The recommendations concerning food additives presented by the Council of Europe are not mandatory, whereas those of the European Economic Community are binding to its member nations.

FUTURE TRENDS IN REGULATION OF CARCINOGENS

Earlier, it was stated that considerable controversy has arisen in recent years concerning the Delaney Clause to the 1958 Amendment to the Federal Food, Drug and Cosmetic Act (Section 409[c][3][A]). This section of the Act prohibits the addition of any substance that has been shown to " . . . induce cancer . . . in man or animal . . . ." The apparent rigidity in this regulation has been criticized both within the scientific community and within the industries whose products are thereby regulated. Criticism has become particularly outspoken as the complexities of the carcinogenesis process become better understood.

In general, "proof" of carcinogenic activity has been obtained by feeding experimental animals (usually rats and/or mice of both sexes) varying doses of the test chemical for a two-year period. As with any chronic toxicity test, records are kept on growth, feeding, and general health until sacrifice of the animals at the termination of the study. In particular, data are obtained on tumor development. These data may be expressed as percent of tumor-bearing animals, numbers of tumors per animal, time to tumor development, size of tumors, and type of tumor tissue. When a statistically significant increase in tumor activity in the test animals is produced, "carcinogenicity" is generally considered to have been established. This conclusion is greatly strengthened if there is a good dose-response relationship and if the tumors are unique when compared with the yield of tumors "spontaneously" arising in the control animals. Supporting data from other types of studies may include the presence of mutagenic activity or evidence of increased cancer risk in exposed humans. Whereas the experimental animal bioassay was originally thought to be straightforward, the fact that cancer is now known to be a multifactorial, multistaged, and multimechanistic disease raises important questions as to which of the multiple factors are most relevant for tumor potential and, therefore, which of these factors should be regulated in as rigorous a fashion as the Delaney Clause stipulates. When chemicals are shown to be mutagenic, form covalent adducts with DNA *in vivo*, and induce cancer in a dose-dependent manner in animals, they are generally regarded as important carcinogens because they initiate the disease, as stipulated by the somatic mutation theory. However, the dose-response relationship may be readily altered when the intake of factors modifying the progression of the disease (promoters and inhibitors) are altered. In fact, recent research has shown that these promoters and inhibitors may be considerably more important as risk determinants than is the dose of the initiator. The use of certain promotion stimuli may even increase tumor yield when no initiators are given. For example, feeding a diet higher in protein or calories may increase the incidence of "spontaneous" tumors whose initiating factors are not known. Thus, if an experiment is designed to test for the "carcinogenicity" of protein or calories, the conclusion that must be drawn—according to the Delaney Clause—is that these nutrients are "carcinogenic." Whereas that conclusion may be initially regarded as rather incredulous, epidemiologic data would be supportive, thus strengthening the original conclusion.

Other concerns that confound a strict interpretation of the Delaney Clause are (1) that for many carcinogens, it is virtually impossible to eliminate every trace of the "carcinogen" without outright banning of the food, (2) that an inconsistency exists between the regulation of direct additives and indirect additives and other adventitious residues, and (3) that the resources devoted to imposition of the Clause for varying substances may not correlate with priorities based on public health relevance. Perhaps one of the most serious concerns is the fact that the traditional bioassays in rats and mice yield data that cannot be effectively extrapolated to humans. Quantitative risk assessment procedures are ineffective in interpolating high-dose to low-dose responses and in extrapolating species-to-species response (Campbell, 1980).

These issues are presently under considerable discussion and are likely to lead to a change in the law. Eventually, the law that effectively and efficiently minimizes cancer risk will have to be one that (1) economizes regulatory resources, (2) recognizes feasibility in the marketplace, (3) establishes priorities based on public health relevance, (4) is consistent for diverse substances, and (5) becomes independent of the ever-changing analytic capabilities. Similar concepts will also be required for any substances that lead to a progressive, irreversible disease (Campbell, 1981). The present proposals to use "levels of concern" and "sensitivity of method" analyses appear to be steps in the right direction.

TOXICOLOGIC SAFETY (HAZARD) ASSESSMENT OF FOOD ADDITIVES

Before the advent of national legislation concerning food safety, the potential for adverse health effects from the consumption of food additives could be assumed to have been relatively high. This risk was especially high when foods containing various substances to disguise their poor quality and to add bulk were consumed. It is difficult to retrospectively evaluate the effect of these foods on public health because of a lack of epidemiologic studies and acceptable health and food consumption records. The passage of the Pure Food and Drug Act of 1906, followed by the establishment of the Food and Drug Administration, began the era when the safety of food was put under close scrutiny. This resulted in marked improvements in food safety. The 1958 revision of the legislation, combined with the development of the science of toxicology as an independent discipline and the overall improvement of toxicologic assessment, led to further improvement in food safety. If one considers overall human exposure to toxicants, including both the natural and synthetic chemicals introduced into the human environment, then the current safety record for food additives must rank this group of substances as one of the lowest risk categories (Doll and Peto, 1981; Select Committee on GRAS Substances, 1977). This is true despite the perceptions of the consumer and consumer activist groups and even the perceptions of health scientists in areas not related to food safety.

A consideration of the toxicologic safety assessment of food additives is complicated by their legal division into various categories, as previously discussed. Safety assessment criteria vary both between and within the different categories of food additives. For this reason, the safety assessment of food additives will be divided into categories representing different classes of food additives.

Safety Assessment of GRAS Substances

As previously discussed, the Food, Drug and Cosmetic Act of 1958 exempted a large number of food additives that had been used before January 1, 1958 from the regulatory requirements. This exclusion "grandfathered" the bulk of food additives in use at that time. This group of substances became known as GRAS for "generally regarded as safe." The FDA compiled a GRAS list containing approximately 600 substances. As admitted by the FDA, this list was far from complete but it served to illustrate substances that the agency considered GRAS. Since the law did not forbid groups other than the FDA from developing GRAS lists, several organizations developed these lists independent of the FDA. The major criterion for addition to the GRAS list was that "experts qualified by scientific training and experience . . . evaluate its safety." An example of a non-FDA-proposed GRAS list is that proposed by the Flavor and Extract Manufacturers' Association (FEMA). The FEMA list contains over 1000 flavoring ingredients approved by their expert committee. The FDA has accepted the FEMA list and it has become a part of the Code of Federal Regulations.

It is important to realize that the GRAS list is not static, and at any time when the safety of a substance is questioned it can be reviewed and removed from GRAS by the FDA. A major problem associated with the GRAS list is that substances were included on the list before modern methods and concepts of toxicologic evaluation were developed; only their historic use without evidence of adverse health effects was noted. However, it is difficult to assign to a particular substance the specific responsibility for an adverse health effect in the human population, particularly with respect to a chronic effect. These problems, among others, led to a 1968 presidential directive to the FDA to review the status of substances listed as GRAS.

In part, the review of GRAS substances was sparked by the discovery of the suspected carcinogenicity of the artificial sweetener cyclamate. This produced concern that other GRAS substances may also have unrecognized toxicities. Thus began the largest toxicologic review in history. Initially the FDA requested scientific literature reviews and unpublished data on the safety of GRAS substances. Data on the current level of usage and estimated daily consumption were obtained through an FDA contract to the National Academy of Sciences, National Research Council. Another contract was given to the Life Sciences Research Office of the Federation of American Societies for Experimental Biology to evaluate this mass of data in terms of safety. To undertake this formidable task, a Select Committee on GRAS Substances (SCOGS), consisting of nongovernmental and nonindustry experts in the fields of toxicology and food safety, was convened. The following procedure was followed for safety approval of a GRAS substance, or group of closely related substances: (1) SCOGS provided the FDA with the initial review of the substance; (2) FDA then made the report public and announced a call for any additional data on the substance that had bearing on its safety; (3) if required, a public hearing with SCOGS could be held on the substance; and (4) with the benefit of any additional data collected, a final report was prepared and made public. The GRAS substances were then placed in the following categories: (1) reaffirmation of GRAS status; (2) reaffirmation of GRAS status at current levels of use; (3) reaffirmation of safety but additional research required; (4) insufficient information to reaffirm safety; and (5) insufficient information to judge safety (Select Committee on GRAS Substances, 1977). The FDA interpretation of these various categories is as follows: (1) Category One and Two substances are reaffirmed as GRAS; (2) Category Three may remain GRAS for a prescribed period of time while additional toxicologic tests are conducted; and (3) Categories Four and Five require the establishment of either safe usage conditions or additional toxicologic data without which the GRAS status is rescinded defining the substance as a food additive. This results in the requirement for the sponsor to provide toxicologic data suitable for safety assessment.

Although this procedure for the assessment of the public health hazard of GRAS substances is not as rigorous as an assessment based on carefully conducted toxicologic studies utilizing current methodology, it is considered justifiable in view of the total number of compounds involved. SCOGS has published an excellent review of their evaluation methods (Select Committee on GRAS Substances, 1977). To ensure that new toxicologic data still support the GRAS status of specific substances, the FDA plans cyclic reviews on their safety. It was the concensus of the SCOGS committee that its work was transitory between the concept of GRAS substances being "evaluated for lack of evidence of hazard" to the inclusion of these substances as food additives "evaluated for the evidence of safety."

Toxicologic Safety Assessment of Direct Food Additives

Food additives, legally defined as those substances which are added to food for a particular technologic purpose and which are not GRAS, must be proven to be without toxicologic hazard at the intended level and condition of usage by the sponsor who wants approval for use. Since the 1958 revision of the Food, Drug and Cosmetic Act, scientific data from toxicologic tests are required to prove safety. The desire of the consumer for greater numbers of "convenience foods" and for a constant year-round supply of specific foods, coupled with the interest in a greater variety of foods, has increasingly led to the need for additional food additives. The ability of the food technologist to take foods apart and recombine them in unique manners has increased the number of substances classified as food additives. The ability of the analytic chemist to analyze and purify specific active components of natural materials used for flavoring, etc. has also led to an increase in the number of food additives. The need to perform safety assessment studies on those compounds which have been given temporary GRAS status, and thus are pseudofood additives, has added to the load of food additives that must be toxicologically evaluated. Taken together these factors have resulted in a great number of specific compounds that require toxicologic evaluation. This has led to the innovative development of approaches to toxicologic assessment of food safety.

One such approach, which placed toxicologic assessment procedures within a broader context, was proposed by the industry supported Food Safety Council (Scientific Committee of the Food Safety Council, 1978). This "decision tree" approach was developed in response to (1) the increasing number and uses of substances as food additives; (2) the limitation of the toxicology community to undertake the number of extensive tests required; (3) the length of time required to complete a comprehensive toxico-

logic evaluation; and (4) the high cost of a comprehensive toxicologic evaluation. The approach begins with simple, inexpensive tests of short duration and works toward the long-term test. At each step within the testing tier, the data are carefully analyzed and a decision is made either to end the testing at that point owing to the potential hazard of the substance or to continue the testing to the next level. In this manner, unnecessary testing is minimized and time, facilities, and finances are conserved for the evaluation of more favorable and relevant substances.

Figure 24–1 represents the decision tree approach to food safety assessment proposed by the Food Safety Council. The Council suggests that this be used as an outline only and that the particular steps may be varied depending on the individual substance under study. Quantitative risk assessment may be performed at various intervals along the tree to determine the utility of proceeding to the next step. The principal value of this system is that it is applicable to risk determination for a wide majority of substances ingested with food such as natural toxicants, pesticides, packaging constituents, etc. and not just for food additives.

For those substances requiring toxicologic evaluation, the decision of exactly what to test is not always clear. Food additives cover the spectrum from simple salts to synthetic organic chemicals to highly complex mixtures of substances obtained from biologic origins. The Food Safety Council has suggested that the substance tested should be that which will be specifically utilized in commerce. This decision may not represent a problem for the easily prepared mineral salts, but may present difficulties with respect to additives of either synthetic or biologic origin. For instance, a synthetic chemical used in commerce is not an absolutely pure compound but will contain impurities, however minute, resulting from the manufacturing process. Therefore, the toxicity of not only the active test substance, but also its impurities, must be considered. Since the test substance may be manufactured by different companies utilizing different synthetic processes, different batches may contain different impurities. Substances of biologic origin may also differ depending not only on the extraction methodology but also on the source. For instance, a plant extract may vary chemically depending on the particular source of the plant and its growing conditions. All these factors must be considered in selecting the specific substance to be tested. The main criterion, however, is that the test substance be representative of the material to be marketed for food use.

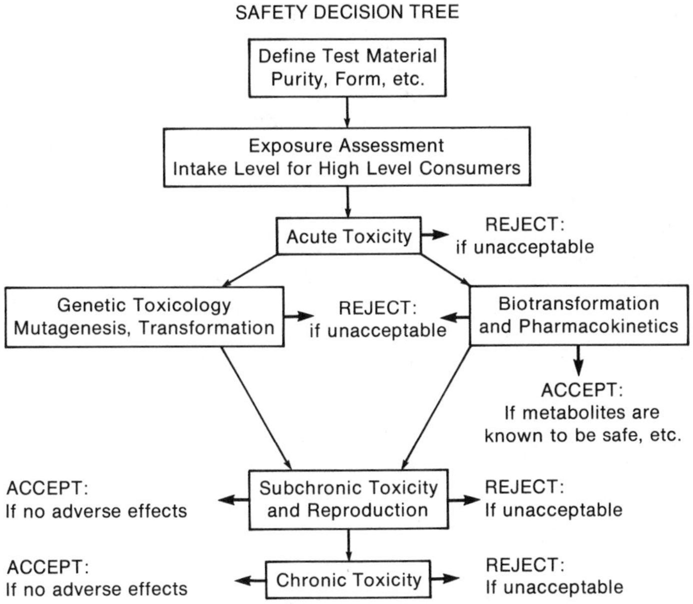

SAFETY DECISION TREE

Figure 24–1. Safety decision tree as recommended by the Scientific Committee of the Food Safety Council, 1978.

Modification of production and marketing practices after toxicologic evaluation may require retesting of the substance.

The next step within the decision tree is an assessment of human exposure to the test substance. This is an essential step in the hazard evaluation of a food additive since an estimate of the expected human dose must be determined. The toxicity finally produced is a combination of the toxicologic potency of the substance and its dose. Determination of the potential human dose of a substance is complicated by many factors, but methods have been developed that yield approximate doses (Filer, 1976). In order to estimate human consumption of a particular food substance, it is necessary to know (1) the levels of the substance in food; (2) the daily intake of each food containing the substance; (3) the distribution of intakes within the population; and (4) the potential consumption of, or exposure to, the substance from nonfood sources.

There are three rather imperfect methods generally used for the determination of human exposure to dietary substances. A "market basket analysis" directly measures the substance in foods purchased in a retail outlet and used to prepare test meals. This method is of no use for a potential food additive not yet appearing in food. The "per capita disappearance" method may be used for both new and previously approved food additives. It consists of determining the total amounts of foods that may contain the

test substance and be sold in the marketplace; the amount of substance thus disappearing is then divided by the number of individuals in the consuming population. This method does not consider the amounts consumed by target groups and may yield misleading data, as illustrated by the case of saccharin. Average per capita consumption of saccharin in 1972 was 23 mg/kg/day, but the major consuming population consisted of low-calorie-soft-drink consumers. In this group the average consumption was 389 mg/kg/day. Another method is the "dietary survey," which consists of interviewing consumers about their dietary habits; however, dietary-recall studies are notoriously inaccurate. The Committee on Food Protection of the National Academy of Sciences has utilized a method that calculates consumption by multiplying the substance's usage level (obtained by survey) by frequency of eating of specific food items (obtained by survey) to determine consumption of specific GRAS substances. A "probablistic method" for estimating consumption has been suggested that may overcome some of the problems associated with the older methods (Subcommittee on GRAS List Survey, Phase III, 1976). This method attempts to determine the probability that a particular substance will occur in an individual food serving. Currently, this method is laborious and has not been applied with many additives. Oser and Hall (1977) have shown that this method shows agreement with certain of the classic methods. Whatever method is employed, consideration must be given to those individuals who consume greater-than-average quantities of specific foods.

Within the Food Safety Council decision tree, the first toxicity test to be performed is the acute toxicity study. This study will provide preliminary data on (1) the clinical manifestations of acute toxicity, (2) information that suggests doses for other tests, and (3) a quantitative measure of acute toxicity (LD50) for comparison with other substances. After the acute toxicity study, the first decision point is reached. At this point a risk analysis is made based on the anticipated consumption level previously determined and the data from the acute toxicity study. Depending on the outcome of this analysis, a decision is made to either discontinue testing at this point or continue to the next testing stage.

Genetic toxicology and biotransformation-pharmacokinetics are the next suggested testing stage. Since these studies can complement each other, they may be performed simultaneously. Both genetic toxicology and biotransformation studies have been previously discussed in this volume (Chapters 4 and 6). The purpose of the genetic toxicology test is to determine whether the test substance exhibits mutagenic activity with and without prior biotransformation. The biotransformation and pharmacokinetic studies should yield data useful in ascertaining the quantitative and qualitative characteristics of the compound's absorption, biotransformation, and excretion and possibly provide evidence of species differences in these parameters. These studies should also provide information on whether the toxicity of significant metabolites needs to be studied in further detail. Particular information on the role of metabolic activation and detoxication pathways may be obtained in the biotransformation studies. The pharmacokinetic studies should yield data on the biologic half-life of the substance, potential for accumulation at specific tissue sites, rates of absorption and excretion, and dose dependency. These studies are not only useful in risk assessment, but also essential for the development of appropriate subchronic and chronic toxicity studies.

If the biotransformation-pharmacokinetic studies indicate that the substance is biotransformed to metabolites with known toxicity, it will be unnecessary to determine their toxicity. However, in cases where metabolites of unknown toxicity are detected, it may be necessary to determine their toxicity. If metabolic activation to products forming covalent adducts is encountered, then the results should be compared with the genetic studies. If the pharmaco-

kinetic studies reveal tissue storage of either the parent compound or its metabolites, this may indicate that the substance is unsuitable as a food additive. Again, a benefit-risk analysis will be supported by the biotransformation and pharmacokinetic data.

Upon completion of these studies, another point of decision is reached. If the genetic toxicology studies reveal negative data, the *probability* is that the substance is not mutagenic and *may* not initiate the process of carcinogenesis. If positive results are obtained within the battery of genetic tests, then a benefit-risk analysis must be made. The Food Safety Council recommends, if the pharmacokinetic studies reveal the production of nontoxic metabolites and the genetic toxicology studies reveal no mutagenicity, that the compound may be accepted at this point. On the other hand, if these studies and the risk assessment leave doubt on the type and extent of risk posed, then the substance is taken to the next level of testing, the subchronic toxicity studies.

The subchronic toxicology series includes a protracted feeding study (usually 90 days) at several dose levels and also includes studies on the potential reproductive toxicity and teratogenicity of the test compound. At the completion of these studies, a risk assessment is made at excessive human exposure levels. The additive is rejected if unacceptable risk is encountered at the estimated consumption level for high consumers. The test substance may be accepted if the consumption level for high consumers is relatively low and no unacceptable risk is encountered at high consumption levels and structure-activity relationships, genetic toxicology, and biotransformation reveal no evidence of carcinogenicity. If any of these criteria are not met, the test substance is moved along to chronic toxicity testing.

Chronic toxicity studies are designed on the basis of all the data collected up to this point. At the conclusion of the chronic toxicity phase of the safety assessment, risk analyses are again performed. If, on the basis of the risk analysis, there are no unacceptable risks from consumption of the compound at the anticipated consumption level of high consumers, the substance is accepted. The decision tree approach proposed by the Food and Safety Council represents a rational approach to toxicity assessment that appears to be efficient in cost and reliable in safety assessment.

With the realization that information on the safety of food additives and colors must be both cost-effective and adequate for regulatory requirements, in 1982 the FDA developed a document suggesting an approach and specifying the data needed to aid in the hazard assessment of food chemicals (Bureau of Foods, 1982). Although this document does not make major changes in the scientific data required for risk determination, it does represent changes in the basic scheme of decision making and priority development. The FDA has stated the safety assessment strategy in the form of four premises: (1) the agency "should possess at least some toxicologic or other biologic safety data for each additive"; (2) the extent of toxicologic evaluation is set by the agency's "concern about potential public health consequences" and may vary from substance to substance; (3) even if no toxicologic data are available, a *level of concern* can still be determined as a function of the level of exposure and the molecular structure correlation with other substances of known toxicity; and (4) the completeness and rigor of the initial safety assessment of a substance can be varied if warranted by the initial series of tests. The new concept of safety assessment of food additives and colors proposed by the FDA is a tier approach based on the concept of *level of concern*. Essentially, this concept is based on the idea that all additives do not possess equivalent potential for adverse public health effects. Therefore, additives can be divided into groups, each of which exhibits a different degree of potential adverse health effects. A *level of concern* can be expressed for each of these groups with the group possessing the highest *level of concern* having the greatest resources devoted to the assessment of its hazards. Ideally, the *level of concern* should be an objective evaluation based on quantitative, empiric data and which is calculatable. In reality, this is not currently possible and the *level of concern* is subjective and based on the best data available. An additive whose use has changed, resulting in an exposure beyond the acceptable level, would have a high level of concern, as would an additive whose latest toxicity data indicate a greater toxicity than originally anticipated. The type of toxicity exhibited by a substance is also important in determining its *level of concern*; i.e., if tests reveal a more severe type of toxicity, then the *level of concern* would be increased regardless of exposure level. *Levels of concern* are divided into three categories, based on three criteria: (1) level of exposure; (2) molecular structural correlation with known compounds, where no toxicologic data are available; and (3) existing toxicologic data.

Categorization according to exposure level is based on criteria previously utilized by the agency. Concern Level III (highest level of concern) contains compounds that contribute more than 1.0 ppm to the total diet. Concern Level II consists of compounds that contribute 0.05 to 1.0 ppm to the diet, and Concern Level I (lowest level of concern) those which contribute below 0.05 ppm to the total diet. Categorization according to molecular structure is based on the association of molecular characteristics with the potential for adverse health effects: Categories A, B, and C reflect molecular structures associated with the potential for low, intermediate, and high toxicity, respectively. Molecular structure information supersedes exposure level information in the assignment of *level of concern*. That is, a compound whose molecular structure places it into Category C would be placed in Concern Level III, even though its potential exposure level would place it in Category I. And finally, categorization of compounds about which some toxicologic data are known can be more accurately undertaken. For example, compounds that are biotransformed to active metabolites would suggest Category III, as would compounds that induce toxicity at low doses and/or after short durations of exposure. Compounds that produce toxic effects only at high doses and whose exposure to humans would be low would be placed in a lower category and would receive less extensive testing. As additional toxicologic data are provided, a particular additive may move from high to lower categories and vice versa. The recommended toxicologic tests for each *level of concern* are listed below.

Concern Level I Substances. These include:
1. Short-term feeding study (at least 28 days) in a rodent species.
2. Short-term test for carcinogenic potential.

Concern Level II Substances. These include:
1. Subchronic feeding study in a rodent species.
2. Subchronic feeding study in a nonrodent species.
3. Multigeneration reproduction in a rodent species employing at least two generations and incorporating a teratology phase.
4. Short-term test for carcinogenic potential.

Concern Level III Substances. These include:
1. Carcinogenicity studies in two rodent species.
2. A chronic feeding study of at least one year in duration in a rodent species (can be incorporated into no. 1, above).
3. A chronic feeding study of at least one year in duration in a nonrodent species.
4. Multigeneration reproduction study in a rodent species employing at least two generations and incorporating a teratology phase.
5. Short-term test for carcinogenic potential that may assist in the evaluation of results from the lifetime studies.

This procedure contains elements of a decision tree approach for hazard assessment. The utility of these suggested approaches will be evaluated with additional evidence, but at the current state of the art and science of toxicology, they appear to be an effective compromise to the requirement of exhaustive toxicity testing for each substance that may be employed as a food additive.

Toxicologic Assessment of Food Colors

The requirements for toxicologic assessment of food colors do not differ from those of other food additives and include specific toxicologic tests and expert evaluation. The goal of this assessment is to determine an acceptable daily intake (ADI) based on appropriate tests and safety factors. Currently, the FDA, World Health Organization, the Joint Expert Committee on Food Additives, and the European Economic Community have set ADIs for various food colors. Presently there is little uniformity internationally with respect to which colors are acceptable and which are unacceptable. Colors legal in some countries are illegal in others.

There is little concern about the acute and subchronic toxicity of the food colors currently in use, but there is considerable concern about their chronic toxicity. Several of the colors approved for use by the Color Amendments have been delisted since 1971, including green 1, green 2, orange B, red 2, red 4, and violet 1. Their delisting occurred owing to concerns over their chronic toxicity, especially carcinogenicity. As previously mentioned, the FDA decided to eliminate the provisional listing of food colors. The color manufacturers were asked to reevaluate the safety of the approved colors. In response, the Certified Colors Manufacturers Association is supporting lifetime studies in the rat and mouse of the listed colors to provide evidence of their lack of harm. Certain of these studies have now been completed and generally indicate that the colors are not hazardous to human health when employed at levels currently in use (Borzelleca et al., 1983). The currently approved and tested colors are (1) the triphenylmethane colors, brilliant blue FCF (blue 1) and fast green FCF (green 3); (2) indigotine (blue 2); (3) the sulfonated naphthalene azo color, sunset yellow FCF (yellow 6), and the related azo, tartrazine (yellow 5); and (4) the xanthene-related erythrosin (red 3).

Controversy still exists on the carcinogenicity of red 3. Erythrosin is a red disodium or dipotassium salt of 2,4,5,7-tetraiodofluorescein. A peer review subcommittee of the National Toxicology Program's Board of Scientific Counselors determined that there was "convincing evidence that red 3 is carcinogenic in male Sprague-Dawley rats" (Food Chemical News, 1983a). Their conclusions were based on evidence of thyroid enlargement, thyroid hyperplasia, and increased incidence of thyroid neoplasms (Food Chemical News, 1983b). Additional studies are presently being undertaken to determine the mechanisms associated with these effects, especially with respect to biotransformation and pharmacokinetic characteristics (Food Chemical News, 1983c).

The ultimate evaluation of the current chronic toxicity studies on the food colors cannot currently be predicted and will take considerable time and effort. It would be surprising if these studies and their evaluations satisfy all the critics of food color usage. A continuing controversy on food color usage may therefore be expected for the foreseeable future.

Owing to current controversies and public concern, two additional areas of toxicologic significance concerning the colors need to be mentioned—hyperactivity in children associated with consumption of the synthetic colors and potential allergenic reactions. Feingold (1968, 1975) proposed that the consumption by children of foods containing artificial colors may be associated with hyperkinesis and learning disabilities. Children generally consume higher levels of food colors than do adults because of the utilization of colors in confections, soft drinks, and snack foods. However, the data indicating that there is an association between food colors and hyperactivity are unconvincing. Several recent studies have not been able to demonstrate this association (Maltes and Gittelman, 1981; Lipton and Mayo, 1983). This controversy is also likely to continue into the foreseeable future.

The uncertainty of the significance of such adverse effects in the general population ought not to be confused with the potential adverse reactions that may develop among a small minority of the population. In particular, adverse reactions associated with immunologic mechanisms (hypersensitivity) need to be better understood. An increased interest appears to be developing among researchers in this field.

Toxicologic Assessment of Unintentional (Indirect) Food Additives

The FDA excluded indirect food additives from its 1982 document on safety assessment of direct food additives and colors. The reasons for this exclusion were the facts that: (1) different and diverse molecular structures were involved; (2) assessments of exposure were unique and difficult to understand; and (3) the levels in food were seemingly negligible. Currently, the toxicologic evaluation of indirect food additives follows the classic safety assessment procedures, although the FDA plans a future document on these substances.

Toxicologic Assessment of Animal Drugs

Animal drugs undergo testing in target species for both efficacy and toxicity. However, a more complex problem exists in the safety assessment of animal drug residues in human food. A determination of the potential human health hazards associated with animal drug residues is complicated by the intervention of animal biotransformation such that the molecular structure, and thus the toxicity, of the drug may be altered. Also, the sensitivity of modern analytic methodologies designed to isolate, detect, qualitate, and quantitate small quantities of drugs and their various metabolites has made the evaluation problem more complex. A typical series of studies used to evaluate the toxicity of animal drugs may include studies on the (1) addition of the drug to the food; (2) consumption and absorption by the target animal; (3) biotransformation of the drug by the target animal; (4) excretion and tissue distribution of the drug and its metabolites in animal products and tissues; (5) consumption of animal products and tissues by humans; (6) potential absorption of the drug and its metabolites by the human; (7) potential biotransformation of the drug and its metabolites by the human; and (8) potential excretion and tissue distribution in humans of the drug, its metabolites, and secondary human metabolites thereof. Thus, the pharmacokinetic and biotransformation characteristics of both the animal and human must be considered in any assessment of the potential human health hazard of an animal drug. Other considerations include the stability of the drug and its metabolites in animal products and tissues, the interaction of the drug and metabolites with the biochemical constituents of the animal products and tissues, and the potential biotransformation of the drug and its metabolites by intestinal microflora. The combination of these factors and the difficulty and expense of determining the parameters that may affect the toxicity of the drug and its metabolites result in complex hazard assessment protocols.

Since some animal drugs can fall under the GRAS category, safety assessment of these compounds is handled as described under the GRAS section. With respect to new animal drugs, hazard assessment is primarily concerned with residues that occur in animal products and edible tissues. The original toxicity determination in the target species should have provided data on the biotransformation and the nature of metabolites, along with data on pharmacokinetics. If this information is not available, then these studies must be performed using the animal species likely to be exposed to the drug. During this phase the parent drug and its metabolites are evaluated both qualitatively and quantitatively in the animal products of concern (eggs, milk, meat, etc.). This may involve the development of sophisticated analytic methodologies. Once these data are obtained, it is then necessary to undertake an exposure assessment to determine potential human exposure to these compounds in the diet and other sources. If adequate toxicity data are available, it will then be possible to undertake a benefit-risk assessment. If the available toxicity data are inadequate, it will be necessary to conduct additional studies. Additional parameters that must be determined are potential human biotransformation of the animal products, as well as the potential for human gastrointestinal flora to convert the animal metabolites to more toxic products. The number of individual compounds involved can be quite large, emphasizing the need to approach their potential hazard along the lines of a decision tree approach.

One approach to the safety assessment of animal drugs and their metabolites is the relay toxicity study. Relay toxicity studies consist of administering the drug to one set of animals and subsequently feeding the products and tissues of this set of animals to a second set. The second set of animals is then utilized to detect any signs of toxicity. Relay studies present problems associated with feeding animals diets that may be different from their natural diets, thus resulting in associated problems of unpalatability, altered digestion, and inadequate nutrition. These studies also have the inherent problems associated with all toxicologic evaluations such as extrapolation of animal data to humans. It is possible to utilize both animal products and tissues in short-term mutagenicity assays to determine mutagenicity and potential carcinogenicity. Overall the hazard assessment associated with animal drugs and their metabolites is a difficult task requiring expertise in several areas.

FOOD CONTAMINANTS

Food is a complex chemical mixture containing not only nutrients, but also a vast diversity of substances of biologic origin. Since all food is of biologic origin, it contains both inorganic and organic molecules important to the survival of the particular plant or animal species from which it was obtained. A certain fraction of these chemicals are identical or very similar to those found in human metabolism or are precursors to normal human tissue constituents. However, other chemicals are unique to the plant or animal species from whence they were produced and therefore they are xenobiotic (foreign) to human biochemistry. These foreign compounds are more likely to produce adverse reactions in humans, especially when the capacity for detoxication and disposition of such compounds by human tissue is exceeded and/or otherwise compromised. Such chemicals are generally referred to as "toxic constituents of foods," as opposed to food contaminants. Although these compounds are "natural" and may have always been components of human foods, it cannot be assumed that adverse reactions will always be unlikely or negligible. The responsiveness of human tissue to such compounds is less likely to reflect the evolutionary time during which exposure occurred and appropriate response mechanisms were thereby produced. Food sources change. For example, tomatoes and potatoes are relatively recent additions to the human food supply, as is the relatively high meat content of Western diets. Intentional modification of plant genotypes by plant geneticists may lead to altered production of certain of these substances, which may present new problems of toxicologic assessment, as might occur when a natural pesticide or fungicide was to be reduced in content, thereby allowing contamination by new or increased levels of insect or fungal products.

Organisms neither live alone nor do they die alone, but are part of complex biologic ecologic systems. Therefore, foods contain not only chemicals unique to a particular food source, but also chemicals that are components of organisms which may become associated with that food source, either in life or in death. Generally, these chemicals are considered as food contaminants. Examples include mycotoxins and bacterial toxins in various foods, which either may have been deposited during the growth of the food product or may have become a component of the food during the postharvest period. In some cases, the food contaminant may be living organisms such as molds, bacteria, viruses, and parasites. Other contaminants that may occur in food include insects and insect parts, as well as rodent hair and feces. These materials are generally termed "filth" and, when found above certain levels, indicate improper storage and handling practices.

Food products may also be contaminated with various synthetic chemicals not directly related to the methods of production, harvesting, processing, and storage. These contaminants may find their way into food by various means, including general environmental pollution, irrigation with contaminated water, chemical spills, etc. Therefore, such substances are not considered to be indirect food additives. Food preparation may result in the production of new chemi-

cal entities that may have the potential to produce adverse human health effects. The process of cooking has been shown to produce highly mutagenic substances from the pyrolysis of proteins and amino acids (Krone and Iwaoka, 1983; Pariza et al., 1983). These pyrolyzed amino acids appear to be carcinogenic to rodents (Sugimura and Nagao, 1982; Sugimura and Sato, 1983). The nature and levels of these substances are dependent on the type of cooking (frying, roasting, boiling, etc.) as well as the temperature and cooking time employed. Cooking also leads to the caramelization of sugars and the reaction of amino acids and sugars to produce various browning products considered by many to enhance the appearance of certain foods. This browned material contains several products that are capable of producing DNA damage and may substantially increase the mutagen burden in humans (Stich et al., 1982).

In many cases the presence and levels of contaminants can be controlled by proper agricultural production methods, proper storage, and adherence to good manufacturing practices. In other cases, the presence and levels of specific contaminants are dependent on growing conditions and are not under human control.

The number of synthetic chemicals introduced into the human environment during the last century appears to be overwhelming and is often cited as primary evidence for the need to expand toxicologic studies. However, when this number is compared with the number of naturally occurring chemicals, the list becomes less impressive (Ames, 1983). Even though there have been intensive efforts to isolate and identify natural products, the number of *unidentified* natural chemicals still vastly exceeds the number of those which have been identified. Therefore, toxicologic assessment and regulation of substances not yet identified would be an enormous problem if the current concepts and methodologies were to be implemented. That being irrational, toxicologic assessment must therefore be considered in the broader context of general health care. Also, toxicologic assessment of foods and food substances should proceed from a systematic evaluation of the whole food through its varied chemical and physical fractions to the responsible individual compounds, after evidence of adverse effects of the whole food are carefully documented. Future research efforts in toxicologic assessment will need to be placed in a broad health context.

Regulation and Control of Food Contaminants

Toxicologic evaluation and safety assessment of food contaminants do not significantly differ from those of other food chemicals. What does differ are the concepts and procedures used for regulation. There are many reasons for this, some of the most important of which are: (1) the variable occurrence of certain contaminants with the growing season, the geographic locality, and the specific genotype; (2) the difficulties and cost of obtaining testable quantities of the contaminant; (3) the difficulties of identifying with certainty the specific contaminants; (4) the lack of sufficient epidemiologic data on public health significance; and (5) the lack of adequate toxicologic data. It is often difficult to control the levels of specific contaminants in food, other than banning the food. Therefore, regulation procedures and concepts are entirely different from those for food additives.

The regulation of these substances is generally performed by the FDA, but other agencies, such as the Department of Agriculture, may become involved. Legally based "action levels," which establish the maximal levels of a contaminant allowed in food and feeds, are generally used. Action levels are subject to change as more adequate toxicologic data become available. For the reasons discussed above, food contaminants are regulated with much broader margins of safety than are the food additives. This does not indicate that the food contaminants have less potential for adverse public health effects, for, in many cases, the opposite may be true. Rodricks and Pohland (1981) have suggested that if the same margin of safety applied to food additives were applied to solanine, a natural toxic glycoalkaloid in potatoes, it could not be added to foods at the level of its natural occurrence. This is probably true of many of the food contaminants, particularly those which may be either mutagenic or carcinogenic (Ames, 1983).

As mentioned above, control of the quantities of contaminants that occur in foods is more difficult than control of additives. In some cases, such as with bacteria and bacterial toxins, control may be handled by good production, processing, and storage practices. In other cases, such as with the mycotoxins, total control is virtually impossible; thus, certain food lots are rejected for human consumption. Control measures can be as varied as the mechanisms by which specific contaminants find their way into food products. Contaminants that enter food through soils and water may be controlled by banning the use of contaminated water for irrigation, by prohibiting the harvesting of aquatic foods from contaminated waters, by limiting the use of certain fertilizers such as heavy-metal-containing sewage sludge, and by forbidding the production of food crops on contaminated soils.

A good example of some of the difficulties in regulating food contaminants is the aflatoxin problem. The current action level is 20 ppb, although a proposal has been made by FDA to reduce it to 15 ppb. Although aflatoxin contamination of corn and peanuts can be controlled by proper storage conditions, contamination that occurs in the field before harvest cannot be effectively controlled. The development of plant strains resistant to mold infestation may help. Certain processing technologies that destroy aflatoxin are also being tested and may be usable for animal feeds. Their efficacy for human food, however, may be questioned because of the need to carefully evaluate the potential adverse effects that might be elicited by the new product being produced. Action levels for food contaminants, therefore, will depend on multicomponent economic considerations, availability and feasibility of technology procedures, and toxicologic risk assessment.

Bacteria, Bacterial Products, and Viruses

Food is also a vehicle for the consumption of a vast array of microorganisms including many that are either pathogenic or produce toxic metabolites. These microorganisms may originate from the soil, water, air, animals, insects, processing, and packaging equipment, as well as from humans involved in food processing and preparation. Illness may be associated with consumption of food containing microbial toxins (food poisoning), with the bacteria themselves (food infection), and with consumption of food containing bacteria that subsequently produce toxins after consumption. Considering the potential, it is not surprising that a major source of human disease is through the consumption of microbial-contaminated food. Although the yearly number of reported illnesses related to consumption of contaminated food in the United States is only a few thousand, various estimates of the total number of cases vary between 5 and 10 million. In less developed countries these figures are probably much higher. A major problem encountered with illnesses associated with food-borne microorganisms is the lack of identity of both the organisms and the associated food in the majority of cases. These factors have made the protection of food from microbial adulteration a major goal of the food industry, ranging from agricultural production to food preparation. In the United States these efforts have resulted in an excellent record, and attempts at improvements are constantly underway. The two areas currently needing the most improvement are food service establishments and the home. A major problem in both these areas is a lack of education in proper food-handling methodology. The major problems contributing to bacterial contamination of foods during preparation appear to be (1) improper cooling of cooked foods; (2) preparation of food a day or more before serving; (3) inadequate cooking; (4) preparation of food by infected individuals; (5) inadequate reheating; (6) improper hot storage; (7) cross-contamination of cooked and raw foods; and (8) inadequate cleaning of equipment (Marth, 1981).

The bacteria most commonly associated with foodborne illnesses are *Staphlococcus aureus, Clostridium botulinum, Clostridium perfringens, Salmonella* species, *Bacillus cereus, Vibrio parahaemolyticus, Vibrio cholera, Shigella* species, *Escherichia coli, Brucella* species, *Yersinia enterocolitica,* and *Campylobacter* species (Marth, 1981). The Federal Center for Disease Control in Atlanta, Georgia maintains records of foodborne disease, and their data indicate that the patterns associated with the number of outbreaks of foodborne illness and the specific type of bacteria appear to change with time. The two bacteria associated with the greatest number of outbreaks are *S. aureus* and *Salmonella,* followed by *C. perfringens* and *C. botulinum.* It should be emphasized that this information is based on confirmed reported outbreaks. Most cases do not get reported, and in more than 60 percent of the reported cases in 1979 the etiology was unknown. Meat appears to be most often associated with outbreaks of foodborne illness with pork being implicated in the largest number of outbreaks, followed by beef and poultry.

Staphlococcus aureus is one of the two most frequent bacterial agents associated with foodborne disease. Cases of *Staphlococcus* poisoning are most often associated with the consumption of meat and animal products, although vegetable preparations containing these products may also be a source. Milk and other dairy products may become contaminated from cows with *S. aureus*–associated udder mastitis or from the animal's exterior, as well as from animal handlers. Meats can be contaminated during slaughter and handling. A problem associated with *S. aureus* is that it is a poor competitor with other bacteria, and processes that destroy these other bacteria may lead to the rapid growth of *S. aureus.* For instance, pasteurized milk supports *S. aureus* growth better than raw milk because of the elimination of a large number of competing bacteria. Prevention of contamination is best carried out by careful hygienic practices, holding products at reduced temperatures and maintaining a pH below 4.5, when possible.

The first evidence that *S. aureus*–associated illness was produced by a metabolite instead of the bacteria itself was presented by Dack *et al.* (1930), who found that volunteers administered a sterile filtrate from *S. aureus* cultures became ill. Currently five enterotoxins produced by *S. aureus* have been identified. These enterotoxins are single polypeptide chains with different physical properties consisting of 239 to 296 amino acid residues. These polypeptides are resistant to heat and are destroyed only by prolonged boiling. Upon consumption of these enterotoxins the onset of toxicity symptoms occurs within one to six hours, depending on amount of toxin consumed. Symptoms generally consist of nausea, vomiting, abdominal cramps, and diarrhea. In cases of high consumption, symptoms may include headache, muscle cramps, chills and fever, and a possible drop in blood pressure. Recovery is dependent on severity of symptoms, but usually averages one to three days. Mortality is usually not associated with *S. aureus* entertoxins (Bergdoll, 1979).

Salmonella species produce three types of illness: (1) enteric or typhoid fever, (2) gastroenteritis, and (3) organ-specific pathology accompanied by septicemia. Again, meats appear to be a major source of this organism. Poultry appears to be the major source, followed closely by red meat, with a smaller percentage of infection occurring from eggs and dairy products. Nonfood sources of *Salmonella* include human-to-human contact and human-to-pet contact. The major sources of outbreaks of salmonellosis have been food service establishments and the home. These outbreaks generally result from improper food handling, including inadequate cooking of food, incomplete reheating, storage of hot foods at too low a temperature, cross-contamination, contaminated raw ingredients, and poor sanitation.

Symptoms associated with *Salmonella* infection depend both on the specific bacteria and on various host factors. Gastroenteritis is usually associated with a 12- to 24-hour incubation period with symptoms consisting of nausea, vomiting, abdominal cramps, and diarrhea. The disease can be accompanied by fever, faintness, and muscular weakness and may include drowsiness, spasmodic twitching, and restlessness. The severity of the disease is related to the type of bacteria consumed as well as the total number of organisms consumed and the immunologic resistance of the host. Severity of the disease can range from mild diarrhea to death, with mortality occurring in less than 1 percent of the cases. Recovery may be from several days to months in the most severe cases. *Salmonella*-associated septicemias yield high remittent fever, and the bacteria may concentrate in any organ yielding a variety of symptoms ranging from abscesses to meningitis. Mortality is higher than for gastroenteritis, ranging from 5 to 20 percent. Typhoid fever generally requires a longer incubation time than other forms of salmonellosis (7 to 14 days) and begins with a loss of appetite and headache. These symptoms usually precede the high fever and lowered pulse rate and include rose-colored spots. The course of the disease may last up to three weeks and relapses can occur. Mortality rates as high as 10 percent can occur in untreated patients. Although individuals infected with any salmonellae may become carriers, this is most likely with typhoid, with as many as 3 percent of infected individuals becoming carriers.

Salmonellosis appears to be associated with an infection as opposed to enterotoxins. Upon reaching the small intestine, salmonellae appear to invade the lumen and multiply. Lymphoid follicles can enlarge and ulcerate and mesenteric nodes enlarge. If the mucosal wall and lymphatic system are penetrated, the bacteria may penetrate the bloodstream, producing septicemia (Bryan *et al.*, 1979).

Clostridium perfringens is another bacterial species that is a source of foodborne disease. Animal products are the major source for *C. perfringens*, with beef and beef-containing products being the food most commonly infected, followed by poultry and, to a minor extent, other meat products. Infection normally takes place during poor food handling at food service establishments. The major problem appears to be holding foods at too low a temperature and slow cooling of cooked foods. *C. perfringens* food poisoning generally results in diarrhea, accompanied by abdominal cramps. The onset of symptoms usually occurs within 8 to 24 hours after ingestion of infected foods and persists for 12 to 24 hours (Hobbs, 1979). Illness is produced by a heat-labile protein entertoxin with a molecular weight of 36,000.

Clostridium botulinum contamination of food is a major concern of those involved in the food industry, not because of a high rate of incidence but because of the extremely toxic nature of the entertoxin produced by this bacterium, which is generally regarded as the most acutely toxic chemical known. The majority of reported cases of botulism have been associated with the consumption of inadequately processed home-canned vegetables. Other major sources have been fish and fish products, followed by fruits and various condiments. The development of *C. botulinum* and its toxin in food products is dependent on complex interactions between several factors such as the storage conditions of the food product, product preparation, especially temperatures employed, and certain intrinsic properties of the food, including pH, salt concentration, water activity, oxidation-reduction potentials, and the presence of certain preservatives. There have been cases of botulism reported far back in history, and even today, with the advances in food technology, problems still

arise. A recent and much publicized case was the discovery of *C. botulinum* in a few cans of salmon. This finding resulted in the recall of large numbers of canned salmon and in significant economic loss to the salmon industry. Contamination of a few cans appears to have resulted from postprocessing contamination due to faulty cans. This incident sparked the formation of a joint task force between the National Food Processors' Association and the Can Manufacturers' Institute to study the risk of botulism attributable to faulty containers and to study how the production of faulty containers could be minimized (Froday, 1983). This group reported that the risk of botulism related to faulty containers was greatest with those products which were most susceptible to postprocessing contamination, products in which detection of spoilage by odor was unlikely and where consumption occurs without heating sufficiently to destroy the *C. bolulinum* toxin. Problems have also been produced in canned foods owing to inadequate heating during processing. Although botulism is commonly thought to be associated with sealed containers, since *C. botulinum* is an anaerobe, the recent cases of botulism from potato salad indicate that this is not always the case (Center for Disease Control, 1969; Seals *et al.*, 1981; Sugiyama *et al.*, 1981). The incidents appear to have been created by the utilization of foil-wrapped potatoes that had been baked and held at room temperature for several days prior to the preparation of potato salad. Apparently microenvironments existed with low enough oxygen tension to allow the growth of *C. botulinum*. Only small packets of bacterial growth are required to yield a toxic food product.

The initial symptoms of botulism occur between 12 and 36 hours after consumption of the toxin and include nausea, vomiting, and diarrhea. Neurologic symptoms occur somewhat later and include lassitude, weakness, blurred vision, weakness of facial muscles, and difficulty with speech and swallowing, among others. Progression of the toxicity leads to neuroparalysis of the respiratory muscles and diaphragm, resulting in death by respiratory failure (Smith, 1977). Between 1899 and 1977 there were 766 reported incidents of botulism in the United States involving approximately 1961 individuals (Gunn, 1979). Home-processed foods accounted for 71.5 percent of these cases with commercially processed foods representing 8.6 percent, and the remaining 19.8 percent being of unknown etiology. Mortality among untreated cases can be as high as 60 percent, but the introduction of an antitoxin has reduced mortality. *C. botulinum* toxins consist of at least seven types labeled A through G. Types A, B, and E are generally associated with human botulism. The toxins are proteins with molecular weights in the range of 200,000 to 400,000, consisting of a toxic and nontoxic polypeptide. These proteins are heat labile and can be inactivated in a time-dependent manner between 80° and 100°C (Sakaguchi, 1979). They apparently produce their toxicity by inhibiting the release of acetylcholine at the neuromuscular junction.

The bacteria discussed above have received most of the attention with respect to foodborne bacteria illness. However, there is increasing evidence that certain other bacteria may also be important, including pathogenic strains of *E. coli*, *Bacillus cerew*, *Vibrio*, *Yersinia*, *Campylobacter*, and *Staphylococcus*. For example, *Campylobacter jejuni* can be recovered as frequently from patients with gastroenteritis as salmonellae. This species occurs in the intestine of poultry and livestock and can contaminate meat products at the time of slaughter. Exposure normally occurs from the consumption of undercooked meats. Procedures employed to prevent *Salmonella* infections should also prevent infection by *C. jejuni*.

Food may also be a vector for the transmission of viral infections (Cliver, 1978). However, more research is needed before the scope of foodborne viral infections is understood. A major problem associated with determinations of the potential transmission of viruses via food is the difficulty in isolation of the viruses. Viruses with potential human pathogenicity have been isolated from dairy products, meats, salads, and seafoods such as oysters, clams, and crabs. Contamination of food with these viruses appears to result from contaminated food handlers or from sewage-contaminated water being used in irrigation or as the growth matrix. Since many viruses can be inactivated by heat, thorough cooking can decrease the chance of viral infection, but in some instances, such as seafoods, traditional eating habits may lead to consumption of significant levels of viruses. Infectious hepatitis is an example of a food-transmitted virus. Between 1973 and 1975 there were 6135 cases of hepatitis from consumption of raw shellfish alone, and other foods such as tossed salads, sandwiches, and hamburger are potential vehicles for hepatitis transmission (Centers for Disease Control, 1977). Apparently contamination occurred through collection of shellfish grown in sewage-polluted water and through infection of foods by food handlers. Control of foodborne hepatitis A can be obtained by eliminating collection of seafood from contaminated waters, not utilizing contaminated waters for irrigation, and careful control of the personal hygiene practices of food handlers.

Although it is possible to transmit several parasites via food, in the United States the major foodborne parasite is *Trichinella sprialis*. The majority of cases, which average about ten per year in the United States, result from the consumption of undercooked pork.

CONTAMINANTS ASSOCIATED WITH FOODS OF BOTANICAL ORIGIN

Mycotoxins

Whereas the molds have provided various fungal metabolites with important medicinal uses, they also produce secondary metabolites with the potential to produce severe adverse human health effects. Mycotoxins represent a diverse group of species-specific chemicals that can occur in a variety of plant foods. They can also occur in animal products derived from animals consuming contaminated feeds. The current interest in mycotoxicoses was generated by a series of reports in 1960–1963 that cited the death of turkeys in England and ducklings in Uganda because of the consumption of feeds containing mold products produced by *Aspergillus flavus* and occurring in peanut meal (Stoloff, 1977). The discovery of these aflatoxin metabolites led to more intensive studies of mycotoxins and to the identification of a variety of these compounds associated with adverse human health effects, both retrospectively and prospectively. Moldy foods are consumed throughout the world during times of famine, as a matter of taste and through ignorance of adverse health effects. Epidemiologic studies designed to ascertain either the acute or chronic effects of such consumption are few. Data from animal studies indicate that the consumption of food contaminated with mycotoxins has a high potential to produce a variety of human diseases.

Aflatoxins. Among the various mycotoxins, the aflatoxins have received the most intensive research because of the extremely potent hepatocarcinogenicity and toxicity of aflatoxin B_1 in the rat. Epidemiologic studies conducted in Africa and Asia indicate that it is a human hepatocarcinogen, and various other reports have implicated the aflatoxins in incidences of human toxicity (Peers *et al.*, 1973; Krishnamachari *et al.*, 1975). Several investigations have associated Reye's syndrome with the ingestion of aflatoxin, an association that deserves more intensive research (Hogan *et al.*, 1978; Siraj *et al.*, 1981).

Generally, aflatoxins occur in susceptible crops as mixtures of aflatoxins B_1, B_2, G_1, and

G_2, with only aflatoxin B_1 and G_1 demonstrating carcinogenicity. A carcinogenic, hydroxylated metabolite of aflatoxin B_1 (termed aflatoxin M_1) can occur in the milk from dairy cows consuming contaminated feed. Aflatoxins may occur in a number of susceptible commodities and products derived from them, including edible nuts (peanuts, pistachios, almonds, walnuts, pecans, Brazil nuts), oil seeds (cottonseed, copra), and grains (corn, grain sorghum, millet) (Stoloff, 1977). In tropical regions aflatoxins can be produced in unrefrigerated prepared foods. The two major sources of aflatoxin contamination of commodities are field contamination, especially during times of drought and other stress which allow insect damage that opens the plant to mold attack, and inadequate storage conditions. Since the discovery of their potential human health hazard, progress has been made in decreasing the level of aflatoxin in specific commodities. Control measures include ensuring adequate storage conditions and careful monitoring of susceptible commodities for aflatoxin level and the banning of lots that surpass the action level for aflatoxin B_1. Currently, reduction of the action levels to near zero would result in the loss of certain important commodities as a human food source.

Aflatoxin B_1 is acutely toxic in all species studied with LD50 ranging from 0.5 mg/kg for the duckling to 60 mg/kg for the mouse (Wogan, 1973). Death typically results from hepatotoxicity. It is also highly mutagenic, hepatocarcinogenic, and possibly teratogenic. A problem in extrapolating animal data to humans is the extremely wide range of species susceptibility to aflatoxin B_1. For instance, while B_1 appears to be the most hepatocarcinogenic compound known for the rat, the adult mouse is essentially totally resistant to its hepatocarcinogenicity.

Aflatoxin B_1 is an extremely biologically reactive compound altering a number of biochemical systems. Although the mechanisms associated with the acute toxicity of aflatoxin B_1 are poorly understood, those associated with its carcinogenicity are being elucidated by a number of laboratories. As previously discussed in Chapter 5, the hepatocarcinogenicity of aflatoxin B_1 is associated with its biotransformation to a highly reactive, electrophilic epoxide, which forms covalent adducts with DNA, RNA, and protein. Damage to DNA is thought to be the initial biochemical lesion resulting in the expression of the pathologic lesion (Miller, 1978). Species differences in response to aflatoxin may be due, in part, to differences in biotransformation and susceptibility to the initial biochemical lesion (Campbell and Hayes, 1976).

Although the aflatoxins have received the greatest attention among the various mycotoxins owing to their hepatocarcinogenicity in certain species, there is currently no evidence that they have the greatest potential to produce adverse human health effects among the various mycotoxins. Table 24–3 lists a number of mycotoxins with potential human health significance, their source, and commodities most often contaminated. It must be emphasized that mycotoxins

Table 24–3. SELECTED MYCOTOXINS PRODUCED BY VARIOUS MOLDS

MYCOTOXIN	SOURCE	COMMODITIES CONTAMINATED
Aflatoxins B_1, B_2, G_1, G_2	*Aspergillus flavus*	Corn, peanuts, and others
Aflatoxin M_1	Metabolite of AFB_1	Milk
Trichothecenes	*Fusarium, Myrothecium,*	Cereal grains, corn
T-2 toxin	*Trichoderma,*	
Trichodermin	*Cephalosporium,*	
Verrucarol	*Stachybotrys,*	
Nivalenol	*Verticimonosporium,*	
Trichothecin	and possibly others	
Vertisporin,		
among others		
Zearalenones	*Fusarium*	Corn, grains
Citreoviridin	*Penicillum citreoviride*	Rice
Cytochalasins E, B, F, H	*Phoma* and others	Grains (possibly)
Ochratoxins A, B, C	*Aspergillus* and	Corn, cereal grains
	Penicillium	
Sterigmatocystin	*Aspergillus versiolar*	Corn
Pennicillic acid	*Penicillium cyclopium*	Grains
Griseofulvin	*Penicillium urticae*	Grains
Rubratoxins A, B	*Penicillium rubrum*	Corn
Patulin	*Penicillium*	Apple and apple products

are generally not consumed as independent toxins, but in combination with other mycotoxins as well as other types of toxic chemicals. It appears that certain mycotoxins, when consumed in combination with others, interact to synergize their toxicity. Other xenobiotics may also modify their toxicity.

Trichothecenes. These mycotoxins represent a group where it is likely that several forms may be consumed concomitantly. They represent over 40 different chemical entities containing the tricholthecene nucleus and are produced by a variety of commonly occurring molds including *Fusarium, Myrothecium, Trichoderma,* and *Cephalosporium,* among others. The trichothecenes were first discovered during attempts to isolate antibiotics, and while some show antibiotic activity, their toxicity has precluded their use pharmacologically. Trichothecenes most often occur in moldy cereal grains. There have been many reported cases of trichlothecene toxicity in farm animals and a few in humans. One of the more famous cases of presumed human toxicity associated with the consumption of tricothecenes occurred in Russia during 1944 around Orenburg, near Siberia. Disruption of agriculture caused by World War II resulted in millet, wheat, and barley being overwintered in the field. Consumption of these commodities resulted in vomiting, skin inflammation, diarrhea, and multiple hemorrhage, among other symptoms fatal to over 10 percent of the individuals consuming the moldy grain (Ueno, 1977). The extent of toxicity in humans and farm animals associated with the tricothecenes is currently unknown owing to the number of entities in this group and the difficulty of assaying for these compounds. The acute LD50s of the tricothecenes range from 0.5 to 70 mg/kg, and though there are reports of possible chronic toxicity associated with certain members of this group, more research is needed before the magnitude of their potential to produce adverse human health effects is understood (Sato and Ueno, 1977).

Another mycotoxin produced by *Fusarium* is zearalenone. It was first discovered during attempts to isolate an agent from feeds that produced a hyperestrogenic syndrome in swine characterized by a swollen and edematous vulva and actual vaginal prolapse in severe cases (Stob *et al.*, 1962). Zearalenone can occur in corn, barley, wheat, hay, and oats as well as other agricultural commodities (Mirocha *et al.*, 1977). Zearalenone consumption can decrease the reproductive potential of farm animals, especially swine. Its human health effects have not been ascertained, although its possible mutagenicity

emphasizes the need for further research concerning this mycotoxin.

Natural Toxic Constituents of Plants

Although the naturally occurring toxic constituents of foods are out of the context of food additives and contaminants, they deserve at least brief mention in any discussion of food safety. These chemicals are part of the natural biochemistries of various plants, but represent xenobiotics with respect to human biochemistry. This group of compounds represents one of the most chemically diverse groups that occur in foods. Some of them have relatively high acute toxicity although the greatest concern with respect to human health effects is their chronic toxicity. The advent of short-term mutagenicity assays has allowed the testing of a number of these chemicals and has indicated that more than a few have mutagenic potential (Ames, 1983).

Safrole and related compounds are found as constituents of several edible plants and have been shown to be mutagenic and carcinogenic in rodents (Miller *et al.*, 1979). Sassafras has been used as a flavoring agent in sarsaparilla root beer and contains high levels of safrole. Black pepper contains smaller amounts of safrole and relatively large amounts of the related compound piperine. Extracts of black pepper have been shown to produce tumors in various sites in mice (Concon *et al.*, 1979). Celery, parsnips, and other members of the Umbelliferae family contain furacoumarins that are mutagenic and carcinogenic. The psoralens, members of this group, are activated by sunlight to produce damage to DNA (Ashwood-Smith and Poulton, 1981). The pyrrolizitine alkaloids represent a group of compounds that occur in a large number of plant species and have been shown to be mutagenic, carcinogenic, and teratogenic. Humans can be exposed to these compounds through consumption of herbs and herbal teas, and human toxicity has been reported (Clark, 1982). White potatoes may contain relatively high levels of the steroidal glycoalkaloids solanine and choconine, which are potent cholinesterase inhibitors. Potatoes that have been exposed to light, resulting in greening, and those that are diseased or bruised may contain levels of glycoalkaloids resulting in illness in humans. These are just a few of the numerous components of plants that pose potential adverse health effects in humans (Committee on Food Protection, 1973). The large number of plant constituents known to possess potential toxicity probably represent a small percentage of those that actually exist. It should be anticipated that more research in this area will yield additional toxic compounds. It must be emphasized that plants also contain various chemicals that may possess anticarcinogenic activity, such as β-carotene and vitamin E. It is interesting to keep in mind the potential adverse health effects of these naturally occurring chemicals while considering the potential adverse health effects of the synthetic food additives.

CONTAMINANTS ASSOCIATED WITH FOODS OF ZOOLOGIC ORIGIN

Botanic Xenobiotics in Animal Tissues and Products

As previously mentioned, either xenobiotics of botanic origin that occur in animal feeds or their metabolites may end up in animal tissues and products. Aflatoxin M_1, which occurs in milk of dairy cows consuming aflatoxin B_1, is an example of this process. Although the transfer of aflatoxins from feeds to animal tissues and products has been studied, there is still much to learn, and nothing is known about the transfer of many of the toxic constituents of plants. Rodricks and Pohland (1981) have pointed out an interesting historic case of transfer of a toxic botanic chemical from an animal to humans, which was first identified by Hall (1979). It is found in the Bible in the book of Numbers, Chapter 11, verses 31 to 33:

"Then a wind from the Lord sprang up; it drove quails in from the west, and they were flying all around the camp for a day's journey, three feet above the ground. The people were busy gathering quails all that day, all night, and all the next day, and even the man who got least gathered ten omers. They spread them out to dry all about the camp. But the meat was scarcely between their teeth and they had not so much as bitten it, when the Lord's anger broke out against the people and he struck them with a deadly plague."

Hall speculated that the quail consumed various poisonous berries, including hemlock, while they overwintered in Africa. The hemlock berry contains coniine, a neurotoxic alkaloid, to which quail are resistant and which can accumulate in their tissue. Humans are not resistant to coniine, and consumption of large quantities of quail tissue containing the neurotoxin could result in death as described in the Biblical scripture.

The potential for adverse human health effects from the consumption of animal tissue and products containing residues of plant xenobiotics is generally unknown. This area is certainly worthy of more intensive research efforts.

Marine Toxins

Coastal dwellers have utilized the sea as a source of food since prehistory and organisms suitable for human consumption have been accepted and those unsuitable have been rejected. Yet consumption of certain seafoods on occasion results in human poisoning. These "occasional" poisonings can be traced to specific toxins that can occur in certain types of seafoods (see also Chapter 22).

Consumption of shellfish sometimes results in symptoms of poisoning, which include either tingling or numbness in the lips, face, and neck and dizziness, headache, and nausea in mild cases, accompanied by muscular paralysis, respiratory difficulty, and death in severe cases. The responsible agent has been termed "paralytic shellfish poison." Schantz et al. (1975) were able to isolate and determine the structure of a major component of this poison. This complex alkaloid, termed saxitoxin, occurs along with various analogs termed gonyantoxins. The ratios of these various components of paralytic shellfish poisons vary with source. Shellfish accumulate saxitoxin through consumption of dinoflagellates, a benthic phytoplankton. Only a few of the more than 1200 species of dinoflagellates produce saritoxin and its analogs. During certain times of the year, under the appropriate environmental factors, these saxitoxin-producing dinoflagellates may undergo a rapid period of reproduction and growth, resulting in a bloom consisting of great numbers. These blooms have been termed "red tide" because the seawater takes on a red hue due to the large number of dinoflagellates. Shellfish feeding in areas with red tide may accumulate the toxins and are apparently resistant to their toxicity. Consumption of shellfish from such waters can result in illness and even death. However, shellfish living in waters with no evidence of red tide may also carry significant levels of the toxins, possibly from consumption of resting cysts of the dinoflagellates (Yentisch and Mague, 1957). Control of paralytic shellfish poisoning is carried out through monitoring for the toxins during harvest and the banning of harvesting from waters where either red tide or evidence of the toxins has been found.

Ingestion of normally safe fish can occasionally result in symptoms of toxicity, including gastrointestinal disorders and signs of neurotoxicity, which can lead to death. This illness has been termed ciguatera, and no specific toxin has yet been associated with it (Hashimoto, 1979). Ciguatoxic fish are tropical saltwater species, which are usually bottom dwellers or fish that feed on bottom dwellers. There are several theories as to how these fish become ciguatoxic, including (1) the consumption of blue-green algae that may contain the responsible toxins, (2) the consumption of certain species of dinoflagellates, or (3) toxins either produced by gut bacteria in the fish or living in association with the blue-green algae (Hashimoto, 1979). Control has consisted mainly of attempts to educate the public as to which fish may be ciguatoxic in a particular geographic region and suggesting that larger fish, which have higher potential to be ciguatoxic, not be consumed and warnings against consumption of the internal organs.

Scombroid poisoning probably represents the greatest number of seafood-related illness. The disease is rarely fatal and resembles an allergic response to histamine. The poisoning obtained its name because it is generally associated with consumption of fish from the family Scombroidae, such as tunas, wahoo, mackerels, and sardines. In this case, the toxicity is thought to result from events that occur after death of the fish instead of during life. Bacterial decarboxylation of muscle histidine produces histamine in the tissue. Apparently another as-yet-unidentified compound acts to synergize the histamine to result in the symptoms of poisoning (Model and Scrimshaw, 1979).

Tetrodotoxin is an extremely toxic compound found in certain organs of the puffer fish, considered a delicacy in Japan. The neurotoxin is quick acting, and death results from respiratory paralysis. To help control the potential health hazard associated with tetradotoxin, Japan allows only specially trained and licensed individuals to prepare puffers for human consumption.

REFERENCES

Ames, B. N.: Dietary carcinogens and anticarcinogens: oxygen radicals and degenerative diseases. *Science*, **221**:1256–64, 1983.

Anonymous: Saccharin. Where do we go from here? *FDA Consumer*, **12**:16–21, 1978.

Bergdoll, M. S.: Staphylococcal intoxications. In Riemann, H., and Bryan, F. L. (eds.): *Food-Borne Infections and Intoxications*, 2nd ed. Academic Press, Inc., New York, 1979, pp. 443–94.

Borzelleca, J. F.; Hallagan, J.; and Reese, C.: Food, drug, and cosmetic colors: toxicological considerations. In Finley, J. W., and Schwass, D. E. (eds.): *Xenobiotics in Foods and Feeds*. American Chemical Society, Washington, D.C., 1983, pp. 311–32.

Bryan, F. L.; Fanelli, M. J.; and Riemann, H.: *Salmonella* infections. In Riemann, H., and Bryan, F. L. (eds.): *Food-Borne Infections and Intoxications*, 2nd ed. Academic Press, Inc., New York, 1979, pp. 73–130.

Bureau of Foods, U.S. Food and Drug Administration: *Toxicological Principles for the Safety Assessment of Direct Food Additives and Color Additives Used in Food*. U.S. Food and Drug Administration, Washington, D.C., 1982.

Campbell, T. C.: Chemical carcinogens and human risk assessment. *Fed. Proc.*, **39**:2467–84, 1980.

———: A decision tree approach to the regulation of food chemicals associated with irreversible toxicities. *Reg. Tox. Pharm.*, **1**:193–201, 1981.

Campbell, T. C., and Hayes, J. R.: The role of aflatoxin metabolism in its toxic lesion. *Toxicol. Appl. Pharmacol.*, **35**:199–222, 1976.

Centers for Disease Control: Common source outbreak, type A botulism. *Morbid. Mortal. Weekly Rep.*, **18**:121, 1969.

———: *Hepatitis Surveillance Report*, No. 39. Centers for Disease Control, Atlanta, Ga.

Clark, A. M.: Endogenous mutagens in green plants. In Klekowski, E. J., Jr. (ed.): *Environmental Mutagenesis, Carcinogenesis and Plant Biology*, Vol. 1. Praeger, New York, 1982, pp. 97–132.

Cliver, D. O.: Viral infections. In Riemann, H., and Bryan, F. L. (eds.): *Food-Borne Infections and Intoxications*, 2nd ed. Academic Press, Inc., New York, 1978, pp. 299–342.

Committee on Animal Health and Committee on Animal Nutrition, Board on Agriculture and Renewable Resources, National Research Council: *Antibiotics in Animal Feeds: The Effect on Human Health of Subtherapeutic Use of Antimicrobials in Animal Feeds*. National Academy Press, Washington, D.C., 1980.

Committee on Food Protection: *Food Colors*. National Academy of Sciences, Washington, D.C., 1971.

———: *Toxicants Occurring Naturally in Foods*. National Academy of Sciences, Washington, D.C., 1973.

Dack, G. M.; Cary, W. E.; Woolpert, O.; and Wiggers, H.: An outbreak of food poisoning proved to be due to a yellow hemolytic staphylococcus. *J. Prev. Med.*, **4**:167–75, 1930.

Doll, R., and Peto, R.: *The Course of Cancer: Quantitative Estimates of Avoidable Risk of Cancer in the United States Today*. Oxford University Press, New York, 1981.

Federal Food, Drug and Cosmetic Act, As Amended. U.S. Government Printing Office, Washington, D.C., 1979.

Feingold, B. F.: Recognition of food additives as a course of symptoms of allergy. *Ann. Allergy*, **26**:309–13, 1968.

———: *Why Your Child Is Hyperactive*. Random House, New York, 1975.

Filer, L. J.: Patterns of consumption of food additives. *Fd. Technol.*, **30**:62–74, 1976.

Food Chemical News: FD and C red 3 is carcinogenic in rats, NTP peer reviewers conclude. *Fd. Chem. News*, **25**(34):50–51, 1983a.

———: FD and C red 3 questions on carcinogenicity sent by FDA to NTP. *Fd. Chem. News*, **25**(32):44–46, 1983b.

———: FD and C red 3 study planned to determine carcinogenic mechanisms. *Fd. Chem. News*, **25**(35):45, 1983c.

Froday, R.: *Progress Report on the NFPA/CMI Container Integrity Program*. Presented at the 76th Annual Convention of the National Food Processors Association, Feb. 8, 1983.

Gunn, R. A.: *Botulism in the United States, 1899–1977*. Center for Disease Control, Atlanta, 197 .

Hall, R. L.: *Proceedings of Marabou Symposium on Foods and Cancer*. Caslan Press, Stockholm, 1979.

Hashimoto, Y.: *Marine Toxins and Other Bioactive Marine Metabolites*. Japan Scientific Societies Press, Tokyo, 1979.

Hayes, J. R., and Borzelleca, J. F.: Biodisposition of xenobiotics in animals. In Beitz, D. C., and Hanson, R. (eds.): *Animal Products in Human Nutrition*. Academic Press, Inc., New York, 1982, pp. 225–59.

Hobbs, B. D.: *Clostricium perfringens* gastroenteritis. In Riemann, H., and Bryan, F. L. (eds.): *Food-Borne In-*

fections and Intoxications, 2nd ed. Academic Press, Inc., New York, 1979, pp. 131–71.

Hogan, G. R.; Ryan, N. J.; and Hayes, A. W.: Aflatoxin B_1 and Reye's syndrome. Lancet, 1:561, 1978.

Jaggi, W.; Lutz, W. K.; Luthy, J.; Zweifel, Y.; and Schlatter, C. H.: In vivo covalent binding of aflatoxin metabolites isolated from animal tissue to rat liver DNA. Food Cosmet. Toxicol., 18:257–60, 1980.

Kilgore, W. W., and Li, M. Y.: Food additives and contaminants. In Doull, J.; Klaassen, C. D.; and Amdur, M. O. (eds.): Casarett and Doull's Toxicology: The Basic Science of Poisons, 2nd ed. Macmillan Publishing Co., New York, 1980, pp. 593–607.

Krishnamachari, K. A. V. R.; Bhat, R. V.; Nagarajan, V.; and Tilak, T. B. G.: Hepatitis due to aflatoxicosis. Lancet, pp. 1061–63, 1975.

Krone, C. A., and Iwooka, W. T.: Mutagen formation in processed foods. In Finley, J. W., and Schwass, D. E.: Xenobiotics in Foods and Feeds. American Chemical Society, Washington, D.C., 1983, pp. 117–27.

Larkin, T.: Exploring food additives. FDA Consumer, 10:4–10, 1976.

Lehmann, P.: More than you ever thought you would know about food additives. Part 1. FDA Consumer, 13:10–12, 1979.

Lipton, M. A., and Mayo, J. P.: Diet and hyperkinesis—an update. J. Am. Diet. Assoc., 83(2):132–34, 1983.

Marth, E. H.: Foodborne hazards of microbial origin. In Roberts, H. R. (ed.): Food Safety. John Wiley & Sons, New York, 1981, pp. 15–65.

Mattes, J. A., and Giltelman, R.: Effects of artificial food colorings in children with hyperactive symptoms. A critical review and results of a controlled study. Arch. Gen. Psychiatry, 38:714–18, 1981.

Miller, E. C.: Some current perspectives on chemical carcinogenesis in humans and experimental animals: presidential address. Cancer Res., 38:1479–96, 1978.

Miller, E. D.; Swanson, A. B.; Phillips, D. H.; Fletcher, T. L.; Liem, A.; and Miller, J. A.: Structure-activity studies of the carcinogenicities in the mouse and rat of some naturally occurring and synthetic alkenylbenzene derivatives related to safrole and estragole. Cancer Res., 43:1124–34, 1983.

Minor, T. E., and Marth, E. H.: Staphylococci and Their Significance in Foods. Elsevier, Amsterdam, 1976.

Mirocha, C. J.; Pathre, S. V.; and Christensen, C. M.: Zearalenone. In Rodricks, J. V.; Hesseltine, C. W.; and Mehlman, M. A. (eds.): Mycotoxins in Human and Animal Health. Pathtox Publishers, Park Forest South, Ill., 1977.

Motil, K. J., and Scrimshaw, N. S.: The role of exogenous histamine in scombroid poisoning. Toxicol. Lett., 3:219–23, 1979.

National Academy of Sciences: Food Chemicals Codex, 2nd ed. National Academy Press, Washington, D.C., 1972.

————: Food Safety Policy: Scientific and Societal Considerations. Committee for a Study of Saccharina and Food Safety Policy, Report No. 2. National Academy Press, Washington, D.C., 1978.

————: Food Safety Policy: Scientific and Societal Considerations. National Academy Press, Washington, D.C., 1979.

————: The Effects on Human Health of Subtherapeutic Use of Antimicrobials in Animal Feeds. National Academy Press, Washington, D.C., 1980.

Office of Technology Assessment, U.S. Congress: Drugs in Livestock Feed, Vol. 1. Technical Report, Publication No. 79-600094, U.S. Government Printing Office, Washington, D.C., 1979.

Oser, B. L., and Hall, R. L.: Criteria employed by the expert panel of FEMA for the GRAS evaluation of fla-

vouring substances. Fd. Cosmet. Toxicol., 15:457–66, 1977.

Pariza, N. W.; Loretz, L. J.; Storkson, J. M.; and Holland, N. C.: Mutagens and modulator of mutagenesis in fried ground beef. Cancer Res., 43(suppl.):2444, 1983.

Peers, F. G.; Gilman, G. A.; and Linsell, C. A.: Dietary aflatoxins and human liver cancer. A study in Swaziland. Int. J. Cancer, 17:167–76, 1976.

President's Science Advisory Committee: Chemicals and Health. National Science Foundation, Washington, D.C., 1973.

Rodricks, J. V., and Pohland, A. E.: Food hazards of natural origin. In Roberts, H. R. (ed.): Food Safety. John Wiley & Sons, New York, 1981, pp. 181–237.

Sakaguchi, G.: Botulism. In Riemann, H., and Bryan, F. L. (eds.): Food-Borne Infections and Intoxications, 2nd ed. Academic Press, Inc., New York, 1979, pp. 389–442.

Sato, N., and Ueno, Y.: Comparative toxicities of trichothecenes. In Rodricks, J. V.; Hesseltine, C. W.; and Mehlman, M. A. (eds.): Mycotoxins in Human and Animal Health. Pathtox Publishers, Park Forest South, Ill., 1977.

Schantz, E. J.; Mold, J. B.; Stanger, D. W.; Shavel, J.; Bowden, J. P.; Lynch, J. M.; Wyler, R. S.; Riegel, B.; and Sommer, H.: Paralytic shellfish poison. VI. A procedure for the isolation and purification of the poison from toxic clam and mussel tissues. J. Am. Chem. Soc., 79:5230–35, 1957.

Scientific Committee of the Food Safety Council: Proposed system for food safety assessment. Fd. Cosmet. Toxicol., 16(2):1–136, 1978.

Seals, J. E.; Snyder, J. D.; Edell, T. A.; Hatheway, C. L.; Johnson, C. J.; Swanson, R. C.; and Hughes, J. M.: Restaurant-associated type A botulism: transmission by potato salad. Am. J. Epidemiol., 113:436–44, 1981.

Select Committee on GRAS Substances: Evaluation of health aspects of GRAS food ingredients: lessons learned and questions unanswered. Fed. Proc., 36(11):2519–62.

Sirgi, M. Y.; Hayes, A. W.; Unger, P. D.; Hogan, G. R.; Ryan, N. J.; and Wray, B. B.: Analysis of aflatoxin B_1 in human tissues with high-pressure liquid chromatography. Toxicol. Appl. Pharmacol., 58:422–30, 1981.

Smith, L. D.: Botulism: The Organism, Its Toxins, the Disease. Charles C Thomas, Pub., Springfield, Ill., 1977.

Stich, H. F.; Rosin, M. P.; Wu, C. H.; and Powrie, W. D.: The use of mutagenicity testing to evaluate food products. In Heddle, J. A. (ed.): Mutagenicity: New Horizons in Genetic Toxicology. Academic Press, Inc., New York, 1982, pp. 117–42.

Stob, M.; Baldwin, R. S.; Tuite, J.; Andrews, F. N.; and Gillette, K. G.: Isolation of an anabolic, uterotropic compound from corn infected with Gibberella zeae. Nature, 196:1318, 1962.

Stoloff, L.: Aflatoxins—an overview. In Rodricks, J. V.; Hesseltine, C. W.; and Mehlman, M. A. (eds.): Mycotoxins in Human and Animal Health. Pathtox Publishers, Park Forest South, Ill., 1977.

Subcommittee on GRAS List Survey (Phase III): Estimating Distribution of Daily Intakes of Certain GRAS Substances. Food and Nutrition Board, National Research Council, National Academy of Sciences, Washington, D.C., 1976.

Sugimura, T., and Nagao, M.: The use of mutagenicity tests to evaluate carcinogenic hazards in our daily life. In Heddle, J. A. (ed.): Mutagenicity: New Horizons in Genetic Toxicology. Academic Press, Inc., New York, 1982, pp. 77–88.

Sugimura, T., and Sato, S.: Mutagens-carcinogens in foods. Cancer Res. 43 (suppl.):2415s, 1983.

Sugiyama, H.; Woodburn, M.; Yang, K. H.; and Mov-roydis, C.: Production of botulinum toxin in inoculated pack studies of foil-wrapped baked potatoes. *J. Food Protect.*, **44**:896–901, 1981.

Tannahill, R.: *Food in History*. Stein & Day, New York, 1973.

Ueno, Y: Trichothecenes: Overview address. In Rodricks, J. V.; Hesseltine, C. W.; and Mehlman, M. A. (eds.): *Mycotoxins in Human and Animal Health*. Pathotox Publishers, Park Forest South, Ill., 1977.

Wogan, G. N.: Aflatoxin carcinogenesis. In Busch, H.: *Methods in Cancer Research*. Academic Press, Inc., New York, 1973, pp. 309–44.

Yentsch, C. M., and Mague, F. C.: Motile cells and cysts: two probable mechanisms of intoxication of shellfish in New England water. In Taylor, D. L., and Saliger, H. H. (eds.): *Toxic Dinoflagellate Blooms*. Elsevier/North Holland, New York, 1957, pp. 127–30.

Chapter 25

AIR POLLUTANTS

Mary O. Amdur

INTRODUCTION

Pollution of the atmosphere has been an undesirable spinoff of human activities presumably since the cavemen first lit fires. These problems increased in magnitude with increasing urbanization. People dug coal from the ground and used it to heat their clustered dwellings, thus creating an atmosphere of sulfurous smoke and filth above the cities. From the thirteenth century onward periodic efforts were made to forbid the burning of coal in London, but on the whole people resigned themselves to acceptance of a polluted atmosphere as a part of urban life. Industrialization and technologic development added a second dimension to pollution of the atmosphere. Power plants burned fossil fuel to generate electricity to light homes and operate machines. Steel mills grew up along river banks and lake shores. Oil refineries rose in port cities or near oil fields. Smelters roasted and refined metals in areas near great mineral deposits. Synthetic chemistry came of age, and factories were built to produce the raw materials needed to manufacture the many things we now take for granted in our daily lives.

In the process of these developments too little thought was given to the effect of waste products on the environment. Some people even went so far as to equate pollution and prosperity, pointing with pride to belching stacks as a symbol of economic development. Cities sprawled and grew, as those who could afford it moved to more desirable areas and commuted daily to the heart of the city. The automobile thus came to add a third dimension to pollution of the atmosphere. "Smog" is really an old word, coined to describe the mixture of smoke and fog that hung over cities like London. In current parlance, however, it has come to refer to the eye-irritating photochemical reaction products of auto exhaust that blanket cities such as Los Angeles when meteorologic conditions produce a stagnant air mass. Over 20 years ago there was already evidence that the date of appearance of plant damage typical of photochemical smog near great cities of the world could be correlated with the date on which the consumption of gasoline passed a critical value.

Air pollution is thus by no means a new problem, although it is a problem of vital current interest. The realization has dawned that a polluted atmosphere is not just another nuisance we must sit back and accept. Efforts have been made on a national as well as on an international level to arrive at air quality standards as a rational basis for control measures. In order to do this it is necessary to integrate and interpret the results of research in many disciplines.

Chemistry provides methods for the determination of concentrations of pollutants in the atmosphere and information on their chemical interactions with one another. Meteorology gives information on conditions causing stagnant air masses in which pollutants can accumulate and studies the dispersion of pollutants from their sources. Engineering supplies the developments in technology needed to control pollution at the source. Toxicology provides information on the physiologic, biochemical, and pathologic effects of known concentrations of pollutants on experimental animals or human subjects. Epidemiology provides information to correlate the health of populations with the known levels of pollution to which they are exposed. Plant pathology yields information on the effects of various pollutants on vegetation, either under field growing conditions or under experimental exposures in greenhouse conditions. Economics attempts, on the one hand, to assess the cost of pollution in terms of corrosion of materials, the loss of income from damaged crops and other effects on the economy, and, on the other hand, to evaluate the cost of pollution control.

TYPES AND SOURCES OF POLLUTANTS

In terms of tons of material emitted annually into the air, five major pollutants account for close to 98 percent of the pollution. These are carbon monoxide (52 percent), sulfur oxides (18 percent), hydrocarbons (12 percent), particulate matter (10 percent), and nitrogen oxides (6 percent). In individual localities the picture would vary widely from these figures. In the vicinity of a smelter, for example, sulfur oxides would be the major pollutant. Downwind from a steel mill, particulate matter would account for a greater percentage of the total pollution than suggested here. In areas where the automobile is the main source of pollution, carbon monoxide, hydrocarbons, and nitrogen oxides would be higher and sulfur dioxide would be lower than indicated.

In discussing air pollution, the distinction is often made between two general types of pollution. The first is characterized by sulfur dioxide and smoke resulting from incomplete combustion of coal and by conditions of fog and cool temperatures. It is the sort of pollution typified by Dickens's "London particular." Because of its chemical nature it is termed reducing type of pollution. The second is characterized by hydrocarbons, oxides of nitrogen, and photochemical oxidants. It results from the atmospheric reaction products of automobile exhaust and occurs with particular frequency and intensity in areas such as the Los Angeles basin, where intense sunlight causes photochemical reactions in polluted air masses trapped by a meteorologic inversion layer. Because of its chemical nature it is termed oxidizing type of pollution. It is also called photochemical air pollution.

In terms of tons of material emitted annually, five major sources account for about 90 percent of the pollution. These are transportation (60 percent), industry (18 percent), electric power generation (13 percent), space heating (16 percent), and refuse disposal (3 percent). Again, these figures would be subject to wide variation depending on local sources of pollution. They do emphasize the importance of the automobile, an integral part of our American way of life, as a major pollution source.

ACUTE HEALTH EFFECTS OF AIR POLLUTION

From time to time there have been situations in which the level of air pollution has risen to concentrations that are definitely hazardous to human health and life. In rare instances, such incidents have involved the accidental release of a specific chemical.

One such incident involved the accidental release of chlorine gas into the subway tunnels of Brooklyn. Another, in Poza Rico, Mexico, involved the release of lethal concentrations of hydrogen sulfide from a malfunction of a new installation in an oil refinery. One case was of a chronic rather than an acute nature. Sufficient beryllium was released from a manufacturing plant to cause beryllium disease in persons residing near the plant. In these incidents the relationship of cause and effect is straightforward. A single chemical was present at a concentration known to be toxic.

The most recent as well as the most disastrous of such incidents occurred the night of December 3, 1984, at Bhopal, India, when approximately 40 tons of methyl isocyanate was released into the atmosphere from a pesticide manufacturing plant. At least 2000 people died and many more became ill. A further discussion of this incident is found in Chapter 12.

In general, when we refer to "acute episodes" of air pollution we have in mind three classic incidents. The first occurred in the Meuse Valley in Belgium in 1930, the second in Donora, Pennsylvania, in 1948, and the third in London in 1952. These incidents have much in common. Meteorologic conditions were those of inversion: the normal situation, in which the lower layers of the atmosphere are warmer than the upper layers, becomes inverted, and the mixing and dilution that occurs as warm air rises and cold air falls cannot take place. The result is an essentially stagnant air mass to which multiple sources continue to add pollutants. The analogy is often made to a "pot with the lid on it." These conditions prevailed for three or four days, during which time the concentration of pollutants rose well above the normal levels for these heavily polluted areas. The Meuse Valley and Donora are industrial areas and in them, as in London, coal was the main fuel for domestic heating. The pollution was therefore of the reducing type, characterized by smoke and sulfur dioxide. In the Meuse Valley and in Donora no measurements were made of the actual levels of pollution. During the London fog the instruments that routinely recorded daily averages of smoke and sulfur dioxide indicated that on the worst day the concentration of smoke was 4.5 mg/m^3 and of sulfur dioxide was 1.34 ppm. Since these are daily averages, short-term peak concentrations would have reached higher levels. Concentrations of neither pollutant are in the range the toxicologist would consider lethal. In the Meuse Valley 65 people died. In Donora 20 people died. In London 4000 deaths were attributed to the fog incident. It is ironic to note that 16 years earlier the prediction was made that if an incident like that in the Meuse Valley were to occur in London, some 3200 deaths would occur.

In all three incidents many people became ill as a result of the pollution. The mortality and morbidity occurred mainly among the elderly and among those with preexisting cardiac and/or respiratory disease. These persons were unable to cope adequately with the added stress imposed by breathing the heavily polluted air. Retrospective investigation suggests the occurrence of earlier acute incidents in these localities. There have been more recent incidents in which meteorologic inversion over polluted urban areas has led to increases in mortality and morbidity. Studies in England led to the suggestion that when concentrations of smoke and sulfur dioxide reach values of 0.75 mg/m^3 for smoke and 0.25 ppm for sulfur dioxide, excess mortality is observed.

There is also clear-cut evidence that more ordinary day-by-day fluctuations in pollution levels have adverse effects on sick people. By giving chronic bronchitic patients a very simple diary in which they recorded whether they felt better or worse than usual, and then relating these entries to daily air pollution data in London, a striking correlation was obtained. It was plain that the patients felt worse on days of greater pollution. These studies were continued after the British Clean Air Act had reduced the levels of both pollutants. It was then possible to conclude that when the 24-hour mean concentrations for smoke and sulfur dioxide were respectively below 0.25 mg/m^3 and 0.19 ppm, the patients showed no response (Lawther, 1975).

The acute effects discussed have been associated with the reducing type of pollution. Less clear-cut evidence exists to associate the photochemical oxidant type of pollution with acute effects on human health. There is, of course, no question of the ability of this type of pollution to produce severe eye irritation that can be correlated with the concentration of pollution present. Studies made of daily mortality among persons 65 and over in Los Angeles County indicated that this was strongly influenced by a heat wave but was not altered consistently by variations in oxidant concentrations. There has been no adequately demonstrated relationship between daily hospital admissions and variations in concentrations of photochemical oxidants. Admissions for conditions considered "highly relevant" (allergic disorders, inflammatory disease of the eye, acute upper respiratory infections, influenza, and bronchitis) were, however, found to show significant correlations with oxidant levels, carbon monoxide, and ozone. It is possible to show a high degree of correlation between diminished performance of high-school cross-country track runners and increased oxi-

dant levels occurring in the hour before the meet.

CHRONIC HEALTH EFFECTS OF AIR POLLUTION

Ambient air pollution can contribute to the occurrence and/or aggravation of disease in urban populations. The diseases that fall into this category are the following: acute nonspecific upper respiratory disease (i.e., the "common cold"), chronic bronchitis, chronic obstructive ventilatory disease, pulmonary emphysema, bronchial asthma, and lung cancer.

Chronic bronchitis is characterized by excessive mucus secretion in the bronchial tree and a chronic or recurrent productive cough. There appears to be little question of a relationship between chronic bronchitis and both cigarette smoking and air pollution. The effect of smoking is by far the greater of the two as a contributing factor to respiratory disease. Unless careful data are included on smoking histories, it is impossible to assess the contribution made by air pollution. This does not mean, however, that air pollution makes no contribution. The following indices of air pollution have been shown to be associated with chronic bronchitis mortality: population size of the community, amounts of fuel burned in large cities, levels of annual sulfur dioxide, levels of dust-fall as well as airborne dust levels, decreased visibility. The following have been shown to be associated with aggravation of symptoms of chronic bronchitis: decreased visibility, outdoor ambient air as contrasted with less polluted indoor air, temporal changes in concentrations of smoke, and sulfur dioxide.

In chronic obstructive ventilatory disease the movement of air in and out of the lungs is impeded by partial closure of the airways. After elimination of the smoking factor, it was found that residents of a polluted area showed lower values for one-second forced expiratory volume (FEV_1) than did residents of an area of low pollution. The difference was small but measurable and was attributed to air pollution. Japanese studies have shown that the airway resistance of schoolchildren living in polluted areas is greater than that of similar children living in nonpolluted areas.

The fact that pulmonary emphysema seems to be increasing, especially in urban areas, points toward air pollution as a possible etiologic factor. If patients with emphysema are placed in a room in which the smog typical of Los Angeles can be removed from the air, after 24 hours they have both subjective relief and objective improvement, which can be measured by pulmonary function tests. Such patients have less oxygen need when they are breathing cleansed air than when they are breathing untreated community air.

Bronchial asthma is produced by many aeroallergens of natural origin that are dispersed by natural forces rather than from human activities. Sometimes these natural allergens can be introduced by man as air pollutants, for example, castor bean dust from factories processing the material, or material from grain handling and milling. Various studies have suggested that asthmatic attacks are associated with higher levels of pollution.

The cause of cancer is, as far as we know, a multiplicity of factors. Among the compounds known to occur as urban air pollutants are some that have known carcinogenic potency. The adsorption of carcinogenic substances on inert particulate material could prolong residence time at sensitive sites in the respiratory tract. Many air pollutants have an irritant action on the mucous membranes of the respiratory tract. There is experimental evidence that when benzopyrene is inhaled by rats whose respiratory tracts have chronic irritation (produced by chronic sulfur dioxide inhalation), bronchogenic carcinoma results (Kuschner, 1968). Experimental evidence also exists that when ozonized gasoline was inhaled by mice that had been infected with influenza virus, epidermoid carcinomas were produced (Kotin and Falk, 1963). There is an urban-rural gradient in incidence of lung cancer that is real when corrected for the effects of cigarette smoking. Kotin and Falk say, "Chemical, physical and biological data unite to form a constellation that strongly implicates the atmosphere as one dominant factor in the pathogenesis of lung cancer."

REDUCING-TYPE POLLUTION

The acute air pollution incidents made plain that under certain meteorologic conditions the reducing-type pollution characterized by sulfur dioxide and smoke was capable of producing disastrous effects. This stimulated toxicologic research on experimental animals and human subjects. Special emphasis, too much for too long, was given to studies of sulfur dioxide alone. Recognition of the critical importance of interactions among components of the sulfurous pollution complex was long overdue when it finally found general acceptance.

The burning of fossil fuels and the smelting of metals emit a variety of particles as well as sulfur dioxide into the atmosphere. Many of these particles are capable of promoting the conversion of sulfur dioxide to the more irritant sulfuric acid. Particles of a submicrometer size are of particular importance. They have a large surface area and are enriched in metals such as zinc and vanadium. These metals can convert sulfur dioxide to sulfuric acid, which is then present as a layer on the surface of the fine particles. Sulfur dioxide is thus the source of atmospheric particulate sulfates such as sulfuric acid, ammonium, sulfate, and ammonium bisulfate. These fine sulfate aerosols may be transported long distances in the atmosphere. In addition to posing a direct hazard to health, they contribute to acid rain, which has become a major ecologic problem in many areas of the northeastern United States, Canada, and Scandinavia.

The EPA, in their revision of the criteria documents, issued a combined *Air Quality Criteria for Particulate Matter and Sulfur Oxides* (EPA, 1982) to replace the original two separate documents. By so doing they acknowledged the fact that it makes little sense to attempt to evaluate the effects of sulfur dioxide without also considering the coexisting particulate matter. The purpose of the criteria documents is to summarize the database available for the setting of the Air Quality Standards by the EPA Administrator. The document thus provides a very comprehensive and up-to-date review of the literature on the reducing-type pollution complex.

Sulfur Dioxide

Mortality and Lung Pathology. Early studies of the mortality produced by sulfur dioxide utilized mice, rats, guinea pigs, and insects. The concentrations required to kill animals are so high that these studies have little relevance to air pollution problems.

Chronic exposure of animals to sulfur dioxide produces a thickening of the mucous layer in the trachea and a hypertrophy of goblet cells and mucous glands, which resembles the pathology of chronic bronchitis. The important point is that such changes can be produced by irritant exposure alone without the intermediary of infection. Infection is of unquestioned importance in the etiology of chronic bronchitis, but experimental evidence indicates that it is not an essential factor in the development of the excessive mucous cells characteristic of this disease. An excellent discussion of the respiratory mucous membrane and its response to irritant agents by Jeffrey and Reid (1977) is recommended reading for students interested in pulmonary toxicology.

In experiments done by Dalhamn (1956), daily exposures of rats to 10 ppm sulfur dioxide for 18 to 67 days produced a thickening of the mucous layer in the trachea of rats. This layer, normally about 5 μm, increased in the exposed animals to about 25 μm. The rate of transport of the mucous layer was decreased and remained so for a month after the end of the exposure. In acute *in vivo* exposures of the trachea of rats to sulfur dioxide, 12 ppm caused cessation of the ciliary beat in four to six minutes. The cilia regained mobility a few minutes after the exposure ceased. In the chronic exposures, however, the frequence of the beat of the cilia was normal but they were unable to move the thickened mucous layer efficiently. Normally beating cilia under a mucous blanket too thick for them to move almost suggests the end result of a self-defeating protective mechanism.

Mawdesley-Thomas *et al.* (1971) exposed rats for ten periods of six hours to 50, 100, 200, and 300 ppm and examined them 72 hours postexposure. The highest dose produced considerable epithelial damage in the trachea and almost complete destruction of goblet cells. A dose-related increase in goblet cells, however, occurred at lower concentrations in the trachea and at all concentrations in the bronchiolus. Excess mucus that reaches the alveolar spaces must be removed by the alveolar macrophages. Exposure to sulfur dioxide did not increase the number of macrophages but did increase their metabolic activity, as indicated by a dose-related increase in acid phosphatase. This increase could be detected at a concentration of 25 ppm.

Daily exposures of dogs to 1 ppm for a year produced a slowing of tracheal mucous transport (Hirsch *et al.*, 1975). In rats, daily exposures to a total of 70 to 170 hours to 0.1, 1.0, and 20 ppm interfered with the clearance of inert particles. The most marked effects were seen with lower doses administered over a longer period of time (Ferin and Leach, 1973).

Following continuous exposure of guinea pigs or monkeys for periods of up to a year or more to concentrations of 0.1 to 5 ppm, no evidence of pulmonary pathology was detected (Alarie *et al.*, 1972, 1975). Unfortunately, the more sensitive techniques discussed above for evaluation of alterations in respiratory mucous membranes were not included in the protocol of these studies.

Absorption and Distribution. On the basis of its solubility in water, one would predict that sulfur dioxide would be readily removed during passage through the upper respiratory tract. This prediction can be tested experimentally by making measurements of the drop in sulfur dioxide concentration when an airstream passes through the upper respiratory tract of larger animals, such as dogs or rabbits, or in human subjects. Indirect assessment of this factor may be made by comparison of the response to given sulfur dioxide concentrations inhaled through the nose or through a tracheal cannula in animals or by comparison of the response to nose and mouth breathing in human subjects.

By the use of $^{35}SO_2$, Strandberg (1964) was able to examine the absorption by the upper respiratory tract of rabbits over a concentration range of 0.05 to 700 ppm. At higher concentrations removal was 90 percent or greater; this is in agreement with the findings of other workers on dogs and human subjects. At concentrations below 1 ppm, however, only 5 percent or less was removed by the upper respiratory tract. These data fit with the observation that guinea pigs breathing through a tracheal cannula to bypass removal by the upper respiratory tract showed an increased response to concentrations of 2, 20, or 100 ppm but no difference at a concentration of 0.4 ppm (Amdur, 1966). This fitting together of data obtained by different methods on different species makes a strong case for the fact that at levels pertinent to air pollution, sulfur dioxide is not efficiently removed by the upper respiratory tract.

The penetration of sulfur dioxide to the lungs is greater during mouth breathing than during nose breathing. An increase in flow rate markedly increases the penetration. In dogs breathing orally, 99 percent of 1 ppm was removed orally at a flow rate of 3.5 liters/min. Increasing the flow rate tenfold decreased the removal efficiency to 33 percent (Frank *et al.*, 1969). These data are of significance in connection with increased uptake in persons exercising and/or mouth breathing during incidents of heavy pollution.

Studies using $^{35}SO_2$ have shown that inhaled sulfur dioxide is readily distributed throughout the body. This also occurs when only an isolated segment of the trachea or the upper airways is exposed. Systemic absorption occurs from these sites, although to a lesser extent than when the lungs are exposed. It is possible that the lungs release some of the gas absorbed in this manner, since radioactivity could be detected in exhaled air samples collected at the carina or below when the lungs had had no sulfur dioxide exposure (Frank *et al.*, 1967). The gas was presumably carried to the lungs from the pulmonary capillaries.

Inhaled sulfur dioxide is only slowly removed from the respiratory tract. Radioactivity can be detected in the respiratory system for a week or more following exposure. Some of the ^{35}S appears to be bound to protein.

Pulmonary Function. The basic physiologic response to inhalation of sulfur dioxide is a mild degree of bronchial constriction, which is reflected in a measurable increase in flow resistance. This increase in resistance has been demonstrated in guinea pigs, dogs, cats, and human subjects. A method for studying the response of guinea pigs (Amdur and Mead, 1958) provides a biologic assay for examining such factors as dose-response relationships, comparison of irritant potency of pollutants, and the effects of aerosols on the response to irritant gases. The method is sufficiently simple that data on many animals exposed only once can be readily obtained. This eliminates the need for reexposure following "recovery," which is an understandable part of the protocol of experiments that use complicated physiologic preparations of larger animals. Unless repeated exposure is the factor being tested, reuse of an experimental animal is not sound toxicologic practice. Studies on larger animals permit the use of more elaborate methods of respiratory physiology that shed light on the mechanisms underlying the changes.

Exposure of guinea pigs to sulfur dioxide produces a dose-related increase in flow resistance. The lower curve in Figure 25–1 shows a dose-response curve relating increase in resistance to sulfur dioxide concentration. Because the figure is designed primarily to demonstrate comparative irritant potency of sulfuric acid and sulfur dioxide, the concentrations are plotted as milligrams of sulfur per m^3 (1 ppm sulfur dioxide = 1.3 mg S/m^3). In exposures to 100 ppm or less of sulfur dioxide alone the resistance returns to control values by the end of a one-hour postexposure period.

Dogs also respond to inhalation of sulfur dioxide with an increase in resistance (Frank and Speizer, 1965). The gas was given to anesthetized dogs by nose, by tracheal cannula, and by

exposing an isolated segment of the trachea to sulfur dioxide while the lungs were ventilated with air. The response was greatest when the gas was introduced directly into the lungs via a tracheal cannula and least when only a segment of trachea was exposed. The fact that resistance increased by exposure of only the tracheal segment suggests a referred reflex constriction of the bronchi. Nasal resistance also increased in a manner roughly proportional to sulfur dioxide concentration. These changes probably reflect mucosal swelling and/or increased secretion of mucus.

The mechanisms of bronchoconstriction produced by sulfur dioxide has been studied in cats (Nadel et al., 1965). Anesthetized cats were ventilated with a pump via a tracheal cannula. Sulfur dioxide gas was delivered either to the lungs or to the upper airways. Total pulmonary resistance increased during the first breath when sulfur dioxide was delivered to the lower airways and lungs during a single inflation cycle. It returned to control values within one minute. Exposing only the upper airways also produced an increase in resistance. An intravenous injection of atropine or cooling of the cervical vagosympathetic nerves abolished these effects; rewarming of the nerve reestablished the response. The rapidity of the response and its reversal suggests that changes in smooth muscle tone are the cause of the bronchoconstriction. The response depends on intact parasympathetic pathways.

The cough reflex in cats is elicited when sulfur dioxide is given through an endobronchial catheter to the lungs and smaller bronchi without coming in contact with the trachea (Widdicombe, 1954). The response produced in this

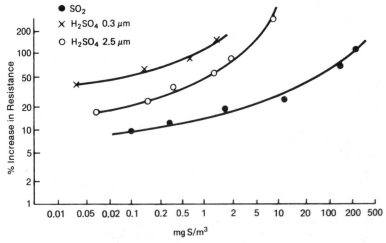

Figure 25–1. Dose-response curves of increase in pulmonary flow resistance produced in guinea pigs exposed for one hour to sulfur dioxide or sulfuric acid.

way was stronger than that produced when sulfur dioxide contacted only the trachea and main bronchi. After several inhalations, the cats became completely refractory to sulfur dioxide but still gave normal response to mechanical stimulation of the trachea. Procaine solution sprayed into the trachea blocked the mechanical cough reflex but failed to affect the response to sulfur dioxide. These data suggest that the receptors for the mechanical stimulus and the sulfur dioxide stimulus are distinct.

This was further confirmed in elegant experiments in which single vagal fibers that were excited by inflation of the lungs were dissected for study (Widdicombe, 1954). One group of these fibers, distributed throughout the lower trachea and main bronchi, was sensitized then inhibited by sulfur dioxide. These fibers were not inhibited by procaine. Another group of fibers was sensitive to mechanical stimulation but not to sulfur dioxide. Vagal temperatures of 7 to 10°C blocked the fibers sensitive to sulfur dioxide. Sulfur dioxide acts via the sympathetic nervous system as well as via the vagus nerve. The group of fibers sensitive to sulfur dioxide sends fibers to the sympathetic trunk.

Human subjects exposed for brief periods to sulfur dioxide also show alterations in pulmonary mechanics. Measurements can be made without interrupting exposure to sulfur dioxide. Frank et al. (1962) exposed 11 subjects to 1, 5, and 13 ppm sulfur dioxide for periods of ten minutes. At 1 ppm only one individual showed an increase in flow resistance. It is of interest to note that this was the individual with the highest control resistance of the group. At a concentration of 5 ppm the average increase in resistance for the group was 39 percent above control values. Nine out of the group showed a statistically significant increase in resistance. At 13 ppm the resistance of all subjects increased, with an average increase for the group of 72 percent. It is thus possible by meticulous attention to experimental protocol and by the use of sensitive physiologic methods to demonstrate a dose-response relationship in human subjects. Studies by other investigators have confirmed this basic finding that the majority of subjects respond to concentrations of 5 ppm or higher, whereas only an occasional sensitive individual responds to 1 ppm. With exercise during exposure, however, a concentration of 1 to 3 ppm increases airway resistance in normal individuals. This effect is no longer seen at 0.5 ppm (Linn et al., 1980).

Lawther et al. (1975) found that airway resistance increased when subjects inhaled 1 to 3 ppm deeply by mouth. There was a dose-response relationship between the number of breaths taken (up to 32) and the observed increase in resistance. Although concentrations of 3 ppm are unlikely as daily or hourly averages, they could be encountered briefly as pockets of pollution from local sources. The fact that few deep breaths will produce increased airway resistance could be of significance to individuals with diseased lungs. The relationship between ventilation and perfusion could be further disturbed with undesirable clinical consequences. Although the subjects used in these studies were normal, healthy individuals, 3 out of 25 showed a greater change that persisted for a longer period after exposure was discontinued.

Clear-cut evidence has recently been obtained that asthmatic individuals are especially sensitive to sulfur dioxide. Sheppard et al. (1981) observed increases in airway resistance in subjects with clinically defined mild asthma during exposure to 0.25 to 0.5 ppm. The subjects were mouth breathing and performing moderate exercise. Koenig et al. (1981) found that in adolescent subjects exposed to 1 ppm with moderate exercise, the degree of response was related to the severity of asthma. They studied three groups: extreme asthmatics, atopics (allergic individuals with no clinical symptoms of asthma), and normals. As examples, airway resistance increased 67, 41, and 3 percent and forced expiratory volume (FEV) decreased 23, 18, and 6 percent for the three groups, respectively. The degree of sensitivity to SO_2 thus appears to depend on the magnitude of preexisting airway hypersensitivity.

The changes we have been discussing were observed in animals or human subjects exposed for short periods of an hour or less to sulfur dioxide. Alarie et al. (1970) exposed guinea pigs to 0.13, 1.01, and 5.72 ppm sulfur dioxide continuously for a year. When compared with a comparable control group breathing clean air, no evidence was found of adverse effects on the mechanical properties of the lung. Measurements included tidal volume, respiratory rate, minute volume, flow resistance, and work of breathing. Monkeys (groups of nine animals) were exposed continuously for 78 weeks to 0.14, 0.64, and 1.28 ppm sulfur dioxide (Alarie et al., 1972). No detrimental alterations in pulmonary function were detected. A fourth group had been started at a level of about 5 ppm. After 30 weeks, there was an accidental high exposure for an hour to somewhere between 200 and 1000 ppm. These animals received no further exposure to sulfur dioxide, but pulmonary function measurements were made according to protocol over the remainder of the 78-week period. Following the overexposure, these animals showed a definite deterioration in pulmonary function, which was shown clearly by the change in the distribution of ventilation.

Lewis *et al.* (1969) exposed dogs to levels of 5 ppm sulfur dioxide about 21 hours a day for 225 days. One group of dogs was normal and the other had had lung impairment produced by prior exposure to nitrogen dioxide (191 days at 26 ppm). The exposure to sulfur dioxide produced about a 50 percent increase in resistance and about a 16 percent decrease in compliance. In general, the adverse effects were less in the dogs with impaired function from previous nitrogen dioxide exposure, which might suggest that a lung previously remodeled by a toxicant may be more difficult to alter physiologically than one which had never been exposed to toxic concentrations of irritant. Vaughan *et al.* (1969) exposed dogs for 16 hours a day for 18 months to a combination of 0.5 ppm sulfur dioxide and 0.1 mg/m^3 sulfuric acid and concluded there was no impairment in pulmonary function.

Well-planned and carefully executed studies of the effect of sulfur dioxide on human subjects exposed continuously for periods of 120 hours were reported by Weir *et al.* (1972). Their subjects lived throughout the exposure period in a 30 m^3 dynamic flow chamber. Daily pulmonary function measurements included airway resistance at varying lung volumes, functional residual capacity, dynamic lung compliance, and total lung volume. In the initial series, 0, 3, 6, and 8 ppm sulfur dioxide were used. Dose-related changes were observed in subjective complaints, clinical evaluations, blood gases, airway resistance, and dynamic lung compliance. The second group of experiments used concentrations of 0.3, 1, and 3 ppm sulfur dioxide. No dose-related changes were observed in subjective complaints, clinical evaluations, or most pulmonary function measurements at these lower concentrations. Significant, but minimal, reversible increases were noted in airway resistance accompanied by a decrease in compliance at high frequencies of breathing at the 3-ppm concentration. Unfortunately, a detailed report of these studies has never been published.

Biochemical Effects. Information on biochemical aspects of the toxicology of sulfur dioxide is very limited. Some early studies indicated that radioactive sulfur persisted in the lung incorporated into protein, but no evidence was presented on the nature of this complex. Work by Gunnison and Palmes (1974) has indicated the presence in plasma of S-sulfonate formed by the reaction of sulfite with the disulfide bond in proteins. This has been found in rabbits and in human subjects. They examined the plasma from subjects exposed in Weir's experiments and found a positive correlation of plasma S-sulfonate levels with exposure concentrations of sulfur dioxide. Most recently they have found S-sulfonate present in the plasma and aorta of rabbits infused with sulfite. While the biologic significance is not at present understood, this finding represents the first biochemical alteration observed in target organs.

Sulfuric Acid

The guinea pig is the small mammal most sensitive to sulfuric acid inhalation. Rabbits, rats, and mice are must less sensitive (Treon *et al.*, 1950). Two early studies (Amdur *et al.*, 1952; Pattle *et al.*, 1956) used guinea pigs to examine the lethal effects of eight-hour exposures to sulfuric acid. The concentration required to kill the animals ranged from 18 to 60 mg/m^3. Animals were more sensitive at one to two months of age than at 18 months. Particles of 2.7 μm were more toxic than 0.8-μm particles when mortality was the criterion of response. This is probably because the larger particles deposited in areas of the respiratory tract where major spasm of the airways would be rapidly lethal. Dropping the temperature to 0°C significantly increased the toxicity of the sulfuric acid, probably owing to the cold stress on a tropical animal. Sufficient ammonium carbonate in the chamber to provide an excess of ammonia protected against the effects of sulfuric acid.

The pathologic findings in the lungs were similar in the two investigations. The cause of death in animals that succumbed rapidly appeared to be bronchoconstriction and laryngeal spasm. Animals dying after a longer exposure showed gross pulmonary pathology, including hemorrhage, capillary engorgement, and some edema. The animals surviving the exposure showed spotty areas of old hemorrhage and areas of consolidation, especially around the hilar regions. Such damage is repaired only slowly.

Extending the exposure time to 72 hours did not increase the mortality beyond that observed for eight-hour exposures, but did increase the lung pathology (Amdur *et al.*, 1952). The mortality was related to concentration of sulfuric acid, and the degree of lung pathology was related to the total dose (concentration × time). This suggests that sulfuric acid has two actions. First, it promotes laryngeal spasm and bronchospasm, which are the causes of death. These actions are related primarily to concentration and individual sensitivity. Sulfuric acid can also cause parenchymal lung damage, and this action is related to the total dosage.

Sulfuric acid produces an increase in flow resistance in guinea pigs, the magnitude of which is related to both concentration and particle size

(Amdur, 1958; Amdur *et al.*, 1978a). In the following discussion, particle size is expressed as mass median diameter (MMD). Particles of 7 μm produced only a slight increase in resistance even at very high concentration (30 mg/m^3). Since these particles would not penetrate beyond the upper respiratory tract, this response was probably a referred reflex or an increase in nasal resistance. Particles of 2.5 μm gave a response that was slow in onset and accompanied by a major decrease in compliance. These mechanical changes were suggestive of closure of large areas of the lung due to constriction or obstruction with mucous secretions. Particles of 1 μm or below produced a swift response similar to that observed with irritant gases. Irritant potency increased with decreasing particle size. At concentrations below 1 mg/m^3 the response was greater for 0.3-μm than for 1-μm particles (Amdur *et al.*, 1978a). Elevated flow resistance produced by sulfuric acid is much slower to return to control values than is the increase produced by sulfur dioxide. The action of irritant particles deposited on the lung surface is more prolonged than that of a gas, which is rapidly cleared from the lungs when exposure ceases.

Dose-response curves shown in Figure 25–1 indicate that at a given concentration of sulfur, sulfuric acid produces a greater response than sulfur dioxide. Even the less irritant 2.5-μm particles produce a two- and threefold greater response than the equivalent amount of sulfur dioxide.

There is evidence that on a chronic basis as well, sulfuric acid is a more potent irritant than sulfur dioxide (Alarie *et al.*, 1972, 1975). These studies involved the exposure of monkeys to either sulfur dioxide or sulfuric acid for periods of 78 weeks. Table 25–1 indicates some of the changes observed. When compared on the basis of mg S/m^3, it is evident that far higher levels of

sulfur administered as sulfur dioxide had no effect on the animals.

The effect of sulfuric acid (0.3 to 0.6 μm) on tracheobronchial mucociliary clearance of radioactively tagged ferric oxide particles has been studied in the donkey (Schlesinger *et al.*, 1978). Previous studies have shown that the donkey is a good experimental model, as clearance changes are consistent with and quantitatively comparable to similar data obtained in human subjects. Three out of four animals demonstrated short-term slowing of clearance as a result of single, one-hour exposures to 194 to 1364 μg/m^3. Two of the four animals showed a more persistent slowing of control clearance values as the series of weekly exposures progressed. Sulfur dioxide affected clearance only at concentrations of 300 ppm or greater. This is another piece of evidence indicating the greater toxicity of sulfuric acid as compared to sulfur dioxide.

Comparative studies in donkey and human subjects done by these investigators are of great practical significance. The effects of single short-term exposures to sulfuric acid on mucociliary clearance are similar in the two species. In donkeys, repeated exposure to low levels of sulfuric acid has a profound effect on clearance rates. It is neither ethical nor practical to do such repeated exposures in human subjects. It is, however, reasonable to assume that the chronic effects in humans would resemble those seen in the donkey. This is further strengthened by the similar response of the two species to cigarette smoke. The misguided chronic self-exposure of humans to cigarette smoke clearly documents the potential for development of chronic bronchitis. The assumption is thus reasonable that chronic exposure of humans to sulfuric acid at levels of 100 μg/m^3 or above would also lead to impaired clearance and chronic bronchitis as seen in donkeys.

Table 25–1. COMPARATIVE TOXICITY OF SO$_2$ AND H$_2$SO$_4$: PULMONARY FUNCTION OF MONKEYS EXPOSED TWO YEARS

COMPOUND	CONCENTRATION	mg S/M^3	ALTERATIONS		
SO$_2$	1 ppm	1.31	None		
			Histopathology	*Distribution of Ventilation*	*Arterial O$_2$*
H$_2$SO$_4$ (2.15 μm)	0.38 mg/m^3	0.12	Slight	0	0
H$_2$SO$_4$ (3.60 μm)	2.43 mg/m^3	0.80	Moderate	Moderate	Slight
H$_2$SO$_4$ (0.73 μm)	4.79 mg/m^3	1.57	—	Slight	0
H$_2$SO$_4$ (0.54 μm)	0.48 mg/m^3	0.16	Moderate to severe	Moderate	Moderate

Particulate Sulfates

The irritant potency of zinc ammonium sulfate, which was reported as a constituent of the Donora fog, was studied at four particle sizes, from 0.29 to 1.4 μm, at concentrations from 0.25 to 3.6 mg/m^3 (Amdur and Corn, 1963). The lowest concentration is of the order of magnitude of what might have occurred during the fog incident. All concentrations tested produced an increase in flow resistance in guinea pigs. The irritant potency increased as the particle size decreased. The slope of the dose-response curves also steepened as the particle size decreased, so that a smaller increment in concentration produced a larger increment in response. This paper points out the utter inadequacy of relying on information about mass concentration alone when attempting to assess the irritant potency of particulate matter. Information on particle size can be equally critical.

Nadel et al. (1967) found that zinc ammonium sulfate produced a response similar to, but lesser in degree than, that produced by histamine. The experiments were made on anesthetized cats artificially ventilated with a pump. The aerosol was submicron in size and the concentration was 40 to 50 mg/m^3. The response to a three-minute inhalation included increased pulmonary resistance, decreased compliance and increased end-expiratory transpulmonary pressure. Isoproterenol prevented the changes, suggesting that they were due to smooth muscle contraction. Cardiac arrest during histamine inhalation did not prevent the changes. This suggests that the action was directly on the airway smooth muscle and was not dependent on circulation. To correlate with the physiologic responses, anatomic studies were made after rapid deep freezing of the lungs in the open thorax. The principal sites of constriction were the alveolar ducts and terminal bronchioles. Bronchi and bronchioles larger than 400 μm were not constricted. Physiologic responses and anatomic data combine to indicate the locus of action of the submicron particles.

The sulfate ion per se is not irritant; therefore, sulfates vary widely in irritant potency. For comparison, the increase in flow resistance can be calculated per microgram of sulfate. Data were obtained with 0.3-μm aerosols (Amdur et al., 1978b). Table 25–2 expresses the response to the sulfate salts as a percentage of the corresponding response to sulfuric acid. Pharmacologic studies also indicate differences among sulfates. Ammonium sulfate causes histamine release by guinea pig lungs, whereas sodium sulfate does not. The removal of intratracheally injected sulfate from the lung is markedly influenced by the cation present (Charles et al.,

Table 25–2. RELATIVE IRRITANT POTENCY OF SULFATES

Sulfuric acid	100
Zinc ammonium sulfate*	33
Ferric sulfate†	26
Zinc sulfate*	19
Ammonium sulfate	10
Ammonium bisulfate	3
Cupric sulfate	2
Ferrous sulfate	0.7
Sodium sulfate‡	0.7
Manganous sulfate†	−0.9§

* Data of Amdur and Corn, 1963.
† Data of Amdur and Underhill, 1968.
‡ Particle size: 0.1 μm.
§ Resistance decreased; change N.S.

1977). Greater effects were seen with ferric iron than with zinc, and manganese did not enhance sulfate uptake. The potency of the various metal cations was thus in general agreement with the ranking based on increased airway resistance. The pharmacologic and pulmonary function changes are probably related.

By other criteria, the potency of sulfate salts shows a different ranking. Mice were exposed for three hours to various sulfate salts and then challenged with S. pyrogens (Ehrlich et al., 1978). Based on the concentrations causing a 20 percent enhancement of bacterial-induced mortality, the sulfates ranked Cd > Cu < Zn < Al > Zn-NH$_4$ > Mg. No effect at all was produced by NH$_4$, Na, and Fe^{3+}. Other workers (Skornik and Brain, 1983) examined in hamsters the effect of sulfate salts on the ability of pulmonary macrophages to clear particles from the lung. Their ranking was Cu > Zn > Fe^{3+} > Zn-NH$_4$, which is in general agreement with data from the S. pyrogens infectivity model. Effects on pulmonary macrophages would be closely related to bacterial clearance.

These data indicate that irritant sulfates should not be ranked in potency on the basis of only one of their possible effects on the lung. They also make clear that an air quality standard based on "suspended sulfate" without further characterization would be entirely inappropriate; the term is toxicologically meaningless.

Effect of Aerosols on the Response to Sulfur Dioxide

Measurement of flow resistance in the guinea pig is a bioassay of sufficient sensitivity to detect quantitatively the potentiation of irritant gases by aerosols. The aerosols are "inert," in that they do not affect resistance when used alone. The dose-response curve for sulfur dioxide plus the aerosol can be compared with the dose-response curve for sulfur dioxide alone.

Early studies with sodium chloride delineate several factors affecting the potentiation (Amdur, 1961). Particle size of the aerosol is important. Submicron particles potentiate, but 2.5-μm particles do not. Concentration of the aerosol is important. At a relatively humidity of 50 percent, 10 mg/m^3 potentiates but 4 mg/m^3 does not. Postexposure resistance values remain elevated (typical of irritant aerosols) and can be related directly to total aerosol dose. The potentiation is relatively slow to develop; at ten minutes the response is the same as that to sulfur dioxide alone (Amdur, 1961; Amdur and Underhill, 1968). Relative humidity (RH) is also important (McJilton et al., 1973). At 80 percent RH 1 mg/m^3 is as effective as 10 mg/m^3 at 50 percent RH. At high humidities the potentiation occurs rapidly.

The aerosols that have produced a major potentiation of the response to sulfur dioxide are soluble salts of such metals as manganese, ferrous iron, and vanadium (Amdur and Underhill, 1968). These materials form droplets that can dissolve sulfur dioxide; the metal ions then promote oxidation to sulfuric acid. These aerosols potentiate the response about threefold when present at a concentration of 1 mg/m^3 at 50 percent RH. This is far greater than the potentiation produced by sodium chloride except at a high relative humidity. At a sulfur dioxide concentration of 0.2 ppm, about 10 percent of the sulfur was converted to sulfuric acid. When this amount of sulfuric acid was added to 0.2 ppm sulfur dioxide, the response to the gas plus metal aerosol could be duplicated (Amdur, 1974).

Coal combustion produces both an ultrafine (<0.1 μm) aerosol and sulfur dioxide. The ultrafine fraction contains metals, such as zinc, capable of promoting the conversion of sulfur dioxide to sulfuric acid, which is then present as a surface layer on the particles. Short-term (three-hour) exposure of guinea pigs to ultrafine zinc oxide generated at combustion temperatures in the presence of sulfur dioxide and water vapor produces major functional and morphologic alterations in the lung at concentrations of 1 ppm sulfur dioxide and 2.5 to 5 mg/m^3 zinc oxide (Lam et al., 1982; Conner et al., 1982). Decreased lung volumes and CO-diffusing capacity are correlated with microscopic evidence of edema and biochemical criteria of damage to epithelial and endothelial cells. The changes persist for 24 to 72 hours following a single exposure. Neither sulfur dioxide nor zinc oxide alone alters any of these parameters.

At a constant concentration of sulfur dioxide (1 ppm) the magnitude of the changes increases with increasing concentrations of zinc oxide. For example, CO-diffusing capacity is 25 percent below that of air control animals at 2.5 mgm^3 and 54 percent below control at 5 mg/m^3 zinc oxide. Chemical studies of these atmospheres indicate that a surface layer of sulfuric acid is present on the zinc oxide aerosol. Thus, when more aerosol particles are present, more sulfuric acid is carried to the lung. These biologic and chemical data suggest the need for control of such ultrafine aerosols. Even though the actual mass concentration of sulfuric acid is very low (at most about 40 μg/m^3), it is carried to the sensitive alveolar regions of the lung on the surface of the ultrafine particles. Because it is on the surface, it is readily available to cause the observed irritant effects. (Amdur, 1985; Amdur et al., 1986).

Results of studies of flow resistance in human subjects exposed to sulfur dioxide alone and in combustion with sodium chloride aerosol are conflicting. Frank et al. (1964) exposed human subjects to 1, 5, and 15 ppm sulfur dioxide alone and with the addition of sodium chloride aerosol. In an initial series of experiments the exposures were given in sequence with a 15- to 20-minute recovery period between them. Whether the gas alone or the combination was given first was randomized. The only consistent finding was that the resistance increase to the second exposure was less than that evoked by the first exposure. The series was repeated, allowing the lapse of a month between exposures. No difference could be detected between the responses to the sulfur dioxide alone and the response to sulfur dioxide plus the aerosol. Although the paper does not so indicate in the discussion, the response of the same individual on different occasions to the same concentration of sulfur dioxide alone is greater than the potentiating effect of sodium chloride observed in guinea pigs. Burton et al. (1969) tested the effect of about 2 mg/m^3 sodium chloride aerosol on the response of ten subjects to 1 to 3 ppm sulfur dioxide. As would have been predicted on the basis of experiments with guinea pigs, at this gas concentration and 4 mg/m^3 sodium chloride, no potentiation was observed.

Toyama (1962) reported that sodium chloride did potentiate the response of human subjects to sulfur dioxide. The dose-response curves for sulfur dioxide alone and plus aerosol resemble strikingly data on guinea pigs. The major toxicologic problem in accepting these results is the fact that the exposures were given in sequence and the second exposure was always to the sulfur dioxide plus aerosol. If data were given on responses of a similar number of subjects to sequential exposures to sulfur dioxide alone, the results could be properly interpreted. As was indicated above, Frank *et al.* (1964) found a lesser response to a second exposure given in sequence, which is the reverse of these findings. Sequential exposures are a toxicologic trap into which unwary physiologists fall.

Toyama and Nakamura (1964) observed potentiation by an aerosol of hydrogen peroxide, which would be a liquid droplet and also oxidize sulfur dioxide to sulfuric acid. Again, there is the problem of sequential exposures. No published data exist on the effect of the soluble metal salts on the response of human subjects to sulfur dioxide. The techniques of the experimental toxicologist, who can use many animals exposed only once, may be more suitable for the elucidation of potentiation responses than are the techniques of the physiologist, who can expose only a few human subjects.

COMPONENTS AND FORMATION OF PHOTOCHEMICAL AIR POLLUTION

Photochemical air pollution arises from a series of atmospheric reactions. The main components are ozone, oxides of nitrogen, aldehydes, peroxyacetyl nitrates, and hydrocarbons. From the point of view of a discussion of the toxicology of air pollutants, the hydrocarbons as such do not concern us. The concentrations in ambient air do not reach levels high enough to produce any toxic effect. They are important because they enter into the chemical reactions that lead to the formation of photochemical smog.

The chemical reactions that lead to the formation of this particular mixture of pollutants in the atmosphere are extremely complex. A detailed discussion and review of this subject, as well as of the toxicology of ozone, was released by the National Academy of Sciences Committee on Medical and Biological Effects on Environmental Pollutants (1977).

The oxidant found in the largest amounts in polluted atmospheres is ozone (O_3). Several miles above the earth's surface there is sufficient short-wave ultraviolet light to convert O_2 to O_3 by direct absorption, but these wavelengths do not reach the earth's surface. Of the major atmospheric pollutants, nitrogen dioxide is the most efficient absorber of the UV light that does reach the earth's surface. This absorption of UV light by NO_2 leads to a complex series of reactions, which may be simplified as follows:

$$NO_2 \xrightarrow{\text{UV}} NO + O \quad\quad (1)$$
$$O + O_2 \longrightarrow O_3 \quad\quad (2)$$
$$O_3 + NO \longrightarrow NO_2 + O_2 \quad\quad (3)$$

Since NO_2 is regenerated by the reaction of the NO and O_3 formed, the overall result is a cyclic reaction, which can be perpetuated.

This NO_2 photolytic cycle serves to explain the initial formation of O_3 in polluted atmospheres, but cannot explain the development of concentrations of O_3 as great as those which have been measured. If no additional mechanisms were involved, most of the O_3 would be broken down by reaction with the NO formed, and in steady-state conditions, O_3 and NO would be formed and destroyed in equal quantities. The hydrocarbons, especially olefins and substituted aromatics, become of importance by providing the necessary added reactants. Oxygen atoms attack the hydrocarbons. The resulting oxidized compounds and free radicals react with NO to produce more NO_2. Thus, the balance of the reactions shown in equations 1 to 3 is upset so that NO_2 and O_3 levels build up while NO levels are depleted. These reactions are very complex and involve the formation of intermediate free radicals that are very reactive and undergo a series of changes.

Aldehydes are major products in the photooxidation of hydrocarbons, and in the reactions of hydrocarbons with ozone, oxygen atoms, or free radicals. Formaldehyde and acrolein have been specifically identified in urban atmospheres. About 50 percent of the total aldehyde is present as formaldehyde and about 5 percent as acrolein.

Peroxyacetyl nitrate, often referred to as PAN, is most likely formed in the atmosphere from the reaction of the peroxyacetyl radical with NO_2. Its chemical formula is CH_3COONO_2. Higher homologs are probably also present, but PAN is the one that has been positively identified as present in urban atmospheres.

Ozone

A variety of toxic effects occur in experimental animals exposed to concentrations of ozone that can occur in urban areas with photochemical pollution. These effects include morphologic, functional, and biochemical alterations. An excellent summary of current knowledge on all aspects of ozone toxicity is available in the proceedings of an international symposium (Lee *et al.*, 1983).

Mortality and Lung Pathology. Ozone is a deep lung irritant capable of causing death from pulmonary edema. The early studies, many of them from his own research group, have been well reviewed by Stokinger (1965). The LC50 following three-hour exposures varies from about 50 ppm for guinea pigs to about 20 ppm for mice. The lethality of ozone is influenced by factors other than concentration and length of exposure. Young mice are more susceptible. Elevated ambient temperature or exercise increases the toxicity. Intermittent exposures are much less toxic than the same total dose administered continuously. Rats exposed to 2 ppm for three hours showed an increased water content of the lung. More sensitive techniques, which utilize recovery of radiolabeled blood albumin in lung lavage fluid, indicate that the threshold for edema formation in rats is 0.25 to 0.5 ppm for six hours (Alpert *et al.*, 1971).

Boatman *et al.* (1974) reported desquamation of the ciliated epithelium throughout the ciliated airways of cats exposed four to six hours to 0.25, 0.5, and 1.0 ppm. The degree of damage was dose related. Alveolar damage included swelling and denudation of the cytoplasm of type I cells, swelling or rupture of the capillary endothelium, and lysis of erythrocytes. In rats, Stephens *et al.* (1974) observed degenerative changes in type I alveolar cells after three-hour exposure to concentrations as low as 0.2 ppm. These are replaced by type II cells beginning a day after exposure.

Rats and monkeys exposed for eight hours a day on seven consecutive days to 0.2, 0.5, or 0.8 ppm showed mild but significant morphologic lesions at the lowest concentrations. When exposure of rats was extended continuously, lesions reached a peak in three to five days and then diminished. After 90 days at 0.8 ppm there was obvious damage, but this was less severe than at seven days (Dungworth, 1976). In monkeys ozone inhalation establishes a new balance between cell loss and replacement in the respiratory bronchioles (Eustis *et al.*, 1981). It is important to note that in the case of ozone, pulmonary pathology has been observed in experimental animals following relatively short exposures to concentrations that can occasionally be attained for short periods in polluted urban areas.

Early studies suggested that long-term exposure to ozone results in effects on morphology and function of the lung and acceleration of lung tumor formation and of aging. Chronic bronchitis, bronchiolitis, fibrosis, and emphysematous changes were observed in a variety of species exposed to ozone concentrations slightly above 1 ppm.

Electron microscopy has been used to document morphologic changes in the lungs of dogs exposed to 1 to 3 ppm ozone for up to 18 months (Stephens *et al.*, 1973). Daily exposure times were 8, 16, or 24 hours. The effects increased in severity in a manner related more to concentration than to duration of exposure. A thickening of the terminal and respiratory bronchioles was accompanied at the highest concentration by an infiltration of cells that reduced the caliber of the small airways. Young rats exposed for up to three weeks to 0.5 to 0.9 ppm showed morphologic lesions in respiratory bronchioles, distal portions of the terminal bronchiolar epithelium, the alveolar duct, and alveoli (Stephens *et al.*, 1974). It is thus evident that damage from ozone occurs in peripheral areas of the lung.

Tolerance. Early studies (Stokinger, 1965) indicated that a single one-hour exposure to 0.3 ppm ozone would protect against subsequent exposure to otherwise lethal concentrations. Tolerance lasted four to six weeks in rats and up to 14 weeks in mice. Water content of the lungs remained normal and there was less histopathologic damage. Lung alkaline phosphatase and glutathione levels remained normal in tolerant animals. Cross-tolerance was found between ozone and other edema-producing irritants such as nitrogen dioxide and phosgene. The tolerance protects against pulmonary edema but not against alterations in pulmonary function. More recent evidence indicates that the antibacterial defense mechanisms of the lung are not protected (Gardner *et al.*, 1972).

Pulmonary Function. Exposure to ozone produces alterations in respiration, the most characteristic of which are shallow, rapid breathing and a decrease in pulmonary compliance. Alterations in resistance occur only at high concentrations. This pattern is typical of materials that have their site of action in the smaller airways and peripheral portions of the lung.

In two-hour exposures of guinea pigs to 0.34 to 1.35 ppm (Murphy *et al.*, 1964b), the earliest effects detected were an increase in frequency and a decrease in tidal volume that were observed at all concentrations. Higher concentrations produced a greater change, which was present earlier in the exposure period. Higher concentrations also produced an increase in flow resistance. These changes were reversible during a 90-minute recovery period. Concentrations of 1.3 to 1.8 ppm will reduce pulmonary compliance by about 50 percent. A lesser change in compliance was produced by 0.4 ppm, but not by 0.2 ppm (Amdur *et al.*, 1978c).

Ozone exposure increases the sensitivity of the lung to bronchoconstrictive agents such as histamine, acetylcholine, and allergens. Easton and Murphy (1967) found an increased respiratory response to histamine injected s.c. in guinea pigs two hours after a two-hour exposure to 1 to 5 ppm ozone. Increased mortality from higher levels of histamine could be produced by as little as 0.5 to 1 ppm ozone. The increased susceptibility persisted up to 12 hours after a two-hour exposure to 5 ppm ozone. More recent studies on dogs (Lee *et al.*, 1977) have shown an increased respiratory response to an aerosol of histamine following exposure to 1 ppm ozone.

This sensitivity can persist for 7 to 28 days. These studies raise important questions in regard to the possibility of ozone sensitizing an individual to subsequent exposure to other pollutants.

Alterations in pulmonary function have also been observed in human subjects when intermittent exercise is superimposed on exposure. This entire area, including emphasis of points critical to appropriate experimental design, is discussed at length in the 1977 National Academy of Sciences monograph and in the international symposium proceedings references earlier (Lee *et al.*, 1983).

At ozone concentrations of 0.3 ppm and above, the results of a number of studies clearly indicate effects on pulmonary function of human subjects exposed for short (one- to two-hour) periods. These changes included decreases in vital capacity, forced expiratory flows, and tidal volume. At the current National Ambient Air Quality Standard of 0.12 ppm, some investigators found small changes but others found no effect.

A recent study (Lippmann *et al.*, 1983) reported that ozone exposures below 0.12 ppm produced decrements in pulmonary function in active children. The children were measured while participating in the program of a summer camp. When the peak one-hour ozone exposure was 0.10 ppm, values for forced vital capacity and forced expiratory volume in one second were lower on days than when the peak was below 0.08 ppm.

Susceptibility to Bacteria. Exposure to ozone prior to challenge with aerosols of infectious agents produces a higher incidence of infection than seen in control animals (Coffin and Blommer, 1967). It is assumed that this results from inhibition of clearance mechanisms, either mucociliary streaming or phagocytosis. Exposure of mice to concentrations as low as 0.08 ppm ozone for three hours enhanced the mortality from subsequent exposure to a bacterial aerosol of streptococcus (Group C). The susceptibility of mice and hamsters to *Klebsiella pneumoniae* aerosol was increased by prior exposure to ozone, as indicated by a higher mortality, shorter survival time, and lower LD50 for *K. pneumoniae* in ozone-exposed animals as compared with controls.

It has been shown that exposure to ozone reduced the number as well as the *in vitro* phagocytic ability of pulmonary macrophages in rabbits. This could help to explain the increased survival time of bacteria observed in the lungs of animals preexposed to ozone. More recent studies (Witz *et al.*, 1983) indicate that membrane damage in macrophages from rats exposed to

ozone impairs production of bactericidal superoxide anion radical.

Biochemical Effects. The similarity of some effects of ozone to those of radiation suggested that ozone toxicity might result from the formation of reactive free-radical intermediates. Stokinger (1965) and Menzel (1970) have reviewed the evidence on this subject. Ozone and x-irradiation are nearly additive in producing chromosomal aberrations in plants and animals. Antioxidant and radical trapping agents such as quinones, ascorbic acid, and α-tocopherol protect against ozone toxicity. Ozone-induced free radicals may be derived from interaction with sulfhydryls and/or from oxidative decomposition of unsaturated fatty acids. It is likely that more than one radical is formed either directly from ozone or from its interaction with normal cellular constituents. Further research is needed to determine the exact radicals produced by ozone *in vivo*.

Various investigators have noted protection from ozone by sulfhydryl compounds. Ozone exposure decreases lung glutathione and succinic dehydrogenase. Exposure of rats to 2 ppm for four to eight hours produced a decrease in both protein and nonprotein lung sulfhydryl groups. Peak oxidation of nonprotein sulfhydryl groups did not occur until 25 hours after exposure and recovery was evident by 48 hours (DeLucia *et al.*, 1975).

Ozone exposure alters the metabolism of lung tissue. Cell injury and/or death produces a depression of enzyme activity. This overlaps with and is followed by a reparative phase in which enzyme activities are elevated. These biochemical changes are temporally correlated with observed turnover of cell populations following ozone exposure.

These metabolic alterations are discussed in a paper by Mustafa *et al.* (1983). When rats were exposed to 0.2, 0.5, or 0.8 ppm O_3 continuously for seven days, enzyme activities rose to their maximum in three days and then remained constant. The magnitude of change was dose related. When exposure ceased, the values reverted to control levels within a week. When animals were reexposed, the enzyme levels rose as in initial exposures.

Incubation of human red cells *in vitro* with ozone or ozonides provides evidence for a role of lipid peroxidation in cellular damage from ozone. Incubation with ozonized liposomes (Tiege *et al.*, 1974) or with ozonized serum (Menzel *et al.*, 1975) was more damaging than incubation with ozone itself. Lung toxicity similar to that seen after ozone exposure was produced in rats by intravenous injection of fatty acid hydroperoxides or ozonides (Cortesi and

Privett, 1972). Conjugated diene bonds were found in extracts of lungs of mice exposed to 0.4 to 0.7 ppm ozone for four hours (Goldstein *et al.*, 1969).

One piece of indirect evidence for a role of lipid peroxidation is the finding that animals deficient in vitamin E were more susceptible to ozone (Goldstein *et al.*, 1970). Data on the protective effect of added supplements of vitamin E are conflicting. Menzel *et al.* (1975) found that oral administration of vitamin E did protect against Heinz body formation in cells incubated *in vitro* with ozonides.

Alterations in the protein fraction of lung tissue have been observed in rabbits following one-hour exposure to 1 ppm ozone (Buell *et al.*, 1965). A variety of aldehydes and ketones were identified. The aldehydes formed may bring about an intra- or intermolecular cross-linking of proteins that would alter normal lung structure. There was also evidence of oxidative degradation of hyaluronic acid, which would suggest alterations in the ground substance of the lungs. Since the ground substance serves as a lubricant and matrix for the fibers of the lung, a decreased slippage and flexibility of elastic protein molecules could result. This could be enhanced by cross-linking of aldehydes with fibers of elastic protein molecules. The authors suggest that these alterations may help explain the increased sensitivity of ozone-exposed animals to bacterial infection because a breakdown of ground substance by ozone exposure would facilitate penetration of bacteria into the lung tissue. More recent studies indicate increased collagen synthesis in lungs of exposed animals.

Extrapulmonary Effects. Various studies have reported effects other than those directly related to the lung in laboratory animals exposed to ozone at a concentration as low as 0.2 ppm. Included are reduction of voluntary activity in mice, chromosomal aberrations in circulating lymphocytes of hamsters, and increased neonatal mortality as well as incidence of jaw abnormalities in offspring of mice exposed to ozone. The National Academy of Sciences Monograph reviews and documents these and other studies.

Nitrogen Dioxide

Mortality and Lung Pathology. Nitrogen dioxide, like ozone, is a deep lung irritant capable of producing pulmonary edema if inhaled in sufficient concentrations. This is a practical problem to farmers, as sufficient amounts can be liberated from ensilage to produce the symptoms of pulmonary damage known as silo-fillers' disease.

Even over short time intervals, Haber's law does not hold for nitrogen dioxide. This law states that $C \times T = K$, where C is the concentration of the toxic material, T is time, and K is a constant. For example, for a 15-minute exposure, 420 ppm nitrogen dioxide kills 50 percent of the animals (Gray *et al.*, 1954). Applying Haber's law, one would predict that 105 ppm for one hour or 26 ppm for four hours would kill 50 percent of the animals so exposed. Experimental results indicate, however, that the rats exposed for longer times can withstand higher concentrations than predicted. The LC50 values found for one-hour and four-hour exposures were 166 and 88 ppm, respectively. Even short exposure to the higher concentration was sufficient to produce overwhelming pulmonary edema and death.

Some earlier work in which animals were allowed to remain in an atmosphere of nitrogen dioxide until they died suggested a low toxicity. Because death from pulmonary edema is delayed, not immediate, the animals unquestionably received multilethal doses of nitrogen dioxide. In the case of irritant agents that produce delayed edema, the experimental design that measures survival time under continuous exposure will underestimate the lethal dose.

Damage to mast cells in the lungs of rats was produced by exposure to as little as 0.5 ppm for four hours or 1 ppm for one hour. The damage, which was repaired within 24 hours, was interpreted as the potential onset of an acute inflammatory reaction. More prolonged alterations in lung collagen were produced in rabbits by exposure to 0.25 ppm four hours a day for six days. Damage was still evident seven days after the final exposure (Mueller and Hitchcock, 1969).

In rats exposed to 2 ppm nitrogen dioxide, changes in cell proliferation in the lung were estimated by determining the proportion of cells that could be labeled with tritiated thymidine. A dose-related increase was found, which peaked on the second day of exposure and had returned to control levels by the fifth day. This occurred in terminal bronchioles and alveoli and represented an increased turnover rate of type II alveolar cells. Type I cells are damaged, slough off, and are replaced by cuboidal cells that have some of the characteristics of type II cells.

Exposure of squirrel monkeys for two hours to 10 to 50 ppm nitrogen dioxide produced primary lesions in the alveoli (Henry *et al.*, 1969). The degree of damage was related to the concentration of nitrogen dioxide. At 10 ppm, there were many septal breaks and the alveoli were markedly expanded. In some areas there were large air vesicles with very thin septal walls. At 15 ppm, the alveolar tissue was expanded with minimal wall thinning and patchy interstitial infiltration with lymphocytes. The bronchioles were normal. At 35 ppm, some lung areas were collapsed and alveolar septa had become very basophilic. In other areas the alveoli were expanded and had thin septal walls. The bronchi were moderately inflamed with some showing epithelial proliferation. Frank edema was produced by 50 ppm. The lungs of these monkeys showed extreme vesicular dilatation or total collapse of alveoli with lymphocyte infiltration. The bronchi showed epithelial surface erosion and the absence of cilia.

Over the past several years the pathologic effects of chronic exposure of rats to nitrogen dioxide have received extensive and meticulous study with both light and electron microscopy (Freeman et al., 1972). The emphysematous nature of the changes observed makes these studies extremely pertinent to cigarette smoking as well as to air pollution. Cigarette smoke contains nitrogen dioxide and increases the incidence of emphysema.

Rats grew normally and survived their natural life-spans in atmospheres containing 0.8 or 2 ppm nitrogen dioxide. They showed moderate tachypnea without apparent distress. The lungs were grossly normal except for slight bloating. They were able to contract on exposure to the atmosphere, although lungs from the rats exposed to 2 ppm retained some air and weighed about 20 percent more than control lungs. The lungs of the rats exposed to 2 ppm showed histologic alterations in the bronchiolar epithelium. The cells were broader and more uniform than controls. The cilia were either reduced or absent. The possibility exists that such a deficiency in ciliary cleansing mechanisms could lead to increased residence time of materials such as carcinogenic hydrocarbons. The group exposed to 0.8 ppm occasionally showed similar cellular alterations, which were not seen in controls of the same age. A 16-week exposure to 4 ppm produced no gross changes in lung volume. The terminal bronchiolar epithelium was tall and hypertrophied. Exposure to 10 and 25 ppm produced large, air-filled heavy lungs without edema or increased blood volume. The animals died of respiratory failure. The development of emphysemalike lungs was accompanied by enlargement of the thoracic cage with dorsal kyphosis.

The terminal bronchiolar lumen of the "emphysematous" lungs was narrowed owing to hypertrophy of the epithelium and to amorphous proteinaceous material, fibrin strands, and alveolar macrophages accumulated at the junctions with alveolar ducts. Such obstructive lesions may have led to the distension of the lungs and to the broken alveolar septa.

Lungs from rats exposed for 20 weeks to 18 ppm nitrogen dioxide were stained appropriately for detection of collagen and elastic tissue. In the exposed lungs both materials stained more prominently and were thicker and more prevalent, especially at the level of the alveolar ducts. The lengthwise elastic tissue fibers were often replicated and fractured into straighter and shorter pieces than could be found in control lungs. Such changes very likely contributed to the increased lung weight and to the reduction observed in pulmonary compliance.

Rats exposed for a lifetime to 15 ppm had voluminous, dry lungs with a large functional residual capacity. At maximal standard pressure the lung volume was greater than in control animals. Terminal bronchioles and alveolar ducts showed loss of cilia, epithelial hypertrophy, and narrowing. Alveoli were distended, and exposed animals had approximately one-third the number of alveoli of control animals with a resultant reduction in ventilatory surface. Arterial oxygen tension was reduced and secondary polycythemia was evident. The disease state resembled human emphysema.

Emphysemalike lesions were also produced in the lungs of beagle dogs exposed for six months to 25 ppm nitrogen dioxide (Riddick et al., 1968). The lungs of one of six exposed dogs showed bullous emphysema. The lungs of the other five exposed dogs showed increased firmness with scattered small bullae. The lungs of all dogs exposed showed a diffuse increase in collagen.

Pulmonary Function. Experimental exposure of animals or human subjects to nitrogen dioxide can cause measurable alterations in pulmonary function. The pattern of changes produced is in general similar to the pattern produced by ozone. This is an increase in respiratory frequency, with a decrease in compliance as the predominant alteration in mechanical behavior of the lungs. Pulmonary flow resistance is minimally altered.

Exposure of guinea pigs for periods of two to four hours at nitrogen dioxide concentrations of 5 to 13 ppm caused an increase in respiratory frequency and a decrease in tidal volume (Murphy et al., 1964b). The overall minute volume remained the same. The magnitude of the changes in frequency and tidal volume was related to the concentration of nitrogen dioxide. In addition, the time at which the maximum response was reached was shorter at higher concentrations. At 5 ppm the respiratory frequency continued to increase and the tidal volume continued to decrease for three hours. After this no further change was produced by an additional hour of exposure. At a concentration of 13 ppm, the maximum change was reached in one hour and no further alteration was noted during a second hour of exposure. The values for respiratory frequency and tidal volume had returned to preexposure values by four hours after the end of exposure. The method used for studying pulmonary mechanics in this investigation did not measure compliance. There is, however, little doubt that there was an accompanying decrease in compliance.

In the long-term studies of rats by Freeman's group, an increase in frequency and a decrease in compliance were observed as chronic effects. In the studies of squirrel monkeys discussed earlier, exposure for two hours to 10 or 15 ppm caused a decrease in tidal volume and minute volume, but no increase in respiratory frequency. Recovery was complete within 24 to 48 hours after exposure. Concentrations of 35 to 50 ppm for two hours caused an increase in respiratory frequency and a decrease in tidal volume that was completely reversible in 72 hours. Similar changes were produced by two-month exposure to 5 ppm.

Abe (1967) exposed five human subjects for ten minutes to 5 ppm nitrogen dioxide. He observed a mean increase in airway resistance of 92 percent. This response was delayed and did not become apparent until 30 minutes after the exposure ended. The mean value of pulmonary compliance was 40 percent below control levels by 30 minutes after the exposure. There was a marked reduction in three subjects and no change in the other two. No indication is given of the time interval over which these delayed effects would be reversed.

In the late 1970s a number of investigators examined the response of human subjects to nitrogen dioxide. The results on the whole are more conflicting and less definitive than those obtained in similar studies of sulfur dioxide or ozone. There seems little doubt that alterations of pulmonary function can be produced in normal, healthy subjects by exposure to 2 to 3 ppm and above. There is also the suggestion in these data that a concentration of 5 ppm may render normal subjects more sensitive to bronchoconstrictive agents and that similar effects may occur at far lower (0.1 ppm) concentrations in some asthmatic subjects (Orehek et al., 1976). Children may also be especially sensitive to nitrogen dioxide. Some studies suggest that decrements in pulmonary function occur in children living in homes with gas cooking stoves that emit nitrogen dioxide. This and other problems related to indoor air pollution have been reviewed by Spengler et al. (1983).

Susceptibility to Respiratory Infection. Data obtained on a variety of species of experimental animals (mice, hamsters, rabbits, squirrel monkeys) suggest that either short-term or long-term exposures to nitrogen dioxide can increase susceptibility to respiratory infection by bacterial pneumonia or influenza virus. The evidence for this effect falls into three categories: (1) increased mortality rates; (2) reduced survival time; and (3) reduced ability to clear pathogenic organisms from the lung, as indicated by the number of viable organisms that can be cultured.

Coffin et al. (1976) tested the effect of varying both concentration and time of exposure on the mortality of mice exposed to *Streptococcus pyrogenes*. A $C \times T$ value of 7 ppm-hours was used with exposures from 14 ppm for 0.5 hour to 1 ppm for seven hours. The concentration was more critical than time in increasing the mortality from infection. In other experiments, 1.5 ppm for 18 hours increased mortality by 25 percent but a two-hour exposure to 14.5 ppm caused a 65 percent increase.

Exposures of two hours to 5 ppm nitrogen dioxide reduced the rate of clearance of *K. pneumoniae* from the lungs of mice and hamsters. The bacterial challenge took place one hour after the irritant exposure. The number of bacteria in the lungs was measured one, three, five, six, seven, and eight hours after infection. In control animals the bacterial population was markedly reduced during the six hours postinfection. The bacterial count then increased, reaching its initial concentration in about eight hours. In the exposed animals the initial period of clearance was reduced to 4.5 (mice) or 5 hours (hamsters), and the original concentration was reestablished in less than seven hours. In rabbits there is evidence that short-term exposure (three hours) to nitrogen dioxide will inhibit phagocytic activity (Gardner et al., 1969).

Both increased mortality and reduced clearance rates of *K. pneumoniae* from the lungs were observed in mice exposed chronically to 0.5 ppm nitrogen dioxide (Ehrlich and Henry, 1968). Statistically significant increases in mortality following infection were observed in mice exposed continuously for three months and after six months of daily 6- or 18-hour exposures. The clearance rate of bacteria from lungs was reduced by exposure for 6 or 18 hours a day for nine months. These effects were more pronounced after 12 months of exposure. When exposure was continuous, a reduced capacity to clear bacteria from the lung was observed after six months as well as at 9 and 12 months.

Increased mortality was seen in squirrel monkeys exposed for short periods of two hours to 50 ppm nitrogen dioxide or for periods of one or two months to 10 or 5 ppm when they were infected with *K. pneumoniae* (Henry et al., 1970). Monkeys exposed to 10 ppm nitrogen dioxide for two hours and then infected had viable bacteria present in their lungs up to 50 days after challenge. Squirrel monkeys were infected with nonlethal levels of A/PR-8 influenza virus and then exposed continuously to 5 or 10 ppm nitrogen dioxide. All six monkeys exposed to 10 ppm died within three days and one out of three exposed to 5 ppm died. Other experiments suggested that exposure of squirrel monkeys for five months to 5 ppm nitrogen dioxide depressed the formation of protective antibody against this influenza virus.

Biochemical Effects. Both acute and chronic exposure to nitrogen dioxide can cause biochemical alterations in the configuration of collagen and elastin in the lungs of rabbits (Buell *et al.*, 1966). Differential ultraviolet spectrophotometry showed molecular alterations in both collagen and elastin in animals killed immediately after exposure. The changes were not observed in an animal killed 24 hours after exposure, which demonstrated the reversibility of the change. It may be remembered that the structural changes in collagen produced by repeated exposures were not reversible up to at least seven days after the final exposure. One might speculate that repeated denaturation of the sort observed here can lead to irreversible structural change.

It is interesting to note that hydroxylysine glycosides, probably originating from the degradation of collagen, were found in the urine of the Apollo crew of the Apollo-Soyuz mission. They had been exposed to an average of 250 ppm nitrogen dioxide for four to five minutes. Pulmonary damage was evident on roentgenograms.

Nitrogen dioxide, like ozone, can cause lipid peroxidation. Four-hour exposures to 1 ppm produced evidence of lipid peroxidation in extracts of lipids from rat lung (Thomas *et al.*, 1968). Peroxidation was maximum 24 hours after exposure and lasted for at least 24 hours longer. When six daily exposures were given, lipid peroxidation increased. This suggests a cumulative effect. Rats fed a diet deficient in vitamin E showed more peroxidation in surfactant and tissue lipids than rats fed a diet normal in vitamin E content.

Aldehydes

Various aldehydes in polluted air are formed as reaction products in the photooxidation of hydrocarbons. The two aldehydes of major interest are formaldehyde and acrolein. These materials probably contribute to the odor of and eye irritation produced by photochemical smog. Formaldehyde accounts for about 50 percent of the estimated total aldehydes in polluted air. Acrolein, the more irritant of the two, may account for about 5 percent of the total aldehydes. A recent study by Kane and Alarie (1978) indicates that these aldehydes act as competitive agonists. Irritation would not be related to "total aldehyde" but to specific concentrations of acrolein and formaldehyde.

Formaldehyde. Formaldehyde is a primary irritant. Because it is very soluble in water, it irritates mucous membranes of the nose, upper respiratory tract, and eyes. Concentrations of 0.5 to 1 ppm are detectable by odor, 2 to 3 ppm produce mild irritation, and 4 to 5 ppm are intolerable to most people.

The effect of low concentrations of formaldehyde on the respiration of guinea pigs has been studied (Amdur, 1960). A one-hour exposure to concentrations of 0.3 ppm and above produced an increase in pulmonary flow resistance accompanied by a lesser decrease in compliance. The respiratory frequency and minute volume decreased, but changes in these factors did not become statistically significant until concentrations of 10 ppm and above were used. The overall pattern of respiratory response to formaldehyde is similar to that produced by sulfur dioxide. A concentration of 0.05 ppm caused no alterations in any of the respiratory criteria used. Below concentrations of 50 ppm the alterations were reversible within an hour after the exposure.

The response to a given concentration of formaldehyde was greater when the gas was inhaled through a tracheal cannula, which bypassed the scrubbing effect of the upper respiratory tract and permitted a greater concentration of the irritant to reach the lungs. The response in these animals was also readily reversible, and the flow resistance values had returned to preexposure levels by one hour after the end of exposure.

The response to formaldehyde was potentiated by the simultaneous administration of a sodium chloride aerosol of submicron particles. The values for pulmonary resistance remained above preexposure levels for one hour after the end of exposure when the gas-aerosol combination was used. This prolonged response, which is typical of the response of irritant aerosols, suggests that the potentiation is brought about by the attachment of formaldehyde to the particles to form an irritant aerosol. This hypothesis is further supported by the fact that when 3, 10, and 30 mg/m^3 concentrations of sodium chloride were used, the potentiation increased with the increasing concentration of particles. The response to a given concentration of formaldehyde plus aerosol breathed by nose was greater than the response to the gas alone breathed through a tracheal cannula. This indicates that the increment added by the aerosol is not due to the transfer of an additional amount of formaldehyde gas as such to the lungs, since it was greater than could be accounted for by the transfer of the full concentration of formaldehyde to the lungs.

The particles of Los Angeles–type smog are capable of carrying a consisderable amount of formaldehyde. This suggests that the biologic data obtained may have some practical significance.

Two aspects of formaldehyde toxicology have recently brought it from relative obscurity to the forefront of the news. One is its presence in indoor atmospheres, especially in homes with improperly installed urea-formaldehyde foam insulation. This aspect is discussed at length in a review article (Spengler et al., 1983). The other is the finding of nasal cancers in rodents chronically exposed to concentrations of 3.5 to 15 ppm formaldehyde. The initial data from Chemical Industries Institute of Toxicology have been confirmed by investigators at New York University.

Had they been obtained on a new chemical, the animal data would have led to a ban on its widespread use in industry and in consumer products. Formaldehyde, however, has been so used for a very long time. If the animal data had relevance to practical exposures, should we not have had evidence of increased incidence of nasal cancer in exposed workers? Because of the animal data, epidemiologists are now looking; meanwhile the typical controversy rages between industrial groups and environmental/ consumer groups on appropriate regulatory action.

Acrolein. Because it is an unsaturated aldehyde, acrolein is much more irritant than formaldehyde. Concentrations below 1 ppm cause irritation of the eyes and mucous membranes of the respiratory tract.

The effect of acrolein on the respiratory function of guinea pigs has been studied (Murphy et al., 1963a). Exposure to 0.6 ppm and above increased pulmonary flow resistance, increased tidal volume, and decreased respiratory frequency. The effects were reversible when the animals were returned to clean air. In the case of irritants of this type, flow resistance is increased by concentrations below those which cause a decrease in frequency. This suggests that flow resistance increases would be produced by far lower concentrations of acrolein than were tested. Atropine, aminophylline, isoproterenol, and epinephrine partially or completely reversed the changes. Pyrilamine and tripelennamine were without effect. The mechanism of increased resistance appears to be bronchocon-

striction mediated through reflex cholinergic stimulation.

Inhalation of acrolein also has effects on various rat liver enzymes (Murphy, 1965). Elevated alkaline phosphatase activity occurred in the liver following 40 hours of continuous exposure to acrolein at concentrations as low as 2.1 ppm. Exposure to higher concentrations for shorter times also increased the enzyme activity, but the effect was not constant with a constant CT (concentration × time). Continuous exposure to 4 ppm acrolein for 4, 8, and 20 hours resulted in liver AP values that were 135, 222, and 253 percent of their respective controls. When a constant CT of 80 ppm-hours was given as 4 ppm for 20 hours, 2 ppm for 40 hours, and 1 ppm for 80 hours, the increases in alkaline phosphatase were 233, 146, and 103 percent of control values, respectively. This suggests that a threshold level of irritation must be reached to initiate processes that result in elevated enzyme activity. Liver alkaline phosphatase and tyrosine-ketoglutarate transaminase activities were markedly increased in rats 5 to 12 hours after injection or inhalation of acrolein. These effects could be prevented or substantially reduced by prior adrenalectomy or hypophysectomy or by pretreatment of the animals with chemicals that inhibit protein synthesis. The data suggest that the irritant action of acrolein stimulates the pituitary-adrenal system, leading to hypersecretion of glucocorticoids, which act to induce or stimulate the synthesis of increased amounts of the enzyme by the liver.

Carbon Monoxide

Carbon monoxide would be classed toxicologically as a chemical asphyxiant, and its toxic action stems from its formation of carboxyhemoglobin. The fundamental factors of the toxicology of carbon monoxide and the physiologic factors that determine the level of carboxyhemoglobin reached in the blood at various atmospheric concentrations of carbon monoxide are dealt with in Chapter 12. A monograph from the New York Academy of Sciences (Coburn, 1970) gives an excellent discussion of all aspects of the toxicology of carbon monoxide.

The normal concentration of carboxyhemoglobin (COHb) in the blood of nonsmokers is about 0.5 percent. This is attributed to endogenous production of CO from such sources as heme catabolism. Uptake of exogenous CO increases blood COHb in proportion to the concentration in the air as well as the length of exposure and the ventilation rate of the person. Continuous exposure of human subjects to 30 ppm CO leads to an equilibrium value of 5 percent COHb. About 80 percent of this value is approached in four hours and the remaining 20 percent is approached slowly over the next eight hours. It can be calculated that continuous exposure to 20 ppm CO gives an equilibrium COHb value of about 3.7 percent and 10 ppm CO gives an equilibrium value of 2 percent COHb. The equilibrium values are generally reached after eight or more hours of exposure. The time required to reach equilibrium can be shortened by physical activity.

Analysis of data from air-monitoring programs in California indicates that eight-hour average values, which may be exceeded for 0.1 percent of the time, ranged from 10 to 40 ppm CO. Depending on location within a community, CO concentrations can vary widely. Concentrations predicted inside the passenger compartments of motor vehicles in downtown traffic were almost three times those for central urban areas and five times those expected in residential areas. Occupants of vehicles traveling on expressways had CO exposures somewhere between those in central urban areas and in downtown traffic. Concentrations above 87 ppm have been measured in underground garages, in tunnels, and in buildings over highways.

No human health effects have been demonstrated for COHb levels below 2 percent. Above 2 percent COHb in nonsmokers (the median value for smokers is of the order of 5 percent COHb) it has been possible to demonstrate effects on the central nervous system. At COHb levels of 2.5 percent resulting from about 90-minute exposure to about 50 ppm CO, there is an impairment of time-interval discrimination; at approximately 5 percent COHb there is an impairment of other psychomotor faculties. Cardiovascular changes may be produced by exposure sufficient to yield over 5 percent COHb. These include increased cardiac output, A-V oxygen difference, and coronary blood flow in patients without coronary disease. Decreased coronary sinus blood PO_2 occurs in patients with coronary heart disease. Impaired oxidative metabolism of the myocardium may occur. These changes could produce an added burden on patients with heart disease. Some adaptation to chronic low levels of CO may occur through such mechanisms as increased hematocrit, hemoglobin, and blood volume.

Auto Exhaust and Synthetic Smog

Many investigators have studied the effect of atmospheres designed to simulate photochemical smog. These have included irradiated and nonirradiated auto exhaust or ozonized gasoline. The observed effects are those of a mixture of components, some of which are known, others unknown. Such experiments have the advantage of being a step closer to actual urban air pollution than studies of individual specific chemicals and the disadvantage that it is difficult to determine which of the many substances present are critical for the observed effects.

Short-Term Exposures. Exposures of two to three hours to heavy Los Angeles smog containing 0.4 ppm total oxidant, or synthetic smog containing 0.5 ppm total oxidant, produced ultrastructural changes in alveolar tissue of mice ranging in age from 5 to 21 months (Bils and Romanovsky, 1967). The severity of the damage increased with increasing age. No change was detectable in the youngest animals. In eight- to nine-month-old animals there were definite alterations, but by 14 to 18 hours after exposure there was no detectable difference from control animals. In animals 15 months of age alterations were still present 24 hours after exposure. The endothelial cells were seriously affected, but the lining epithelium and basement membrane were intact. In the oldest animals changes that could be interpreted as edemalike occurred in the lining epithelium. The alterations were still present 18 hours after exposure. The implication is clear that loss of regenerative capacity of alveolar tissue following damage is one result of aging.

Exposure of A-strain and C_{57} black mice to 1 to 3.8 ppm ozonized gasoline produced an increased incidence of lung tumors (Kotin and Falk, 1956; Kotin et al., 1958). True carcinomas have been produced in C_{57} black mice by combined exposure to ozonized gasoline and influenza virus.

Mice were exposed for four hours to auto exhaust containing 0.08 to 0.67 ppm oxidant and 12 to 100 ppm CO for four hours (Coffin and Blommer, 1967). Immediately following this exposure the mice were exposed to a bacterial aerosol of Streptococcus (group C) at the rate of 100,000 organisms per mouse. When the exhaust contained 0.35 to 0.67 ppm oxidant and 100 ppm CO, there was enhanced mortality from streptococcal pneumonia: 53 percent among the exposed and 11 percent among the controls. The mortality was not enhanced by exhaust containing 0.12 ppm oxidant and 25 ppm CO. The increased mortality was probably related to the oxidant content. The levels involved are well below peak concentrations reported for heavy pollution.

The respiratory function of guinea pigs exposed to irradiated and nonirradiated auto exhaust has been measured (Murphy et al., 1963a). Increases in flow resistance were produced by 150:1 dilutions of irradiated exhaust but not by similar dilutions of nonirradiated exhaust. This was attributed to the formation of aldehydes, nitrogen dioxide, and total oxidant by irradiation. The nature of the response suggests aldehyde as the most likely component responsible for the observed change.

Chronic Exposures. In an extensive experiment designed to assess the long-term effects of auto exhaust, beagle dogs were exposed daily for 16 hours for a total of 68 months (Lewis *et al.*, 1974). A variety of pulmonary function studies were made at intervals throughout the exposure years. At the end of the exposure period the dogs were moved from the EPA laboratory in Cincinnati to the college of Veterinary Medicine at Davis, California. There a series of physiologic measurements were made both on arrival and two years after the exposure had terminated. The dogs were then sacrificed and extensive morphologic examination by light and electron microscopy was made of the lungs. These experiments thus provided an opportunity to correlate physiologic and morphologic observations.

One hundred and four dogs were divided into eight groups. One group included 20 dogs that served as controls and were exposed in similar chambers to clean air. The seven experimental groups each contained 12 dogs. The exposures were to: (1) nonirradiated auto exhaust; (2) irradiated auto exhaust; (3) sulfur dioxide plus sulfuric acid; (4) and (5) the two types of exhaust plus the sulfur mixture; and (6) and (7) a high and low level of nitrogen oxides. The irradiated exhaust contained oxidant (measured as ozone) at about 0.2 ppm and nitrogen dioxide at about 0.9 ppm. The raw exhaust contained minimal concentrations of these materials and about 1.5 ppm nitric oxide. Both forms of exhaust contained close to 100 ppm carbon monoxide.

The values for physiologic tests done on the control dogs showed no change between the end of exposure and two years after. All other exposure groups had pulmonary function values different from controls and had more functional abnormalities at the end of the two-year post-exposure period. Pulmonary function tests suggested that auto exhaust exposure injured the airways and parenchyma while oxides of sulfur or nitrogen injured the parenchyma.

Two important exposure-related pulmonary lesions were observed. Enlargement of air spaces and loss of interalveolar septa in proximal acinar regions were most severe in dogs exposed to oxides of nitrogen, oxides of sulfur, or the latter with irradiated exhaust. Hyperplasia of nonciliated bronchiolar cells was most severe in dogs exposed to raw auto exhaust alone or with oxides of sulfur.

These studies indicate that alterations in function that are reflected by morphologic injury are persistent in nature following exposure to quite realistic levels of mixed pollution.

CONCLUSIONS

Since this chapter was written for a textbook of toxicology, it has discussed mainly the results of experimental studies related to specific compounds that occur as pollutants of urban air. Data of this kind are among the factors considered in the practical deliberations on the development of air quality criteria and standards.

The Clean Air Act sets forth the legal steps leading to the establishment of air quality standards. The initial step in this process is the preparation of an air quality criteria document that sets forth the state of knowledge in regard to the effects of the substance on animals, humans, plants, and materials. It is in this step that the availability of pertinent toxicologic data is of prime importance. This has been and should continue to be an incentive to toxicologists to develop sensitive methods capable of assaying the response to low concentrations of materials that occur as air pollutants.

REFERENCES

Abe, M.: Effects of mixed NO_2-SO_2 gas on human pulmonary functions. Effects of air pollution on the human body. *Bull. Tokyo Med. Dental Univ.*, **14**:415–33, 1967.

Alarie, Y. C.; Ulrich, C. E.; Busey, W. M.; Swann, H. E., Jr.; and MacFarland, H. N.: Long-term continuous exposure of guinea pigs to sulfur dioxide. *Arch. Environ. Health*, **21**:769–77, 1970.

Alarie, Y. C.; Ulrich, C. E.; Busey, W. M.; Krumm, A. A.; and MacFarland, H. N.: Long-term continuous exposure to sulfur dioxide in cynomolgus monkeys. *Arch. Environ. Health*, **24**:115–28, 1972.

Alarie, Y. C.; Krumm, A. A.; Busey, W. M.; Ulrich, C. E.; and Kantz, R. J., Jr.: Long-term exposure to sulfur dioxide, sulfuric acid mist, fly ash, and their mixtures. Results of studies in monkeys and guinea pigs. *Arch. Environ. Health*, **30**:254–62, 1975.

Alpert, S. M.; Schwartz, B. B.; Lee, S. D.; and Lewis, T. R.: Alveolar protein accumulation. A sensitive indicator of low level oxidant toxicity. *Arch. Intern. Med.*, **128**:69–73, 1973.

Amdur, M. O.: The respiratory response of guinea pigs to sulfuric acid mist. *A.M.A. Arch. Ind. Health*, **18**:407–14, 1958.

———: The response of guinea pigs to inhalation of formaldehyde and formic acid alone and with a sodium chloride aerosol. *Int. J. Air Pollut.*, **3**:201–20, 1960.

———: The effect of aerosols on the response to irritant gases. In Davies, C. N. (ed.): *Inhaled Particles and Vapours.* Pergamon Press, Oxford, 1961, pp. 281–92.

———: Respiratory absorption data and SO_2 dose-response curves. *Arch. Environ. Health*, **12**:729–32, 1966.

———: 1974 Cummings Memorial Lecture. The long road from Donora. *Am. Ind. Hyg. Assoc. J.*, **35**:589–97, 1974.

———: The 1984 Henry F. Smyth, Jr. Lecture. When one plus zero is more than one. *Am. Ind. Hyg. Assoc. J.*, **46**:467–75, 1985.

Amdur, M. O., and Corn, M.: The irritant potency of zinc ammonium sulfate of different particle sizes. *Am. Ind. Hyg. Assoc. J.*, **24**:326–33, 1963.

Amdur, M. O., and Mead, J.: Mechanics of respiration in unanesthetized guinea pigs. *Am. J. Physiol.*, **192**:364–68, 1958.

Amdur, M. O., and Underhill, D. W.: The effect of various aerosols on the response of guinea pigs to sulfur dioxide. *Arch. Environ. Health,* 16:460–68, 1968.

Amdur, M. O.; Schultz, R. Z.; and Drinker, P.: Toxicity of sulfuric acid mist to guinea pigs. *A.M.A. Arch. Ind. Hyg. Occup. Med.,* 5:318–29, 1952.

Amdur, M. O.; Dubriel, M.; and Creasia, D. A.: Respiratory response of guinea pigs to low levels of sulfuric acid. *Environ. Res.,* 15:418–23, 1978a.

Amdur, M. O.; Bayles, J.; Ugro, V.; and Underhill, D. W.: Comparative irritant potency of sulfate salts. *Environ. Res.,* 16:1–8, 1978b.

Amdur, M. O.; Ugro, V.; and Underhill, D. W.: Respiratory response of guinea pigs to ozone alone and with sulfur dioxide. *Am. Ind. Hyg. Assoc. J.,* 39:958–61, 1978c.

Amdur, M. O.; Sarofim, A. F.; Neville, M.; Quann, R. J.; McCarthy, J. F.; Elliott, J. F.; Lam, H. F.; Rogers, A. E.; and Conner, M. W.: Coal combustion aerosols and SO$_2$: an interdisciplinary analysis. *Environ. Sci. Tech.,* 20:139–45, 1986.

Bils, R. F., and Romanovsky, J. C.: Ultrastructural alterations of alveolar tissue of mice. II. Synthetic photochemical smog. *Arch. Environ. Health,* 14:844–58, 1967.

Boatman, E. S.; Sato, S.; and Frank R.: Acute effects of ozone on cat lungs. II. Structural. *Am. Rev. Respir. Dis.,* 110:157–69, 1974.

Buell, G. C.; Tokiwa, Y.; and Mueller, P. K.: Potential crosslinking agents in lung tissue. Formation and isolation after *in vivo* exposure to ozone. *Arch. Environ. Health,* 10:213–19, 1965.

——— : Lung collagen and elastin denaturation *in vivo* following inhalation of nitrogen dioxide. Paper No. 66-7, *59th Air Pollution Control Association Meeting,* San Francisco, June, 1966.

Burton, G. G.; Corn, M.; Gee, J. B. L.; Vasallo, C.; and Thomas, A. P.: Response of healthy men to inhaled low concentrations of gas-aerosol mixtures. *Arch. Environ. Health,* 18:681–92, 1969.

Charles, J. M.; Gardiner, D. E.; Coffin, D. L.; and Menzel, D. B.: Augmentation of sulfate absorption from the rat lung by heavy metals. *Toxicol. Appl. Pharmacol.,* 42:531–38, 1977.

Coburn, R. F. (ed.): Biological effects of carbon monoxide. *Ann. N.Y. Acad. Sci.,* 174(Art. 1):1–430, 1970.

Coffin, D. L., and Blommer, E. J.: Acute toxicity of irradiated auto exhaust. Its indication by enhancement of mortality from streptococcal pneumonia. *Arch. Environ. Health,* 15:36–38, 1967.

Coffin, D. L.; Gardner, D. E.; and Blommer, E. J.: Time-dose response for nitrogen dioxide exposure in an infectivity model system. *Environ. Health Perspect.,* 13:11–15, 1976.

Conner, M. W.; Rogers, A. E.; and Amdur, M. O.: Response of guinea pig respiratory tract to inhalation of submicron zinc oxide particles generated in the presence of sulfur dioxide and water vapor. *Toxicol. Appl. Pharmacol.,* 66:434–42, 1982.

Cortesi, R., and Privett, O. S.: Toxicity of fatty ozonides and peroxides. *Lipids,* 7:715–21, 1972.

Dalhamn, T.: Mucous flow and ciliary activity in the trachea of health rats and rats exposed to respiratory irritant gases (SO$_2$, H$_3$N, HCHO). A functional and morphologic (light microscopic and electron microscopic) study, with special reference to technique. *Acta Physiol. Scand.,* 36(suppl. 123):1–161, 1956.

DeLucia, A. J.; Mustafa, M. G.; Hussain, M. Z.; and Cross, C. E.: Ozone interaction with rodent lung. III. Oxidation of reduced glutathione and formation of mixed disulfides between protein and nonprotein sulfhydryls. *J. Clin. Invest.,* 55:794–802, 1975.

Dungworth, D. L.: Short-term effects of ozone on lungs of rats, mice and monkeys (abstr.). *Environ. Health Perspect.,* 16:179, 1976.

Easton, R. E., and Murphy, S. D.: Experimental ozone pre-exposure and histamine. Effect on the acute toxicity and respiratory function effects of histamine in guinea pigs. *Arch. Environ. Health,* 15:160–66, 1967.

Ehrlich, R., and Henry, M. C.: Chronic toxicity of nitrogen dioxide. I. Effect on resistance to bacterial pneumonia. *Arch. Environ. Health,* 17:860–65, 1968.

Ehrlich, R.; Findlay, J. C.; and Gardner, D. E.: Susceptibility to bacterial pneumonia in animals exposed to sulfates. *Toxicol. Lett.,* 1:325–30, 1978.

Eustis, S. L.; Swartz, L. W.; Kosch, P. C.; and Dungworth, D. L.: Chronic bronchiolitis in nonhuman primates after prolonged ozone exposure. *Am. J. Pathol.* 105:121–27, 1981.

Ferin, J., and Leach, L. J.: The effect of SO$_2$ on lung clearance of TiO$_2$ particles in rats. *Am. Ind. Hyg. Assoc. J.,* 34:260–63, 1973.

Frank, N. R., and Speizer, F. E.: SO$_2$ effects on the respiratory system in dogs. Changes in mechanical behavior at different levels of the respiratory system during acute exposure to the gas. *Arch. Environ. Health,* 11:624–34, 1965.

Frank, N. R.; Amdur, M. O.; Worchester, J.; and Whittenberger, J. L.: Effects of acute controlled exposure to SO$_2$ on respiratory mechanics in healthy male adults. *J. Appl. Physiol.,* 17:252–58, 1962.

Frank, N. R.; Amdur, M. O.; and Whittenberger, J. L.: A comparison of the acute effects of SO$_2$ administered alone or in combination with NaCl particles on the respiratory mechanics of healthy adults. *Int. J. Air Water Pollut.,* 8:125–33, 1964.

Frank, N. R.; Yoder, R. E.; Yokoyama, E.; and Speizer, F. E.: The diffusion of ^{35}SO$_2$ from tissue fluids into the lungs following exposure of dogs to ^{35}SO$_2$. *Health Phys.,* 13:31–38, 1967.

Frank, N. R.; Yoder, R. E.; Brain, J. D.; and Yokoyama, E.: SO$_2$ (^{35}S labeled) absorption by the nose and mouth under conditions of varying concentration and flow. *Arch. Environ. Health,* 18:315–22, 1969.

Freeman, G.; Crane, S. C.; Furiosi, N. J.; Stephens, R. J.; Evans, M. J.; and Moore, W. D.: Covert reduction in ventilatory surface in rats during prolonged exposure to subacute nitrogen dioxide. *Am. Rev. Respir. Dis.,* 106:563–79, 1972.

Gardner, D. E.; Holzman, R. S.; and Coffin, D. L.: Effects of nitrogen dioxide on pulmonary cell population. *J. Bacteriol.,* 98:1401–1403, 1969.

Gardner, D. E.; Lewis, T. R.; Alpert, S. M.; Hurst, D. J.; and Coffin, D. L.: The role of tolerance in pulmonary defense mechanisms. *Arch. Environ. Health,* 25:432–38, 1972.

Goldstein, B. D.; Lodi, C.; Collinson, C.; and Balchum, O. J.: Ozone and lipid peroxidation. *Arch. Environ. Health,* 18:631–35, 1969.

Goldstein, B. D.; Buckley, R. D.; Cardenas, R.; and Balchum, O. J.: Ozone and vitamin E. *Science,* 169:605–606, 1970.

Gray, E. L.; Patton, F. M.; Goldberg, S. B.; and Kaplan, E.: Toxicity of the oxides of nitrogen. II. Acute inhalation toxicity of nitrogen dioxide, red fuming nitric acid, and white fuming nitric acid. *A.M.A. Arch. Ind. Hyg. Occup. Med.,* 10:418–22, 1954.

Gunnison, A. F., and Palmes, E. D.: *S*-Sulfonates in human plasma following inhalation of sulfur dioxide. *Am. Ind. Hyg. Assoc. J.,* 35:288–91, 1974.

Henry, M. C.; Ehrlich, R.; and Blair, W. H.: Effect of nitrogen dioxide on resistance of squirrel monkeys to *Klebsiella pneumoniae* infection. *Am. Ind. Hyg. Assoc. J.,* 18:580–87, 1969.

Henry, M. C.; Findlay, J.; Spengler, J.; and Ehrlich, R.: Chronic toxicity of NO$_2$ in squirrel monkeys. III. Effect on resistance to bacterial and viral infection. *Am. Ind. Hyg. Assoc. J.,* 20:566–70, 1970.

Hirsch, J. A.; Swenson, E. W.; and Wanner, A.: Tracheal mucous transport in beagles after long-term exposure to 1 ppm sulfur dioxide. *Am. Ind. Hyg. Assoc. J.,* **30**:249–53, 1975.

Jeffrey, P. K., and Reid, L. M.: The respiratory mucous membrane. In Brain, J. D.; Proctor, D. F.; and Reid, L. M. (eds.): *Respiratory Defense Mechanisms,* Part I. Marcel Dekker, New York, 1977.

Kane, L. E., and Alarie, Y.: Evaluation of sensory irritation from acrolein-formaldehyde mixtures. *Am. Ind. Hyg. Assoc. J.,* **39**:270–74, 1978.

Koenig, J. Q.; Pierson, W. E.; Horike, M.; and Frank, R.: Effects of SO_2 plus NaCl aerosol combined with moderate exercise on pulmonary function in asthmatic adolescents. *Environ. Res.,* **25**:340–48, 1981.

Kotin, P., and Falk, H. L.: The experimental induction of pulmonary tumors in strain-A mice after their exposure to an atmosphere of ozonized gasoline. *Cancer (Philadelphia),* **9**:910–17, 1956.

——— : Atmospheric factors in pathogenesis of lung cancer. *Adv. Cancer Res.,* **7**:475–514, 1963.

Kotin, P.; Falk, H. L.; and McCammon, C. J.: The experimental induction of pulmonary tumors and changes in the respiratory epithelium of C57BL mice following their exposure to an atmosphere of ozonized gasoline. *Cancer (Philadelphia),* **11**:473–81, 1958.

Kuschner, M.: The J. Burns Amberson Lecture. The causes of lung cancer. *Am. Rev. Respir. Dis.,* **98**:573–90, 1968.

Lam, H. F.; Peisch, R.; and Amdur, M. O.: Changes in lung volumes and diffusing capacity in guinea pigs exposed to a combination of sulfur dioxide and submicron zinc oxide mixed in a humidified furnace. *Toxicol. Appl. Pharmacol.,* **66**:427–33, 1982.

Lawther, P. J.: Air pollution and public health—a personal appraisal. *Edwin Stevens Lectures for the Laity,* Royal Society of Medicine, 1975.

Lawther, P. J.; MacFarlane, A. J.; Waller, R. E.; and Brooks, A. G. F.: Pulmonary function and sulphur dioxide, some preliminary findings. *Environ. Res.,* **10**:355–67, 1975.

Lee, L. Y.; Bleeker, E.; and Nadel, J. A.: Ozone-induced airway hyperirritability in dogs. *Fed. Proc.,* **36**:616, 1977.

Lee, S. D.; Mustafa, M. G.; and Mehlman, M. A. (eds.): *International Symposium on the Biomedical Effects of Ozone and Related Photochemical Oxidants.* Vol. V, *Advances in Modern Environmental Toxicology.* Princeton Sci. Publishers, Princeton, N.J., 1983.

Lewis, T. R.; Campbell, K. I.; and Vaughan, T. R., Jr.: Effects on canine pulmonary function. Via induced NO_2 impairment, particulate interaction, and subsequent SO_x. *Arch. Environ. Health,* **18**:596–601, 1969.

Lewis, T. R.; Moorman, W. J.; Yang, Y. Y.; and Stara, J. F.: Long-term exposure to auto exhaust and other pollutant mixtures. *Arch. Environ. Health,* **21**:102–106, 1974.

Linn, W. S.; Jones, M. P.; Bailey, R. M.; Kleinman, M. T.; Spier, C. E.; Fischer, R. D.; and Kackney, J. D.: Respiratory effects of mixed nitrogen dioxide and sulfur dioxide in human volunteers under simulated ambient exposure conditions. *Environ. Res.,* **22**:431–38, 1980.

Lippmann, M.; Lioy, P. J.; Leikauf, G.; Green, K. B.; Baxter, D.; Morandi, M.; Pasternack, B. S.; Fife, D.; and Speizer, F. E.: Effects of ozone on the pulmonary function of children. In Lee, S. D.; Mustafa, M. G.; and Mehlman, M. A. (eds.): *International Symposium on the Biomedical Effects of Ozone and Related Photochemical Oxidants.* Vol. 5, *Advances in Modern Environmental Toxicology.* Princeton Sci. Publishers, Princeton, N.J., 1983, pp. 423–46.

Mawdesley-Thomas, L. E.; Healey, P.; and Barry, D. H.: Experimental bronchitis in animals due to sulphur dioxide and cigarette smoke. An automated quan-

titative study. In Walton, W. H. (ed.): *Inhaled Particles and Vapours, III.* Unwin Brothers Ltd., Old Woking, Surrey, England, 1971.

McJilton, C.; Frank, N. R.; and Charlson, R. E.: Role of relative humidity in the synergistic effect of a sulfur dioxide-aerosol mixture on the lung. *Science,* **182**:503–504, 1973.

Menzel, D. B.: Toxicity of ozone, oxygen, and radiation. *Annu. Rev. Pharmacol.,* **10**:379–94, 1970.

Menzel, D. B.; Slaughter, R. J.; Bryant, A. M.; and Jauregui, H. O.: Heinz bodies formed in erythrocytes by fatty acid ozonides and ozone. *Arch. Environ. Health,* **30**:296–301, 1975.

Mueller, P. K., and Hitchcock, M.: Air quality criteria—toxicological appraisal for oxidants, nitrogen oxides, and hydrocarbons. *J. Air Pollut. Control Assoc.,* **19**:670–76, 1969.

Murphy, S. D.: Mechanism of the effect of acrolein on rat liver enzymes. *Toxicol. Appl. Pharmacol.,* **7**:833–43, 1965.

Murphy, S. D.; Klingshirn, D. A.; and Ulrich, C. E.: Respiratory response of guinea pigs during acrolein inhalation and its modification by drugs. *J. Pharmacol. Exp. Ther.,* **141**:79–83, 1963.

Murphy, S. D.; Ulrich, C. E.; Frankowitz, S. H.; and Xintaras, C.: Altered function in animals inhaling low concentrations of ozone and nitrogen dioxide. *Am. Ind. Hyg. Assoc. J.,* **25**:246–53, 1964.

Mustafa, M. G.; Elsayed, N. M.; Graham, J. A.; and Gardner, D. E.: Effects of ozone exposure on lung metabolism: influence of animal age, species and exposure conditions. In Lee, S. D.; Mustafa, M. G.; and Mehlman, M. A. (eds.): *International Symposium on the Biomedical Effects of Ozone and Related Photochemical Oxidants.* Vol. V, of *Advances in Modern Environmental Toxicology.* Princeton Sci. Publishers, Princeton, N.J., 1983, pp. 57–73.

Nadel, J. A.; Salem, H.; Tamplin, B.; and Tokiwa, Y.: Mechanism of bronchoconstriction during inhalation of sulfur dioxide. *J. Appl. Physiol.,* **20**:164–67, 1965.

Nadel, J. A.; Corn, M.; Zwi, S.; Flesch, J.; and Graf, P.: Location and mechanism of airway constriction after inhalation of histamine aerosol and inorganic sulfate aerosol. In Davies, C. N. (ed.): *Inhaled Particles and Vapours, II.* Pergamon Press, Oxford, 1967, pp. 55–66.

National Academy of Sciences, Committee on Medical and Biologic Effects of Environmental Pollutants: *Ozone and Other Photochemical Oxidants.* National Academy of Sciences, Washington, D.C., 1977.

Orehek, J.; Massari, J. P.; Gayrard, P.; Grimaud, C.; and Charpin, J.: Effect of short-term, low-level nitrogen dioxide exposure on bronchial sensitivity of asthmatic patients. *J. Clin. Invest.,* **57**:301–307, 1976.

Pattle, R. E.; Burgess, F.; and Cullumbine, H.: The effects of a cold environment and of ammonia on the toxicity of sulphuric acid mist to guinea pigs. *J. Pathol. Bacteriol.,* **72**:219–32, 1956.

Riddick, J. H., Jr.; Campbell, K. I.; and Coffin, D. L.: Histopathologic changes secondary to nitrogen dioxide exposure in dog lungs. *Am. J. Clin. Pathol.,* **49**:239, 1968.

Schlesinger, R. B.; Lippmann, M.; and Albert, R. E.: Effects of short-term exposures to sulfuric acid and ammonium sulfate aerosols upon bronchial airway function in the donkey. *Am. Ind. Hyg. Assoc. J.,* **39**:275–86, 1978.

Sheppard, D. A.; Saisho, A.; Nadel, J. A.; and Boushey, H. A.: Exercise increases sulfur dioxide induced bronchoconstriction in asthmatic subjects. *Am. Rev. Respir. Dis.,* **123**:486–91, 1981.

Skornik, W. A., and Brain, J. D.: Relative toxicity of inhaled metal sulfate salts for pulmonary macrophages. *Am. Rev. Respir. Dis.,* **128**:297–303, 1983.

Spengler, J. D., and Sexton, K.: Indoor air pollution: a public health perspective. *Science, 221*:9–17, 1983.

Stephens, R. J.; Freeman, G.; Stara, J. F.; and Coffin, D. L.: Cytologic changes in dog lungs induced by chronic exposure to ozone. *Am. J. Pathol., 73*:711–18, 1973.

Stephens, R. J.; Sloan, M. F.; Evans, M. J.; and Freeman, G.: Early response of lung to low levels of ozone. *Am. J. Pathol., 74*:31–57, 1974.

Stokinger, H. E.: Ozone toxicology. A review of research and industrial experience: 1954–1964. *Arch. Environ. Health, 10*:719–31, 1965.

Strandberg, L. G.: SO_2 absorption in the respiratory tract. Studies on the absorption in rabbits, its dependence on concentration and breathing pace. *Arch. Environ. Health, 9*:160–66, 1964.

Thomas, H. V.; Mueller, P. K.; and Lyman, R. L.: Lipoperoxidation of lung lipids in rats exposed to nitrogen dioxide. *Science, 159*:532–34, 1968.

Tiege, B.; McManus, T. T.; and Mudd, J. B.: Reaction of ozone with phosphatidylcholine liposomes and the lytic effect of products on red blood cells. *Chem. Phys. Lipids, 12*:153–71, 1974.

Toyama, T.: Studies on aerosols. 1. Synergistic response of the pulmonary airway resistance on inhaling sodium chloride aerosols and SO_2 in man. *Jpn. J. Ind. Health, 4*:86–92, 1962.

Toyama, T., and Nakamura, K.: Synergistic response of hydrogen peroxide aerosols and sulfur dioxide to pulmonary airway resistance. *Ind. Health, 2*:34–45, 1964.

Treon, J. F.; Dutra, F. R.; Cappel, J.; Sigmon, H.; and Younker, W.: Toxicity of sulfuric acid mist. *A.M.A. Arch. Ind. Hyg. Occup. Med., 2*:716–34, 1950.

U.S. Environmental Protection Agency: *Air Quality Criteria for Particulate Matter and Sulfur Oxides,* December, 1982.

Vaughan, T. R., Jr.; Jennelle, L. F.; and Lewis, T. R.: Long-term exposure to low levels of air pollutants. Effects on pulmonary function in the beagle. *Arch. Environ. Health, 19*:45–50, 1969.

Weir, F. W.; Stevens, D. H.; and Bromberg, P. A.: Pulmonary function studies of men exposed for 120 hours to sulfur dioxide. *Toxicol. Appl. Pharmacol., 22*:319, 1972.

Widdicombe, J. G.: Respiratory reflexes from the trachea and bronchi of the cat. *J. Physiol., 123*:55–70, 1954.

Witz, G.; Amoruso, M. A.; and Goldstein, B.: Effect of ozone on alveolar macrophage function: Membrane dynamic properties. In Lee, S. D.; Mustafa, M. G.; and Mehlman, M. A. (eds.): *International Symposium on the Biomedical Effects of Ozone and Related Photochemical Oxidants.* Vol. V, of *Advances in Modern Environmental Toxicology.* Princeton Sci. Publishers, Princeton, N.J., 1983, pp. 263–72.

Chapter 26

WATER AND SOIL POLLUTANTS

Robert E. Menzer and *Judd O. Nelson*

INTRODUCTION

The ultimate sinks for most chemicals produced and used by humans are water and soil. Three-quarters of the earth's surface is covered by water, and the remainder that is not covered by asphalt or concrete is covered by soil. Although water and soil are usually considered as separate ecologic systems, one needs to realize that suspended soil particles in water represent an interface between the two systems and serve as a mechanism for contamination of the one by the other. In reality it is impossible to consider any component of the world in isolation from any other, as illustrated in Figure 26–1. For our purposes, however, we shall consider the presence, fate, and effects of chemicals in water and in soil as separate systems, as far as that is possible.

Systems of water may be compartmentalized based on their natural occurrence and the use made of them. One may consider separately the naturally occurring bodies of water: marine systems, fresh water systems, and the interface between them, the estuarine systems. One may also consider these systems on the basis of the use made of water removed from them for drinking purposes or other domestic consumption. Water systems are also the recipients of the products of domestic and industrial sewage systems. Bodies of water, including rivers, lakes, ponds, and the ground water, are also the recipients of runoff from agricultural and urban areas, which greatly modifies their capability to support life and their usefulness for other purposes.

Although water can be ultimately purified to a specific, definite chemical entity, soil has no commonly accepted compositional definition. Soils are composed of inorganic and organic constituents. The inorganic are silt, sand, and clay in varying ratios. These inorganic particles are coated and admixed with organic constituents, living and dead. The behavior of soil to a major degree is determined by the size and shape of the particles of which it is composed. Soil particles range in size from less than

0.002 mm to about 2.0 mm in diameter. Soils are classified according to particle size ranges as follows: clay, <0.002 mm; silt, 0.002 to 0.02 mm; find sand, 0.02 to 0.20 mm; and coarse sand, 0.2 to 2.0 mm. The most important use of soil is for agriculture. Soil is the ultimate support of man's sources of most food and much fiber. In addition, the soil has been the final disposal site for much of the industrial and urban waste generated by human societies.

The interface between soil and water is an intimate one. Virtually all water systems contain suspended soil particles, and virtually all soil contains at least a small amount of water. The sediment that is the end product of soil erosion is by volume the greatest single pollutant of surface waters and is the principal carrier of most pollutants found in water. In a joint study the United States Department of Agriculture and the Environmental Protection Agency have estimated that potential annual water erosion losses range from negligible to more than 100 tons of soil per acre. About 20 percent of the 438 million acres of crop land in the United States averages more than 8 tons of soil loss per acre per year; 30 percent averages less than 3 tons; and the other 50 percent between 3 and 8 tons (Stewart *et al.*, 1975). In fact, the sedimentary materials in water resulting from soil erosion accumulate more than 700 times more than those derived from sewage discharges (Weber, 1972). Thus, any treatment of the environmental toxicology of soil and water must consider each as a two-phase system, each containing the other and interacting through the water-sediment system.

Sources of Chemicals in the Environment

Chemicals in the environment may be classified in a variety of ways. In this chapter we have chosen to consider chemicals primarily according to their use; secondarily, by chemical properties. Thus, we will consider chemicals by their source as follows: (1) industrial, (2) agricultural, (3) domestic and urban, and (4) naturally occurring. No matter what use is made of chemicals,

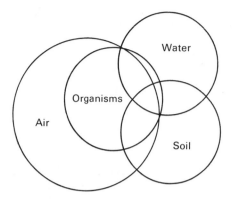

Figure 26–1. Overlapping relationships of environmental compartments.

contamination of the environment may be either from point sources or from nonpoint sources. The results of point source pollution are generally easy to identify and the remedies are frequently more attainable. Nonpoint source pollution, on the other hand, is generally less dramatic in its initial effects, but is more difficult to contain or correct.

The production, use, and disposal of industrial chemicals all lead to contamination of soil and water. Production activities lead to soil and water contamination when by-product chemicals are not properly conserved during manufacturing processes. For example, in various smelting operations toxic chemicals present in ores may not be properly controlled. Naturally occurring arsenic in copper ores, for example, frequently finds its way into soil and water. Accidental spillage of industrial chemicals may also result in contamination, sometimes dramatically, of soil and water. Careless manufacturing practices in a small chemical firm in Hopewell, Virginia, led to serious contamination of the James River and Chesapeake Bay by the pesticide Kepone. Even though these practices have now ceased, the contamination of the estuarine system will be present for many decades. Another example is the contamination of the Ohio River with carbon tetrachloride resulting from an accidental dumping of the material from a chemical plant. Such incidents of point source contamination of water can generally be prevented or controlled by the appropriate use of technology. The result, however, of not controlling such point source pollution is frequently a very high cost for decontamination, where that is even possible, and frequently both acute and chronic detrimental effects on organisms.

The use of chemicals for their intended purpose often leads to contamination, sometimes undesirably, of soil and water. Lead contamination of soils and occasionally water near high-

ways results from the use of tetraethyl lead as an antiknock component of gasoline for automobiles. Although a commitment was made to reduce the use of this compound in gasoline, the many years during which it was used and the nonpoint source nature of the contamination have resulted in concentrations of lead that will remain for many years in soils and water. A chemical that is intentionally added to water for therapeutic purposes is fluorine. The use of water fluoridation to prevent tooth decay is well known and has been practised in the United States for many years. Excessive concentrations of fluorine, however, can result in undesirable effects in teeth, manifested primarily by their mottling and discoloration. Careful attention must be paid to the use of fluorine to prevent overfluoridation with its undesirable side effects.

The disposal of industrial chemicals following their use presents a major problem in several industries. Detergents used in clothes laundering are discharged into sewage systems and ultimately into rivers, lakes, and streams. Phosphate detergents then serve as nutrients for algae and other organisms that can cause major difficulties in these bodies of water. The green scum resulting from algal blooms is a familiar sight in some areas. The contamination of rivers resulting from discharge of water containing organic mercurials used in paper manufacturing presents a problem in some local situations. Other chemicals resulting from paper making can also present serious water pollution problems. Asbestos tailings resulting from mining operations have also contaminated water systems in some parts of the United States, and this has resulted in concern over the potential health effects of the material that then finds its way into drinking-water systems.

The use of chemicals in agriculture results in contamination of soil and water, including groundwater, through the direct use of pesticides and fertilizers. Pesticides are, of course, applied directly to the soil in some cases to control insects, weeds, and plant diseases. Some of these chemicals can persist for many years and thereby cause concern about their potential movement from soil into water systems and from both soil and water into organisms that live in and on water and soil. The effects of pesticides in the food chain are now generally familiar. Likewise, fertilizers applied to the soil to promote plant growth and productivity can leach or run off from soil and find their way into natural water systems, causing an upset in the ecologic balance to the degree that organisms living in those systems can be either enhanced or otherwise affected.

The domestic and urban use and disposal of chemicals also result in the contamination of soil and water. Domestic wastes are concentrated in sewage systems and landfill operations. Frequently, large buildups of heavy metals occur as a result. Pesticides and fertilizers used in suburban and some urban situations for lawn and home garden purposes or pest control in other situations also are serious problems when improperly used. Detergents may also cause difficulties as referred to above. The discovery that the process of purifying water can result in the chlorination of certain organic chemicals to produce chlorinated hydrocarbons that are potential carcinogens has generated concern. In some parts of the country concentrations of such chemicals above levels considered to be safe have been found in drinking-water systems.

Finally, metals, minerals, and plant or animal toxins are found in the environment as natural components of water and soil systems. Although they have always been there and always will be, human activities frequently result in excessive production or movement of such chemicals found naturally occurring in the environment and can result in concentrations detrimental to human or other organisms. Furthermore, the possibility of interaction of synthetic chemicals and pollutants with naturally occurring metals, minerals, and toxins must be considered.

Transport, Mobility, and Disposition

The fate and distribution of chemicals in the environment are determined by several variables that can interact in numerous ways. An analogy between pharmacodynamics and chemodynamics can be drawn to illustrate some basic similarities in each approach. First, one must appreciate the physicochemical properties of a chemical, such as water solubility, lipid solubility, partitioning behavior, vapor pressure, pKa for ionic species, chemical stability, etc., if one is to predict the behavior of a chemical in a system—be it human or an ecosystem. Second, the processes that act within the system must be considered. Transport, via serum proteins versus suspended sediments; circulation, via the circulatory system versus the hydrologic cycle; degradation, in liver versus soil microorganisms; and excretion, via urine, feces, and expired air versus dilution in water and air to nondetectable levels or deposition in ultimate sinks such as deep ocean sediments, are all processes that act on chemicals to determine the mobility and final disposition of a chemical in a system. The analogy can be carried one step further to include target organs or tissues affected by the chemical in comparison with the susceptible species of an ecosystem. The fundamental difference in this consideration is one of scale, in both time and dimension, which then requires models of varying scale. Several mathematical models have become available in recent years to predict the transport and fate of organic chemicals and metals in both aquatic and soil systems (Dickson *et al.*, 1982). The soil models are divided into unsaturated and saturated systems while other models deal with runoff and the transport of toxicants in surface waters. The value of such models is in understanding the properties that are most important in determining the environmental fate of a chemical under given conditions. A second objective is to predict exposure of various organisms through time to various toxicants and thus aid regulatory agencies in decision making.

Water Solubility. The water solubility and latent heat of solution are critical properties of a chemical that affect its environmental fate. Many environmental toxicants are hydrophobic, having solubilities in the parts-per-million (ppm, mg/l) to parts-per-billion (ppb, μg/l) range. Reported solubility values vary with the method used for determination (Gunther *et al.*, 1968). Water solubilities are affected by pH (for ionizable chemicals), presence of dissolved salts and organics, and temperature.

Soil Adsorption. Adsorption to particulate matter is a major mechanism by which chemicals are removed from solution. Adsorbent materials in soils and sediments can be divided into clay minerals and soil organic matter. Clay minerals include various hydrous silicates, oxides, and layer silicates. The clay minerals have been extensively studied and are characterized by physical structure or layering type, either 1:1 or 2:1, swelling ability, cation exchange capacity, and specific surface (m^2/g) (Weber, 1972). These parameters are important considerations in the behavior of organic cations, polar organic molecules, and metal ions in soils. High specific surface is associated with small particle size; therefore, the colloidal fraction of the soil is a dominant factor in chemical-soil interactions. Cation exchange capacity of the inorganic fraction is a function of the magnitude and distribution of the structural charge. Exchangeability is dependent on the adsorbed cations, usually sodium, potassium, or calcium, and the nature of the replacing cations.

The water associated with clay plays an important role in defining its characteristics. Adsorbed water on clay surfaces is more ordered than free water. Water on the clay surface may also be more ionized than otherwise. Thus, the hydrogen ion concentration of the clay surface is high. The effect of pH on the adsorption of classes of chemicals has been summarized by Hamaker and Thompson (1972) (Table 26–1).

Adsorption data for chemicals in soils is usually expressed by the Freundlich isotherm, $x/m = KC^n$; x/m is the amount of chemical sorbed per weight of the adsorbent, C is the equilibrium concentration of the chemical, and K and n are constants. The constant K represents the extent of adsorption while the value n sheds light on the nature of the adsorption mechanism and the role of the solvent, water.

Soil organic matter usually ranges from 0.1 to 7.0 percent and serves as the most important sorptive surface for nonionic chemicals. Above a few percent organic matter, all the soil mineral surfaces are effectively blocked and thus no longer function as adsorbents. Soil organic matter can be divided into two main groups: (1) nonhumic substances, which are fresh or incompletely decomposed plant and animal material, and (2) humic substances, which are more or less completely altered or resynthesized materials. The former serve as a source for the latter. Nonhumic materials include well-known organic chemical groups with definite characteristics: proteins, carbohydrates, organic acids, sugars, fats, waxes, resins, lignins, pigments, and low-molecular-weight compounds. These

materials comprise 10 to 15 percent of the soil organic matter. Their composition and residence times are quite variable. Humic substances account for 85 to 90 percent of soil organic matter and their nature is not well understood. Humic substances are fractionated to give fulvic acid, which is soluble in both alkali and acid; humic acid, which is soluble in alkali but not in acid; and the humin fraction, which cannot be readily extracted with cold alkali. Humic acid and fulvic acid are aromatic polymers with molecular weights that range from 5000 to 100,000 and from 2000 to 9000, respectively. Functional groups that have been identified on humic substances are carboxyl, phenolic hydroxyl, alcoholic hydroxyl, carbonyl, and methoxy. Heterocyclic rings with oxygen and nitrogen atoms are also present. A hypothetic structure for humic acid has been proposed by Kononova (1966) as shown below.

Vaporization. Vaporization from soil, water, or plant surfaces is a major transport process for many chemicals. The volatility of a chemical is a function of its vapor pressure, but the rate of vaporization also depends on environmental conditions such as temperature, degree of adsorption, soil properties, and soil water content. Airflow over the evaporating surface affects

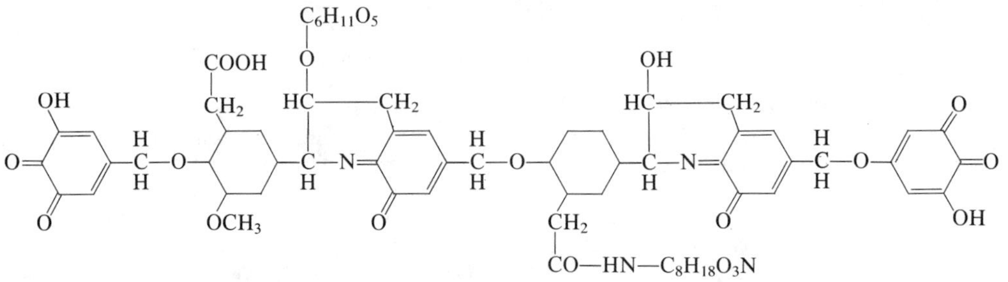

Table 26–1. CLASSES OF MATERIALS RELATED TO THE EFFECT OF pH ON ADSORPTION*

| | | | MOLECULAR FORM | | |
CLASS	EXAMPLE	pK_a	Low pH	High pH	pH Effect
Strong acid	Linear alkylsulfonates		Anion	Anion	Small
Weak acid	Picloram	3.7	Free acid	Anion	Large adsorption; pH approx. pK_a
Strong base	Diquat		Cation	Cation	Decrease at very low pH (18 N H_2SO_4)
Weak base	Ametryne		Cation	Free base	Increasing adsorption to pH approx. pK_a and then decrease
Polar molecules	Diuron		Nonionized	Un-ionized	Small
Neutral molecules	DDT	Nil	Nonionized	Un-ionized	Probably none

* From Hamaker, J. W., and Thompson, J. M.: Adsorption. In Goring, C. A. I., and Hamaker, J. W. (eds.): *Organic Chemicals in the Soil Environment*, Vol. 1. Marcel Dekker, Inc., New York, 1972. Reprinted by courtesy of Marcel Dekker, Inc.

vaporization rate since air movement continuously replaces and mixes air around the evaporating surface. Many chemicals evaporate simultaneously with water, which leads some researchers to believe that chemicals such as DDT "codistill" with water. This phenomenon can be demonstrated in laboratory distillations at 100°C, but does not occur at normal environmental temperatures. Instead, water evaporation and DDT volatilization occur independently. Higher vapor loss from most soil surfaces correlates with pesticide volatilization, but is due to desorption of chemicals from soil adsorption sites by water molecules and the mass flow of chemical to the soil surface by the "wick effect." This phenomenon has been noted with chemicals such as 2,4-D esters, thiolcarbamates, triazines, organochlorine insecticides, and N-methyl-carbamates. Volatility of organic chemicals from water increases with decreasing water solubility. As a result, a chemical with both low vapor pressure in the solid phase and very low water solubility would be much more volatile from aqueous solution than might be expected. DDT is again the example.

Partitioning. The distribution relationships for a chemical between the environmental compartments of air, soil, water, and biota can be expressed by a series of partition coefficients (McCall et al., 1983). The soil sorption constant (K_d) relates the amount of chemical sorbed to soil to the concentration in water (Table 26–2). Since organic matter is a key to the sorption process in many soils, as discussed above, the sorption characteristics of a chemical can be normalized by use of K_{oc}, which relates sorption properties to soil organic matter. Air-water distribution, expressed as K_w from Henry's law, is valid only for dilute solutions, which is the case for most environmental chemicals. The bioconcentration factor (BCF) is actually a measure of the partitioning of a chemical between water and fish but is a suitable indicator for biota in general. This information provides relative rankings of chemicals, although variations will occur among different organisms with respect to bioconcentration. A laboratory measure of the partitioning of a chemical between n-octanol and water provides K_{ow}, which is related to water solubility. K_{ow} values have been correlated with bioconcentration factors and soil sorption constants for a number of organic chemicals. Recently, retention times for chemicals on reversed-phase high-performance liquid chromatography (RP-HPLC) have been used to predict partitioning between the organic and aqueous phases of the environment (Swann et al., 1983). Thus, with just a few measurements of the properties of a chemical (water solubility, vapor pressure, melting point, partitioning parameters, or RP-HPLC retention times) it is possible to guess a chemical's expected environmental distribution.

Bioaccumulation. Bioaccumulation is different from other environmental processes because it concentrates rather than diffuses the chemical in question. This concentration effect is expressed as the ratio of the concentration of a chemical in the organism to that in the medium (usually water). Bioaccumulation refers to both uptake of dissolved chemicals from water (bioconcentration) and uptake from ingested food and sediment residues. The two properties of a chemical that are responsible for high bioaccumulation ratio values are: (1) high partition coefficient, i.e., lipophilic, and (2) recalcitrance

Table 26–2. KEY PHYSICAL AND ENVIRONMENTAL PROPERTIES IN FATE ASSESSMENT*

PROPERTY	DEFINITION
Soil sorption coefficient (K_d)	$\dfrac{\mu g \text{ Chemical soil/g of soil}}{\mu g \text{ Chemical water/g of water}}$
Soil sorption constant (K_{oc})	$\dfrac{K_d}{\% \text{ Organic carbon}} \times 100$
Water-air ratio (K_w)	$\dfrac{\mu g \text{ Chemical/cm}^3 \text{ of water}}{\mu g \text{ Chemical/cm}^3 \text{ of air}}$
n-Octanol-water coefficient (K_{ow})	$\dfrac{\mu g \text{ Chemical/ml } n\text{-octanol}}{\mu g \text{ Chemical/ml of water}}$
Bioconcentration factor (BCF)	$\dfrac{\mu g \text{ of Chemical/g of fish}}{\mu g \text{ of Chemical/g of water}}$

* From Swann, R. L., et al: A rapid method for the estimation of the environmental parameters octanol/water partition coefficient, soil sorption constant, water to air ratio, and water solubility. *Residue Rev.*, **85**:17–28, 1983.

toward all types of degradation. The length of the food chain also determines final concentrations in the top organisms. Bioaccumulation ratios have been determined for a variety of environmental chemicals in laboratory model ecosystems and correlate well with the n-octanol/water partition coefficients.

Degradation. Transformations of chemicals in soil and water occur by chemical, photochemical, and biochemical reactions. Degradation results in the true "disappearance" of a chemical's molecular form, as opposed to transport processes, which merely move chemicals from one environmental compartment to another. However, it must be recognized that transport processes that move chemicals to ultimate sinks, such as deep ocean sediments, for all practical purposes do remove chemicals from the environment.

Chemical transformations are classified as hydrolyses, oxidations, reductions, nucleophilic substitutions involving water, and free radical reactions. These reactions may be catalyzed by the presence of metal ions, metal oxides, clay surfaces, organic compounds, and organic surfaces. The pH of solutions and the effective pH of clay surfaces, which may be quite different from the surrounding aqueous environment, can significantly influence rates of degradation. Other obvious conditions that affect degradation rates are temperature, moisture content in soils, and other environmental processes that alter chemical concentrations. The kinetics of degradation rates are dependent on the mechanism of degradation. Some degradative processes follow first-order kinetics, while others are best described by a "hyperbolic rate model" (Hamaker, 1972).

Photochemical reactions of chemicals occur in air and water but are probably of little or no significance in soils. For a chemical to undergo a photochemical reaction, it must absorb light energy from an appropriate portion of the spectrum or have the light energy transferred through an intermediate substance known as a sensitizer. Ultraviolet light (4- to 400-nm wavelengths) has sufficient energy to break existing chemical bonds, but light above 450 nm, which represents an energy of 65 kcal/mole, is usually not sufficient to initiate reactions. Light of wavelengths shorter than 295 nm does not reach the earth's surface in appreciable amounts. The principal reactions are photo-oxidations and photoreductions which proceed through light-formed free radicals and which then react with molecular oxygen or abstract hydrogen from organic compounds, respectively.

Biologic reactions of chemicals in soil and water are mediated primarily by microorganisms. Microorganisms are quite versatile when confronted with foreign chemicals. The major reactions involved are dehalogenation, hydrolysis, oxidations, reductions, conjugations, and methylations. They are also very important in the natural cycles of many elements, such as mercury and arsenic. These natural cycles can be disturbed by introduction of various forms of metals and can increase formation of toxic species, e.g., methyl mercury. The types and rates of microbiologic reactions are determined by the microbial ecology of any given system. Thus, pH, temperature, redox potential, nutrient availability and microbial interactions will affect the microbial degradation of a chemical.

Chemodynamics. As we have seen above, there are numerous routes by which chemicals enter the environment and many factors to consider in understanding their behavior once they are there. Much of what is known about chemodynamics is derived from studies of pesticides and, to a lesser extent, industrial chemicals and heavy metals. Certainly, pesticide applications, sewage sludge disposal, and industrial waste effluents each present different starting points for a consideration of chemodynamics. We shall deal with environmental processes in the following sections and attempt to relate the (1) physicochemical properties of a chemical and (2) the environmental conditions that serve as modifiers of the processes. Each process has a rate that describes the transport from one component to the next and a rate that describes the degradation of the chemical in question. A complete analysis of all of the rates for entry, transport, and degradation of a chemical will describe its ultimate fate in the water and soil. More detailed discussion of these processes will be found in the monograph by Thibodeaux (1979).

PESTICIDES

The major classes of pesticides have been grouped as "nonpersistent" or "slightly residual," "moderately persistent" or "moderately residual," or "persistent" or "highly residual" (Harris, 1969; Kearney *et al.*, 1969). Persistence times reflect the time required for 75 to 100 percent disappearance of pesticide residues from the site of application. Nonpersistent pesticides have persistence values of 1 to 12 weeks; moderately persistent pesticides, 1 to 18 months; and persistent pesticides, two to five years. Persistence times vary with environmental conditions and the generalizations about the classes are subject to several exceptions by individual pesticides within the class (Figure 26-2).

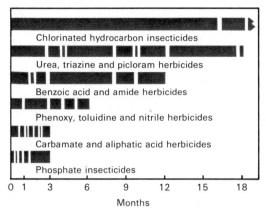

0 1   3   6   9   12   15   18

Months

Figure 26–2. Persistence in soils of several classes of insecticides and herbicides. (From Kearney, P. C.; Nash, R. G.; and Isensee, A. R.: Persistence of pesticide residues in soils. In Miller, M. W., and Berg, G. G. [eds.]: *Chemical Fallout*. Charles C Thomas Pub., Springfield, Ill., 1969.)

Persistent Pesticides

Chlorinated Hydrocarbon Insecticides. This group of chemicals includes DDT, TDE (a major metabolite of DDT), methoxychlor, and related chemicals; the cyclodiene insecticides, aldrin, dieldrin, endrin, heptachlor, chlordane, mirex, and Kepone; the hexachlorocyclohexanes (commonly referred to as BHC) and the purified gamma isomer, lindane; and toxaphene. The technology, application, and biologic and environmental aspects of this class of insecticides have been authoritatively reviewed in a two-volume treatise by Brooks (1974). The persistence of pesticides in the environment has been the subject of numerous books and reviews.

DDT, its major metabolites, DDD (TDE) and DDE (which are collectively referred to as DDT-R), and dieldrin, which is both an insecticide and the major metabolite of the insecticide aldrin, are ubiquitous residues and the prime examples of persistent pesticides. Studies with DDT and dieldrin have elucidated several important concepts in environmental toxicology. First, persistence is not a desirable attribute as originally believed. Second, the transport and disposition of persistent pesticides is affected by physical and biologic processes, which occur from the micro to the global scale. Third, high lipid solubility combined with chemical and biologic stability can lead to biologic magnification of pesticide residues.

Persistence is primarily a function of physicochemical properties of substances. In addition, the sorption/desorption process is one of the important factors controlling the fate of pesticides in soils. Sorption of pesticides in soils has

been reviewed by numerous authors (Goring, 1967; Bailey and White, 1970; Weber, 1972). Chlorinated hydrocarbon insecticides are highly soluble in lipids and most organic solvents, but have low water solubilities and relatively low vapor pressures. Studies of the adsorption of chlorinated hydrocarbons on various soils are difficult because of their low water solubility. However, studies with PCBs, which have many similar physicochemical properties to the chlorinated hydrocarbons, show that adsorption of the hydrophobic chlorinated hydrocarbons depends strongly on the presence of soil organic matter. Once adsorbed, these chemicals do not readily desorb. Two implications are readily apparent: (1) such compounds will not leach or diffuse in soils and (2) transport into the hydrosphere from contaminated soils will be through erosion of soil particles or sediment, not by desorption and dissolution. When chlorinated hydrocarbons are poorly adsorbed, as in sandy soils, the vaporization loss will be significant as compared to that in soils with higher organic matter.

Volatilization of pesticides into the atmosphere from water and soils is also a transport route. The volatility of a chemical from soil or water is a function of its vapor pressure, but the actual vaporization rate depends on several environmental parameters. Temperature, soil properties, soil water content, and other physicochemical properties such as water solubility and degree of adsorption affect the vaporization rate of pesticides from soil. Soil properties such as high organic matter that cause the pesticide to be strongly adsorbed reduce volatility greatly. The importance of soil moisture in volatilization of chlorinated hydrocarbons led to the use of the term "codistillation." DDT codistills with water in the laboratory (Acree *et al.*, 1963). However, the effect observed in soils is more adequately described as displacement of the sorbed pesticide by water molecules, plus a carrier action by water to the soil-air interface. The distribution of a pesticide between water and air is dependent on both water solubility and vapor pressure. As a result, compounds like DDT with very low water solubilities are quite volatile from water.

Degradation of the chlorinated hydrocarbons is quite slow as compared to the other classes of insecticides, and in soil and water is due mainly to the action of microorganisms. To a lesser extent, chemical reactions and photochemical reactions degrade the chlorinated hydrocarbons under certain conditions. A summary of the pathways for DDT emphasizes the importance of dechlorination and dehydrochlorination reactions. Oxidative reactions are only moderately important in this scheme. The formation of DDCN in sewage sludge and lake sediment is an example of the unique reactions carried out by microorganisms. Epoxidations and rearrangement reactions are common among the cyclodiene insecticides. The most thoroughly studied of these reactions is the epoxidation of aldrin to dieldrin and heptachlor to heptachlor epoxide (Lichtenstein and Schulz, 1960). The rearrangement products are mainly complicated "caged" structures that are still toxic. The caged compounds mirex and Kepone undergo very little detectable degradation. Toxaphene and BHC are degraded initially by dechlorinations and dehydrochlorinations.

The bioaccumulation of the chlorinated hydrocarbons DDT and dieldrin is well documented by environmental residue data (Edwards, 1970). Bioaccumulation ratios relate organism residues to environmental residue levels and are higher in aquatic ecosystems as opposed to terrestial ecosystems (Table 26–3). The processes involved in bioaccumulation are quite complex owing to population fluctuations, food web relationships, metabolic capabilities of various species, and numerous other ecologic considerations. However, the physicochemical parameters of lipid solubility, low water solubility, and chemical stability, which characterize the chlorinated hydrocarbons, appear to be most important in bioaccumulation of organic pesticides.

It may be observed that the effects of bioaccumulation of DDT-R and dieldrin are manifest primarily at the tops of food chains. Predatory fish and birds suffer from acute toxicity, chronic toxicity, and reproductive failures. However, significant declines in organochlorine residues in eggs from brown pelicans have been associated with increases in eggshell thickness and reproductive success in a breeding population in South Carolina (Blus, 1982). Behavioral changes in DDT-treated fish have been demonstrated. Thus, the effects can range from obvious toxicity to subtle behavioral changes, but there is evidence that the population effects of these persistent pesticides are reversible with time.

Cationic Herbicides. The two chemicals of importance in this group are diquat and paraquat, which are used in conservation tillage farming. These compounds readily dissolve and dissociate in aqueous solution. As cations, they are strongly adsorbed to soil particles by cation exchange reactions (Weber, 1972):

Table 26–3. **BIOCONCENTRATION OF DDT-R RESIDUES IN PLANTS OR ANIMALS FROM ITS ENVIRONMENT***

ENVIRONMENT	PLANT OR ANIMAL ORGANISM	(DDT-R RESIDUE IN ORGANISM DIVIDED BY RESIDUE IN ENVIRONMENT)	
		Maximum Value Observed	*Minimum Value Observed*
Soil	Earthworm	73	0.67
	Beetles	2.81	0.31
	Slugs	3.70	2.33
	Crop roots	0.13	0.04
	Crop foliage	0.08	—
Water	Sea squirt	1,000,000[†]	200[†]
	Sea hare	178,000[†]	—
	Eastern oyster, clam	70,000[†]	60
	Shrimp	2,800[†]	280
	Crabs	144	—
	Crayfish	97	17
	Snails	1,480[†]	—
	Plankton	16,666[†]	250
	Fish	829,300[†]	5–(1,450)[†]
	Fish (DDD)	9,214[†]	417
	Algae	33	0.34
	Aquatic plants	100,000[†]	0.45
Diet	Pheasant	2.91	—
	Woodcock	4.5	2.6
	Bald eagle		
	Brain	0.1	—
	Liver	1.9	—
	Fat	35.7	—

* Modified from Edwards, C. A.: *Persistent Pesticides in the Environment.* CRC Press, Cleveland, 1970.
† DDT may be present in excess of solubility in water.

Paraquat^{2+} + 2Na-clay $\rightleftharpoons$ Paraquat-clay
+2 Na$^+$

X-ray studies show that these planar molecules interlayer between the parallel silicate sheets of various clays. The adsorption behavior is also related to surface charge densities on various clays. Adsorption isotherms for these cationic compounds indicate a high affinity of the solute for the adsorbent until the cation exchange capacity is reached.

Paraquat and diquat as soil-bound residues are resistant to microbial degradation and photodecomposition. Tightly adsorbed residues are not biologically available and therefore persist indefinitely. In a field test begun in 1967 nearly all of the paraquat applied was still in the soil in 1973. Annual rate of loss was only 10 percent, which results in an estimated half-life in the field of 6.6 years (Hance *et al.*, 1980). Both diquat and paraquat are nonvolatile and are not transported in the vapor phase. Environmental transport is thus tied to sediment transport processes.

Moderately Persistent Pesticides

Triazine Herbicides. The triazines behave as weak bases in aqueous solution with pK_a values that range from 1.1 to 4.3. Water solubilities are therefore determined by the pH level, with the triazines being more soluble at low pH levels. The behavior and fate of triazines in soils has been extensively studied and reviewed (Gunther, 1970). Adsorption of triazines through an exchange process to organic matter and clay minerals is dependent on the pH of the solution and the acidity of the adsorbent surface. Hydrogen bonding and hydrophobic bonding are other mechanisms by which soil organic matter adsorbs triazine herbicides, especially at higher pH levels.

Hydrolysis and oxidation are the general routes of soil metabolism for triazine herbicides. Photodecomposition appears to be minimal on soils. Vapor transport losses of triazines are dependent on vapor pressure and pH of the evaporating surface, since ionized compounds are less volatile. Transport from soil to water occurs in solution and in sediments.

Considerable attention has been focused on the possibility that the observed decline in submersed aquatic vegetation in the Chesapeake Bay was caused by herbicide runoff from agricultural use. The compound of greatest concern was atrazine, one of the triazine herbicides extensively used in Maryland. Laboratory studies (Forney and Davis, 1981) and field measurements and observations (Forney and Davis, 1981; Wu, 1981), however, do not support the conclusion of a relationship between atrazine and the observed decline of the aquatic vegetation.

Phenylurea Herbicides. Between 20 and 25 different substituted phenylurea compounds are presently commercially available as herbicides for the control of annual and perennial grasses in a variety of crops. The phenylureas can be divided into three categories based on their water solubilities, which in turn seem to be related to a number of other properties that the groups have in common (Weber, 1972). Fenuron, the most water soluble of the phenylureas at approximately 2900 to 3850 ppm, is in a category by itself. This compound is also the most mobile in soil systems of all the phenylureas. Fenuron has been shown to move substantially in a lateral direction over the soil surface and in a vertical direction into the subsoil. Its movement is also related to soil texture and organic matter content. Movement was greater in coarse-textured soils and was decreased at higher organic contents.

The middle group of phenylureas in terms of water solubility includes monuron, diuron, linuron, monolinuron, fluometuron, metobromuron, norea, and siduron, in which water solubilities range from 18 to 580 ppm. Compounds in this category are moderately mobile in the soil; their relative movement decreases as the water solubilities decrease. Movement of the compounds also decreases as organic matter content of the soil increases, and in turn, the herbicidal activity of the phenylureas decreases as the compounds are bound to the soil organic matter.

The least soluble of the phenylureas are neburon and chloroxuron, where water solubilities range from 2.0 to 4.8 ppm. These compounds are rather immobile in the soil.

Most of the phenylurea compounds have relatively low vapor pressures and are not very volatile from the soil. Soil pH does not appear to significantly affect adsorption, mobility, or herbicidal activity of the phenylureas. The field persistence of these compounds is moderate, with residues remaining following application for several months at the longest.

The phenylurea herbicides are readily biotransformed by most biologic systems. The combination of their low mammalian toxicity and biodegradability leads to the conclusion that these compounds are not significant factors in the contamination of soil and water systems, and their significance as environmental pollutants seems to be minimal.

Substituted Dinitroanilines. The substituted dinitroanilines are an important group of herbicides, which include trifluralin, oryzalin, pendimethalin, and related materials. These compounds are only slightly soluble in water, have generally low vapor pressures, and are relatively immobile in soil systems, remaining essentially where they are applied. They have been classed among the least mobile of the herbicides. Like many of the herbicides they appear to be readily adsorbed by soil organic matter. Compounds that were the most highly adsorbed were also the least available to growing plants and hence the least effective as herbicides. The dinitroanilines are considered to be moderately persistent herbicides in the soil. They are generally considered to have a very low degree of toxicity to mammals and are degraded in the environment to products without significant adverse effects on organisms.

Nonpersistent Pesticides

Phenoxy and Related Acidic Herbicides. A large group of compounds may be designated as acidic herbicides, since they are chemicals that possess carboxyl or phenolic functional groups and which ionize in aqueous systems yielding pK_a's of <4. The behavior of these chemicals is closely correlated with their acid character. The most significant factor with respect to mobility of these compounds is the organic matter content of the soil. Various adsorption studies have shown that the compounds are readily adsorbed by soil organic matter. Furthermore, in acidic systems these compounds are also adsorbed by clay particles. A number of these compounds are commercially available in either the acid form or as esters. The behavior of the esters might be expected to be considerably different from that of the acid forms.

Included within this group of herbicides are several important herbicide classes. The phenoxyacetic acids, including 2,4-D and its esters, were introduced following World War II for their high activity against many broad-leaved weeds. The chlorinated aliphatic acids include dalapon and trichloroacetic acid, compounds used against perennial weeds. The benzoic acid herbicides include chloramben, dicamba, diclobenil, and several other compounds. This is a very heterogeneous group of herbicides used for a variety of purposes. The dinitrophenols are a group of broad-spectrum herbicides, the most common of which is dinitro-o-cresol (DNOC).

Phenylcarbamate and Carbanilate Herbicides. The phenylcarbamate herbicides are much more water soluble than the substituted anilines. In spite of this, however, they are very immobile in soil systems. Again, these compounds have been shown to be inactivated by adsorption to soil organic matter. Compounds in this group include propham, chlorpropham, barban, ter-

butol, and dichlormate. The mechanism of adsorption to soil organic matter is thought to involve hydrogen bonding between the carboxyl groups of the organic matter and the nitrogen and carbonyl oxygen of the carbamate.

Ethylenebisdithiocarbamate Fungicides. The metal derivatives of the ethylene*bis*dithiocarbamates are one of the most important groups of fungicides currently used in agriculture. The principal compounds in this group are the manganese and zinc derivatives, maneb and zineb, and the disodium derivative, nabam (see Chapter 18). A closely related group is dithiocarbamates, represented by ferbam, ferric dimethyldithiocarbamate, and ziram, zinc dimethyldithiocarbamate. From a toxicologic standpoint these compounds have caused concern because of the common contaminant, degradation product, and metabolite, ethylenethiourea, a known carcinogen. This group is thoroughly considered in a two-volume treatise on antifungal compounds (Siegel and Sisler, 1977).

These compounds may be used as seed protectants and foliar fungicides. Only small quantities find their way into the soil, and once there, are rapidly degraded. In soil ethylenethiourea, ethylenethiuram monosulfide, CS_2, and H_2S result from treatment with nabam, zineb, and maneb. Ethylenethiourea is further degraded to ethyleneurea. Plants growing on treated soil will take up residues of ethylenethiourea, which are translocated and further biotransformed. The ethylene*bis*-dithiocarbamates decompose rather rapidly in water.

Because of the carcinogenic activity of ethylenethiourea, its residues found in soils, plants, and food are of concern. Although the residues of ethylenethiourea itself may be small, it has been shown that cooking vegetables containing residues of ethylene*bis*dithiocarbamates release ethylenethiourea. Hence, the toxicologic significance of residues of these chemicals in soil, once thought to be of little consequence, is now a matter of considerable attention.

Synthetic Pyrethroids. The synthetic pyrethroid insecticides are examples of optimized insecticidal activity, selectivity, and tailored environmental persistence. These compounds are modeled after natural pyrethrins, which possess the first two properties but are insufficiently stable under agricultural use conditions to be commercially viable. Through modifications of both the acid and alcohol portions of these esters (Figure 26–3) compounds of desired residual activity have been synthesized while maintaining the biodegradable ester linkage. Thus, this group of insecticides, which has been actively

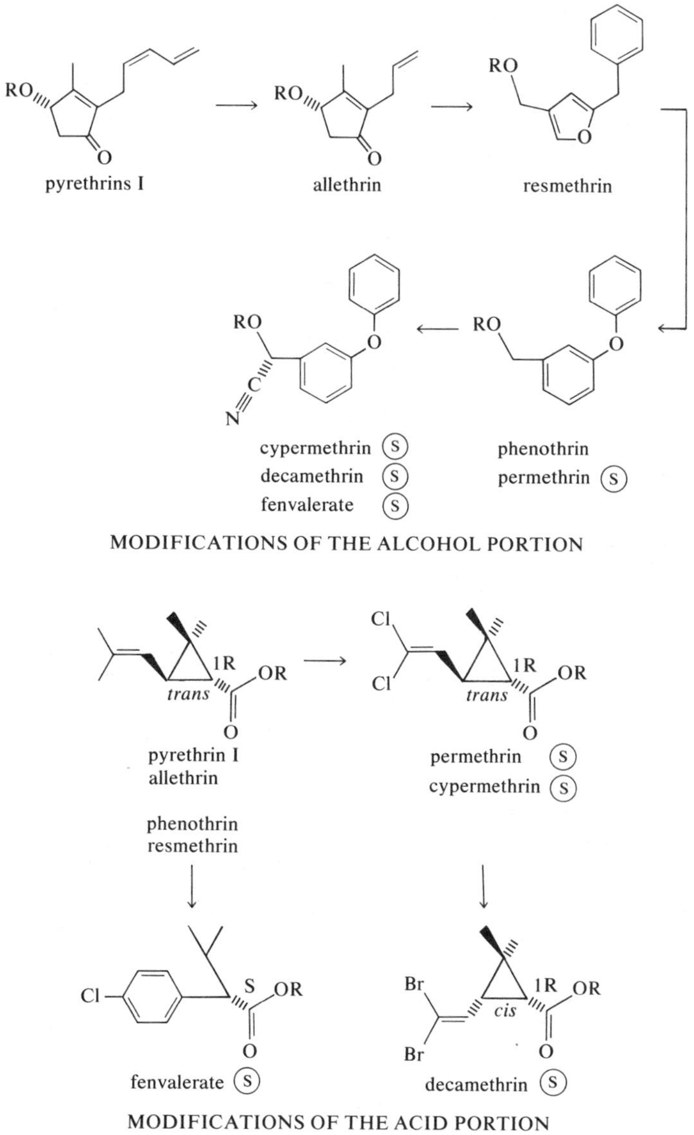

Figure 26–3. Development of synthetic pyrethroid insecticide structures leading to stable compounds (S) that can be used on field crops. (Modified from Elliot, 1977; Casida, 1980.)

researched since the mid-1970s, represents an enlightened approach to the tradeoff between environmental persistence versus residual activity. These compounds are generally very toxic to fish in laboratory aquarium bioassays. However, under field conditions the residues are tightly bound to sediment, and the toxicity is greatly reduced.

Organophosphorus and Carbamate Insecticides. In contrast to the persistent insecticides, particularly the chlorinated hydrocarbons, the organophosphorus and carbamate insecticides are relatively nonpersistent in the environment.

They are typically applied to crops, sometimes directly to the soil as systemic insecticides, for the control of phytophagous pests. These chemicals generally persist from only a few hours through several weeks to months. Only in rare instances are organophosphorus or carbamate residues found in crops beyond the growing season during which they were applied. These chemicals have generally replaced the chlorinated hydrocarbon insecticides as the principal weapons in the arsenal of American agriculture against the invasion of the pests that compete with humans for food and fiber. More than half

(57 percent in 1971) of the total volume of insecticides applied in the United States is made up of members of this group of chemicals. These compounds have been comprehensively reviewed by Eto (1974) and Kuhr and Dorough (1976).

The organophosphates and carbamates used as insecticides are neutral esters of phosphoric and carbamic acids. A large number of these compounds representing a variety of chemical, physical, and biologic properties are presently in commercial use, allowing their specific application to be tailored to particular needs. They act as anticholinesterase agents by phosphorylating or carbamylating acetylcholinesterase freeing in the process a leaving group, which is generally easily further degraded (see Chapter 18). This reaction may take place as well in the environment by chemical or photochemical mechanisms. Thus, these compounds do not generally represent a serious problem as contaminants of soil and water. Their breakdown products are usually nontoxic, being composed of low-molecular-weight, volatile molecules that are easily degraded and utilized by organisms.

The rate of chemical and biochemical transformation of the organophosphorus and carbamate insecticides depends on the specific properties of the individual compounds. Some of these compounds are relatively soluble in water. Being esters, they are also susceptible to hydrolysis. The half-lives of a number of common organophosphorus insecticides at various temperatures and pH values are given in Table 26–4. Most organophosphorus and carbamate compounds are stable at acid pH values. However, under alkaline conditions hydrolysis is rapid, the breakdown rate increasing approximately tenfold for each pH unit above 7. An increase of $10°$ of temperature will increase the hydrolysis rate approximately fourfold (Mühlmann and Schrader, 1957).

Organophosphorus and carbamate insecticides may contaminate soils by either direct application or through runoff from applications to crops. When these compounds are present in the soil, their disappearance is influenced by their interaction with the physical characteristics of the soil, the water content of the soil, and the microflora present. They may be tightly bound in certain types of soils, even to the point where they are unavailable for biologic decomposition. Under such conditions very little movement takes place even though water may be running through the soil or over its surface. The combination of interaction with soil components and rapid chemical and biochemical degradation in the soil results in minimal contamination of water supplies and soil to which compounds have not been applied.

A notable exception to this generalization was the discovery that the carbamate insecticide aldicarb has leached into the ground water aquifers that constitute the major source of drinking water on Long Island, New York. This acutely

Table 26–4. EFFECT OF TEMPERATURE AND pH ON THE HYDROLYSIS IN WATER OF SOME ORGANOPHOSPHORUS INSECTICIDES*

TEMP. (°C)[†]	HALF-LIFE						
	Parathion	Paraoxon	Methyl Parathion	Disulfoton	Trichlorofon	Dichlorvos	Azinphos-methyl
Days							
10	3,000	1,200	760	4,830	2,400	240	1,070
20	690	320	175	1,110	526	61.5	240
30	180	93	45	290	140	17.3	61.5
40	50	29	12.5	78	41	5.8	18
50	15	9.6	4.0	24	10.7	1.66	5.46
60	4.75	3.2	1.34	7.8	3.2	0.58	1.9
70	1.65	1.2	0.47	2.7	1.13	0.164	0.61
Hours							
70							
pH 1	34	18.5	15.4	62	32	2.3	24
3	21	23	11.2	62	33	3.4	9
5	19.5	24.4	10.7	60	15.3	2.8	8.9
7	7.8	11.5	6.9	27.6	0.7	0.45	4.8
9	2.7	2.1	1.5		0.1		

* Data from Mühlmann, R., and Schrader, G.: Hydrolyse der insektiziden Phosphorsäureester. *Z. Naturforsch.*, **12b**:196–208, 1957.
† At pH 1 to 5.

toxic compound provided effective control of potato insects, but the particularly sandy, porous soil and the climactic conditions on eastern Long Island resulted in its unexpected movement through the soil into ground water. Estimates of the length of time during which aldicarb would be present in the ground water above the New York State advisory guideline of 7 ppb range up to 20 years (Cornell University, 1983), although the estimates are based on models whose reliability has not been thoroughly tested and on monitoring data that are incomplete. Subsequently, aldicarb has been found in ground water in other locations.

The detection of organophosphorus and carbamate insecticides in soil can be difficult. Their interaction with soil components renders them unavailable to exert their toxic action on organisms and makes them difficult to remove by conventional solvent extraction techniques. Hence, methods that depend on removal of residues from soil particles often underestimate the presence of these compounds. The analysis of organophosphorus and carbamate residues in water, on the other hand, is relatively uncomplicated and easily done. Extraction of large quantities of water with organic solvents and subsequent analysis provides a very sensitive assay for small quantities of organophosphorus and carbamate insecticides in water, although other water pollutants may complicate the analyses when they are coextracted with the insecticide.

When organophosphates or carbamates reach the soil, their subsequent disposition is influenced by interaction with the mineral components of the soil, soil organic matter, soil pH, and soil moisture. In addition, the flora and fauna present in the soil are responsible for the degradation of these insecticides into innocuous breakdown products. After treatment of soil with organophosphorus compounds in laboratory or controlled field studies, extraction of the material from the soil is increasingly difficult as time progresses (Duff and Menzer, 1973; Menzer et al., 1971).

The persistence of these compounds is, at least in part, a function of interactions with the mineral components of soil. Metallic ions in soils interact with organophosphorus insecticides. Malathion, for example, is quickly incorporated into the montmorillonite clay interlayer region, where it is adsorbed as a double layer. The mechanism was shown to be hydrogen binding between carbonyl oxygen atoms and the hydration water shells of cations. In this case adsorption was so strong that no degradation of the malathion was observed (Bowman et al., 1970). Similarly, Saltzman and Yaron (1972) have shown a strong affinity of parathion for sodium

montmorillonite. On the other hand, diazinon and chlorpyrifos were decomposed rapidly on contact with copper(II)-montmorillonite (Mortland and Raman, 1967).

Binding of organophosphorus and carbamate insecticides correlates well with the organic matter content of soils (Edwards, 1966). It has been shown, for example, that the amount of mevinphos bound by soils increased with increasing organic matter content. Furthermore, the absorption of phorate from the soil by plants appeared to be in competition with the binding of the compound with the organic matter content of the soil.

In a kinetic study of the adsorption of carbaryl to soil organic matter surfaces, Leenheer and Ahlrichs (1971) found that carbaryl was more readily adsorbed to acid soils than to neutral or alkaline soils. This may be due to decreased displacement of the carbamate from the active sites by water at lower pH values.

Soil moisture has a major influence on the availability and extractability of residues of organophosphorus and carbamate insecticides, apparently because of competition between the insecticides and water for the adsorption sites on the soil particles. Harris (1964) has shown, for example, that diazinon, parathion, trichlorfon, and mevinphos are 135-fold, 28-fold, 20-fold, and 1.4-fold, respectively, more active in moist soils than in dry soils. Analytic procedures for the recovery of residues from soils generally recommend the addition of water for the desorption of the residues from soil particles before extraction with an organic solvent. However, even though there is a major interaction between these insecticides and water, they do not appear to move freely in soils with water, and loss by leaching does not appear to be a major factor in the disappearance of these compounds from soils, with some notable exceptions.

The fact that microorganisms exert a major influence on the behavior of pesticide residues in soil has been demonstrated by observing the effect of soil sterilization on the breakdown of a number of compounds. Getzin (1968) showed that zinophos degraded faster in nonautoclaved soil, although the decomposition of diazinon was unaffected by autoclaving. Getzin and Rosefield (1968) showed that malathion, Ciodrin, dichlorvos, mevinphos, parathion, methyl parathion, Supracide, dimethoate, and chlorpyrifos were all degraded faster in nonsterile soils. Lichtenstein et al. (1968) showed that both sodium azide treatment and autoclaving reduced soil bacteria and resulted in an increased persistence of parathion. Bro-Rasmussen et al. (1968) reported that sterilization extensively affected diazinon degradation in loam and sandy loam soils. The effect of sterilization of soil on pesticide degradation may appear to be somewhat ambiguous because of changes other than the destruction of soil microorganisms that would have an effect on the degradation of compounds applied. In general, however, there is at least strong evidence that microorganisms exert a major influence on the degradation of pesticides in soils.

There is little data on the effects of organophosphates and carbamates on organisms living in water and soil. In general, only minute amounts of residues of the insecticides and their toxic degradation products are found in natural water systems. Thus, their biologic effect seems to be minimal. In soil, however, there is greater likelihood of the presence and buildup of toxic residues. Several studies have shown that some compounds can cause reduction in bacterial populations. Garretson and San Clemente (1968) showed that parathion inhibited nitrifying chemolithotrophic bacteria, although malathion did not. Sommer (1970) showed that organophosphates had little effect, while carbamates markedly inhibited nitrification. In studies to assess the effect of diazinon on soil microorganisms Gunner and co-workers (Gunner et al., 1966; Gunner, 1970) showed that the compound exerted a selective effect on both soil and rhizosphere microflora expressed as selective enrichment of coccoidal rods. In another instance the microflora that arose in response to diazinon belonged primarily to one species of *Arthrobacter*. Similar results were obtained by Stojanovic et al. (1972) with carbaryl as the test insecticide. Various studies show that these insecticides may cause a variety of effects on the soil flora and fauna not always expressed as directly toxic effects.

Glyphosate. This compound is an important nonselective, postemergence herbicide for control of deep-rooted perennial species and some biennial and annual grasses. It is very mobile in soil and water and is readily translocated in plants, even downward (Marquis et al., 1981), as demonstrated in Sago pond weed when the compound applied to the shoots was translocated to the roots. Even at low temperatures, glyphosate is degraded in soil (Mueller et al., 1981) and would not be expected to persist from one growing season to the next.

NONPESTICIDAL ORGANIC CHEMICALS

In a continuing data-gathering program, the U.S. Environmental Protection Agency monitors organic chemicals in the drinking water of the United States. The list was begun in 1973; 253 different organic chemicals were detected through November 1975. In an updated report issued in 1976, the number had increased to 309; in 1978, the number was over 700. Undoubtedly the number will continue to increase as monitoring programs increase in their sophistication and extent of coverage. The list of chemicals detected includes both aliphatic and aromatic hydrocarbons, pesticides, industrial chemicals, plasticizers, and solvents. Many of these materials are halogenated, and some are produced by chlorination of the water during the purification process, including trihalomethanes and halogenated carboxylic acids (Johnson et al., 1982). Others appear through industrial and municipal discharges, urban and rural runoff, natural sources, and sewage purification practices.

The principal objective of the nationwide survey of organic chemicals in drinking water made by the Environmental Protection Agency is to determine the extent and significance of the occurrence of suspected carcinogens in water (Symons et al., 1975). These data were considered in a series of reports on the potential health effects of chemicals in drinking water that have been produced by the National Academy of Sciences (National Research Council, 1977–83) under mandate of the Safe Drinking Water Act of 1974.

Low-Molecular-Weight Halogenated Hydrocarbons

Of particular concern is the production of low-molecular-weight chlorinated hydrocarbons through the use of chlorination for water purification. This concern focuses principally on the four trihalomethanes, chloroform, bromodichloromethane, dibromochloromethane, and bromoform; and carbon tetrachloride and 1,2-dichloroethane. A study was conducted by the Environmental Protection Agency to ascertain the presence of these chemicals in water, and whether they were produced by chlorination. A National Organics Reconnaissance Survey (NORS) was conducted in November 1974 for this purpose (Symons et al., 1975) and was followed by the National Organics Monitoring Survey (NOMS) in 1976 (Brass et al., 1977). The results are summarized in Table 26–5. It was noted that all of these materials were found in drinking water and most were found in the raw water before chlorination. Several conclusions can be drawn from these and subsequent studies (National Research Council, Vol. 3, 1980). Chloroform, bromodichloromethane, dibromochloromethane, and bromoform do result from chlorination of precursors, particularly naturally occurring humic substances, in the raw water. On the other hand, carbon tetrachloride, meth-

Table 26–5. ORGANICS DETECTED IN WATER IN THE EPA NATIONAL ORGANICS RECONNAISSANCE SURVEY*

| | RAW WATER ANALYSIS | | FINISHED WATER ANALYSIS | | |
| | | | | Concentration | |
COMPOUND	No. of Locations Where Detected	Concentration Range (μg/l)	No. of Locations Where Detected	Range (μg/l)	Median
Chloroform	49	<0.1–0.9	80	<0.1–311	21
Bromodichloromethane	7	<0.2–0.8	78	0.3–116	6
Dibromochloromethane	1	3	72	<0.4–110	1.2
Bromoform	0	—	26	<0.8–92	5
Carbon tetrachloride	4	<2–4	10	<2–3	—
1,2-Dichloroethane	11	<0.2–3	26	<0.2–6	—

* Data derived from *Preliminary Assessment of Suspected Carcinogens in Drinking Water, Report to Congress.* U.S. Environmental Protection Agency, Washington, D.C., 1975.

ylene chloride, and 1,2-dichloroethane do not appear to be produced chemically during the treatment process. Raw water with low turbidity generally yields finished water low in trihalomethanes. There appears to be a correlation between chloroform, dibromochloromethane, bromodichloromethane, and bromoform concentrations. The ratio between the four chemicals appears to be relatively constant in all waters examined, indicating the probability of a common precursor or group of precursors for these halogenated hydrocarbons.

Studies have been conducted to compare the rate and extent of trihalomethane formation when chlorine was added to raw river water, filtered water, and activated-carbon treated water (National Research Council, Vol. 3, 1980). When sufficient chlorine is added to satisfy the chlorine demand, chlorination of raw river water yields approximately seven times as much chloroform as chlorination of filtered water and approximately 80 times as much as chlorination of activated carbon-treated water. Concentrations of humic materials are probably reduced during coagulation, settling, and filtration, thereby reducing the rate and extent of chloroform formation by chlorination. Thus, it may be possible to reduce the quantity of chlorinated hydrocarbons formed during chlorination by altering the water purification process so that chlorination is performed following the removal of humic materials through filtration and coagulation steps.

As yet, there is no generally accepted substitute for the use of chlorine as a disinfectant in water purification. However, the confirmation that chlorination produces a number of halogenated hydrocarbons has stimulated an extensive investigation of other chemicals that could be used for this purpose, such as chloramines, chlorine dioxide, ozone, bromine, and iodine (National Research Council, Vol. 3, 1980).

Concern about low-molecular-weight halogenated hydrocarbons in drinking water came to public attention in the mid-1970s when it was reported that the drinking water supply of New Orleans, Louisiana, contained more chlorinated hydrocarbons than untreated Mississippi River water (Dowty *et al.*, 1975). In addition, these workers reported the presence of chlorinated hydrocarbons, including carbon tetrachloride, in blood plasma collected from human volunteers in New Orleans. Following that report, Page *et al.* (1976) reported a statistical correlation between the incidence of certain types of cancer among the New Orleans population and the source of the water supply. While later studies (Gottlieb *et al.*, 1982) have not confirmed all of the earlier conclusions with respect to cancer incidence, a case-control cancer mortality study showed a definite association between surface chlorinated water in southern Louisiana and significant risk of rectal cancer. No increased risk of colon cancer and no effect on bladder cancer from water was detected. There was a significant association between chlorine levels in water and breast cancer incidence. A similar case-control study was conducted to determine the possible association of drinking water with cancer incidence in Wisconsin (Kanarek and Young, 1982). It was concluded that colon cancer in Wisconsin was related to the combination of chlorination and organic contamination. Chlorinated ground water was also responsible for elevated colon cancer. Presently, it is generally accepted that it is highly likely that there is a relationship between rectal, colon, and bladder cancer and water quality (Crump and Guess, 1980; Cantor, 1982). However, it appears that the increases in cancer risks lie near the lower limit of what can be reliably detected by epidemiologic methods. Clearly, however, there is cause for concern about the exposure of a very large percentage of the population to these chemicals in drinking water.

In addition to the possibility of a relationship between trihalomethanes and cancer, there is also concern about other chronic effects of these chemicals in drinking water. Studies in mice (Munson *et al.*, 1982) have shown increased liver weights, elevations of SGOT and SGPT, decreased spleen weights, and a decreased number of splenic IgM antibody-forming cells in a 14-day gavage treatment at one-tenth of the LD50 dose. The enzyme changes, however, were not observed in a 90-day study, indicating that there may be the development of tolerance to the chemicals over a longer term of exposure.

Aromatic Halogenated Hydrocarbons

In recent years a number of halogenated aromatic compounds have engendered increasing concern about their effects as environmental pollutants. The polychlorinated biphenyls (PCB) have appeared as ubiquitous contaminants of soil and water. Chlorophenols used for a variety of purposes have been detected in surface waters and drinking water. The extremely toxic 2,3,7,8-tetrachlorodibenzo-*p*-dioxin (TCDD) has contaminated large areas of both water and soil through industrial accidents, improper waste disposal, wide-scale application of herbicides containing small quantities of the chemical as a contaminant, and as a trace byproduct of combustion.

Polychlorinated Biphenyls. PCBs are very stable materials of low flammability, which contain from 12 to 68 percent chlorine. They are exceptionally persistent in the environment, some even more persistent than the chlorinated hydrocarbon insecticides, with which they often have been confused in analytic studies of environmental samples. They have been used as insulating materials in electrical capacitors and transformers, plasticizers in waxes, in paper manufacturing, and for a variety of other industrial purposes. The diversity of their use patterns, the large quantities used, and their stability has led to widespread occurrence of these compounds in soil and water. Fish from the upper Hudson River and Lake Ontario have been found to contain PCB concentrations from 5 to 20 ppm. Fish from a number of other rivers throughout the United States have also been found to contain comparable quantities of PCBs. Waterfowl have also accumulated high concentrations of PCBs. These examples of PCB pollution have occurred in spite of efforts to restrict and eventually eliminate the release of such compounds into the environment.

The health effects of PCBs are well established. Investigations have shown that PCBs interfere with reproduction in phytoplankters (Masser *et al.*, 1972). Other observed effects in mammals and birds include microsomal enzyme induction, porphyrogenic action, tumor promotion, estrogenic activity, and immunosuppression (Bitman 1972; Vos, 1972). Other adverse effects are possible since the PCBs are lipophilic, a property, along with their stability, that leads to bioaccumulation and the possibility of long-term effects that have not been completely identified.

Chlorophenols. Pentachlorophenol has been used in significant quantities since 1936 as a wood preservative. As a result of this use surface water and treated drinking water have been found to contain as much as 0.70 and 0.06 ppb, respectively, pentachlorophenol (Buhler *et al.*, 1973). Hexachlorophene 2,2'-methylene-*bis*-(3,4,6-trichlorophenol) has been widely used as an antibacterial agent in a number of consumer products, including soaps and deodorants. It has been detected in surface waters as high as 48 ppb and in drinking water at 0.01 ppb (Buhler *et al.*, 1973). Hexachlorophene is resistant to biotransformation and tends to persist in the environment and bioaccumulates in food chains (Sims and Pfaender, 1975).

Pentachlorophenol has a fairly high acute toxicity and has been shown to cause reproductive failures in rats. The acute toxicity of hexachlorophene is also quite high. The compound has exhibited neurotoxicity in dogs, sheep, and rats. One of the concerns about these chemicals is their possible contamination by the very toxic polychlorinated dibenzo-*p*-dioxins and dibenzofurans. The presence of these chemicals and their contaminants in water needs to be closely monitored because of their high toxicity and the possibility of adverse health effects in man.

2,3,7,8-Tetrachlorodibenzo-*p*-dioxin. What was probably the most dramatic and catastrophic occurrence of environmental pollution by a toxic chemical occurred in Seveso, Italy, July 10, 1976. On that date a safety disk in a reaction vessel being used to manufacture 2,4,5-trichlorophenol, an intermediate in the production of hexachlorophene and 2,4,5-trichlorophenoxyacetic acid (2,4,5-T), ruptured, releasing a chemical cloud over the region. The cloud contained predominantly 2,4,5-trichlorophenol. However, an estimated 3 to 16 kg of 2,3,7,8-tetrachlorodibenzo-*p*-dioxin (TCDD, also improperly called simply "dioxin"), a potent teratogen, was also released. The area was thus contaminated with the greatest concentration of TCDD ever found in the environment, up to 51.3 ppm in some samples.

TCDD is extremely toxic to some animal species as indicated by its acute oral LD50 reported between 0.6 and 115 μg/kg (National Research Council, 1977). It causes degenerative changes in the liver and thymus, chloracne, porphyria, altered serum enzyme concentrations, loss of body weight, induction of microsomal enzymes, and is a potent carcinogen in rats. Thymic atrophy is a very sensitive index of TCDD exposure in many animals while chloracne is the most prominent symptom for human exposures. To date, there have been no known human deaths from TCDD exposure.

The significance of TCDD as an environmental pollutant lies in (1) its extreme biologic potency and potential chronic effects, (2) the ability of analytic methods to detect trace quantities of TCDD in environmental samples, and (3) the inability of toxicologists to agree on the significance of exposure to these trace residues. Confounding the scientific questions are the emotional aspects of unknowing exposure to TCDD through Agent Orange spraying in Vietnam, TCDD-contaminated soils in Times Beach, Missouri, and industrial accident exposure in Seveso, Italy. Indeed, TCDD has become a household word, much like DDT in the 1960s.

Phthalate Ester Plasticizers

The phthalate ester plasticizers are used in virtually every major product category, including construction, automotive, household products, apparel, toys, packaging, and medical products, resulting in the widest possible distribution of these materials. The industry today comprises ten major suppliers who produce approximately 1 billion pounds of over 25 different compounds. The two most abundantly produced phthalate ester plasticizers are di-2-ethyl-hexylphthalate (DEHP) (400 million pounds in 1977) and di-*n*-butylphthalate (DBP).

The phthalate esters are now known to be ubiquitously distributed in the environment. They have been found complexed with the fulvic acid components of humic substances in soil (Ogner and Schnitzer, 1970) and in both marine and estuarine waters. Fulvic acid apparently functions as a solubilizer for the rather insoluble phthalate esters and thus serves to mediate the mobilization, transport, and immobilization of these materials in soil and water. Hites (1973) reported the presence of phthalate esters in the Charles and Merrimack Rivers in Massachusetts. In the Charles River, concentration of phthalate esters at river mile 7 was approximately 1.9 ppb, while at the mouth of the river concentrations had decreased to 0.97 ppb. In another study (Giam *et al.*, 1978), phthalate ester plasticizers were detected in the open ocean environment of the Gulf of Mexico and the North Atlantic. DEHP and DBP were found in almost all samples analyzed, including a deep-sea jellyfish, *Atolla*, from 1000-m depths in the North Atlantic (Morris, 1970),

Atlantic herring, and mackerel (Musial *et al.*, 1981). Concentrations of DEHP in surface water ranged from 4.9 to 130 ng/liter. DBP ranged from a nondetectable level to 95 ng/liter. Lower levels of both compounds were found in sediment. It has become clear that the phthalate ester plasticizers are general contaminants of virtually all soil and water ecosystems; it has become very difficult to analyze any soil or water sample without detecting the presence of phthalate esters.

Because of the widespread occurrence of these compounds, their toxicity is of concern. In general, the phthalate esters have low acute toxicity. The intraperitoneal LD50 dose in mice ranges from 1.5 to 14.2 g/kg (Rubin and Jaeger, 1973). Ninety-day and two-year feeding studies of DEHP in rats and one-year feeding studies in guinea pigs and dogs indicated a low order of chronic toxicity. However, recent studies have demonstrated the carcinogenicity of DEHP in Fischer 344 rats and B6C3F1 mice. At both the maximally tolerated dose and one-half of the maximally tolerated dose, liver tumors were produced in both sexes (Kluwe *et al.*, 1982a, 1982b, 1983). A conference on phthalates, convened in 1981, evaluated these results and concluded that the weight of evidence on the carcinogenicity of DEHP was very strong (Conference on Phthalates, 1982). At the conference it was also noted that the experiments reported prior to the report of Kluwe and co-workers were not properly designed to permit the evaluation of the carcinogenicity of phthalates in mice or rats (Wilbourn and Montesano, 1982). It has also been pointed out that much more testing is desirable on this class of compounds; the report on carcinogenicity did not permit an analysis of the mechanism, which appeared to be nongenetic. There is obviously a need for further testing of other phthalates as well.

Other subtle chronic toxic effects of DEHP have been reported (Rubin and Jaeger, 1973). As little as 4 μg/ml in the culture medium was lethal to 97 to 98 percent of cultured beating chick embryo heart cells. This concentration could be reached in human blood stored in vinyl plastic bags for a period of one to two days. Considerable interest in the chronic toxicity of low levels of phthalate esters has been evident over the last several years. The reader is referred to a series of papers on a number of possible toxic effects published in Volume 45 of *Environmental Health Perspectives* (1982), which were reported at the 1981 Conference on Phthalates.

Data reported by Mayer and Sanders (1973) indicate that DEHP and DBP may also be detrimental to the reproduction of some aquatic organisms at low concentrations. *Daphnia magna* reproduction was decreased by approximately 80 percent by continuous exposure of 30 μg/l DEHP for up to 21 days. Reproduction in zebra fish and guppies was also decreased by low concentrations of DEHP.

Although the concentrations of phthalate esters in soil and water are quite low, the recent report of carcinogenicity and the continuing reports of the ubiquitous presence of residues in the environment led to concern about the potential for human health effects. Because phthalates have been found to occur in drinking water in the United States (Brass et al., 1977) and are present in food, that concern is reinforced.

METALS

The toxicology of metals, including their use, occurrence, and effects, has already been presented in Chapter 19. In this section we will deal only with some aspects of the natural cycles of elements and conditions that alter the process involved. It is necessary to limit this treatment to the best-studied examples of environmentally important elements: mercury, cadmium, lead, arsenic, and selenium. (Note: arsenic and selenium are not metals, but the term will be used to include these metalloids.)

Mercury. Methyl mercury pollution of Minimata Bay and the subsequent human poisoning from consumption of contaminated seafood has stimulated much research on the origin and fate of methyl mercury. An important theme throughout the discussion of metals is the question of chemical species. Mercury, for example, exists in the inorganic form as free mercury, $Hg°$, mercury ion in salts and complexes, Hg^{2+}; or as organic mercury compounds, such as phenylmercuric salts, which have been used as fungicides and herbicides, and the alkyl-mercury compounds including methyl mercury. In natural systems, a dynamic equilibrium that is determined by the physiochemical and biologic conditions of the soil-water system exists between the various chemical species. Some organic forms of mercury are man-made, such as the phenylmercuric compounds, while methyl mercury is produced by humans, sediment microorganisms, nonbiologically in sediments, and possibly by some fish. As expected, each species of mercury has its own set of physical, chemical, and toxicologic properties.

Mercury is transported to aquatic ecosystems via surface runoff and through the atmosphere. It is complexed or tightly bound to both organic and inorganic particles. Sediments with high sulfur content will strongly bind mercury. Organic acids such as fulvic and humic acid are usually associated with the mercury that is not bound to particles.

Methylation of mercury by microorganisms is a detoxication response that allows the organism to dispose of heavy metal ions as small organometallic complexes. Conditions for methylation by sediment microorganisms are strict and occur only within a narrow pH range. The rate of synthesis of methyl mercury also depends on the redox potential, composition of the microbial population, availability of Hg^{2+}, and temperature. Vitamin B_{12} derivatives are believed to be the methylating agents, since mechanistically they are the only methyl carbanion and methyl radical donating coenzymes known (Ridley et al., 1977). An understanding of the biomethylation reaction mechanisms together with oxidation-reduction chemistry of elements allows predictions of the environmental conditions necessary for the biomethylation of mercury and several other metals. However, the best conversion rate for inorganic mercury to methyl mercury under ideal conditions is less than 1.5 percent per month (Jensen and Jernelov, 1969).

Little or no methyl mercury is found in sediments. Conversion of inorganic mercury to methyl mercury results in its desorption from sediment particles at a relatively fast rate. Demethylation by sediment microorganisms also occurs at a rapid rate when compared to methylation. Methyl mercury released in surface waters can undergo photodecomposition to inorganic mercury. However, methyl mercury can also be bioaccumulated by plankton algae and fish. In fish, the rate of absorption of methyl mercury is faster than that for inorganic mercury, and the clearance rate is slower with a net result of high methyl mercury concentrations in the muscle tissue. Selenium, which is present in seawater and seafood, readily complexes with methyl mercury and is believed to have an important protective action against the toxic effects of methyl mercury. In summary, the danger of methyl mercury poisoning, as occurred in Minimata, arises from direct methyl mercury contamination rather than methylation of environmental sources of inorganic mercury.

Cadmium. Cadmium has long been recognized as a toxic element. Its importance as an environmental contaminant was demonstrated in the outbreak of itai-itai disease caused by smelter wastes that contaminated rice paddies in Japan (see Chapter 19). Cadmium deposits are found as sulfides with zinc, copper, and lead deposits, and cadmium is recovered as a by-product of smelting processes for those metals. A major environmental source of cadmium is vapor emissions that contaminate surrounding soil and water through fallout during smelting. Natural soil concentrations of cadmium are less than 1 ppm and average about 0.4 ppm. Sewage sludge is often contaminated with cadmium, which then concentrates in plants grown on contaminated soils. The problem of heavy-metal contamination, especially cadmium, has been one of the most serious concerns impeding the use and disposal of domestic sewage sludge on agricultural lands. Cadmium also enters agricultural soils as a contaminant of phosphate fertilizers. There is some evidence for the leaching of cadmium in soils.

Among the metals, cadmium is one of the most readily absorbed and accumulated in plants grown on contaminated soil. The significance of this phenomenon is readily apparent in the relationship of cadmium concentrations in rice with the incidence of itai-itai disease. Although there is some question about the specific etiology of this disease, there is ample evidence from many studies of a positive correlation between rice cadmium content and the incidence of the disease in Japan (see, for example, Nogawa et al., 1982, 1983).

Cadmium concentrations in fresh waters are usually less than 1 ppb, while concentrations in seawater range from 0.05 to 0.2 ppb and average about 0.15 ppb (Fleischer et al., 1974). Higher concentrations of cadmium in surface water are usually due to metallurgical plants, plating operations, cadmium pigments, batteries, plastics manufacture, or from sewage effluent. Mine drainage and mineralized areas also contribute significantly to cadmium fluxes in the Mississippi River in the Missouri-Tennessee-Kentucky area.

Drinking water in soft-water areas can serve as a source of cadmium through corrosion of plumbing. However, this source is estimated to be small in relation to food intake. As in the association of selenium and mercury, there appears to be a protective effect with zinc and calcium against cadmium toxicity.

Lead. The use of lead, its mining, and its processing date back several centuries. Changing usage patterns rather than increased consumption determine present environmental inputs from man's use of lead. Batteries, gasoline additives, and paint pigments are major uses, but combustion of gasoline additives is the major source of environmental pollution by lead. Thus, lead is primarily an atmospheric pollutant that enters soil and water as fallout, a process determined by physical form and particle size. The net result is a buildup of lead near heavily traveled roads. In a study in Massachusetts, there was a close concordance between the use of leaded gasoline and umbilical cord blood lead levels. This suggests that further reductions in leaded gasoline usage would result in lower human exposure levels (Rabinowitz and Needleham, 1983).

Lead enters aquatic systems from runoff or as fallout of insoluble precipitates and is found in sediments. Typical fresh-water concentrations lie between 1 and 10 μg/l while natural lead concentrations in soil range from 2 to 200 ppm and average 10 to 15 ppm. Deep ocean waters, below 1000 m, contain lead at 0.02 to 0.04 μg/kg concentrations, but surface waters of the Mediterranean Sea and Pacific Ocean contain 0.20 and 0.35 μg/kg levels (National Academy of Sciences, 1972). Drinking water concentrations of lead may be greatly increased in soft-water areas through corrosion of lead-lined piping and connections. However, average drinking-water intake is considerably less than food sources.

The biologic methylation of inorganic lead to tetramethyl lead by lake sediment microorganisms has been demonstrated (Wong et al., 1975), but the significance of this observation remains unknown. It has not been possible to detect tetramethyl lead, trimethyl lead, or dimethyl lead in sediments or water that have high lead levels.

Arsenic. Arsenic is widely distributed in the environment. Man's input of arsenic into the global cycle occurs through smelting, coal burning, and the use of arsenical pesticides. Speciation of arsenic is an important consideration in the fate, movement, and action of this element. The chemical and biochemical transformations of arsenic include oxidation, reduction, and methylation, which affect the volatilization, adsorption, dissolution, and biologic disposition of the arsenic species involved.

Arsenic contamination of soils from point sources such as copper smelters or coal-burning power plants is easier to control than the dispersive use of arsenical pesticides, resulting in non-point-source pollution. Various forms of arsenic are used as pesticides. Chromated copper arsenate continues to grow in usage as a wood preservative (Fitzgerald, 1983). Arsenic acid (H_3AsO_4) is a leaf desiccant used in cotton production, lead and calcium arsenates were used as insecticides, and organic arsenicals, which include methanearsonic acid and its sodium salts as well as dimethyl arsenic acid (cacodylic acid), are used as postemergence herbicides. The transport of arsenic in the environment is largely controlled by adsorption/desorption processes in soil and sediments. Therefore, sediment movement is responsible for transfer of arsenic soil residues to their ultimate sinks in deep ocean sediments. The clay fraction, plus ferrous and aluminum oxides that coat clay particles, adsorbs arsenicals as depicted in Figure 26–4. The reactions of arsenicals in soil include oxidation, reduction, methylation, and demethylation. Conversion of arsenic to volatile alkylarsines leads to air transport loss from soils. The transformation processes of arsenic and its transport processes are intimately linked.

Arsenic concentrations in water are generally much lower than in sediments. In Lake Michigan, the concentrations in water range from 0.5 to 2.3 μg/liter while sediment concentrations range from 7.2 to 28.8 mg/kg (Seydel, 1972). Inorganic arsenic exists in water in different oxidation states, depending on the pH and E_h of the water. Arsenate is apparently reduced by bacteria to arsenite in marine environments since the

ratio of arsenate to total arsenic is much lower than is predicted thermodynamically. Methylation of arsenic occurs in both freshwater and marine systems and where arsenic is detected as arsenate, arsenite, methanearsonic acid, and dimethylarsinic acid (Braman and Foreback, 1973).

Bioaccumulation of arsenic species occurs readily in some aquatic organisms. Some seaweeds, freshwater algae, and crustaceans accumulate significant amounts of arsenic. Some arsenic in *Daphnia magna* and algae occurs as arsenoanalogs of phospholipids, indicating the mistaken accumulation and utilization of arsenate in place of phosphate. Crabs, lobsters, and other marine organisms accumulate organoarsenicals along the food chain. Man can alter the concentration of arsenicals in environmental

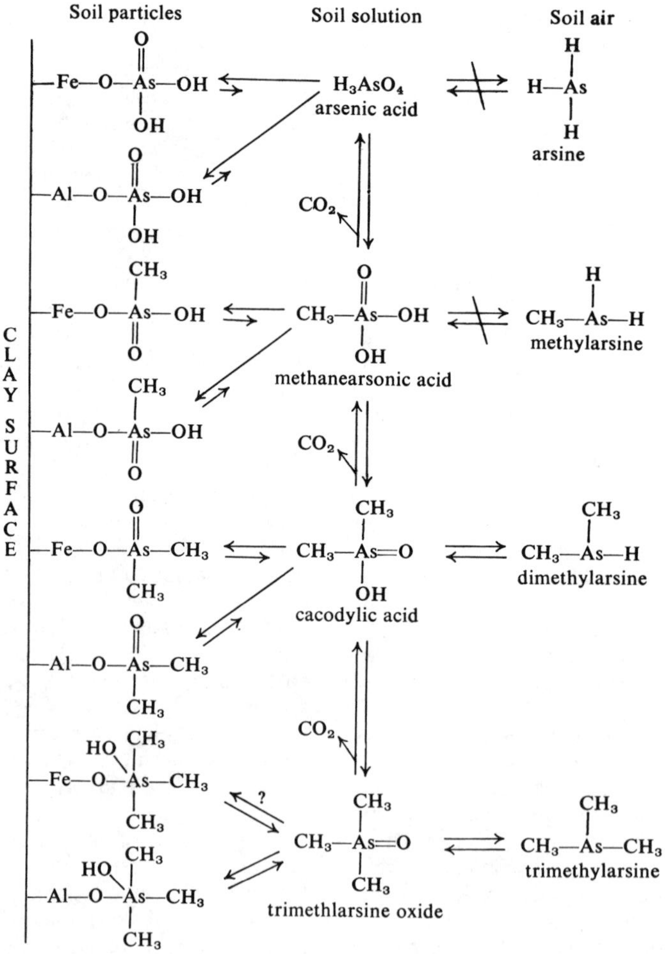

Figure 26–4. Dissolution and reactions of arsenicals within the soil environment. (From Woolson, E. A.: Fate of arsenicals in different environmental substrates. *Environ. Health Perspect.*, **19**:73–81, 1977.)

components in a very localized area, but there is little evidence that this affects the global-scale arsenic cycle (Woolson, 1983).

Selenium. Selenium is an interesting and controversial element. Early concerns about its toxicity to cattle and carcinogenicity have given way to recognition of its beneficial properties. Selenium is now thought to have an anticarcinogenic function. It also protects against the toxicity of heavy metals such as cadmium, mercury, and silver. Deficiency of selenium in the diet has been associated with an increased incidence of heart disease. Although the biochemical mechanisms are not yet understood, it appears that selenium is an essential element (Schnell and Angle, 1983).

Selenium concentrations in natural waters depend largely on the occurrence of seleniferous soils. Feeding on plants from seleniferous soils has been the cause of toxic effects in livestock. Average concentrations for selenium in natural waters are less than 10 μg/liter, but can reach several hundred micrograms per liter in certain areas of some Western states. Dietary sources of selenium are usually more important than drinking-water sources. Environmental redistribution of selenium through human activities is due to copper smelting; lead, zinc, phosphate, and uranium mining and processing; manufacturing of glass ceramics and pigments; and burning of fuels.

Selenium can be methylated as also demonstrated for mercury, arsenic, lead, and tin. Sediment microorganisms are responsible for the production of dimethyl selenide and dimethyl diselenide from both inorganic and organic selenium compounds and contribute to its biogeochemical cycling (Chau, 1976).

INORGANIC IONS

Nitrate, phosphate, and fluoride are inorganic ions that have caused considerable concern over their environmental effects. With nitrates and fluorides the concern is principally human health, but nitrates and particularly phosphates also cause eutrophication of lakes and ponds, a process that is considered environmentally undesirable. Midsummer algal blooms are a familiar sight in some parts of the United States.

Nitrates. Man has altered the nitrogen cycle through his agricultural and technologic practices. Changing patterns in agriculture, food processing, urbanization, and industrialization have had an impact on the accumulation of nitrate in the environment. Intensive agricultural production has consumed an increasing amount of nitrogen-based fertilizers, particularly with corn,

vegetables, other row crops, and forages. Nitrogenous wastes from livestock and poultry production as well as urban sewage treatment have contributed nitrogenous wastes to the soil and water environments. Nitrate and nitrite are used extensively for color enhancement and preservation of processed meat products. These practices inevitably lead to increased exposure of humans and animals to significant nitrate levels in food, feed, and water (National Academy of Sciences, 1981).

The nitrate form of nitrogen is of concern because of the high water solubility of this ion and consequent leaching, diffusion, and environmental mobility in soil and water. Nitrate can contaminate ground water to unacceptable levels. Gradual increases in nitrate levels in many surface and ground water sources of drinking water have been reported. It is estimated that United States drinking water averages 1.3 mg nitrate/liter, contributing thereby 2.0 mg/person/ day to total daily intake of nitrate. This amount is considered to be negligible compared to the estimated total daily intake of 75 mg/person/day from all sources. However, estimates of exposure to nitrate in areas of high nitrate in water are 160 mg/person/day. Nitrite is formed from nitrate or ammonium ion by certain microorganisms in soil, water, sewage, and the alimentary tract. Thus, the concern with nitrate in the environment relates to its conversion by biologic systems to nitrite.

Methemoglobinemia is caused by high levels of nitrite, or indirectly from nitrate, in humans. It results in difficulties in the oxygen transport system of the blood. Poisoning of infants from nitrate in well water was first reported in the United States in 1944. Cases numbering in the thousands have now been reported, mostly from rural areas and mostly involving poisonings in infants.

Of more recent concern is the production of nitrosamines in food by the reaction of nitrite with secondary amines. Other nitroso compounds can result from the analogous reactions of nitrites with amides, ureas, carbamates, and other nitrogenous compounds. Nitrosamines have been shown to produce liver damage, hemorrhagic lung lesions, convulsions, and coma in rats, and teratogenic effects in various experimental animals. N-nitroso compounds represent a major class of important chemical carcinogens and mutagens. The induction of tumors by single doses of N-nitroso compounds testifies to their potency. While it is difficult to extrapolate animal carcinogenicity data to humans, the data strongly suggest that these compounds are also human carcinogens. The health effects of nitrite, nitrate, and N-nitroso compounds has been comprehensively reviewed by the National Academy of Sciences (1981).

Phosphates. Although the principal problem of phosphates in the environment is not directly related to human health, there is considerable concern about the effects of phosphorus from various sources on water quality. Phosphate fertilizers and agricultural practices are a major contributor to the levels of phosphates found in water as are phosphate detergents and other phosphates from sewage treatment effluents.

Phosphorus applied to the soil as fertilizer moves primarily by erosion because phosphate adsorbs strongly on soil particles. However, some soluble phosphorus compounds do move in runoff water. The total phosphorus content of soils ranges from 0.01 to 0.13 percent (Stewart *et al.*, 1975). The phosphorus fertilizers applied as soluble orthophosphate soon revert to insoluble forms in soil. This conversion limits leaching and leads to a higher phosphorus concentration in sediments than in the original soil since phosphorus seems to be associated with finer particles. Decaying plant material and animal wastes are a significant source of phosphates in runoff water from fields especially when the ground is frozen and snow covered. Control of phosphate pollution from agriculture will result from efforts to reduce erosion and sediment loss by modified agricultural practices (Taylor and Kilmer, 1980).

The contribution to water of phosphorus from detergents is likely to be associated with the degree of urbanization. Some states and local areas have restricted or banned the use of phosphate detergents completely. In some areas secondary treatment of sewage waste results in the precipitation and removal of phosphates from the effluent before discharge.

Phosphate is a major cause of the eutrophication process in lakes and ponds (Thomas, 1973). Phosphorus is an essential plant nutrient and is usually the limiting nutrient for blue-green algae. The observer of a lake undergoing eutrophication notices first an extraordinarily rapid growth of algae in the surface water. This occurs when phosphorus concentrations exceed about 50 ppb. Planktonic algae cause turbidity and flotation films. Shore algae cause ugly muddying, films, and damage to reeds. Decay of these algae causes oxygen depletion in the deep water and in shallow water near the shore. This process is self-perpetuating because the anoxic condition at the sediment/water interface causes the release of more adsorbed phosphates from the sediment. This rapid growth of algae gives rise to a number of undesirable effects on treatment of the water for consumption, on fisheries, and on the use of lakes for recreational purposes.

Fluorides. The beneficial effects of low levels of fluorides in preventing dental caries have led to the extensive use of fluoride in drinking water. Most public water supplies of the 100 largest cities in the United States are fluoridated, but the levels were less than 1 mg/liter in 92 percent of the cases in the 1969 Community Water Supply Survey. Fluoride contents ranged from 0.2 to 4.4 mg/liter. Most water supplies that were not intentionally fluoridated contained fluoride at less than 0.3 mg/liter (National Research Council, Vol 1, 1977; Vol. 3, 1980). Fluoride in drinking water represents the largest single component of the element's daily intake, although there is some exposure in pharmaceutical products, from industrial sources, and in the soil and atmosphere (Miller, 1982).

While small amounts of fluoride are now generally conceded to have a beneficial effect in the reduction of dental caries, especially in children, two forms of chronic toxic effects may be caused by intake of excessive fluoride over a long period of time, dental fluorosis, and skeletal fluorosis. The most sensitive effect, tooth mottling, may occur at fluoride concentrations as low as 0.8 to 1.6 mg/liter. These observations were made a number of years ago, however, and there have been no recent studies to determine whether these levels are still causing this effect. Crippling skeletal fluorosis may result from high levels of chronic fluoride ingestion. While the precise levels are not well defined, it is estimated that daily ingestion of 2 to 80 mg fluoride for more than ten years will cause the effect (National Research Council, Vol. 3, 1980).

ASBESTOS

Asbestos is a general term applied to a family of silicate minerals that have a number of properties in common that render them useful for several commercial purposes. These minerals are fibrous in structure and have electrical and thermal insulating properties as well as being sufficiently flexible that they can be woven into fabrics. The production and use of such materials has been described by Rosato (1959). Approximately 88 percent of asbestos use has been in the construction industry, including cement products, floor tile, paper products, and paint and caulking, with the remainder being used in transportation, textiles, and plastics industries (May and Lewis, 1970).

The definition of asbestos listed in the *Glossary of Geology* is as follows:*

"(a) a commercial term applied to a group of highly fibrous silicate minerals that readily sepa-

---

* From American Geological Institute: *Glossary of Geology*. The Institute, Washington, D.C., p. 41, 1972.

rate into long, thin, strong fibers of sufficient flexibility to be woven, are heat resistant and chemically inert, and possess a high electric insulation, and therefore are suitable for uses (as in yarn, cloth, paper, paint, brake linings, tiles, insulation cement, fillers, and filters), where incombustible, nonconducting, or chemically resistant material is required.

"(b) a mineral of the asbestos group, principally chrysotile (best adapted for spinning) and certain fibrous varieties of amphibole (example: tremolite, actinolite, and crocidolite)."

The mineral fibers that comprise the asbetos group are the serpentine: chrysotile; and the amphiboles: actinolite, amosite (a cunningtonite-grunerite mineral), anthophyllite, crocidolite, and tremolite. Asbestos minerals are mined in Canada and the United States, where chrysotile accounts for about 95 percent of the production. Amosite and crocidolite make up most of the remainder. The largest chrysotile deposit in the world is found between Danville and Chaudiere, Quebec, Canada. Other deposits are found in northern Ontario, northern British Columbia, and Newfoundland in Canada, and in California, Vermont, Arizona, and North Carolina in the United States.

Asbestos is made up of fibrils of individual tubes of single crystals that bind together to produce a fiber. The size of the individual fibers varies greatly for the various minerals making up the asbestos group. Minimum fiber widths range between 0.06 μm for crocidolite to 0.25 μm for anthophylite. Fiber lengths in general range between 0.2 and 2.0 μm. Occasional longer fibers up to 100 μm are found, although these are much rarer in the general environment than in occupational situations (Rendall, 1970).

Solubility is an important consideration in assessing the presence and impact of chemicals in soil and water. Asbestos minerals are soluble in acid solution to varying degrees (Choi and Smith, 1971). The isoelectric point of the various minerals differs widely; chrysotile has an isoelectric point of 11.8 while the amosite isoelectric point falls between 5.2 and 6.0 (Parks, 1967). As the pH of an aqueous medium falls below the isoelectric point, the charge of suspended asbestos particles will become more positive, thereby attracting other dissolved minerals that can interact with them. Therefore, the mobility, transport, disposition, and biologic properties of asbestos will vary widely depending on the mineral involved, the pH of the medium, and the presence of other materials with which the asbestos may interact.

A major difficulty in assessing the environmental impact of asbestos is the difficulty in detecting and analyzing it. Since asbestos is a very heterogeneous material, its detection is also difficult. A number of methods have been proposed for the identification and quantitation of asbestos in air, water, and biologic materials. Optical and electron microscopy, x-ray diffraction, and differential thermal analysis have all been proposed. Analytic problems are complicated by the difficulty of distinguishing between asbestos fibers and other fibers and particles of minerals that may be present in the same sample with them. The quantities present in environmental samples, furthermore, are generally quite small, and the particles present may exist in a wide range of sizes, making identification difficult and greatly complicating the quantitation of the mineral present. It is generally felt that transmission electron microscopy is the most satisfactory method for the detection of asbestos. A useful summary of the advantages, disadvantages, possibilities, and difficulties of various analytic techniques that have been investigated is given by Langer (1974) and Langer et al. (1974)

Asbestos is found ubiquitously in the environment. Chrysotile asbestos is a common air pollutant in most large urban areas in the United States (Selikoff et al., 1972). In fact, because of the industrial use of asbestos the highest concentrations found in air and water are generally in metropolitan areas (Cunningham and Pontefract, 1971; Kay, 1973).

Drinking water in the United States is known to be contaminated with asbestos fibers resulting from mining operation, geologic erosion, the disintegration of asbestos cement pipe, and atmospheric sources. Asbestos contamination of domestic water supplies was first reported in 1973–74 when the Lake Superior situation was described:*

Duluth, Minnesota, drew its water directly from Lake Superior, about 60 miles Southwest of an iron ore mining company located at Silver Bay, Minnesota. The tailings from the mining operation were discharged directly into the lake at approximately 70,000 tons per day. These tailings were the residue from the processing of taconite ore into pellets and were predominately of the amosite type of asbestos. Bottom currents carry some of this material to the Duluth area. The water in Duluth was shown to contain numerous amphibole fibers and pieces as well as other crystalline material. The concentration of verified asbestos mineral fibers in the Duluth water ranged from approximately 20×10^6 fi-

* From Nicholson, W. J.: Analysis of amphibole asbestiform fibers in municipal water supplies. *Environ. Health Perspect.*, 9:165–72, 1974.

bers/liter of water. This corresponds to 5 to 30 μg of asbestos fibers per liter of water.

Since that time numerous analyses of domestic water supplies have been conducted (Millette et al., 1980, 1983). In addition to the Lake Superior locations, where fiber counts as high as 200 × 10^6 fibers/liter have been detected, locations in Kentucky, California, Washington, South Carolina, Florida, and Pennsylvania were detected with asbestos contamination from a variety of sources. A summary of the distribution of reported asbestos concentrations in the drinking water in the United States is given in Table 26–6.

The health effects of asbestos in water have so far been incompletely ascertained. Occupational exposure to inhaled asbestos is known to lead to asbestosis characterized primarily by pulmonary fibrosis, the formation of pleural plaques, a greatly increased risk of bronchogenic carcinoma, pleural mesothelioma, and peritoneal mesothelioma, as discussed elsewhere in this book. It is not clear, however, whether the ingestion of asbestos-contaminated food or water will have an adverse impact on health. Most studies with experimental animals have been negative in the detection of tumors of the gastrointestinal tract (Craighead and Mossman, 1982). Experiments in both rats (Hilding et al., 1981) and hamsters (Smith et al., 1980) have been conducted by administering both highly controlled samples of asbestos preparations and samples drawn from practical situations, such as taconite tailings. The only positive result from such studies was an indication of squamous cell carcinomas of the forestomach in hamsters treated with a preparation of amosite asbestos.

Epidemiologic studies have been conducted in areas of natural exposure to asbestos: San Fran-

cisco (Kanarek et al., 1980; Conforti et al., 1981; Kanarek, 1983), Puget Sound, Washington (Polissar et al., 1982, 1983, 1984), and Duluth (Sigurdson et al., 1981). The San Francisco study showed a positive relationship between chrysotile asbestos content of drinking water and some esophageal, stomach, digestive organ, and pancreatic cancers. The mortality rates of Duluth compared with Minneapolis–St. Paul were higher for pancreatic and gastrointestinal cancer for comparable periods of time when water levels of asbestos were highest in Duluth. In the Puget Sound area, odds ratios for tumors of the small intestine were consistently elevated. These results give sufficient positive correlation of a relationship between ingested asbestos and cancer that there is growing demand to take steps to remove asbestos from drinking water (Hills, 1979). However, experiments with long-term, high-level ingestion of various types of asbestos fibers in more than one animal species have failed to produce a definitive, reproducible, organspecific carcinogenic effect (Condie, 1983).

CHEMICAL WASTE DISPOSAL

The sources of hazardous chemical wastes are numerous and widely scattered throughout the United States. Industry, the federal government, agriculture, and institutions such as laboratories, hospitals, and universities are all sources of materials that need to be discarded when they are no longer useful. These materials take the form of solids, sludges, liquids, and gases, and are classified as toxic chemical, flammable, radioactive, explosive, and biologic. Often such materials are directly hazardous to human health or to other organisms, but also contamination of soil and both surface and ground water leads to more subtle and long-lasting toxicologic problems (Environmental Protection Agency, 1974). In 1970 it was estimated that 9 million metric tons of nonradioactive hazardous wastes were generated by industrial sources, practically all of which is categorized as toxic for regulatory purposes. A large proportion of hazardous wastes, 90 percent in one estimation, are disposed of in an unsound manner, 48 percent in surface impoundments, 30 percent in inadequate landfills, 10 percent by improper burning, and 2 percent by other means (Neely et al., 1981).

The Environmental Protection Agency's report to Congress on the storage and disposal of hazardous wastes as mandated by the Solid Waste Disposal Act (PL 89-272) is a catalog of environmental assaults (Environmental Protection Agency, 1974). Improper arsenic disposal in

Table 26–6. DISTRIBUTION OF REPORTED ASBESTOS CONCENTRATIONS IN DRINKING WATER FROM 406 CITIES IN 47 STATES, PUERTO RICO, AND THE DISTRICT OF COLUMBIA, USA*

HIGHEST ASBESTOS CONCENTRATION, 10^6 FIBERS/LITER	NUMBER OF CITIES	PERCENTAGE
Below detectable limits	117	28.8
Not significant (<0.5)	103	25.4
< 1	113	27.8
1–10	33	8.1
> 10	40	9.9
Total	406	100

* From Millette, J. R.; Clark, P. J.; Pansing, M. F.; and Twyman, J. D.: Concentration and size of asbestos in water supplies. *Environ. Health Perspect.*, **34**:13–25, 1980.

Minnesota, lead waste hazard in the San Francisco Bay area, cyanide and phenol disposal in Texas, insecticide dumping in Missouri, discharge of hydrocarbon gases into a river in Mississippi—the list goes on and on. The most dramatic example of improper chemical waste disposal—Love Canal—has become a household word in the United States. An estimated 20,000 metric tons, composed of at least 300 different chemicals, were buried in an abandoned canal in Niagara County, New York. Subsequently, families living in homes built many years later on the site were forced to abandon their homes permanently when toxic chemicals seeped up through the ground into basements. The EPA has identified, as of 1980, 151 hazardous waste sites that pose a threat to human health or the environment. Other studies indicate that the number may be much larger (Environmental Protection Agency, 1980).

A symposium entitled "Research Needs for Evaluation of Health Effects of Toxic Chemical Waste Dumps" was held in 1981 under the sponsorship of the National Institute of Environmental Health Sciences. The proceedings were published in Volume 48 of *Environmental Health Perspectives*. The conference highlighted some of the particularly salient problem areas involving hazardous chemical wastes: the central question of exposure of humans to waste chemicals, the problem of mixtures, the lack of toxicologic information on a significant portion of the chemicals found in dumps, and the psychosocial and legal aspects of the problem. Another summary of the conference and an assessment of the problem has appeared (Maugh, 1982a, 1982b). Specific reports range from an assessment of individual chemical effects on organ systems to epidemiologic studies of populations exposed to waste dumps. Particularly important are the papers addressing questions of the methodology that should be used in approaching this issue. Clearly, we are seeing now only the beginnings of what must become a concerted, well-coordinated attack on this serious environmental, potential public health problem.

IMPACT OF CHEMICALS ON SOIL AND WATER SYSTEMS

The traditional view of the environment embodied in the phrase "balance of nature" represents an outmoded conceptualization of the forces that control environmental processes. There is, in fact, no simple balance of nature. The environment is composed of many systems and subsystems, each internally balanced in a dynamic way and influenced by many external processes that tend to interact and influence the structure and function of the whole system. The thrust of nature's "balance" is an evolutionary movement toward greater diversity, greater speciation, and more complex structure.

The course of evolution has been influenced by man's activities through technologic advances in agriculture and industry. A side effect of a number of these advances is the introduction of chemicals resulting from agricultural and industrial practices to the soil and water ecosystems and the resulting impact of these chemicals on organisms residing there. The effects of chemical pollution are threefold (Woodwell, 1970; Stickel, 1974): (1) a tendency toward simplification of communities through the elimination of more sensitive species and their replacement by larger populations of tolerant species, (2) the change in species relationships within communities, whereby the species that earlier might have enjoyed only a minor niche dominated by other species are allowed to expand into a dominant role in the ecosystem by the disappearance of the control species, and (3) alterations in nutrient cycles, which may have a long-lasting effect on the basic composition of the ecosystem. Alteration of nutrient cycles may lead in turn to permanent changes in an ecosystem through erosion and leaching, which in turn change the basic physical structure.

Effects of pollutants are seen primarily at the tops of food chains and are observed usually as changes in population levels of predator species. The chlorinated hydrocarbon pesticides and industrial chemicals, for example, may cause reproductive difficulties in birds, such as the peregrine falcon. Mink are highly sensitive to methylmercury, while apparently other mammals are not so sensitive. Contamination with methylmercury can thus alter the diversity and dominance characteristics of the ecosystem.

Disturbances in the ecosystem can be detected in nutrient cycling even though no effects are measured in the diversity or population of the community. Several studies have now shown that changes in nutrients, such as nitrates, are more sensitive than biologic parameters to chemical stress (O'Neill *et al.*, 1977; Jackson *et al.*, 1977). This results from the fact that changes in nutrient pools must eventually directly affect the productivity of the entire ecosystem, even though the effects may not be measurable in biologic terms until a number of years later.

The net effect of decreased diversity in an ecosystem is a more unstable system. Such communities are subject to wide fluctuations in populations of organisms and are more easily influenced by outside pressures such as chemical pollutants. This leads in turn to the necessity for man's further intervention in an attempt to stabilize the system, a process that historically has sometimes been self-defeating.

The effect of the reduction in species diversity in the ecosystem on man is yet to be understood. Changes in the dominance characteristics of ecosystems will have a major effect on man's activities as they cause him to change strategies of pest control, alter his use of water systems, and change his perceptions of the aesthetic quality of the environment. Changes in nutrient cycling lead to the expenditure of resources to correct resulting imbalances. As man changes the agricultural ecosystem to his advantage it is necessary to add nutrients in the form of phosphate and nitrate fertilizers, frequently leading to additional imbalances in managing the contamination of water systems.

To understand the effect of chemicals on organisms other than man, one must study the responses of those organisms in their own environments. Considerable effort is now being directed toward such studies (Cairns et al., 1978; Eaton et al., 1980; Maki et al., 1980; Branson and Dickson, 1981; Dickson et al., 1982). The effect of chemicals on man is known in many instances only indirectly through laboratory experimentation with test organisms, such as laboratory animals, at high doses. The same chemicals in the environment will not necessarily affect man in the same direct ways since they are always found in the presence of other chemicals with which they may interact. Furthermore, the mobility, transport, availability, disposition, and toxicologic effect of a chemical in the environment must be considered in assessing its interactions with biologic systems.

REFERENCES

Acree, F., Jr.; Beroza, M.; and Bowman, M. C.: Codistillation of DDT with water. *J. Agric. Food Chem.*, 11:278–80, 1963.

American Geological Institute. Gary, M.; McAfee, R., Jr.; and Wolf, C. L. (eds.): *Glossary of Geology*. The Institute, Washington, D.C., 1972.

Bailey, G. W., and White, J. L.: Factors influencing the adsorption, desorption and movement of pesticides in soil. *Residue Rev.*, 32:29–92, 1970.

Bitman, J.; Cecil, H. C.; and Harris, S. J.: Biological effects of polychlorinated biphenyls in rats and quail. *Environ. Health Perspect.*, 1:145–49, 1972.

Blus, J. J.: Further interpretation of the relation of organochlorine residues in brown pelican eggs to reproductive success. *Environ. Pollut.*, 28A:15–33, 1982.

Bowman, B. T.; Adams, R. S., Jr.; and Fenton, S. W.: Effect of water on malathion adsorption onto five montmorillonite systems. *J. Agric. Food Chem.*, 18:723–27, 1970.

Braman, R. S., and Foreback, C. C.: Methylated forms of arsenic in the environment. *Science*, 182:1247–49, 1973.

Branson, D. R., and Dickson, K. L. (eds.): *Aquatic Toxicology and Hazard Assessment*. Special Technical Publication 737, American Society for Testing and Materials, Philadelphia, 1981.

Brass, H. J.; Feige, M. A.; Halloran, T.; Mello, J. W.; Munch, D.; and Thomas, R. F.: The national organic monitoring survey: samplings and analyses for purgeable organic compounds. In Pojasek, R. B., (ed.): *Drinking Water Quality Through Source Protection*. Ann Arbor Science Publishers, Ann Arbor, Mich., 1977, pp. 393–416.

Brooks, G. T.: *Chlorinated Insecticides*, Vols. I and II. CRC Press, Cleveland, 1974.

Bro-Rasmussen, F.; Noddegaard, E.; and Voldum-Clausen, K.: Degradation of diazinon in soil. *J. Sci. Food Agric.*, 19:278–81, 1968.

Buhler, D. R.; Rasmusson M. E.; and Nakaue, H. S.: Occurrence of hexachlorophene and pentachlorophenol in sewage and water. *Environ. Sci. Technol.*, 7:929–34, 1973.

Cairns, J., Jr.; Dickson, K. L.; and Maki, A. W. (eds.): *Estimating the Hazard of Chemical Substances to Aquatic Life*. Special Technical Publication 657, American Society for Testing and Materials, Philadelphia, 1978.

Cantor, K. P.: Epidemiological evidence of carcinogenicity of chlorinated organics in drinking water: *Environ. Health Perspect.*, 46:187–95, 1982.

Casida, J. E.: Pyrethrum flowers and pyrethroid insecticides. *Environ. Health Perspect.*, 34:189–202, 1980.

Chau, Y. K.; Wong, P. T. S.; Silverberg, B. A.; Luxon, P. L.; and Bengert, G. A.: Methylation of selenium in the aquatic environment. *Science*, 192:1130–31, 1976.

Choi, I., and Smith, R. W.: Kinetic study of dissolution of asbestos fibers in water. *J. Colloid Interface Sci.*, 40:253–62, 1971.

Condie, L. W.: Review of published studies of orally administered asbestos. *Environ. Health Perspect.*, 53:3–9, 1983.

Conference on Phthalates: Discussion and summary remarks. *Environ. Health Perspect.*, 45:149–53, 1982.

Conforti, P. M.; Kanarek, M. S.; Jackson, L. A.; Cooper, R. C.; and Murchio, J. C.: Asbestos in drinking water and cancer in the San Francisco Bay area, California, USA. *J. Chronic Dis.*, 34:211–24, 1981.

Cornell University, Institute for Comparative and Environmental Toxicology: A toxicological evaluation of aldicarb and its metabolites in relation to the potential human health impact of aldicarb residues in Long Island ground water. January 1983.

Craighead, J. E., and Mossman, B. T.: The pathogenesis of asbestos-associated diseases. *N. Engl. J. Med.*, 306:1446–55, 1982.

Crump, K. S., and Guess, H. A.: Drinking water and cancer: review of recent findings and assessment of risks. Prepared for the Council on Environmental Quality, Washington, D.C., 1980.

Cunningham, H. M., and Pontefract, R.: Asbestos fibers in beverages and drinking water. *Nature*, 232:332–33, 1971.

Dickson, K. L.; Maki, A. W.; and Cairns, J., Jr.: *Modeling the Fate of Chemicals in the Aquatic Environment*. Ann Arbor Science, Ann Arbor, Mich., 1982.

Dowty, B.; Carlisle, D.; and Laseter, J. L.: Halogenated hydrocarbons in New Orleans water and blood plasma. *Science*, 187:75–77, 1975.

Duff, W. G., and Menzer, R. E.: Persistence, mobility, and degradation of ^{14}C-dimethoate in soils. *Environ. Entomol.*, 2:309–18, 1973.

Eaton, J. G.; Parrish, P. R.; and Hendricks, A. C. (eds.): *Aquatic Toxicology*. Special Technical Publication 707, American Society for Testing and Materials, Philadelphia, 1980.

Edwards, C. A.: Insecticide residues in soils. *Residue Rev.*, 13:83–132, 1966.

———: *Persistent Pesticides in the Environment.* CRC Press, Cleveland, 1970.

Elliot, M.: Synthetic Pyrethroids. In Elliot, M. (ed.): *Synthetic Pyrethroids.* Symposium Series 42, American Chemical Society, Washington, D.C., 1977, pp. 1–28.

Environmental Protection Agency: *Disposal of Hazardous Wastes: Report to Congress.* Publication SW-115, Washington, D.C., 1974.

———: *Preliminary Assessment of Suspected Carcinogens in Drinking Water: Report to Congress.* Washington, D.C., 1975.

———: *Research Summary: Controlling Hazardous Wastes.* Publication EPA-600/8-80-017, Washington, D.C., 1980.

Eto, M.: *Organophosphorus Pesticides: Organic and Biological Chemistry.* CRC Press, Cleveland, 1974.

Fitzgerald, L. D.: Arsenic sources, production and application in the 1980's. In Lederer, W. H., and Fensterheim, R. J. (eds.): *Arsenic—Industrial, Biomedical, Environmental Perspectives.* Van Nostrand Reinhold, New York, 1983, pp. 3–9.

Fleischer, M.; Sarofim, A. F.; Fasset, D. W.; Hammond, P.; Shacklette, H. T.; Nisbet, I. C. T.; and Epstein, S.: Environmental impact of cadmium: a review by the panel on hazardous trace substances. *Environ. Health Perspect.,* 7:253–323, 1974.

Forney, D. R., and Davis, D. E.: Effects of low concentrations of herbicides on submersed aquatic plants. *Weed Sci.,* 29:677–85, 1981.

Garretson, A. L., and San Clemente, C. L.: Inhibition of nitrifying chemolithotrophic bacteria by several insecticides. *J. Econ. Entomol.,* 61:285–88, 1968.

Getzin, L. W.: Persistence of diazinon and zinophos in soil: effects of autoclaving, temperature, moisture, and acidity. *J. Econ. Entomol.,* 61:1560–65, 1968.

Getzin, L. W., and Rosefield, I.: Organophosphorus insecticide degradation by heat-labile substances in soil. *J. Agric Food Chem.,* 16:598–601, 1968.

Giam, C. S.; Chan, H. S.; Neff, G. S.; and Atlas, E. L.: Phthalate ester plasticizers: a new class of marine pollutant. *Science,* 199:419–21, 1978.

Goring, C. A. I.: Physical aspects of soil in relation to the action of soil fungicides. *Ann. Rev. Phytopathol.,* 5:285–318, 1967.

Gottlieb, M. S., and Carr, J. K.: Case-control cancer mortality study and chlorination of drinking water in Louisiana. *Environ. Health Perspect.,* 46:169–77, 1982.

Gunner, H. B.: Microbial ecosystem stress induced by an organophosphate insecticide. *Mededelingen Faculteit Landbouwwetenschappen Gent,* 35:581–97, 1970.

Gunner, H. B.; Zuckerman, B. M.; Walker, R. W.; Miller, C. W.; Deubert, K. H.; and Longley, R. E.: The distribution and persistence of diazinon applied to plant and soil and its influence on rhizosphere and soil microflora. *Plant Soil,* 25:249–64, 1966.

Gunther, F. A. (ed.): The triazine herbicides. *Residue Rev.,* 32:1–413, 1970.

Gunther, F. A.; Westlake, W. E.; and Jaglan, P. S.: Reported solubilities of 738 pesticide chemicals in water. *Residue Rev.,* 20:1–148, 1968.

Hamaker, J. W., and Thompson, J. M.: Adsorption. In Goring, C. A. I., and Hamaker, J. W. (eds.): *Organic Chemicals in the Soil Environment,* Vol. 1. Marcel Dekker, Inc., New York, 1972, pp. 49–143.

Hance, R. J.; Byast, T. H.; and Smith, P. D.: Apparent decomposition of paraquat in soil. *Soil Biol. Biochem.,* 12:447–48, 1980.

Harris, C. R.: Influence of soil moisture on the toxicity of insecticides in a mineral soil to insects. *J. Econ. Entomol.,* 57:946–50, 1964.

———: Laboratory studies on the persistence of biological activity of some insecticides in soils. *J. Econ. Entomol.,* 62:1437–41, 1969.

Hilding, A. C.; Hilding, D. A.; Larson, D. M.; and Aufderheide, A. C.: Biological effects of ingested amosite asbestos, taconite tailings, diatomaceous earth and Lake Superior water in rats. *Arch. Environ. Health,* 36:298–303, 1981.

Hills, J. P.: Asbestos in public water supplies: discussion of future problems. *Ann. N.Y. Acad. Sci.,* 330:573–78, 1979.

Hites, R. A.: Phthalates in the Charles and the Merrimack Rivers. *Environ. Health Perspect.,* 3:17–21, 1973.

Jackson, D. R.; Washburne, C. D.; and Asmus, B. S.: Loss of Ca and NO_3-N from terrestrial microcosms as an indicator of soil pollution. *Water, Air, Soil Pollut.,* 8:279–84, 1977.

Jensen, S., and Jernelov, A.: Biologic methylation of mercury in aquatic organisms. *Nature,* 223:753–54, 1969.

Johnson, J. D.; Christman, R. F.; Norwood, D. L.; and Millington, D. S.: Reaction products of aquatic humic substances with chlorine. *Environ. Health Perspect.,* 46:63–71, 1982.

Kanarek, M. S.: The San Francisco Bay epidemiology studies on asbestos in drinking water and cancer incidence: relationship to studies in other locations and pointers for further research. *Environ. Health Perspect.,* 53:105–106, 1983.

Kanarek, M. S.; Conforti, P. M.; Jackson, L. A.; Cooper, R. C.; and Murchio, J. C.: Asbestos in drinking water and cancer incidence in the San Francisco Bay area. *Am. J. Epidemiol.,* 112:54–72, 1980.

Kanarek, M. S., and Young, T. B.: Drinking water treatment and risk of cancer death in Wisconsin. *Environ. Health Perspect.,* 46:179–86, 1982.

Kay, G.: Ontario intensifies search for asbestos in drinking water. *J. Water Pollut. Control Fed.,* 3:33–35, 1973.

Kearney, P. C.; Nash, R. G.; and Isensee, A. R.: Persistence of pesticide residues in soils. In Miller, M. W., and Berg, G. G. (eds.): *Chemical Fallout.* Charles C Thomas, Pub., Springfield, Ill., 1969, pp. 54–67.

Kluwe, W. M.; Haseman, J. K.; Douglas, J. F.; and Huff, J. E.: The carcinogenicity of dietary di(2-ethylhexyl) phthalate (DEHP) in Fischer 344 rats and B6C3Fl mice. *J. Toxicol. Environ. Health,* 10:797–815, 1982a.

Kluwe, W. M.; McConnell, E. E.; Huff, J. E.; Haseman, J. K.; Douglas, J. F.; and Hartwell, W. V.: Carcinogenicity testing of phthalate esters and related compounds by the National Toxicology Program and the National Cancer Institute. *Environ. Health Perspect.,* 45:129–33, 1982b.

Kluwe, W. M.; Haseman, J. K.; and Huff, J. E.: The carcinogenicity of di(2-ethylhexyl) phthalate (DEHP) in perspective. *J. Toxicol. Environ. Health,* 12:159–69, 1983.

Kononova, M. M.: *Soil Organic Matter.* Pergamon Press, New York, 1966.

Kuhr, R. J., and Dorough, H. W.: *Carbamate Insecticides: Chemistry, Biochemistry, and Toxicology.* CRC Press, Cleveland, 1976.

Langer, A. M.: Approaches and constraints to identification and quantitation of asbestos fibers. *Environ. Health Perspect.,* 9:133–36, 1974.

Langer, A. M.; Mackler, A. D.; and Pooley, F. D.: Electron microscopical investigation of asbestos fibers. *Environ. Health Perspect.* 9:63–80, 1974.

Leenheer, J. A., and Ahlrichs, J. L.: A kinetic and equilibrium study of the adsorption of carbaryl and parathion upon soil organic matter surfaces. *Soil Sci. Soc. Am. Proc.,* 35:700, 1971.

Lichtenstein, E. P., and Schulz, K. R.: Epoxidation of aldrin and heptachlor in soils as influenced by autoclaving, moisture, and soil types. *J. Econ. Entomol.,* 53:192–97, 1960.

Lichtenstein, E. P.; Fuhreman, T. W.; and Schulz,

K. R.: Effect of sterilizing agents on persistence of parathion and diazinon in soils and water. *J. Agric. Food Chem.*, 16:870–73, 1968.

Maki, A. W.; Dickson, K. L.; and Cairns, J., Jr. (eds.): *Biotransformation and Fate of Chemicals in the Aquatic Environment.* American Society for Microbiology, Washington, D.C., 1980.

Marquis, L. Y.; Comes, R. D.; and Yang, C. P.: Absorption and translocation of fluridone and glyphosate in submersed vascular plants. *Weed Sci.*, 29:229–36, 1981.

Masser, J. L.; Fisher, N. S.; Teng, T.-C.; and Wurster, C. F.: Polychlorinated biphenyls: toxicity to certain phytoplankters. *Science*, 175:191–92, 1972.

Maugh, T. H.: Just how hazardous are dumps? *Science*, 215:490–93, 1982a.

——: Biological markers for chemical exposure. *Science*, 215:643–47, 1982b.

May, T. C., and Lewis, R. W.: Asbestos. In *Mineral Facts and Problems. U.S. Bureau of Mines Bull.*, 650:851–65, 1970.

Mayer, F. L., and Sanders, H. O.: Toxicology of phthalic acid esters in aquatic organisms. *Environ. Health Perspect.*, 3:153–57, 1973.

McCall, P. J.; Laskowski, D. A.; Swann, R. L.; and Dishburger, H. J.: Estimation of environmental partitioning of organic chemicals in model ecosystems. *Residue Rev.*, 85:231–44, 1983.

Menzer, R. E.; Iqbal, Z. M.; and Boyd, G. R.: Metabolism of *O*-ethyl *S,S*-dipropyl phosphorodithioate (Mocap) in bean and corn plants. *J. Agric. Food Chem.*, 19:351–56, 1971.

Miller, I. J.: Fluorides and dental fluorosis. *Int. Dent. J.*, 32:135–47, 1982.

Millette, J. R.; Clark, P. J.; Pansing, M. F.; and Twyman, J. D.: Concentration and size of asbestos in water supplies. *Environ. Health Perspect.*, 34:1325, 1980.

Millette, J. R.; Clark, P. J.; Stober, J.; and Rosenthal, M.: Asbestos in water supplies of the United States. *Environ. Health Perspect.*, 53:45–48, 1983.

Morris, R. J.: Phthalic acid in the deep sea jellyfish *Atolla. Nature*, 227:1264, 1970.

Mortland, M. M., and Raman, K. V.: Catalytic hydrolysis of some organic phosphate pesticides by copper (II). *J. Agric. Food Chem.*, 15:163–67, 1967.

Mueller, M. M.; Rosenberg, C; Siltanen, H.; and Wartiovaara, T.: Fate of glyphosate and its nitrogen-cycling in two Finnish agriculture soils. *Bull. Environ. Contam. Toxicol.*, 27:724–30, 1981.

Mühlmann, R., and Schrader, G.: Hydrolyse der insektiziden Phosphorsaureester. *Z. Naturforsch.*, 12b:196–208, 1957.

Munson, A. E.; Sain, L. E.; Sanders, V. M.; Kauffmann, B. M.; White, K. L., Jr.; Page, D. G.; Barnes, D. W.; and Borzelleca, J. F.: Toxicology of organic drinking water contaminants: trichloromethane, bromodichloromethane, dibromochloromethane, and tribromomethane. *Environ. Health Perspect.*, 46:117–26, 1982.

Musial, C. J.; Uthe, J. F.; Sirota, G. R.; Burns, B. G.; Gilgan, M. W.; Zitko, V.; and Matheson, R. A.: Di-*n*-hexyl phthalate, a newly identified contaminant in Atlantic herring (*Clupea harengus harengus*) and Atlantic mackerel (*Scomber scombrus*). *Can J. Fish Aquat. Sci.*, 38:856–59, 1981.

National Academy of Sciences: *Lead: Airborne Lead in Perspective.* National Academy of Sciences, Washington, D.C., 1972.

——: *The Health Effects of Nitrate, Nitrite, and N-Nitroso Compounds.* National Academy Press, Washington, D.C.; 1981.

National Research Council: *Drinking Water and Health.* National Academy of Sciences, Washington, D.C. Vol. 1, 1977; Vol. 2, 1980; Vol. 3, 1980; Vol. 4, 1982; Vol. 5, 1983.

Neely, N.; Gillespie, D.; Schauf, F.; and Walsh, J.: Remedial actions at hazardous waste sites, survey and case studies. Report 430/9-81-05, Environmental Protection Agency, Washington, D.C., 1981.

Nicholson, W. J.: Analysis of amphibole asbestiform fibers in municipal water supplies. *Environ. Health Perspect.*, 9:165–72, 1974.

Nogawa, K.; Konoi, S.; and Kato T.: Toxicity of cadmium. III-2. Occurrence of the itai-itai disease in relation to cadmium contamination in rice. *Kenkyo Hoken Repoto*, 48:149–51, 1982.

Nogawa, K.; Kawano, S.; Kato, T.; and Sakamoto, M.: The prevalence of itai-itai disease and the mean cadmium concentration in rice produced by individual villages. *Nippon Eiseigaku Zasshi*, 37:843–47, 1983.

Ogner, G., and Schnitzer, M.: Humic substances: Fulvic acid-dialkyl phthalate complexes and their role in pollution. *Science*, 170:317–18, 1970.

O'Neill, R. V.; Ausmus, B. S.; Jackson, D. R.; Van Hook, R. I.; Van Voris, P.; Washburne, C.; and Watson, A. P.: Monitoring terrestrial ecosystems by analysis of nutrient export. *Water, Air, Soil Pollut.*, 8:271–77, 1977.

Page, T.; Harris, R. H.; and Epstein, S. S.: Drinking water and cancer mortality in Louisiana. *Science*, 193:55–57, 1976.

Parks, G. A.: Aqueous surface chemistry of oxides and complex oxide minerals. In Stumm, W. (ed.): *Equilibrium Concepts in Natural Water Systems.* Adv. Chem. No. 67, American Chemical Society, Washington, D.C., 1967, pp. 121–60.

Polissar, L.; Severson, R. K.; Boatman, E. S.; and Thomas, D. B.: Cancer incidence in relation to asbestos in drinking water in the Puget Sound region (Washington, USA). *Am. J. Epidemiol.*, 116:314–28, 1982.

Polissar, L.; Severson, R. K.; and Boatman, E. S.: Cancer risk from asbestos in drinking water: summary of a case-control study in western Washington. *Environ. Health Perspect.*, 53:57–60, 1983.

——: Case-control study of asbestos in drinking water and cancer risk. *Am. J. Epidemiol.* 119:456–71, 1984.

Rabinowitz, M., and Needleman, H. L.: Petrol lead sales and umbilical cord blood lead levels in Boston, Massachusetts. *Lancet*, 1:Iss. 8314–15, 63, 1983.

Rendall, R. E. G.: The data sheets on the chemical and physical properties of the UICC standard reference samples. In Shapiro, H. A. (ed.): *Pneumoconiosis.* Oxford University Press, London, 1970.

Ridley, W. P.; Dizikes, L. J.; and Wood, J. M.: Biomethylation of toxic elements in the environment. *Science*, 197:329–32, 1977.

Rosato, D. V.: *Asbestos, Its Industrial Applications.* Reinhold, New York, 1959, p. 214.

Rubin, R. J., and Jaeger, R. J.: Some pharmacologic and toxicologic effects of di-2-ethylhexyl phthalate (DEHP) and other plasticizers. *Environ. Health Perspect.*, 3:53–59, 1973.

Saltzman, S., and Yaron, B.: Parathion adsorption from aqueous solutions as influenced by soil components. In Tahori, A. S. (ed.): *Pesticide Chemistry.* Vol. VI, *Proc. 2nd Intern. IUPAC Congr.* Gordon & Breach, London, 1972, pp. 87–100.

Schnell, R. C.; and Angle, C. R.: Selenium—toxin or panacea. *Fundam. Appl. Toxicol.*, 3:409–10, 1983.

Selikoff, I. J.; Nicholson, W. J.; and Langer, A. M.: Asbestos air pollution. *Arch. Environ. Health*, 25:1, 1972.

Seydel, I. S.: Distribution and circulation of arsenic through water, organisms and sediments of Lake Michigan. *Arch. Hydrobiol.*, 71:17–30, 1972.

Siegel, M. R., and Sisler, H. D.: *Antifungal Compounds*, 2 Vols. Marcel Dekker, Inc. New York, 1977.

Sigurdson, E. R.; Levy, B. S.; Mandel, J.; McHugh, R.; Michienzi, L. J.; Jagger, H.; and Pearson, J.: Cancer morbidity investigations: lessons from the Duluth study of possible effects of asbestos in drinking water. *Environ. Res.*, **25**:50–61, 1981.

Sims, J. L., and Pfaender, F. K.: Distribution and biomagnification of hexachlorophene in urban drainage areas. *Bull. Environ. Contam. Toxicol.*, **14**:214–20, 1975.

Smith, W. E.; Hubert, D. D.; Sobel, H. J.; Peters, E. T.; and Doerfler, T. E.: Health of experimental animals drinking water with and without amosite asbestos and other mineral particles. *J. Environ. Pathol. Toxicol.*, **3**:277–300, 1980.

Sommer, K.: Effect of various pesticides on nitrification and nitrogen transformation in soils. *Landwirtsch. Forsch. Sonderh.*, **25**:22–30, 1970.

Stewart, B. A.; Woolhiser, D. A.; Wischmeier, W. H.; Caro, J. H.; and Frere, M. H.: *Control of Water Pollution from Cropland*. USDA/EPA, Report No. ARS-H-5-1/EPA-600/2-75-026a, Washington, D.C., 1975.

Stickel, W. H.: Some effects of pollutants in terrestrial ecosystems. In McIntyre, A. D., and Mills, C. F. (eds.): *Ecological Toxicology Research: Effects of Heavy Metal and Organohalogen Compounds*. Plenum Press, New York, 1975, pp. 25–74.

Stojanovic, B. J.; Kennedy, M. V.; and Shuman, F. L., Jr.: Edaphic aspects of the disposal of unused pesticides, pesticide wastes, and pesticide containers. *J. Environ. Qual.*, **1**:54, 1972.

Swann, R. L.; Laskowski, D. A.; McCall, P. J.; Vander Kuy, K.; and Dishburger, H. J.: A rapid method for the estimation of the environmental parameters octanol/water partition coefficient, soil sorption constant, water to air ratio, and water solubility. *Residue Rev.*, **85**:17–28, 1983.

Symons, J. M.; Bellar, T. A.; Carswell, J. K.; Demarco, J.; Kropp, K. L.; Robeck, G. C.; Seeger, D. R.; Slocum, C. J.; Smith, B. L.; and Stevens, A. A.: National organic reconnaissance survey for halogenated organics. *J. Am. Water Works Assoc.*, **67**:634–47, 1975.

Taylor, A. W., and Kilmer, V. J.: Agricultural phosphorus in the environment. In Khasawneh, F. E.; Sample, E. C.; and Kanparth, E. J. (eds.): *The Role of Phosphorous in Agriculture*. American Society of Agronomy, Madison, Wisc., 1980, pp. 545–57.

Thibodeaux, L. J.: *Chemodynamics, Environmental Movement of Chemicals in Air, Water and Soil*. John Wiley & Sons, Inc., New York, 1979.

Thomas, E. A.: Phosphorus and eutrophication. In Griffith, E. J.; Beeton, A.; Spencer, J. M.; and Mitchell, D. T. (eds.): *Environmental Phosphorus Handbook*. John Wiley & Sons, New York, 1973, pp. 585–611.

Vos, J. G.: Toxicology of PCBs for mammals and for birds. *Environ. Health Perspect.* **1**:105–17, 1972.

Weber, J. B.: Interaction of organic pesticides with particulate matter in aquatic and soil systems. In Gold, R. F. (ed.): *Fate of Organic Pesticides in the Aquatic Environment*. American Chemical Society, Washington, D.C., 1972, pp. 55–120.

Wilbourn, J., and Montesano, R.: An overview of phthalate ester carcinogenicity testing results: the past. *Environ. Health Perspect.*, **45**:127–28, 1982.

Wong, P. T. S.; Chau, Y. K.; and Luxon, P. L.: Methylation of lead in the environment. *Nature*, **253**:263–64, 1975.

Woodwell, G. M.: Effects of pollution on the structure and physiology of ecosystems. *Science*, **168**:429–33, 1970.

Woolson, E. A.: Fate of arsenicals in different environmental substrates. *Environ. Health Perspect.*, **19**:73–81, 1977.

———: Man's pertubation of the arsenic cycle. In Lederer, W. H., and Fensterheim, R. J. (eds.): *Arsenic—Industrial, Biomedical, Environmental Perspectives*. Van Nostrand Reinhold, New York, 1983, pp. 393–408.

Wu, T. L.: Atrazine in estuarine water and the aerial deposition of atrazine into Rhode River, Maryland. *Water, Air, Soil Pollut.*, **15**:173–84, 1981.

UNIT V
APPLICATIONS OF TOXICOLOGY

Chapter 27

ANALYTIC TOXICOLOGY

Irving Sunshine

INTRODUCTION

The analytic toxicologist's potential to resolve questions related to poisoning episodes is a function of his prowess in analytic chemistry. His ability to use the cutting edge of modern instrumental analysis enables him to detect the very small concentrations of the many varied chemical substances that are today's hazards. Granted ability and the requisite expensive instrumentation, all of which will be discussed later, the results he evolves require interpretation (McCarron, 1983a). Therein lies the crux of all his dilligence and competence. From the finite analytic results he produces comes the presumption that they portend dire consequences. Dioxin, pentachlorophenol, lead, mercury—the list is extensive. As one substance fades into oblivion another appears, just as day follows night. Consequently, the analytic toxicologist is beholden to complement his analytic skill with a solid background in toxicology such that he can make a proper evaluation of the analytic results.

Space limitations being what they are for this treatise, only four aspects of analytic toxicology will be presented in some detail. These concern acute poisoning, therapeutic drug monitoring, drugs subject to abuse, and forensic toxicology and are similar in that they utilize similar analytic techniques. They differ in their analysis time requirements, the quanta and type of proof needed, and the type of available specimens. The first three usually deal with living people (clinical toxicology) whereas the fourth deals primarily but not exclusively with postmortem material (forensic toxicology).

ACUTE POISONING

Clinical toxicology has two major divisions, based on the identity of the analyte in question. When it is unknown (acute poisonings, preemployment testing, parole violation, rehabilitation programs), the challenge is both qualitative and quantitative. On the other hand, if the question is "What is the plasma concentration of ———?" (therapeutic drug monitoring), a quantitative analysis of a known analyte is required. In this instance straightforward available quantitative procedures can be utilized because the analyte is identifiable. In contrast, the quest for drugs involved in acute poisonings provides a greater challenge to the analyst because the scope of the required effort must include many analytes. There are so many potentially toxic substances that no one can provide a comprehensive result encompassing them all. Hence, a decision of what should be included is needed, requiring extensive introspection. Two key words are "diagnostic" (Is my patient poisoned?) and "prognostic" (When will my patient recover?). Answers to the first question need to be rapid and simple, whereas the second requires time, equipment, and technical and scientific expertise.

Diagnostic needs are usually served by providing reliable data that indicate exogeneous chemical substances are or are not present. Simple positive or negative results suffice, bearing in mind that "negative" translates into "not detectable by the methods used or not present in concentrations consistent with toxic symptoms" (McCarron, 1983b). These data are best accumulated by analyzing the patient's urine. Positive urine results should then be followed with quantitative analyses of the patient's blood. This has prognostic value, if all the active agents are identified and quantified. This task is not simple and requires significant effort from well-qualified personnel.

Many argue that the toxicology laboratory contributes little to the care of poisoned patients because (1) therapy must be initiated immediately, (2) the laboratory data do not influence therapy, and (3) the laboratory data are usually misleading and unreliable (Hepler *et al.*, 1982). Surely no one can disagree that poisoned patients must be treated promptly, but therapy is usually supportive. For only a relatively few substances is specific therapy available. Triage of poisoned patients is improved significantly by prompt reliable reporting of toxicologic findings. Although a poisoned patient's therapy may be minimally affected by a positive laboratory report, since only a few drugs have true antidotes (Thompson, 1980), such a positive result may obviate other and expensive diagnostic tests. On the other hand, a "negative" report suggests that other diagnoses must be considered to ensure proper patient care or that another analyte, not included in the routine testing, may be present.

Reports indicating that laboratory data are unreliable present nothing novel about laboratory performance in laboratory medicine. There will always be some laboratories that cannot perform well. It is the responsibility of the user to ensure that the laboratory he chooses can and will provide him with the quality data he requires for his purposes (Ingelfinger, *et al.*, 1981). Eternal vigilance is essential. Users should periodically submit to the laboratory they use specimens of known analyte content and check the reliability of the reported results.

Role of the Clinician

A clinician must initiate the toxicologist's role. A major problem both face is one of communication (Bailey, 1983). With the recognition that mutual supportive activities are essential comes the necessary initial interchanges that ensure reliable, prompt laboratory service. The limitations of the laboratory, the scope of its activities, the timing of its reports, the substances to be encompassed—all these topics need detailed discussions by involved clinicians, laboratory personnel, and administrators before any toxicology program is started. This group must reach a consensus on which tests the toxicologist should be expected to perform (Walberg, 1983a). This decision must be based on the anticipated needs of the physician and the qualifications of the toxicology staff, equipment, and expertise (Walberg, 1983a), and must be cost effective (Lundberg, 1983). Once a decision on the extent of the program is made, additional tests can be envisioned but should be implemented only if, again, a consensus of the interested parties is obtained.

Having agreed on a given toxicology protocol, all clinicians who are expected to use it must be made aware of its scope and their related responsibilities. Of those unit operations involved in toxicologic analysis (Table 27–1) the physician has responsibility for the first four. All these must be completed before any laboratory analysis can start. Samples must be obtained. It is not sufficient to order that this be done; it is essential, particularly for a stat request, that the clinicians see to it that his orders have been executed effectively. A request slip should accompany the properly labeled specimens (10 ml of unclotted blood, 25 to 50 ml of urine, any gastric aspirate or vomitus obtained). This request should identify the patient, what medications the patient had been self-administering or had been given therapeutically, when this occurred, when was the patient last conscious, and a simple statement of the patient's major presenting symptoms. Obviously, the laboratory cannot function until these labeled specimens are received. Resolving this transportation problem should be another of the attending physician's responsibilities. After the necessary specimens have been sent to the laboratory, it is desirable that the physician phone the toxicologist to discuss the patient's problem(s). This helps focus the analytic procedure so that those analytes suspected to be involved receive precedence. However, despite the history or the symptoms, the entire previously discussed comprehensive analytic program should be undertaken. Polypharmacology prevails, and many poisonings involve more than one substance. In a study of the incidence of acute poisonings (Bailey and Manoguerra, 1980), 25 percent of the patients used an unsuspected drug, and in 16 percent another drug, other than the suspected one, was found. This is only one of the many studies that indicate the desirability of a broad testing program when a poisoning is suspected.

Once the laboratory receives the specimens, the actual analysis must be performed in real time. Many procedures are available (Sunshine, 1981; Baselt, 1983). Which should be used will have been determined by the established protocol. All the results obtained should be reported promptly to the attending physician. The result-

---

Table 27–1.   UNIT OPERATIONS INVOLVED IN TOXICOLOGIC ANALYSES

1. Ordering test	5. Separation of analytes	7. Timely reporting to clinician
2. Collection of adequate specimens	6. Analysis of the isolated analytes	8. Evaluation of data in terms of a patient
3. Identification of patient and problem		9. Action ensuring patient care
4. Transportation of specimens to laboratory		

ing discussion should elaborate whether or not the laboratory results contribute to a reasonable explanation of the patient's illness. Should they not, the clinician must consider other alternative diagnoses. If necessary, one alternative could be a repeat analysis. The probability of laboratory error, however small, always exists and, depending on the circumstances, discrepant results should be checked by a repeat analysis of another specimen. It should be apparent to all concerned that the toxicologic protocol does not include a comprehensive analysis. If the history or symptoms suggest a substance not in the usual scheme, consideration should be given to the use of a reliable reference laboratory or to whether the toxicology laboratory can and should encompass the unusual substance. Only a frank discussion of the laboratory report will serve the patient's best interests.

Another obligation the physician assumes is to inform the laboratory promptly if the need for a "stat" analysis has been obviated. If another diagnosis was established or, as sometimes happens, the patient is discharged or "signs himself out," then the laboratory should be informed so that their emergency measures can be moderated.

Previous discussion related to establishing a set of analytes that will satisfy most clinician's requests and are within the scope of the laboratory's facilities. Many previous studies (Bailey and Guba, 1979; National Institute on Drug Abuse, 1981) of the incidence of toxic substances in acute poisonings have indicated that 80 to 90 percent of all poisonings involve about 20 analytes (Table 27–2A, Table 27–2B). The number of analytes that occasionally contribute to a poisoning that are not included in these tables is legion, and their detection and quantitation are beyond the scope of all but the most comprehensive reference laboratories. Fishing in these uncharted waters is only productive

when done by experienced, skilled analysts possessing the most modern equipment. Hence, the stress on a limited "menu" that is within the capability of the local group.

Many roads lead to Rome. Roaming through the literature one uncovers many different procedures for a given analyte. Each professes to be optimal. Well it may be in the hands of its originator. In a given situation the described equipment, technical expertise, time requirements, frequency, as well as many other factors, will dictate which procedures are most compatible with a laboratory's facilities. Using compilations (Sunshine, 1981; Baselt, 1983) that present various recipes may simplify the search for a suitable procedure. The literature abounds with many more. Achieving a successful result requires that any described procedure be followed explicitly. Modifications and revisions should be contemplated only after the original has been successfully used and found wanting. Those who modify a published procedure first and decry its results do not do the progenitor justice.

THERAPEUTIC DRUG MONITORING

Therapeutic drug monitoring (TDM) was given first impetus by neurologists (Krall *et al.*, 1978). Faced with the dilemma of selecting which of the many antiepileptic agents would best benefit their patients, they sought laboratory support. Chemists met these challenges with gas chromatographic procedures that could simultaneously quantitate most of the then commonly used antiepileptic drugs and their metabolites (Pesh-Iman *et al.*, 1979). The neurologists explored the relationship between the resulting blood drug concentrations and their patients' clinical conditions. In many instances reasonable correlations were developed when proficient analysts collaborated with alert clinicians (Pippenger *et al.*, 1978). Not infrequently seem-

Table 27–2A.   FREQUENTLY FOUND DRUGS (1982) LISTED IN ORDER OF DECREASING FREQUENCY

	CORONER'S LAB		
POLICE LAB	*All Cases*	*Poisonings*	REFERENCE LAB
Cannabis	Ethanol	Benzodiazepines	Benzodiazepines
Triplennamine	Benzodiazepines	Carbon monoxide	Ethanol
Pentazocine (Talwin)	Lidocaine	Ethanol	Barbiturates
Cocaine	Acetaminophen	Tricyclic antidepressants	Acetaminophen
Benzodiazepines	Salicylate	Opiates	Salicylate
Phencyclidine (PCP)	Tricyclic antidepressants	Barbiturates	Sympathomimetic amines
	Barbiturates	Acetaminophen	Phenothiazines
	Opiates		Tricyclic antidepressants
	Carbon monoxide		Opiates

Table 27–2B.   RESULTS OF TOXICOLOGIC ANALYSES, 1982: OCCURRENCE/100 CASES

SUBSTANCE	POLICE LAB OCCURRENCE/100 CASES (# OCCUR)	CORONER'S OFFICE POSITIVE OCCUR/100 (# OCCUR)	POISONINGS OCCUR/100 (# OCCUR)	REFERENCE LAB OCCUR/100 (# OCCUR)
Acetaminophen		10.5	10	16.6
Barbiturates (total)	(.7)	(7.2)	(10)	(24.4)
Amobarbital		0.2		3.1
Butabarbital		0.2	2	0.7
Butalbital		0.2		2.7
Pentobarbital		0.5		1.1
Phenobarbital		5.3	2	12.0
Secobarbital		0.7	6	4.9
Benzodiazepines (total)		(20.6)	(48)	(45.5)
Diazepam	2.7	10.6	22	} 31.8
N-desmethyldiazepam		8.4	18	
N-desalkylflurazepam		0.9	2	—
Flurazepam		0.5	4	3.8
Oxazepam		0.2	2	
Chlordiazepoxide				10.0
Brompheniramine		0.2		1.8
Cannabis	55.3			
Carbon monoxide		5.3	44	
Chlorpheniramine		0.2		3.6
Chlorpropamide		0.9	2	—
Cimetidine		0.7		—
Cocaine	4.8	0.7	2	1.1
Corrosives		0.5	4	—
Cyclizine		0.2	2	—
Dextromethorphan	0.4			0.4
Diphenhydramine		0.2		3.6
Disopropamide		0.2		—
Doxylamine		0.5		—
Fentanyl		0.2	2	—
Glutethimide		0.2	2	0.7
Heroin	2.0			
Lidocaine		15.1	6	2.0
LSD	1.0			
Meperidine	.8	1.7	4	2.7
Meprobamate				3.3
Methaqualone	.5	0.5	2	1.1
Methadone		2.2	6	.2
Methadone metabolite		0.5		
Methprylon				1.6
Normeperidine		1.2	4	
Norpropoxyphene		2.4	6	
Opiates (total)		(5.7)	(24)	(8.2)
Codeine		2.2	10	5.1
Hydromorphone	1.5	0.7	10	
Morphine		2.9	4	3.1
Oxycodone	2.1			
Pentazocine	9.1	0.9	2	2.2
Phencyclidine	2.7	0.9	2	1.8
Phenothiazines (total)		(1.9)	(6)	(10.0)
Chlorpromazine		0.7		
Thioridazine		0.5	4	
Mesoridazine		0.2	2	
Others		0.5		
Phenytoin		3.1	2	8.0
Placidyl		0.5	2	2.0
Propoxyphene		2.2	6	6.0
Primadone		0.5		

Table 27–2B. *(continued)*

SUBSTANCE	POLICE LAB OCCURRENCE/100 CASES (# OCCUR)	CORONER'S OFFICE POSITIVE OCCUR/100 (# OCCUR)	CORONER'S OFFICE POISONINGS OCCUR/100 (# OCCUR)	REFERENCE LAB OCCUR/100 (# OCCUR)
Quinidine		0.7	4	
Quinine		0.9		1.3
Tricyclic antidepressants (total)		(7.2)	(28)	9.2
Amitriptyline		2.2	8	6.5
Amoxapine		0.5	2	
Desipramine		0.5	2	
Doxepin		0.9	4	2.0
Imipramine		0.2		0.7
Nordoxepin		0.7	4	
Nortriptyline		2.2	8	
Salicylate		7.4	6	13.8
Sympathomimeticamines (total)	2.1	(3.1)	(2)	13.1
Amphetamine		0.2		0.7
Methamphetamine		0.2		0.4
Ephedrine		1.2		4.7
Phenmetrazine	2.3	0.2		
Phenylpropanolamine		1.2	2	7.3
Theophylline		0.5		
Toluene	2.3			
Tripelennamine	10.0	1.2	2	
Volatiles (total)		(65.0)	(42)	44.4
Methanol		0.2	2	0.2
Ethanol		26.6	40	27.3
Isopropanol				0.2
Acetone				2.6
Total occurrences	602	756	142	1029

ing disparities were reported. These tended to deprecate the laboratory's ability to contribute to patient care. A study of laboratory performance revealed that grossly aberrant results were reported by many laboratories (Pippenger *et al.*, 1976). As a consequence, the Epilepsy Foundation of America encouraged Dr. Charles Pippenger to initiate an innovative proficiency testing program that helped participating laboratories discover how reliable (or unreliable) their methods were. When those analytic procedures found deficient were corrected, more reliable laboratory data resulted. TDM became commonplace for neurologists. Clinical pharmacologists and clinical pharmacists also contributed to the development and propagation of this program. Their success indicated a need for a similar approach to other common therapeutic agents. The consequent extensive investigative activities extended the scope of TDM to theophylline, all antiepileptic agents, aminoglycosides, tricyclic antidepressants, methotrexate, procainemide, and lidocaine (Cross *et al.*, 1982). Other commonly therapeutic agents are slowly being added as innovative analytic methods permit detection of the relatively low blood concentration consistent with daily use of medications.

Therapeutic drug monitoring (TDM) has become a growing part of clinical laboratory medicine. Physicians, clinical pharmacists, and drug analysts are gathering and using plasma drug concentrations to optimize a patient's therapeutic regimen. In doing so they have done much to improve patient care and drug monitoring programs.

TDM should be used if:

1. A drug has a narrow therapeutic range.
2. A patient's compliance is in question.
3. Toxic side effects are noted.
4. Efficacy is not apparent.
5. Drug utilization may be altered by secondary disease processes or hereditary metabolic deficiencies.
6. Drug interactions are suggested or different dose formulations are noted and do not produce similar results (lack of bioequivalence or altered bioavailability).
7. Therapeutic effects cannot be monitored by clinical observation.
8. Anyone presumes that a standard dose for a standard patient will give a specific serum concentration.
9. Medicologic verification of treatment.

How should drugs be monitored? Thanks

to the ingenuity and creativity of many investigators, excellent procedures are available. Although most laboratories employ immunoassays (Cross *et al.*, 1982), gas chromatography (GC) and high-pressure liquid chromatography (HPLC) have their proponents (Scoggins *et al.*, 1980). These chromatographic techniques can process a large number of specimens automatically and accurately and they are cost effective. Reasonable justification of the use of any one of these three techniques can be made. The major argument in favor of GC and HPLC is their ability to determine several substances during one procedure; e.g., this is a forcible argument in its favor when several antiepileptic drugs are in concomitant use or if one wants to determine the tricyclics and their metabolites simultaneously (Pesh-Iman *et al.*, 1979). In favor of the immunoassays is their versatility—many systems (TDX®, ICM®, Stratus®, Multistat®) now compete with the commonly accepted homogeneous enzyme immunoassay (EMIT®) developed by Syva. An advantage of the EMIT® system is its significant cost savings by the use of centrifugal analyzers (Scoggins *et al.*, 1982). These allow significant dilution of the recommended reagent volumes with little loss in sensitivity or accuracy.

Equipped with modern automated units, many clinical laboratories are generating a large number of TDM results with a minimal demand on staff time or expertise. Their major problem is interpretative. Particularly for TDM, basic data about the patient *must* be known if a reliable interpretation is to be made (Boeckx, 1983). These data include (1) age, weight, sex; (2) the time specimen was drawn; (3) the time, amount, route, and form of the administered dose; and (4) the patient's kidney or renal disease, genetic traits, and tolerance to the drugs involved. All these facts should be known if one is to interpret the analytic results correctly. Many times all these required data are not available. Under this circumstance reliable interpretation is not feasible. When attempted, inconsistencies appear that may be attributed to inadequate laboratory performance. This is usually not the case, hence the need for a cooperative team effort to ensure that all the necessary information is optimal and available. Seldom can one person do this.

Some aspects of the proper time to obtain samples need amplification. The patient should be at steady state when the sample is drawn; i.e., a constant amount of the drug should have been administered for more than four to five half-lives of the drug. Depending on the pharmacokinetics of the drug, samples should be drawn at trough periods (just before administration of the next dose) or at peak periods 15 to 30 min-

utes after intravenous administration, one to two hours after intramuscular administration, i. m., or $1\frac{1}{2}$ to 6 hours after oral use (Werner, 1982).

If all these conditions are met, therapeutic plasma drug concentrations can be established (Table 27–3). If the results are beyond these critical values, the laboratory has an obligation to inform the attending physician very promptly. At that time all concerned should be well aware of the many previously cited factors that influence proper interpretation, the most important among these being age, genetic variability, and the patient's pathophysiology. Dosage regimens need major modifications when excretion is limited by renal disease or biotransformation is impaired because of compromised liver function. The very young and the elderly have peculiar modifying factors, as does the patient who has been taking a medication routinely for a long time.

The preceding discussion emphasizes that therapy must be individualized based on competent observation of the patient. If the desired effect is achieved at a lower concentration than is usual, there is no need to increase the dose to achieve a so-called optimal concentration; conversely higher-than-optimal concentrations may be required for others to achieve the same therapeutic effect. Vive la différence, and be aware of it.

In some instances the desired correlation between serum drug concentration and clinical condition is not apparent. Some theorize that only the free drug is the active agent and the analyst should report that value, not the value which usually included both free and protein bound drug-total drug content. Classically free drug was separated by dialysis. This tedious procedure, which would limit the use of the approach, was vitiated by the application of Millipore filters (Pippenger and Garlock, 1979). This ingenious unit separates free from bound drug in serum and thus permits quantitation of the free drug. All that is required to make this effective is even more sensitive analyses that would detect the much lower concentrations found as free drug. These challenges have been met, and the future will reveal the value of this approach.

"Spit is a horrid word." However, a serious hypothesis today is that saliva is a noninvasive specimen whose concentration may reflect free drug in serum (Toback *et al.*, 1982). Research is proceeding apace, and preliminary data give some support to this preposition. Considerably more data are required before it can be accepted. This is underway.

The future for increased use of TDM is bright, with reasonable anticipation of continued and significant growth in the variety as well as the

Table 27-3. THERAPEUTIC DRUG LEVELS

DRUG	THERAPEUTIC RANGE	CRITICAL VALUE
Acetaminophen	5–20 μg/ml	150 μg/ml
Amikacin	15–25 μg/ml (peak)	> 35 μg/ml (peak)
Amitriptyline	120–250 ng/ml	400 ng/ml
Carbamazepine	6–10 μg/ml	> 20 μg/ml
Chloramphenicol	15–25 μg/ml (peak)	> 60 μg/ml (peak)
Desipramine	150–300 ng/ml	400 ng/ml
Digoxin	0.5–2.0 ng/ml	2.5 ng/ml
Digitoxin	10–32 ng/ml	35 ng/ml
Disopyramide	2–5 μg/ml	> 7 μg/ml
Doxepin	150–300 ng/ml	400 ng/ml
Ethosuximide	40–100 μg/ml	> 200 μg/ml
Gentamicin	4–10 μg/ml (peak)	> 12 μg/ml (peak)
Imipramine	150–300 ng/ml	400 ng/ml
Lidocaine	1.6–5.0 μg/ml	> 9 μg/ml
Nortriptyline	50–150 ng/ml	200 ng/ml
Phenobarbital	15–30 μg/ml	> 60 μg/ml
Phenytoin	10–20 μg/ml	> 40 μg/ml
Primidone	8–12 μg/ml	> 24 μg/ml
Procainamide	4–8 μg/ml	> 12 μg/ml
Procainamide and N-acetyl procainamide	10–30 μg/ml	> 30 μg/ml
Protriptyline	50–150 ng/ml	200 ng/ml
Quinidine (double extraction method)	2.3–5.0 μg/ml	> 10 μg/ml
Salicylate	20–25 mg/dl	30 mg/dl
Theophylline	10–20 μg/ml	> 25 μg/ml
Tobramycin	4–10 μg/ml (peak)	> 12 μg/ml (peak)
Valproic acid	50–100 μg/ml	> 200 μg/ml

number of tests requested. As physicians gain familiarity with TDM, they can be expected to request this service, because it helps them to avoid prescribing blindly (Koch-Wiser, 1981). A major obstacle is the lack of appreciation of the value of TDM by most physicians. As this is recorded in the scientific literature, and as workshops and training programs provide the necessary background, we will see increasing use of TDM and of the toxicology laboratory.

DRUGS SUBJECT TO ABUSE

One of the by-products of the Vietnam War was the reincarnation of the drug abuse ogre. The then prevalent opinion was that a majority of the U.S. contingent was resorting to the abuse of illicit drugs and that this abuse problem was serious enough to warrant a major effort to uncover those involved. The number of specimens anticipated was staggering. The then existing technology was inadequate. Thin-layer chromatographic (TLC) procedures were available that could serve the need (Davidow et al., 1966; Mulé et al., 1969). These were used with decreasing effectiveness in some laboratories. TLC requires considerable diligence, careful at-

tention to procedural processes, and extensive experience with the nuances of the shades and colors of the reactions to the spray reagents. Although many developed the necessary skills and produced reliable results, slothful, nonconscientious personnel could incorrectly interpret the resulting spots. These individuals may be small in number, but their disparate reports could cause serious problems.

Hence, there arose a significant demand for a simple, objective procedure that would obviate the problems related to TLC. The rewards for an adequate solution were great, financially and professionally. The response was a major thrust forward for analytic chemists—the application of immunologic techniques to the detection of chemically related analytes (Rubinstein, 1972). Originally radioactive tags were used to follow the reaction (Skelly et al., 1973). This required separation of the bound and unbound moities. With the advent of homogeneous immunoassays, which obviated the separation step, came greater ease and significant decrease in the time required for a single analysis (Schneider et al., 1973).

One of the first homogeneous immunoassays (EMIT), and still the most popular of these, used an enzyme, which acted on a specific added substrate in the system, as the marker. Currently many alternative "markers" have been developed. These utilize fluorescence (Bund, 1979), nephelometry (Deaton et al., 1981), and fluorescence polarization (Lu-Steffs et al., 1981) and are now strong competitors of the EMIT system.

The immunoassays are a reliable complement to TLC. They are available for each of the drugs subject to abuse, are very sensitive to chemically related drugs, are automatable, and do provide objective answers. Although theoretically each laboratory so inclined can produce its own antibodies, most prefer to purchase them from vendors, whose kits are costly but reliable. The high reagent cost is counterbalanced by significantly lower time demands on the laboratory staff. Further savings are realized in some systems if centrifugal analyzers are used. Any one of these units requires about one-fifth of the usual volume of reagents, thus permitting a significant cost reduction (Cross et al., 1982).

By using immunoassays one could avoid the tedium and technical demands of the alternative procedure—thin-layer chromatography (TLC). This is not to decry the power of TLC. TLC has been, and is, an excellent technique for the qualitative identification of drugs (Bastos et al., 1970). It is relatively inexpensive, permits the simultaneous analysis of up to 20 samples on each chromatogram, is a nondestructive separation technique so that any suspicious spots can be eluted and tested by another technique, and is relatively simple and well within the capability of most laboratory personnel. Also, it is painstaking, labor intensive, requires careful attention to details, is time consuming, and requires extensive practical experience before its fullest potential can be realized. It is very subjective and beyond a color blind person. During the heyday of the testing programs for drug abuse, it was not unusual to see a large number of sprayed plates racked up on a large wall for interpretation and review. When a properly motivated staff did this work, reliable data were developed. When motivation was poor, the results could be very unreliable.

Either of the two techniques (immunoassay or TLC) may be used effectively. The major problem is the use to which the results are put. This will determine the quanta of proof required before a definitive report can be made. Basically this depends on whether or not the person tested is in a punitive situation.

Most participants in rehabilitation programs are required to submit periodic urine specimens for control analysis. These results are used by the counselors to evaluate their clients' statements about abstinence. Patients are not discharged from the program if they relapse to former undesirable practices, but efforts are redoubled to encourage their avoidance of use of substances subject to abuse. In such a nonpunitive program, the laboratory can provide unconfirmed results by a single test. This is economical and effective. On the other hand, if the testing program is punitive, i.e., a positive result jeopardizes continuance in the rehabilitation program (or parole or employment), then corroborative tests using a second technique are essential. The laboratory must be reasonably sure which substance is involved—e.g., an opiate present is an inadequate answer. One must be able to indicate that the positive result, e.g., an opiate, is due to a therapeutic agent or to an illicit agent such as codeine, morphine, or some other narcotic. TLC is a good presumptive indicator but must be followed by a confirmatory test. The corresponding immunoassay is frequently used for this purpose. By itself the later too is nonspecific. However, when coupled with the TLC result, a measure of reliability is achieved. Whether this is adequate needs serious consideration. Most laboratories prefer to confirm the TLC and/or the immunoassay with additional chromatographic techniques. Of course, any one chromatographic procedure is subject to coelution problems. If more certainty is required, then gas chromatography coupled with mass spectrophotometry (GC/MS) should be considered as a confirmatory test procedure (Foltz et al., 1980).

Since GC/MS is expensive (instrument cost) and demanding (laboratory personnel's expertise), seldom is it used for drug abuse programs. The one exception to this is marijuana (Hawks, 1982). Currently this substance poses a major problem. Preliminary testing by immunoassay produces a reasonable result that yields presumptive identification. At this writing there are no other simple techniques for confirming these except GC/MS. In the wings are both HPLC and TLC. Preliminary experiments suggest that TLC is sufficiently sensitive and specific methods will be forthcoming.

This review does not encompass the details of the many analytic procedures discussed. Their limitations in terms of specificity and sensitivity are of interest and these are recorded in Table 27–4. References in this section and elsewhere in this review indicate where the readers may find descriptions of detailed analytic procedures.

FORENSIC TOXICOLOGY

Forensic toxicology poses a great challenge to the analytic toxicologist. The variety of analytes is large, the quantity and quality of available

Table 27–4. **REPORTED SENSITIVITIES AND SPECIFICITIES OF IMMUNOASSAYS FOR DRUGS SUBJECT TO ABUSE**

ASSAY	DRUG OR METABOLITES DETECTED	DETECTION LIMITS (μg/ml)*	
		EMIT®†	ABUSCREEN®‡
Amphetamine	Amphetamine	0.3	1.0
	Methamphetamine	$\leq$1.0	
	d,l-Ephedrine	$\geq$1.0	
	Isoxsuprine	$\geq$6.0	
	Mephentermine	$\geq$0.5	
	Nylidrin	$\geq$2.0	
	Phenmetrazine	$\geq$1.0	
	Phentermine	$\geq$0.5	
	Phenylpropanolamine	$\geq$1.0	
Barbiturates	Secobarbital	0.3	0.2
	Amobarbital	$\leq$2.0	
	Aprobarbital		$\leq$1.0
	Butabarbital	$\leq$1.0	$\leq$1.0
	Pentobarbital	$\leq$1.0	$\leq$1.0
	Phenobarbital	$\leq$3.0	$\leq$4.0
Benzodiazepines	Oxazepam	0.3	
	Chlordiazepoxide	3.0	
	Diazepam	2.0	
	N-Desalkylflurazepam	2.0	
	N-Desmethyldiazepam	2.0	
	Flurazepam	2.0	
	Lorazepam	3.0	
Cannabinoid	Δ^9-THC metabolite	0.2	0.075
Cocaine and/or metabolite	Benzoylecognine	0.3	$\leq$1.0
	Cocaine	>25.0	0.75
	Ecgonine	$\geq$5.0	
Methadone	Methadone	0.3	0.5
	Dextromethorphan	>300	
	Diphenhydramine	>100	
	Promethazine	>75	
Methaqualone	Methaqualone	0.30	0.75
	Mecloqualone	1.0	
	3' and 4'-Hydroxy metabolite	1.0	$\leq$0.75
	6'-Hydroxy metabolite	*	3.0
Opiate	Morphine	0.3	0.04
	Morphine-glucuronide	$\leq$3.0	$\leq$0.05
	Codeine	$\leq$1.0	$\leq$0.04
	Hydromorphone	$\leq$3.0	
	Meperidine	520	
Phencyclidine	Phencyclidine	0.75	0.025
	TCP	1.0	
	PCP metabolites	1.0–3.0	
Propoxyphene	Propoxyphene	2.0	

* As specified by manufacturer.
† Emit—Syva Corp., Palo Alto, Calif. 94303.
‡ Abuscreen—Roche Diagnostics, Nutley, N.J. 07110.

material may be very limited (especially from putrified, mumified, or severely burned bodies), the artifacts encounted may be significant, the quanta of proof of identity are high, and the results of the analytes may have far-reaching consequences, sometimes pertaining to other than the person from whom the specimens were obtained. More often than not, the analyst must be prepared to defend his data in court, and withstand vigorous cross-examination. Although physically and scientifically forensic and clinical toxicologists have comparable skills, equipment, procedures, and expertise, this need of the forensic toxicologist to satisfy legal processes sharply distinguishes them.

Previously, in the discussion of clinical toxicology, the recommendation was made that the scope of a toxicologic analysis should be finite and limited. The forensic toxicologist might prefer to do likewise, but his examination perforce has to be as all-inclusive as possible. His need for functional, state-of-the-art equipment is real. He must have these in sufficient variety, quantity, and quality so that the necessary analyses can be performed "in house." His staff has to include trained scientists who can use and maintain these instruments. Not only must they then be able to interpret their results, but they must be competent to defend these data if cross-examined in court. The required quanta of proof are high, necessitating several different methods that qualitatively and quantitatively determine any exogeneous substances purported to be involved.

The forensic toxicologist is also a member of the health care team. His efforts are applied not only to criminal or civil juridical matters but also to improving the general well-being of the community. A few examples illustrate this point. Demonstrating that a person found "dead in bed" succumbed to carbon monoxide from an unsuspected source may uncover an unsuspected leak in a chimney or gas appliance. Repairing these ensures that others will not succumb in a similar manner. By unmasking industrial chemicals that contribute to a worker's demise, the toxicologist can lead to institution of suitable remedial measures. By comparing regional and national experiences, misuse of therapeutic agents can be uncovered. Two such surveys led to the realization by the medical profession that Valium® and Darvon® were being used injudiciously and that more rigid controls were essential to ensure that this misuse did not continue (Finkle et al., 1976). The resulting controls led to a marked decrease in deaths due to propoxyphene.

Although every result the forensic toxicologist generates may lead eventually to a court appearance, this is not general practice. Most forensic toxicologists are in a governmental medicolegal agency, and the results of that agency's staff are admissible in evidence without presentation by those who developed the results. Only when the defense or prosecution feels a need to question the data does the toxicologist go to court, and the frequency of court appearances varies with each agency.

The two situations that most often result in a forensic toxicologist's court appearance are the blood analyses related to charges of driving while under the influence of alcohol and/or drugs and the urinalysis related to the use of marijuana (tetrahydrocannabinol). The former concerns a driver's privilege to continue to drive, which is usually jeopardized for a significant period of time if a conviction is obtained. It also may involve a mandatory jail stay. Hence many of these cases are contested, and this seldom re-

volves about the scientific data. Rather they concern peripheral activities of everyone involved in the analysis. The chain of evidence and the sampling process are suspect and, if vulnerable, may vitiate the laboratory test and spare the defendant. The toxicologist must learn how to spar with defense attorneys who are intent on invalidating an accurate laboratory result by challenging these related activities that do not concern analytic procedures (Kogan, 1981).

Cannabinoids pose a different problem. There are now reasonably reliable presumptive tests that will indicate, if positive, that the urine specimen probably contains a metabolite of THC (Hawks, 1982). Since one probative test is not sufficient to make a positive statement in court, as previously noted, a confirmatory test is essential. A GC/MS can perform this with reasonable certainty. TLC can also be used effectively. Gas chromatographic methods have been used (Whiting and Manders, 1982), but their sensitivity and reliability have been questioned. Since most laboratories still do not have a GC/MS, confirmatory results are difficult to obtain. When they can be obtained, their interpretation is difficult. Marijuana, once used, will be excreted in the urine for up to 14 days later (Hunt and Jones, 1980). To testify when the person with a positive urine test used the marijuana is well nigh impossible. Thus, ensuring that justice is done on the basis of the laboratory data is difficult and a challenge that present knowledge does not guarantee.

Because some forensic toxicologists perforce develop reasonable ease in courtroom procedure and because they acquire expertise in the evaluation of chemical hazards, some are sought out as consultants in untoward occupational and environmental exposures. If their experience warrants, they may develop the necessary chemical data, evaluate the extent of an exposure, assess the potential for damage, and present their findings and opinion to the court. Not every forensic toxicologist becomes so involved, but those who have the competence contribute significantly.

Another integral part of forensic toxicology may include teaching and scientific research. Many governmental forensic agencies have medical school affiliations that require these pursuits. The number of formal academic training programs in analytic toxicology is small, but growing (Lynch, 1981). Most educational activity programs are tutorial on the job programs, rewarding to the individuals involved, but not compatible with developing the quantity and quality of professional personnel required. As the demand grows (and it is markedly), suitable educational programs may develop.

ANALYTIC PROCEDURES*

Previously we mentioned procedures relevant to each of the topics presented. The following review is designed to familiarize the reader with the growth and development of these relevant analytic procedures.

Looking backward permits an assessment of one's present position. Looking forward may reveal the future prospect. Initially we will focus on the mid-twentieth century, then view the rapidly accelerating growth of analytic toxicology to the present, and speculate on what the future may bring. Since Adam's fall, the first documented poisoning, man has tasted the forbidden fruits that surround him, to his peril and sometimes his death. The commonplace poisons in previous time were harmful plants and simple chemicals. As scientists have developed and produced new agents, these have been misused and abused, sometimes with dire consequences. Today the array of potentially harmful substances is frightening, and each year brings with it many new hazardous products. Poisonings are a direct function of the number of available dangerous substances, and their incidence has increased significantly.

How does the analytic toxicologist fit into this ever-expanding scene? Many debate this question and some suggest that patient care is not improved by the toxicologist's results and that there is no need for his laboratory's services (Dinoro and Gottschalk, 1976; Teitelbaum *et al.,* 1977; Ingelfinger *et al.,* 1981). Those who have negative feelings about the toxicologist's role have seldom had the aid of an effective, reliable laboratory group. When prompt, accurate toxicologic analyses are available, they have proven to be very helpful to the health care team. These results have helped guide therapy for acutely poisoned patients, have facilitated adjustments in drug therapy, and have provided reliable evidential information for rehabilitation, probation, and medicolegal programs (Walberg *et al.,* 1979; Bailey and Manoguerra, 1980; Ungerleider *et al.,* 1980; Micozzi, 1982).

Historically (Gettler, 1956), only forensic problems concerned the toxicology pioneers. They were concerned primarily with arsenicals, mercurials, and some few naturally occurring toxicants, opiates, nux vomica (strychnine), and belladonna (atropine). Their laboratory procedures reflected the status of early twentieth-

century analytic chemistry. They used the tedious, laborious Stas Otto technique to separate organic poisons from tissues. The toxicants in the resulting residues were identified by a series of chromophores that were produced by many chemical reagents devised by a host of ingenious investigators—Marquis, Froede, Mandelin, Trinder, Dragendorff, to mention only a few. Their efforts produced procedures that even today's esoteric equipment cannot top. Trinder's (1954) test for salicylate, the purple color produced when a salicylate reacts with ferric ion, is state of the art today.

The various chromophores produced by the Dragendorff's reagent, Mandelin's reagent, iodoplatinate characterized many of the ingredients of the waxy residues resulting from the Stas Otto ethanol extraction procedure (Umberger, 1954). These reagents are still used in modern thin-layer chromatography (TLC) (Bastos *et al.,* 1970). Without them TLC would not be the powerful tool that it is.

The analysis for ethanol, separated by distillation and assayed by redox reactions, as suggested by Nicloux (1913) and modified by Widmark (1922), Kozelka-Hine (1941) and Dubowski-Withrow (1952), is still the standard approach prescribed by legal codes in many countries. Although tedious, it does produce very accurate results. It is still used today in those small laboratories where expendable glassware is the mainstay.

Arsenicals and mercurials posed many forensic problems, reliable answers to which were devised by Reinsch (1841, see Kaye, 1975) and by Marsh (1836, see Kaye, 1975). Even today the fastest, most effective method for determining whether one of these compounds caused a poisoning is to place a tube containing a freshly cleaned copper coil in an acidified mixture of the specimen and heat it in a boiling water bath for 10 to 15 minutes. If elements below copper in the EMF series are present, they will deposit on the wire's surface. The discoloration is readily apparent, and Kaye has summarized the series of subsequent wet chemical reactions that can be used to characterize the substance involved (Kaye, 1975).

The advent of a reliable spectrophotometer in 1940–1950 permitted new approaches to new problems—barbiturates, antimalarials. Brodie and Udenfriend (1945) developed their methyl orange technique for the analysis of organic bases. (Today we call it ion pairing.) Recognizing that organic solvents would extract organic material from biologic specimens, they coupled the extracted organic compound with methyl orange to form organic soluble helianthates. The decomposition of this ion pair by an acid solu-

---

* Modified from Sunshine, I.: Clinical toxicology—growth and development. *Therapeutic Drug Monitoring and Emergency Toxicology Continuing Education and Quality Control Program.* American Association for Clinical Chemistry, Washington, D.C., Vol. 6, No. 8, July, 1984.

tion yielded a chromophore that reflected the concentration of the drug. Reliable quantitation was achieved. Gettler and Sunshine (1951) extended this technique to the analysis of tissues, enhancing its potential for forensic problems.

During this period, another application of spectrophotometry was developed, the analysis for barbiturates. These sedatives were then the chief causes of acute and fatal poisonings. Specific therapeutic procedures were devised to cope with the acutely barbiturate-intoxicated patients. Alkalinization, hemodialysis—these depended on proper identification and quantification of the barbiturate involved. Several ingenious procedures for the acidic sedatives were developed in a two- to three-year span. The one that was commonly accepted was described by Goldbaum (1952), and it is still an effective procedure in reasonable use today. Jatlow (1968) has updated this procedure so that it now encompasses a host of drugs developed since then, the benzodiazepines, the antidiabetics such as chlorpropamide and tolbutamide, and methaqualone, to mention a few. The major criticism of this approach was that it did not provide desirable qualitative identification of the barbiturate involved. Many efforts were made to remedy this, including acid hydrolysis (Broughton, 1956), alkaline hydrolysis, selective extraction (Stephenson, 1961). These were effective for pure drugs, but drugs separated from a biologic matrix contained coextracted artifacts, which made qualitative interpretation difficult. Stephenson (1961) developed a selective extraction procedure that very effectively differentiated long- from short-acting barbiturates, which distinction was clinically significant and sufficient. However, little publicity was given to this simple, but effective, technique, and it received little use despite its value. Walberg (1981) recently published this information, which, it is hoped, will now be used by those who still use these ultraviolet spectrophotometric procedures.

Just as the barbiturates posed a major problem for adults, so did lead for one- to four-year-olds (Jacobzinner and Raybin, 1962). Although lead poisonings are now a relatively minor problem, in the mid-1950s it was routine practice to request a lead determination on specimens obtained from young children whose financially underprivileged families lived in poorly maintained homes. Elevated lead concentrations were commonplace and were used to initiate preventive measures or therapy (Newill et al., 1963). The absorbances of various dithizone extracts following wet digestion were used to measure the lead concentrations (Sunshine, 1968). These spectrophotometric procedures were diagnostic and contributory.

Other applications of UV spectrophotometry were to the analysis of alkaline extracts of biologic specimens. Urines were more amenable than bloods. Following a double extraction (alkaline urine into organic solvent into acid, which was then made alkaline and reextracted into organic solvent and then into acid again), UV analysis of the acid extract detected some organic bases (Siek, 1974, 1975, 1976). As with the barbiturates, these UV absorption curves were not specific, since several related drugs yield similar UV absorption curves (Siek, 1974, 1975, 1976). Nonetheless, this was progress beyond Brodie's methyl orange analyses (Brodie and Udenfriend, 1945) and the nonspecific color tests.

A harbinger of things to come was Stolman's excellent separation of opiates using Fluorisil columns (Stolman and Stewart, 1949). His data indicated the separation potential of column chromatography. Unfortunately, his work failed to attract attention, and the principle lay dormant until recently. Admittedly Fluorisil is not the absorbent of choice today. The nonionic Amberlite resin XAD-2 was used extensively, but has yielded, in recent years, to ClinElut®, Bondelut®, and a host of other absorbents that have been found more suitable for the isolation of toxicants in the blood or urine specimens currently processed (Bastos et al., 1973). Nonetheless, Stolman's research pointed a way that neither he nor his contemporaries had the foresight to exploit further. His efforts were before their time.

The next major step forward, in the late 1950s, was the introduction and effective use of thin-layer chromatography. Kirchner (1951) and Stahl (1956) were prime movers who found supporters in Switzerland, Germany, Austria, Italy, England, and the United States. These innovators investigated many different drugs and produced a bounteous harvest of very practical methods. With the highly expanded pharmacopeia and the increased use of therapeutic agents, this novel technique made it possible to analyze for a multitude of drugs simultaneously and to process many samples (up to 20 on one 20 × 20 cm plate) simultaneously. The analytic challenge was great; the response was fantastic. Many developing solvent mixtures were explored. Visualization techniques were uncovered such that functional group reactions could be successively applied to a given chromatogram (Bastos et al., 1970). The resulting color responses at given Rf values were used to make tentative identifications. Using several plates, each developed in solvents of differing solubilities, reasonably positive qualitative identifications could be made by TLC alone (Sunshine et al., 1966).

By coupling the TLC data with UV absorption data, toxicologists could produce qualitative and quantitative data. A spectacular improvement had been achieved in less than a decade. No doubt a good deal of progress in TLC came as a response to the demand for analyses of urine specimens taken from servicemen suspected to be misusing drugs subject to abuse. Oceans of urine flowed through many large laboratory units especially set up to perform this high volume of work (Bastos *et al.,* 1973; Sunderman, 1973). TLC was the only effective tool at the time. It did a very efficient job and provided methodology that is still used today in attacking problems related not only to drug abuse but to acute poisonings (Bastos *et al.,* 1973).

In the middle and late 1960s the death knell of spectrophotometry began to sound. Its last gasp produced a puff of smoke that came from a graphite furnace or a Delves cup that was then automatically analyzed by atomic absorption spectrophotometry (Sunderman, 1973).

The old order "yielded place to the new" chromatographic procedures. Gas chromatographic (GC) equipment was modified and applied to toxicologic problems (Barrett, 1971). Small volumes of samples could now be used because GC methodologies were very sensitive. No longer were the 500 g of tissue required for the Stas Otto procedure needed. Ten milliliters of blood or 25 ml of urine would do, even less as GC methods and detectors improved (Finkle *et al.,* 1971). Now qualitative and quantitative data were obtained simultaneously. The previously described extracts of TLC spots could be analyzed by gas chromatography (Reynolds, 1975), thus providing confirmatory data previously lacking. Surely all one could desire was now achieved.

Not so. The press for greater sensitivity, specificity, and accuracy produced new GC methodology, derivatization techniques (Ahiya, 1976) that permitted the use of electron-capture detectors and nitrogen phosphorus detectors so sensitive to the nitrogenous compounds in question that only 50 μl of serum was required for a comprehensive analysis for most of the antiepileptic drugs then in use (Bente, 1978). A flood of innovative techniques were developed such that by 1970 reliable GC methods were available for most drugs (Finkle *et al.,* 1971). Thus, acquisition of quantitative data on many drugs became a reality. This paved the way for an increased prognostic value for the laboratory data as correlations between drug concentrations in blood and patients' clinical conditions were developed.

This success did not discourage further innovation. On the contrary, it was encouraged. As more methods were developed and applied, as clinicians began to appreciate the laboratory support available to them, their demands for service increased.

A grand step forward was taken in the early seventies with the application of immunologic techniques to analytic toxicology. Responding to the need for more sensitive tests for drugs subject to abuse, a group of very innovative scientists applied principles developed by Yalow and Berson (1960). They injected an immunogen, a drug coupled to a carrier protein, into animals that thereupon developed antibodies to the drug. In the presence of a specimen containing the drug used to form the immunogen, an antigen-antibody reaction will ensue. If, in the same system, a specimen is introduced that contains a labeled derivative of the drug in question, a competitive reaction occurs between the labeled and unlabeled drug. The amount of drug in the specimen can then be determined as a function of this competitive reaction.

Originally, radioactive labels were used (Shelly *et al.,* 1973), and separation steps were necessary to measure the free or bound drug. With the introduction of the enzyme multiplied immunoassay technique (EMIT), which uses an enzyme's reaction on a substrate as the marker, the procedure was simplified because no separation techniques were required. An analysis needs only 50 μl, the time required is short, 45 seconds, the method is objective, producing a printed number representing an absorbance difference for the time interval involved, the results are accurate and precise, the technique is very simple, the equipment costs are nominal—all significant attributes that have led to the general acceptance and use of this technique. Its limitations, lack of specificity, and relative high cost of reagents are the calculated debits one must balance against the procedure's very positive credits. Tremendous use has been made of these immunologic procedures. By 1980, reagents existed for more than 65 substances, applicable to blood, urine, and other biologic specimens. In the last several years additional labels have been used such that fluorescence (Burd, 1979), nephelometric inhibition (Finley, 1981), and fluorescent polarization (Watson *et al.,* 1976) are now competing with the initial techniques, more or less successfully. Automation has been achieved (Caron *et al.,* 1983), costs per test have been reduced, and these innovative techniques are now feasible for any laboratory's use.

Armed with all these reliable procedures one might expect a plateau in the development of new approaches. Not so. The 1980s have been replete with more developments that complement those already described. High-pressure liquid chromatography has entered the field like an express train highballing down a clear, level, straight track. Instrumentation has advanced from individual components carefully selected to meet particular needs to more complex comprehensive units with automatic sampling, control of analytic parameters, and computer calculations, all under microprocessor control. Methods have been developed for the sedatives (Szabo and Sunshine, 1982), the benzodiazepines (Sutheimer and Sunshine, 1982), the antiepileptics (Pesh-Iman et al., 1979), theophylline by HPLC (Adams et al., 1976), the antiarrhythmics (Kabra et al., 1981), the tricyclics (Scoggins et al., 1980), and the opiates (Jane and Taylor, 1975). The last were achieved by use of a novel electrochemical detector, which permits accurate analyses of drugs such as morphine, codeine, hydromorphone, and oxycodone. Previous opiate methodologies using immunoassay (Schneider et al., 1973), fluorescence (Kupferberg et al., 1964), or gas chromatography (Nakamura and Way, 1975) gave some results but lacked either sensitivity, specificity, or accuracy for these compounds. Many drugs involved in acute poisonings can be analyzed by HPLC methods. The biggest gap at this time are those organic bases used as stimulants and antihistamines, but in time the methods for these will also be developed. New developments in this field include smaller columns of smaller-mesh column materials that permit very rapid analyses with separations comparable to those of the longer columns (Novotny, 1981). Coupled to this are detectors that will provide UV absorption spectra of the eluting material so that more positive identification can be made using the UV absorption data.

The gas chromatographers, in the face of the onslaught by HPLC, have not yielded the field. Armed with the practical experience of Costello et al. (1974), Fensilau (1972), and Finkle et al. (1974), and aided by strides in the development of more elegant equipment and microprocessor handling of data, gas chromatography coupled to mass spectroscopy has become the most elegant, sensitive, specific method for analysis of biologic specimens purported to contain exogeneous chemical agents. Despite the complexity of the equipment and the difficulties of maintenance unless a very knowledgeable scientist is a staff member, the GC/MS procedures are relatively simple to perform. They can easily be mastered by technicians who, by using this technology, already process effectively many samples daily (Ullucci et al., 1978). GC/MS offers definitive analyses of complex mixtures, isolating drugs and metabolites with relative ease.

Using GC/MS may help resolve some of the seeming anomalous relationship between serum drug concentration and a patient's clinical condition. With separation of the active drug and metabolites from the chemically similar inactive metabolites, better insights into the clinical correlation are possible. At this time, GC/MS is not in routine use in most laboratories and probably will not be so for some time. Its lack of cost effectiveness is a partial explanation. Most administrators are loath to put up the high-dollar investment for the present relatively small workload. However, when the critical volume of work is reached, or when research interests require this support, GC/MS will become standard laboratory equipment. Another factor that will influence its future use is the development of simpler, rugged less expensive units. Ingenious manufacturers, sensing significant sales, have made this a reality.

As the heavy artillery masses to confound the naive tyro in the field, so efforts have increased to produce simple techniques that will provide reasonable preliminary data that are significant to attending physicians. Their diagnostic problems require very rapid qualitative or semiquantitative data. To this end two significant approaches have been developed, a rapid TLC procedure, TOXI-LAB® (Michaud and Jones, 1980), and an almost instantaneous immunologic one, EMIT$_{ST}$® (Sutheimer et al., 1982). Each of these is remarkably easy to carry out. Well-trained technicians can produce qualitative data in about one hour using the TOXI-LAB TLC procedure. In this procedure many reference drug compounds are prespotted on a preprocessed chromatogram into which the technician places a small disk that is dried in the organic solvent extract of a urine specimen. This chromatogram is successively dipped into visualization reagents. The response of the sample is compared to those of the simultaneously analyzed reference compounds already impregnated in the chromatogram and to a comprehensive reference file of typical chromatograms supplied by the manufacturer: this procedure enables a tentative identification. This analysis is remarkably simple to perform since all the required materials are available at reasonable cost. A major problem is in the interpretation of the chromatogram. A color-blind technician would be distraught and ineffectual! Those not so afflicted acquire the necessary competence with time. There is no substitute for experience. Once this experience is acquired, that person can be remarkably effective.

Paralleling this development have been Syva's Single Test Units (Sutheimer et al., 1982). These are vials that contain the lyophilized reagents required for a test. All the operator need do is dispense an aliquot of the specimen into one vial and an identical volume of a cutoff calibrator, containing the test drug at a known concentration, into a second vial. These solutions dissolve the lyophilized reagents and initiate the test reaction. Placing the tubes into a specially designed photometer starts the time sequence, and 90 seconds later a printout of the difference in absorbance of the two tubes is obtained. Although not recommended by the manufacturer at this time, this absorbance difference can be used to semiquantitate the result, particularly if calibrators are used that bracket the absorbance difference of the specimen. Simple to use, requiring simple, relatively inexpensive, rugged equipment, this procedure is a very powerful tool for all laboratories concerned with acute emergency toxicology. Its limitations must be recognized. To be effective the entire but limited battery of tests must be used. The relatively high reagent cost is offset by the low labor cost. The results are class specific. To identify which particular drug in the class is the offending agent is beyond the procedure's potential. Nonetheless, one must bear in mind the question to be answered, "Has my patient taken an exogeneous chemical agent that will cause his presenting condition?" In many cases, the relatively nonspecific single test result and that obtained by the TOXI-LAB procedure will suffice. What many laboratories have not recognized is the synergistic potential that results from coupling these two procedures. By using both, better and corroborated qualitative and even semiquantitative data are obtained. Some cost containment may be achieved if the results of the TLC procedure are used to select the appropriate single test units that could confirm the TLC data. Those attempting this approach must consider the relative sensitivities of each method for each drug in question. Seemingly disparate data may be explained by these sensitivity differences.

Where do we go from here? Upward and onward at a dizzying pace. The number of interested creative scientists is growing. They are frenetically generating new approaches. Negative-ion GC/MS (Brandenberger, 1978), second derivative UV absorption spectrophotometry (O'Haver, 1981), inductively coupled plasma jet for simultaneous multielement analysis (Fessel, 1979), ion-specific electrodes involving simple enzyme systems (Martin and Frieser, 1980), monoclonal antibodies (Geltosky, 1983)—all these are in the pot, simmering away. What will distill out is to be seen. Surely many more advances should be expected in the near future.

What does all this mean to the bench analyst beset by the question of "Should I attempt to do some toxicologic analysis in response to clinicians' demands?" An emphatic "yes" should be the response. In consultation with concerned physicians, an adequate laboratory program should be devised based on the available or procurable equipment and expertise. The laboratory should have procedures for those analytes for which prompt therapy is available and essential, acetaminophen, methanol, and salicylates (Thompson, 1980).

Qualitative or semiquantitative data should be available for those drugs commonly used in a particular area. These are relatively few, easily defined, but subject to change as local mores change. The menu should be specified and its limits defined, and that should be the primary toxicology laboratory product. Exceptions should be rare and then only by mutual consent. Responses should be forthcoming within two to four hours after the receipt of blood *and urine* specimens. Urine specimens are essential because they are the basis for many simple qualitative tests. The results of these tests can then be used as a guide to the necessary quantitative blood assay. These responses should be made to the clinician involved and interpretation, if needed, should be provided by senior laboratory staff.

Many procedures can be used (Hepler, 1982). The simplest would utilize an alcohol dehydrogenase (ADH) based method for ethanol, photometric analyses for salicylate, acetaminophen, and several other commonly used drugs, and homogeneous immunoassays paired with TLC for other drugs. If more sophisticated personnel and equipment are available, they could complement the above with HPLC for the sedative (acid neutral) drugs (Szabo and Sunshine, 1982) and gas chromatography (Wu Chen *et al.,* 1983) for the many organic bases. If this expertise and equipment are not available, a *reliable, tested* reference laboratory should be considered. The timeliness of its response may determine its value to patient care. In large cities where such reference laboratories exist, they may satisfy the time factor, but the cost effectiveness of the referral needs critical evaluation.

The thesis is that there is a role for the laboratory in acute poisonings. With a reasonable effort and at realistic costs, clinical laboratories can implement procedures that most technicians can utilize to furnish reasonable laboratory results in the time required to be clinically significant. Those willing to make these efforts will be rewarded by their increased ability to help provide better health care for the community.

COLLECTION AND PRESERVATION OF SPECIMENS

Specimens for toxicologic analysis should be properly obtained, placed in appropriate containers, sealed, signed, dated, and taken to the laboratory. All toxicologic specimens should be stored at 4°C or −20°C until analyzed.

In forensic cases, the toxicologist should sign or initial the seal on each container and record the hour and date received. The chain of possession, in all cases, must be intact, guaranteeing complete chronologic accountability of the samples in the expectation of judicial proceedings.

Postmortem Specimens

Inasmuch as it is usually impossible to determine at autopsy what tissues the toxicologist will need in his analysis, adequate samples of all tissues should be taken. These can be disposed of later if not required, whereas the possibility for disinterment of a body is remote (Curran, 1971).

Blood. Great care should be exercised in collection of the blood sample to ensure freedom from contamination. Heart blood is preferred, and peripheral blood is acceptable. Under no circumstances should the sample be "scooped up" from the body cavity since this blood may be contaminated with fluids from the viscera and/or the stomach contents. A 100-ml sample will usually suffice for routine studies. The storage vessel should contain fluoride and oxalate as preservative and anticoagulant.

Urine. All available urine should be collected, and if the bladder appears empty, the bladder should be submitted intact. A small amount of urine will be present in the empty bladder, and this can be utilized either for a micro sugar and acetone determination or for immunologic determination. Postmortem blood sugar levels are of little or no value, but the urinalysis may give evidence of diabetes. Urine often provides a concentrated, relatively unadulterated form of a poison and its metabolites and is applicable to a variety of preliminary screening tests.

Bile. The gallbladder should not be opened at the time of autopsy but, rather, should be removed intact and placed into a separate container. Biliary excretion is an important route of elimination for a number of foreign compounds, including drugs such as morphine, methadone, and glutethimide.

Vitreous. Aspirate the vitreous fluid and replace it with normal saline.

Brain. At least 50 g should be collected. This tissue is especially useful in the demonstration of alcohol and other volatile poisons.

Kidney. The equivalent of one kidney should be taken. This is the tissue of choice for most metals and sulfonamides.

Liver. A sample of 100 g is a minimal requirement. The liver is the site of biotransformation for the majority of toxicants, and the levels found in this tissue may be up to several hundred times higher than those found in the blood. In many instances, the liver may be the only tissue in which the toxic substance will be found in sufficiently high concentration for absolute identification and quantitation.

Lung. At least 100 g of lung should be obtained. This tissue will be especially useful in fatalities due to substance inhalation. It may likewise be a strategic tissue in certain instances of injection or ingestion of a poison. In acute deaths resulting from the intravenous injection of heroin, morphine, the principal biotransformation product, is found in significant concentrations in the blood and lungs and may not be present at detectable levels in other tissues.

Bone. Bone should be collected if there is any indication that a pesticide or metal is suspected. A total of 100 g should prove adequate.

Hair and Fingernails. These specimens should be taken if chronic metal poisoning is suspected.

Adipose. A minimum sample of 50 g should be taken routinely. In cases in which the victim has survived some days following ingestion of an unknown poison, or if pesticides or insecticides are suspected, adipose tissue should be analyzed. Among the drugs that will accumulate in the fat are thiopental, glutethimide, and ethchlorvynol.

Antemortem Specimens

The specimens of choice depend on the clinical situation. The requirements for each of the several toxicologic situations discussed previously are listed below.

Acute poisoning:	Blood, unclotted (fluoride and/or oxalate, EDTA): 10 ml Urine: 25–50 ml Gastric aspirate: all available. Emesis: all available
TDM:	Blood, unclotted: 10 ml (adults) 2–5 ml (children)
Drugs subject to abuse:	Urine: 50 ml (close supervision of the sampling process is essential)

INTERPRETATION OF FINDINGS

Already stressed many times in this chapter has been the thesis that no matter how reliable the laboratory strives to make its results, their ultimate value lies in their interpretation and application to patient care.

An approach to the problem of interpretation usually begins with a review of data abstracted from the literature or culled from previous cases investigated by the toxicologist and his colleagues. The former often supplies information concerning blood levels resulting from therapeutic administration of a drug or from overdosage in which the patient survived (Baselt and Cravey, 1977). The latter concerns statistical data on body distribution studies from fatalities known to have arisen from a particular compound. An experienced analyst will usually have available a substantial body of information that greatly enhances his ability to evaluate toxicologic findings. Information from well-documented and well-investigated cases that the toxicologist personally obtains is of the foremost value in understanding toxic and fatal levels. In evaluating data received from outside sources, one must bear in mind that there is no uniformity or standardization of toxicologic procedures among clinical and forensic laboratories. Methods for isolating, identifying, and quantitating toxic substances from tissues often differ greatly in their degree of specificity, sensitivity, and accuracy.

Recovery alone poses a problem since drug-protein complexes formed in plasma and other tissues may be difficult to break down without substantial loss of the drug. Thus, the values reported are indicative only of the amount of a compound recovered and do not necessarily reflect the amount actually present in the tissue.

Since for the majority of drugs and chemicals the blood or plasma level most clearly reflects the clinical state of the patient, it is this level that is most often cited in the toxicologist's report as the deciding factor in a case of possible overdosage. It is certainly true that in clinical studies involving naïve subjects, individuals do not vary significantly with respect to the pharmacologic effects produced by certain well-defined blood concentrations of most drugs (Vesell and Passananti, 1971). However, in interpreting levels exceeding these therapeutic concentrations the toxicologist should be aware of modifying factors likely to be encountered.

Factors Affecting the Clinical State at a Given Blood Concentration of a Drug

Tolerance, a state of decreased responsiveness to a drug, is a result of prior exposure, usually long term, to a given drug or its congener.

Cellular adaptation is one type of tolerance in which ever-increasing blood concentrations of a drug are required in order to maintain a certain pharmacologic response. This situation is exemplified by the methadone maintenance patient who may be receiving a daily oral dose of 100 mg of methadone hydrochloride. This same dose, although it produces no noticeable narcotic effects in the tolerant patient, could easily prove fatal if ingested by a nontolerant individual. While it is tempting, the toxicologist should refrain from classifying a blood level as consistent with death according to literature values until the decedent's history of drug usage has been determined.

The problem of drugs in combination is a frequent obstacle to interpretation of toxicologic findings. The possibility of antagonism of one drug by another, although rare, should not be overlooked. More often the additive or synergistic effects produced by the interaction of two or more depressant drugs may result in coma or death, although none of the drugs is present in toxic levels. The combination of alcohol and secobarbital is commonly employed for purposes of intoxication or as a means of suicide.

Unfortunately, the effects of many other drug combinations are not known. A significant number of coroner's cases are those revealing no pathologic changes, in which the toxicologist has isolated several drugs, each in relatively low levels. In these cases only previous reports can help elaborate on whether the effect created is that of addition, synergism, untoward reaction to one or more of the drugs, or some other mechanism. However, if the chemical findings constitute the only positive findings in a case in which a complete autopsy and investigation have been performed, it may be reasonable to conclude that the terminal episode was produced by the chemicals found. However, this conclusion occasionally is not justified.

A further, possibly obvious, factor in the interpretation of blood levels is the likelihood of the analyst determining a pharmacologically inactive metabolite along with a parent drug and thus recording an inaccurate and high test result. While this problem is usually avoided with the newer chromatographic techniques used in toxicologic analysis, many of the traditional visible and ultraviolet spectrophotometric methods are less specific and will yield positive results with certain products of drug biotransformation.

Factors Affecting Blood Concentrations of Drugs

There are many variations of this theme, but in essence it requires an assumption on the part of the toxicologist that there exist for this drug both a well-defined dose-blood concentration relationship and pharmacokinetic constants for its rates of biotransformation and excretion. Any estimate of dosage or of time until death on this basis is at best a gross approximation, and the toxicologist should approach this field of speculation with great caution.

The primary factor determining blood concentration produced by a given amount of most drugs (assuming standardization as to weight of the subject and route of administration) is the rate of drug biotransformation. This is largely controlled genetically and is subject to significant individual variation. For instance, administration of a standard dose of isoniazid to 267 subjects resulted in a very broad distribution pattern of plasma levels of the drug (Figure 27–1). This type of individual variation may be an important cause of idiosyncratic drug reactions, although disease conditions can certainly predispose individuals in these unpredictable responses.

Aside from genetic differences, there are the factors of induction and inhibition of the drug-metabolizing enzymes found in the liver. Many drugs can inhibit the metabolic inactivation of other drugs and thus cause an increased pharmacologic response (Mannering, 1968). Of more practical importance is the phenomenon of enzyme induction, or metabolic tolerance, a condition of accelerated drug biotransformation attributable to chronic administration of the same drug, its analogs, or a nonspecific inducing agent. Among these nonspecific agents are such ubiquitous compounds as phenobarbital and ethanol, which can enhance the biotransformation of many other drugs and endogenous compounds (Mannering, 1968; Rubin and Lieber,

1971). Of special relevance to the forensic toxicologist is ethanol, which is known to induce its own biotransformation (Figure 27–2). This action may serve in part to explain the tolerance of chronic users to large amounts of alcohol, although there is certainly a cellular adaptation vector present as well (Newman, 1941).

The rate of urinary excretion of unchanged drugs may also have an important influence on the establishment of their blood concentrations. Although this may be kept relatively constant under controlled conditions, it is theoretically possible to effect a tenfold change in the rate of clearance of weakly acidic and basic drugs for every unit change of urinary pH (Milne, 1967). This pH-dependent excretion has been demonstrated for a number of psychotropic drugs, including amphetamine (Beckett and Rowland, 1965) and methadone (Baselt and Casarett, 1972).

In certain instances other parameters than blood concentrations may be used to affix the time of survival following a drug overdose. Wright (1955) originally suggested that when death supervenes after the ingestion of a barbiturate, the concentration of the drug is significantly higher in the liver than in the blood. This observation was extended by Curry and Sunshine (1960), who showed that for the majority of cases the liver/blood barbiturate ratio is greater than four when death occurs within five hours of ingestion and less than four when the time interval exceeds five hours.

Other Factors Bearing on Interpretation of Findings

The route of administration of a drug must also be considered in interpreting fatal cases. Most cases of overdosage in the past have in-

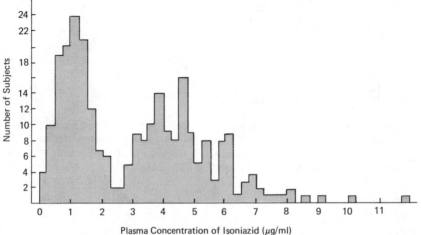

Figure 27–1. Plasma concentrations of isoniazid in 267 human subjects six hours after oral administration of the drug at a dose of 9.8 mg/kg. (From Evans, D. A. P.; Manley, K. A.; and McKusick, V. C.: Genetic control of isoniazid metabolism in man. *Br. Med. J.,* 2:485–91, 1960.)

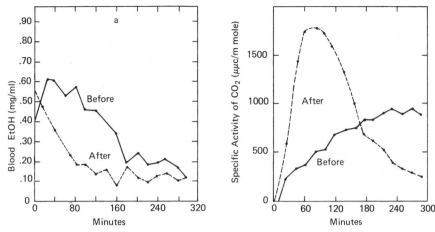

Figure 27–2. Blood alcohol concentations and expiration of $^{14}CO_2$ in a human subject after a test dose of ^{14}C-ethanol, before and after a seven-day period of ethanol administration (3.2 g/kg/day). (From Mendelson, J. H.; Stein, S.; and Mello, N. K.: Effects of experimentally induced intoxication on metabolism of ethanol-l-^{14}C in alcoholic subjects. *Metabolism*, **14**:1255–66, 1965. Reproduced by permission.)

volved administration by the oral, buccal, or inhalation routes, whereas in recent years the parenteral, and especially the intravenous mode has increased in popularity among abusers of narcotics, barbiturates, and amphetamines. Due to the rapidity with which the drug enters the circulation after intravenous administration and the high initial concentrations that are produced, toxic effects may occur that would not be expected after administration of the same dose orally. Additionally, acute allergic responses are more likely to be observed following intravenous administration than by other routes. Therefore, levels in fatal cases due to intravenous injection may be quite low compared with levels found after oral ingestion. Table 27–5 compares amphetamine levels in fatal cases following both routes of administration. A review of further miscellaneous factors that may affect interpretation of toxicologic results is to be found in Gonzales and co-workers (1954).

Table 27–5 TISSUE AMPHETAMINE LEVELS IN FOUR VICTIMS OF FATAL OVERDOSAGE*

ROUTE OF ADMINISTRATION	TISSUE CONCENTRATIONS, μg/g			
	Blood	*Brain*	*Kidney*	*Liver*
Intravenous	1.1	1.6	0.4	0.7
Intravenous	0.1	0.4	1.8	0.8
Intravenous	0.1	0.3	—	0.7
Oral	40.0	144.0	87.0	206.0

* Data from Cravey and Baselt, 1968; Cravey and Reed, 1970.

REFERENCES

Adams, R. F.; Vandemark, F. L.; and Schmidt, G. F.: More sensitive high pressure liquid chromatographic determination of theophylline in serum. *Clin. Chem.*, **22**:1903–06, 1976.

Ahuja, S. A.: Derivativization in gas chromatography. *J. Pharm. Sci.*, **65**:163–81, 1976.

Bailey, D. N.: The role of the laboratory in treatment of the poisoned patient. *J. Anal. Toxicol.*, **7**:136–41, 1983.

Bailey, D. N., and Guba, J. J.: Survey of emergency toxicology screening in a university medical center. *J. Anal. Toxicol.*, **3**:133–36, 1979.

Bailey, D. N., and Manoguererra, A. S.: Survey of drug-abuse patterns and toxicology analysis in an emergency room population. *J. Anal. Toxicol.*, **4**:199–203, 1980.

Barrett, J. M.: An integrated gas chromatographic program to drug screening in serum and urine. *Clin. Chem. Newsletter*, **3**(1):1, 1971.

Baselt, R. C.: *Disposition of Toxic Drugs in Man.* Biomedical Publications, Davis, Calif., 1983.

Baselt, R. C., and Casarett, L. J.: Urinary excretion of methadone in man. *Clin. Pharmacol. Ther.*, **13**:64–71, 1972.

Baselt, R. C., and Cravey, R. H.: A compendium of therapeutic and toxic concentrations of toxicologically significant drugs in human biofluids. *J. Anal. Toxicol.*, **1**:81–103, 1977.

Bastos, M. L.; Jakofsky, D.; and Mulé, S. J.: Routine identification of drugs of abuse in human urine. *J. Chromatogr.*, **81**:93–98, 1973.

Bastos, M. L.; Kananen, G. E.; Young, R. M.; Monforte, J. P.; and Sunshine, I.: Detection of basic organic drugs and their metabolites in urine. *Clin. Chem.*, **16**:931–40, 1970.

Beckett, A. H., and Rowland, M.: Urinary excretion kinetics of amphetamines in man. *J. Pharm. Pharmacol.*, **17**:628–39, 1965.

Bente, H. B.: Nitrogen selective detectors: application to quantitation of antiepileptic drugs. In Pippenger, C. E.; Perry, J. K.; and Kutt, H. (ed.): *Antiepileptic Drugs: Quantitative Analysis and Interpretation.* Raven Press, New York, 1978, pp. 139–45.

Boeckx, R. L.: Therapeutic drug monitoring: the hidden factors. *Lab. Management*, **21**:29–34, 1983.

Brandenberger, H.: Present state and future trends of negative ion M/S in toxicology, forensic and environmental chemistry. Recent devel. in M/S, *Biochem. Med.*, **2**:227–55, 1979.

Brodie, B. R., and Udenfriend, S.: The estimation of basic organic compounds and technique for the appraisal of specificity. *J. Biol. Chem.*, **158**:705–14, 1945.

Broughton, P. M. G.: U.V. method for the determination and identification of barbiturates. *Biochem. J.*, **63**:207–13, 1956.

Burd, J. F.: Substrate-labeled fluorescent immunoassays (SLFIA) for measuring therapeutic drug levels in human serum. *Clin. Chem.*, **25**:1077A, 1979.

Caron, G.; Salmon, J.; and Sheehan, M.: Semi-automated and automated enzyme immunoassays for ethosuximide. *Clin. Chem.*, **29**:1239A, 1983.

Costello, C. E.: Routine use of GC/MS to identify drugs and their metabolites in body fluids. *Clin. Chem.*, **20**:225–67, 1974.

Cross, R. E.; Wojcieszyn, O. A.; Conrad, P.; and Parker, N. C.: Therapeutic drug monitoring: a rapid combined system. *Lab. Management*, **20**:57–63, 1982.

Curry, A. S., and Sunshine, I.: The liver:blood ratio in cases of barbiturate poisoning. *Toxicol. Appl. Pharmacol.*, **2**:602–606, 1960.

Davidow, B.; Petri, N. L.; and Quame, B.: A TLC procedure for identifying drugs of abuse. *Am. J. Clin. Pathol.*, **50**:714–19, 1968.

Deaton, C. D.; Derry, C. K.; and Decker, M. J.: Performances of a nephelometric immunoassay for therapeutic drugs. *Clin. Chem.*, **27**:1091A, 1981.

Dinovo, E. C., and Gottschalk, L. A.: Results of a nine laboratory survey of forensic toxicology proficiency. *Clin. Chem.*, **22**:843–46, 1976.

Done, A. K.: The toxic emergency: asking for laboratory backup. *Emerg. Med.*, **9**:91–98, 1977.

Dubowski, K. M., and Withrow, I. R.: A photometric microdetermination method for ethyl alcohol in biological materials. *Proc. Am. Acad. Forensic Sci.*, **2**:323–36, 1952.

Fensilau, C.: Applications of MS to pharmacological problems. In Chignell, C. F. (ed.): *Methods in Pharmacology*, Vol. 2. Appleton-Century-Crofts, New York, 1972, pp. 401–42.

Fessel, V. A.: Simultaneous or sequential determination of the elements at all concentration levels—the renaissance of an old approach. *Anal. Chem.*, **51**:1290A–1308A, 1979.

Finkle, B. S.; Cherry, E. J.; and Taylor, D. M.: A GLC based system for the detection of poisons, drugs, and human metabolites encountered in forensic toxicology. *J. Chromatogr. Sci.*, **9**:393–419, 1971.

Finkle, B. S.; Foltz, R. L.; and Taylor, D. M.: A comprehensive GC/MS reference data system for toxicological and biomedical purposes. *J. Chromatogr. Sci.*, **12**:304–29, 1974.

Finkle, B. S.; McCloskey, K. L.; and Goodman, L. S.: Diazepam and associated deaths. *JAMA*, **242**:429–34, 1979.

Finkle, B. S.; McCloskey, K. L.; Kiplinger, G. F.; and Bennett, I. F.: A national assessment of propoxyphene in postmortem legal investigation, 1972–1975. *J. Forensic Sci.*, **21**:706–42, 1976.

Finley, P. R.: Rate nephelometric inhibition immunoassay of phenobarbital and phenytoin. *Clin. Chem. News.*, **27**:405–409, 1981.

Geltosky, J. E.: Production of monoclonal antibodies to theophylline for clinical use. *Clin. Chem.*, **29**:1201A, 1983.

Gettler, A. O.: The historical development of toxicology. *J. Forensic Sci.*, **1**:3–25, 1956.

Gettler, A. O., and Sunshine, I.: Colorimetric determination of alkaloids in tissues by means of methyl orange. *Anal. Chem.*, **23**:779–81, 1951.

Goldbaum, L. R.; Williams, M. A.; and Kopanyi, R.: Analytical determination of barbiturates. *Anal. Chem.*, **24**:1600–1604, 1952.

Gonzales, T. A.; Helpern, M.; and Umberger, C.: *Legal Medicine, Pathology and Toxicology*. Appleton-Century-Crofts, New York, 1954.

Hawks, R. L.: *The Analysis of Cannabinoids in Biological Fluids*. NIDA Research Monograph 42, NIDA, Rockville, Md., 1982.

Hepler, B. R.; Sutheimer, C. A.; Sebrosky, G. F.; and Sunshine, I.: Combined enzyme immunoassay-LCEC method for the identification, confirmation and quantitation of opiates in biological fluids. *J. Anal. Toxicol.*, **8**:78–90, 1984.

Hepler, B. R.; Sutheimer, C. A.; and Sunshine, I.: The role of the toxicology laboratory in emergency medicine. *J. Toxicol. Clin. Toxicol.*, **19**:353–65, 1982.

Hunt, C. A., and Jones, R. T.: Tolerance and disposition of THC in man. *J. Pharmacol. Expl. Ther.*, **215**:35–44, 1980.

Ingelfinger, J. A.; Isakson, G.; Shine, D.; Costello, L.; and Goldman, P.: Reliability of the toxic screen in drug overdose. *Clin. Pharmacol. Ther.*, **29**:570–75, 1981.

Jacobzinner, H., and Raybin, H.: Lead poisoning in infancy and young children. *N.Y. State J. Med.*, **79**:72–76, 1962.

Jane, I., and Taylor, T.: Characteristics and quantitation of morphine in urine using high pressure liquid chromatography with fluorescence detection. *J. Chromatogr.*, **109**:37–42, 1975.

Jatlow, P.: UV spectrophotometry for sedative drugs frequently involved in overdose emergencies, In Sunshine, I. (ed.) *Methodology for Analytical Toxicology*, Vol. 1. CRC Press, Boca Raton, Fl., 1975, pp. 414–20.

Kabra, P. M.; Chen. S.-H.; and Marton, L. J.: Liquid chromatographic determination of antidysrhythmic drugs: procainamide, lidocaine, quinidine, disopyramide and propanolol. *Ther. Drug Monit.*, **3**:91–101, 1981.

Kaye, S.: Heavy Metals. In Sunshine, I. (ed.): *Methodology for Analytical Toxicology*, Vol. 1. CRC Press, Boca Raton, Fl., 1975, pp. 395–98.

Kirchner, J. G.: Separation and identification of some terpenes by a new chromatographic technique. *Anal. Chem.*, **23**:420–27, 1951.

Koch-Wiser, J.: Serum drug concentrations in clinical prospective. *Ther. Drug Monit.*, **3**:3–16, 1981.

Kogan, J. D.: Expert testimony. In Baselt, R. L., and Cravey, R. (eds.): *Introduction to Forensic Toxicology*. Biomedical Publications, Davis, Calif., 1981, pp. 247–57.

Kozelka, F. L., and Hine, C. H.: Method for determination of ethyl alcohol for medicolegal purposes. *Ind. Eng. Chem., Anal. Ed.*, **13**:905–907, 1941.

Krall, R. L.; Perry, J. K.; White, B. G.; Kupferberg, H. J.; and Swinyard, E. A.: Antiepileptic drug development. II. Anticonvulsant drug screening. *Epilepsia*, **19**:409–28, 1978.

Kupferberg, H. J.; Burkalter, A.; and Leong-Way, E.: A sensitive fluorometric assay for morphine in plasma and brain. *J. Pharmacol. Exp. Ther.*, **145**:247–51, 1964.

Lundberg, G.: Operations management in emergency toxicology. *J. Anal. Toxicol.*, **7**:152–54, 1983.

Lu-Steffes, M.; Jolley, M.; Pittluck, G.; Panes, H.; Olive, D.; Wang, C. J.; Nystrom, D.; and Strorepe, S.: Fluorescence polarization immunoassays of phenytoin and phenobarbital. *Clin. Chem.*, **27**:1093A, 1981.

Lynch, V.: Training in forensic toxicology. In R. L. Baselt, and Cravey, R. (eds.): *Introduction to Forensic Toxicology*. Biomedical Publications, Davis, Calif., 1981, pp. 275–88.

Mannering, G. J.: Significance of stimulation and inhibition of drug metabolism. In Burger, A. (ed.): *Selected Pharmacological Testing Methods*. Marcel Dekker, Inc., New York, 1968, pp. 51–119.

Marsh, J.: Method for separating small quantities of arsenic. *London Med. Gazette*, 18:650–54, 1836.

Martin, C. R., and Freiser, H.: Ion-selective electrode for the determination of phencyclidine. *Anal. Chem.*, 52:1772, 1980.

McCarron, M. M.: The role of the laboratory in treatment of the poisoned patient: clinical perspective. *J. Anal. Toxicol.*, 7:142–45, 1983a.

McCarron, M. M.: The use of toxicology tests in emergency room diagnosis. *J. Anal. Toxicol.*, 7:131–35, 1983b.

Michaud, J. D., and Jones, D. W.: TLC for broad spectrum drug detection. *Am. Lab.*, 12:104–107, 1980.

Micozzi, M. S.: Psychotropic and anticonvulsent drug monitoring. *Lab. Management*, 20:45–54, 1982.

Mulé, S.: Identification of narcotics, barbiturates, amphetamines, tranquilizers and psychotomimetics in human urine. *J. Chromatogr.*, 39:302–11, 1969.

Nakamura, G. R., and Way, E. L.: Determination of morphine and codeine in postmortem samples. *Anal. Chem.*, 47:775–778, 1975.

National Institute of Drug Abuse: Foltz, R. L.; Fentiman, A. F.; and Foltz, R. B. (eds.): *GC/MS Assay of Abused Drugs in Body Fluids*. National Institute of Drug Abuse, Rockville, Md., 1980.

————: *Drug Use Motivation Differentials in Emergency Room Episodes*. DHHS Publication No. (ADM) 83-1272, Rockville, Md., 1983, p. 9.

Newill, V. A.; Sunshine, I.; Griggs, R. C.; Buchanan, S.; and Herman, W.: Lead poisoning in children. *Med. Sci.*, 13:367–73, 1963.

Newman, H. W.: Acquired tolerance to ethyl alcohol. *Q. J. Stud. Alcohol*, 2:453–63, 1941.

Nicloux, M.: Sur le dosage et la distillation de trace alcohol ethylique. *C. R. Soc. Biol. (Paris)*, 74:267–70, 1913.

Novotny, M.: Microcolumns in liquid chromatography. *Anal. Chem.*, 53:1294A–1308A, 1981.

O'Haver, T. C.: Potential clinical applications of derivative and wavelength modulation spectormetry. *Clin. Chem.*, 25:1548–53, 1981.

Pesh-Iman, M.; Fretthold, D. W.; Sunshine, I.; Kumar, S.; Terrentine, S.; and Willis, C. E.: High pressure liquid chromatography for simultaneous analysis of anticonvulsants: comparison with EMIT system. *Ther. Drug Monit.*, 1:289–299, 1979.

Pippenger, C. E.: Interlaboratory variability in the determination of plasma antiepileptic drug concentrations. *Arch. Neurol.*, 33:351–55, 1976.

Pippenger, C. E.; Kutt, H.; and Perry, J. H.: *Antiepileptic Drugs: Quantitative Analysis and Interpretation*. Raven Press, New York, 1978.

Pippenger, C. E., and Garlock, C. M.: A rapid ultrafiltration technique for the determination of free drug concentration in plasma. *Clin. Chem.*, 25:1117A, 1979.

Reinsch, H.: *J. Prakt. Chem.*, 24:244–47, 1841.

Reynolds, P.: In Sunshine, I. (ed.): *Methodology for Analytical Toxicology*. CRC Press, Boca Raton, Fl., 1975, pp. 143–44.

Rubin, E., and Lieber, C. S.: Alcoholism, alcohol, and drugs. *Science*, 172:1097–1102, 1971.

Rubinstein, K. E.; Schneider, R. S.; and Ullman, E. F.: Homogeneous enzyme immunoassay. *Biochem. Biophys. Res. Commun.*, 47:846–51, 1972.

Schneider, R. S.; Lingquist, P.; Tong-in-Wong, E.; Rubinstein, K. E.; and Ullman, E. F.: Homogeneous immunoassay for opiates in urine. *Clin. Chem.*, 19:821–25, 1973.

Scoggins, B. A.; Maguire, K. P.; Norman, T. R.; and Burrows, G. D.: Measurement of tricyclic antidepressants. Part 1. A review of methodology. *Clin. Chem.*, 26:5–17, 1980.

Siek, T. J.: Identification of drugs and other toxic compounds from UV spectra. *J. Forensic Sci.*, 19:193–208, 1974; 20:18–37, 1975; 21:525–45, 1976.

Skelly, D. S.; Brown, L. P.; and Besch, P. K.: Radioimmunoassay. *Clin. Chem.*, 19:146–86, 1973.

Stahl, E.: Thin layer chromatography. *Pharmazie*, 11:633–37, 1956.

Stephenson, G.: Spectrophotometric determination of blood barbiturates. *Anal. Chem.*, 33:1374–78, 1961.

Stolman, A., and Stewart, C. P.: Isolation and determination of opiates from visera and body fluids by absorption. *Analyst*, 74:536–43, 1949.

Sunderman, Jr., F. W.: Atomic absorption spectrophotometry of trace metals. *Human Pathol.*, 4:549–82, 1973.

Sunshine, I.: Lead in biological materials, In Sunshine, I. (ed.): *Methodology for Analytical Toxicology*. CRC Press, Boca Raton, Fl., 1968, pp. 204–206.

Sunshine, I. (ed.): *Methodology in Analytical Toxicology*, Vol. 1. CRC Press, Boca Raton, Fl., 1975.

Sunshine, I., and Jatlow, P. (eds.): *Methodology in Analytical Toxicology*, Vol. 2. CRC Press, Boca Raton, Fl., 1981.

Sunshine, I.; Fike, W.; and Landesman, H.: Identification of therapeutically significant organic bases by TLC. *J. Forensic Sci.*, 11:428–39, 1966.

Sutheimer, C., and Sunshine, I.: Benzodiazepines by reversed phase HPLC. In Sunshine, I., and Jatlow, P. (eds.): *Methodology in Analytical Toxicology*. CRC Press, Boca Raton, Fl., 1982, pp. 25–30.

Szabo, E., and Sunshine, I.: Analysis of neutral and acidic drugs by gas chromatography and reversed phase high pressure liquid chromatography. In Sunshine, I. and Jatlow, P. (eds.): *Methodology in Analytical Toxicology*. CRC Press, Boca Raton, Fl., 1982, pp. 11–18.

Teitelbaum, D. T.; Morgan, J.; and Gray, G.: Noncordance between clinical impression and laboratory findings in clinical toxicology. *Clin. Toxicol.*, 10:417–22, 1977.

Thompson, W. L.: Poisoning: the twentieth century black death. In Shoemaker, W. C., and Thompson, W. (eds.): *Critical Care*. Society of Critical Care Medicine, Anaheim, Calif., 1980, p. 1.

Tobak, T. W.; Gal, P.; Erkan, V.; Roop, C.; and Robinson, H.: Usefulness of theophylline saliva levels in neonates. *Ther. Drug Monit.*, 5:185–89, 1983.

Trinder, P.: Determination of salicylate in biological materials. *Biochem. J.*, 57:301–303, 1954.

Ullucci, P. A.; Cadoret, B.; Stasiowski, P. D.; and Martin, H. F.: A comprehensive GC/MS drug screening procedure. *J. Anal. Toxicol.*, 2:33–38, 1978.

Umberger, C. J.: In Gonzales, T. A.; Vance, M.; Helpern, M.; and Umberger, C. J. (eds.): *Legal Medicine, Pathology and Toxicology*, 2nd ed. Appleton-Century-Crofts, New York, 1954.

Ungerleider, T. J.; Lundberg, G. M.; Sunshine, I.; and Walberg, C. B.: The drug abuse warning (DAWN) network. *Arch. Gen. Psychiatry*, 37:106–109, 1980.

Vesell, E. S., and Pasananti, G. T.: Utility of clinical chemical determinations of drug concentrations in biological fluids. *Clin. Chem.*, 17:851–66, 1971.

Walberg, C. B.: An ultraviolet spectorphotmetric procedure for differentiation and quantitation of barbiturates. *Clin. Toxicol.*, 18:879–85, 1981.

————: Comprehensive approaches to emergency toxicology. *J. Anal. Toxicol.*, 7:146–48, 1983a.

————: Training of personnel for emergency toxicology. *J. Anal. Toxicol.*, 7:155–57, 1983b.

Walberg, C. B.; Lundberg, G. D.; and Pantlik, V. A.: Emergency hospital toxicology. *J. Chromatogr. Sci.*, 12:225–36, 1974.

Watson, R. A. A.; Landon, J.; Shaw, E. J.; and Smith, D. S.: Polarization fluoroimmunoassay of gentamicin. *Clin. Chim. Acta.,* **73**:51–55, 1976.

Werner, M.: Drug assays vs. formulas. *Med. Lab. Observer,* **14**:55–66, 1982.

Whitney, J. D., and Manders, W. W.: Confirmation of a THC metabolite in urine by GC. *J. Anal. Toxicol.,* **6**:49–52, 1982.

Widmark, E. M. P.: Eine Mikromethode zur bestummung von athylalkohol um blut. *Biochem. Z.,* **131**:473–84, 1922.

Wright, J. T.: The value of barbiturate estimations in the diagnosis and treatment of barbiturate intoxication. *Q. J. Med.,* **24**:95–108, 1955.

Wu Chen, N.; Schaffer, M. I.; Reng-Lang, L.; Kurland, M. L.; Donoghue, E. R.; and Stein, R. J.: The general unknown. I. The systematic approach. *J. Forensic Sci.,* **28**:391–97, 1983.

Yalow, R. S., and Berson, S.: Immunoassay of endogenous plasma insulin in man. *J. Clin. Invest.,* **39**:1157–75, 1960.

Chapter 28

CLINICAL TOXICOLOGY

Barry H. Rumack and Frederick H. Lovejoy, Jr.

INTRODUCTION

Treatment of the poisoned patient based on pharmacologic principles promotes the institution of rational methods most beneficial to recovery. Unfortunately the communication of these principles and methods has not always been appropriate, and some current reference sources still recommend procedures that are antiquated and should be contraindicated.

The material presented in this chapter provides a framework for the approach to the poisoned patient exposed to drugs, chemicals, plants, or other situations that confront the clinical toxicologist. This chapter reviews some of the principles of clinical management, as well as specific current theory and treatment of frequently encountered toxic situations.

TOXICOKINETICS

The basic application of pharmacokinetics to the toxic substance exposure is often useful in monitoring the severity and course of the poisoning and determining therapeutic maneuvers. The ability to calculate a body burden of a drug, its half-life, route of excretion, and other kinetic characteristics will aid in decisions such as use of diuresis, dialysis, or hemoperfusion. However, it must be recognized that most pharmacokinetic data are based on the therapeutic evaluation of drugs, and significant changes in kinetic parameters may occur in overdoses. For example, it is well known that salicylate peak blood levels are prolonged up to six hours from the normal values of one or two hours and that its half-life increases from two to four hours to 25 to 30 hours in significantly overdosed patients (Done, 1960). Theophylline overdose results in a prolongation of serum half-life from three to four hours to ten hours (Gaudreault *et al.*, 1983). Conversely, digoxin half-life may be shortened to one-third its expected value in overdose (Rumack *et al.*, 1974). Thus, it is critical for the clinician to determine that the data on which decisions are to be based are related to overdose rather than therapeutic information.

LD50 and MLD

The LD50 and MLD (median lethal dose) values are considered important to many clinicians in formulating a plan for dealing with the poisoned patient. Unfortunately they are rarely of practical value clinically.

First, these values are obtained from various animal trials that establish a dose that will statistically kill half of a group or some other predetermined number. Differences in biotransformation between humans and animal species are remarkable, and linear correlation or extrapolation of animal biotransformation data to humans is rarely possible.

Second, the clinician obtains a *history* of overdose and attempts to relate the amount ingested by history with the LD50. This disregards factors such as the accuracy of history (which is often accurate less than 50 percent of the time), rate and extent of absorption of agent, biotransformation/disposition of the agent, the clinical response of the patient, and the effect of other drugs simultaneously ingested.

Consequently, the generally accepted recommendation is to disregard LD50 and MLD data on a particular poison and to determine the expected toxicology of the drug followed by appropriate monitoring to determine if the patient demonstrates the predicted clinical findings. The adage "Treat the patient not the *poison*" represents the most basic and important principle in clinical toxicology.

Half-Life

The half-life is a measure of rate for the time required to eliminate one half of a quantity of a chemical in the body. For drugs exhibiting first-order kinetics the half-life can be calculated with the use of the following equation where *Kel* is the elimination rate constant.

$$t_{1/2} = \frac{0.693}{Kel}$$

Clinically it is estimated simply by plotting at least three concentration values of the chemical against time on semilogarithmic paper. Once several values have been plotted, a straight line should be evident, and the amount of time that it takes for the drug concentration to decrease by half from any point on the line can be determined.

The clinical value of determining a patient's half-life during the course of a poisoning is to see the rate at which a patient is approaching therapeutic levels of a drug and whether methods of therapy being employed are effective. For some drugs, half-life values in the overdose situation are prolonged over values seen in normal dose. Therefore, measures to enhance elimination to shorten drug half-life are desirable. With digoxin, however, the $t_{1/2}$ has been reported to be shorter in overdose than in therapeutic situations (Rumack *et al.*, 1974). In such cases supportive rather than elimination-enhancing measures are more practical.

Kinetic Relationships

The volume of distribution is the apparent space in which an agent is distributed following absorption and subsequent distribution in the body. Salicylate is distributed in total body water or about 60 percent of body mass. Digoxin, on the other hand, has an enormous volume of distribution of 500 liters or more in a 70-kg human (approximately 7 liters/kg). Since this is impossible practically, the term *apparent* volume of distribution is utilized. While this is the apparent volume based on the measured value of the drug in the blood, the drug is concentrated or sequestered somewhere out of the blood, i.e., tissue compartments (see Chapter 3).

Some useful mathematic relationships are

$$Vd = \frac{D}{Cp} \qquad Cp = \frac{D}{Vd} \qquad D = Cp \cdot Vd$$

Where Vd = value of distribution
D = dose administered
Cp = plasma concentration (at zero time)

$$Cl = Kel \cdot Vd$$

Where Cl = clearance of drug
Kel = elimination rate constant

$$Kel = \frac{0.693}{t_{1/2}}$$

Thus, if the history is that of a 25-kg child who was estimated to have consumed 500 mg of phenobarbital and the Vd for phenobarbital is approximately 60 percent body weight, then the estimated blood level would be 33.3 μg/ml. This approximates phenobarbital's high therapeutic range.

Example calculations:

25 kg $\times$ 0.60 liters/kg = 15 liters = Vd
500 mg/15 liters = 33.3 mg/liters or 33.3 μg/ml

In this case, the decision would be made clinically that the maximum possible dose by history, assuming total absorption could produce toxicity, and, therefore, the child probably needs to be seen and observed by medical personnel.

MEASURES TO ENHANCE ELIMINATION

Once a patient has been observed clinically to be in a seriously toxic state, then it must be determined whether or not the agent can be eliminated more rapidly, thereby shortening the duration of coma and lessening toxic manifestations. Procedures to enhance elimination are indicated in severely poisoned patients.

Diuresis

The basic principles of diuresis are ion trapping and increasing urine flow. The ion-trapping phenomenon occurs when the pK_a of the agent is such that, after glomerular filtration in the renal tubules, alteration of the pH of the urine can ionize and "trap" the agent. Once the toxin is ionized, then reabsorption from the renal tubules is impaired and the result is that more of the drug is excreted in the urine. Salicylates and phenobarbital elimination is significantly enhanced by forced alkaline diuresis, while phencyclidine, and amphetamine elimination is hastened in an acid urine. Even though a drug's pK_a may indicate that the drug might be successfully eliminated by this method, other factors, such as high lipid solubility and large volume of distribution, may render this method ineffective (see Table 28–1).

For some drugs urine flow rate is important. Normal urine output is 1 to 2 ml/kg/hour. Forced diuresis results in a urine flow rate of 3 to 6 ml/kg/hour. In theory, for drugs whose renal elimination is flow dependent, increasing urine output by the use of fluids or diuretics may enhance drug or toxin elimination. Risks of fluid diuresis include pulmonary edema and cardiac arrhythmias or failure.

Dialysis

The dialysis technique, either peritoneal or hemodialysis, relies on passage of the toxic agent through a semipermeable dialysis membrane so it can equilibrate with the dialysate and subsequently be removed. This is in part dependent on the molecular weight of the compound. Some drugs such as phenobarbital can

Table 28-1. TOXICOKINETIC DATA OF DRUGS AND TOXINS
(NUMBERS EXPRESSED AS A MEAN OR AS A RANGE)

AGENT	pk_a	vd l/kg	THER. $t_{1/2}$ hrs	O.D. $t_{1/2}$ hrs	DIURESIS	DIALYSIS	SPECIFIC THERAPY
Acetaminophen	9.5	0.75	2	4	No	No	N-Acetylcysteine
Amitriptyline	9.4	40+	36	72	No	No	Physostigmine
Amobarbital	7.9	2.4	16	36+	No	No	
Amphetamine	9.8	0.60	8–12	18–24	Acid	Yes	Chlorpromazine
Bromide	—	40+	300	300	Yes	Yes	
Caffeine	13	0.75	3.5	4–120	No	No	
Chloral hydrate	—	0.75	8	10–18	No	No	
Chlorpromazine	9.3	40+	16–24	24–36	No	No	
Codeine	8.2	3	2	2	No	No	Naloxone
Coumadin	5.7	0.1	36–48	36–48	No	No	Vitamin K
Desipramine	10.2	50+	18	72	No	No	Physostigmine
Diazepam	3.3	1–2	36–72	48–144	No	No	
Digoxin	—	7–10	36	13	No	No	Fab antibodies
Diphenhydramine	8.3	—	4–6	4–8	No	No	Physostigmine
Ethanol	—	0.6	2–4	—	No	No	
Ethchlorvynol	8.7	3–4	1–2	36–48	No	No	
Glutethimide	4.5	20–25	8–12	24+	No	No	
Isoniazid	3.5	0.60	2–4	6+	No	Yes	Pyridoxine
Methadone	8.3	6–10	12–18	12–18	No	No	Naloxone
Methicillin	2.8	0.60	2–4	2–4	Yes	Yes	
Pentobarbital	8.11	2.0	10–20	50+	No	No	
Phencyclidine	8.5	—	—	12–48	Acid	Yes	
Phenobarbital	7.4	0.75	36–48	72–120	Alkaline	Yes	
Phenytoin	8.3	0.60	24–30	36–72	No	No	
Quinidine	4.3, 8.4	3	7–8	10	No	No	
Salicylate	3.2	0.1–0.3	2–4	25–30	Alkaline	Yes	
Tetracycline	7.7	3	6–10	6–10	No	No	
Theophylline	0.7	0.46	4.5	6+	No	Yes	

readily cross these membranes and go from high concentrations in plasma to a lower concentration in the dialysate. Since the volume of distribution of phenobarbital is 75 percent of the body weight, there is a reasonable opporrnity for enough drug to be removed from total body burden that the technique is valuable in serious cases. Conversely, drugs with large volumes of distribution would be expected to be poorly dialyzable. Similarly, drugs that are highly serum protein bound are not expected to be well removed by dialysis (see Watanabe, 1977).

Lipid dialysis has been suggested for lipid-soluble drugs (like glutethimide) that do not readily concentrate in aqueous dialysate. Unfortunately, most lipophilic drugs have extremely large volume of distribution, and consequently even with four to six hours of dialysis only a small percentage may be removed (see Table 28-2).

Hemoperfusion

Passing blood through a column of charcoal or adsorbent resin is the newest technique of extracorporeal drug/toxin removal. While some agents are better removed by this technique be-cause of the adsorptive capacity of the column, the volume of distribution of an agent may limit removal in a similar manner to hemodialysis. If the drug is highly tissue bound such as in fat stores and only a small proportion is presented via the blood compartment to a device, then only the proportion that is in blood is available for removal. To date there are few agents that are able to significantly displace toxins from either fat stores or tissue binding, sites. The application of digoxin Fab antibodies in digoxin overdose represents one such chemically useful example (Smith *et al.*, 1982).

APPROACH TO THE POISONED PATIENT

Telephone management of the pediatric patient, especially under the age of five, comprises 85 percent of this patient population's treatment. Epidemiologic data demonstrate that the peak age of ingestion is two years of age, which is consistent with the ambulatory growth and development of children. Most children suffer *ingestion* rather than poisoning with fewer than 1 percent becoming symptomatic. In fact, the

Table 28–2. DRUG TOXIN REMOVAL BY DIALYSIS, INTENSIVE SUPPORTIVE CARE, AND USE OF ACTIVATED CHARCOAL

Dialysis Indicated on Basis of Condition Of Patient

Amphetamines	Meprobamate (Equanil,
Anilines	Miltown)
Antibiotics	Paraldehyde
Boric acid	Phencyclidine
Bromide	Phenobarbital
Calcium	Potassium
Chloral hydrate	Quinidine
Fluorides	Salicylates
Iodides	Strychnine
Isoniazid	Thiocynates

Dialysis Not Indicated Except for Support in the Following Poisons; Therapy Is Intensive Supportive Care

Antidepressants (tricyclic and MAO inhibitors also)
Antihistamines
Chlordiazepoxide (Librium)
Digitalis and related
Diphenoxylate (Lomotil)
Ethchlorvynol (Placidyl)
Glutethimide (Doriden)
Hallucinogens
Heroin and other opiates
Methaqualone (Quaalude)
Noludar (Methyprylon)
Oxazepam (Serax)
Phenothiazines
Synthetic anticholinergics and belladonna
  compounds

Well Adsorbed by Activated Charcoal

Amphetamines	Nicotine
Antimony	Opium
Antipyrene	Oxalates
Atropine	Parathion
Arsenic	Penicillin
Barbiturates	Phenol
Camphor	Phenolphthalein
Cantharides	Phenothiazine
Cocaine	Phosphorus
Digitalis	Potassium permanganate
Glutethimide	Quinine
Iodine	Salicylates
Ipecac	Selenium
Malathion	Silver
Mercuric chloride	Stramonium
Methylene blue	Strychnine
Morphine	Sulfonamides
Muscarine	

major traumatic event associated with a pediatric ingestion is the emesis that results from the therapeutic administration of syrup of ipecac. Poison centers, therefore, have adopted standard protocols for dealing with these childhood accidents so as to preclude missing those that actually become symptomatic (Rumack *et al.,* 1978). In addition, it is prudent for the clinician

to become familiar with the local and regional poison control centers for consultative toxicology services. (Chafee-Bahamon *et al.,* 1983).

Key Steps in Telephone Management

When dealing with a potential ingestion, the history represents the first step in determining the necessity for instituting therapeutic measures. The following represent critical history points and subsequent measures.

1. Telephone number, name, address, age, weight
2. Time of ingestion, route, agent
3. Assessment of severity
4. Assessment of reliability of history
5. Determination of safety of home therapy
6. Instructions in home therapy—emesis, catharsis, charcoal
7. Follow-up
1 hour—Determine success of therapy, usually emesis, and assess condition of patient
4 hours—Determine condition of patient
24 hours—Determine condition of patient, suggest psychiatric services, social services, or visiting nurses service if appropriate. Basically, if the status changes or if it seems that more than these calls need to be made, then the patient should be seen. A rule of thumb in most poison centers is that children under six months of age should be seen or referred to a physician regardless of history. Child abuse should be considered in any repeat poisoning case (Rumack, 1978; Kressel *et al.,* 1982).

Evaluation of the Patient

The decision that determines whether or not the patient should be hospitalized is based on an evaluation of the severity of the potential poisoning. If it is apparent that the patient is in no danger, hospital referral in most cases is not necessary. Poison control center experience indicates that a vast majority of these situations can be appropriately handled at home. However, if it is judged that the patient's life is in immediate or potential danger, the patient should be brought or taken by ambulance to the nearest hospital or emergency room. Initial emergency room contact requires determining if the patient is breathing and/or is in shock with immediate life support instituted as necessary. Clinical evaluation, in addition to the usual physical examination of the poisoned patient, includes several widely used scoring systems for coma, hyperactivity, and withdrawal. They are not only useful to assess the condition of the patient but also as a reminder to check certain key clinical points. They serve as a useful monitoring parameters to follow and to determine if the patient's condition is improving or deteriorating. Finally, they serve as a useful method for quantitating response to therapy. Table 28–3 identifies these scoring methods and criteria.

Emesis

Syrup of ipecac in appropriate doses (30 ml, adult; 10 to 15 ml, pediatric) has been shown to be a safe and effective means of producing emesis (Eason and Lovejoy, 1979). While apomorphine has a more rapid onset of action than ipecac syrup, the average percent recovery of ingested toxin is the same. Apomorphine in ther-

---

Table 28–3. SCORING SYSTEMS FOR COMA, HYPERACTIVITY, AND WITHDRAWAL

Classification of Coma

0   Asleep, but can be aroused and can answer questions.
1   Comatose, does withdraw from painful stimuli, reflexes intact.
2   Comatose, does not withdraw from painful stimuli, most reflexes intact, no respiratory or circulatory depression.
3   Comatose, most or all reflexes are absent but without depression of respiration or circulation
4   Comatose, reflexes absent, respiratory depression with cyanosis, circulatory failure or shock.

Classification of Hyperactivity

1+   Restlessness, irritability, insomnia, tremor, hyperreflexia, sweating, mydriasis, flushing.
2+   Confusion, hyperactivity, hypertension, tachypnea, tachycardia, extrasystoles, sweating, mydriasis, flushing, mild hyperpyrexia.
3+   Dilirium, mania, self-injury, marked hypertension, tachycardia, arrhythmias, hyperpyrexia.
4+   Above plus: convulsions, coma, circulatory collapse.

Classification of Withdrawal

Score the following finding on a 0-, 1-, 2-point basis:

Diarrhea	Hypertension	Restlessness
Dilated pupils	Insomnia	Tachycardia
Gooseflesh	Lacrimation	Yawning
Hyperactive bowel sounds	Muscle cramps	

    1–5, mild
    6–10, moderate
    11–15, severe
Seizures indicate severe withdrawal regardless of the rest of the score.

---

apeutic dose is toxic in children, producing central nervous system depression. This effect may persist past the reversal action of naloxone administered to counteract the toxicity of this emetic. In addition, apomorphine may result in protracted vomiting, which is often unresponsive to narcotic antagonist intervention. Emesis with ipecac syrup or apomorphine 60 minutes after ingestion produces recovery of approximately 30 percent of ingested toxin.

Emesis is generally contraindicated when the patient is comatose, convulsing, or without the gag reflex. Strong acid or base ingestion is another reason for not inducing emesis since this will reexpose the patient's esophagus to these agents, thus contributing to further damage. While petroleum distillate hydrocarbons have been a contraindication in the past, they are no longer considered an absolute contraindication to emesis in many cases (Subcommittee on Accidental Poisoning, 1976).

Lavage

Gastric lavage with a large-bore tube is a rapid and effective way to empty the stomach. While there has been criticism in the past of this technique, most comparative studies were performed with small-bore (16-French) lavage tube. Proper lavage with large (36- to 40-French) tubes utilizing 10 to 20 liters of warm-saline in an adult or 5 to 10 liters of ½N saline in a child is the method of choice to empty the stomach if a contraindication to emesis exists or if the patient is obstructed or comatose (Matthew and Lawson, 1975).

Cathartics

The rationale for the administration of cathartics in the poisoned patient is to hasten the toxin through the gastrointestinal tract, thereby minimizing its absorption. Preliminary controlled data suggest clinical efficacy of cathartic agents. They are indicated in several situations, including ingestion of enteric-coated tablets, when the lag time since ingestion is greater than one hour, and when decreased bowel motility slows passage of the ingested toxin through the gastrointestinal tract. Preferred agents are the saline cathartics (sodium sulfate, magnesium sulfate, citrate, or phosphates), which have a relatively prompt onset of action and lower toxicity than the oil-based cathartics, which have attendant aspiration risks.

Charcoal

The classic paper of Corby and Decker (1970) demonstrates the value of administration of sufficient quantities of charcoal to bind toxin that has not been removed by emesis or lavage.

Although concern has been raised that charcoal cannot "catch up" with drugs and other agents once they have passed through the pylorus, there is ample evidence to show that administration of charcoal-following methods to empty the stomach will result in lower plasma levels than if emesis or lavage alone is used. Concomitant administration of activated charcoal with syrup of ipecac often renders the ipecac ineffective.

Repeated doses of activated charcoal given every four to six hours for three or four doses have found recent use in an effort to interupt hepatoenteric circulation of a drug. Evidence exists for the efficacy of this procedure where hepatic metabolism and biliary excretion of active drug into the small bowel exists (tricyclic antidepressants and digitoxin) (Crome *et al.*, 1977). More recently repetitive activated charcoal given every four hours for 24 to 48 hours has been shown to shorten half-life and enhance clearance of phenobarbital and theophylline when given intravenously. On therapeutic doses to volunteers (Berg *et al.*, 1982), this method of "gastrointestinal dialysis" in experiencing active clinical investigation as well as use in the overdose setting.

Laboratory

Measurement of plasma, urine, or gastric levels of drugs or toxins when done in appropriate relationship to time following ingestion and clinical status can have a significant impact in the clinical management of the poisoned patient. Qualitative screens on blood and urine are helpful to identify ingested toxin(s) while quantiative analyses are useful in determining appropriate therapy with selected toxins (e.g., methanol, iron, acetaminophen). When a toxic screen is requested, the clinician must be aware of which drugs are actually being examined. Too often the clinician interprets a negative toxic screen to mean that there are no toxic agents on board. Interpretation of a patient's levels should be related to the therapeutic levels from the same laboratory. Statements such as "lethal level" are not relevant since toxicologists assume that most patients arriving alive in the emergency department will eventually recover. Specific relationships of blood levels will be presented with each drug discussed in the next sections of this chapter (Curry, 1974).

ACETAMINOPHEN

Acetaminophen has been utilized as an analgesic and antipyretic since the mid-1950s and has become more prominently recognized as a potential hepatotoxin in the overdose situation since the original British reports in the late 1960s (Proudfoot and Wright, 1970). Recent work on the mechanism of liver toxicity of the drug has provided a theoretic basis for therapy (Mitchell *et al.*, 1973).

Acetaminophen in normal individuals is inactivated by sulfation (approximately 52 percent) and by glucuronide conjugation (42 percent). About 2 percent of the drug is excreted unchanged. The remaining 4 percent is biotransformed by the cytochrome P-450 mixed-function oxidase system. This P-450 metabolic process results in a potentially toxic metabolite that is detoxified by conjugation with glutathione and excreted as the mercapturate. Evidence extrapolated from animals indicates that when 70 percent of endogenous hepatic glutathione is consumed, the toxic metabolite becomes available for covalent binding to hepatic cellular components. The ensuing hepatic necrosis would be expected to take place after absorption of 15.8 g of acetaminophen, the amount needed to deplete glutathione in a normal 70-kg human. Other factors may alter this figure. Ingestion of 15.8 g may not produce toxicity if all of the dose is not absorbed, if the history is inaccurate, if the patient has a biotransformation inhibitor on board such as piperonyl butoxide, or if he suffers from anorexia nervosa. On the other hand, patients on long-term biotransformation enhancers (microsomal enzyme inducers) such as phenobarbital may produce more than 4 percent of the toxic metabolite. The range of metabolic response and the difficulty of estimating accurately the amount ingested and absorbed precludes making therapeutic decisions on a historic predictive basis alone (Peterson and Rumack, 1978).

The clinical presentation of these patients is also sufficiently confusing in some cases to make waiting for appearance of symptoms inadequate for diagnosis. The usual patient presents in the following stages:

Stage I—2 to 24 hours
Anorexia, nausea, vomiting
A general feeling of malaise not unlike the common cold or flu.
Stage II—Improvement; the patient begins to feel better—may become hungry and willing to get out of bed. At this same time the SGOT, SGPT, bilirubin, and prothrombin time become abnormal. Right upper quadrant pain may occur.
Stage III—three to five days
Hepatic necrosis with peak abnormalities of hepatic function.
Stage IV—seven to eight days
Return to normal of hepatic functions and general clinical improvement.
Follow-up liver biopsy studies of patients who

have recovered three months to a year after hepatotoxicity have demonstrated no long-term sequelae or chronic toxicity (Clark *et al.*, 1973). A very small percentage (0.25 percent) of patients in the national multiclinic study conducted in Denver may progress to hepatic encephalopathy with subsequent death. The clinical nature of the overdose is one of a sharp peak of SGOT by day 3 and with recovery to less than 100 IU/liter by day 7 or 8. Patients with SGOT levels as high as 20,000 IU/liter have shown complete recovery and no sequelae one week after ingestion (Arena *et al.*, 1978).

Laboratory evaluation of the potentially poisoned patient is crucial in terms of both hepatic measures of toxicity and plasma levels of acetaminophen. Accurate estimation of acetaminophen in the plasma, preferably by high-pressure liquid chromatography or gas chromatography, should be done on samples drawn three to four hours after ingestion when peak plasma levels can be expected. While *p*-aminophenol was once considered an adequate urine screening test, it is no longer indicated for this purpose since acetaminophen does not produce this metabolite in significant measurable quantities.

Once an accurate plasma level is obtained, it should be plotted on the Rumack-Matthew nomogram to determine whether therapy is or is not indicated (see Figure 28–1). This nomogram is based on a series of patients with and without hepatotoxicity and their corresponding blood levels. While half-life was once considered an accurate way to determine potential acetaminophen hepatotoxicity, it is no longer considered adequate since the toxic metabolite comprises only about 4 percent of the total biotransformation. Similarly, back extrapolation of data to the zero-hour axis may not accurately reflect initial levels since the slope of excretion curve does not necessarily reflect hepatic toxicity.

Treatment should be instituted in any patient with a plasma level in the potentially toxic range. Standard support with gastric lavage should be followed by oral administration of *N*-acetylcysteine (Mucomyst). A major national multiclinic open study has demonstrated a protective effect of *N*-acetylcysteine in acetaminophen poisoning when contrasted to controls not receiving antidotal therapy (Rumack *et al.*, 1981). Activated charcoal, unless administered within a few minutes of ingestion, should be avoided because of its potential adsorptive capacity for *N*-acetylcysteine (NAC). Because NAC is most effective if given prior to 16 hours, postingestion patients in whom blood levels cannot be obtained should have NAC treatment instituted and therapy terminated only if levels are nontoxic. The dosing regimen for NAC is a loading dose of 140 mg/kg orally, followed by 70 mg/

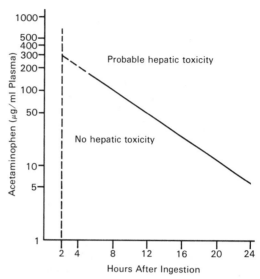

SEMILOGARITHMIC PLOT
OF PLASMA ACETAMINOPHEN LEVELS VS. TIME

Figure 28–1. Rumack-Matthew nomogram for acetaminophen poisoning. Cautions for use of chart: (*1*) The time coordinates refer to time of ingestion. (*2*) Serum levels drawn before four hours may not represent peak levels. (*3*) The graph should be used only in relation to a single acute ingestion. (*4*) A half-life of greater than four hours indicates a high likelihood of significant hepatic injury. (From Rumack, B. H., and Matthew, H.: Acetaminophen poisoning and toxicity. *Pediatrics*, **55**:871, 1975. Copyright American Academy of Pediatrics 1975.)

kg orally for 17 additional doses (Peterson and Rumack, 1977). Methionine has been shown to be less effective than NAC or cysteamine (Prescott *et al.*, 1976).

Children less than 9 to 12 years of age have a lower incidence of hepatotoxicity following overdose than do adults (Rumack, 1984).

Daily SGOT, SGPT, bilirubin, and prothrombin time should be monitored, as well as constructional dyspraxia. Chronic ethanol ingestion is additive in its hepatotoxicity when acetaminophen poisoning is superimposed, while acute ethanol ingestion as a simple ingestion concomitantly with acetaminophen is protective (Rumack, 1981). The same effect occurs in children (Rumack, 1984).

Chronic toxicity is unlikely with acetaminophen because of its lack of accumulative kinetics (Peterson and Rumack, 1978).

ACIDS

Acids such as hydrochloric acid, nitric acid, sulfuric acid, and sodium bisulfate are commonly found around the home in products such as toilet bowl cleaners, automobile batteries, swimming pool cleaning agents, and other such products. Despite the fact that these agents have various degrees of toxicity, even a very small amount (milliliters) can result in serious sequelae that can occasionally progress to death, for example, if the caustic acid agent is aspirated. Clinically, the patient may present with irritation and crying, in association with inability to swallow, pain upon swallowing, mucous membrane burns, circumoral burns, hematemesis, abdominal pain, respiratory distress (secondary to epiglottal edema), shock, and renal failure. Once the patient has been treated through the initial stages of the ingestion, residual sequelae may occur with lesions of the esophagus and gastrointestinal tract that may progress to scarring and strictures. Ingestion of concentrated acids has led to necrosis of esophageal tissue, with death occurring one to five days postingestion.

The use of emetics and lavage are absolutely contraindicated. Dilution or therapy with water or milk immediately following ingestion represents the treatment of choice since these substances do not result in an exothermic chemical reaction. Despite labeling of many acid-containing products, alkaline substances or carbonate preparations are contraindicated since, when administered, they may produce increased amounts of heat and carbonates may form carbon dioxide gas, which presents an unacceptable risk of gastric perforation. In addition, immediate irrigation with copious amounts of water should be instituted to the exposed areas of skin, mucous membranes, and other affected areas. Olive oil is not indicated and may interfere with further therapy. Analgesics, administered by the parenteral route, may be indicated. Development of shock requires appropriate treatment with fluid therapy and pressor agents as indicated. Development of laryngoedema may require placement of an endotracheal tube, and esophagoscopy should be considered in all patients with significant symptoms indicating extensive burn involvement. Acids are more likely to produce gastric burns than esophageal burns. The value of corticosteroid therapy for the prevention of stricture and scar formation with acid burns is unclear at this time.

ALKALIES

Strong alkaline substances are found in such products as Drano, Liquid Plum'r, and Clinitest Tablets, all of which contain compounds such as sodium hypochlorite, sodium hydroxide, or potassium hydroxide. Experience has shown that strongly basic substances such as these are more likely to produce more severe injuries than are seen with acidic caustic ingestions. Recent ex-perience has determined that the chlorinated bleaches, which contain a 3 to 6 percent concentration of sodium hypochlorite, are not as toxic as formerly thought. Following an ingestion of sodium hypochlorite, this compound interacts with the acidic milieu of the stomach, producing hypochlorous acid, which is an irritant to the mucous membranes and skin but does not cause stricture formation. More serious problems are presented following ingestions of compounds such as Drano, which can cause burns of the skin, mucous membranes, and eyes almost immediately on contact. However, the absence of evidence of burns, irritation, erythema, or other such signs in the oral or circumoral area does not necessarily indicate that esophageal injury does not exist (Gaudreault et al., 1983). There have been cases demonstrating the absence of oral involvement with subsequent esophagoscopy proving esophageal burns. Edema of the epiglottis may result in respiratory distress, and inhalation of fumes may result in pulmonary edema or pneumonitis. Shock may occur. Recent experience has shown that "button" batteries, containing concentrated solutions of sodium or potassium hydroxide, represent a serious risk for leakage, corrosion, and perforation when lodged in the esophagus (Litovitz, 1983).

Alkaline caustic exposures require immediate irrigation of the affected areas with large amounts of water. Exposures to the eyes require irrigation for a minimum of 20 to 30 minutes and may require instillation of a local anesthetic to treat the blepharospasm. Oral ingestions require immediate dilution therapy with water or milk. Antiquated antidotes such as vinegar or lemon juice are absolutely contraindicated. Ingestion of chlorinated bleaches does not necessarily require esophagoscopy unless a highly concentrated solution has been ingested or the patient is demonstrating symptoms or signs of esophageal burns. Institution of a three-week course of corticosteroids such as dexamethasone, in a dose of 10 mg initially followed by 1 mg every four hours, is indicated when esophageal burns are demonstrated. Bougienage (passage of a cannula) has been reported to be of some benefit for subsequent dilation of strictures of the esophagus. Antibiotic therapy should be instituted if mediastinitis occurs. Further information on the treatment of alkaline poisoning can be found in the following publications: Leape et al., 1971; Haller et al., 1971; Burrington, 1974; Rumack et al., 1977.

AMPHETAMINE AND RELATED DRUGS

Stimulant drugs such as amphetamine, methylphenidate, and others can produce anxiety, hyperpyrexia, hypertension, and severe

CNS stimulation. A paranoid psychosis is not uncommon, especially as the patient begins to come off the "high." These tablets and capsules are used as "diet" pills even though they are clearly not effective as anorexic agents after two weeks of therapy. Street "speed" or "crystal" may contain in addition to or in lieu of amphetamine such compounds as caffeine, strychnine, or phencyclidine (PCP).

Therapy of the severely agitated patient should be directed toward tranquilization with chlorpromazine and acid diuresis to ion-trap and promote excretion (Espelin and Done, 1968). The dose of chlorpromazine should be 1 mg/kg in pure amphetamine overdose and 0.5 mg/kg if the amphetamine has been mixed with a barbiturate. A major problem with this therapy is the interaction of chlorpromazine with several street drugs such as STP, MDA, or DMT, which may produce dramatic hypotension. If the history is not definitive for amphetamine, then diazepam at 0.1 to 0.3 mg/kg as a starting intravenous dose should be administered.

Acid diuresis may be instituted with sufficient intravenous fluids to produce a urine flow of 3 to 6 ml/kg/hour. Ammonium chloride, at 75 mg/kg/dose administered intravenously four times per day, to a maximum of 6 g total dose per day, may be used. This will produce a urine with a pH range of 4.5 to 5.5. Rhabdomyolysis (myoglobinuria) seen with phencyclidine poisoning is a contraindication to acid diuresis.

ANTICHOLINERGICS

A number of agents may produce anticholinergic toxicity following acute overdose, and these agents include drugs such as antihistamines (e.g., Benadryl, Dramamine, Chlortrimeton), atropine, homatropine, over-the-counter sleeping medications (which contain both antihistamines and belladonna-like agents), and certain plants (e.g., jimsonweed, deadly nightshade) (Mikolich et al., 1975; Rumack et al., 1974; Bryson et al., 1978). Antihistamines are readily available in many common nonprescription products as well as prescription medications. Plants containing belladonna alkaloids such as jimsonweed are frequently used in folk medicine cures for the common cold or as an hallucinogen by thrill seekers. Patients with anticholinergic toxicity may present with atropinic symptoms including dry mouth; thirst; fixed, dilated pupils; flushed face; fever; hot, dry, red skin; and tachycardia. Speech and swallowing may be impaired in association with blurred vision. In infants, particularly those ingesting antihistamines, paradoxic excitement may occur subsequently followed by a more characteristic central nervous depression. Severe overdoses can present with hallucination-like delirium, tremors, convulsions, coma, respiratory failure, or cardiovascular collapse. Potentially fatal doses of most antihistamines have been estimated to be approximately 25 to 30 mg/kg.

Immediate treatment should include instituting emesis, with syrup of ipecac or lavage, followed by administration of activated charcoal and saline cathartics. In ingestions of antihistamines related to the phenothiazines or in massive ingestions, induced emesis may be ineffective. Development of severe symptoms such as convulsions, coma, or hypotension presents an immediate indication for physostigmine therapy in a dose of 0.5 to 2 mg, administered intravenously which can be repeated every 30 minutes as needed (Rumack, 1973). Physostigmine dramatically reverses the central and peripheral signs of anticholinergic toxicity, which are usually not seen with other cholinergic antagonists such as neostigmine because they do not cross the blood-brain barrier and enter the central nervous system (Rumack, 1973). Measures such as forced diuresis and dialysis have not yet been shown to be effective in treating severe anticholinergic poisonings.

BENZODIAZEPINES

Benzodiazepine agents are widely prescribed in the treatment of anxiety and nervousness. In fact, in 1976 and 1977, the no. 1 prescribed drug in the United States was diazepam (Valium). A large number of congeners have been marketed by the pharmaceutical industry with little, if any, significant differences between the agents. Available products include chlordiazepoxide (Librium), clonazepam (Clonopin), flurazepam (Dalmane), lorapezam (Atvian), and oxazepam (Serax). Although their pharmacologic effects do not differ greatly in terms of their clinical application, there are some differences in their major routes of biotransformation, volumes of distribution, and half-lives with respect to their pharmacokinetics in overdose. Chlordiazepoxide and oxazepam have shorter half-life values than the other agents such as diazepam and flurazepam. Following acute overdose, clinical symptoms or manifestations may include sleepiness, which, following larger overdose, can range from stage-zero to stage-one coma. Initially, excitement may be seen as a result of the disinhibition effects of these drugs, which then progresses to central nervous system depression, hypotension, respiratory depression, and coma (Welch et al., 1977). On occasion, anticholinergic symptoms such as dry mouth, tachycardia, dilated pupils, and absent bowel sounds may be seen. Patients who have been receiving or ingesting benzodiazepines on a chronic basis

(40 to 80 mg or more per day for one to two months or more) may exhibit mild to moderate symptoms of withdrawal, with severe withdrawal symptoms seen in patients taking the drug for many months to years. Symptoms may include jitteriness, nervousness, anxiety, agitation, confusion, hallucinations, and seizures. Patients exhibiting withdrawal symptoms should be restarted on benzodiazepine, and slowly withdrawn over a period of several months (Rifkin and Floyd, 1976). In most cases, ingestions of a benzodiazepine agent alone of up to 1.5 g results in only minor toxicity, i.e., CNS depression. Fatality, following oral ingestion, is rare unless a combination of drugs is taken with the benzodiazepine (Greenblatt et al., 1978). Therapeutic levels of diazepam or chlordiazepoxide are reported to be about 0.5 mg/100 ml.

Treatment of benzodiazepam overdose is primarily supportive. Establishment of respiration with assisted ventilation if necessary should be instituted immediately. Emesis should be considered unless the patient is comatose, convulsing, or has lost his gag reflex. If these contraindications exist, the patient may be intubated and lavaged followed by administration of activated charcoal and a saline cathartic such as sodium or magnesium sulfate. Hypotension should be treated initially with fluid. Institution of vasopressor agents should be used only if the patient is unresponsive to other measures. Physostigmine has been reported to be effective in treating diazepam overdose; however, since this type of drug overdose has been associated with only morbidity and essentially no mortality, there is no clinical indication for the use of physostigmine unless the patient has also ingested anticholinergic substances and is demonstrating cardiac arrhythmias or hypertension. Forced diuresis and dialysis are of no value in the treatment of benzodiazepine overdoses.

CYANIDE

Cyanide is commonly found in certain rat and pest poisons, silver and metal polishes, photographic solutions, and fumigating products. Compounds such as potassium cyanide can also be readily purchased from chemical stores. Cyanide is readily absorbed from all routes, including the skin, mucous membranes, and by inhalation, although alkali salts of cyanide are toxic only when ingested. Death may occur with ingestion of even small amounts of sodium or potassium cyanide and can occur within minutes to several hours depending on route of exposure. Inhalation of toxic fumes represents a potentially rapidly fatal type of exposure. Sodium nitroprusside (Smith and Kruszyna, 1974) and apricot

seeds (Sayre and Kaymakcalan, 1964) have also caused cyanide poisoning. A blood cyanide level of greater than 0.2 µg/ml is associated with toxic manifestions. Lethal cases have usually had levels above 1 µg/ml. Clinically, cyanide poisoning is reported to produce a bitter, almond odor on the breath of the patient; however, approximately 20 percent of the population is genetically unable to discern this characteristic odor. Typically, cyanide has a bitter, burning taste, and following poisoning, symptoms of salivation, nausea without vomiting, anxiety, confusion, vertigo, giddiness, lower jaw stiffness, convulsions, opisthotonos, paralysis, coma, cardiac arrhythmias, and transient respiratory stimulation followed by a respiratory failure may occur. Bradycardia is a common finding, but in most cases heartbeat usually outlasts respirations (Wexler et al., 1947). A prolonged expiratory phase is considered to be characteristic of cyanide poisoning.

Artificial respiration with 100 percent oxygen should be started immediately in patients with respiratory difficulty or apnea. Administration of 1 to 2 ampules of amyl nitrite by inhalation to the patient for 15 to 30 seconds every minute should be instituted concurrently while preparing sodium nitrite for intravenous administration (Chen and Rose, 1952). Amyl nitrite has the ability to induce methemoglobin, which has a higher affinity for cyanide than hemoglobin; however, amyl nitrite alone is able to produce only a 5 percent methemoglobin level (Stewart, 1974). The Lilly cyanide kit (Lilly stock no. M76) contains ampules of amyl nitrite, sodium nitrite, and sodium thiosulfate with appropriate instructions. Sodium nitrite, 300 mg intravenously, should be administered to adults to attain a desired methemoglobin level of approximately 25 percent. However, doses this high should not be administered to children, as potentially fatal methemoglobinemia may result (Berlin, 1970). Children weighing less than 25 kg must be dosed on the basis of their hemoglobin levels and weight. In the absence of immediate serum hemoglobin levels, a dose of 10 mg/kg is considered safe (Berlin, 1970). Once intravenous sodium nitrite is administered, sodium thiosulfate should be immediately given. Thiosulfate combines with available cyanide to form thiocyanate, which is then readily excreted in the urine (Stewart, 1974; Chen and Rose, 1952). Oxygen should also be given since it increases the effectiveness of the nitrites and the thiosulfate. Oxygen therapy should be maintained during and after thiosulfate therapy to ensure adequate oxygenation of the blood. A methemoglobin level of greater than 50 percent is an indication for exchange transfusion or administration of blood.

Since cyanide toxicity may reoccur, the patient should be observed for no less than 24 to 48 hours, and reoccurrence is an indication for retreatment with sodium nitrite and sodium thiosulfate in one-half the recommended doses. Some data indicate that the use of cobalt compounds such as hydroxocobalamin or dicobalt edetate (Kelocyanor) may be of value in the treatment of cyanide poisoning (Hillman et al., 1974; Bain and Knowles, 1967; Paulet, 1965; Posner et al., 1976). However, experience in the United States with these compounds is limited due to lack of availability. Further clinical experience is required to evaluate the role of these agents in the treatment of cyanide poisoning.

DIGITALIS GLYCOSIDES

Digitalis glycosides are available in prescription medications as digoxin (Lanoxin) and digitoxin as well as through a number of plant sources (oleander, foxglove). Many ingestions of digitalis occur in infants who inadvertently get into a grandparent's heart medication, although the drug has been used on occasion by persons with suicidal intent. Acute toxic manifestations of the digitalis glycosides represent extensions of the compound's vagal effects. Clinical manifestations seen in the acute overdose include nausea, vomiting, bradycardia, heart block, cardiac arrhythmia, and cardiac arrest. Younger individuals without significant heart disease tend to present with bradycardia and heart block, while other patients may present with ventricular arrhythmias, with or without heart block (Ekins and Watanabe, 1978). While hypokalemia is a frequent hallmark associated with chronic digitalis poisoning, in the acute-overdose situation hyperkalemia is more frequently found. Serum digoxin levels in excess of 5 μg/liter (ng/ml) are often seen.

Emesis or lavage is indicated followed by administration of activated charcoal with saline cathartics. Potassium administration is contraindicated unless there is documented hypokalemia since potassium administration with unsuspected concurrent digitalis-induced hyperkalemia in the overdose situation may result in heart block progressing to sinus arrest. Patients should be monitored by ECG and antiarrhythmics instituted for the treatment of arrhythmias. Phenytoin (Dilantin) is considered to be the antiarrhythmic of choice for ventricular arrhythmia (Rumack et al., 1974), while atropine has been shown to be useful in the treatment of severe bradycardia. Pacemaker therapy may be required in refractory cases. The use of resin-binding agents such as cholestyramine (Cuemid, Questran) or colestipol has been recommended to minimize absorption of cardiac glycosides as well as to interrupt enterohepatic circulation of these compounds. A recent advance in the treatment of digitalis poisoning is the use of Fab fragments for digoxin's specific antibodies (Lloyd and Smith, 1978). Preliminary clinical experience with this method is not available and suggests its efficacy for digoxin and digitoxin overdose (Smith et al., 1982).

ETHANOL

Excessive consumption of ethanol produces a depressed state that may be additive if other depressants such as sedatives, hypnotics, or tranquilizers have also been consumed. The following tabulation summarizes clinical findings at various blood levels.

BLOOD ETHANOL

50–150 mg/100 ml:	Incoordination, slow reaction time, and blurred vision
150–300 mg/100 ml:	Visual impairment, staggering, and slurred speech; marked hypoglycemia, especially in children
300–500 mg/100 ml:	Marked incoordination, stupor, hypoglycemia, and convulsion
500 mg and over/100 ml:	Coma and death, except in tolerant individuals (Lambecier et al., 1968).

One patient who was reported to exhibit a peak level of 780 mg/100 ml was capable of holding a normal conversation at 520 mg/100 ml and related a history of chronic alcoholism (Hammond et al., 1973). Hypoglycemia occurring as ethanol levels are falling is a complication of ethanol poisoning in children.

Absorption of ethanol from the gastrointestinal tract is rapid, particularly in the fasting state with peak blood levels attained within 30 to 60 minutes after ingestion. Metabolism in adults will eliminate 7 to 11 g of ethanol per hour, which is equivalent to ½ to 1 oz of 50-proof beverage per hour. A rule of thumb is that 1 ml of absolute ethanol per kilogram of body weight results in a level of 100 mg/100 ml in one hour (Elbel, 1956). Although ethanol is considered to be biotransformed according to zero-order kinetics (Wilkinson et al., 1976), some patients at high levels have been found to have ethanol metabolism demonstrating first-order kinetics (Hammond et al., 1973).

Treatment of ethanol overdose consists of intensive supportive care. Attention must be directed toward hypoglycemia and ketoacidosis.

Chronic alcoholics may experience delirium tremens. During ethanol withdrawal, conservative management and benzodiazepines or other sedatives can adequately control these symptoms and prevent convulsions. Dialysis is rarely indicated unless the patient is unable to dispose of the ethanol because of hepatic or renal failure.

HYDROCARBONS-PETROLEUM DISTILLATES

Hydrocarbons or petroleum distillates are available in a wide variety of forms, including motor oil, gasoline, kerosene, red seal oil, and furniture polish, and in combination with other chemicals as a vehicle or solvent. The toxicity of hydrocarbons is generally indirectly proportional to the agent's viscosity, with products having high viscosity (150 to 250) such as heavy greases and oils considered to have only limited toxicity. Products with viscosity in the 30 to 35 range or lower present an extreme aspiration risk and include such agents as mineral seal oil, which is found in furniture polishes. It is important to realize that even small amounts of a low-viscosity material, once aspirated, can involve a significant portion of the lung and produce a chemical pneumonitis. Oral ingestion of hydrocarbons is often associated with symptoms of mucous membrane irritation, vomiting, and CNS depression. Cyanosis, tachycardia, and tachypnea may appear as a result of aspiration, with subsequent development of chemical pneumonitis. Other clinical findings include albuminuria, hematuria, hepatic enzyme derangement, and cardiac arrhythmias. Doses as low as 10 ml orally have been reported to be potentially fatal, while other cases have survived ingesting 60 ml of petroleum distillates (Rumack, 1977). A history that presents with coughing or choking in association with vomiting strongly suggests aspiration and hydrocarbon pneumonia. Hydrocarbon pneumonia is an acute hemorrhagic necrotizing disease that can develop within 24 hours of the ingestion. Pneumonia may require several weeks for complete resolution.

Although controversial, emesis is indicated in some hydrocarbon ingestions, where absorption may produce systemic effects. Agents such as asphalt, tar, heavy lubricants, Vaseline®, and mineral oil are considered to be relatively nontoxic and do not require removal. Chlorinated hydrocarbon solvents, gasoline, kerosene, or any hydrocarbon or petroleum distillate with a potentially dangerous additive (camphor, pesticide, heavy metals) should be considered for vomiting. Petroleum naphtha and mineral seal oil (or signal oil) as found in furniture polish or oil polishes produce severe and prolonged chemical pneumonitis. (Rumack, 1977). These compounds are maximally absorbed from the stomach and, if absorbed, produce mild CNS toxicity (Bratton and Haddow, 1975). Saline cathartics such as magnesium or sodium sulfate should be administered and are preferable to oil-based cathartics. Oil administration may result in a higher incidence of pneumonia (Beaman et al., 1976). Gastric lavage is not indicated for hydrocarbon ingestion due to the risk of aspiration should the patient vomit around the lavage tube (Ng, 1974). X-rays taken early in the course of ingestion may not demonstrate chemical pneumonia and, even if demonstrated, the clinical severity does not correlate will with the degree of x-ray findings. However, x-rays should be repeated on follow-up to detect development of pneumonitis or demonstrate pneumatoceles (Bergson, 1975). Patients who arrive coughing probably already have aspirated and should be monitored closely for development of pneumonitis. The decision for hospitalization should be based on clinical criteria (e.g., cyanosis, respiratory distress) rather than on x-ray findings alone (Anas et al., 1981). Steroid therapy may be harmful (Marks et al., 1972; Brown et al., 1974). Antibiotics, oxygen, and positive end-expiratory pressure should be instituted as indicated (Rumack, 1977, 1978; Steele et al., 1972).

INSECTICIDES

Chlorinated Hydrocarbons

Chlorinated hydrocarbon insecticides are stable lipophilic chemicals and are usually contained in various organic solvents or as petroleum distillates. Often the petroleum distillates or organic solvents used as vehicles for the chemicals are as toxic as the pesticides themselves and, in the event of a significant ingestion, the vehicle toxicity should be considered as well (i.e., hydrocarbon pneumonitis). Many of the chlorinated hydrocarbon insecticides are rapidly absorbed and produce central nervous system toxicity. Because of the halogenated nature of these organic compounds, hepatoxicity, renal toxicity, and mycardial toxicity may also occur. Examples of chlorinated hydrocarbons include chlordane, DDT, dieldrin, Kepone, lindane, toxaphene, and paradichlorobenzene. Clinical manifestations following ingestion include apprehension, agitation, vomiting, gastrointestinal upset, abdominal pain, and CNS depression. Convulsions may occur at higher doses and may be preceded by symptoms of ataxia, muscle spasms, and fasciculations.

In cases of ingestion, emesis is indicated unless the patient is comatose, convulsing, or has lost the gag reflex. Emesis should be followed by administration of activated charcoal and saline cathartics. Oil-based cathartics such as castor oil or other substances including fats or oils should be avoided since these compounds may tend to enhance the absorption of the chlorinated hydrocarbon from the gastrointestinal tract. Epinephrine is contraindicated since it may induce ventricular fibrillation due to the sensitization effects of the myocardium by the chlorinated hydrocarbons. Convulsions may be treated with diazepam in a dose of 0.1 mg/kg, administered intravenously, to a maximum of 10 mg. Methods to enhance elimination have not been successful other than as a supportive measure for hepatic and renal failure. Cholestyramine, which has been shown to bind chlordecone (Kepone) in the intestinal tract, may offer a means to treat chronic Kepone poisoning and, pending further study, may have application to other agents (Boylan *et al.*, 1978).

Organophosphates

Organophosphate insecticides such as diazinon, malathion, parathion, TEPP, and DFP are potent cholinesterase enzyme inhibitors that act by interfering with the metabolism of acetylcholine, which results in accumulation of acetylcholine at neuroreceptor transmission sites. Exposure produces a broad spectrum of clinical effects indicative of massive overstimulation of the chlorinergic system, including muscarinic effects (parasympathetic), nicotinic effects (sympathetic and motor), and CNS effects (Namba, 1971). These effects present clinically as feelings of headache, weakness, dizziness, blurred vision, psychosis, respiratory difficulty, paralysis, convulsions, and coma. Typical findings are given by the mnemonic "SLUD," which stands for salivation, lacrimation, urination, and defecation. A small percentage of patients may fail to demonstrate miosis, a classic diagnostic hallmark (Mann, 1967). Onset of clinical manifestation of organophosphate poisoning usually occurs within 12 hours of exposure. Measurement of red cell cholinesterase is usually diagnostic; when there is a reduction to 50 percent or less of control values this indicates significant poisoning and is an indication for institution of 2-PAM (Protopam, pralidoxime), a cholinesterase-regenerating agent. Efforts must be made to ensure that the patient does not become reexposed through such means as contaminated clothing or reexposure to the contaminated environment. Decontamination may be achieved by using soap washings followed by alcohol-soap washings using tincture of green soap. Rescuers and medical personnel should

also be protected from contamination by use of rubber gloves and aprons.

Maintaining adequate respiratory function should be the first treatment measure taken. In cases of ingestion, emesis is indicated unless the patient is comatose, convulsing, or has lost the gag reflex. This should be followed by administration of activated charcoal and sodium or magnesium sulfate as a cathartic. Atropine is the drug of first choice (especially in patients with respiratory problems) and should be administered until signs of atropinism occur, i.e., dry mouth, tachycardia. In some cases, large doses (up to 2 g of atropine) may be required in order to reverse cholinergic excess. The presence of significant cholinesterase depression in red blood cells requires treatment with 2-PAM in conjunction with atropine. In an adult a dose of 1 g intravenously administered at a rate of 500 mg/minute should be given and repeated every 8 to 12 hours. After administration of three doses of 2-PAM, the drug is not likely to be of any additional benefit. The pediatric dose is 250 mg/dose administered slowly by the intravenous route and repeated every 8 to 12 hours. The use of aminophylline/theophylline, succinylcholine, physostigmine, and morphine is contraindicated.

Carbamates

Carbamate insecticides include agents such as aminocarb, carbaryl (Sevin), and landrin. These insecticides are reversible inhibitors of cholinesterase, whose actions are often enhanced by formulating them with pyrethrin or piperonyl butoxide. Clinical manifestations are those seen with cholinesterase inhibition but may not be identical to the signs and symptoms seen with organophosphate poisoning. However, with carbamate exposure the degree of toxicity is considered less severe due to the rapid reversal of the cholinesterase inhibition. Symptoms such as headache, blurred vision, weakness, sweating, myosis, chest pain or tightness, salivation, lacrimation, nausea, vomiting, urination, abdominal cramps, and diarrhea may occur. More severe exposure may result in muscle cramps, fasciculations, pulmonary edema, areflexia, and convulsions. Blood cholinesterase activity can be measured but may not show significant depression unless blood samples are drawn and assayed immediately due to rapid cholinesterase regeneration. Atropine in large doses for maintenance of airway and respiration is the treatment of choice, dosed initially at 2 mg intravenously in an adult and 0.05 mg/kg intravenously in a child, with the drug repeated at five- to ten-minute intervals if needed. The patient should be thoroughly decontaminated and other measures instituted to prevent absorption. Again care must be exercised to protect rescuers and medical personnel from exposure. 2-PAM is usually not needed due to the rapid regeneration of cholinesterase and is considered to be contraindicated in certain carbamate poisonings, e.g., carbaryl. Data for this contraindication are questionable.

IRON

Iron is available in a wide variety of preparations including iron supplement tablets (ferrous sulfate, ferrous gluconate, ferrous fumarate), multiple-vitamin preparations, and prenatal vitamin preparations. As described on the labels of these preparations, the amount of iron given may be calculated in terms of a milligram amount of the salt form (e.g., ferrous sulfate 300 mg or ferrous gluconate 320 mg) or by the actual amount of elemental iron. It is important to note that iron toxicity relates to the amount of *elemental* iron and, therefore, for the salt forms the actual elemental iron content must be calculated.

SALT FORM	% ELEMENTAL IRON
Ferrous fumarate	33
Ferrous gluconate	12
Ferrous sulfate (exsiccated)	30
Ferrous sulfate	20

Clinically, there are generally five phases of toxicity subsequent to ingestion of iron (Jacobs *et al.*, 1965). The first phase lasts from 30 minutes to two hours after ingestion and may be characterized by symptoms of lethargy, restlessness, hematemesis, abdominal pain, and bloody diarrhea. Necrosis of the gastrointestinal mucosa is a result of the direct corrosive effect of iron on tissue and may result in severe hemorrhagic necrosis with development of shock. Iron absorbed through intact mucosa may also cause shock. The second phase presents as an apparent recovery period, which then progresses into the third phase. This third phase occurs 2 to 12 hours after the first phase and is characterized by the onset of shock, metabolic acidosis, cyanosis, and fever. Acidosis results from the release of hydrogen ion from the conversion of ferric (Fe + 3) to ferrous (Fe + 2) ion forms and accumulation of lactic and citric acids. The fourth phase occurs two to four days after ingestion and is sometimes characterized by the development of hepatic necrosis, which is thought to be due to a direct toxic action of iron on mitochondia. The fifth phase occurs from two to four weeks after ingestion and is characterized

by gastrointestinal obstruction, which is secondary to gastric or pyloric scarring and healed tissue. Oral ingestion of iron is a potentially fatal occurrence, and ingestions of over 30 mg/kg body weight should be considered for hospital admission for observation depending on clinical symptoms and findings (Stein *et al.*, 1976). Qualitative methods for determining the injestion of iron include: (a) a consistent history and physical examination, (b) a positive abdominal x-ray for iron tablets, and (c) a semiquantitative color change demonstrable when gastric aspirate containing iron is mixed with deferoxamine (McGuigan *et al.*, 1979). Quantitative methods used in iron overdose include: (a) a white blood cell count of greater than 15,000 or a blood sugar greater than 150 mg/dl obtained within six hours of injestion (Lacouture *et al.*, 1981), (b) a positive urinary deferoxamine challenge (excretion of a very rose color), and (c) an elevated serum iron level (Lacouture *et al.*, 1981).

Emesis or lavage with a large-bore tube is indicated. Abdominal x-rays may reveal full tablets or tablet fragments in the gastrointestinal fract since they are radiopaque. Fleet phosphate enema solution is the preferred lavage solution since when given orally and diluted in a 1:4 concentration this will result in the formation of a nonabsorbable iron phosphate complex. However, excessive use (more than 60 ml) of the enema solution may result in hypernatremia, hyperphosatemia, and hypokalemia. The use of deferoxamine is considered somewhat controversial since this drug may induce severe hypotension following oral doses. When used, the dose is 2 to 10 g of deferoxamine dissolved in 25 ml of lavage fluid followed by a second dose of 50 percent of the initial dose in four hours and a similar third dose in 8 to 12 hours. If free iron is present in serum, or if the patient is exhibiting shock, or coma, or if the serum iron is greater than 350 mcg/ml intravenously, deferoxamine should be administered at a rate not to exceed 15 mg/kg/hour for eight hours followed by 5 mg/kg/hour if needed (Stein *et al.*, 1976; Lovejoy, 1982). If the patient is not in shock, deferoxamine may be administered intramuscularly (20 mg/kg every four to six hours), depending on the clinical condition. Shock with dehydration should be treated with appropriate fluid therapy (Robertson, 1971).

LOMOTIL

Lomotil is a frequently prescribed antidiarrheal preparation that contains 2.5 mg of the narcotic diphenoxylate and 0.025 mg of atropine per tablet or 5 ml of liquid. The atropine is allegedly included in the dosage form to discourage abuse since the dose per tablet or teaspoon is essentially homeopathic. However, in the overdose situation, the clinical picture is often a mixture of that seen for narcotics and atropine overdosage, with early findings primarily due to atropine toxicity. The atropinic symptoms seen may include flushing, lethargy, hyperpyrexia, tachycardia, urinary retention, reduced bowel motility, and hallucinations. Mydriasis, although expected, is often not seen due to the overriding narcotic effects of diphenoxylate, and thus pinpoint pupils are noted. Cyclic coma has been seen in some cases and is probably due to changes in gastrointestinal motility with subsequent absorption of the drug (Snyder *et al.,* 1973). In many cases, there may be a delay in the onset of toxicity and/or coma of up to 6 to 12 hours even in the face of appropriate initial therapy such as emesis and activated charcoal. Patients, particularly pediatric patients, should be monitored for a minimum of 12 to 24 hours, depending on the history of the ingestion (Rumack and Temple, 1974; Rosenstein *et al.,* 1973).

Establishment of respiratory support as necessary and measures to prevent absorption should be instituted immediately. If the patient is comatose or convulsing, endotracheal intubation should be instituted followed by gastric lavage and administration of activated charcoal and saline cathartics. Forced diuresis does not enhance the elimination of diphenoxalate (Rumack and Temple, 1974) and fluid should be administered cautiously to avoid pulmonary or cerebral edema. Naloxone in a dose of 0.03 mg/kg administered intravenously is the drug of choice, and it should be administered at frequent intervals in order to maintain a therapeutic effect since the duration of naloxone's effect is less than that of the opiate. In some cases, up to 11 to 13 doses of Narcan have been administered in order to reverse opiate effects (Rumack and Temple, 1974). Physostigmine is rarely needed because signs of atropine poisoning are generally mild.

MERCURY

Mercury in its various forms is available widely in the forms of metallic mercury (thermometers, Miller-Abbot tubes, fungicides, all hearing aid and watch batteries, paints, mercurial drugs, and antiquated cathartics and ointments). Poisoning may occur from either chronic or acute exposure to such agents or through the food chain (Eyl, 1971; Teitelbaum and Ott, 1969). Toxicity of the mercury is primarily related to its form (see Chapter 19) since metallic mercury is relatively nontoxic unless it is converted to an ionized form, such as occurs

on exposure to acids or strong oxidants. In general, the mercuric salts are more soluble and produce more serious poisoning than do the mercurous salts (Goldwater, 1957; Shoemaker, 1957). Inorganic forms of mercury are corrosive and produce symptoms of metallic taste, burning, irritation, salivation, vomiting, diarrhea, upper gastrointestinal tract edema, abdominal pain, and hemorrhage. These effects are seen acutely and may subside with subsequent lower gastrointestinal ulceration (Goldwater, 1957). Large ingestions of the mercurial salts may produce kidney damage, which may present with nephrosis, oliguria, and anuria. Ingestion of organic mercurials such as ethylmercury may produce symptoms of nausea, vomiting, abdominal pain, and diarrhea, but in most cases the main toxicity is neurologic involvement presenting with paresthesias, visual disturbances, mental disturbances, hallucinations, ataxia, hearing defects, stupor, coma, and death. Symptoms may occur for several weeks after exposure. Exposure and poisoning can occur following ingestion of mercury-contaminated seafood, grains, or inhalation of vaporized organomercurials. Chronic inorganic mercury poisoning may occur following repeated environmental exposure and may present with a neurologic syndrome often described as the "mad hatter syndrome."

Therapy should be initiated with emesis or lavage followed by administration of activated charcoal and a saline cathartic. Milk may be administered to help precipitate the mercury compound. Blood and urine levels of mercury may be of value in determining the indication of administration of chelating agents such as D-pencillamine or dimercaprol (BAL) (Kark, 1971). D-Penicillamine is administered in a dose of 250 mg orally four times a day in adults, 100 mg/kg/day in children, to a maximum recommended dose of 1 g per day for three to ten days with continuous monitoring of mercury urinary excretion. In patients who cannot tolerate penicillamine, BAL can be administered in a dose of 3 to 5 mg/kg/dose every four hours by deep intramuscular injection for the first two days followed by 2.5 to 3 mg/kg/dose intramuscularly every six hours for two days followed by 2.5 to 3 mg/kg/dose every 12 hours intramuscularly for one week. Adverse reactions associated with BAL administration such as urticaria can often be controlled with antihistamines such as diphenhydramine. The development of renal failure contraindicates penicillamine therapy since the kidney is the main route of renal excretion for penicillin. BAL therapy can be used cautiously in spite of renal failure since BAL is excreted in the bile; however, BAL toxicity, which consists of fever, rash, hypertension, and CNS stimulation, must be closely monitored. Dialysis does not remove either chelated or free mercury metal (Robillard *et al.*, 1976).

NARCOTIC OPIATES

Narcotic overdose may occur in a number of different situations, such as in the newborn infant, in addition to drug addiction. Accidental or intentional overdoses frequently involve Lomotil, Darvon, Talwin, morphine, or dextromethorphan. Acute overdoses of any narcotic drug may result in respiratory arrest and coma with an initial clinical presentation of pinpoint pupils, hypertension, bradycardia, and respiratory depression, urinary retention, muscle spasm, and itching. Propoxyphene overdose has been associated with convulsions (Lovejoy *et al.*, 1974). Other signs such as leukocytosis, hyperpyrexia, and pulmonary edema may occur, particularly in drug abusers injecting street drugs intravenously. Ingestions of methadone or propoxyphene may have a prolonged or protracted clinical course lasting 24 to 48 hours or more (Lovejoy *et al.*, 1974). Chronic narcotic use is often associated with skin abscesses, cellulitis, endocarditis, myoglobinuria, cardiac arrhythmias, tetanus, and thrombophlebitis. Lomotil ingestion is frequently complicated by the presence of atropine in the proprietary dosage forms with a resultant mixed picture of narcotic and anticholinergic symptoms (Rumack and Temple, 1974).

Emesis or lavage should always be performed since delayed gastric emptying is common following narcotic ingestions (Rumack and Temple, 1974). Emesis can be induced in the alert patient; however, if seizures or coma exist, intubation and gastric lavage with a large-bore (28-French or larger) Ewald tube should be carried out. Activated charcoal, five or ten times the estimated weight of ingested drug (minimum of 10 g), as well as a nonabsorbable saline cathartic (sodium sulfate or magnesium sulfate, 250 mg/kg of body weight) should be instilled following emesis or lavage. The cathartic should be repeated every three to four hours until stooling has occurred. Other basic supportive measures should be provided as needed. Naloxone at a dose of 0.03 mg/kg in the child or 1.2 mg in the adolescent or adult intravenously is the drug of choice for all narcotic ingestions including pentazocine and propoxyphene as well as methadone, morphine, and codeine (Martin, 1976). In some cases doses of naloxone as high as 0.1 mg/kg in the child or 2 to 4 mg in the adolescent or adult may be required for those failing to respond to the initial dose, and there is little evidence that such doses of naloxone are associated with any ill effects (Moore *et al.*, 1980). Due to the short duration of action of naloxone (60 to 90 minutes) (Evans *et al.*, 1974), repeated doses of naloxone may be necessary until the narcotic is biotransformed particularly in the treatment of methadone overdoses (Aranol *et al.*, 1972; Frand *et al.*, 1972; Lovejoy *et al.*, 1974). In some cases of narcotic overdose, up to 20 mg of naloxone may be required (Moore *et al.*, 1980). Other narcotic antagonists such as nalorphine (Nalline) and levallorphan (Lorfan) possess narcotic antagonistic effects, i.e., respiratory depressant effects (Foldes *et al.*, 1969), and are no longer recommended.

PHENCYCLIDINE (PCP)

Phencyclidine, which is commonly called PCP, was originally developed as an anesthetic for humans but was abandoned due to its postoperative side effects, i.e., hallucinations and agitation. It is now legally available as a verterinary medication for use as an animal tranquilizer. It is also known by various street names: angel dust, dust, embalming fluid, elephant or horse tranquilizer, killer weed, super weed, monkey dust, peace pill, rocket fuel, and hog. It is frequently sold as THC (tetrahydrocannabinol), but may appear also as mescaline, psilocybin, LSD, amphetamine, and cocaine. It is closely related to the anesthetic ketamine (Ketalar), and both agents produce what has been called disassociative anesthesia. Due to the availability and ease of manufacture, there has been an increased use of PCP, particularly in the teenage population where it is ingested orally, smoked, or snorted. Intravenous use is less common but on occasion has been reported. Clinical manifestations from phencyclidine use include symptoms of excitation with marked paranoid or aggressive behavior, which is frequently characterized as self-destructive. Characteristically, miosis, nystagmus, both horizontal and vertical, is noted in association with ataxia, impaired speech, bizarre behavior, tachycardia, hypertension that may progress to later stages of hypotension, increased reflexes, seizures, respiratory depression, and coma (Bolter, 1970; Linden *et al.*, 1975; Tong *et al.*, 1975). The sensations that the user may feel subsequent to PCP ingestion are feelings of depersonalization, distortion of body image, a sense of distance and estrangement from the environment in association with time expansion, and slowed body movements. Phencyclidine can be analyzed in serum, urine, and gastric contents.

Initial management of phencyclidine ingestion requires isolation of the patient from all sensory stimuli such as noise, lights, and touch (Stein, 1973). Provision of a quiet, supportive, and non-threatening environment may help reduction of psychotomimetic effects from bad trips. Therapy by talking the patient down with continual verbal reassurance in many cases may be all that is required. Extremely agitated or convulsing patients should be protected from self-inflicted harm and given diazepam intravenously in 2- to 3-mg increments. In severe cases with hypotension, PCP should be treated with use of plasma expanders before vasopressors are attempted. Diazoxide has been used with good success in hypertensive crisis secondary to phencyclidine (Eastman and Cohen, 1975). Gastric lavage or gastric dialysis has been suggested to be of benefit in capturing PCP excreted into the stomach. Acidification of the urine in association with forced diuresis may hasten renal elimination of phencyclidine (Done et al., 1977). Myoglobinuria is a contraindication to the use of acid diuresis.

PHENOTHIAZINES

The phenothiazine class of antipsychotic agents includes a broad class of drugs with similar therapeutic effects. Individual agents depending on the class of phenothiazine (aliphatic, piperidine, or piperazine) differ primarily in their milligram potencies and their tendencies to produce extrapyramidal symptoms, sedation, and hypotension. Agents such as fluphenazine (Prolixin) and trifluoperazine (Stelazine) have a high tendency to produce extrapyramidal effects, while chlorpromazine (Thorazine) and thioridazine (Mellaril) have a lesser tendency to produce extrapyramidal effects but a higher tendency to produce sedation and hypotension. Two other classes of antipsychotic drugs that are nonphenothiazine-related include butyrophenones such as haloperidol (Haldol) and the thioxanthine class such as chlorprothixene (Taractane) and thiothixene (Navane). These non-phenothiazine-class drugs have a higher tendency to produce extrapyramidal symptoms over sedation and hypotension. These drugs possess significant anticholinergic, alpha-adrenergic blocking, quinidine-like, and extrapyramidal ·effects. In addition, phenothiazines also lower the seizure threshold (Logothetis, 1967). Overdose with these drugs may result in CNS depression, which can present initially with reduced activity, emotional quieting, and affective indifference, although such patients may also exhibit a period of agitation, hyperactivity, or convulsions prior to the depressed state (Hollister, 1966). Hyperthermia or hypothermia may develop due to phenothiazine's effects on the

temperature-regulating mechanisms at the hypothalamus. Tachycardia with hypotension as a result of anticholinergic and alpha-blocking effects may occur. In addition, widening of the QRS complex due to the "quinidine-like" effect of these drugs can occur and may result in ventricular tachycardia. Extrapyramidal symptoms, present as torticollis, stiffening of the body, spasticity, impaired speech, and opisthotonos, may occur (Gupta et al., 1967). These symptoms may frequently occur in children who have been administered prochlorperazine (Compazine) in the treatment of nausea and vomiting.

Emesis or lavage is indicated, followed by administration of activated charcoal and a saline cathartic. Phenothiazines are radiopaque, and unabsorbed drug in the form of full or partial tablets may be visualized in the gastrointestinal tract by abdominal x-ray (Barry et al., 1973). Development of convulsions should be treated with intravenous diazepam in a dose of 0.1 to 3 mg/kg in pediatric patients and 5 to 10 mg in an adult. Hypotension requires the use of a pure alpha agonist such as norepinephrine (levarterenol or Levophed) since administration of epinephrine may cause hypotension. Dialysis is ineffective in removing phenothiazine since these drugs are highly tissue bound. Cardiac arrhythmias may respond to the use of phenytoin (Dilantin) or lidocaine; in patients with refractory arrhythmias a cardiac pacemaker may be required. Extrapyramidal reactions are usually adequately treated by the use of intravenous diphenhydramine (Benadryl) in a dose of 1 to 2 mg/kg (Gupta et al., 1967; Davies 1970). Hypothermia or hyperthermia should be treated appropriately. Drugs that can potentiate the depressant effect on phenothiazine, such as barbiturates, sedatives, alcohol, narcotics, and anesthetics, are best avoided.

SALICYLATES

Accidental or intentional ingestion of salicylates by children and adults continues to represent a major poisoning problem due to the high incidence of use of these compounds, their widespread availability, their numerous proprietary and nonproprietary products and preparations, and their mass promotion through advertising media. Most salicylate poisonings involve the use of aspirin or acetylsalicylic acid, although other serious salicylate exposures may result from such compounds as oil of wintergreen (methylsalicylate). Generally, ingestion of doses larger than 150 mg/kg (or 70 mg/lb) can produce toxic symptoms such as tinnitus, nausea, and vomiting. Serious toxicity can be seen with ingestions greater than 400 mg/kg (approximately 180 mg/lb), with severe vomiting, hyperventilation, hyperthermia, confusion, coma, convulsions, hyper- or hypoglycemia, and acid-base disturbances such as respiratory alkalosis or metabolic acidosis (Gabow et al., 1978; Pierce, 1974). In severe cases, the clinical course may progress to pulmonary edema, hemorrhage, acute renal failure, or death (Anderson et al., 1976). It is important to note that the salicylate-overdoses patient can progress to a more serious condition over time as additional drug is absorbed from the gastrointestinal tract. Chronic salicylism presents clinically in a similar fashion to the acute situation, although it is often associated with a higher morbidity and mortality as well as more pronounced hyperventilation, dehydration, coma, seizures, and acidosis (Gaudreault et al., 1982). Although acute overdoses may be associated with salicylate levels of 25 to 35 mg/100 ml or more, chronic salicylism can result in death at lower salicylate levels, i.e., as low as 10 to 15 mg/100 ml. It is important to remember that the kinetics of salicylates are dose dependent, and at higher serum concentrations of salicylate the drug's half-life may be prolonged, i.e., 15 to 30 hours. The Done nomogram (Figure 28–2) can be utilized as an aid in interpreting a given salicylate level as long as the blood sample was not drawn prior to six hours after ingestion. In addition, the Done nomogram is not useful in cases of chronic salicylism. Salicylates are exceptionally sensitive to pH changes, with resulting ionization changes having a pronounced effect on disposition in the body. Acidosis, which is a common finding in acute salicylate overdose, can result in a larger percentage of the drug distributing into the central nervous system. Similarly, alkalinization of the urine results in ion trapping of salicylate in the kidney tubule, causing greater urinary excretion (Hill, 1973).

Emesis should be initiated unless the patient is comatose, convulsing, or has lost the gag reflex. If these contraindications exist, intubation should proceed with gastric lavage, using a large-bore tube such as a 36 French. Subsequently, activated charcoal should be administered followed by saline cathartics to hasten the elimination of any unabsorbed drugs through the gastrointestinal tract. Alkalinization of the urine can result in a tenfold increase in a drug's excretion by increasing urinary pH from 6.5 to 7.5. Hypokalemia secondary to respiratory alkalosis induced by salicylate poisoning should be corrected, since this condition may make alkalinization of urine difficult.

Acetazolamide (Diamox) is not indicated for urine alkalization since this drug may contribute to metabolic acidosis. Hemodialysis, peritoneal dialysis, exchange transfusion, and hemoperfu-

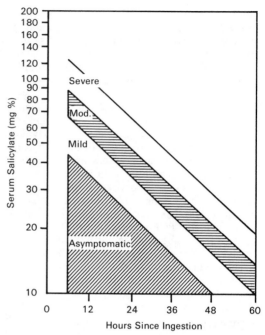

Figure 28–2. Done nomogram for salicylate poisoning. Cautions for use of chart: (*1*) The patient has taken a single acute ingestion and is not suffering from chronic toxicity. (*2*) The blood level to be plotted on the nomogram was drawn six hours after *ingestion*. (*3*) Levels in the toxic range drawn before six hours should be treated. (*4*) Levels in the nontoxic range drawn before six hours should be repeated to see if the level is increasing. (From Done, A. K.: *Pediatrics,* 26:805, 1960. Copyright American Academy of Pediatrics, 1960.)

sion can be effective in removing salicylate from blood compartments but are indicated in only the most severe cases or when alkalinization of the urine is ineffective or contraindicated. Adequate fluid therapy should be instituted to prevent dehydration and to correct electrolyte imbalances. Systemic acidosis should be corrected promptly with sodium bicarbonate. Should hemorrhagic complications in association with a prolonged prothrombin time occur, vitamin K_1 or phytonadione is indicated. It is important to note that salicylate may cause coagulation defects due to platelet effects that will not be responsive to vitamin K administration (Pierce, 1974). The patient's serum electrolytes, renal function, and cardiac status should be monitored. If hyperpyrexia occurs, appropriate treatment measures should be instituted (Hill, 1973).

SEDATIVE-HYPNOTICS

Sedative hypnotics include a wide range of pharmacologic agents used in the treatment of anxiety, nervousness, and sleep disorders. The most widely known agents are the barbiturates (short acting and long acting), benzodiazopines, chloral hydrate, ethchlorvynol (Placidyl), meprobamate (Miltown), methyprylon (Noludar), glutethimide (Doriden), and methaqualone (Quaalude). These agents have the propensity following chronic overuse or abuse to cause physical addiction, and the possibility of physical withdrawal symptoms should be considered in the treatment of patients overdosed on sedative-hypnotics. Table 28–4 compares some of the different pharmacokinetic properties of the more commonly used agents. Patients presenting with sedative-hypnotic overdose may manifest symptoms of confusion, poor coordination, ataxia, respiratory distress, apnea, and coma. Barbiturate overdose cases may present characteristically with "barb burns" on clear vesicular bullous skin lesions appearing on the hands, buttocks, and between the knees (Groschel et al., 1970). Glutethimide may present with a clinical course characterized by an unusually prolonged coma or cyclic coma with periods of alternating unconsciousness and wakefulness (Decker et al., 1970). Much of the severity of this drug's toxicity is related to its biotransformation to and accumulation of a metabolite, 4-hydroxyglutethimide, that has a long half-life and is twice as potent as the parent drug (Hansen et al., 1975). Gastric drug mass or drug bezoar formation has been reported, particularly in association with sedative-hypnotic agents that are poorly soluble in water (Schwartz, 1976). In such cases, gastrotomy has been required to surgically remove drug bezoars.

In the vast majority of sedative-hypnotic overdoses, conservative treatment represents the most successful approach to managing such patients. If the patient is conscious, vomiting may be indicated, although in many cases gastric lavage followed by administration of activated charcoal and saline cathartics is required to terminate the exposure. Maintaining a patent airway, providing adequate ventilation, and control of hypotension and other supportive measures are the mainstays of therapy. In some cases, such as with phenobarbital, forced alkaline diuresis has been shown to be of benefit to hasten elimination of the drug. For lipid-soluble drugs such as glutethimide, methaqualone, and ethchlorvynol, dialysis procedures have not been shown to be effective. Some data suggest that meprobamate may be adequately treated in severe cases with the use of diuresis and/or dialysis, while chloral hydrate may be significantly removed by hemodialysis (Stalker et al., 1978). Analeptics or other stimulants (e.g., caffeine) have never been shown to be of any value and are therefore contraindicated. In sedative-hypnotic overdose, patients may develop pulmonary edema or shock that should be treated appropriately.

TRICYCLIC ANTIDEPRESSANTS

The tricyclic antidepressants are available in a wide variety of brands, including amitriptyline (Elavil), doxepin (Sinequan), and imipramine (Tofranil), and in combination with phenothiazine drugs in Triavil and Etrafon. Tricyclic antidepressants have three primary pharmacologic actions, including anticholinergic effects, reuptake blockade of catecholamines at the adrenergic neuronal site, and quinidine-like effects on the cardiac tissue. The newer tricyclic depressants, such as amoxapine, have a significantly higher incidence of seizures and lower incidence of cardiac arrhythmias than the older tricyclic antidepressants. Tricyclic antidepressant overdose represents a life-threatening episode. Initial symptoms seen are those of central nervous system depression with manifestations of lethargy, disorientation, ataxia, respiratory depression, hypothermia, and agitation. Severe toxicity may be associated with hallucinations, deep tendon reflex loss, muscle twitching, coma, and convulsions. Anticholinergic or atropinic effects of these drugs include dry mouth, hyperpyrexia, dilated pupils, urinary retention, tachycardia, and reduced gastrointestinal motility, which may result in marked delay of the onset of symptoms but also allows for the institution of emesis and lavage long after ingestion to still be effective. Life-threatening sequelae of the tricyclic antidepressants are the cardiovascular effects, resulting in cardiac arrhythmias such as supraventricular tachycardia, premature ventricular contractions, ventricular tachycardia, ventricular flutter, and ventricular fibrillation that progresses to hypotension and shock. The electrocardiogram characteristically demonstrates prolonged PR interval, widening of the QRS complex, QT prolongation, T-wave flattening or inversion, ST segment depression, and varying degrees of heart block progressing to cardiac standstill (Tobis and Das, 1976). Widening of the QRS complex has been reported to correlate well with the severity of the toxicity following acute overdose ingestions (Biggs et al., 1977). Widening of the QRS complex past 100 milliseconds or greater within the first 24 hours is an indication of severe toxicity.

Emesis and lavage are indicated as appropriate, followed by administration of activated charcoal and a saline cathartic such as sodium or magnesium sulfate. Patients admitted with tricyclic antidepressant overdose but without symptoms should be monitored for a minimum of six hours to detect any possible delayed symptom onset. Vital signs and the electrocardiogram

Table 28–4. SEDATIVE HYPNOTICS

DRUG	vd (% BODY WEIGHT)	PROTEIN BINDING, (%)	pKₐ	PEAK CONCERN TIME, (hr)	$t_{1/2}$, (hr)	THERAPEUTIC BLOOD LEVEL	MAJOR ROUTE OF ELIMINATION	DIURESIS	DIALYSIS	HEMO-PERFUSION
Long-acting barbiturates										
Phenobarbital	75	20	7.41	1–6	48–96 (overdose)	10–20 μg/ml	20–40% excreted unchanged; remainder biotransformed	Alkaline	Yes	Yes
Short-acting barbiturates										
Pentobarbital	200–300	30	8.1	0.5–2	36	50 μg/ml	Biotransformed	No	No	No
Secobarbital	200–300	45	7.9	0.5–2	24					
Benzodiazepines										
Diazepam	100–200	90			25–30	<0.5 mg/100 ml	Biotransformed to active	No	No	Yes
Chlordiazepoxide	25	90			7–15					
Chloral hydrate	25	40–80 for trichlor-ethanol	6.8		6–9	10–15 μg/ml	Biotransformed metabolite	No	No	Yes
Ethchlorvynol	600	50	8.7	1	100 (overdose)	<100 μg	Biotransformed	No	No	No
Glutethimide	—	—	4.52	—	40 (overdose)	—	Biotransformed to active metabolite	No	No	?
Meprobamate	75	10–20	9.2	1–2	8	<4 mg/100 ml	Biotransformed with 25–50% excreted unchanged	Yes	Yes	Yes
Methyprylon	>100	?	7.1	½–1	3–6	<1 mg/100 ml	Biotransformed	No	No	?
Methaqualone	100–200	?	—	1–4	2–3	<2 mg/100 ml	Biotransformed	No	?	Yes

Wexler, J.; Whittenberger, J. L.; and Dumke, P. R.: The effect of cyanide on the electrocardiogram of man. *Am. Heart J.*, **34**:163–73, 1947.

should be monitored for 48 hours in symptomatic patients since fatal cardiac arrhythmias have occurred late in the course. Hypotension should be treated with fluids and a vasopressor such as levarterenol (Levophed) administered as needed. The development of severe hallucinations, hypertension, and sinus tachycardia is an indication for physostigmine use, administered intravenously in adults in a therapeutic trial of 2 mg slowly followed by 1 to 2 mg. For pediatric patients that trial dose is 0.5 mg, administered slowly by the intravenous route, followed by the lowest total effective trial (Rumack, 1973). Physostigmine should be administered with caution in the presence of asthma, gangrene, cardiovascular disease, and mechanical obstructions of the gastrointestinal or urogenital tract. Adjustment of blood pH with bicarbonate to pH 7.45, coupled with appropriate antiarrhythmia drugs (lidocaine, phenytoin, etc.), is the primary approach to therapy of cardiac arrhythmias. Arrhythmias other than sinus tachycardia, as well as seizures and hypotension, are poorly responsive to physostigmine. Seizures are responsive to phenytoin, diazepam, or barbiturates (Bigger et al., 1977).

REFERENCES

Anas, N.; Namasonthi, V.; and Ginsburg, C. M.: Criteria for hospitalizing children who have ingested products containing hydrocarbons. *JAMA*, **246**:840–43, 1981.

Anderson, R. J.; Potts, D. E.; Gabow, P. A.; Rumack, B. H.; and Schrier, R. W.: Unrecognized adult salicylate intoxication. *Ann. Intern. Med.*, **85**:745–48, 1976.

Arena, J. M.; Rourke, M. H.; and Sibrach, C. D.: Acetaminophen: report of an unusual poisoning. *Pediartrics*, **61**:68–72, 1978.

Aronow, R.; Shashi, D. P.; and Wooley, P. V.: Childhood poisoning and unfortunate consequences of methadone availability. *JAMA*, **219**:321–24, 1972.

Bain, J. T. B., and Knowles, E. L.: Successful treatment of cyanide poisoning, *Br. Med. J.*, **2**:763, 1967.

Baldochin, B. J., and Melmed, R. N.: Clinical and therapeutic aspects of kerosene poisoning: a series of 200 cases. *Br. Med. J.*, **2**:28–30, 1964.

Barry, D.; Meyskens, F. L., Jr.; and Becker, C. E.: Phenothiazine poisoning: a review of 48 cases. *Cal. Med.*, **118**:1, 1973.

Beamon, R.; Seigel, C.; and Landers, G.: Hydrocarbon ingestion in children: a six year retrospective study. *JACEP*, **5**:771–75, 1976.

Berg, M. J.; Berlinger, W. G.; Goldberg, M. J.; Spector, R. and Johnson, G. F.: Acceleration of the body clearance of phenobarbital by oral activated charcoal. *N. Eng. J. Med.*, **307**:642–43, 1982.

Bergson, F.: Pneumatocoeles following hydrocarbon ingestion. *Am. J. Dis. Child.*, **129**:49–54, 1975.

Berlin, C. M., Jr.: The treatment of cyanide poisoning in children. *Pediatrics*, **46**:793, 1970.

Bigger, J. T.: Is physostigmine effective for cardiac toxicity of tricyclic antidepressant drugs? *JAMA*, **273**:1311, 1977.

———: Tricyclic antidepressant overdose: incidence of symptoms, *JAMA*, **238**:135–38, 1977.

Bolter, A.: Phencyclidine (PCP) abuse. *West. J. Med.*, **127**:80, 1970.

Boylan, J. L.; Egle, J. L.; and Guzelian, P. D.: Cholestyramine: use as a new therapeutic approach forchlordecone (Kepone) poisoning. *Science*, **199**:893–95, 1978.

Brown, J.; Burke, B.; and DaJanias, C.: Experimental kerosene pneumonia: evaluation of some therapeutic regimens. *J. Pediatr.*, **84**:396–401, 1974.

Bryson, P. D.; Watanabe, A. S.; Rumack, B. H., and Murphy, R. C.: Burdock root tea poisoning: case report involving a commercial preparation. *JAMA*, **239**:2157, 1978.

Burrington, J. P.: Clinitest burns of the esophagus. *Ann. Thorac. Surg.*, **20**:400, 1974.

Chafee-Bahamon, C., and Lovejoy, F. H., Jr.: The effectiveness of a regional poison center in reducing excess emergency room visits for children's poisonings. *Pediatrics*, **73**:164–69, 1983.

Chen, K. K., and Rose, C. L.: Nitrite and thiosulfate therapy in cyanide poisoning. *JAMA*, **149**:113, 1952.

Clark, R.; Borirakchanyavat, V.; Davidson, A. R.; Thompson, R. P. H.; Widdop, B.; Goulding, R.; and Williams, R.: Hepatic damage and death from overdose of paracetamal. *Lancet*, **1**:66, 1973.

Clemmesen, C., and Nilsson, E.: Therapeutic trends in the treatment of barbiturate poisoning: the Scandinavian method. *Clin. Pharmacol. Ther.*, **2**:220–29, 1961.

Corby, D. G., and Decker, W. J.: Activated charcoal for sedative overdosage. *Pediatr. Clin. North. Am.*, **17**:620, 1970.

Crome, P.; Dawling, S.; Braitwaite, R. A.; Masters, J.; and Walkey, R.: Effect of activated charcoal on absorption of nortriptyline. *Lancet*, **2**:1203–1205, 1979.

Curry, A. S.: *The Poisoned Patient: The Role of the Laboratory.* Elsevier, Amsterdam, 1974.

Davies, D. M.: Treatment of drug-induced dyskinesias. *Lancet*, **1**:567, 1970.

Decker, W. J.: Gluthethimide rebound. *Lancet*, **1**:778, 1970.

Done, A. K.; Aronow, R., and Miceli, J. N.: Pharmacokinetic observation in the treatment of phencyclidine poisoning. In Rumack, B. H., and Temple, A. R. (eds.): *Management of the Poisoned Patient.* Science Press, Princeton, N.J., 1977.

Eason, J. M., and Lovejoy, F. H., Jr.: Efficacy and safety of gastrointestinal decontamination in the treatment of oral poisoning. *Pediatr. Clin. North Am.*, **26**:827–36, 1979.

Eastman, J. W., and Cohen, S. N.: Hypertensive crisis and death associated with phencyclidine poisoning. *JAMA*, **231**:270–71, 1975.

Ekins, B. R., and Watanabe, A. S.: Acute digoxin poisoning: review of therapy. *Am. J. Hosp. Pharm.*, **35**:268–77, 1978.

Elbel, H., and Schleyer, F.: In *Blutalkatal: Die Wissenschaftlichen Grudlagen der Beruteilung von Blutalkoholbefunden bei Strassenverke-Msdelkien Stuttgart.* Georg Thieme, Heidelberg, 1956, p. 226.

Espelin, D. E., and Done, A. K.: Amphetamine poisoning: effectiveness of chlorpromazine. *N. Engl J. Med.*, **278**:1361–65, 1968.

Evans, J. M.; Hogg, M. I. J.; Lynn, J. N.; and Rosen, M.: Degree and duration of reversal by naloxone of effects of morphine in conscious subjects. *Br. Med. J.*, **2**:589–91, 1974.

Eyl, T. B.: Organic-mercury food poisoning. *N. Engl. J. Med.*, **284**:706, 1971.

Fischer, D. S.; Parkman, R., and Finch, S. C.: Acute iron poisoning in children. *JAMA*, **218**:1179–84, 1971.

Foldes, F. F.; Duncalf, D., and Kuwabara, S.: The respiratory, circulatory, and narcotic antagonistic effects of nalorphine, levallorphan, and naloxone in anesthetized subjects. *Can. Anaesth. Soc. J.*, **16**:151–61, 1969.

Frand, U. I.; Chang, S. S.; and Williams, M. H., Jr.: Methadone induced pulmonary edema. *Ann. Intern. Med.*, **76**:975–79, 1972.

Gabow, P. A.; Anderson, R. J.; and Potts, D. E.: Acid-based disturbances in the salicylate-intoxicated adult. *Arch. Intern. Med.*, **138**:1481–84, 1978.

Gaudreault, P.; Temple, A. R.; and Lovejoy, F. H., Jr.: The relative severity of acute versus chronic salicylate poisoning in children. *Pediatrics*, **70**:566–69, 1982.

Gaudreault, P.; Wason, S.; and Lovejoy, F. H., Jr.: Acute theophylline overdose: a summary of 28 cases. *J. Pediatr.*, **102**:474–76, 1983.

Gaudreault, P.; Parent, M.; McGuigan, M. A.; Chicoine, L., and Lovejoy F. H., Jr.: Predictability of esophageal injury from signs and symptoms: a study of caustic ingestion in 378 children. *Pediatrics*, **71**:767–70, 1983.

Ginsburg, C. M.: Lomotil intoxication. *Am. J. Dis. Child.*, **925**:241–42, 1973.

Greenblatt, D. J.: Rapid recovery from massive diazepan overdose. *JAMA*, **240**:872–74, 1978.

Groschel, D.; Gerstein, A. R.; and Rosenbaum, J. M.: Skin lesions as a diagnostic aid in barbiturate poisoning, *N. Engl. J. Med.*, **403**:409–10, 1970.

Gupta, J. M., and Lovejoy F. H., Jr.: Acute phenothiazine toxicity in children. *Pediatrics*, **71**:890–94, 1967.

Haller, J. A., Jr.: Pathophysiology and management of acute corrosive burns of the esophagus. *J. Pediatr. Surg.*, **6**:578, 1971.

Hammond, R. B; Rumack, B. H.; and Rodgerson, D. O.: Blood ethanol: a report of unusually high levels in a living patient. *JAMA*, **226**:63–64, 1973.

Hansen, A. R.; Kennedy, K. A.; Ambre, J. J.; and Fischer, L. J.: Glutethimide poisoning—a metabolite contributes to morbidity and mortality. *N. Engl. J. Med.*, **292**:250–52, 1975.

Hill, J. B.: Salicylate intoxication. *N. Engl. J. Med.*, **2–8**:1110, 1113, 1973.

Hillman, B.; Bardham, K. D.; and Bain, J. T. B.: The use of dicobalt edetate (Kelocyanor) in cyanide poisoning. *Postgrad. Med. J.*, **50**:171–74, 1974.

Jacobs, J.; Greene, H.; and Gendel, B. R.: Acute ironintoxication. *N. Engl. J. Med.*, **273**:1124–27, 1965.

Kark, R. A. P.: Mercury poisoning and its treatment with N-acetyl-D,L-penicillamine. *N. Engl. J. Med.*, **285**:1, 1971.

Kressel, J. J.; Lovejoy, F. H., Jr.; Boyle, W. E., and Easom, J. M.: Comparison of two child resistant containers. *Clin. Toxicol.*, **19**(4):377–84, 1982.

Lacouture, P. G.; Wason, S.; Temple, A. R.; Wallace, D. K.; and Lovejoy, F. H., Jr.: Emergency assessment of severity in iron overdose. *J. Pediatr.*, **99**:89–91, 1981.

Lambecier, M. R., and DuPan, R. M.: L'intoxication alcoolique aigue et les accidents d'automobile. *Schweiz. Med. Wochenschr.*, **76**:395–98, 421–28, 1968.

Leape, L. L.; Ashcraft, K. W.; Scarpelli, D. G.; and Holder, T. M.: Hazards to your health, liquid lye. *N. Engl. J. Med.*, **284**:578–84, 1971.

Linden, C. B.; Lovejoy, F. H., Jr.; and Costello, C.: Phencyclidine. *JAMA*, **234**:513–16, 1975.

Litovitz, T. L.: Button battery intestions. *JAMA*, **249**:2495, 1983.

Lloyd, B. L., and Smith, T. W.: Contrasting rates of reversal of digoxin toxicity by digoxin specific IgG and Fab fragments. *Circulation*, **58**:280–83, 1978.

Logothetis, J.: Spontaneous epileptic seizures and EEG changes in the course of phenothiazine therapy. *Neurology*, **17**:869–77, 1967.

Lovejoy, F. H., Jr.: Chelation therapy in iron poisoning. *Clin. Toxicol.*, **19**:871–74, 1982.

Lovejoy, F. H., Jr.; Mitchel, A. A.; and Goldman, P.: Management of propoxyphene poisoning. *J. Pediatr.*, **85**:98–100, 1974.

Lovejoy, F. H., Jr.; Lee, K. D.; and Haddow, J. E.: Childhood methadone intoxication, *Clin. Pediatr.*, **13**:36–38, 1974.

Mann, J. B.: Diagnostic aids in organophosphate poisoning. *Ann. Intern. Med.*, **67**:905–906, 1967.

Marks, M. I.; Chicoine, L.; and Legere, G.: Adrenocorticosteroid treatment of hydrocarbon pneumonia in children—a cooperative study. *J. Pediatr.*, **81**:366–69, 1972.

Martin, W. R.: Naloxone. *Ann. Intern. Med.*, **85**:765, 1976.

Matthew, H., and Lawson, A. A.: *Treatment of Common Acute Poisoning*, 3rd ed. Livingston, London, 1975.

McGuigan, M.; Lovejoy, F. H., Jr.; Marino, S.; Propper, R. D.; and Goldman, P.: Qualitative deferoxamine test for iron ingestion. *J. Pediatr.*, **94**:940–42, 1979.

Mikolich, J. R.; Paulson, G. W.; and Cross, C. J.: Acute anticholinergic syndromes due to jimson weed ingestion. *Ann. Intern. Med.*, **83**:321, 1975.

Mitchell, J. R.; Jollow, D. J.; Potter, W. Z.; Davis, D. C.; Gillette, J. R.; and Brodie, B. B.: Acetaminophen induced hepatic necrosis. *J. Pharmacol. Exp. Ther.*, **187**:185, 1973.

Moore, R. A.; Rumack, B. H.; Conner, C. S.; and Peterson, R. G.: Naloxone: underdosage after narcotic poisoning. *Am. J. Dis. Child.*, **134**:156–58, 1980.

Namba, T.: Poisoning due to organophosphate insecsticides: acute and chronic manifestations. *Am. J. Med.*, **50**:475–92, 1971.

Ng, R.; Darwich, H.; and Stewart, D. A.: Emergency treatment of petroleum distillate and turpentine ingestion. *CMA Journal*, **111**:538, 1974.

Paulet, G.: Intoxication cyanhydrique et chelater de cobalt. *J. Physiol. Path. Gen.*, **50**:438, 1958.

Peterson, R. G., and Rumack, B. H.: Treating acute acetaminophen poisoning with acetylcysteine. *JAMA*, **237**:2406–2407, 1977.

Pierce, A. W.: Salicylate poisoning. *Pediatrics*, **54**:342–47, 1974.

Posner, M. A.; Tobey, R. E.; and McElroy, H.: Hydraoxocobalamine therapy of cyanide intoxication in guinea pigs. *Anesthesiology*, **44**:157, 1976.

Prescott, L. E.; Sutherland, G. R.; and Park, J.: Cysteamine, methionine and penicillamine in the treatment of paracetamol poisoning. *Lancet*, **2**:109–13, 1976.

Proudfoot, A. T., and Wright, N.: Acute paracetamol poisoning. *Br. Med. J.*, **2**:557, 1970.

Rifkin, A.; Quitkin, F.; and Klein, D. F.: Withdrawal reaction to diazepan. *JAMA*, **236**:2172–73, 1976.

Robertson, W. O.: Treatment of acute iron poisoning. *Mod. Treat.*, **8**:552–60, 1971.

Robillard, J. E.; Rames, L. K.; Jensen, R. L.; and Roberts, R. J.: Peritoneal dialysis in mercurial-diuretic intoxication. *J. Pediatr.*, **88**:79–81, 1976.

Rosenstein, G.; Freeman, M.; Standard, A. L.; and Westen, N.: Warning: the use of Lomotil in children. *Pediatrics*, **51**:132–34, 1973.

Rumack, B. H.: Anticholinergic poisonings: treatment with physostigmine. *Pediatrics*, **52**:449, 1973a.

——: Anticholinergic poisonings: treatment with physostigmine. *Pediatrics*, **2**:449, 1973b.

——: Management of acute poisoning and overdose. In Cozzetto, E. J. and Brettell, H. R.: *Topics in Family Practice*. Symposia Specialists Medical Books, New York, 1976.

——: Hydrocarbon ingestions in perspective. *JACEP*, **6**:4, 1977.

——: Acetaminophen overdose in young children: treatment and effects of alcohol and other additional ingestants in 417 cases. *Am. J. Dis. Child.*, **138**:428–33, 1984.

——: *Poisindex*. Micromedex, Inc., Denver, 1986.

Rumack, B. H.; Anderson, R. H.; Wolfe, R.; Fletcher, E. C.; and Vestal, B.: Ornade and anticholinergic toxicity: hypertension, hallucination and arrhythmias. *Clin. Toxicol.*, **7**:573–81, 1974.

Rumack, B. H.; Wolfe, R. R.; and Gilfrich, H.: Diphenylhydantoin treatment of massive digoxin overdose. *Br. Heart J.,* **36**:405–408, 1974.

Rumack, B. H., and Burrington, J. P.: Antidotal therapy of caustic reactions. *Clin. Toxicol.,* **11**:27, 1977.

Rumack, B. H.; Ford, P.; Sbarbaro, J.; Bryson, P.; and Winokur, M.: Regionalization of poison centers—a rational role model. *Clin. Toxicol.,* **12**(3):367–75, 1978.

Rumack, B. H., and Matthew, H.: Acetaminophen poisoning and toxicity. *Pediatrics,* **55**:871, 1975.

Rumack, B. H., and Temple, A. R.: Lomotil poisoning. *Pediatrics,* **53**:495–500, 1974.

Rumack, B. H., and Temple, A. R. (eds.): *Management of the Poisoned Patient.* Science Press, Princeton, N.J., 1977.

Rumack, B. H.; Wolfe, R. R.; and Gilfrich, H.: Phenytoin treatment of massive digoxin overdose. *Br. Heart J.,* **36**:405–408, 1974.

Rumack, B. H.; Peterson, R. C.; Koch, G. G.; and Amara, I. A.: Acetaminophen overdose: 662 cases with evaluation of oral acetylcysteine treatment. *Arch. Intern. Med.,* **141**:380–85, 1981.

Sayre, J. W., and Kaymakcalen, S.: Cyanide poisoning from apricot seeds among children in central Turkey. *N. Engl. J. Med.,* **270**:1113, 1964.

Schwartz, H. S.: Acute meprobamate poisoning with gastrostomy and removal of a drug contained mass. *N. Engl. J. Med.,* **295**:1177, 1976.

Smith, T. W.; Haber, E.; Yeatman, L.; and Butler, V. P., Jr.: Reversal of advanced digoxin intoxication with Fab fragments of digoxin-specific antibodies. *N. Engl. J. Med.,* **294**:797–800, 1976.

Smith, T. W.; Butler, V. P.; Haber, E., *et al.:* Treatment of life-threatening digitalis intoxication with digoxin-specific Fab antibody fragments. *N. Engl. J. Med.,* **307**:1357–62, 1982.

Snyder, R.; Mofenson, H.; and Greensher, J.: Toxicity from Lomotil. *Clin. Pediatr.,* **12**:47, 1973.

Stalker, N. E.; Gamertoglio, J. G.; Fukumitsu, C. J.; et al: Acute massive chloral hydrate intoxication treated with hemodialysis: a clinical pharmacokinetic analysis. *J. Clin. Pharmacol.,* **18**:136–42, 1978.

Steele, R. W.; Conklin, R. H.; and March, H. M.: Corticosteroids and antibiotics for the treatment of fulminant hydrocarbon aspiration. *JAMA,* **219**:1434–37, 1972.

Stein, J. L.: Phencyclidine induced psychosis: the need to avoid unnecessary sensory influx. *Milit. Med.,* **138**:590, 1973.

Stein, M.; Blayney, D.; Feit, T.; Goergen, T. G.; Micik, S.; and Nyhan, W. L.: Acute iron poisoning in children. *West. J. Med.,* **125**:289–97, 1976.

Stewart, R.: Cyanide poisoning. *Clin. Toxicol.,* **7**:561, 1974.

Subcommittee on Accidental Poisoning: Kerosene and related petroleum distillates. In *Handbook of Common Poisonings in Children.* FDA-76-7004, U.S. Department of HEW, Rockville, Md., 1976.

Thompson, D. F.; Trammel, H. L.; Robertson, N. J.; and Reigart, J. R.: Evaluation of regional and nonregional poison centers. *N. Engl. J. Med.,* **308**:191–94, 1983.

Tobis, J., and Das, B. N.: Cardiac complications in amitriptyline poisoning—successful treatment with physostigmine. *JAMA,* **234**:1474–76, 1976.

Tong, T. G.; Benowitz, N. L.; Becker, C. E.; Forni, P. J.; and Boerner, U.: Phencyclidine poisoning. *JAMA,* **234**:512–13, 1975.

Victor, M., and Adams, R. D.: Barbiturate. In *Harrison's Principles of Internal Medicine.* McGraw-Hill Book Co., New York, 1977, Chap. 120.

Watanabe, A. S.: Pharmacokinetic aspects of the dialysis of drugs. *Drug Intell. Clin. Pharmacol.,* **11**:407–16, 1977.

Wexler, J.; Whittenberger, J. L.; and Dumke, P. R.: The effect of cyanide on the electrocardiogram of man. *Am. Heart J.,* **34**:163–73, 1947.

Wilkinson, P. K.: Blood ethanol concentrations during and following constant rate IV infusion of alcohol. *Clin. Pharmacol. Ther.,* **19**:213, 1976.

Chapter 29

OCCUPATIONAL TOXICOLOGY

Robert R. Lauwerys

INTRODUCTION

The main objective of industrial toxicology is the prevention of health impairments in workers handling or exposed to industrial chemicals. This objective can only be reached if conditions of exposure or work practices are defined that do not entail an unacceptable health risk. With the possible exception of carcinogenic substances, for which it is still debatable whether "safe" conditions of exposure can presently be defined, this implies in practice the definition of permissible levels of exposure to industrial chemicals. These levels can be expressed either in terms of allowable atmospheric concentrations (maximum allowable concentrations—MAC; threshold limit values—TLV; time-weighted averages—TWA; threshold limit value-ceiling—TLV-C; short-term exposure limits—STEL) or in terms of permissible biologic levels for the chemicals or their metabolites (biologic TLV). To evaluate with some degree of confidence the level of exposure at which the risk of health impairment is negligible, a body of toxicologic information is required that derives from two main sources: experimental investigations on animals and clinical surveillance of exposed workers (including retrospective studies on previously exposed workers). In some circumstances, limited investigations on volunteers can also be considered.

The large-scale use of any chemical in industry should be preceded by certain types of toxicologic investigations on animals in order to establish a tentative "no-adverse-effect" level (see Chapter 2). Other important information that may also be derived from these investigations concerns methods of biologic monitoring of exposure and early health effects and preexisting pathologic states that may increase the susceptibility to the chemical. Animal testing can provide only an estimate of the toxicity of a chemical for humans. For example, there is a great risk of missing allergic reactions in testing new materials in animals. Thus, when the compound is actually handled in industry, monitoring of the workplaces and careful clinical surveillance of the workers are essential. The design of these clinical surveys will to a large extent depend on the information collected during the first experimental phase of the investigations. The main objectives of the clinical work are (1) to test the validity of the provisional permissible level of exposure based on animal experiments; (2) to detect as early as possible hypersensitive reactions unpredictable from animal investigations; and (3) to confirm the usefulness of biologic methods of monitoring workers. One must, however, recognize that for many chemicals toxicologic investigations on animals have not been performed before the chemicals' use in industry. In that case, clinical work (retrospective epidemiologic studies; historic prospective studies) is aimed at defining the no-adverse-effect level directly in humans.

In some circumstances exposure of volunteers can be considered when the information, e.g., threshold for upper-respiratory-tract irritation, is not easily obtainable by other means and when the experiments entail no risk for the volunteers (which means that extensive biologic information should already be available before any experiments on volunteers are undertaken). Experimental investigations on animals and clinical studies on workers or volunteers are closely related, and the material below will illustrate how collaboration between disciplines or approaches helps accomplish more rapid progress in the field of industrial toxicology.

PRELIMINARY TESTING ON ANIMALS

It is evident that certainty as to the complete safety of a chemical can never be obtained, whatever the extent of toxicologic investigations performed on animals. Nevertheless, some basic requirements can be suggested to estimate with some degree of confidence the level of exposure at which the risk of health impairment is negligible and thus acceptable. We are excluding from the following considerations chemicals that have only very limited use, as in a research laboratory, and can be handled by a limited number of skilled persons in a way that prevents any exposure.

General guidelines for assessing experimentally the toxicologic hazards of industrial chemicals have been recommended (Lauwerys, 1976). Their principles do not differ much from the investigations presently required for evaluating the toxicity of substances to which the general public can be exposed (drugs, food additives, pesticides residues, etc.) (NAS, 1975). These tests include local and systemic acute toxicity tests, skin sensitization tests, toxicity following repeated exposure, short-term tests for detecting potential mutagens and carcinogens, studies of effect on reproduction and of teratogenic activity, investigations of metabolism and mechanism of action, interaction studies, etc., and have been extensively described in previous chapters. The following discussion stresses a few points that are important or more relevant to the field of industrial toxicology.

The need for performing some (or all) of those investigations should be carefully evaluated for any industrial chemical to which workers will be exposed. The toxicologist is guided in selecting the studies most relevant for safety evaluation by an understanding of the physicochemical properties of the chemical; the conditions of use and degree of exposure, including the possibility of generating toxic derivatives when the chemical is submitted to various chemical and physical factors (heat, pH change, etc.); the type of exposure, which may be continuous or accidental; and possibly toxicologic information already available on other chemicals with similar chemical structure and reactive chemical groups. It should be stressed that conclusions drawn from any toxicologic investigation are valid only if the exact composition (e.g., nature and concentration of impurities or degradation products) of the tested preparation is known precisely. The assessment of the toxicity of 2,4,5-T illustrates this point. Its teratogenic hazard is estimated differently depending on the content of the highly toxic impurity 2,3,7,8-tetrachlorodibenzodioxin in the preparation tested (Courtney and Moore, 1971; Emerson et al., 1971). Accurate methods of analysis of the chemical in air and in biologic material should also be available. Flexibility of approach is essential in deciding the duration of tests necessary to establish a reasonable no-effect level for occupational exposure. This depends mainly on the type of toxic action that is suspected, but it is generally recognized that subacute and short-term toxicity studies are usually unsatisfactory for proposing permissible exposure levels. Subacute and short-term toxicity tests are usually performed to find out whether the compound exhibits some cumulative toxic properties and to select the doses for long-term exposure and the kind of tests that may be most informative when applied during long-term exposures. Several studies have recently drawn attention to the fact that the reproductive system may also be the target organ of industrial chemicals (e.g., anesthetic gases, monochlorodibromopropane, vinyl chloride). Studies designed to evaluate reproductive performance and teratogenic action should therefore also be considered during routine toxicologic testing of industrial chemicals.

Information derived from similar exposure routes (skin, lung) to those sustained by workers is clearly most relevant. For airborne pollutants, inhalation exposure studies provide the basic data on which provisional permissible levels are based. Experimental methodology is certainly much more complicated for inhalation studies than for oral administration experiments. For example, in the case of exposure to aerosol, particle size distribution should be estimated and the approximate degree of retention in the respiratory tract of the animal species selected should be known. Ideally, particle size should be selected according to the deposition pattern of solid or liquid aerosols in the particular animal species used. It should also be kept in mind that the concentration of the material in the air and the duration of exposure do not give a direct estimate of the dose, which is also dependent on the minute volume and percent retention. The appropriateness of other routes of administration (usually oral) in combination with limited data from tests by inhalation or skin application must be scientifically evaluated for each chemical (depending on its main site of action, metabolism, etc.). The morphologic, physiologic, and biologic parameters that are usually evaluated, either at regular intervals in the course of the exposure period or at its termination, have been reviewed (NAS, 1975; Shibko and Flamm, 1975; Lauwerys, 1976). It is evident that investigations that can make use of specific physiologic or biochemical tests based on the knowledge of the "critical" organ or function produce highly valuable information and hence increase confidence in the TLV derived from them. In the field of industrial toxicology, knowledge of the disposition (absorption, distribution, biotransformation, excretion) of the chemical and/or its mechanism of action is of major interest. Indeed, as indicated in the introduction, the main objective of occupational toxicology is to prevent the development of occupational diseases. In this respect the biologic monitoring of workers exposed to various industrial chemicals may play an important role, by detecting excessive exposure as early as possible, before the occurrence of significant biologic disturbances, or at least when they are still reversible or have not yet caused any health impairment. A rational biologic monitoring of exposure and early health effects is possible only when sufficient toxicologic information has been gathered on the mechanism of action and/or the biotransformation of xenobiotics to which workers may be exposed. These studies must be performed first on animals.

OBSERVATIONS ON WORKERS

When a new chemical is being used on a large scale, careful clinical survey of the workers and monitoring of the workplaces should be planned. In addition to the specific actions immediately taken if any adverse effect on the health of the workers is discovered, a clinical survey may have two main general objectives: to evaluate the validity of the "no-adverse-effect" level derived from animal experiments, and to test the validity of a biologic method of monitoring.

Evaluation of the Validity of Animal Experiments

Evaluation of the validity of the no-adverse-effect level derived from animal experiments is certainly the prime objective since, as stated by Barnes (1963), "studies and observations on man will always be the final basis for deciding whether or not a MAC set originally on the basis of tests on animals is, in fact, truly acceptable as one that will not produce any signs of intoxication." This means that behavioral, clinical, biochemical, physiologic, or morphologic tests that are considered to be the most sensitive for detecting an adverse effect of the chemical should be regularly applied to the workers at the same time their overall exposure is evaluated to provide personal monitoring of airborne contaminants.

Since the adverse effects under scrutiny for the early detection of health impairment are subtle, and since individual variations exist in the response to a chemical insult, results can only be evaluated on a statistical basis. This means that the dose-response curves found among exposed workers should always be compared to similar responses in a group of unexposed workers matched for other variables such as age, sex, socioeconomic status, and smoking habits. The importance of selecting a control group that is well matched with the exposed group and that undergoes exactly the same standardized clinical, biologic, or physiologic evaluation at the same time as the exposed

group must be emphasized. Since an employed population is a group selected to a certain degree for health, comparison with the general population is not valid. Since such a survey lasts for several years (prospective survey or observational cohort study), the importance of good standardization of all methods of investigation, such as questionnaires related to subjective complaints, instrumentation, and analytic techniques, must be stressed before the start of the survey.

If labor turnover is too high to allow a typical cohort study (i.e., regular examination of the same exposed and control workers), repeated cross-sectional studies of exposed and matched controls should be undertaken. If exposure is above the threshold level of response, these studies may permit (1) establishment of the relationship between integrated exposure (intensity × time) and frequently of abnormal responses, and consequently (2) a redefinition of the no-adverse-effect level.

When this surveillance program has not been planned before the introduction of a new chemical, it is more difficult to obtain the desired information through investigations designed after the fact. Indeed, in this case, evaluation depends on retrospective cohort studies or, more usually, simple cross-sectional studies. Since the information regarding the past exposure of the workers is often incomplete, a correct evaluation of the no-effect level is much more difficult. Whether or not clinical investigations are planned from the introduction of a new chemical or process, it is essential to keep standardized records of workers' occupational histories and exposure. The need may arise for mortality or case history studies in order to answer an urgent question on a suspected risk. The evaluation of the no-effect level of vinyl chloride in man illustrates this point.

In addition to these clinical surveys, it is useful to report in case studies any particular observations resulting from exposure to the chemicals (e.g., accidental acute intoxications). Although such isolated observations are not helpful for determining the no-effect level in man, they are of interest, mainly for new chemicals. They may indicate whether human symptomatology is similar to that found in animals and hence may suggest the functional or biologic tests that might prove useful for the routine control of exposed workers.

Testing the Validity of a Biologic Method of Monitoring

Experimental work may have suggested a biologic method for monitoring of workers (e.g., evaluation of current exposure, internal load, or early biologic response by measuring a metabolite or the compound itself in urine or blood, or by determining blood enzyme activity). Clinical investigations must then be made to test the applicability of such methods in industrial situations. A brief review of the main biologic monitoring methods presently available for evaluating exposure to some industrial toxicologic hazards is presented at the end of this chapter.

EXPERIMENTAL STUDIES ON VOLUNTEERS

Experimental studies on volunteers are usually designed to answer very specific questions, e.g., time course of metabolite excretion during and after exposure; threshold doses for blood cholinesterase inhibition; evaluation of the threshold concentration for sensory responses (odor, irritation of the nasal mucosa, etc.); acute effect of solvent exposure on perception, vigilance, and the like. For evident ethical reasons, such studies can only be undertaken when the same results cannot be obtained through other means and under circumstances where the risk for the volunteers can reasonably be estimated as nonexistent. The experimentation should comply with the Declaration of Helsinki (1964); i.e., it should be carried out under proper medical supervision on duly-informed volunteers.

COLLABORATION BETWEEN ANIMAL AND CLINICAL INVESTIGATIONS

Perhaps in the field of industrial toxicology more than in other areas of toxicology, close collaboration between experimental investigations on animals and clinical studies on workers plays an important role in explaining the potential risk linked with overexposure to chemicals, and hence in suggesting preventive measures to protect the health of the workers. A few examples will illustrate the complementarity of both disciplines in occupational toxicology.

The firm identification of an occupational carcinogen requires both epidemiologic and experimental evidence; an excess of cancer is found in a group exposed to a known chemical, and tumors can be produced in experimental animals by the same chemical (Higginson and Muir, 1976). The carcinogenicity of vinyl chloride was first demonstrated in rats (Viola, 1971), and a few years later epidemiologic studies confirmed the same carcinogenic risk for humans (Creech and Johnson, 1974; Monson et al., 1974). This observation stimulated several investigations on its biotransformation in animals and on its mutagenic activity in various in vitro systems. Identification of vinyl chloride metabolites led to the conclusion that an epoxy derivative is first formed that is suspected to be the proximate

carcinogen. This report triggered a number of investigations on the biotransformation of structurally related chemicals extensively used in industry, such as trichloroethylene, vinylidene chloride, styrene and 2-chlorobutadiene (chloroprene). It is likely that all give rise to reactive epoxy intermediates (Bonse et al., 1975; Leibman, 1975; Uehleke et al., 1977). Furthermore, several of these chemicals or their metabolites exhibit mutagenic activity in vitro. This observation stimulated the search for chromosomal aberrations in workers. Such anomalies were indeed found in persons exposed to vinyl chloride (Heath et al., 1977), styrene (Andersson et al., 1980), and 2-chlorobutadiene (IARC, 1979). The evidence for carcinogenicity of these chemicals to humans is still inadequate (IARC, 1982). Retrospective epidemiologic studies on persons who are or have been occupationally exposed to these chemicals are therefore indicated.

Dioxane is an industrial solvent with a variety of industrial applications. When it is administered at high doses, the principal toxic effects in rats are centrilobular hepatocellular and renal tubular epithelial degeneration and necrosis and induction of hepatic and nasal carcinoma (Kociba et al., 1974). The major metabolite in rats was identified as either β-hydroxyethoxyacetic acid (HEAA) or p-dioxane-2-one, depending on the acidity and the alkalinity of the solution. It was found, however, that the biotransformation of dioxane to HEAA may be saturated at high doses of dioxane. This observation led Young to suggest that the toxicity of dioxane occurs when doses are given sufficient to saturate the biotransformation pathway for its detoxication (Young et al., 1976a). On the premise that similarity of the biotransformation pathway of dioxane in rats and humans would greatly facilitate the extrapolation of toxicologic data from rats to humans (Young et al., 1976b), the same authors examined the urine of plant personnel exposed to dioxane vapor. In urine of workers exposed to a time-weighted average concentration of 1.6 ppm dioxane for 7.5 hours, they found the same product (HEAA) as was found previously in rats. Furthermore, the high ratio of HEAA to dioxane, 118 to 1, suggests that at a low-exposure concentration dioxane is rapidly biotransformed to HEAA. The authors concluded that since saturation of the biotransformation of dioxane in rats was correlated with toxicity, their results on humans support the hypothesis that low levels of dioxane vapor in the workplace pose a negligible hazard. This conclusion is debatable, however, since dioxane is a carcinogen and the existence of a threshold level for such chemicals is still controversial (Claus et al., 1974; Dinman, 1972; Henschler, 1974). Furthermore, Woo et al. (1977) have reported that p-dioxane-2-one is more toxic than dioxane and its production in vivo may be related to dioxane toxicity and/or carcinogenicity, in view of the fact that a number of lactones with similar structure are known to be carcinogenic. If it can be shown that p-dioxane-2-one is really a proximate carcinogen, workers found to excrete the metabolite will have to be considered at risk.

Dimethylformamide (DMF) is a hepatotoxic solvent extensively used in laboratories and in the production of acrylic resins. Exposure of workers occurs mainly by inhalation of vapor and through skin contact. Its biotransformation was first investigated in rats and dogs in vitro and in vivo (Barnes and Ranta, 1972; Kimmerle and Eben, 1975a). These investigations demonstrated that DMF is rapidly biotransformed in vivo and suggested that N-methylformamide (NMF) was its main urinary metabolite. The animal studies stimulated human studies to evaluate whether in vivo biotransformation could lead to the proposal of a biologic method for monitoring workers exposed to DMF. First, two groups of workers investigated the biotransformation of DMF on volunteers (Kimmerle and Eben, 1975b; Maxfield et al., 1975). Both found that the majority of the absorbed substance is eliminated within 24 hours. As in animals, NMF was considered to be the main urinary metabolite. Its concentration was related to the intensity of exposure. The next logical test was to evaluate the practicability of this biologic monitoring method on workers. A preliminary investigation in an acrylic fiber factory confirmed that NMF in urine is a sensitive biologic indicator of exposure since its presence could be easily detected, even when the average airborne DMF concentration was below the current ACGIH-TLV (30 mg/m^3). Furthermore, in a group of workers, the amount of NMF excreted at the end of the shift seems to reflect the intensity of exposure of the same day (Lauwerys et al., 1975). Measurement of the amount of NMF excreted by workers from an acrylic fiber factory who were examined under different exposure conditions (skin protection with gloves and barrier creams or respiratory tract protection by the use of a self-contained breathing apparatus in the pressure demand mode) demonstrated that skin absorption is more important than inhalation in the overall exposure of the solvent when no personal protective devices are used (Lauwerys et al., 1980).

In order to better understand the relationship between DMF biotransformation and toxicity, the biotransformation of DMF has been recently reexamined in vitro and in vivo in rats and in mice. Surprisingly, it was found that in vitro

formaldehyde is not a metabolic product as previously reported, but methylhydroxymethylformamide is formed, which is measured as NMF owing to the breakdown of the hydroxymethyl group during gas chromatography (Gescher et al., 1982; Scailteur et al., 1984). The analysis of urine of rats treated with DMF confirmed that methylhydroxymethylformamide (and not NMF) constitutes the main urinary metabolite in vivo. The previous reports of NMF detection in urine of rats treated with DMF result from an analytic artifact (transformation of methylhydroxymethylformamide into NMF during gas chromatography). The same observation was confirmed in humans (Scailteur et al., 1983). These examples (vinyl chloride, dioxane, dimethylformamide) demonstrate that the study of the metabolic handling of an industrial chemical in animals is very important because it may lead to the characterization of reactive intermediates, suggesting yet-unsuspected risks, or it may indicate new methods of biologic monitoring, which must first be validated by a field study.

Conversely, clinical observations on workers may stimulate the study of the biotransformation or the mechanism of toxicity of an industrial chemical in animals. This may help in predicting the human response to structurally related compounds or in evaluating the health significance of a biologic disturbance. In 1973, an outbreak of peripheral neuropathy occurred in workers exposed to the solvent methyl butyl ketone (MBK) (Allen et al., 1975; Billmaier et al., 1974; McDonough, 1974). The same lesion was reproduced in animals (Duckett et al., 1974; Mendell et al., 1974; Spencer et al., 1975). Biotransformation studies were then undertaken in rats and guinea pigs (Abdel-Rahman et al., 1974; DiVincenzo et al., 1976, 1977), and some MBK metabolites (2,5-hexanedione, 5-hydroxy-2-hexanone) were also found to possess neurotoxic activity (DiVincenzo et al., 1977; Spencer and Schaumburg, 1975).

Similar oxidation products are formed from n-hexane, the neurotoxicity of which is probably due to the same active metabolite as that produced from MBK. According to DiVincenzo et al. (1977), the most probable active intermediate is 2,5-hexanedione. Since methyl isobutyl ketone and methyl ethyl ketone cannot give rise to 2,5-hexanedione (DiVincenzo et al., 1976), they should preferably replace MBK as solvents. n-Hexane derivatives that are oxidized to 2,5-hexanedione are probably also neurotoxic for humans (DiVincenzo et al., 1977).

Investigations on volunteers and on workers have shown that for the same level of exposure to lead the accumulation of free erythrocyte prophyrin (FEP) is more important in women than in men (Roels *et al.*, 1975; Stuik, 1974). Whether this finding justifies the proposal of different permissible levels of exposure to lead for women and for men is debatable, since its health significance is still unknown. A study on the mechanism of the sex difference could clarify its health significance. A joint experimental and clinical approach seems very promising in being able to yield an understanding of the mechanism of this sex-lead interaction. A difference in the level of the iron pool between men and women was first proposed as the main mechanism of the different susceptibility to lead. A relative iron deficiency in women could synergize the action of lead on the enzyme chelatase in bone marrow. Two arguments, one clinical and one experimental, suggest that the lead-sex interaction may also involve other biologic factors. In women moderately exposed to lead, who did not suffer from iron-deficiency anemia, no correlation was found between FEP and plasma iron, nor between concentration of lead in blood and plasma iron (Roels *et al.*, 1979). Furthermore, it was possible to reproduce the sex difference in FEP response to lead in rats (Buchet *et al.*, 1978). In this species under normal feeding conditions the action of lead on FEP accumulation is apparently independent of the iron pool but is influenced by sex hormones, in particular progesterone. Such hormonal influence is in agreement with the finding that in women a slightly increased excretion of δ-aminolevulinic acid (a heme precursor) is also found during pregnancy and this is associated with a slight increase in plomburia (Lauwerys, unpublished results). The mechanism by which sex hormones interfere with the action of absorbed lead in the heme biosynthetic pathway deserves further investigation. It is possible that sex hormones influence the distribution of lead in blood and increase the proportion of ultrafiltrable lead in plasma. A preliminary clinical observation compatible with this hypothesis is the finding of a greater urinary excretion of lead in women than in men for the same level of lead in blood. Further *in vitro* investigations on lead distribution in plasma and *in vivo* studies on animals under different stages of hormonal impregnation are required to validate this hypothesis.

Cases of glomerulonephritis have been reported after repeated cutaneous application of mercury-containing creams (Becker *et al.*, 1962). Increased urinary excretion of plasma proteins without signs of renal insufficiency has also been detected in a certain percentage of workers exposed to mercury vapor and clinically in good health (Buchet *et al.*, 1980). Attempts were made to develop an animal model in order to understand the mechanism of this toxic effect, which is quite different from the tubular necrosis induced by acute exposure to inorganic mercury salts. It was found that repeated administration of mercuric chloride can induce an immunologically mediated glomerulonephritis in certain strains of rats and in rabbits (Druet *et al.*, 1982). In Brown Norway (BN) rats, cutaneous and intravaginal application of mercurial antiseptics and inhalation of mercury vapor can also induce the same disease. In rats, the susceptibility to the induction of the disease, which is self-limited, seems to be genetically controlled. In BN rats, circulating anti-glomerular basement membrane antibodies (anti-GBM) and immune complexes are detected at certain stages of the disease process, whereas in PVG/C rats circulating antinuclear antibodies are detected, but no-anti-GMB. Epidemiologic studies were designed to test the relevance of these observations to humans. In a first study on 43 workers exposed to elemental mercury in a chloralkali plant and a zinc-mercury amalgam factory, no increased level of circulating immune complexes (assayed with rheumatoid factor and MAG agglutinator) was found even in those workers with biologic signs of mercury-induced renal disturbances (Roels *et al.*, 1982). However, in a second study on 62 male workers moderately exposed to mercury vapour for 5.5 years on the average, circulating antilaminin antibodies (laminin is a noncollagenous glycoprotein isolated from basement membrane) were found in eight of them, but in none of the matched control workers (Lauwerys *et al.*, 1983). Renal function and mercury exposure parameters did not differ significantly between workers without and with circulating antilaminin antibodies. These results suggest that, as previously reported in rats, exposure of humans to moderate concentrations of mercury vapor may lead to immune dysfunction in a certain percentage of the exposed population. It would be very important to determine whether the occurrence of antilaminin antibodies is persistent and whether their finding is predictive of renal impairment if exposure is maintained. The answer to this question will help in deciding whether the analysis of serum for anti-basement membrane antibodies can be proposed for the early detection of mercury workers at risk of immune glomerulonephritis.

Other examples of fruitful collaboration between experimental and clinical studies in the area of industrial toxicology can be found in a review article (Lauwerys *et al.*, 1977). More rapid achievement of the control of occupational hazards can be accomplished if close collaboration between both disciplines is further stimulated.

PRACTICAL APPLICATIONS

We have already stressed three important types of applications of toxicologic investigations, i.e., the proposal of permissible levels of exposure, the development of methods for the biologic evaluation of the intensity of exposure to chemicals and for the early detection of their health effects.

Permissible Levels of Exposure to Airborne Industrial Chemicals

It is a cliché to say that the best practice in occupational hygiene is to maintain concentrations of all atmospheric contaminants as low as is practical, but even this does not always preclude overexposure to toxic levels of chemicals. The industrial physician must have guidelines to judge the potential health hazards of industrial chemicals and to evaluate whether the general preventive methods in use in the factory are adequate or must be improved or must be complemented by the use of personal protective devices. An important objective of experimental and clinical investigations in industrial toxicology is the proposal of "safe" (i.e., acceptable) levels of exposure. Various private and official institutions review regularly the toxicologic information on chemicals in order to propose permissible levels of exposure. Critical evaluation of these data can be found in the following publications: various NIOSH criteria documents on specific chemicals, documentation of TLV's prepared by the American Conference of Governmental Industrial Hygienists, and reports prepared by the Deutsche Forschungsgemeinschaft (Toxikologisch-Arbeitsmedizinische Begründung von MAK-Werten). It is evident that with the accumulation of new information on the toxicity of industrial chemicals, the proposed permissible levels must be reevaluated at regular intervals. It should also be made clear that these levels are only guides and should not take the place of close medical surveillance of the workers.

Biologic Monitoring of Exposure to Industrial Chemicals

Biologic monitoring of exposure to industrial chemicals means evaluation of the internal exposure of the organism to a chemical agent (i.e., the internal dose) by a biologic method. Depending on the chemical and the analyzed biologic parameter, the term internal exposure or internal dose may cover different concepts. It may mean the amount of the chemical recently absorbed, the amount already stored in the organism (body burden), or the amount of the active chemical species bound to the sites of action.

Three types of measurement are usually selected to evaluate the internal dose:

1. The concentration of the substance itself in various biologic media
2. The concentration of its biotransformation products (metabolites) in the same media
3. The determination of nonadverse biologic changes that are the results of the reaction of the organism to exposure.

New biologic monitoring methods of exposure are suggested by animal experiment, but their applicability requires detailed clinical investigations on workers.

The advantages, conditions, and limitations of the principal biologic monitoring methods presently available for detecting individual workers or groups of workers excessively exposed to industrial chemicals have been recently evaluated (Lauwerys, 1983). A summary of this evaluation is presented in Table 29–1, Parts I and II. The chemicals have been subdivided into two categories: those for which there is already some strong indication that a biologic monitoring method may be useful for detecting an excessive internal dose or body burden (Part I) and those for which a biologic monitoring method has been suggested but its usefulness has not yet been studied or is still doubtful (Part II). For each chemical agent, are listed the proposed biologic parameters, their normal values, and, when data were available, the tentative maximum permissible values. The significance of the latter proposals must be kept clearly in mind. They are simply tentative guidelines based on the currently available scientific knowledge. Like the airborne TLV's these guidelines should be subject to regular revision in the light of new scientific data.

Early Detection of Health Effects

A biologic monitoring program designed to evaluate the intensity of exposure of workers to industrial chemicals must always be complemented by a health surveillance program. The objective of the latter is to detect as early as possible any adverse biologic and functional effects in exposed workers (e.g., release of hepatic enzymes into the plasma, increased urinary excretion of specific proteins, bronchoconstriction, etc). Such a program should be implemented even when the results of the environmental or biologic monitoring program of exposure indicate that the latter is probably below the acceptable level. Indeed, this level may sometimes contain a large factor of uncertainty, and furthermore, an internal exposure considered safe according to the present state of knowledge may still cause some harmful effects in susceptible individuals. The proposal of tests capable of detecting early adverse biologic effects of indus-

Table 29-1. SUMMARY—PRACTICAL RECOMMENDATIONS FOR THE BIOLOGIC MONITORING OF EXPOSURE TO INDUSTRIAL CHEMICALS

Part 1: Chemicals for which there is some suggestive evidence that (a) biologic monitoring method(s) may be useful for detecting an excessive internal dose on an individual basis and/or on a group basis*

CHEMICAL AGENT	BIOLOGIC PARAMETER	BIOLOGIC MATERIAL	NORMAL VALUE	TENTATIVE MAXIMUM PERMISSIBLE VALUE	REMARKS
Inorganic and Organometallic Substances					
Inorganic arsenic	Sum of inorganic arsenic, monomethylarsinic acid, cacodilic acid	Urine	<10 μg/g creat.	220 μg/g creat.	No interference of arsenic from marine origin
Cadmium	Cadmium	Urine	<2 μg/g creat.	10 μg/g creat.	
	Metallothionein	Urine			
	Cadmium	Blood	<0.5 μg/100 ml	1 μg/100 ml	
Carbon disulfide	Iodine-azide test	Urine		6.5 (Vasak index)	
	2-Thiothiazolidine-4-carboxylic acid	Urine			
Chromium (soluble compounds)	Chromium	Urine	<5 μg/g creat.	30 μg/g creat.	
Fluoride	Fluoride	Urine	<0.4 mg/g creat.	Preshift: 4 mg/g creat. Postshift: 7 mg/g creat.	
Lead	Lead	Blood	<35 μg/100 ml	60 μg/100 ml	Male workers
	Lead	Urine	<50 μg/g creat.	150 μg/g creat.	
	δ-aminolevulinic acid	Urine	<4.5 mg/g creat.	10 mg/g creat.	
	Coproporphyrin	Urine	<100 μg/g creat.	250 μg/creat.	
	Non-iron-bound porphyrin	Red blood cells	<75 μg/100 ml RBC	300 μg/100 ml RBC	
	Zn-protoporphyrin	Blood	<2.5 μg/g Hb	12.5 μg/g Hb	
Lead tetraalkyl	Lead	Urine	<50 μg/g creat.	100 μg/g creat.	
Mercury inorganic	Mercury	Urine	<5 μg/g creat.	50 μg/g creat.	
	Mercury	Blood	<2 μg/100 ml	3 μg/100 ml	
Mercury (methyl)	Mercury	Blood	<2 μg/100 ml	10 μg/100 ml	
Nickel (soluble compounds)	Nickel	Urine	<5 μg/g creat.	70 μg/g creat.	
	Nickel	Plasma	<1 μg/100 ml	1 μg/100 ml	
Selenium	Urine	Urine	<25 μg/g creat.		
Thallium	Thallium	Urine	<1 μg/g creat.		
Uranium	Uranium	Urine	<0.3 μg/g creat.		
Vanadium	Vanadium	Urine	<1 μg/g creat.	50 μg/g creat.	

* From Lauwerys R. R.: *Industrial Chemical Exposure: Guidelines for Biological Monitoring.* Biomedical Publications, Davis, Calif. 1983.

Table 29–1. *(continued)*

CHEMICAL AGENT	BIOLOGIC PARAMETER	BIOLOGIC NORMAL MATERIAL	TENTATIVE MAXIMUM VALUE	PERMISSIBLE VALUE	REMARKS
Nonsubstituted Aliphatic and Alicyclic Hydrocarbons					
n-Hexane	2-Hexanol	Urine		0.2 mg/g creat.	
	2-5-Hexanedione	Urine		5.3 mg/g creat.	
	n-Hexane	Blood		15 µg/100 ml	During exposure
	n-Hexane	Expired air		50 ppm	During exposure
2-Methyl-pentane	2-Methyl-2-pentanol	Urine			
	2-Methylpentane	Expired air			
3-Methyl-pentane	3-Methyl-2-pentanol	Urine			
	3-Methylpentane	Expired air			
Cyclohexane	Cyclohexanol	Urine		3.2 mg/g creat.	During exposure
	Cyclohexanol	Blood		45 µg/100 ml	During exposure
	Cyclohexane	Expired air		220 ppm	
Nonsubstituted Aromatic Hydrocarbons					
Benzene	Phenol	Urine	<20 mg/g creat.	45 mg/g creat.	
	Benzene	Blood			
	Benzene	Expired air	<0.006 ppm		
Toluene	Hippuric acid	Urine	<1.5 g/g creat.	2.5 g/g creat.	
	O-Cresol	Urine	<0.3 mg/g creat.	1 mg/g creat.	
	Toluene	Blood		0.1 mg/100 ml	During exposure
	Toluene	Expired air		20 ppm	During exposure
Xylene	Methylhippuric acid	Urine		1.5 g/g creat.	
	Xylene	Blood		0.3 mg/100 ml	During exposure
	Xylene	Expired air			
Ethylbenzene	Mandelic acid	Urine		2 g/g creat.	
	Ethylphenol	Urine			
	Ethylbenzene	Blood		0.15 mg/100 ml	During exposure
Isopropylbenzene (cumene)	Dimethylphenylcarbinol	Urine		200 mg/g creat.	
Styrene	Mandelic acid (MA)	Urine		1 g/g creat.	
	Phenylglyoxylic acid (PA)	Urine		350 mg/g creat.	
	Styrene	Blood			
	Styrene	Expired air			
Biphenyl	4-Hydroxybiphenyl	Urine			
Halogenated Hydrocarbons					
Dichloromethane (methylene-chloride)	Methylene chloride	Blood		0.08 mg/100 ml	
	Carboxyhemoglobin	Blood	<1%	5%	Nonsmokers
	Methylene chloride	Expired air		35 ppm	

Substance	Determinant	Medium	Value		Sampling time
Trichloromethane (chloroform)	Chloroform	Blood			
	Chloroform	Expired air			
Tetrachloromethane (carbon tetrachloride)	Carbon tetrachloride	Blood			
	Carbon tetrachloride	Expired air			
1,1,1-Trichloroethane (methylchloroform)	Sum of trichloroethanol and trichloroacetic acid	Urine	50 mg/g creat.		
	Trichloroethanol	Urine			
	Methylchloroform	Blood	30 mg/g creat.		
	Methylchloroform	Expired air	50 ppm		During exposure
Trichloroethylene	Trichloroethanol	Urine	125 mg/g creat.		After 5-day exposure
	Trichloroacetic acid	Urine	75 mg/g creat.		During exposure
	Trichloroethylene	Blood	0.6 mg/100 ml		After 5-day exposure
	Trichloroethanol	Plasma	0.23 mg/100 ml		After 5-day exposure
	Trichloroacetic acid	Plasma	5 mg/100 ml		During exposure
	Trichloroethylene	Expired air	12 ppm		16 hours after exposure
Tetrachloroethylene	Tetrachloroethylene	Blood	<0.5 ppm		16 hours after exposure
	Tetrachloroethylene	Expired air	4 ppm		
Vinyl chloride	Thiodiglycolic acid	Urine		<2 mg/g creat.	
Halothane	Trifluoroacetic acid	Urine	10 mg/g creat.		After 5-day exposure
	Trifluoroacetic acid	Blood	0.25 mg/100 ml		After 5-day exposure
Polychlorinated biphenyl	Polychlorinated biphenyl	Blood			
Amino- and Nitroderivatives					
Ethyleneglycol dinitrate	Ethyleneglycol dinitrate	Urine			
Several aromatic amino- and nitro-compounds (aniline, nitrobenzene, dinitrobenzene, etc)	Methemoglobin	Blood	5%	<2%	
	Diazo-positive metabolites	Urine		<10 mg/g creat.	
	Parent compound (e.g., benzidine, β-naphthylamine)	Urine			
Aniline	p-Aminophenol	Urine	10 mg/g creat.		
	Methemoglobin	Blood	5%	<2%	
Nitrobenzene	p-Nitrophenol	Urine	5 mg/g creat.		
	Methemoglobin	Blood	5%	<2%	
Benzidine-derived azo compounds	Benzidine	Urine			
Monoacetylbenzidine-derived azo compounds	Monoacetylbenzidine	Urine			

Table 29–1. (continued)

CHEMICAL AGENT	BIOLOGIC PARAMETER	BIOLOGIC NORMAL MATERIAL	TENTATIVE MAXIMUM VALUE	PERMISSIBLE VALUE	REMARKS
Alcohols—Glycols and Derivatives					
Methanol	Methanol	Urine		7 mg/g creat.	
	Formic acid	Urine	<2.5 mg/g creat.		
	Formic acid	Blood			
Ethyleneglycol	Methoxyacetic acid	Urine			
	Ethyleneglycol	Serum			
Diethyleneglycol	Oxalic acid	Urine	<100 mg/g creat.		
Ethyleneglycol-monomethylether (methylcellosolve)	Oxalic acid	Urine	<100 mg/g creat.		
Dioxane	Methylcellosolve	Expired air			
	β-Hydroxyethoxyacetic acid	Urine			
Ketones					
Methylethyl ketone	Methylethylketone	Urine		2.6 mg/g creat.	
Methyl *n*-butylketone	2,5-Hexanedione	Urine			
Acetone	Acetone	Urine		20 mg/g creat.	
	Formic acid	Urine	<2 mg/g creat.		
	Acetone	Blood	<0.2 mg/100 ml	2 mg/100 ml	
	Acetone	Expired air			
Aldehydes					
Formaldehyde	Formic acid	Urine			
	Formaldehyde	Blood			
Furfural	Furoic acid	Urine	<65 mg/g creat.	200 mg/g creat.	
Amides					
Dimethylformamide	1. Methylhydroxyme-thylformamide measured as *N*-methylformamide	Urine		40 mg/g creat.	
	2. Dimethylformamide	Blood		0.15 mg/100 ml	
	3. Methylhydroxyme-thylformamide (measured as *N*-methylformamide)	Blood		0.1 mg/100 ml	
	4. Dimethylformamide	Expired air		1 ppm	During exposure

Dimethylacetamide	N-methylacetamide (probably methyl-hydroxymethylacetamide)	Urine	<20 mg/g creat.		
Phenols					
Phenol	Phenol	Urine		300 mg/g creat.	
p-tert-Butylphenol	p-tert-Butylphenol	Urine		2 mg/g creat.	
Asphyxiants					
Carbon monoxide	Carboxyhemoglobin	Blood	<1%	5%	nonsmoker
	Carbon monoxide	Blood	<0.15 ml/100 ml	10 ml/100 ml	nonsmoker
	Carbon monoxide	Expired air	<2 ppm	18 ppm	nonsmoker
Cyanide	Thiocyanate	Urine	<2.5 mg/g creat.		Nonsmoker
	Thiocyanate	Plasma	<0.6 mg/100 ml		Nonsmoker
	Cyanide	Blood			
	Ratio between thiocyanate, urine (mg/g creat.), and carboxyhemoglobin (%)	Urine + blood		3	
Acrylonitrile	Acrylonitrile	Urine			
	Thiocyanate	Urine	<2.5 mg/g creat.		
Methemoglobin-forming agents	Methemoglobin	Blood	<2%	5%	Nonsmoker
Pesticides					
Lindane	Lindane	Blood			
DDT	DDT, DDE, DDD, DDA	Blood			
		Urine			
Hexachlorobenzene	Hexachlorobenzene	Blood		0.03 mg/100 ml	
Dieldrin	Dieldrin	Urine			
	Dieldrin	Blood		15 µg/100 ml	
Endrin	Anti-12-hydroxyendrin	Urine		0.13 µg/g creat.	
	Endrin	Blood		5 µg/100 ml	
Organophosphorus insecticides	Cholinesterase	Plasma		50% inhibition	
	Cholinesterase	RBC		30% inhibition	
	Cholinesterase	Whole blood		30% inhibition	
	Alkylphosphates	Urine			
Parathion	p-Nitrophenol	Urine		2 mg/g creat.	
Carbamate insecticides	Cholinesterase	Plasma		50% inhibition	
	Cholinesterase	RBC		30% inhibition	
	Cholinesterase	Whole blood		30% inhibition	
Carbaryl	1-Naphthol	Urine		10 mg/g creat.	

Table 29–1. (*continued*)

CHEMICAL AGENT	BIOLOGIC PARAMETER	BIOLOGIC MATERIAL	TENTATIVE MAXIMUM VALUE	PERMISSIBLE VALUE	REMARKS
2-Isopropoxyphenyl N-methylcarbamate	Isopropoxyphenol	Urine			
2,4-D	2,4-D	Urine			
2,4,5-T	2,4,5-T	Urine			
DNOC	DNOC	Blood		1 mg/100 ml	
Pentachlorophenol	Pentachlorophenol (free)	Urine		1 mg/g creat.	
Hormones					
Diethylstilbestrol	Diethylstilbestrol		30 mg/g creat.	24-hour urine collection	

Part II: Chemicals for which additional information is required to decide upon the usefulness of the suggested biologic monitoring methods.*

CHEMICAL AGENTS	BIOLOGIC PARAMETER	BIOLOGIC MATERIAL	NORMAL VALUE	TENTATIVE MAXIMUM PERMISSIBLE VALUE	REMARKS
Aluminum	Aluminum	Serum	<2 μg/100 ml		
	Aluminum	Urine			
Antimony	Antimony	Urine	<2 μg/g creat.		Higher values in smokers
Beryllium	Beryllium	Urine	<2 μg/g creat.		
Cobalt	Cobalt	Urine	<2 μg/g creat.		
Manganese	Manganese	Urine	<3 μg/g creat.		
	Manganese	Blood	2 μg/100 ml		
Tellurium	Tellurium	Urine			
α-Methylstyrene	Atrolactic acid	Urine			
Monochloromethane (methylchloride)	S-methylcysteine	Urine			
Monobromomethane (methylbromide)	S-methylcysteine	Urine			
	bromure	Blood			
Nitroglycerine	Nitroglycerine	Blood			
Ethyleneglycol monobutylether	Butoxyacetic acid	Urine			
Mutagenic and carcinogenic substances	Mutagenic activity	Urine			Comparison with control group
	Thioethers	Urine			
	Chromosome analysis	Lymphocytes			
	Spermatozoa analysis	Sperm			
	Alkylated aminoacids in proteins	Blood			
	Modified nucleosides	Urine			

* From Lauwerys, R. R.; *Industrial Chemical Exposure: Guidelines for Biological Monitoring*. Biomedical Publications, Davis, Calif., 1983.

trial chemicals requires a detailed knowledge of their mechanism of action. Unfortunately, for many chemicals, such information is still missing. In this case, the screening tests are frequently too insensitive for detecting health effects at a reversible stage. Further fundamental research on the mechanism of action of industrial chemicals is needed for developing more valid health surveillance program of workers.

CONCLUSION

The working environment will always present the risk of workers' overexposure to various chemicals. It is self-evident that the control of these risks cannot wait until epidemiologic studies have defined the no-adverse-effect level directly in man. However, extrapolation from animal data has its limitations. A combined experimental and clinical approach is certainly the most effective for evaluating the potential risks of industrial chemicals, hence for recommending adequate preventive measures and for applying the most valid screening procedures on workers.

Thus the field of industrial toxicology provides many opportunities for scientists with different backgrounds (physicians, chemists, biologists, hygienists) who are convinced of the usefulness of working in close collaboration to understand and prevent the adverse effects of industrial chemicals on workers' health.

REFERENCES

Abdel-Rahman, M. S.; Hetland, L. B.; and Couri, D.: Toxicity and metabolism of methyl *n*-butylketone. *Am. Ind. Hyg. Assoc. J.*, 37:95–102, 1976.

Allen, N.; Mendell, J. R.; Billmaier, D. J.; Fontaine, R. E.; and O'Neill, J.: Toxic polyneuropathy due to methyl *n*-butyl ketone. *Arch. Neurol.*, 32:209–18, 1975.

Andersson, H. C.; Tranberg, E. A.; Uggla, A. H.; and Zetterberg, G.: Chromosomal aberrations and sister-chromatid exchanges in lymphocytes of men occupationally exposed to styrene in a plastic-boat factory. *Mutat. Res.*, 73:387, 1980.

Barnes, J. M.: The basis for establishing and fixing maximum allowable concentrations. *Trans. Assoc. Ind. Med. Off.*, 13:74–76, 1963.

Barnes, J. R., and Ranta, K. E.: The metabolism of dimethylformamide and dimethylacetamide. *Toxicol. Appl. Pharmacol.*, 23:271–76, 1972.

Becker, C. G.; Becker, E. L.; Maher, J. F.; and Schreiner, G.: Nephrotic syndrome after contact with mercury. A report of five cases, three after the use of ammoniated mercury ointment. *Arch. Intern. Med.*, 110:178–86, 1962.

Billmaier, D.; Yee, H. T.; Allen, N.; Craft, R.; Williams, N.; Epstein, S.; and Fontaine, R.: Peripheral neuropathy in a coated fabrics plant. *J. Occup. Med.*, 16:665–71, 1974.

Bonse, G.; Urban, T.; Reichert, D.; and Henschler, D.: Chemical reactivity, metabolic oxirane formation and biological reactivity of chlorinated ethylenes in the isolated perfused rat liver preparation. *Biochem. Pharmacol.*, 24:1829–34, 1975.

Buchet, J. P.; Roels, H.; and Lauwerys, R.: Influence of sex hormones on free erythrocyte protoporphyrin response to lead in rats. *Toxicology*, 9:249–53, 1978.

Buchet, J. P.; Roels, H.; Bernard, A.; and Lauwerys, R.: Assessment of renal function of workers exposed to inorganic lead, cadmium or mercury vapor. *J. Occup. Med.*, 22:741–50, 1980.

Claus, G.; Krisko, I.; and Bolander, K.: Chemical carcinogens in the environment and in the human diet: can a threshold be established? *Food Cosmet. Toxicol.*, 12:737–46, 1974.

Courtney, K. D., and Moore, J. A.: Teratology studies with 2,4,5-trichlorophenoxyacetic acid and 2,3,7,8-tetrachlorodibenzo-*p*-dioxin. *Toxicol. Appl. Pharmacol.*, 20:396–403, 1971.

Creech, J. L., and Johnson, H. M.: Angiosarcoma of the liver in the manufacture of polyvinylchloride. *J. Occup. Med.*, 16:150–1, 1974.

Dinman, B. D.: "Non-concept" of "no-threshold" chemicals in the environment. *Science*, 175:495–97, 1972.

Divencenzo, G. D.; Kaplan, C. J.; and Dedinas, J.: Characterization of the metabolites of methyl-*n*-butyl ketone, methyl iso-butyl ketone, and methyl ethyl ketone in guinea pig serum and their clearance. *Toxicol. Appl. Pharmacol.*, 36:511–22, 1976.

Divencenzo, G. D.; Hamilton, M. L.; Kaplan, C. J.; and Dedinas, J.: Metabolic fate and disposition of ^{14}C-labeled methyl-*n*-butyl ketone in the rat. *Toxicol. Appl. Pharmacol.*, 41:547–60, 1977.

Druet, P.; Bernard, A.; Hirsch, F.; Weening, J. J.; Gengoux, P.; Mahieu, P.; and Birkeland, S.: Immunologically mediated glomerulonephritis induced by heavy metals. *Arch. Toxicol.*, 50:187–94, 1982.

Duckett, S.; Williams, N.; and Francis, S.: Peripheral neuropathy associated with inhalation of methyl-*n*-butyl ketone. *Experientia*, 30 (11):1283–84, 1974.

Emerson, J. L.; Thompson, D. J.; Strebing, R. J.; Gerbig, C. G.; and Robinson, V. B.: Teratogenic studies on 2,4,5-trichlorophenoxyacetic acid in the rat and rabbit. *Food Cosmet. Toxicol.*, 9:395–404, 1971.

Gescher, A. N.; Gibson, N. W.; Hickman, J. A.; Longdon, S. P.; Ross, D.; and Atassi, G.: *N*-methylformamide: Antitumor activity and metabolism in mice. *Br. J. Cancer*, 45:843–50, 1982.

Heath, C. W.; Dumont, C. R.; Gamble, J.; and Waxweiler, R. J.: Chromosomal damage in men occupationally exposed to vinyl chloride monomer and other chemicals. *Environ. Res.*, 14:68–72, 1977.

Henschler, D.: New approaches to a definition of threshold values for "irreversible" toxic effects? *Arch. Toxicol.*, 32:63–67, 1974.

Higginson, J., and Muir, C. S.: The role of epidemiology in elucidating the importance of environmental factors in human cancer. *Cancer Detection Prevention*, 1:79–105, 1976.

IARC (International Agency for Research on Cancer): *IARC Monographs on the Evaluation of the Carcinogenic Risk of Chemicals to Humans*. Vol. 19, *Some Monomers, Plastics and Synthetic Elastomers, and Acrolein*. IARC Lyn, France, 1979.

——: *IARC Monographs on the Evaluation of the Carcinogenic Risk of Chemicals to Humans*, Suppl. 4. IARC, Lyon, France, 1982.

Kazantzis, G.; Schiller, K. F. R.; Asscher, A. W.; and Drew, R. G.: Albuminuria and the nephrotic syndrome following exposure to mercury and its compounds. *Q.J. Med.*, 31:403–18, 1962.

Kimmerle, G., and Eben, A.: Metabolism studies of *N, N*-dimethylformamide. I. Studies in rats and dogs. *Int. Arch. Arbeitsmed.*, 34:109–26, 1975a.

——: Metabolism studies of *N,N*-dimethylformamide II. Studies in persons. *Int. Arch. Arbeitsmed.*, 14:127–36, 1975b.

Kociba, R. J.; McCollister, S. B., Park, C.; Torkelson, R. T. and Gehring, P. J.: 1,4-Dioxane I. Results of a 2-year ingestion study in rats. *Toxicol. Appl. Pharmacol.*, **30**:275–86, 1974.

Lauwerys, R.: Biological criteria for selected industrial toxic chemicals: a review. *Scand. J. Work Environ. Health*, **1**:139–72, 1975.

———: Experimental and clinical investigations for assessing the toxicological hazards of industrial chemicals. *Proceedings of the Meeting of the Scientific Committee, Carlo Erba Foundation, Occupational and Environmental Health Section*, Milan, 1976, pp. 9–48.

———: *Industrial Chemical Exposure: Guidelines for Biological Monitoring*. Biomedical Publications, Davis, Calif., 1983.

Lauwerys, R.; Buchet, J. P.; Roels, H.; Berlin, A.; and Smeets, J.: Intercomparison program of lead, mercury and cadmium analysis in blood, urine, and aqueous solutions. *Clin. Chem.*, **21**:551–57, 1975.

Lauwerys, R.; Buchet, J. P.; Roels, H.; and Bernard, A.: Industrial toxicology: a collaborative approach to laboratory animal research and clinical field studies. In Duncan, W., and Plaa, G. (eds.): *Proceedings First International Congress in Toxicology*. Academic Press, Inc., Toronto, 1977, pp. 311–26.

Lauwerys, R.; Kivits, A.; Lhoir, M.; Rigolet, P.; Houbeau, D.; Buchet, J. P.; and Roels, H. A.: Biological surveillance of workers exposed to dimethylformamide and the influence of skin protection on its percutaneous absorption. *Int. Arch. Occup. Environ. Health*, **45**:199–203, 1980.

Lauwerys, R.; Bernard, A.; Roels, H.; Buchet, J. P.; Gennart, J. P.; Mahieu, P.; and Foidart, J. M.: Antilaminin antibodies in workers exposed to mercury vapour. *Toxicol. Lett.*, **17**:113–16, 1983.

Leibman, K. C.: Metabolism and toxicity of styrene. *Environ. Health Perspect.*, **11**:115–19, 1975.

Linch, A. L.: *Biological Monitoring for Industrial Chemical Exposure Control*. CRC Press, Cleveland, 1974.

Maxfield, M. E.; Barnes, J. R.; Azar, A.; and Trochimowicz, H. T.: Urinary excretion of metabolite following experimental human exposures to DMF or to DMAC. *J. Occup. Med.*, **17**:506–11, 1975.

McDonough, J. R.: Possible neuropathy from methyl-*n*-butyl ketone. *N. Engl. J. Med.*, **290**:695, 1974.

Mendell, J. R.; Saida, K.; Ganasia, M. F.; Jackson, D. B.; Weiss, H.; Gardier, R. W.; Chrisman, C.; Allen, N.; Couri, D.; O'Neill, J.; Marks, B.; and Hetland, L.: Toxic polyneuropathy produced by methyl-*n*-butyl ketone. *Science*, **185**:787–89, 1974.

Monson, R. R.; Peters, J. M.; and Johnson, M. N.: Proportional mortality among vinyl-chloride workers. *Lancet*, **2**:397–98, 1974.

NAS (National Academy of Sciences): *Principles for Evaluating Chemicals in the Environment*. Washington, D.C., 1975.

Roels, H. A.; Lauwerys, R. R.; Buchet, J. P.; and Vrelust, M. T.: Response of free erythrocyte prophyrin and urinary α-aminolevulinic acid in men and women moderately exposed to lead. *Int. Arch. Arbeitsmed.*, **34**:97–108, 1975.

Roels, H.; Balis-Jacques, M. N.; Buchet, J. P.; and Lauwerys, R.: The influence of sex and chelation therapy on erythrocyte protoporphyrin and urinary 5-aminolevulinic-acid in lead-exposed workers. *J. Occup. Med.*, **21**:527–39, 1979.

Roels, H.; Lauwerys, R.; Buchet, J. P.; Bernard, A.; Barthels, A.; Oversteyns, M.; and Gaussin, J.: Comparison of renal function and psychomotor performance in workers exposed to elemental mercury. *Int. Arch. Occup. Environ. Health*, **50**:77–93, 1982.

Scailteur, V.; de Hoffmann, E.; Buchet, J. P. and Lauwerys, R.: Study on *in vivo* and *in vitro* metabolism of dimethylformamide in male and female rats. *Toxicology*, **29**:221–34, 1984.

Shibko, S. I., and Flamm, W. G. (eds.): Symposium on safety evaluation and toxicological tests and procedures. Jointly sponsored by the AOAC and the Society of Toxicology. *J. Assoc. Off. Anal. Chem.*, **58**:633–93, 1975.

Spencer, P. S.; Schaumburg, H. H.; Raleigh, R. L.; and Terhaar, C. J.: Nervous system degeneration produced by the industrial solvent methyl-*n*-butyl ketone. *Arch. Neurol.*, **32**:219–22, 1975.

Spencer, P. S., and Schaumburg, H. H.: Experimental neuropathy produced by 2,5-hexanedione—a major metabolite of the neurotoxic industrial solvent methyl-*n*-butyl ketone. *J. Neurol. Neurosurg. Psychiatry*, **38**:771–75, 1975.

Stuik, E. J.: Biological response of male and female volunteers to inorganic lead. *Int. Arch. Arbeitsmed.*, **33**:83–97, 1974.

Uehleke, H.; Tabarelli-Poplawski, S.; Bonse, G.; and Henschler, R.: Spectral evidence for 2,2,3-trichlorooxirane formation during microsomal trichloroethylene oxidation. *Arch. Toxicol.*, **37**:95–105, 1977.

Viola, P. L.; Bigotti, A.; and Caputo, A.: Oncogenic response of rat skin, lungs and bones to vinyl chloride. *Cancer Res.*, **31**:516–22, 1971.

Woo, Y. T.; Arcos, J. C.; and Argus, M. F.: Metabolism *in vivo* of dioxane: identification of *p*-dioxane-2-one as the major urinary metabolite. *Biochem. Pharmacol.*, **26**:1535–38, 1977.

Young, J. D.; Braun, W. H.; Lebeau, J. E.; and Gehring, P. J.: Saturated metabolism as the mechanism for the dose dependent fate of 1,4-dioxane in rats. *Toxicol. Appl. Pharmacol.*, **37**:138, 1976a.

Young, J. D.; Braun, W. H.; Gehring, P. J.; Horvath, B. S.; and Daniel, R. L.: 1,4-Dioxane and β-hydroxyethoxyacetic acid excretion in urine of humans exposed to dioxane vapors. *Toxicol. Appl. Pharmacol.*, **38**:643–46, 1976b.

Chapter 30

REGULATORY TOXICOLOGY

Richard A. Merrill

THE ROLES OF SCIENCE AND REGULATION

An understanding of the relationship between toxicology and health regulation begins with an appreciation of the different objectives of scientific inquiry and government decision-making. Readers are probably familiar with colleagues who have expressed exasperation over what they regard as the distortion of scientific principles or experimental data in the regulatory process. While such denunciations are often misguided, there is no question that the regulatory process sometimes mistreats the work of the scientific community. Perhaps no field has been "victimized" as often as toxicology, for its findings have been at the heart of many controversial governmental decisions during the past decade. One need mention only DDT, FD&C red 2, saccharin, cyclamate, nitrite, and formaldehyde to bring this point home.

This chapter does not attempt to justify the uses regulators make of toxicology, but rather to explain how the two activities interrelate. We should begin by remembering a central difference between the objectives of science and the role of government: science investigates and attempts to explain natural phenomenon; it is cautious, incremental, and truth-seeking. Government regulation seeks to affect human behavior and settle human disputes; it is episodic, halting, and seeks resolution rather than truth. The raison d'être of the regulatory decision-making process is to solve problems—on the basis of evidence if possible, but if necessary on the basis of surmise, speculation, or sometimes mere dictate.

A regulator often cannot withhold a decision about a problem even when the facts appear to call for suspension of judgment, for a decision to withhold judgment, e.g., on whether saccharin poses a risk of human cancer, has real world consequences. With saccharin on the market, it means that humans continue to be exposed to a substance that may be harmful, though they enjoy its benefits. If the compound in question is not currently being sold, on the other hand, withholding judgment may prevent enjoyment of its benefits while averting an unknown, but possibly trivial, risk. Because toxicology is continuously investigating the effects of chemicals, though less often reaching definitive conclusions about their cause, magnitude, or duration, the regulator is invariably forced to intervene, i.e., to decide, before knowledge is complete. This imperative often gives regulatory decisions the appearance of prematurity in the eyes of scientists; their exasperation is generally reserved for cases where the gap between what is known and what remains to be discovered seems enormous.

Scientists are often frustrated by another uniquely American feature of regulatory decision-making. As a nation, we accord government officials less discretion, i.e., less room for untrammeled, unreviewed, politically constrained judgment, than any other industrialized society. We believe that government actions affecting private interests must satisfy the "rule of law." At a minimum this means that they be of a kind authorized by the legislature, and that they possess the factual predicate specified by the legislature for such decisions. Furthermore, we observe administrative procedures that force regulators to set forth the facts on which they rely and that allow opponents numerous opportunities to disprove those facts. Participants in the regulatory process start from the assumption that the available knowledge, however thin, can fairly be construed in the light most favorable to their position. This philosophy encourages regulators to overstate the evidence for their decisions, amplifying and sometimes even distorting current knowledge.

A third source of controversy likewise stems from the different functions of science and regulation. Legislators generally pay little attention to what science is capable of determining when they establish criteria for regulatory decision-making. Their goal is to enunciate standards that make sense in political or social terms. Thus, according to Congress, no pesticide may cause "unreasonable adverse effects on health or the environment" (FIFRA, 1972), and "*no* worker" may be put in risk of material health impairment "to the extent [it is] feasible" to prevent it (OSHA, 1970). These standards may be rough approximations of desirable social outcomes, but they are difficult to implement and they may demand more of science than it can provide. A regulator cannot change the law he is given, however, so he may impose unreasonable demands on science or, as often, translate tentative hypotheses into the proven facts he believes legally necessary to support a decision.

RELATIONSHIPS BETWEEN TOXICOLOGY AND REGULATION

The previous observations could apply to any scientific discipline whose investigations support regulatory decision-making. But regulation and toxicology have become intertwined over the past two decades in distinctive ways. The most obvious connection is that regulators of health make increasing use of toxicologic concepts and data in reaching decisions. Whether the decision is to assign priorities among a group of compounds, to approve a new substance, or to restrict an old one, toxicologic data are likely to be studied and relied on.

Regulation is thus an exploiter of toxicology; it relies on this scientific discipline to make social decisions. But regulators are not merely consumers of information that toxicologists generate. Regulatory programs have provided a major impetus for improvements in toxicologic methods and stimulated conduct of toxicologic studies. Some programs, like the Food and Drug Administration's (FDA) programs for drugs and food additives and the Environmental Protection Agency's (EPA) program for pesticides, explicitly demand toxicologic investigations of new, and in some cases marketed, compounds. Such "coerced" toxicology comprises a major part of the discipline's research agenda. But regulation would call forth toxicologic studies even if no agency were officially empowered to demand them. Concern for public health as well as apprehension of liability would lead marketers of new or existing products to turn to toxicology to evaluate their possible health hazards. The line between studies that government has mandated and those that the law has merely encouraged is often difficult to discern.

Regulatory agencies likewise influence the design and conduct of toxicologic studies; i.e., they affect the internal workings of the discipline. Once again, the effects are the product of both official prescription and private foresight.

EPA is empowered by the Toxic Substances Control Act to promulgate standards for different types of toxicologic (and other scientific) investigations required or volunteered for its decision-making (TCSA, 1976), and FDA has long maintained "guidelines" for laboratory studies submitted in support of food additives and drugs. When an agency characterizes a particular study protocol as desirable or uninformative, it has obvious implications for future research because many studies are funded by firms that are interested in government approval.

Communication between government officials and laboratory scientists is bilateral. Government testing standards are powerfully influenced by the prevailing consensus among toxicologists, many of whom work in regulatory agencies. The procedures for adopting such criteria always permit, if they do not always encourage, the expression of views from the discipline. Moreover, those views can have major impact, for an agency is often as interested in establishing *some* fixed measure of performance as in selecting *a particular* measure. Predictability and uniformity enjoy a high value among regulators, sometimes even higher value than accuracy.

Finally, but by no means least, regulators significantly influence the public understanding of toxicologic findings. This influence is often unanticipated and sometimes misguided. There can be no question, however, that FDA's 1977 proposal to ban saccharin, apparently on the basis of a single two-generation bioassay in rodents, generated unprecedented public interest in the use of animal models as predictors of human risk, the statistical interpretation of study findings, and the relationships between dose and effect. No doubt one could find expressions in the media—often editorial-page cartoons—that would cause professionals to cringe, but public understanding of the value of toxicology and of its limits probably increased as a result.

REGULATORY PROGRAMS THAT RELY ON TOXICOLOGY

The balance of this chapter focuses on the first and second of these prominent linkages between toxicology and regulation. This part outlines the legal and administrative contexts in which regulators rely on toxicologic data in making critical social and commercial decisions. The focus in the final part is on government as a regulator of toxicology, i.e., as the source of guidance for the design and conduct of laboratory studies.

The chapter does not purport to provide a comprehensive treatment of legal and regulatory requirements that impinge on toxicology. It does not discuss every program that relies on toxicologic data. And it omits such topics as legislation restricting the use of animals in laboratory research, law and regulations designed to protect workers, legal restrictions on the handling of dangerous substances, or local requirements for the operation of toxicology laboratories. Space simply does not allow discussion of these important, yet ancillary, topics.

Approaches to Toxic Chemical Regulation

This part surveys current federal programs for controlling human exposure to toxic chemicals. While its primary focus is the legal standards that govern agency decision-making, attention is also given to the commercial context and effects of agency decisions. The discussion highlights features of regulatory programs that influence both the quantity and quality of safety data necessary to support an agency's decisions.

One such feature, often overlooked by nonlawyers, is the law's allocation of the "burden of proof," i.e., the responsibility for demonstrating that a substance is safe or dangerous. The range of possible approaches can be observed by comparing laws such as the Food Additives Amendment, which requires users of new substances to prove lack of hazard *before* humans may be exposed, with laws such as the Occupational Safety and Health Act, which require regulators to show that a substance is hazardous *before* exposures can be restricted. The approach chosen by Congress affects both an agency's ability to require comprehensive toxicologic investigation of compounds as well as the quality of data on which decisions ultimately are based.

Another distinction, which becomes important under laws that mandate premarket testing, is that between substances not yet on the market and those approved some time before, on the basis of studies that inevitably become outmoded as investigatory methods improve. Even though the law may specify that the burden of proving safety always rests with the commercial sponsor of a substance, as a practical matter the agency has the burden at least of demonstrating sufficient doubt about safety of an approved substance to justify reexamination.

The following discussion of legal standards suggests a clarity that many statutes in fact lack. Congress often speaks in general terms, leaving regulators to define the criteria they will use. Regulators thus have considerable flexibility— to act or to refrain from acting—in the face of debatable scientific evidence.

Typology of Regulatory Approaches. At least two issues must be resolved to justify government action to regulate human exposure to a chemical. First, it must be determined whether the chemical is capable of harming persons who may be exposed. Second, it must be determined whether humans are likely to be exposed to the chemical in ways that could be harmful. In the absence of affirmative answers to both questions, government intervention to control exposure could not be justified. A very few statutes require only these two findings, but most laws under which chemicals are regulated mandate or permit consideration of other criteria as well, such as the magnitude of the risk posed by a substance and the consequences of regulating it. The criteria embodied in current laws fall into three broad categories. A very few statutes mandate a "no-risk" policy, which for a carcinogen may mean that the agency must attempt to prevent any human exposure. Other laws, either expressly or through administrative construction, direct the agency to eliminate or regulate only significant risks. A larger and more diverse class includes laws that direct the agency to allow other considerations to moderate its efforts to protect human health. These considerations may be limited to the technologic capability of an industry to reduce exposure, but often they include a wider range of consequences of regulation.

Agencies Involved. Four federal agencies are primarily responsible for regulating human exposure to chemicals: the Food and Drug Administration (FDA), the Environmental Protection Agency (EPA), the Occupational Safety and Health Administration (OSHA), and the Consumer Product Safety Commission (CPSC). It has sometimes been said that the nation has no coherent policy toward chemical hazards, and the numerous laws administered by these four agencies do indeed convey different levels of concern about risks to human health and about the weight to be given economic costs (OTA, 1981). This diversity has several explanations. The laws were enacted in different eras. The laws originated with, and remain under the influence of, different political constituencies. Furthermore, statutory standards often reflect real differences in the technical feasibility of controlling different types of exposures and embody different Congressional judgments about their economic and social benefits.

Summary of Current Approaches. With this introduction, let us consider the prototype approaches in more detail.

No Risk. This approach is epitomized by the famous Delaney Clause, enacted in 1958 as part of the Food Additives Amendment, which requires that any food additive be found "safe" before FDA may approve its use (FD&C Act, 1958). The Delaney Clause stipulates that this finding cannot be made for a food additive that has been shown to induce cancer in man or in experimental animals. The statute does not require FDA to make any further inquiry, e.g., to consider whether some level of a carcinogen additive is "safe enough" in light of the benefits of its use. The Delaney Clause has been characterized as a categorical risk-benefit judgment by Congress that no food additive is likely to offer benefits sufficient to outweigh any risk of cancer (Turner, 1973). Although section 112 of the Clean Air Act also ostensibly adopts a "no-risk" standard for toxic air pollutants, such standards are not typical of federal health laws.

Negligible Risk. Because the risk posed by a toxic substance depends on the dose, it is sometimes possible to reduce human exposure to levels low enough that any associated risk is small enough to ignore without considering any other criteria. No current health law mandates such a "negligible" risk approach, but FDA has adopted it administratively for some classes of food constituents. For example, under a 1962 amendment to the Delaney Clause, FDA may approve a carcinogenic drug for use in food-producing animals if "no residue" will be "found" in edible tissues of treated animals (FD&C Act, 1962). FDA has announced that it will calibrate its efforts to search for residues, i.e., its methods of chemical analysis, to the potency of a compound (FDA, 1985). It will approve a carcinogenic drug if the sponsor can provide an analytic method capable of detecting residues large enough to pose a lifetime risk of greater than 1 in 1,000,000, as determined by extrapolation from animal bioassays. FDA has followed essentially the same approach in approving color additives containing carcinogenic contaminants and carcinogenic food packaging materials, concluding on the basis of quantitative risk assessment that the lifetime cancer risk from the trace amounts likely to get into food will not exceed 1 in 1,000,000 (FDA, 1982, 1984).

FDA's "negligible-risk" approach requires data depicting carcinogenic potency. This is not a major problem where the agency can require a product's sponsor to conduct the necessary tests, but programs in which regulation responds to exposures that are already occurring lack such leverage. A "negligible-risk" approach also requires the selection of a method for quantifying the risk associated with low doses of a carcinogen. Furthermore, as a practical matter, the approach can work only where exposures to toxic substances can be reduced to low levels without major sacrifice of other values.

Tradeoff Approaches. This heading embraces several different formulas that have one common feature: each requires the regulatory agency to weigh factors in addition to the health risks posed by substances targeted for regulation. These factors can moderate or occasionally even nullify the desire to prevent human illness. One version is illustrated by the Occupational Safety and Health Act, which directs OSHA, in setting workplace standards for toxic materials, to select the standard "which most adequately assures, to the extent feasible . . . that no employee will suffer material impairment of health or functional capacity" (OSHA, 1970). OSHA has interpreted "feasibility" as requiring it to consider, in addition to the risk posed by a substance, the availability of technology for reducing exposure, and the financial ability of the responsible industries to pay for the necessary controls. The Supreme Court has made clear, however, that the agency need not balance the health benefits of mandated exposure controls against the costs of achieving them (*American Textile Mfgrs. Institute,* 1982).

Another type of "tradeoff" law is the Federal Insecticide, Fungicide, and Rodenticide Act (FIFRA), which requires that any pesticide must be registered by EPA before it can be marketed. EPA is directed to refuse or withdraw registration if it finds that use of a pesticide is likely to result in "unreasonable adverse effects on health or the environment" (FIFRA, 1972). The agency interprets this language as requiring that it weigh all of the effects of a pesticide—its contribution to food production as well as its possible adverse effects on applicators, consumers, and the natural environment—in determining whether, or on what terms, to permit registration. FIFRA is not unique; the Toxic Substances Control Act mandates risk-benefit balancing in more explicit language. EPA's experience in administering FIFRA illustrates both the virtues and disadvantages of such standards. Its decisions explore all effects of pesticide use and generally avoid all-or-nothing outcomes, but its procedures are complex and slow, and its demands for data are enormous.

Current Programs for Regulating Chemical Hazards

Food and Drug Administration. The oldest of the major health regulation laws, the Food, Drug, and Cosmetic Act, was enacted in 1938 and covers foods for humans and animals, human and veterinary drugs, medical devices, and cosmetics.

Food. The original FD&C Act contained two prohibitions addressed to foods containing hazardous constituents; both remain part of the current law. The first forbids the marketing of any food containing "any *added* poisonous or deleterious *substance which may render it injurious* to health," a provision that FDA has interpreted as barring foods presenting any serious risk. The second forbids the marketing of foods containing *nonadded* toxicants, i.e., natural agricultural commodities, which make them *"ordinarily injurious* to health," a standard according preferred status to traditional components of the American diet (FD&C Act § 402(a)). Neither of these original provisions required premarket approval; FDA had the burden of proving that a food was adulterated.

Congress has since amended the Act several times to improve FDA's ability to assure the safety of foods. Each time it identified a class of "added" substances for which it prescribed a form of premarket approval, thus giving FDA the authority not only to evaluate a substance's safety before humans are exposed, but also to prescribe the kinds of studies necessary to obtain approval.

The most important of these amendments was the 1958 Food Additives Amendment. For substances classified as "food additives," the law requires safety to be demonstrated prior to marketing. The critical standard for approval is "reasonably certain to be safe"; no inquiry into the benefits of an additive is undertaken or authorized (Cooper, 1978). But the Amendment does not apply to all food ingredients. Congress excluded substances that are "generally recognized as safe" (GRAS) by qualified scientific experts. In effect, it instructed FDA to pay less attention to ingredients that had been in use for many years without observable adverse effects. If new evidence raises doubts about the safety of a GRAS ingredient, it automatically becomes a "food additive" whose use requires approval. Congress also excepted ingredients "sanctioned" by FDA or by USDA prior to 1958. This category includes some controversial substances, including sodium nitrite used in curing meat products. The practical significance of this exception is that a "prior-sanctioned" ingredient is not subject to the Delaney Clause because it is not a "food additive" in the legal sense.

Three classes of "indirect" food constituents—pesticide residues, animal drug residues, and food contact materials—are subject to distinct regulatory standards. Pesticide residues on raw agricultural commodities are regulated by EPA under a 1954 amendment to the FD&C Act, which requires advance approval, in the form of a tolerance, for any pesticide residue (FD&C Act § 348). The statute instructs the agency to consider both the potential health effects of residues and the value of pesticide uses. Any animal drug residue must be shown to be safe for humans under the same standards that apply to food additives with a notable difference. In 1962, Congress authorized FDA to approve a carcinogen for use in food producing animals "if . . . no residue of the additive will be found (by methods of examination prescribed or approved by [FDA] . . .) in any edible portion of such animal. . . . " A food contact substance is classed as a "food additive" if, when used as intended, it "may reasonably be expected to become a component of food." Thus, a packaging material requires approval by FDA if it is likely to migrate. Furthermore, the Delaney Clause precludes approval if the material induces cancer. Because some important food-packaging materials are carcinogens and apparently migrate at low levels, FDA has attempted to avoid this collision between toxicologic findings and advances in analytic chemistry by holding that carcinogenic migrants whose extrapolated risk does not exceed 1 in 1,000,000 be considered *"de minimus"* and ignored (FDA, 1984).

Environmental contaminants constitute the final category of food constituents of concern to FDA. FDA relies on a provision of the 1938 Act that authorizes the establishment of tolerances for "added poisonous or deleterious substances" that cannot be avoided through good manufacturing practice. In setting such tolerances, FDA weighs three factors: (1) the health effects of the contaminant, usually estimated on the basis of animal data; (2) the ability to measure the contaminant; and (3) the effects of various tolerance levels on the price and availability of the food (FDA, 1974). Because contaminants have no commercial proponents, FDA must assemble its own supporting data from the scientific literature and its own laboratories.

Human Drugs. Toxicologic evidence plays an important role in FDA's regulation of human drugs. The current law requires premarket approval, for both safety and efficacy, of all "new" drugs, a category that as a practical matter embraces virtually all prescription drug entities introduced since 1938 (Merrill and Hutt, 1980). Investigation of therapeutic agents in humans has long been accepted, and consequently the primary evidence of safety comes from clinical and not laboratory studies. However, toxicologic data underpin many FDA decisions during the preclinical stages of drug development. Animal studies are the sole source of information about a substance's biologic effects when human trials are begun and influence not only the decision whether to expose human subjects but also the design of clinical protocols. Chronic animal studies may also be the basis for FDA-mandated warnings in the approved labeling for marketed drugs.

The FD&C Act requires that any marketed drug be proved safe and effective for its labeled indications. While not an explicit mandate to balance risks and benefits, FDA has interpreted this cryptic language as requiring precisely such a balancing—and thus it seeks to characterize all the adverse effects of a drug and compare them with its therapeutic performance in deciding whether to allow marketing. Because the standard for approval is necessarily judgmental, and most drugs pose some risk of adverse effects, FDA has never attempted to define the Act's safety standard more precisely.

Medical Devices. In 1976 Congress overhauled the FD&C Act's requirements for medical devices, according FDA major new authority to regulate their testing, marketing, and use. The elaborate new scheme contemplates three tiers of control, calibrated to the health risks posed by a device, the most restrictive of which is premarket approval similar to that required for new drugs. To obtain FDA approval of a so-called class III device, the sponsor must demonstrate safety and efficacy. The bulk of the data supporting such applications will be derived from clinical investigations but they will also include toxicologic studies of any constituents likely to be absorbed by the patient.

Cosmetics. After foods and human drugs, toxicologic data are probably most important in FDA's regulation of cosmetic safety. The provisions governing cosmetics do not require premarket approval of any product or demand that manufacturers test their products for safety. Most manufacturers routinely do so, however, and FDA has sometimes tested individual ingredients or recommended studies. Furthermore, in 1977 the costmetic industry undertook a comprehensive evaluation of the safety of all cosmetic ingredients in common use.

The basic safety standard for cosmetics is similar to that for food ingredients: no product may be marketed if it contains "a poisonous or deleterious substance which may render it injurious to health" (FD&C Act § 601(a)). The case law establishes that this language, too, precludes distribution of a product posing any significant risk of more than transitory harm when used as intended, but it places on FDA the burden of proving violations (Merrill and Hutt, 1980). FDA has brought few cases under this standard, in part because acute toxic reactions are readily detected and immediately result in abandonment of the offending ingredient. The market would not respond in the same way to marketing of a chronically toxic ingredient, about which FDA has been more concerned. Its current position can be characterized as opposing the use of any ingredient that may cause cancer, unless the calculated risk is so low as to be "insignificant."

While the law does not require premarket proof of safety for cosmetic ingredients gener-

ally, it does mandate safety testing for color additives, several of which are important ingredients in cosmetics (as well as foods and drugs). The scheme enacted by Congress in 1960 (FD&C Act § 706) resembles that for food additives, except that no colors are exempt; every color additive must be shown, with "reasonable certainty," to be safe. FDA's major difficulty in administering this requirement has stemmed from Congress's willingness to allow all previously sanctioned colors to retain "interim" approval until their safety could be confirmed. Several circumstances, including improvements in toxicologic testing, have prevented the FDA from providing this confirmation for several colors, which still remain "interim listed" pending completion of progressively more sophisticated studies sponsored by commercial users.

Environmental Protection Agency. Created by Executive Order only in 1970, EPA became responsible for administering numerous laws protecting human health and the environment. A comprehensive review of EPA's programs is not possible here; the following summary focuses on those EPA activities in which toxicologic evidence plays an important role: pesticide regulation, regulation of toxic chemicals, hazardous waste control, and regulation of toxic pollutants of water and of air.

Pesticides. Congress enacted the first pesticide law in 1925; the current statute has been administered by EPA since 1970. Under FIFRA (the Federal Insecticide, Fungicide, and Rodenticide Act) no pesticide may be marketed unless it has been registered by EPA. The law specifies that a pesticide shall be registered if it is effective, it bears proper labeling, and "when properly used . . . it will not generally cause unreasonable adverse effects on the environment" (FIFRA § 1366). Congress further defined this last criterion as "any reasonable risk to man or the environment, taking into account the economic, social and environmental costs and benefits of the use of any pesticide." Most of the data supporting initial registration—mainly from toxicologic studies—are provided by the sponsor, which ostensibly retains the burden of proving it is safe enough to remain on the market.

EPA engendered considerable controversy in the early 1970s by cancelling registrations for a number of pesticides—including DDT, aldrin, and dieldrin—based primarily on studies suggesting their carcinogenicity for animals. Criticism of its "hair trigger" approach to regulation, coupled with court rulings that the agency was legally obligated to initiate cancellation of any pesticide whose safety came into question, led to important changes in the law and in EPA's implementation. Congress added procedural safeguards for pesticide manufacturers and created a panel of outside scientists to review contemplated actions against toxic pesticides (FEPCA, 1972). EPA itself established a procedure, titled the "rebuttable presumption against registration" (now "special review") process, for public ventilation of disputes over the risks and benefits of pesticides before the formal cancellation process was begun (EPA, 1975).

Under EPA's original "special review" (or RPAR) regulations, a pesticide is presumed unregistrable if the agency concludes that it causes significant acute toxicity in humans or induces cancer "in experimental mammalian species or in man" through oral, pulmonary, or dermal exposure. EPA has published general guidelines for assessing whether a pesticide—or any other substance—poses a cancer risk to humans (EPA, 1976, 1984). Even if a pesticide were convincingly shown to be a human carcinogen, however, FIFRA would permit its registration if EPA determined that its economic benefits outweighed the risk.

Toxic Substances. The Toxic Substances Control Act (TSCA, 1976), represents Congress's most ambitious effort to control chemical hazards. It applies to all chemical substances manufactured or processed in, or imported into, the United States—except for substances already regulated under other laws. A chemical substance is defined broadly as "any organic or inorganic substance of a particular molecular identity." TSCA gives EPA three main powers.

EPA is empowered to restrict the manufacture, processing, distribution, use, or disposal of a chemical substance when there is a "reasonable basis" to conclude any such activity poses an "unreasonable risk of injury to health or environment." In determining whether a chemical substance presents an unreasonable risk, EPA is instructed to consider:

"the effects of such substance or mixture on the health and the magnitude of the exposure of human beings to such substance or mixture;

the effects of such substance or mixture on the environment and the magnitude of the exposure of the environment to such substance or mixture;

the benefits of such substance for various uses and the availability of substitutes; and

the reasonably ascertainable economic consequences of the rule, after consideration of the effect on the national economy, small business, technological innovation, the environment and public health."

EPA must also consider any rule's positive impact on the development and use of substitutes as well as its negative impact on manufacturers or processors of the chemical, and weigh the economic savings to society resulting from reduction of the risk.

If EPA suspects that a chemical *may* pose an unreasonable risk but lacks sufficient data to take action, TSCA empowers it to require testing to develop the necessary data. It may similarly order testing if the chemical will be produced in substantial quantities that may result in significant human exposure whose effects cannot be predicted on the basis of existing data. In either case, EPA must consider the "relative costs of the various test protocols and methodologies" and the "reasonably foreseeable availability of the facilities and personnel" needed to perform the tests. While Congress contemplated that EPA would mandate testing through public rulemaking, the burdens of that process and the desire for flexibility in test selection and design have led to a more informal process in which firms undertake to conduct the tests agreed upon with EPA as necessary to resolve open safety issues (GAO, 1982).

TSCA also creates an Interagency Testing Committee to recommend a list of chemicals that should be tested first. The committee consists of members from EPA, OSHA, CEQ, NIOSH, the National Institute of Environmental Health Sciences, NCI, NSF, and the Department of Commerce. Once a chemical substance is recommended by the ITC, EPA must within 12 months either initiate testing or publish its reasons for not doing so.

Finally, to enable EPA to evaluate chemicals before humans are exposed, TSCA requires the manufacturer of a new chemical substance to notify the agency 90 days prior to production (TSCA § 5(a)(1)). A manufacturer or processor that is obligated to submit a notice to EPA must include any data it possesses that show the substance does not present an unreasonable risk. This authority does not, however, empower EPA to require that manufacturers conduct testing of all new chemicals to permit an evaluation of their risks; Congress declined to confer premarket approval authority of the kind FDA exercises for drugs and food additives.

Hazardous Wastes. Several statutes administered by EPA regulate land disposal of hazardous materials, but the principal one is the Resource Conservation and Recovery Act (RCRA), enacted in 1976. RCRA established a comprehensive federal scheme for regulating hazardous waste, which is defined as any waste material, in solid, liquid, semisolid, or gaseous form, "which because of its quantity, concentration, or physical, chemical, or infectious characteristics may—(a) cause, or significantly contribute to an increase in mortality or an increase in serious irreversible, or incapacitating reversible, illness; or (b) pose a substantial present or potential hazard to human health or to the environment when improperly treated, stored, transported, or disposed of, or otherwise managed."

Directed to promulgate criteria for identifying hazardous wastes, EPA specified ignitability, corrosivity, reactivity, and toxicity, believing these characteristics to be the only ones for which test protocols are available. The agency has proposed a set of accepted test protocols as well as a list of substances whose presence will make waste hazardous.

RCRA also directs EPA to promulgate regulations governing the activities of generators, transporters, and those who treat, store, or dispose of hazardous wastes. The standards applicable to generators and transporters feature a manifest system that is designed to create a paper trail for every shipment of waste, from generator to final destination, to ensure proper handling and accountability.

EPA has the broadest authority over persons who own or operate hazardous waste treatment, storage, or disposal facilities. By statute, the agency must prescribe the methods for treating, storing, and disposing of wastes; specify the location, design, and construction of all facilities; establish contingency plans to minimize negative impacts from such facilities; set qualifications for ownership, training, and financial responsibility; and—most important—require permits for all such facilities. EPA has promulgated specific design and operating standards for permitted facilities and has also proposed "human health and environmental standards."

Under RCRA the standards applicable to generators, transporters, and handlers of hazardous wastes must "protect human health and the environment." Theoretically, economic or technical considerations may not offset this objective. As a practical matter, however, it has proved difficult for EPA to design and implement its regulations without considering costs or technical feasibility.

Toxic Water Pollutants. The 1972 Amendments to the Federal Water Pollution Control Act for several years provided the basis for EPA's efforts to control toxic water pollutants. EPA's problems in implementing the law, however, led first to a judicial rewriting of its responsibilities and later to Congress's revision of the 1972 design. As originally enacted, section 307

required EPA to publish, within 90 days from enactment, and periodically add to a list of toxic pollutants for which effluent standards would then be established. According to the Act:

"The term 'toxic pollutant' means those pollutants, or combination of pollutants, including disease-causing agents, which after discharge and upon exposure, ingestion, inhalation or assimilation into any organism, either directly from the environment or indirectly by ingestion, through food chains, will, on the basis of information available to the Administrator, cause death, disease, behavioral abnormalities, cancer genetic mutations, physiological malfunctions (including malfunctions in reproduction) or physical deformations, in such organisms or their offspring."

In establishing effluent standards for each of pollutants listed, EPA was instructed to consider six factors: (1) toxicity, (2) persistence, (3) degradability, (4) the usual or potential presence of affected organisms in water, (5) the importance of affected organisms, and (6) the nature and effect of the toxic pollutant on such organisms. Section 307(a)(4) specified that each standard should limit effluents to that level which "provides an *ample margin of safety*"—a criterion that places primary emphasis on human health. The 1972 law prescribed a rapid timetable and complex procedure for standard-setting: an effluent standard for each listed pollutant had to be proposed within 180 days; a hearing was required within 30 days, and no more than six months later a final standard was to be promulgated.

EPA's hesitant efforts to comply with these instructions precipitated a series of lawsuits challenging its performance. After being sued for failure to list any pollutants, the agency published a list of nine—four pesticides (DDT, aldrin/dieldrin, toxaphene, and endrin) and five other substances (mercury, cadmium, cyanide, benzidine, and PCBs)—for which it proposed effluent standards. The statutorily mandated public hearing brought forth claims that technology did not exist to monitor or detect the pollutants at low levels and that the limits proposed would shut down major American industries. The proposed standards were withdrawn in 1976, provoking a new round of lawsuits by environmental groups.

EPA eventually reached a judicially sanctioned settlement that fundamentally changed federal regulation of toxic water pollutants. The settlement allowed EPA to act under other provisions of the Act that permit industry-wide effluent standards and mandate consideration of economic costs and technologic feasibility in setting limits. The settlement also simplified the procedures for promulgating standards, and allowed regulated parties three years to comply with industry-wide pollution standards. As part of the settlement the EPA agreed to press ahead with effluent standards for six of the chemicals on its original list and has since completed regulation of all six. Congress incorporated the terms of this settlement in 1977 amendments to the statue, which now mandates technology-based, industry-wide limits on toxic pollutants, but still allows EPA to prescribe more stringent controls when necessary to protect health.

Drinking Water. The Safe Drinking Water Act of 1972 (SDWA) was enacted to assure that public water supply systems "meet minimum national standards for the protection of public health." Under the Act, the EPA is required to regulate contaminants "which may have an adverse effect on human health." In this context, too, EPA has accepted the premise that there is no safe level of exposure to a carcinogen, but it has recognized that the costs of controlling human exposure must be reasonable.

SDWA authorizes EPA to regulate public water systems by either of two methods: the agency may establish a maximum contaminant level (MCL) for a contaminant, and/or it may prescribe a treatment technique for its control. The feasibility of monitoring the level of a contaminant in the water supply largely determines whether a treatment technique will be selected in lieu of establishing an MCL.

The Act proscribes a two-stage process for the promulgation of regulations. EPA was first required to promulgate interim national primary drinking water regulations, whose purpose was to establish quickly uniform minimum standards that would "protect health to the extent feasible . . . (taking costs into consideration)." These interim regulations were later supplanted by revised regulations formulated on the basis of a study by the National Academy of Sciences (NAS). The NAS study recommended the MCL's necessary to protect humans from any known or anticipated adverse health effects. The Act directs EPA to specify MCL's or treatment techniques so as to come as close as is feasible to the levels recommended by the Academy. Since the feasibility of achieving a specified MCL or of implementing a treatment technique may change with technologic advances, the statute also requires continual revision and updating of the primary regulations.

Toxic Air Pollutants. Section 112 of the Clean Air Act (CAA) authorizes EPA to regulate air pollutants that threaten human health. It provides for the listing of pollutants that "cause or contribute to air pollution which may reasonably be anticipated to result in an increase in mortality or an increase in serious irreversible, or incapacitating reversible, illness." The statute requires EPA to establish emissions standards or control requirements for sources that emit any substance listed as a hazardous air pollutant. The standards must provide "an ample margin of safety to protect the public health from such hazardous air pollutants," a criterion that appears oblivious to the costs of emissions control.

EPA proposed a policy for regulating airborne carcinogens in October 1979. The proposed policy recognized that, to maximize the public health benefits obtainable with limited resources, priorities should be established with respect to both the listing procedures and the development of standards. Carcinogenic pollutants should be listed under Section 112 only if there were evidence either of significant public exposure from stationary source emission or of a significant risk to groups most likely to be exposed. Under the proposed policy, risk assessments would determine priorities for source categories that posed significant public health risks. At a minimum, the policy contemplated the use of "best available technology" (BAT) to control emissions from new or existing source categories posing such risks, with more stringent controls to eliminate any remaining "unreasonable residual risks." Thus, although the statute seemed to mandate elimination of all health risks, EPA indicated that it would consider technologic capability and control costs.

The Reagan Administration allowed EPA's proposed policy for carcinogenic air pollutants to die without adoption. By 1986, the agency had become less reluctant to list hazardous pollutants but bolder in reinterpreting the statutory standards for control measures. It declines to propose controls for pollutants whose risk is assessed as not "significant," based on quantitative risk assessment. For pollutants and/or sources warranting control, EPA identifies the level of control achievable with "best available technology," and then considers whether more stringent controls are warranted in light of the residual risks and added costs (ELR, 1986).

Occupational Safety and Health Administration. OSHA administers the Occupational Safety and Health Act, which obligates employers to provide working conditions that are safe for employees, and empowers the agency to prescribe mandatory occupational safety and health standards. OSHA's most controversial standards have dealt with toxic chemicals.

While FDA and EPA have authority to regulate food additives, drugs, and pesticides before the public is exposed, no employer is obligated to obtain approval of new processes or materials or to conduct tests to assure that its operations will jeopardize worker health. Only if it discovers that a material already in use threatens the health of workers may OSHA attempt to control exposure. OSHA health standards typically set maximum limits on employee exposure and prescribe change in employer procedures or equipment to achieve this level. Some standards also require workers to use protective equipment, but this approach historically has been disfavored by the agency, as well as organized labor (OSHA, 1980).

The OSH Act specifies that in regulating toxic chemicals, OSHA shall prescribe the standard "which most adequately assures, to the extent feasible, on the basis of the best available evidence, that no employee will suffer material impairment of health or physical capacity" (OSH Act § 6(b)(5)). The meaning of these delphic, and to some extent contradictory, phrases has been a source of prolonged controversy. Court decisions have made clear that the "best available evidence" does not require proof of causation or positive epidemiologic findings; toxicologic data alone can support regulation of a toxic substance. OSHA must consider whether safeguards are technologically and economically "feasible," but it is not confined to existing methods for worker protection; it may require improvements or even the development of new ones.

For years the most hotly contested issue was the extent of OSHA's obligation to weigh the economic costs of its standards. While the agency acknowledged that it was required to consider technologic achievability and industry survival, it resolutely insisted that it was not obliged to balance health benefits and economic costs (OSHA, 1980). Its costly controls for benzene, lead, and cotton dust precipitated challenges that twice led to the Supreme Court. The Court overturned OSHA's benzene standard on the ground that the agency had not shown that prevailing exposure levels posed a "significant" health risk (*Industrial Union Dep't v. American Petroleum Inst.*, 1980). Shortly after, however, it upheld OSHA's cotton dust standard with the explanation that Congress itself had balanced the benefits and costs of rigorous worker safeguards; the agency was not obligated to revisit these issues in setting individual standards (*American Textile Mfgrs. Institute v. Donovan*, 1982).

OSHA also provoked dispute when it attempted to codify its criteria for regulating substances that pose a cancer risk. Proposed in 1977 and adopted in 1980, OSHA's "generic cancer policy" (OSHA, 1980) was an elaborate discussion of the standards it would use in interpreting human and animal data to determine whether substances posed a cancer risk and a reiteration of its evolving policy of demanding the most protective "feasible" controls for any substance for which the finding was affirmative. The final document was stayed by the Reagan administration.

Because it lacks premarket approval authority and its power to mandate testing has not been confirmed, OSHA generally must rely on data already generated about workplace chemicals. The OSH Act created the National Institutes of Occupational Safety and Health (NIOSH) to serve as OSHA's independent research arm. NIOSH assembled much of the data—and performed some of the epidemiologic studies—on which OSHA relied in its early standards for toxic substances. OSHA itself has not been an initiator of health effects research.

Consumer Product Safety Commission. Of the four agencies, the CPSC has played the least prominent role in federal efforts to control toxic chemicals. The Commission was created in 1972 by the Consumer Product Safety Act (CPSA) with authority to regulate products that pose an unreasonable risk of injury or illness to consumers. "Consumer products" include all articles sold for general or personal use in the home, school, or recreational settings, except products regulated by FDA and EPA. The CPSA empowers the Commission to promulgate safety standards that it finds "reasonably necessary to prevent or reduce an unreasonable risk of injury" associated with a consumer product. If no feasible standard "would adequately protect the public from the unreasonable risk of injury" posed by a consumer product, the CPSC may ban the product from commerce (CPSA § 8). In assessing the need for a standard or ban, the CPSC must balance the likelihood that a product will cause harm and the gravity of the harm against the effect of reducing the risk on the product's utility, cost, and availability to consumers.

The Commission also administers the older Federal Hazardous Substances Act of 1960 (FHSA). The FHSA authorizes the CPSC to regulate products that are toxic, corrosive, combustible, or radioactive or that generate pressure through decomposition, heat, or other means. While labeling and warning requirements constitute the primary forms of regulation under the FHSA, that law also confers authority to ban a substance from use.

The FHSA is unusual among federal health laws on containing detailed criteria for agency evaluation of toxicity. It defines "highly toxic" in terms of a substance's acute effects in specified tests in rodents; substances capable of producing chronic effects, such as cancer, thus fall within the "toxic" category. The FHSA contains another unique provision specifically addressing the relative weight of animal and human data on acute toxicity:

"If the [Commission] finds that available data on human experience with any substance indicates results different from those obtained on animals in the above-named dosages or concentrations, the human data shall take precedence (FHSA § 2(h)(2))."

The law, however, says nothing about the relative weight of human and animal evidence relating to chronic effects.

The CPSC has promulgated several regulations prescribing labeling for products containing substances that may be acutely toxic. It has also acted to ban several substances used in consumer products that pose a cancer risk, including asbestos, vinyl chloride as a propellant, benzene, TRIS, and formaldehyde as a component of foam insulation (Merrill, 1981). The latter action was set aside by a reviewing court in an opinion that is remarkable for its detailed and critical analysis of the agency's handling of toxicologic data. The court particularly faulted the Commission's quantitative estimate of the risk posed by formaldehyde in foam insulation, based in major part on the flaws in its exposure measurements (*Gulf South Insulation v. CPSC*, 1983).

The CPSC obtains most of its data about chemical hazards from other sources, including scientific organizations and sister regulatory agencies. The agency's capacity to test products is limited, and its budget has been shrinking. Furthermore, the agency bears the burden of initiating regulatory proceedings to control any chemical; neither the CPSA nor the FHSA imposes any obligation on manufacturers to notify the Commission of its plans to market a new product or to obtain approval for any design or material.

REGULATORY CONTROLS OVER TOXICOLOGY

The previous discussion has focused on the contexts in which regulators draw on toxicologic data in deciding whether and at what levels to control environmental chemicals. But the regulatory process impinges on the discipline of toxicology in other, more immediate ways. Regulatory agencies often prescribe the content and characteristics of studies that are required to meet regulatory requirements. In this role, they touch directly on the activities of toxicologists.

Ways in Which Regulation Impinges on Toxicology

An agency's power to influence toxicologic investigations depends on the character of its regulatory responsibilities. An agency—like FDA or EPA—that must confirm the safety of new substances before marketing can, as a practical matter, dictate the kinds of tests that manufacturers submit to elicit a finding of safety. By contrast, an agency—like OSHA or CPSC—that lacks premarket approval power has considerably less leverage. These agencies bear the burden of proving that a substance warrants regulation. While such an agency can specify what sorts of evidence will persuade it to regulate, it lacks obvious means to elicit necessary testing. Typically, it must use whatever tests have been reported in the scientific literature. This dichotomy between regulatory laws that place the burden of proving safety on users of chemicals and laws that authorize control only after a determination that a substance or activity is hazardous is the main determinant of an agency's effective authority over the discipline of toxicology.

The terms of legislation do not accurately forecast the content or reach of an agency's power. The FD&C Act does not in so many words authorize FDA to prescribe the kinds of preclinical tests a manufacturer of human drugs must conduct; it says merely that no new drug may be marketed until the manufacture has satisfied FDA, "by all methods reasonably applicable," that it is "safe" (FD&C Act § 505(c)). The Food Additives Amendment similarly focuses on the criterion for approval—safety—without specifically according FDA power to prescribe the studies necessary to permit such a finding. But FDA's clear power to hold up approval when it has doubts about a compound's safety provides the agency the practical leverage necessary to force manufacturers to conduct the sorts of tests agency scientists believe necessary. A few laws, notably TSCA, are more explicit in according authority to mandate and prescribe testing. However, where an agency has the ability to prevent marketing until safety is proved, any doubts about its legal authority to prescribe testing requirements are academic; the important issues are the procedures by which agency requirements are adopted, their scope and scientific support, and their legal effect.

The last issue is important for laboratory scientists and for commercial sponsors of tested compounds, as well as for lawyers. Two significant, if arcane, legal distinctions should be noted. The first is the distinction between requirements that an agency imposes for testing a specific compound and so-called generic standards that it prescribes for all compounds within a class, e.g., direct food additives. An agency could impose its views of appropriate toxicologic testing without ever enunciating any general testing requirements. When a compound's sponsor sought approval it could be told that its tests were inadequate, or individual sponsors could elicit the agency's advice about what tests were necessary before conducting any. The first approach wastes money and testing resources, and the second—unless agency advice is broadly disseminated—fails to guide other potential sponsors and permits inconsistency in the treatment of similar compounds.

For these reasons agencies have moved increasingly toward the establishment of generic standards or guidelines. This trend has focused attention on another legal distinction of some importance: the distinction between binding regulations and advisory guidelines. Any time a regulatory agency wants to provide guidance for behavior, it confronts, at least implicitly, a choice between establishing standards that have the force of law—regulations—and offering its current best judgment of what will satisfy the law—guidelines. A regulation specifies what the law mandates; failure to comply, e.g., the failure to perform a test or to follow a protocol specified in a regulation, constitutes a violation of law just as if the regulation had been enacted by Congress. A guideline describes performance that will meet legal requirements; it is a promise to accept tests that conform to the guideline, but failure to follow the guideline is not automatically forbidden. The agency may accept another approach, e.g., a different set of studies or studies conducted under different protocols, as meeting the law's basic requirements.

An advantage of regulations is that they assure consistency and are more easily enforced than guidelines. But they are potentially more rigid because they bind the agency and the procedures for their adoption are cumbersome. Furthermore, sound regulatory requirements must suit the subject they address. The design and conduct of toxicologic studies, it is argued, require scientific judgment that takes into account the characteristics of the test compound, the end-points to be evaluated, the resources available, and perhaps even laboratory capabilities. More important, accepted standards in toxicology are continually evolving as scientists acquire more knowledge. Test standards embodied in regulations would restrict judgment and impede adaptation. Accordingly, with some exceptions, regulatory agencies have preferred to announce their standards as guidelines, permitting product sponsors and laboratory scientists to consider and sometimes use alternative approaches. This trend is pronounced in agency

standards for particular types of tests, e.g., carcinogencity bioassays in rodents; it is less evident in requirements specifying the types of tests necessary to permit an evaluation of safety.

This last observation is a reminder of the variety of regulatory requirements that impinge on toxicologists. Four kinds can be distinguished. The first is a statement of the types of tests an agency requires before it will consider a compound, e.g., acute toxicity, subchronic, and chronic. An agency might elaborate more detailed requirements within each of these categories, essentially enumerating its "base set" data demands. A second kind of requirement describes methods for executing a particular test, e.g., a bioassay for carcinogenesis, and is the most common form of guideline encountered in the regulatory process. A third kind, which at both FDA and EPA takes the form of regulations, specifies the laboratory procedures for conducting tests required or submitted for regulatory consideration. These good laboratory practice (GLP) regulations enunciate essential but often mundane features of sound laboratory science, such as animal husbandry standards and record-keeping practices (FDA, 1978; EPA, 1979). A fourth kind of directive is an agency's specification of testing requirements for a specific chemical, such as those EPA is empowered to adopt under TSCA.

FDA and EPA Testing Standards

It would serve little purpose to detail here regulatory agency requirements for the design and conduct of toxicologic studies now in place. Whether phrased as regulations or guidelines, these requirements change so frequently that any summary would soon be outdated. This chapter thus attempts only to acquaint the reader with the major regulatory programs under which agencies have attempted to specify standards for toxicity testing and to suggest the features currently applicable requirements are likely to possess. The discussion focuses on FDA and EPA, the two agencies whose regulatory responsibilities provide explicit or implied authority to affect directly the activities of toxicologists.

Food and Drug Administration. FDA exercises premarketing approval authority over several classes of compounds. The most important, for present purposes, are new human drugs and direct and indirect additives to food.

Toxicologic Testing Requirements for Human Drugs. FDA has long exercised control over the testing of compounds investigated as possible therapeutic agents. In 1962 Congress expressly authorized FDA to exempt investigational drugs from the premarket approval requirement so that the drugs could be shipped for use in clinical testing, subject to conditions the agency believed appropriate to protect the safety and integrity of human subjects (FD&C Act, § 505(i)). One such condition was that the drug have first been evaluated in preclinical, i.e., toxicologic studies. This requirement appears in current FDA regulations that amplify, in text and in referenced guidelines, the type of tests that are to be performed and the design they should follow. Thus, FDA mandates the basic features of preclinical studies. Almost invariably, a drug's sponsor will consult further with agency personnel to get a more precise understanding of what sorts of toxicologic studies they expect.

Studies of substances that are candidates for use as human drugs must meet FDA's GLP regulations. These regulations apply to all laboratories—university, independent, and manufacturer-owned—in which such studies are conducted. They were adopted, at Congressional urging, in 1978, following FDA investigations into the integrity of toxicologic studies previously submitted in support of several drugs and food additives. These investigations revealed serious deficiencies in many laboratories, including some instances of fraud.

Testing Requirements for Food Additives. The Food Additives Amendment and the Color Additive Amendments require premarket approval of new additives to human food. Both laws assume that laboratory studies in animals will provide the principal data for evaluating safety. The food additives law requires that a petitioner submit "full reports of investigations made with respect to the safety for use of such additives, including full information as to the methods and controls used . . . " (FD&C Act, § 409(c)). The statute does not explicitly empower FDA to regulate the design or conduct of such studies, but the agency has exercised that authority for several years.

FDA's food additive regulations contained only general statements about the need for, and characteristics of, toxicologic studies. For many years, however, the agency has maintained an advice-giving system in which it prescribes the type and design of tests to be performed, and in 1982 FDA codified its "common law" in *Toxicological Principles for the Safety Assessment of Direct Food Additives and Color Additives Used in Food,* sometimes known as "the Red Book." This publication is the most comprehensive summary of regulatory requirements for toxicologic evaluation of chemicals, but it has not supplanted informal case-by-case advice. The Red Book describes the types of tests FDA believes necessary to evaluate an additive's safety. The agency's requirements—which constitute guidelines rather than regulations—are calibrated to the purposes for which the additive will be used, to estimated levels of human exposure, and to the results of sequential studies. In addition to fulfilling the objectives of the Red Book, tests of food additives must comply with FDA's agency-wide GLP regulations.

Environmental Protection Agency. EPA has for many years exercised premarket approval authority over pesticides, placing it, like FDA, in a position to dictate the design and conduct of many toxicologic studies. In the 1976 Toxic Substances Control Act, Congress explicitly gave EPA additional authority to mandate testing of other chemicals in use or scheduled for introduction and to specify, by regulation, test standards.

Toxicologic Requirements for Pesticides. As noted previously, FIFRA requires that a pesticide be registered with, i.e., approved by, EPA before it may be marketed. One statutory criterion for approval—demonstrated lack of "unreasonable adverse effects" on health—clearly contemplates the submission of toxicologic studies, as well as other types of investigations, to support EPA's evaluation (FIFRA § 1366). FIFRA further requires EPA to "publish guidelines specifying the kinds of information which will be required to support the registration of a pesticide and to revise such guidelines from time to time." In this provision, Congress apparently contemplated that EPA guidelines would both outline the kinds of data required to secure approval and describe the characteristics each study should possess.

EPA's regulations state broadly that pesticide registration depends on evaluation of "all available, pertinent data," which must satisfy the minimum requirements set forth in registration guidelines (EPA, 1978). The agency has issued guidelines outlining the procedures for submission of registration petitions and their basic content (EPA, 1985). Toxicologic studies of pesticides must also comply with EPA's GLP regulations, which were inspired by the same investigations that led FDA to promulgate minimum standards for testing laboratories.

Testing Requirements under TSCA. TSCA is an unusual law because it authorizes EPA to require testing of chemicals and prescribe the required tests, without also giving the agency premarket approval responsibility. TSCA does demand premarket notification of new substances, but this is not a premarket approval requirement; the statute does not demand any specified quantity of safety data but merely requires the disclosure of whatever safety information the distributor possesses. By suggesting the kinds of data it believes an adequate premarket notice should contain, however, EPA will be able to induce some testing and influence the design of whatever tests manufacturers voluntarily undertake.

The primary means by which EPA can mandate the performance of safety tests, i.e., toxicologic investigations, is section 4(a) of TSCA. That provision states that the Administrator "shall by rule require that testing be conducted . . . to develop data with respect to the health and environmental effects for which there is an insufficiency of data and experience" to permit an assessment of whether a substance presents an unreasonable risk. This obligation to order testing is triggered by an administrative finding that a chemical presents a potential risk (based on suspicion of toxicity) or that humans or the environment will be exposed to substantial quantities. Section 4 also establishes a standing committee responsible for recommending substances for testing and obligates EPA to respond to its recommendations within a year.

Section 4 thus creates an ongoing system for the consideration and imposition of requirements to test chemicals. The law contemplates that EPA will impose testing requirements by regulation, but the agency has rarely proceeded in this way. The complications of public rulemaking have led EPA, with the support of the chemical industry, to rely primarily on testing agreements negotiated with the producers and users of the substances in question. Such agreements, which are matters of public record, are likely to continue to be the primary source of testing obligations under TSCA.

The agreements uniformly specify what types of tests are to be done. Their design is governed either by EPA "test methodology guidelines," which have been issued for more than a dozen types of tests, or by the terms of the agreement itself. Section 4 of TSCA contemplates that test rules will specify the manner in which required tests are to be performed, either establishing or incorporating previously established test standards. However, EPA's preference for informal testing agreements rather than binding rules has obviated this approach. The agency's current "standards" for testing under TSCA are thus to be found in published guidelines as incorporated or modified in individual test agreements.

All toxicologic studies submitted to EPA under TSCA must comply with its GLP regulations.

Interagency Testing Criteria and Programs

The foregoing summary of four regulatory programs that require toxicologic tests suggests the potential for inconsistency in government testing standards. The responsible regulatory agencies, including OSHA and the CPSC as well as FDA and EPA, have been concerned about this possibility and since 1978 have worked to avoid it. It is perhaps unrealistic to expect that the agencies will regularly agree on what tests should be performed on substances falling within their joint jurisdiction: use levels may differ widely, varying routes of exposure may dictate different test protocols, and the agencies may become concerned about a substance at different times. Where it is clear that two agencies will be engaged in evaluating the safety of a substance simultaneously, however, they usually seek to ensure that their data demands are at least complementary.

It is more important and more feasible to assure consistency among test standards: a chronic toxicity study performed to obtain FDA approval of a food additive should also satisfy EPA's minimum standards. The former Interagency Regulatory Liaison Group (IRLG) had the goal of securing agreement among the four agencies on the design of standard toxicologic tests. This objective of consistency has persisted. It has led EPA to make sure that any test guidelines under FIFRA parallel those issued under TSCA. FDA has made similar efforts to assure compatibility between the standards for tests of food additives and drugs.

There has been comparable pressure, from within and outside government, to ensure that GLP requirements are consistent. EPA was persuaded to revise proposed GLP regulations to make the final version textually congruent with those previously adopted by FDA. Inconsistency is a greater problem where testing requirements are framed as regulations, because compliance is presumably a matter of legal obligation, not agency choice, and revision is difficult. Despite growing official recognition of the problems caused by inconsistency among testing obligations and test standards, laboratory researchers should not be astonished to discover that sometimes two sister agencies appear to be sending different messages.

There is one notable area in which the agencies have achieved effective collaboration. The National Toxicology Program (NTP) was established in 1978 as an administrative umbrella for coordinating the numerous federal efforts to improve test methods and perform toxicologic studies then underway, primarily in the Department of Health and Human Services. One of NTP's major functions was to take over the NCI bioassay program. In exercising this responsibility, NTP has attempted to involve the regulatory agencies that are most interested in the results of such studies. An NTP committee that includes representatives of all four regulatory agencies is responsible for selecting chemicals to be tested at public expense.

Readers are likely to be aware of efforts to achieve international agreement on test standards as well as on minimum data requirements for new chemicals. Led by the OECD, these efforts have already influenced the content of EPA and FDA test guidelines and of EPA's "base set" of data for new chemicals for which TSCA requires notification. Space does not permit a review of these international standards or an evaluation of their consistency with current requirements of federal agencies. The latter, while no doubt influenced by emerging international consensus, will for some time remain the principal source of governmental guidance for the conduct of toxicologic studies.

REFERENCES

Cases

American Textile Manufacturers Association v. Donovan, 452 U.S. 490, 495 (1980).
Environmental Defense Fund, Inc. v. Environmental Protection Agency, 548 F.2d 998 (D.C. Cir. 1976).
Environmental Defense Fund, Inc. v. Ruckelshaus, 439 F.2d 584 (D.C. Cir. 1971).
Environmental Defense Fund, Inc. and National Audubon Society v. Environmental Protection Agency, 510 F.2d 1292 (D.C. Cir. 1975).
Gulf South Insulation v. CPSC, 701 F.2d 1137 (5th Cir. 1983).
Industrial Union Department, AFL-CIO v. American Petroleum Institute, 448 U.S. 607 (1980).
Industrial Union Department, AFL-CIO v. Hodgson, 499 F.2d 467 (D.C. Cir. 1974).
Monsanto v. Kennedy, 613 F.2d 947 (D.C. Cir. 1979).
NRDC v. Train, 8 E.R.C. 2120 (D.D.C. 1976).
Society of the Plastics Industry, Inc. v. OSHA, 509 F.2d 1301 (2d Cir. 1975).

Secondary Sources

Assessment of Technologies for Determining the Cancer Risks from the Environment. Report by the Office of Technology Assessment. U.S. Government Printing Office, Washington, D.C., June 1981.
Berger, J., and Riskin, S.: Economic and technological feasibility under the Occupational Safety and Health Act. *Ecology L.O., 7*:285, 1978.
Bruser, J.; Harris, R.; and Page, T.: Waterborne carcinogens: an economist's view. In *The Scientific Basis of Health and Safety Regulation.* Brookings Institute, Washington, D.C., 1981.
Cooper, R.: The role of regulatory agencies in risk-benefit decision-making. *Food Drug Cosm. L.J., 33*:755–57, 1978.
Douglas, I.: Safe Drinking Water Act of 1974—history and critique. *Environ. Affairs, 5*:501, 1976.
Drinking Water and Health. Report by the Safe Drinking Water Committee of the National Academy of Sciences. National Academy Press, Washington, D.C., 1977.
EPA Implementation of Selected Aspects of the Toxic Substances Control Act. Report by the U.S. General Accounting Office, Washington, D.C., December 1982.
Horne, C.: EPA's August, 1980 Proposal: Reforms in the rules of practice for cancellation hearings (January 2, 1982) (unpublished paper).

House Interstate and Foreign Commerce Committee Report: *Safe Drinking Water Act,* 93rd Congress, 2nd Session. Report No. 93-1185, December 3, 1974.
Merrill, R.: Regulating carcinogens in food: a legislator's guide to the food safety provisions of the federal Food, Drug, and Cosmetic Act. *Mich. L. Rev., 77*:179–84, 1979.
——— : CPSA regulation of cancer risks in consumer products: 1972–81. *Va. L. Rev., 67*:1261, 1981.
Merrill, R., and Hutt, P. B.: *Food and Drug Law: Cases and Materials.* Foundation Press, Inc., Mineola, N.Y., 1980.
Merrill, R., and Schewel, M.: FDA regulation of environmental contaminants of food. *Va. L. Rev., 66*:1357, 1980.
National Toxicology Program Annual Plan for Fiscal Year 1983. Report by the U.S. Department of Health and Human Services, January 1983.
Page, N. P.: Testing for health and environmental effects: the OECD guidelines. *Toxic Substances J., 4*:135, Autumn 1982.
Reed, P. D.: The trial of hazardous air pollution regulation. *Environ. L. Register, 16*:10066–72, 1986.
Speech by Peter Barton Hutt, partner in the Washington, D.C. law firm of Covington & Burling, at the Symposium on Assessing Health Risks from Chemicals, 1982.
Toxicological Principles for the Safety Assessment of Direct Food Additives and Color Additives Used in Food. Report by the U.S. Food and Drug Administration, 1982.
Turner, J.: The Delaney anticancer clause: A model environmental protection law. *Vand. L. Rev., 24*:889, 1971.
U.S. Environmental Protection Agency's Proposed Policy and Procedures for Identifying, Assessing, and Regulating Airborne Substances Posing a Risk of Cancer. Report by the Regulatory Analysis Review Group, 1980.

Statutes and Regulations

Clean Air Act (1976), 42 U.S.C. § 7401 et seq.
Color Additive Amendments of 1960 to the Federal Food, Drug, and Cosmetic Act, 21 U.S.C. § 706.
Consumer Product Safety Act (1972), 15 U.S.C. § 2051 et seq.
Criteria for determinations of unreasonable adverse effects, 40 C.F.R. § 162.11 (1981).
Data requirements for registration, 40 C.F.R. § 158 (1985).
Drug Amendments of 1962 to the Federal Food, Drug, and Cosmetic Act, 21 U.S.C. § 360(b).
Drugs for Human Use, 21 C.F.R. §§ 310, 312, 314 (1982).
Federal Food, Drug, and Cosmetic Act (1938), 21 U.S.C. § 321 et seq.
Federal Hazardous Substances Act (1976), 15 U.S.C. § 1261 et seq.
Federal Insecticide, Fungicide, and Rodenticide Act (1976), 7 U.S.C. § 135 et seq.
Federal Water Pollution Control Act Amendments of 1972, 33 U.S.C. § 307.
Food Additive Amendments to the Federal Food, Drug, and Cosmetic Act (1958), 21 U.S.C. § 348 et seq.
Food for Human Consumption: Food Additives, 21 C.F.R. § 170 (1983).
Good Laboratory Practice for Nonclinical Laboratory Studies, 21 C.F.R. § 58 (1983).
Good Laboratory Practice Standards for Health Effects: Environmental Protection Agency. *Federal Register, 44*(No. 91):27362, May 9, 1979.
Health Risk and Economic Impact Assessments of Suspected Carcinogens: Environmental Protection Agency. *Federal Register, 41*(No. 102):21402–405, May 25, 1976.
Identification, Classification and Regulation of Potential Occupational Carcinogens: Occupational Safety and

Health Act. *Federal Register*, 45(No. 15):5002, January 22, 1980.

Identification, Classification and Regulation of Potential Occupational Carcinogens: Occupational Safety and Health Act. *Federal Register*, 47(No. 2):187–90, January 5, 1982.

Indirect Food Additives: Polymers; Acrylonitrile/Styrene Copolymers. *Federal Register*, 49(No. 183): 36635–44, September 19, 1984.

Lead Acetate: Listing as a Color Additive in Cosmetics that Color the Hair on the Scalp: Food and Drug Administration. *Federal Register*, 45(No. 213):72112–18, October 31, 1980.

National Emissions Standard for Identifying, Assessing, and Regulating Airborne Substances Posing a Risk of Cancer: Environmental Protection Agency. *Federal Register*, 44(No. 197):58641–70, October 10, 1979.

Occupational Safety and Health Act (1970), 29 U.S.C. § 651 et seq.

Pesticide Residue Amendments to the Federal Food, Drug, and Cosmetic Act (1954), 21 U.S.C. § 348 et seq.

Policy for Regulating Carcinogenic Chemicals in Food and Color Additives; Advanced Notice of Proposed Rulemaking: Food and Drug Administration. *Federal Register*, 47(No. 64):14464–69, April 2, 1982.

Proposed Guidelines for Carcinogen Risk Assessment; Request for Comments. *Federal Register*, 49(No. 227): 46293–301, November 23, 1984.

Proposed Guidelines for Registering Pesticides in the United States: Environmental Protection Agency. *Federal Register*, 43(No. 163):37336, August 22, 1978.

Proposed Health Effects Test Standards for Toxic Substances Control Act Test Rules: Environmental Protection Agency. *Federal Register*, 44(No. 145):44054, July 26, 1979.

Proposed Interim Primary Drinking Water Regulations: Environmental Protection Agency. *Federal Register*, 43(No. 130):29135–37, July 6, 1978 (to be codified at 40 C.F.R. § 141).

Rebuttable Presumption Against Registration (RPAR) Proceedings and Hearings Under Section 6 of the Federal Insecticide, Fungicide, and Rodenticide Act (FIFRA): Environmental Protection Agency. *Federal Register*, 45(No. 154):52628–74, August 7, 1980.

Registration, Reregistration and Classification Procedures: Environmental Protection Agency. *Federal Register*, 40(No. 129):28242–86, July 3, 1975.

Resource Conservation and Recovery Act (1976), 42 U.S.C.A. § 6901.

Safe Drinking Water Act (1976), 42 U.S.C. §§ 300f to 300j-9.

Sponsored Compounds in Food Producing Animals; Proposed Rule and Notice. *Federal Register*, 50(No. 211):45529–56, October 31, 1985.

Toxic Substances Control Act (1976), 15 U.S.C. § 2601.

INDEX*

---

*Page numbers in **boldface** type indicate primary discussion.